Current Pediatric Therapy

18th Edition

ASSOCIATE SECTION EDITORS:

Roger L. Berkow, MD

Professor and Vice-Chair
Department of Pediatrics
University of Alabama at Birmingham
Professor of Pediatrics
Department of Pediatric Hematology/Oncology
University of Alabama at Birmingham–Children's
  Hospital of Alabama
Birmingham, Alabama
Hematology

Leonard G. Feld, MD, PhD

Professor of Pediatrics
University of Medicine & Dentistry of New Jersey–
  New Jersey Medical School
Newark, New Jersey
Chairman, Department of Pediatrics
Goryeb Children's Hospital–Atlantic Health System
Morristown, New Jersey
Symptomatic Care Prior to Diagnosis

Mark L. Helpin, DMD

Section Head, Pediatric Dentistry
Department of Oral Medicine
Carolina's Medical Center
Charlotte, North Carolina
Dental Problems

Peter J. Hotez, MD, PhD

Professor and Chair
Division of Microbiology and Tropical Medicine
The George Washington University
Washington, DC
Infectious Diseases—Helminth Infections

Amy J. Theos, MD

Assistant Professor
Department of Dermatology
University of Alabama at Birmingham
Director of Pediatric Dermatology
Children's Health System
Birmingham, Alabama
Skin

ASSOCIATE EDITOR OF PHARMACOLOGY:

Lea S. Eiland, PharmD, BCPS

Assistant Clinical Professor of Pharmacy Practice
Auburn University Harrison School of Pharmacy
Auburn, Alabama
Clinical Assistant Professor of Pediatrics
University of Alabama at Birmingham, Huntsville
  Regional Medical Campus
Huntsville, Alabama

Current Pediatric Therapy

18th Edition

Fredric D. Burg, MD
SENIOR EDITOR

Professor of Pediatrics
University of Alabama at Birmingham
Birmingham, Alabama
Chair, Alabama Emergency Response Commission on Health Care Crisis
Adjunct Professor of Nursing
University of Alabama at Huntsville
Huntsville, Alabama
Emeritus Professor of Pediatrics
University of Pennsylvania
Philadelphia, Pennsylvania

Julie R. Ingelfinger, MD
Professor of Pediatrics
Harvard Medical School
Senior Consultant in Pediatric
  Nephrology
Department of Pediatrics, Division of
  Pediatric Nephrology
MassGeneral Hospital for Children
  at Massachusetts General Hospital
Boston, Massachusetts

Richard A. Polin, MD
Professor of Pediatrics
Columbia University College of
  Physicians and Surgeons
Director, Division of Neonatology
Morgan Stanley Children's Hospital
  of New York–Presbyterian
New York, New York

Anne A. Gershon, MD
Professor of Pediatrics
Columbia University College of
  Physicians and Surgeons
Attending Physician
Morgan Stanley Children's
  Hospital of New York–
  Presbyterian
New York, New York

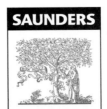

SAUNDERS

ELSEVIER

SAUNDERS

ELSEVIER

1600 John F. Kennedy Blvd.
Ste 1800
Philadelphia, Pennsylvania 19103

CURRENT PEDIATRIC THERAPY

ISBN-13: 978-0-7216-0549-4
ISBN-10: 0-7216-0549-4

Some material previously published.

Notice

Knowledge and best practice in this field are constantly changing. As new research and experience broaden our knowledge, changes in practice, treatment, and drug therapy may become necessary or appropriate. Readers are advised to check the most current information provided (i) on procedures featured or (ii) by the manufacturer of each product to be administered, to verify the recommended dose or formula, the method and duration of administration, and contraindications. It is the responsibility of the practitioner, relying on experience and knowledge of the patient, to make diagnoses, to determine dosages and the best treatment for each individual patient, and to take all appropriate safety precautions. To the fullest extent of the law, neither the Publisher nor the Editors assume any liability for any injury and/or damage to persons or property arising out of or related to any use of the material contained in this book.

The Publisher

Library of Congress International Standard Serial Number 1069–2460

ISBN-13: 978-0-7216-0549-4
ISBN-10: 0-7216-0549-4

Acquisitions Editor: Joanne Husovski
Developmental Editor: Jennifer Shreiner
Publishing Services Manager: Frank Polizzano
Project Manager: Joan Nikelsky
Design Direction: Karen O'Keefe Owens

Printed in the United States of America

Last digit is the print number: 9 8 7 6 5 4 3 2 1

Working together to grow
libraries in developing countries

www.elsevier.com | www.bookaid.org | www.sabre.org

ELSEVIER   BOOK AID International   Sabre Foundation

To my wife, Nancy Burg, *and my children,* Benjamin, Beth, David, Kate, Paul, and Jennifer

FDB

To my husband, Pete, *my children*, Erich, Katy, and Franz, *and my stepchildren*, Sarah and Bill

JRI

To my wife, Helene, *and my children*, Allison, Mitchell, Jessica, and Gregory

RAP

To my husband, Michael Gershon

AAG

Contributors

Elaine J. Abrams, MD
Associate Professor of Clinical Pediatrics and Epidemiology, Department of Pediatrics, Columbia University College of Physicians and Surgeons; Director of Research, Department of Pediatrics, Harlem Hospital Center; Director, MTCT-Plus Initiative, International Center for AIDS Care and Treatment Programs, Columbia University Mailman School of Public Health, New York, New York
NONTUBERCULOUS *MYCOBACTERIUM* INFECTIONS; HUMAN IMMUNODEFICIENCY VIRUS INFECTION

Elias Abrutyn, MD
Associate Provost and Associate Dean for Faculty Affairs, Interim Chief, Infectious Diseases, Department of Medicine; and Professor of Medicine and Public Health, Drexel University College of Medicine, Philadelphia, Pennsylvania
TETANUS NEONATORUM

Thomas C. Abshire, MD
Professor of Pediatrics, Emory University School of Medicine; Staff Physician, Atlas Cancer Center and Blood Disorders Service, Atlanta, Georgia
DISORDERS OF COAGULATION, PLATELET NUMBER, AND FUNCTION

Mark J. Abzug, MD
Professor of Pediatrics (Pediatric Infectious Diseases), University of Colorado School of Medicine; Staff Physician, The Children's Hospital, Denver, Colorado
VIRAL MENINGITIS AND ENCEPHALITIS

Seema Aceves, MD, PhD
Assistant Adjunct Professor, Department of Pediatrics, University of California, San Diego, School of Medicine; Allergist, Division of Allergy and Immunology, Children's Hospital San Diego, San Diego, California
SERUM SICKNESS

Raymond Adelman, MD
Pediatric Nephrologist, Phoenix Children's Hospital, Phoenix, Arizona
FLUID AND ELECTROLYTE THERAPY

Samuel M. Alaish, MD
Assistant Professor of Surgery, Department of Pediatric Surgery, University of Maryland School of Medicine; Assistant Professor of Surgery, Division of Pediatric Surgery, Johns Hopkins University School of Medicine, Baltimore, Maryland
PLEURAL EFFUSION, EMPYEMA, AND CHYLOTHORAX

Mark E. Alexander, MD
Instructor in Pediatrics, Harvard Medical School; Assistant in Cardiology, Arrhythmia Service, Department of Cardiology, Children's Hospital, Boston, Massachusetts
SYNCOPE

Julian Lewis Allen, MD
Professor of Pediatrics, University of Pennsylvania School of Medicine; Chief, Division of Pulmonary Medicine and Cystic Fibrosis Center, and Robert Gerard Morse Endowed Chair in Pulmonary Medicine, The Children's Hospital of Philadelphia, Philadelphia, Pennsylvania
BRONCHITIS AND BRONCHIOLITIS

Uri S. Alon, MD
Professor of Pediatrics, University of Missouri at Kansas City School of Medicine; Pediatric Nephrologist, Children's Mercy Hospital, Kansas City, Missouri
URINARY TRACT INFECTION AND PERINEPHRIC/INTRANEPHRIC ABSCESS

Blanche P. Alter, MD, MPH
Expert, Clinical Genetics Branch, Division of Cancer Epidemiology and Genetics, National Cancer Institute, Department of Health and Human Services, Rockville, Maryland
INHERITED FORMS OF APLASTIC ANEMIA: THE INHERITED BONE MARROW FAILURE SYNDROMES; ACQUIRED APLASTIC ANEMIA

R. Peter Altman, MD
Professor of Surgery, Columbia University College of Physicians and Surgeons; Surgeon in Chief, Morgan Stanley Children's Hospital of New York–Presbyterian, New York, New York
PLEURAL EFFUSION, EMPYEMA, AND CHYLOTHORAX

Richard C. E. Anderson, MD
Assistant Professor of Neurosurgery and Pediatric Neurosurgery, College of Physicians and Surgeons; Pediatric Neurosurgeon, Childrens Hospital of New York, New York
DIAGNOSIS AND MANAGEMENT OF CHIARI I MALFORMATION; DIAGNOSIS AND MANAGEMENT OF HYDROCEPHALUS

Sharon Phillips Andreoli, MD
Professor of Pediatrics, Indiana University College of Medicine; Staff Physician, James Whitcomb Riley Hospital for Children, Indianapolis, Indiana
HEMOLYTIC UREMIC SYNDROME

Richard J. Antaya, MD
Assistant Professor of Dermatology and Pediatrics, Yale University School of Medicine; Staff Physician, Departments of Dermatology and Pediatrics, Yale–New Haven Hospital, New Haven, Connecticut
DISORDERS OF THE HAIR AND SCALP

Robert J. Arceci, MD, PhD
Director and King Fahd Professor of Pediatric Oncology, Department of Oncology, Johns Hopkins University School of Medicine; Professor of Oncology and Pediatrics, Sidney Kimmel Comprehensive Cancer Center at Johns Hopkins, and Director of Pediatric Oncology, Johns Hopkins Hospital, Baltimore, Maryland
HISTIOCYTOSIS

Marc S. Arkovitz, MD
Assistant Professor of Surgery, Columbia University College of Physicians and Surgeons; Attending Pediatric Surgeon, Children's Hospital of New York–Presbyterian, New York, New York
PNEUMOTHORAX AND PNEUMOMEDIASTINUM

Carola A. S. Arndt, MD
Associate Professor and Division Chair, Pediatric Hematology/Oncology, Department of Pediatric and Adolescent Medicine, Mayo Clinic and Foundation, Staff Physician, Mayo Clinic, Rochester, Minnesota
NEUROBLASTOMA

David P. Ascher, MD, MBA
Professor of Pediatrics, Virginia Commonwealth University School of Medicine, Richmond; Chairman, Department of Pediatrics, Inova Fairfax Hospital for Children, Fairfax, Virginia
INTESTINAL PROTOZOA

Lee I. Ascherman, MD, MPh
Director, Division of Child and Adolescent Psychiatry, Department of Psychiatry, University of Alabama at Birmingham School of Medicine; Chief of Service, Child and Adolescent Psychiatry, The Children's Hospital of Alabama, Birmingham, Alabama
PSYCHIATRC DISORDERS AND MENTAL HEALTH DISORDERS IN CHILDREN AND ADOLESCENTS

Jane T. Atkins, MD
Hospital Epidemiologist, Methodist Children's Hospital of South Texas, San Antonio, Texas
INTESTINAL PROTOZOA

Diego H. Aviles, MD
Associate Professor, Department of Pediatrics, Louisiana State University School of Medicine at New Orleans; Pediatric Nephrologist, Children's Hospital, New Orleans, Louisiana
TREATMENT OF GLOMERULONEPHRITIS

Felicia B. Axelrod, MD
Carl Seaman Family Professor of Dysautonomia Treatment and Research, Department of Pediatrics, and Professor of Neurology, New York University School of Medicine; Attending, Department of Pediatrics, and Director, Dysautonomia Treatment and Evaluation Center,

Department of Pediatrics and Neurology, NYU Medical Center, New York, New York
FAMILIAL DYSAUTONOMIA

Estanislao Bachrach, PhD
Research Associate, Genetics Department, Harvard Medical School and Genomics Program, Children's Hospital Boston, Boston, Massachusetts
MUSCULAR DYSTROPHIES

Terry M. Baird, MD
Assistant Professor of Pediatrics, Case School of Medicine; Director, Normal Newborn Nurseries, Rainbow Babies and Children's Hospital, Cleveland, Ohio
APNEA OF PREMATURITY

Carol J. Baker, MD
Professor and Head, Division of Pediatric Infectious Diseases, Departments of Pediatrics and Molecular Virology and Microbiology, Baylor College of Medicine; Attending Physician, Division of Pediatric Infectious Diseases, Texas Children's Hospital; Medical Director, Infection Control, Woman's Hospital of Texas, Houston, Texas
GROUP B STREPTOCOCCAL INFECTIONS

Ma. Victoria F. Balagon, MD
Assistant Chief, Epidemiology Branch, Leonard Wood Memorial Center for Leprosy Research, Cebu City, Philippines
LEPROSY (HANSEN DISEASE)

Robert S. Baltimore, MD, FAAP
Professor of Pediatrics and Epidemiology, Department of Pediatrics, Yale University School of Medicine; Attending Physician, Yale–New Haven Children's Hospital, New Haven, Connecticut
CELLULITIS

Gina-Marie Barletta, MD
Staff, Pediatric Nephrology and Transplantation, DeVos Children's Hospital, Grand Rapids, Michigan
DIALYTIC THERAPIES

Joel L. Bass, MD
Associate Clinical Professor of Pediatrics, Harvard Medical School, Boston; Chair, Department of Pediatrics, Newton-Wellesley Hospital, Newton; Attending Pediatrician, Massachusetts General Hospital for Children, Boston; Adjunct Clinical Professor of Pediatrics, Boston University School of Medicine, Boston, Massachusetts
PREVENTING CHILDHOOD INJURIES

David A. Bateman, MD
Associate Professor of Clinical Pediatrics, Columbia University College of Physicians and Surgeons; Director of Network Nurseries, Department of Pediatrics/Neonatology, New York–Presbyterian Hospital, New York, New York
HYDROPS FETALIS

Eraka Bath, MD
Assistant Clinical Professor of Psychiatry, Division of Child and Adolescent Psychiatry, New York University School of Medicine; Clinical Director, ACS–Bellevue Mental Health Service, NYU Child Study Center, New York, New York
PSYCHOSOMATIC ILLNESS

L. Arturo Batres, MD
Assistant Professor of Pediatrics, Eastern Virginia Medical School; Staff Physician, Division of Pediatric Gastroenterology and Nutrition, Department of Pediatrics, The Children's Hospital of the King's Daughters, Norfolk, Virginia
HELICOBACTER PYLORI INFECTION

Mark L. Batshaw, MD
Professor and Chair, Department of Pediatrics, George Washington University School of Medicine and Health Sciences; Chief Academic Officer, Children's National Medical Center; Director, Children's Research Institute, Washington, DC
MENTAL RETARDATION

Eric D. Baum, MD
Clinical Instructor, Department of Otorhinolaryngology, Head and Neck Surgery, University of Pennsylvania School of Medicine; Senior Fellow, Department of Otolaryngology, The Children's Hospital of Philadelphia, Philadelphia, Pennsylvania
BACTERIAL INFECTIONS OF THE NECK

Leslie Baumann, MD
Associate Professor of Dermatology, University of Miami Miller School of Medicine, Miami, Florida
SUN PROTECTION IN THE PEDIATRIC PATIENT

Stephen Baumgart, MD
Professor of Pediatrics, George Washington University School of Medicine and Health Sciences; Staff Physician, Department of Neonatology, Children's National Medical Center, Washington, DC
WATER AND ELECTROLYTE BALANCE IN LOW-BIRTH-WEIGHT INFANTS

Brook Belay, MD, MPh
Assistant Professor of Pediatrics, Temple University School of Medicine; Staff Physician, Temple University Children's Medical Center, Philadelphia, Pennsylvania
CHRONIC KIDNEY DISEASE

Mark R. Benfield, MD
Professor of Pediatrics, University of Alabama at Birmingham School of Medicine; Director, Pediatric Nephrology, Department of Pediatrics, Children's Health System of Alabama, Birmingham, Alabama
MANAGING END-STAGE RENAL DISEASE

Latanya T. Benjamin, MD
Pediatric Dermatology Clinical Research Fellow, Department of Dermatology and Cutaneous Surgery Division of Pediatric Dermatology, University of Miami Miller School of Medicine; Staff Physician, Jackson Memorial Hospital, Miami, Florida
SUN PROTECTION IN THE PEDIATRIC PATIENT

Suzanne Beno, MD
Instructor, Department of Pediatrics University of Pennsylvania School of Medicine; Fellow, Pediatric Emergency Medicine, The Children's Hospital of Philadelphia, Philadelphia, Pennsylvania
ANAPHYLAXIS

Abbey L. Berg, PhD
Assistant Professor, Communication Studies/Division of Communication Sciences and Disorders, Pace University; Staff, Otolaryngology/Head and Neck Surgery, Children's Hospital of New York; Assistant Professor of Otolaryngology/Head and Neck Surgery, College of Physicians and Surgeons, New York, New York
HEARING LOSS

Joel Howard Berg, DDS, MS
Lloyd and Kay Chapman Chair for Oral Health and Professor, Department of Pediatric Dentistry, University of Washington School of Medicine, Seattle, Washington
ORAL HEALTH

Roger L. Berkow, MD
Professor and Vice-Chair, Department of Pediatrics, University of Alabama at Birmingham School of Medicine; Staff Physician, Pediatric Hematology/Oncology, Children's Hospital of Alabama, Birmingham, Alabama
HEMOLYTIC ANEMIAS

Jonathan Berman, MD, PhD, FAAP
Director, Office of Clinical and Regulatory Affairs National Center for Complementary and Alternative Medicine, National Institutes of Health, Bethesda, Maryland
LEISHMANIASIS, AMERICAN TRYPANOSOMIASIS, AFRICAN TRYPANSOSOMIASIS

David I. Bernstein, MD, MA
Albert Sabin Professor of Pediatrics, University of Cincinnati College of Medicine; Director, Division of Infectious Diseases, Cincinnati Children's Hospital Medical Center, Cincinnati, Ohio
ROTAVIRUS INFECTIONS

Gerard T. Berry, MD
Professor of Pediatrics
Jefferson Medical College of Thomas Jefferson University, Philadelphia, Pennsylvania
METABOLIC EMERGENCIES IN THE NEWBORN

Jeffrey M. Bethony, MS, PhD
Assistant Professor, Department of Microbiology, Immunology, and Tropical Medicine, George Washington University School of Medicine and Health Sciences, Washington, DC
SOIL-TRANSMITTED HELMINTH INFECTIONS

Katherine Biagas, MD
Assistant Professor, Department of Pediatrics, Columbia University College of Physicians and Surgeons; Staff Physician, New York–Presbyterian Hospital, New York, New York
DROWNING AND NEAR DROWNING: SUBMERSION INJURY

Robert James Bidwell, MD
Associate Professor of Pediatrics
University of Hawaii John A. Burns School of Medicine; Director of Adolescent Medicine, Department of Pediatrics, Kapiolani Medical Center for Women and Children, Honolulu, Hawaii
ISSUES OF SEXUAL ORIENTATION AND GENDER IDENTITY

John J. Bissler, MD
Associate Professor of Pediatrics, Division of Nephrology and Hypertension, University of Cincinnati College of Medicine; Staff Physician, Children's Hospital Medical Center, Cincinnati, Ohio
HEMATURIA AND PROTEINURIA

Steven Black, MD
Clinical Professor of Pediatric Infectious Disease, Department of Pediatrics, Stanford University School of Medicine, Stanford; Co-Director, Kaiser Permanente Vaccine Study Center, Oakland, California
MENINGOCOCCAL DISEASE

Ronald E. Blanton, MD, MS
Associate Professor of International Health, Center for Global Health and Diseases, Case School of Medicine, Cleveland, Ohio
SCHISTOSOMIASIS

Nathan J. Blum, MD
Associate Professor of Pediatrics, University of Pennsylvania School of Medicine; Director, Section of Behavioral Pediatrics, Division of Child Development and Rehabilitation, The Children's Hospital of Philadelphia, Philadelphia, Pennsylvania
BREATH-HOLDING SPELLS

Amy Eldridge Bobrowski, MD
Fellow, Department of Pediatrics, Division of Kidney Diseases, Northwestern University McGaw School of Medicine and Children's Memorial Hospital, Chicago, Illinois
NEPHROLITHIASIS

Mark Boguniewicz, MD
Professor of Pediatrics University of Colorado School of Medicine; Staff Physician, Department of Pediatrics, National Jewish Medical and Research Center, Denver, Colorado
ATOPIC DERMATITIS

William Borkowsky, MD
Professor of Pediatrics, New York University School of Medicine, New York, New York
WEST NILE VIRUS; HUMAN PAPILLOMAVIRUS

Caroline D. Boyd, MD
Fellow, Pediatric Critical Care, Department of Anesthesiology and Critical Care Medicine, Alfred I. duPont Hospital for Children, Wilmington, Delaware
ACUTE RESPIRATORY DISTRESS SYNDROME

John Timothy Boyle, MD
Professor of Pediatrics, University of Alabama at Birmingham School of Medicine; Chief, Pediatric Gastroenterology and Nutrition, Children's Hospital of Alabama, Birmingham, Alabama
ACUTE ABDOMINAL PAIN

Darla J. Bradshaw, RD, CNSD, LDN
Nutrition Support Dietitian, Pediatric Intensive Care Unit, Department of Clinical Nutrition, The Children's Hospital of Philadelphia, Philadelphia, Pennsylvania
NUTRITION SUPPORT OF THE VERY ILL PEDIATRIC PATIENT

Brian E. Brigman, MD
Assistant Professor of Surgery, Division of Orthopaedic Surgery, Duke University School of Medicine, Durham, North Carolina
MALIGNANT TUMORS OF BONE AND LIMB SALVAGE

Michael Briones, DO
Assistant Professor, Division of Pediatric Hematology and Oncology, Emory University School of Medicine; Staff, AFLAC Cancer Center and Blood Disorder, Children's Healthcare of Atlanta, Atlanta, Georgia
DISORDERS OF COAGULATION, PLATELET NUMBER, AND FUNCTION

Kenneth Bromberg, MD, FAAP
Professor of Pediatrics, Weill Medical College of Cornell University, New York; Chairman of Pediatrics, The Brooklyn Hospital Center, Brooklyn, New York
GONOCOCCAL INFECTIONS

Itzhak Brook, MD, MSc
Professor of Pediatrics, Georgetown University School of Medicine; Attending, Department of Pediatrics, Georgetown University Medical Center, Washington, DC; Consultant, Infectious Diseases, Department of Pediatrics, Naval Medical Center, Bethesda, Maryland
ANAEROBIC INFECTIONS

Simon Brooker, DPhil
Senior Lecturer, Department of Infectious and Tropical Diseases, London School of Hygiene and Tropical Medicine, London, United Kingdom
SOIL-TRANSMITTED HELMINTH INFECTIONS

Lawrence W. Brown, MD
Associate Professor of Neurology and Pediatrics, University of Pennsylvania School of Medicine; Staff Physician, The Children's Hospital of Philadelphia, Philadelphia, Pennsylvania
REYE SYNDROME; TOURETTE SYNDROME

Rachel E. Brown, MD
Neonatal-Perinatal Fellow, Department of Pediatrics, University of Florida College of Medicine, Gainesville, Florida
NECROTIZING ENTEROCOLITIS

Terri Brown-Whitehorn, MD
Attending Physician, Division of Allergy and Immunology, The Children's Hospital of Philadelphia, Philadelphia, Pennsylvania
ANAPHYLAXIS

Robert L. Buka, MD, JD
Mount Sinai School of Medicine; Assistant Attending, Pediatric Dermatology, Mount Sinai Hospital, New York, New York; Director of Pediatric and Adolescent Dermatology, The Dermatology Group, Verona, New Jersey
NEVI AND NEVOID TUMORS

Timothy E. Bunchman, MD
Director, Pediatric Nephrology and Transplantation, DeVos Children's Hospital, Grand Rapids, Michigan
DIALYTIC THERAPIES

Michael R. Bye, MD
Professor of Clinical Pediatrics, Columbia University College
of Physicians and Surgeons; Acting Director, Pediatric
Pulmonary Medicine, Children's Hospital of New York–
Presbyterian, New York, New York
ASPIRATION SYNDROMES

Carrie L. Byington, MD
Associate Professor of Pediatrics and Infectious Diseases,
University of Utah School of Medicine; Salt Lake City, Utah
ENTEROVIRUSES

Mitchell S. Cairo, MD
Professor of Pediatrics, Medicine, and Pathology; Director,
Division of Pediatric Hematology and Bone Marrow
Transplantation, Department of Pediatrics, Columbia
University College of Physicians and Surgeons, New York,
New York
NEONATAL AND CHILDHOOD NEUTROPENIA; BLOOD AND MARROW
TRANSPLANTATION

Diane P. Calello, MD
Instructor of Pediatrics, University of Pennsylvania School of
Medicine; Attending Physician, Department of Pediatrics,
Division of Emergency Medicine, The Children's Hospital of
Philadelphia, Philadelphia, Pennsylvania
ACUTE POISONING

Melissa S. Camp, MD
Resident, General Surgery, Johns Hopkins Hospital,
Baltimore, Maryland
PERITONITIS

Joshua Cappell, MD
Assistant Professor of Neurology and Pediatrics, Columbia
University College of Physicians and Surgeons; Assistant
Attending Physician, Departments of Neurology and
Pediatrics, Children's Hospital of New York–Presbyterian,
New York, New York
PSEUDOTUMOR CEREBRI SYNDROME

Michael Cappello, MD
Professor of Pediatrics and Epidemiology and Public Health,
Yale University School of Medicine; Director, Program in
International Child Health, Yale Child Health Research
Center, New Haven, Connecticut
TRICHINELLOSIS (TRICHINOSIS)

Joseph A. Carcillo, MD
Associate Professor of Critical Care Medicine and Pediatrics,
University of Pittsburgh School of Medicine; Associate
Director, Pediatric ICU, Children's Hospital of Pittsburgh,
Pittsburgh, Pennsylvania
MANAGEMENT OF SEPSIS AND SEPTIC SHOCK

K. Robin Carder, MD
Assistant Professor of Dermatology and Pediatrics, The
University of Texas Southwestern Medical School, Dallas,
Texas
SKIN DISEASES OF THE NEONATE, INCLUDING DIAPER DERMATITIS

Ivan Cardona, MD
Allergy/Immunology Fellow, Department of Pediatrics,
University of Colorado Health Sciences Center, and National
Jewish Medical and Research Center, Denver, Colorado
ATOPIC DERMATITIS

Thomas O. Carpenter, MD
Professor of Pediatrics, Yale University School of Medicine;
Attending Physician, Department of Pediatrics,
Yale–New Haven Hospital, New Haven, Connecticut
DISORDERS OF THE PARATHYROIDS, HYPOCALCEMIA,
AND HYPERCALCEMIA

Christopher L. Case, DMD, MD
Associate Director, Pediatric Cardiology Unit, Cook
Children's Medical Center, Fort Worth, Texas
CARDIAC DYSRHYTHMIAS

Jacqueline Casillas, MD, MSHS
Assistant Professor of Pediatrics, David Geffen School of
Medicine at UCLA; Staff Physician, Division of Hematology/
Oncology Mattel Children's Hospital at UCLA, Los Angeles,
California
THE CHILD CURED OF CANCER

N. John Cavuto, MD
Fellow, Pediatric Gastroenterology and Nutrition Unit,
Massachusetts General Hospital, Boston, Massachusetts
CIRRHOSIS AND PORTAL HYPERTENSION

Roland V. Cellona, MD, DPH (Lond), FPDS
Assistant Professor, Department of Medicine, Section of
Dermatology, Cebu Institute of Medicine; Chief
Epidemiologist Department of Dermatology,
Cebu Skin Clinic, American Leprosy Foundation,
Cebu City, Philippines
LEPROSY (HANSEN DISEASE)

Samuel Chachkin, MD
Instructor of Pediatrics, University of Pennsylvania
School of Medicine; Attending Physician,
The Children's Hospital of Philadelphia,
Philadelphia, Pennsylvania
ERYTHEMA NODOSUM

James C. M. Chan, MD
Professor of Pediatrics, University of Vermont College of
Medicine, Burlington, Vermont; Director of Research, The
Barbara Bush Children's Hospital, Portland, Maine
THE NEPHROTIC SYNDROME

Manju M. Chandra, MD
Professor of Pediatrics, New York University School of
Medicine, New York; Staff Physician, Division of Pediatric
Nephrology, Schneider Children's Hospital, New Hyde Park;
Physician in Charge, Urodynamics Laboratory, North Shore
University Hospital, Manhasset, New York
ENURESIS AND VOIDING DYSFUNCTION

**Anne Bernadette Chang, MBBS, FRACP,
MPHTM, PhD**
Associate Professor of Paediatrics and Child Health,
University of Queensland Faculty of Medicine; Attending,
Division of Respiratory Medicine, Royal Children's Hospital,
Brisbane, Queensland, Australia
COUGH

R. Victoria Chen, MD, MPH
Pediatrician, Kaiser Permanente, Fontana, California
NEONATAL SEIZURES

Judy W. Cheng, MPAS, PA-C
Dermatology Associates Medical Group Beverly Hills,
California
ERYTHEMA NODOSUM

James D. Cherry, MD, MSc
Professor of Pediatrics, David Geffen School of Medicine at
UCLA; Los Angeles, California; Member, Division of
Infectious Diseases Department of Pediatrics, Mattel
Children's Hospital at UCLA, Los Angeles, California
BORDETELLA PERTUSSIS (WHOOPING COUGH)

Russell W. Chesney, MD
LeBonheur Professor and Chair, Department of Pediatrics,
University of Tennessee Health Science Center, College of
Medicine; Attending, LeBonheur Children's Medical Center,
Memphis, Tennessee
AN APPROACH TO THE TREATMENT OF METABOLIC DISEASE

Robert L. Chevalier, MD
Professor and Chair, Department of Pediatrics, University of
Virginia School of Medicine; Pediatrician-in-Chief,
University of Virginia Health System, Charlottesville,
Virginia
OBSTRUCTIVE UROPATHY

Michael F. Chiang, MD
Assistant Professor, Department of Ophthalmology,
Columbia University College of Physicians and Surgeons;
Assistant Attending, Department of Ophthalmology,
New York–Presbyterian Hospital, New York, New York
RETINOPATHY OF PREMATURITY

Claudia A. Chiriboga, MD, MPH
Associate Professor of Clinical Neurology and Clinical
Pediatrics, Division of Pediatric Neurology, Department of
Neurology, Columbia University College of Physicians and
Surgeons; Associate Attending, Department of Neurology,
Columbia University Medical Center, New York, New York
ACUTE ATAXIA

Abraham M. Chutorian, MD
Professor of Neurology and Pediatrics
Weill Medical College of Cornell University; Attending
Neurologist/Pediatrician, New York–Presbyterian Hospital;
Attending Pediatrician, Lennox Hill Hospital, New York;
Consultant Pediatric Neurologist, Blythedale Children's
Hospital, Valhalla, New York
HEADACHES

William L. Clarke, MD
Genentech Professor of Pediatrics, University of Virginia
School of Medicine, Charlottesville, Virginia
HYPOGLYCEMIA

Thomas G. Cleary, MD
Professor of Pediatrics, University of Texas Medical School;
Professor, Center for Infectious Diseases/University of Texas
School of Public Health, Houston, Texas
CAMPYLOBACTER; NONTYPHOIDAL *SALMONELLA*; SHIGELLOSIS;
TYPHOID FEVER

Dennis A. Clements, MD, PhD
Professor of Pediatrics and Infectious Diseases, Duke
University School of Medicine; Staff Physician, Duke
Children's Hospital, Durham, North Carolina
INFECTIONS IN DAYCARE ENVIRONMENTS

Susan E. Coffin, MD, MPH
Assistant Professor of Pediatrics, Division of Infectious
Diseases, University of Pennsylvania School of Medicine;
Medical Director, Department of Infection Prevention and
Control, The Children's Hospital of Philadelphia,
Philadelphia, Pennsylvania
ABSCESS IN THE CENTRAL NERVOUS SYSTEM

George J. Cohen, MD
Clinical Professor of Pediatrics, George Washington
University School of Medicine; Attending Pediatrician,
Children's National Medical Center, Washington, DC;
Academic Staff, Department of Pediatrics, Holy Cross
Hospital, Silver Spring, Maryland
CHILDREN OF DIVORCING PARENTS

Steven D. Colan, MD
Professor of Pediatrics, Harvard Medical School; Chief,
Division of Noninvasive Cardiology, Children's Hospital
Boston, Boston, Massachusetts
MYOCARDITIS AND PERICARDITIS

John J. Collins, MBBS, PhD, FRACP
Head, Pain and Palliative Care Service, Children's Hospital
at Westmead, Sydney, New South Wales, Australia
END-OF-LIFE CARE FOR PEDIATRIC PATIENTS

Elizabeth Alvarez Connelly, MD
Departments of Pediatrics and Medicine (Dermatology),
University of California, San Diego, School of Medicine; Staff
Pediatrician, Children's Hospital and Health Center–San
Diego, San Diego, California
FUNGAL INFECTIONS OF THE SKIN, HAIR, AND NAILS; SUN PROTECTION IN
THE PEDIATRIC PATIENT

Alex R. Constantinescu, MD
Associate Professor–Voluntary, Department of Pediatrics,
University of Miami Miller School of Medicine, Miami;
Director, Pediatric Nephrology Division, Joe DiMaggio
Children's Hospital, Hollywood, Florida
RENAL TUBULOPATHIES

Arthur Cooper, MD, MS
Professor of Surgery, Columbia University College of Physicians
and Surgeons; Director of Trauma and Pediatric Surgical
Services, Harlem Hospital Center, New York, New York
STABILIZING THE INJURED CHILD

Karoll J. Cortez, MD
Staff Clinician, Immunocompromised Host Section, Pediatric
Oncology Branch, National Cancer Institute, National
Institutes of Health, Bethesda, Maryland
THE IMMUNOCOMPROMISED HOST

Andrew T. Costarino Jr., MD
Chairman, Department of Anesthesiology and Critical Care
Medicine, Alfred I. duPont Hospital for Children,
Wilmington, Delaware
ACUTE RESPIRATORY DISTRESS SYNDROME

Robert A. Cowles, MD
Assistant Professor of Surgery, Division of Pediatric Surgery,
Columbia University College of Physicians and Surgeons;
Assistant Attending Surgeon, Division of Pediatric Surgery,
Morgan Stanley Children's Hospital of New York–
Presbyterian, New York, New York
ABDOMINAL WALL DEFECTS AND DISORDERS OF THE UMBILICUS

Susan E. Crawford, MD
Instructor, Department of Pediatrics, Northwestern
University Feinberg School of Medicine; Staff, Children's
Memorial Hospital; Research Associate, Department of
Pediatric Infectious Diseases, University of Chicago Pritzker
School of Medicine, Chicago, Illinois
STAPHYLOCOCCAL INFECTIONS

James T. Cullinan, DO
Assistant Professor, Department of Psychiatry and
Behavioral Neurobiology, Division of Child and Adolescent
Psychiatry, University of Alabama at Birmingham School of
Medicine; Inpatient Medical Director, Child and Adolescent
Psychiatry, Children's Hospital of Alabama, Birmingham,
Alabama
PSYCHIATRIC DISORDERS AND MENTAL HEALTH DISORDERS IN
CHILDREN AND ADOLESCENTS

Ilan Dalal, MD
Senior Lecturer in Medicine, Sackler Faculty of Medicine, Tel
Aviv University, Tel Aviv; Staff Physician, Pediatric Allergy/
Clinical Immunology Unit, Department of Pediatrics, Edith
Wolfson Medical Center, Holon, Israel
URTICARIA AND ANGIOEDEMA

David A. Dasher, MD
Resident Physician, Department of Internal Medicine UNC
Hospital, Chapel Hill, North Carolina
PSORIASIS AND OTHER PAPULOSQUAMOUS DISORDERS

Robert S. Daum, MD, CM
Professor of Pediatrics and Professor, Committee on
Microbiology and Professor, Committee on Molecular
Medicine, University of Chicago Pritzker School of Medicine;
Section Chief , Pediatric Infectious Diseases, University of
Chicago Children's Hospital, Chicago, Illinois
INFECTIVE ENDOCARDITIS; STAPHYLOCOCCAL INFECTIONS

Gustavo H. Dayan, MD
Medical Epidemiologist, National Immunization Program,
Centers for Disease Control and Prevention, Atlanta,
Georgia
RUBELLA

Peter S. Dayan, MD, MSc
Assistant Professor of Clinical Pediatrics, Columbia
University College of Physicians and Surgeons; Assistant
Attending, Department of Pediatrics, Division of Pediatric
Emergency Medicine, Morgan Stanley Children's Hospital of
New York–Presbyterian, New York, New York
MAMMALIAN BITES AND BITE-RELATED INFECTIONS

Dorr G. Dearborn, PhD, MD
Mary Ann Swetland Professor of Environmental Health
Science, Department of Pediatrics,
Case School of Medicine; Staff Physician, Pulmonary
Division, and Rainbow Babies Children's Hospital,
Cleveland, Ohio
DIFFUSE ALVEOLAR HEMORRHAGE (PULMONARY SIDEROSIS)

Gustavo Del Toro, MD
Assistant Professor of Pediatrics, Columbia University
College of Physicians and Surgeons; Clinical Director,
Pediatric Bone Marrow Transplantation, Morgan Stanley

Children's Hospital of New York–Presbyterian, New York,
New York
BLOOD AND MARROW TRANSPLANTATION

Gail J. Demmler, MD
Professor of Pediatrics, Baylor College of Medicine; Director,
Diagnostic Virology Laboratory, and Attending Physician,
Infectious Diseases Service, Texas Children's Hospital,
Houston, Texas
CYTOMEGALOVIRUS INFECTIONS

Catherine L. Dent, MD
Assistant Professor of Pediatrics, University of Cincinnati
College of Medicine; Staff Physician, Division of Pediatric
Cardiology, Cincinnati Children's Hospital Medical Center,
Cincinnati, Ohio
PULMONARY HYPERTENSION IN CHILDREN

Lianne M. deSerres, MD, MS
Assistant Professor of Otolaryngology–Head and Neck
Surgery, Columbia University College of Physicians and
Surgeons; Attending, Physician, Otolaryngology–Head and
Neck Surgery, Division of Pediatric Otolaryngology,
New York–Presbyterian Hospital, New York, New York
TONSILLECTOMY AND ADENOIDECTOMY

James G. H. Dinulos, MD
Assistant Professor of Medicine and Pediatrics
(Dermatology), Dartmouth Medical School; Attending
Pediatrician, Dartmouth-Hitchcock Medical Center,
Lebanon New Hampshire
MANAGEMENT OF GENETIC SKIN DISORDERS

Mary Beth Dinulos, MD
Assistant Professor of Pediatrics, Dartmouth Medical School;
Attending Pediatrician, Dartmouth-Hitchcock Medical
Center, Lebanon, New Hampshire
MANAGEMENT OF GENETIC SKIN DISORDERS

Samuel R. Dominguez, MD, PhD
Staff Physician, Department of Pediatric Infectious Diseases,
The Children's Hospital, Denver, Colorado
INFECTIVE ENDOCARDITIS

Marc E. Dovey, MD
Assistant Professor of Pediatrics, Joan and Sanford I. Weill
Medical College of Cornell University; Chief, Division of
Pediatric Pulmonology, Allergy, and Immunology,
Department of Pediatrics, New York–Presbyterian Hospital,
New York, New York
CYSTIC FIBROSIS

J. Scott Doyle, MD
Assistant Professor of Orthopaedic Surgery, University of
Alabama at Birmingham School of Medicine; Pediatric
Orthopaedic Surgeon, The Children's Hospital of Alabama,
Birmingham, Alabama
DISORDERS OF THE SPINE AND SHOULDER GIRDLE

Amy L. Drendel, DO, MS
Assistant Professor of Pediatrics, Medical College of
Wisconsin; Attending Physician, Department of Pediatric
Emergency Medicine, Children's Hospital of Wisconsin,
Milwaukee, Wisconsin
ROTATIONAL ORTHOPEDIC PROBLEMS OF THE EXTREMITIES

Alistair J. A. Duff, MD
Consultant Clinical Psychologist and Head of Paediatric Psychology Services, Department of Clinical and Health Psychology, Leeds Teaching Hospitals NHS Trust, Leeds, United Kingdom
ADHERENCE TO TREATMENT IN CHILDREN AND ADOLESCENTS LIVING WITH CHRONIC ILLNESS

Morven S. Edwards, MD
Professor of Pediatrics, Baylor College of Medicine; Attending Physician, Department of Pediatrics, Texas Children's Hospital, Houston, Texas
GROUP B STREPTOCOCCAL INFECTIONS

Lisa M. Elden, MD
Assistant Professor, Department of Otolaryngology, University of Pennsylvania School of Medicine; Associate, Pediatric Otolaryngology, The Children's Hospital of Philadelphia, Philadelphia, Pennsylvania
BACTERIAL INFECTIONS OF THE NECK

Wafaa M. El-Sadr, MD, MPH
Professor of Clinical Medicine and Epidemiology, Mailman School of Public Health and College of Physicians and Surgeons, Columbia University; Chief, Division of Infectious Diseases, Harlem Hospital Center, New York, New York
TUBERCULOSIS

S. Jean Emans, MD
Professor of Pediatrics, Harvard Medical School; Chief, Division of Adolescent/Young Adult Medicine, Department of Medicine, Children's Hospital Boston, Boston, Massachusetts
ADOLESCENT GYNECOLOGY

Moshe Ephros, MD, FAAP
Senior Lecturer in Pediatrics
Faculty of Medicine, Technion-Israel Institute of Technology; Senior Pediatrician and Consultant in Infectious Diseases, Department of Pediatrics, Carmel Medical Center, Haifa, Israel
CAT-SCRATCH DISEASE

Jacquelyn R. Evans, MD
Clinical Professor of Pediatrics, University of Pennsylvania School of Medicine; Medical Director, Newborn Infant Center, Department of Pediatrics, The Children's Hospital of Philadelphia, Philadelphia, Pennsylvania
PATENT DUCTUS ARTERIOSUS

Avroy A. Fanaroff, MB, BCh
Professor and Chair, Department of Pediatrics, Case School of Medicine; Eliza Henry Barnes Chair of Neonatology, Department of Pediatrics, and Physician-in-Chief, Rainbow Babies and Children's Hospital, Cleveland, Ohio
PERINATAL CARE AT THE THRESHOLD OF VIABILITY

Stephen A. Feig, MD
Professor of Pediatrics, David Geffen School of Medicine at UCLA; Chief Division of Hematology/Oncology, Department of Pediatrics, Mattel Children's Hospital at UCLA, Los Angeles, California
THE CHILD CURED OF CANCER

Leonard G. Feld, MD, PhD
Professor of Pediatrics, UMDNJ–New Jersey Medical School, Newark; Chairman, Department of Pediatrics, Goryeb Children's Hospital–Atlantic Health System, Morristown, New Jersey
FEVER IN INFANTS AND CHILDREN FROM BIRTH TO 3 YEARS

Heidi M. Feldman, MD, PhD
Professor of Pediatrics, University of Pittsburgh School of Medicine; Staff Physician, Child Development Unit, Children's Hospital of Pittsburgh, Pittsburgh, Pennsylvania
ATTENTION DEFICIT HYPERACTIVITY DISORDER

Neil A. Feldstein, MD
Assistant Professor of Clinical Neurological Surgery, Department of Neurological Surgery, New York–Presbyterian Hospital; Children's Hospital of New York–Presbyterian, New York, New York
EPIDURAL AND SUBDURAL HEMATOMAS; DIAGNOSIS AND MANAGEMENT OF CHIARI I MALFORMATION; DIAGNOSIS AND MANAGEMENT OF HYDROCEPHALUS

Polly J. Ferguson, MD
Assistant Professor of Pediatrics, University of Iowa Lucille A. and Roy J. Carver College of Medicine, Iowa City, Iowa
PEDIATRIC SYSTEMIC LUPUS ERYTHEMATOSUS

William S. Ferguson, MD
Professor of Pediatrics, St. Louis University School of Medicine; Director of Hematology-Oncology, Cardinal Glennon Children's Hospital, St. Louis, Missouri
VISCERAL TUMORS

Dorothy Fielding, MSc, PhD, ABPsS
Visiting Professor, Department of Psychology, Leeds University; Head of Psychological Services, Department of Clinical and Health Psychology, Leeds Teaching Hospitals Trust–St. James's University Hospital, Leeds, United Kingdom
ADHERENCE TO TREATMENT IN CHILDREN AND ADOLESCENTS LIVING WITH CHRONIC ILLNESS

Neil N. Finer, MD
Professor of Pediatrics and Director, Division of Neonatology, Department of Pediatrics, University of California, San Diego, School of Medicine; Associate, Department of Neonatology, Children's Hospital San Diego, San Diego, California
PERSISTENT PULMONARY HYPERTENSION OF THE NEWBORN

Richard S. Finkel, MD
Clinical Associate Professor of Pediatrics and Neurology, University of Pennsylvania School of Medicine; Director, Neuromuscular Program, The Children's Hospital of Philadelphia, Philadelphia, Pennsylvania
MYASTHENIA GRAVIS

Lewis R. First, MD, MS
Professor and Chair, Department of Pediatrics, and Senior Associate Dean for Medical Education, University of Vermont College of Medicine; Chief of Pediatrics, Vermont Children's Hospital at Fletcher Allen Health Care, Burlington, Vermont
SCREENING IN THE NEWBORN INFANT: HEARING LOSS, RISK OF SEVERE HYPERBILIRUBINEMIA, CONGENITAL HEART DISEASE; FOREIGN BODIES IN THE GASTROINTESTINAL TRACT

John T. Flynn, MD
Anne S. Cohen, Professor of Pediatric Ophthalmology,
Department of Ophthalmology, Columbia University College
of Physicians and Surgeons; Attending, Department of
Ophthalmology, New York–Presbyterian Hospital,
New York, New York
RETINOPATHY OF PREMATURITY

Marc D. Foca, MD
Assistant Professor of Pediatrics, Columbia University
College of Physicians and Surgeons; Assistant Attending,
Department of Pediatrics, Morgan Stanley Children's
Hospital of New York–Presbyterian, New York, New York
PNEUMONIA; CATHETER-ASSOCIATED INFECTIONS

Thomas P. Foley Jr., MD
Emeritus Professor of Pediatrics and Epidemiology, School
of Medicine and Graduate School of Public Health,
University of Pittsburgh; Emeritus Staff, Department of
Pediatrics, Children's Hospital of Pittsburgh, Pittsburgh,
Pennsylvania
THYROID DISORDERS

John W. Foreman, MD
Professor of Pediatrics, Duke University School of Medicine;
Chief, Division of Pediatric Nephrology, Department of
Pediatrics, Duke University Medical Center, Durham, North
Carolina
THE NEPHROTIC SYNDROME

Anna Keating Franklin, MD
Instructor, Department of Pediatrics, Memorial Sloan-
Kettering Cancer Center, New York, New York
ACUTE LEUKEMIA

Lisa M. Frenkel, M.D.
Professor of Pediatrics and Laboratory Medicine, University
of Washington School of Medicine; Associate, Department of
Infectious Disease, Children's Hospital and Regional Medical
Center, Seattle, Washington
ANTIVIRAL THERAPIES

Sheila Fallon Friedlander, MD
Clinical Professor of Pediatrics and Medicine (Dermatology),
University of California, San Diego, School of Medicine;
Attending Staff, Department of Pediatrics, Children's
Hospital and Health Center–San Diego, San Diego,
California
FUNGAL INFECTIONS OF THE SKIN, HAIR, AND NAILS

Sandeep Gangadharan, MD
Clinical Instructor in Pediatrics, Columbia University
College of Physicians and Surgeons, New York, New York;
Attending Physician, Department of Pediatrics, Children's
Hospital of New York, New York, New York
RESPIRATORY FAILURE

Soren Gantt, MD, PhD
Pediatric Infectious Disease Fellow, Department of
Pediatrics, Children's Hospital and Regional Medical Center/
University of Washington School of Medicine, Seattle,
Washington
ANTIVIRAL THERAPIES

Samuel J. Garber, MD
Clinical Associate, Division of Neonatology, Department of
Pediatrics, University of Pennsylvania School of Medicine,
Philadelphia, Pennsylvania
NEONATAL SEPSIS

Mark C. Gebhardt, MD
Frederick W. and Jane M. Ilfeld Professor of Orthopaedic
Surgery, Harvard Medical School; Chief, Orthopaedic
Surgery, and Orthopaedic Surgeon-in-Chief, Beth Israel
Deaconess Medical Center, Boston, Massachusetts
MALIGNANT TUMORS OF BONE AND LIMB SALVAGE

Robert H. Gelber, MD
Clinical Professor of Medicine and Dermatology, University
of California, San Francisco, School of Medicine, San
Francisco, California; Scientific Director, Epidemiology
Branch, Leonard Wood Memorial Center for Leprosy
Research, Cebu City, Philippines
LEPROSY (HANSEN DISEASE)

Andrew R. Gennery, MD
Senior Lecturer, Paediatric Immunology and Bone Marrow
Transplantation, Department of Clinical Medical Sciences
(Child Health), University of Newcastle upon Tyne;
Honorary Consultant, Paediatric Immunology and Bone
Marrow Transplantation, Children's BMT Unit, Newcastle
General Hospital, Newcastle upon Tyne, United Kingdom
PRIMARY IMMUNODEFICIENCY SYNDROMES

Michael A. Gerber, MD
Professor of Pediatrics, University of Cincinnati College of
Medicine; Attending Physician, Division of Infectious
Diseases, Cincinnati Children's Hospital Medical Center,
Cincinnati, Ohio
GROUP A STREPTOCOCCAL INFECTIONS

Karen I. Gerber-Vecsey, MD
Fellow, Division of Pediatric Nephrology, University at
Buffalo SUNY School of Medicine and Biomedical Sciences
and The Women and Children's Hospital of Buffalo, Buffalo,
New York
RHABDOMYOLYSIS

Sezelle Gereau, MD
Assistant Professor, Department of Pediatric
Otolaryngology, Columbia University College of Physicians
and Surgeons; Attending Otolaryngologist, Department of
Pediatric Otolaryngology, Children's Hospital of New York,
New York, New York
DISORDERS OF THE NECK AND PAROTID

John A. Germiller, MD, PhD
Assistant Professor of Otorhinolaryngology, University of
Pennsylvania School of Medicine; Staff Physician, Division of
Otolaryngology, The Children's Hospital of Philadelphia,
Philadelphia, Pennsylvania
LABYRINTHITIS

Anne A. Gershon, MD
Professor of Pediatrics, Columbia University College of
Physicians and Surgeons; Attending Physician, Department
of Pediatrics, Morgan Stanley Children's Hospital of
New York–Presbyterian, New York, New York
VARICELLA-ZOSTER INFECTIONS

Fred E. Ghali, MD
Private Practice, Pediatric Dermatology of North Texas, P.A.,
Grapevine, Texas
ALLERGIC CONTACT DERMATITIS

Saadi Ghatan, MD
Assistant Professor of Neurological Surgery, Columbia
University College of Physicians and Surgeons; Attending
Pediatric Neurosurgeon, Children's Hospital of New York–
Presbyterian, New York, New York; Valley Hospital,
Ridgewood, New Jersey; and Northern Westchester Hospital,
Mt. Kisco, New York
MYELOMENINGOCELE

Eric Gibson, MD
Associate Professor of Pediatrics, Jefferson Medical College
of Thomas Jefferson University, Philadelphia, Pennsylvania;
Staff Pediatrics, Alexis I. duPont Hospital for Children,
Wilmington, Delaware
SUDDEN INFANT DEATH SYNDROME

Michael Giladi, MD, MSc
Director, Infectious Disease Unit and Bernard Pridan
Laboratory for Molecular Biology of Infectious Diseases, Tel
Aviv Medical Center, Tel Aviv, Israel
CAT-SCRATCH DISEASE

Neelam Giri, MD
Staff Clinician, Clinical Genetics Branch, Division of Cancer
Epidemiology and Genetics, National Cancer Institute,
Department of Health and Human Services, Rockville,
Maryland
ACQUIRED APLASTIC ANEMIA

Wallace A. Gleason Jr., MD
Professor and Assistant Dean, Department of Pediatrics,
University of Texas–Houston Medical School; Chief,
Pediatric Gastroenterology, Hepatology, and Nutrition,
Memorial Hermann Children's Hospital and Lyndon B.
Johnson General Hospital, Houston, Texas
CONJUGATED AND UNCONJUGATED HYPERBILIRUBINEMIA AND
DISORDERS OF THE BILIARY TREE

Benjamin D. Gold, MD
Associate Professor of Pediatrics and Director, Division of
Pediatric Gastroenterology and Nutrition, Department of
Pediatrics, Emory University School of Medicine; Chief of
Gastroenterology Service, Egleston Children's Hospital
Campus, Department of Pediatric Medicine, Children's
Healthcare of Atlanta, Atlanta, Georgia
HELICOBACTER PYLORI INFECTION

Eric F. Grabowski, MD, DrEngrSci
Associate Professor of Pediatrics, Harvard Medical School;
Pediatrician and Director, Program in Pediatric Hemostasis
and Thrombosis, and Director, Cardiovascular Thrombosis
Laboratory, MassGeneral Hospital for Children at
Massachusetts General Hospital; Chairman, New England
Retinoblastoma Group, Boston, Massachusetts
DEEP VENOUS THROMBOSIS WITH AND WITHOUT PULMONARY EMBOLISM;
INTRAOCULAR AND EXTRAOCULAR RETINOBLASTOMA

Philip L. Graham III, MD, MS
Assistant Professor of Pediatrics, Columbia University
College of Physicians and Surgeons; Assistant Attending

Physician, Department of Pediatrics, New York–
Presbyterian Hospital, Children's Hospital of New York–
Presbyterian, New York, New York
HEALTH CARE–ASSOCIATED INFECTIONS

David E. Green, MD
Director and Associate Professor of Obstetrics and
Gynecology, University of Alabama at Birmingham School of
Medicine–Huntsville Regional Medical Campus, Huntsville,
Alabama
ADOLESCENT CONTRACEPTION

Rebecca P. Green, MD, PhD
Department of Pediatrics, Division of Pediatric
Endocrinology, Washington University School of Medicine in
St. Louis; Staff Physician, Department of Pediatrics,
St. Louis Children's Hospital and Barnes-Jewish Hospital,
St. Louis, Missouri
DIABETES INSIPIDUS, SIADH, AND CEREBRAL SALT WASTING

Robert A. Green, MD
Assistant Professor of Clinical Medicine, Department of
Emergency Medicine, Columbia University College of
Physicians and Surgeons; Associate Director,
Department of Emergency Medicine,
New York–Presbyterian Hospital/Columbia University
Medical Center, New York, New York
MAMMALIAN BITES AND BITE-RELATED INFECTIONS

Donald E. Greydanus, MD, FAAP, FSAM, FIAP(H)
Professor of Pediatrics and Human Development
Michigan State University College of Human Medicine,
Kalamazoo and East Lansing; Program Director,
Department of Pediatrics, MSU/Kalamazoo Center for
Medical Studies, Kalamazoo, Michigan
SEXUALLY TRANSMITTED DISEASES IN ADOLESCENTS

Eli Grunstein, MD
Resident Physician, Department of Otolaryngology–Head
and Neck Surgery, New York–Presbyterian Hospital,
New York, New York
DISORDERS OF THE NECK AND PAROTID

Warren G. Guntheroth, MD
Professor of Pediatrics (Cardiology), University of
Washington School of Medicine; Attending Physician,
University of Washington Medical Center, Division of
Pediatric Cardiology, Seattle, Washington
CONGENITAL HEART DISEASE

Hector H. Gutierrez, MD
Associate Professor of Pediatrics, University of Alabama at
Birmingham School of Medicine, Birmingham, Alabama
PULMONARY SARCOIDOSIS

David H. Gutmann, MD, PhD
Professor of Neurology, Washington University in St. Louis
School of Medicine; Staff Pediatrician, St. Louis Children's
Hospital, St. Louis, Missouri
NEUROFIBROMATOSIS TYPE I

Joseph Haddad, Jr., MD
Professor and Vice Chairman, Department of
Otolaryngology/Head and Neck Surgery, Columbia

University College of Physicians and Surgeons; Lawrence Savetsky Chair and Director, Pediatric Otolaryngology/Head and Neck Surgery, Children's Hospital of New York–Presbyterian, New York, New York
DISORDERS OF THE LARYNX; CHOANAL ATRESIA

Sophie Hambleton, MRCP, DPhil
Postdoctoral Research Fellow, Department of Pediatrics, Pediatric Infectious Disease Division, Columbia University College of Physicians and Surgeons, New York, New York
PRIMARY IMMUNODEFICIENCY SYNDROMES

Margaret R. Hammerschlag, MD
Professor of Pediatrics and Medicine and Director, Division of Pediatric Infectious Diseases, Department of Pediatrics, State University of New York Downstate Medical Center College of Medicine, Brooklyn, New York
CHLAMYDIAL INFECTIONS

Catherine A. Hansen, MD
Clinical Instructor in Pediatrics, Columbia University College of Physicians and Surgeons; Director, Neonatal Services, Department of Pediatrics, Harlem Hospital Center, New York, New York
HYDROPS FETALIS

William G. Harmon, MD
Assistant Professor of Pediatrics, Divisions of Pediatric Cardiology and Critical Care, University of Rochester School of Medicine and Dentistry, Rochester, New York
KAWASAKI DISEASE

Mary Catherine Harris, MD
Associate Professor of Pediatrics (Neonatology), University of Pennsylvania School of Medicine; Staff Physician, Department of Neonatology, The Children's Hospital of Philadelphia, Philadelphia, Pennsylvania
NEONATAL SEPSIS

Rick E. Harrison, MD, FAAP
Professor of Pediatrics, David Geffen School of Medicine at UCLA; Staff Physician, Mattel Children's Hospital at UCLA, Los Angeles, California
BORDETELLA PERTUSSIS (WHOOPING COUGH)

Meeghan A. Hart, MD
Assistant Professor of Pediatrics, Case School of Medicine; Pediatric Pulmonologist, University Hospitals of Cleveland—Rainbow Babies and Children's Hospital, Cleveland, Ohio
DIFFUSE ALVEOLAR HEMORRHAGE (PULMONARY SIDEROSIS)

Robert H. A. Haslam, MD, FAAP, FRCPC
Emeritus Professor and Chairman, Department of Pediatrics, Professor of Medicine (Neurology), University of Toronto Faculty of Medicine; Emeritus Pediatrician-in-Chief, The Hospital for Sick Children, Toronto, Ontario, Canada
DEGENERATIVE DISEASES OF THE CENTRAL NERVOUS SYSTEM

Sarmistha B. Hauger, MD
Medical Director, Pediatric Infectious Diseases, Children's Hospital of Austin, Austin, Texas
YERSINIA ENTEROCOLITICA

William C. Heird, MD
Professor of Pediatrics, Baylor College of Medicine; Children's Nutrition Research Center, Houston, Texas
NUTRIENT REQUIREMENTS OF TERM AND PRETERM INFANTS

Mellissa R. Held, MD
Department of Pediatrics, Division of Infectious Diseases, Yale University School of Medicine, New Haven, Connecticut
TRICHINELLOSIS (TRICHINOSIS)

Mark A. Helfaer, MD
Professor of Anesthesia, University of Pennsylvania School of Medicine; Anesthesiologist, Hospital of the University of Pennsylvania, and Department of Anesthesia and Critical Care Medicine, The Children's Hospital of Philadelphia, Philadelphia, Pennsylvania
DISORDERS OF TEMPERATURE CONTROL

Mark L. Helpin, DMD
Section Head, Pediatric Dentistry, Department of Oral Medicine, Carolinas Medical Center, Charlotte, North Carolina
ORAL HEALTH

Karen D. Hendricks-Muñoz, MD, MPH
Associate Professor, Department of Pediatrics, New York University School of Medicine; Director of Neonatology, Tisch Hospital and Bellevue Hospital, New York, New York
INFANTS OF DIABETIC MOTHERS

Theresa A. Hennessey, MD
Resident, Division of Pediatric Orthopaedics, Rainbow Babies and Children's Hospital, University Hospitals of Cleveland, Cleveland, Ohio
THE LIMPING CHILD

Erick Hernandez, MD
Assistant Professor of Clinical Pediatrics, Department of Pediatric Gastroenterology, University of Miami Miller School of Medicine; Pediatric Gastroenterologist, Jackson Memorial Hospital, Miami, Florida
INFLAMMATORY BOWEL DISEASE

Barry A. Hicks, MD
Professor of Surgery, Department of Pediatric Surgery, The University of Texas Southwestern Medical Center College of Medicine; Chief, Surgical Services, Children's Medical Center of Dallas, Dallas, Texas
BLUNT ABDOMINAL TRAUMA

Lee M. Hilliard, MD
Associate Professor, Division of Pediatric Hematology and Oncology, Department of Pediatrics, University of Alabama at Birmingham School of Medicine, Birmingham, Alabama
SICKLE CELL DISORDERS

David Henry Hiltzik, MD
Resident, Department of Otolaryngology—Head and Neck Surgery, Columbia University, New York, New York
TONSILLECTOMY AND ADENOIDECTOMY

Philip G. Holtzapple, MD
Professor of Pediatrics, State University of New York Health Science Center, Syracuse, New York
CIRRHOSIS AND PORTAL HYPERTENSION

Kord Honda, MD
Resident Physician, Department of Medicine, Division of
Dermatology, University of Washington, Medical Center,
Seattle, Washington
DISORDERS OF PIGMENTATION

Maria-Arantxa Horga, MD
Mount Sinai School of Medicine,
Department of Pediatric Infectious Diseases, New York,
New York
RESPIRATORY SYNCYTIAL VIRUS

Duane R. Hospenthal, MD, PhD
Associate Professor of Medicine, F. Edward Hébert School of
Medicine, Uniformed Services University of the Health
Sciences, Bethesda, Maryland; Chief, Infectious Disease
Service, Brooke Army Medical Center, Fort Sam Houston,
Texas; Clinical Associate Professor, Department of Medicine,
University of Texas Medical School at San Antonio, San
Antonio, Texas
HISTOPLASMOSIS

Peter J. Hotez, MD, PhD
Professor and Chair, Division of Microbiology and Tropical
Medicine, George Washington University School of Medicine
and Health Sciences, Washington, DC
SOIL-TRANSMITTED HELMINTH INFECTIONS

Thomas H. Howard, MD
Professor and Director, Division of Pediatric Hematology and
Oncology, Department of Pediatrics, University of Alabama
at Birmingham School of Medicine, Birmingham, Alabama
SICKLE CELL DISORDERS

Jimmy W. Huh, MD
Assistant Professor of Anesthesiology and Critical Care,
University of Pennsylvania School of Medicine; Staff
Physician, The Children's Hospital of Philadelphia,
Philadelphia, Pennsylvania
DISORDERS OF TEMPERATURE CONTROL

Janice Hutchinson, MD, MPH
Assistant Professor of Psychiatry and Pediatrics, Howard
University College of Medicine, Washington, DC
SUICIDE

Joshua E. Hyman, MD, FAAP
Assistant Professor of Octhopaedic Surgery, Columbia
University College of Physicians and Surgeons; Attending
Surgeon, Division of Orthopaedic Surgery, Children's
Hospital of New York–Presbyterian, New York,
New York
ORTHOPEDIC TRAUMA

Lisa Imundo, MD
Director, Pediatric Rheumatology, and Assistant Clinical
Professor of Pediatrics, Department of Pediatrics, Columbia
University College of Physicians and Surgeons; Staff
Pediatrician, Children's Hospital of New York–Presbyterian,
New York, New York
IDIOPATHIC PAIN SYNDROMES AND CHRONIC FATIGUE SYNDROME;
JUVENILE RHEUMATOID ARTHRITIS AND SPONDYLOARTHROPATHY
SYNDROMES

Julie R. Ingelfinger, MD
Professor of Pediatrics, Harvard Medical School;
Senior Consultant in Pediatric Nephrology, Department
of Pediatrics, Division of Pediatric Nephrology,
MassGeneral Hospital for Children at Massachusetts
General Hospital, Boston, Massachusetts
SOLID ORGAN TRANSPLANTATION

Esther Jacobowitz Israel, MD
Assistant Professor of Pediatrics Harvard Medical School;
Associate Chief, Pediatric Gastroenterology and Nutrition,
MassGeneral Hospital for Children at Massachusetts
General Hospital, Boston, Massachusetts
GASTRITIS AND PEPTIC ULCER DISEASE

Ian N. Jacobs, MD
Associate Professor of Otorhinolaryngology–Head and Neck
Surgery, University of Pennsylvania School of Medicine;
Attending, Division of Pediatric Otolaryngology, The
Children's Hospital of Philadelphia, Philadelphia,
Pennsylvania
CROUP AND EPIGLOTTITIS

Richard F. Jacobs, MD, FAAP
Horace C. Cabe, Professor of Pediatrics, University of
Arkansas for Medical Sciences College of Medicine; Chief,
Pediatric Infectious Diseases, Arkansas Children's Hospital,
Little Rock, Arkansas
TULAREMIA

Peggy F. Jacobson, PhD, CCC-SP/L
Assistant Professor, Department of Speech, Communication
Sciences, and Theatre, St. John's University, Queens,
New York
EVIDENCE-BASED PRACTICE IN COMMUNICATION DISORDERS: LANGUAGE,
SPEECH, AND VOICE DISORDERS

Elka Jacobson-Dickman, MD
Clinical and Research Fellow, Department of Pediatric
Endocrinology, Harvard Medical School and Massachusetts
General Hospital, Boston, Massachusetts
GONADAL DISORDERS

Shirley Jankelevich, MD
Medical Officer, Division of AIDS, (National Institute
of Allergy and Infectious Diseases, National Institutes
of Health, Bethesda, Maryland
MUCORMYCOSIS

Renée R. Jenkins, MD
Professor and Chair, Department of Pediatrics and Child
Health, Howard University College of Medicine; Chair,
Department of Pediatrics, Howard University Hospital,
Washington, DC
SUICIDE

Chandy C. John, MD, MS
Associate Professor of Pediatrics University of Minnesota
Medical School; Director, Global Pediatrics Program,
Pediatrics (Division of Pediatric Infectious Diseases),
University of Minnesota Children's Hospital–Fairview,
Minneapolis, Minnesota
MALARIA

Jeffrey L. Jones, MD, MPH
Medical Epidemiologist, Division of Parasitic Diseases,
National Center for Infectious Disease, Centers for Disease
Control and Prevention, Atlanta, Georgia
TOXOPLASMOSIS

S. Anne Joseph, MBBS
Assistant Clinical Professor of Neurology, Medical College of
Wisconsin; Staff Physician, Neuroscience Center, Children's
Hospital of Wisconsin, Milwaukee, Wisconsin
CEREBROVASCULAR DISEASE

Harald W. Jüppner, MD
Associate Professor of Pediatrics, Harvard Medical School;
Chief, Pediatric Nephrology, Endocrine Unit, MassGeneral
Hospital for Children at Massachusetts General Hospital,
Boston, Massachusetts
DISORDERS OF THE PARATHYROIDS, HYPOCALCEMIA, AND
HYPERCALCEMIA

Angela Kadenhe-Chiweshe, MD
Resident, General Surgery, Columbia University College of
Physicians and Surgeons, New York, New York
NEONATAL INTESTINAL OBSTRUCTION

Jessica A. Kahn, MD, MPH
Associate Professor of Pediatrics, University of Cincinnati
College of Medicine; Staff Physician, Division of Adolescent
Medicine, Cincinnati Children's Hospital Medical Center,
Cincinnati, Ohio
ADOLESCENT GYNECOLOGY

Philip J. Kahn, MD
Fellow in Pediatrics, Morgan Stanley Children's Hospital of
New York–Presbyterian, New York, New York
JUVENILE RHEUMATOID ARTHRITIS AND SPONDYLOARTHROPATHY
SYNDROMES

Daniel S. Kamin, MD
Clinical Fellow, Department of Pediatrics, Children's
Hospital Boston, Boston, Massachusetts
ACUTE AND CHRONIC HEPATITIS

Peter B. Kang, MD
Instructor in Neurology, Harvard Medical School; Assistant
in Neurology, Children's Hospital Boston; Research
Associate, Howard Hughes Medical Institute, Boston,
Massachusetts
MYASTHENIA GRAVIS

Gaurav Kapur, MD
Fellow in Pediatric Nephrology, Department of Pediatrics,
Wayne State University School of Medicine and Children's
Hospital of Michigan, Detroit, Michigan
ACUTE RENAL FAILURE

Manoochehr Karjoo, MD
Abu Dabi, United Arab Emirates
CIRRHOSIS AND PORTAL HYPERTENSION

Frederick J. Kaskel, MD, PhD
Professor of Pediatrics and Vice Chair, Affiliate and Network
Relations, Albert Einstein College of Medicine of Yeshiva
University; Chief, Section of Nephrology, Children's Hospital
at Montefiore, Bronx, New York
CHRONIC KIDNEY DISEASE

Ben Z. Katz, MD
Associate Professor of Pediatrics, Northwestern University,
Feinberg School of Medicine; Attending Physician, Division
of Infectious Diseases, Children's Memorial Hospital,
Chicago, Illinois
INFECTIOUS MONONUCLEOSIS

Joseph D. Kay, MD
Assistant Professor of Adult and Pediatric Cardiology,
University of Colorado School of Medicine, Denver, Colorado
CONGESTIVE HEART FAILURE

Ken Kazahaya, MD, MBA
Assistant Professor, Department of Otorhinolaryngology–
Head and Neck Surgery, University of Pennsylvania
School of Medicine; Director, Pediatric Skull Base Surgery,
and Associate Medical Director, Cochlear Implant Program,
Division of Pediatric Otolaryngology, The Children's Hospital
of Philadelphia, Philadelphia, Pennsylvania
LABYRINTHITIS

James P. Keating, MD, MSc
W. McKim Marriott Professor of Pediatrics, Washington
University in St. Louis School of Medicine; Staff Pediatrician,
St. Louis Children's Hospital, St. Louis, Missouri
MALABSORPTION; INTUSSUSCEPTION

Jeffrey L. Keller, MD, FACS, FAAP
Assistant Clinical Professor, Department of Otolaryngology,
Mount Sinai School of Medicine; Attending Physician,
Department of Otolaryngology, Mount Sinai Hospital,
New York; Northern Westchester Hospital Center,
and Mount Kisco Medical Group, Mount Kisco, New York
PEDIATRIC RHINITIS AND ACUTE AND CHRONIC SINUSITIS

Kent R. Kelley, MD
Assistant Professor of Clinical Neurology and Pediatrics,
Department of Pediatric Neurology, Northwestern
University Feinberg School of Medicine; Attending in
Clinical Pediatrics and Neurology, Children's Epilepsy
Center, Children's Memorial Hospital, Chicago, Illinois
MOVEMENT DISORDERS

Leila M. Khazaeni, MD
Assistant Professor, Department of Ophthalmology,
Loma Linda University School of Medicine; Attending
Physician, Department of Opthalmology, Loma Linda
University Health Care, Loma Linda, California
AMBLYOPIA; STRABISMUS; NASOLACRIMAL DUCT OBSTRUCTION; RED EYE

Todd J. Kilbaugh, MD
Fellow, Department of Anesthesia, Critical Care Medicine
and Pediatrics, University of Pennsylvania School of
Medicine, and Department of Anesthesia and Critical Care
Medicine, The Children's Hospital of Philadelphia,
Philadelphia, Pennsylvania
DISORDERS OF TEMPERATURE CONTROL

Brigid K. Killelea, MD, MPH
Research Fellow, International Center for Health Outcomes
and Innovation Research, College of Physicians and
Surgeons and Mailman School of Public Health,
Columbia University; Pediatric Surgeon, New York–
Presbyterian Hospital, New York, New York
PNEUMOTHORAX AND PNEUMOMEDIASTINUM

David W. Kimberlin, MD
Associate Professor of Pediatrics, University of Alabama at Birmingham School of Medicine, Birmingham, Alabama
HERPES SIMPLEX VIRUS

T. Bernard Kinane, MD
Associate Professor of Pediatrics, Harvard Medical School; Staff Physician, Massachusetts General Hospital for Children, Boston, Massachusetts
ASTHMA

Ronald E. Kleinman, MD
Professor of Pediatrics, Harvard Medical School; Chief, Division of Pediatric Gastroenterology and Nutrition, MassGeneral Hospital for Children at Massachusetts General Hospital, Boston, Massachusetts
NAUSEA AND VOMITING; CONSTIPATION; ACUTE AND CHRONIC HEPATITIS; CIRRHOSIS AND PORTAL HYPERTENSION

Alex Kline, MD
Neonatal Fellow, Jefferson Medical College of Thomas Jefferson University, Philadelphia, Pennsylvania
SUDDEN INFANT DEATH SYNDROME

Martin Kluckow, MBBS, PhD
Senior Lecturer in Obstetrics and Gynaecology, University of Sydney Faculty of Medicine; Senior Neonatologist, Royal North Shore Hospital, Sydney, New South Wales, Australia
HYPOTENSION IN THE NEONATE

William C. Koch, MD
Associate Professor of Pediatrics, Division of Infectious Diseases, Virginia Commonwealth University School of Medicine; Attending Physician, Children's Medical Center, Medical College of Virginia Hospitals, Richmond, Virginia
PARVOVIRUS INFECTION

Linda M. Kollar, RN, MSN
Director of Clinical Services, Division of Adolescent Medicine, Cincinnati Children's Hospital Medical Center, Cincinnati, Ohio
ADOLESCENT GYNECOLOGY

Peter J. Koltai, MD, FACS, FAAP
Professor of Pediatric Otolaryngology, Stanford University School of Medicine; Chief, Division of Pediatric Otolaryngology, Department of Otolaryngology, Stanford Hospital and Clinics, Stanford, California
FACIAL AND MIDDLE EAR TRAUMA

Susan Konek, MA, RD, CSP, LDN
Inpatient Clinical Nutrition Manager and Nutrition Support Coordinator, Department of Clinical Nutrition, The Children's Hospital of Philadelphia, Philadelphia, Pennsylvania
VITAMIN DEFICIENCIES AND EXCESSES

Harold S. Koplewicz, MD
Arnold & Debbie Simon Professor of Child and Adolescent Psychiatry and Vice Chairman, Department of Psychiatry; Professor of Pediatrics, Department of Pediatrics, New York University School of Medicine; Director, NYU Child Study Center, New York, New York
PSYCHOSOMATIC ILLNESS

Christian M. Korff, MD
Fellow, Epilepsy Center, Neurology Service, Children's Memorial Hospital, Chicago, Illinois
STATUS EPILEPTICUS

Paul R. Krakovitz, MD
Pediatric surgeon, Section of Pediatric Otolaryngology, Department of Otolaryngology, The Cleveland Clinic, Cleveland, Ohio
FACIAL AND MIDDLE EAR TRAUMA

Peter J. Krause, MD
Professor of Pediatrics, University of Connecticut School of Medicine, Farmington; Chief, Division of Infectious Diseases, Connecticut Children's Medical Center, Hartford, Connecticut
BABESIOSIS

Paul Krogstad, MD
Professor of Pediatrics and Molecular and Medical Pharmacology, David Geffen School of Medicine at UCLA, Los Angeles, California
OSTEOMYELITIS; SEPTIC ARTHRITIS

Christine J. Kubin, PharmD, BCPS
Assistant in Medicine, Department of Medicine, Division of Infectious Diseases, Columbia University College of Physicians and Surgeons; Clinical Pharmacist, New York–Presbyterian Hospital, New York, New York; Affiliate Assistant Clinical Professor, College of Pharmacy, St. John's University, Queens, New York
CANDIDIASIS; ADVERSE DRUG REACTIONS

Taco W. Kuijpers, MD, PhD
Professor and Staff Physician, Department of Pediatric Hematology, Immunology, and Infectious Disease, Emma Children's Hospital, Amsterdam, The Netherlands
COMPLEMENT DISORDERS AND LECTIN PATHWAY

Louis M. Kunkel, PhD
Professor of Pediatrics and Genetics, Department of Genetics, Harvard Medical School; Director, Program in Genomics, Department of Medicine, Children's Hospital Boston; Investigator, Howard Hughes Medical Institute, Boston, Massachusetts
MUSCULAR DYSTROPHIES

Lori M. B. Laffel, MD, MPH
Associate Professor of Pediatrics, Harvard Medical School; Staff, Pediatric and Adolescent Unit, Behavioral Research and Mental Health Section/Genetics and Epidemiology Section, Joslin Diabetes Center; Staff Physician, Department of Medicine, Children's Hospital Boston, Boston, Massachusetts
DIABETES MELLITUS IN CHILDREN AND ADOLESCENTS

Craig B. Langman, MD
Isaac A. Abt, MD, Professor of Kidney Diseases Department of Pediatrics, Northwestern University Feinberg School of Medicine; Division Head, Kidney Diseases, Children's Memorial Hospital, Chicago, Illinois
NEPHROLITHIASIS

Marc R. Laufer, MD
Associate Professor of Obstetrics, Gynecology, and
Reproductive Biology, Harvard Medical School; Chief,
Division of Pediatric/Adolescent Gynecology, Reproductive
Medicine/Gynecologic Surgery, Brigham and Women's
Hospital; Chief of Gynecology/Associate in Surgery/Co-
Director Center for Young Women's Health, Department of
Gynecology, Children's Hospital Boston; Active Medical
Staff, Department of Gynecology, Dana-Farber Cancer
Institute, Boston, Massachusetts
ADOLESCENT GYNECOLOGY

Jane M. Lavelle, MD
Associate Professor of Pediatrics, University of Pennsylvania
School of Medicine; Attending, Division of Pediatric
Emergency Medicine, The Children's Hospital of
Philadelphia, Philadelphia, Pennsylvania
EPISTAXIS AND NASAL TRAUMA

William V. La Via, MD
Assistant Professor of Clinical Pediatrics, Keck School of
Medicine of USC; Attending Physician, Division of Infectious
Diseases, Department of Pediatrics, Childrens Hospital Los
Angeles, Los Angeles, California
CRYPTOCOCCUS NEOFORMANS

Jane S. Lee, MD, MPH
Assistant Professor of Pediatrics, Columbia University
College of Physicians and Surgeons; Attending
Neonatologist, Children's Hospital of New York–
Presbyterian, New York, New York
MANAGEMENT OF THE INFANT IN THE DELIVERY ROOM

Mary Min-Chin Lee, MD
Professor of Pediatrics, University of Massachusetts Medical
School; Director, Pediatric Endocrine and Diabetes Division,
Department of Pediatrics, UMass Memorial Medical
Center, Worcester, Massachusetts
DISORDERS OF THE ADRENAL GLAND

Beth A. Leeman, MD
Clinical and Research Fellow, Department of Neurology,
Massachusetts General Hospital, Boston, Massachusetts
NEUROFIBROMATOSIS TYPE I

Leslie E. Lehmann, MD
Assistant Professor in Pediatrics, Harvard Medical School;
Interim Director, Pediatric Stem Cell Transplantation,
Department of Pediatric Oncology, Dana-Farber Cancer
Institute and Children's Hospital Boston, Boston,
Massachusetts
BURKITT LYMPHOMA

Kevin V. Lemley, MD, PhD
Consultant in Nephrology, Stanford University School of
Medicine, Stanford, California
RENAL VEIN THROMBOSIS

Tina A. Leone, MD
Assistant Professor of Pediatrics, University of California,
San Diego, School of Medicine; Neonatologist,
University of California, San Diego, Medical Center,
San Diego, California
PERSISTENT PULMONARY HYPERTENSION OF THE NEWBORN

Donald Y. M. Leung, MD, PhD
Professor of Pediatrics, University of Colorado School of
Medicine; Head, Division of Pediatric Allergy and
Immunology, Department of Pediatrics, National Jewish
Medical and Research Center, Denver, Colorado
ATOPIC DERMATITIS

Lynne L. Levitsky, MD
Associate Professor of Pediatrics, Harvard Medical School;
Chief, Pediatric Endocrine Unit, MassGeneral Hospital for
Children at Massachusetts General Hospital, Boston,
Massachusetts
DISORDERS OF THE ADRENAL GLAND

John C. Lin, MD
Adjunct Assistant Professor, Division of Pediatric Critical
Care Medicine, University of Pittsburgh School of Medicine;
Staff Physician, Children's Hospital of Pittsburgh,
Pittsburgh, Pennsylvania; Staff Pediatric Intensivist,
Department of Pediatrics, Wilford Hall Medical Center, San
Antonio, Texas
MANAGEMENT OF SEPSIS AND SEPTIC SHOCK

Steven E. Lipshultz, MD
Professor and Chairman, Department of Pediatrics;
Professor of Epidemiology and Public Health; and Professor
of Medicine (Oncology), University of Miami Miller School of
Medicine; Chief-of-Staff, Holtz Children's Hospital of the
University of Miami–Jackson Memorial Medical Center;
Director, Batchelor Children's Research Institute; Associate
Director, Mailman Institute for Child Development; and
Member, Sylvester Comprehensive Cancer Center, Miami,
Florida
KAWASAKI DISEASE

Irene M. Loe, MD
Fellow, Developmental-Behavioral Pediatrics, University of
Pittsburgh School of Medicine and Children's Hospital of
Pittsburgh, Pittsburgh, Pennsylvania
ATTENTION DEFICIT HYPERACTIVITY DISORDER

Anthony M. Loizides, M.D.
Assistant Professor of Pediatrics, Division of Pediatric
Gastroenterology, Albert Einstein College of Medicine of
Yeshiva University; Attending Physician, Department of
Pediatrics, Division of Pediatric Gastroenterology, Children's
Hospital at Montefiore and Bronx-Lebanon Medical Center,
Bronx, New York
ALLERGIC GASTROINTESTINAL DISORDERS

Sarah S. Long, MD
Professor of Pediatrics, Dreyel University College of
Medicine; Chief, Section of Infectious Diseases,
St. Christopher's Hospital for Children, Philadelphia,
Pennsylvania
INFANT BOTULISM

Naomi L. C. Luban, MD
Interim Executive Director, Center for Cancer and Blood
Disorders; Chair, Laboratory Medicine and Pathology, and
Director, Transfusion Medicine/The Edward J. Miller Donor
Center, Children's National Medical Center; Vice Chair for
Academic Affairs, Department of Pediatrics, and Professor,
Departments of Pediatrics and Pathology, George
Washington University School of Medicine and Health
Sciences, Washington, DC
COMPLICATIONS OF BLOOD TRANSFUSION

Jon F. Lucas, MD
Instructor in Pediatric Cardiology, Medical University
of South Carolina College of Medicine, Charleston,
South Carolina
INNOCENT MURMURS

Jeffrey Lukish, MD
Assistant Professor of Surgery and Pediatrics, Department of
Surgery, F. Edward Hebert School of Medicine; Uniformed
Services University of the Health Sciences; Pediatric
Surgeon, National Naval Medical Center, Bethesda,
Maryland; Pediatric Surgeon, Walter Reed Army Medical
Center and Children's National Medical Center,
Washington, DC
BURNS

G. Reid Lyon, PhD
Executive Vice President for Research and Evaluation, Best
Associates and Whitney University, Dallas, Texas
DYSLEXIA (SPECIFIC READING DISABILITY)

Christopher M. Makris, MD, MPH
Associate Professor of Pediatrics, University of Alabama at
Birmingham School of Medicine; Medical Director, Sleep
Disorder Center, Children's Hospital, of Alabama,
Birmingham, Alabama
COMMON SLEEP DISORDERS

Michael A. Manfredi, MD
Clinical Fellow in Pediatrics, Harvard Medical School;
Clinical Fellow in Medicine, Children's Hospital Boston; and
Clinical Fellow in Pediatrics, MassGeneral Hospital for
Children at Massachusetts General Hospital, Boston,
Massachusetts
GASTRITIS AND PEPTIC ULCER DISEASE

John F. Marcinak, MD
Associate Professor of Pediatrics, University of Chicago
Pritzker School of Medicine, Chicago, Illinois
BLASTOMYCOSIS: RECOGNITION, DIAGNOSIS, AND MANAGEMENT

David Markenson, MD, FAAP
Director, Center for Disaster Medicine/New York Medical
College School of Public Health; Chief, Pediatric Emergency
Medicine, Maria Fareri Children's Hospital at Westchester
Medical Center/Emergency Medical Associates; Assistant
Professor of Pediatrics, New York Medical College,
Valhalla, New York
BIOTERRORISM

Richard J. Martin, MBBS, FRACP
Professor, Department of Pediatrics, Reproductive Biology,
Physiology, and Biophysics, Case School of Medicine;
Director, Division of Neonatology, Department of Pediatrics,
Rainbow Babies and Children's Hospital, Cleveland, Ohio
APNEA OF PREMATURITY

Maria R. Mascarenhas, MBBS
Associate Professor of Pediatrics, University of Pennsylvania
School of Medicine; Director, Nutrition Support Service;
Assistant Director, Cystic Fibrosis Center; Attending
Gastroenterologist and Section Chief, Division of
Gastrointestinal and Nutrition, Department of Pediatrics,
The Children's Hospital of Philadelphia, Philadelphia,
Pennsylvania
VITAMIN DEFICIENCIES AND EXCESSES

Joelle Mast, PhD, MD
Assistant Clinical Professor of Pediatrics and Neurology,
Weill Medical College of Cornell University, New York; Vice
President, Chief Medical Officer, Chief of Pediatrics, and
Attending Neurologist, Blythedale Children's Hospital,
Valhalla; Assistant Attending Pediatrician, New York–
Presbyterian Hospital, New York, New York
CEREBRAL PALSY

Tej K. Mattoo, MD, DCH, FRCP(UK)
Professor of Pediatrics, Wayne State University School of
Medicine; Chief, Pediatric Nephrology, Children's Hospital of
Michigan, Detroit, Michigan
ACUTE RENAL FAILURE

Dominic J. Maxwell, MD
Assistant Professor of Psychiatry, Division of Child and
Adolescent Psychiatry, University of Alabama at
Birmingham School of Medicine, Birmingham, Alabama
PSYCHIATRIC DISORDERS AND MENTAL HEALTH DISORDERS IN CHILDREN
AND ADOLESCENTS

Lynnette J. Mazur, MD, MPH
Professor of Pediatrics, University of Texas Medical School at
Houston, Houston, Texas
DIARRHEA; GASTROESOPHAGEAL REFLUX

Erin E. McGintee, MD
Fellow, Department of Allergy and Immunology, The
Children's Hospital of Philadelphia, Philadelphia,
Pennsylvania
ANAPHYLAXIS

Marianne McPherson, MD
Resident in Pediatrics, Children's National Medical Center,
Washington, DC
IRON DEFICIENCY ANEMIA

Denise W. Metry, MD
Assistant Professor of Dermatology and Pediatrics, Baylor
College of Medicine; Chief, Pediatric Dermatology Clinic,
Texas Children's Hospital, Houston, Texas
CHRONIC, NONHEREDITARY BULLOUS DISEASES OF CHILDHOOD

Francisca Okolo MgBodile, MD
Assistant Professor of Psychiatry and Behavioral Neurobiology
University of Alabama at Birmingham School of Medicine;
Assistant Professor, Child and Adolescent Psychiatry,
University of Alabama Health Service Foundation;
Attending Physician, Child and Adolescent Psychiatry,
Children's Hospital of Alabama, Birmingham, Alabama
PSYCHIATRIC DISORDERS AND MENTAL HEALTH DISORDERS IN
CHILDREN AND ADOLESCENTS

William Middlesworth, MD
Assistant Professor of Surgery and Pediatric Surgery
(Pediatrics), Columbia University College of Physicians and
Surgeons; Assistant Assending Surgeon, Children's Hospital
of New York–Presbyterian, New York, New York
NEONATAL INTESTINAL OBSTRUCTION

Monte D. Mills, MD
Assistant Professor of Ophthalmology, University of
Pennsylvania School of Medicine; Chief of Ophthalmology,
The Children's Hospital of Philadelphia, Philadelphia,
Pennsylvania
AMBLYOPIA; STRABISMUS; NASOLACRIMAL DUCT OBSTRUCTION; RED EYE

Madhusmita Misra, MD, MPH
Assistant Professor of Pediatrics, Harvard Medical School;
Assistant in Pediatrics and Assistant in Biology, Pediatric
Endocrine and Neuroendocrine Units, MassGeneral Hospital
for Children at Massachusetts General Hospital, Boston,
Massachusetts
DISORDERS OF PUBERTY; GONADAL DISORDERS

Mark Mitsnefes, MD, MS
Assistant Professor of Pediatrics, Cincinnati College of
Medicine; Staff Physician, Division of Nephrology and
Hypertension, Cincinnati Children's Hospital Medical
Center, Cincinnati, Ohio
SYSTEMIC HYPERTENSION AND THE CHILD AT RISK FOR
CARDIOVASCULAR DISEASE

Laura Montgomery-Barefield, MD
Assistant Professor of Psychiatry, University of Alabama at
Birmingham School of Medicine; Medical Director of
Outpatient Services, Division of Child Psychiatry,
Department of Children's Behavioral Health, Children's
Health System, Birmingham, Alabama
PSYCHIATRIC DISORDERS AND MENTAL HEALTH DISORDERS IN
CHILDREN AND ADOLESCENTS

Cynthia W. Moore, PhD
Instructor in Psychiatry, Harvard Medical School; Child
Psychologist, Division of Child and Adolescent Psychiatry,
Massachusetts General Hospital, Boston, Massachusetts
THE CHILD AND THE DEATH OF A LOVED ONE

Derek W. Moore, MD
Resident, Department of Orthopaedic Surgery, New York–
Presbyterian Hospital, New York, New York
ORTHOPEDIC TRAUMA

Dean S. Morrell, MD
Assistant Professor of Dermatology, University of North
Carolina at Chapel Hill School of Medicine, Chapel Hill,
North Carolina
PSORIASIS AND OTHER PAPULOSQUAMOUS DISORDERS

Erin Morris, RN, BSN
Clinical Research Nurse, Department of Pediatrics,
Columbia University College of Physicians and Surgeons;
Clinical Research Nurse, Department of Pediatrics, Morgan
Stanley Children's Hospital of New York–Presbyterian,
New York, New York
NEONATAL AND CHILDHOOD NEUTROPENIA; BLOOD AND
MARROW TRANSPLANTATION

Anne Moscona, MD
Professor of Pediatrics and Microbiology and Immunology,
Department of Pediatrics, Weill Medical College at Cornell
University; Attending Physician and Vice Chair for
Research, Department of Pediatrics, New York–Presbyterian
Hospital, New York, New York
SEVERE ACUTE RESPIRATORY SYNDROME (SARS); RESPIRATORY SYNCYTIAL
VIRUS

Scott Moses, MD
Family Physician/Staff Physician, Fairview Lakes Regional
Medical Center, Wyoming, Minnesota; Family Physician,
Fairview Lino Lakes Clinic, Fairview Health Systems, Lino
Lakes, Minnesota
PRURITUS

Louis J. Muglia, MD, PhD
Associate Professor of Pediatrics, Washington University in
St. Louis School of Medicine; Director, Division of
Endocrinology and Metabolism, St. Louis Children's
Hospital, St. Louis, Missouri
DIABETES INSIPIDUS, SIADH, AND CEREBRAL SALT WASTING

Karen F. Murray, MD
Associate Professor of Pediatrics, University of Washington
School of Medicine; Director, Hepatobiliary Program,
Department of Pediatrics, Division of Gastroenterology,
Children's Hospital and Regional Medical Center, Seattle,
Washington
VIRAL HEPATITIS

Karna Murthy, MD
Fellow, Division of Pediatric Neonatology, The Children's
Hospital of Philadelphia, and University of Pennsylvania
School of Medicine, Philadelphia, Pennsylvania
PATENT DUCTUS ARTERIOSUS

Erich N. Mussak, BS
Medical Student, Weill Medical College of Cornell
University, New York, New York
CHOANAL ATRESIA

Sharon A. Nachman, MD
Professor of Pediatrics, Stony Brook University School of
Medicine, Stony Brook, New York
LISTERIOSIS; ASPERGILLOSIS

Martin A. Nash, MD
Professor of Clinical Pediatrics, Department of Pediatrics,
Columbia University College of Physicians and Surgeons;
Director of Pediatric Nephrology, Morgan Stanley Children's
Hospital of New York–Presbyterian, New York, New York
HYPERTENSIVE EMERGENCIES

Herbert L. Needleman, MD
Professor of Psychiatry and Pediatrics, University of
Pittsburgh School of Medicine, Pittsburgh, Pennsylvania
LEAD TOXICITY

Josef Neu, MD
Professor of Pediatrics, University of Florida College of
Medicine; Staff Pediatrician, Shands Hospital at University
of Florida, Gainesville, Florida
NECROTIZING ENTEROCOLITIS

Natalie Neu, MD
Associate Clinical Professor of Pediatrics, Division of
Pediatric Infectious Diseases, Columbia University College
of Physicians and Surgeons; Attending, Department of
Pediatrics, Morgan Stanley Children's Hospital of New York–
Presbyterian, New York, New York
IMMUNIZATION PRACTICES; CANDIDIASIS

Jesica A. Neuhart, MD
Resident in Pediatrics, Louisiana State University Health
Science Center, New Orleans, Louisiana
CHOLERA

Yoram Nevo, MD
Director, Neuropediatric Unit, Hadassah, Hebrew
University Medical Center, Jerusalem, Israel
ACUTE AND CHRONIC IMMUNE-MEDIATED POLYNEUROPATHY

Jane W. Newburger, MD, MPH
Professor of Pediatrics, Harvard Medical School; Associate Cardiologist-in-Chief, Children's Hospital Boston, Boston, Massachusetts
KAWASAKI DISEASE

Peter Ngo, MD
Clinical and Research Fellow in Pediatrics, Division of Pediatric Gastroenterology and Nutrition, Harvard Medical School and Massachusetts General Hospital, Boston Massachusetts
NAUSEA AND VOMITING; CONSTIPATION

Douglas R. Nordli, Jr., MD
Associate Professor of Clinical Neurology and Clinical Practice, Department of Neurology, Northwestern University Feinberg School of Medicine; Director, Epilepsy Center, Department of Neurology, Children's Memorial Hospital, Chicago, Illinois
STATUS EPILEPTICUS; FEBRILE SEIZURES

Robert L. Norris, MD, FACEP
Associate Professor of Surgery, Stanford University School of Medicine; Chief, Emergency Medicine, Stanford Hospital and Clinics, Stanford, California
VENOMOUS SNAKEBITE

Melvin D. Oatis, MD
Assistant Professor of Clinical Psychiatry, Department of Child Psychiatry, New York University School of Medicine; Director of Pediatric Consultation Liaison Services, Tisch Hospital, New York, New York
PSYCHOSOMATIC ILLNESS

Theresa J. Ochoa, MD
Assistant Professor of Pediatrics, Universidad Peruana Cayetano Heredia, Lima, Peru
CAMPYLOBACTER; NONTYPHOIDAL *SALMONELLA*; SHIGELLOSIS; TYPHOID FEVER

Alfred T. Ogden, MD
Resident in Neurological Surgery, Neurological Institute, New York–Presbyterian Hospital, and Children's Hospital of New York–Presbyterian, New York, New York
EPIDURAL AND SUBDURAL HEMATOMAS

David P. Olson, MD, PhD
Instructor in Medicine, Department of Medicine, Division of Endocrinology, Harvard Medical School; Staff, Children's Hospital Boston, Boston, Massachusetts
GYNECOMASTIA

Walter A. Orenstein, MD
Professor of Medicine and Pediatrics and Director, Vaccine Policy and Development, Emory University School of Medicine, Atlanta, Georgia
MEASLES; RUBELLA

David Osborn, MBBS, MM, FRACP
Neonatologist, RPA Newborn Care, Royal Prince Alfred Hospital, Sydney, New South Wales, Australia
HYPOTENSION IN THE NEONATE

Eugenia K. Pallotto, MD, MSCE
Assistant Professor of Pediatrics, Department of Pediatrics, Section of Neonatal-Perinatal Medicine, University of Missouri–Kansas City School of Medicine; Attending Neonatologist, Children's Mercy Hospitals and Clinics, Kansas City, Missouri
HYPOGLYCEMIA IN THE NEWBORN INFANT

Howard B. Panitch, MD
Associate Professor of Pediatrics, University of Pennsylvania School of Medicine; Senior Physician, Department of Pediatrics, Division of Pulmonary Medicine, The Children's Hospital of Philadelphia, Philadelphia, Pennsylvania
EMPHYSEMA

Robert H. Pass, MD
Assistant Professor of Pediatrics, Department of Pediatrics, Division of Pediatric Cardiology, Columbia University College of Physicians and Surgeons; Attending Physician and Director of Pediatric Arrhythmia Service, Department of Pediatrics, New York–Presbyterian Hospital, Morgan Stanley Children's Hospital of New York–Presbyterian, New York, New York
STABILIZATION OF THE NEONATE WITH CONGENITAL HEART DISEASE

Dilip R. Patel, MD, FAAP, FAACPDM, FACSM, FSAM
Professor, Department of Pediatrics and Human Development, Michigan State University College of Human Medicine; Staff, Kalamazoo Center for Medical Studies, Kalamazoo, Michigan
SEXUALLY TRANSMITTED DISEASES IN ADOLESCENTS

Marc C. Patterson, MD, FRACP
Professor of Clinical Neurology and Pediatrics and Head, Division of Pediatric Neurology, Departments of Neurology and Pediatrics, Columbia University College of Physicians and Surgeons; Director of Pediatric Neurology, Departments of Neurology and Pediatrics, Morgan Stanley Children's Hospital of New York–Presbyterian, New York, New York
PSEUDOTUMOR CEREBRI SYNDROME

Richard H. Pearl, MD, FACS, FAAP, FRCSC
Professor of Surgery and Pediatrics, Department of Surgery, University of Illinois College of Medicine; Surgeon-in-Chief, Children's Hospital of Illinois, Peoria, Illinois
BLUNT ABDOMINAL TRAUMA

Antonio Luis Perez, AB
Medical Student, Harvard Medical School, Boston, Massachusetts
MUSCULAR DYSTROPHIES

Elizabeth A. Perkett, MD
Professor of Pediatrics, University of New Mexico School of Medicine, Albuquerque, New Mexico
BRONCHOPULMONARY DYSPLASIA IN THE NEONATE

Jeffrey M. Perlman, MB, ChB
Professor of Pediatrics, Weill Medical College of Cornell University; Division Chief, Newborn Medicine, New York–Presbyterian Hospital, New York, New York
NEONATAL SEIZURES; INTRACRANIAL HEMORRHAGE IN THE NEWBORN

Robert T. Perry, MD MPH
Medical Epidemiologist, Global Measles Branch, National
Immunization Program, Centers for Disease Control and
Prevention, Atlanta, Georgia
MEASLES

Robert H. Pfister, MD
Instructor, Department of Pediatrics, Division of
Neonatology, University of Vermont College of Medicine;
Fellow of Neonatal-Perinatal Medicine, Vermont Children's
Hospital, Burlington, Vermont
RESPIRATORY DISTRESS SYNDROME

Jeanette R. Pleasure, MD
Clinical Professor of Pediatrics, Division of Neonatology,
University of California, Davis, School of Medicine, Davis;
Attending Neonatologist, Children's Hospital of UCDavis,
Sacramento California
TETANUS NEONATORUM

Ronald L. Poland, MD
Professor of Pediatrics, University of New Mexico School of
Medicine, Albuquerque, New Mexico
TREATMENT OF NEONATAL HYPERBILIRUBINEMIA

Rajani Prabhakaran, MD
Clinical and Research Fellow, Division of Pediatric
Endocrinology, MassGeneral Hospital for Children, and
Harvard Medical School, Boston, Massachusetts
DISORDERS OF PUBERTY

Alice Prince, MD
Professor of Pediatrics and Pharmacology, Columbia
University College of Physicians and Surgeons; Attending
Pediatrician, Childrens Hospital of New York, New York,
New York
BACTERIAL MENINGITIS; ANTIFUNGAL THERAPIES

Naveen Qureshi, MD
Pediatric Hematology-Oncology Fellow, Children's
Hospital and Research Center at Oakland, Oakland,
California
THALASSEMIA

Malcolm Rabie, MBBCh(Wits), FCP(SA) Neurol
Staff Physician, Neuropediatric Unit, Hadassah, Hebrew
University Medical Center, Jerusalem, Israel
ACUTE AND CHRONIC IMMUNE-MEDIATED POLYNEUROPATHY

Sally Radovick, MD
Professor of Pediatrics, Department of Pediatrics, Johns
Hopkins University School of Medicine; Chief, Division of
Endocrinology, Johns Hopkins Medical Institutes, Baltimore,
Maryland
HYPOPITUITARISM AND GROWTH HORMONE THERAPY

Sujatha Rajan, MD
Assistant Professor of Pediatrics, Albert Einstein College of
Medicine of Yeshiva University, Bronx; Staff Physician,
Division of Pediatric Infectious Diseases, Schneider
Children's Hospital at North Shore, Long Island Jewish
Health System, Manhasset, New York
IMMUNIZATION PRACTICES

David I. Rappaport, MD
Department of Pediatrics, Jefferson Medical College of
Thomas Jefferson University, Philadelphia, Pennsylvania;
Staff Physician, Division of General Pediatrics, Alfred I.
duPont Hospital for Children, Wilmington, Delaware
INTESTINAL PROTOZOA

Paula K. Rauch, MD
Assistant Professor of Psychiatry, Harvard Medical School;
Director, Child Psychiatry Consultation Service,
Massachusetts General Hospital, Boston, Massachusetts
THE CHILD AND THE DEATH OF A LOVED ONE

Saran Anne Rawstron, MBBS
Adjunct Assistant Professor of Pediatrics and Medicine, State
University of New York Downstate Medical Center College of
Medicine; Pediatric Residency Program Director, The
Brooklyn Hospital Center, Brooklyn, New York
SYPHILIS

Irwin Redlener, MD
Associate Dean and Director, National Center for Disaster
Preparedness, Columbia University Mailman School of
Public Health, New York, New York; President & Co-founder
The Children's Health Fund New York, NY
BIOTERRORISM

Michael D. Reed, PharmD, FCCP, FCP
Professor of Pediatrics, Case School of Medicine; Director,
Pediatric Clinical Pharmacology/Toxicology, Rainbow Babies
and Children's Hospital, Cleveland, Ohio
APNEA OF PREMATURITY

Susan E. Reef, MD
Medical Epidemiologist, National Immunization Program,
Centers for Disease Control and Prevention, Atlanta, Georgia
RUBELLA

**Michael J. Rieder, MD, PhD, FRCPC, FAAP,
FRCP (Glasgow)**
Professor of Paediatrics, Physiology and Pharmacology, and
Medicine, University of Western Ontario Schulich School of
Medicine and Dentistry, London, Ontario, Canada
DRUG REACTIONS AND THE SKIN

Steven Alan Ringer, MD, PhD
Assistant Professor of Pediatrics, Harvard Medical School;
Chief, Division of Newborn Medicine, Brigham and Women's
Hospital, Boston, Massachusetts
HEMOLYTIC DISEASES OF THE NEWBORN

James J. Riviello, Jr., MD
Professor of Neurology, Harvard University Medical School;
Director, Epilepsy Program, Division of Epilepsy and Clinical
Neurophysiology, Department of Neurology, Children's
Hospital Boston, Boston, Massachusetts
GENERAL CONCEPTS IN SEIZURE MANAGEMENT

E. Steve Roach, MD
Professor of Neurology and Director, Comprehensive
Epilepsy Center, Department of Neurology, Wake Forest
University School of Medicine, Winston-Salem,
North Carolina
TUBEROUS SCLEROSIS COMPLEX

Jennifer L. Robbins, MD
Fellow in Pediatric Endocrinology, University of Chicago
Pritzker School of Medicine, Chicago, Illinois
HYPOPITUITARISM AND GROWTH HORMONE THERAPY

Lisa-Gaye Robinson, MD
Assistant Professor of Clinical Pediatrics, Department of
Pediatrics, Columbia University College of Physicians and
Surgeons; Assistant Attending, Department of Pediatrics,
Harlem Hospital Center, New York, New York
NONTUBERCULOUS MYCOBACTERIUM INFECTIONS; TUBERCULOSIS

Peter N. Robinson, MD
Institute of Medical Genetics, Charité University Hospital
and Humboldt University, Berlin, Germany
MARFAN SYNDROME

Lauren M. Robitaille, PharmD
Clinical Pharmacy Manager, Department of Pharmacy,
New York–Presbyterian Hospital, New York,
New York
ADVERSE DRUG REACTIONS

Richard M. Rosenfeld, MD, MPH
Professor of Otolaryngology, State University of New York
Downstate Medical Center College of Medicine; Director,
Pediatric Otolaryngology, Long Island College Hospital and
University Hospital of Brooklyn, Brooklyn, New York
OTITIS MEDIA

Joel R. Rosh, MD, FAAP, FACG
Associate Professor of Pediatrics, University of Medicine and
Dentistry–New Jersey Medical School; Director, Pediatric
Gastroenterology, Atlantic Health System, Morristown, New
Jersey
ABDOMINAL PAIN: APPROACH TO A DIAGNOSIS

N. Paul Rosman, MD
Professor of Pediatrics and Neurology, Boston University
School of Medicine; Senior Neurologist, Department of
Pediatrics, Boston Medical Center, Boston, Massachusetts
HEAD INJURY

Philip Roth, MD, PhD
Associate Professor of Pediatrics, State University of
New York Downstate Medical Center College of Medicine,
Brooklyn; Director of Neonatology and Associate Chairman,
Department of Pediatrics, Staten Island University Hospital,
Staten Island, New York
BIRTH INJURIES

Benjamin D. Roye, MD, MPH
Assistant Professor and Division Chief, Pediatric
Orthopaedics, Department of Orthopaedic Surgery, Mount
Sinai School of Medicine, New York, New York
TORTICOLLIS

David P. Roye, MD
St. Giles Professor of Pediatric Orthopaedic Surgery,
Columbia University College of Physicians and Surgeons;
Chief, Division of Pediatric Orthopaedic Surgery, Morgan
Stanley Children's Hospital of New York–Presbyterian,
New York, New York
TORTICOLLIS

Shehzad A. Saeed, MD, FAAP
Assistant Professor of Pediatrics and Nutrition Sciences,
Division of Pediatric Gastroenterology and Nutrition,
University of Alabama at Birmingham School of Medicine;
Staff Physician, The Children's Hospital of Alabama,
Birmingham, Alabama
ACUTE ABDOMINAL PAIN

Lisa Saiman, MD, MPH
Professor of Clinical Pediatrics, Department of Pediatrics,
Columbia University College of Physicians and Surgeons;
Staff Pediatrician, New York–Presbyterian Medical Center
and Children's Hospital of New York–Presbyterian,
New York, New York
ANTIBACTERIAL THERAPIES

Howard W. Sander, MD
Associate Professor of Clinical Neurology,
Department of Neurology, Weill Medical College of Cornell
University; Associate Director, Peripheral Neuropathy
Center, New York–Presbyterian Hospital, New York,
New York
ACUTE AND CHRONIC IMMUNE-MEDIATED POLYNEUROPATHY

J. Philip Saul, MD
Professor of Pediatrics and Chief, Pediatric Cardiology,
Department of Pediatrics, Medical University of South
Carolina College of Medicine; Medical Director, Department
of Pediatrics, MUSC Children's Hospital, Charleston,
South Carolina
INNOCENT MURMURS

Jeffrey R. Sawyer, MD, FAAOS, FAAP
Assistant Professor of Orthopaedics, University of
Tennessee–Campbell Clinic; Head, Limb Deformity
Program, Department of Orthopaedic Surgery,
Le Bonheur Children's Hospital; Attending Orthopaedic
Surgeon, St. Jude's Children's Hospital, Memphis,
Tennessee
ROTATIONAL ORTHOPEDIC PROBLEMS OF THE EXTREMITIES

Lawrence A. Schachner, MD
Interim Chairman and Professor, Department of
Dermatology and Cutaneous Surgery, Division of Pediatric
Dermatology, University of Miami Miller School of Medicine;
Staff Physician, Pediatric Dermatology, Jackson Memorial
Hospital, Miami, Florida, USA
SUN PROTECTION IN THE PEDIATRIC PATIENT

Richard J. Schanler, MD
Professor of Pediatrics, Albert Einstein College of Medicine of
Yeshiva University, Bronx; Chief, Neonatal-Perinatal
Medicine, Schneider Children's Hospital at North Shore,
North Shore University Hospital, Manhasset,
New York
RATIONALE FOR BREASTFEEDING AND MANAGEMENT ISSUES

William Seth Schechter, MD, MS, FAAP
Associate Clinical Professor of Anesthesiology and
Pediatrics, Columbia University College of Physicians and
Surgeons; Director, Pediatric Pain Medicine Program,
Morgan Stanley Children's Hospital of New York–
Presbyterian, New York, New York
PEDIATRIC PAIN MANAGEMENT

Frances L. V. Scheffler, PhD
Assistant Professor, Communication Sciences Program, Hunter College of the City University of New York, New York, New York
EVIDENCE-BASED PRACTICE IN COMMUNICATION DISORDERS: LANGUAGE, SPEECH, AND VOICE DISORDERS

Mark S. Scher, MD
Professor of Pediatrics and Neurology, Department of Pediatrics, Case School of Medicine; Division Chief, Pediatric Neurology, and Director, Pediatric Sleep/Epilepsy and Fetal/Neonatal Neurology Programs, Rainbow Babies and Children's Hospital, University Hospitals of Cleveland, Cleveland, Ohio
INFANTILE SPASMS: WEST SYNDROME

Charles L. Schleien, MD
Professor of Pediatrics and Anesthesiology and Vice Chair for Finance, Columbia University College of Physicians and Surgeons; Medical Director, Pediatric Critical Care Medicine, Morgan Stanley Children's Hospital of New York–Presbyterian, New York, New York
RESPIRATORY FAILURE

Jay J. Schnitzer, MD, PhD
Associate Professor of Surgery, Division of Pediatric Surgery, Harvard Medical School; Associate Visiting Surgeon, Pediatric Surgery, Massachusetts General Hospital, Boston, Massachusetts
HERNIAS AND HYDROCELES

Andrew L. Schwaderer, MD
Assistant Clinical Professor, Department of Pediatrics, The Ohio State University College of Medicine and Public Health, Columbus, Ohio
ACID–BASE DISORDERS

George J. Schwartz, MD
Professor and Chief of Nephrology, Department of Pediatrics, University of Rochester School of Medicine and Dentistry; Attending Physician, Department of Pediatrics, Golisano Children's Hospital at Strong, Rochester, New York
ACID–BASE DISORDERS

Jeffrey H. Schwartz, MD
Pediatric Hematologist/Oncologist, Nemours Children's Clinic, Pensacola, Florida
HEMOLYTIC ANEMIAS

Richard G. Schwartz, MS, PhD
Presidential Professor, Ph.D. Program in Speech and Hearing Sciences, The Graduate Center of the City University of New York, New York, New York
EVIDENCE-BASED PRACTICE IN COMMUNICATION DISORDERS: LANGUAGE, SPEECH, AND VOICE DISORDERS

Christina V. Scirica, MD
Instructor in Pediatrics, Harvard Medical School; Clinical Fellow, Pediatric Pulmonary Unit, MassGeneral Hospital for Children; Research Fellow, Channing Laboratory, Brigham and Women's Hospital, Boston, Massachusetts
ASTHMA

Dorry L. Segev, MD
Instructor in Surgery, Johns Hopkins University School of Medicine, Baltimore, Maryland
PERITONITIS

Kavita S. Seth, DO
Assistant Clinical Instructor and Fellow of Pediatric Infectious Diseases, Department of Pediatrics, Division of Pediatric Infectious Diseases, Stony Brook University School of Medicine, Stony Brook, New York
LISTERIOSIS; ASPERGILLOSIS

Suken A. Shah, MD
Assistant Professor of Orthopaedic Surgery, Jefferson Medical College of Thomas Jefferson University, Philadelphia, Pennsylvania; Attending Pediatric Orthopaedic Surgeon, Alfred I. duPont Hospital for Children, Wilmington, Delaware
THE HIP

Udayan K. Shah, MD, FAAP, FACS
Assistant Professor of Otorhinolaryngology–Head and Neck Surgery, University of Pennsylvania School of Medicine; Attending Surgeon, Pediatric Otolaryngology, The Children's Hospital of Philadelphia, Philadelphia, Pennsylvania
TUMORS AND POLYPS OF THE NOSE; FOREIGN BODIES IN THE EAR, NOSE, AND PHARYNX

Bruce K. Shapiro, MD
Associate Professor of Pediatrics, Johns Hopkins University School of Medicine; Vice President, Training, Kennedy Krieger Institute, Baltimore, Maryland
MENTAL RETARDATION

Eugene D. Shapiro, MD
Professor, Departments of Pediatrics and Epidemiology and Investigative Medicine, Yale University School of Medicine; Attending Pediatrician, Children's Hospital at Yale–New Haven, New Haven, Connecticut
LYME DISEASE; ERHLICHIOSIS (ANAPLASMOSIS)

Bennett A. Shaywitz, MD
Professor of Pediatrics and Neurology and Chief, Division of Child Neurology, Department of Pediatrics, Yale University School of Medicine; Co-Director, Yale Center for the Study of Learning, Reading, and Attention, New Haven, Connecticut
DYSLEXIA (SPECIFIC READING DISABILITY)

Sally E. Shaywitz, MD
Professor of Pediatrics, Yale University School of Medicine; Co-Director, Yale Center for the Study of Learning, Reading, and Attention, New Haven, Connecticut
DYSLEXIA (SPECIFIC READING DISABILITY)

Ziad M. Shehab, MD
Professor of Clinical Pediatrics and Pathology, University of Arizona School of Medicine; Attending Physician, Departments of Pediatrics and Pathology, University Medical Center; Attending Physician, Department of Pediatrics, Tucson Medical Center, Tucson, Arizona
COCCIDIOIDOMYCOSIS

Henry R. Shinefield, MD
Clinical Professor of Pediatrics and Dermatology, University of California, San Francisco, School of Medicine, San Francisco, California
MENINGOCOCCAL DISEASE

Mark G. Shrime, MD
Resident, Department of Otolaryngology/Head and Neck Surgery, Columbia University College of Physicians and Surgeons, New York, New York
PEDIATRIC RHINITIS AND ACUTE AND CHRONIC SINUSITIS

Robert Sidbury, MD
Assistant Professor, Department of Pediatrics, Division of Dermatology, University of Washington School of Medicine; Staff Physician, Children's Hospital and Regional Medical Center, Seattle, Washington
DISORDERS OF PIGMENTATION; ACNE VULGARIS

Eric Jon Sigel, MD, CPH
Associate Professor of Pediatrics, University of Colorado School of Medicine; Clinic Director, Adolescent Medicine Center, Children's Hospital, Denver, Colorado
CONDUCT DISORDER, AGGRESSION, VIOLENCE, AND DELINQUENCY IN YOUTH AND ADOLESCENTS

Nanette B. Silverberg, MD
Clinical Assistant Professor of Dermatology, Columbia University College of Physicians and Surgeons; Director, Pediatric Dermatology, St. Luke's–Roosevelt Hospital Center, New York, New York
WARTS AND MOLLUSCUM IN CHILDREN

Rebecca A. Simmons, MD
Assistant Professor of Pediatrics, University of Pennsylvania School of Medicine; Staff Physician, The Children's Hospital of Philadelphia, Philadelphia, Pennsylvania
HYPOGLYCEMIA IN THE NEWBORN INFANT

Eric Small, MD, FAAP
Assistant Clinical Professor of Pediatrics, Orthopedics, and Rehabilitation Medicine, Mount Sinai School of Medicine; Medical Director, Family Sports Medicine and Nutrition, New York, New York
THE SPORTS PHYSICAL

Holly D. Smith, MD
Assistant Professor of Pediatrics, University of Texas Medical College at Houston; Staff Physician, Divisions of Internal Medicine and Pediatrics, Memorial Hermann Hospital and Lyndon B. Johnson Hospital, Houston, Texas
GASTROESOPHAGEAL REFLUX

Roger F. Soll, MD
Professor of Pediatrics, University of Vermont College of Medicine; Director, Neonatal Intensive Care, Department of Children's Services, Vermont Children's Hospital of Fletcher Allen Health Care, Burlington, Vermont
RESPIRATORY DISTRESS SYNDROME

F. Meridith Sonnett, MD
Associate Professor of Clinical Pediatrics, Department of Pediatrics, Columbia University College of Physicians and Surgeons; Acting Director, Division of Pediatric Emergency Medicine, Morgan Stanley Children's Hospital of New York–Presbyterian, New York, New York
MAMMALIAN BITES AND BITE-RELATED INFECTIONS

Steven P. Sparagana, MD
Assistant Professor of Neurology, University of Texas Southwestern Medical School; Pediatric Neurologist, Texas Scottish Rite Hospital for Children, Dallas, Texas
TUBEROUS SCLEROSIS COMPLEX

Bonnie A. Spear, PhD, RD
Associate Professor of Pediatrics, University of Alabama at Birmingham School of Medicine; Co-Director, Eating Disorder Clinic, Department of Adolescent Medicine, The Children's Health Systems, Birmingham Alabama
EATING DISORDERS AND OBESITY

Lawrence M. Stankovits, MD
Assistant Professor of Orthopaedic Surgery, UMDNJ–Robert Wood Johnson Medical School, New Brunswick; Staff Surgeon, Department of Orthopaedic Surgery, Bristol-Meyers-Squibb Hospital for Children, New Brunswick, and Monmouth Medical Center, Long Branch, New Jersey
THE HIP

Barbara W. Stechenberg, MD
Professor of Pediatrics, Tufts University School of Medicine, Boston; Vice Chairman and Director, Pediatric Infectious Diseases, Baystate Medical Center Children's Hospital, Springfield, Massachusetts
DIPHTHERIA

Russell W. Steele, MD
Professor and Vice-Chairman, Department of Pediatrics, Louisiana State University School of Medicine; Division Head, Pediatric Infectious Diseases, Children's Hospital and University Hospital, New Orleans, Louisiana
CHOLERA

Ruth E. K. Stein, MD
Professor of Pediatrics, Albert Einstein College of Medicine of Yeshiva University; Attending, Children's Hospital at Montefiore, Bronx, New York
THE CHILD WITH A SERIOUS ONGOING CONDITION

Sarah L. Stein, MD
Assistant Professor of Medicine and Pediatrics, Section of Dermatology, University of Chicago Pritzker School of Medicine, Chicago, Illinois
ERYTHEMA MULTIFORME

Peter G. Steinherz, MD
Professor in Pediatrics, Weill Medical College of Cornell University; Attending Pediatrician, Department of Pediatrics, and Member, Memorial Hospital, Memorial Sloan-Kettering Cancer Center; Attending Pediatrician, Department of Pediatrics, New York–Presbyterian Hospital—New York Cornell Campus; New York, New York
ACUTE LEUKEMIA

John Stirling, MD
Consultant Physician, Regional Child Abuse Consultation Network, University of Washington Medical Center, Seattle; Staff Physician, Department of Pediatrics, Southwest

Washington Medical Center, Vancouver; Chair, Department of Pediatrics, The Vancouver Clinic, Vancouver, Washington
CHILD MALTREATMENT

Charles J. H. Stolar, MD
Professor of Surgery and Pediatrics, Columbia University College of Physicians and Surgeons; Staff Physician, Morgan Stanley Children's Hospital of New York–Presbyterian, New York, New York
ABDOMINAL WALL DEFECTS AND DISORDERS OF THE UMBILICUS

William B. Strong, MD
Emeritus L.H. Charbonnier Professor of Pediatrics, Medical College of Georgia; Chief, Section of Pediatric Cardiology, and Director, Georgia Institution for the Prevention of Human Disease and Accidents, Atlanta, Georgia
ACUTE RHEUMATIC FEVER

Marsha S. Sturdevant, MD
Associate Professor of Pediatrics, Division of General Pediatrics and Adolescent Medicine, University of Alabama at Birmingham School of Medicine; Medical Director, Division of Adolescent Medicine, Children's Hospital of Alabama, Birmingham, Alabama
EATING DISORDERS AND OBESITY

Steven Stylianos, MD
Professor of Surgery, University of Miami Miller School of Medicine; Chief, Department of Pediatric Surgery, Miami Children's Hospital, Miami, Florida
BLUNT ABDOMINAL TRAUMA

Maria Luisa Sulis, MD
Assistant Professor of Pediatrics, Columbia University College of Physicians and Surgeons, New York, New York
NEONATAL AND CHILDHOOD NEUTROPENIA

Gautham K. Suresh, MD, DM, MS
Assistant Professor of Pediatrics, Medical University of South Carolina College of Medicine, Charleston, South Carolina
SCREENING IN THE NEWBORN NURSERY: HEARING LOSS, RISK OF SEVERE HYPERBILIRUBINEMIA, CONGENITAL HEART DISEASE

David L. Suskind, MD
Assistant Professor of Pediatrics, University of Washington School of Medicine; Staff Pediatrician, Seattle Children's Hospital and Regional Medical Center, Seattle, Washington
VIRAL HEPATITIS

Britta M. Svoren, MD
Harvard Medical School; Fellow in Endocrinology, Pediatric and Adolescent Unit, Genetics and Epidemiology Section, Joslin Diabetes Center, and Department of Medicine, Children's Hospital Boston, Boston, Massachusetts
DIABETES MELLITUS IN CHILDREN AND ADOLESCENTS

Ilona S. Szer, MD
Professor of Clinical Pediatrics, University of California, San Diego, School of Medicine; Director, Pediatric Rheumatology, Childrens Hospital and Health Center, San Diego, California
TREATMENT OF JUVENILE DERMATOMYOSITIS

Nancy J. Tarbell, MD
C.C. Wang Professor of Radiation Oncology, Harvard Medical School; Head, Pediatric Radiation Oncology, Massachusetts General Hospital; Director, Center for Faculty Development, Massachusetts General Hospital, Boston, Massachusetts
PEDIATRIC BRAIN TUMORS

Jennifer Tender, MD
Assistant Professor of Pediatrics, George Washington University School of Medicine and Health Sciences; Staff Pediatrician, Children's National Medical Center, Washington, DC
IRON DEFICIENCY ANEMIA

Andrew M. Tershakovec, MD
Medical Director, U.S. Human Health, Merck & Co., Inc., Horsham, Pennsylvania
NUTRITION SUPPORT OF THE VERY ILL PEDIATRIC PATIENT

Amy J. Theos, MD
Assistant Professor of Dermatology, University of Alabama at Birmingham School of Medicine; Director, Pediatric Dermatology, Children's Health System, Birmingham, Alabama
SCABIES AND PEDICULOSIS

George H. Thompson, MD
Professor of Orthopaedic Surgery and Pediatrics, Case School of Medicine; Director, Pediatric Orthopaedics, Rainbow Babies and Children's Hospital, Cleveland, Ohio
THE LIMPING CHILD

John F. Thompson, MD
Director, Division of Pediatric Gastroenterology and Nutrition, and Professor, Department of Pediatrics, University of Miami Miller School of Medicine; Staff Physician, Jackson Memorial Hospital and Baptist Hospital, Miami, Florida
INFLAMMATORY BOWEL DISEASE

Lawrence W. C. Tom, MD
Associate Professor of Otorhinolaryngology–Head and Neck Surgery, University of Pennsylvania School of Medicine; Associate Surgeon, Division of Otolaryngology, The Children's Hospital of Philadelphia, Philadelphia, Pennsylvania
TUMORS AND POLYPS OF THE NOSE; FOREIGN BODIES IN THE EAR, NOSE, AND PHARYNX

Helen M. Towers, LRCP&SI, MB, BCh
Assistant Professor of Pediatrics, Columbia University Medical Center College of Physicians and Surgeons; Associate Medical Director, NICU, Department of Pediatrics, Morgan Stanley Children's Hospital of New York–Presbyterian, New York, New York
ANEMIA OF PREMATURITY AND WHEN TO TRANSFUSE; CIRCUMCISION

Martin H. Ulshen, MD
Professor of Pediatrics, Duke University School of Medicine; Chief, Division of Pediatric Gastroenterology and Nutrition, Duke University Medical Center, Durham, North Carolina
INTESTINAL MALFORMATIONS

Reena Moza Vaid, MD
Resident in Pediatrics, Texas Childrens Hospital, Houston, Texas
CHRONIC, NONHEREDITARY BULLOUS DISEASES OF CHILDHOOD

Jon A. Vanderhoof, MD
Chief of Pediatric Gastroenterology and Nutrition, Department of Pediatrics and Internal Medicine, University of Nebraska Medical Center, Omaha, Nebraska; Vice President, Global Medical Affairs, Mead-Johnson Nutritionals, Evansville, Indiana
HIRSCHSPRUNG DISEASE

René G. VanDeVoorde III, MD
Clinical Fellow, Pediatric Nephrology and Hypertension, Cincinnati Children's Hospital Medical Center, Cincinnati, Ohio
HEMATURIA AND PROTEINURIA

V. Matti Vehaskari, MD, PhD
Professor of Pediatrics and Director of Pediatric Nephrology, Department of Pediatrics, Louisiana State University School of Medicine; Director of Pediatric Nephrology, Children's Hospital, New Orleans, Louisiana
RENAL HYPOPLASIA AND DYSPLASIA

Charles P. Venditti, MD, PhD
Director, Organic Acid Research Unit, National Human Genome Research Institute, and Attending Physician, Mark O. Hatfield Clinical Research Center, National Institutes of Health, Bethesda, Maryland
METABOLIC EMERGENCIES IN THE NEWBORN

Elliott Vichinsky, MD
Medical Director, Department of Hematology/Oncology, Children's Hospital and Research Center at Oakland, Oakland, California
THALASSEMIA

Yskert von Kodolitsch, DrMed
Professor of Cardiology, Universitäres Herzzentrum gGmbH; Klinik und Poliklinik für Kardiologie/Angiologie, Medizinische Klinik III, Universitätsklinikum Hamburg-Eppendorf, Hamburg, Germany
MARFAN SYNDROME

Thomas J. Walsh, MD
Senior Investigator and Head, Immunocompromised Host Section, Pediatric Oncology Branch, National Cancer Institute, National Institutes of Health, Bethesda, Maryland
THE IMMUNOCOMPROMISED HOST

Juan N. Walterspiel, MD, FAAP
Assistant Clinical Professor of Pediatrics, Yale University School of Medicine; Attending Physician, Yale–New Haven Children's Hospital, New Haven, Connecticut; Adjunct Associate Clinical Professor of Pediatrics, Emory School of Medicine, Atlanta, Georgia
CELLULITIS

Valerie J. Waters, MD, MSc
Assistant Professor of Pediatrics, Division of Infectious Diseases, University of Toronto Faculty of Medicine; Staff Physician, Division of Infectious Diseases, The Hospital for Sick Children, Toronto, Ontario, Canada
ANTIFUNGAL THERAPIES

Kristi L. Watterberg, MD
Professor and Chief, Division of Neonatology, Department of Pediatrics, University of New Mexico School of Medicine, Albuquerque, New Mexico
BRONCHOPULMONARY DYSPLASIA IN THE NEONATE

Wayne R. Waz, MD
Associate Professor of Clinical Pediatrics, University at Buffalo SUNY School of Medicine and Biomedical Sciences; Chief, Division of Pediatric Nephrology, Women and Children's Hospital of Buffalo, Buffalo, New York
RHABDOMYOLYSIS

Marc Weissbluth, MD
Professor of Clinical Pediatrics, Department of Pediatrics, Northwestern University Feinberg School of Medicine; Active Attending, Department of Pediatrics, Children's Memorial Hospital, Chicago, Illinois
COLIC

Steven L. Werlin, MD
Professor of Pediatrics, Medical College of Wisconsin; Staff Physician, The Children's Hospital of Wisconsin, Milwaukee, Wisconsin
PANCREATIC DISEASES

Barry K. Wershil, MD
Professor of Pediatrics, Albert Einstein College of Medicine of Yeshiva University; Section Chief, Pediatric Gastroenterology and Nutrition, The Children's Hospital at Montefiore, Bronx, New York
ALLERGIC GASTROINTESTINAL DISORDERS

L. Joseph Wheat, MD
Mira Vista Diagnostics & Mira Bella Technologies, Indianapolis, Indiana
BLASTOMYCOSIS: RECOGNITION, DIAGNOSIS, AND MANAGEMENT

A. Clinton White, Jr., MD
Professor of Medicine, Division of Infectious Diseases, Baylor College of Medicine; Staff Physician, Division of Infectious Diseases, Ben Taub General Hospital, Houston, Texas
CYSTICERCOSIS

Robert W. Wilmott, MD
IMMUNO Professor and Chair, Department of Pediatrics, Saint Louis University School of Medicine; Pediatrician-in-Chief, Cardinal Glennon Children's Hospital, St. Louis, Missouri
BRONCHIETASIS

Joseph I. Wolfsdorf, MB, BCh
Associate Professor of Pediatrics, Harvard Medical School; Senior Associate in Medicine (Endocrinology), Children's Hospital Boston, Boston, Massachusetts
GYNECOMASTIA

Susan H. Wootton, MD
Clinical Research Fellow, Department of Pediatrics, Division of Infectious and Immunological Diseases, University of

British Columbia, and BC Children's Hospital, Vancouver, British Columbia, Canada
CYSTICERCOSIS

Albert C. Yan, MD
Assistant Professor of Pediatrics and Dermatology, University of Pennsylvania School of Medicine; Director, Section of Dermatology, The Children's Hospital of Philadelphia, Philadelphia, Pennsylvania
ERYTHEMA NODOSUM

Linda S. Yancey, MD
Infectious Disease Fellow, Department of Medicine, Baylor College of Medicine, Houston, Texas
CYSTICERCOSIS

Yih-Ming Yang, MD
Professor of Pediatrics, Emory School of Medicine; Attending Physician, Aflac Cancer Center and Blood Disorders Service, Children's Health Care of Atlanta, Atlanta, Georgia
MEGALOBLASTIC ANEMIA

Robert J. Yetman, MD
Director, Division of Community and General Pediatrics, Department of Pediatrics, University of Texas Medical School at Houston, Houston, Texas
DIARRHEA

Torunn I. Yock, MD, MCH
Harvard University; Department of Radiation Oncology, Massachusetts General Hospital, Boston, Massachusetts
PEDIATRIC BRAIN TUMORS

Rosemary J. Young, MS, RN
Clinical Nurse Specialist, Pediatric Gastroenterology Division, University of Nebraska Medical Center, Omaha, Nebraska
HIRSCHSPRUNG DISEASE

Thomas W. Young, MD
Attending Pediatric Cardiologist, Ochsner Clinic Foundation, New Orleans, Louisiana
ACUTE RHEUMATIC FEVER

Nader N. Youssef, MD
Assistant Professor of Pediatrics, University of Medicine and Dentistry–New Jersey Medical School; Staff, Center for Pediatric Irritable Bowel and Motility Disorders, Goryeb Children's Hospital–Atlantic Health System, Morristown, New Jersey
ABDOMINAL PAIN: APPROACH TO A DIAGNOSIS

Ditza A. Zachor, MD
Assistant Professor of Pediatrics (Medicine), Tel-Aviv University School of Medicine; Director, Autism Center, Department of Pediatrics, Assaf Harofeh Medical Center, Tel-Aviv, Israel
AUTISM

Kenneth M. Zangwill, MD
Professor of Clinical Pediatrics, David Geffen School of Medicine at UCLA; Staff Pediatrician, Harbor-UCLA Medical Center, Los Angeles, California
INFLUENZA VIRUS

Heather J. Zar, MD, PhD
Associate Professor, Department of Pediatric Pulmonology, School of Child and Adolescent Health, University of Cape Town Faculty of Medicine; Pediatric Pulmonologist, Red Cross Children's Hospital, Cape Town, South Africa
PNEUMOCYSTIS JIROVECI PNEUMONIA (PCP)

Christa M. H. Zehle, MD
Clinical Assistant Professor, Department of Pediatrics, University of Vermont College of Medicine; Clinical Assistant Professor/Pediatric Hospitalist, Vermont Children's Hospital at Fletcher Allen Health Care, Burlington, Vermont
FOREIGN BODIES IN THE GASTROINTESTINAL TRACT

Mary L. Zupanc, MD
Professor and Division Chief, Department of Neurology and Pediatrics, Medical College of Wisconsin; Director, Pediatric Epilepsy Center, Department of Neurology, Children's Hospital of Wisconsin, Milwaukee, Wisconsin
CEREBROVASCULAR DISEASE

Preface

Throughout its many editions, *Current Pediatric Therapy* has become the standard text in its field, consistently providing practicing clinicians with practical approaches to the management of pediatric disease. The experience and expert opinions of the leading physicians and scientists who have contributed to this textbook have played an indispensable role in its continued relevance and utility. With the renewed focus on evidence-based medicine in recent years, we thought it time to merge this rich and valued history with a critical examination of outcomes and practices. Of course, such evidence without benefit of clinical experience is an insufficient guide for clinicians. Therefore, we asked each author to develop new content that would not only discuss the evidence supporting each recommendation but also provide practical management recommendations based on their own clinical experience.

The aim of this book has always been to improve the quality of clinical care. We have endeavored to present the best possible treatment options in our pages by reviewing the prevailing patterns of practices, providing evidence from the literature, addressing differences of opinion and approach, and synthesizing the information to enhance the reader's ease of use. All of the chapters in this new edition follow a similar format, beginning with a list of "Key Concepts" for the management of each disease discussed. This is followed by sections on "Expert Opinion on Management," "Common Pitfalls," and "Communication and Counseling." It is our hope that the more uniform presentation in this new edition will enhance the functionality of the work. A better organizational understanding of treatment options can only improve the overall quality of care.

The key to this edition is the quality of our contributors. We have found the best and the brightest health care providers in all areas of pediatrics to contribute. We surveyed department chairs and leaders of pediatrics programs throughout the world, asking them to recommend clinicians who are considered excellent teachers and writers in their fields. In addition, we used our own experience in the field to select appropriate contributors for the book. As a result, we have amalgamated what we believe to be the most authoritative and complete volume of *Current Pediatric Therapy* to date.

Because the focus of this book is on management, we asked the contributors to help the reader understand why a particular treatment is used for a given condition. The contributors also were requested to describe their approach to management on the basis of their own experience and expertise and to consider both the quality and the cost of care. This book does *not* promise easy, inexpensive shortcuts—just the state of the art in the practice of pediatrics.

We believe that many disciplines should be involved in modern pediatric practice so that the highest quality of care is provided to children. With this aim in mind, we invited psychologists, general surgeons, cardiac surgeons, neurosurgeons, orthopedic surgeons, urologists, otorhinolaryngologists, dentists, and ophthalmologists to contribute. We think you will find the sections developed by these specialists to be helpful for understanding the reasons that various approaches are used in the management of certain pediatric problems.

We learned from previous editions that tables are helpful to the reader, and thus we encouraged their use in this edition. We also have been more liberal with the use of references with annotations, while working hard to maintain the manageable size of the book. Finally, we have sought to enhance the psychosocial content of the book—something that we believe to be of great importance in the practice of pediatrics.

We would like to thank the contributors to this edition; the completion of their chapters made it possible for us to go to press in a timely manner. We also would like to thank Heidi Kleinbart of Columbia University for her editorial support and assistance in the preparation of this work. Thanks also to Jennifer Shreiner, developmental editor, Joan Nikelsky, project manager, and the rest of the key staff at Elsevier for their help in producing yet another quality edition of *Current Pediatric Therapy*. As we prepare to begin work on the 19th edition, we ask once again that those of you who are teachers, writers, and experts in your fields come forth and let us know how you may contribute to the next edition. Please write to Rebecca Gaertner at *r.gaertner@elsevier.com*.

Fredric D. Burg

Julie R. Ingelfinger

Richard A. Polin

Anne A. Gershon

Contents

SECTION 4
Communication in Therapy

SECTION 5
Special Problems in the Infant and Neonate

SECTION **6**
Special Problems in the Adolescent

SECTION **7**
Nervous System

SECTION 11
Nephrology and Genitourinary Tract

SECTION 12
Infectious Diseases

Foci of Infection

Bacterial Infections

SECTION 15
Metabolic Disorders

SECTION 16
Musculoskeletal System and Connective Tissue

SECTION 17
Skin

SECTION 22
Mental Development and Behavioral Disorders

SECTION 23
Dental Problems

Symptomatic Care Prior to Diagnosis

Cough

Anne Bernadette Chang

KEY CONCEPTS

- All children with cough should be carefully evaluated and managed differently from adults with cough because the etiologic factors and treatment in children are significantly different.

- Most children with acute cough (<2 weeks) have acute upper respiratory tract infection. They should be assessed for inhalation of foreign body, pneumonia, and other lower respiratory tract infection and other less common causes of cough.

- Children with subacute or chronic cough should be assessed for presence of specific cough pointers, and those with chronic cough should have, at a minimum, a chest radiograph and spirometry (if age appropriate). When specific cough is present, further testing is usually warranted, except when asthma is the cause.

- In children with nonspecific cough, the cough usually spontaneously resolves, but children should be evaluated for emergence of specific cough pointers. In some children a short (2- to 4-week) trial of 400 µg per day of beclomethasone equivalent may be warranted. However, most children with isolated cough do not have asthma. If the cough does not resolve, the medication should be withdrawn and another diagnosis should be considered.

- In all children with cough, exacerbation factors such as environmental tobacco smoke exposure should be sought and intervention options for cessation initiated. Parent expectations and specific concerns should be sought and addressed.

- Children with cough should not be treated with medications (such as over-the-counter medications for cough) for symptomatic relief of cough. Treatment, if any, should be based on etiology.

Cough, an essential defense mechanism for lung health, is the most common symptom of children treated by physicians. It is a symptom that is representative of disease of the entire respiratory system, from minor respiratory tract infections (RTIs) to major illnesses such as cystic fibrosis (CF), and it is rarely a symptom of extrapulmonary disease. Although most coughs in children are minor and often trivialized, cough has a significantly negative impact on parents and children.

Clinicians should be cognizant of some general issues regarding cough. Cough is essential for airway clearance, and suppression of cough may be harmful. Well children occasionally cough, and children without a preceding upper RTI (URTI) (within the last 4 weeks) might cough numerous times in a 24-hour period. Even though cough is a very common symptom, it can exacerbate anxiety and lead to unnecessary medical therapy. In one of the few randomized, controlled trials of medications for cough in children, irrespective of medicines (drug, placebo, or no treatment) received, parents who wanted pharmacologic treatment were more likely to report improvement at follow-up. The benefit of placebo treatment for cough is as high as 85%, and non–placebo-controlled intervention studies need to be interpreted with caution. Finally, cough is affected by psychological influences because cough is cortically modulated; children are more likely to cough in certain psychological settings.

Pediatric cough can be classified based on time frame, etiology, and/or characteristic (moist vs. dry), with a degree of overlap. The time frame is divided into acute (<2 weeks), subacute (2 to 4 weeks), and chronic (>4 weeks) cough (Fig. 1). Cough related to a URTI resolves within 10 days in 50% of children and by 25 days in 90%; arguably, childhood chronic cough should be defined as persistent daily cough after 4 weeks. Chronic cough is subdivided into specific cough (cough associated with other symptoms and signs that are suggestive of an associated or underlying problem) and nonspecific cough (dry cough in the absence of any identifiable respiratory disease or known etiology). These classifications are not mutually exclusive.

Expert Opinion on Management Issues

ACUTE COUGH

Although acute URTIs are the most common cause of acute cough in children, all children should be assessed for symptoms and signs of a more serious etiology (Table 1). Acute URTI may coexist with an underlying disorder, and 8% to 12% of children with URTI develop complications. Children with fever and chest findings are more likely to have URTI with a complication requiring treatment (e.g., antibiotics).

In the majority of children, acute cough is self-limiting, and treatment, if any, should be directed at the etiology rather than the symptom of cough. Over-the-counter (OTC) medications for cough confer no

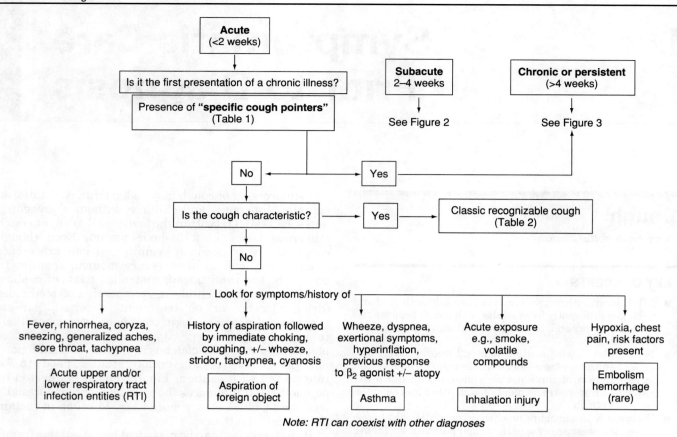

FIGURE 1. Pathway for acute cough. These pathways are a guide to the approach of a child with a cough. The suggested approach is dependent on the length of cough and whether any symptoms and/or signs are present ("specific cough pointers" listed in Table 1). Symptoms and signs can be age-dependent, and thus the child's age and severity of illness must also be considered when assessing a child with cough. It would not be possible to factor the various combinations in these pathways. RTI, respiratory tract infection. (From Chang AB, Asher MI: A review of cough in children. J Asthma 38:299–309, 2001. Copyright 2001. Reproduced by permission of Taylor & Francis Group, LLC., http://www.taylorandfrancis.com.)

TABLE 1 Specific Cough Pointers
Auscultatory findings
Cardiac abnormalities
Chest pain
Dyspnea or tachypnea
Chest wall deformity
Digital clubbing
Daily moist or productive cough
Exertional dyspnea
Failure to thrive
Feeding difficulties
Hemoptysis
Hypoxia/cyanosis
Immune deficiency
Neurodevelopmental abnormality
Recurrent pneumonia

benefit in the symptomatic control of cough or on the sleep pattern of children or parents and might cause harm. Steam inhalation, vitamin C, zinc, and echinacea for URTI have little benefit for symptomatic relief of cough. Systematic reviews have reported that oral or inhaled β_2-agonists confer no benefit in children with acute cough without evidence of airflow obstruction.

Antimicrobial agents are not beneficial in acute cough associated with viral infections.

SUBACUTE AND CHRONIC COUGH

There are no prospective studies on the follow-up of well children with acute cough beyond 25 days. A retrospective review showed that 3 weeks following an acute URTI, 5% to 10% of preschool-age children still coughed. Children with subacute cough should be evaluated for first presentation of an underlying pulmonary disorder (Fig. 2). Clinical signs and symptoms that suggest an underlying pulmonary or systemic disorder are termed *specific cough pointers* (see Table 1). When any of these pointers are present, the cough is referred to as *specific cough*. If specific cough pointers are present, further investigations and management of the primary pulmonary pathology is usually warranted. If not, a counsel-watch-wait-and-review approach is suggested. Diagnoses with simple treatment options (e.g., asthma and complications of URTIs such as sinusitis and bronchitis), may be considered. However the evidence for the association between asthma and upper airway disorders and cough is not as straightforward in children as it is in adults.

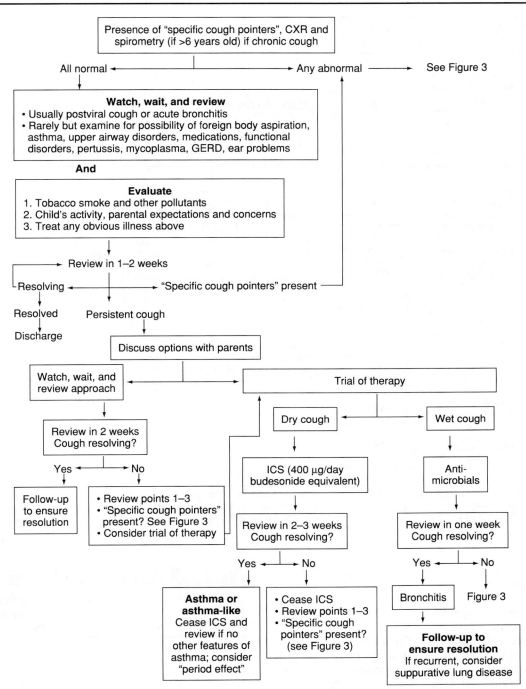

FIGURE 2. Pathway for subacute and nonspecific chronic cough. CXR, chest x-ray; GERD, gastroesophageal reflux disease; ICS, inhaled corticosteroid. (From Chang AB, Asher MI: A review of cough in children. J Asthma 38:299–309, 2001. Copyright 2001. Reproduced by permission of Taylor & Francis Group, LLC., http://www.taylorandfrancis.com.)

The use of isolated cough as a marker of asthma is controversial with newer evidence (clinical and community epidemiologic studies) showing that in most children, isolated cough does not represent asthma.

Children with chronic cough (Fig. 3) should:

■ Be reviewed for possible exacerbation factors (environmental tobacco smoke [ETS] exposure, etc.) irrespective of presence of other etiology.

■ Have spirometry (if age appropriate) and chest radiograph performed.

■ Be carefully evaluated, especially for symptoms and signs of an underlying respiratory or systemic disease (termed *specific cough pointers*, [see Table 1]).

In some instances, particular characteristics of cough may be recognizable and suggestive of specific etiology

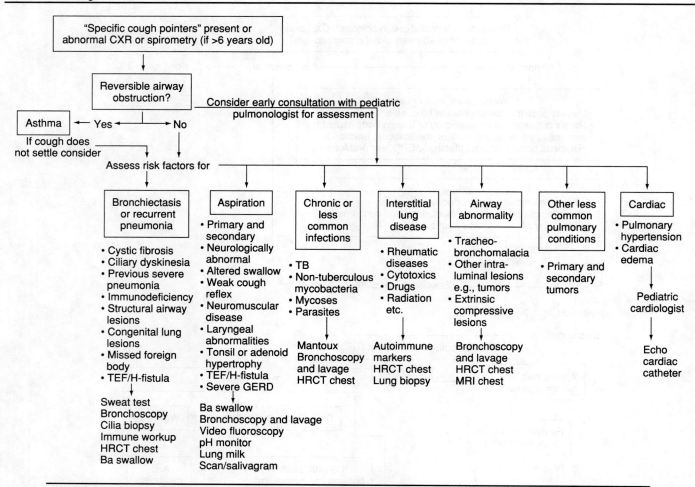

FIGURE 3. Chronic cough pathway. GERD, gastroesophageal reflux disease; HRCT, high-resolution computed tomography scan; MRI, magnetic resonance imaging; TB, tuberculosis; TEF, tracheoesophageal fistula. (From Chang AB, Asher MI: A review of cough in children. J Asthma 2001;38:299–309. Copyright 2001. Reproduced by permission of Taylor & Francis Group, LLC., http://www.taylorandfrancis.com.)

(Table 2); chronic productive purulent cough is always pathologic. Figure 2 outlines an approach to children with nonspecific cough.

Table 3 summarizes problems in relating etiologic factors in nonspecific cough.

Treatment for subacute and chronic cough should be based on etiology; specific cough therapy is beyond the scope of this article. Table 4 summarizes evidence (or lack of) in treatment trials for nonspecific cough. Significant morbidity and mortality from OTC cough therapy can occur, and these therapies are commonly ingested unintentionally by children younger than 5 years of age. Cochrane Reviews reports that symptomatic treatment of cough by diphenhydramine is not beneficial for pertussis-related cough, that chromones and anticholinergics have little, if any, role in nonspecific chronic childhood cough, and that 10 days of antimicrobial therapy reduces persistent cough in children with chronic nasal discharge, although benefits are modest.

Antimicrobial agents may be indicated for subacute/ chronic moist cough; two randomized, controlled trials showed predominance of *Moraxella catarrhalis*. A meta-analysis of antimicrobial therapy for acute bronchitis in

TABLE 2 Classical Recognizable Cough	
Cough Characteristic	**Suggested Underlying Etiology or Contributing Factor**
Barking or brassy	Croup, tracheomalacia, habit cough
Cough productive of casts	Plastic bronchitis
Honking	Psychogenic
Paroxysmal (with/without whoop)	Pertussis and parapertussis
Staccato	Chlamydia in infants

older children (>8 years of age), and adults showed a small benefit of 0.58 days but a rise in significant adverse events. Systematic review of uncomplicated sinusitis in children showed that the clinical improvement rate was 88% with antibiotic therapy and 60% without antimicrobial treatment. There are only two published randomized, controlled trials on inhaled corticosteroids for nonspecific cough in children, and both studies

TABLE 3 Major Points and Pitfalls in Diagnosis of Chronic Cough

Etiology	Key Briefs; Look For:	Major Pitfalls
Nonspecific Cough		
Asthma	Exertional dyspnea, recurrent wheeze, eczema, allergic rhinitis, parental asthma, eosinophilia (>4%), and possibly nocturnal cough. Asthma-associated cough (without a coexistent RTI) is usually dry. Signs include Harrison sulci, wheeze, hyperinflation, eczema.	Spirometry is valuable in the diagnosis of reversible airway obstruction in children with chronic cough. However, spirometry is relatively insensitive, and a normal spirometry does not exclude underlying respiratory abnormality. Objective monitoring has shown that cough associated with asthma is more common during the day and that nocturnal cough is unreliably reported.
Bronchitis/postviral cough	Preceding URTI, persistent wet or mixed cough.	Although this term is often used, there is little information on its pathophysiology.
Upper airways disorders Allergic rhinitis Sinusitis Tonsil-adenoid hypertrophy	Nasal discharge and cough reported as the two most prominent symptoms in children with chronic sinusitis. Examination findings.	Supportive evidence of cause and effect in children is less convincing than in adults. The relationship between nasal secretions and cough is more likely linked by common etiology (infection or inflammation causing both) or caused by clearing of secretions reaching the larynx.
Pertussis and parapertussis	Contact, character of cough, vaccination history.	Both can cause persistent cough not associated with other symptoms; cough is not necessarily spasmodic. Other infections such as chlamydia, *Mycoplasma*, and RSV can also cause spasmodic cough in selected age groups.
Mycoplasma	History of contact, other symptoms of RTI.	Associated symptoms may be absent.
Medications	Timing with commencement of medication; cough associated with ACE inhibitors resolves within 3–7 days after medication withdrawal.	Asthma medications and omeprazole used to treat nonspecific cough can also cause cough.
Functional respiratory disorder	Typical honking cough is more common in adolescent females. Habitual cough is more common in boys.	Habitual cough or cough as a "vocal tic" may be transient or chronic.
Otogenic causes	Can cause cough if Arnold ear-cough reflex is present (2.3%–4.2% of people).	Ear problems are common in children, and Arnold ear reflex is uncommon. Difficult to elucidate if ear disease, if present, is the cause of cough.
Environmental toxicants, e.g., ETS exposure	Exposure history.	Under-reporting of cough in parents who smoke may bias history.
Eosinophilic bronchitis and allergy	Cough probably represents an overlap with asthma, eosinophilic bronchitis, allergic rhinitis, and adenoid tonsillar hypertrophy.	Not a well-recognized entity in children. Atopic cough only described in Japan. Inconsistent findings regarding cough and atopy in literature.
Foreign body inhalation	History of choking, unilateral wheeze.	Absent history does not indicate absence of foreign body.
GERD	Symptoms of GERD (halitosis, vomiting, irritability with feeds, poor weight gain, dysphagia, abdominal or substernal pain).	Although GER has been associated with chronic cough, cough can also cause GER. There is little evidence of GERD as a common cause of cough in otherwise well children.
Treatment side effect	History of chronic vagus nerve stimulation.	A rare etiology.
Selected Causes of Specific Cough		
Airway lesions, e.g., tracheobronchomalacia	Monophonic wheeze, recurrent infections, risk factors such as cardiac anomalies, pectus excavatum, connective tissue disease.	How commonly airway lesions are found in asymptomatic children is unknown.
Aspiration	Neurodevelopmental problems, bulbar or pseudobulbar palsy, coughs or chokes on drinking thin fluids.	The gold standard is undefined. Increased lipid laden macrophage index and video fluoroscopy are often used.
Chronic suppurative lung disease or bronchiectasis	Chronic productive or moist cough, history of immune deficiency, recurrent pneumonia, clubbing, hyperinflation.	Cough may be dry initially. In aboriginal and developing world settings, bronchiectasis is likely the most common cause of chronic cough.
Parenchymal lung disease	Combination of symptoms and signs (see Table 1).	

ACE, angiotensin-converting enzyme; ETS, environmental tobacco smoke; GER, gastroesophageal reflux; GERD, gastroesophageal reflux disease; RSV, respiratory syncytial virus; RTI, respiratory tract infection; URTI, upper respiratory tract infection.

cautioned against its prolonged use. In the guidelines of the North American Society for Pediatric Gastroenterology and Nutrition (NASPGN), the conclusion on cough and gastroesophageal reflux disease (GERD) was that "there is insufficient evidence and experience in children for a uniform approach to diagnosis and treatment."

Cough is reported as an adverse event to omeprazole in adults, although there are no similar reports in children. A randomized controlled trial of ketotifen revealed no beneficial effect in the treatment of 113 infants and children with chronic cough and/or wheeze. However, in another randomized, controlled trial of 20 children

TABLE 4 Suggested Therapies Used for Nonspecific Cough

Therapy	Time to Response*	Pitfall or Limitation
Antihistamines	1 week	Inconclusive data, adverse events
Antimicrobials	1–2 weeks	Adverse events
Asthma therapy		
Chromones	2 weeks	Single open trial only
Anticholinergics		No trials in children
Inhaled corticosteroids	2–4 weeks	Small benefit if any, adverse event
Oral corticosteroids		No RCTs, adverse events
Beta$_2$-agonist (oral or inhaled)		Nonbeneficial; adverse events
Theophylline	1–2 weeks	No RCTs, adverse events
GERD* therapy		
Motility agents		No benefit in single controlled trial
Acid suppression	2–8 weeks (adult data)	No RCT, adverse events
Food thickening or antireflux formula	1 week	Inconclusive data, one RCT reported increase in cough and a second significant reduction
Fundoplication		No RCT, adverse events
Herbal therapy		No RCTs
OTC cough medications		Nonbeneficial; adverse events
Physical therapies steam, vapor, rubs		No RCTs, adverse events, e.g., burns

*Time to response is the expected improvement or resolution in cough severity if treatment is effective.
GERD, gastroesophageal reflux disease; OTC, over-the-counter; RTC, randomized, controlled trial.

with cough associated with pollen allergy, cetirizine reduced cough subjectively, and the effect was evident by 1 week of treatment.

Common Pitfalls

There are many pitfalls in diagnosis and management of childhood cough; Tables 3 and 4 list major ones. Moist or productive cough may initially manifest as dry cough, and there is an overlap between specific and nonspecific cough; hence re-evaluation is important. The most likely etiology depends on the setting, selection criteria of children studied, follow-up rate and depth of clinical history, and examination and investigations performed. Clinical trial data on management of childhood cough are relatively sparse.

Communication and Counseling

In contrast to adult data, there are no quality-of-life studies for parents and children with chronic cough. However, parents taking children to U.S. and British doctors for cough have significant concerns—fear of their child dying from choking, asthma attack, sudden death, and permanent chest damage; disturbed sleep; and relief of discomfort. These concerns are often not appreciated by health professionals, and exploration of parental expectations and fears is valuable in the management of cough. As with other medical information, the Internet provides incorrect advice on the home management of cough in children. When evaluating any child with cough, irrespective of the etiology, exacerbation factors should be explored even though no clinical trials have examined the effect of cessation of environmental pollutants on cough. The policy of the American Academy of

Pediatrics (AAP) on tobacco includes recommendations for tobacco cessation. Providing parents with information on the expected time length of resolution of RTI may reduce anxiety in parents and the need for medication use. Parental and professional expectations and physicians' perception of patients' expectations often influences consulting rates and prescription of medications in RTI. Education is best performed with consultation about the child's specific condition because written information without consultation has only modest benefits in changing perceptions and behavior.

SUGGESTED READINGS

1. Arroll B, Kenealy T: Antibiotics for the common cold and acute purulent rhinitis. Cochrane Database Syst Rev 3:CD000247, 2005.
2. Berlin CM, McCarver-May DG, Notterman DA, et al: Use of codeine- and dextromethorphan-containing cough remedies in children. Pediatrics 99:918–919, 1997. **American Academy of Pediatrics guidelines on over-the-counter medicines for cough.**
3. Chang AB: State of the art: Cough, cough receptors, and asthma in children. Pediatr Pulmonol 28:59–70, 1999. **A review of main concepts of cough physiology and application to children.**
4. Chang AB, Asher MI: A review of cough in children. J Asthma 38:299–309, 2001. **A more detailed review of cough in children. Paper also discusses limitations of extrapolation of common causes of chronic cough in adults to children and their controversies.**
5. Chang AB, Gaffney J, Connor F, Garske LA: Gastro-oesophageal reflux treatment for prolonged non-specific cough in children and adults. Cochrane Database Syst Rev 2:CD004823, 2005. **Cochrane reviews on cough-related treatment.**
6. Chang AB, McKean M, Morris P: Inhaled anti-cholinergics for prolonged non-specific cough in children. Cochrane Database Syst Rev, 1:CD004358, 2004. **Cochrane reviews on cough-related treatment.**
7. Chang AB, Marchant JM, McKean M, Morris P: Inhaled cromones for prolonged non-specific cough in children. The Cochrane Database Syst Rev, 1:CD004358, 2004. **Cochrane reviews on cough-related treatment**.

8. Cochrane Library 2004;Issue 1, 2004. Chichester, UK: John Wiley & Sons. **Cochrane reviews on cough-related treatment.**

9. Hay AD, Wilson A, Fahey T, Peters TJ: The duration of acute cough in pre-school children presenting to primary care: a prospective cohort study. Fam Pract 20:696–705, 2003. **A prospective study examining the symptom of cough in children with URTI. This paper follows the group's previous systematic review of duration of cough in children. However paper does not describe how many children subsequently developed complications of URTI and when these occurred.**

10. Hutton N, Wilson MH, Mellits ED, et al: Effectiveness of an antihistamine-decongestant combination for young children with the common cold: A randomized, controlled clinical trial. J Pediatr 118:125–130, 1991. **One of the first randomized, controlled trials on cough treatment in children. This study examined the effect of antihistamine-decongestant, placebo, and no treatment on cough. The authors also uniquely reported on the effect of parental expectations or beliefs on cough reporting.**

11. Kelly LF: Pediatric cough and cold preparations. Pediatr Rev 25:115–123, 2004. **The latest review of cough and cold preparations for children.**

12. Morris P, Leach A: Antibiotics for persistent nasal discharge (rhinosinusitis) in children. Cochrane Database Syst Rev, 4: CD001094, 2002. **Cochrane reviews on cough-related treatment.**

13. Pillay V, Swingler G: Symptomatic treatment of the cough in whooping cough. Cochrane Database Syst Rev 4:CD003257, 2003. **Cochrane reviews on cough-related treatment.**

14. Schroeder K, Fahey T: Over the counter medications for acute cough in children and adults in ambulatory settings. Cochrane Database Syst Rev, 4:CD001831, 2004. Cochrane reviews on cough-related treatment.

Diarrhea

Robert J. Yetman and Lynnette J. Mazur

KEY CONCEPTS

- Perform a complete history and physical examination with particular attention to signs and symptoms of dehydration.
- Evaluate the child for evidence of serious or chronic disease; further evaluation and testing should be directed based on the history and physical examination.
  - Findings observed with more serious causes of diarrhea include pallor, poor growth, edema, rashes or stomatitis, digital clubbing, evidence of respiratory infections or opportunistic infections, joint swelling or pain, and/or thyromegaly.
- Determine if the patient requires laboratory testing. Most instances of diarrhea are infectious in etiology, are self-limited, and require no testing.
  - Measurement of electrolytes for patients with moderate or severe dehydration should be considered.
  - Stool studies (enzyme-linked immunoabsorbent assay) can confirm rotavirus disease, but the result rarely alters therapy in the patient with mild, acute diarrhea. Results of stool for guaiac, fecal leukocytes, and culture rarely alter conservative therapy unless the patient has severe disease or associated symptoms (such as high fever, pallor, or seizures). Polymorphonuclear cells in the stool may be helpful to predict a bacterial stool pathogen.
  - Complete blood counts with differentials and erythrocyte sedimentation rates are neither sensitive nor specific tests, especially for the patient with mild

disease. Urine for specific gravity may assist in confirming dehydration coupled with a properly performed history and physical examination.
- For chronic or more severe diarrhea, depending on the history and physical examination, evaluations may include serum albumin, sweat chloride, lactose tolerance tests, urinalysis and urine culture, and more extensive stool studies (ova and parasites, pH, reducing substances, fat stains, *Clostridium difficile* toxin) based on the clinical findings.

Although short-lived diarrhea in the otherwise healthy child is most likely to be acute, self-limited, infectious gastroenteritis, a variety of other conditions could be the culprit if the diarrhea was unusually severe or prolonged. The history, physical examination (H&PE), and, if needed, some basic laboratory testing may be helpful in identifying children with diarrhea for whom an alternative explanation should be considered.

A wide variety of *infectious agents* can cause diarrhea, and specific treatment for each of these conditions can be found elsewhere in this text. Ingestion of antibiotics can result in diarrhea, although pseudomembranous colitis should be considered in the patient who has recently been prescribed antibiotics (especially clindamycin, cephalosporins, or amoxicillin) and is experiencing fever, tenesmus, bloody stools, and abdominal pain with the diarrhea. Infectious processes, other than in the gastrointestinal (GI) tract, can result in diarrhea; evidence for such entities as otitis media and urinary tract infection (UTI) can be considered.

Noninfectious conditions can cause diarrhea. Overfeeding, typically with fruit juices, may result in osmotic diarrhea in younger infants. Allergic diarrhea, often discussed but rarely found, can be considered in the patient who has a strong personal or family history of atopic disease, has prolonged moderate to severe symptoms of colitis, has occult blood in the stool, or who has hypoproteinemia. A double-blind oral challenge with the suspected offending agent is often diagnostic. A wide variety of malabsorption syndromes including conditions such as cystic fibrosis, carbohydrate malabsorption, immune deficiencies, short bowel, and endocrinopathies can cause diarrhea. In general these syndromes are unusual, may occur with a family history of similar illness, manifest with prolonged and watery diarrhea, or are found associated with symptoms of failure to thrive, intermittent fevers, or rashes.

Expert Opinion on Management Issues

Oral rehydration therapy (ORT) is the initial treatment of choice for most patients (see Fluid and Electrolyte Therapy in Section 2). Patients who are not dehydrated and who refuse the salty taste of the ORT are more appropriately managed with a regular diet; patients who have ileus, altered mental status, shock, or severe dehydration require intravenous fluid therapy. Occasionally, persistent or severe vomiting precludes adequate resuscitation with ORT in moderately dehydrated patients; in these cases initial intravenous (IV) therapy with transition to ORT is often used. Alternatively, nasogastric infusions of the rehydration fluid can also be considered.

Early return to regular, age-appropriate diet (especially those containing complex carbohydrates, lean meats, yogurt, fruits, and vegetables) modestly reduces the duration of diarrhea while providing improved nutrition as compared to ORT or IV therapy alone. Previous recommendations of slowly reintroducing into the diet milk-based formulas or cow's milk and BRAT diets (bananas, rice, applesauce, and toast) are to be avoided.

Although ORT is recommended for most cases of dehydration (except as outlined above), the costs and benefits of IV therapy must be considered. Initial IV therapy for patients with shock or near-shock is vigorous, aimed at improving cardiovascular perfusion, with weaning to ORT delayed until the medical condition permits. Some argue that ORT therapy can be time-consuming, especially in a patient with frequent vomiting, and advocate the use of IV fluids initially with transition to ORT when possible; others counter that ORT is neither more labor-intensive nor time-consuming. Regardless of the route chosen, the response to therapy must be monitored and adjusted accordingly.

Common Pitfalls

- Failure to adequately assess hydration status of the child.
- Failure to offer in most cases ORT as an initial treatment option.
- Reliance on treatments in which the side effects exceed the benefits:
  - Medications to alter intestinal motility including loperamide, difenoxin/atropine, diphenoxylate/atropine, and tincture of opium.
  - Medications to alter intestinal secretion including various bismuth compounds.
  - Use of toxins and water absorbants including kaolin-pectin, fiber, activated charcoal, and attapulgite.
  - Experimental agents such berberine, nicotinic acid, clonidine, chloride channel blockers, calmodulin inhibitors, octreotide acetate, and nonsteroidal anti-inflammatory drugs (NSAIDs).

Communication and Counseling

Probably the most effective means to prevent diarrheal illness is with primary prevention:

- Adequate hand washing.
- Excluding children with diarrhea from daycare until resolution of symptoms.
- Avoiding traveler's diarrhea by using bottled water, eating only steaming hot foods, and avoiding items potentially exposed to contaminated water, such as fresh fruits and vegetables with the exception of those that can be peeled, such as bananas and citrus fruits.

A previous version of a rotavirus vaccine, although successful in preventing serious diarrhea, caused intussusception and is no longer available. Newer agents are being developed and are currently undergoing clinical investigations; early results appear to be promising.

Potential therapies are:

- Probiotic therapy, the use of saccharolytic bacteria (*Lactobacillus*, *Bifidobacteria* species, *Streptococcus thermophilus*, *Saccharomyces boulardii*) to ferment unabsorbed carbohydrates thereby reducing the pH in the intestine, has been proposed by some clinicians. The reduced gut pH results in increased production of short-chain fatty acids; these fatty acids are more easily absorbed in the colon, improve absorption of water, and deter intestinal pathogens. Although not recommended by the American Academy of Pediatrics (AAP), some meta-analyses have suggested benefit of this treatment and reported no side effects.
- Zinc supplementation curtails the severity of acute diarrheal episodes in developing countries; its value in the treatment for acute diarrhea in developed areas is unknown.
- Homeopathy is commonly used. Although a meta-analysis of unknown homeopathic agents demonstrated a small but statistically significant treatment effect (improved symptoms by 0.66 days), the exact role of this treatment modality remains unclear.

SUGGESTED READINGS

1. American Academy of Pediatrics: Practice parameter: The management of acute gastroenteritis in young children. Pediatrics 97:424–433, 1996. **The AAP statement on acute gastroenteritis outlining diagnosis and treatment options.**
2. American Academy of Pediatrics: Rotavirus. In Pickering LK (ed): Red Book: 2003. Report of the Committee on Infectious Diseases, 26th ed. Elk Grove Village, IL: American Academy of Pediatrics, 2003, pp 534–536. **A review of rotavirus disease.**
3. Atherly-John YC, Cunningham SJ, Crain EF: A randomized trial of oral vs intravenous rehydration in a pediatric emergency department. Arch Pediatr Adolesc Med 156:1240–1243, 2001. **Randomized trial suggesting that ORT in the emergency department is superior to intravenous therapy for the treatment of dehydration.**
4. Cremonini F, Di Caro S, Nista EC, et al: Meta-analysis: the effect of probiotic administration on antibiotic-associated diarrhoea. Aliment Pharmacol Ther 16:1461–1467, 2002. **A meta-analysis of probiotic use in acute childhood diarrhea demonstrating modest improvement in diarrhea symptoms.**
5. DeWitt TG, Humphrey KF, McCarthy P: Clinical predictors of acute bacterial diarrhea in young children. Pediatrics 76:551–556, 1985. **Outlines sensitivity and specificity of commonly used tests in the diagnosis of diarrhea.**
6. D'Souza AL, Rajkumar C, Cooke J, et al: Probiotics in prevention of antibiotic associated diarrhoea: meta-analysis. BMJ 324: 1361–1366, 2002. **A meta-analysis of probiotic use in acute childhood diarrhea demonstrating modest improvement in diarrhea symptoms.**
7. Huang JS, Bousvaros A, Lee JW, et al: Efficacy of probiotic use in acute diarrhea in children: a meta-analysis. Dig Dis Sci 47:2625–2634, 2002. **A meta-analysis of probiotic use in acute childhood diarrhea demonstrating modest improvement in diarrhea symptoms.**
8. Moineau G, Newman J: Rapid intravenous rehydration in the pediatric emergency department. Pediatr Emerg Care 6:186–188, 1990. **Case series suggesting that IV therapy in the emergency department obviates hospitalization.**

9. Nager AL, Brink JA, Wang VJ: Comparison of nasogastric and intravenous methods of rehydration in pediatric patients with acute dehydration. Pediatrics 45:566–572, 2002. **This study suggests that nasogastric rehydration is safe and efficacious as compared to IV rehydration. Also, suggests that laboratory testing in most cases of dehydration is of limited value.**

10. Reid SR, Bonadio WA: Outpatient rapid intravenous rehydration to correct dehydration and resolve vomiting in children with acute gastroenteritis. Ann Emerg Med 28:319–323, 1996. **Case series suggesting that IV therapy should be considered in the emergency department more often as a treatment for dehydration.**

Fever in Infants and Children from Birth to 3 Years

Leonard G. Feld

KEY CONCEPTS

- Perform a complete history and physical examination with particular attention to evaluation and management criteria, including:
  - Has the infant been previously healthy?
  - Term gestation.
  - No perinatal infections or unexplained hyperbilirubinemia.
  - No history of previous hospitalizations or surgeries.
  - Laboratory values:
    - Peripheral blood white blood cells 5000 to 15,000/mm^3.
    - Absolute band form count <1500/mm^3.
    - Fewer than 10 white blood cells per high power field on spun urine specimen.
    - Fewer than 5 white blood cells on a stool smear (if infant has diarrhea).
  - Lumbar puncture based on clinical evaluation.
- If the febrile infant younger than 90 days of age is ill or appears toxic, admit to hospital, perform sepsis evaluation, and treat.
- If the febrile child 3 to 36 months of age is ill or appears toxic, admit to hospital, perform sepsis workup, and treat.
- If the febrile child 3 to 36 months of age is well or does not appear toxic, workup and management is based on the duration of temperature elevation and history of pneumococcal conjugate vaccines.

Fever is an elevation of the body temperature above the normal range secondary to a modification of the thermoregulatory center (hypothalamus) set point of the body. Despite the variety of methods (rectal, oral, axillary, tympanic) used to measure temperature, fever is defined as a rectal temperature above 100.4°F (38°C). Even though the cause is identified in many children (pneumonia and urinary tract infections) or is presumed to be of viral origin, the concern remains about occult bacterial infections and the associated risk of serious invasive disease. The approach to the infant and child with a fever without a source has evolved based on evidence-based

medicine. New clinical research trials, effectiveness of the *Haemophilus influenzae* type b conjugate (Hib) and the heptavalent pneumococcal conjugate vaccines (PCV) in reducing invasive bacterial infections (meningitis, pneumonia, sepsis, bacteremia), and the different practice patterns between office-based primary care practitioners and the emergency medicine physicians have influenced the shift in the practice parameters. Despite the expected (70%) reduction of pneumococcal infections such as pneumonia, meningitis, and bacteremia with the introduction of PCV in 2000, prospective surveillance is required to monitor for antibiotic resistance and new virulent serotypes. Review of the clinical fever practice guidelines will be based on the evolution of additional medical evidence.

Expert Opinion on Management Issues

MANAGEMENT OF INFANTS YOUNGER THAN 3 MONTHS OF AGE

Because of the increased proportion of serious or invasive bacterial infections in infants younger than 3 months with fever, practice management guidelines are less controversial. The debate is whether the well-appearing child with low-risk criteria and/or a low observation score should receive empirical antibiotics. Based on the majority of studies, expectant management is reasonable with a scheduled clinical reassessment in 24 hours (Fig. 1). The rate of bacteremia is about 2% to 3% in all febrile infants younger than 2 to 3 months of age. In infants younger than 28 days of age, studies indicate that the low-risk criteria may fail to identify up to 10% of infants with bacteremia. This factor coupled with the clinician's inability to confidently discriminate the ill from the well infant leads to a very conservative and encompassing treatment plan (Box 1).

MANAGEMENT OF INFANTS AND CHILDREN AGED 3 TO 36 MONTHS OF AGE

In 1993, a consensus panel published practice guidelines for the management of fever in children 0 to 36 months of age. Over the past decade, many commentaries and articles addressed the bias of the panel, amalgamation of randomized, controlled and observational studies, and lack of true consensus by the general pediatric community with these guidelines. The practice guidelines were modified in December 2000 to consider a less-aggressive approach for a child who received the PCV. The impact of the PCV could be substantial. With the expected risk of bacteremia because of *Streptococcus pneumoniae* estimated to be approximately 3% in febrile children without a focus of infections but with a white blood cell (WBC) count greater than 15,000 cells/mm^3 and a temperature above 102.2°F (39°C), PCV should reduce the risk of serious infections in this group by approximately 70%. PCV could also reduce the expected risk to 0.3%

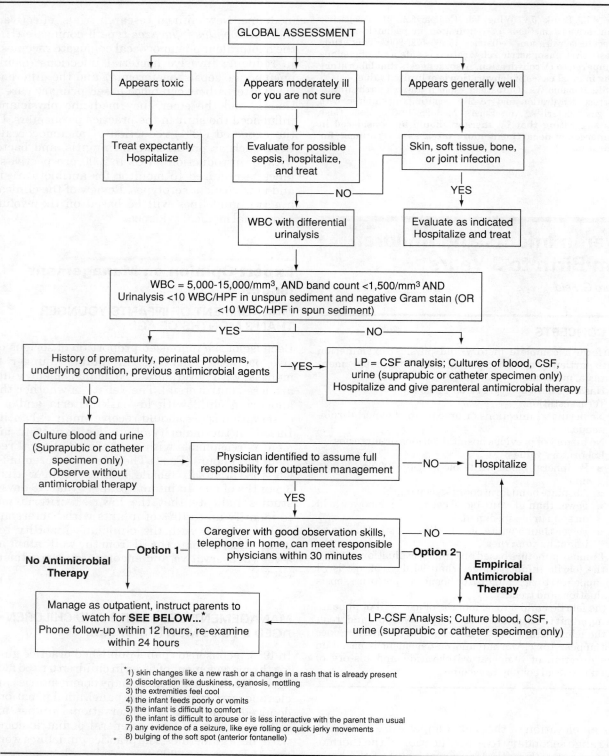

FIGURE 1. Evaluation and management of the febrile infant younger than 60 days of age. CSF, cerebrospinal fluid; HPF, high-power field; WBC, white blood cell. From Meltzer AJ, Powell KR, Avner JR: Fever in infants and children. In Feld LG, Hyams JS (eds): Consensus in Pediatrics. Evanston, IL, Mead Johnson & Company, 2005, p13.

with less than 0.02% of untreated children developing *S. pneumoniae* meningitis. Vaccination of healthy infants would prevent 53,000 cases of pneumonia, 1 million cases of otitis media, 12,000 cases of meningitis and bacter- emia, and 116 deaths because of *S. pneumoniae* infection. If PCV achieves the success of the Hib vaccination, the decision process for the older infants and toddlers with fever should be a nonentity.

BOX 1 Rochester Criteria*

- Infant appears generally well—negative impression of sepsis.
- Infant has been previously healthy:
    - Born at term (37 weeks' gestation)
    - Did not receive perinatal antimicrobial therapy
    - Was not treated for unexplained hyperbilirubinemia
    - Had not received and was not receiving antimicrobial agents
    - Had not been previously hospitalized
    - Had no chronic or underlying illness
    - Was not hospitalized longer than mother
- No evidence of skin, soft tissue, bone, joint, or ear infection
- Laboratory values:
    - Peripheral blood WBC count 5000 to 15,000/mm^3
    - Absolute band form count less than 1500/mm^3
    - <10 WBC per hpf on spun urine specimen
    - <5 WBC on a stool smear (if infant has diarrhea)

*All must be present to classify an infant as *low-risk*. *High-risk* infants have one or more of the above historical information, clinical impression, or a laboratory value that is out of range or remarkable.

ESR, erythrocyte sedimentation rate; hpf, high power field; WBC, white blood cell.

From Jaskiewicz JA, McCarthy CA, Richardson AC, et al: Febrile infants at low risk for serious bacterial infection—an appraisal of the Rochester criteria and implications for management. Febrile Infant Collaborative Study Group. Pediatrics 94:390–396, 1994. Reproduced with permission from Pediatrics 94:391, Table 1, 1994. Copyright 1994.

OUTPATIENT MANAGEMENT OF ALL WELL-APPEARING CHILDREN WITH URINE CULTURES

The practice patterns of non–emergency room physicians suggest that adherence to sound practice principles achieves compliance with instructions for home monitoring and that follow-up minimizes adverse outcomes. However, the concern is blood or urine contamination. Urine culture contamination occurs frequently with the bag collection method, and blood culture contamination is reported as high as 40%. If these children did not receive antibiotics, the following are reasonable directives:

- If the urine culture shows multiple organisms or a single growth of a likely contaminant, repeat the culture.
- Consider using the urine nitrite and leukocyte esterase (LE) to screen children for urine culture and antibiotics. The recommendations strengthen the argument that the combined use of age, urinalysis, selective urine cultures, and antibiotic therapy will decrease admissions and complications (renal scarring, etc.) in young children. If the urinalysis shows no pyuria, bacteria, nitrites, or LE, then it is reasonable to hold off until a urine culture result is available. If the bag specimen is used, only a negative result is reliable in an infant or young child.

OUTPATIENT MANAGEMENT OF ALL WELL-APPEARING CHILDREN WITH POSITIVE BLOOD CULTURE

Despite the added expense, inconvenience, and spontaneous resolution of occult bacteremia, repeat blood cultures are suggested. The decision to start antibiotics

TABLE 1 Suggested Antipyretic Therapy

Medication	Dose
Acetaminophen	10–20 mg/kg/dose PR every 4–6 hours (as needed)
	10–15 mg/kg/dose PO every 4–6 hours (as needed)
Ibuprofen (6 months to 12 years)	Temperature <102.5°F: 5 mg/kg/dose every 6–8 hours
	Temperature >102.5°F: 10 mg/kg/dose every 6–8 hours
	Maximum daily dose: 40 mg/kg/day

in a well-appearing, afebrile child with a positive blood culture is an individual decision.

URGENT INTERVENTIONS

It is inherently obvious that any ill-appearing or toxic child younger than 36 months with a fever without a source requires immediate intervention. The child should be admitted with age-appropriate evaluation and empirical antibiotics (see Fig. 1 and Table 2).

RECOMMENDATION OF CEFTRIAXONE FOR OUTPATIENT THERAPY

Ceftriaxone is prescribed for lower respiratory tract infections, meningitis, sepsis, and UTIs. In the case of a child vaccinated with PCV, there is no support for antibiotic therapy. The controversy is whether any antibiotic should be prescribed pending culture results in an unvaccinated child and if so, is ceftriaxone (except for convenience—parenteral and once-a-day dosing) superior to high-dose regimens of amoxicillin or other antibiotics. In three studies evaluating the use of antibiotics for occult bacteremia, there was no beneficial effect of ceftriaxone over amoxicillin on the rate of persistent bacteremia or serious invasive disease.

Common Pitfalls and Errors

- Failure to adequately classify the child as toxic versus nontoxic.
- Variability of the method to measure temperature (use rectal thermometer).
- Vaccination schedule that is not up-to-date. With the increased cost of vaccines and reduced insurance reimbursement, these factors have the potential to reduce PCV immunizations.
- Parental pressure to limit ancillary testing, admissions, and antibiotic use.
- Empirical use of antibiotics without obtaining blood or urine cultures.
- Failure to collect urine properly.
    - Antibiotic treatment based on urinalysis without obtaining the gold standard—urine culture.
- Obtaining a chest radiograph without clinical evidence of pulmonary process.

TABLE 2 Suggested Intravenous Therapy for High-risk Infants or Low-risk Infants with Positive Cultures*

Medication	Dose
Ampicillin	100–200 mg/kg/24 hr divided every 6 hours
Cefotaxime	100–200 mg/kg/24 hr divided every 6–8 hours

*Therapy is based on clinical information. Modify medication choice and dosage based on source of infection, community standards and antimicrobial resistant patterns, and culture/sensitivity results. Consider the addition of acyclovir for infants younger than 30 days of age. If CSF abnormalities suggest meningitis, higher dosages of ampicillin and cefotaxime should be considered.

Communication and Counseling

Regardless of the clinical setting (private practice office, hospital or community clinic, or emergency room), it is imperative to provide clear instructions to the family that delineate your expectations for notification if there are changes in the child's condition that signal a toxic state.

A prepared fact sheet with specific instructions will avoid confusion and provide a "pseudo-contract" between the family and the physician. Some suggested key elements include:

- Instructions on how to take a temperature with a rectal thermometer.
- How to administer antipyretic medication, frequency, dosage.
- Issues regarding substitutions of antipyretics (acetaminophen and ibuprofen).
- Contraindications on the use of ice water and alcohol sponging.
- When to call for problems and concerns.
- Plans for phone or office follow-up in 24 hours.

ANTICIPATORY GUIDANCE

As part of anticipatory guidance it is important to educate the patient on the general principles of fever rather than in the setting of an acute illness. Some important tips and education points about fever phobia for families and physicians are as follows:

- Fever is a normal physiologic response and may be viewed as an appropriate body defense response.
- Fever is not a disease, only one symptom suggestive of a disease process.
- Fever can continue for days after appropriate antibiotic therapy.
- Fever does not always require treatment (especially low-grade elevations in older infants and children).
- Physicians may reduce *fever phobia* by avoiding certain phrases or unintentional instructions:
  - "Call me for any fever."
  - "Go ahead and give antipyretics. What do you have around the house?"

SUGGESTED READINGS

1. Alpern ER, Alessandrini EA, Bell LM, et al: Occult bacteremia from a pediatric emergency department: Current prevalence, time to detection, and outcome. Pediatrics 106:505–511, 2000. **The prevalence of occult bacteremia in the post–*Haemophilus influenzae* type b (Hib) era is lower than previously reported.**

2. Avner JR, Baker MD: Management of fever in infants and children. Emerg Med Clin North Amer 20:46–67, 2002. **A broad perspective on the evaluation and management of fever in young children, with an emphasis on the use of clinical judgment.**

3. Baker MD, Bell LM, Avner JR: The efficacy of routine outpatient management without antibiotics of fever in selected infants. Pediatrics 103:627–631, 1999. **The Philadelphia protocol for outpatient management without antibiotics for low-risk febrile infants 29 to 60 days of age.**

4. Baraff LJ: Management of fever without source infants and children. Ann Emerg Med 36:602–614, 2000. **Despite these new guidelines, the conjugate *Streptococcus pneumoniae* vaccine may limit the need for extensive screening.**

5. Baraff LJ, Bass JW, Fleisher GR, et al: Practice guideline for the management of infants and children 0 to 36 months of age with fever without a source. Pediatrics 82:1–12, 1993. **These are proposed guidelines by the authors and do not constitute Practice Guidelines by the American Academy of Pediatrics.**

6. Baraff LJ, Oslund SA, Schriger DL: Probability of bacterial infections in febrile infants less than three months of age: A meta-analysis. Pediatr Infect Dis J 11:257–265, 1992. **Infants younger than 8 weeks of age who are not low-risk should be admitted and treated with parenteral antibiotics.**

7. Crain EF, Gershel JC: Which febrile infants younger than two weeks of age are likely to have sepsis? A pilot study. Pediatr Infect Dis 7:561–564, 1998. **Although based on a small cohort, the data suggest that sepsis and meningitis may not be different in neonates younger than 15 days of age compared to infants younger than 8 weeks of age.**

8. Dagan R, Owell KR, Hall CB, et al: Identification of infants unlikely to have serious bacterial infection although hospitalized for suspected sepsis. J Pediatr 107:855–860, 1985. **Previously healthy infants younger than 3 months with an acute illness are unlikely to have serious bacterial infection if they have no findings consistent with ear, soft tissue, or skeletal infections and have normal WBC and band counts and normal urine findings.**

9. Kramer MS, Shapiro ED: Management of the young febrile child: A commentary on recent practice guidelines. Pediatrics 100: 128–134, 1997. **Young febrile children should be carefully assessed for bacterial foci of infection. If the physician is concerned about the adequacy of parental follow-up, repeated observation over time in the office or emergency department is often helpful, and hospital admission may occasionally be necessary.**

10. Lee GM, Fleisher GR, Harper MB: Management of febrile children in the age of conjugate pneumococcal vaccine: A cost-effectiveness analysis. Pediatrics 108:835–844, 2001. **A complete blood count (CBC) and a selective blood culture and treatment with a WBC cutoff of 15,000/mm³ is cost-effective based on the current rate of pneumococcal bacteremia.**

11. Lieu TA, Ray GT, Black SB, et al: Projected cost-effectiveness of pneumococcal conjugate vaccination of healthy infants and young children. JAMA 283:1460–1468, 2000. **Pneumococcal conjugate vaccine should be assessed based on the value of preventing mortality and morbidity from the disease.**

12. Lin PL, Michals MG, Janosky J, et al: Incidence of invasive pneumococcal disease in children 3 to 36 months of age at a tertiary care pediatric center 2 years after licensure of the pneumococcal conjugate vaccine. Pediatrics 111:896–899, 2003. **The incidence of invasive pneumococcal disease in children 3 to 36 months decreased from 220 to 40 per 100,000 at this center.**

13. Slater M, Krug SE: Evaluation of the infant without source: An evidence based review. Emergency Medicine Clinics of North America 17:1:98–1261, 1999. **A combination of detailed history, physical examination, and selected laboratory tests allows the clinician to discern which infants are at lower risk for bacterial illness.**

14. Whitney CG, Farley MM, Hadler J, et al: Decline in invasive pneumococcal disease after the introduction of protein-polysaccharide conjugate vaccine. NEJM 348:1737–1746, 2003. **In children younger than 2 years of age, invasive pneumococcal disease decreased by 69% in the United States with the conjugate vaccine.**

15. Wittler RR, Cain KK, Bass JW: A survey about management of febrile children without source by primary care physicians. Pediatr Infect Dis J 17:271–277, 1998. **Pediatrician's use of outpatient antibiotics increased threefold for a 7-week old infant from 1991/1992 to 1997.**

Pediatric Pain Management

William Seth Schechter

KEY CONCEPTS

- Proper pain assessment is age specific and remains the key to appropriate pain treatment.
- For acute, severe pain, titrate intravenous opioids to clinical effect beginning with a low dose rather than using a large fixed dose. Most intravenous opioids can be redosed under your observation every 10 minutes until the patient is comfortable.
- Do not assume that pain is because of inadequate amounts of analgesic. This is especially true if there is a change in the quality, intensity, location, or duration of pain. Always perform a careful interval examination to rule out treatable causes of pain.
- Pain treatment is frequently multimodal.
- Pain treatment must always include an appreciation of the psychosocial domain.

The International Association for the Study of Pain (IASP) has defined pain as "an unpleasant sensory experience associated with actual or potential tissue damage." Pain is a subjective experience that should always be believed. Frequently, pediatric patients cannot verbally describe sensations of pain, as is obviously the case for neonates and some intellectually impaired children. For these patients and for others, the presence of pain can frequently be inferred from the clinical context. Proper pain assessment is the cornerstone of appropriate treatment. Table 1 describes assessment tools that are appropriate for age and condition of the patient.

Pain treatment should be painless. This is a basic tenet of pediatric pain management, which is sacrosanct except for the most extraordinary circumstances. Intramuscular injections to treat pain should therefore be avoided. It has been said that children would rather "suffer in silence" than receive a painful "shot." Within the hospital environment, safe venues where children know they will have respite from painful procedures should be available.

Proper pain management implies a continuum of care. It begins at the onset of a painful illness or before a procedure or operation and includes teaching to provide a realistic explanation to both the parent and child of what can be expected. Sedation or anesthesia should be available for all painful or frightening procedures if it is needed. Postprocedural pain control then naturally follows. Supportive, aggressive treatment of chronic pain should be available. End-of-life care represents the final stage of this continuum.

Expert Opinion on Management Issues

NONPHARMACOLOGIC APPROACHES TO MANAGING PAIN

Pain management does not necessarily require pharmacologic therapy. Before surgery, explanation and the use of tours and videos can go a long way toward relieving

TABLE 1 Clinically Useful Pain Assessment Tools

Behavioral Indicators

Facial grimacing: The Neonatal Facial Coding System* uses several facial actions that may be indicators of pain. Pain is characterized by a bulging brow with tight creases in between, tightly closed eyelids, a deeply furrowed nasolabial groove, a horizontal, wide opened mouth, and a taut tongue that may be quivering along with the chin.

Crying: May be an indicator of pain.

Activity: Withdrawal or immobilization of a limb may be an indicator of pain.

Response to comfort measures: Feeding, swaddling, holding, and ensuring that the infant is neither wet nor cold may help to discriminate between pain and other conditions.

Physiologic indicators: Alterations in heart rate, blood pressure, SpO_2, respiratory rate, or alterations in pattern of respiration may be nonspecific indicators of pain.

Multidimensional Instrument

FLACC[†] Scoring System: May be used in preverbal, mechanically ventilated, or cognitively impaired patients; it is an acronym that includes five indicators, each scored as a 0, 1, or 2 that forms a ten-point composite scale with a range from "0" (no pain) to "10" (worst pain).

FLACC: Score each category between 0 and 2. The total score may be any number from 0 to 10.

Score:	0	1	2
Face	No expression	Occasional action	Frequent action
Legs	Normal	Restless or tense	Kicking, legs withdrawn
Activity	Quiet	Shifting or tense	Rigid, arched, jerking
Cry	None	Moan, whimper	Steady crying, screaming, sobbing, or frequent complaints
Consolability	Content	Consolable	Inconsolable

Self-Report of Pain

Categorical description: Toddlers or young children are asked to say if they are having "a little bit," a "middle amount," or "a lot" of pain.

Faces Scales[‡]: Children who do not have an appreciation of ordinal numbering are asked to rate their pain based upon cartoons depicting facial indicators of distress.

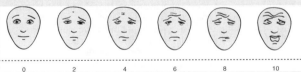

0	2	4	6	8	10

NRS[§]: Older children and teenagers are asked to rate their pain on a scale of "0" (no pain) to "10" (worst pain).

VAS[§]: Children or teenagers are asked to move an indicator along a mechanical slide to depict the level of pain; the clinician reads a number along a 10-cm indicator on the back to determine the numeric score.

---

*Grunau RV, Craig KD: Pain expression in neonates: Facial action and cry. Pain 28:395–410, 1987.

†Voepel-Lewis T, Merkel S, Tait AR, et al: The reliability and validity of the Face, Legs, Activity, Cry, Consolability observational tool as a measure of pain in children with cognitive impairment. Anesth Analg 95(5):1224–1229, 2002.

‡The Faces Pain Scale—Revised (FPS-R). Copyright © 2001 International Association for the Study of Pain (IASP). Bieri D, Reeve RA, Champion GD, et al: The FACES Pain Scale for the self-assessment of the severity of pain experienced by children: Development, initial validation, and preliminary investigation for ratio scale properties. Pain 41:139–150, 1990, www.painsourcebook.ca; Whaley L, Wong DL: Nursing Care of Infants and Children, (3rd ed). St. Louis: CV Mosby, 1987.

§Price DD, Bush FM, Long S, et al: A comparison of pain measurement characteristics of mechanical visual analogue and simple numerical rating scales. Pain 56:217–226, 1994.

NRS, numerical rating scale; VAS, visual analog scale.

the anxiety that heightens pain perception. The use of distraction, guided imagery, focused breathing, biofeedback, meditation, and hypnosis can help decrease the pain associated with procedures. The presence of a parent or other supportive caregiver during a procedure may at times be very helpful. Both transcutaneous electrical nerve stimulation (TENS) and percutaneous electrical nerve stimulation (PENS) have been used as adjuncts in the treatment of chronic pain, as have traditional methods of acupuncture.

PHARMACOLOGIC APPROACHES TO MANAGING PAIN

Box 1 outlines the general pharmacologic issues in pediatric pain management. Box 2 outlines some common pitfalls in management.

Medications Used in the Treatment of Nociceptive Inflammatory Pain

Salicylates

Aspirin is no longer recommended for use in the treatment of pain because of its association with Reye disease. However, aspirin therapy is used in the treatment of certain inflammatory diseases such as Kawasaki disease and various arthritides. Aspirin irreversibly binds to platelets, functionally inactivating them for their lifetime, and may contribute to the development of a hemorrhagic diathesis. A minimum of 10 to 14 days is recommended between discontinuance of aspirin therapy and major invasive procedures or surgery. The dosage of aspirin is 10 to 15 mg/kg given orally every 4 hours up to a maximum dose of 90 mg/kg/day in children or 4 g/day in adults. Some evidence suggests that choline-magnesium trisalicylate is less likely to contribute to a hemorrhagic diathesis than acetylsalicylic acid.

Nonsteroidal Anti-inflammatory Drugs

Nonsteroidal anti-inflammatory drugs (NSAIDs) include commonly prescribed drugs such as ibuprofen, indomethacin, naproxen, and ketorolac, which inhibit both cyclooxygenase 1 (COX–1) and 2 (COX–2) nonspecifically (Table 2). NSAIDs have both anti-inflammatory and analgesic properties. NSAIDs functionally inactivate platelets for 48 to 72 hours after administration.

BOX 1 Pharmacology of Analgesics in Children

Neonates

- Have a decreased clearance of many drugs because of immature hepatic and renal systems; therefore, less frequent dosing intervals may be required.
- Have a greater volume of distribution for hydrophilic drugs; therefore, a higher initial drug dose may be required.
- Have a lower plasma concentration of proteins that bind drugs (α1 acid glycoprotein, albumin); hence they may have an increased free fraction of drug and potential for greater drug effect or toxicity.
- Have immature enzyme systems. Postgestational maturation of P-glycoprotein transport systems may limit drug entry into the brain, hence its central effect. Some enzyme systems mature with postgestational age (e.g., CYP2D6), limiting conversion of a prodrug to its active form early in life.
- Have immature receptor and second messenger systems.

Older Children (In Contrast)

- Have an increased liver-mass-to-body-weight ratio compared to adults and mature enzyme systems; therefore, they may have higher rates of clearance of many drugs than adults. More frequent drug dosing may be required.

Summary

- There is tremendous variability with respect to opioid pharmacology in pediatric patients, especially in the very young.

From Berde CB, Sethna NF: Drug treatment: Analgesics in the treatment of pain in children. N Engl J Med 347:1094–1103, 2002.

BOX 2 General Pain Management Caveats

- Children who have been on opioids or benzodiazepines at high doses or for prolonged periods (approximately >5 days) are at risk for withdrawal with abrupt discontinuation of medication. Dose should be tapered slowly: no more than 25% of the initial dose on the first day and no greater than 10% to 15% on each subsequent day.
  - Never use a fentanyl patch in an opioid-naive patient or in the setting of acute pain. It creates a depot of drug that is long lasting and difficult to titrate, and its effect may last for 24 hours after removing the patch. It is for the treatment of chronic pain in the opioid-tolerant patient when enteral administration of opioid is not feasible.
  - Opioids given together with benzodiazepines may cause severe hypotension, especially in the hypovolemic patient. Be aware that the risk of respiratory depression and upper airway obstruction increases unpredictably when opioids are combined with anxiolytics, antihistamines, or other sedating drugs.
  - Most opioid complications are caused by dosing errors. Be especially cautious when drugs are ordered in microgram doses, when converting between drugs, and when changing the route of administration. When making dose calculations, be careful about decimal point errors.
- Toxicity of local anesthetic is related to total dose and site of injection (injection into a vascular area results in rapid uptake and higher plasma levels). Toxicities include:
  - Seizures: Support airway and circulation. Treat seizure with a benzodiazepine, phenytoin or appropriate barbiturate. Because acidosis will increase toxicity, treat metabolic and respiratory acidosis promptly.
  - Dysrhythmias: Support airway and circulation. Dysrhythmias may be especially malignant with bupivacaine, may be refractory to treatment, and require prolonged cardiopulmonary support such as CPR, ECMO, or CPB until the drug is cleared. Lidocaine or mexiletine *should not* be used to treat local anesthetic–induced dysrhythmias.
  - Methemoglobinemia or hemolysis: The former is seen with prilocaine, the latter is seen with prilocaine in patients with G6PD deficiency. Methemoglobinemia may also be seen when excessive quantities of benzocaine are used.
- DO NOT USE THE FOLLOWING DRUGS TOGETHER:
  - Methylphenidate and clonidine (dysrhythmia potential)
  - Tramadol and SSRIs or TCADs (serotonergic syndrome)
  - Meperidine and MAOIs (hyperpyrexia, seizures, adrenergic syndrome)

CPB, cardiopulmonary bypass; CPR, cardiopulmonary resuscitation; ECMO, extracorporeal membrane oxygenation; MAOI, monoamine oxidase inhibitor; SSRI, selective serotonin reuptake inhibitor; TCAD, tricyclic antidepressant.

TABLE 2 Commonly Used NSAID Analgesic Dosing Guidelines

Drug	Dosage and Route of Administration
Acetylsalicylic acid (aspirin)	10–15 mg/kg PO/PR q4h. Maximum recommended daily dose in children: 90 mg/kg/day. Adult maximum: 4 g/day.
Choline magnesium trisalicylate	10–15 mg/kg PO q6h (dose based on total salicylate content). Hypermagnesemia may develop in patients with renal failure.
Acetaminophen	10–15 mg/kg PO q4h. See text for maximum doses.
Ibuprofen	10 mg/kg PO q6h. Adult maximum 3.2 g/day.
Indomethacin	0.5–1 mg/kg PO q8h. Maximum dose 4 mg/kg/day in the child or 200 mg/day in the adult. Available as a 50-mg rectal suppository for adult dosing.
Naproxen	5–7 mg/kg PO q12h.
Ketorolac	Adult maximum 120 mg/day. 0.25–0.5 mg/kg IV q6h. Limit therapy to 5 days.
Diclofenac	1–2 mg/kg PO q6–8h. The maximum adult dosage is from 100–200 mg/day.

IV, intravenously; NSAID, nonsteroidal anti-inflammatory drug; PO, orally; PR, rectally; q, every.

Cyclooxygenase enzymes catalyze the conversion of arachidonic acid to the prostaglandins, which play a role in inflammation and pain generation. COX–1 is a constitutive enzyme that engages in many "housekeeping activities" to maintain cell function and integrity. Inhibition of COX–1 may therefore result in organ-specific toxic effects such as gastritis, renal insufficiency, hepatic dysfunction, and increased airway reactivity. COX–2 is an inducible enzyme system that may be activated by mediators of inflammation.

All the NSAIDs exhibit a ceiling effect; above a certain dose, no further increase in analgesia is observed, but adverse effects, such as gastropathy, hepatic dysfunction, or renal insufficiency may increase in incidence or severity. Toxic effects may also increase when these drugs are administered concomitantly with other nephrotoxic drugs or under conditions of decreased splanchnic perfusion.

NSAIDs are very effective analgesic agents when administered either alone or in combination with opioids. As a class, NSAIDs may be particularly helpful in treating bladder and ureteral spasm. NSAIDs are also particularly helpful for the treatment of bone pain, although there is some question about whether treatment with NSAIDs may inhibit bone fusion.

Acetaminophen

Acetaminophen has been a safe and effective analgesic and antipyretic when administered in proper dosage and has been used for many years. Although its mechanism of action is incompletely understood, it acts, in part, to mildly inhibit cyclooxygenase activity both centrally and peripherally. The currently recommended oral or rectal dose is 10 to 15 mg/kg every 4 hours. For postoperative pain relief, a higher single rectal dose (30 to 40 mg/kg administered once intraoperatively with the first subsequent oral dose of 10 to 15 mg/kg being given no sooner than 6 hours later) has been recommended. Rectal absorption is erratic and may be delayed. Rectal suppositories should not be divided because acetaminophen may not be evenly distributed within the matrix of a suppository.

Acetaminophen is a potentially hepatotoxic drug and is present in a wide variety of over-the-counter (OTC) preparations. Toxicity may inadvertently occur when several drugs administered together have not been recognized by the practitioner or parent to individually contain acetaminophen. Toxicity may be further enhanced by concomitant administration of drugs, which are inducers of acetaminophen metabolism (N-hydroxylation) via cytochrome P450 2E1 (CYP2E1). Care should be taken to not exceed the maximum recommended daily dose. For adults, the maximum oral daily dose is 4 g/day. For pediatric patients, Berde recommends the following maximum dosages: 90 mg/kg/day for children, 60 mg/kg/day for infants and for neonates; provisional recommendations are not to exceed 30 to 40 mg/kg/day. This dosage recommendation can be followed, in part, by limiting the number of doses to no more than five per 24-hour period.

Opiates and Opioids

This class of drugs remains the mainstay of postoperative pain management. The considerable synergy among NSAIDS, acetaminophen, and opioids may enable a decrease in total opioid dose. This is termed the *opioid-sparing effect* and may be of considerable benefit in decreasing opioid-related side effects. Opioids exhibit no ceiling effect; the dose may be increased to achieve adequate pain control, as long as the respiratory drive is not compromised and other adverse effects such as sedation, pruritus, nausea, and vomiting are well controlled. In general, sedation is an antecedent to respiratory depression and should never be ignored. Increases in opioid requirement may occur because of the development of tolerance or progression of the primary disease. A change in the quality, intensity, duration, or location of pain requires a physical examination and a thorough medical or surgical evaluation, not simply a reflexive increase in opioid dose. For example, an apparent increase in pain expression may be the result of an evolving compartment syndrome, an acute abdominal or cardiorespiratory process, a full bladder, or simply an infiltrated intravenous catheter.

Morphine remains the gold standard to which all other drugs are compared. Other opioids that are commonly prescribed by pediatricians include hydromorphone, meperidine, fentanyl, methadone, codeine, oxycodone, and hydrocodone.

Morphine's onset of action is rapid following intravenous administration. Morphine is approximately 30% protein-bound in the adult and 20% protein-bound in neonates; therefore, the free fraction is increased in the young. This increased free fraction coupled with an immature neonatal blood–brain barrier implies that the tissue concentration of morphine within a neonate's brain may be higher after a single dose. Some data also suggest that the ratios of various opioid receptor subtypes to one another may be different in the infant brain from those ratios in the adult brain. This coupled with an immature respiratory control mechanism may therefore place infants, especially premature infants, at a greater risk of respiratory depression.

Morphine is *N*-demethylated and conjugated by the mature liver to the primary metabolites morphine-6-glucuronide (M6G) and morphine-3-glucoronide (M3G). M6G is an active metabolite and may accumulate in young infants (who have a decreased glomerular filtration rate up to 3 months of postgestational age) and in patients who have renal insufficiency and thus lead to increased sedation or respiratory depression. M3G accumulation may lead to central excitation characterized by agitation or heightened perception of pain. Clearance of morphine is highly dependent on hepatic blood flow and may consequently be prolonged following some abdominal operations. Clearance takes longer in the premature infant and full-term neonate than in adults because of the incomplete maturation of the hepatic enzyme systems. Data suggest that following a single dose in the young infant, a higher plasma concentration of drug will be observed and it will decline more slowly than in older patients.

Morphine clearance is highly variable in the young, especially during the first week of life. Its elimination increases with postnatal age. After several months, morphine clearance may exceed adult values partly because of a relative increase in hepatic blood flow and efficient use of both glucuronidation and sulfonation pathways.

Morphine and all the other opioids may cause nausea, vomiting, constipation, and urinary retention. Additionally, morphine causes release of histamine, which may result in pruritus or an urticarial rash. Pruritus, as a symptom, frequently occurs in biliary disease, renal failure, and graft-versus-host disease and may be treated similarly with variable efficacy.

Pruritus and nausea can be as distressing as pain, if not more so. Pruritus can be treated by administration of an antihistamine, such as diphenhydramine, either orally or intravenously (Table 3); caution is advised, however, because increased sedation and occasionally airway obstruction may occur. Other approaches to the treatment of pruritus or nausea include the following:

- Changing to a different opioid may be helpful because these effects may be idiosyncratic.
- A 5-hydroxyhistamine$_3$ antagonist such as ondansetron may be administered. Ondansetron has been approved as an antiemetic and is without the adverse extrapyramidal side effects seen with some other antiemetics. It may also help relieve itching (an effect of the drug shown to be helpful for pruritus secondary to hyperbilirubinemia).
- The partial agonist–antagonist nalbuphine may also be effective in treating pruritus associated with intra-axial administration of opioids, especially the opioid fentanyl. Rapid administration of high doses may precipitate acute withdrawal.

TABLE 3 Management of Opioid-Induced Adverse Effects

Respiratory Depression

Naloxone: 0.01–0.02 mg/kg up to a full reversal dose of 0.1 mg/kg. May be given IV, IM, SC, or ET. The full reversal dose should initially be used for apnea in opioid-naive patients. In opioid-tolerant patients, a reduced dose should be given and titrated up slowly to treat symptoms but prevent acute withdrawal. Ventilation may need to be supported during this process. May repeat dose every 2 minutes to a total of 10 mg. Adult maximum dose is 2 mg/dose. Give with caution to patients who are receiving chronic opioids as it may precipitate acute withdrawal. Duration of effect is 1–4 hours; therefore, close observation for renarcotization is essential.

Excessive Sedation without Evidence of Respiratory Depression

Methylphenidate*: 0.3 mg/kg per dose PO (typically 10 to 20 mg/dose to a teenager) before breakfast and lunch. Do not administer to patients on clonidine because dysrhythmias may develop.
Dextroamphetamine: 2.5 to 10 mg on awakening and at noon. Not for use in young children or in patients with cardiovascular disease or hypertension.
Modafinil: Pediatric dose not established. May be useful in selected patients. Typical adult dose: 50 to 200 mg/day.
Change opioid or decrease the dose.

Nausea and Vomiting

Metoclopramide†: 0.15 mg/kg IV up to 10 mg/dose q6–12h for 24 h.
Trimethobenzamide: PO or PR if less than 15 kg, 100 mg q6h; if greater than 15 kg, 200 mg q6h. (NB: Suppository contains benzocaine 2%.) Not for use in newborn infants or premature infants.
5-HT$_3$ blockers:
  Ondansetron: 0.15 mg/kg up to 8 mg IV q6–8h not to exceed 32 mg/day (also available as a sublingual tablet).
  Granisetron: 10 to 20 μg/kg IV q12–24h.
  Prochlorperazine* (Compazine): >2 yr or 20 kg, 0.1 mg/kg per dose q8h IM or PO up to 10 mg/dose.
Change opioid.

Pruritus

Diphenhydramine: 0.5 mg/kg IV or PO q6h.
Hydroxyzine: 0.5 mg/kg PO q6h.
Nalbuphine: 0.1 mg/kg IV q6h for pruritus caused by intraaxial opioids, especially fentanyl. Administer slowly over 15 to 20 min. May cause acute reversal of systemic μ-receptor effects and leave κ-agonism intact.
Naloxone: 0.003 to 0.1 mg/kg/h IV infusion (titrate up to decrease pruritus and reduce infusion if pain increases).
Cyproheptadine†: 0.1 to 0.2 mg/kg PO q8–12h. Maximum dose 12 mg.
Change opioid.

Constipation

Encourage water consumption, high-fiber diet, and vegetable roughage.
Bulk laxatives: Metamucil, Maltsupex.
Lubricants: Mineral oil 15 to 30 mL PO qd as needed (not for use in infants because of aspiration risk).
Surfactants: Sodium docusate (Colace):
  <3 yr: 10 mg PO q8h
  3 to 6 yr: 15 mg PO q8h
  6 to 12 yr: 50 mg PO q8h
  >12 yr: 100 mg PO q8h
Stimulants:
Bisacodyl suppository (Dulcolax): <2 yr, 5 mg PR qhs; >2 yr 10 mg PR qhs.
Senna syrup (218 mg/5mL): >3 yr, 5 mL qhs.
Enema: Fleet's hypertonic phosphate enema (older children; risk of hyperphosphatemia).
Electrolytic/osmotic: Milk of magnesia; for severe impaction: polyethylene glycol (GoLYTELY, MiraLax).

Urinary Retention

Straight catheterization, indwelling catheter.

---

*Avoid in patients on monoamine oxidase inhibitors.
†May be associated with extrapyramidal side effects, which may be more commonly seen in children than in adults.

ET, endotracheally; IM, intramuscularly; IV, intravenously; PO, orally; PR, rectally; q, every; qd, daily; qhs, at bedtime; SC, subcutaneously.

- Naloxone, infused in very low doses, may decrease itching without appreciably interfering with analgesia.
- Cyproheptadine, a 5-HT$_{2A}$ antagonist with mild anticholinergic effects, has been used in the treatment of the itching associated with cold urticaria and may play a role in refractory cases of pruritus.

Morphine increases venous capacitance and, as a consequence, may cause hypotension and reflex tachycardia. Morphine may be administered orally, intravenously, or intramuscularly. It is available, orally, in liquid and in pill forms.

For years it was suggested that meperidine is less likely than morphine to result in respiratory depression in the young. Data indicate that at equal analgesic doses, morphine and meperidine are equally depressant. The liver metabolizes meperidine to normeperidine. This metabolite is excitatory; consequently, meperidine administration has been associated with seizures when given in repeated or high doses. The adverse effect profile of meperidine is not significantly different from that of morphine and the drug offers no distinct advantages. It cannot be combined with monoamine oxidase (MAO) inhibitors because severe adverse reactions, including hyperpyrexia and seizures, may occur. It is structurally similar to atropine, and its administration is associated with tachycardia, not bradycardia. In addition to μ-receptor agonism, it is purported to have some local anesthetic effects. It has been used to treat postoperative shivering and the rigors associated with the administration of blood products or certain drugs such as amphotericin B. It may be used cautiously in patients with renal insufficiency because some of the metabolites may contribute to neuroexcitation.

Hydromorphone is similar to morphine but more potent. It may have a more benign side effect profile in certain patients. It is glucuronidated by the liver and has no active metabolites with analgesic activity. It may be used cautiously in patients with renal insufficiency without increased risk of oversedation because of metabolites.

Methadone is a potent opioid that has a long duration of action and may accumulate with fixed repetitive doses over time. A dose reduction is commonly required after 2 or 3 days of treatment. It is unique among opioids in that it is a racemic mixture; the L-isomer binds to μ-receptors, and the D-isomer binds to *N*-methyl-D-aspartate (NMDA) receptors. The latter action antagonizes the effect of excitatory neurotransmitters such as glutamate. Because of this property, (1) it may have a special role in the treatment of neuropathic pain, and (2) tolerance to methadone may develop more slowly than to other opioids. As a consequence, there is less need to escalate the dose rapidly over the course of therapy than with other opioids. Its long duration of action makes it a most important drug in the treatment of chronic pain.

Although it is an important drug, methadone should be used only by clinicians very familiar with its pharmacokinetics because of the possibility of delayed respiratory depression. Methadone may also increase the QT$_c$ interval and so its use should be avoided in patients with electrocardiogram (ECG) evidence of baseline prolongation of the QT$_c$ interval. Methadone is the only long-acting opioid available in liquid form.

The synthetic opioid fentanyl, and its congeners sufentanil, alfentanil, and remifentanil, are highly potent and are administered in microgram doses. Fentanyl produces little cardiovascular effect, although it may cause a relative decrease in heart rate as a consequence of both central sympatholysis and by causing an increase in vagal tone. In patients whose cardiac output is heart rate dependent (fixed or decreased stroke volume), such as neonates, patients with stenotic valvular disease, and those with decreased stroke volume because of severe cardiomyopathy, a dose-dependent decrease in blood pressure may be observed with the use of fentanyl. If fentanyl or any other opioid is administered along with a benzodiazepine, hypotension may develop, especially in the hypovolemic- or catecholamine-depleted patient.

Fentanyl may be associated with fewer side effects than those seen with morphine but this is largely idiosyncratic. Pruritus following fentanyl administration is mediated by a direct mechanism (μ-receptor mediated), not by histamine release. If given in a large dose or administered rapidly, fentanyl may cause axial muscle rigidity. Although this can be observed with all opioids, it is particularly well described with fentanyl and its congeners. Administering a paralytic agent and the application of bag-valve-mask ventilation may be necessary should axial muscle rigidity occur.

Fentanyl is highly bound to α-1-acid-glycoprotein, which is reduced in the infant. This reduction in glycoprotein results in an increased free fraction of this drug. Fentanyl exhibits an increase in context-sensitive half-life after multiple doses or after continuous infusions; like morphine, its clearance may be decreased under conditions of decreased hepatic blood flow as is seen following major abdominal procedures or in conditions associated with decreased cardiac output. Inactive fentanyl metabolites are cleared by both the biliary system and the kidney. Fentanyl is commonly used with midazolam for analgesia and sedation of the ventilated patient in the intensive care unit (ICU) setting. Because both are metabolized by CYP3A4, competitive inhibition is likely, hence the clearance of both drugs may be decreased.

Fentanyl is highly lipophilic, as opposed to morphine and hydromorphone, which are hydrophilic drugs. This property is exploited when it is administered epidurally; it tends to bind to μ-receptors at the level of the spinal cord where it is infused and exhibits little spread to supraspinal structures, thereby maximizing analgesia and minimizing adverse effects such as sedation and respiratory depression.

In addition to the intravenous route, fentanyl is currently available as a transdermal patch in doses of 25, 50, 75, and 100 μg/h. The patch is applied to the skin and changed every 72 hours, although a small number of patients may need the patch changed every 48 hours for maximum efficacy. A dermal pool of drug remains available for 12 to 18 hours after the patch has been removed. It is, therefore, a drug delivery system that cannot be easily titrated and the dose cannot be rapidly reduced. For these reasons transdermal fentanyl is not to be used in the setting of acute pain or in the opiate-naive patient. Tachyphylaxis in response to fentanyl may develop rapidly over time, necessitating higher doses for efficacy. The fentanyl patch should be used by chronic pain patients who can not tolerate oral opioids. It is not approved for use in children at the time of this writing; however, a 12.5 μg/h patch has undergone pharmacokinetic study in pediatric patients.

Codeine, hydrocodone, and oxycodone are less-potent analgesics that are frequently prescribed orally in combination with acetaminophen. All are potentially emetogenic and highly constipating, especially codeine. They, like all other opioids, should always be administered with a stool lubricant or softener and a stimulant if needed. Instruction should be given to the patient to drink copious amounts of water while taking opioids and to consume foods high in fiber content. Several of these opioids have active metabolites that may significantly accumulate in patients with renal failure.

Codeine is a prodrug that requires conversion by CYP2D6 to morphine. The activity of this enzyme system is reduced in young infants and in 7% to 10% of the general population, rendering codeine less effective than other oral analgesics. Oxycodone does not require metabolism for efficacy. It is metabolized to noroxycodone, which is also a weak analgesic and small amounts of oxymorphone are also formed by a CYP2D6-dependent mechanism; these metabolites and their conjugates are excreted by the kidney. Hydrocodone undergoes a complex metabolism of demethylation and keto reduction to a variety of hydroxymetabolites before elimination.

Tramadol is a unique drug that has μ-agonist activity but also blocks serotonin and norepinephrine reuptake. It is occasionally prescribed for both somatic and neuropathic pain symptoms. Tramadol has a variety of interactions with other drugs, including the serotonin re-uptake inhibitors, and has the potential to cause seizures when combined with MAO inhibitors.

Procedural Pain and Discomfort

The pain and anxiety associated with repetitive needle sticks and procedures such as lumbar puncture, bone marrow aspiration and biopsy, endoscopic procedures, repetitive wound debridement, and dressing changes are commonly cited by children as being worse than pain associated with disease itself. Nonpainful but frightening examinations such as an MRI or CT or treatments such as radiation therapy can also produce considerable anxiety. This can be addressed nonpharmacologically with hypnosis and other cognitive/behavioral techniques in selected children. In the special circumstance of infants younger than 3 months of age who are undergoing brief, nonpainful procedures such as CT scanning, withholding a nap before the procedure followed by feeding and swaddling just before the examination is frequently all that is needed to enable an infant to fall asleep. Sucking on a pacifier dipped in a solution of 24% sucrose has been demonstrated to reduce the response to pain in infants undergoing routine circumcision.

Often, pharmacologic sedation may be necessary for these frightening but mildly uncomfortable procedures.

It is well recognized that the first procedural experience that the child endures affects behavior during subsequent procedures. It is therefore most important that the first procedure be as comfortable and nonthreatening as possible.

Topical Application and Subcutaneous Injection of Local Anesthetics

A eutectic mixture consists of a biphasic emulsion of solvents that allows for a higher concentration of solutes than would otherwise be possible. A eutectic mixture of local anesthetics (EMLA) is an emulsion of oil and water in a 50:50 mixture of 2.5% lidocaine and 2.5% prilocaine. This high concentration of local anesthetic allows for dermal penetration. It is generally applied to intact skin and the site covered by an occlusive dressing. The EMLA cream should be applied 1 hour prior to the procedure for optimal effect. It is particularly useful for intravenous catheter placement, port access, lumbar puncture, and infant circumcision.

Pediatricians may use a variety of local anesthetics for tissue infiltration or for peripheral nerve block. They all act by blocking transmembrane sodium conductance. Amide local anesthetics are metabolized by the liver to para-amino acid derivatives. Ester local anesthetics are hydrolyzed by plasma cholinesterases and, in general, have shorter half-lives. Epinephrine at a concentration of 5 μg/mL (1:200,000) is frequently added to the local anesthetic to decrease vascular absorption thus decreasing toxicity and increasing the duration of action. Epinephrine containing local anesthetic should never be administered into regions such as the digits or penis that are supplied by end arteries. A mixture of lidocaine, epinephrine, and tetracaine (LET) may be useful for suturing lacerations. Table 4 lists the maximum recommended doses of commonly administered local anesthetics. Exceeding the maximal dose may be associated with seizures, dysrhythmias, and myocardial depression. Bupivacaine is long-acting and can cause life-threatening dysrhythmias at doses far less than that shown to be associated with neurotoxicity. Prilocaine is metabolized to O-toluidine, which contributes to methemoglobinemia; thus, the use of prilocaine should be limited to restricted dermal application in neonates and other patients susceptible to methemoglobinemia. Mucosal and pleural absorption of local anesthetic may be rapid; large doses of local anesthetic in the vicinity of

TABLE 4 Toxic Doses of Local Anesthetics

Drug	Dose without Epinephrine (mg/kg)	Dose with Epinephrine (mg/kg)
Lidocaine	5	7
Bupivacaine	2	2.5
Mepivacaine	5	6
Chloroprocaine	8	10
Prilocaine	5	7
Procaine	7	8.5
Ropivacaine	2.5	4

major blood vessels may also result in rapid absorption and enhanced toxic effects. One should always use the lowest concentration of drug necessary to obtain a sensory block and inject slowly, with frequent aspiration of the syringe to ensure that an intravascular injection is avoided.

Local anesthetics are used for nerve blocks, subarachnoid block (spinal analgesia), and epidural block. Commonly used local anesthetics employed for this purpose include lidocaine, procaine, 2-choroprocaine, bupivacaine, and a newer agent, ropivacaine, which may have an improved toxicity profile over bupivacaine. The time to onset of action (10 to 20 minutes) for bupivacaine is substantially longer than either lidocaine or procaine (several minutes).

POSTOPERATIVE PAIN MANAGEMENT

General Principles

Computerized or preprinted postoperative order forms designed to decrease the risk of medication, computational, decimal point, and unit errors contribute to safety. Nursing education and collaboration with the unit nursing staff in the establishment of practical pain management guidelines that can be easily followed is of paramount importance. Policies and procedures must take into account the needs and resources of each unit within the hospital. Electronic monitoring, although important, can never substitute for frequent interval evaluations of respiratory rate and depth, degree of sedation, and pain score. The need for specific categories of electronic monitoring must be established on the basis of the premorbid condition and the age of the patient, the nature of the surgery, and the modality of analgesia. Postoperative and chronic pain are most effectively managed using a team approach involving the primary service, unit nursing, child life personnel, and a dedicated pain management team. Often during treatment of chronic pain, input from experts in developmental pediatrics, physical therapy, child psychology, and child psychiatry, in addition to anesthesiology, can be of great benefit.

There is evidence that postoperative pain is undertreated in children. As-needed scheduling of opioids is frequently interpreted as "give as little as possible." Orders for enteral or intravenous bolus doses of opioids should be written on an around-the-clock (ATC) schedule. The patient should be evaluated carefully prior to administering the next dose. A dose should be withheld if the patient is asleep or difficult to arouse, shows evidence of respiratory depression, or is not in pain. Low-dose continuous infusions may be given postoperatively, but it may be difficult to determine where within the therapeutic window the plasma level of opioid may be at any given point. Continuous infusions necessitate extra vigilance; in infants, such vigilance is especially appropriate. Alternatively, intermittent bolus doses of opioid may be administered but also necessitate frequent interval evaluations of pain score, level of sedation, and vital signs. Parenteral opioids should be prescribed until the patient is able to take liquids adequately and then switched to oral medications.

Patient-Controlled Analgesia

In addition to oral administration, bolus injection by hospital staff, and continuous infusion, opioids can be administered by patient-controlled analgesia (PCA) devices. The prescription, typically ordered by an anesthesiologist, includes the bolus dose, a lockout time interval (which will prevent the machine from delivering subsequent doses if the button is repeatedly pressed) and a 1- or 4-hour total dose limit. The total dose administered and the patient's pattern of use can be reviewed and the prescription logically adjusted. Often a low-dose basal infusion is prescribed. This approach is especially useful on the first postoperative night or if the patient is in severe continuous pain.

The inherent safety of this technique is that the child becomes sedated and unable to press the button before respiratory rate decreases to an unacceptable level. Studies have demonstrated decreased opioid use and improvement in pain scores when the patient is empowered with this means of control over pain. Because most postoperative pain is incidental and related to movement, coughing, or respiratory toilet, the patient should be encouraged to use the PCA device in anticipation of such maneuvers. In general, a PCA device is appropriate for any child capable of playing a video game and who has been instructed preoperatively in its use. Such children may be as young as 6 years old.

Some institutions allow PCA devices to be operated by adults for children incapable of using the device by themselves. Nurse-controlled analgesia or parent-controlled analgesia allows the nurse or parent to press the PCA button. This strategy must be used with the utmost care because the major safety mechanism (the child) is being bypassed. After establishment of a specific educational module and with strict dosing and monitoring guidelines in place, it may be considered. Parent-controlled analgesia should be reserved for a carefully selected group of parents who have been instructed in the use of the PCA device.

Epidural Analgesia

Caudal, lumbar, or thoracic epidural nerve blocks may be administered by placing a catheter intraoperatively and continuously infusing one of several preservative-free solutions: either local anesthetic alone, an opioid alone, or a mixture of local anesthetic and opioid solutions during the postoperative period. Preservative-free clonidine has also been used epidurally to increase the intensity and duration of the block. In a manner similar to the PCA, patient-controlled epidural analgesia (PCEA) enables the patient to administer small bolus doses if the initial epidural infusion rate is inadequate to maintain good postoperative pain control.

The purported advantages of epidural mixtures over intravenous opioids include an improved side-effect profile, less sedation, and improved pulmonary function. There is some evidence that preemptive analgesia—that is, administration of local anesthetic before the initial painful stimulus of surgery—may decrease the perception of pain postoperatively and thus decrease the requirements for pain medication. Hence, many anesthesiologists begin an epidural infusion before incision and continue this infusion into the postoperative period. Phantom limb pain or sensations may be ablated if a continuous local anesthetic block is initiated before the amputation.

In infants, epidural catheters may be threaded as high as the thoracic region from the entry point at the sacral hiatus. This technique may be particularly beneficial for infants undergoing thoracotomies for lung surgery, tracheoesophageal fistula repair, or correction of diaphragmatic hernia or for infants having upper abdominal incisions for such procedures as fundoplication and repair of omphalocele or gastroschisis. Often, a single shot of local anesthetic is administered, for procedures below the umbilicus, via the caudal canal. This may provide postoperative analgesia for as long as 6 to 8 hours, which is enough time to allow the child to recover from surgery and begin pain treatment with NSAIDs, acetaminophen, or enteral opioids.

One problem related to epidural catheter placement is improper positioning of the catheter. In general, the catheter must be placed at the dermatomal level of maximal expected discomfort. If the catheter is inadvertently placed within the subarachnoid space, or in the unlikely event that it erodes into that position, infusion of local anesthetic is likely to result in total spinal anesthesia and cause paralysis of the motor nerves innervating both the diaphragm (C_3–C_5) and intercostal muscles (T_1–T_{12}). Ventilation would need to be immediately supported until the anesthetic effect subsides.

A high thoracic epidural block may cause bradycardia as a result of inhibition of the cardiac accelerator fibers at T_1–T_4. Blockade of sympathetic outflow commonly causes a decrease in blood pressure in older children that may necessitate additional fluid administration. This problem is not commonly seen in infants and young children.

Patients may also complain of tingling or numbness of the hands and fingers in a C_8–T_1 distribution (medial forearm, fourth and fifth digits). This complaint should be considered a warning sign that the level may be too high and that respiratory problems may ensue. In such cases, the infusion should be stopped until the level regresses; when the infusion is resumed a lower infusion rate should be prescribed.

If the catheter migrates into an epidural blood vessel, signs of systemic toxicity will become manifest, such as tinnitus, lightheadedness, diffuse tingling, and a complaint of a metallic taste. Seizures, dysrhythmias, or cardiovascular collapse may ensue. Treatment of systemic absorption or inappropriately high spinal levels requires immediate cessation of the infusion and appropriate supportive intervention.

Peripheral Nerve Blocks

These blocks may be administered intraoperatively and can provide postoperative analgesia. Examples include the dorsal penile nerve block or ring block, which are useful for pain relief after circumcision, and iliohypogastric and ilioinguinal nerve block, which are used to relieve the pain of hernia repair. A variety of other blocks may be performed involving both the upper and lower extremities. On occasion, an indwelling catheter is positioned adjacent to a nerve or plexus for prolonged postoperative infusion of dilute local anesthetic such as a brachial plexus block.

Special Postsurgical Problems

Orthopedic patients, especially those who have had a history of spasticity, may suffer from muscle spasm in the postoperative period. This side effect frequently responds to adjuvants such as the benzodiazepines. Diazepam given orally at a dose of 0.1 to 0.15 mg/kg every 6 hours may be quite effective.

Urology patients may have postsurgical ureteral or bladder spasms that may respond to treatment with NSAIDs or benzodiazepines. Oxybutynin (Ditropan), a muscarinic receptor antagonist, may also be useful. The dose in children older than 5 years is 5 mg/kg orally three times daily. Phenazopyridine (Pyridium), a local analgesic, given at a dose of 4 mg/kg orally three times a day, may be given to the older child who has bladder irritation secondary to infection or the presence of a urinary catheter. It should not be given to children in renal failure or for longer than 48 hours.

SPECIFIC CONDITIONS

The Neonate

Data indicate that neonates and even premature infants are capable of sensing pain. Indeed, because excitatory ascending pathways develop earlier than descending inhibitory pathways, some speculate that premature infants may have a heightened perception of pain. Lower pain thresholds, shorter latency periods, and prolonged hypersensitivity to painful stimuli have been demonstrated in neonatal animal models in comparison to adult animals. Pain experienced in early infancy is a form of learning; it may result in long-term changes in the structure and function of the central nervous system (CNS) and may influence behavior later in life. Neonates whose pain is not effectively treated may demonstrate an exaggerated stress response that may adversely affect outcome and even survival. This response has been suggested in a cohort of infants undergoing cardiovascular surgery.

Sickle Cell Disease

Sickle cell disease is a model of both chronic and recurrent acute pain. Vaso-occlusive crisis may result in dactylitis (pain in the distal end of extremities); acute chest syndrome; and severe back, abdominal, and extremity pain. Stroke may be associated with the subsequent development of central pain syndromes. Multiple bone infarctions can result in chronic bone pain. Prevention and treatment of those crises requires a comprehensive program of care. Hydroxyurea is now used in many centers to help prevent crisis by increasing hemoglobin F synthesis.

Most painful crises can be treated at home with oral hydration, acetaminophen, or NSAIDs, and oral opioid analgesics such as codeine, hydrocodone, or oxycodone.

This approach is not always completely effective, and many patients with sickle cell disease come to the hospital as a last resort, complaining of severe "10/10" pain. Their pain should not be doubted. They may require hospitalization, intravenous hydration, and parenteral opioid treatment. Parenteral opioids are best administered by PCA. Ketorolac or other NSAIDs may decrease the dose of opioid that is required for effective management of vaso-occlusive painful crises. Many of these patients require substantial doses of opioids for several days until the painful crisis resolves. The role of long-acting oral opioids in the treatment of chronic sickle cell pain and in the prevention of crises needs further investigation.

Childhood Arthritides

Primary therapy with NSAIDs, steroids, or other chemotherapeutic agents along with maintenance of physical and psychosocial function is the key to successful management. Typically, rheumatologists prescribe higher, anti-inflammatory doses of NSAIDs than are commonly prescribed by pain management physicians.

Cancer

The most common cause of pain in cancer patients is the pain associated with procedures. Neuropathies may develop as a consequence of progression of disease and nerve compression and metabolic disturbances. Chemotherapeutic agents such as vincristine and tamoxifen, for example, may also be neurotoxic. Mucositis is common and is managed by using topical treatments such as "magic mouthwash" (usually a mixture of Maalox, diphenhydramine [Benadryl], and viscous 2% lidocaine mixed in equal volumes) and by systemic opioid treatment with a PCA device. The pain of bone metastasis may be relieved in some cases by intranasal calcitonin or intravenous pamidronate and NSAIDs, steroids, opioids, or radiotherapy. Table 5 shows the World Health Organization's (WHO) analgesic ladder, which is an effective guide to the step-wise management of cancer pain. Symptoms related to complications of the disease, chemotherapy, or radiation treatment such as nausea, vomiting, pruritus, air hunger, neuropathy, or excessive sedation must be aggressively treated. Lack of energy and sleeping disturbances must also be addressed. Long-acting oral opioids should be used to achieve maximal pain control.

TABLE 5 Adaptation of the World Health Organization Analgesic Ladder	
Step 1:	Nonopioid analgesics, nonpharmacologic interventions
Step 2:	Weak opioids given orally ± adjuvants
Step 3:	Strong opioids given parenterally ± adjuvants
Step 4:	Invasive techniques:
	Neurolysis
	Radiofrequency ablation
	Intraspinal electrical stimulation
	Intrathecal medication infusions

Modified from World Health Organization: Cancer Pain and Palliative Care in Children. Geneva: World Health Organization, in association with the International Association for the Study of Pain, 1998.

Massive dose escalation over time may be required. Oral transmucosal fentanyl citrate may be helpful for sudden severe breakthrough pain of short duration. Transdermal fentanyl patches may be effective in older patients who cannot take oral opioids. Intra-axial infusions (either epidural or subarachnoid) with local anesthetics and opioids can be highly efficacious. Long-term infusions of opioid combined with clonidine via tunneled catheters may relieve pain that would otherwise be refractory to therapy. Orally administered tetrahydrocannabinol has been occasionally used as an appetite stimulant, antiemetic, and analgesic adjuvant. Occasionally chemical neurolysis or radiofrequency ablation may be used to relieve pain associated with the terminal stages of disease. Anxiolysis, treatment of depression, and psychosocial support are also an integral part of this process.

Burn Patients

Like cancer patients, burn patients are subject to the distress of having to endure multiple painful procedures such as debridement, contracture release, and grafting. Many of these patients suffer severe pruritus during the healing phase that can be extremely distressing. Burn patients may have lost loved ones and so they are at risk for both acute stress and post-traumatic stress disorders. Disfigurement may lead to further depression, which may exacerbate the perception of pain. Anxiety, depression, and sleep disorders must be appropriately addressed along with aggressive pain treatment. On occasion, children who have been burned may be victims of their own fire-setting behavior. Premorbid psychosocial dysfunction may complicate long-term pain therapy and so early involvement with behavioral or psychiatric specialists is needed.

Neuropathic Pain

Neuropathic pain is diagnosed when one or more of the following sensations are present:

- Hyperalgesia (intense, prolonged, severe pain to mildly painful stimulation).
- Allodynia (pain in response to otherwise nonpainful phenomena such as mild mechanical or thermal stimulation; examples include pain evoked by gentle stroking of the skin and intense pain evoked by the application of droplets of cool water).
- Paresthesias (disturbing although not necessarily painful sensations, such as the pins and needles feeling experienced as a limb "falls asleep").
- Dysesthesias (painful paresthesias such as intense burning, stinging, or lancinating pain).
- Hyperpathia (intensely increasing pain following repetitive stimuli, such as stroking of the skin).

Neuralgias constitute a neuropathic process in which the pain follows the distribution of a specific nerve and is usually described as shock-like, or lancinating. It is important to obtain a thorough pain history to determine whether a neuropathic pain component is present, because neuropathic pain is often treated differently from inflammatory nociceptive pain.

Chronic regional pain syndrome (CRPS) 1, formerly known as reflex sympathetic dystrophy (RSD) is a poorly understood syndrome that may occur as a consequence of an otherwise insignificant injury. Pain is most often maintained by sympathetic nervous system drive but may, in some circumstances, be sympathetically independent; that is, sympatholysis will not relieve the pain. If not appropriately treated, it can lead to disuse of an extremity and severe, crippling, trophic changes. CRPS 2, formerly known as causalgia, is neuropathic pain secondary to a nerve lesion or transection.

Neuropathic pain may also result from CNS processes such as those involved with thalamic disease, and it may also follow spinal cord injury or transection. Infection with human immunodeficiency virus (HIV) and other viruses such as varicella or herpes may result in severe and difficult-to-treat forms of neuropathic pain. Painful metabolic and toxic neuropathies are rarely encountered in children but should be considered in the differential diagnosis.

In the case of CRPS the primary goals are to maintain function of the limb and to prevent atrophy and contractures. A program of aggressive physical or occupational therapy and psychological counseling is necessary to prevent development of handicaps and social disability.

Medications and Techniques used in the Treatment of Neuropathic Pain

Gabapentin may be effective in the treatment of neuropathic pain and it has an excellent side-effect profile. Patients may initially complain of somnolence or lightheadedness but will usually adapt to these side effects. Gabapentin has no active metabolites and is excreted by the kidneys. Tricyclic antidepressants such as amitriptyline or nortriptyline may also be effective. Because of the degree of sedation associated with tricyclic antidepressants, they are usually given as a single nighttime dose and the dose is gradually increased. They should not be administered to children with a history of dysrhythmias or long QT syndrome. Other drugs that have been used in the treatment of neuropathic pain include other anticonvulsants and local anesthetics such as systemically administered mexiletine.

Centrally acting α_2 agonists such as clonidine may also be helpful in the treatment of sympathetically maintained pain.

Often, peripheral nerve blocks, epidural blockade, or sympathetic nerve blocks are needed to break the cycle of pain and allow for effective physical therapy. Children with neuropathic pain syndromes are best treated in a multidisciplinary pediatric pain treatment center.

Children with Intellectual Disability Who Are in Pain

Children with intellectual disabilities have been excluded from most pain studies despite a high prevalence of pain in this population. Assessment is still largely observational, although some children with mild cognitive impairment may be able to use numeric rating scales and body maps to more effectively communicate about their pain.

These children may have a wide variety of painful conditions and frequently require corrective surgery. Examples include children with

- Trisomy 21, who may require corrective surgery for complex congenital heart disease, intestinal atresias, or hip dysplasias.
- Fragile X syndrome, who may have ocular problems or require scoliosis surgery.
- Mental retardation of various etiologies.
- Cerebral palsy, who may have painful joint contractures, muscle spasms, or spasticity in addition to problems with skin ulceration.

Common causes of pain in this group of patients include esophagitis secondary to gastric reflux, decubitus ulcers, joint dislocations, and occult fractures secondary to severe osteopenia.

Some children with severe neurologic impairment are said to suffer "neural agony" and may moan or scream interminably. Despite extensive evaluation for a cause, the cause may never be identified in some of these children. Simple measures such as orthotics, a different chair, improved padding, or a different feeding regimen may make a dramatic difference in their degree of suffering. Benzodiazepines may play a role in treatment if muscle spasm is a contributing factor. Baclofen, a γ-aminobutyric acid B-receptor (GABA$_B$) agonist, and botulinum toxin may play a role in the treatment of spasticity. A therapeutic trial of pain medication, including the opiates, given under conditions of close observation, may be indicated in selected patients.

Functional Abdominal Pain

"Recurrent abdominal pain of childhood" or functional abdominal pain is defined by Rome II criteria as pain, usually periumbilical, occurring intermittently or continuously for at least 12 weeks. (Rome II is a working group formed by attendees of the International Congress of Gastroenterology to establish diagnostic criteria for the functional gastrointestinal disorders.) There is no convincing relationship between pain and physiologic events such as eating, defecating, activity, or the menstrual cycle. There is usually a sleep disturbance associated with the pain.

If the child with functional abdominal pain has a normal pattern of growth and physical examination, it is extremely unlikely that an extensive workup will reveal the etiology of the child's pain. Many of these patients are "hypervigilant" and their perception of pain is amplified.

Most of these children, however, undergo an extensive medical workup and multiple medical evaluations. Initially, a thorough evaluation is quite justifiable. It is theoretically possible that some of these children suffer from occult infection, a metabolic disorder, visceral neuropathy, or dysfunction of the enteric nervous system; however, the etiology of "functional" abdominal pain remains largely unknown. Psychosocial evaluation is a key element in the treatment process.

Functional abdominal pain, as a syndrome, has become recognized as part of a spectrum of diseases, which include chronic daily headache, chronic fatigue syndrome, the fibromyalgia and myofascial syndromes, irritable bowel syndrome, and reflex sympathetic dystrophy. These conditions may lead to a "social disability of childhood," heralded by school avoidance and progressive social isolation. Treatment must be prompt, multimodal, multidisciplinary, and supportive of both the family and child. Some studies now suggest the use of complementary and alternative medicine therapies.

Common Pitfalls

OPIOID TOLERANCE AND WITHDRAWAL

Tolerance to opioids may develop rapidly in children and is commonly observed in the pediatric intensive care unit. This may necessitate an increase in dose to achieve similar levels of pain control. Physical dependence may also occur, particularly if the opioid is administered in high dose or for periods exceeding 5 to 7 days. Signs and symptoms of withdrawal may develop if opioids are abruptly discontinued. Patients who are taking opioids should be warned not to discontinue such medication suddenly, but to do so only under the care of a physician.

Signs and symptoms of opioid withdrawal include diarrhea, flushing, myalgias, piloerection, nasal congestion, agitation, tremor, tachycardia, hypertension, and dysrhythmias. Tapering the opioid slowly, perhaps by 25% on the first day and 10% to 15% on subsequent days can usually prevent this. Occasionally, some patients require a slower weaning regimen. Withdrawal is treated by readministration of the opioid, supportive care measures, and a longer, slower weaning period. Clonidine may be helpful in ablating the autonomic signs and symptoms of opioid withdrawal during the tapering period. Clonidine may be administered either orally (2 to 4 µg/kg every 6 hours) or by transdermal patch, which is appropriate for use in adolescents. A dose of 0.1 mg/day delivered as a transdermal patch is usually sufficient. Addiction, or psychological dependence, is rarely, if ever, encountered when opioids are administered for treatment of acute pain in children.

OPIOID CONVERSIONS

Conversion from the intravenous route to the oral route of administration or vice versa depends on the patient's condition and medical progress. In general, once a patient can reliably take fluids by mouth, enteral opioids can be tolerated. A higher dose of opioid may be needed when administration is switched from the intravenous route to the oral route, if the opioid undergoes considerable first-pass hepatic metabolism.

Occasionally, a patient may be rotated from one opioid to another if untreatable adverse effects ensue or excessive tolerance develops. If the decision is made to switch from one opioid to a different opioid, the *equianalgesic dose* of the new drug must first be determined (Tables 6 and 7). The equianalgesic dose, which is empirically derived, should serve only as an initial dosing guideline. In general, the dose of the first drug is converted to an intravenous morphine dose equivalent; the equianalgesic dose of the new drug is then calculated from the intravenous morphine dose. This calculation does not take into account the important issue of incomplete cross-tolerance between opioids. *Incomplete cross-tolerance* may occur because of differential downregulation of µ-receptor isoforms after chronic opioid exposure and from differences in opioid avidity of the remaining functional receptors. It is not uncommon for clinicians to calculate the equianalgesic dose and then reduce that dose by a considerable proportion initially—say 25% to 50%—for safety. For conversions to the long-acting opioid methadone, it is not uncommon to decrease the equivalent dose by 75% to 90% initially. If a higher dose of methadone is needed, one should titrate the dose up no more often than every 2 to 3 days because of its long half-life.

Until such time as the clinician is thoroughly familiar with the pharmacology of opioid conversions, consultation with a pain management physician is advised to prevent overdose or withdrawal.

CONTROVERSIAL INTERVENTIONS

The use of long-acting opioids in patients with chronic, nonmalignant pain has become very controversial because they have become highly publicized drugs of

TABLE 6 Approximate Equianalgesic Doses of Common Opioids

Drug	Intravenous Equianalgesic Dose (mg)	Oral Equianalgesic Dose (mg)
Morphine	10	30
Hydromorphone	1.5	7.5
Meperidine	100	200
Fentanyl	0.1	PO dosing not applicable since fentanyl undergoes significant first-pass metabolism. The hourly transdermal dose is equivalent to the hourly IV dose.
Methadone	10	10–20
Oral codeine	Not recommended	120
Oral hydrocodone	Not available; oral route only	12
Oral oxycodone	Not available; oral route only	10

Conversion from one drug to another may require consultation with a pain management physician. Doses of fentanyl are conventionally in micrograms; thus, 10 mg of morphine ≡ 100 µg of fentanyl. IV, intravenously; PO, orally.

TABLE 7 Equivalent Opioid Ratios and Starting Doses

Drug	Parenteral/Oral Equivalent Dose Ratio	Starting Dosages and Routes of Administration
Morphine	1:3	PO: 0.3 mg/kg q3–4h. IV bolus: 0.05–0.1 mg/kg q2–4h. IV PCA continuous infusion: 0.015 mg/kg/h. IV PCA bolus: 0.015–0.030 mg/kg/dose q10min.
Hydromorphone	1:5–7	PO:0.02–0.1 mg/kg q3–4h. IV bolus: 0.015mg q2–4h. IV PCA continuous infusion: 0.003–0.006 mg/kg/h. IV PCA bolus: 0.003 mg/kg q10min.
Meperidine	1:2	PO: 2 mg/kg q3–4h. IV bolus: 1 mg/kg q4h. IV for treatment of rigors: 0.1 mg/kg. PCA use not recommended.
Fentanyl	1:1 (IV/transdermal)	*Oral transmucosal:* 5–15 µg/kg per dose to a maximum of 400 µg/dose; may require careful monitoring for respiratory depression and salivation; associated with a high incidence of nausea and vomiting. *Transdermal patch:* Not currently recommended for children. IV titration for sedation: 0.5–3 µg/kg. IV PCA continuous infusion: 0.5–2 µg/kg/h. IV PCA bolus: 0.5–2 µg/kg.
Methadone	1:1–2	PO: 0.1–0.2 mg/kg q4–8h PRN for pain. IV bolus: 0.1 mg/kg q4–8h PRN for pain. May have a very long half-life; a dose reduction may be needed after 48–72 h. Use with caution and monitor for delayed sedation. Withhold in the presence of sedation, decreased respiratory rate for age, lack of pain; may need to decrease the dose or increase the dosing interval if these occur. If administered on a PRN basis, assess the patient before each dose. If the drug is prescribed via the PO route chronically, the usual dose interval is 8–12 h. A q 4-h sliding scale dosage regimen has also been recommended as follows: No Pain: withhold dose Mild pain: 25 µg/kg Moderate pain: 50 µg/kg Severe pain: 75 µg/kg
Codeine	Not recommended intravenously	PO: 1 mg/kg PO q4–6h. Available as both an elixir and oral solution at a concentration of 120 mg acetaminophen + 12 mg codeine/5mL. Frequently given in combination with 300 mg of acetaminophen per tablet as: Tylenol and Codeine #1: 7.5 mg Tylenol and Codeine #2: 15 mg Tylenol and Codeine #3: 30 mg Tylenol and Codeine #4: 60 mg Do not exceed maximum recommended acetaminophen dose.
Hydrocodone	Orally administered	PO: 0.1 mg/kg q3–4h. Only fixed combinations available with acetaminophen.
Oxycodone	Orally administered	PO: 0.1 mg/kg q3–4h. Fixed combinations available with acetaminophen

These are guidelines to be followed in the acute setting; actual dosages must be individualized for each patient. IV, intravenously; PCA, patient controlled analgesia; PO, orally; PRN, as needed; q, every.

abuse. However, they remain valuable pharmacotherapy for selected patients, particularly those with cancer.

A variety of continuous release preparations (dosing every 8 to 12 hours) such as MS Contin (morphine) and OxyContin (oxycodone) or sustained release preparations of morphine (dosing every 12 to 24 hours) such as Oramorph SR and Kadian are available. In addition to greater convenience, these preparations allow for a sustained systemic level of opioid, which is most appropriate for use in patients who are in severe chronic pain. To determine the correct dose, the amount of short-acting opioid required over a span of several days or weeks is quantified; then the average 24-hour consumption of short-acting opioid is totaled and divided into the appropriate interval for the long-acting oral drug chosen (every 8, 12, or 24 hours). For reasons of safety, the initial dosage of long-acting medication must be a conservative estimate of the total daily requirement.

Long-acting preparations cannot be chewed. Kadian is in the form of a capsule that may be opened and whose contents may be sprinkled on puddings or in applesauce for adolescent patients who cannot swallow capsules. Some clinicians believe that tolerance develops more slowly in patients who are on long-acting opioids when compared to those who are chronically treated with short-acting drugs alone.

Long-acting opioids should not be used on an as-needed basis, but they may be used along with a short-acting drug given every 3 to 4 hours for the treatment of acute breakthrough or incidental pain. Patients taking long-acting opioids *should* occasionally require breakthrough pain medication; if they do not, the dose of long-acting medication may be too high.

Communication and Counseling

Barriers to proper therapy include incomplete knowledge of the pharmacokinetics and pharmacodynamics of the drugs used, fear of respiratory depression and other adverse physiologic effects, irrational fear of addiction or of regulatory agencies, inadequate parental instruction, inappropriate modes of drug administration, economic concerns, and lack of confidence in non-pharmacologic techniques.

Ideally, optimal pain treatment should relieve suffering and improve outcome. The latter goal may be attained either by improving survival, as a result of decreasing the stress response to pain in acute models of pain management, or by improving quality of life (decreased handicap) in chronic pain management models. Although pain can be effectively and safely managed in the vast majority of patients, it can not yet be entirely eliminated in all patients. Substantial research and education is still needed to improve the quality, safety, and availability of pain management for children. Pediatricians should educate parents, nurses, and other caregivers, and the lay public and should advocate for proper pain treatment for children of all ages.

SUGGESTED READINGS

1. Anand KJ: Effects of perinatal pain and stress. Prog Brain Res 122:117–129, 2000. **A review of neonatal pain and its possible consequences.**
2. Anand KJ, Hickey PR: Halothane-morphine compared with high-dose sufentanil for anesthesia and perioperative analgesia in neonatal cardiac surgery. N Engl J Med 326:1–9, 1992. **The first article to suggest that pain treatment may alter outcome in this cohort of patients.**
3. Cote CJ, Karl HW, Notterman DA, et al: Adverse sedation events in pediatrics: Analysis of medications used for sedation. Pediatrics 106:633–644, 2000. **Critical incident analysis of adverse events related to sedation medication.**
4. Cote CJ, Notterman DA, Karl HW, et al: Adverse sedation events in pediatrics: A critical incident analysis of contributing factors. Pediatrics 105:805–814, 2000. **A review of factors related to adverse sedation events.**
5. Drossman DA: Rome II: The Functional Gastrointestinal Disorders, 2nd ed. Lawrence, Kan: Degnon Associates, 2000. **Standard reference in the field of functional bowel diseases.**
6. Greco CD, Berde CB: Pain management in children. In Behrman RE, Kliegman RM, Jenson HJ (eds): Nelson's Textbook of Pediatrics, 16th ed. Philadelphia: WB Saunders, 2000, pp 306–312. **General review of pediatric pain management.**
7. Schechter NL, Berde CB, Yaster M: Pain in Infants, Children and Adolescents. Baltimore. Lippincott, Williams & Wilkins, 2003. **General review of pediatric pain management.**
8. Yaster M: Acute Pain in Children. Pediatric Clinics of North America. Philadelphia: WB Saunders, 2000. **General review of pediatric pain management.**
9. Yaster M, Krane EJ, Kaplan RF, et al: Pediatric Pain Management and Sedation Handbook. St. Louis: Mosby, 1997.

Pruritus
Scott Moses

KEY CONCEPTS

- Reassuring findings suggestive of nonorganic cause include recent onset, localized itch, pruritus limited to exposed skin, household members also with pruritus, and recent travel history.
- Red flag symptoms that suggest organic cause include growth failure, anorexia, fatigue, associated bowel or bladder changes, and nighttime awakenings because of pruritus.
- Pruritus is usually self-limited and responds well to nonspecific measures such as liberal use of skin lubricants and avoidance of provocative factors. Antihistamines are not uniformly effective in reducing itch.
- Left untreated, itch and its associated persistent scratch risks impetigo and cellulitis in the short term and lichen simplex chronicus and prurigo nodularis in chronic cases.

As pruritus is the most common symptom in dermatology, clinicians are frequently asked to reduce its distressing effect on comfort and sleep. Left untreated, itch and its associated persistent scratch will risk chronic skin changes and secondary infection. Pruritus distribution is often the best clue to its etiology (Fig. 1). Although pruritus in children is most often due to a dermatologic condition, it may also represent a sign of underlying systemic disease (Table 1).

The sensation of itch starts in the skin's free nerve endings, travels via unmyelinated C fibers to the spine, and finally travels via the spinothalamic tract to the brain. Histamine, commonly associated with allergic rhinitis and urticaria, is only one of several chemical mediators of pruritus. Serotonin is integral to the pruritus of uremia, cholestasis, polycythemia vera, lymphoma, and morphine-associated pruritus. In atopic dermatitis, proinflammatory mediators (e.g., cytokines) are released in an immune-mediated response.

Expert Opinion on Management Issues

Pruritus is usually self-limited and responds well to nonspecific measures such as liberal use of skin lubricants and avoidance of provocative factors (Table 2). Oral antihistamines are not uniformly effective in all causes of pruritus. Specific management of dermatitis, as with atopic dermatitis, scabies, and contact dermatitis, will offer relief of symptoms. In the atypical case, in which these measures fail, a systemic condition may be uncovered. In these patients, the itch should be alleviated by treating the underlying condition, as with thyroid replacement in hypothyroidism or iron supplementation in iron deficiency anemia. Uremia and cholestasis-related pruritus have established effective therapies beyond treating the causative chronic renal or hepatic insufficiency (Table 3).

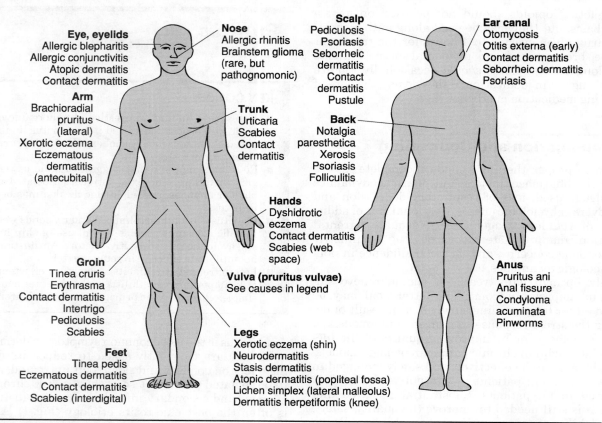

Eye, eyelids
Allergic blepharitis
Allergic conjunctivitis
Atopic dermatitis
Contact dermatitis

Nose
Allergic rhinitis
Brainstem glioma
(rare, but
pathognomonic)

Scalp
Pediculosis
Psoriasis
Seborrheic
dermatitis
Contact
dermatitis
Pustule

Ear canal
Otomycosis
Otitis externa (early)
Contact dermatitis
Seborrheic dermatitis
Psoriasis

Arm
Brachioradial
pruritus
(lateral)
Xerotic eczema
Eczematous
dermatitis
(antecubital)

Trunk
Urticaria
Scabies
Contact
dermatitis

Back
Notalgia
paresthetica
Xerosis
Psoriasis
Folliculitis

Hands
Dyshidrotic
eczema
Contact dermatitis
Scabies (web
space)

Groin
Tinea cruris
Erythrasma
Contact dermatitis
Intertrigo
Pediculosis
Scabies

Vulva (pruritus vulvae)
See causes in legend

Anus
Pruritus ani
Anal fissure
Condyloma
acuminata
Pinworms

Feet
Tinea pedis
Eczematous dermatitis
Contact dermatitis
Scabies (interdigital)

Legs
Xerotic eczema (shin)
Neurodermatitis
Stasis dermatitis
Atopic dermatitis (popliteal fossa)
Lichen simplex (lateral malleolus)
Dermatitis herpetiformis (knee)

FIGURE 1. Localized pruritus causes. *Pruritus vulvae causes: In prepubertal girls they are poor hygiene, streptococcus, *Escherichia coli*, pinworms, scabies, contact dermatitis; in young women they are vaginitis, contact dermatitis, hidradenitis suppurativa, lichen simplex chronicus.

TABLE 1 Systemic Pruritus Causes[1,2,3,4]

Cholestasis[5,6]	Intense itching worse at night; affects hands, feet, and pressure sites. Reactive hyperpigmentation spares midback (butterfly appearance).
Chronic renal failure	Severe paroxysms of generalized itching, worse in summer.
Delusions of parasitosis	Focal erosions on exposed areas of arms and legs.
HIV[7]	Pruritus is a common presenting symptom resulting from secondary causes. Causes: Eczema, drug reaction, eosinophilic folliculitis, seborrhea.
Hodgkin lymphoma[8]	Prolonged generalized pruritus often precedes diagnosis.
Hyperthyroidism[9,10]	Skin is warm and moist; pretibial edema may be present. Onycholysis, hyperpigmentation, and vitiligo have been associated. Other dermatologic signs include glossitis and angular cheilitis.
Iron deficiency anemia[11]	Intermittent head and neck flushing with explosive diarrhea.
Malignant carcinoid	Elderly with bone pain, headache, cachexia, anemia, and renal failure.
Multiple myeloma	Bouts of intense itching that may awaken patient from a sound sleep.
Neurodermatitis or neurotic excoriations[12]	Affects scalp, neck, wrist, extensor elbow, outer leg, ankle, perineum.
Parasitic infection	*Usually in returning travelers or immigrants.*
Filariasis	Tropical parasite responsible for lymphedema.
Schistosomiasis	Fresh water exposure in Africa, Mediterranean, South America.
Onchocerciasis	Transmitted by black fly in Africa, Latin America.
Trichinosis	Undercooked pork, bear, wild boar, or walrus meat.
Parvovirus B19	Slapped cheek appearance in children; arthritis in some adults.
Peripheral neuropathy	
Brachioradial pruritus	Affects lateral arm of white patients in the tropics.[13]
Notalgia paresthetica	Midback pruritus with hyperpigmented patch.[2]
Herpes zoster	Accompanies painful prodrome 2 days before rash.

TABLE 1 Systemic Pruritus Causes—cont'd

Polycythemia rubra vera[14]	Pricking-type itch persists for hours after hot shower or bath.
Scleroderma	Nonpitting extremity edema, erythema, and intense pruritus.
	Edema phase with pruritus precedes fibrosis of the skin.
Urticaria	Response to allergen, cold, heat, exercise, sunlight, or direct pressure.
Weight loss (rapid) in eating disorders[15]	Other signs include hair loss or fine lanugo hair on back and cheeks.
	Also, yellow skin discoloration and petechiae.

[1]Parker F: Structure and function of skin. In Goldman L, Bennett JC (eds): Cecil Textbook of Medicine, 21st ed. Philadelphia: WB Saunders, 2000, p 2266.

[2]Krajnik M, Zylicz Z: Understanding pruritus in systemic disease. J Pain Symptom Manage 21:151–168, 2001.

[3]Shellow WVR: Evaluation of pruritus. In Goroll AH, Mulley AG (eds): Primary Care Medicine, 4th ed. Philadelphia: Lippincott Williams & Wilkins, 2000, pp 1001–1004.

[4]Habif TP: Clinical Dermatology, 3rd ed. Chicago: Mosby, 1996

[5]Ghent CN: The pruritus of cholestasis. Hepatology 29:1003–1006, 1999.

[6]Gelfand JM, Rudikoff D: Evaluation and treatment of itching in HIV-infected patients. Mt Sinai J Med 68:298–308, 2001.

[7]Callen JP, Bernardi DM, Clark RAF, et al: Adult-onset recalcitrant eczema: A marker of noncutaneous lymphoma or leukemia. J Am Acad Dermatol 43:207–210, 2000.

[8]Tormey WP, Chambers JPM: Pruritus as the presenting symptom in hyperthyroidism. Br J Clin Pract 48:224, 1994.

[9]Heymann WR: Chronic urticaria and angioedema associated with thyroid autoimmunity: Review and therapeutic implications. J Am Acad Dermatol 40:229–32, 1999.

[10]Valsecchi R, Cainelli T: Generalized pruritus: A manifestation of iron deficiency. Arch Dermatol 119:630, 1983.

[11]Cyr PR, Dreher GK: Neurotic excoriations. Am Fam Physician 64:1981–1984, 2001.

[12]Veien NK, Hattel T, Laurberg G, et al: Brachioradial pruritus. J Am Acad Dermatol 44:7045, 2001.

[13]Diehn F, Tefferi A: Pruritus in polycythaemia vera: prevalence, laboratory correlates and management. 115:619–621, 2001.

[14]Gupta MA, Gupta AK, Voorhees JJ: Starvation-associated pruritus: A clinical feature of eating disorders. J Am Acad Dermatol 27:118–120, 1992.

[15]Harrigan E, Rabinowitz LG: Atopic dermatitis. Immunol Allergy Clin North Am 19:383–396, 1999.

HIV, human immunodeficiency virus.

TABLE 2 Nonspecific Management of Pruritus[1,2,3,4,5]

Use skin lubricants liberally.	Petrolatum or skin lubricant cream at bedtime.
	Apply alcohol-free, hypoallergenic lotions frequently during day.
Avoid excessive bathing.	Briefly pat dry after bath and immediately apply skin lubricants.
	Decrease bath frequency.
	Limit bathing to brief exposure to tepid water.
Limit soap use.	Use mild, unscented, hypoallergenic soap 2–3 times per week.
	Daily use of soap only in groin and axilla; spare legs, arms, and torso.
Minimize dryness.	Humidify dry indoor environment (especially in winter).
Choose clothing that does not irritate the skin.	Doubly rinsed cotton clothes and silk are best.
	Add bath oil (e.g., Alpha Keri) to rinse cycle when washing sheets.
	Avoid heat-retaining fabrics (synthetics).
	Avoid wool and smooth-textured cotton clothes.
Avoid vasodilators.	Avoid caffeine, alcohol, spices, hot water, and excessive sweating.
Avoid provocative topical medications.	Avoid prolonged topical corticosteroids (risk of skin atrophy).
	Avoid topical anesthetics and antihistamines.
	May sensitize exposed skin and risk contact dermatitis.
Standard antipruritic topical agents	Menthol and camphor (e.g., Sarna Lotion).
	Oatmeal baths (e.g., Aveeno).
	Pramoxine (e.g., PrameGel, Pramosone).
	Calamine lotion (use on weeping lesions only, not on dry skin).
Antipruritic topical agents for refractory cases (used in severe atopic dermatitis)	Doxepin 5% cream (Zonalon) applied 4 times a day for up to 8 days.*
	Burow solution (wet dressings).
	Unna boot.
	Tar emulsion.
Systemic antipruritic agents (used in allergic and urticarial disease)	Doxepin (Sinequan) 1 mg/kg up to 25 mg qhs (Level A).*†
	Hydroxyzine (Atarax) 0.5 mg/kg up to 25 to 50 mg qhs.
	Nonsedating antihistamines (e.g., Fexofenadine, Level A)[3]
Prevent complications of scratching.	Keep fingernails short and clean.
	Rub skin with palms if urge to scratch is irresistible.

[1]Krajnik M, Zylicz Z: Understanding pruritus in systemic disease. J Pain Symptom Manage 21:151–168, 2001.

[2]Shellow WVR: Evaluation of pruritus. In Goroll AH, Mulley AG (eds): Primary Care Medicine, 4th ed. Philadelphia: Lippincott Williams & Wilkins, 2000, pp 1001–1004.

[3]Finn AF, Kaplan AP, Fretwell R, et al: A double-blind, placebo-controlled trial of fexofenadine HCl in the treatment of chronic idiopathic urticaria. J Allergy Clin Immunol 103:1071–1078, 1999.

[4]Robinson-Bostom L, DiGiovanna JJ: Cutaneous manifestations of end-stage renal disease. J Am Acad Dermatol 43:975–986, 2000.

[5]Bender BG: Sedation and performance impairment of diphenhydramine and second-generation antihistamines: A meta-analysis. J Allergy Clin Immunol 111:770–776, 2003.

*Studies have not addressed use in children.

†FDA black box warning regarding antidepressants and suicidality in children.

qhs, at bedtime.

TABLE 3 Specific Management of Pruritic Conditions*

Cholestasis[1,2,3]	Cholestyramine 240 mg/kg/day divided tid (up to 6 g/day) Level B
	Ondansetron (Level B)
	Opiate receptor antagonist (Level A)
	Rifampin 10 mg/kg per day divided bid (max: 300 mg bid) (Level B)
	Bile duct stenting from extrahepatic cholestasis (Level A)
	Bright light therapy (Level B)
Neurotic excoriation[4,5]	Pimozide (Orap) for delusions of parasitosis
	Selective serotonin reuptake inhibitor (SSRI)[†]
Notalgia paresthetica[6]	Capsaicin applied 4–6 times per day for several weeks (Level B)
Polycythemia vera[7]	Aspirin: Do not use in acute febrile illness in children. (Level B)
	Selective serotonin reuptake inhibitors (e.g., paroxetine, Level B)[†]
	Interferon-α (Level B)
Spinal opioid-induced pruritus[8]	Ondansetron concurrent with opioid (Level A)
	Mixed opioid agonist–antagonist (Level B)
	Capsaicin 0.025% cream applied to localized pruritus 4–6 times per day (adults, children older than age 2 years)
Uremia[9,10]	UV B phototherapy twice weekly for 1 month (Level A)
	Activated charcoal (adults use 6 g/day) (Level A)[‡]
	Topical capsaicin 0.025% cream to localized areas (Level A)
	Ondansetron and naltrexone are not efficacious in uremia (Level A)

Levels of Evidence:
   Level A: Evidence from high-quality randomized, controlled clinical trials or meta-analyses
   Level B: Evidence from nonrandomized clinical studies or nonquantitative systematic reviews
   Level C: Based on consensus viewpoint or expert opinion

[1]Krajnik M, Zylicz Z: Understanding pruritus in systemic disease. J Pain Symptom Manage 21:151–168, 2001.
[2]Ghent CN: The pruritus of cholestasis. Hepatology 29:1003–1006, 1999.
[3]Gelfand JM, Rudikoff D: Evaluation and treatment of itching in HIV-infected patients. Mt Sinai J Med 68:298–308, 2001.
[4]Veien NK, Hattel T, Laurberg G, et al: Brachioradial pruritus. J Am Acad Dermatol 44:7045, 2001.
[5]Gupta MA, Gupta AK, Voorhees JJ: Starvation-associated pruritus: A clinical feature of eating disorders. J Am Acad Dermatol 27:118–120, 1992.
[6]Goroll AH, Mulley AG: Evaluation of vulvar pruritus. In Goroll AH (ed): Primary Care Medicine, 4th ed. Philadelphia: Lippincott Williams & Wilkins, 2000.
[7]Lidofsky S, Scharschmidt BF: Jaundice. In Feldman M, Scharschmidt BF, Sleisenger MH (eds): Sleisenger and Fordtran's Gastrointestinal and Liver Disease, 6th ed. Philadelphia: WB Saunders, 1998, pp 230–231.
[8]Correale CE, Walker C, Lydia M, et al: Atopic dermatitis: A review of diagnosis and treatment. Am Fam Physician 60:1191–210, 1999.
[9]Koblenzer CS: Itching and atopic skin. J Allergy Clin Immunol 104:S109-S113, 1999.
[10]Tennyson H: Neurotropic and psychotropic drugs in dermatology. Dermatol Clin 19:179–197, 2001.
*These medications are off-label use, directed by expert opinion.
[†]FDA black box warning regarding antidepressants and suicidality in children.
[‡]Dosing not available for this drug in children.
bid, twice daily; tid, three times per day.

Common Pitfalls

Itch and the scratch it induces are not benign. If scratching is left unchecked, fingernails introduce bacteria into abraded skin, with impetigo or cellulitis ensuing. Lichen simplex chronicus and prurigo nodularis are chronic skin changes seen with long-term scratching and in particular with atopic dermatitis. Medications to treat pruritus are also not without adverse effects. Antihistamines may affect alertness and learning if used during the day, and with chronic use, the associated dry mouth may predispose to tooth decay.

Communication and Counseling

General measures to treat pruritus should be reviewed at each visit. Consistent practice of these simple home strategies can prevent sleepless nights, frequent evaluations, unnecessary medications, and the complications of scratching.

SUGGESTED READINGS

1. Koblenzer CS: Itching and atopic skin. J Allergy Clin Immunol 104: S109–S113, 1999. **Dr. Koblenzer specifically addresses pruritus in atopic dermatitis. This is one of seven articles on atopic dermatitis in this supplemental issue.**
2. Krajnik M, Zylicz Z: Understanding pruritus in systemic disease. J Pain Symptom Manage 21:151–168, 2001. **A thorough literature review of the systemic causes of pruritus, their pathophysiology, and specific management strategies.**
3. Leung AKC: Pruritus in children. J R Soc Health 118:280–286, 1998. **Dr. Leung authors an excellent article that generally reviews an approach to pruritus in children.**
4. Moses S: Pruritus. Am Fam Physician 68:1135–1146, 2003. **A review of pruritus evaluation and management in adults and children.**

Headaches
Abraham M. Chutorian

KEY CONCEPTS

- The physical examination of a child with headache should always include a neurologic exam and funduscopy.
- Paroxysmal headaches with intervals of well-being are nearly always migraines.
- Headaches exacerbated by recumbency or by Valsalva maneuvers and that are increasing in frequency, associated with nausea and/or vomiting, and/or are persistently focal, require investigation for symptomatic headache.
- Treatment of acute headache involves judicial use of abortive, analgesic, sedative, and antiemetic agents.

- Both migraine and tension-type headaches are exacerbated by stress and adverse emotional factors, requiring careful attention to environmental and emotional issues as well as to pharmacologic options.
- Treatment of very frequent and severe or refractory headache warrants prophylaxis.
- Tension-type headache and migraine may coexist in the same child. Treatment issues are often similar.
- The first choice of pharmacologic agent chosen to treat acute or chronic and recurrent headache should be based on an optimal mix of efficacy, tolerability, and ease of administration. For example, prophylaxis with amitriptyline and propranolol has similar efficacy and tolerability, but amitriptyline is administered in a single daily dose.
- Treatment of excruciating, protracted headache that is refractory to abortive, analgesic, and other oral medications may require emergency treatment with unusual measures such as the administration of corticosteroids or intravenous dihydroergotamine. This treatment should be carried out by clinicians experienced in the use and application of these agents and is beyond the scope of this chapter.

Most children with chronic recurring headache have either migraine or tension-type headaches. Epidemiologic studies suggest that the migraine is at least as frequent in children as in adults, although the so-called classic migraine is probably less common in children and occurs in less than 5% of cases of recurrent headaches. Nevertheless, the migraine is an appropriate designation for many children with recurrent, severe headache, and it may affect more than 5% of all prepubertal children. Perhaps more frequent than the migraine is the tension-type headache, formerly called "muscle contraction headache" and believed by some to be psychogenic.

The term *mixed headache* commonly refers to the coexistence of migraine and tension-type headaches in the same patient, although some patients with chronic daily headache lasting many months may have any mix of a migraine, tension-type headache, and psychogenic headache, particularly when associated with depression.

The type of headache that requires imaging of the head and other urgent neurodiagnostic interventions (too frequently performed for migraine and tension-type headache and often under the urging of an anxious parent) will be addressed later. However, the myriad other types of headache that recur and are recognizable clinical conditions, such as sinus-related headache, febrile headache, headache secondary to dental malocclusion, and others, will not be discussed in this article.

Expert Opinion on Management Issues

MIGRAINE

The pathogenesis of a migraine is complex. Triggers include diet and stress, although predisposition is hereditary (usually autosomal dominant). Activation of the trigeminal ganglion and pontine centers mediates both a spreading cortical depression and trigeminal nerve transmission, triggering vascular events, with release of vasoactive peptides and resultant vasospasm with pain mediated by specific 5-hydroxytryptamine (5-HT) receptors. Recent evidence also implicates a nontrigeminal site of action, the periaqueductal gray matter, as evidenced by the inhibition of dural nociception by injection of naratriptan, a 5-HT antagonist, into the periaqueductal gray matter.

The best-recognized classification of migraine has three categories:

1. Classic migraine
2. Common migraine
3. Complicated migraine.

Classic migraine is preceded by an aura, often in the form of visual scintillation, and followed by frontal unilateral pain of such a moderate to severe degree that the migraine frequently causes nausea and vomiting in association with photophobia and phonophobia. Pain builds in intensity from a lower grade over a period of as long as an hour. Its duration is usually several hours, at times clustering over a span of 1 day to several days. Relief is obtained by sleep in a dark, quiet room and the use of analgesic drugs and nonanalgesic pharmacotherapeutic agents designed to arrest the headache. Figure 1 lists preventive medications.

Common migraine differs from classic migraine by virtue of the absence of an aura. Often a pediatric headache and a common migraine are generalized rather than focal, and nausea may not be associated with vomiting.

Complicated migraine occurs when the attack is associated with acute hemiparesis, hemisensory symptoms, ophthalmoplegia, dimming of vision, or a global confusional state. Frequently hemisensory or hemiparetic symptoms occur in a premonitory manner and disappear as the headache appears and increases in severity. These symptoms and signs occur in a significant minority of children with migraine and are virtually always transient. Particularly uncommon are hemiplegia,

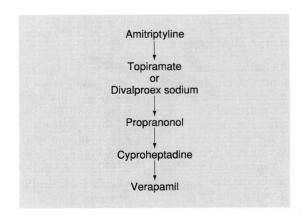

FIGURE 1. Prevention of headache. The arrows indicate descending order of preferred therapy for optimal efficacy, ease of administration, and tolerance.

ophthalmoplegia, and a global confusional state. No evidence has indicated that treatment in children with complicated migraine requires a different approach from that for classic or common migraine.

Precipitants or triggers of migraine headache include eating certain foods (e.g., nitrate-containing substances), stress, or fatigue. Girls may experience menstrual migraine or migraine associated with oral contraceptives. An increased predilection for migraine has been noted in children with benign paroxysmal vertigo, benign paroxysmal torticollis, and motion sickness. Migraine develops in some children with cyclic vomiting, or they may respond to antimigraine pharmacotherapy during episodes of cyclic vomiting, or to prophylaxis to prevent cyclic vomiting.

TENSION-TYPE HEADACHE

This classification applies to subjects with steady rather than throbbing or pulsatile pain, bilateral headache, slight to moderate intensity, and protracted duration—usually days, weeks, or months. Occasionally the headache is chiefly suboccipital and associated with chronic cervical muscle contraction, which can be relieved by injection of botulinum toxin. Stress plays a more prominent role in children with tension-type headache. Another major precipitant of this type of headache is the overuse of analgesic, especially with recurrent "rebound" headache. Unilateral headache, aura, and vomiting are notably absent, although nausea is not an uncommon complaint.

MIXED HEADACHE

Some patients who complain of severe attacks of migraine have more protracted periods of chronic transfrontal headache that are better characterized as tension type. It is important to separate these headaches historically so that pharmacotherapy, if indicated, can be appropriately chosen and the results of treatment selectively appreciated. Typically the migrainous episodes are paroxysmal and more severe, with an admixture of milder, more persistent, and generalized headaches.

CHRONIC DAILY HEADACHE

Chronic daily headache is defined by more than 15 days per month of headache for several months or longer. Chronic daily headache and tension-type headache are at times not easily differentiated and will be discussed jointly in regard to management issues. It is often difficult to determine whether emotional factors preceded or followed the development of this type of headache. Because social, psychological, and emotional factors are paramount in this type of headache, a tactful approach to the treatment of the whole child is necessary to avoid perceived humiliation on the part of the patient, or lack of parental cooperation. In these situations endless studies and examinations are often undertaken; however, the child will remain refractory to treatment with virtually

the entire headache pharmacopeia until the underlying issues are addressed. It is important to note that at times the use of pharmacotherapeutic agents of a psychotropic type are warranted (e.g., mood elevation for depression), but at the same time it must also be realized that the phenomenon known as a "rebound headache" may be responsible for some of the persistent headaches as a result of the use of innumerable drugs over a protracted period of time. This possibility emphasizes the need for spacing appropriate intervals between pharmacotherapeutic efforts.

CLUSTER HEADACHE

This type of headache, which used to be referred to as a "histamine headache," evokes nasal congestion, rhinorrhea, and tearing of the eye, with excruciating focal pain. It is very rare in children and requires special treatment considerations that are not within the scope of this chapter.

HEADACHE CAUSED BY INTRACRANIAL STRUCTURAL LESIONS

Headache associated with structural intracranial pathology is usually intermittent but typically progresses in frequency and severity. Recumbency aggravates the headache by virtue of increasing traction on pain-sensitive structures, including the leptomeninges and basal blood vessels, either directly or by raising intracranial pressure. Thus headache, often associated with vomiting, is worse on waking in the morning, may be aggravated by Valsalva maneuvers (even causing reflex constipation in some children), and tends to be associated with a variety of focal neurologic deficits and other symptoms suggestive of raised intracranial pressure (diplopia) or personality change. The term "traction headache" is applied because of a perception that traction on pain-sensitive perivascular and parameningeal structures is responsible for the headache. The fact that drainage (in which intracranial pressure is actually below normal) caused by, for example, leakage of cerebrospinal fluid after lumbar puncture or overshunting of cerebrospinal fluid can cause severe headache provides support for this belief. Treatment of symptomatic headache, whether caused by an intrastructural lesion or not, addresses the specific cause.

THERAPY

General Measures

It is vital to consider social and psychological factors that address the needs of both children and parents. In the absence of evidence of secondary symptomatic headache, reassurance is important. Moderation is needed in all aspects of lifestyle, academic and social. School attendance should be strongly encouraged whenever possible to forestall habitual absence. Communication with the school nurse or infirmary may be needed to provide optimal management while at school. Precipitants of headache include pharmacologic agents, stress, and diet. These factors need to be specifically addressed, which may often require parental documentation over an extended period. Treatment of the different types of headache, of course, depends on accurate classification. Failure of response to sequential approaches or pharmacotherapeutic measures should prompt reassessment of the diagnosis.

Treatment of Migraine

Treatment depends on the desired effect and includes abortive measures, symptomatic relief, and prophylaxis. Tables 1 and 2 list the pharmacologic agents, dosage, and common side effects for prophylaxis of migraine and of tension-type (and chronic daily) headache. Table 3 indicates the same features for the treatment of acute headache. Combinations of drugs may be used for refractory headache. For treatment of acute headache, for example, treatment might warrant the combined use of analgesic, anti-inflammatory, sedative, or anti-emetic drugs. A combination of agents for prophylactic treatment is not routinely advisable, but it deserves consideration in refractory headache. In addition, treatment of acute headache that breaks through prophylactic treatment justifies the addition of a drug more appropriate for treatment of the acute attack. At times, treatment of

excruciating protracted headache that is refractory to all treatment modalities requires an emergency department or hospital setting in which parenteral corticosteroids or parenteral ergotamine tartrate can be administered. Details of treatment with these agents are beyond the scope of this chapter.

Abortive Treatment

Ergot compounds may be used at any age but are generally avoided in preadolescents. Rectal and sublingual compounds, often combined with caffeine, are available in addition to oral preparations, which are unsuitable in children whose headaches are soon followed by vomiting. Ergot preparations should be given only for treatment of acute severe headache and as soon as possible after onset of the headache (or oral where applicable) for optimal abortive and symptomatic effect. The dose may be repeated once if needed after 1 hour. It is best to treat no more than one headache per week with ergot compounds.

A number of triptans are available for abortive or symptomatic treatment of migraine, the first of which was sumatriptan (Imitrex). Sumatriptan has been used extensively, usually with favorable results. Children 8 to 10 years of age or older often tolerate 25 mg of the oral

TABLE 1 Prophylactic Treatment of Migraine

Generic Name (Trade Name)	Dosage, Route, Regimen	Maximum Dose	Dose Formulation	Common Adverse Reactions	Comments
Tricyclics					
Amitriptyline (Elavil)	25–75 mg/day in qd dosing 2-wk intervals between dosage increases	100 mg per day	Tablet: 10 mg, 25 mg, 50 mg, 75 mg, 100 mg	Dry mouth, sedation	Contraindicated in cardiac disease or with MAO inhibitor
β-Blockade					
Propranolol (Inderal)	1–3 mg/kg/day in tid dosing Weekly intervals between dosage increases	3 mg/kg/day	Tablet: 10 mg, 20 mg, 40 mg, 60 mg, 80 mg	Bradycardia, postural hypotension, depression, fatigue	Contraindicated in asthma and heart block
Calcium Channel Blockade					
Verapamil	3–5 mg/kg/day in bid dosing, increased by 10 mg/kg/day for headache recurrence	350 mg/kg/day	Tablet: 40 mg, 80 mg, 120 mg	Dizziness, constipation	Contraindicated in some cardiovascular disorders
Neuroprotective (Antiepileptic)					
Divalproex sodium	20–30 mg/kg/day in bid dosing	40 mg/kg/day	Tablets: 250 mg, 500 mg Syrup: 250 mg/5 mL, Sprinkle: 125 mg	Hair loss, nausea, tremor, somnolence, weight gain	
Topiramate (Topimax)	1–4 mg/kg/day in bid dosing; increase 25 mg bid for headache recurrence	200 mg/day	Tablet: 25 mg, 50 mg, 200 mg Sprinkles: 15 mg, 25 mg	Impaired cognition, anorexia, weight loss, fatigue, dizziness	Rare ureteral calculi; encourage hydration
Other					
Cyproheptadine	0.2 mg/kg/day	0.2 mg/kg/day	Liquid: 2 mg/5 mL Tablets: 4 mg	Sedation, blurred vision, fatigue, dry mouth	

bid, twice daily; MAO, monoamine oxidase; od, once daily; tid, three times daily.

TABLE 2 Prophylactic Treatment of Tension-Type Headache

Generic Name (Trade Name)	Dosage, Route, Regimen	Maximum Dose	Dose Formulation	Common Adverse Reactions	Comments
Neuroprotective (Antiepileptic)					
Divalproex sodium	20–30 mg/kg/day in bid dosing	40 mg/kg/day	Tablets: 250 mg, 500 mg Syrup: 250 mg/5 mL Sprinkles: 125 mg	Hair loss, nausea, tremor, somnolence, weight gain	
Topiramate (Topimax)	1–4 mg/kg/day in bid dosing; increase 25 mg bid for headache recurrence	200 mg/day	Tablet: 25 mg, 50 mg, 100 mg, 200 mg Sprinkles: 15 mg, 25 mg	Impaired cognition, anorexia, weight loss, fatigue, dizziness	Rare ureteral calculi; encourage hydration
Gabapentin (Neurontin)	750–2700 mg/day in tid dosing	3600 mg/day	Capsule: 100 mg, 300 mg, 400 mg Liquid: 250 mg/5 mL Tablet: 100 mg, 300 mg, 400 mg, 600 mg, 800 mg	Fatigue, lethargy, dizziness	
Tricyclics					
Amitriptyline (Elavil)	25–75 mg/day in qd dosing 2-wk intervals between dosage increases	100 mg per day	Tablet: 10 mg, 25 mg, 50 mg, 75 mg, 100 mg	Dry mouth, sedation	Contraindicated in cardiac disease or with MAO inhibitor
SSRI					
Fluoxetine (Prozac)	10–20 mg/day in od dosing q AM	20 mg	Capsule: 10 mg, 20 mg	Nausea, insomnia, lethargy, anxiety	Potentiates epilepsy Do not use if MAO inhibitor taken

bid, twice daily; MAO, monoamine oxidase; od, once daily; SSRI, selective serotonin reuptake inhibitor; tid, three times daily.

preparation, which should be given as soon as possible after onset of headache or prodromal symptoms. The dose may be advanced to 50 mg with the next attack if the response is inadequate. More rapidly effective but sometimes less well tolerated is sumatriptan nasal spray available in 5-mg and 20-mg doses for insufflation. The rare child with cardiac disease and migraine should not be treated with sumatriptan because of the potential coronary constrictive effects of the drug. Rizatriptan benzoate (Maxalt) may be more effective in some children. Doses of 5 and 10 mg of rizatriptan benzoate are equivalent in dosage to 25 and 50 mg of sumatriptan, respectively. The same cardiac contraindications apply. For children who vomit soon after the onset of the attack, injectable preparations of sumatriptan are available in addition to the nasal spray, although obviously the latter is ordinarily preferable. A dose of 5 mg may be administered by spray into one nostril. The next incremental increase in dose if ineffective would be a dose of a 5-mg spray in each nostril. Older adolescents and postpuberal children may take the 20-mg nasal spray. The mechanism of action is by attachment to 5-hydroxytryptamine receptors.

Prophylactic Treatment

Most parents are understandably reluctant to permit a regimen of daily medication to prevent headache, unless the headaches are frequent and severe. A chronic treatment regimen designed to prevent a headache every 3 months would be highly questionable. In addition a mild to moderate headache recurring on a weekly basis may not be sufficient to warrant prophylaxis. Prophylaxis is warranted only when headaches are refractory to abortive measures and to measures designed to alleviate the acute attack (symptomatic treatment). The prophylactic drugs commonly used for refractory migraine are amitriptyline, propranolol, selected antiepileptic or neuroprotective drugs, and cyproheptadine.

As illustrated in Figures 1 and 2, a gradual increase in the dosage of each prophylactic drug is warranted as long as one adheres to monitoring guidelines and suggested maximal dosage schedules. For example, dosage increases for tizanidine and propranolol should be monitored by pulse and blood pressure measurements after each increase to avoid precipitating orthostatic hypotension.

Some children with migraine have contraindications to the use of one or more of these agents. For example, the use of propranolol and cyproheptadine is contraindicated in a child with asthma, whereas a cardiac arrhythmia or other cardiac contraindication may restrict the use of amitriptyline or the triptans.

Complete control of headache may be an unrealistic goal. Treatment of acute episodes is not incompatible with continuing prophylaxis. A minimum of several weeks at maximally tolerated doses of the prophylactic drug should be mandated before treatment is considered a failure. Often, gradual withdrawal of prophylactic treatment is successful after only a few months of treatment.

The use of biofeedback/relaxation therapy is considered controversial by many, but more than modest success is claimed in a number of publications. This approach could be considered in children with refractory

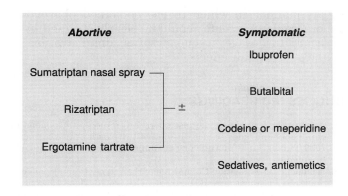

FIGURE 2. Treatment of acute headache. ±, with or without.

migraine who respond neither to pharmacotherapy nor to the usual social and psychological interventions.

Symptomatic Treatment

Symptomatic treatment should address the common associated symptoms such as photophobia and phonophobia by prescribing rest in a darkened and quiet room. The use of cold frontal compresses is a time-honored treatment, whatever the mechanism of action. Analgesics that may be effective include acetyl salicylate (aspirin) and acetaminophen. Nonsteroidal anti-inflammatory drugs (NSAIDs) are often sufficiently effective to preclude the need for other compounds. Ibuprofen has been most frequently used and must often be given in greater amounts than usual, as much as 300 to 400 mg at 6- to 8-hour intervals in the average child older than 5 years. In postpuberal children as much as 600 to 800 mg at 8-hour intervals may be required for efficacy. Liberal fluid intake must be insured if these doses are required. If a child receiving ibuprofen is known to suffer secondary gastritis, the preadministration or coadministration of omeprazole (Prilosec), 20 mg daily, may be preventive.

TABLE 3 Symptomatic Treatment of Acute Headache

Generic Name (Trade Name)	Dosage, Route, Regimen	Maximum Dose	Dose Formulation	Common Adverse Reactions	Comments
Analgesics					
Acetaminophen (Tylenol)	10–15 mg/kg/dose q4h	500 mg q4h	Tablets: 325 mg, 500 mg		Hepatic damage in acute overdose
Ibuprofen	10 mg/kg/dose q4h	800 mg q8h	Tablets: 50 mg, 100 mg, 200 mg, 400 mg, 600 mg, 800 mg Syrup: 100 mg/5 mL	Gastric irritation	Hydrate well
Naproxen sodium (Aleve)	5–7 mg/kg/dose q8–12h	7 mg/kg q8h	Tablets: 250 mg, 375 mg, 500 mg	Gastric irritation	Hydrate well
Acetaminophen, caffeine, butalbitol (Fioricet)	1 tablet per dose q4–6h	6 tablets per day	Tablet	Sedation	Use in children older than 10 years of age
Sedatives and Muscle Relaxants					
Diazepam (Valium)	<30 kg: 0.1 mg/kg/day >30 kg: 0.2–0.3 mg/kg/day q4–6h dosing	0.3 mg/kg/day	Tablets: 2 mg, 5 mg, 10 mg	Sedation	
Tizanidine (Zanaflex)	1 mg tid; increase prn to 2 mg tid	3 mg tid	Tablets: 2 mg, 4 mg, 6 mg	Sedation, postural hypotension, elevated liver enzymes	Dosage limited by deep sedation or postural hypotension
Antiemetics					
Trimethobenzamide (Tigan)	5 mg/kg/dose by rectal suppository in tid or qid dosing	600 mg/day	Suppositories: 100 mg, 200 mg	Sedation, extrapyramidal symptoms	Diphenhydramine (Benadryl) alleviates extrapyramidal symptoms
Odansetron (Zofran)	6–12 years: 8 mg q8h >12 years: 12 mg q8h	36 mg/day	Oral disintegrating tablets (melt): 4 mg, 8 mg	Headache, diarrhea, elevated liver enzymes	

bid, twice daily; MAO, monoamine oxidase; od, once daily; prn, as needed; qid, four times daily; tid, three times daily.

Treatment of Tension-Type Headache

Treatment of tension-type headache is designed to alleviate anxiety, tension, or depression. Therefore the use of pharmacotherapeutic agents should be highly selective and combined with psychotherapy, regardless of whether the patient is referred for psychotherapy on a formal basis. The limiting factor in the use of so-called muscle relaxants, including diazepam, is drowsiness and, occasionally, a paradoxical increase in tension. Some of the compounds effective for the treatment of migraine are appropriate for tension-type headache, including analgesics, NSAIDs, and amitriptyline. Tizanidine has been used effectively in tension-type headache, although it is unknown whether this muscle relaxant is effective as a result of its antispastic or antinociceptive properties. It is an α-adrenergic agent, and the chief dose-limiting factor is sedation.

Overuse of these drugs is a risk if the physician fails to recognize that "rebound headache" requires a drug-free period rather than the immediate reintroduction of a new analgesic or sedative drug. This practice at times promotes or aggravates the occurrence of refractory, chronic daily headache.

Prognosis

An optimistic outlook for headache control or spontaneous remission is justified in all varieties of nonsymptomatic headache in children, although some will require dedicated effort for optimal control.

Common Pitfalls

- Under- or overemphasis of social and psychological issues.
- Under- or overuse of ancillary studies such as cranial neuroimaging. If migraine is strongly suspected, a trial of therapy is warranted. If abortive and/or prophylactic treatment is ineffective, investigation for symptomatic headache should be more complete, not withstanding the apparent diagnosis.
- Failure to use adequate dosage of therapeutic drugs is common. Adolescents frequently tolerate higher doses, such as the 20-mg dose of sumatriptan nasal spray, or as much as 200 mg per day of propranolol.
- Failure to use combinations of drugs in refractory headache with associated symptoms.

Communication and Counseling

- A headache diary provides an objective account of the number and duration of headaches and the other vital diagnostic features.
- The patient should clearly be instructed when to call or revisit if atypical features develop or if the child fails to respond well to treatment.
- The dosage of medication, the frequency of administration, and the possible side effects should be clearly delineated.

- The manner in which to use combined pharmacotherapeutic agents should be clearly outlined in regard to dosage, frequency of coadministration, and possible side effects.

SUGGESTED READINGS

1. Anequin D, Tourniaire B, Massiou H: Migraine and headache in childhood and adolescence. Pediatr Clin North Am 47:617–631, 2000. **This is a useful and very readable discussion of pediatric headache.**
2. Headache Classification Committee of the International Headache Society: Classification and Diagnostic Criteria for Headache Disorders, Cranial Neuralgias and Facial Pain. Cephalalgia 8(Suppl 7):9–73, 1988. **The International Headache Society classification provides the widely accepted basis for the study and management of different types of headache.**
3. Hermann C, Kim M, Blanchard EB: Behavioral and prophylactic pharmacologic intervention studies of pediatric migraine: An exploratory meta-analysis. Pain 60:239–256, 1994. **Analysis of the validity and usefulness of studies of pharmacologic and non-pharmacologic management of pediatric migraine.**
4. Hershey AD, Powers SW, Vockell AL, et al: Effectiveness of topiramate in the prevention of childhood headaches. Headache 42:810–818, 2002. **This study indicates the efficacy of topiramate, an antiepileptic and neuroprotective drug, for the prevention of pediatric migraine.**
5. Lewis DW, Diamond S, Scott D, et al: Prophylactic treatment of childhood migraine. Headache 44:230–237, 2004. **A general overview of various recorded approaches to the prophylaxis of childhood migraine.**
6. Lewis DW, Kellstein D, Dahl G, et al: Children's ibuprofen suspension for the acute treatment of pediatric migraine. Headache 42:780–786, 2002. **The time-honored efficacy of ibuprofen for the treatment of acute headache in children is vindicated.**
7. Millichap JG, Yee MM: The diet factor in pediatric and adolescent migraine (Review). Ped Neurol 28:9–15, 2003. **Description of a variety of perceived, often undocumented, dietary features of migraine.**
8. Rothner AD, Winner P, Webster CJ, et al: Adolescent migraine sumatriptan nasal spray is effective and well tolerated. Ann Neurol 56(Suppl 8):S87, 2004. **This work established sumatriptan nasal spray as the treatment of choice for abortive treatment of acute migraine in children.**
9. Seradoglu G, Erhan E, Tekgul H, et al: Sodium valproate prophylaxis in childhood migraine. Headache 42:819–822, 2002. **Documentation of a role for valproate in the prevention of pediatric migraine.**
10. Silberstein SD, Neto W, Schmitt J, et al: MIG–001 study group topiramate in migraine prevention: Results of a large controlled trial. Arch Neurol 61:490–495, 2004. **Good evidence for the efficacy of topiramate for migraine prophylaxis.**
11. Tepper SJ, Rapaport AM, Sheftell FD: Mechanisms of action of the 5-HT$_{1b-1d}$ receptor agonists. Arch Neurol 59:1084–1088, 2002. **This paper provides evidence for the manner in which 5-HT receptor agonists function to provide for headache relief.**
12. Victor S, Ryan SW: Drugs for preventing migraine headaches in children (Review). Cochrane Database Syst Rev 4:CD002761, 2003. **A review of drugs used for migraine prophylaxis in children.**
13. Winner P, Lewis D, Visser WH, et al: Rizatriptan 5 mg for the acute treatment of migraine in adolescents: A randomized, double blind, placebo controlled study. Headache 42:49–55, 2002. **Rizatriptan is effective in aborting acute headache in children.**
14. Winner P, Rothner AD (eds): Headache in children and adolescents, London: BC Decker, 2001. **The experience and reason of Drs. Winner and Rothner make for an excellent overview of pediatric headache in regard to classification, recognition, and management.**
15. Winner P, Rothner AD, Saper J: A randomized, double blind, placebo controlled study of sumatriptan nasal spray in the treatment of acute migraine in adolescents. Pediatrics 106:989–997, 2000. **A controlled study of sumatriptan nasal spray indicates that this treatment effectively aborts acute pediatric migraine.**

The Limping Child

George H. Thompson and Theresa A. Hennessey

KEY CONCEPTS

- Limping is a common childhood complaint.
- Evaluation begins with a history and physical examination. Radiographic studies of the injured or painful area are usually necessary. Occasionally, advanced imaging such as a CT or MRI are necessary. Hematologic studies are necessary for suspected infectious, neoplastic, or inflammatory disorders.
- The differential diagnosis of limping is extensive but can be condensed based on whether the limp is painful (antalgic) or painless (Trendelenburg) and the age of the patient (toddler, child, or adolescent).
- Appropriate treatment is dependent on an accurate diagnosis.

A limp in a child is a common complaint in a pediatrician's office. Evaluation begins with a thorough history, followed by a physical examination and usually radiographic studies. Occasionally, hematologic laboratory studies are also necessary. Most causes of limping in children involve the lower extremity. However, spinal disorders, such as intervertebral discitis, can also produce limping or difficulty walking (Box 1).

An antalgic gait due to pain in the lower extremity, and occasionally the spine or pelvis, is the most common cause of limping. The limp is characterized by a shortened stance phase on the affected limb. In an effort to minimize pain, the child will spend as little time as possible standing or weight bearing on the involved extremity. Simultaneously, the swing phase of the unaffected extremity will be quickened. The source of the pain may be at any location in the extremity—bones, muscles, soft tissue, or joints. Painful limping is predominantly due to acute processes, such as trauma, infection, neoplasia, and rheumatologic disorders.

Painless limping, or a Trendelenburg gait, is characteristic of weakened hip abductor muscles. The hip abductor muscles on the involved side cannot effectively support the weight of the body, resulting in the characteristic waddle with a truncal lean toward the affected side. Because this type of limping is painless, the stance and swing phases are normal. This type of limping is commonly observed with congenital or developmental disorders, such as developmental dysplasia of the hip (DDH), congenital coxa vara, or neuromuscular disorders. Children with cerebral palsy (spastic hemiplegia or diplegia) may have an associated painless limp caused by muscle spasticity and concomitant weakness of the antagonist muscles. Lower extremity length discrepancies (LELD) are another common cause of Trendelenburg gait. These are usually well compensated until the difference exceeds 2 centimeters, at which point a toe-walking or equinus gait develops. Box 2 presents the differential diagnosis of LELD.

BOX 1 Differential Diagnosis of Limping

Toddler (1 to 3 years)
- Painful Limp
  - Septic arthritis and osteomyelitis—hip and knee
  - Transient monoarticular synovitis of the hip
  - Occult trauma—toddler's fracture of the tibia
  - Neoplasia—benign and malignant lesions
- Painless Limp
  - Developmental dysplasia of the hip (DDH)
  - Neuromuscular disorder
  - Cerebral palsy
  - Lower extremity length discrepancies (LELD)

Child (3 to 10 years)
- Painful Limp
  - Septic arthritis and osteomyelitis—hip and knee
  - Transient monoarticular synovitis of the hip
  - Trauma
  - Rheumatologic disorders—juvenile rheumatoid arthritis (JRA)
  - Intervertebral discitis
  - Legg-Calvé-Perthes disease (LCPD)
  - Neoplasia—benign and malignant lesions
- Painless Limp
  - Developmental dysplasia of the hip (DDH)
  - Legg-Calvé-Perthes disease (LCPD)
  - Lower extremity length discrepancies (LELD)
  - Neuromuscular disorder
  - Cerebral palsy
  - Muscular dystrophy

Adolescent (11 years to skeletal maturity)
- Painful Limp
  - Septic arthritis and osteomyelitis
  - Trauma
  - Rheumatologic disorders—juvenile rheumatoid arthritis
  - Intervertebral discitis
  - Spondylolysis/spondylolisthesis
  - Slipped capital femoral epiphysis (SCFE)
  - Neoplasia—benign and malignant lesions
  - Tarsal coalition
- Painless Limp
  - Slipped capital femoral epiphysis (SCFE)
  - Developmental dysplasia of the hip, acetabular dysplasia
  - Lower extremity length discrepancies (LELD)
  - Neuromuscular disorder

Adapted from Thompson GH: Gait disturbances. In Kliegman RM, Greenbaum LA, Lye PS (eds): *Practical Strategies in Pediatric Diagnosis and Therapy*, 2nd ed. Philadelphia: Elsevier, 2004, pp 823–843.

However, it is possible for certain developmental disorders to have both painful and painless limping during different phases of the disease process. Legg-Calvé-Perthes disease (LCPD) and slipped capital femoral epiphysis (SCFE) may produce painful limping early in the disease process and a painless limp following resolution. The latter are commonly because of a LELD.

Expert Opinion on Management Issues

The most important aspect of management of the child with limping is establishing the correct diagnosis. A careful history, physical examination using the categories of painful and painless limp, and the age of

---

BOX 2 Common Causes of Lower Extremity Length Discrepancy

Congenital
- Proximal femoral focal deficiency (PFFD)
- Coxa vara
- Hemiatrophy and hemihypertrophy
- Skeletal dysplasia

Developmental
- Developmental dysplasia of the hip (DDH)
- Legg-Calvé-Perthes disease (LCPD)
- Slipped capital femoral epiphysis (SCFE)
- Neoplasia

Neuromuscular
- Poliomyelitis
- Cerebral palsy (spastic hemiplegia)
- Myelodysplasia

Infectious—Inflammation
- Pyogenic osteomyelitis with physeal damage
- Rheumatologic disorders

Trauma
- Physeal injury with premature closure
- Overgrowth
- Malunion

Tumor
- Physeal destruction
- Radiation-induced physeal injury
- Overgrowth

---

the patient will usually allow a relatively accurate tentative diagnosis. The final diagnosis can usually be confirmed with appropriate radiographic evaluation and possibly hematologic laboratory studies.

Common Pitfalls

The major pitfall in the management of a child with limping is delaying or making an erroneous diagnosis. Although transient monarticular synovitis of the hip is probably the most common cause of limping in children, there are numerous other causes of limping. Each child must be carefully and individually evaluated. Referred pain is also a major problem. It must be remembered that nontraumatic anterior thigh and knee pain is most likely because of hip pathology. The hip must be carefully evaluated clinically and radiographically in this situation.

Communication and Counseling

All toddlers, children, and adolescents with a limp, particularly one that is acute in onset, should be evaluated by a orthopedic surgeon. They are most familiar with the causes of limping and the appropriate diagnostic tests and treatment. Some of these will require emergent surgical intervention, such as acute osteomyelitis or septic arthritis involving the hip joint. Many will require only observation and symptomatic treatment, although others may be managed medically, particularly those with rheumatologic disorders.

Causes of chronic limping may require involvement from other specialists, particularly for confirmation of the diagnosis. In particular, neuromuscular disorders may require a pediatric neurology evaluation and possibly a genetic evaluation.

SUGGESTED READINGS

1. Copley L, Dormans JP: Benign Pediatric Bone Tumors. Pediatr Clin North Am 43:949–966, 1996. **Differential diagnosis, evaluation, and treatment of benign musculoskeletal neoplasms in children.**
2. Early SD, Kay RM, Tolo VT: Childhood diskitis. J Am Acad Orthop Surg 11:413–420, 2003. **Discusses variable presenting symptoms, evaluation, and treatment of children with disc space infections.**
3. Himelstein BP, Dormans JP: Malignant bone tumors of childhood. Pediatr Clin North Am 43:967–984, 1996. **Differential diagnosis, evaluation, and treatment of malignant musculoskeletal neoplasms in children.**
4. Kocher MS, Zurakowski D, Kasser JR: Differentiating between septic arthritis and transient synovitis of the hip in children: An evidence based clinical prediction algorithm. J Bone Joint Surg Am 81:1662–1670, 1999. **Identifies four independent multivariate clinical predictors to differentiate between septic arthritis and transient synovitis of the hip. These include fever, non–weight-bearing, erythrocyte sedimentation rate greater than 40 mm/h, and white blood cell count greater than 12,000 per mm³.**
5. Leet AI, Skaggs DL: Evaluation of the acutely limping child. Am Fam Phys 61:1011–1018, 2000. **Discusses the differential diagnosis, evaluation, and treatment of the child with an acute onset limp.**
6. Myers M, Myers MT, Thompson GH: Imaging the child with a limp. Pediatr Clin North Am 44:637–658, 1997. **Discusses the indications for imaging studies in the child with a limp.**
7. Thompson GH: Gait disturbances. In Kliegman RM, Greenbaum LA, Lye PS (eds): Practical Strategies in Pediatric Diagnosis Therapy, 2nd ed. Philadelphia: Elsevier, 2004, pp 823–843. **Extensive review of gait disturbances in children including torsional variations (in-toeing and out-toeing), toe-walking (equinus gait), and limping.**

Syncope

Mark E. Alexander

KEY CONCEPTS

- Typical neurocardiogenic syncope is exceptionally common. It is characterized by a prodrome of dizziness, warmth, and visual changes prior to transient loss of consciousness and recovery, with residual symptoms of fatigue, headache, and nausea. This episode is typically associated with marked pallor. Events are generally associated with standing or a clear trigger.
- There are frequently less severe presyncopal symptoms between events that may dominate the presentation. These symptoms often include dizziness and palpitations from heart rate swings.
- Multiple systemic illnesses and some medications may predispose to neurocardiogenic syncope. These are generally apparent on initial evaluation.
- Prolonged periods of "loss of consciousness" with reasonable vital signs while supine are not consistent with either cardiac syncope or neurocardiogenic syncope.
- Event history, past medical history, family history of syncope and cardiac events, supine and standing heart rate

and blood pressures, physical examination, and electrocardiogram provide an effective initial screen.

- With both a limited ability to recreate symptoms and an excessive potential to induce faints in normal adolescents, head-up tilt testing is not needed to make a diagnosis of neurocardiogenic syncope.
- A 5- to 10-minute period of resting either supine or with legs up will allow effective recovery in most patients. Early standing may trigger repeated episodes.
- The vast majority of patients with neurocardiogenic syncope respond to fluids, education, and prevention. Medication is needed in only a small minority.
- Syncope associated with an active arrhythmia should be managed using standard emergency algorithms.
- Initial evaluation is focused as much on excluding serious but rare cardiac syncope as confirming the presumptive diagnosis of neurocardiogenic syncope.
- Any of the following symptoms—history of exercise as a trigger of syncope, associated injury or incontinence, a past history of heart disease, a family history of sudden death at younger than 40 years of age, a family history of cardiomyopathy, long QT syndrome or related diseases, an abnormal cardiac exam, or abnormal electrocardiogram—should trigger cardiology referral.

Both common *neurocardiogenic syncope* (NCS), which is fainting, and rare, potentially life-threatening episodes of *cardiac syncope*, are abrupt and transient losses of consciousness that result from decreased blood pressure and decreased cerebral blood flow. The presentations of each type of syncope can be similar. In addition the presentation of syncope can overlap with those of seizure disorders or other neurologic events, some metabolic and endocrine disturbances, and hysterical or psychogenic spells.

Neurocardiogenic syncope occurs in as many as 25% of the population, with a peak incidence in adolescent females. This common and typically benign physiology has many synonyms, each of which describes a subgroup of patients. NCS, as the name suggests, represents the interaction of the voluntary and involuntary nervous system with the heart and blood vessels in controlling heart rate, blood pressure, and hence brain blood flow. The orthostatic stress of standing induces a coordinated series of responses: venous pooling, which decreases blood pressure and cardiac filling, followed by sympathetic activation, and decreased vagal or parasympathetic nervous activity. Together these responses will mildly increase blood pressure and heart rate stabilizing both at effective levels. Exaggerated or ineffective responses at any of those mechanical and reflex levels can lead to a cyclic loss of effective homeostasis and syncope. Marked and inappropriate vagal activation leads to bradycardia, and a decrease in catecholamine stimulation can result in hypotension and collapse. Partially effective responses to this physiology can result in symptoms of dizziness and sometimes palpitations and near-syncope. Rather than viewing NCS as a specific disorder of one aspect of the physiology, it is more accurate to view NCS as a usually temporary derangement of cardiovascular control.

The clinical presentation of typical NCS is a transient collapse that usually starts with the patient upright and is preceded by presyncopal symptoms of dizziness, visual changes of visual spots or visual dimming, diaphoresis, and pallor. This presentation rarely progresses to abrupt collapse with myoclonic jerks, and almost never includes urinary or fecal incontinence. Recovery is prompt, although residual symptoms of headache and fatigue are typical.

Cardiac syncope is the result of hemodynamic collapse secondary to combinations of pathologic arrhythmia and mechanical obstruction or myopathy. Specific patient history and physician examination increase the probability that an episode represents cardiac syncope, really a self-limited life-threatening event. Although rare, those episodes require prompt evaluation. Any of the following symptoms—history of exercise as a trigger of syncope, associated injury or incontinence, a past history of heart disease, a family history of sudden death at younger than 40 years of age, a family history of cardiomyopathy, long QT syndrome or related diseases, an abnormal cardiac exam, or abnormal electrocardiogram (ECG)—should trigger a cardiology referral.

Expert Opinion on Management Issues

The majority of patients do not require referral (Table 1). Initial evaluation consists of a careful event, past medical, and family medical history; orthostatic (supine and standing, without sitting) heart rate and blood pressure; detailed cardiac examination and screening neurology examination; and an ECG. A typical history and normal physical examination, family history, and ECG suggest the diagnosis of NCS. The majority of children should be followed in their primary care setting without additional testing. When the presentation is highly suggestive of either a specific cardiac or neurologic diagnosis appropriate referrals should be facilitated. When cardiac syncope is suspected the child should be restricted from sports until evaluated.

School-age children and adolescents have a high degree of orthostatic intolerance. Even without a history of syncope, up to 40% to 80% of adolescents will have syncope or marked presyncope induced with tilt-table testing. With this poor specificity, tilt testing should be reserved for selected patients in which there is diagnostic uncertainty.

PREVENTIVE MEASURES

Specific counseling on behavioral maneuvers to prevent neurally mediated syncope may prevent future spells. If patients modify episodes, the subsequent course will further inform the diagnosis. The principles of nonpharmacologic management include increased hydration, increased but not excessive sodium intake, awareness of presyncopal symptoms, and learning isometric and other antigravity maneuvers. Fluid intake should be sufficient to keep the urine relatively dilute, typically about 2 liters/day for an adolescent. Patients can be shown how to squat or perform isometric leg contractions or isometric tightening of the shoulder muscles while palpating the radial pulse to give immediate feedback. Each of these physical countermaneuvers permits

TABLE 1   Referral with Pediatric Spells

Cardiology	Known heart disease
	Family history of heart disease
	Exercise trigger
	Abnormal ECG
	Abnormal cardiac examination
	Abrupt onset/offset
	Injury/incontinence without sustained seizures
	Repeated episodes with negative neurology evaluation
Neurology	Focal onset
	Sustained motor seizures
	Repeated episodes with negative cardiology evaluation
Psychiatry	Repeated/bizarre episodes without physiologic correlate
	Refractory syncope with reasonable drug therapy
	Severe situational syncope
No referral needed	Toddler or adolescent
	Infrequent
	Typical syncope
	Prodrome
	No injury
	Negative family history
	Normal examination
	Normal ECG
	Acute illness

ECG, electrocardiogram.

rapid increases in blood pressure and may abort a subsequent faint. Weight-bearing aerobic exercise may further decrease chronic symptoms.

DRUGS AND OTHER THERAPY

A small minority of patients with repeated syncope benefit from drug therapy (Table 2). Data, particularly pediatric data, supporting pharmacologic management are limited. Popular choices include the mineralocorticoid fludrocortisone, which enhances sodium retention; β-blockers, which may blunt excessive reflex response; and the short-acting peripheral α-agonist midodrine hydrochloride, which increases vascular resistance. Pediatric experience suggests fludrocortisone and β-blockers are comparable in efficacy.

A small minority of patients with significant sinus pauses from pallid breath-holding spells or convulsive neurally mediated syncope will benefit from permanent pacemakers. Those patients may not achieve complete resolution of their symptoms.

For cardiac syncope, therapy is directed at the specific clinical substrate.

Common Pitfalls

NCS is a benign and almost always self-limited event. Patients with recurrent episodes will return to their

TABLE 2   Popular Therapy Options for Neurally Mediated Syncope in Adolescents and Older Children

Therapy	Specific Guidelines	Comments
Hydration	↑ Sodium intake	Aiming for dilute urine
	↑ Fluids (water)	No cost
	↓ Caffeine	No side effects
	Possibility of a prescription	Empowers patient
Physical countermaneuvers	Demonstrate in office:	Advantages as above
	Squatting	Rapid ↑ blood pressure
	Leg tensing	Transient effects
	Shoulder tensing	
Fludrocortisone	0.1 mg qd to start	Pure mineralocorticoid
		Once daily
		Low side effects
		Slow onset
		Mixed data
		At higher doses:
		↓ K$^+$
		↑ Blood pressure
β-blockers	Variable	Complex logic
		Mixed data
		Mixed side effects
Midodrine hydrochloride	5 mg every 4 h when awake	Peripheral α-agonist
	May titrate up	Rapid (30-min) effect
		Short (4–6 hr) duration
		Need motivated patient
		Most measurable drug therapy
Pacemaker	Dual chamber if possible	Rarely needed
		Often only partially effective
		Repeated correlation with sinus pauses

qd, every day.

primary care physician; hence there is little risk in under-managing a single typical syncopal event.

Although rare, sudden death does occur in children. Serious and occult conditions may manifest with syncope. Modern therapy options may prevent many of these events. Failure to consider those pathologic diagnoses in the initial history and evaluation misses an opportunity to identify important disease. History, family history, physical examination, and ECG will identify the overwhelming majority of patients who require further evaluation.

The dramatic nature of initial syncopal events may provoke excessive anxiety in families. Appropriate reassurance and education may limit this anxiety.

Some patients with infrequent true syncopal events (or even no fainting episodes) will have frequent presyncope that benefits from therapy. They often demonstrate orthostatic tachycardia without orthostatic hypotension.

Communication and Counseling

When the evaluation suggests that the syncopal spell is self-limited, specific reassurance that the episodes are not life-threatening is useful. It is important to understand the specific fears the family has regarding the symptoms. Several hours of rest and decreased activity, although not always required, is reasonable after a syncopal spell. Subsequently, activity can return to normal. Patients with high-risk presentations of syncope should generally avoid competitive athletics until evaluated by a cardiologist.

The adolescent who is driving should be cautioned to pull over if dizzy or presyncopal. Patients with more abrupt symptoms, possible seizures, or potential cardiac syncope should avoid driving until further evaluation. In some states they are unlicensed for several months after an event.

Follow-up for isolated or infrequent NCS is generally flexible. Specific guidelines to seek additional care focus on the presence of repeated spells, with exercise, sustained palpitations, injury, and incontinence increasing frequency of symptoms.

SUGGESTED READINGS

1. Alexander ME, Walsh EP, Saul JP, et al: Value of programmed ventricular stimulation in patients with congenital heart disease. J Cardiovasc Electrophysiol 10:1033–1044, 1999. **In patients with congenital heart disease and syncope or other serious symptoms, detailed cardiac testing helps stratify future risk of mortality and life-threatening arrhythmia.**
2. DiVasta AD, Alexander ME: Fainting freshmen and sinking sophomores: Cardiovascular issues of the adolescent. Curr Opin Pediatr 16:350–356, 2004. **Up-to-date review of pediatric and adolescent syncope including focus on problematic patients who are athletes, struggle with fatigue, or have eating disorders.**
3. Driscoll DJ, Jacobsen SJ, Porter CJ, Wollan PC: Syncope in children and adolescents. J Am Coll Cardiol 29:1039–1045, 1997. **Population-based study on the incidence of children seeking care for syncope in Olmstead County.**
4. Morris JA, Blount RL, Brown RT, et al: Association of parental psychological and behavioral factors and children's syncope. J Consult Clin Psychol 69:851–857, 2001. **In patients who had recurrent syncope, the frequency and intensity of their symptoms was strongly associated with parental factors.**
5. Salim MA: Effectiveness of fludrocortisone and salt in preventing syncope recurrence in children: A double-blind, placebo-controlled, randomized trial. J Am Coll Cardiol 45:484–488, 2005. **When multiple treatments are suggested, the role of placebo and supportive care may be considerable. In a small, double-blind study of adolescents with syncope and positive head-up tilt tests, patients treated with 0.1 mg/day of fludrocortisone and salt had more recurrent syncope than those treated with placebo.**
6. Scott WA, Pongiglione G, Bromberg BI, et al: Randomized comparison of atenolol and fludrocortisone acetate in the treatment of pediatric neurally mediated syncope. Am J Cardiol 76:400–402, 1995. **Both atenolol and fludrocortisone seem effective, yet neither is perfect (and neither may be needed).**
7. Stewart JM: Orthostatic intolerance in pediatrics. J Pediatr 140:404–411, 2002. **A thorough summary of the current understanding of symptomatic and asymptomatic orthostasis.**

Abdominal Pain: Approach to a Diagnosis

Nader N. Youssef and Joel R. Rosh

KEY CONCEPTS

- Acute abdominal pain should be rapidly evaluated to exclude emergent surgical pathology.
- Chronic abdominal pain can have many etiologies that are broadly divided into organic and functional categories.
- Chronic or recurrent abdominal pain in children and adolescents is common and should be approached through a model that considers biologic, psychological, and social factors.
- On the basis of a detailed history and physical examination augmented by judicious use of laboratory testing, one can usually diagnose the cause of chronic abdominal pain thereby minimizing the need for invasive testing.
- Treatment strategies for most organic causes of chronic abdominal pain are better defined than those for functional etiologies. This can lead to frustration on the part of families and care providers in cases of chronic functional abdominal pain.
- A history and physical examination are usually adequate to differentiate functional abdominal pain from organic disease processes.
- Sudden onset of abdominal pain that manifests with other worrisome signs including fever, vomiting, or change in bowel habits should be evaluated in an urgent manner no matter what the age of the patient.
- Persistent abdominal pain after a recent gastroenteritis or a course of antibiotics is not uncommon and may indicate a "sensitized" intestinal tract with a lower threshold for pain perception.
- Children with abdominal pain should not be treated with medications (e.g., over-the-counter antacids) for symptomatic relief of abdominal pain. Treatment, if any, should be based on etiology.

This chapter is intended to cover the essentials of the diagnostic approach to abdominal pain in children. Correct decisions when managing abdominal pain are based on careful clinical assessment. An accurate history and a detailed examination will provide more information than a multitude of tests and investigations. When a thorough history and physical examination are performed, focused laboratory and imaging evaluation can aid in differentiating organic and nonorganic causes for abdominal pain and guide further management. The causes of painful intraabdominal conditions vary with age of the child, and serious cases are relatively rare. Congenital gastrointestinal disorders occur in 1 of 5000 live births. Appendicitis, the most common cause of serious abdominal emergency, has a lifetime risk of 8.6% in male patients and 6.7% in female patients, but only 0.1% of children annually require an operation. In contrast, approximately 15% to 20% of school-age children are brought to the physician because of abdominal pain of indeterminate origin.

Expert Opinion on Management Issues

Abdominal pain is a broad topic that covers both medical and surgical disease processes. A carefully taken history is the key to establishing a diagnosis (Box 1).

Emphasis must be placed on the parents' interpretation of the child's symptoms, particularly for the very young infant. However, one should never neglect to ask the child directly for additional facts to confirm the history obtained from the parents. Older children should be allowed to provide their own history, with the parents contributing and elaborating as required.

DIFFERENTIATING ETIOLOGY OF ABDOMINAL PAIN BY HISTORY

Organic

The onset of abdominal pain may be acute or insidious. Sudden-onset severe pain may appear with acute ischemic events such as volvulus, intussusception, and testicular or ovarian torsion. Progressive pain may be associated with appendicitis or constipation. Localization of pain is important. Visceral pain (colic, obstruction) is referred to the region of the somatic segments of the viscus involved (epigastrium for foregut, umbilicus for midgut, hypogastrium for hindgut). This finding is less reliable in young children, who invariably point to the umbilicus. Older children usually are able to localize the pain with more accuracy. Parietal peritoneal pain specifically localizes to the site of the irritation and indicates persistent inflammation with guarding on examination.

The pattern and nature of the pain can vary enormously. It may be intermittent, continuous, or colicky. Several illnesses, especially appendicitis, begin with vague abdominal discomfort. Respiration or movement of the child often increases the pain, indicating generalized peritoneal inflammation and parietal peritoneal pain. Pelvic inflammation may result in painful micturition and vague lower abdominal discomfort that occasionally may be relieved after defecation. Aggravating and relieving factors such as lying down and vomiting are important. The child's activity level can aid in establishing the diagnosis. Writhing may be suggestive of colic; a quiet, still child may have peritonitis.

Night pain or pain on awakening can suggest a peptic origin, although pain that occurs in the evening or during dinner is a feature of constipation. Children often do not complain of heartburn, but other features of peptic disease include early satiety, nausea, and the supra-esophageal or respiratory complications of gastroesophageal reflux. A diary that lists diet, symptoms, and associated features for 3 to 7 days is invaluable because it will indicate potential causes of the symptoms, such as exposure to lactose or the failure to have a normal bowel movement. The diary also should include any intervention initiated by the child or the parents.

The review of systems should focus on features that may be related to abdominal pain, such as documented weight loss or gain, linear growth, fever, joint complaints, oral sores, and rash. The presence of one or more of these signs suggests an inflammatory process such as seen in inflammatory bowel disease or celiac disease. The respiratory complications of gastroesophageal reflux, including chronic cough, reactive airway disease, or persistent laryngitis, may be more prominent than emesis or chest pain. Box 2 lists the key clues ("red flags") to potential organic pathology for abdominal pain.

A careful review of recent medications may turn up potential side effects, for example, antibiotics may predispose the patient to intestinal bacterial overgrowth, acne medications may induce esophagitis, and tricyclic antidepressants may cause constipation.

A family history of peptic disease, irritable or inflammatory bowel disease, pancreatitis, biliary disease, or migraine should be sought.

The chronology of symptoms should also be noted in the history. When abdominal pain, diarrhea and/or vomiting are present, try to determine which symptoms appeared first. If abdominal pain is the first symptom followed by other gastrointestinal symptoms, a "surgical

---

BOX 1 Approach to Abdominal Pain: Key Considerations in History Taking

- How long have you had the pain?
- What were you doing when the pain started?
- Did the pain start suddenly or develop gradually?
- How severe is your pain? Rate your pain on a scale of 1 to 10.
- Is your pain generalized or localized? If you have localized pain, where is it located?
- How would you describe your pain—cramping, a steady ache, burning, or tearing sensation?
- Have you had other symptoms, such as nausea, vomiting, constipation, diarrhea, a change in urination, or fever?
- Have you had this type of pain before? If so, did you see a health professional?
- What makes the pain better? What makes the pain worse?
- Have you recently traveled outside of the United States?
- Have you had any untreated well, stream, or lake water?
- Have you taken any antibiotics recently?

abdomen" may need to be ruled out. Organic causes for both gastrointestinal and nongastrointestinal causes for abdominal pain are provided Table 1.

Whenever possible, a few minutes should be taken alone with adolescents to address concerns in the absence of parents and to elicit honest answers about sexual issues, psychological fears, and any disruption to lifestyle caused by the parents' interventions. The influence of pain on the child's daily activities can be assessed through questions about school attendance, athletic endeavors, and peer relationships.

Nonorganic

Nonorganic, chronic abdominal pain, previously termed recurrent abdominal pain is often associated with a functional bowel disorder (FBD). This is abdominal pain that is continuous, persistent, or intermittent over a period of a few months to years. The pain may wax and wane, with some days being better than others. This is abdominal pain that is not associated with worrisome signs (see Box 2). Diagnostic criteria known as *Rome II*, which were developed in a consensus meeting of experts in

Rome in 1998, have been established for abdominal pain associated with functional gastrointestinal disorders. The most common functional causes of abdominal pain include irritable bowel syndrome (IBS), nonulcer dyspepsia, and functional abdominal pain. Symptoms consistent with IBS are one of the most common FBDs, occurring in 14% of all high school students and 6% of all middle school students.

There is evidence that the pain and discomfort of IBS can be because of hyperalgesia and allodynia of the gut. Although in hyperalgesia a painful stimulus is perceived as even more painful, in allodynia a nonpainful stimulus becomes painful. A noxious stimulus applied to a particular area of the gut may sensitize primary afferent fibers and nociceptors of adjacent areas resulting in painful sensations with a low-intensity stimulus.

EXAMINATION OF THE CHILD WITH ABDOMINAL PAIN

The overall appearance of the patient can be quite helpful. Although a patient with ureteral lithiasis will writhe in agony, the patient with an intestinal perforation and diffuse peritonitis will usually lie very still. Patients who are relieved by leaning forward may have pancreatitis. The facial expression of the patient may signal whether the pain is crampy or constant in nature.

Examination of the whole patient is mandatory to evaluate the patient with abdominal pain. The head and neck should be examined for intraoral lesions, scleral icterus,

---

BOX 2 Avoiding Pitfalls: "Red Flags" in Association with Organic Abdominal Pain

- Age younger than 5 years
- Pain further away from the umbilicus
- Fever
- Emesis
- Weight loss
- Growth deceleration
- Pain awakening the child at night
- Blood in stool
- Perianal disease
- Elevated erythrocyte sedimentation rate
- Elevated white count
- Hypoalbuminemia
- Anemia
- Dysuria, hematuria
- Joint involvement
- Family history of inflammatory bowel disease
- Family history of celiac disease

TABLE 1 Causes for Organic Abdominal Pain

Gastrointestinal	Nongastrointestinal
Enteric infection/mesenteric adenitis	Renal calculi
Constipation/acute fecal impaction	Pyelonephritis
Carbohydrate malabsorption/bloating	Acute hydronephrosis
Intestinal ileus	Mononucleosis
Gastritis/peptic ulcer disease	Nephritis
Appendicitis	Ovarian or testicular
Hepatitis	torsion
Cholelithiasis/cholecystitis	Psoas abscess
Intussusception	Tubo-ovarian abscess
Pancreatitis	Ectopic pregnancy
Celiac disease	Pneumonia
Inflammatory bowel disease	Sickle cell crisis
Vasculitis/Henoch-Schönlein purpura	Lymphoma
Porphyria	Trauma
Intestinal abnormalities (malrotation, volvulus, hernia, adhesions)	

TABLE 2 Investigations in the Evaluation of Organic Abdominal Pain and "Red Flags"

Investigation	Working Diagnosis
Complete blood count	Anemia-associated inflammatory bowel disease or celiac disease
Comprehensive metabolic panel	Hypoalbuminemia indicating malabsorption seen with inflammatory bowel disease and celiac disease
Urinalysis	Urinary tract infection, nephritis, renal stones
Tissue transglutaminase, anti-endomysial antibodies, total IgA level	Celiac disease
Stool studies for bacteria and protozoa	Bacterial infection, *Giardia*, *Clostridium difficile*
Lactose breath test	Carbohydrate malabsorption
Amylase and lipase	Pancreatitis
Obstructive liver enzymes	Gallbladder dysfunction/gall stones
Abdominal x-ray (flat plate)	Occult constipation/renal stones
Abdominal ultrasound	Evaluation for organomegaly, gallstones, hydronephrosis, ascites
Upper gastrointestinal series (contrast study)	Intestinal anomalies including malrotation, volvulus, and duplication cysts
Small bowel series (contrast study)	Intestinal abnormalities associated with obstruction/malabsorption (Crohn disease)

IgA, immunoglobulin A.

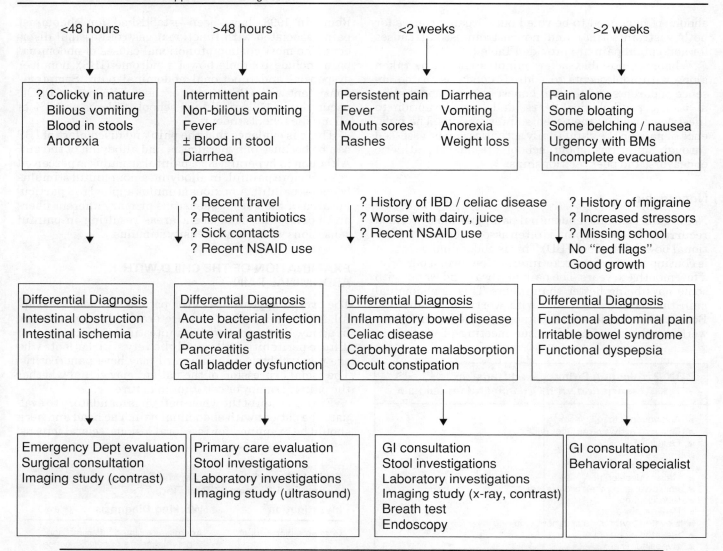

FIGURE 1. Evaluation of the child with abdominal pain. BM, bowel movement; Dept, department; GI, gastrointestinal; IBD, inflammatory bowel disease; NSAID, nonsteroidal anti-inflammatory drug.

and cervical adenopathy. The chest should be examined for patterns of movement and tenderness of the ribs and costochondral junctions. Pneumonia and pleuritic inflammation can manifest as upper abdominal pain. Therefore auscultation of all lobes listening for rhonchi, rales, or pleuritic rubs is essential. The skin of the abdomen and thorax should be examined for evidence of unusual rash or bruising. The flank should be palpated to elicit the tenderness of pyelonephritis or other musculoskeletal causes of abdominal pain.

The abdomen should be examined with the patient as comfortable as possible. *Visual inspection* is begun by looking for distension, hernias, abdominal pulsation, mass effect, and the pattern of movement and respiration. *Auscultation* of the abdomen gives information about bowel sounds (hyper/hypoactive) and the presence or absence of abdominal bruits and may help diagnose vascular problems. *Palpation* of the abdomen should always begin away from the area of maximal tenderness. All quadrants and the epigastrium should be examined carefully. Muscular tone, organomegaly, and the presence of

hernias, warmth, and pulsation should be noted. Shifting dullness on percussion of the abdomen may indicate the presence of ascites, although loss of hepatic dullness suggests free intraperitoneal air.

No abdominal examination is complete without inspection of the perianal region and a digital rectal examination. Evaluation of the perianal region may reveal evidence consistent with inflammatory bowel disease such as fistulas and skin tags. It may reveal evidence for hemorrhoids consistent with chronic constipation. Rectal examination can allow detection of a pelvic floor collection or mass. It is particularly helpful in the patient with a rigid abdomen. Stool should be inspected for the presence of gross and microscopic blood.

DIAGNOSTIC EVALUATION

When indicated, an organic condition can be excluded using inexpensive and easily available diagnostic tests in a directed manner (Table 2; Fig. 1). In patients with chronic abdominal pain and with no red flag symptoms, the ROME II criteria have a positive predictive value of approximately 98%, with additional diagnostic tests providing a yield of 2% or less.

Common Pitfalls

- Failure to appreciate the etiologic differences between acute and chronic abdominal pain.
- Managing chronic abdominal pain as if it was acute pain, leading to unnecessary interventions including surgery and automatic use of opioid analgesics.
- Overemphasis on finding an organic diagnosis or fear of missing such a diagnosis in cases of chronic abdominal pain. As a result, there becomes an over-reliance on imaging studies and invasive testing such as endoscopic procedures.
- When first meeting a patient with chronic abdominal pain, overemphasizing the need for a diagnosis rather than addressing the pain and its social impact including missed activities such as school.
- Considering a functional diagnosis to be one of "exclusion" rather than actively using symptom-based criteria to "rule in" a functional diagnosis and using red flag symptoms to dictate the need for further clinical investigation.
- Reluctance to openly discuss the well-established coincidence of anxiety and/or depression in children and adolescents with chronic abdominal pain.
- Failure to reassure patients and their families that chronic abdominal pain is common and can be addressed in a timely and effective manner with a minimum of invasive testing.

Communication and Counseling

- Focus will be on chronic abdominal pain.
- Reassurance at the first encounter that in addition to establishing a diagnosis, pain relief and a return to social function will be the prime goal of the doctor-patient relationship.
- Use of a pain diary to establish frequency, pattern, and associated symptoms and activity of the pain.
- The patient and family should be encouraged to call and, preferably, be seen promptly if new medical or psychosocial symptoms develop.
- The manner in which to use combination therapies should be clearly outlined in regard to dosage, frequency of co-administration, and possible side effects.

In contrast to adult data, there are no quality-of-life studies for parents and children with chronic abdominal pain. However, parents presenting their children for treatment of abdominal pain have significant concerns: fear of the child dying from cancer, frequent missed school, disturbed sleep, and relief of discomfort. Health professionals often do not appreciate these concerns, and exploration of parental expectations and fears is often valuable in the management of chronic abdominal pain. It is also known that the Internet provides confusing information on chronic abdominal pain in children. When reviewing any child with abdominal pain irrespective of the etiology, exacerbation factors should be explored. Providing parents with information and education regarding the pathogenesis of chronic abdominal pain may reduce anxiety in parents and the need for medication.

SUGGESTED READINGS

1. American Academy of Pediatrics Subcommittee on Chronic Abdominal Pain and the North American Society for Pediatric Gastroenterology, Hepatology, and Nutrition: Chronic abdominal pain in children: A technical report of the American Academy of Pediatrics and the North American Society for Pediatric Gastroenterology, Hepatology and Nutrition. Pediatrics Mar; 115(3):e370–e381, 2005. **The subcommittee examined the diagnostic and therapeutic value of a medical and psychological history, diagnostic tests, and pharmacological and behavioral therapy.**
2. D'Agostino J: Common abdominal emergencies in children. Em Med Clin N Amer 20:139–153, 2002. **This article emphasizes the point that repeated examinations and observation are useful tools. Physicians should listen carefully to parents and their children, respect their concerns, and honor their complaints.**
3. Gauderer MLW: When to operate immediately and when to observe. Surg Clin N Amer 74–80, 1997. **This article emphasizes that the acute abdomen is a clinical diagnosis. Other diagnostic modalities have merely supporting roles.**
4. Kohli R, Li BU: Differential diagnosis of recurrent abdominal pain: New considerations. Pediatr Ann 33:113–122, 2004. **This article describes differential diagnosis as extensive and growing but dominated by functional disorders for which there are new diagnostic criteria despite the lack of specific confirmatory laboratory markers.**
5. Pollack ES: Pediatric abdominal surgical emergencies. Pediatr Ann 25:448–457, 1996. **This article emphasizes that the early involvement of surgical consultants in the care of pediatric patients who have significant gastrointestinal symptoms or findings is always appropriate.**
6. Spitz L, Kimber C: The History. Sem Pediatr Surg 6:58–61, 1997. **This article outlines a structured approach to history taking and details the common causes of acute abdomen in childhood.**
7. Rasquin-Weber A, Hyman PE, Cucchiara S, et al: Childhood functional gastrointestinal disorders. Gut 45(Suppl 2):60–68, 1999. **This article attempts to define criteria for pediatric functional gastrointestinal disorders.**

Acute Abdominal Pain

Shehzad A. Saeed and John Timothy Boyle

KEY CONCEPTS

- A *sick* general appearance suggests a late stage of acute abdominal disease.
- Acute abdominal pain may herald catastrophic events including generalized peritonitis, intestinal infarction, or infarction of the ovaries or testes. Such complications may follow blunt or penetrating trauma; high-grade intestinal obstruction (intussusception); closed loop intestinal obstruction (volvulus, incarcerated hernia); testicular or ovarian torsion; and perforation secondary to peptic

- ulcer, intestinal foreign body, gallbladder hydrops, or acute cholecystitis.
- Vomiting usually precedes or occurs simultaneously with the onset of pain in acute gastroenteritis. In acute appendicitis, pain almost always precedes vomiting.
- Fever usually precedes or occurs simultaneously with the onset of pain in acute gastroenteritis. Fever is unusual in the early stages of an acute surgical abdomen (appendicitis, intestinal obstruction).
- The first symptom of acute appendicitis is usually epigastric or periumbilical abdominal pain.
- The differential diagnosis of acute right lower quadrant (RLQ) abdominal pain includes appendicitis, Crohn disease, small bowel obstruction, pyelonephritis, renal colic, acute salpingitis, ovarian torsion, dysmenorrhea, ruptured ovarian cyst, mittelschmerz, typhlitis, ectopic pregnancy, and mesenteric adenitis.
- *Mesenteric adenitis* is a term commonly used to describe clustering of lymph nodes in the region of the terminal ileum in patients undergoing abdominal CT or at the time of appendectomy. Mesenteric adenitis should not be considered a separate diagnosis but rather a sequela of viral or bacterial gastroenteritis.
- Acute abdominal pain may be a presenting symptom of extraintestinal medical conditions including pneumonia, sickle crisis, diabetic ketoacidosis, porphyria, urinary tract infections, and poisoning.

Acute abdominal pain refers to complaints of abdominal discomfort of recent onset that prompt an urgent evaluation by a primary care or an emergency department physician. Acute abdominal pain accounts for approximately 5% of unscheduled pediatric visits. In patients who present with acute abdominal pain to a primary care practice or an emergency department, the frequency of diseases requiring surgical intervention may be as low as 1%. The majority of patients have self-limiting acute viral syndromes (upper respiratory infection, pharyngitis, viral gastroenteritis, and mesenteric adenitis) or more intense flares of chronic, functional medical conditions including functional abdominal pain, constipation, or intestinal gas. The major challenge is to make a timely diagnosis of an acute surgical abdomen and to diagnose medical conditions that may require specific therapies or hospitalization. Clinical presentation and physical examination may guide the physician in assessing the need for further evaluation including imaging studies and surgical consultation. A consistent approach is important to address key diagnostic categories and to provide parents with guidelines to recognize warning signs requiring re-evaluation.

Expert Opinion on Prioritizing Differential Diagnoses

The sequence and timing of the progression of symptoms provide important diagnostic clues (Table 1).

An acute viral syndrome (upper respiratory infection, pharyngitis, gastroenteritis) is the most common cause of acute abdominal pain beyond the neonatal period. When multiple symptoms—including fever, vomiting, diarrhea, decreased appetite, headache, cough, sore throat, and rhinorrhea—occur simultaneously with the onset of diffuse crampy abdominal pain, the first thought should be "viral syndrome." The abdomen is generally soft and not distended, palpation elicits generalized pressure tenderness without rebound, and bowel sounds are normal or hyperactive. The keys to management are reassurance and education of parents about signs and symptoms of dehydration and need for re-evaluation if pain progresses or localizes in the next 24 to 36 hours.

A significant number of children who present with acute abdominal pain are experiencing a flare of chronic functional abdominal pain. A history of chronic pain, normal physical examination, and absence of alarm signals (weight loss, growth deceleration, fever, significant vomiting or diarrhea, guaiac-positive stools) suggests a flare of functional abdominal pain. In the absence of confirming history and a rectum full of stool by digital examination, a child with acute abdominal pain should not be treated for acute constipation if an abdominal flat plate x-ray, performed to screen for obstruction, shows a moderate or large amount of stool. An abdominal plain film also has low specificity for diagnosing excessive intraluminal gas. In the absence of a history of excessive air swallowing and distension, caution should be exercised in attributing acute abdominal pain to excessive intestinal gas.

The first symptom of appendicitis is usually epigastric or periumbilical pain. A common presentation of acute appendicitis is a previously well child awakening with acute abdominal pain. Temperature is usually normal but may rise to 100°F (37.8°C) to 100.5°F (37.1°C) within a few hours, often associated with vomiting. Characteristically, over time, pain shifts to the right lower quadrant. If the appendix is retrocecal, pain may localize to the lateral abdomen or flank. An appendix pointing to the left lower quadrant may manifest with suprapubic tenderness. Leukocytosis (up to 17,000 per mm^3) is seen in 80% of patients, but its specificity is noted to be poor. Unless the conventional plain abdominal radiograph reveals a calcified fecalith (seen in 10% of patients with appendicitis), it is nonspecific in the diagnosis of appendicitis. Imaging with high resolution ultrasonography or CT scan of the abdomen improves the accuracy of diagnosis and decreases the need for hospitalization in patients with suspected, but a low probability of, appendicitis. Many cases of appendicitis, especially in very young children, progress to perforation before localization of pain or onset of vomiting. Immediately following perforation, abdominal pain may improve. However, within 1 to 2 hours the patient develops generalized or localized rebound tenderness accompanied by frequent vomiting, pallor, tachycardia, and fever above 101°F (38.3°C). Profuse secretory diarrhea may be predominant if the inflammatory mass rests against the sigmoid colon. Abdominal CT is more sensitive and specific and less operator-dependent than ultrasound for diagnosing perforated appendix

The symptoms of intestinal obstruction depend on the location of the obstruction. Dull, crampy abdominal pain is usually present from the onset and frequently occurs in bouts and spasms. In acute intestinal obstruction, the

TABLE 1 Clinical Scenarios to Help Differentiate the Various Causes of Acute Abdominal Pain

Specific Disease Process	Sequence and Timing of Acute Pain
Viral gastroenteritis, "viral syndrome," mesenteric adenitis	Symptoms of fever, vomiting, diarrhea, or respiratory illness precede or occur simultaneously with onset of diffuse, crampy abdominal pain.
Bacterial enterocolitis, food poisoning	Abrupt onset of fever, diffuse abdominal pain, followed shortly by diarrhea. Small volume, bloody, mucous diarrhea with fecal leukocytes suggests bacterial rather than viral etiology. Acute presentation of ulcerative colitis and, rarely, Crohn disease.
Acute gastritis, duodenitis, peptic ulcer	Epigastric pain and vomiting, most commonly during eating or postprandially. Diagnosis suggested by history of predisposing causes: acute viral syndrome, acute stress, ingestion of NSAIDs, family history of *Helicobacter pylori* or peptic ulcer.
Pneumonia	Acute abdominal pain with fever, chills, tachypnea out of proportion to fever, cough, decreased breath sounds, and inspiratory rales.
Pyelonephritis	Diffuse abdominal/flank pain, urinary urgency, dysuria.
Urolithiasis	Excruciating colicky abdominal/flank pain with hematuria.
Pelvic inflammatory disease	Lower abdominal pain and fever in an adolescent female who has just completed a menstrual period.
Mittelschmerz	Unilateral abdominal pain at midpoint of menstrual cycle with or without spotty vaginal bleeding.
Ectopic pregnancy	History of amenorrhea, lower quadrant abdominal pain, and vaginal bleeding. Urine or serum pregnancy test should be performed in adolescent females with acute lower abdominal pain.
Fecal impaction	Left-sided or suprapubic abdominal pain antedated by absent or very small bowel movements for several days.
Acute presentation of inflammatory bowel disease	May mimic presentation of acute bacterial enterocolitis.
Biliary colic	Frequently follows a meal; sustained right upper quadrant, epigastric, or periumbilical pain, which may be referred to back near right scapula, rises to plateau over 5–20 min, then gradually resolves over 1 to 4 h. Nausea and vomiting are common. A common bile duct stone should be considered if the patient is jaundiced. Cholangitis should be suspected in a patient who has right upper quadrant pain, shaking chills, and spiking fever greater than 102.2°F (39°C)
Acute cholecystitis	Biliary colic that persists for greater than 30 min, more generalized in upper quadrants, intensity increased by deep palpation.
Pancreatitis	Progression of epigastric pain over several hours, knife-like or boring in quality, referred to left scapula. Vomiting may be severe or protracted, bowel sounds decreased, low-grade fever (<101.3°F [38.5°C]) present. The abdomen may be distended but is rarely rigid. Rebound tenderness is rare. Bowel sounds may be decreased. Child prefers to lie still.
Hepatitis	Five- to 7-day prodrome of progressive epigastric or right upper quadrant pain, accompanied by flulike symptoms including low-grade fever, anorexia, nausea, vomiting, and fatigue, associated with tender hepatomegaly.
Perihepatitis (Fitz-Hugh-Curtis syndrome)	Severe right upper quadrant pain and tenderness in adolescent females in proximity to menstrual cycle. Fever may or may not be present. The syndrome has been associated with both *Neisseria gonorrhoeae* and *Chlamydia trachomatis*.
Henoch-Schönlein purpura	Diffuse abdominal pain with or without hematochezia may precede skin involvement by 1 week. Suspect if there is associated joint pain, hematuria, or proteinuria.
Diabetic ketoacidosis	Antecedent history of polydipsia, polyuria, and weight loss. Exquisite abdominal tenderness with guarding and rigidity may mimic peritonitis. Smell of ketones on breath, deep breathing reflect ketoacidosis.
Veno-occlusive crisis in sickle cell disease	Signs of peritonitis. Patient describes symptoms that are distinctly different from usual painful crises.
Primary peritonitis	Rare, complication of ascites, most commonly in children with nephrosis or cirrhosis. Suggested by rebound tenderness.
Appendicitis	Epigastric or periumbilical pain followed by vomiting and low-grade fever followed by shift of pain to right lower quadrant. Pain localizing to lateral abdomen or flank suggests retrocecal appendix.
Perforated appendix	Signs of generalized peritonitis, pallor, dyspnea, tachycardia, and high fever. Child prefers to lie still.
Closed loop intestinal obstruction (volvulus)	Frequent emesis (initially gastric contents, becoming bilious) beginning soon after onset of epigastric pain suggests high intestinal obstruction. Obstruction in the distal intestine or colon begins with crampy abdominal pain and nausea followed later by vomiting first gastric contents, then bilious and then feculent vomit. Feculent vomiting is diagnostic of distal intestinal obstruction.
Intussusception	Symptoms of viral gastroenteritis followed by crampy abdominal pain followed by progressive irritability, anorexia, vomiting. Gastrointestinal bleeding is a late sign suggesting incipient bowel infarction.
Incarcerated inguinal hernia	Irritability, vomiting, and occasionally abdominal distention. Can be missed if whole abdomen is not observed, especially in obese patients. A firm, discrete mass can be palpated at internal inguinal ring. Testes may appear dark, blue.
Torsion of testis	Usually sudden onset of scrotal pain radiating to abdomen, accompanied by nausea and vomiting. Testis is swollen and diffusely tender.

NSAIDs, nonsteroidal anti-inflammatory drugs.

temperature is usually normal. Frequent bilious emesis, beginning soon after onset of epigastric pain, suggests high obstruction from malrotation with Ladd bands. If the obstruction is in the distal small bowel or colon, nausea is constant from onset with vomiting as a late symptom. Bilious vomiting becoming feculent (foul-smelling) is diagnostic of low intestinal obstruction. Intussusception occurs most often in infants 6 to 18 months of age, frequently follows a viral syndrome, and is usually ileocolic in location. Evidence of gastrointestinal (GI) blood loss is a late symptom of intussusception, frequently indicating ischemic bowel. Barium contrast upper GI series is the test of choice to evaluate high obstruction. Abdominal CT has significantly advanced the evaluation of distal obstruction, especially strangulating obstruction. The abdominal CT diagnosis of high-grade obstruction requires a dilated proximal small bowel and collapsed distal bowel. CT may miss partial obstruction secondary to Crohn disease or postsurgical adhesions, but such situations rarely result in bowel strangulation.

Epigastric pain, right upper quadrant pain, or epigastric pain radiating to the right upper quadrant should suggest hepatobiliary disease, pancreatitis, or peptic ulcer disease. Screening tests include serum transaminases, alkaline phosphatase, γ-glutamyl transferase (GGT), amylase, and lipase, and possibly abdominal ultrasound and hepatobiliary scintigraphy.

Common Pitfalls

■ A "honeymoon" stage, in which abdominal pain, vomiting, and fever lessen or resolve, may precede onset of shock and peritonitis in catastrophic events such as intestinal perforation or infarction. Sending the patient home or admitting the patient to a subacute care hospital ward can have disastrous consequences because this stage is soon followed by a shock-like picture accompanied by high fever, abdominal distension, GI bleeding, and shock.

■ Rebound tenderness may or may not be a sign of a surgical abdomen. Rebound has been associated with severe gastroenteritis, pneumonia, Henoch-Schönlein purpura, and lead poisoning.

■ Beware of ascribing acute abdominal pain to paralytic ileus. Paralytic ileus may be associated with viral gastroenteritis, drugs that interfere with GI motility, post-traumatic shock, hypokalemia, uremia, and lead poisoning. Paralytic ileus commonly manifests with minimal abdominal pain, increasing abdominal distention, nausea, infrequent vomiting, increased flatus, and diarrhea.

■ Beware of diagnosing constipation as the cause of abdominal pain based on plain films of the abdomen in the absence of a positive history or rectal exam.

■ *Helicobacter pylori* gastritis in the absence of peptic ulcer rarely manifests with acute abdominal pain.

Communication and Counseling

Although most children with acute abdominal pain have self-limiting conditions, the pain may herald a serious medical or surgical emergency. Although it is often impossible to be sure of the exact diagnosis, a working diagnosis needs to be established early in children who present with acute abdominal pain. Parents need to be informed that the sequence and timing of the progression of symptoms provide important diagnostic clues. The importance of periodic re-examination cannot be overstated, because many disorders become obvious only by observing their natural history.

SUGGESTED READINGS

1. Anderson RE, Hugander AP, Ghazi SH, et al: Diagnostic value of disease history, clinical presentation, and inflammatory parameters of appendicitis. World J Surg 23:133–140, 1993. **Discusses the diagnostic value and comparison of elements of history, presentation, and various inflammatory markers of advanced appendicitis and recommends using them as part of the diagnostic workup.**
2. del Pozo G, Albillos J, Tejedor D: Intussusception: US findings with pathologic correlation—the crescent-in-doughnut sign. Radiology 199:688–692, 1996. **Describes the characteristic ultrasound findings of intussusception and its different radiographic components.**
3. Frager D: Intestinal obstruction: Role of CT. Gastroenterol Clin North Am 31:777–799, 2002. **Describes the utility of CT scan in diagnosis of various types of small-bowel and colonic obstruction.**
4. Scholer SJ, Pituch K, Orr DP, Dittus RS: Clinical outcomes of children with acute abdominal pain. Pediatrics 98:680–685, 1996. **Describes a cohort of patients seen for an unscheduled visit with complaint of atraumatic abdominal pain and the eventual outcomes.**
5. Silen W: Cope's Early Diagnosis of the Acute Abdomen, 18th ed. Oxford University Press, New York, 1991. **Describes in detail various presentations, diagnostic evaluations, examination, and etiologies of acute abdominal pain, including the initial description of the entity by Sir Zachary Cope.**
6. Vignault F, Filiatrault D, Brandt ML, et al: Acute appendicitis in children: Evaluation with US. Radiology 176:501–504, 1990. **Describes in detail the pattern of characteristic ultrasound findings consistent with acute appendicitis and the predictive values of positive findings.**

Nausea and Vomiting

Peter Ngo and Ronald E. Kleinman

KEY CONCEPTS

■ Age, context, and duration of symptoms determine the need for investigation beyond the history and physical examination.

■ Bilious vomiting and abdominal distention at any age may indicate intestinal obstruction and typically necessitates further investigation.

■ Antiemetic agents should be used with caution when the underlying process is not clear; they are inappropriate in a child who may require abdominal surgery.

■ Gastroesophageal reflux is common in infants; it is uncommon to find a serious disease process in the well-appearing, thriving baby who appears untroubled by "spit-ups."

■ Recurrent episodes of vomiting may represent cyclic vomiting syndrome, but the diagnosis requires excluding structural and metabolic causes of vomiting.

■ The use of antiemetics for self-limited infectious gastroenteritis is typically unnecessary, and its use to prevent further dehydration must be balanced against the risk of side effects.

Nausea and vomiting are common, sporadic, and usually self-limited symptoms in infants and children. The age at

TABLE 1 Conditions Frequently Associated with Nausea and Vomiting

Condition	Examples
Intestinal infections	Rotavirus, Norwalk virus, staphylococcal toxin ingestion, bacterial gastroenteritis
Extraintestinal infections	Pyelonephritis, meningitis
Surgical emergencies	Appendicitis, obstructive cholelithiasis, intussusception, volvulus, testicular torsion, ureteropelvic junction obstruction, nephrolithiasis
Toxin/drug ingestion	Ipecac, acetaminophen overdose, phenytoin
Metabolic disorders	Mitochondrial dysfunction, urea cycle disorders
Endocrine disorders	Diabetic ketoacidosis, adrenal infarction, adrenogenital syndrome
Central nervous system disorders	Increased intracranial pressure (neoplasms, pseudotumor cerebri), encephalitis, migraine headaches
Cancer chemotherapy and radiation therapy	Cisplatin, cyclophosphamide, doxorubicin
Postanesthesia status	Certain procedures are more commonly associated with emesis, e.g., strabismus surgery
Disorders of gastrointestinal motility	Gastroparesis, chronic intestinal pseudo-obstruction syndrome
Psychological disorders	Bulimia

initial evaluation and the context and duration of these symptoms help determine the need for further investigation beyond the history and physical. For example, intermittent effortless vomiting of recently ingested food is not unusual behavior in a 3-week old infant, but it is definitely abnormal in a 16-year old adolescent.

Nausea and vomiting (the forceful expulsion of stomach contents) can be provoked by stimulation of one or more pathways in the central or peripheral nervous system. For example, stimulation of the vestibular apparatus leads to nausea and stimulation of the chemoreceptor trigger zone in the brain stem by a number of drugs causes vomiting. Both nausea and vomiting may be accompanied by signs of increased autonomic activity, such as increased perspiration and pallor, and a decrease in appetite. Nausea generally precedes vomiting, but vomiting does not invariably follow nausea. Multiple afferent and efferent nerve pathways are involved in vomiting. In particular, the chemoreceptor trigger zone located in the area postrema in the floor of the fourth ventricle and an area in the medulla known as the *nucleus tractus solitarius* respond to humoral factors such as drugs, neurotransmitters, and toxins to coordinate the vomiting reflex. Efferent signals to various motor nuclei produce a sequence of somatic and visceral muscle contractions and relaxations that lead to the expulsion of gastric contents out of the mouth by forceful contraction of the abdominal wall musculature and a subsequent decrease in intrathoracic pressure. Simultaneous relaxation of the gastroesophageal sphincter and closure of the glottis also take place.

Nausea and vomiting are important not just for the distress that they cause; they are also associated with a wide variety of diseases. In determining the significance of nausea, with or without vomiting, clinical assessment is paramount. A history of nonbilious projectile vomiting in a 7-week old baby who is clinically dehydrated and has lost weight suggests pyloric stenosis, whereas another 7-week old baby who spits up milk after each feeding but appears to be well and thriving suggests gastroesophageal reflux. Therefore the age of the child, duration of symptoms, and the occurrence of associated symptoms such as weight loss, irritability, fever, and diarrhea are critical

elements of the history. It is also important to establish the appearance, quantity, frequency, and character of the emesis, in particular, whether it is bloody, bilious, or projectile. It is crucial to identify any medications the child may be taking. If the onset of vomiting is acute, any medications or toxins the child may have had access to should be identified. Food and travel history should be elicited as well as any ill contacts. Table 1 lists of some of the many conditions associated with nausea and vomiting.

Expert Opinion on Management Issues

Management of nausea and vomiting depends in large part on identifying the cause or causes of the symptoms. In some cases, efforts will be directed only at the management of these symptoms, whereas in others, treatment is focused on management of the underlying disorder. Despite gaps in understanding of the neurophysiology of nausea and vomiting, effective antiemetics are available for use in infants and children. Table 2 lists the most frequently used agents and medications.

DRUG THERAPY

Histamine Type 1 Receptor Antagonists

Histamine type 1 (H_1) receptor antagonists with prominent anticholinergic effects, such as diphenhydramine, have modest antiemetic properties. Stimulation of the vestibular apparatus, as occurs in motion sickness, sends an afferent signal to the chemoreceptor trigger zone. Thus the effectiveness of this class of medication to treat motion sickness is a result of blockade of the muscarinic receptor. Although this practice is somewhat controversial, promethazine given via a rectal suppository is the most widely used antiemetic by pediatricians and emergency physicians for the symptomatic relief of vomiting associated with acute gastroenteritis. The predictable and manageable side effect of sedation contributes to its preferential use over some of the other available antiemetics.

TABLE 2   Medications for Nausea and Vomiting

Drug Name (Trade name)	Dosage/Route/Regimen	Maximum Dose	Dosage Formulation
Histamine (H_1) Receptor Antagonists			
Diphenhydramine (Benadryl) OTC	PO: 1–1.5 mg/kg q4–6h (adult dose 25–50 mg). IV/IM: 5 mg/kg/day divided in 4 doses. GFR <50: increase dose interval q6–12h.	300 mg/day	Tablet/capsule: 25, 50 mg Chew tab: 12.5 mg, 50 mg Elixir: 12.5 mg/5 mL Injection: 50 mg/mL
Promethazine (Phenergan) Rx	>2 yr: 12.5–25 mg or 1.1 mg/kg PO/PR every q4–6h prn. Motion sickness: 12.5–25 mg PO/PR bid.	<17 yrs IV dose: 0.5 mg/kg per dose (25 mg)	Tablet: 10, 25, 50 mg Syrup: 6.25 mg/5 mL 10 mg/5 mL Suppository: 12.5, 25, 50 mg Injection: 25, 50 mg/mL
Dopamine Antagonists			
Prochlorperazine (Compazine) Rx	>2 yrs: 0.4–0.6 mg/kg/day divided three or four times per day, prn.	Max doses: <20 kg: 10 mg/day 20–40 kg: 15 mg/day	Tablet: 5, 10 mg Syrup: 5 mg/5 mL Suppository: 5 mg, 25 mg
Metoclopramide (Reglan) Rx	GERD: Infants: 0.1 mg/kg PO tid-qid. Postoperative N/V: 0.25 mg/kg per dose IV q6–8h prn. CrCl <50 mL/min: 50%–75% dose.	Max dose: infants: 0.75 mg/kg per day	Tablet: 5, 10 mg Syrup: 1 mg/mL Injection: 5 mg/mL Concentrate solution: 10 mg/mL
Trimethobenzamide (Tigan) Rx	<14 kg: 100 mg PR three or four times per day; 14–41 kg: 100–200 mg PR three or four times per day.		Suppository: 100 mg Caps: 100, 250, 300 mg (not approved for PO/IV use in children)
5-HT$_3$ Serotonin Antagonists			
Ondansetron (Zofran) Rx	Chemotherapy-induced N/V: 4–18 yr: 0.15 mg/kg IV 30 min prior to chemo, repeated 4 and 8 h after first dose then every 8 h for 1–2 days. Postoperative N/V: 2–12 yr <40 kg: 0.1 mg/kg IV; >40 kg: 4 mg IV; >12 yr: adult dosing (8 mg PO/dose).		Tablet: 4, 8 mg (available as orally disintegrating tablet [ODT]). Injection: 2 mg/mL, 32 mg/50 mL solution for injection Oral solution: 4 mg/5 mL
Granisetron (Kytril) Rx	Chemotherapy induced N/V: >2 yr: 10–40 µg/kg IV 30 min prior to chemo. Adult PO dose: 2 mg prior to chemo/radiation.		Tablet: 1 mg Oral solution: 4 mg/5 mL Injection: 1 mg/mL solution for injection
Anticholinergic Agents (Antimuscarinic Effects)			
Scopolamine (Transderm Scop) Rx	Motion sickness: Children >13 yr: 1 transdermal patch behind ear 4 h before needed, replace every 3 days prn.		Transdermal patch: 1.5 mg

bid, twice daily; Cr Cl: creatinine clearance; GERD, gastroesophageal reflux disease; GFR, glomerular filtration rate; GI, gastrointestinal; IM, intramuscularly; IV, intravenously; N/V, nausea and vomiting; OTC, over-the-counter medication; PO, orally; PR, rectally; prn, as needed; pts, patients; q, every; qid, four times daily; Rx, prescription; tid, three times per day.

Common Adverse Reactions	Comments
Sedation, drowsiness, dry mouth, dizziness, dyskinesias	For motion sickness prophylaxis, give full dose 30 min prior to exposure to motion and further doses before meals and at bedtime.
Sedation, drowsiness, dry mouth, extrapyramidal symptoms	Not for use in children <2 yr.
Extrapyramidal symptoms, blurred vision, dizziness, drowsiness, dry mouth, constipation, blood dyscrasias (rare)	Not for use in children <2 yr or 20 lb; not for use following pediatric surgery, or pts with bone marrow suppression/blood dyscrasias. For use only with severe nausea and vomiting.
Drowsiness, dystonic reactions, sedation, constipation	Dystonic reactions can occur in children at therapeutic doses. Most effective 10–30 min before meals and at bedtime. Contraindicated with GI obstruction or hemorrhage. Avoid use in patients with seizure disorders.
Anticholinergic effects, drowsiness, hypotension, extrapyramidal symptoms (rare)	
Headache, constipation, diarrhea, dry mouth, elevated liver function tests	Very effective and few side effects; however, cost is often prohibitive for common self-limited illnesses. May be more effective as a scheduled antiemetic versus a rescue/prn agent. Can mask ileus in patients following abdominal surgery or chemotherapy.
Headache, constipation, diarrhea, somnolence	See notes for ondansetron.
Drowsiness, dry mouth, blurred vision	Used for prophylaxis of motion sickness. The transdermal patch releases medication for 3 days.

Dopamine Receptor Antagonists

Dopamine receptor antagonists (phenothiazines, butyrophenones, and benzamides) act primarily by antagonizing the dopamine type 2 (D_2) receptors in the area postrema in the midbrain and are antiemetic at lower doses than those used for antipsychotic purposes. These medications have a direct action on the chemoreceptor trigger zone. However, dopaminergic receptors are found in the stomach and the central nervous system (CNS), and inhibition of these receptors prevents the decrease in gastric motility that is found during emesis. The prokinetic effects of the benzamide metoclopramide, which enhances gastric emptying and increases lower esophageal sphincter tone, can be useful in conditions such as gastroparesis. The main side effect of the dopamine receptor antagonists is extrapyramidal symptoms such as dystonia.

Selective Serotonin Type 3 Antagonists

Selective serotonin type 3 ($5\text{-}HT_3$) antagonists such as ondansetron (Zofran) and granisetron (Kytril), are very effective agents that have largely replaced the use of other classes of antiemetics in the treatment of vomiting associated with moderate to highly emetogenic chemotherapeutic agents. These agents may act both centrally in the chemoreceptor trigger zone and peripherally on $5\text{-}HT_3$ receptors in the vagus nerve. Multiple studies show that these agents are the most effective available agents for postoperative nausea and vomiting, especially for strabismus surgery, which is commonly associated with nausea and vomiting. Although these agents are effective and have few side effects, their high cost is somewhat prohibitive for more widespread use in common causes of nausea and vomiting.

Miscellaneous Agents

Cannabinoids (e.g., Marinol) show superiority to placebo in adults and are most useful with emetogenic cancer chemotherapy. However, their use is rare now with the availability of more effective antiemetics with fewer adverse CNS side effects. Benzodiazepines (lorazepam) as single agents are relatively weak antiemetics and their mechanism of action is poorly understood. They appear to be most useful as adjunctive agents, especially with chemotherapy, with some benefits coming from their anxiolytic action. Erythromycin enhances gastric emptying and can be useful in gastric motility disorders such as gastroparesis. Corticosteroids are useful agents for vomiting associated with chemotherapy and are frequently used in conjunction with $5\text{-}HT_3$ antagonists.

Antiemetic agents should be used with caution when the underlying process is not clear. In fact their use is inappropriate in a child who may require abdominal surgery because observation of signs and symptoms often dictates the timing of operative intervention. The converse holds that these agents have their highest utility in clinical scenarios that are known to produce emesis, such as administration of chemotherapeutic agents and after strabismus surgery.

CAUSES OF NAUSEA AND VOMITING

Gastroenteritis

The management of nausea and vomiting associated with self-limited acute infectious gastroenteritis is typically supportive, with efforts focusing mainly on maintaining hydration with either oral rehydration solutions or intravenous fluids. Although such illnesses are typically best managed without the use of antiemetic pharmacotherapy and its accompanying side effects, there are situations in which use of antiemetics can be considered. In a survey of pediatricians and emergency medicine and pediatric emergency medicine specialists, over 50% of responders from all three specialties reported using antiemetics at least once in the prior year for pediatric patients with acute gastroenteritis. In these cases, rectal promethazine was most frequently used. In addition to the prokinetics mentioned for use in gastroparesis, a change in eating habits to small frequent meals can also enhance gastric emptying and bring symptomatic relief.

Recurrent Vomiting

Children with rumination, the frequent and effortless regurgitation of small amounts of food that may either be spit out or reswallowed, may respond to a behavior modification program. Specialized psychotherapy is required for children with disorders such as bulimia nervosa.

Cyclic vomiting syndrome is characterized by recurrent episodes of continuous, repeated vomiting, often over a period of several days, separated by symptom-free intervals that can range from several weeks to a year. It is a condition of unknown pathogenesis that in some children is accompanied by generalized autonomic dysfunction and, in others, by migraine headaches. It has an average age of onset of 5.2 years. Treatment during episodes focuses on maintaining hydration, often with intravenous fluids, and abortive or symptomatic pharmacotherapy. Ondansetron in combination with the antiemetic anxiolytic lorazepam is a commonly used combination. Various antimigraine agents can also be used to prevent or abort episodes. Neuroleptics and gastrointestinal (GI) prokinetic agents have been used with varying degrees of success. Cyclic vomiting syndrome can be diagnosed only after a thorough evaluation has excluded other causes of recurrent vomiting, such as metabolic disorders or structural abnormalities of the GI or urinary tracts.

Other important conditions in the differential diagnosis of recurrent vomiting include peptic disease, gastric and intestinal motility disorders, CNS abnormalities, familial pancreatitis, adrenal insufficiency, and diabetes mellitus.

Inborn Errors of Metabolism

A number of inborn errors of metabolism may manifest with vomiting as a prominent symptom. In addition to vomiting, clinical features are often nonspecific but may include lethargy, failure to thrive, seizures, and disturbances of motor tone. Electrolyte abnormalities, metabolic acidosis, or ketonuria may be seen and serum and urine amino acid and organic acid analysis may be helpful in securing a diagnosis.

Infantile Gastroesophageal Reflux

When the well-appearing and thriving infant presents with gastroesophageal reflux (GER) it is most important to reassure parents that this is extremely common, albeit frustrating, in healthy infants and that in most cases the regurgitation decreases in frequency after 6 months of age and resolves in many by the first birthday. However, infants with gastroesophageal reflux disease (GERD) may have esophagitis causing irritability, failure to thrive, or apneic episodes that can be treated with acid-suppressing medications, such as ranitidine (5 to 10 mg/kg/day divided twice a day), omeprazole (1 mg/kg/day) or lansoprazole (1 mg/kg/day).

The clinical efficacy of various prokinetic agents in the treatment of infantile GERD has not been confirmed consistently and the most efficacious prokinetic, cisapride (Propulsid), is no longer available because of concerns of serious cardiac side effects associated with a prolongation of the QT interval. For infants with GERD who fail to respond to acid blockade, a trial of a diet free of cow's milk or soy protein may be helpful. Although cow's milk and soy protein colitis almost always present in healthy-appearing young infants as blood-streaked or heme-positive stools, irritability and vomiting are typically seen with allergic gastroenteropathy or esophagitis.

Common Pitfalls

- The failure to recognize the surgical emergency in a patient presenting with nausea and vomiting can have severe consequences. Patients may have signs of obstruction with bilious vomiting, abdominal distention, and the ill appearance one would see with intestinal malrotation and volvulus. However, more subtle presentations of surgical conditions can occur, as in the patient who feels better immediately following the rupture of an acute appendicitis. Plain films of the abdomen are often useful and immediate surgical consultation is warranted if appendicitis, bowel obstruction, or bowel perforation is suspected.
- Pediatricians should have a low threshold for suspecting pregnancy. The adolescent patient may not have considered pregnancy or may present with vague complaints and a "hidden agenda" of suspected pregnancy.
- Although increased intracranial pressure from conditions such as intracranial masses or pseudotumor cerebri typically are associated with headache, nausea and vomiting can be the predominant features. When patients present with "red flag" symptoms of such neurologic abnormalities—vomiting that awakens a child from sleep or a prolonged history of progressively worsening vomiting—an intracranial process must be considered, especially in the absence of signs of an infectious cause such as fever and diarrhea.
- Chronic vomiting, significant weight loss, severe abdominal pain, or GI bleeding should be considered abnormal and an etiology should always be sought.

Communication and Counseling

Most episodes of nausea and vomiting in pediatric patients represent self-limited illnesses. When the history and physical do not point to more serious or long-standing conditions, it is important to stress to parents that supportive care including maintenance of hydration is the mainstay of therapy. When the thriving, healthy-appearing infant with physiologic GER presents with frequent spit-ups, reassurance becomes the most important therapy for parents. Although most children outgrow their GER by their first birthday, children may not improve, or may have increased spitting up between 4 and 6 months of age.

Dopaminergic agents, such as metoclopramide, can produce irritability and dystonic reactions in children even at therapeutic doses and so should be used with caution. Although effective antidotes are available (diphenhydramine), a dystonic reaction is very upsetting for the child and family alike. Therefore, counseling parents in advance about this possibility is advised.

SUGGESTED READINGS

1. Fleisher DR, Matar M: The cyclic vomiting syndrome: A report of 71 cases and literature review. J Pediatr Gastroenterol Nutr 17 (4):361–369, 1993. **This review outlines the clinical features of cyclic vomiting syndrome, considerations in the differential diagnosis, and management.**
2. Kwon KT, Rudkin SE, Langdorf MI: Antiemetic use in pediatric gastroenteritis: A national survey of emergency physicians, pediatricians, and pediatric emergency physicians. Clin Pediatr (Phila) 41(9):641–652, 2002. **In this survey, a majority of responders from all three specialty groups reported use of antiemetics for pediatric gastroenteritis within the prior year.**
3. Longstreth GF, Hesketh PJ: Characteristics of antiemetic drugs. In Rose BD (ed): Wellesley, Mass, 2004. **A review of available antiemetic drugs is presented, including mechanisms of action, side effects, and common uses.**
4. Rudolph CD, Mazur LJ, Liptak GS, et al: Guidelines for evaluation and treatment of gastroesophageal reflux in infants and children: recommendations of the North American Society for Pediatric Gastroenterology and Nutrition. J Pediatr Gastroenterol Nutr 32 (Suppl 2):S1–S31, 2001. **These clinical practice guidelines, which are endorsed by the American Academy of Pediatrics, provide recommendations for management of gastroesophageal reflux by the primary care provider, including evaluation, initial treatment, follow-up, and indications for consultation with a specialist. Recommendations for management by the pediatric gastroenterologist are also included.**

Constipation

Peter Ngo and Ronald E. Kleinman

KEY CONCEPTS

- A history and physical examination is usually adequate to differentiate idiopathic functional constipation from organic disease processes.
- Hirschsprung disease should be considered in patients with delayed passage of meconium after birth or constipation "since birth."
- Patient and parental commitment to the treatment strategy are essential.

Constipation, the infrequent passage of hard stools with or without fecal soiling, accounts for up to 25% of patient visits in pediatric gastroenterology subspecialty practices. Approximately 10% of all children present to their pediatricians at some time with the complaint of constipation. The toll on families and children can be considerable, especially when encopresis (retentive fecal soiling) is also a problem. Parents generally consider that their infant or child is constipated when bowel movements are infrequent, painful, very large, or hard. Normal patterns of stooling can vary dramatically between infancy and childhood and also with diet. The mean number of bowel movements for infants 2 to 20 weeks of age is three per day for breastfed infants and two per day for formula-fed infants. Older children have a stooling frequency similar to that of adults, with a broad range from three times a week to three times a day. Because there is such variability in the frequency of normal stooling, it is important to differentiate the infant or child that stools infrequently but has soft, comfortable bowel movements from the child with hard, painful stools or fecal soiling.

The frequency, size, and consistency of stools are important questions to ask in the medical history. Parents of children with constipation often describe the stool as looking too big to have been passed by the child. Conversely, children with constipation and encopresis may only pass frequent, small amounts of fecal fluid that may soil their clothing, making it difficult for parents to believe that their child is in fact constipated. It is important to ask older children these questions directly because they usually do not talk about their bowel movements with their parents. A child may, on questioning, state that defecation is painful and those children with soiling may say they are unaware of passing stool. Many will deny constipation or soiling despite the fact that it is obvious to others. The presence of fresh red blood on toilet paper after wiping, or blood coating the stool, suggests a distal traumatic injury such as a fissure in ano, often seen with large hard stools. Stool-withholding behavior such as retentive posturing should be sought, as well as symptoms suggesting obstruction, such as vomiting, abdominal pain, and distention.

The history is extremely helpful in identifying factors that make an organic etiology more likely. In the child younger than 1 year of age, or in the child with "constipation since birth," the age at passage of meconium is important. Ninety-eight percent of newborns pass meconium by 48 hours of age. In those who do not, Hirschsprung disease and cystic fibrosis (CF) must be considered. Infants with meconium ileus secondary to CF generally have signs of small bowel obstruction, such as a distended abdomen and bile-stained vomitus, whereas infants with Hirschsprung disease may have signs of large-bowel obstruction, such as feculent vomiting. The rectum in infants with Hirschsprung disease is usually empty, but digital rectal exam often leads to a spurt of meconium and feces. Paradoxically, children with malabsorption disorders such as CF or celiac disease can also have constipation.

Constipation is often seen in children with neuromuscular disorders such as cerebral palsy and myelomeningocele (Table 1). Medications that a child is taking may also cause constipation. In particular, various psychotropic and opiate-containing medications frequently cause constipation. Although it is a commonly held belief that the administration of iron supplementation causes constipation in children, blinded, randomized, controlled trials do not support this. A family history may reveal other family members with constipation. Delayed development may be a clue to hypothyroidism or lead poisoning.

Expert Opinion on Management Issues

Successful treatment of idiopathic functional constipation begins by explaining the factors leading to constipation and describing the treatment to the child and parents. Treatment of constipation will not work without the commitment of the family, and the support of a teacher if the child is old enough to attend school. Such cooperation is dependent on the family understanding that

TABLE 1 Conditions Frequently Associated with Constipation

Condition	Important Features
Hirschsprung disease	Constipation "since birth," delayed passage of meconium, passage of liquid stool following digital rectal examination.
Cystic fibrosis	Associated with meconium ileus in the newborn with signs of small bowel obstruction.
Celiac disease	May have accompanying abdominal pain, may alternate with diarrhea.
Hypothyroidism	Associated with growth failure, decreased energy, delayed deep tendon reflexes. It is unlikely that constipation will be the sole presenting symptom.
Opiate, anesthetic, and antidepressant agents	Constipation commonly in the postoperative period because of combination of opiate use and immobility.
Spina bifida and spinal cord lesions	Associated colonic dysfunction and immobility predispose to constipation. Spinal and neurologic exams are frequently abnormal.

the treatment process and resolution of the problem will take time. Pharmacologic therapy is only one part of the treatment of constipation, which also includes behavioral, dietary, and sometimes psychological interventions.

Initial treatment of constipation usually requires clearing the bowel and rectum of accumulated solid feces around which liquid stool can leak and produce soiling or encopresis. Unless the colon and rectum can be emptied successfully at the start of treatment, other measures are unlikely to work. Disimpaction can be achieved by the use of medications given either orally or per rectum. In severe and refractory cases, nasogastric lavage solutions or manual disimpaction under anesthesia may be necessary. Occasionally, hospitalization with nasogastric lavage of large amounts of polyethylene glycol with electrolytes (GoLYTELY) for 2 to 3 days may be needed to achieve a full clean-out. Because most children better tolerate oral medications for disimpaction, this method is typically preferred in the nonacute setting. Table 2 lists the common medications for use in constipation.

Pharmacologic agents can be categorized as stimulants, osmotic agents, and lubricants. Osmotic agents, which keep fluid within the bowel lumen, are the most frequently used medications for oral disimpaction. The dosage used for disimpaction may be several-fold higher than that for daily maintenance therapy. For example, the prescription medication polyethylene glycol powder for solution (MiraLax) is typically given as a single daily maintenance dose ranging from 0.5 to 1.0 g/kg/day; however, for initial disimpaction in the moderate to severely constipated child this dose is often doubled for several days to first achieve loose stools then titrated down to a suitable maintenance dose. Studies examining its use for bowel preparations prior to colonoscopy in children have found that these doses are well tolerated without significant electrolyte disturbances. The addition of a stimulant, such as a chewable chocolate form of senna, can be useful, in addition to osmotic agents for initial disimpaction. Magnesium citrate is widely available over the counter as a 10-ounce bottle and can be given at a dosage of 1 ounce per year of age (to a maximum of 10 ounces) in two divided doses as an initial disimpaction regimen. Although it is less palatable than polyethylene glycol powder for solution (which is easily dissolvable and nearly undetectable in most fluids), oral magnesium citrate is a very effective disimpaction agent for the more cooperative child.

Although disimpaction is extremely important for the severely constipated child, many children may have very mild intermittent constipation that can be treated with a combination of dietary and behavioral modifications such as frequent toilet sitting and increased fluid, fruit, vegetable, and fiber intake. The child's age in years plus 5 g provides an estimate of daily fiber needs. Additionally, many children with constipation can be started on a maintenance dose of osmotic laxatives. Children with moderate to severe constipation often require consistent, daily maintenance therapy. The goal of maintenance therapy is a comfortable, soft, daily bowel movement. Especially in children with a history of fecal impactions and encopresis, it is better to err on the side of "borderline loose" stools than to allow these children to lapse back into a frustrating pattern of constipation with fecal soiling that will require a repeat disimpaction.

Although stimulant medications are effective at producing bowel movements, they play a lesser role in daily maintenance because of the possibility of dependence on pharmacologic stimulation for effective colonic contraction. Stimulants can be useful as "rescue" agents for the constipated child who goes several days without a bowel movement despite maintenance therapy. Typically, to achieve long-term success, maintenance therapy is needed for at least 3 months. If toilet training has not yet been successful, continuing therapy through this period is advised because of the high likelihood of recurrent symptoms during the toilet training period. Maintenance therapy can be difficult to sustain in children who are no longer constipated and therefore reluctant to take daily medication. Scheduled follow-up and repeated explanation of the need for treatment greatly improve compliance.

Common Pitfalls

- Failure to explain to parents and children that constipation does not have a "quick fix" and that relapse of symptoms is very common when parents do not remain vigilant and committed to treatment.
- Inadequate initial clean-outs, especially in the child with retentive fecal soiling or encopresis.
- Inadequate duration of pharmacologic maintenance therapy in the constipated child, especially in the toilet training period. Laxatives should not be weaned until a normal bowel habit is maintained.
- Laxatives should be weaned slowly over 1 to 2 months and doses increased in strength, if regular bowel movements cannot be maintained or symptoms recur.
- Setting inadequate goals for patients: the goal of treatment for the constipated child is a soft, comfortable daily bowel movement. It is better to err on the side of borderline loose stools and slowly titrate medication doses back than to allow patients to become comfortable with an inadequate dose.
- Poor follow-up is a common cause for relapse. Approximately 50% of children with chronic constipation require treatment and close follow-up for at least 6 to 12 months.
- For children who do not respond to a standard treatment plan, the history and examination should be reviewed with key questions directed at whether an organic condition has been missed, compliance has been optimal, and medications are the correct agents and doses.

Communication and Counseling

It is crucial for both the child and the parents that the physician alleviates feelings of guilt and shame. Explaining that soiling is a consequence of a full rectum and using a positive nonaccusatory approach is typically accepted

TABLE 2 Medications for Constipation

Drug Name (Trade name)	Dosage/Route/Regimen	Maximum Dose
Stimulants (Stimulate colonic contraction and passage of stool without softening stool)		
Bisacodyl (Dulcolax, Fleet Laxative, Correctol) OTC	PO: 3–12 yr: 0.3 mg/kg/day or 5–10 mg qd >12 yr: 5–15 mg qd Supp: <2 yr: 5 mg PR qd >2 yr 5–10 mg qd	
Sennosides (Ex-Lax, Senokot) OTC	PO: 2–6 yr: 0.5–1 chocolate square qd 6–12 yr: 15 mg or 1 chocolate square once or twice daily >12 yr: 30 mg or 2 chocolate squares qd or bid	
Osmotic Agents (Nonabsorbable agents that draw water into the intestinal lumen via osmotic gradients)		
Polyethylene Glycol (MiraLax) Rx Including electrolytes (GoLYTELY) Rx	Maintenance PO: 0.5–1 g/kg/day in 8 oz fluid (one capful or 17 g for children >20 kg) NG lavage: Solution with electrolytes 20 mL/kg/h	
Lactulose (Kristalose, Cephulac, Chronulac) Rx	Infants: PO: 1–3 mL/kg/day Children: 7.5 mL or 5 g/day after breakfast	Max: 60 mL/day
Magnesium Citrate OTC	PO: >5 yr: 100–150 mL of 6% solution (1 oz/yr of age for disimpaction)	Max: 10 oz/day
Magnesium Hydroxide (Phillips' Milk of Magnesia) OTC	PO: Infants: 0.5 mL/kg/day 2–5 yr: 1–3 tsp (5–15 mL)/day 5–11 yr: 1–2 Tbs (15–30 mL)/day >11 yr: 2–4 Tbs (30–60 mL)/day	
Phosphosoda (Fleet) OTC	PO: 5–9 yr: 5 mL 10–12 yr: 10 mL >12 yr: 20–30 mL Rectal: 6 mL/kg up to 135 mL	
Lubricants (Nonabsorbable agents that reduce friction and ease passage of stool)		
Mineral oil (Fleet mineral oil enema, etc.) OTC	6–12 yr: 5–15 mL PO qhs >12 yr: 15–45 mL PO at bedtime 1–3 mL/kg/day Enema: 2–11 yr: 59 mL PR qd >12 yr: 118 mL PR qd	Max PO dose: 45 mL/day

bid, twice daily; NG, nasogastric; OCT, over the counter; PO, orally; PR, rectally; qd, daily; qhs, at bedtime; Rx, prescription.

Dosage Formulation	Common Adverse Reactions	Comments
Tablets: 5 mg Supp: 10 mg (can break in half)	Cramping, abdominal pain, diarrhea, possible dependence with chronic use.	Stimulants do not have a role as a daily maintenance medication for functional constipation; however, they can be useful as occasional adjunctive agents and to aid in initial disimpaction.
Tablets: 8.6 mg, 15 mg Chewable chocolate squares: one square = 15 mg	Cramping, abdominal pain, diarrhea, possible dependence with chronic use.	Stimulants do not have a role as a daily maintenance medication for functional constipation; however, they can be useful as occasional adjunctive agents and to aid in initial disimpaction.
Powder for solution: 255- to 527-g bottles Capful (i.e., line midway up cap) = 17 g	Abdominal cramping, bloating, flatulence.	Electrolyte-free powder for solution has become most widely used agent among pediatric gastroenterologists for treatment of chronic constipation in children because of effectiveness, low side effects, and excellent palatability and compliance. (Studies of use >1 yr in children show no significant long-term adverse events.) Dose can be titrated down to maintain 1–2 soft comfortable stools/day.
Solution: 10 g/15 mL Packets for solution: 10, 20 g/packet Solution: 10-oz bottles	Abdominal cramps, flatulence, bloating, nausea, and vomiting.	Lactulose is a fermentable sugar, allowing colonic bacteria to produce gaseous products that may cause discomfort—these symptoms typically respond to decreased doses. Effective for disimpaction, poorly palatable.
Solution: 400 mg/5 mL Chew tablet: 311 mg Concentrate liquid: 800 mg/5 mL	Abdominal cramps, hypermagnesemia (especially in infants).	
Oral solution: 3-oz bottle (combination of monobasic and dibasic sodium phosphate) Enemas: 4.5-oz bottle	Cramping, bloating, diarrhea, nausea and vomiting, hyperphosphatemia.	Very poorly palatable.
Liquid: 30 mL/30 mL Enema: 118 mL	Mineral oil can leak from anus and stain clothes. Prolonged use can result in malabsorption of fat-soluble vitamins.	Mineral oil is a complex mixture of hydrocarbons derived from petroleum. Not suitable for children who cannot protect their airway because of aspiration risk. Poorly palatable. Not approved for oral administration in children <6 yr.

1

with relief by both the child and parents. Acknowledging possible setbacks but explaining that the prognosis is excellent will help greatly in compliance. A combination of oral laxatives, frequent toilet sitting (for 5 to 10 minutes approximately 30 minutes after meals) and parental praise and reward is more successful than laxatives alone. Some parents and children find that a "sticker" or "star" calendar documenting days with successful bowel movements or absence of soiling provides a positive way to encourage behavioral modifications. Small rewards can be given for consecutive days with stickers, and, as bowel movements become more regular, rewards can be spaced out to longer durations of success.

SUGGESTED READINGS

1. Baker SS, Liptak GS, Colletti RB, et al: Constipation in infants and children: Evaluation and treatment. J Pediatr Gastroenterol Nutr 29(5):612–626, 1999. **This article presents clinical practice guidelines developed by the North American Society for Pediatric Gastroenterology and Nutrition for the management of pediatric constipation.**
2. Loening-Baucke V: Chronic constipation in children. Gastroenterology 105(5):1557–1564, 1993. **A review of the diagnosis, evaluation, and management of chronic constipation in children.**
3. Pashankar DS, Loening-Baucke V, Bishop WP: Safety of polyethylene glycol 3350 for the treatment of chronic constipation in children. Arch Pediatr Adolesc Med 157(7):661–664, 2003. **This study assesses the biochemical and clinical safety profile of long-term polyethylene glycol for oral solution in children. Eighty-three children (mean dose of 0.75 g/kg per day and mean duration of 8.7 months) were studied. Polyethylene glycol (PEG) was well tolerated, with minimal adverse events.**
4. Reeves JD, Yip R: Lack of adverse side effects of oral ferrous sulfate therapy in 1-year-old infants. Pediatrics 75(2):352–355, 1985. **This placebo-controlled, randomized study found no increase in constipation compared to placebo in 278 healthy 1-year-olds given 3 mg/kg/day supplemental iron for 3 months.**
5. Weaver LT, Ewing G, Taylor LC: The bowel habit of milk-fed infants. J Pediatr Gastroenterol Nutr 7(4):568–571, 1988. **A prospective study of the bowel habits of 240 breast- and formula-fed infants 2 to 20 weeks of age showing large variation in normal stooling with softer, more frequent stools among breast-fed infants.**
6. Youssef NN, Di Lorenzo C: Childhood constipation: evaluation and treatment. J Clin Gastroenterol 33(3):199–205, 2001. **This article discusses the evaluation and management options available for practitioners treating children with chronic constipation. It includes a practical approach and a useful evaluation and management flowchart.**

Colic

Marc Weissbluth

KEY CONCEPTS

- All newborns have a propensity to exhibit increasing and then decreasing amounts of fuss/cry behavior during the first 3 to 4 months of age.
- Because all babies have some degree of fuss/cry behavior, all parents should receive counseling to help them understand and learn to cope.
- When counseling parents, distinguish between helping parents better soothe their infant to reduce their infant's fuss/cry behavior and helping parents cope well.

Wessel and associates studied 98 healthy children, of whom 48 (49%) were defined as "fussy" because they had "paroxysms of irritability, fussing, *or* crying lasting for a total of more than three hours a day and occurring on more than three days in any one week." Also, for 26% of the 98 infants, "25 were considered to be seriously fussy in that their paroxysms continued to recur for more than three weeks or became so severe that the pediatrician thought that medication was indicated." In a footnote, the authors state that these 25 "seriously fussy" infants would be classified as "colicky" by most pediatric observers. Many other studies on colic show a similar prevalence rate of approximately 20%, but studies using different diagnostic criteria report different prevalence rates.

The emphasis on fussing as opposed to crying behavior is important to note both in the title of Wessel's paper and his concept of seriously fussy because a child might fulfill Wessel's criteria and cry very little or not at all. That is, if parents spend more than 3 hours per day, more than 3 days per week, for more than 3 weeks successfully soothing their fussy newborn to prevent crying (which would have otherwise occurred if the parents' soothing efforts were less or absent), the child is labeled "colicky." Fussing is an unsettled, irritable, not continuous, low-level distress vocalization or a precry state that would lead to crying if soothing efforts were not forthcoming. Crying is intense and continuous vocalization signifying apparent distress.

The proclivity to fuss or cry is observed in all newborns in every culture studied and follows a predictable pattern. Shortly after 40 weeks from conception, a transition occurs from a quiet sleepy state to a more active wakeful state followed by increasing amounts of unexplained fussing and crying that peaks at approximately 46 weeks and then decreases over the next several weeks. This pattern occurs mostly independent of the gestational age at birth. Parenting practices such as constantly carrying infants, sleeping with infants, or feeding infants at a high frequency may be associated with decreased duration of the bouts of crying/fussing but not a decrease in the frequency of bouts of crying/fussing. The bouts of fussing/crying usually start when the infant is awake and stop when the infant falls asleep. At their peak, the bouts tend to be highly focused in the evening hours. Because measurements of crying/fussing show no discontinuities, it is incorrect to describe two distinctly different populations of infants, those with and those without unexplained crying/fussiness. The onset, peak, and disappearance linked to postconceptual age, universality, circadian occurrence, and state specificity all suggest that fuss/cry behavior is caused by a developmental physiologic process showing a range of intensity and duration rather than a pathologic condition.

These are healthy infants with normal weight gain and no diagnosed disease, but because they behave as if they are in distress, they stress the parents. Because of its highly predictable pattern and universality, this crying/fussiness most likely represents a developmental phase of normal behavior. Colic is not a medical problem that requires medical treatment.

High responsivity, defined as crying after stimulation, such as undressing or putting down, that persists for longer durations and continues despite soothing intervention measured at 1 week is associated with increased crying in general. These measured individual differences and home observations strongly suggest that the *onset* of early infant crying is not caused by suboptimal parental care. Infant crying in general appears to be modifiable by parent care. In infants with the greatest amounts of fussing/crying related to colic, it is questionable whether parent care is responsible for maintaining or capable of modifying the course of infant crying. The responsivity of the newborn may be a congenital trait, but the magnitude or intensity of what appears to be the infant's proclivity to distress may be viewed as a combination of factors within the child and the parents' ability to soothe their infant.

Distress during pregnancy as a risk factor for colic has been studied. It is unclear whether prenatal general distress (financial circumstances, housing conditions, work situation, relationship to partner, family, or friends, pregnancy, own health, illness among family or friends) or psychological distress (fearful, hopeless about the future, constantly under strain, nervous, blue, edgy, tense, or keyed up) has a causal relationship to colic, causes a postnatal reporting bias, or is a postnatal impaired maternal coping response to a crying infant.

Expert Opinion on Management Issues

- It is important to discuss fuss/cry behavior with all parents because there is no clinical way to determine which newborns will have high levels of fussing/crying.
- Counseling is more effective if started early (anticipatory guidance) and if the father or other family members (grandparents) are involved. Direct contact with the parents is best.
- Repetition is necessary because of parental sleep deprivation and anxiety. Parents need to understand that they do not cause this behavior, but they may be able to modify fuss/cry behavior, especially the duration of individual fuss/cry bouts.

This approach must be modified for families from different social or cultural backgrounds and is further individualized based on the family's resources for soothing their infant. Resources or items that make soothing easier include the presence of father; involvement of relatives, neighbors, or friends; agreements between parents regarding child-rearing issues such as breast-feeding or family bed; the absence of marital discord, postpartum depression, other children requiring attention, medical problems of family members, or financial pressure requiring the mother to have a short maternity leave; ease of breast-feeding; number of bedrooms; and ability to afford housekeeping or child-care help.

Soothing infants to reduce fuss/cry behavior involves the following strategies:

- Encourage sucking: Breast, fist, wrist, fingers, pacifier.
- Provide rhythmic rocking: Swing, rocking chair, car ride, jogger, bouncing, walking, dancing.
- Try gentle pressure: Swaddling, massage, snuggling in a soft cloth front carrier.
- Provide sounds: Loud rough mechanical sounds, lullabies, shushing, womb- or heartbeat-recorded sounds, humming, sounds from nature (running water, birds, waves crashing).
- Meet the infant's five needs: Feed, sleep, hold, suck, and stimulate.
- Reduce stimulation: Think dark, quiet, and motionless.
- Provide supplemental carrying: Carry more even when not fussing/crying. (Published studies show that supplemental carrying reduces crying in unselected infants but does not reduce crying in infants selected for colic.)
- Feed frequently: Shorten the interval between feeding.
- Avoid the overtired state: Try to nap the infant during the day within 1 to 2 hours of wakefulness.
- Consider behavioral interventions as involving the reframing of crying as an unmet need, not pain. Respond quickly to meet the five needs and try not to let the infant cry. Gather detailed data regarding fussing, crying, and sleeping to formulate a support system and a clear daily routine emphasizing external regulation of internal behaviors, either reducing overstimulation or increasing understimulation; attempting to encourage infant's ability to self-soothe; and attempting to become more attuned to discriminate between reasons for crying. Emphasize day and night differences in the environment; make nighttime as uninteresting as possible for the infant to encourage sleeping by providing minimal interaction and stimulation. (Behavioral interventions alone appear more powerful than empathy alone.)

Helping parents to cope well involves these strategies:

- Provide empathy with extra reassurance and support. Continue to try any and all methods that help, even if only temporarily. Understand the mother, share her feelings of distress, reassure her that the infant's behavior is not her fault, take away feelings of self-blame, make her feel better, make her feel more confident, combat feelings of loneliness and isolation, encourage her to take breaks from the infant. Breaks away from the infant are framed as a benefit for the infant, not selfish for the parent, because they allow the mother to recharge her batteries and become better able to resume soothing activities. Parents need to be explicitly and repeatedly told that they cannot spoil their infant by giving their infant too much attention during the first several weeks of life. (Empathy alone is not more effective than control groups receiving standard pediatric care. Empathy is necessary but not sufficient.)
- Provide educational handouts or books on infant fussing/crying/sleeping. (Education alone is not

more effective than control groups receiving standard pediatric care.)

- When the infant is approximately 4 months old, teach parents how to prevent postcolic sleep problems and motivate them to change how they handle their child's fussing, crying, and wakefulness.

Prenatal Visit. Prepare the family for the 6-week peak of fussing or crying and wakefulness. Fathers or other caregivers are encouraged to take off a few days from work at approximately 6 weeks of age or come home early to help soothe their babies and give their partners a break. Fathers are encouraged to learn how to soothe babies by learning lullabies and infant massage, and they are requested to spend time soothing in the evening or at night. Mothers are encouraged to allow fathers to become involved in soothing to prevent crying in the evening and soothing to sleep at night or in the middle of the night.

Maternity Hospital, Day 1. All the information at the prenatal visit is repeated. Written information describing soothing techniques and newborn crying and sleeping patterns is given to the father to read and to share with his partner. The father is explicitly included and encouraged to take an active role. He has more energy because he is not postpartum or lactating.

First Office Visit, Days 3 through 5. All the information at the prenatal visit is repeated. Because the parents are exhausted at the maternity hospital, they often do not have time or energy to read the original handout or they misplace it. Therefore, the same handout given at the maternity hospital is again reviewed and given to the father to share with his partner. The family is told about the increasing fussiness, crying, and wakefulness that will develop over the next 5 weeks, and a second handout is given to the father that discusses practical coping and management strategies for this anticipated shift in behavior. Again, the father is explicitly included and encouraged to take an active role.

Second Office Visit, Week 2. All the preceding information is reviewed and clarified. After this time period and before the next office visit, the parents are encouraged to call regarding fussing, crying, and wakefulness. The office staff should provide reassurance over the telephone and encourage the parents to review handouts for soothing techniques.

Third Office Visit, Month 2. Information is presented to anticipate the evolving earlier bedtime and the need to learn how to help the colicky infant slowly learn self-soothing skills for sleep over the next 2 months. A third handout is given that discusses the emerging circadian sleep patterns to help prevent postcolic sleep problems by anticipating the emergence of an earlier bedtime and attempting to put the child to sleep at night drowsy but awake.

Using Wessel's exact criteria, an estimated 20% of the parents receiving this approach in my office report their child has colic-based fussing behavior but there has been almost no crying. Because the families are not stressed by many hours of crying and they understand the peak of fussing has passed, they are now more willing to change their parenting style slowly to help make the transition from a parent-soothed infant to a self-soothed infant.

Fourth Office Visit, Month 4. The sleep schedule is reviewed in detail and an individualized behavioral management plan is discussed to prevent postcolic sleep problems. Details of this plan are presented in the Suggested Readings.

Common Pitfalls

- The major error in management is to trivialize the parents' complaint on the basis of the supposition that colic is a transitory condition with no known morbidity or complications.
- Some busy practitioners, knowing there is no cure for colic, simply attempt to buy time by suggesting one unproven remedy after another, such as switching formulas, but this produces persistent parental stress until the natural peak of fussing/crying passes.
- Behavioral interventions appear to reduce parental stress but this is accomplished successfully only if the parents trust the pediatrician. It takes more time to build trust than to simply give a handout, order some medical tests, or recommend switching formulas or herbal teas. If the parents do not trust the caregiver, there may be unnecessary maternal self-blame and heightened anxiety. Also, lack of trust contributes to the failure to recognize and manage postcolic sleep problems. This occurs, in part, because the parents are now unwilling to try new strategies because the old recommendations failed. This attitude may result in postcolic sleep problems causing enduring sleep deprivation in the child and parents long after 3 to 4 months of age.

Communication and Counseling

Treatment progresses when parents know their pediatrician is an ally, they know what to expect regarding fussing and crying, they know not to waste their energy and upset their emotional stability on unproven remedies, and they feel unlucky but not guilty. Parents have to be told repeatedly that the crying is not their fault.

To alleviate unnecessary guilt and prevent misdirected therapies focused on parental psychological factors, pediatricians should inform parents that no sound scientific evidence suggests their inexperience, anxiety, or parenting practices are directly causing the fussing/crying. Self-doubt, feelings of inadequacy of parenting skills, or failure to nurse well should be discussed openly because all parents blame themselves for the fussing/crying. Parents should be told that treatments with formula switching, fiber-enriched formulas, sedatives, hypnotics, antiflatulents, antacids, antihistamines, alcohol, gripe water, or spinal manipulation are no better than a placebo. The physician should be patient, sympathetically supportive, and appropriately tentative when offering advice. The physician should perform a thorough examination, sometimes repeatedly, because it reassures the parents that their child is healthy and is being looked after by someone who really cares.

Parents want expertise, but they dislike so-called experts who they think are too quick to judge them. Thus it is important to consider how to gain the trust of the parents. Brief or rushed visits or phone calls are of little value. Parents need someone to listen to them. They tend to see their child as suffering. They need a way to alleviate that suffering, so they need someone to acknowledge their infant's distress sympathetically and seriously. They want to be believed and sincerely told they are not to blame. They need reassurance that their infant is not ill and the crying will eventually stop. Sharing your understanding of the experience helps parents overcome the feelings of isolation. By listening to what they have to say, you are respecting the parents, which builds trust. Trust permits the parents to be more willing to consider behavioral interventions. If parents trust you when you tell them that they are not to blame, they are more able to cope. If you focus only on the parents' emotional response and exhaustion, they are less likely to trust you.

SUGGESTED READINGS

1. Dihigo SH: New strategies for the treatment of colic: Modifying the parent/infant interaction. J Pediatr Health Care 12:256–262. **Nonblind, randomized control study of 23 infants at approximately 6 weeks showing that behavioral intervention reduced crying more than being empathetic.**
2. Sondergaard C, Olsen J, Friis-Hasche E, et al: Psychosocial distress during pregnancy and the risk of infantile colic: A follow-up study. Acta Paediatr 92:811–816, 2003. **Stressors associated with colic; how prenatal general or psychological distress might cause colic, a biased postnatal report, or an impaired postnatal maternal coping response to infant crying.**
3. St. James-Roberts I, Goodwin J, Peter B, et al: Individual differences in responsivity to a neurobehavioral examination predict crying patterns of 1-week-old infants at home. Dev Med Child Neurol 45:400–407, 2003. **Infants at 8 days who are most upset by undressing, putting down, and sustained handling are likely to cry more. Early infant crying is a "graded signal" that conveys the degree of an infant's distress rather than its specific cause. The developmental view of early infant crying implies that it does not require a medical cure.**
4. St James-Roberts I, Sleep J, Morris S, et al: Use of a behavioral programme in the first 3 months to prevent infant crying and sleeping problems. J Paediatr Child Health 37:289–297, 2001. **Nonblind, randomized control study on 610 infants studied at 3, 6, 9, and 12 weeks showing that behavioral intervention, but not an education intervention, reduced subsequent requests for help regarding crying or sleeping problems and increased the number of infants sleeping through the night at 12 weeks.**
5. Weissbluth M: Healthy Sleep Habits, Happy Child. New York: Ballantine Books, 2003. **How to correct postcolic sleep problems.**
6. Weissbluth M: The Northwestern Children's Practice online. Sleeping & crying. Available at http://www.sweetbabies.com. **A parent guide describing the development of sleeping and crying from birth to 2 months.**
7. Weissbluth M: The Northwestern Children's Practice online. Sleeping at about 2 months; Available at http://www.sweetbabies.com. **A parent guide advising different ways to help infants sleep at 2 months.**
8. Weissbluth M: The Northwestern Children's Practice online. Sleeping at about 4 months; Available at http://www.sweetbabies.com. **A parent guide describing sleep patterns at 4 months.**
9. Weissbluth M: Healthy Sleep Habits, Happy Child. New York: Ballantine, 2003. **How to correct postcolic sleep problems.**
10. Weissbluth M: Your Fussy Baby: How to Soothe Your Newborn. New York: Ballantine, 2003. **Review of colic literature, advice to parents on coping; how to prevent postcolic sleep problems.**
11. Weissbluth M: Sleep in infants with colic. In Sheldon S, Dahl R, Kryger M, Ferber R (eds): Principles and Practice of Pediatric Sleep Medicine. Philadelphia: WB Saunders, 2005. **Discussion of the association between colic and wakefulness and how postcolic sleep problems might develop.**

1

General Maintenance

Management of the Infant in the Delivery Room

Jane S. Lee

KEY CONCEPTS

- An ongoing evaluation-decision-action approach during neonatal resuscitation enables simultaneous integration of resuscitative measures by delivery team members.
- Establishment of effective positive-pressure ventilation (PPV) is the critical step in cardiopulmonary resuscitation of the compromised infant.
- If respiratory depression persists despite tactile stimulation (secondary apnea), assisted ventilation with 100% oxygen should be started immediately. If oxygen is unavailable, resuscitation with room air assisted ventilation may be provided.
- In the presence of meconium-stained amniotic fluid of any consistency, direct endotracheal intubation and suctioning is recommended for infants who are not vigorous immediately after birth as demonstrated by the presence of poor respiratory effort, poor muscle tone (lack of spontaneous movement or flexion of extremities), and heart rate less than 100 beats per minute (bpm) as well as for vigorous infants who subsequently exhibit signs of respiratory distress after initial assessment and stabilization.
- Chest compressions should be initiated in newly born infants who exhibit severe bradycardia (heart rate less than 60 bpm) despite a minimum of 30 seconds of effective PPV.
- Epinephrine may be administered to infants with severe bradycardia unresponsive to a minimum of 30 seconds of coordinated ventilation and chest compressions.
- Noninitiation of neonatal resuscitation is appropriate under special circumstances, such as birth weight less than 400 g, confirmed gestation less than 23 weeks, anencephaly, and confirmed trisomy 13 or 18.
- Discontinuation of resuscitation may be appropriate if no return of spontaneous circulation occurs within 15 minutes of initiation of adequate resuscitative efforts.

In the United States, more than 4 million infants are born each year. For the overwhelming majority of these newly born infants, the transition to the extrauterine environment occurs effortlessly. However, in approximately 10% of infants, active intervention is required in the delivery room. In at least 1%, extensive resuscitation may be necessary to sustain life. Because optimal resuscitative measures may reduce the risk of subsequent morbidity and mortality, the American Academy of Pediatrics (AAP) and the American Heart Association (AHA) established national guidelines for resuscitation. These recommendations serve as the core of the neonatal resuscitation program (NRP). Since its inception, more than 1.4 million health care providers have learned the NRP. Despite NRP's becoming the standard of care, however, the efficacy of neonatal resuscitation as outlined in the NRP has never been validated. As research in this area expands, ongoing modifications of these guidelines continue. The current recommendations offer substantive changes in the execution of resuscitative techniques from earlier publications and represent a critical, systematic evaluation of neonatal resuscitation practices based on the available scientific evidence.

Expert Opinion on Management Issues

RECOMMENDED INTERVENTIONS

Figure 1 illustrates the NRP algorithm for neonatal resuscitation, as recommended in the AAP/AHA International Guidelines 2000 for Cardiopulmonary Resuscitation and Emergency Cardiovascular Care: International Consensus on Science. At every delivery, medical staff capable of performing neonatal resuscitation should be present. Immediately upon birth, the infant must undergo a rapid assessment to determine if any meconium is present; to evaluate the quality of respirations, heart rate, and color; and to ascertain overall maturity. If this initial assessment reveals no abnormalities, the infant only requires routine care, consisting of drying, warming, positioning, and possibly clearing the airway. Suctioning the mouth and nose with either a bulb syringe or suction catheter, if performed, should be brief, with an applied negative pressure not exceeding 100 mm Hg. Compromised infants may require additional repositioning, supplemental oxygen, tactile stimulation, assisted ventilation, and chest compressions.

In any resuscitation, the most crucial action is establishing adequate ventilation. Use of 100% oxygen, preferably heated and humidified, at a flow rate between 5 and 10 L per minute via a flow-inflating ventilator

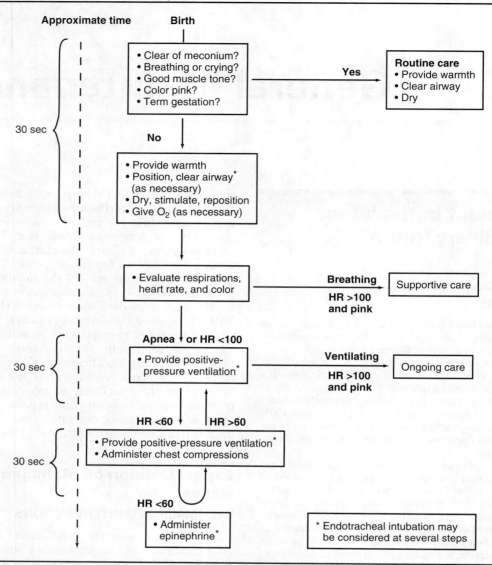

FIGURE 1. Neonatal Resuscitation Program algorithm for resuscitation of the newly born infant. From Niermeyer S, Kattwinkel J, Van Reempts P, et al: International Guidelines for Neonatal Resuscitation: An excerpt from the Guidelines 2000 for Cardiopulmonary Resuscitation and Emergency Cardiovascular Care: International Consensus on Science. Contributors and Reviewers for the Neonatal Resuscitation Guidelines. Pediatrics 106:E29, 2000.

bag-and-mask device, oxygen mask, or hand cupped around oxygen tubing is indicated in cyanotic infants who have adequate respiratory effort and sustained heart rate above 100 beats per minute (bpm). If respiratory effort is absent or irregular, tactile stimulation should be initiated. Positive-pressure ventilation (PPV) with 100% oxygen is recommended if apnea or gasping respirations persist despite tactile stimulation, heart rate is less than 100 bpm, or central cyanosis persists despite administration of 100% oxygen. Although substantial amounts of animal data support the use of room air resuscitation, there is insufficient data from clinical trials in neonates to change the current recommendation. In situations where oxygen is unavailable, however, room air resuscitation should be started.

When assisted ventilation is initiated, the lowest inflation pressures sufficient to result in adequate chest rise should be employed. Most infants require higher inflation pressures with the initial breaths. Variations in distending pressures and inflation times are not studied extensively enough at this time to recommend a universal approach. The recommended ventilation rate is 40 to 60 breaths per minute or 30 breaths per minute if chest compressions are also required. If ventilation is inadequate, repositioning, clearing of any residual airway secretions, and increasing inflation pressures may be necessary. PPV may be gradually reduced and withdrawn if spontaneous respirations are present and heart rate is sustained at more than 100 bpm.

Endotracheal intubation is indicated in the setting of ineffective or prolonged bag-mask ventilation, administration of medications, and special situations, such as meconium staining, congenital diaphragmatic hernia, and extreme prematurity. Free-flow oxygen should be

TABLE 1 Neonatal Resuscitation Program Suggested Guidelines for Endotracheal Tube Size and Insertion Depth

Birth Weight	Gestational Age	Tube Size (ID)	Insertion Depth	Blade Size (no.)
<1000 g	<28 wk	2.5 mm	6.5–7.0 cm	0
1000–2000 g	28–34 wk	3.0 mm	7–8 cm	0
2000–3000 g	34–38 wk	3.5 mm	8–9 cm	0 or 1
>3000 g	>38 wk	3.5–4.0 mm	>9 cm	1

From Niermeyer S, Kattwinkel J, Van Reempts P, et al: International Guidelines for Neonatal Resuscitation: An excerpt from the Guidelines 2000 for Cardiopulmonary Resuscitation and Emergency Cardiovascular Care: International Consensus on Science. Contributors and Reviewers for the Neonatal Resuscitation Guidelines. Pediatrics 106:E29, 2000.

administered throughout the procedure, and each attempt should be limited to less than 20 seconds. Appropriate choice of blade and endotracheal tube size is based on the infant's birth weight and gestational age (Table 1). If the vocal cord guide at the distal tip of the endotracheal tube (ETT) is advanced slightly beyond the vocal cords, theoretically the tip should lie between the vocal cords and the carina. Appropriate placement should be confirmed by clinical evaluation (i.e., equal breath sounds on auscultation, vital sign improvement) and position on chest radiograph.

Meconium-stained amniotic fluid (MSAF) occurs in approximately 10% to 15% of all deliveries. Although it is rarely seen in infants born before 37 weeks' gestation, MSAF may occur in more than 30% of pregnancies that extend beyond 42 weeks' gestation. Between 5% and 12% of these infants may exhibit respiratory distress consistent with meconium aspiration syndrome (MAS). Intubation and mechanical ventilation may be necessary in as many as 50% of infants who develop MAS. Although in utero aspiration is suspected in up to 20% to 30% of meconium-stained infants, the current obstetric management is to perform intrapartum suctioning of the hypopharynx and nose with either bulb syringe or DeLee suction catheter prior to delivery of the infant's shoulders. This recommendation will most likely be revised given the recently published prospective multicenter randomized, controlled trial by Vain and colleagues that demonstrates no significant difference in incidence of meconium aspiration with intrapartum oropharyngeal and nasopharyngeal suctioning.

After delivery, all vigorous infants should receive expectant care regardless of the consistency of the meconium. *Vigor* is defined as the presence of spontaneous respirations, reasonable muscle tone (some degree of extremity flexion or visible spontaneous movements of the extremities), and heart rate above 100 bpm. In their prospective multicenter randomized, controlled trial, Wiswell and colleagues show that expectant management is just as efficacious as routine intubation and suctioning in preventing meconium aspiration syndrome in vigorous infants. However, intubation and direct suctioning should still be performed in infants who are nonvigorous at birth or who subsequently develop respiratory distress after initial assessment. Wall suction should be set at a negative pressure between 80 and 100 mm Hg. Continuous suctioning by means of a meconium aspirator should be applied for 3 to 5 seconds as the tube is removed. Repeat intubation and suctioning is recommended until

no further meconium is recovered or until significant bradycardia indicates that resuscitation must proceed.

Most infants respond to effective assisted ventilation. However, chest compressions should be initiated in infants who remain bradycardic (heart rate below 60 bpm) despite a minimum of 30 seconds of effective PPV. Based on animal studies, a relative compression depth of approximately one third of the anterior-posterior diameter of the chest is necessary to generate a palpable pulse. Ventilation and chest compressions should be coordinated in a 3:1 ratio. As resuscitation progresses, heart rate must be continually reassessed by either palpating pulsations at the base of the umbilical cord or auscultation of the precordium. Once the heart rate rises above 60 bpm, chest compressions can be discontinued. PPV should be continued until the infant has regular spontaneous respirations.

Fortunately, medications are used in only a small minority of resuscitations. The medications available for use in the delivery room are epinephrine, volume expanders, naloxone, and sodium bicarbonate (Table 2). The current recommendations for their use are based primarily on extrapolations from experimental studies and human studies in the older pediatric and adult populations. Although the intratracheal (IT) route is the most accessible route, intravenous (IV) administration by the umbilical vein is the preferred route of drug administration. Under sterile conditions, the umbilical venous catheter (UVC) should be inserted until blood flow is obtained. Alternatively, peripheral venous cannulation can also be attempted. If appropriate intravenous access cannot be obtained, intraosseous (IO) administration is acceptable. Umbilical arterial catheter (UAC) use is not recommended because of potential complications related to infusion of vasoactive or hypertonic medications.

The administration of epinephrine is recommended in infants who have sustained bradycardia (less than 60 bpm) despite adequate coordinated ventilation and chest compressions lasting at least 30 seconds. It may be particularly useful in infants who are asystolic at birth. The current recommended dose for epinephrine is 0.01 to 0.03 mg/kg; use of higher doses is not currently supported. Although adult data demonstrate improved myocardial and cerebral perfusion pressures with high-dose epinephrine, pediatric clinical data and neonatal animal models do not reveal any clear benefit in return of spontaneous circulation (ROSC), survival, or neurologic outcomes. Instead, the evidence indicates potentially more adverse effects associated with the higher dose. Research is also

TABLE 2 Medications Available for Neonatal Resuscitation

Medications	Route/Dosage/Regimen	Dosage Formulations	Potential Adverse Reactions	Comments
Epinephrine	IV/IT. 0.01–0.03 mg/kg (0.1–0.3 mL/kg) Repeat q3–5 min as indicated	Solution: 1:10,000 (0.1 mg/mL) Preparation: 3 mL, 10 mL ampoules	Hypertension, tachycardia, arrhythmia, intracranial hemorrhage	Administer rapidly; 0.5–1.0 mL saline flush is recommended Do *not* infuse through UAC; infuse over 5-10 min
Isotonic Crystalloid	IV/IO 10 mL/kg Repeat as indicated	Solution: normal saline (0.9%); lactated Ringer's	Pulmonary edema, intracranial hemorrhage	If acute blood loss is suspected, consider O-negative red blood cells; 5% albumin is *not* recommended
Naloxone	IV/IT/IO/IM/SC. 0.1 mg/kg (0.1 mL/kg). Repeat q3–5 min as indicated	Solution: 0.4 mg/mL (1-mL ampoule), 1.0 mg/mL (2-mL ampoule)	Acute withdrawal, seizures (in narcotic-habituated infant)	*Contraindicated* in infants born to mothers with narcotic addiction or on methadone maintenance Delayed onset if given by IM/SC route
Sodium Bicarbonate	IV/IO 1-2 mEq/kg (4 mL/kg) Repeat as indicated	Solution: 4.2% (0.5 mEq/mL) Preparation: 10-mL ampoules	Hypernatremia, hypocalcemia, intracranial hemorrhage	Confirm adequate ventilation *prior* to use Infuse *slowly* over 2 min; minimum rate is 1 mEq/kg/min. Do *not* infuse with other medications

IM, intramuscular; IO, intraosseous; IT, intratracheal; IV, intravenous; SC, subcutaneous; UAC, umbilical arterial catheter.
From Kattwinkel J (ed): Textbook of Neonatal Resuscitation, 4th ed. Elk Grove Village, Ill: American Academy of Pediatrics/American Heart Association, 2000.

contradictory regarding the effectiveness of IT administration; however, epinephrine continues to be given by this route because of its easy accessibility.

In the setting of acute blood loss or shock, the fluid of choice for volume expansion is an isotonic crystalloid solution such as normal saline or lactated Ringer's. If large blood loss is anticipated, O-negative red blood cells may also be considered. However, albumin is no longer recommended for use in initial volume expansion because of the infectious risk and increased mortality associated with albumin use and clinical data demonstrating the efficacy of crystalloid solution in treatment of hypotension.

Naloxone continues to be recommended for use in infants who exhibit respiratory depression following maternal opioid analgesia within the preceding 4 hours prior to delivery. This recommendation is based on experimental evidence displaying its benefit in reversing narcotic-induced apnea. No neonatal studies are available to evaluate its effect on establishing effective respirations, comparing the various modes of administration, or defining its long-term sequelae. Naloxone remains contraindicated in infants born to mothers with a suspected narcotic addiction or on methadone maintenance because it could potentially induce withdrawal symptoms and seizures in this subgroup. When naloxone is used, repeat doses may be required given the shorter half-life of naloxone compared to opioid agents.

Sodium bicarbonate administration in the delivery room is cautiously recommended for use only in prolonged cardiopulmonary arrests unresponsive to other therapies. Adequate ventilation and circulation must be established prior to administration. However, there is an obvious lack of scientific evidence showing any benefit to its use; specifically, no neonatal studies demonstrate any improvement in acid-base status, ROSC, or survival. Additional studies are necessary to address these clinically meaningful outcomes if it is to remain in the collection of medications available for use in the delivery room setting.

CONTROVERSIAL INTERVENTIONS

Although direct laryngoscopy and visualization is the gold standard for confirmation of endotracheal intubation, confirmation by capnography or colorimetric CO_2 detector use is increasing, especially when clinical assessment is equivocal. Current application of these newer tools in the delivery room is limited because of reduced sensitivity (false negatives) in the setting of low lung volumes or low cardiac output as seen in extremely premature infants and congenital heart disease. False-positive results are also reported when the ETT is positioned improperly in the pharynx. Therefore, these devices are currently recommended only for secondary confirmation of ETT placement.

The use of a laryngeal mask airway (LMA) in neonatal resuscitation is recognized as a potential alternative method in establishing an airway when bag-mask ventilation is ineffective or endotracheal intubation is not successful. In fact, it may be lifesaving in a subset of infants with severe congenital airway abnormalities. However, LMA use remains classified as "indeterminate class" because of the paucity of neonatal data in the delivery room setting. Although one of its advantages is the ease of use, a recent survey reveals a current low level of competence and use of this device. The usefulness of the LMA may be limited in smaller preterm infants or infants of low birth weight and in situations where high airway pressures or IT administration of resuscitative medications are required. There are also no data compiled in the setting of meconium staining. Further studies are required before its routine use in the delivery room can be recommended.

Respiratory management continues to be an area of active debate in preterm infants, who represent the largest subgroup requiring resuscitation. Although the evidence supports early prophylactic administration of surfactant in extremely premature infants born at less than 28 weeks' gestation, wide practice variation exists in its application. Controversy persists regarding the acceptable window for prophylactic surfactant administration, the use of continuous positive airway pressure during delivery room resuscitation, as well as the parameters for ventilatory support (i.e., gentle ventilation).

Another focus for current research is the use of cerebral hypothermia. Experimental data suggest that cerebral hypothermia may reduce the risk of reperfusion injury associated with perinatal asphyxia. Selective head cooling with mild systemic hypothermia for up to 72 hours appears safe in term asphyxiated infants. Preliminary data presented at a recent national meeting suggests that cerebral hypothermia may improve intact survival in asphyxiated infants with moderately suppressed amplitudes on electroencephalography (EEG). Yet insufficient clinical evidence is available regarding long-term outcomes to support its routine application in this subpopulation of infants. Until definitive data are established, infants should be maintained in an isothermic environment. At present, the Cool Cap device (Olympic Medical, Seattle, WA) is under consideration for FDA approval in moderately to severely asphyxiated infants.

As obstetric management and neonatal intensive care continue to improve, ethical dilemmas are increasingly more prevalent. There is little consensus on noninitiation and discontinuation of resuscitative measures in the delivery room. The AAP and AHA are intentionally vague on this matter; offering only broad suggestions (Box 1). Noninitiation of resuscitation is appropriate in limited situations in which extreme prematurity or lethal congenital anomaly is confirmed. Discontinuation of resuscitative measures may be considered if asystole persists for longer than 15 minutes despite appropriate intervention. Population-based data indicate a low likelihood of intact survival if ROSC does not occur within 10 minutes of active resuscitation. More specific recommendations regarding the duration and extent of resuscitation in other situations, such as prolonged or refractory bradycardia, are not available.

Common Pitfalls

- In addition to NRP (neonatal resuscitation program) certification, supervised training in actual delivery room resuscitations is necessary until hands-on competence is clearly demonstrated.
- Use of resuscitative medications not in accordance to NRP guidelines should be avoided.
- In nonvigorous infants born through meconium-stained amniotic fluid, numerous endotracheal intubations for tracheal suctioning of meconium may result in delays in implementing further resuscitative measures.
- NRP guidelines defer decisions regarding discontinuation of resuscitative measures to local institutional boards.

Communication and Counseling

The extent and duration of delivery room resuscitation depends on the infant's gestational age, birth weight, and clinical status upon birth, as well as subsequent response to resuscitative measures. Among those who require active intervention, extremely premature infants pose a unique ethical dilemma. The current lower limit of viability suggested by many professional organizations is approximately 23 to 25 weeks' gestation. Despite improving survival of infants born in this gray zone, outcome studies continue to report a 30% to 50% incidence of moderate or severe disability among the survivors. In this subset in which prognosis is uncertain, obstetrical and neonatal providers must provide parents with consistent and accurate counseling. These discussions need to include available information on survival from local and national data, the spectrum of possible outcomes and treatment options, and the potential risks associated with the available therapies. Once resuscitation is initiated, full resuscitative measures should be provided until the infant improves or medical support is withdrawn. Similarly, infants born with congenital anomalies also require an individualized approach. The severity of the malformations should not affect the delivery room management unless a diagnosis of a lethal congenital anomaly is previously confirmed. Again, if the diagnosis is uncertain, resuscitative efforts should continue until an accurate diagnosis is established.

BOX 1 Neonatal Resuscitation Program Suggested Guidelines for Endotracheal Tube Size and Insertion Depth

Noninitiation

- Birth weight <400 g
- Confirmed gestational age <23 weeks
- Anencephaly
- Confirmed trisomy 13 or 18

Discontinuation

- No return of spontaneous circulation after 15 min of asystole

From Niermeyer S, Kattwinkel J, Van Reempts P, et al: International Guidelines for Neonatal Resuscitation: An excerpt from Guidelines 2000 for Cardiopulmonary Resuscitation and Emergency Cardiovascular Care: International Consensus on Science. Contributors and Reviewers for the Neonatal Resuscitation Guidelines. Pediatrics 106:E29, 2000.

SUGGESTED READINGS

1. Cochrane Injuries Group Albumin Reviewers: Human albumin administration in critically ill patients: Systematic review of randomized controlled trials. BMJ 317:235–240, 1998. **A meta-analysis revealing an increased mortality associated with albumin use.**

2. Kattwinkel J (ed): Textbook of Neonatal Resuscitation, 4th ed. Elk Grove Village, Ill. American Academy of Pediatrics/American Heart Association, 2000. **Provides details of current neonatal resuscitative measures recommended by the AAP and the AHA.**

3. Lorenz JM: Management decisions in extremely premature infants. Semin Neonatol 8:475–482, 2003. **Discusses the range of medical management provided to extremely premature infants.**

4. MacDonald H, and the Committee on Fetus and Newborn: Perinatal care at the threshold of viability. Pediatrics 110:1024–1027, 2002. **Report describing the counseling and support that should be provided to families of extremely premature infants.**

5. McGuire W, Fowlie PW: Naloxone for narcotic exposed newborn infants: Systematic review. Arch Dis Child Fetal Neonatal Ed 88: F308–F311, 2003. **A meta-analysis finding no study examining naloxone use and the need for subsequent assisted ventilation.**

6. Niermeyer S, Kattwinkel J, Van Reempts P, et al: International Guidelines for Neonatal Resuscitation: An excerpt from the Guidelines 2000 for Cardiopulmonary Resuscitation and Emergency Cardiovascular Care: International Consensus on Science. Pediatrics 106:E29, 2000. **Provides algorithm for neonatal resuscitation and detailed recommendations from the AAP and AHA.**

7. Saugstad OD, Rootwelt T, Aalen O: Resuscitation of asphyxiated newborn infants with room air or oxygen: An international controlled trial: The Resair 2 study. Pediatrics 102:E1, 1998. **Prospective, international, multicenter, quasi-randomized, nonblind trial in asphyxiated infants that demonstrated no difference in overall survival or development of hypoxic ischemic encephalopathy between infants resuscitated with room air or 100% oxygen.**

8. So KW, Fok TF, Ng PC, et al: Randomised controlled trial of colloid or crystalloid in hypotensive preterm infants. Arch Dis Child 76: F43–F46, 1997. **Study demonstrating efficacy of isotonic saline in treatment of acute hypotension.**

9. Vain N, Szyld EG, Prudent LM, et al: Oropharyngeal and nasopharyngeal suctioning of meconium-stained neonates before delivery of their shoulders: Multicentre, randomised controlled trial. Lancet 364:597–602, 2004. **Prospective randomized controlled trial revealing no reduction in incidence of MAS with use of intrapartum suctioning.**

10. Wiswell TE, Gannon CM, Jacobs J, et al: Delivery room management of the apparently vigorous meconium-stained neonate: Results of the multicenter, international collaborative trial. Pediatrics 105:1–7, 2000. **Prospective randomized, controlled trial showing no difference between routine tracheal intubation and suctioning versus expectant management in the incidence of MAS for vigorous infants born through MSAF.**

Nutrient Requirements of Term and Preterm Infants

William C. Heird

KEY CONCEPTS

- Breast-feeding for the first 6 months of life or longer is recommended for term infants.
- If breast-feeding is impossible or the mother decides against it, a standard term infant formula is a reasonable option.

- Breast-fed and formula-fed infants should receive complementary foods starting between 4 and 6 months of age.
- The order of introduction of complementary foods is of little importance unless there is a strong family history of food allergy or atopic disease, in which case breast-feeding should be continued through the first year and allergenic foods (e.g., eggs, cow's milk, meats) should not be introduced until approximately 1 year of age; only one new food should be introduced at a time with a spacing of 2 to 4 days between foods.
- Mothers of preterm infants should be encouraged, but not coerced, to provide breast milk for feeding their infants, but it should be fortified by one of the available human milk fortifiers.
- Preterm infants who cannot be fed immediately should receive parenteral nutrients starting within 24 hours of birth and continuing until the infant tolerates a formula or fortified human milk intake of at least 120 mL/kg/day.
- Formula-fed preterm infants should be given a post-discharge (transitional) formula rather than a standard term formula.
- Preterm infants can be started on complementary foods at approximately the same postconceptional age as recommended for term infants.
- Neither term nor preterm infants should receive whole cow's milk until after 1 year of age.

Growth of the healthy breast-fed term infant is the most widely accepted standard for growth from birth through 4 to 6 months of age. Thus it is logical to assume that the amounts of each nutrient ingested by the breast-fed term infant during this period are adequate, and the most recent dietary reference intakes for the 0- to 6-month-old term infant (Table 1) reflect the amount of each nutrient in the average volume of human milk ingested by 0- to 6-month-old breast-fed infants (i.e., 780 mL per day). Currently available term formulas provide even greater amounts of most nutrients. Thus, unless there is an underlying condition that limits intake, interferes with absorption, or increases nutrient needs, most breast-fed infants receive adequate amounts of all nutrients for the first 4 to 6 months of life, and formula-fed infants receive adequate intakes for even longer.

There is no equally satisfactory standard for growth of preterm infants. Rather, the nutrient requirements of these infants are usually defined as the amounts necessary to support intrauterine rates of growth as well as nutrient accretion. Table 2 summarizes the requirements proposed in 1985 by the American Academy of Pediatrics Committee on Nutrition. Unfortunately, considering the many advantages of human milk (e.g., fewer common infections; better neurodevelopmental outcomes), the rate of growth of preterm infants fed unsupplemented human milk is lower than the intrauterine growth rate. Further, even if the total protein, calcium, phosphorus, sodium, and, perhaps, zinc contents of a reasonable volume of human milk were absorbed and completely retained, the amounts retained would not be sufficient to support intrauterine rates of accretion.

If the requirements for supporting intrauterine rates of growth and nutrient deposition are provided from birth onward, the infant of low birth weight (LBW), in theory, should continue to grow as if birth had not

TABLE 1 Daily Reference Intakes of Nutrients for Normal Infants*

Nutrient	Reference Intake per Day	
	0–6 Months (6 kg)	7–12 Months (9 kg)
Energy (kcal (kJ)	550 (2310)	720 (3013)
Fat (g)	31	30
Linoleic acid (g)	4.4	4.6
α-Linolenic acid (g)	0.5	0.5
Carbohydrate (g)	60	95
Protein (g)	9.3	11[†]
Water (mL)	700	800
Electrolytes and minerals		
Calcium (mg)	210	270
Phosphorus (mg)	100	275
Magnesium (mg)	30	75
Sodium (mg)	120[†]	370[†]
Chloride (mg)	180[†]	570[†]
Potassium (mg)	400[†]	700[†]
Iron (mg)	0.27	11[†]
Zinc (mg)	2	3[†]
Copper (μg)	200	220
Iodine (μg)	110	130
Selenium (μg)	15	20
Manganese (μg)	3	600
Fluoride (μg)	10	500
Chromium (μg)	0.2	5.5
Molybdenum (μg)	2	3
Vitamins		
Vitamin A (μg)	400	500
Vitamin D (μg)	5	5
Vitamin E (mg α-tocopherol)	4	6
Vitamin K (μg)	2.0	2.5
Vitamin C (mg)	40	50
Thiamine (mg)	0.2	0.3
Riboflavin (mg)	0.3	0.4
Niacin (mg niacin equivalent)	2	4
Vitamin B_6 (μg)	0.1	0.3
Folate (μg)	65	80
Vitamin B_{12} (μg)	0.4	0.5
Biotin (μg)	5	6
Pantothenic acid (mg)	1.7	1.8
Choline (mg)	125	150

*Adequate intake (AI) unless indicated otherwise.
[†]Recommended daily allowance (RDA).

intervened. However, few LBW infants make a successful transition to enteral intake until some time after birth. Most lose a minimum of 10% of initial weight during the first week of life and do not regain it until 1 to 3 weeks later. Some of this weight loss, approximately half, reflects loss of excess extracellular fluid and is of little importance to the infant, but the remainder reflects primarily loss of lean body mass and may have serious consequences for the infant.

Even if intakes sufficient to support intrauterine rates of nutrient accretion are provided, few infants regain birth weight before at least 2 weeks of age. Further, providing these intakes throughout the remainder of hospitalization does not prevent the infant from weighing less than a fetus of the same postconceptional age, and, at discharge, approximately 90% weigh less than the 10th percentile of intrauterine standards.

A likely contributor to this growth retardation at discharge is failure of the protein and energy intakes that support intrauterine rates of weight gain and protein accretion to replenish any loss of lean body mass prior to the infant's regaining birth weight. Doing so requires an additional allowance for catch-up growth, which varies considerably from infant to infant and is additional to the needs for supporting intrauterine rates of growth and nutrient accretion. These differing needs for catch-up growth make it difficult to define appropriate nutrient requirements for all preterm infants. Rather, each infant has a unique requirement consisting of the need for maintaining intrauterine rates of growth and nutrient retention plus the need for catch-up.

Expert Opinion on Management Issues

TERM INFANTS

Most authorities advocate breast-feeding of the normal term infant. However, if this is not possible or if the mother chooses not to do so, modern infant formulas are a

TABLE 2 Recommended Nutrient Intakes for Infants of Low Birth Weight

Nutrient	Recommended Intake*
Macronutrients	*Amount per 100 kcal*
Protein (g)	2.7–3.1
Fat (g)	(300 mg essential fatty acids)
Carbohydrate	—
Electrolytes and minerals	*Amount per 100 kcal*
Sodium (mEq)	2.3–2.7
Potassium (mEq)	1.8–1.9
Calcium (mg)	140–150
Magnesium (mg)	6.5–7.5
Phosphorus (mg)	95–108
Chloride (mEq)	2–2.4
Trace minerals	*Amount per 100 kcal*
Zinc (mg)	0.5
Copper (μg)	90
Manganese (μg)	5
Iodine (μg)	5
Vitamins	*Amount per Day*
A (IU)	1400
D (IU)	500
E (IU)	5–25 (1.0 IU/g linoleic acid)
C (mg)	35
Thiamine (μg)	300
Riboflavin (μg)	400
Niacin (mg)	6
B_6 (μg)	300 (15 μg/g protein)
Folic acid (μg)	0.3
B_{12} (μg)	2
Pantothenic acid (mg)	25
Biotin (μg)	35

Data from Committee on Nutrition, American Academy of Pediatrics: Pediatrics 75:976–986, 1985.

*Lower values are the recommended intakes for smaller infants (birth weight <1250 g).

cereals other than rice, eggs, and other particularly allergenic foods should not be introduced until after 1 year of age. Only one new food should be introduced at a time, and it should be given for approximately 3 days before another food is introduced. Either home-prepared or commercial strained foods can be used.

By 1 year of age, most infants are ready for at least some table food. By this time, they should be receiving approximately two to three servings of cereal, one serving of meat, and three to five servings of fruits and vegetables. Breast milk or infant formula should be continued through at least the first 12 months of life after which regular cow's milk can be introduced. Most infants decrease their intake of breast milk and/or formula as complementary foods are introduced. Those who do not should be watched carefully to assure that weight gain is not excessive.

PRETERM INFANTS

Preterm/LBW infants are usually fed either supplemented human milk or formulas derived from cow's milk that contain more protein (2.71 to 3 g per 100 kcal), calcium (165 to 180 mg per 100 kcal), and phosphorus (83 to 100 mg per 100 kcal) than human milk or term infant formulas. Fat provides approximately 50% of the nonprotein energy of both human milk and LBW infant formulas. Although poorer fat absorption by LBW versus term infants is reported and attributed to a deficiency of pancreatic lipase and bile salts, modern LBW formulas contain primarily unsaturated long-chain triglycerides and medium-chain triglycerides, both of which are well absorbed. Because of concern that the LBW infant may have difficulty digesting lactose secondary to a developmental lag in intestinal mucosal lactase activity, LBW infant formulas contain a mixture of lactose and glucose polymers.

Although the immunologic properties of human milk, both cellular and humoral, are a distinct advantage, evidence that human milk is nutritionally superior to available LBW formulas is lacking. In fact, growth rates of LBW infants fed their own mothers' milk (which has a 20% to 25% higher protein concentration than term milk for the first 3 to 4 weeks of lactation) are lower than those of infants fed LBW infant formulas. In addition, the calcium and phosphorus contents of human milk are insufficient to support adequate skeletal mineralization; thus the LBW infant fed human milk is at risk for developing rickets as well as fractures. Supplementation of human milk with commercially available human milk fortifiers that provide protein, calcium, phosphorus, and sodium appears largely to overcome these nutritional inadequacies.

In general, a mother who wishes to provide milk for her LBW infant should be encouraged to do so. This provides the infant with the non-nutritional advantages of human milk, provides potential psychological benefits for the mother, and may help ensure eventual success with breast-feeding. Infants whose mothers elect not to provide milk should be fed LBW infant formula. Many LBW infants are switched to unsupplemented human milk or formulas designed for term infants when ready

good second choice. Exclusive breast-feeding provides adequate amounts of all needed nutrients for the first 4 to 6 months of life and also confers some protection against common infections. There is some disagreement about the optimal duration of exclusive breast-feeding; some authorities advocate 6 months; others advocate 4 to 6 months. This is because the content of some nutrients in breast milk become limiting sometime between 4 and 6 months of age, requiring the initiation of complementary foods. Although modern formulas provide adequate amounts of all nutrients for at least the first year of life, formula-fed infants also need complementary foods at approximately the same age as breast-fed infants for experience with different flavors and textures.

Few infants are ready developmentally for complementary foods before approximately 4 months of age. By this age, digestive and metabolic capacities are near those of the adult and the infant is beginning to sit without support. Because the nutrient most needed from complementary food is iron, foods rich in iron (e.g., iron-fortified rice cereal, strained meats) are usually the first foods introduced. The order of introduction of other foods is not particularly important unless there is a strong family history of food allergies or atopic disease, in which case

TABLE 3 Composition of Parenteral Nutrition Infusates for Central Vein Infusion and Peripheral Vein Infusion

Component	Central Vein (amount/kg/day)	Peripheral Vein (amount/kg/day)
Crystalline amino acids (g)	3–4	2.5–3.0
Glucose (g)	20–30	12–15
Lipid emulsion (g)	0.5–3.0	0.5–3.0
Sodium (mEq)	3–4	3–4
Potassium* (mEq)	2–4	2–4
Calcium (mg)	40–80	40–80
Magnesium (mEq)	0.25	0.25
Chloride (mEq)	3–4	3–4
Phosphorus* (mmol)	1–2	1–2
Zinc (µg)	300	300
Copper (µg)	20	20
Other trace minerals[†]		
Iron[‡]		
Vitamins (M.V.I. Pediatric)§ (mL)	1.5	1.5–2
Total volume (mL)	120–130	120–150

*Hyperphosphatemia frequently develops if phosphorus intake exceeds 3 mmol/kg/day—the amount given with a daily potassium intake of 3 mEq/kg as a mixture of KH_2PO_4 and K_2HPO_4. If a potassium intake of more than 2 mEq/kg/day is required, the additional potassium should be given as KCl.

†See text.

‡Iron dextran (Imferon) can be added to the infusate of patients requiring prolonged parenteral nutrition therapy; we arbitrarily limit the dose to 0.1 mg/kg/d. Alternatively, the indicated intramuscular dose can be used intermittently, either as the sole source of iron or as an additional dose.

§M.V.I. Pediatric is a lyophilized product. When reconstituted as directed, 5 mL added to the daily infusate provides 80 mg vitamin C, 700 µg vitamin A, 10 µg vitamin D, 1.3 mg thiamine, 1.4 mg riboflavin, 1.0 mg pyridoxine, 17 mg niacin, 5 mg pantothenic acid, 7 mg vitamin E, 20 µg biotin, 140 µg folic acid, 1 µg vitamin B_{12}, and 200 µg vitamin K_1.

for discharge, but use of a postdischarge formula may aid catch-up growth.

Larger LBW infants without significant lung disease can be started on enteral feedings within the first 24 hours of life. A number of randomized studies show that early minimal enteral feedings given along with parenteral nutrition may improve tolerance of subsequent enteral feeding and shorten the time necessary to achieve full enteral intake. Thus early minimal feedings (approximately 1 mL/kg/hour) are usually recommended.

Infants born before 34 weeks' gestation usually cannot be fed by nipple and require gavage feedings. These can be given either intermittently or continuously by a nasogastric or an orogastric catheter. Because nasal tubes may affect pulmonary mechanics, oral tubes are usually preferred, especially if the infant is fed intermittently. If the tube is to be left in place, a nasogastric tube is easier to secure. Continuous feedings can be infused directly into the stomach or into the duodenum (transpyloric feeding). In general, if intermittent feedings are not tolerated, a trial of continuous nasogastric feedings should be attempted before instituting transpyloric feedings. Transpyloric feedings (e.g., nasojejunal feedings) may result in fat malabsorption, probably because salivary and gastric lipases are bypassed. It also may result in intestinal perforation; thus radiographic confirmation of the position of the catheter is important.

Few LBW infants tolerate an adequate enteral intake until 2 or 3 weeks after birth and hence require parenterally delivered nutrients, which can be delivered by either a central or a peripheral vein. Regimens delivered by either route can provide sufficient amounts of all nutrients to prevent further catabolism, but central vein delivery is usually necessary to provide energy intakes exceeding 80 kcal/kg/day. However, this energy intake plus

adequate intakes of amino acids, electrolytes, minerals, and vitamins supports some growth. As a general rule, infants who seem likely to tolerate adequate enteral intakes within approximately 2 weeks should receive the parenteral nutrition infusate by peripheral vein, but infants who are not expected to tolerate enteral feeds within this period are candidates for nutritional delivery by central vein.

The nutritional infusate, whether for peripheral or central vein delivery, should include nitrogen and energy as well as sufficient electrolytes, minerals, and vitamins. Table 3 shows the compositions of infusates suitable for both routes of delivery.

Several amino acid mixtures are available for use as the nitrogen source for parenteral nutrition. Some were designed specifically for the pediatric patient and result in more optimal plasma amino acid concentrations than mixtures intended for adults. An amino acid intake of 2.5 g/kg/day supports nitrogen retention comparable to that of the enterally fed term infant, but an intake of 3 to 4 g/kg/day is required to achieve intrauterine rates of nitrogen retention. Many clinicians provide an initial amino acid intake of as little as 1 g/kg/day or less and gradually increase intake over the next several days. However, no evidence indicates such a graded increase in amino acid intake is necessary. In contrast, there is abundant evidence that an intake as high as 3 g/kg/day, starting within 24 hours of birth, is well tolerated and supports reasonable rates of growth and nitrogen accretion.

Glucose is the predominant energy source of parenteral nutrition regimens. Most infants do not tolerate initial intakes greater than 12 to 15 g/kg/day, and the very small LBW infant (<1000 g) may only tolerate a rate of infusion of 10 g/kg/day or less. In these infants, it is wise to begin with a glucose intake of only 5 to 8 g/kg/day and increase intake as tolerated by the infant, usually by 2 to 5 g/kg/day.

LBW infants who receive fat-free parenteral nutrition regimens develop essential fatty acid deficiency within a few days, which can be prevented by parenteral lipid emulsions. Emulsions of either soybean oil (Intralipid, Travamulsion, McGaw IV Fat Emulsion) or a mixture of safflower and soybean oils (Liposyn II) are available in both 10% and 20% concentrations. Although the ability to metabolize intravenous fat emulsions is related directly to maturity, most LBW infants can tolerate the small doses required to prevent essential fatty acid deficiency (0.5 to 1.0 g/kg/day). The 20% soybean oil emulsion appears to be cleared more rapidly than the 10% emulsion. After tolerance of small doses is obvious, intake can be increased as tolerated (usually by approximately 0.5 g/kg/day) to a maximal intake of 2 to 3 g/kg/day.

Because electrolyte and mineral requirements vary considerably from infant to infant, adjustments are usually required. These should be made on the basis of close monitoring. The chemical incompatibility of calcium and phosphorus often makes it impossible to provide the amounts of these minerals necessary to ensure optimal skeletal mineralization. Zinc and copper should be added to the parenteral nutrition infusate of any infant who is likely to require parenteral nutrition for more than a week. Other trace elements (e.g., selenium, chromium, manganese, molybdenum) should be considered for patients who require parenteral nutrition for a longer period. A pediatric multivitamin preparation should be used to provide the recommended amounts of vitamins.

The parenteral nutrition infusate should be delivered at a constant rate using an infusion pump. Use of a 0.22-μm membrane filter between the catheter and the administration tubing is recommended, but the lipid emulsion must be piggybacked to the infusate beyond the filter.

The complications associated with parenteral nutrition result from the technique per se (catheter related) or from the infusate (metabolic). The major catheter-related complication is infection, typically not caused by contamination of the infusate but rather due to the inadequate care of the catheter exit site. The most common complications of peripheral venous infusions are thrombophlebitis and skin or subcutaneous sloughs related to infiltration of the infusate. Metabolic complications may be related to the limited metabolic capacity of the infant or to the infusate itself. Some of the metabolic complications encountered in the early days of parenteral nutrition (metabolic acidosis, hyperammonemia) were related to the amino acid mixtures available at that time. Most metabolic complications related to the limited metabolic capacity of the infant (hyperglycemia, electrolyte or mineral abnormalities) can be avoided by close monitoring. The major concern is hepatic disorders (cholestasis) associated with parenteral nutrition.

Enteral feedings should be introduced as soon as they are tolerated and advanced as tolerated by the infant. During the period of combined enteral and parenteral nutrition, care should be taken to ensure that the infant's tolerance for both fluids and nutrients is not exceeded. This requires careful attention to the total (enteral plus parenteral) intake and frequent adjustments downward of the parenteral intake as the enteral intake increases. When enteral intakes of approximately 120 mL/kg/day (approximately 100 kcal/kg/day) are achieved, parenteral nutrition can be discontinued. Enteral feedings should then be advanced as tolerated by the infant.

Common Pitfalls

TERM INFANTS

A major pitfall in feeding term infants is the low prevalence of breast-feeding, particularly exclusive breast-feeding, beyond the first few weeks of life. Another problem is introduction of whole cow's milk before a year of age. Yet another is the relatively high proportion of children receiving calorie-rich and/or salty snacks before 1 year of age. Of these, the infrequency of exclusive breast-feeding for the first 6 or the first 4 to 6 weeks of life is likely the most difficult to remedy. For example, although up to 75% of mothers initiate breast-feeding, the number who continue to do so drops precipitously after discharge, particularly after the mother returns to work. A major factor is the relative lack of child-care services and breast-pumping facilities at the workplace.

The number of infants fed whole cow's milk before 1 year of age and the number receiving calorie-dense and/or salty snacks has decreased over the past decade and, with parental education, is likely to continue to do so. Considering the high cost of infant formula, it is easy to understand why so many infants are switched to whole cow's milk before 1 year of age. However, this milk provides excessive protein and sodium but inadequate iron.

PRETERM INFANTS

The major pitfall in nutritional management of preterm/LBW infants is failure to provide the necessary nutrients either because the necessary amounts are not ordered or the amounts ordered are not administered. Remedying these problems requires more careful attention to these infants' nutrient needs and, particularly, to the amounts actually received. Specific problems include failure to start parenteral nutrients until after several days of life and, then to start with lower amounts of some nutrients (e.g., amino acids) than needed and shown to be well tolerated by most infants. The same degree of attention to nutrition as currently given to other neonatal problems is likely to improve nutritional management of these vulnerable infants.

Communication and Counseling

Attempts to increase the prevalence of breast-feeding and the duration of exclusive breast-feeding for both term and preterm infants are warranted. This is particularly true for term infants in whom there are no disadvantages to breast-feeding. Unsupplemented human milk does not support optimal rates of growth of LBW infants, but these infants are likely to benefit more than term infants from the many non-nutritional properties of human milk. Moreover, fortification of human milk makes it nutritionally similar to LBW infant formulas.

It is not clear to whom attempts to increase the prevalence of breast-feeding and the duration of exclusive breast-feeding should be addressed. Certainly parents should be made aware of the advantages of breast-feeding, and mothers with any inclination to do so should be supported to the greatest extent possible. However, doing so requires that physicians be aware both of the reasons to increase the prevalence of breast-feeding and how to address parents' questions and concerns. Removing the barriers to breast-feeding imposed by current maternity leave policies and lack of child care and/or pumping facilities in the workplace is a more formidable problem that possibly will require political action. Yet this cannot be expected in the absence of evidence that the changes are needed.

SUGGESTED READINGS

1. Butte N, Cobb K, Dwyer J, et al: The start healthy feeding guidelines for infants and toddlers. J Am Diet Assoc 104:442–454, 2004. **Evidence-based guidelines for feeding infants and toddlers based on a project sponsored jointly by Gerber Products Company and the American Dietetic Association.**
2. Food and Nutrition Board, Institute of Medicine: Dietary Reference Intakes for Water, Potassium, Sodium, Chloride, and Sulfate. Washington, DC: National Academy Press, 2004. **Rationale for Dietary Reference Intakes of electrolytes proposed by the Food and Nutrition Board, Institute of Medicine.**
3. Heird WC: Nutritional requirements. In Behrman RE, Jenson HB, Kliegman RM (eds): Nelson Textbook of Pediatrics. 17th ed. Philadelphia: Saunders, 2004. **Discussion of nutritional needs of infants and young children.**
4. Heird WC: The feeding of infants and children. In Behrman RE, Kliegman RM, Jenson HB (eds): Nelson Textbook of Pediatrics. 17th ed. Philadelphia: Saunders, 2004. **Discussion of how and what to feed infants and young children.**
5. Kashyap S, Heird WC: Protein requirements of low birthweight, very low birthweight, and small for gestational age infants. In Räihä N.C.R. (ed): Protein Metabolism during Infancy. Nestlé Nutrition Workshop Series, vol. 33. New York: Nestec, Vevey/Raven Press, 1994, pp 133–146. **Summary of the author's studies of protein and energy needs of LBW infants.**
6. Panel on Dietary Antioxidants and Related Compounds, Subcommittees on Upper Reference Levels of Nutrients and Interpretation and Uses of Dietary Reference Intakes, and the Standing Committee on the Scientific Evaluation of Dietary Reference Intakes, Food and Nutrition Board, Institute of Medicine: Dietary Reference Intakes for Vitamin C, Vitamin E, Selenium and Carotenoids. Washington, DC: National Academy Press, 2000. **Rationale for Dietary Reference Intakes of vitamins C and E, selenium, and carotenoids proposed by the Food and Nutrition Board, Institute of Medicine.**
7. Panel on Macronutrients, Subcommittees on Upper Reference Levels of Nutrients and of Interpretation and Use of Dietary Reference Intakes, and the Standing Committee on the Scientific Evaluation of Dietary Reference Intakes, Food and Nutrition Board, Institute of Medicine: Dietary Reference Intakes for Energy, Carbohydrate, Fiber, Fat, Fatty Acids, Cholesterol, Protein and Amino Acids. Washington, DC: National Academy Press, 2002. **Rationale for Dietary Reference Intakes of protein and energy proposed by the Food and Nutrition Board, Institute of Medicine.**
8. Panel on Micronutrients, Subcommittees on Upper Reference Levels of Nutrients and of Interpretation and Use of Dietary Reference Intakes, and the Standing Committee on the Scientific Evaluation of Dietary Reference Intakes, Food and Nutrition Board, Institute of Medicine: Dietary Reference Intakes for Vitamin A, Vitamin K, Arsenic, Boron, Chromium, Copper, Iodine, Iron, Manganese, Molybdenum, Nickel, Silicon, Vanadium, and Zinc. Washington, DC: National Academy Press, 2001. **Rationale for Dietary Reference Intakes of several micronutrients proposed by the Food and Nutrition Board, Institute of Medicine.**
9. Standing Committee on the Scientific Evaluation of Dietary Reference Intakes, Food and Nutrition Board, Institute of Medicine: Dietary Reference Intakes for Calcium, Phosphorus, Magnesium, Vitamin D and Fluoride. Washington, DC: National Academy Press, 1997. **Rationale for Dietary Reference Intakes of B vitamins proposed by the Food and Nutrition Board, Institute of Medicine.**
10. Standing Committee on the Scientific Evaluation of Dietary Reference Intakes and Its Panel on Folate, Other B Vitamins and Choline and Subcommittee on Upper Reference Levels of Nutrients, Food and Nutrition Board, Institute of Medicine: Dietary Reference Intakes for Thiamin, Riboflavin, Niacin, Vitamin B_6, Folate, Vitamin B_{12}, Pantothenic Acid, Biotin and Choline. Washington, DC: National Academy Press, 1998. **Rationale for Dietary Reference Intakes of calcium, phosphorus, magnesium, vitamin D, and fluoride proposed by the Food and Nutrition Board, Institute of Medicine.**
11. Thureen P, Heird WC: Protein and energy requirements of the preterm/low birthweight (LBW) infant. Pediatr Res 57:95R–98R, 2005. **Discussion of research needs related to protein and energy needs of LBW infants.**

Rationale for Breastfeeding and Management Issues

Richard J. Schanler

2

KEY CONCEPTS

- Human milk is the model for infant nutrition.
- Breastfeeding is recommended as the exclusive diet for infants during the first 6 months of age.
- Breastfeeding provides benefits to mothers as well as infants.
- Hospital policies must facilitate breastfeeding.
- Few contraindications for breastfeeding exist.
- Most medications are compatible with breastfeeding.

The American Academy of Pediatrics (AAP) and the Canadian Paediatric Society strongly recommend breastfeeding for full-term infants. Human milk is advised as the exclusive nutrient source for feeding full-term infants during the first 6 months after birth and should be continued, with the addition of complementary foods, at least through the first 12 months. The recommendation for human milk feeding stems from its acknowledged benefits with respect to infant nutrition, gastrointestinal function, host defense, and psychological well-being. Favorable outcomes of breastfeeding are reported both for infants and mothers. The incidence of breastfeeding in the United States increased during the 1970s, peaked in the mid-1980s, slowed for a short while, and then began to rise in the 1990s. Nationwide figures for 2003, collected by the Centers for Disease Control and Prevention National Immunization Survey, indicate that 70.9% of U.S. women "ever" breastfed their newborns in the hospital; "any" breastfeeding was reported for 36.2% at 6 months and 17.2% at 12 months.

Benefits of Breastfeeding for the Infant

NUTRITIONAL SOURCE

Many of the components in human milk have dual roles, one as a nutrient source or facilitator of nutrient absorption, and the other as an enhancer of host defense or gastrointestinal function. The composition of human milk also is remarkable for its variability because the content of certain nutrients changes during lactation or throughout the day or differs among women. This variability in component composition probably adapts the nutrient composition specifically to meet the needs of the infant, and the lack of homogeneity possibly allows better acceptance of new flavors and foods.

Protein (Nitrogen)

In the first few weeks after birth, the total nitrogen content of milk from mothers who deliver premature infants (preterm milk) is greater than milk obtained from women delivering full-term infants (term milk). Usually beyond the first few weeks of lactation, the total nitrogen content in both milks declines similarly to approach what we call *mature milk*. Despite the decline in content, the protein status of breastfed infants is normal at 1 year of age. Approximately 20% of the total nitrogen is in the form of nonprotein nitrogen-containing compounds, such as free amino acids and urea, in contrast to infant formula, which has less than 5% nonprotein nitrogen. The nonprotein nitrogen compounds can be used by the infant.

Whey proteins remain soluble after exposure to gastric acid. The caseins are proteins that precipitate in acid media. Human milk protein is 70% whey and 30% casein. The whey fraction is more easily digested and tends to promote more rapid gastric emptying. The whey protein fraction also contributes to lower concentrations of phenylalanine, tyrosine, and methionine and higher concentrations of taurine characteristic of human milk. The pattern of amino acids in the plasma of breastfed infants is used as a reference in infant nutrition. As such, potentially toxic imbalances in the levels of various amino acids are avoided. The whey and casein fractions in infant formula have variable proportions, and each fraction contains proteins that differ from those found in human milk.

Lipid

The lipid system in human milk, responsible for providing approximately 50% of the calories in the milk, is structured to facilitate superior fat digestion and absorption. The lipid system is composed of an organized milk fat globule, a pattern of fatty acids (high in palmitic 16:0, oleic 18:1, and the essential fatty acids, linoleic 18:2ω6, and linolenic 18:3ω3) characteristically distributed on the triglyceride molecule (the major fatty acid, 16:0, esterified at the 2-position of the molecule), and bile salt–stimulated lipase. Because the lipase is heat labile, the superior fat absorption from human milk

is reported only when unprocessed milk is fed. Most manufacturers of infant formulas attempt to modify their fat blends to mimic the fat absorption in human milk. Thus the content of fatty acids in infant formulas, generally derived from vegetable oils and containing a greater quantity of medium-chain fatty acids, differs from that in human milk.

Of the macronutrients in human milk, fat is the most variable in content. The fat content rises slightly throughout lactation, changes over the course of 1 day, increases within feed, and varies from mother to mother. The interindividual variation tracks through lactation, and although not affected by diet, it may be affected directly by maternal fat stores.

The pattern of fatty acids in human milk also is unique in its composition of very long-chain fatty acids, arachidonic acid (20:4ω6) and docosahexaenoic acid (22:6ω3), which functionally are associated with improved cognition, growth, and vision.

Carbohydrate

The carbohydrate composition of human milk is important as a nutritional source of lactose, the major carbohydrate in milk, and for the presence of oligosaccharides. Although studies in full-term infants demonstrate a small proportion of unabsorbed lactose in the feces, the presence of lactose is assumed to be a normal physiologic effect of feeding human milk. A softer stool consistency, more nonpathogenic bacterial fecal flora, and improved absorption of minerals are attributable to the presence of small quantities of unabsorbed lactose from human milk feeding.

Mineral and Trace Elements

The concentration of calcium and phosphorus in human milk is significantly lower than in infant formula. The content of these macrominerals is relatively constant through lactation. In human milk, the minerals are bound to digestible proteins and also present in complexed and ionized states, which improve their bioavailability compared with the relatively insoluble salts added to infant formula. Thus, despite differences in mineral intake, the bone mineral content of breastfed infants is similar to that of infants fed formula.

The concentrations of iron, zinc, and copper decline through lactation. The concentrations of copper and zinc, despite their decline through lactation, appear adequate to meet the infant's nutritional needs. The concentration of iron, however, may not meet the infant's needs beyond 6 months of breastfeeding. Therefore, iron-containing foods should be introduced after 6 months.

Vitamins

Maternal vitamin status may affect the content of vitamins in the milk. Generally, maternal deficiency may result in low concentrations in milk that increase in response to dietary supplementation. This is more common for water-soluble than fat-soluble vitamins. Vitamin K deficiency may be a concern in the breastfed infant.

Bacterial flora is responsible for providing adequate vitamin K. The intestinal flora of the breastfed infant makes less of the vitamin, and the content of vitamin K in human milk is low. Therefore, to meet vitamin K needs, a single dose of vitamin K is given at birth. Rickets caused by vitamin D deficiency may occur if there is inadequate sunlight exposure. Because human milk provides only a small quantity of vitamin D and parents are reluctant to expose infants to the sun unless they apply sunscreen, the AAP recommends that all infants receive a vitamin D supplement by 2 months of age (Table 1).

BODY COMPOSITION

Although lower concentrations of calcium and phosphorus are observed in human milk compared with formula, measures of bone mineralization are similar between full-term infants fed human milk or formula during the first year of life. Children who were breastfed had nearly half the prevalence of obesity than children fed formula, and the prevalence of obesity was related positively to the dose of human milk the infant received.

GASTROINTESTINAL FUNCTION

The numerous factors, enzymes, and hormones in human milk promote the development and maturation of the gastrointestinal tract. Gastric emptying is faster following the feeding of human milk than with infant formula. The clinical impression is that large gastric residual volumes are reported less frequently in premature infants fed human milk.

ACUTE INFECTIOUS DISEASE

Numerous studies delineate the protective effects of breastfeeding. To some degree, the mechanisms for the protective effects of human milk are explained by the functions of the bioactive factors in human milk (Table 2). In developing areas, the incidence of gastroenteritis and respiratory disease and overall morbidity and mortality are lower in breastfed infants than infants fed milk substitutes. In developed countries, such as in the United States, breastfed infants have lower rates of diarrhea, lower respiratory tract illness, acute and recurrent otitis

TABLE 1 Dietary Supplements for Breastfed Infants

Vitamin K	Birth	**To prevent bleeding from vitamin K deficiency** Fecal flora maintains vitamin K sufficiency. Breastfed infants' fecal flora produces less vitamin K. Human milk has low content of vitamin K.
Vitamin D	2 mo	**To prevent rickets from vitamin D deficiency** Sunshine exposure determines vitamin D status. Difficult to quantitate sunshine exposure. Parents avoid sunshine exposure for infants. Sunscreen used. Human milk has low content of vitamin D.
Iron	6 mo	**To prevent iron deficiency** Iron absorption from human milk is excellent. Iron content declines during lactation. Breastfed infants need iron supplement beyond 6 mo. Iron-containing foods: good source.

TABLE 2 Protective Factors in Human Milk

Secretory IgA	Specific antigen-targeted anti-infective action
Lactoferrin	Antibacterial by binding iron, trophic for intestinal growth
Lysozyme	Lysis of bacterial cell walls
Casein	Antiadhesive, bacterial flora
Oligosaccharides	Mimics bacterial receptors, blocks attachment
Cytokines	Anti-inflammatory, epithelial barrier function
Growth factors	
Epidermal growth factor	Luminal surveillance, repair of intestine
Transforming growth factor	Promotes epithelial cell growth Immunomodulation
Nerve growth factor	Growth, innervation
Enzymes	
PAF acetylhydrolase	Blocks action of platelet-activating factor (PAF)
Glutathione peroxidase	Prevents lipid oxidation
Nucleotides	Enhance antibody responses, bacterial flora
Vitamins A, E, C	Antioxidants
Amino acids	
Glutamine	Intestinal cell fuel, immune responses
Taurine	Intestinal growth
Lipids	Anti-infective properties
Hormones	Cortisol, somatomedin C, insulin-like growth factors, insulin, thyroid hormone
Gastrointestinal mediators	Neurotensin, motilin

TABLE 3 Human Milk Protects Against Acute and Chronic Illnesses in Infants, Children, and Young Adults

Protection from acute illnesses

Diarrhea
Otitis media
Recurrent otitis media
Respiratory tract illnesses
Urinary tract infection
Necrotizing enterocolitis
Late-onset sepsis in premature infants

Reduced number of hospitalizations
Long-term reduction in chronic disorders

Asthma
Celiac disease
Childhood cancer
Lymphoma
Leukemia
Crohn disease
Hypercholesterolemia
Type 1 diabetes mellitus
Obesity

media, and urinary tract infection (Table 3). Not only is the attack rate lower, but the duration and severity of illness appear to be shortened in the breastfed infant. Most recently, breastfeeding is attributed to a reduction in U.S. infant mortality through the first year.

The enteromammary and bronchomammary immune pathways may partially explain the protective effects of breastfeeding against gastrointestinal and respiratory illnesses. The secretory IgA (sIgA) antibody is synthesized by plasma cells against specific foreign antigens after their introduction via the gastrointestinal and/or respiratory tracts. The mother produces sIgA antibodies when exposed to foreign antigens. The plasma cells traverse the lymphatic system and are secreted at mucosal surfaces, including the mammary gland. Ingestion of milk, therefore, provides the infant with passive sIgA antibody against the offending antigen. The systems are active in infants against a variety of antigens.

CHRONIC DISEASE IN PEDIATRICS

Epidemiologic evidence suggests that certain chronic pediatric disorders have a lower incidence in children who were breastfed as infants (see Table 3). Several of these relationships eventually may be explained by the immunomodulating effects of human milk.

NEUROBEHAVIORAL ASPECTS

Maternal-infant bonding is enhanced during breastfeeding. In addition, improved long-term cognitive and motor abilities in full-term infants are directly correlated with the duration of breastfeeding. Even when adjusted for socioeconomic status and parent education, at 3, 4, and 5 years of age, there were significant increments in a limited set of cognitive test scores that paralleled the duration of breastfeeding. Improved long-term cognitive development in premature infants also is correlated with the receipt of human milk during their hospitalization.

A series of studies indicates that human milk fed to full-term and premature infants improves visual function compared with infants not receiving human milk. Breastfeeding during painful procedures in neonates provides an analgesic effect not seen with other modes of feeding.

Benefits of Breastfeeding to the Mother

Recovery from childbirth is accelerated by oxytocin's action on uterine involution. Although breastfeeding should not be considered an entirely reliable means of contraception, it does prolong the period of postpartum anovulation and promote child spacing. Frequency, intensity, and timing of feeds affect the endocrinologic responses that modulate ovulatory status.

Prolonged breastfeeding may confer some advantage in terms of weight loss. Bone demineralization occurs during lactation, with a compensatory remineralization after weaning. Lactation confers a protective effect against osteoporosis and bone fracture in later life, but this is not confirmed in all studies.

A protective effect of breastfeeding against breast cancer is found in a number of studies. The effects were even greater in premenopausal women who had a cumulative total of 24 months of breastfeeding or who were 20 years of age or younger when they first lactated.

Expert Opinion on Management Issues

PRENATAL CONSIDERATIONS

The successful management of lactation begins during pregnancy. The prenatal office visit is an ideal time to inquire about choice of infant feeding and to provide information so families can make an informed choice about the benefits of breastfeeding. Although some studies show that infant feeding decisions are made before the third trimester, choices may be influenced by certain misconceptions or fears held by the expectant mother or father, such as the following:

- Fear of inadequate milk supply because of small breast size
- Possible loss of sexual breast activity during lactation
- Cosmetic breast changes as a result of lactation
- Fear of failing at breastfeeding
- Beliefs that breast milk is "not rich enough"
- Difficulties in learning how to breastfeed
- Disapproval of the spouse
- Poor public acceptance
- Possible loss of freedom or spontaneity

Because decisions generally are made early, and few women have pediatric office visits prenatally, the early obstetric visit must take advantage of the opportunity to discuss and promote breastfeeding. As such, during the initial breast examination at an early obstetric visit, the mother should be commended on her choice of breastfeeding and told that her breasts will pose no problems.

TABLE 4   Ten Steps to Successful Breastfeeding

Every facility providing maternity services and care for newborn infants should:

1. Have a written breastfeeding policy that is routinely communicated to all health care staff.
2. Train all health care staff in skills necessary to implement this policy.
3. Inform all pregnant women about the benefits and management of breastfeeding.
4. Help mothers initiate breastfeeding within one hour of birth.
5. Show mothers how to breastfeed and how to maintain lactation even if they should be separated from their infants.
6. Give newborn infants no food or drink other than breastmilk, unless *medically* indicated.
7. Practice rooming-in – allow mothers and infants to remain together 24 hours a day.
8. Encourage breastfeeding on demand.
9. Give no artificial teats or pacifiers to breastfeeding infants.
10. Foster the establishment of breastfeeding support groups and refer mothers to them on discharge from the hospital or clinic.

From World Health Organization & UNICEF. Evidence for the Ten Steps to Successful Breastfeeding, 1998. Geneva, Switzerland: World Health Organization; 1998. For more information, contact Baby-Friendly USA, 327 Quaker Meeting House Road, E. Sandwich, MA 02537. (508)888-8092. Fax (508)888-8050. E-mail: info@babyfriendlyusa.org.

GETTING STARTED IN THE HOSPITAL

The early days of lactation are critical to the establishment of a good milk supply and effective letdown reflex. The Baby-Friendly Hospital Initiative (BFHI) outlines 10 steps to ensure breastfeeding success in the hospital (Table 4). Postpartum units must maintain a written policy on breastfeeding that is communicated to the entire staff. All health care staff must be trained in the implementation of this policy. Pregnant women should be informed of the benefits of breastfeeding. Breastfeeding should commence within 1 hour of birth unless medically contraindicated. Health care staff must be able to demonstrate appropriate breastfeeding skills to mothers. Infants should be given nothing but breast milk unless medically indicated. There is no reason to supply water, glucose water, or formula to the exclusively breastfed infant who is otherwise healthy. If the appetite or the sucking response is partially satiated by water or formula, the infant takes less from the breast, causing diminished milk production that may lead to lactation failure. Water and glucose water supplements may exacerbate hyperbilirubinemia because they prevent adequate milk (calorie) intake and gastrocolic stimulation. Unconjugated (indirect) bilirubin is not water soluble, must be eliminated in the feces, and is not excreted in the urine.

Mother and infant should not be separated unless it is medically indicated. Rooming-in for 24 hours per day should be practiced to allow unrestricted breastfeeding. The mother should be offered as much assistance as necessary in positioning herself comfortably and facilitating the infant's proper grasp of the breast. Enough of the areola should be in the infant's mouth to permit the tongue to compress the areola against the hard palate. This provides a good seal and proper emptying or milking of the collecting ducts. After suckling at the first breast, the infant is repositioned on the second breast. It is appropriate to alternate the side used to initiate the feeding and to equalize the time spent at each breast in a day's feedings.

The time for suckling should be unrestricted. Infants should be nursed approximately 8 to 12 times every 24 hours until satiety, usually 10 to 15 minutes at each breast. Breastfeeding should continue when the infant is wakeful and at least every 2 to 3 hours to stimulate milk production and facilitate bilirubin excretion. A normal infant is alert and attentive and should root, grasp, and suckle well. But some infants may not demand feed in the first few days; parents should be instructed to wake these infants for feedings. In the first weeks, infants should go no longer than 4 hours between feedings. The use of a pacifier in the early weeks also should be avoided so any need for sucking is satisfied with breastfeeding.

Hospital staff should formally evaluate breastfeeding at least twice daily and document their findings in the medical record. Families should have access to expert information on breastfeeding. They should be encouraged to keep in touch with physicians if questions arise. In the case of early hospital discharge, signs of hydration and the adequacy of feeding should be monitored. All breastfed infants should be seen by a knowledgeable health care professional at 2 to 5 days of age to avoid potential problems of dehydration and severe jaundice. Each hospital should establish breastfeeding support groups or work with organized community support groups so families have a resource when they leave the hospital.

ASSESSMENT OF ADEQUACY OF MILK INTAKE

Fear that the infant is not receiving enough milk is a reason many mothers discontinue breastfeeding. Moreover, newspaper headlines have identified isolated tragedies associated with breastfeeding causing catastrophic cases of dehydration. To alleviate these possibilities, mothers, as well as health care professionals, should be taught simple methods to monitor the hydration status and milk intake of the breastfed infant.

In the first few weeks after birth, an infant is adequately nourished if at least 8 to 12 feedings are received every 24 hours and the infant sleeps contentedly between feedings. The adequacy of milk intake can be assessed daily by counting the number of wet diapers, the number and quantity of stools, and weight gain (body weight loss of more than 7% should be avoided). In the first 24 hours after birth, the infant should have at least one wet diaper and one stool. On day 3, breastfed infants usually have three to four wet diapers and one to two stools that no longer look like meconium but are beginning to appear yellow. Later in the first week after birth, there should be six pale yellow diapers per day and a yellow stool with each feeding. Later in the month, the stool frequency may diminish to three per day. Families or health care professionals can maintain a written record to assess the adequacy of milk intake, but it should not take the place of the physical examination of the infant if any concerns arise.

Because lactogenesis stage 2 (milk "coming-in") may not peak until day 4, the usual hospital discharge (at

48 hours) poses a concern for monitoring the breastfed infant. A knowledgeable health care professional should see the infant between 3 and 5 days of age (depending on age at hospital discharge). This first visit should assess the adequacy of hydration, milk intake, and body weight, the presence of jaundice, and the state of the mother (anxiety, concerns). Breastfeeding should be observed during this first visit. Telephone contact should be encouraged if further questions arise. Families should be made aware of the availability of community, office, and/or hospital lactation resources.

BREAST CHANGES AND CARE

Lactogenesis stage 2, or the onset of milk secretion, which usually occurs on the second to fourth postpartum day, is associated with engorgement or swelling of the breasts. Engorgement can cause the nipple areola junction to be tense and convex, making it difficult for the infant to grasp correctly. Manual or mechanical (breast pump) expression of milk prior to nursing softens the areola area and facilitates the infant's latch-on.

Breast engorgement is an uncomfortable and sometimes painful swelling caused by increased blood and lymph flow to the breast at the onset of lactogenesis. Poor or infrequent emptying of the breast exacerbates this condition. Fortunately, the condition is easily managed by frequent emptying of the breast through feeding or milk expression through manual or mechanical methods.

The initial grasp and suck of the nipple may cause pain during the first few days of lactation. This sensation is the result of negative pressure on the empty ductules. Sore nipples can be exacerbated by incorrect latch-on or impaired milk letdown. Usually this condition begins during the first few days of feeding and is greatest at the onset of feeding. Once lactation is well established, the tenderness diminishes.

Cracked or fissured nipples are usually the result of improper latch-on, improper disengagement, or the use of abrasive soaps or alcohol on the breast. Because the Montgomery glands provide the best lubrication for the areola and nipple throughout pregnancy, no additional lubricants are needed. Occasional application of milk, allowed to dry on the nipple, may assist the healing process.

Chronically sore nipples, a burning pain throughout the breast, may be caused by *Candida* infection. There often is concomitant thrush or fungal diaper rash in the infant. Treatment of both maternal and infant sources of infection with topical antifungal agents is needed.

Localized areas of breast discomfort may be caused by plugged ducts. These are focal areas of breast engorgement caused by milk stasis. The condition results from irregular nursing, skipped feedings, and inadequate breast emptying. This condition of localized tenderness and mass in an area of the breast should be differentiated from mastitis. The plugged duct may be a precursor of mastitis. Treatment of a plugged duct involves starting consecutive feedings on the affected side and changing nursing position to facilitate emptying different lobes of the breast. Additional relief is provided by gently massaging the affected area during nursing or pumping while applying moist heat. Frequent nursing is recommended.

Mastitis is a cellulitis of the interlobar connective tissue of the breast. Affected women experience pain, swelling, erythema, fever, and generalized flu-like symptoms. The infection is usually caused by *Staphylococcus aureus* and occasionally by *Streptococcus* species. Predisposing factors to mastitis include cracked nipples, incomplete breast emptying, plugged ducts, and breast trauma. The treatment for mastitis is antibiotic therapy, which should be instituted promptly and offer coverage against staphylococcal bacteria. The treatment duration usually is 10 days. Bed rest and analgesics may be necessary. Breastfeeding should not be stopped during therapy, especially because breast emptying may facilitate the healing process. The mother may find it more comfortable to initiate nursing on the unaffected side and then move to the affected breast once letdown is triggered. Occasionally, letdown becomes difficult. An electric breast pump may help facilitate milk expression from the affected breast.

JAUNDICE IN BREASTFED INFANTS

Jaundice because of unconjugated hyperbilirubinemia may be associated with breastfeeding in two circumstances: during the first week and beyond the first week of age. In the first week after birth, the entity *breastfeeding jaundice* is related to inadequate milk intake and poor lactation performance. The treatment is aimed at decreasing the enterohepatic recirculation of bilirubin by increasing milk intake through an increase in the frequency of breastfeeding. By increasing the frequency of breastfeeding, milk supply increases and jaundice diminishes. If hyperbilirubinemia is advanced and milk production is low, formula may be given to the infant after each breastfeeding while the mother uses a manual or mechanical method for milk expression to stimulate milk production. Alternatively, supplemental formula can be fed by other means (e.g., through a tube or cup) during the breastfeeding or soon after. This entity may be avoided by appropriate lactation counseling early after delivery and appropriate follow-up of infants after hospital discharge.

The classical entity *breast milk jaundice* usually begins insidiously and peaks after the first week of age. In this condition the infant is thriving and appears healthy but remains jaundiced despite adequate maternal lactation performance. This entity may be related either to one or more factors in human milk or to a combination of specific milk factors and a susceptible recipient infant that perpetuate the enterohepatic recirculation of bilirubin. In extreme circumstances, usually when the serum bilirubin concentration exceeds 20 mg/dL, the hyperbilirubinemia can be reduced by interrupting breastfeeding for 2 to 4 days. If this course is chosen, the mother must be encouraged to maintain her milk supply with a manual or mechanical method while the infant receives formula. When breastfeeding resumes, the serum bilirubin may rise slightly, but once the cycle is interrupted, recurrence of the jaundice is unlikely.

MEDICATIONS AND BREASTFEEDING

A number of drugs may be secreted into human milk, but only a few are considered problematic for the breastfeeding infant and/or mother (see Pitfalls). These include chemotherapeutic agents, radioactive isotopes, drugs of abuse, and drugs that suppress lactation. In addition, anticonvulsants, antihistamines, sulfa drugs, and salicylates may have minor effects on some breastfeeding infants. Potential exposures from environmental agents also should be considered. Caffeine may enter milk, but maternal consumption of one or two caffeine-containing beverages per day is usually not associated with significant manifestations in the infant. Some studies indicate that alcohol may affect infant behavior adversely. Cigarette smoking may affect milk volume.

Secretion of medications into milk is affected by dose schedule and duration, feeding pattern of the infant, and the infant's total diet and age. The timing of breastfeeding should avoid peak blood concentrations of selected medications. For some medications, the stage of lactation (age of the infant) determines the safety of the agent. The mother should be encouraged to discuss any medication with her physician, and the physician should substitute potentially problematic medications with those acknowledged to have better safety profiles.

CONTRAINDICATIONS TO BREASTFEEDING

In certain situations, breastfeeding is not in the best interest of the infant. These include infants with galactosemia, infants of mothers using illicit drugs, infants of mothers with active miliary tuberculosis, and infants born to mothers positive for HIV. In cases of HIV, the benefit of breastfeeding versus unavailability of other modes of infant feeding may be greater than the risks of acquiring HIV. Although mothers with active miliary tuberculosis should not breastfeed, mothers who are seroconverters or receiving antituberculosis therapy may breastfeed their infants.

Maternal herpes infections localized to the perineal area or the oral mucosa do not pose a risk to the breastfed infant. Maternal herpetic lesions localized to the areola, however, do pose a risk, and the infant should not be breastfed while these lesions remain. Cytomegalovirus excretion is common in human milk when the mother is seropositive for cytomegalovirus. In the full-term infant, this is not a concern with respect to breastfeeding. Maternal rubella or maternal rubella immunization does not increase the risk of disease in the breastfed infant. To date, most authorities recommend breastfeeding for mothers exposed to and infected with the hepatitis viruses. It also is appropriate to recommend breastfeeding to the mother who has mastitis and undergoing treatment for the condition.

Common Pitfalls

- Lack of an expensive ad campaign to educate the public
- Lack of physician expertise
- Inability to teach sustained lactation adequately in hospital
- Inadequate training of physicians and nurses
- Variable backgrounds and expertise of paraprofessional consultants
- Work obstacles to lactation
- BFHI and other similar programs not sought, principally because of lobbying by the formula industry
- Medications and breastfeeding poorly understood and search for safe medications seldom done

Communication and Counseling

The benefits of breastfeeding should be communicated to all families, so parents can make an informed choice about infant feeding. Once parents choose breastfeeding, they should receive as much reassurance as possible. Before delivery, any maternal risk factors that would impede breastfeeding (e.g., surgery) should be sought and discussed. At delivery, the experience of skin-to-skin contact in the delivery room is critical. Mothers should be reassured that being with their infant throughout the transition period and "rooming-in" are appropriate practices to facilitate maternal-infant bonding and breastfeeding. Practitioners should teach parents how to assess milk intake and the hydration status of the infant. A visit with a knowledgeable health care professional at 3 to 5 days of age further reassures the family that breastfeeding is going well. That visit is primarily important to detect any potential problems with breastfeeding. Throughout the series of pediatric office visits, mothers should be praised for their breastfeeding accomplishments. Some offices supply certificates to mothers. The office also should support breastfeeding by allowing mothers to breastfeed and by providing appropriate breastfeeding literature and visual aids.

SUGGESTED READINGS

1. American Academy of Pediatrics & Committee on Drugs: The transfer of drugs and other chemicals into human milk. Pediatrics 108:776–789, 2001. **Provides lists of medications that are safe and problematic for breastfeeding.**
2. American Academy of Pediatrics, Section on Breastfeeding: Breastfeeding and the use of human milk. Pediatrics (in press). **Describes benefits of breastfeeding and recommendations for pediatric care.**
3. Blanc B: Biochemical aspects of human milk—comparison with bovine milk. World Rev Nutr Diet 36:1–89, 1981. **Tabulates and describes characteristics of the nutrient composition of human milk.**
4. Centers for Disease Control and Prevention online. http://www.cdc.gov/breastfeeding/. **Provides current rates of breastfeeding by geographic local and maternal demographics.**
5. Chen A, Rogan WJ: Breastfeeding and the risk of postneonatal death in the United States. Pediatrics 113:E435–E439, 2004. **Describes the new finding of the effect of breastfeeding on the reduction in U.S. infant mortality.**
6. Gartner LM, Lee K: Jaundice in the breastfed infant. Clin Perinatol 26:431–445, 1999. **Describes the characteristics and treatment for jaundice in breastfed infants.**
7. Hamosh M: Bioactive factors in human milk. Pediatr Clin North Am 48:69–86, 2002. **Describes immune and nonimmune protective factors in human milk.**

8. Naylor AJ: Baby friendly hospital initiative: Protecting, promoting, and supporting breastfeeding in the twenty-first century. Pediatr Clin North Am 48:475–484, 2001. **Describes the BFHI.**

9. Neifert MR: Prevention of breastfeeding tragedies. Pediatr Clin North Am 48:273–298, 2001. **Discusses how to assess the adequacy of hydration in the breastfed infant.**

10. Schanler RJ: The use of human milk for premature infants. Pediatr Clin North Am 48:207–220, 2001. **Describes the benefits and use of human milk in the neonatal intensive care unit.**

11. Wight NE: Management of common breastfeeding issues. Pediatr Clin North Am 48:321–344, 2001. **Describes common breastfeeding problems in mothers and infants and their management.**

Acid–Base Disorders

Andrew L. Schwaderer and George J. Schwartz

KEY CONCEPTS

- Successful treatment of metabolic acidosis and metabolic alkalosis depends on identifying and treating the underlying condition responsible for the altered acid–base homeostasis. Treatment with acid or alkali is recommended only for severe cases.

- Fomepizole is a safe and effective alternative to ethanol for use as an alcohol dehydrogenase inhibitor in ethylene glycol and methanol ingestions.

- Patients with chloride-responsive metabolic alkalosis are usually volume contracted, have low urine chloride levels, and are treated with saline infusion. Patients with chloride-unresponsive metabolic alkalosis have a normal or high urine chloride, are volume expanded, and are treated by addressing the source of excess mineralocorticoid.

- Loop and thiazide diuretics can cause a metabolic alkalosis, and potassium-sparing diuretics and acetazolamide inhibitors can cause a metabolic acidosis.

The normal pH of arterial blood is 7.4 and is maintained within narrow limits. *Acidemia* is defined as an arterial pH less than 7.36, and *alkalemia* occurs when the arterial pH is greater than 7.44. *Acidosis* refers to processes that can cause acid to accumulate; *alkalosis* refers to processes that cause base to accumulate. Altered acid–base homeostasis can impair cardiovascular, respiratory, metabolic, and cerebral function and, in pediatrics, growth.

Acid–base regulation involves chemical buffering, respiratory compensation, and renal compensation. Chemical buffering occurs within minutes and includes intracellular and extracellular buffers, of which bicarbonate (HCO_3^-) is the most important. Respiratory compensation, which controls the partial pressure of carbon dioxide (PCO_2), begins within an hour and is completed within 24 hours. Renal compensation, which takes a few days to complete, controls the serum bicarbonate by increases in renal acid secretion. The proximal tubule reabsorbs 85% of filtered bicarbonate, and the rest is reabsorbed by the distal nephron. In the collecting duct, excreted acid combines with buffers in the tubularb lumen, allowing the regeneration of additional bicarbonate.

The patient's acid–base status is determined by the ratio of bicarbonate to carbon dioxide (CO_2) concentration as expressed by the Henderson–Hasselbalch equation:

$$pH = 6.1 + \log \frac{[HCO_3^-]}{(0.03 \times PCO_2)}$$

Respiratory acidosis or alkalosis results from a primary increase or decrease in PCO_2, and metabolic acidosis or alkalosis results from a primary increase or decrease in the serum bicarbonate. Acid–base disorders can be simple, such as metabolic alkalosis, or mixed, such as combined metabolic alkalosis and respiratory acidosis. Definition of the acid–base disorders requires knowledge of the magnitude of the compensatory response. A normal pH in the setting of abnormal arterial PCO_2 and serum bicarbonate suggests a mixed disorder.

METABOLIC ACIDOSIS

Metabolic acidosis is one of the cardinal acid–base disorders (Table 1). It is defined as an acid–base disturbance in which plasma bicarbonate is reduced because of the net loss of bicarbonate or gain of hydrogen ions. Arterial pH is below 7.36, resulting from increased acid production or ingestion, decreased renal acid excretion, or increased bicarbonate loss from the gastrointestinal tract or the kidneys. The calculation of the anion gap (Table 2) separates this entity into two groups: normal anion gap (hyperchloremic) and high anion gap (normochloremic) (Box 1). This separation is valuable both in differential diagnosis and in making decisions about treatment.

Etiology

NORMAL ANION GAP METABOLIC ACIDOSIS

A normal anion gap metabolic acidosis may result from gastrointestinal or renal loss of bicarbonate, surgical procedures that expose urine to ileal or sigmoid mucosa, defective renal acid excretion out of proportion to changes in the glomerular filtration rate, or drainage of alkaline pancreatic or biliary secretions.

HIGH ANION GAP METABOLIC ACIDOSIS

A high anion gap metabolic acidosis occurs in the setting of increased organic acid production, toxic ingestions, inborn errors of metabolism, or decreased excretion of acid with renal failure. The overproduction of ketoacids in ketoacidosis and decreased use of excess lactate in lactic acidosis leads to the high anion gap. Lactic acidosis can be divided into type A, which results from tissue hypoxia or hypoperfusion, and type B, which results from systemic disease, drugs, toxins, and inborn errors of mitochondrial metabolism (congenital lactic acidosis). Lactic acidosis, which often occurs with life-threatening illnesses, is associated with a high mortality rate. Ethylene glycol, methanol, and paraldehyde produce an osmolar gap in addition to an anion gap, such that the

TABLE 1 Cardinal Acid–Base Disturbances with Their Secondary Responses

Disorder	Primary Change	Compensatory Response
Metabolic acidosis*	Decreased [HCO_3^-]	1.2-mm decrease in $Paco_2$ for 1 mEq/L decrease in HCO_3^-
Metabolic alkalosis*	Increased [HCO_3^-]	0.7 mm increase in $Paco_2$ for 1 mEq/L increase in HCO_3^-
Respiratory acidosis	Increased $Paco_2$	
Acute		1 mEq/L increase in HCO_3^- for 10-mm increase in $Paco_2$
Chronic		3.5 mEq/L increase in HCO_3^- for 10-mm increase in $Paco_2$
Respiratory alkalosis	Decreased $Paco_2$	
Acute		2 mEq/L decrease in HCO_3^- for 10 mm decrease in $Paco_2$
Chronic		4 mEq/L decrease in HCO_3^- for 10-mm decrease in $Paco_2$

From Rose BD, Post TW: Clinical Physiology of Acid–Base and Electrolyte Disorders, 5th ed. New York, McGraw-Hill, 2001, p 543.
*With the metabolic disturbances, the change in $Paco_2$ is an adaptive response to the rise in plasma bicarbonate concentration and takes approximately 24 to 72 hours to reach its peak.

TABLE 2 Diagnostic Calculations

Measurement	Calculation	Importance
Serum anion gap	$Na^+ - (Cl^- + HCO_3^-)$; normal value <12	Used to help identify cause of a metabolic acidosis.
Calculated serum osmolality	$2 \times$ (serum Na^+) + (serum glucose/18) + (BUN/2.8)	Used in the calculation of an osmolal gap.
Osmolal gap	Measured osmolality – calculated osmolality; normal value <10 mOsm/L	Unmeasured solutes such as ethylene glycol are not included in this formula and would account for an elevated osmolal gap.
Urine net charge	Urine Na^+ + urine K^+ – urine Cl^-; during metabolic acidosis, the normal value is <0 mEq/L	Because ammonium (an unmeasured cation) accompanies chloride in acidic urine, the concentration of chloride should be greater than the sum of the sodium and potassium, resulting in a negative net charge. A positive net charge indicates impaired distal acid secretion because no ammonium is in the urine.
Urine ammonium	$0.5 \times$ {urine osmolality – [$2 \times$ (urine Na^+ + urine K^+) + urine urea/2.8 + urine glucose/18]}	The absence of ammonium in the setting of metabolic acidosis indicates impaired distal acid secretion.

Note: All electrolytes measured in mEq/L; glucose, urine urea, and blood urea nitrogen (BUN) are measured in mg/dL.

BOX 1 Causes of Metabolic Acidosis Based on Anion Gap

Normal Anion Gap

- **B**icarbonate loss (diarrhea, ureteroenterostomy, small bowel and pancreatic fistula)
- **R**enal tubular acidosis, proximal or distal types
- **A**cid load (NH_4Cl, arginine hydrochloride, hyperalimentation)
- **D**ilution (rapid intravenous hydration with 0.9% $NaCl$)
- **P**osthypocapnea
- **A**ldosterone deficiency
- **C**arbonic anhydrase inhibitors (acetazolamide)

High Anion Gap

- **L**actic acidosis (tissue hypoxia, muscular exercise, ethanol ingestion, systemic disease, congenital lactic acidosis)
- **U**remic acidosis
- **K**etoacidosis (diabetic ketoacidosis, starvation, ethanol intoxication)
- **I**ngestions (salicylate, methanol, ethylene glycol, paraldehyde)
- **E**rrors of metabolism (e.g., propionicacidemia, methymalonicacidemia, other organic acidemias)

Note: **BRAD PAC** is a suitable mnemonic for normal anion gap acidosis, and **LUKIE** is a suitable mnemonic for high anion gap acidosis.

measured osmolality exceeds the calculated osmolality by greater than 10 mOsm/kg (see Table 2). When the glomerular filtration rate is below 25 mL/min/1.73 m^2 in acute or chronic renal failure, the reduced ability to excrete the organic acids generated from metabolism results in a metabolic acidosis with a high anion gap.

Diagnosis

Symptoms of acidemia may include labored breathing, nausea, vomiting, abdominal pain, anorexia, fatigue, weakness, lethargy, and peripheral arterial vasodilation and vasoconstriction. Chronic metabolic acidosis can result in growth failure and osteomalacia. Severe acute metabolic acidosis may cause depression of myocardial contractility, cardiac arrhythmias, stupor, and coma. The urine net charge or a modification of the urine osmolal gap can be used to demonstrate reduced urine ammonium excretion (see Table 2). Hyperkalemia is often seen with acidosis and is caused by a shift of potassium out of the cell, but persistence of hyperkalemia suggests type IV or hyperkalemic type I renal tubular acidosis (RTA). Patients with an acidosis caused by diarrhea generally have a negative urine net charge and a urine pH of less than 6.5. Phosphorous, blood urea nitrogen (BUN), and creatinine levels are elevated in uremic acidosis. An elevated serum osmolal gap in the setting of high anion gap metabolic acidosis suggests ethylene glycol, alcohol, or methanol intoxication. Glucosuria and ketosuria in the setting of hyperglycemia suggests diabetic ketoacidosis.

Expert Opinion on Management Issues

Therapy for metabolic acidosis varies depending on the etiology responsible (Table 3). The underlying cause of the metabolic acidosis should be treated whenever possible. Correction of underlying volume and electrolyte deficiencies, removal of toxins, and treatment of sepsis should be given priority. If diarrhea is the underlying etiology, the discontinuation of oral feeds should be considered.

RENAL TUBULAR ACIDOSIS

In distal renal tubular acidosis, 4 mEq/kg/day of potassium citrate salts is usually sufficient to normalize the serum bicarbonate and allow for catch-up growth. Polycitra provides 2 mEq of potential alkali, 1 mEq with Na^+ and 1 mEq with K^+ per milliliter; Polycitra-K provides all of the citrate with K^+. In proximal tubular acidosis, 10 to 25 mEq/kg/day is usually required for optimal growth. Doses are divided into two to four a day.

KETOACIDOSIS

Treatment of diabetic ketoacidosis consists of expansion of extracellular volume followed by correction of insulin and electrolyte deficiencies. Hypophosphatemia is a potential complication of diabetic ketoacidosis and should be addressed if present; however, the majority of randomized, controlled trials do not demonstrate any clinical benefit of routine phosphate therapy. The use of bicarbonate in diabetic ketoacidosis is controversial because retrospective studies do not show a conclusive benefit. It is currently recommended to treat if the pH remains below 7.0 after 1 hour of hydration. Administration of saline is generally adequate for treatment of alcoholic ketoacidosis.

LACTIC ACIDOSIS

Therapy for lactic acidosis focuses on restoring adequate tissue oxygenation and treating the underlying cause. Neither bicarbonate nor dichloroacetate (a medication that promotes the metabolism of pyruvate, the precursor of lactate) is effective in improving patient outcome. One study suggests that dichloroacetate might be useful in the treatment of congenital lactic acidosis. Dichloroacetate rapidly decreases lactate in children with malaria-associated lactic acidosis and improves survival in a rat model, providing the only intervention that has a favorable effect on survival.

INGESTIONS

Neither ethylene glycol nor methanol is highly toxic, but each is metabolized to toxic metabolites. Ethylene glycol ingestion can lead to acidosis, renal failure, damage to the central nervous system, and cardiovascular instability; methanol ingestion can lead to metabolic acidosis, blindness, and cardiovascular instability. Ethanol and fomepizole are alcohol dehydrogenase inhibitors used to reduce the formation of toxic metabolites.

Fomepizole, unlike ethanol, is easy to administer and does not cause hypoglycemia, hyperosmolality, or altered mental status. The current dosing regimen is 15 mg/kg intravenously followed by 10 mg/kg every 12 hours (every 4 hours during hemodialysis). Indications for hemodialysis include high anion gap metabolic acidosis and deteriorating clinical status with renal failure or metabolic abnormalities unresponsive to standard therapies. Traditionally, an ethylene glycol level greater than 50 mg/dL was an indication for hemodialysis; however, recent experience suggests that fomepizole alone suffices as long as the patient is not acidotic and has normal renal function. Unlike ethylene glycol, methanol is not significantly cleared by the kidney and therefore requires hemodialysis even if fomepizole is used.

Treatment for salicylate ingestion includes gastrointestinal decontamination with activated charcoal. Urinary alkalization (urine pH more than 7.5) prevents reabsorption of salicylates from the urine. In severe cases, hemodialysis is required.

SEVERE METABOLIC ACIDOSIS

Assuming an adequate ventilatory response, an acute acidosis is severe when the arterial pH is less than 7.1 or the serum bicarbonate is less than 8 mEq/L. At this level of acidemia, cardiac depression is observed in experimental studies. In severe acidosis, exogenous bicarbonate is recommended by some to increase the arterial pH to 7.2 or the bicarbonate to 10 mEq/L. Sodium bicarbonate is usually infused over several minutes to a few hours, with boluses only used in extreme cases. The clinical effects of the therapy may be judged approximately 30 minutes after completion of the infusion. A biologically inert amino acid, tromethamine (THAM), is used as an alternative to bicarbonate in severe acidosis but rarely employed in pediatrics because of complications associated with its use, including hypoglycemia, hypokalemia, respiratory suppression, sclerosis, and venous irritation.

Common Pitfalls

Several complications may occur with the treatment of acidosis, particularly with bicarbonate therapy, including overshoot alkalosis, volume overload, and exacerbation of hypokalemia. Hypokalemia results from reentry of potassium into the intracellular compartment with correction of the acidosis and/or infusion of insulin (in diabetic ketoacidosis). Diluting 100 mEq/L of sodium bicarbonate in 0.25% NaCl to render a nearly isotonic solution can reduce the risk of hypernatremia and

TABLE 3 Rationale for Treatment Options of Metabolic Acidosis

Diagnosis	Study Design	Treatment Regimen	Results	Reference
Idiopathic distal renal tubular acidosis	Prospective study, 8 children; mean age 9.7 ± 1.2 yr	Potassium citrate, 4 mEq/kg/day given PO in three divided doses	Dose sufficient to normalize the serum bicarbonate, correct hypokalemia and hypocitraturia, and normalize the calcium oxalate but not the calcium phosphate supersaturation.	Am J Kidney Dis 39:383–391, 2002
Distal renal tubular acidosis	Prospective trial, 10 children	Alkali therapy with maximum requirement ranging from 4.8 to 14.1 mEq/kg/day given PO	Patients with bicarbonate wasting needed increased amounts of bicarbonate for optimal growth; each patient achieved normal height with corrected serum bicarbonate.	J Clin Invest 61:509–527, 1978
Severe lactic acidosis	Prospective controlled study of 10 patients	Administered bicarbonate (1 mEq/kg IV) or equal volume of sodium chloride and observed for 60 min	No change in hemodynamic parameters despite an increase in arterial pH and Pco_2.	Crit Care Med 19:1352–1356, 1991
Severe lactic acidosis	Multicenter, placebo-controlled study of 252 adults	Dichloroacetate, 50 mg/kg/dose IV, infused over 30 min and repeated after 2 h (126 patients); placebo (126 patients)	Dichloroacetate treatment resulted in statistically significant improvement in serum lactate levels and pH but failed to improve either hemodynamics or survival.	N Engl J Med 327:1564–1569, 1992
Congenital lactic acidosis	Case series, 53 patients; mean age 5.4 yr	Dichloroacetate, 25–100 mg/kg/day given PO/IV	Reduced lactate in 76% of patients; clinical improvement in 38% of patients.	Arch Dis Child 77:535–541, 1997
Lactic acidosis caused by severe malaria	Randomized, double blind, placebo-controlled study of 124 children	Dichloroacetate, 50 mg/kg IV, given at the same time as a dose of IV quinine	Dichloroacetate significantly increased the rate and degree of fall in serum lactate levels.	J Clin Pharmacol 43:386–396, 2003
Severe diabetic ketoacidosis	Retrospective study of 106 children	57 patients with $NaHCO_3$ treatment and 49 without $NaHCO_3$ treatment	No difference in the blood glucose and acidosis recovery rates or in complications.	Ann Emerg Med 31:41–48, 1998
Ethylene glycol ingestion	Prospective trials, 19 patients, mean age of 41 yr with a range of 19–73 yr; ethylene glycol levels >20 mg/dL and acidosis in 15 of 20 patients	Fomepizole, 15 mg/kg IV followed by 10 mg/kg q12h for 48 h; hemodialysis if severe acidosis, renal failure, or ethylene glycol concentration >59 mg/dL	Fomepizole prevented renal injury by inhibiting the formation of toxic metabolites of ethylene glycol ingestion, with few adverse effects attributable to fomepizole.	N Engl J Med 340:832–838, 1999
Ethylene glycol ingestion	Case report, 8-month-old infant	Fomepizole, 15 mg/kg IV followed by 10 mg/kg q12h with the interval decreased to q4h during hemodialysis	First case report of fomepizole administration for ethylene glycol ingestion in an infant; fomepizole appeared to prevent the metabolism of ethylene glycol to toxic acids.	Pediatrics 106:1489–1497, 2000
Methanol ingestion	Multicenter, prospective trial; 11 patients; mean age 40 yr with a range of 18–61 yr	Fomepizole, 15 mg/kg IV, followed by 10 mg/kg q12h; hemodialysis if patient was acidotic, had visual disturbances or had a methanol level >50 mg/dL	Fomepizole was safe and effective in the treatment of methanol poisoning and reduced plasma formic acid levels in all patients.	N Engl J Med 344:424–429, 2001
Methanol ingestion	Case report, 5-year-old child	Fomepizole, 15 mg/kg IV, followed by hemodialysis	Patient had no visual abnormalities or evidence of methanol toxicity; fomepizole averted the use of IV ethanol infusion.	Pediatrics 108:77–80, 2001

IV, intravenous; PO, by mouth; q, every.

2

hyperosmolality. Rapid correction can lead to an increased Pco_2 of the cerebrospinal fluid with deterioration of neurologic status. Care must be taken to avoid overtreatment, transitioning the patient to alkalemia. Because treatment of acidosis depends on the underlying etiology, failure to identify the correct diagnosis could adversely affect the patient.

METABOLIC ALKALOSIS

Metabolic alkalosis denotes a disturbance initiated by an elevation in plasma bicarbonate concentration. It is also characterized by an arterial pH above 7.44 and elevated arterial $Paco_2$ (see Table 1). A metabolic alkalosis is generated by one of three situations:

1. Loss of acid from the extracellular fluid
2. Functional addition of new bicarbonate (either through increased intake or decreased excretion)
3. Volume contraction around a constant amount of extracellular bicarbonate (sometimes referred to as a "contraction alkalosis")

A normal kidney would rapidly excrete a large amount of bicarbonate, correcting the alkalosis. Therefore, a metabolic alkalosis must be generated and then sustained by impaired renal bicarbonate excretion. Causes of impaired bicarbonate excretion are a decreased glomerular filtration rate, which occurs with volume contraction or renal insufficiency, and increased tubular bicarbonate reabsorption and acid secretion. The latter occurs through decreased effective circulating volume, which results in increased proximal tubular bicarbonate reabsorption and stimulation of the renin-angiotensin-aldosterone system. Aldosterone stimulates acid secretion in the collecting ducts. In addition, chloride depletion inhibits bicarbonate secretion by the cortical collecting duct.

Etiology

For diagnostic and therapeutic reasons, conditions that cause metabolic alkalosis are divided into chloride-responsive and chloride-unresponsive groups (Box 2). A low urinary chloride (less than 10 mEq/L) characterizes the chloride-responsive group, and a normal to high urinary chloride level (more than 10 mEq/L) characterizes the chloride-unresponsive group.

CHLORIDE-RESPONSIVE METABOLIC ALKALOSIS

Gastrointestinal loss of acid occurs with loss of gastric secretions, with chronic nasogastric suctioning or recurrent vomiting seen in pyloric stenosis or bulimia. The kidneys respond with a bicarbonate diuresis associated with increased sodium and potassium losses, resulting in hypokalemia and volume depletion, which maintains the alkalosis. Congenital chloridorrhea causes a metabolic alkalosis because of a defect in intestinal chloride reabsorption and bicarbonate secretion leading to

---

BOX 2 Causes of Metabolic Alkalosis

Chloride Responsive (Urinary Chloride <10 mEq/L)
- Gastrointestinal causes
  - Vomiting
  - Nasogastric suction
  - Chloride-wasting diarrhea
  - Villous adenoma: colon
  - Laxative abuse

- Diuretic therapy
- Posthypercapnea
- Penicillin
- Cystic fibrosis

Chloride Responsive (Urinary Chloride >10 mEq/L)
- Adrenal disorders
  - Hyperaldosteronism
  - Cushing syndrome

- Exogenous steroid
  - Gluco- or mineralocorticoid
  - Licorice ingestion

- Alkali ingestion
- Refeeding alkalosis
- Bartter syndrome
- Gitelman syndrome

Adapted from Hanna JD, Scheinman JI, Chwan JM: The kidney in acid–base balance. Pediatr Clin North Am 46:1365–1395, 1995; and Narins RG, Emmet M: Simple and mixed acid–base disorders: A practical approach. Medicine 59:161–187, 1980.

---

excessive chloride loss in the stool. Laxative abuse in the setting of hypokalemia can also cause a metabolic alkalosis. Cystic fibrosis is associated with sodium and chloride losses from sweat and volume depletion from diarrhea, both of which can lead to metabolic alkalosis.

Inadequate intake of chloride was seen in the late 1970s in infants fed chloride-deficient soybean formula. Loop and thiazide diuretics can generate and sustain a metabolic alkalosis by causing hypovolemia, which stimulates secondary hyperaldosteronism and leads to hypokalemia. Diuretic-induced metabolic alkalosis is often seen in neonates with bronchopulmonary dysplasia who receive aggressive diuretic therapy for lung fluid accumulation. Chronic respiratory acidosis stimulates increased renal acid secretion. Treatment with mechanical ventilation lowers the Pco_2 but leaves the bicarbonate elevated. Penicillin acts as a nonreabsorbable anion, resulting in the exchange of protons and potassium for sodium.

CHLORIDE-UNRESPONSIVE METABOLIC ALKALOSIS

Renal acid loss with primary mineralocorticoid excess promotes acid secretion in the collecting duct, and the hypokalemia induced by concomitant urinary potassium loss plays a major role in sustaining the metabolic alkalosis. Other uncommon conditions that cause metabolic alkalosis are the primary renal hypokalemic tubulopathies, such as the Bartter and Gitelman syndromes.

TABLE 4 Rationale for the Treatment of Metabolic Alkalosis

Diagnosis	Study Type	Treatment Regimen	Conclusions	Reference
Refractory metabolic alkalosis	Retrospective study involving 17 patients, ages 21 to 88 yr	0.1 N hydrochloric acid calculated from base excess infused through a central vein.	IV administration of hydrochloric acid used to treat patients with refractory alkalosis is safe and effective, even in patients with renal failure or hepatic dysfunction.	Am Surg 46:140–146, 1980
Metabolic alkalosis resistant to fluid or KCl	Randomized, double-blind, placebo-controlled trial of 40 adults mechanically ventilated with asthma or COPD	Acetazolamide, one dose of 500 mg IV, compared to 250 mg IV q6h for a total of four doses.	A single 500-mg dose of acetazolamide reversed metabolic alkalosis as effectively as multiple doses of 250 mg.	Crit Care Med 27:1257–1261, 1999
Congenital chloride diarrhea	Case series of 21 children diagnosed from birth to 2 yr of age	The oral Cl^- needed to maintain normal serum electrolytes was approximately 5 mEq/kg/day, given as a 0.7% NaCl and 0.3% KCl solution, until 3 yr of age, then given as a 1.8% NaCl and 1.9% KCl solution.	With adequate substitution, patients with congenital chloride diarrhea exhibit normal mental and physical development.	Arch Dis Child 127:566–570, 1974
Bartter syndrome	Reviews of 20 patients with mean age of diagnosis 10.5 mo, all with failure to thrive	5% KCl with indomethacin or spironolactone added to medical regimen if the hypokalemia was severe.	Linear growth and body weight increased substantially in all patients but remained less than the third percentile.	Pediatr Nephrol 11:296–301, 1997
Postgastroplasty metabolic alkalosis unresponsive to ranitidine	Case report, 4-year-old boy with renal failure	Omeprazole, 5 mg twice daily (0.2 mg/kg/dose).	Successful management of alkalosis with omeprazole.	J Urol 147:435–437, 1992

COPD, chronic obstructive pulmonary disease; IV, intravenous; q, every.

2

Diagnosis

Symptoms of metabolic alkalosis are usually minimal or related to volume depletion (weakness, muscle cramps, postural dizziness) or hypokalemia (polyuria, polydipsia, muscle weakness). Patients with primary mineralocorticoid excess tend to be volume expanded and hypertensive. Patients with Bartter syndrome are volume contracted and prone to failure to thrive, short stature, polydipsia, and polyuria during early childhood. Children with Gitelman syndrome are likely to have febrile seizures, muscle weakness, and hypomagnesemic tetany, which occur later in life.

An arterial pH is needed to distinguish among a respiratory, metabolic, or mixed alkalosis. A mixed respiratory acidosis and metabolic alkalosis is seen in infants with bronchopulmonary dysplasia treated with diuretics. Serum potassium levels are often decreased when mineralocorticoid excess is present.

Expert Opinion on Management Issues

Treatment of metabolic alkalosis is directed at the underlying mechanisms causing and sustaining the alkalosis. Accordingly, treatment is dictated by whether the alkalosis is chloride responsive or chloride resistant. Most information used to guide the treatment of alkalosis is obtained from case reports and series (Table 4).

CHLORIDE-RESPONSIVE METABOLIC ALKALOSIS

In the chloride-responsive group of metabolic alkalosis, cases caused by vomiting, nasogastric suction, or diuretics, the urinary chloride is low and the extracellular volume is contracted. Correction of the volume contraction with saline and the potassium depletion with potassium chloride (KCl) usually promotes a brisk bicarbonate response and corrects the alkalemia. Vomiting can be treated with antiemetics, and gastric acid loss can be reduced by the use of H_2 receptor blockers and/or gastric proton pump inhibitors. Loop or thiazide diuretic doses may be decreased or coupled with a potassium-sparing diuretic. Therapies that contain bicarbonate and bicarbonate precursors, such as lactate, citrate, and acetate, or drugs that have mineralocorticoid activity should have their indication and dosage reassessed. Patients with congestive heart failure, cirrhosis, or nephrotic syndrome, who might not tolerate saline infusion, can be treated with acetazolamide, hydrochloric acid, or dialysis with a low bicarbonate bath.

Correction of the metabolic alkalosis over a few days with restoration of extracellular fluid and replacement of the potassium losses is necessary in infants with pyloric stenosis because an unstable acid–base status heightens the risk of complications during anesthesia.

Congenital chloride diarrhea is usually treated with approximately 4 to 5 mEq/kg of chloride (0.7% [121 mEq/L] NaCl and 0.3% [40 mEq/L] KCl), with the dose adjusted to achieve normal serum pH and electrolytes and maintain some chloride in the urine. In infants with alkalosis secondary to bronchopulmonary dysplasia and treated with diuretics, administration of sodium could worsen respiratory failure; 3 to 7 mEq/kg/day of KCl is the treatment of choice.

CHLORIDE-UNRESPONSIVE METABOLIC ALKALOSIS

With a chloride-unresponsive metabolic alkalosis, administration of saline is counterproductive because edema rather than volume contraction is present. Therapy is directed at the source of the mineralocorticoid (removal of the tumor, correction of the renal artery stenosis, or discontinuation of any mineralocorticoid-sustaining substance such as licorice). Medical management includes the use of a potassium-sparing diuretic, such as spironolactone or amiloride.

Potassium supplementation divided in three to four doses and titrated (up to 10 mEq/kg/day) to correct the serum value is the mainstay of therapy for the Bartter and Gitelman syndromes. The addition of potassium-sparing diuretics is associated with increased growth rates in children. Prostaglandin inhibitors, such as indomethacin (1.5 to 2.5 mg/kg/day in two to three divided doses), may improve the polyuria and hypokalemia of Bartter syndrome. Because hyperprostaglanduria is not present in Gitelman syndrome, prostaglandin inhibitors are not indicated, but magnesium supplementation is usually required.

SEVERE METABOLIC ALKALOSIS

In the presence of an appropriate ventilatory response, an alkalosis is severe when the serum bicarbonate is greater than 45 mEq/L or the pH is greater than 7.55. Several studies demonstrate increased mortality in the intensive care unit (ICU) directly correlated with blood pH rising, particularly above 7.55. Acidifying agents should be considered in the setting of a severe alkalosis with the goal of preventing the potential adverse effects, which include impaired cardiac, respiratory, metabolic, and cerebral function. Hydrochloric acid (100 mmol/L) can be safely infused through a central line and dosed based on the bicarbonate space (see Table 3). To avoid vascular sclerosis, it should be infused at a rate of no more than 0.2 mmol/kg/hour. Hydrochloric acid generators, ammonium chloride (20 g/L, 374 mmol/L of potential acid), or 10% arginine monohydrochloride (100 g/L, 475 mmol/L of potential acid) are sometimes used. Infusion through a central line is usually recommended because both are hyperosmotic solutions; however, 5 mL/kg of a 10% solution of arginine monohydrochloride (500 mg/kg) infused peripherally over 30 minutes is used safely in the measurement of growth hormone reserve in children. Ammonium chloride must be used cautiously with liver failure because it can raise serum ammonia levels, and arginine monohydrochloride can induce severe hyperkalemia when used with impaired renal function. Both ammonium chloride and arginine monohydrochloride require hepatic conversion for full activity.

Severe chloride-resistant alkalosis is rare but usually responds to aggressive potassium repletion; however, the basis of the therapy should be geared toward treating the underlying cause. When the cause of the mineralocorticoid excess cannot be treated, symptomatic relief can be provided with moderate restriction of sodium chloride coupled with potassium-sparing diuretics.

Common Pitfalls

Treatment of severe chloride-responsive metabolic alkalosis can be challenging in patients who are prone to pulmonary edema, such as those with severe cardiac disease or pulmonary capillary leak syndrome. Acetazolamide, infusions of hydrochloric acid, or hemodialysis with a reduced bicarbonate concentration of the standard dialysate are alternative therapies to consider when the associated fluid load of standard therapy is problematic. Because the treatment is different for a respiratory alkalosis than a metabolic alkalosis, reviewing the patient's clinical condition and performing an arterial blood gas is important to distinguish among the diagnoses. Alkalosis can lower serum ionized calcium and serum potassium levels, thereby requiring the clinician to be aware of these changes during the diagnosis and treatment of alkalosis.

Communication and Counseling

Because adequate treatment of chronic acid–base disorders such as renal tubule acidosis and Bartter syndrome improves growth, compliance with treatment regimens cannot be overemphasized. Most patients with mild acid–base disorders recover uneventfully once the underlying condition is addressed; however, severe acid–base disorders can be life-threatening. Parents should be given realistic expectations when optimal treatments are not available, such as in severe lactic acidosis.

SUGGESTED READINGS

1. Adrogue HJ, Madias NE: Management of life threatening acid base disorders, first of two parts. N Engl J Med 338:26–34, 1998. **Overview of the treatment of severe acidosis.**
2. Adrogue HJ, Madias NE: Management of life threatening acid base disorders, second of two parts. N Engl J Med 338:107–111, 1998. **Overview of the treatment of severe alkalosis.**
3. Brown MJ, Shannon MW, Woolf A, et al: Childhood methanol ingestion treated with fomepizole and hemodialysis. Pediatrics 108:77–80, 2001. **Case report of fomepizole use in a pediatric patient.**
4. Chabali R: Diagnostic use of anion and osmolal gaps in pediatric emergency medicine. Ped Emerg Care 13:204–210, 1997. **Overview of anion and osmolal gap in regard to pediatrics.**
5. Domrongkitchaiporn S, Khositseth S, Stitchantrakul W, et al: Dosage of potassium citrate in the correction of urinary abnormalities in pediatric distal renal tubular acidosis patients. Am J Kidney Dis 39:383–391, 2002. **Study evaluating efficacy of potassium citrate therapy in distal renal tubular acidosis.**
6. Greenberg A: Diuretic complications. Am J Med Sci 319:10–24, 2000. **Summary of the complications that might arise with diuretics that both cause and are used to treat acid–base disorders.**
7. Hanna JD, Scheinman JI, Chwan JM: The kidney in acid–base balance. Pediatr Clin North Am 46:1365–1395, 1995. **In-depth summary of acid–base disorders in pediatrics.**

8. Kraut JA, Kurtz I: Use of base in the treatment of severe acidemic states. Am J Kidney Dis 38:703–727, 2001. **In-depth review of the evidence in the literature both for and against the use of base in severe acidosis.**

9. Rose BP, Post TW: Metabolic alkalosis. In Rose BD, Post TW (eds): Clinical Physiology of Acid–Base and Electrolyte Disorders. New York: McGraw-Hill, 2001, pp 551–577. **Excellent reference for the pathophysiology of metabolic alkalosis.**

10. Rose BP, Post TW: Metabolic alkalosis. In Rose BD, Post TW (eds): Clinical Physiology of Acid–Base and Electrolyte Disorders. New York: McGraw-Hill, 2001, pp 578–646. **Excellent reference for the pathophysiology of metabolic acidosis.**

11. Shaer A: Inherited primary renal tubular hypokalemic alkalosis: A review of Gitelman and Bartter syndromes. Am J Med Sci 322:316–332, 2001. **Description of the genetics, clinical characteristics, pathophysiology, and treatment of the Gitelman and Bartter syndromes.**

Water and Electrolyte Balance in Low-Birth-Weight Infants

Stephen Baumgart

KEY CONCEPTS

- In premature neonates of extremely low birth weight (ELBW: less than 1000 g birth weight), poor epidermal barrier function at birth results in severe transcutaneous evaporation, dehydration, and electrolyte disturbances. The fragile skin also presents a poor barrier to infections.
- In these infants (and in premature infants of very low birth weight [VLBW: less than 1500 g]), pulmonary edema formation with a patent ductus arteriosus (PDA) can result from overzealous fluid replacement therapy. Increased lung water may contribute to bronchopulmonary dysplasia (BPD), leading to the present controversy of fluid restriction versus replenishment in prescribing fluid maintenance therapy.
- Associations are now described between electrolyte disturbances occurring early in life and subsequently adverse neurodevelopmental outcomes.

A gelatinous neonatal skin permits large transepidermal evaporation that is highest on day 1 of life (estimated 100 to 170 mL/kg/day) and diminishes unpredictably. Thus a large reservoir of sodium-enriched extracellular fluid is exposed to evaporation, leading to hypernatremia (Figure 1). Maintenance fluid therapy may require between 80 and 160 mL/kg/day (or more), depending on incubator temperature, humidity, and radiant warming. Electrolyte replacements must be balanced several times daily against changing estimates of transepidermal fluid and measured renal losses. Serial urine volume and serum *and* urine electrolyte determinations every 8 to 12 hours from days 1 to 3 are probably more helpful than daily weights in judging replacement therapy. Hyperkalemia may occur early on as sodium leaks into cells, displacing potassium into the extracellular compartment. Titrating insulin (0.01 to 0.1 U/kg/hour) and glucose (usually 5 to 10 mg/kg/minute) infusions to maintain serum potassium concentrations below

6.7 mEq/L is part of routine fluid management in these infants.

Artificial Barriers to Prevent Transcutaneous Evaporation

Incubator humidity regulated to provide 40% to 80% relative humidity may promote better fluid balance. Petroleum-based ointments used as skin emollients have received much attention; however, because of an increased incidence of bacterial infections in a large randomized trial, we do not recommend this practice. The use of Saran plastic blankets and adherent polyurethane skin dressings (Opsite or Tegederm) are effective in reducing evaporation; however, the skin of extremely low-birth-weight (ELBW) infants can be easily damaged.

Preventing Pulmonary Edema

After the first 5 to 7 days of life, the risk for dehydration in extremely premature babies diminishes as epidermal keratin forms. During weeks 2 and 3, many investigators now describe water overload contributing to the pathogenesis of lung injury and edema and probably resulting from overzealous fluid replenishment therapy continued past the first week to compensate for excessive weight loss (Figure 2).

FLUID RESTRICTION

Bell and Acarregui reported a meta-analysis of four randomized, controlled trials of high- and low-fluid replacement therapy (Table 1). Fluid intakes ranged from as low as 50 mL/kg/day to as high as 200 mL/kg/day. All four studies were conducted primarily in very-low-birthweight (VLBW) (and not ELBW) populations, and only two of the studies demonstrated significant differences in the occurrences of PDA, congestive heart failure, BPD, necrotizing enterocolitis (NEC), or death in the high-fluid groups. The meta-analysis favored low-fluid volume infusions in VLBW infants. We recommend giving the minimum volume required to maintain serum sodium concentration below 150 mEq/L in both VLBW and ELBW infants.

DIURETICS

Although widely used, diuretic therapy to treat pulmonary edema is controversial. A Cochrane Database analysis in 2002 reported six randomized trials for the combination of spironolactone and thiazide for 3 weeks or longer, with limited success in the treatment of chronic lung edema in BPD. However, a previous Cochrane Database analysis in 2001 described six randomized trials for the use of furosemide to treat pulmonary edema in respiratory distress syndrome (RDS). Furosemide was associated with the development of PDA, and some cases developed hypovolemia requiring fluid volume resuscitation. We conclude that furosemide should not be used for treating RDS, and that thiazide and spironolactone may be used for limited periods from 1 to 3 weeks in BPD.

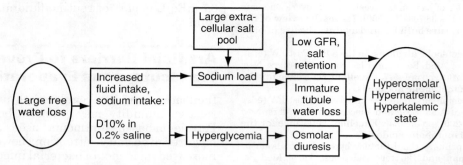

FIGURE 1. Large free water loss replacement, usually adding sodium to match anticipated urinary sodium excretion, contributes to a sodium load presented to an immature kidney. Added to this load is the large sodium reservoir residing in the extracellular space. The low glomerular filtration rate (GFR) of the fetal kidney results in salt retention, and immature tubular function (with poor concentrating ability) wastes additional free water. An osmolar diuresis may occur with the hyperglycemia common in this population. By 48 to 72 hours, a hyperosmolar, hypernatremic state evolves. This state contributes to the development of life-threatening hyperkalemia as sodium enters the cell, promoting potassium leak. (From Burg F, Polin RA (eds): Workbook in Practical Neonatology. Philadelphia, WB Saunders, 1983, pp 25–39. Reproduced with permission.)

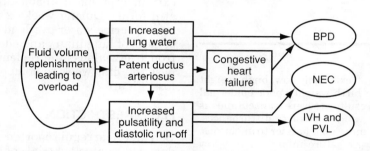

FIGURE 2. Fluid replenishment volume when administered too aggressively may result in increased lung water and contribute to the pathogenesis of bronchopulmonary dysplasia (BPD). High fluid intake is also associated with development of clinically significant patent ductus arteriosus (PDA), congestive heart failure, necrotizing enterocolitis (NEC), periventricular leukomalacia (PVL), and intraventricular hemorrhage (IVH). (From Burg F, Polin RA (eds): Workbook in Practical Neonatology. Philadelphia, WB Saunders, 1983, pp 25–39. Reproduced with permission.)

TABLE 1 Meta-Analysis of Four Studies Evaluating High Versus Low Fluid Volume Intake Strategies for Maintenance Therapy in Infants of Very Low Birth Weight

Reference*	Study Design	Weights and Gestations	High-Fluid/Low-Fluid Volume Limits	Outcomes
Bell et al: N Engl J Med 302:598–604, 1980	170 sequential matched pairs, 30 days	1.41 kg; 31 wk	122/169 mL/kg/day	PDA, CHF, NEC in high-fluid group
Von Stackhauser, et al: Klin Pediatr 192:539–546, 1980	56 random pairs, 3 days	1.9/2.0 kg; 34.6/34.2 wk	60/150 mL/kg/day	No differences
Lorenz, et al: J Pediatr 101:423–432, 1982	88 random matched pairs, 5 days	1.20 kg; 29 wk	60–85 mL/kg/day 80–140 mL/kg/day	No differences
Tammela, et al: Acta Paediatr 81:207–212, 1992	100 random pairs, 28 days	1.30 kg; 31 wk	50–150 mL/kg/day 80–200 mL/kg/day	Death, BPD in high-fluid group

Note: Patent ductus arteriosus (PDA), congestive heart failure (CHF), and necrotizing enterocolitis (NEC) were significantly more common with high-fluid volumes administered. Adapted from Bell EF, Acarregui MJ: Restricted versus liberal water intake for preventing morbidity and mortality in preterm infants. Cochrane Database of Systematic Reviews 3:CD000503, 2001.

BPD, bronchopulmonary dysplasia; CHF, congestive heart failure, NEC, necrotizing enterocolitis; PDA, patent ductus arteriosus.

*Complete references for table:

Bell EF, Warburton D, Stonestreet BS, Oh W: Effect of fluid administration on the development of symptomatic patent ductus arteriosus and congestive heart failure in premature infants. N Engl J Med 302:598–604, 1980.

Lorenz JM, Kleinman LI, Kotagal UR, Reller MD: Water balance in very low-birth-weight infants: relationship to water and sodium intake and effect on outcome. J Pediatr 101:423–432, 1982.

Tammella OKT, Koivisto ME: Fluid restriction for preventing bronchopulmonary dysplasia. Reduced fluid intake during the first weeks of life improves the outcome of low-birth-weight infants. Acta Paediatr 81:207–212, 1992.

von Stockhausen HB, Struve M: Die Auswirkungen einer stark unterschiedlichen parenteral en Flussigkeitszufuhr bei Fruh- und Neugeborenen in den ersten drei Lebenstagen. Klin Padiatr 192: 539–546, 1980.

TABLE 2 Published Studies Suggesting Hyponatremia Is Associated with Adverse Neurodevelopmental Outcomes

Reference*	Study Design	Population	Developmental Deficits
Leslie et al: J Paediatr Child Health 31:312–316, 1995.	Case controls	ELBW	Sensorineural hearing loss
Murphy et al: BMJ 314:404–408, 1997.	Case controls	VLBW	Cerebral palsy
Ertl et al: Biol Neonate 79:109–112, 2001.	Multivariate analysis, case controls	VLBW	Sensorineural hearing loss

*Complete references for table:
Leslie GI, Kalaw MB, Bowen JR, Arnold JD: Risk factors for sensorineural hearing loss in extremely premature infants. J Paediatr Child Health 31:312–316, 1995.
Murphy DJ, Hope PL, Johnson A: Neonatal risk factors for cerebral palsy in very preterm babies: Case-control study. BMJ 314:404–408, 1997.
Ertl T, Hadzsiev K, Vincze O, et al: Hyponatremia and sensorineural hearing loss in preterm infants. Biol Neonate 79:109–112, 2001.

CORTICOSTEROIDS

Omar, Lorenz, and colleagues reported higher urine output during the first 2 days of life in infants receiving prenatal corticosteroids, by maturing renal development in ELBW infants. They speculated that natriuresis might result from better mobilization of lung fluid by augmenting Na^+,K^+-ATPase (adenosine triphosphatase) in the pulmonary epithelium. Results of postnatal studies on corticosteroids and fluid balance remain highly speculative, however, and no recommendations for routine therapy can be made.

Electrolyte Imbalance and Poor Neurodevelopment

HYPONATREMIA

Bhatty and colleagues (personal communication, 1997) described hyponatremia (serum sodium concentration less than 125 mEq/L) in ELBW infants who subsequently developed a higher occurrence of cerebral palsy, hypotonia, and sensorineural hearing loss. Other studies suggest an association between hyponatremia and neurodevelopmental problems (Table 2).

HYPERNATREMIA

An association between hypernatremia and central nervous system disruptions is not yet closely examined. Simmons and Battaglia (1974) suggested restricting hypertonic sodium bicarbonate use because of an association of hypernatremia with significant intraventricular hemorrhage (IVH). Little is reported on the occurrence of these problems in the VLBW and ELBW populations in which hypernatremia occurs most often, and developmental follow-up is most needed.

Expert Opinion on Management Issues

CORRECTION OF HYPONATREMIA

Bhatty and colleagues (1997) evaluated the duration, severity, and recovery from hyponatremia. These investigators found that only speed of recovery from hyponatremia correlated to poor neurodevelopmental outcomes. They recommend that correction should proceed at a slow rate, no more than 0.4 mEq/L/hour, or at most 10 mEq/L/day.

SUPPLEMENTING SODIUM INTAKE

Al-Dahhana and colleagues reported that sodium-supplemented infants of low birth weight and less than 32 weeks' gestation assigned to a replenishment protocol of 4 to 5 mEq/kg/day and lasting from 4 to 14 days of life had at 10 years of age better performance intelligence quotients (IQs), better motor and memory indexes, and improved behavioral assessments. However, confirmation of this finding should be sought before universal recommendations are made. We recommend that minimum sodium be given to achieve sodium *balance*, replacing measured urine sodium losses (except in the first few days of life when there is an obligate contraction of the extracellular fluid space) and providing sodium for growth (1 to 2 mEq/kg/day).

Common Pitfalls

- Routinely replacing large amounts of sodium-free water during the first days of life invites iatrogenic fluid overload (PDA, pulmonary edema, hyponatremia), particularly as the infant's skin matures rapidly over the first week of life.
- Insulin and glucose infusions for treating hyperkalemia should be monitored closely with serial plasma glucose and serum electrolyte concentrations.
- Humidity in incubators should be invisible—any appearance of mist or condensation (rainout) should be avoided.
- We recommend no more than 80% relative humidity for the smallest infants, but only for 1 to 2 weeks until skin keratin has formed.
- Removing adherent polyurethane skin dressings (Opsite or Tegederm) poses the risk of debriding the delicately developing epidermis underneath. This technique depends on expert nursing for application and removal.
- Fluid restriction to prevent PDA-related morbidity is not yet investigated in the ELBW infant population. These infants may suffer serious dehydration and electrolyte disturbances if restricted to less than 80 to 100 mL/kg/day. A better strategy to prevent PDA and pulmonary edema is to attempt to reduce transcutaneous evaporation to more

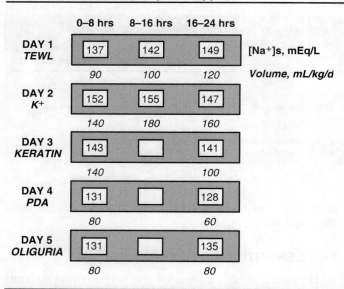

	0–8 hrs	8–16 hrs	16–24 hrs	
DAY 1 *TEWL*	137	142	149	[Na+]s, mEq/L
	90	100	120	Volume, mL/kg/d
DAY 2 *K+*	152	155	147	
	140	180	160	
DAY 3 *KERATIN*	143		141	
	140		100	
DAY 4 *PDA*	131		128	
	80		60	
DAY 5 *OLIGURIA*	131		135	
	80		80	

FIGURE 3. Concepts for timely fluid volume management for low-birth-weight infants during the first week of life. Volume intake is adjusted frequently according to measured serum electrolytes. Pathologic events that are likely to occur are shown at the left. Numerical values shown here are for a fictitious patient. PDA, patent ductus arteriosus; TEWL, transepidermal water loss. (From Sridhar S, Baumgart S: Water and electrolyte balance in newborn infants. In Hay WW, Thureen PJ (eds): Neonatal Nutrition and Metabolism, 2nd ed. New York, Cambridge University Press, 2005. Reprinted with permission.)

controllable volumes, easing the need for large parenteral fluid volume replacement.

Communication and Counseling

Avoiding fluid and electrolyte disturbances in VLBW and ELBW infants requires clinical vigilance (Figure 3). Practitioners should be wary of applying cookbook practices such as fluid restriction, sodium supplementation, and humidification for all premature babies. Rather, an individual infant's developmental appearance at birth should be observed, the effect of the infant's environment on fluid losses critically evaluated, and then strict fluid volume, and sodium and potassium *balances* should be assessed with frequent serum and urine chemistry measurements. Therapeutic decisions should weigh known risks of each intervention strategy against proven benefits.

SUGGESTED READINGS

1. Al-Dahhana J, Jannoun L, Haycock G: Developmental risks and protective factors for influencing cognitive outcome at 5½ years of age in very low birth weight children. Dev Med Child Neurol 44:508–516, 2002. **Presents an intriguing theory that routine sodium supplementation in premature babies (less than 32 weeks' gestation) may improve IQ and other developmental parameters.**
2. Bell EF, Acarregui MJ: Restricted versus liberal water intake for preventing morbidity and mortality in preterm infants. Cochrane Database of Systematic Reviews 3:CD000503, 2001. **Four randomized trials comparing low (50 to 120 mL/kg/day) and high (85 to 200 mL/kg/day) daily maintenance fluid volumes and morbidity in VLBW infants are summarized.**
3. Brion LP, Sol RF: Diuretics for respiratory distress syndrome in preterm infants. Cochrane Database of Systematic Reviews 2: CD001454; PMID:10796265, 2000. **Furosemide used to treat RDS acutely in six randomized trials was associated with the development of PDA, and some patients developed hypovolemia requiring fluid volume resuscitation. Furosemide is not recommended for treating RDS.**
4. Brion LP, Primhak RA, Ambrosio-Perez I: Diuretics acting on the distal renal tubule for preterm infants with (or developing) chronic lung disease. Cochrane Database of Systematic Reviews 3: CD001817; PMID:10908511, 2000. **Six randomized trials demonstrated limited success for the combination of spironolactone and thiazide for 3 weeks or longer in the treatment of chronic lung edema in BPD.**
5. Costarino AT, Gruskay JA, Corcoran L, et al: Sodium restriction vs. daily maintenance replacement in very low birth weight premature neonates, a randomized and blinded therapeutic trial. J Pediatr 120:99–106, 1992. **Neither routine sodium restriction nor supplementation reliably avoids electrolyte disturbances in this population. Measured sodium *balance* is a key to appropriate management in preventing electrolyte disturbances.**
6. Edwards WH, Conner JM, Soll RF, and Vermont Oxford Network Neonatal Skin Care Study Group: The effect of prophylactic ointment therapy on nosocomial sepsis rates and skin integrity in infants with birth weights of 501–1000 g. Pediatrics 113:1195–1203, 2004. **Multicenter randomized trial of prophylactic ointment applied to the skin of VLBW infants to reduce water loss reports increased nosocomial sepsis with use.**
7. Gaylord MS, Wright K, Lorch K, et al: Improved fluid management utilizing humidified incubators in extremely low birth weight infants. J Perinatol 21:438–443, 2001. **Humidification of incubators works to prevent electrolyte disturbances but at the cost of bacterial colonization and potential infections.**
8. Omar SA, Decristofaro JD, Agarwal BI, et al: Effects of prenatal steroids on water and sodium homeostasis in extremely low birth weight neonates. Pediatrics 104:482–488, 1999. **Prenatal corticosteroid prophylaxis may reduce postnatal pulmonary edema by acting directly on pulmonary epithelium sodium transport.**
9. Simmons MA, Adcock EW, III, Bard H, Battaglia FC: Hypernatremia and intracranial hemorrhage in neonates. New Engl J Med 291:6–10, 1974. **Hypernatremia is associated with IVH in premature infants receiving hypertonic bicarbonate infusions.**

Fluid and Electrolyte Therapy

Raymond Adelman

KEY CONCEPTS

- Intracellular and extracellular osmolality are the same; a rapid fall in extracellular water (ECF) osmolality causes a shift in water to intracellular water (ICF) and cell swelling.
- Maintenance fluids, given every 24 hours, are independent of deficit replacement. Never correct deficit by simply increasing maintenance fluids.
- Isotonic solution is used in all types of dehydration. Always monitor clinical response to make sure adequate fluid is provided.
- Correct hyponatremia and hypernatremia gradually to avoid rapid changes in osmolality; symptomatic hyponatremia can be treated with 3% hypertonic saline until symptoms abate.

Our bodies are largely composed of water and chemicals. The goal of fluid and electrolyte therapy is to restore and maintain the volume and composition of bodily fluids safely and efficiently. Total body water (TBW) per kilogram of body weight is highest in the newborn: 80 mL/kg in the term infant and 90 mL/kg in the preterm infant, falling to 65 mL/kg by 1 year of age. Because most body water is in lean body mass and not fat, obese individuals have a smaller percentage of their body weight as water. Fluid and medications given to obese individuals need to be adjusted accordingly, based on estimated lean body mass (50th percentile weight for height). TBW consists of intracellular water (ICF), which is approximately 40% of body weight, and extracellular water (ECF), which is 45% of body weight for the newborn, falling to the adult 25% of body weight by 1 year of age. ECF consists of plasma as well as transcellular water, interstitial fluid, connective tissue, and bone. ECF maintains the integrity, constancy, and function of cell systems by acting as a buffer between cells and the exterior. Changes in fluid volume and composition that are severe and remain uncorrected impair cellular function and may lead to cellular injury and death.

The composition of ECF is quite different from that of ICF. The major ECF cation is sodium and the major anion is chloride. In ICF, the major cation is potassium and the major anion is phosphate. Chemical analysis of plasma (or more precisely serum) reflects changes in ECF fluid compartments. Such is not the case for intracellular constituents. Indeed, by the time hypokalemia or hypophosphatemia is detected in serum, dramatic intracellular deficits have already taken place.

Intracellular osmolality and extracellular osmolality are roughly equal; hence dramatic changes in extracellular osmolality, precipitated, for example, by a fall in serum sodium, trigger a rapid corrective adjustment, initially by movement of water into cells, to lower ICF osmolality and to raise ECF osmolality until osmolar equivalence is met. Such dramatic shifts in water can cause acute cell swelling, which can have serious, even lethal, consequences. The correct use of maintenance and rehydration fluids by the physician is critical to mitigate pathophysiologic insults to the body and to avoid iatrogenic complications that may be more dangerous than the presenting illness.

Expert Opinion on Management Issues

MANAGEMENT OF MAINTENANCE FLUIDS

Maintenance fluids and electrolytes are those required daily to maintain homeostasis in an otherwise normal individual unable to take fluids orally. Maintenance fluids are *never* used to restore deficits. It is easiest to think of maintenance requirements for water, sodium, and potassium in terms of caloric requirements. This approach is physiologic because insensible water loss is linked to metabolic rate; it is also easy to use and applicable over a wide range of weights, from a 3-kg infant to a 70-kg adolescent.

The standard Holliday-Segar approach estimates calories used per kilogram of body weight and then provides

TABLE 1 Calculation of Maintenance Fluids

Weight	Calories	Water
0–10 kg	100 cal/kg	100 mL/100 cal
10–20 kg	1000 cal + 50 cal/kg	100 mL/100 cal
20–70 kg	1500 cal + 20 cal/kg	100 mL/100 cal

Formula adjustment: Multiply total mL × 0.8 = total mL administered.
Example: A 15-kg child needs 1000 calories + 5 × 50 calories = 1250 calories. Total fluid is 100 mL/100 calories, or 1250 mL. Multiply 1250 × 0.8 (correction factor) = 1000 mL, which is the actual amount to be administered.
Adapted from Holliday MA, Segar WE: The maintenance need for water in parenteral fluid therapy. Pediatrics 19:823–832, 1957.

for 100 mL of water for each 100 calories metabolized. Because of overestimations of water needs, we recommend only 80% of calculated water actually be given to the patient, with appropriate adjustments in the face of abnormal insensible or urinary water requirements (Table 1).

Water requirements include insensible losses, 50 mL per 100 calories (two thirds of which is respiratory and one third cutaneous), and urinary losses, 65 mL per 100 calories. Because approximately 15 mL of water is generated through oxidation of nutrients, net insensible loss is 35 mL per 100 calories.

Insensible water loss is greater with hyperpnea, such as in asthma, and in the premature infant where losses can exceed 100 mL/kg/day or more. Insensible losses are decreased if humidified ventilator air is provided.

Urinary water loss is estimated as what is necessary to provide a comfortable excretion of a solute load in a child with normal renal concentrating ability. Urinary water losses may be higher in patients with a solute diuresis, such as diabetic ketoacidosis or after mannitol, or with a serious concentrating defect, such as diabetes insipidus. Patients with reduced urinary losses include those with acute anuric renal failure in which no water for urinary losses is required or with the syndrome of inappropriate antidiuretic hormone (SIADH) in which total fluids are halved. As discussed later, severe hyponatremia can occur when SIADH goes unrecognized and water provided for urinary losses is not appropriately reduced. In contrast, patients with concentrating defects, such as those with sickle cell disease or obstructive uropathy, may become seriously dehydrated if increased fluids are not provided for increased urinary water losses.

MANAGEMENT OF MAINTENANCE ELECTROLYTES

Sodium is the chief cation in ECF. Normally the kidney has an extraordinary ability to both conserve sodium in face of sodium deficiency and excrete sodium in the presence of sodium excess. Maintenance sodium requirements can conveniently be linked to water requirements, providing 2 to 4 mEq of sodium per 100 mL of water or 20 to 40 mEq/L (0.25 normal saline has 38.5 mEq/L). No sodium is needed when there is anuric renal failure. Reduced sodium, approximately 1 to 2 mEq per 100 mL of water, is provided in sodium-excess states such as

TABLE 2 Clinical Assessment of Severity of Dehydration

Signs and Symptoms	Mild	Moderate	Severe
Body weight lost	3%	5%–7%	10% or more
General appearance	Alert	Thirsty, lethargic, irritable	Lethargic to limp, cyanosis, cold
Pulse	Normal	Rapid and weak	Rapid, feeble, impalpable
Respiration	Normal	Deep	Deep and rapid
Anterior fontanelle	Normal	Sunken	Sunken
Blood pressure	Normal	Normal to low	Low, may be unrecordable
Skin turgor	Normal	Slow pinch retraction	Very slow pinch retraction
Eyes	Normal	Slightly sunken	Very sunken
Tears	Normal	Reduced	Absent
Mucous membranes	Moist	Dry	Very dry
Urine flow	Normal	Reduced	Anuria, severe oliguria
Capillary refill	Normal	≤2 sec	>3 sec

edema secondary to cardiac, renal, or hepatic disease. Additional sodium may be required with excess gastrointestinal, genitourinary, or cutaneous losses. Premature infants of very low birth weight may require added maintenance sodium because of poor tubular retention of sodium.

Potassium is the chief ICF cation. One may provide 2 to 3 mEq per 100 mL or 20 to 30 mEq/L of potassium to the normal child on parenteral fluids. No potassium is given with acute renal failure or adrenal insufficiency; potassium is often reduced with chronic renal insufficiency. Increased potassium may be needed in conditions with increased gastrointestinal, genitourinary, or cutaneous losses of potassium. There may be profound ongoing hypokalemia in patients receiving total parenteral nutrition (TPN) for nutritional support because of a large intracellular uptake of potassium and in patients with potassium-losing tubulopathies as a consequence of chemotherapeutic or antimicrobial agents.

Maintenance fluids and electrolytes are given every 24 hours and are *independent of fluids* administered for resuscitation. One *never* corrects fluid deficits simply by increasing the amount of maintenance fluids administered. The common practice of treating dehydration with 1.5 or 2 times maintenance is unphysiologic, careless, and may be dangerous. Finally, maintenance fluids are based on mL per calories metabolized per day, not on mL per kilogram body weight per day. Giving maintenance fluids based on mL/kg/day can lead to administration of excessive fluids, which can have serious consequences.

MANAGEMENT OF FLUID RESUSCITATION

Diarrheal Dehydration

The most common need for fluid resuscitation is dehydration caused by gastroenteritis. Because acute changes in body weight predominantly reflect fluid losses, dehydration is described as percentage of body weight lost and primarily affects the ECF compartment. Table 2 describes physical findings associated with percentage of body weight lost. Minimal dehydration in which signs and symptoms are mild or even undetectable is 3%; moderate dehydration in which signs and symptoms are clearly present is 5% to 7%; and severe dehydration in which

profound changes are evident is 10%. Infants have a greater percentage of body weight as fluid. Mild dehydration in infants is 5%; moderate, 10%; and severe, 15% of body weight lost. In patients with chronic diarrheal disease, some of the body weight change represents intracellular fluid losses because of loss of lean body mass.

Studies show that the extent of dehydration tends to be overestimated by physicians; the average degree of dehydration seen in emergency departments is 5% to 6% or less, or approximately 50 to 60 mL of ECF per kilogram. The signs and symptoms of dehydration (see Table 1) suffer from observer bias as well. Several studies suggest that poor skin turgor, delayed capillary refill, dry mucous membranes, labored respiratory rate, and sunken eyeballs may be among the more valid clinical signs.

Although the extent of dehydration is estimated as the percentage of body weight lost, the type of dehydration is determined by serum sodium: hyponatremic (Na less than 130 mEq/L) or hypotonic; hypernatremic (Na more than 150 mEq/L) or hypertonic; and isonatremic (Na 130 to 150 mEq/L) or isotonic. Isonatremic dehydration constitutes approximately 80% of patients with dehydration; hypernatremic and hyponatremic dehydration constitute approximately 10% each.

The history and physical findings may help identify the different types of dehydration, although the type and volume of initial rehydration fluid is the same regardless of the type of dehydration. Patients with chronic gastrointestinal losses whose intake mostly consists of water are more likely to present with hyponatremia. These patients often are quite ill, appear very hypovolemic, and tend to require more resuscitation fluid to achieve hemodynamic stability. Conversely, patients with hypernatremic dehydration are often infants with high fevers, increased insensible water loss, and lack of access to fluids. They have doughy skin, warm extremities, and marked irritability.

Over the last 50 years, deficit therapy was recommended to be administered gradually, over 24 to 48 hours. Recent approaches suggest this is both unnecessary and illogical. Rapid restoration of deficit restores cardiovascular stability and facilitates restorative processes through the pulmonary and renal systems. Hence full deficit replacement can take place over a few hours. One should give only an isotonic solution for deficit replacement, such as normal saline or lactated Ringer's, at a rate of 20 to 30 mL/kg/hour. Larger volumes may be indicated if hemodynamic stability is not achieved. However, because most diarrheal dehydration represents losses of 50 to 60 mL/kg or less, full correction of deficit can be achieved in 2 to 3 hours. Some advocate larger volumes and more rapid administration, but insufficient data in the literature show this to be either safe or necessary.

Many studies show that oral rehydration is just as effective as parenteral rehydration in patients with mild to moderate dehydration who are able to take fluids either orally or by nasogastric tube. The time to recovery, subsequent toleration of oral feeds, and percentage of patients eventually hospitalized do not differ between cases treated enterally or parenterally. A number of oral solutions are available, such as Infalyte, Naturalyte, Pedialyte, and WHO ORS. All provide sodium and potassium well in excess of that in fruit juices, sodas, and athletic hydration drinks such as Gatorade, and they have a sugar content that optimizes sodium uptake. Patients should be given 5 to 10 mL every 5 to 10 minutes, which may be increased as tolerated. Zofran may be given initially to reduce the likelihood of emesis. Obviously, patients who refuse oral rehydration, have persistent emesis, or are critically ill require intravenous hydration.

Shock

Patients with profound hypovolemia, such as those in uncompensated shock from sepsis, hemorrhage, or massive fluid losses, need large volumes of ECF replacement, 40 mL or more per kg per hour. One should rapidly provide as much as is needed to achieve cardiovascular stability as reflected by a normal blood pressure and normal capillary refill.

In all forms of parenteral rehydration, isotonic solution must be used. Clinical response must be monitored carefully to ensure adequate fluid is provided to correct deficits. One must not be content to rely solely on calculated losses because these are, at best, coarse estimates. Finally, overcorrecting deficits must be avoided because it may lead to complications, especially in patients with renal or cardiac disease.

Hyponatremia

Hyponatremia, a serum sodium of less than 130 mEq/L, may be seen as a result of true sodium depletion (as in gastroenteritis), an excess of water (as in SIADH), or a combination of the two (Box 1). Low sodium may also be seen in terminally ill conditions or may be artifactual, as seen with diabetic ketoacidosis and the nephrotic syndrome. SIADH is perhaps the most common cause of hyponatremia in the hospitalized patient. This occurs when excess antidiuretic hormone is secreted, resulting in fluid retention and a dilutional hyponatremia. SIADH is common after surgery, with pain, and with the use of medications such as opiates. Although hyponatremia is also seen with meningitis, asthma, and bronchiolitis, it may not represent true SIADH. In these conditions, antidiuretic

---

BOX 1 Causes of Hyponatremia

Sodium Deficit with Sodium Depletion

- Renal losses
  - Prematurity
  - Acute tubular necrosis, recovery phase
  - Diuretics
  - Renal salt wasting
  - Mineralocorticoid deficiency
  - Osmotic diuresis
  - Renal tubular acidosis
  - Cerebral salt wasting
- Extrarenal losses
  - Vomiting and diarrhea
  - Third spacing
  - Nasogastric drainage
  - Cystic fibrosis
  - Excess sweating
  - Burns
- Nutritional deficits
  - WIC syndrome
  - Inadequate sodium in parenteral fluids

Water Excess with Water Gain

- Syndrome of inappropriate ADH (SIADH)
- Glucocorticoid deficiency
- Hypothyroidism
- Drugs
- Excess parenteral fluid
- Psychogenic polydipsia
- Tap water enemas

Excess Sodium and Water

- Nephrotic syndrome
- Cirrhosis
- Cardiac failure
- Renal failure

ADH, antidiuretic hormone; SIADH, syndrome of inappropriate antidiuretic hormone; WIC, Women, Infants, and Children Program (see text for explanation).

---

hormone (ADH) may be appropriately increased in response to hypovolemia.

Symptoms of hyponatremia depend on both the rate of fall in serum sodium and the absolute level achieved. Patients with chronic hyponatremia developing over months may appear surprisingly well. Acutely ill patients are often symptomatic with levels under 120 mEq/L, with symptoms that can include lethargy, convulsions, shock, disorientation, and emesis. Hyponatremia is a major cause of convulsions in infants younger than 6 months of age because of the WIC syndrome, so called because mothers receiving infant formula through the WIC (Women, Infants, and Children) government aid program may dilute formula excessively to make the supply last longer.

Clinical evaluation of the patient and measurement of urinary sodium may help determine etiology of hyponatremia. True sodium deficiency is apparent from clinical signs of hypovolemia and by reduced urinary excretion of sodium (less than 10 mEq/L), except in cases of renal salt wasting or chronic renal insufficiency. Isotonic saline should be administered in these situations. Patients with both salt and water excess and hyponatremia, such as those with edematous states, are generally treated

---

BOX 2   **Causes of Hypernatremia**

Primary Sodium Excess
- Improperly mixed formula
- Excess sodium bicarbonate during resuscitation
- Hypertonic saline administration
- High breast-milk sodium
- Salt poisoning

Primary Water Deficit
- Diabetes insipidus (central, nephrogenic)
- Diabetes mellitus
- Gastroenteritis
- Inadequate breast-feeding
- Increased insensible loss
- Adipsia
- Intentional withholding of water

BOX 3   **Causes of Hypokalemia**

Renal Losses
- Renal tubular acidosis
- Diuretic use
- Fanconi syndrome
- Bartter syndrome
- Antibiotic use
- Chemotherapy
- Diabetic ketoacidosis
- Excess mineralocorticoid
- Cushing syndrome
- Renovascular disease
- Amphotericin

Nonrenal Losses

Cutaneous
- Gastrointestinal
- Enema abuse
- Laxative abuse
- Anorexia

Hypokalemia without Deficits
- Alkalosis
- Insulin therapy
- Familial hypokalemia paralysis

---

with water and sodium restriction, although care must be taken not to reduce effective plasma volume by an overvigorous approach. Patients with excess water, such as with SIADH, do not have signs of volume depletion, have increased body weight, and have urinary sodium exceeding 20 mEq/L. Such patients generally respond to fluid restriction. In severe cases, furosemide may be helpful in augmenting urinary water loss.

The failure to recognize SIADH and to reduce maintenance fluids, the inappropriate use of maintenance fluids, rather than isotonic fluids, for rehydration therapy, and the miscalculation of maintenance fluids on a per-kilogram rather than per 100 calories basis leads to water intoxication with profound hyponatremia and death. In patients for whom SIADH is anticipated, maintenance fluids should be halved.

Treatment of symptomatic hyponatremia consists of administration of hypertonic saline, only to raise serum sodium to a value of approximately 125 mEq/L, at which time symptoms should abate; 6 mL/kg of 3% sodium chloride solution raises serum sodium by approximately 5 mEq/L. Too rapid correction of hyponatremia should be avoided since it may cause central pontine myelinosis, a condition manifesting with disturbed sensorium, quadriplegia, and pseudo bulbar palsy. Sodium should not rise more than 8 to 10 mEq per 24 hours during the correction phase. Total sodium deficit can be calculated as follows:

140 − actual serum sodium × weight in kilogram × total body weight (0.8 in infant, 0.6 in child and adolescent)

MANAGEMENT OF HYPERNATREMIA

Hypernatremia may result from a primary sodium excess, such as salt poisoning or improperly mixed formula, or from a primary water deficit, as in inadequate breast milk volume and increased insensible water loss in febrile infants (Box 2). Hypernatremia is associated with a high mortality, especially if severe. Salt poisoning with serum sodium more than 200 mEq/L is best treated with dialysis. Hypernatremia due to other etiologies is treated with an isotonic solution, such as normal saline with 40

mEq/L of potassium and calcium as needed. The rate of fall of sodium is critical and should not exceed 10 to 12 mEq/L in 24 hours. Too precipitous a fall leads to a shift of water into cells, leading to brain cell edema and increased intracranial pressure, and it can result in herniation and death. Because such falls in serum sodium can take place quickly, often with irreversible cellular consequences, serum electrolytes must be measured frequently. Abrupt changes in ECF osmolality from other causes, such as too-rapid correction of diabetic hyperglycemia, may lead to the same consequences.

MANAGEMENT OF HYPOKALEMIA

Hypokalemia may be seen because of severe gastrointestinal losses, as in gastroenteritis; urinary losses, as in the Bartter syndrome; renal tubulopathies associated with chemotherapeutic agents, amphotericin, and aminoglycosides; or cutaneous losses, as in cystic fibrosis. Hypokalemia without true losses may occur with alkalosis or after insulin therapy (Box 3).

Symptoms of hypokalemia include muscle weakness, myalgia, thirst, ileus, decreased peristalsis, and flat or absent T waves and U waves on electrocardiogram (ECG). Patients may present with frank paralysis and respiratory failure. Chronic hypokalemia can cause permanent renal injury.

The treatment of hypokalemia is limited by the necessity of potassium to traverse the ECF to reach the ICF. Too much potassium leads to hyperkalemia and cardiac irregularities. In general, no more than 3 mEq/kg/day are provided for potassium deficit. If larger amounts are needed, as in the Bartter syndrome or massive urinary losses from chemotherapy, they should be given carefully and with appropriate monitoring. The potassium losses seen in acute diarrheal diseases may be substantial, but

---

BOX 4 Causes of Hyperkalemia

Potassium Excess
- Renal failure
- Hypoaldosteronism
- Potassium-sparing diuretics
- Spitzer syndrome
- Adrenal insufficiency
- Excess parenteral potassium

Hyperkalemia without Excess Potassium
- Cell breakdown
- Leukocytosis
- Thrombocytosis
- Metabolic acidosis
- Blood hemolysis
- Rhabdomyolysis

---

total repletion usually takes place over several days after oral feeds are reintroduced.

MANAGEMENT OF HYPERKALEMIA

Hyperkalemia, defined as potassium more than 5.5 mEq/L in the older child and more than 5.9 mEq/L in the newborn, can occur with true potassium excess, such as in acute renal failure, adrenocortical deficiency, and excess parenteral administration of potassium. Hyperkalemia may be seen after a redistribution of potassium, such as cell lysis from chemotherapy and severe metabolic acidosis (Box 4). Excess potassium can also come from hidden sources, such as medications. The consequences of severe hyperkalemia are mainly cardiovascular, with peaking of T waves, lengthening of the P-R interval, widening of the QRS, and then ventricular fibrillation leading to death. These findings generally do not occur with mild hyperkalemia, which can be treated with reduced potassium intake and use of sodium polystyrene. Levels above 6.5 to 7.0 mEq/L, especially if accompanied by ECG changes, must be treated promptly. The presence or absence of ECG changes may be helpful in deciding when and how to initiate therapy.

Rapid intravenous administration of sodium bicarbonate (1 to 3 mEq/kg) and glucose and insulin (0.5 to 1.0 g glucose per kilogram with 1 IU crystalline insulin per 3 g of glucose) results in movement of potassium into cells. Sodium bicarbonate alone has limited usefulness except in the presence of significant metabolic acidosis. Insulin and glucose can be repeated in 30 to 60 minutes. Salbutamol, given intravenously at 5 µg/kg over 15 minutes, or albuterol, given by nebulizer at 2.5 to 5.0 mg, are very effective in lowering potassium for up to 2 to 4 hours, although individual responses may vary. Intravenous calcium gluconate (up to 1.0 mL of a 10% solution per kilogram), given slowly over 3 to 5 minutes, helps counter the cardiotoxicity of hyperkalemia. Calcium gluconate may be repeated in 10 minutes. None of these measures removes significant quantities of potassium from the body. They are temporary until potassium is removed by ion exchange resins, such as Kayexalate (1 g/kg given orally or rectally with sorbitol every 6 to 12 hours), or by dialysis. The effectiveness of Kayexalate in removing potassium is modest and probably mostly because of the effect of sorbitol. If there is good renal function, increased urinary losses of potassium can be effected through diuretics such as furosemide.

Common Pitfalls

- Maintenance fluids are always based on milliliters per 100 calories metabolized daily. Adjust the Holliday-Segar formula by providing 80% of calculated fluids per 100 calories. Never provide maintenance fluids on a milliliter-per-kilogram basis.
- Fluid and electrolytes given to obese individuals should be adjusted to estimated kilograms of lean body mass.
- Maintenance fluids are never used to restore deficits. Use appropriate oral rehydration fluids or intravenous isotonic solution at 20 to 30 mL/kg/hour or more if the patient is severely dehydrated or in shock.
- Failure to recognize SIADH, inappropriate use of maintenance fluids for rehydration, and miscalculation of maintenance fluids on a per-kilogram basis can lead to severe and even fatal hyponatremia.

SUGGESTED READINGS

1. Adelman RD, Solhaug MJ: Pathophysiology of body fluids and fluid therapy. In Behrman RE, Kliegman RM, Jensen HB (eds): Nelson's Textbook of Pediatrics, 16th ed. Philadelphia: WB Saunders, 2000, pp 189–224. **Excellent, comprehensive discussion of the pathophysiology and management of fluid and electrolyte disorders.**
2. Gerigk M, Gnehm HE, Rascher W: Arginine vasopressin and renin in acutely ill children: Implication for fluid therapy. Acta Paediatr 85:550–553, 1996. **Examines the role of volume depletion in hyponatremia in acutely ill children.**
3. Hanna S, Tibby SM, Durward A, Murdoch IAS: Incidence of hyponatremia and hyponatremic seizures in severe respiratory syncytial virus bronchiolitis. Acta Paediatr 92:430–434, 2003. **Hyponatremia is very common in children with respiratory syncytial virus (RSV) bronchiolitis.**
4. Holliday MA, Segar WE: The maintenance need for water in parenteral fluid therapy. Pediatrics 19:823–832, 1957. **The classic paper on fluid and electrolyte recommendations for the hospitalized child.**
5. Holliday MA, Friedman AL, Segar WE, et al: Acute hospital induced hyponatremia in children: A physiologic approach. J Pediatr 145:584–587, 2004. **A review of the fundamental concepts of fluid and electrolyte therapy and approaches to avoid hospital-induced hyponatremia.**
6. Hoorn EJ, Geary D, Robb M, et al: Acute hyponatremia related to intravenous fluid administration in hospitalized children: An observational study. Pediatrics 113:1279–1284, 2004. **The most important cause of hospital-acquired hyponatremia is excessive hypotonic fluid.**
7. Phin SJ, McCaskill ME, Browne GJ, Lam LT: Clinical pathway using rapid rehydration for children with gastroenteritis. J Paediatr Child Health 39:343–348, 2003. **Demonstrates safety and efficacy of rapid intravenous rehydration.**
8. Spandorfer PR, Alessandrini EA, Joffe MD, et al: Oral versus intravenous rehydration of moderately dehydrated children: A randomized controlled trial. Pediatrics 115:295–301. **Study showing safety and efficacy of oral rehydration.**
9. Stenier MJ, DeWalt DA, Byerley JS: Is this child dehydrated? JAMA 291:2746–2754, 2004. **Analysis of the validity of clinical assessment tools for dehydration.**

Nutrition Support of the Very Ill Pediatric Patient

Darla J. Bradshaw and Andrew M. Tershakovec

KEY CONCEPTS

- Assess nutritional needs early.
- Adjust nutritional needs for special circumstances.
- Assess the most appropriate method of delivery for nutrition.
- Reassess nutritional status and delivery of nutritional support as disease state evolves.
- Use enteral nutrition whenever possible.

Nutrition management of the critically ill child presents unique challenges for even the most experienced health care practitioner. The goal of nutrition support includes supporting the patient during the hypermetabolic phase commonly associated with severe illness or injury, supporting basic body function and structural integrity, promoting healing, supporting normal immune function to fight and prevent infection, preventing catabolism, and promoting positive nitrogen balance and ultimately growth after the acute phase of the illness or injury passes. Enteral nutrition support should be considered as early as possible. If enteral feeding is not possible, parenteral nutrition can be used.

Expert Opinion on Management Issues

NUTRITION ASSESSMENT

A nutrition assessment is a comprehensive review of the medical history that includes a complete review of systems, as well as a nutrition history highlighting feeding history, formula type, preparation and route of feeding, typical intake, change in eating habits, food aversions, allergies or intolerances, weight and growth history, swallowing difficulties, and the use of vitamin, mineral, herbal, and other supplements. Physical exam should include assessment of growth and anthropometric measurements such as weight, height or recumbent length, head circumference, body mass index (BMI) (for child older than 2 years), midarm circumference, and triceps skinfold. Midarm circumference and triceps skinfold can be measured monthly as an estimate of response to therapy and to assess total body fat and protein stores, although significant edema may skew these measurements. The height, weight, head circumference, and BMI data are plotted on the National Center for Health Statistics (NCHS) growth charts. Specialized growth charts, such as those for prematurity, Down syndrome, or Turner syndrome, should be used when appropriate. Weights are frequently unavailable in the intensive care unit; therefore these anthropometric measurements, along with laboratory values, are relied on to monitor response to

therapy. No one single measurement can completely assess a child's nutritional status. Additionally, an assessment of physical signs of nutritional excesses and/or deficiencies should also be completed, including an examination of hair, skin, nails, eyes, and assessment of the oral cavity.

Biochemical laboratory data are also important in the evaluation of nutritional status and should include serum electrolytes, blood urea nitrogen (BUN), creatinine, calcium, magnesium, phosphorus, prealbumin, C-reactive protein, liver function tests, transaminases, γ-glutamyltransferase (GGT), and triglycerides. These lab values should be checked daily to weekly on initiation of nutrition support and weekly to monthly once the patient is stabilized. Some laboratory values can be affected by non-nutritional variables. Serum albumin is widely used in the assessment of nutritional status; however, its long half-life and susceptibility to change with hydration status make it less reliable as an assessment measure for acute changes in nutritional status. In contrast, prealbumin has a short half-life and responds quickly to acute changes in nutritional status; thus prealbumin is a better choice in the acute-care setting. Prealbumin can be depressed during times of stress because the liver prioritizes for the synthesis of acute-phase reactants. Additionally, serum proteins can be affected by hepatic and renal disease, neoplastic disease, the body's response to infection or inflammation, and medications, such as steroids. C-reactive protein is an indicator of inflammation and used to help differentiate if an inflammatory response or inadequate nutrition support is causing a low prealbumin concentration.

In the assessment of the critically ill child, a registered dietitian (RD) should be involved to help perform a nutrition assessment, assess nutritional requirements, and provide recommendations of the most appropriate composition and method of nutrition support. Continued monitoring of nutrition status and ongoing assessment of nutritional requirements helps ensure that the patient's optimal nutrition support goals are met for different conditions as each phase of the illness changes. Table 1 lists the nutritional considerations for selected conditions.

ASSESSMENT OF ENERGY REQUIREMENTS

Assessment of energy requirements for the critically ill child is important because overfeeding can cause hyperglycemia, hypertriglyceridemia, fatty liver, excessive nitrogen delivery and elevated BUN, excessive weight gain, and increased carbon dioxide (CO_2) production that may necessitate prolonged mechanical ventilation. Underfeeding can lead to catabolism, depressed immunity, impaired organ function, delayed wound healing, prolonged morbidity, and increased mortality. Energy needs are reduced with mechanical ventilation, sedation, paralysis, and loss of lean body mass, and they are increased with fever, infection, postsurgery, trauma/injury, cardiac disease, traumatic brain injury, and other hypermetabolic states. In addition, metabolism can be affected by severe illnesses, as demonstrated by hyperglycemia and hypertriglyceridemia, commonly seen in critically ill children.

TABLE 1 Selected Diseases/Conditions and Selected Nutritional Considerations

Disease/Condition	Nutritional Considerations
Liver disease	Ascites/edema can mask malnutrition.
	Decreased serum hepatic proteins.
	Malabsorption.
	Fluid and sodium restriction for end-stage disease.
	Fat-soluble vitamin/multivitamin supplementation.
	Protein restriction only with encephalopathy.
	Increase energy requirements for growth.
	Enteral formulas containing MCT oil.
	Prevention of essential fatty acid deficiency.
	Prevention of fat-soluble vitamin deficiency.
	Monitor copper, manganese, and selenium and adjust in PN.
Renal disease	Fluid, sodium, phosphorus, and potassium restriction may be indicated.
	Increased serum proteins.
	Phosphate binders.
	Calcium, vitamin D supplementation.
	Provide minimum RDA for protein and more if patient is undergoing hemodialysis (HD).
	Monitor trace mineral supplementation in PN and adjust accordingly.
Cardiac disease	Elevated energy requirements.
	Fluid restriction.
	Long-term enteral feedings may be required for adequate growth.
Mechanically ventilated	Decreased energy requirements to REE if sedated/paralyzed.
	Sedation/pain medications can decrease gut motility.
Traumatic brain injury	Elevated energy requirements up to 120% to 130% above predicted; however, consideration must be given to sedatives, neuromuscular blockage, and mechanical intubation, which significantly lower energy requirements
	Elevated protein requirements.
	Sedation/pain medications can decrease gut motility.
Extracorporeal membrane oxygenation (ECMO)	PN often administered through ECMO circuit.
	IV fat emulsion administered via peripheral venous access.
	Sedation/pain medications can decrease gut motility.
	Decreased energy requirements.

IV, intravenous; MCT, medium-chain triglyceride; RDA, recommended dietary allowance; REE, resting energy expenditure; PN, parenteral nutrition.

TABLE 2 Guide to Estimating Resting Energy Expenditure (REE) in Pediatric Patients

Age	1–3 yr	3–10 yr	10–18 yr
Male	60.9 kg − 54	22.7 kg + 495	17.5 kg + 651
Female	61 kg − 51	22.5 kg + 499	12.2 kg + 746

Adapted from World Health Organization (WHO) Technical Report Series 724:711, 1985: Energy and protein requirements.

TABLE 3 Application of Activity/Stress Adjustment Factors*

REE × 1.3	Well nourished at bed rest with mild to moderate stress
REE × 1.5	Normally active with mild to moderate stress, inactive with severe stress, minimal activity and malnutrition requiring catch-up growth
REE × 1.7	Active requiring catch-up growth or active with severe stress

*Multiply REE above × adjustment factor for estimated daily energy requirements.

Energy requirements are estimated using standard predictive equations such as the 1985 World Health Organization (WHO) equations (Table 2) to calculate resting energy expenditure (REE). REE is adjusted using activity and stress factors (Table 3), dependent on type of illness and current medical treatment and procedures, to estimate total energy expenditure. For obese patients (more than 120% ideal body weight) and patients with failure to thrive, the Schofield height and weight equation is often used as a more accurate predictor of energy requirements (Table 4). Attention should also be given to macronutrient distribution (Table 5). Much has been written about the estimation of energy requirements, and numerous studies demonstrate the inaccuracy of predictive equations. These REE equations were developed for healthy children and often lead to overestimation of energy requirements and the provision of inappropriate nutrition support. Recent research on pediatric intensive care patients suggests that energy needs are not as dependent on severity of illness as once thought but rather are related to the particular phase of illness and recovery. Because research shows these predictive equations can be relatively imprecise for critically ill children, however, indirect calorimetry should be used to measure REE more directly whenever possible.

ASSESSMENT OF PROTEIN REQUIREMENTS

For the critically ill child, protein requirements can increase up to 2.5 times the recommended dietary

TABLE 4 Predicting Resting Energy Expenditure (REE) in Children (0–18 yr): Schofield Height and Weight Equation (kcal/day)

	0–3 yr	3–10 yr	10–18 yr
Female	16.252W + 1023.2H −413.5	16.969W + 161.8H + 371.2	8.265W + 465H + 200
Male	0.167W + 1517.4H = 617.6	19.59W + 130.3H + 414.9	16.25W + 137.2H = 515.5

H, height in cm; W, weight in kg.
Adapted from Schofield WN: Predicting basal metabolic rate: New standards and review of previous work. Hum Nutr Clin Nutr 39(Suppl 1):5–41, 1985.

TABLE 5 Acceptable Macronutrient Distribution Ranges for Healthy Children

Macronutrient	Range (percentage energy) Children, 1–3 yr	Range (percentage energy) Children, 4–18 yr
Fat	30–40	25–35
N–6 polyunsaturated fatty acids (linoleic acid)	5–10	5–10
N–3 polyunsaturated fatty acids (linolenic acid)	0.6–1.2	0.6–1.2
Carbohydrate	45–65	45–65
Protein	5–20	10–30

Adapted from Institute of Medicine: Dietary Reference Intakes for energy, carbohydrates, fiber, fat, fatty acids, cholesterol, protein and amino acids. Part I. Washington, DC: National Academies Press, 2001.

TABLE 6 Protein Guidelines for Critically Ill Pediatric Patients

Age (yrs)	Protein (g/kg)
0–1	2–3.5
1–6	2–2.5
>6	1.5–2

Adapted from Eichelberger M: Pediatric Trauma, Prevention, Acute Care, and Rehabilitation. St. Louis: Mosby–Year Book, 1993.

TABLE 7 Fluid Requirements

100 cc/kg for the first 10 kg
1000 cc + 50 cc/kg for every kg over 10 kg (for a child 10–20 kg)
1500 cc + 20 cc/kg for every kg over 20 kg (for a child over 20 kg)

Adapted from Holliday MA, Seger WE: The maintenance need for water in parenteral fluid therapy. Pediatrics 19:825–832, 1957.

allowance (RDA). Trauma predisposes pediatric patients to a negative nitrogen balance that can peak in 2 to 3 days but gradually normalizes once the stress response has subsided. Table 6 lists the guidelines for protein requirements. The critically ill child is also at risk for further protein depletion secondary to drainage from chest tubes, drains, fistulas, and so on. In such instances, protein losses in drainage fluids can be measured and this amount of protein added to the child's calculated protein needs. It is also important to supply adequate calories from carbohydrate and fat to ensure proper use of protein.

ASSESSMENT OF FLUID REQUIREMENTS

It can be difficult to provide adequate nutrition to the critically ill child when fluids are significantly restricted. In such cases, concentrated enteral formulas with 1.2, 1.5, or 2 kcal/mL for children older than 1 year can be provided. Parenteral nutrition can also be concentrated, provided that adequate central venous access is available. Table 7 lists fluid requirements.

ENTERAL AND PARENTERAL NUTRITION

Enteral nutrition involves the delivery of nutrients directly to the gastrointestinal tract and can include nutrients ingested orally as well as those delivered to the stomach or intestine by a tube. Nutrient delivery to the intestine minimizes gut atrophy and decreases the risk of bacterial translocation. Early initiation of enteral nutrition within 48 to 72 hours of injury or surgery promotes the integrity of the gastrointestinal (GI) tract and reduces the risk of infectious complications. Additionally, enteral nutrition can reduce the risk of hepatic complications associated with total parenteral nutrition (TPN) and can reduce the risk of infectious complications sometimes seen with parenteral nutrition and prolonged venous access.

Enteral feedings are typically administered directly into the stomach through a nasogastric tube (NGT), when they are considered short term, or a gastrostomy tube, when feedings are expected for longer than 2 to 3 months. When gastroesophageal reflux or aspiration are a concern, feeding tubes can be passed into the jejunum or duodenum. Enteral nutrition can be delivered by a variety of methods, including continuous, bolus, or intermittent feeds. Feeding tolerance must always be monitored, and symptoms of intolerance can include

TABLE 8 Guidelines for Initiation and Advancement of Total Parenteral Nutrition in Children Older Than 1 Year*

	Children (1–10 yr)	Adolescents (11–18 yr)
Initial dose	Dextrose: up to 10%[†] Protein: as required Lipids: 1–1.5 g/kg	Dextrose: up to 10[†] Protein: as required Lipids: 0.5–1 g/kg
Daily dose advancement	Dextrose: 5% daily to goal as tolerated[‡] Protein: as required Lipids: 0.5–1 g/kg to goal of 1.5–3 g/kg per day maximum recommended	Dextrose: 5% daily to goal as tolerated[‡] Protein: as required Lipids: 0.5–1 g/kg to goal of 0.5–1 g/kg per day maximum recommended

*Evaluate for potential lipid allergies before initiation.
[†]Higher if already receiving D10 intravenous fluids.
[‡]D12.5 maximum concentration with peripheral access.

abdominal distention, emesis, or diarrhea. Signs of feeding intolerance can also be caused by medications (e.g., those medications delivered in a sorbitol-containing suspension) and infections such as *Clostridium difficile*; therefore, the most prudent approach is to investigate the cause before assuming the child is not tolerating the feedings. The use of a probiotic, such as Lactobacillus GG, can be beneficial in the treatment of diarrhea caused by bacterial overgrowth.

Formula selection for pediatric patients is determined by a number of factors, including age, GI function, fluid limitations, and osmolality, caloric density, and composition of the formula. Pediatric formulas are designed to meet the needs of children 1 to 10 years of age and include intact protein and elemental and semielemental formulas. These formulas usually contain 1.0 or 1.2 kcal/mL. Some formulas are available in a variety of flavors both with and without fiber, although flavoring significantly increases the osmolality of the formula. For children with a functioning GI tract and no malabsorption issues, a standard intact protein formula with long-chain fats and complex carbohydrates is indicated. For a patient with malabsorption or allergies, often a semielemental formula consisting of peptides or an elemental formula containing free amino acids is indicated. These formulas often contain some medium-chain triglycerides as a fat source. For children older than 10 years, an adult enteral formula may be used. As with the pediatric formulas, available adult formulas include standard intact protein, elemental and semielemental formulas, both with and without fiber. These formulas typically contain 1.0, 1.2, 1.5, or 2 kcal/mL.

Parenteral nutrition is indicated for patients who are unable to meet nutritional requirements solely by the enteral route. Because of the potential for complications, such as infection or electrolyte imbalance associated with parenteral nutrition, it should only be used when indicated.

Parenteral nutrition is composed of macronutrients (dextrose, amino acids, and lipid emulsions) and micronutrients (multivitamins and trace minerals), as well as electrolytes and additives, such as insulin or ranitidine, as needed. TPN is provided through a central venous catheter; peripheral parenteral nutrition (PPN) is provided through peripheral access. TPN is indicated when administration is anticipated for greater than 7

days; PPN is indicated for short-term use of 5 to 7 days. The dextrose concentration is limited in PPN to 10% to 12.5% to reduce the risk of thrombophlebitis. Parenteral nutrition should be administered as a continuous infusion over 24 hours until the patient is stable and demonstrates tolerance at goal calorie delivery. At this point, it is appropriate to begin to transition the parenteral nutrition over a period of 2 to 4 days to a 8- to 12-hour cycle. Table 8 shows the steps in initiating parenteral nutrition.

Glucose is provided in the form of dextrose, which yields 3.4 kcal/g and contributes most of the osmolality in the parenteral nutrition solution. Glucose should contribute 50% to 65% of total calories in parenteral nutrition and at a minimum provided to prevent hypoglycemia. The glucose infusion rate (GIR) should be generally maintained at less than 10 mg/kg/minute, although higher rates are sometimes necessary, especially for younger children. Providing insulin as a continuous infusion should be considered if significant glucose intolerance occurs that limits the provision of adequate calories.

Protein is provided in parenteral nutrition as crystalline amino acids and yields approximately 4 kcal/g and should contribute 10% to 15% of total calories in parenteral nutrition. Specialized amino acid solutions are available for children with renal and hepatic disease, but strong evidence is lacking to substantiate their advantage over a standard amino acid solution. Additionally, specialized amino acid solutions are also available for specific metabolic disorders, such as maple syrup urine disease (MSUD). Children who are well hydrated and demonstrate normal renal function can safely receive optimal protein intake when TPN is initiated. Gradually increasing the protein delivery over several days only postpones the delivery of adequate nutrition.

Intravenous fat emulsions are a concentrated source of calories and are provided in parenteral nutrition to prevent essential fatty acid deficiency. Fat emulsions contain soybean oil and/or safflower oil and are available as 10%, 20%, and 30% solutions (1.1, 2.0, or 3.0 kcal/mL, respectively), although the 20% solution is most commonly used. Ideally, intravenous fat should contribute less than 30% of total calories in parenteral nutrition, although in some instances up to 50% of calories may be necessary for the short term. For the pulmonary patient on mechanical ventilation, it may be prudent to provide a higher fat-to-carbohydrate ratio to limit CO_2 production, although some believe higher fat delivery may negatively affect pulmonary function. Longer infusion times (e.g., over a 24-hour period) may be considered to prevent or limit significant hypertriglyceridemia. Serum triglyceride (TG) levels should be measured to monitor the clearance of lipids. Ideally, TG levels should be measured 4 hours after starting or increasing an intravenous fat infusion. The American Gastroenterological Association recommends an upper limit of serum triglycerides of 400 mg/dL, although limited data support this specific recommendation.

Monitoring parenteral nutrition tolerance involves checking the laboratory values previously described as well as intake and output, weight, and respiratory function and monitoring the patient's venous access. A complication sometimes seen in pediatric patients receiving long-term parenteral nutrition is hepatic cholestasis. This may occur more frequently with prematurity, sepsis, overfeeding, and limited biliary stimulation from lack of enteral nutrition. When possible, the provision of trophic enteral feeds, cycling parenteral nutrition, and minimizing the delivery of protein may help decrease the risk of hepatic dysfunction.

Common Pitfalls

- Delayed nutrition secondary to frequent nothing-by-mouth status for tests and feeding intolerance
- Limited availability of weights and anthropometric measurements for accurate nutritional assessment
- Fluid limitations limiting nutrient delivery
- Altered metabolism (e.g., hyperglycemia, hypertriglyceridemia)
- Difficulty interpreting anthropometrics secondary to edema
- Difficulty interpreting laboratory values secondary to edema, stress response (which can decrease prealbumin), altered renal or hepatic function

Communication and Counseling

Nutrition support in the critically ill child requires strict attention to provision of appropriate macro- and micronutrients. Nutritional requirements in this population vary widely and depend on clinical factors as well as phase of injury. Children with critical illness are at risk for malnutrition, and a nutrition assessment should be completed to develop a nutritional plan that best meets their needs, with repeated evaluation to assess their response to nutritional therapy. When possible, indirect calorimetry should be used to determine energy requirements, although if calorimetry is not feasible, energy requirements should be based on phase of illness, and overfeeding should be avoided. Enteral nutrition is preferred over parenteral nutrition when possible. A multidisciplinary team, including dietitians, physicians, and nurses, should participate in the planning and implementation of a nutrition care plan for each child.

SUGGESTED READINGS

1. Bettler J, Roberts KE: Nutrition assessment of the critically ill child. AACN Clin Issues 11(4):498–506, 2000. **A review article describing how to complete a nutritional assessment of a critically ill child.**
2. Chwals WJ: Overfeeding the critically ill child: Fact or fantasy? Pediatr Crit Care Med 2(2):147–155, 1994. **A discussion of the potential consequences of overfeeding the critically ill child.**
3. Coss-Bu JA, Klish WJ, Walding D, et al: Energy metabolism, nitrogen balance, and substrate utilization in critically ill children. Am J Clin Nutr 74:664–669, 2001. **A description of the energy expenditure, nitrogen balance, and substrate utilization as assessed in ventilated critically ill children receiving parenteral nutrition.**
4. Fung EB: Estimating energy expenditure in critically ill adults and children. AACN Clin Issues 11(4):480–497, 2000. **A review article describing methods to assess the energy expenditure of critically ill adults and children.**
5. Horn D, Chaboyer W: Gastric feeding in critically ill children: A randomized controlled trial. Am J Crit Care 12(5):461–468, 2003. **A study comparing continuous and intermittent gastric feedings in critically ill children.**
6. Irving SY, Simone SD, Hicks FW, et al: Nutrition for the critically ill child: Enteral and parenteral support. AACN Clin Issues 11(4):541–558, 2000. **A review article describing and comparing enteral and parenteral nutritional support for the critically ill child.**
7. Kaplan AS, Zemel BS, Neiswender KM, et al: Resting energy expenditure in clinical pediatrics: Measured versus prediction equations. J Pediatr 127:200–205, 1995. **A study documenting the use of the Schofield height and weight equation to predict resting energy expenditure in critically ill children.**
8. Kirby DF, Delegge MH, Fleming CR: American Gastroenterological Association technical review on tube feeding for enteral nutrition. Gastroenterology 108(4):1282–1301, 1995. **A review of enteral nutrition and common clinical practice recommendations. Also includes a review of clinical use of enteral nutrition.**
9. Koretz RL, Lipman TO, Klein S: AGA technical review on parenteral nutrition. Gastroenterology 121:970–1001, 2001. **A review of randomized controlled trials evaluating the efficacy of parenteral nutrition on mortality, morbidity, duration of hospitalization, or cost. Also includes a review of clinical use of parenteral nutrition.**
10. Martin CM, Doig GS, Heyland DK, et al: Multicentre, cluster-randomized clinical trial of algorithms for critical-care enteral and parenteral therapy (ACCEPT). CMAJ 170(2):197–204, 2004. **A study demonstrating that the use of evidence-based patient care algorithms for nutrition support resulted in improved provision of nutrition support and improved patient outcomes in an adult intensive care unit.**
11. Martinez JLV, Martinez-Romillo PD, Sebastian JD, et al: Predicted versus measured energy expenditure by continuous, online indirect calorimetry in ventilated, critically ill children during the early postinjury period. Pediatr Crit Care Med 5(1):19–27, 1994. **A study of mechanically ventilated critically ill children in which energy expenditure is compared using predictive equations and measured indirect calorimetry during the early postinjury period.**
12. Mascarenhas MR, Zemel B, Stallings VA: Nutritional assessment in pediatrics. Nutrition 14(1):105–113, 1998. **A review article summarizing the parameters of a complete nutritional assessment of a pediatric patient.**
13. Maxvold NJ, Smoyer WE, Custer JR, et al: Amino acid loss and nitrogen balance in critically ill children with acute renal failure: A prospective comparison between classic hemofiltration and hemofiltration with dialysis. Crit Care Med 28(4):1161–1165, 2000. **Description and assessment of amino acid losses and nitrogen balance with hemofiltration in critically ill children.**
14. McCall M, Jeejeebhoy K, Pencharz P, et al: Effect of neuromuscular blockade on energy expenditure in patients with severe head injury. JPEN J Parenter Enteral Nutr 27(1):27–35, 2003. **An assessment of the associations among neuromuscular blockade, severe head injury, and energy expenditure.**

15. Rodriguez G, Moreno LA, Sarria A, et al: Resting energy expenditure in children and adolescents: Agreement between calorimetry and prediction equations. Clin Nutr 21(3):255–260, 2000. **A study assessing the accuracy of predictive equations in obese and nonobese children and adolescents.**

16. Rogers EJ, Gilbertson HR, Heine RG, Henning R: Barriers to adequate nutrition in critically ill children. Nutrition 19:865–868, 2003. **This study documents the inadequacy of caloric delivery to critically ill children and identifies barriers to the delivery of adequate nutrition.**

17. Shulman RJ, Phillips S: Parenteral nutrition in infants and children. J Pediatr Gastroenterol Nutr 36:587–607, 2003. **A review article discussing common misconceptions regarding parenteral nutrition as well as a discussion regarding components of parenteral nutrition.**

18. Taylor RM, Cheeseman P, Preedy V, et al: Can energy expenditure be predicted in critically ill children? Pediatr Crit Care Med 4(2):176–180, 2003. **A study evaluating the decreased metabolic rate in critically ill children and the accuracy of predicted equations in estimating their energy requirements.**

19. Taylor RM, Preedy VR, Baker AJ, et al: Nutritional support in critically ill children. Clin Nutr 22(4):365–369, 2003. **A retrospective survey of the adequacy of nutritional support provided to critically ill children, with specific emphasis on the differences between parenteral and enteral nutrition.**

20. Verger JT, Bradshaw DJ, Henry E, et al: The pragmatics of feeding the pediatric patient with acute respiratory distress syndrome. Crit Care Nurs Clin North Am 16(3):431–443, 2004. **An article highlighting the nutritional implications of acute respiratory distress syndrome (ARDS) with discussions on nutritional assessment and relevant considerations for enteral and parenteral nutrition for the pediatric patient with ARDS.**

21. Wells JCK, Mok Q, Johnson AW, et al: Energy requirements and body composition in stable pediatric intensive care patients receiving ventilatory support. Food Nutr Bull 23(3):95–98, 2002. **An assessment of the energy requirements and body composition of children receiving long-term ventilatory support.**

22. White MS, Shepherd RW, McEniery JA: Energy expenditure in 100 ventilated, critically ill children: Improving the accuracy of predictive equations. Crit Care Med 28(7):2307–2312, 2000. **An assessment of the accuracy of existing energy expenditure equations for critically ill ventilated children and a description of a more accurate, newly developed equation.**

23. Zaloga GP: Early enteral nutritional support improves outcome: Hypothesis or fact? Crit Care Med 27:259–261, 1999. **A review of early enteral nutrition on improving outcome in critically ill patients.**

24. Zaloga GP, Roberts P: Permissive underfeeding. New Horiz 2(2):257–263, 1994. **A discussion on the potential benefit of restricted nutrient intake for the critically ill patient.**

Vitamin Deficiencies and Excesses

Susan Konek and Maria R. Mascarenhas

KEY CONCEPTS

- Requirements for vitamins change and are based on life stage and gender groups. Variability in growth and development through childhood is factored into criteria for reference intakes.
- An evaluation of vitamin intake for an individual child requires consideration of dietary sources as well as supplements used.
- Complementary medicine in the form of vitamin supplements is increasing and extends to the pediatric population.
- Levels to determine vitamin adequacy/excesses should be used for at-risk populations as well as a guide to medication therapy.
- A careful diet history and evaluation of food consumed over time are useful in identifying an individual's risk for deficiency before blood levels drop or deficiency disease symptoms are evident.
- Fat-soluble vitamins are not excreted; rather they are stored in the body. This property can lead to overdose when supplementation exceeds the upper limit.
- Water-soluble vitamins must be consumed daily because there is limited storage in the body and amounts in excess of current metabolic needs are excreted in the urine. Only vitamin B_{12} is stored efficiently in the body.
- Deficiencies of water-soluble vitamins are rarely seen in healthy infants and children consuming adequate calories from a variety of foods.
- Water-soluble vitamins are excreted when levels exceed the body's requirements. For these vitamins, overdose and toxic levels are less likely.
- Concentration of water-soluble vitamins (except folate) in human milk is quite strongly related to the mother's dietary intake of these vitamins and, to a lesser extent, her vitamin status. For this reason, in populations at high risk for maternal depletion, complementary foods, used in the second half of the first year, are recommended to provide adequate amounts of B vitamins.

Vitamins, dietary factors obtained from organic sources, are essential to life. Determining the optimal or adequate level of vitamin intake for infants, children, and adolescents is difficult because data on age-based requirements are not available and the levels that produce toxic effects vary considerably. The recent development of the dietary reference intakes (DRIs) expands and replaces the series of recommended dietary allowances (RDAs) in the United States as well as the recommended nutrient intakes (RNIs) in Canada as the guide for planning the nutrition of groups and individuals. The DRIs provide evidence-based recommendations for all vitamins as well as upper limits for their use. Table 1 lists the recommendations for vitamins for infants and children, as well as tolerable upper levels.

The references include RDAs—the dietary intake level that meets the nutrient requirement of nearly all healthy individuals (97% to 98%) based on life stage and gender. Adequate intakes (AIs)—the recommended intake value based on observed or experimentally determined approximation of intake by a group of healthy people—are assumed sufficient. The AI is used when the RDA cannot be determined. RDAs for children older than infants are based on extrapolation from recommendations based on adult evidence. Tolerable upper level (UL) of intake is the highest level of nutrient intake that is likely to pose no risk of adverse health effects for almost all individuals in the general population. These values have particular use when considering dosage for fat-soluble vitamins. Estimated average requirements (EARs) are the nutrient intake value estimated to meet the requirements of half the apparently healthy individuals in a life stage and

TABLE 1 *Dietary Reference Intakes: Recommended Intakes for Individuals and Tolerable Upper Levels of Intake

Life Stage Group	Vitamin A (μg/day)	Vitamin C (mg/day)	Vitamin D (μg/day)	Vitamin E (mg/day)	Vitamin K (μg/day)	Thiamine (mg/day)	Riboflavin (mg/day)	Niacin (mg/day)	Vitamin B6 (mg/day)	Folate (μg/day)	Vitamin B12 (μg/day)	Pantothenic Acid (mg/day)
Infants												
0–6 mo	400 (600)	40 (ND)	5 (25)	4 (ND)	2.0 (ND)	0.2 (ND)	0.3 (ND)	2 (ND)	0.1 (ND)	65 (ND)	0.4 (ND)	1.7 (ND)
7–12 mo	500 (600)	50 (ND)	5 (25)	5 (ND)	2.5 (ND)	0.3 (ND)	0.4 (ND)	4 (ND)	0.3 (ND)	80 (ND)	0.5 (ND)	1.8 (ND)
Children												
1–3 yr	**300** (600)	**15** (400)	5 (50)	**6** (200)	30 (ND)	**0.5** (ND)	**0.5** (ND)	**6** (10)	**0.5** (30)	**150** (300)	**0.9** (ND)	2 (ND)
4–8 yr	**400** (900)	**25** (650)	5 (50)	**7** (300)	55 (ND)	**0.6** (ND)	**0.6** (ND)	**8** (15)	**0.6** (40)	**200** (400)	**1.2** (ND)	3 (ND)
Boys												
9–13 yr	**600** (1700)	**45** (1200)	5 (50)	**11** (600)	60 (ND)	**0.9** (ND)	**0.9** (ND)	**12** (20)	**1.0** (60)	**300** (600)	**1.8** (ND)	4 (ND)
14–18 yr	**900** (2800)	**75** (1800)	5 (50)	**15** (800)	75 (ND)	**1.2** (ND)	**1.3** (ND)	**16** (30)	**1.3** (80)	**400** (800)	**2.4** (ND)	5 (ND)
Girls												
9–13 yr	**600** (1700)	**45** (1200)	5 (50)	**11** (600)	60 (ND)	**0.9** (ND)	**0.9** (ND)	**12** (20)	**1.0** (60)	**300** (600)	**1.8** (ND)	4 (ND)
14–18 yr	**700** (2800)	**65** (1800)	5 (50)	**15** (800)	75 (ND)	**1.0** (ND)	**1.0** (ND)	**14** (30)	**1.2** (80)	**400** (800)	**2.4** (ND)	5 (ND)

*This table (adapted from the DRI reports; see www.nap.edu) presents recommended dietary allowances (RDAs) in bold type and adequate intakes (AIs) in regular type. Tolerable upper levels (ULs) of intake appear in parentheses after each DRI value. ND, not determinable because of lack of data of adverse effects in this age group and concern with regard to lack of ability to handle excess amounts. Source of intake should be from food only to prevent high levels of intake.

Adapted from the Food and Nutrition Board, Institute of Medicine publications showing dietary reference intakes for these nutrients. See Suggested Readings for specific references.

gender group. To use the DRIs to evaluate individual children, the average of several typical days of food intake should be reviewed and compared to the reference intakes for adequacy. This provides an estimate of the risk of nutrient deficiencies.

Vitamin deficiencies occur in these situations:

- Intakes are inadequate.
- Physiologic requirements are high.
- Losses are excessive.
- Nutrient-nutrient or drug-nutrient imbalances reduce efficacy.

Although vitamin-deficiency diseases are rare today in developed countries, health care professionals must be aware of the individual patient's risk and be able to recognize the symptoms of a specific vitamin deficiency. This is especially true for patients with absorptive defects, limited food choices, and illnesses that necessitate the use of medications that affect nutrients. Table 2 reviews the diagnosis of vitamin deficiencies as well as food sources for vitamins.

Excessive vitamin intakes that may produce toxic effects must also be recognized, especially because some vitamins are used for therapeutic purposes, not just to maintain health. In such instances, the vitamins are considered drugs because the dosages are in the pharmacologic range. Table 3 outlines the treatment of vitamin deficiencies.

Expert Opinion on Management Issues

FAT-SOLUBLE VITAMINS

The fat-soluble vitamins are vitamin A (retinol, retinal, retinoic acid), vitamin D (cholecalciferol, ergosterol), vitamin E (primarily α-tocopherol), and vitamin K (menaquinone, phytonadione). Absorption and transport of these vitamins are associated with lipid absorption and transport. The presence of bile salts is required for adequate absorption. The fat-soluble vitamins are not excreted but stored in the body in varying amounts. This storage allows for accumulation of these vitamins and eliminates the need for daily ingestion. It also creates the potential for toxicity when increased amounts are ingested over time. Because these vitamins are readily available in the diets of children, hazards of vitamin A and D toxicity from routine prophylaxis use in well-fed healthy infants and children may be greater than that of deficiency.

Vitamin A

The term *vitamin A* refers to retinol and its derivatives, the primary compounds of which are retinol, retinal (retinaldehyde), retinoic acid, and retinyl esters. The functions of vitamin A are maintenance of vision, epithelial integrity and regulation of glycoprotein synthesis, and cell differentiation. Vitamin A occurs in the diet as retinyl esters from animal sources (liver and fish, liver oils, dairy products, kidney, and eggs) and provitamin A

carotenoids (mainly β-carotene) distributed widely in green and yellow vegetables.

Vitamin A deficiency symptoms in children are growth failure, skeletal abnormalities, poor visual adaptation to darkness (night blindness), conjunctival and corneal xerosis and ulceration (xerophthalmia), hyperkeratosis, increased susceptibility to infections, and keratinization of epithelial cells of the respiratory tract and other organs. A deficiency can result from fat malabsorption with gastrointestinal and liver diseases or from inadequate intake. Vitamin A activity is expressed as retinol activity equivalents (RAEs; 1 µg of all-*trans*-retinol = 1 RAE = 3.3 IU vitamin A activity; 1 µg of all-*trans*-retinol = 12 µg of all-*trans*-β-carotene = 24 µg of other provitamin A carotenoids). Large amounts of β-carotene are needed to achieve vitamin A requirements, compared to preformed vitamin A. The AI for infants is 400 µg RAE for 0 to 6 months of age and 500 µg of RAE for 7 to 12 months of age. These requirements are readily met because human milk, cow's milk, and infant formulas are excellent sources of vitamin A. The ULs are set for vitamin A for all life stages, beginning with 600 µg per day for infants.

Ingestion of high doses of vitamin A may result in toxicity. Signs usually appear after long-term daily intakes exceeding 20,000 IU. Vitamin A–related toxicity signs include headache, bone abnormalities, alopecia, vomiting, dryness of the mucous membranes, and liver damage. Large doses of vitamin A are used to treat acne and to prevent infection. Serious toxic effects are seen in children with as little as 6000 µg RAE per day. Recently published studies suggest a correlation between ingestion of large amounts of preformed vitamin A and fractures caused by stimulation of bone resorption and inhibition of bone formation. The carotenoids (vitamin A precursors) do not produce toxic effects, even at high doses, although they are absorbed into the subcutaneous fat, in continued large doses, causing yellow discoloration of the skin. This discoloration disappears when large doses are withheld. Consumption of excess vitamin A (including derivatives such as retinoic acid) is teratogenic. Teenagers who may become pregnant should be informed of the dangers of vitamin A use in the treatment of acne. Strict vegetarians (vegans) are challenged to meet vitamin A requirements. Preformed vitamin A is found only in animal-derived foods. Although carotenoids are found in green leafy vegetables and many fruits, it takes 12 µg of dietary β-carotene to provide 1 RAE. Therefore, a large amount of fruit and vegetables is needed to achieve the vitamin A requirement.

Vitamin D

Vitamin D functions in the body to maintain serum calcium and phosphorus levels within the normal range by increasing the small intestine's absorption of these minerals from the diet. Vitamin D comes in many forms; the two most physiologically active are vitamin D_2 (ergocalciferol) and vitamin D_3 (cholecalciferol). Vitamin D is obtained from endogenous synthesis of cholecalciferol (D_3) in the skin by action of ultraviolet light on 7-dehydrocholesterol and from the diet (in the form of

TABLE 2 Diagnosis of Vitamin Deficiencies

Vitamin	Diagnostic Test	Predisposing Condition	Clinical Features	Food Sources
Vitamin A	Serum retinol levels	Prematurity Total parenteral nutrition Malnutrition Fat malabsorption Liver disease	Night blindness Xerophthalmia Xerosis Blindness Follicular hyperkeratosis Pruritus Growth retardation Skeletal abnormalities Anemia	Liver, fish, dairy products, kidney, eggs, and green and yellow vegetables from provitamin A carotenoids
Vitamin D	Serum 25-hydroxy vitamin D levels	No exposure to sun Children consuming milk not fortified with vitamin D Fat malabsorption Hepatic and renal disease Inborn errors of metabolism	Rickets Osteomalacia Craniotabes Rachitic rosary Pigeon breast Bowed legs Delayed eruption of teeth Bone pain Fractures Anorexia Weakness	Vitamin D–fortified dairy products (present as cholecalciferol from animal sources and ergocalciferol, or vitamin D_2, from plants and fungi)
Vitamin E	Serum vitamin E levels	Prematurity Liver disease Pancreatic insufficiency Short bowel syndrome Abetalipoproteinemia	Hemolytic anemia Progressive neurologic disorder Ophthalmoplegia and retinal dysfunction	Vegetable oil, cereal, grains, sardines, butter, liver, and egg yolk
Vitamin K	Prothrombin time, plasma PIVKA II levels	Newborns who do not receive vitamin K Drugs (nonabsorbable), antibiotics, and anticoagulants Fat malabsorption	Hemorrhage Easy bruisability Mucosal bleeding	Leafy vegetables, soybean oil, fruits, seeds, pork, and liver
Thiamin (B_1)	Whole blood thiamine/erythrocyte transketolase levels	Breast-fed infants of malnourished or alcoholic mothers Total parenteral nutrition Malnutrition Prematurity	Anorexia Irritability Vomiting Constipation Cardiac symptoms Peripheral paralysis Neuropathy Edema	Whole-grain products and refined-grain products fortified with thiamin
Riboflavin (B_2)	Serum riboflavin RBC glutathione reductase levels	Malnutrition Prematurity Total parenteral nutrition	Cheilosis Angular stomatitis Glossitis Dermatitis Photophobia	Milk, milk drinks, bread products, and fortified cereals
Pyridoxine (B_6)	Plasma PLP or pyridoxal 5'-phosphate levels	Drugs: isoniazid (INH), L-dopa, oral contraceptive pill Prematurity Vitamin B_6 dependency syndromes Alcoholism	Seborrheic dermatitis Microcytic anemia seizures Depression Confusion	Fortified ready-to-eat cereals, meat, fish, poultry, white potatoes, starchy vegetables, noncitrus fruits, beef liver, organ meats, soy-based meat substitutes
Niacin	Urinary excretion of N1-methyl-2-pyridone-5-carboxamide and N1-methyl-nicotinamide	Prematurity High-maize diets	Dermatitis Vomiting Constipation Diarrhea Glossitis Depression Apathy Headache Fatigue Loss of memory	Meat, fish, poultry, enriched whole-grain breads and bread products, fortified ready-to-eat cereals, liver
Biotin	Urinary biotin and 3-hydroxy-isovaleric acid excretion	Biotinidase deficiency, anticonvulsants, pregnancy, ingestion of large quantities of raw egg white	Dermatitis Conjunctivitis Alopecia Central nervous system abnormalities	Liver

TABLE 2—cont'd

Vitamin	Diagnostic Test	Predisposing Condition	Clinical Features	Food Sources
Folate (folic acid and folacin)	Serum or erythrocyte folate levels	Prematurity Breast-fed infants of folate-deficient mothers Kwashiorkor Chronic hemolytic anemia Diarrhea Malignancies Hypermetabolic states Malabsorption Drug (sulfasalazine) Infants consuming goat's milk	Megaloblastic anemia Glossitis Diarrhea Growth failure Thrombocytopenia Neutropenia	Folate-fortified cereal, grains, vegetables such as green beans and peas
Cyanocobalamin (vitamin B_{12})	Serum vitamin B_{12} levels, plus plasma methylmalonic acid (MMA) levels	Breast-fed infants of vegetarian mothers or mothers with latent pernicious anemia Terminal ileal disease Malabsorption	Megaloblastic anemia Memory loss Paresthesias Confusion	Animal products such as red meat, poultry, fish, eggs, and dairy, as well as cereals fortified with vitamin B_{12}
Vitamin C	Plasma vitamin C levels	Breast-fed infants of vitamin C–deficient mothers or mothers who smoke	Scurvy Dyspnea Edema Weakness Fatigue Depression Anemia Impaired bone growth	Fruits and vegetables, especially citrus fruits, tomatoes, tomato juice, potatoes, broccoli, kiwi, yams, strawberries, melons

PIVKA, prothrombin induced by vitamin K absence or antagonist-II; RBC, red blood cell.

cholecalciferol from animal sources and ergocalciferol [D_2] from plants and fungi).

The vitamin D deficiency disease in infants and children is rickets, characterized by poor bone mineralization, resulting in skeletal deformities. Rickets, thought to be rare in the United States, is seeing a resurgence (at least in the literature), in part because of the protection of infants and children from ultraviolet light by the use of sunscreens. To obtain adequate sunlight exposure to form vitamin D in the skin, white infants require an estimated unprotected 30 minutes per week clothed in a diaper or 2 hours per week fully clothed with face and head exposed. Rickets is an example of extreme vitamin D deficiency with a deficient state present months prior to overt symptoms. Symptoms may include hypocalcemia, hypophosphatemia, tetany, osteomalacia, and rickets. Infants who are breast-fed without supplementation are at risk for developing rickets, in particular African American infants with limited exposure to the sun. For this reason, the American Academy of Pediatrics (AAP) recommends that exclusively breast-fed infants receive vitamin D supplementation of 200 IU per day. Other children at risk for deficiency include those with chronic fat malabsorption and those with nephritic syndrome.

Clinical features of rickets include craniotabes (in children younger than 1 year of age), a persistently open fontanelle in children older than 18 months of age, and bone abnormalities in the chest, such as rachitic rosary, frontal bossing, and bowed legs. Characteristic long bone radiographic changes are seen in the epiphyseal areas of rapidly growing bones with flaring and cupping of the epiphysis, ground-glass appearance of the shaft, and generalized demineralization of all bones. The diagnosis of vitamin D deficiency may be confirmed from a low serum 25-hydroxy vitamin D level.

Medications that may interfere with the use of vitamin D should be considered when estimating a patient's requirement. Glucocorticoids and seizure medications, including phenobarbital and phenytoin (Dilantin), interfere with vitamin D function. Included in are treatment doses for vitamin D deficiency. Length of therapy for this deficiency is usually up to 4 months or until the elevated serum alkaline phosphatase associated with vitamin D deficiency normalizes. Adequate calcium intake must be ensured to prevent hypocalcemia, which may occur when newly available vitamin D drives serum calcium into the bone. After successful treatment of rickets, adequate dietary intake of calcium and vitamin D should be maintained.

Toxicity from ingestion of excessive amounts is more common with vitamin D than with any other vitamin. Clinical features of toxicity include vomiting, hypertension, anorexia, renal failure, and failure to thrive. Hypercalcemia and hypercalciuria may lead to deposition of calcium in various soft tissues, with renal and cardiovascular damage often irreversible. For these reasons, the ULs have been set.

Vitamin E

Vitamin E is believed to function primarily as a chain-breaking antioxidant that prevents propagation of lipid peroxidation. Through this function, it protects cell membranes and thiol-rich protein and nucleic acids from oxidant damage of free-radical reactions. Vitamin E is required for maintenance of structure and function of the human nervous system, retina, and skeletal muscles. Overt deficiency is rare and seen most often in individuals unable to absorb fat (patients with cystic fibrosis, biliary atresia, other liver diseases, and lipid transport

TABLE 3 Treatment of Vitamin Deficiencies

	Clinical Features	Suggested Doses
Vitamin A	Severe deficiency with xerophthalmia	Infants: 7500–15,000 U/day IM, followed by oral 5000–10,000 U/day for 10 days. Children 1–8 yr of age: oral 5,000–10,000 U/kg/day for 5 days or until recovery. Children >8 yr of age and adults: oral 500,000 U/day for 3 days; then 50,000 U/day for 14 days; then 10,000–20,000 U/day for 2 mo.
	Deficiency without corneal changes	Infants <1 yr of age: 100,000 U/day orally, q4-6mo. Children 1-8 yr of age: 200,000 U/day orally, q4-6mo. Children >8 yr and adults: 100,000 U/day for 3 days, followed by 50,000 U/day for 10 days.
	Deficiency	IM given only to those patients with malabsorption in whom oral dosing is not possible. Infants: 7,500–15,000 U/day for 10 days. Children 1–8 yr of age: 17,500–35,000 U/day for 10 days. Children >8 yr of age and adults: 100,000 U/day for 3 days, then 50,000 U/day for 14 days. Give follow-up oral multivitamin which contains vitamin A: LBW infants: no dose established, children ≤8 years of age: 5,000–10,000 U/day, children >8 yr of age and adults: 10,000–20,000 U daily.
	Malabsorption syndrome (prophylaxis)	Children >8 yr of age and adults: oral 10,000–50,000 U/day of water-miscible product.
	Cystic fibrosis	1,500–10,000 U/day prophylaxis (CF Foundation).
	Measles	WHO recommendations: single dose, repeating the dose next day and at 4 wk for children with eye findings: 6 mo to 1 yr of age: 100,000 U; >1 yr of age: 200,000 U.
Vitamin D	Liver disease	4,000–8,000 U/day ergocalciferol.
	Malabsorption	1000 U/day ergocalciferol
	Nutritional rickets and osteomalacia	Ergocalciferol: Children and adults with normal absorption: 1,000–5,000 U/day. Children with malabsorption: 10,000–25,000 U/day. Adults with malabsorption: 10,000–300,000 U/day.
	Renal disease and failure	Ergocalciferol: child: 4,000–40,000 U/day; adults: 20,000 U/day.
	Cystic fibrosis	Ergocalciferol: 400–800 U/day PO (CF Foundation).
	Hypoparathyroidism	Children: 50,000–200,000 U/day ergocalciferol and calcium supplements. Adults: 25,000–200,000 U/day ergocalciferol and calcium supplements.
	Vitamin D–dependent rickets	Children: 3000–5000 U/day ergocalciferol; max: 60,000 U/day. Adults: 10,000–60,000 U/day ergocalciferol.
	Vitamin D–resistant rickets	Children: initial 40,000–80,000 U/day with phosphate supplements, daily dosage is increased at 3- to 4-mo intervals in 10,000–20,000 U increments. Adults: 10,000–60,000 U/day with phosphate supplements.
Vitamin E	Premature infant, neonates, infants of low birth weight	D-α-tocopherol: 25–50 U/day for 1 wk orally.
	Fat malabsorption and liver disease	10–25 U/kg/day of water-miscible vitamin E preparation.
	Cystic fibrosis	<1 yr of age: 25–50 U/day; 1–2 years of age: 100 U/day; >2 yr of age: 100 U/day bid or 200 U daily orally (CF Foundation).
	Sickle cell disease	450 U/day orally.
	β-Thalassemia	750 U/day orally.
Vitamin K	Hemorrhagic disease of the newborn	Phytonadione: 0.5–1.0 mg SC or IM as prophylaxis within 1 hr of birth, may repeat 6–8 hours later; 1–2 mg/day as treatment.
	Deficiency	Infants and children: 2.5–5 mg/day orally, or 1–2 mg/dose SC, IM, IV as a single dose; adults: 5–25 mg/day or 10 mg IM, IV.
	Cystic fibrosis	2.5 mg, twice a week (CF Foundation).
Folate, folic acid, and folacin	Deficiency	Infants: 50 μg daily. Children 1–10 yr of age: 1 mg/day initially, then 0.1–0.4 mg/day as maintenance. Children >11 yr of age and adults: 1 mg/day initially, then 0.5 mg/day as maintenance.
	Hemolytic anemia	May require higher doses than those listed previously.
Niacin	Pellagra	Children: 50–100 mg tid. Adults: 50–100 mg/day, max 100 mg/day.
Pyridoxine (B$_6$)	Seizures	Neonates and infants: initial 50–100 mg/day orally, IM, IV, SC.
	Drug-induced deficiencies	Children: 10–50 mg/day as treatment, 1–2 mg/kg/day as prophylaxis. Adults: 100–200 mg/day as treatment, 25–100 mg/day as prophylaxis.
	Dietary deficiency	Children: 5–25 mg/day for 3 wk, then 1.5–2.5 mg/day in a multivitamin product. Adults: 10–20 mg/day for 3 wk.
Riboflavin (B$_2$)		Children: 2.5–10 mg/day in divided doses. Adults: 5–30 mg/day in divided doses.
Thiamine (B$_1$)	Beriberi: critically ill	Children: 10–25 mg/day IM or IV. Adults: 5–30 mg/dose IM, IV tid, then 5–30 mg/day orally in a single or three divided doses for 1 mo.
	Beriberi: not critically ill	Children: 10–50 mg/day orally for 2 wk, then 5–10 mg/day for 1 mo.
	Metabolic disease	Adults: 10–20 mg/day orally.
	Wernicke encephalopathy	Adults: initially 100 mg IV, then 50–100 mg/day IM/IV until eating a balanced diet.

TABLE 3—cont'd

	Clinical Features	Suggested Doses
Cyanocobalamin (B$_{12}$)	Nutritional deficiency	Intranasal gel: 500 µg once a wk. Orally: 25–250 µg/wk.
	Anemia	Give IM or deep SC; oral route not recommended because of poor absorption and IV route not recommended because of more rapid elimination.
	Pernicious anemia	If evidence of neurologic involvement in neonates and infants (congenital), 1000 µg/day IM, SC, for at least 2 wk, and then maintenance, 50–100 µg/mo or 100 µg/day for 6–7 days. If clinical improvement, give 100 µg every other day for 7 doses, then every 3–4 days for 2–3 wk, followed by 100 µg/mo for life. Administer with folic acid if needed (1 mg/day for 1 mo concomitantly). Children: 30–50 µg/day for 2 or more wk (total dose of 1000 µg) IM, SC, then 100 µg/mo as maintenance. Adults: 100 µg/day for 6–7 days; if improvement, administer same dose on alternate days for 7 doses, then every 3–4 days for 2–3 wk. Once hematological values are normal, give maintenance doses of 100 µg/mo parenterally.
	Hematologic remission	No evidence of neurologic involvement: use intranasal gel: 500 µg per wk.
	Vitamin B$_{12}$ deficiency	Children with neurologic signs: 100 µg/day for 10–15 days (total dose of 1–1.5 mg), then 1–2/wk for several mo and taper to 60 µg/mo. Children with hematological signs: 10–50 µg/day for 5–10 days, followed by 100–250 µg/day every 2–4 wk. Adults: 30 µg/day for 5–10 days, followed by maintenance doses of 100–200 µg/mo.
Ascorbic acid	Scurvy	Children: 100–300 mg/day in divided doses orally, IM, IV, or SC for several days. Adults: 100–250 mg/day one to two times/day.

bid, two times per day; CF, cystic fibrosis; IM, intramuscular; IV, intravenous; LBW, low birth weight; q, every; SC, subcutaneous; tid, three times per day; WHO, World Health Organization.

Data from Lexi-Comp Inc., Hudson, Ohio, 2004. Available at http://online.lexi.com/crlsql/servlet/crlonline

abnormalities). Vitamin E absorption from the intestinal lumen depends on biliary and pancreatic secretions, micelle formation, uptake into enterocytes, and chylomicron secretion. Defects in any step lead to impaired absorption.

Vitamin E deficiency is seen most often in premature infants and those with very low birth weight (VLBW). Vitamin E occurs in vegetable oil and cereal grains as well as sardines, butter, liver, and egg yolk. Current dietary patterns appear adequate to prevent deficiency symptoms such as peripheral neuropathy. Deficiency states result in neurologic defects and hemolytic anemia. Anemia is related to the relationship of vitamin E and dietary polyunsaturated fatty acids (PUFAs). As intake of PUFAs increases, the requirement for vitamin E increases or peroxidation of lipids occurs. Most of the dietary oils that supply PUFAs are also good sources of vitamin E. Toxic effects from excessive oral intake of vitamin E are not substantiated. Pharmacologic doses given in treatment regimens over long periods do not result in serious side effects, although the symptoms of nausea, headache, and fatigue are reported. Because no known childhood health benefits are associated with vitamin E supplementation, it is not recommended for well-nourished children. Vitamin E toxicities should be avoided because risks include impaired resistance to infections from decreased leukocyte function and increased bleeding in individuals deficient in vitamin K.

The DRI for vitamin E is based on α-tocopherol only because this form is preferentially secreted by the liver into plasma. The AI for infants 0 to 6 months of age is determined by the average content (4.9 mg/L) of α-tocopherol in 780 mL per day of human milk (mean volume for this age). The AI for 7 to 12 months of age is set at 5 mg per day. The ULs are set, varying from not determinable (ND) in infants to 1000 mg per day in adolescents.

Vitamin K

Vitamin K is sometimes defined as the antihemorrhagic vitamin because it is necessary for the synthesis of factors required for blood coagulation. Also important is the role of vitamin K in synthesis of a group of proteins involved in calcium homeostasis. These proteins are critical in bone mineralization, both early skeletal development and later maintenance. Infants are at risk for vitamin K deficiency because milk-based products are a poor source. The newborn infant is usually given vitamin K soon after birth prophylactically to protect against hemorrhagic disease of the newborn, now known as vitamin K deficiency bleeding (VKDB). Vitamin K should be given as a single intramuscular dose of 0.5 to 1 mg. In response to concerns raised in a study in England that large-dose vitamin K injections may be related to increased incidence of leukemia, oral vitamin K dosing is now used in some European countries. The AAP at present accepts intramuscular (IM) vitamin K prophylaxis as safe. Because vitamin K content depends on the mother's vitamin K status, exclusively breast-fed infants and infants delivered at home require special attention. Vitamin K is present in most cow's milk formulas. It is stored primarily in the liver. A regular supply of vitamin K is needed because it is not stored in significant quantities. Other infants and children at risk for vitamin K deficiency are those who malabsorb fat and those treated with anticoagulant drugs, including aspirin, or long-course broad-spectrum antibiotics (which destroy the normal gut flora that make vitamin K).

Humans use several forms of vitamin K. Phylloquinone (vitamin K_1) is obtained from leafy vegetables, soybean oil, fruits, seeds, pork, and liver. Menaquinone (vitamin K_2) is synthesized in the gut by intestinal bacteria. Menadione (vitamin K_3) is synthesized chemically and has better water solubility than the two natural forms. The absorption of vitamin K depends on its incorporation into mixed micelles in the intestinal lumen, thus requiring the presence of bile acids and pancreatic enzymes. The AI for infants is 2 μg per day of phylloquinone or menaquinone for the first 6 months of life and 2.5 μg per day for the second 6 months. No ULs are established for vitamin K intake. Excessive amounts of the natural forms of vitamin K do not cause toxic effects, but the synthetic form (menadione), when ingested in large amounts, produces toxic effects in neonates and patients with glucose–6-phosphatase deficiency. These effects are manifested as hemolytic anemia and hyperbilirubinemia.

WATER-SOLUBLE VITAMINS

The water-soluble vitamins include the B vitamins (thiamine, riboflavin, niacin, pyridoxine, cyanocobalamin, folate, biotin, and pantothenic acid) and vitamin C. The B complex vitamins generally function as coenzymes in metabolic processes. Vitamin C functions as an antioxidant as well as a cofactor in enzymatic processes.

Thiamine

Thiamine is a coenzyme in the metabolism of carbohydrates and branched chain amino acids. Requirements are directly related to total calorie intake and the proportion of calories as carbohydrate. A deficiency of thiamine results in beriberi, a well-described disease characterized by mental confusion, muscle weakness, anorexia, peripheral paralysis, muscle wasting, tachycardia, and cardiomegaly. The occurrence of beriberi in the United States is extremely rare because thiamine is abundant in whole-grain products and refined grain products are fortified with thiamin. Wernicke-Korsakoff syndrome, a type of beriberi related most frequently to alcoholism, is reported in children in some high-risk groups, notably cancer patients and those with gastrointestinal (GI) disease. This syndrome manifests with a clinical triad of ocular abnormalities, mental status changes, and ataxia. Adequate supplementation of these patient groups is recommended to prevent thiamine deficiency. Infantile beriberi occurs in babies breast-fed by mothers with a history of alcoholism or poor dietary intake. Symptoms include cardiac failure, aphonia, anorexia, vomiting, and irritability. The aphonia is related to recurrent laryngeal nerve paralysis or vocal cord edema. Older infants may have a pseudomeningitic type of infantile beriberi with seizures, fever, and ocular findings. Patients with congenital heart disease, before and after corrective surgery, are at risk for thiamine deficiency. No reports are available of adverse effects from consumption of excess thiamine in food and supplements. No UL is set. There

are reports of sensitivity or toxicity related to large amounts in parenteral solutions, however. Pharmacologic doses of thiamine are used in the treatment of some inborn errors of metabolism (e.g., maple syrup urine disease and thiamine-responsive lactic acidosis).

Riboflavin

Riboflavin functions as a coenzyme in numerous redox reactions and energy production. This is accomplished as a component of the coenzymes flavin mononucleotide (FMN) and flavin adenine dinucleotide (FAD). No specific deficiency disease is attributed to a lack of riboflavin, although symptoms are sometimes referred to as *ariboflavinosis*. Clinical symptoms of deficiency include angular stomatitis, cheilosis, glossitis, sore throat, seborrheic dermatitis, scrotal skin changes, and normochromic anemia or normocytic anemia. Riboflavin deficiency is most often seen with other nutrient deficiencies. Because riboflavin is used in the metabolism of niacin and pyridoxine, some deficiency symptoms may result from failure of metabolic processes that require these nutrients. Cancer, cardiac diseases, and diabetes may precipitate or compound riboflavin deficiency. Pediatric patients with intensive chemotherapy are found deficient. Food sources for riboflavin are numerous because most plant and animal tissues contain at least small amounts of riboflavin, with the largest amounts found in milk, milk drinks, bread products, and fortified cereals. Riboflavin loss occurs if it is exposed to light. Although neonates receiving high doses may develop hemolysis, no adverse effects associated with riboflavin consumption from food or regular dose supplements are reported. An upper limit cannot be derived.

Niacin

Niacin functions in many biologic redox reactions via coenzymes nicotinamide adenine dinucleotide (NAD) and nicotinamide adenine dinucleotide phosphate (NADP). The requirement for niacin (nicotinic acid and nicotinamide) is complicated because much of the need for niacin is provided by the conversion of the amino acid tryptophan to niacin. Pellagra, the niacin-deficiency disease, is characterized by diarrhea, dermatitis, dementia, glossitis, and death. It was seen in Europe and in the United States in the early 20th century, in areas where corn and maize were the main dietary staple. These two grains are low in niacin and tryptophan. Currently, it is seen in alcoholics, in individuals with disorders involving tryptophan metabolism, in patients with anorexia, and in underdeveloped countries. Large doses of nicotinic acid (more than 3 g per day) may cause flushing or vasodilation, hepatitis, jaundice, glucose intolerance, and ocular effects. The adverse effects on excess niacin intake are more prominent in individuals with liver disease, gout, peptic ulcer disease, cardiac arrhythmias, migraines, alcoholism, and inflammatory bowel disease. Pharmacologic doses of niacin are used in treating hypercholesterolemia. The UL is based on the dose at which flushing results in the patient choosing to reduce niacin intake.

Pyridoxine (Vitamin B₆)

Pyridoxine acts as a coenzyme for many enzymes involved in amino acid metabolism. Deficiency of pyridoxine rarely occurs in isolation. It tends to occur instead in conjunction with deficiencies of other B complex vitamins. In addition, the need for vitamin B_6 is closely related to the amount of dietary protein ingested: As protein intake increases, the deficiency symptoms of pyridoxine are exacerbated. Symptoms of deficiency in infants and children include seizures, abdominal distress, anemia, dermatitis, and hyperirritability. No toxicity from excessive intake in infants and children is documented; however, some adults treated with pharmacologic doses show symptoms of skin lesions and sensory neuropathy. Pyridoxine is used in large therapeutic doses to treat a variety of general symptoms (depression, carpal tunnel syndrome, premenstrual syndrome, morning sickness, and impaired glucose tolerance) without consistent documented efficacy. No benefit from pyridoxine supplements in the well-nourished child is documented. The UL is based on the dose at which sensory neuropathy develops.

Biotin

Biotin is a coenzyme in carboxylation reactions. Deficiency states are produced by ingesting large amounts of raw egg whites, which contain avidin, a biotin binder. Rare cases of biotin deficiencies are described in infants and children within 3 to 6 months of receiving biotin-free parenteral nutrition and in those with biotinidase deficiency. Some early evidence suggests marginal biotin deficiency in the first trimester of pregnancy. The symptoms of biotin deficiency include dry scaly dermatitis, alopecia, conjunctivitis, and central nervous system (CNS) abnormalities. There are no documented instances or reports of toxicity from ingestion of excessive amounts of biotin. A UL cannot be described.

Pantothenic Acid

Pantothenic acid is a component of coenzyme A and widely distributed in foods. Deficiency of this vitamin is seen in individuals fed a semisynthetic diet or those ingesting pantothenic acid antagonists. Irritability, fatigue, malaise, sleep disturbances, muscle cramps, hypoglycemia, and an increased sensitivity to insulin are some of the symptoms seen in deficiency states. The burning feet syndrome described in malnourished prisoners of war may be a form of pantothenic deficiency. Pantothenic acid is abundant in foodstuffs, making deficiency states unlikely to develop. In addition, no toxic effects of this vitamin are reported.

Folate (Folic Acid and Folacin)

Folate functions as a coenzyme in single-carbon transfers in the metabolism of nucleic and amino acids. This vitamin is essential in development of the CNS. Insufficient folate activity at the time of conception and early pregnancy can result in congenital neural tube defects. In addition, the results of Canadian fortification of flour with folic acid led to the suggestion that the decreased incidence of neural tube defects is a positive outcome of supplementation during pregnancy. Inadequate folate leads to a decrease in erythrocyte folate concentrations, a rise in homocysteine concentration, and megaloblastic changes in the bone marrow and other tissues. The effects of high homocysteine levels in children was studied. Although it is unclear that increased levels may lead to the adult link with arterial disease and dementia, pediatric patients with renal transplant, having high homocysteine levels, are treated with folate supplementation.

The deficiency diseases of macrocytic and megaloblastic anemias caused by folate deficiency are rare in infants and children because human and cow's milk are excellent sources of folate. The U.S. mandatory fortification of all cereal grains in 1998 increased the folate available to the general population. Commonly eaten vegetables, such as green beans and peas, are an excellent source. Deficiencies of both folate and vitamin B_{12} cause megaloblastic anemia. Levels of both vitamins must be evaluated to determine the proper diagnosis and treatment. When anemia becomes moderate to severe, the symptoms of weakness, fatigue, and shortness of breath occur, as well as difficulty concentrating. Excessive intake of folic acid may inhibit the therapeutic effects of the anticonvulsant drug phenytoin. This calls for caution in administering supplemental folic acid in children with seizure disorders. Thus supplemental folate should not be given in large amounts. A UL was determined for folate use in adults based on suggestive evidence that excessive folate intake may precipitate an increase in neuropathy in vitamin B_{12}–deficient individuals. Infants should receive folate only from food sources (no UL). Extrapolation of the 1000 µg/day UL for adults is used to set the UL for children 1 to 18 years of age.

Cyanocobalamin (Vitamin B₁₂)

Two cobalamin-dependent enzymatic reactions occur in humans. Cobalamin is a cofactor in the conversion of methylmalonyl-coenzyme A to succinyl CoA. Also, cobalamin is a cofactor in the synthesis of methionine from homocysteine. Therefore, deficiency of B_{12} results in increased levels of methylmalonic acid (MMA) and homocysteine as normal metabolic pathways are interrupted. Vitamin B_{12} is found in many food sources, all of animal origin, such as red meat, poultry, fish, eggs, and dairy. Foods derived from plants lack the vitamin unless they are fortified, such as cereals. For this reason, infants and young children in families practicing total vegetarianism (vegans) may be at risk for vitamin B_{12} deficiency. Breast-fed infants of vegetarian mothers with low levels of vitamin B_{12} have low serum levels and symptoms of deficiency, such as macrocytic or megaloblastic anemias. Infants fed by unsupplemented mothers may show signs of deficiency by 4 months of age. The degree of deficiency may be related to the length of time that mothers practice unsupplemented vegetarianism. For these reasons, breast-fed infants of vegan mothers may require supplementation. Other symptoms of vitamin B_{12} deficiency are skin hypersensitivity, glossitis, and neurologic signs caused by demyelination in the central and peripheral nervous systems. The duration of B_{12} deficiency may affect the ability to recover from neurologic complications. Cases of pediatric vitamin B_{12} deficiency are rare; most are the result of poor vitamin B_{12} absorption secondary to terminal ileal disease or resection. Other causes may be gastric dysfunction, which interferes with intrinsic factor (IF) availability (IF is required for B_{12} absorption). In adults, use of acid-lowering agents and cholestyramine causes B_{12} deficiency. A more subtle deficiency of B_{12} in pediatrics is seen in studies that found homocysteine levels in children increase with age through childhood, corresponding with decreases in B_{12} and folate during the same period. These investigators suggest that B_{12} and folate intake should be supplied in adequate amounts to prevent increased homocysteine levels. No toxic effects of excessive amounts of vitamin B_{12} is reported. No UL is determined. In addition, no benefits from giving nondeficient children large amounts of B_{12} are documented.

Vitamin C

Vitamin C is an antioxidant important in collagen, carnitine, and neurotransmitter biosynthesis, and deficiency results in capillary fragility. Scurvy, the clinical manifestation of vitamin C deficiency, is characterized by anemia, swollen or bleeding gums, petechial hemorrhages, joint pain with tenderness and swelling of extremities, and bone demineralization. Fatigue and loss of appetite are common in affected older children. With supplementation in the forms of fruit juices and drinks and the amount of vitamin C that naturally occurs in fresh fruit and vegetables, the incidence of scurvy is rare in children who follow a varied diet. Infants fed evaporated or boiled cow's milk (heat destroys vitamin C) without vitamin C supplementation may develop infantile scurvy. Deficiency states are seen in children on severely restricted diets secondary to developmental delays and psychiatric problems. Clinical evidence of a deficiency state can appear within an estimated 2 to 4 months of inadequate intake. Response to supplementation is usually quick. Toxic effects of vitamin C in children are not reported, although nausea and vomiting may occur in adults with large does. There is disagreement about the beneficial effects, if any, of larger doses of vitamin C on general health. Pharmacologic doses are prescribed to enhance absorption of heme iron and as an antioxidant to prevent oxidative destruction of fat-soluble vitamins A and E.

Common Pitfalls

All patients with vitamin deficiencies and excesses should have their levels closely monitored. In general, blood values should be checked at regular intervals once supplementation is initiated or stopped in deficiency or excess states, respectively. This prevents toxicities or excess states, especially of the fat-soluble vitamins where the margin of safety is narrow. All patients with vitamin deficiencies should also have their blood levels monitored during therapy and at regular intervals thereafter to prevent a recurrence of a deficiency state once supplementation

stops. A search should be made for the causes of the deficiency or toxicity state to prevent a recurrence. In some instances, vitamin levels may not truly reflect the vitamin status of the patient and functional tests may need to be performed to better assess vitamin status.

Communication and Counseling

Because of the narrow range of safe levels of intake of most vitamins and the lack of a clear benefit of supplementation beyond recommended intakes, routine supplementation is not recommended for infants and children. Only infants and children at risk for vitamin deficiency or who show clinical signs of deficiency disease require supplementation. Thus parents should be cautioned against supplementation with vitamins. If vitamins are used in pharmacologic doses, the health care provider must carefully monitor blood levels, physical symptoms, and side effects. Care should be exercised when certain medications are used that are known to cause vitamin-deficiency states (e.g., isoniazid and pyridoxine).

SUGGESTED READINGS

1. Dharmarajan TS, Norkus EP: Approaches to vitamin B_{12} deficiency. Postgrad Med 110:99–105, 2001. **Screening for vitamin B_{12} deficiency is discussed, including predisposing conditions, some with application in children. Treatment is outlined.**
2. Food and Nutrition Board, Institute of Medicine: Dietary reference intakes for calcium, phosphorus, magnesium, vitamin D and fluoride. Washington, DC: National Academies Press, 1997, pp 250–287. **Complete review of the development of DRIs for vitamin D.**
3. Food and Nutrition Board, Institute of Medicine: Dietary reference intakes for thiamin, riboflavin, niacin, B_6, folate, vitamin B_{12}, pantothenic acid, biotin and choline. Washington, DC: National Academies Press, 1998, pp 58–389. **Complete review of the development of DRIs for the included water-soluble vitamins.**
4. Food and Nutrition Board, Institute of Medicine: Dietary reference intakes for vitamin A, vitamin K, arsenic, boron, chromium, copper, iodine, iron, manganese, molybdenum, nickel, silicon, vanadium and zinc. Washington, DC: National Academies Press, 2001, pp 82–196. **Complete review of the development of DRIs for vitamins A and K.**
5. Food and Nutrition Board, Institute of Medicine: Dietary reference intakes for vitamin C, vitamin E, selenium and carotenoids. Washington, DC: National Academies Press, 2000, pp 95–382. **Complete review of the development of DRIs for vitamins C and E.**
6. Gartner LM, Greer FR, Section on Breastfeeding Committee on Nutrition: Prevention of rickets and vitamin D deficiency: New guidelines for vitamin D intake. Pediatrics 111:908–910, 2003. **Update on recommendation to supplement breast-fed babies with vitamin D.**
7. Holick MF: Evolution and function of vitamin D. Recent Results Cancer Res 164:3–28, 2003. **Reviews present knowledge of vitamin D and its many functions.**
8. Krinsky NI: Human requirements for fat-soluble vitamins, and other things concerning these nutrients. Mol Aspects Med 24:317–324, 2003. **Excellent overview of the fat-soluble vitamins, their minimum requirements, maximum safe amounts, and their use as supplements.**
9. Michaelsson K, Lithell H, Vessby B, Melhus H: Serum retinol levels and the risk of fracture. N Engl J Med 348:287–294, 2003. **Reported large study in adults of the correlation of high vitamin A intake and increased bone fragility.**
10. Vasconcelos MM, Silva KP, Vidal G, et al: Early diagnosis of pediatric Wernicke's encephalopathy. Pediatr Neurol 20:289–294, 1999. **Reports cases in the literature in which pediatric patients present with thiamin deficiency in the classic form of Wernicke encephalopathy. The most frequent underlying disorder leading to this condition was malignancy.**

Immunization Practices

Sujatha Rajan and Natalie Neu

KEY CONCEPTS

- Active and passive immunization interact to help protect the body against disease.
- All health care providers should review changes in the vaccination recommendations annually.
- Health care providers who deliver vaccinations should have policies and procedures created for informed consent, administration, and reporting of adverse events.
- Discussing parental concerns about vaccines helps ensure adherence to immunization recommendations.
- Advances in vaccine research lead to the development of combination vaccines and new vaccines against common childhood pathogens.

During the 20th century, substantial achievements were made in controlling many vaccine-preventable diseases. Immunization of children has had the most profound impact in decreasing diseases and represents the most efficacious and cost-effective way to prevent disease. Currently in the United States, the immunization schedule provides for protection against 13 diseases through the administration of 10 different vaccines.

Expert Opinion on Management Issues

TYPES OF IMMUNIZATION

The main purpose of the immune system is to identify and eliminate foreign substances, called *antigens,* from the body. Immunization is the process of artificially inducing immunity or providing protection from disease. The immune system defends the body against antigens by making proteins called *antibodies,* which help eliminate antigens. This system is also involved in inactivating viruses, microbes, and bacteria, as well as remembering prior interactions with these agents to mount a stronger response upon next exposure.

There are two types of immunity: active and passive. *Active immunity* is obtained by natural disease or vaccination. *Vaccines* are defined as agents that induce an immune response in the host. There are two types of vaccines; live attenuated and inactivated forms. *Live attenuated vaccines* are produced by modifying a bacterium or virus so it can replicate and produce immunity without causing disease. *Inactivated vaccines* are made of bacteria or viruses that are modified or killed with heat or chemicals. These microbes are not alive, nor can they replicate or cause disease in the recipient. Active immunity confers immunologic memory so that when an individual is exposed to the antigen again, memory B cells replicate and produce antibodies to reinstate protection. Immunization can result in antitoxin, antiadherence, anti-invasive, or neutralizing activity or other types of

protective humoral or cellular response in the recipient. *Passive immunity* provides an individual temporary immunity, either by transmission of antibody from mother to fetus or through administration of parenteral antibodies. Passive immunity is short-lived.

ROUTINE CHILDHOOD VACCINES

Childhood immunization schedules used in the United States are defined jointly by the Advisory Committee on Immunization Practices (ACIP) of the U.S. Public Health Service, the Committee on Infectious Diseases (COID) of the American Academy of Pediatrics (AAP), and the American Academy of Family Physicians (AAFP). The schedule in Figure 1 represents a consensus for routine childhood immunizations in the year 2005. This schedule is issued annually in January to incorporate new vaccines and revised recommendations. The schedule specifies both the timing and the acceptable range of timing recommended for each dose of universally recommended vaccines. Special attention should be given to footnotes on the schedule because they summarize major recommendations for childhood immunizations. Physicians and other health care providers should always ensure they are following the most up-to-date schedules, which are available from the Centers for Disease Control and Prevention (CDC) National Immunization Program website at http://www.cdc.gov/nip

Some of the recently incorporated changes in the immunization schedule since 2000 are as follows:

- Hepatitis A virus vaccine (HAV) was recommended in states with high HAV incidence rates.
- Conjugated pneumococcal vaccine was recommended for all children 2 to 23 months of age.
- In 2004, influenza vaccine was recommended for all children 6 to 23 months of age as a routine vaccination (because of increased risk of hospitalization) in addition to those children traditionally considered at high risk (asthma, cardiac disease, sickle cell, HIV, and diabetes).
- Meningococcal polysaccharide conjugate vaccine was recommended for 11- to 55-year-olds in 2005.
- Two tetanus toxoid, reduced diphtheria toxoid, and acellular pertussis (TDaP) vaccines were licensed in 2005 as single booster vaccines for adolescents.

CATCH-UP IMMUNIZATIONS OR UNKNOWN/UNCERTAIN STATUS

The vaccine schedule can be resumed regardless of the time span that has elapsed since the last dose administered. Tables 1 and 2 provide the guidelines for resumption of lapsed immunizations. When the documentation or history of vaccination is of questionable validity, children and adolescents should generally be considered susceptible to disease, and appropriate vaccines should be administered. Persons already immune are not harmed (other than experiencing pain during injection) by administration of any currently recommended childhood vaccine.

Vaccine	Birth	1 mo	2 mos	4 mos	6 mos	12 mos	15 mos	18 mos	24 mos	4–6 yrs	11–12 yrs	13–14 yrs	15 yrs	16–18 yrs
Hepatitis B[1]	HepB	HepB		HepB[1]		HepB					HepB series			
Diphtheria, tetanus, pertussis[2]			DTaP	DTaP	DTaP		DTaP			DTaP	Tdap			Tdap
Haemophilus influenzae type b[3]			Hib	Hib	Hib[3]	Hib								
Inactivated poliovirus			IPV	IPV		IPV				IPV				
Measles, mumps, rubella[4]						MMR				MMR		MMR		
Varicella[5]						Varicella					Varicella			
Meningococcal[6]											MCV4		MCV4	
										MPSV4			MCV4	
Pneumococcal[7]			PCV	PCV	PCV	PCV				PCV	PPV			
Influenza[8]					Influenza (yearly)						Influenza (yearly)			
Hepatitis A[9]						HepA series					HepA series			

Vaccines within broken line are for selected populations

☐ Range of recommended ages   ▨ Catch-up immunization   ■ Assessment at age 11-12 years

FIGURE 1. Recommended childhood and adolescent immunization schedule by vaccine and age. This schedule indicates the recommended ages for routine administration of currently licensed childhood vaccines, as of December 1, 2005, for children through age 18 years. Any dose not given at the recommended age should be given at any subsequent visit when indicated and feasible. The lightest shaded areas indicate age groups that warrant special effort to administer those vaccines not previously given. Additional vaccines may be licensed and recommended during the year. Licensed combination vaccines may be used whenever any components of the combination are indicated and the vaccine's other components are not contraindicated and if approved by the Food and Drug Administration for that dose of the series. Providers should consult respective Advisory Committee on Immunization Practices (ACIP) statements for detailed recommendations. Clinically significant adverse events that follow immunization should be reported to the Vaccine Adverse Event Reporting System (VAERS). Guidance about how to obtain and complete a VAERS form can be found on the Internet: www.vaers.hhs.org or by calling 800–822–7967.

[1]*at birth:* All newborns should receive monovalent HepB soon after birth and before hospital discharge. *Infants born to mothers who are hepatitis B surface antigen (HBsAg)-positive* should receive HepB and 0.5mL of hepatitis B immune globulin (HBIG) within 12 hours of birth. *Infants born to mothers whose HBsAg status is unknown* should receive HepB within 12 hours of birth. The mother should have blood drawn as soon as possible to determine her HBsAg status; if HBsAg-positive, the infant should receive HBIG as soon as possible (no later than age 1 week). *For infants born to HBsAg-negative mothers,* the birth dose can be delayed in rare circumstances but only if a physician's order to withhold the vaccine and a copy of the mother's original HBsAg-negative laboratory report are documented in the infant's medical record.

following the birth dose: The HepB series should be completed with either monovalent HepB or a combination vaccine containing HepB. The second dose should be administered at age 1–2 months. The final dose should be administered at age ≥24 weeks. Administering four doses of HepB is permissible (e.g., when combination vaccines are administered after the birth dose); however, if monovalent HepB is used, a dose at age 4 months is not needed. *Infants born to HBsAg-positive mothers* should be tested for HBsAg and antibody to HBsAg after completion of the HepB series at age 9–18 months (generally at the next well-child visit after completion of the vaccine series).

[2]The fourth dose of DTaP may be administered as early as age 12 months, provided 6 months have elapsed since the third dose and the child is unlikely to return at age 15–18 months. The final dose in the series should be administered at age ≥4 years. *Tetanus toxoid, reduced diphtheria toxoid, and acellular pertussis vaccine (Tdap adolescent preparation)* is recommended at age 11–12 years for those who have completed the recommended childhood DTP/DTaP vaccination series and have not received a tetanus and diphtheria toxoids (Td) booster dose. Adolescents aged 13–18 years who missed the age 11–12-year Td/Tdap booster dose should also receive a single dose of Tdap if they have completed the recommended childhood DTP/DTaP vaccination series. *Subsequent Td* boosters are recommended every 10 years.

[3]Three Hib conjugate vaccines are licensed for infant use. If PRP-OMP (PedvaxHIB® or ComVax® [Merck]) is administered at ages 2 and 4 months, a dose at age 6 months is not required. DTaP/Hib combination products should not be used for primary immunization in infants at ages 2, 4, or 6 months but may be used as boosters after any Hib vaccine. The final dose in the series should be administered at age ≥12 months.

[4]The second dose of MMR is recommended routinely at age 4–6 years but may be administered during any visit, provided at least 4 weeks have elapsed since the first dose and both doses are administered at or after age 12 months. Children who have not previously received the second dose should complete the schedule by age 11–12 years.

[5]Varicella vaccine is recommended at any visit at or after age 12 months for susceptible children (i.e., those who lack a reliable history of varicella). Susceptible persons aged ≥13 years should receive 2 doses administered at least 4 weeks apart.

[6]Meningococcal conjugate vaccine (MCV4) should be administered to all children at age 11–12 years as well as to unvaccinated adolescents at high school entry (age 15 years). Other adolescents who wish to decrease their risk for meningococcal disease may also be vaccinated. All college freshmen living in dormitories should also be vaccinated, preferably with MCV4, although *meningococcal polysaccharide vaccine (MPSV4)* is an acceptable alternative. Vaccination against invasive meningococcal disease is recommended for children and adolescents aged ≥2 years with terminal complement

TABLE 1 Catch-up* Immunization Schedule for Children Ages 4 Months to 6 Years

Vaccine	Minimum Age for Dose 1	Minimum Interval between Doses			
		Dose 1 to Dose 2	Dose 2 to Dose 3	Dose 3 to Dose 4	Dose 4 to Dose 5
DTaP	6 wk	4 wk	4 wk	6 mo	6 mo[1]
IPV	6 wk	4 wk	4 wk	4 wk[2]	
HepB[3]	Birth	4 wk	8 wk (and 16 wk after first dose)		
MMR	12 mo	4 wk[4]			
Varicella	12 mo				
Hib[5]	6 wk	4 wk if first dose administered at age <12 mo. 8 wk (as final dose) if first dose administered at age 12–14 mo. No further doses needed if first dose administered at age ≥15 mo	4 wk[6] if current age < 12 mo. 8 wk (as final dose)[6] if current age ≥12 mo and second dose administered at age <15 mo. No further doses needed if previous dose administered at age ≥15 mo.	8 wk (as final dose). This dose is only necessary for children ages 12 mo to 5 yr who received 3 doses before age 12 mo.	
PCV[7]	6 wk	4 wk if first dose administered at age <12 mo and current age <24 mo. 8 wk (as final dose) if first dose administered at age ≥12 mo or current age 24–59 mo. No further doses needed for healthy children if first dose administered at age ≥24 mo.	4 wk if current age <12 mo. 8 wk (as final dose) if current age ≥12 mo. No further doses needed for healthy children if previous dose administered at age ≥24 mo.	8 wk (as final dose). This dose is only necessary for children ages 12 mo to 5 yr who received 3 doses before age 12 mo.	

*For children and adolescents who start late or are more than 1 month behind.

Note: A vaccine series does not require restarting, regardless of the time that has elapsed between doses.

[1]The fifth dose is not necessary if the fourth dose was given after the fourth birthday.

[2]For children who received an all-IPV or all-oral poliovirus (OPV) series, a fourth dose is not necessary if third dose was given at age ≥4 years. If both OPV and IPV were given as part of a series, a total of 4 doses should be given, regardless of the child's current age.

[3]Administer the 3-dose series to all persons aged < 19 yr if they were not previously vaccinated.

[4]The second dose of MMR is recommended routinely at age 4–6 years but may be given earlier if desired.

[5]Vaccine is not generally recommended for children aged ≥5 years.

[6]If current age <12 months and the first 2 doses were PRP-OMP (PedvaxHIB or ComVax [Merck]), the third (and final) dose should be given at age 12–15 months and at least 8 weeks after the second dose.

[7]Vaccine is not generally recommended for children aged ≥5 years.

DTaP, diphtheria, tetanus, acellular pertussis; HepB, hepatitis B vaccine; Hib, *Haemophilus influenzae* type b; IPV, inactivated polio vaccine; MMR, measles, mumps, and rubella; OPV, oral polio vaccine; PCV, pneumococcal vaccine.

(From Centers for Disease Control and Prevention: Recommended Childhood and Adolescent Immunization Schedule—United States, 2006. MMWR 2005: 54 [Nos. 51&52]: Q1–Q4.)

2

deficiencies or anatomic or functional asplenia and for certain other high risk groups (see *MMWR* 2005;54[No. RR-7]); use MPSV4 for children aged 2–10 years and MCV4 for older children, although MPSV4 is an acceptable alternative.

[7]The hepatavalent *pneumococcal conjugate vaccine* (PCV) is recommended for all children aged 2–23 months and for certain children aged 24–59 months. The final dose in the series should be administered at age ≥12 months. *Pneumococcal polysaccharide vaccine (PPV)* is recommended in addition to PCV for certain high-risk groups. See *MMWR* 2000;49(No. RR-9).

[8]Influenza vaccine is recommended annually for children aged ≥6 months with certain risk factors (including, but not limited to, asthma, cardiac disease, sickle cell disease, human immunodeficiency virus infection, diabetes, and conditions that can compromise respiratory function or handling of respiratory secretions or that can increase the risk for aspiration), health-care workers, and other persons (including household members) in close contact with persons in groups at high risk (see *MMR* 2005;54[No. RR-8]). In addition, healthy children aged 6–23 months and close contacts of healthy children aged 0–5 months are recommended to receive influenza vaccine because children in this age group are at substantially increased risk for influenza-related hospitalizations. For healthy, nonpregnant persons aged 5–49 years, the intranasally administered, live, attenuated influenza vaccine (LAIV) is an acceptable alternative to the intramuscular trivalent inactivated influenza vaccine (TIV). See *MMWR* 2005;54(No. RR-8). Children receiving TIV should be administered an age-appropriate dosage (0.25 mL for children aged 6–35 months or 0.5 mL for children aged ≥3 years). Children aged ≤8 years who are receiving influenza vaccine for the first time should receive 2 doses (separated by at least 4 weeks for TIV and at least 6 weeks for LAIV).

[9]HepA is recommended for all children at age 1 year (i.e., 12–23 months). The 2 doses in the series should be administered at least 6 months apart. States, counties, and communities with existing HepA vaccination programs for children aged 2–18 years are encouraged to maintain these programs. In these areas, new efforts focused on routine vaccination of children aged 1 year should enhance, not replace, ongoing programs directed at a broader population of children. HepA is also recommended for certain high risk groups (see *MMWR* 1999;48[No. RR-12]).

(From Centers for Disease Control and Prevention: Recommended Childhood and Adolescent Immunization Schedule—United States, 2006. MMWR 2005: 54 [Nos. 51&52]: Q1–Q4.)

TABLE 2 Catch-up* Immunization Schedule for Children and Adolescents Ages 7 to 18 Years Who Start Late or Are More Than 1 Month Behind

Vaccine	Minimum Interval between Doses		
	Dose 1 to Dose 2	Dose 2 to Dose 3	Dose 3 to Booster Dose
Td[1]	4 wk	6 mo	6 mo[1] if first dose administered at age <12 m and current age <11 yr; otherwise 5 yr
IPV[2]	4 wk	4 wk	
HepB	4 wk	8 wk (and 16 wk after first dose)	
MMR	4 wk		
Varicella[3]	4 wk		

Note: A vaccine series does not require restarting, regardless of the time that has elapsed between doses.

[1]Adolescent preparation may be substituted for any dose in a primary catch-up series or as a booster if age appropriate for Tdap. A 5-year interval from the last Td dose is encouraged when Tdap is used as a booster dose. See ACIP recommendations for additional information.

[2]Vaccine is not generally recommended for persons aged ≥18 years.

[3]Give 2-dose series to all susceptible adolescents aged ≥13 years.

HepB, hepatitis B vaccine; Hib, *Hemophilus influenzae* type b; IPV, inactivated polio vaccine; MMR, measles, mumps, and rubella; Td, tetanus and diphtheria.

Adapted from Centers for Disease Control and Prevention: Recommended Childhood and Adolescent Immunization Schedule—United States, 2006. MMWR 2005: 54 [Nos. 51&52]: Q1–Q4.

IMMUNIZATIONS RECEIVED OUTSIDE THE UNITED STATES

Most vaccines used worldwide are produced with appropriate quality control and are reliable. Written documentation of administration of vaccines from many countries, however, is suspect. Currently, written vaccination records from Central and South America are generally considered reliable, provided the vaccines, dates of administration, number of doses, age at doses, and interval between doses are comparable to the current recommended schedule in the United States. Records from Eastern Europe, the countries of the former Soviet Union, and China may not reflect the immune status of the child accurately (especially children from orphanages). In situations in which the immunization history is absent or questionable, it is advisable to begin immunization series even if this risks total reimmunization. Alternatively, antibody levels against infectious agents contained in the various vaccines can be obtained.

ADMINISTRATION OF VACCINES

Administration of vaccines should employ sterile technique. Recommended routes of injection and needle length are always given by the manufacturer and are part of the research on the vaccine. For infants, the anterolateral aspect of the thigh should be used for injection. For toddlers and older children, the deltoid may be used if muscle mass is adequate and if institutional policies permit.

MINIMUM AGES AND MINIMUM INTERVALS BETWEEN DOSES

Vaccination providers are encouraged to adhere as closely as possible to the recommended childhood immunization schedule. Clinical studies report that recommended ages and intervals between doses of multidose antigens provide optimal protection or have the best evidence of efficacy. Figure 1 provides the recommended vaccines and recommended intervals between doses.

ROLE OF COMBINATION VACCINES

Combination vaccines offer many potential advantages: fewer injections and associated risks, less pain and anxiety, simplified schedule and inventory, better compliance, and decreased administration costs. Protecting children from a wider spectrum of illnesses while reducing the number of shots children must receive is the ultimate goal toward a more effective way of reducing infections. Immunogenicity also does not appear to be affected adversely except in specific circumstances, for example, with the mixture of measles, mumps, and rubella (MMR) with varicella vaccine (MMRV). There is some concern that responses to the varicella component are diminished, presumably because measles virus replication interferes with replication of the varicella component. ProQuad (Merck), an MMRV vaccine not yet licensed, overcomes this problem by increasing the amount of varicella in the mixture.

Based on the potential for improved coverage rates, reduced costs, and facilitation of introduction of new vaccines, the ACIP, AAP, and the AAFP issued a joint statement in 1999 indicating a clear preference for combination vaccines as opposed to separate injections of monovalent compounds. The joint statement concludes that combination vaccines may be used whenever any component is indicated and other components are not contraindicated. It is recognized that this may result in unnecessary doses of a given component, but the benefits in terms of timely coverage probably outweigh the risks. Table 3 lists the currently licensed and to-be-licensed combination vaccines.

NEW VACCINES

Quadrivalent Meningococcal Conjugate Vaccine

The vast majority of the cases of invasive meningococcal disease in the United States are sporadic. Five major serogroups (A, B, C, W135, and Y) are known to cause

TABLE 3 Combination Vaccines: Currently Licensed and Future Vaccines

	Company (Licensure Date)	Recommendations
Current Combination Vaccines (Components)		
TriHIBit (DTaP2 and Hib as ActHib)	Aventis Pasteur (1996)	Not for use in infants. Licensed for 15–18 mo as a fourth dose of Hib and DTaP.
COMVAX (hepatitis B and Hib as PRP-OMP)	Merck (1996)	Must be administered after 6 wk of age. May be used to complete hepatitis series if monovalent hepatitis B given at birth. Four doses of vaccine are acceptable if birth dose given. Dosing schedule: 2, 4, 15–18 mo. Minimal interval between doses: 4 wk between first and second dose; 8 wk between second and third dose.
PEDIARIX (DTaP3, hepatitis B, and IPV)	GlaxoSmithKline (2002)	Must be administered after 6 wk of age. Do not administer to children older than 7 yr of age. Dosing schedule: three-dose series at 8-wk intervals (e.g., 2, 4, 6 mo). Can be used to complete series for hepatitis B or IPV. *Cannot* be used to complete series for DTaP.
TWINRIX (hepatitis A and hepatitis B)	GlaxoSmithKline (2001)	Indicated for persons 18 yr of age and older. Dosing schedule: three-dose series given at 0, 1, 6 mo
Future Combination Vaccines		
PENTACEL (Hib [as PRP-T], DTaP5, and IPV)	Aventis Pasteur	Used in Canada since 1997. Five vaccines in one injection. Dosing schedule: 2, 4, 6, 18 mo, and 4–6 yr.
ProQuad (MMR and varicella)	Merck	Acceptable combination because both vaccines may be given at 1 year of age. May need varicella booster in the future.

DTaP, diphtheria-tetanus-acellular pertussis; MMR, measles, mumps, and rubella; Hib, *Haemophilus influenzae* type b; IPV, inactivated polio vaccine.

2

human disease. Meningococcal disease occurs in three clinical forms—meningitis (49% of cases), blood infection (33% of cases), and pneumonia (9% of cases)—and in other forms. Onset can be abrupt with a fulminant course and is associated with a case fatality rate between 9% and 12%, despite advances in medical management and continued sensitivity of *Neisseria meningitidis* to penicillin and various other antibiotics. The quadrivalent meningococcal vaccine currently licensed for use in the United States contains group-specific (A, C, W135, and Y) polysaccharide antigens against *N. meningitidis*. This meningococcal vaccine does not induce long-acting, T-cell–dependent immunologic memory; hence it is poorly immunogenic in children, especially those younger than 24 months of age.

A new meningococcal quadrivalent (groups A, C, Y, W135), a diphtheria toxoid conjugate vaccine called Menactra (Aventis Pasteur), was licensed in January 2005. This vaccine contains 4 μg each of A, C, Y, and W135 polysaccharide conjugated to 48 μg of diphtheria toxoid and has acceptable safety and immunogenicity in adolescents and adults. The conjugated vaccine has seroconversion rates and serum bactericidal responses that are comparable with or superior to the polysaccharide vaccine. A single dose of vaccine is recommended by the AAP and ACIP for use in children 11 to 12 years of age, teens entering high school, and college students living in dormitories and other high-risk groups between 11 and 55 years of age. The optimal timing of booster vaccination is not clear.

Tetanus, Diphtheria, and Acellular Pertussis

Parents or other household members are the contact sources for most pediatric pertussis cases. Vaccine protection wanes by 11 to 15 years of age, and thus illness in adults, which is often mild, may be the source for young infant contacts. Current data support the use of booster doses of vaccine as the next step in an effort to reduce the incidence of disease in children. Two vaccines are now FDA approved and available for the booster dose in adolescents and adults against tetanus, diphtheria, and pertussis: BOOSTRIX (GlaxoSmithKline) and Adacel (Aventis Pasteur). Numerous studies include vaccines containing one to five components of pertussis vaccine using concentrations of antigen that are equal or lower than in currently available pediatric products. Vaccines are well tolerated in all studies, with systemic symptoms occurring no more frequently among those subjects receiving vaccine and those receiving a placebo control.

Rotavirus Vaccines

Rotavirus affects virtually all children during the first 5 years of life, causing severe gastroenteritis worldwide and even death in young children in developing countries because of dehydration. In the United States, rotavirus is a common cause of hospitalization, clinic visits, and considerable health costs. Because of this large burden of disease, a live oral tetravalent, rhesus-based rotavirus vaccine, RotaShield (Wyeth-Ayerst Laboratories), was studied and licensed for use in August 1998. A year later this vaccine was withdrawn because of the occurrence of 15 cases of intussusception that had a strong temporal and specific relation to the vaccine. Two other vaccine candidates for rotavirus are currently undergoing extensive clinical trials both in the United States and abroad. One is a live attenuated monovalent human strain derived vaccine called Rotarix (GlaxoSmithKline). The other is a multivalent vaccine called RotaTeq (Merck & Co.), which has a bovine gene backbone and five human rotavirus genes coding for five serotypes: G1, G2, G3, G4, and P1a.

Preliminary studies for both vaccines found efficacy greater than 75%, with no adverse events. The total number of cases of intussusception was not significantly different compared to the placebo group, and no temporal clustering has so far been found. Rotarix is already licensed in Mexico and is expected to be in clinical use in several Latin American countries in 2006.

Human Papillomavirus Vaccine

Human papillomavirus (HPV) infection is a widespread problem associated with significant morbidity and mortality in terms of its association with genital warts and the development of cervical cancer. HPV vaccines are based on the L1 protein, the major protein of the viral capsule. HPV L1 virus-like particles (VLPs) assemble into a particle that resembles the wild-type virion, but because these particles are DNA free, they are not infectious. VLPs are very immunogenic and safe in clinical trials. Two companies, GlaxoSmithKline and Merck, currently have phase III clinical trials using a quadrivalent product that includes VLPs from HPV–16 and HPV–18 (the oncogenic types) as well as HPV–6 and HPV–11 (the types that cause warts). HPV vaccine trials show efficacy in women. Trials are ongoing in the male population. Issues currently surrounding the HPV vaccines include when to initiate vaccination (optimally presexual debut), efficacy and utility in the male population, and the expense of the vaccine (especially for developing nations, which shoulder a large burden of HPV disease).

General Issues

INFORMED CONSENT AND RECORD KEEPING

Health care providers are required to provide specific information to parents before administering vaccines. Review of the vaccine information statements (VIS) detailing the potential benefits and risks of each vaccine should be done for all vaccines covered by the National Childhood Vaccine Injury Act (NCVIA). Copies of the VISs may be obtained from the CDC National Immunization Program, the AAP, or state health departments. The CDC additionally requires physicians to record the date on which the VIS was provided and discussed with the parent/caregiver and/or patient. Parent/caregiver signatures are not required in the record or on the VIS. The patient's medical record, date of administration, vaccine manufacturer, the lot number, and the name and business address of the provider should be recorded. The site and route of administration and vaccine expiration date should also be recorded.

ADVERSE EVENTS AND REPORTING

All vaccines licensed in the United States are largely safe and effective, but no agent is completely safe or always effective. Common side effects are generally mild to moderate in severity and resolve without permanent injury. Fever and injection site inflammation and pain are the most common side effects. Mild forms of disease can occur with live-attenuated vaccines. Suspected adverse events temporally related to vaccinations should be reported to the Vaccine Adverse Events Reporting System (VAERS) (1–800–822–7967 or www.vaers.org). Submission of reports does not necessarily imply a cause-and-effect relationship between the vaccine and the event. VAERS staff follow up on the condition of the patient both 60 days and 1 year after the date of the apparent adverse event. Reports are evaluated for indications of previously unrecognized adverse events. Patient confidentiality is maintained. For the very rare patients who suffer an injury or death as a result of administration of covered vaccines, the Vaccine Injury Compensation Program (VICP) established a no-fault compensation system. These events can be accessed at the VAERS website (http://www.vaers.org). The program provides prompt and fair compensation to the families of children who are affected and has reduced lawsuits against health care professionals and manufacturers, which in turn has helped maintain a stable vaccine supply and marketplace.

VACCINE CONTRAINDICATIONS AND PRECAUTIONS

Knowledge of vaccine contraindications and precautions is an important aspect of immunization practice. A *contraindication* indicates that the vaccine should not be administered. A *precaution* specifies a circumstance in which a vaccine may be indicated if the benefit to an individual is judged to outweigh the risk and consequences of an adverse event. General contraindications and precautions for all vaccines (DTP, DTaP, OPV, IPV, MMR, Hib, hepatitis B) include anaphylactic reaction to a vaccine or a vaccine component. Further doses of vaccine or vaccines containing that substance should be avoided. Specific relevant information for individual vaccines may be found in the package inserts for each vaccine product, in the Red Book, and at http://www.cdc.gov/nip/recs/contraindications.htm

Before vaccine administration, inquiry must be made regarding the child's current state of health, possible contraindications, precautions, and any previous adverse events in response to vaccine administration. Vaccines produced in chick embryo tissue culture, including measles and mumps vaccine, contain insignificant amounts of egg protein, and skin testing before administering these vaccines is no longer indicated for children with true egg hypersensitivity. However, inactivated influenza and yellow fever vaccines are produced in eggs, and true hypersensitivity to egg protein is a contraindication to these vaccines. Skin testing with yellow fever vaccine is recommended before administration to those with a history of systemic anaphylactic reaction to egg protein.

Hypersensitivity reactions to constituents of vaccine products are rare. However, in all settings in which vaccines are administered, the necessary personnel, therapeutic agents, and supportive equipment should be available for treating severe immediate hypersensitivity reactions. Patients should be observed for 15 to 20 minutes after vaccination whenever possible.

Common Pitfalls

Vaccines are sometimes delayed by health care workers for conditions regarded as relative contraindications. This results in missed opportunities to complete immunizations. The following are considered pitfalls and are not contraindications; hence, vaccines may be administered:

- Mild to moderate local reaction (soreness, redness, swelling) following a dose of an injectable antigen
- Mild acute illness with our without low-grade fever
- Current antimicrobial therapy
- Convalescent phase of illnesses
- Prematurity (same dosage and indications as for normal full-term infants)

VACCINE HANDLING AND STORAGE

Vaccines should be handled and stored as recommended in the manufacturers' package inserts; the expiration date for each vaccine should be noted. Temperatures at which vaccines are stored and transported should be monitored and recorded twice daily. Vaccine failure can result from failure to observe the precise conditions required for storing, handling, and administration of a product. Storage requirements are provided in the product package inserts. For a concise compilation of storage requirements and the duration of stability of commonly used vaccines, see the Red Book.

INTERCHANGEABILITY OF VACCINE PRODUCTS

Different brands of the same vaccine may differ in their components and elicit different immune responses; hence it is generally preferable to use the same vaccine product for all required doses. When this is not feasible, other brands of the currently used vaccines can be used to complete the recommended dose series. Interchangeability data are limited, but this flexibility is allowed for immunization with all currently licensed *Haemophilus influenza* B conjugate vaccines, hepatitis A and B vaccines, and diphtheria-tetanus-acellular pertussis (DTaP) vaccines. For acellular pertussis vaccines, the same product should be used for the three-dose primary series when possible. Any product then can be used for the fourth and fifth doses. However, if the specific DTaP product received previously is not known or the previously administered product is not readily available, any licensed product may be used. Providers must closely monitor recommendations on interchangeability.

SIMULTANEOUS ADMINISTRATION OF MULTIPLE VACCINES

The ability to administer multiple vaccines at the same visit is key to maintaining and improving immunization rates. Studies show that immune responses to one vaccine generally do not interfere with those to other vaccines administered in separate anatomic sites. Hence multiple vaccines can be given simultaneously, provided each is given properly. Each injected vaccine should be administered with a separate syringe at a different anatomic site. At least five injections may be needed at a single visit to comply with current recommendations. With combination vaccines and boosters, children may receive more doses of the antigen than the standard immunization schedule requires. This is usually not a problem; however, some children may experience reactogenicity events such as limb swelling or erythema at the injection site, most commonly with the polyvalent pneumococcal vaccine, DTaP, and tetanus (Td). There is no consensus about the cause of these events, and reactions usually resolve spontaneously without sequelae.

VACCINES IN SPECIAL CIRCUMSTANCES

High-risk medical conditions may be the result of infection with HIV, hematologic or generalized malignancies, chemotherapeutic or immunosuppressive agents, radiation, steroids, functional or anatomic asplenia, and complement or immunoglobulin deficiencies. Recommendations of vaccinations in these groups vary according to the degree and cause of immunodeficiency.

Human Immunodeficiency Virus Infection

Children and adolescents with asymptomatic or symptomatic HIV infection should receive all inactivated vaccines, including DTaP, inactivated polio vaccine (IPV), hepatitis B, *H. influenzae* type b (Hib), and pneumococcal conjugate vaccines, according to the recommended schedule. Annual influenza immunization of HIV-infected people is recommended. Because the ability of HIV-infected children to respond to vaccine antigens likely is related to the degree of immunosuppression at the time of immunization and may be inadequate, these children should be considered potentially susceptible to vaccine-preventable diseases, even after appropriate immunization. Hence passive immunoprophylaxis or chemoprophylaxis after exposure to these diseases should be considered, even if the child previously has received the recommended vaccines. Specific guidelines for use of MMR and varicella vaccine in HIV-infected children are provided in the Red Book. In general, MMR and varicella vaccination can be given to HIV-infected children who are not severely immunosuppressed. Household members of HIV-infected persons should be immunized with MMR vaccine unless they are known to be immune or have a contraindication of their own.

Severe Immunocompromise without HIV Infection

Individuals can be severely immunocompromised as a result of hematologic or general malignancy, chemotherapy, radiation therapy, high doses of corticosteroids (generally the equivalent of 20 mg/day of prednisone for longer than 2 weeks), or other immunosuppressive therapies. The degree of immunocompromise should be evaluated individually. Steroids given for less than 2 weeks—alternate-day therapy with short-acting, low-dose preparations; physiologic replacement doses; topical preparations used for either skin, eye, or lung; or injections into joints—are not considered immunosuppressive for the purpose of vaccination decisions with live-virus vaccines. For patients receiving high-dose corticosteroids for more than 2 weeks, live-virus vaccines should be given 1 month after discontinuation of the drug. If the duration of the high-dose corticosteroid use is less than 2 weeks, waiting 2 weeks may suffice.

Ideally, any vaccination should precede chemotherapy or radiation therapy by more than 2 weeks and should be avoided during chemotherapy because of a potential suboptimal response. The interval between vaccination and cessation of immunosuppression varies with the intensity and type of immunosuppressive therapy, radiation therapy, underlying disease, and other factors. Hence it is often not possible to make a definitive recommendation for an interval after cessation of immunosuppressive therapy. This interval varies from 3 months after chemotherapy to 2 years after bone marrow transplant. In vitro testing of immune function and antibody titers may provide useful guidance to ensure safe timing of live-virus vaccines in these children. In general, inactivated viral or bacterial vaccines and toxoids are safe for all severely immunocompromised patients. Live vaccines are contraindicated unless the immunocompromised state is reversible (steroids, chemotherapy, radiation therapy, or other immunosuppressive therapy) and an appropriate interval has elapsed between discontinuation of therapy and administration of live vaccine.

Asplenic Patients

Asplenic states results from surgical removal of the spleen; certain diseases, such as sickle cell disease (functional asplenia); or congenital asplenia. These patients are at increased risk of fulminant bacteremia, with high mortality. *Streptococcus pneumoniae, N. meningitidis,* and *H. influenzae* are the most common causes of bacteremia. *Escherichia coli, Staphylococcus aureus,* and gram-negative bacilli are less common causes. These patients should have routine immunizations. Quadrivalent meningococcal polysaccharide vaccine should be given to children 2 years of age and older. Older children who did not receive the conjugate pneumococcal vaccine should be immunized with either the conjugate or the polysaccharide vaccine.

Preterm Infants

The immune response to vaccination is a function of postnatal rather than gestational age. Prematurity does not increase the incidence of vaccine-related adverse events. Hence preterm infants, including those of very low birth weight, should be vaccinated at the same chronologic age as full-term infants and according to the routine childhood immunization schedule (see Figure 1). One exception to this recommendation is hepatitis B vaccination of infants of low birth weights (2 kg) who were born of hepatitis B surface antigen (HBsAg)-negative mothers. Initiation of vaccination in this case should be delayed until the infant is 1 month of age. Vaccine in conjunction with hepatitis B immunoglobulin (HBIG) should be given at birth to all preterm infants and infants of low birth weight born of HBsAg-positive mothers, but the vaccine dose is not counted in the completion of a three-dose primary hepatitis B vaccine schedule. The dose for preterm infants should not be reduced for any vaccine.

Household Members of Immunocompromised Hosts

The presence of immunosuppressed contacts in a patient's household is a contraindication only for oral polio vaccine (OPV), which is currently not recommended for routine use in the United States. MMR vaccine virus strains do not spread from recipients to contacts. Varicella vaccine can be administered to susceptible persons with immunosuppressed household contacts.

Foreign Travel

Children and adults traveling to foreign countries should have their routine recommended vaccination history reviewed and updated. In addition, they may require specific vaccines and chemoprophylaxis depending on the destination and type of travel (urban vs. rural, short vs. extended stays). Excellent sources of information include the current edition of the Red Book, Health Information for International Travel (the CDC Yellow Book), and the CDC website (http://www.cdc.gov/travel/index.htm).

Parents should be advised of state laws pertaining to school or child-care entry, which might require that unimmunized children stay home from school during outbreaks. Documentation of such discussions of risk in the child's record may help reduce any legal liability should an unimmunized child acquire a vaccine-preventable disease.

Passive Immunization

Passive immunization involves the administration of preformed antibodies given to prevent or treat infectious diseases. The different preparations include intramuscular immunoglobulin, intravenous immunoglobulin (IGIV), hyperimmune globulins (concentrations of specific antibody against a particular pathogen), monoclonal antibodies against a specific pathogen, and specific antitoxins (human and animal derived). Table 4 lists the names of the various products and indications.

In general, passive immunization is used for a variety of clinical conditions:

TABLE 4 Agents Used in Passive Immunity: Immune Globulins, Antibodies, and Antitoxins

Immunobiologic	Indication
For Intramuscular Administration	
Immune globulin (human)	Hepatitis A pre- and postexposure prophylaxis; measles postexposure prophylaxis
Hepatitis B immune globulin (human)	Hepatitis B postexposure prophylaxis
Rabies immune globulin (human)	Rabies postexposure management of people not previously immunized with rabies vaccine
Tetanus immune globulin (human)	Treatment of tetanus; postexposure prophylaxis of people not adequately immunized with tetanus toxoid
Varicella-zoster immune globulin (human)	Postexposure prophylaxis of susceptible immunocompromised people, certain susceptible pregnant women, and perinatally exposed newborn infants
Diphtheria antitoxin (equine)	Treatment of respiratory diphtheria
For Intravenous Administration	
Immune globulin intravenous (human)	Replacement therapy for antibody deficiency disorders; immune thrombocytopenic purpura; hypogammaglobulinemia in chronic lymphocytic leukemia; Kawasaki disease
Cytomegalovirus immune globulin intravenous (human) (CytoGam, MedImmune)	Prophylaxis for bone marrow and kidney transplant recipients
Botulinum antitoxin (human-derived botulism immune globulin intravenous) (BabyBIG, California Department of Health Services)	Treatment of botulism (Infant Botulism Treatment and Prevention Program, California Department of Health Services, 510–540–2646)
Humanized monoclonal antibody-palivizumab (Synagis, MedImmune)	Prophylaxis for high-risk children <2 yr of age against serious complications of respiratory syncytial virus (RSV) disease

BOX 1 Common Misconceptions and Concerns

- Measles, mumps, and rubella (MMR) vaccine and autism.
- Thimerosal and vaccines.
- Multiple immunizations and immune dysfunction.
- Hepatitis B vaccine and demyelination neurologic disorders.
- Simian virus–40 contamination of poliovirus vaccine and cancer.
- Vaccinations and sudden unexpected death.
- Influenza vaccine and neurologic complications.
- Diseases had already begun to disappear before vaccines were introduced because of better hygiene and sanitation.
- The majority of people who get disease are vaccinated.
- There are *hot lots* of vaccine associated with more adverse events and deaths than others. Parents should find the numbers of these lots and not allow their children to receive vaccines from them.
- Vaccines cause many harmful side effects, illnesses, and even death—not to mention possible unknown long-term effects.
- Vaccine-preventable diseases are virtually eliminated in the United States, so there is no need for my child to be vaccinated.
- Giving a child multiple vaccinations for different diseases at the same time increases the risk of harmful side effects and can overload the immune system.

- Treatment of primary and, in certain cases, secondary immunodeficiency.
- As prophylaxis against infections in high-risk patients exposed to certain diseases who have not been immunized against the disease in question and at high risk of severe complications. (e.g., a child with leukemia exposed to varicella or measles).
- Therapeutically, when a disease is already present, antibodies may help in suppressing the effects of a toxin (e.g., foodborne or wound botulism, diphtheria, or tetanus) or suppress the inflammatory response (e.g., Kawasaki syndrome).

Immunoglobulin preparations and other antibody-containing blood products do not interfere with the immune response to inactivated vaccines, but they do interfere with the antibody response to live vaccines, with the exception of oral typhoid and yellow fever vaccine. Because the immune response to a live vaccine occurs 1 to 2 weeks after vaccination, any immunoglobulin-containing product should be given 2 weeks after an MMR or 3 weeks after varicella vaccine. The time interval between administering an immunoglobulin-containing product and a live-virus vaccine appears to be dose dependent. The suggested time intervals are given in detail in the Red Book.

Communication and Counseling

ADDRESSING MISCONCEPTIONS AND CONCERNS

Concerns related to the safety of vaccines are becoming increasingly common. Many studies indicate that lower immunization rates in children are correlated with concern regarding vaccine-related side effects, superiority of natural immunity, and vaccine safety, confusing vaccination schedules, vaccine expense, religious objection to vaccination, and frequent illness in the child. Box 1 lists common parental concerns about vaccines. The CDC and National Institutes of Health Commissioned the National Academy of Sciences Institute of Medicine (IOM) to convene an Immunization Safety Review Committee. Details of this review can be found online (http://www.iom.edu/project.asp?id=4705). Overall, no studies establish a causal link between vaccines and the concerns just

TABLE 5 Selected Sources of Vaccine Information

Name	Website Address
American Academy of Family Physicians (AAFP)	www.familydoctor.org
American Academy of Pediatrics (AAP)	www.aap.org www.cispimmunize.org
American Medical Association (AMA)	www.ama-assn.org
Centers for Disease Control and Prevention (CDC)	www.cdc.gov/travel/vaccinat.htm
National Center for Infectious Diseases (NCID)	www.cdc.gov/ncidod
National Immunization Program (NIP)	www.cdc.gov/nip/publications
National Institute of Allergy and Infectious Diseases (NIAID)	www.niaid.nih.gov/dmid/vaccines
World Health Organization	www.who.int/vaccines
Allied Vaccine Group	www.vaccine.org
Immunization Action Coalition	www.immunize.org www.vaccineinformation.org

described. Health care professionals should discuss the specific concerns and provide factual information, using appropriate language. Effective, empathetic vaccine risk communication is essential in responding to misinformation and concerns, recognizing that for certain persons, risk assessment and decision making is difficult and confusing. Their concerns should then be addressed in the context of this information, using the VISs and offering other resource materials (e.g., information available on the National Immunization Program website).

PROVIDING SOURCES OF VACCINE INFORMATION

Numerous sources of information about vaccinations are available to practitioners and parents. Having good resources available for parents is increasingly important because growing numbers of parents in the United States have fears about vaccine side effects that, although generally scientifically unfounded, create resistance to having their children immunized. Table 5 lists a selection of these resources, including Internet sites.

SUGGESTED READINGS

1. American Academy of Pediatrics: Active and passive immunization. In Pickering LK (ed): Red Book: Report of the Committee on Infectious Diseases, 26th ed. Elk Grove Village, Ill: American Academy of Pediatrics, 2003, pp 1–98. **An excellent summary of pertinent infectious diseases in pediatrics with descriptions of clinical manifestations, etiology, epidemiology, diagnosis, treatment, and prevention of the disease.**
2. Cohn A, Broder K, Pickering L: Immunizations in the United States: A rite of passage. Pediatr Clin North Am 52:669–693, 2005. **Reviews the U.S. immunization program and highlights new vaccines and new vaccine recommendations.**
3. Maloney S, Weinberg M: Prevention of infectious diseases among international pediatric travelers: Considerations for clinicians. Semin Pediatr Infect Dis 15:137–149, 2004. **Offers concise information about vaccinations for pediatric travelers and other information to give to parents traveling with children.**
4. Marchant C. (guest ed): Pertussis: Increasing incidence and the need for booster vaccination in adolescents. Pediatric Infect Dis J, 24(Suppl. 6), 2005. **Contains several articles specifically about**

pertussis but also contains information that can be generalized to all vaccines about immunity, adverse events, and the economics of vaccine delivery.

Screening in the Newborn Nursery: Hearing Loss, Risk of Severe Hyperbilirubinemia, Congenital Heart Disease

Gautham K. Suresh and Lewis R. First

Screening for Hearing Loss

KEY CONCEPTS

- Hearing loss is present in 1 to 3 per 1000 newborns at birth and can also be acquired in the neonatal period. Risk factors include infections, use of aminoglycosides, hyperbilirubinemia, and neonatal intensive care.
- Universal screening of newborn infants for hearing loss is widespread in most developed countries to ensure early identification of hearing loss and timely intervention, thereby ensuring normal language development.
- Newborns should be screened prior to hospital discharge.
- Either evoked otoacoustic emissions (EOAE) or automated auditory brainstem responses (AABR) can be used for screening. Repeat testing of infants who fail the screen can reduce the number of false positives.
- Infants suspected to have hearing loss based on screening should be referred for detailed audiologic evaluation.
- Screening and follow-up programs should aim to detect all newborns with hearing loss by 3 months of age, and intervention such as amplification should be ensured by 6 months of age.

On average, 1 to 3 per 1000 newborns are born with hearing loss, which is genetic in origin (predominantly nonsyndromic) in approximately 50% of cases. Neonatal hearing loss can also result from exposure of a neonate to ototoxic factors such as aminoglycosides, high levels of bilirubin, hypoxia, meningitis, and cytomegalovirus infection. An estimated 2 to 4 per 100 newborns managed in the intensive care unit have hearing loss. Hearing loss that is undetected and untreated can result in permanent impairment of language development and have adverse social, academic, and vocational effects. Without early detection, the age of identification of neonatal hearing loss is as high as 18 to 30 months of age or greater. Early detection of neonatal hearing loss and intervention prior to 6 months of age increases the likelihood of normal language development in infants. To ensure such early detection and intervention, neonatal hearing screening is performed. The earlier practice of screening only neonates with risk factors can miss up to 50% of infants with hearing loss (Box 1). Therefore, universal neonatal hearing screening is now widespread in the United

States and other developed countries, with the goals of screening at least 95% of all newborns, universal detection of hearing loss before 3 months of age, and appropriate intervention by 6 months of age.

Expert Opinion on Management Issues

Hearing screening of newborns in the well infant nursery should be done prior to hospital discharge. The methodology used should detect all infants with significant bilateral hearing impairment (i.e., those with hearing loss more than 35 decibels in the better ear) and should not miss any infants with significant hearing loss (with a false-negative rate of zero). Two methods of screening can be used: evoked otoacoustic emissions (EOAE) and automated auditory brainstem responses (AABR). In EOAE, a small probe placed in the external ear canal records inaudible sounds produced in the cochlea in response to audible click or tone stimuli. With hearing loss, emissions are absent. EOAE screening is quicker and less expensive than AABR, but debris in the external ear or fluid in the external or middle ear can lead to false-positive results. It also can miss auditory nerve or brainstem auditory pathway dysfunction, especially with associated cochlear outer hair cell dysfunction. With AABR, electroencephalographic waves generated in response to audible clicks are recorded by scalp electrodes. With hearing loss the waves are diminished, absent, or delayed. This test is not affected by debris or fluid in the ear and is the preferred test when auditory neuropathy is a possibility, as in infants who are treated in the neonatal intensive care unit. It does require the infant to be quiet or asleep during testing.

With either method of testing, when an ear fails initial testing, retesting the same ear can decrease the incidence of false positives. Infants who fail the initial EOAE screen can be retested with EOAE or with AABR. Retesting of infants who initially undergo AABR screening should be with AABR. Infants who fail retesting should be referred for an audiologic evaluation for confirmation of hearing loss and assessment of its severity and type. The referral rate for audiologic testing after screening should not exceed 4%. The presence of risk factors for hearing loss (see Box 1) should lower the threshold for audiologic evaluation.

Common Pitfalls

- Inadvertent omission of hearing screening before hospital discharge
- Omission of testing in infants born at home
- Difficulty in scheduling infants for audiologic evaluation
- Lack of access to audiology services
- Lack of insurance coverage for audiologic evaluation and amplification
- Parental noncompliance with audiology appointments
- Parental noncompliance with therapeutic interventions, such as amplification

---

BOX 1 Risk Factors for Hearing Loss in Infants

- Family history of permanent childhood sensorineural hearing loss
- Infections
  - In utero fetal infection (e.g., cytomegalovirus, toxoplasmosis, rubella, syphilis, herpes)
  - Bacterial meningitis
  - Recurrent or persistent otitis media
- Perinatal hypoxia
  - Perinatal asphyxia
  - Persistent pulmonary hypertension
  - Extracorporeal membrane oxygenation
  - Severe respiratory distress
- Severe hyperbilirubinemia
- Malformations and syndromes
  - Craniofacial anomalies, including those with morphologic abnormalities of the pinna and ear canal
  - Syndromes and other congenital disorders known to include hearing loss
  - Conditions associated with progressive hearing loss: neurofibromatosis, osteopetrosis, Usher syndrome
- Neurodegenerative disorders, such as mucopolysaccharidoses, sensorimotor neuropathies
- Head trauma
- Intracranial hemorrhage
- Illness or condition requiring neonatal intensive care for 48 hours or longer
- Parental or caregiver concern regarding hearing, language, or general development

---

- In infants who have a normal newborn hearing screen, failure to realize that hearing loss can still be present or develop later.

All hospitals that deliver newborn infants should establish programs for universal newborn hearing screening that are responsible for developing a screening protocol, training staff, ensuring accurate screening technique, providing parental education and support, documenting and communicating the results of screening, and encouraging compliance with follow-up and intervention services. Regionwide, adequate health services should be developed so patients are not lost to follow-up, audiology services are available, and timely management is ensured in the form of amplification, early intervention, parental education, and, in selected cases, cochlear implants. Finally, in all infants with normal results on hearing screening prior to hospital discharge, parents and pediatric health care providers should remain vigilant for signs of hearing loss and impaired language development, especially if an infant has risk factors for hearing loss (see Box 1).

Communication and Counseling

Parental anxiety and stress can result when a newborn hearing screening test results in referral for diagnostic audiologic evaluation, especially in the period between referral and evaluation. Screening program personnel should minimize parental anxiety by reducing false-positive rates, ensuring adequate communication with parents, and conducting comprehensive, culturally sensitive counseling and education of parents. Some parents can have too little concern, which can result in noncompliance with follow-up appointments and with therapy.

Screening for Risk of Severe Unconjugated Hyperbilirubinemia

> ## KEY CONCEPTS
>
> - Physiologic jaundice is common and benign in newborn infants.
> - Severe neonatal hyperbilirubinemia can cause bilirubin encephalopathy, or kernicterus, resulting in neurodevelopmental disabilities.
> - Prevention of kernicterus requires identification of at-risk infants, parental education, adequate feeding, and timely institution of effective therapy, such as phototherapy.
> - Pregnant women and, when necessary, their babies, should be screened for the presence of hemolytic disorders such as Rh incompatibility and ABO (blood group system of groups A, AB, B, and O) incompatibility.
> - Glucose-6-phosphate dehydrogenase deficiency is an important cause of unconjugated neonatal hyperbilirubinemia.
> - All newborns should be assessed for risk factors for severe hyperbilirubinemia, such as hemolysis, onset of jaundice in the first 24 hours of life, cephalhematoma, East Asian race, and sibling with jaundice.
> - Visual inspection should not be relied on to assess the degree of jaundice. A serum or a transcutaneous bilirubin should be obtained.
> - All newborns should be evaluated by a health care provider within 48 hours of hospital discharge.

Jaundice occurs in approximately 60% of full-term healthy newborns and in most cases is physiologic and self-limiting. It results from:

- A high production of bilirubin (a product of heme catabolism) because of a high red cell mass and a short red cell life span in the neonate
- Immature mechanisms of bilirubin elimination (i.e., hepatocyte uptake and conjugation);
- Increased enterohepatic circulation in the neonate.

In rare cases, especially in the presence of conditions that cause a rapid or severe increase in bilirubin levels, the hyperbilirubinemia places the infant at risk for bilirubin encephalopathy, or kernicterus. Such conditions include hemolysis, extravascular blood collections, polycythemia, and sepsis. Two conditions particularly pose an increased risk of severe hyperbilirubinemia and are commonly under-recognized: mild prematurity (gestation of 35 to 36 weeks) and glucose-6-phosphate dehydrogenase (G6PD) deficiency. In addition, Gilbert syndrome is increasingly recognized as a cause of neonatal jaundice. Finally, suboptimal breast-feeding with dehydration in the first few days of life commonly predisposes to severe hyperbilirubinemia.

Although rare, cases of kernicterus continue to occur in the United States, and they usually result in lifelong severe neurodevelopmental disabilities or death.

Prevention of kernicterus requires early identification of infants at risk, proper parental education prior to newborn discharge, adequate feeding (preferably breast-feeding), and timely institution of effective treatment, such as phototherapy and exchange transfusion. A recent clinical practice guideline from the American Academy of Pediatrics (AAP) provides comprehensive recommendations for the management of hyperbilirubinemia in newborns of 35 or more weeks of gestation.

Expert Opinion on Management Issues

SCREENING FOR HEMOLYTIC DISORDERS

All pregnant women should be tested for ABO and Rh blood types and screened for unusual isoimmune antibodies. In the absence of such testing, or if the mother is Rh negative, the infant's umbilical cord blood should be sent for a direct Coombs test, blood type, and Rh type. Infants of mothers whose blood type is O and Rh positive need not routinely be tested for blood type or the Coombs test, provided other mechanisms are in place for timely identification and treatment of jaundice (discussed later).

RISK ASSESSMENT

After delivery and prior to hospital discharge, newborns should be inspected periodically for jaundice in adequate daylight. Because visual estimation of the degree of jaundice can be erroneous, a low threshold should be used to measure the total serum bilirubin. A total serum bilirubin should be checked in any infant who is jaundiced before 24 hours of life and in any infant whose jaundice seems excessive for age. Transcutaneous bilirubinometers can provide measurements that are within 2 to 3 mg/dL of the serum bilirubin, but their accuracy in patients with a bilirubin level above 15 mg/dL is not established. All infants should also be assessed for the presence of risk factors for development of severe hyperbilirubinemia (Box 2). Routine measurement of predischarge serum or transcutaneous bilirubin is used to assess risk before discharge, but the effectiveness and false-negative rate of this approach are not established, and it can lead to a significant increase in health care costs.

DISCHARGE PREPARATION AND FOLLOW-UP

Ensuring appropriate follow-up of the newborn after hospital discharge, either in a physician's office or with a home nurse visit, is critical. Newborns discharged before 24 hours of age should be seen by 72 hours, those discharged after 24 and before 48 hours should be seen by 96 hours, and those discharged between 48 and 72 hours should be seen by 120 hours. Earlier or more frequent follow-up should be provided for those who have risk factors (see Box 2). If the infant has risk factors and adequate follow-up cannot be ensured, delaying hospital discharge is prudent. At follow-up, the infant should be assessed for adequacy of intake, urine and stool output, weight change since birth, and jaundice. Again, visual assessment should not be relied on, and a low threshold should be used for measuring a serum or transcutaneous bilirubin.

BOX 2   Risk Factors for Development of Severe Hyperbilirubinemia in Infants of 35 or More Weeks' Gestation

- High serum or transcutaneous bilirubin level prior to discharge
- Jaundice observed before discharge, especially in the first 24 hours of life
- Evidence of possible hemolytic disease, such as blood group incompatibility, positive direct antiglobulin test, glucose-6-phosphate dehydrogenase (G6PD) deficiency, or other conditions
- Polycythemia
- Gestational age 38 weeks or less, especially if 35 to 36 weeks
- Previous sibling with jaundice, especially if phototherapy or exchange transfusion was required
- Cephalohematoma or significant cutaneous bruising
- Exclusive breast-feeding, particularly if baby is feeding poorly and losing excessive weight
- East Asian maternal race
- Macrosomic infant of a diabetic mother
- Maternal age 25 years or greater
- Male gender
- Maternal oxytocin therapy

Management of Hyperbilirubinemia

Figure 1 provides the recommended bilirubin levels for institution of phototherapy in infants of different risk categories. Intensive phototherapy should be used when the total serum bilirubin exceeds the indicated level for each category. The risk factors listed in Figure 1 are conditions that can increase the risk of bilirubin encephalopathy by altering albumin binding of bilirubin, the blood–brain barrier, and the susceptibility of the brain cells to bilirubin-induced damage. Infants who are started on phototherapy and those whose bilirubin is rapidly rising without an obvious cause should undergo laboratory testing for the cause of hyperbilirubinemia and the assessment of risk. Tests to be considered, if not already done, are blood type, Coombs test, complete blood count, peripheral blood smear, reticulocyte count, G6PD levels, serum albumin, and direct bilirubin. Infants with an elevated direct bilirubin should undergo urinalysis and urine culture, and, if suggestive clinical features are present, they should be evaluated for sepsis. Exchange transfusion is recommended in any infant with significant hyperbilirubinemia who has signs of acute bilirubin encephalopathy or if the total serum bilirubin level is more than 25 mg/dL. The threshold for exchange transfusion is lowered in the presence of factors that increase the risk of bilirubin encephalopathy (see Figure 1) and if the infant is younger than 96 hours of age. In isoimmune

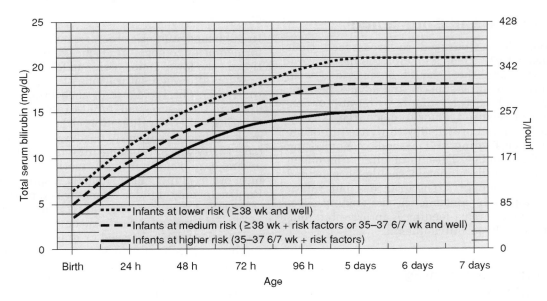

- Use total bilirubin. Do not subtract direct reacting or conjugated bilirubin.
- Risk factors: isoimmune hemolytic disease, G6PD deficiency, asphyxia, significant lethargy, temperature instability, sepsis, acidosis, or albumin <3.0 g/dL (if measured).
- For well infants 35–37 6/7 wk can adjust TSB levels for intervention around the medium risk line. It is an option to intervene at lower TSB levels for infants closer to 35 wks and at higher TSB levels for those closer to 37 6/7 wk.
- It is an option to provide conventional phototherapy in hospital or at home at TSB levels 2–3 mg/dL (35–50 mmol/L) below those shown, but home phototherapy should not be used in any infant with risk factors.

FIGURE 1. Guidelines for phototherapy in hospitalized infants of 35 or more weeks' gestation. G6PD, glucose–6-phosphate dehydrogenase; TSB, total serum bilirubin. (From American Academy of Pediatrics Clinical Practice Guideline: Subcommittee on Hyperbilirubinemia. Management of hyperbilirubinemia in the newborn infant 35 or more weeks of gestation. Pediatrics 114:297–316, 2004. Used with permissinon of the American Acadamy of Pediatrics.)

hemolytic disease, intravenous immunoglobulin therapy is recommended if the total serum bilirubin is rising despite phototherapy or it is approaching a level requiring an exchange transfusion.

Common Pitfalls

- Failure to identify risk factors for severe hyperbilirubinemia prior to hospital discharge can place the infant at risk for severe hyperbilirubinemia.
- Failure to provide adequate parental education about jaundice prior to discharge (discussed later) can also be dangerous. With current newborn discharge practices, the parents are often the primary persons to observe and assess jaundice in their newborn.
- Failure to follow up on newborns adequately after hospital discharge is a major cause of delays in identification and treatment of severe hyperbilirubinemia.
- Parental lack of access to health care providers, particularly on weekends, can lead to delays in assessment and treatment.
- Delays can occur in health care providers responding to parental concern about jaundice, in scheduling office appointments, in the evaluation of infants in emergency rooms, and in the institution of phototherapy or exchange transfusion.

Communication and Counseling

Mothers should be encouraged to breast-feed their infants at least 8 to 12 times a day for the first several days after birth, and they should be provided with appropriate breast-feeding support and advice. Routine supplementation of breast-fed infants with water or dextrose water is not required. Prior to discharge, parents should be educated and provided with written information about jaundice, feeding, and methods of monitoring the newborn for jaundice. Parents of infants managed for significant hyperbilirubinemia should be provided with psychological support, reassurance about infant bonding, and support for continued breast-feeding, especially in cases where breast-feeding is interrupted temporarily to decrease hyperbilirubinemia.

Pulse Oximetry Screening for Neonatal Congenital Cardiovascular Malformations

KEY CONCEPTS

- Critical congenital cardiovascular malformations occur in 2.7 per 1000 live births and are often undetected until after discharge home.
- Routine pulse oximetry of newborns prior to hospital discharge can potentially lead to early identification and treatment of such lesions and decreased neonatal mortality and morbidity.

- In published studies, 1% of newborns or less had low postductal oxygen saturations (ranging from less than 90% to less than 95%) and were evaluated by echocardiograms. Almost all had a congenital cardiovascular malformation. Some had significant noncardiac disorders.
- Although pulse oximetry screening is promising, further research is required to establish its effectiveness in improving neonatal outcomes and its feasibility in nonacademic medical centers, before it can be recommended.

The incidence of critical congenital cardiovascular malformations is 2.7 per 1000 live births. A significant number of newborn infants continue to die from undetected congenital heart disease or suffer morbidity from its late detection. Findings suggestive of congenital heart disease may be missed or absent on routine newborn examination prior to hospital discharge. With the current practice of discharging newborns prior to 48 to 72 hours of life, symptoms and signs of heart disease commence after discharge, at home. Thus routine screening of newborns prior to hospital discharge for the presence of a critical congenital cardiovascular malformation has the potential to decrease neonatal mortality and morbidity. Routine fetal or neonatal echocardiography is expensive and not widely available, so pulse oximetry is being tested as a screening tool for congenital heart disease prior to newborn hospital discharge.

Expert Opinion on Management Issues

In published studies, screening pulse oximetry was performed prior to hospital discharge in a postductal location on the lower limbs. Criteria for failure ranged from postductal oxygen saturations of less than 90% to less than 95%. The incidence of such failures ranged from 0.04% to 1% of screened infants. Infants with low oxygen saturation were evaluated by echocardiograms and almost all had a congenital cardiovascular malformation (specificity was 99%). Some infants with low saturations and no cardiovascular malformation were discovered to have other significant (primarily respiratory) disorders. Routine neonatal pulse oximetry is a promising screening method to ensure the detection and early treatment of critical congenital cardiovascular malformations that might otherwise be missed or diagnosed late. However, further research is required to demonstrate its effectiveness in reducing neonatal morbidity and mortality, as well as its feasibility in nonacademic centers before widespread implementation.

Common Pitfalls

Routine pulse oximetry does not detect all cases of neonatal congenital heart disease and can miss newborns with acyanotic lesions (sensitivity was 50% to 60% in published studies). This emphasizes the continued need for a careful physical examination of the newborn prior to discharge, in a quiet environment under good lighting, to detect signs such as cyanosis, hyperdynamic precordium, abnormal intensity of the second heart sound, wide splitting of the second heart sound, single second heart sound, cardiac murmurs, diminished or absent femoral pulses, and the presence of noncardiac anomalies associated with congenital heart disease. In centers with easily available pediatric cardiology services, newborns with abnormal pulse oximetry readings can undergo echocardiography relatively quickly to confirm or rule out congenital heart disease. However, performing routine pulse oximetry in centers without readily available pediatric cardiology support can lead to dilemmas about transferring the newborn to a tertiary center for echocardiography, with the associated logistic difficulties of transfer.

Communication and Counseling

Parental education prior to newborn discharge should include instructions to call the primary care physician if the newborn does not feed well, develops respiratory distress, is lethargic, cries excessively, becomes blue, or develops other signs of heart disease. Although many newborns evaluated for heart disease have benign heart lesions, such as a ventricular septal defect or a patent foramen ovale, the possibility of serious heart disease can cause significant parental anxiety during the process of cardiac evaluation. Adequate counseling and support should be provided to parents during this phase.

SUGGESTED READINGS

1. American Academy of Pediatrics Clinical Practice Guideline: Management of hyperbilirubinemia in the newborn infant 35 or more weeks of gestation. Pediatrics 114:297–316, 2004. **Comprehensive recommendations for risk assessment and management of neonatal jaundice.**
2. Barratt A, Irwig L, Glasziou P, et al: Users' guides to the medical literature: XVII. How to use guidelines and recommendations about screening. Evidence-Based Medicine Working Group. JAMA 281 (21):2029–2034, 1999. **Describes how to evaluate the usefulness of screening tests and programs rationally and critically.**
3. Dennery PA, Seidman DS, Stevenson DK: Neonatal hyperbilirubinemia. N Engl J Med 344(8):581–590, 2001. **Review of neonatal jaundice.**
4. Kenna MA: Neonatal hearing screening. Pediatr Clin North Am 50:301–313, 2003. **Overview and description of evolution of universal hearing screening.**
5. Keren R, Helfand M, Homer C, et al: Projected cost-effectiveness of statewide universal newborn hearing screening. Pediatrics 110 (5):855–864, 2002. **Provides estimates of costs and emphasizes need for timely intervention prior to 6 months of age.**
6. Koppel RI, Druschel CM, Carter T, et al: Effectiveness of pulse oximetry screening for congenital heart disease in asymptomatic newborns. Pediatrics 111(3):451–455, 2003. **Provides estimates of number of cases of congenital heart disease detected by routine pulse oximetry screening of newborns.**
7. Maisels MJ, Newman TB: Jaundice in full-term and near-term babies who leave the hospital within 36 hours. Clin Perinatol 25:295–302, 1998. **Discussion of how problems with newborn follow-up after discharge place infants at risk for severe hyperbilirubinemia.**
8. Suresh GK, Clark RE: Cost-effectiveness of strategies that are intended to prevent kernicterus in newborn infants. Pediatrics 114:917–924, 2004. **Describes the cost implications and uncertainties involved in routine predischarge bilirubin testing.**
9. Thompson DC, McPhillips H, Davis RL, et al: Universal newborn hearing screening: Summary of evidence. JAMA 286:2000–2010, 2001. **Summary of the literature on universal newborn hearing screening.**
10. White KR: Early hearing detection and intervention programs: Opportunities for genetic services. Am J Med Genet 130A:29–36, 2004. **Describes the genetic and syndromic causes of hearing loss and management implications.**

2

Emergencies

Neonatal Seizures

R. Victoria Chen and Jeffrey M. Perlman

KEY CONCEPTS

- Neonatal seizures differ from those in the older child, often manifesting with subtle activity.
- The most frequent cause of neonatal seizures is hypoxia-ischemia.
- No consistent relationship exists between clinical and electroencephalogram (EEG) seizures; approximately 30% to 50% of neonatal seizures are expressed as EEG seizures only.
- There is a lack of consensus regarding the appropriate treatment of EEG seizures.
- Phenobarbital remains the initial anticonvulsant of choice.
- Duration of anticonvulsant therapy depends on the cause of the seizures, the neurologic examination, and the interictal EEG.

Neonatal seizures are poorly classified phenomena that often suggest underlying neurologic disease in the newborn. The presentation differs from that in the older child and can be difficult to recognize as well as treat. Thus neonates are unable to sustain generalized tonic-clonic activity; rather, the manifestations are often subtle (i.e., oral-buccal-lingual movements). The latter may be secondary to relatively advanced cortical development in limbic structures and the connections to the diencephalons and the brainstem. It is only after programmed synaptogenesis, apoptosis, and myelination have progressed that classical adult-type seizures are observed.

Classification

The diagnosis of seizures in neonates can be challenging and should include both clinical and electrographic criteria for diagnosis. Clinical subtypes originally described by Volpe (Table 1) include subtle seizures, clonic seizures categorized as focal or multifocal, tonic seizures categorized as focal or generalized, and myoclonic seizures. More current classifications focus on the association of the clinical events just described with an electroencephalographic (EEG) correlate of seizures, and they group them as follows: clinical seizures without EEG seizures, electroclinical dissociation (i.e., the same clinical events occurring with or without electrographic seizures), and electroclinical seizures (i.e., electrographic seizures without clinical accompaniments). Indeed, studies indicate that from 30% to 50% are expressed only as EEG seizures, particularly in infants paralyzed for ventilatory control or those receiving antiepileptic medications.

Etiology

The etiology is multifactorial, but most commonly seizures result from hypoxic-ischemic injury. Indeed, 50%

TABLE 1 Relationship between Clinical Seizures and Simultaneous EEG Findings

Type of Seizure	Clinical Manifestation	EEG Findings	Origin
Subtle seizure	Bicycling, lip smacking, apnea, eye deviations, staring, chewing, tongue thrusting	Typically no EEG correlation unless associated with tonic eye deviations.	Subcortical
Clonic seizure	Nonordered clonic movements that may be focal or multifocal	EEG rhythmic seizure activity.	Cortical
Tonic seizure	Tonic extension of all limbs that may be generalized or focal (i.e., eye deviation)	Focal seizures usually have EEG correlation.	Cortical
Myoclonic seizure	Single or multiple jerks of flexion of upper or lower limbs	May or may not have EEG correlation.	Cortical

EEG, electroencephalogram.

to 60% of all neonatal seizures are related to this mechanism. Other less-common etiologies include neonatal stroke or focal cerebral infarction; intracranial hemorrhage, including subarachnoid, intraventricular, or intraparenchymal hemorrhage; metabolic disorders, including hypocalcemia, hypomagnesemia, or hypoglycemia; central nervous system infections; brain malformations; drug withdrawal; and in some cases no cause that can be delineated.

Evaluation

The evaluation of a neonate suspected of seizures should include a clinical assessment, video EEG recording, metabolic evaluation (i.e., determination of calcium, magnesium, glucose levels, spinal tap, if clinically indicated, neuroimaging (i.e., cranial sonogram, usually useful as a screen), CT scan, and MRI. Additional studies depend on specific clinical findings.

Expert Opinion on Management Issues

The purpose of treating neonatal seizures is to prevent recurrence and consequently minimize the pathophysiologic and metabolic abnormalities provoked by this process. Controversy persists with respect to when and for how long to treat the neonate with seizures. Some advocate treatment when clinical seizures are recognized but believe that brief electrographic seizures do not routinely require intervention. As an alternative strategy, others argue that the experimental evidence of long-term deleterious effects of repetitive electrographic seizures on brain structure demands a more aggressive approach, that is, the elimination of all EEG seizures. This approach can require very high anticonvulsant levels that may sedate the infant and interfere with neurologic assessment, as well as compromise cardiorespiratory status.

The single most important factor in determining treatment of neonatal seizures relates to the underlying etiology of the event. Thus, if there is an identified metabolic disturbance, such as hypoglycemia or hypocalcemia, the prompt correction of the abnormality should eliminate the seizures. If correction of the metabolic disturbance does stop the seizures, antiepileptic medications may be required.

Phenobarbital and phenytoin remain the most widely prescribed anticonvulsants for the initial treatment of neonatal seizures (Table 2). If seizures persist, 20 mg/kg of phenobarbital should be administered intravenously (IV) over 10 to 15 minutes. This dose is necessary to achieve a blood level of 20 µg/mL, a level that clearly exhibits measurable anticonvulsant effect in the neonate. If seizures persist, additional 5 mg/kg boluses should be administered every 5 minutes until a maximum dose of 40 mg/kg is reached or all clinical and EEG seizures cease. This is followed by a daily maintenance dose of 3 to 4 mg/kg initiated 12 to 24 hours after the loading dose is given. In neonates, the half-life of phenobarbital ranges from 40 to 175 hours. The variation can be explained in part on the basis of hepatic metabolism, such as p-hydroxylation of the phenyl ring and renal elimination enhanced in alkaline urine. Both weight and gestational age do not appear to influence the blood level appreciably. To achieve comparable blood levels when given intramuscularly, the dose needs to be increased by 10% to 15%. Although there is no agreed-on therapeutic level, in

TABLE 2 Anticonvulsants to Treat Neonatal Seizures

Anticonvulsants	Dose/Route	Side Effect	Other
Phenobarbital	Loading dose: 20 mg/kg IV given slowly over 10 to 15 min Refractory seizures: Additional 5 mg/kg doses up to a total of 40 mg/kg Maintenance: 3 to 4 mg/kg/day, beginning 12 to 24 hr after the load	Sedation at serum concentration 40 µg/mL. Respiratory depression: >60 µg/mL.	Therapeutic serum concentration 15–40 µg/mL; half-life: 45–175 h
Phenytoin	Loading dose: 15 to 20 mg/kg IV infusion over 30 min Maintenance: 4–8 mg/kg every 12–24 hr via slow IV infusion	Bradycardia, arrhythmia, and hypotension during rapid infusion. Tissue inflammation and necrosis, with extravasations.	Incompatible in dextrose-containing solutions; infusion should be >0.5 mg/kg/h
Lorazepam	Dose: 0.05 to 0.1 mg/kg per dose via slow infusion; repeat doses are based on the clinical response	Respiratory depression.	Half-life: ~40 hr
Diazepam	Dose load: 0.5 mg/kg Refractory seizures: Continuous infusion: 0.3 mg/kg/h	Respiratory depression Displacement of bilirubin from albumin	

IV, intravenous.

general the target is between 15 and 40 µg/mL. Respiratory depression is usually not observed until serum concentrations reach 60 µg/mL. The efficacy of phenobarbital in the treatment of clinical seizures relates to the primary process causing the seizures (ranging from 45% to 85%); consequently, a second antiepileptic medication sometimes needs to be added. When initiating a second agent, approximately 30% of phenobarbital is protein bound, and concurrent use of other antiepileptic medications (particularly phenytoin and valproate) may increase serum concentrations. When single therapy with phenobarbital is not sufficient, a second medication, usually phenytoin or fosphenytoin, is added. The loading dose of phenytoin is 15 to 20 mg/kg IV over at least 30 minutes to avoid cardiovascular side effects that can occur when administered rapidly. Thus bradycardia, arrhythmias, and hypotension may be seen if the infusion rate is greater than 0.5 mg/kg/minute. A maintenance dose of 4 to 8 mg/kg is administered 24 hours after the loading dose. Fosphenytoin, a phosphate ester prodrug of phenytoin, has major advantages to the newborn because it is an aqueous solution that is soluble in glucose-containing solutions, and thus it can be administered more quickly than phenytoin without causing soft-tissue necrosis. Maintenance therapy for both medications is difficult to achieve consistently because of nonlinear kinetics and rapid decrease in elimination rates in the first weeks of life. Hence the therapeutic range is 6 to 15 µg/mL in the first few weeks of life and increases to 10 to 20 µg/mL thereafter. The serum half-life is 18 to 60 hours, and 85% to 90% of phenytoin is protein bound.

If the infant has seizures refractory to the antiepileptic medications just listed, a benzodiazepine should be considered. Both lorazepam and diazepam are used for this purpose. Both enter the brain very rapidly and produce an anticonvulsant effect within 5 minutes. But lorazepam is less lipophilic than diazepam and thus does not redistribute from the brain as rapidly. The duration of action is generally from 3 to 24 hours. Lorazepam has a long half-life of approximately 40 hours in the asphyxiated term neonate. The effective dose is 0.05 mg/kg to 0.1 mg/kg repeated based on the clinical response. The recommended initial IV dose of diazepam is 0.5 mg/kg, although the drug is most effective as a continuous IV infusion.

Additional anticonvulsants used in the neonate with refractory seizures include primidone, lidocaine, valproic acid, and carbamazepine.

Duration of Therapy

The optimal duration of therapy of the infant with seizures should be based on the likelihood of recurrence of seizures should the anticonvulsants be discontinued. Discontinuation of the medications prior to discharge should be a goal. Three factors need to be considered in this decision-making process: the neonatal neurologic examination, the cause of the seizures, and the interictal EEG. If the neurologic examination is abnormal at discharge, the risk for recurrent seizures is approximately 50%, whereas it is very low with a normal examination.

The cause of the seizures is highly relevant to the risk for recurrences (i.e., the risk following hypoxia ischemia is approximately 30%, whereas it is almost universal with migrational defects) and almost never follows hypocalcemic-related seizures. The interictal EEG is a valuable adjunct in determining the risk of recurrence. Thus if the pattern is normal, the risk for recurrence is rare, whereas it is up to 40% in an infant whose EEG shows marked suppression of activity.

If the decision is made to discontinue therapy, phenytoin and other second-line antiepileptic medications are usually stopped first. This is followed by weaning of phenobarbital, which can be accomplished over a period of a few weeks.

Communication and Counseling

Parents need to be educated about duration and discontinuation of therapy (see earlier) as well as the prognosis following neonatal seizures. The latter appears to be related to two major factors. The first is linked to the neuropathologic process that underlies the seizures. Thus the potential for normal outcome for infants with seizures secondary to hypoxia-ischemia is approximately 50%, whereas it is invariably favorable following seizures related to a subarachnoid hemorrhage, and it is universally poor for infants with developmental defects. The second is linked to the interictal EEG. Thus with a normal EEG the outcome is favorable; when there is a burst suppression pattern, the outcome is always unfavorable.

SUGGESTED READINGS

1. Holmes GL, Gairsa JL, Chevassus-Au-Louis N, Ben-Ari Y: Consequences of neonatal seizures in the rat: Morphological and behavioral effects. Ann Neurol 44:845–857, 1998. **This study demonstrates that recurrent brief seizures during the neonatal period have long-term detrimental effects on behavior, seizure susceptibility, and brain development.**
2. Mizrahi EM, Kellaway P: Characterization and classification of neonatal seizures. Neurology 37:1837–1847, 1987. **This study points out the inconsistency between clinical and electrographic seizures.**
3. Painter MJ, Scher MS, Stein AD, et al: Phenobarbital compared with phenytoin for the treatment of neonatal seizures. N Engl J Med 341:485–489, 1999. **This study compares phenobarbital versus phenytoin in the treatment of neonatal seizures. Seizures were controlled in 43% of 30 neonates assigned to receive phenobarbital and 45% of 29 neonates assigned to receive phenytoin. When combined treatment was considered, seizure control was achieved in 57% of the neonates assigned to receive phenobarbital first and 62% of those assigned to receive phenytoin first. The severity of the seizures was a stronger predictor of the success of treatment than was the assigned agent.**
4. Scher MS, Aso K, Beggarly ME, et al: Electrographic seizures in preterm and full term neonates: Clinical correlates, associated brain lesions and risk for neurologic sequelae. Pediatrics 91:128–134, 1993. **This study shows that electrographic seizures are more common than electroclinical seizures in both preterm and term infants.**
5. Volpe JJ: Neonatal seizures. In Volpe JJ (ed): Neurology of the Newborn, 4th ed. Philadelphia: WB Saunders, 2001, pp 178–214. **This chapter reviews the causes of seizures, the debate of who to treat, and the current treatment approach, including duration of therapy.**

3

Status Epilepticus

Christian M. Korff and Douglas R. Nordli, Jr.

KEY CONCEPTS

- Status epilepticus (SE) is an important neurologic emergency, common in childhood.
- Its definition and classification are subject to controversy.
- The most important determinant of outcome is etiology.
- The management of SE relies on general resuscitation measures and the use of a benzodiazepine as first-choice medication.
- Current thought is leading toward the rapid use of general anesthesia after the failure of two agents.
- Treatment should be initiated as soon as possible.

Status epilepticus (SE) is a potentially fatal condition, common in childhood. The International League against Epilepsy (ILAE) defines it as "a seizure that persists for a sufficient length of time or is repeated frequently enough that recovery between attacks does not occur." Most authors consider 30 minutes as the necessary duration to establish SE, based on observations that neuronal damage occurs in certain animal models at a later point.

The application of this rationale to humans is questioned by others, who consider the relation between the duration of the seizure and neuronal damage in humans complex and believe that this conclusion is lacking in convincing data. It seems clear that neuronal injury, systemic complications, and mortality increase dramatically after 1 to 2 hours of seizure activity, and treatment is aimed at preventing these complications. The time at which the benefits of treatment outweigh its own risks remains unknown.

Considering these observations and the fact that the overall duration of secondary generalized seizures rarely exceeds 5 minutes, Lowenstein and colleagues propose an operational definition of generalized convulsive SE in adults and in children older than 5 years. These authors diagnose SE if a seizure lasts continuously for more than 5 minutes or if two or more seizures occur over 5 minutes or more without complete recovery of consciousness. They excluded younger children from this definition because conclusive data regarding seizure duration for this group were missing.

A prospective study of 407 children, 1 month to 19 years of age with a first unprovoked seizure, showed that seizures lasted more than 5 minutes in 50% of cases and more than 30 minutes in 12% of cases. The likelihood of a seizure stopping spontaneously decreased after 5 minutes and was minimal after 15 minutes. These data support the initiation of treatment after 5 to 10 minutes and the current definition of SE in childhood as seizure activity lasting more than 30 minutes.

Expert Opinion on Management Issues

CLASSIFICATION

Classifying SE into different subtypes can help its management (Table 1). An ideal classification would precisely define groups of patients with SE who could be managed similarly. The usual subdivision is based on clinical and electrographic findings, and it separates SE into convulsive and nonconvulsive, generalized and partial categories. This classification is controversial because important prognostic factors, such as etiology and age, are not considered, and by grouping diverse conditions under the heading of nonconvulsive status epilepticus (NCSE), specificity is sacrificed. For example, absence SE usually has a good prognosis (and responds to treatment), whereas myoclonic SE has a poor prognosis and is often refractory to treatment. Attempts to include these aspects in a revised form of classification of SE have been made but remain to be approved. As with the previously described issues regarding the definition of SE, this lack of uniformity in its classification reflects the limited understanding of the pathophysiologic mechanisms underlying this condition.

Convulsive Status Epilepticus

Convulsive status epilepticus (CSE) is characterized by continuous or repeated jerks of the extremities. Generalized convulsive status epilepticus (GCSE) implies loss of consciousness and generalized abnormal features on the electroencephalogram (EEG). Partial convulsive status epilepticus (PCSE) applies to the cases in which the convulsive activity is confined to one side of the body and does not imply a complete alteration of the state of consciousness; the EEG shows epileptiform activity on the contralateral side of the brain. Myoclonic status epilepticus (MSE) is a rare presentation of SE that can be observed in patients with conditions such as juvenile myoclonic epilepsy, progressive myoclonic epilepsy, Dravet syndrome (severe myoclonic epilepsy of infancy), myoclonic-astatic epilepsy (as described by Doose), or Angelman syndrome, among others. MSE in patients with coma is usually associated with acute anoxic, toxic, or metabolic damage.

A small proportion of pediatric patients develop refractory status epilepticus (RSE) despite adequate initial

TABLE 1 Types of Status Epilepticus

- Convulsive
- Generalized
- Partial
- Myoclonic
- Nonconvulsive
- Typical absence
- Complex partial
- In patients with learning difficulties
- In patients with coma

treatment. Twenty-two such children were identified over an 8-year period at Children's Hospital in Boston. It is generally agreed that the longer the seizure lasts, the more difficult it is to treat.

Nonconvulsive Status Epilepticus

NCSE consists of very heterogeneous syndromes observed in ambulatory as well as in comatose patients. It is defined as "an epileptic state lasting more than 30 minutes with some clinically evident change in mental status or behavior from baseline and ictal activity on EEG" (Brenner, 2002). Walker divided it into the following four entities:

1. Typical absence SE, characterized by prolonged absence attacks and 3-Hz spike and waves in patients with generalized epilepsy
2. Complex partial SE, defined as a prolonged confusional state with variable clinical symptoms and recurrent focal electrographic epileptiform discharges originating in any cortical region
3. Nonconvulsive SE in patients with learning difficulties, including those with electrical status epilepticus during sleep (ESES), such as in Landau-Kleffner syndrome; atypical absence SE; and tonic SE, mostly observed in patients with Lennox-Gastaut syndrome
4. Nonconvulsive SE in coma, which sometimes follows CSE

Other classification proposals are based on the level of consciousness of the patient, as follows: "minimally impaired with the patient able to talk, and interactive; lethargic, but following commands; comatose" (Kaplan, 2000). This latter classification is more easily applied to daily use, but a definite consensus remains to be found.

The diagnosis of NCSE is difficult, regardless of its presentation, and it strongly relies on EEG findings. These can be confusing, and there is disagreement on the origin of several electrographic patterns that can be observed in comatose patients, such as triphasic waves or periodic lateralized epileptiform discharges (PLEDs). According to several authors, the definition of NCSE should therefore include "unequivocal electrographic seizure activity, rhythmic electrographic discharges with clinical seizures, and clinical or electrographic response to treatment" (Walker, 2003).

ETIOLOGY

An estimated 33% to 62% of pediatric patients do not have a prior history of epilepsy at the time of their first episode of SE. According to a large prospective epidemiologic study, the etiologies most often associated with SE in childhood were infection with fever (52% of the pediatric cases); chronic central nervous system (CNS) disorder (39%); and noncompliance with antiepileptic drugs (AEDs) (21%) in epileptic patients. Stroke, metabolic disturbances, and hypoxic brain injuries were also observed but less frequently. No etiology was found in 4% of the pediatric cases.

MORBIDITY AND MORTALITY

After a certain time, CSE provokes neurologic and systemic effects. Initial systemic effects include low pH, high plasmatic lactate and glucose levels, high blood pressure, and tachycardia. In its second phase, temperature elevation and respiratory compromise can be observed. Potential causes for death include cardiac arrhythmias, high pulmonary vascular pressure resulting in pulmonary edema, rhabdomyolysis, and renal insufficiency. Most of these complications are usually attributed to the elevation of plasmatic catecholamines found during SE. Damage to the brain after SE is demonstrated in animal studies. Cerebral edema and neuronal cell death are the major concerns. Importantly, most adverse neuronal effects were observed in the absence of systemic complications (which were experimentally controlled), understating the possibility of direct brain damage by seizure activity itself, such as in NCSE. This was also suggested by the demonstration that neuron-specific enolase, a marker of neuronal damage in humans, was elevated in blood and cerebrospinal fluid (CSF) in patients with subclinical electrographic SE.

SE is estimated to cause between 22,000 and 42,000 deaths per year in the United States, most often because of the systemic effects previously discussed. Overall, the mortality rate is much lower in children than in adults (3% to 4%). The most important determinant of outcome of SE is etiology. Acute symptomatic SE carries much higher morbidity and mortality rates than SE occurring in epileptic or in febrile nonepileptic patients. In children, hypoxic/anoxic events, encephalitis, cerebral hemorrhage, stroke, or CNS toxins are associated with a poor prognosis. In two series (Sillanpaa, et al., and Maytal, et al.), almost all pediatric deaths were observed in children with severe underlying neurologic disabilities or acute symptomatic etiologies. In the latter study, the duration of seizure activity was a determinant of outcome only in the acute symptomatic group. Moreover, neither deaths nor neurologic sequelae were observed in children with unprovoked or febrile SE, whatever their duration. Thus, more than a specific isolated factor, it is the combination of an injured brain and prolonged seizure activity that seems to be the primary determinant for morbidity and mortality in SE. Accordingly, refractory status epilepticus (RSE) in childhood carries a particularly bad prognosis. The mortality rate was 32% in a series of 22 children, and none of the survivors returned to baseline, all but one of them having developed intractable epilepsy. The children who had the worst prognosis were the very young, which also reflected the fact that symptomatic etiologies were more frequently diagnosed in this group. Long-term neurologic sequelae occur in up to 57% of pediatric patients with RSE, according to a meta-analysis, and consist mainly of cognitive or motor dysfunction.

In the series by Maytal and colleagues, one third of patients with SE developed subsequent epilepsy, and 9.1% of patients had new motor or cognitive deficits following SE. The risk for subsequent seizures, therefore, is not higher than if the first seizure was short. The incidence of new deficits was a function of age, with most sequelae occurring in the youngest patients. Again, the age only reflected the underlying etiology because most of these patients belonged to the acute symptomatic group or had a progressive encephalopathy. Controversial data exist regarding possible brain damage, particularly mesial temporal sclerosis caused by prolonged febrile seizures. Studies of the cause and effect between mesial temporal sclerosis and febrile SE are in progress.

The prognosis of NCSE depends on its diagnostic subtype. As mentioned, comatose patients with continuous electrical epileptic activity have a very poor prognosis because of their severe underlying condition. However, some types of NCSE, including absence status, cause no cognitive sequelae. ESES is associated with cognitive decline in a certain number of children diagnosed with Landau-Kleffner syndrome, which can persist even when seizures are controlled and EEG features have normalized.

TREATMENT OF CONVULSIVE STATUS EPILEPTICUS

The goals of SE management apply to both partial and generalized forms and can be summarized as cardiopulmonary and temperature stabilization, termination of seizure activity and identification of a possible underlying etiology, prevention of seizure recurrences, and minimizing treatment-related morbidity (Table 2). For practical reasons, it is recommended that treatment be started after 5 minutes of seizure activity.

Benzodiazepines are the first-line medications for CSE. They penetrate the brain rapidly and almost immediately activate the γ-aminobutyric acid (GABA)-mediated inhibitor system. Their efficacy is recognized in numerous studies. Potential side effects include sedation, respiratory depression, and cardiovascular compromise, but their safety as prehospital treatment for SE

was demonstrated in adults and in children. When intravenous (IV) access is available, lorazepam is the agent of choice and usually administered as 0.1 mg per kg at a rate of 2 mg per minute. When compared to IV diazepam, IV lorazepam showed a similar efficacy, safety, and cost profile but a lower seizure recurrence rate. Rectal diazepam gel can be used when IV access is not available. This route of administration is safe and rapidly effective. It can be used by parents and other caregivers, such as teachers and paramedics. Recommended doses are 0.5 mg/kg/dose for patients 2 to 5 years of age, 0.3 mg/kg/dose for patients 6 to 11 years of age, and 0.2 mg per kg for patients older than 12 years, to a maximum of 20 mg. Fosphenytoin or phenytoin should be administered next in sequence, particularly if SE has not stopped. In patients who respond to treatment with a benzodiazepine, a load of phenytoin or fosphenytoin need not automatically follow. In particular, those patients known to have epilepsy and already taking medication may not need an additional IV medication if status stabilizes following benzodiazepine treatment. In many such cases, it is more efficient, effective, and safe simply to give an additional or supplemental dose of the patient's routine medication. Fosphenytoin is preferred whenever available. It is a phosphorylated precursor of phenytoin and can be administered via IV or intramuscularly (IM). Fosphenytoin is water soluble and has a normal pH that allows more rapid administration with less vein irritation, less risk of necrosis with extravasation, and less hypotension. Phenytoin should not be mixed with glucose/dextrose and should not be given IM. Potential systemic side effects include hypotension, cardiac arrhythmias, sedation, respiratory depression, and pruritus. The recommended IV dose of fosphenytoin is 20 mg/kg of phenytoin equivalent (PE) at a rate of 3 mg PE/kg/minute.

Phenobarbital is being progressively replaced as second-line treatment for SE. It has a relatively slow onset of action and carries higher risks for side effects than the previously mentioned agents, among them deep and prolonged sedation, respiratory depression, and hypotension.

Some authors recommend the administration of 100 mg IV pyridoxine (vitamin B_6) to children younger than 2 years in SE.

TREATMENT OF REFRACTORY CONVULSIVE STATUS EPILEPTICUS

Once patients with SE have failed to respond to two medications, it is highly unlikely they will respond to a third conventional agent. Current recommendations (see Table 2) support general anesthesia, intubation, and transfer to an intensive care unit as the next phase of SE management. EEG monitoring is also recommended for diagnosis and treatment at this stage. The presence of NCSE should be evaluated once apparent seizures have stopped. Electrographic burst suppression is often considered the endpoint for treatment at this stage. Supposedly, it represents disconnection between the gray and white matter and can be induced with conventional anesthetic agents. However, the required degree of anesthesia carries a high risk of hypotension, and one published meta-analysis of the management of RSE in adults

---

TABLE 2 Treatment Recommendations for Status Epilepticus

- *A*irway
- *B*reathing
- *C*irculation
- *D*rugs
  - No IV access: diazepam, rectal, 0.2–0.5 mg/kg (see text)
  - IV access established: lorazepam, IV, 0.1 mg/kg at 2 mg/min
    followed by
  - Fosphenytoin, IV, 20 mg PE/kg at 3 mg/kg/min (max rate: 150 mg/min)*
  - If seizures are refractory: intubation, anesthesia
  - Midazolam, IV, 0.2 mg/kg, then continuous infusion 1–10 µg/kg/min
    or
  - Pentobarbital, IV, 5–15 mg/kg, then continuous infusion 1–5 mg/kg/h
- *E*valuation: Remainder of vital signs, history, physical, and selected laboratory tests

---

* If fosphenytoin is not effective, and as an alternative to anesthesia, consider valproic acid, IV, 20–40 mg/kg, then continuous infusion 5 mg/kg/h (in nonconvulsive SE) *or* phenobarbital, IV, 20 mg/kg, then additional 10 mg/kg boluses (particularly in neonatal SE).

IV, intravenous; max, maximum; PE, phenytoin equivalent; SE, status epilepticus.

showed that burst suppression did not influence the overall poor outcome but was associated with fewer breakthrough seizures. Therefore, we prefer to aim for termination of electrographic ictal activity. Treatment is generally interrupted after 12 to 48 hours, to evaluate the progression of the condition. Although no consensus exists, the medications discussed next are frequently used in RSE.

Midazolam is water soluble and becomes highly lipophilic at physiologic pH. This transformation allows easy administration and rapid transfer across the blood–brain barrier. Side effects include hypotension and tachyphylaxis, with significant progressive prolongation of half-life with continuous administration. The half-life for midazolam is very short, and relapses frequently occur after bolus injections. Its small volume of distribution makes it less prone to accumulation than other agents. It is usually administered as a single IV loading dose of 0.2 mg/kg, followed by an IV infusion of 1 to 10 µg/kg/minute. Continuous infusion is effective and safe, terminating seizure activity in more than 90% of patients, without major side effects. The efficacy and rapidity of response of midazolam and diazepam are comparable, but midazolam is associated with more seizure recurrences. Pentobarbital, thiopentone, and phenobarbital are all very effective in controlling seizures and achieving burst suppression. They have an anesthetic action at high doses. Pentobarbital is the most frequently used agent in RSE. Potential side effects include respiratory depression, persistent hypotension, prolonged sedation (because of its long half-life and its tendency to accumulate), myocardial depression, immune suppression, and ileus. Pentobarbital is associated with less seizure recurrence when compared to midazolam and propofol, but it provokes more hypotension. Thiopental has a more rapid effect but produces more hypotension than the two other agents. Pentobarbital is administered with an IV loading dose of 5 to 15 mg/kg followed by an IV infusion of 1 to 5 mg/kg/hour.

Propofol is a nonbarbiturate lipophilic anesthetic agent with a high potential for rapid seizure control. Recovery following discontinuation is very quick, making its use convenient in neurologic intensive care. It has a large volume of distribution and therefore carries a potential risk for accumulation with prolonged use. A retrospective study comparing propofol and midazolam in adults with RSE found similar profiles regarding efficacy and safety for both drugs. However, major side effects are reported with long-term continuous administration of propofol, such as multiorgan failure, pancreatitis, lipidemia, acidosis, and rhabdomyolysis, particularly in young children, in whom its use is discouraged. The recommended dosage is 1 to 2 mg/kg as IV loading dose, followed by an IV infusion of 2 to 10 mg/kg/hour, but the association with multiorgan failure in young children virtually precludes its use.

Emerging Options

Valproate is increasingly recognized as an efficient and safe therapeutic option for RSE. Its IV form allows rapid and convenient administration. Moreover, it does not cause any sedation or respiratory depression, and its transition to oral maintenance treatment is usually successful. A meta-analysis showed efficacy in 83% of adults and children with RSE. Hypotension was a rare side effect. Considering the limited data currently available, IV valproate should be reserved as a third- or fourth-line option in RSE or in patients who expressed their desire not to be ventilated mechanically. In one study, valproate was effective in 78% of patients, and a response was observed in less than 6 minutes in 65.9%. No systemic side effects were reported. The recommended dosage is 20 to 40 mg/kg as IV loading dose administered over 1 to 5 minutes, followed by an IV infusion of 5 mg/kg/hour.

Topiramate is an antiepileptic drug with multiple modes of action that is efficient when administered as a suspension via nasogastric tube in a small series of adults with RSE. Its use in children with RSE is limited.

TREATMENT OF NONCONVULSIVE STATUS EPILEPTICUS

Absence SE treatment options (see Table 2) include oral or IV benzodiazepines, such as lorazepam at 0.05 to 0.1 mg/kg/dose. IV valproate or acetazolamide can be considered if benzodiazepines fail. Because brain damage is unlikely to result from this condition, aggressive treatment is not recommended.

Complex partial SE is treated with benzodiazepines as first-line options (e.g., oral clobazam and rectal diazepam) and IV benzodiazepine or phenytoin in case of resistance. ESES is usually treated with oral benzodiazepines, such as clobazam and clonazepam. If this fails, oral steroids are considered. Surgery is reserved for the most severe refractory cases. Carbamazepine, phenytoin, and phenobarbital should be avoided, considering their potential for worsening the condition.

Continuous electrographic seizure activity in coma with or without subtle convulsive movements should be treated aggressively with the previously mentioned agents for CSE when it is part of the evolution of CSE. Electrographic SE from other causes without overt clinical manifestations should probably be treated as well "in the hope that it may improve outcome" (Walker, 2003), but this remains hypothetical.

Common Pitfalls

Failure to recognize nonepileptic events mimicking status epilepticus is a common pitfall. The diagnosis of GCSE is usually obvious. Care must be taken, however, not to misdiagnose SE in patients who present with clinically similar nonepileptic events, such as psychogenic or pseudo–status epilepticus. This condition belongs to the group of conversion disorders and is seen in children as young as 5 years of age, who often have coexistent epilepsy. In specialist practice it may be more common than true SE. It can clinically resemble any type of seizures but most often mimics primarily or secondarily generalized CSE and is not associated with any abnormal ictal or postictal electrographic features. An ictal EEG is mandatory to make the diagnosis when such an event is suspected. Lack of guidelines for treatment are often cited as causes for treatment response delay or failure. Clear and updated recommendations should be readily available in every health care facility to improve the management of patients in SE.

Communication and Counseling

Despite ongoing controversies on its definition, classification, and potential deleterious effects, treatment of SE should be initiated as soon as possible. The initial management includes stabilization of vital signs and antiseizure medications. The current evidence supports the use of a benzodiazepine as first choice, such as rectal diazepam or IV lorazepam. RSE should be treated aggressively with continuous IV antiseizure medications. Nonconvulsive status should be treated individually.

ACKNOWLEDGMENTS

Dr. Korff is the recipient of a scholarship from the Eugenio Litta Foundation, Vaduz, Liechtenstein.

SUGGESTED READINGS

1. Alldredge BK, Gelb AM, Isaacs SM, et al: A comparison of lorazepam, diazepam, and placebo for the treatment of out-of-hospital status epilepticus. N Engl J Med 345(9):631–637, 2001. **Compares lorazepam, diazepam, and placebo for out-of-hospital treatment of SE in adults.**
2. Alldredge BK, Wall DB, Ferriero DM: Effect of prehospital treatment on the outcome of status epilepticus in children. Pediatr Neurol 12(3):213–216, 1995. **The outcome of SE in children depends on etiology and duration. Supports the use of diazepam as prehospital treatment.**
3. Arzimanoglou A, Guerrini R, Aicardi J: Status epilepticus. In Arzimanoglou A, Guerrini R, Aicardi J (eds): Aicardi's Epilepsy in Children, 3rd ed. Philadelphia: Lippincott Williams & Wilkins, 2004, pp 241–261. **Review and controversies about SE in children.**
4. Bassin S, Smith TL, Bleck TP: Clinical review: Status epilepticus. Crit Care 6(2):137–142, 2002. **Epidemiologic data on status epilepticus in the United States; review of pathophysiology and treatment options for SE.**
5. Bleck TP: Management approaches to prolonged seizures and status epilepticus. Epilepsia 40(Suppl. 1):S59–S63, discussion S64–S66, 1999. **Mentions the emerging consensus for a 5- to 10-minute limit to diagnose SE; complex partial status should be treated aggressively.**
6. Brenner RP: Is it status? Epilepsia 43(Suppl. 3):103–113, 2002. **Diagnosis, treatment, and prognosis of NCSE.**
7. Claassen J, Hirsch LJ, Emerson RG, et al: Treatment of refractory status epilepticus with pentobarbital, propofol, or midazolam: A systematic review. Epilepsia 43(2):146–153, 2002. **Meta-analysis that compares the efficacy of midazolam, propofol, and pentobarbital in RSE.**
8. Cock HR, Schapira AH: A comparison of lorazepam and diazepam as initial therapy in convulsive status epilepticus. QJM 95(4):225–231, 2002. **Compares lorazepam and diazepam for CSE. First choice is lorazepam.**
9. DeLorenzo RJ, Hauser WA, Towne AR, et al: A prospective, population-based epidemiologic study of status epilepticus in Richmond, Virginia. Neurology 46(4):1029–1035, 1996. **Epidemiologic prospective study of SE in Virginia.**
10. Duane DC, Ng YT, Rekate HL, et al: Treatment of refractory status epilepticus with hemispherectomy. Epilepsia 45(8):1001–1004, 2004. **Case report, hemispherectomy in refractory localization-related SE.**
11. Gilbert DL, Gartside PS, Glauser TA: Efficacy and mortality in treatment of refractory generalized convulsive status epilepticus in children: A meta-analysis. J Child Neurol 14(9):602–609, 1999. **RSE in children can be managed with different equally effective drugs. Midazolam shows no mortality.**
12. Hirsch LJ, Claassen J: The current state of treatment of status epilepticus. Curr Neurol Neurosci Rep 2(4):345–356, 2002. **Emphasis on electroencephalography and future needs regarding treatment and prognosis of status epilepticus.**
13. Hodges BM, Mazur JE: Intravenous valproate in status epilepticus. Ann Pharmacother 35(11):1465–1470, 2001. **IV valproate is safe and effective in children and adults with SE.**
14. Holtkamp M, Masuhr F, Harms L, et al: The management of refractory generalized convulsive and complex partial status epilepticus in three European countries: A survey among epileptologists and critical care neurologists. J Neurol Neurosurg Psychiatry 74(8):1095–1099, 2003. **Shows the variability in the management of SE in three European countries.**
15. Kahriman M, Minecan D, Kutluay E, et al: Efficacy of topiramate in children with refractory status epilepticus. Epilepsia 44(10):1353–1356, 2003. **Topiramate is possibly effective for RSE in children; three case reports.**
16. Kaplan PW: Prognosis in nonconvulsive status epilepticus. Epileptic Disord 2(4):185–193, 2000. **Classification of NCSE based on the state of consciousness.**
17. Koul R, Chacko A, Javed H, et al: Eight-year study of childhood status epilepticus: Midazolam infusion in management and outcome. J Child Neurol 17(12):908–910, 2002. **Continuous IV infusion of midazolam is effective in pediatric RSE and NCSE.**
18. Lothman E: The biochemical basis and pathophysiology of status epilepticus. Neurology 40(5, Suppl. 2):13–23, 1990. **Complete review of the pathophysiology of SE.**
19. Lowenstein DH: Status epilepticus: An overview of the clinical problem. Epilepsia 40(Suppl. 1):S3–S18; discussion S21–S22, 1999. **Historic overview of the definition of SE; proposes an operational definition.**
20. Lowenstein DH, Bleck T, Macdonald RL: It's time to revise the definition of status epilepticus. Epilepsia 40(1):120–122, 1999. **Treatment should be started after 5 minutes of seizure activity.**
21. Maytal J, Shinnar S, Moshe SL, et al: Low morbidity and mortality of status epilepticus in children. Pediatrics 83(3):323–331, 1989. **The mortality and incidence of sequelae of SE in children is low and primarily a function of etiology.**
22. Mitchell WG: Status epilepticus and acute serial seizures in children. J Child Neurol 17(Suppl. 1):S36–S43, 2002. **Review of SE in children.**
23. Ng YT, Kim HL, Wheless JW: Successful neurosurgical treatment of childhood complex partial status epilepticus with focal resection. Epilepsia 44(3):468–471, 2003. **Case report, multiple subpial transsections, and focal cortical resection for refractory complex partial SE.**
24. Papavasiliou A, Vassilaki N, Paraskevoulakos E, et al: Psychogenic status epilepticus in children. Epilepsy Behav 5(4):539–546, 2004. **Six case reports of psychogenic SE in children.**
25. Prasad A, Worrall BB, Bertram EH, et al: Propofol and midazolam in the treatment of refractory status epilepticus. Epilepsia 42(3):380–386, 2001. **Compares the efficacy and tolerability of midazolam and propofol for RSE.**
26. Proposal for revised clinical and electroencephalographic classification of epileptic seizures: From the Commission on Classification and Terminology of the International League against Epilepsy. Epilepsia 22(4):489–501, 1981. **So-called official classification of epileptic seizures.**
27. Sahin M, Menache CC, Holmes GL, et al: Outcome of severe refractory status epilepticus in children. Epilepsia 42(11):1461–1467, 2001. **Shows that RSE in children has a worse outcome than nonrefractory status. A seizure-free state is unlikely in children with refractory status.**
28. Shinnar S, Berg AT, Moshe SL, et al: How long do new-onset seizures in children last? Ann Neurol 49(5):659–664, 2001. **A subgroup of patients is predisposed to prolonged seizures. Long-lasting seizures are frequent in children. Supports the current definition of SE in children of a duration of more than 30 minutes.**
29. Shinnar S, Pellock JM, Berg AT, et al: Short-term outcomes of children with febrile status epilepticus. Epilepsia 42(1):47–53, 2001. **The outcome of febrile SE in children overall is good.**

30. Shorvon S: The management of status epilepticus. J Neurol Neurosurg Psychiatry 70(Suppl. 2):II22–II27, 2001. **Review. Pseudostatus is frequent and a cause of medication failure.**

31. Sillanpaa M, Shinnar S: Status epilepticus in a population-based cohort with childhood-onset epilepsy in Finland. Ann Neurol 52 (3):303–310, 2002. **Risk factors for SE; identification of a subgroup of patients with prolonged seizures.**

32. The Status Epilepticus Working Party: The treatment of convulsive status epilepticus in children. Arch Dis Child 83(5):415–419, 2000. **Evidence-based and experience-based guidelines for the treatment of SE.**

33. Towne AR, Garnett LK, Waterhouse EJ, et al: The use of topiramate in refractory status epilepticus. Neurology 60(2):332–334, 2003. **Six case reports: topiramate is safe and effective in convulsive and nonconvulsive RSE.**

34. Towne AR, Pellock JM, Ko D, et al: Determinants of mortality in status epilepticus. Epilepsia 35(1):27–34, 1994. **Shows that duration, etiology, and increasing age are correlated to high mortality in adults with SE.**

35. Uberall MA, Trollmann R, Wunsiedler U, et al: Intravenous valproate in pediatric epilepsy patients with refractory status epilepticus. Neurology 54(11):2188–2189, 2000. **IV valproate is safe and effective in pediatric RSE.**

36. Ulvi H, Yoldas T, Mungen B, et al: Continuous infusion of midazolam in the treatment of refractory generalized convulsive status epilepticus. Neurol Sci 23(4):177–182, 2002. **Continuous IV midazolam is safe and effective for RSE.**

37. Walker MC: Diagnosis and treatment of nonconvulsive status epilepticus. CNS Drugs 15(12):931–939, 2001. **Review of NCSE.**

38. Walker MC: Status epilepticus on the intensive care unit. J Neurol 250(4):401–406, 2003. **Management of SE in the intensive care unit.**

39. Wheless JW: Acute management of seizures in the syndromes of idiopathic generalized epilepsies. Epilepsia 44(Suppl. 2):22–26, 2003. **Treatment of SE: first choice is lorazepam; valproate is first choice for the prevention of recurrent absence status.**

40. Wheless JW: Treatment of status epilepticus in children. Pediatric Ann 33(6):377–383, 2004. **Review, status in children, with guidelines for management.**

41. Winston KR, Levisohn P, Miller BR, et al: Vagal nerve stimulation for status epilepticus. Pediatr Neurosurg 34(4):190–192, 2001. **Case report; vagal nerve stimulator for SE.**

42. Yu KT, Mills S, Thompson N, et al: Safety and efficacy of intravenous valproate in pediatric status epilepticus and acute repetitive seizures. Epilepsia 44(5):724–726, 2003. **IV valproate is safe and effective for children in SE.**

Respiratory Failure

Sandeep Gangadharan and Charles Schleien

KEY CONCEPTS

■ The pediatric respiratory system has significant anatomic and developmental disadvantages that increase its risk for developing respiratory distress and failure.

■ To achieve adequate gas exchange, the work of the respiratory system is determined by the sum of its elastic and frictional resistance.

■ Excessive resistive load in the setting of insufficient power leads to respiratory failure because the system cannot meet physiologic demand.

■ Early recognition of respiratory insufficiency is critical, and therapy should be directed toward decreasing total resistance and supporting the innate power of the system while treating the underlying disease.

Acquired and congenital respiratory diseases are among the most common causes of pediatric medical encounters, and respiratory failure is the most common life-threatening process in children. The fundamental functions of the respiratory system are to provide oxygen for aerobic function and to remove carbon dioxide, its primary waste product. Failure of the respiratory system to provide gas exchange to meet metabolic demand results in clinically significant hypoxemia and hypercarbia, which may result in organ system dysfunction, cardiovascular instability, and electrolyte imbalance that can progress to serious morbidity and even death.

Respiratory failure occurs when the demand for gas exchange exceeds the capacity of the respiratory system to support metabolic function (Fig. 1). The primary consequence of respiratory failure is impaired gas exchange. The pathophysiologic mechanisms of hypoxemia are ventilation–perfusion ($\dot{V}/\dot{Q}$) mismatch, diffusion defect, low inspired oxygen tension, severe hypoventilation, and intrapulmonary or intracardiac shunt. The mechanisms of hypercarbia are hypoventilation and $\dot{V}/\dot{Q}$ mismatch.

Infants and children are at greater risk than adults for clinically significant respiratory illness. Immature respiratory and immune systems predispose infants and children to repeated infectious respiratory illnesses. Infants consume substantial amounts of energy relative to body weight to maintain body temperature. The greater energy demands increase basal oxygen requirements and carbon dioxide excretion load. Infants are limited in their ability to increase gas exchange substantially during illness compared to adults.

The anatomy and physiology of the pediatric respiratory system further predispose children to clinically significant respiratory illness and failure (Tables 1 and 2). The pediatric airway is small relative to the adult airway; airway resistance is inversely proportional to the fourth power of the radius with laminar flow and the fifth power with turbulent flow. Therefore, small changes in the radius in a small airway result in substantial increases in total airway resistance.

Clinically significant upper airway obstruction is common in children. The nasal passages, nasopharynx, and oropharynx contribute to half of the total resistance to airflow. Nasal obstruction can cause clinically significant respiratory distress in infants because they are obligate nasal breathers for the first several months of life. The subglottic cricoid ring is the narrowest portion of the pediatric extrathoracic airway. Its narrow conical shape, in comparison to the cylindrical adult airway, makes it more prone to obstruction. Fixed upper airway obstruction can be caused by malformed tissue, extrinsic compression, or subglottic edema. Dynamic obstruction of the upper airway can occur, although it is far more common in the intrathoracic airways that lack cartilaginous support. Loss of pharyngeal muscle tone in obstructive apnea and laryngeal tracheomalacia results in dynamic obstruction of the upper airway.

The intrathoracic small airway is also commonly implicated in clinically significant obstruction. Small changes in diameter from mucus, bronchospasm, or external compression can result in airway obstruction as

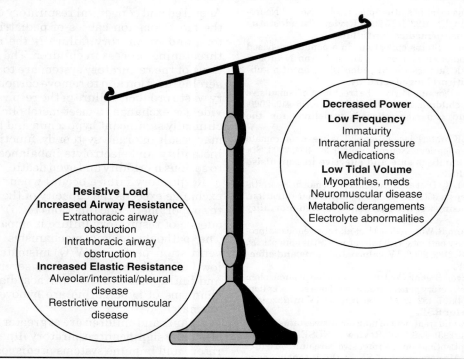

FIGURE 1. Respiratory failure—the balance between resistive load and power.

TABLE 1 Summary of Developmental Differences in Pediatric Airway Anatomy

Extrathoracic Airway	Intrathoracic Airway	Respiratory Pump
Large tongue	Fewer alveoli	Immature drive
Small oropharynx	Smaller alveoli	Horizontal rib orientation
Cephalad larynx	Collateral ventilation	Diaphragm less apposed to ribs
Conically shaped airway	Less well developed	Less-developed musculature
Larger floppy epiglottis	Less cartilaginous support	Early fatigue of diaphragm
Narrow subglottic area		
Obligate nasal		

predicted by the Hagen-Poiseuille law. The intrathoracic bronchiolar tree can have both fixed and dynamic obstruction, resulting in a significant increase in resistive load. The Bernoulli law predicts that partially obstructed small airways without cartilaginous support will collapse on exhalation from decreased intraluminal pressure. Dynamic small airway obstruction from asthma or bronchiolitis remains the most common cause of abnormal respiratory mechanics in pediatric patients.

Intrathoracic small airway obstructions (e.g., asthma, bronchiolitis) increase airway resistance and cause dynamic hyperinflation, atelectasis, $\dot{V}/\dot{Q}$ mismatch, and increased work of breathing. Hypercarbia associated with small airway disease is an ominous sign. With mild to moderate small airway disease, children normalize arterial carbon dioxide tension with tachypnea. Patients often present with hypocarbia and respiratory alkalosis from hypoxemia. The associated increase in work of breathing requires large increases in energy consumption, accelerating both the demand for oxygen and supply of carbon dioxide. Eventually, the compensatory

mechanisms are overwhelmed by the increased demands for gas exchange, and respiratory failure ensues.

Infants and children are also at a greater risk for developing significant alveolar collapse leading to $\dot{V}/\dot{Q}$ mismatch. Infants possess a fraction of the total alveoli present in the adult lung and increase alveolar gas exchange surface area by more than tenfold in the first 8 years of life. Children lack pores of Kohn between adjacent alveoli and channels between bronchioles that allow for collateral distribution of ventilation. Collateral ventilation is important in limiting the progression of heterogeneous lung disease such as atelectasis or acute respiratory distress syndrome (ARDS).

The respiratory pump is immature and mechanically disadvantaged in early childhood. Apnea is common in young infants before the central respiratory control center matures. The anteroposterior diameter of the thorax is relatively large because of horizontal displacement of the ribs, limiting its capacity to increase tidal volume. The slow-twitch fibers of the diaphragm are immature, predisposing infants to diaphragmatic fatigue earlier

TABLE 2 Anatomic Differential Diagnosis of Pediatric Respiratory Insufficiency

Intrathoracic Airway and Lung	Extrathoracic Airway	Respiratory Pump
Asthma	**Acquired lesions**	**Chest wall**
Aspiration		Diaphragm eventration
Bronchiolitis	*Infections*	Diaphragmatic hernia
Bronchomalacia	Retropharyngeal abscess	Flail chest
Lung contusion	Ludwig angina	Kyphoscoliosis
Near drowning	Laryngotracheobronchitis	**Respiratory muscles**
Pneumonia	Bacterial tracheitis	Infant botulism
Pulmonary edema	Peritonsillar abscess	Poliomyelitis
Sepsis		Spinal cord trauma
	Traumatic	Spinal muscular atrophy
	Postextubation croup	**Central control**
	Thermal burns	Intoxication
	Foreign body aspiration	Sleep apnea
		Central nervous system infection
	Other	
	Hypertrophic tonsils, adenoids	
	Congenital lesions	
	Subglottic stenosis	
	Subglottic web, cyst	
	Laryngomalacia	
	Tracheomalacia	
	Vascular ring	
	Cystic hygroma	
	Craniofacial anomalies	
	Hypocalcemia	

From Priestley MA, Costarino AT Jr: Pediatric respiratory failure. In Burg FD, Ingelfinger JR, Polin RA, Gershon AA (eds): Gellis and Kagan's Current Pediatric Therapy, 17th ed. Philadelphia, WB Saunders, 2002.

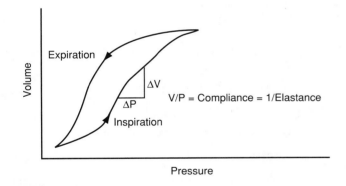

FIGURE 2. Respiratory system compliance. (From Taussig LM, Landau LI: Pediatric Respiratory Medicine. St. Louis: Mosby, 1999, p. 100.)

than seen in adults. A very compliant chest wall poorly opposes the inherent tendency of the lung to collapse, leaving infant lungs with a low functional residual capacity and an increased likelihood of atelectasis.

Respiratory illness that decreases lung compliance (e.g., interstitial edema, inflammation, or fibrosis) or chest wall compliance (e.g., kyphoscoliosis) results in tidal breathing at low lung volumes. Low lung volumes result in atelectasis because alveoli with low volumes have an inherent tendency to collapse. Collapsed alveoli require greater effort and pressure generation to recruit them. Atelectasis results in hypoxemia from inadequate ventilation to perfused areas of the lung $\dot{V}/\dot{Q}$ mismatch). Tidal breathing at low, less-compliant lung volumes increases the work of breathing as well (Fig. 2).

Expert Opinion on Management Issues

DIAGNOSIS

Obtaining a detailed history of length and severity of antecedent illness and comorbid conditions is of paramount importance. The physical examination should be thorough, with specific attention to detailed examination of the respiratory and cardiovascular systems. A careful assessment of the patient's mental status can be helpful in determining the severity of disease because both hypoxemia and hypercarbia can cause impairment in orientation or level of alertness. The salient features of the respiratory exam include the rate, rhythm, and quality of effort. Percussion and auscultation of lung fields can be helpful in localizing disease.

Children with extrathoracic airway obstruction tend to breathe slowly, with larger-than-normal tidal volumes, thereby minimizing turbulent flow and decreasing relative airway resistance and resistive work. Intrathoracic airway obstruction from dynamic collapse of bronchioles results in a shallow, rapid respiratory pattern that helps stent airways open and minimizes collapse.

Musical sounds auscultated in respiratory illness are caused by turbulent airflow. Turbulent flow is more likely in obstructed airways that increase airflow velocity. Turbulent flow produces stridor in the extrathoracic airway and wheezing in the intrathoracic airway. Stridor is present on inspiration with extrathoracic airway obstruction because velocity is greater in that phase of respiration. However, very severe narrowing of the extrathoracic airway can result in turbulent flow and stridor during expiration as well. Wheezing, in small airway disease, is largely a consequence of dynamic airway constriction causing turbulent airflow during exhalation when intrathoracic airways are at their narrowest.

Inspiratory crackles can be heard when collapsed atelectatic alveoli are opened by flow of inspired air. Consolidated collapsed lung from pneumonic processes or pleural fluid can result in decreased breath sounds, dullness to percussion, and egophony. An inspiratory rub may suggest fluid in the pleural space.

The stigmata of respiratory distress, such as retractions, grunting, nasal flaring, and paradoxical abdominal breathing, should alert the clinician that the system is severely stressed and, although temporarily compensated, is no longer in homeostasis. Suprasternal retractions are an effort to stent the upper airway open and suggest the presence of significant obstruction.

Intercostal and subcostal retractions are evidence of accessory muscle recruitment in an effort to increase anteroposterior thoracic diameter, open collapsed lungs, and increase tidal volume. Grunting is a premature termination of exhalation against a closed glottis, an attempt to decrease dynamic airway and alveolar collapse at end expiration. Nasal flaring decreases nasal impedance and reduces total airway resistance. Paradoxical abdominal breathing is an ominous sign and suggests diaphragmatic fatigue and recruitment of abdominal muscles to aid inspiratory effort. In this setting, tachycardia, diaphoresis, and hypertension are caused by sympathetic stimulation from hypoxemia or hypercarbia.

Pulse oximetry is a safe and noninvasive means to assess effective oxygenation and is indicated for all patients with significant respiratory illness. It uses two wavelengths of light (red and near-infrared) to measure the relative amounts of oxyhemoglobin to

---

TABLE 3 Evidence-Based Review of Respiratory Insufficiency Strategies

Strategy	EBM Evidence	Consensus
Humidified Air		
Extrathoracic airway obstruction	Anecdotal. Case reports suggest symptomatic improvement.	Minimal risk intervention for mild disease.
Racemic Epinephrine		
Extrathoracic airway obstruction	Anecdotal, case reports.	Commonly used; no evidence of efficacy.
Intrathoracic airway obstruction	Prospective RCT: no change in vitals, distress, LOS.[1]	Commonly used; no evidence of efficacy.
Heliox		
Extrathoracic airway obstruction	Case reports, anecdotal evidence suggest significant symptomatic improvement.	Common ICU use; do not use if Fio_2 >30%.
Intrathoracic airway obstruction	Review of six small prospective RCTs.[2] No conclusive difference in PFTs.	*Not* indicated as first-line management.
Noninvasive Ventilation		
Extrathoracic airway obstruction	Case reports of success with dynamic obstruction.	Common use in dynamic diagnoses; no evidence.
Intrathoracic airway obstruction	One RCT (no patients required intubation).[3] Three case series (decreased intubation).[4]	Suggestive, not compelling evidence.
Alveolar/interstitial pleural disease	One RCT (not statistically significant decrease in intubation) ICU LOS: Pneumonia: 7 case series, not statistically significant. ARDS: 5 case series, not statistically significant. Pulmonary edema: 1 RCT; insufficient evidence.	Commonly used. Insufficient evidence.
Systemic Steroids		
Extrathoracic airway obstruction	Evidence varies with etiology.	Commonly used with inflammatory diagnosis.
Intrathoracic airway obstruction	Evidence varies with etiology.	Equivocal evidence with bronchiolitis.
Alveolar/interstitial pleural disease	Evidence depends on etiology.	Suggestive evidence with late ARDS of improved outcome.
Empirical antibiotics	Evidence varies with etiology.	Choice of antibiotics.

[1]Wainwright C, Altamirano L, Cheney M, et al: A multicenter, randomized, double-blind, controlled trial of nebulized epinephrine in infants with acute bronchiolitis. N Engl J Med 349(1):27–35, 2003.
[2]Rodrigo G, Pollack C, Rodrigo C, Rowe BH: Heliox for nonintubated acute asthma patients. Cochrane Database Syst Rev 4:CD002884, 2003.
[3]Kramer N, Meyer TJ, Meharg J, et al: Randomized, prospective trial of noninvasive positive pressure ventilation in acute respiratory failure. Am J Respir Crit Care Med 151(6):1799–1806, 1995.
[4]Mehta S, Hill NS: Noninvasive ventilation. Am J Respir Crit Care Med 163(2):540–577, 2001.
ARDS, acute respiratory distress syndrome; EBM, evidence-based medicine; ICU, intensive care unit; LOS, length of stay; PFT, pulmonary function test; RCT, randomized controlled trial.

deoxyhemoglobin, and it is most accurate above 75% oxygen saturation. Virtually all of the oxygen in blood is bound to hemoglobin, with insignificant amounts dissolved because of oxygen's low solubility. Therefore, pulse oximetry provides an accurate estimate of the patient's arterial oxygen content. Accurate pulse oximetry assumes a normal hemoglobin concentration and the absence of dyshemoglobinemias such as carboxyhemoglobinemia and methemoglobinemia. If hypercarbia is suspected or pulse oximetry cannot be relied upon, an arterial blood gas sample should be obtained.

Chest radiographs are often the most useful diagnostic imaging modality for respiratory failure. Anteroposterior and lateral radiographs of the neck can help confirm airway narrowing. If anatomic detail is necessary for diagnostic or therapeutic decisions, more sophisticated imaging such as CT or MRI is warranted. If the disease is dynamic, as in the case of laryngomalacia or bronchomalacia, or if lavage specimens are necessary, bronchoscopy is required. Diagnosis of diaphragmatic paralysis requires either ultrasound or fluoroscopy. Continuous multimodal monitoring, such as a sleep study, may be useful in evaluating disorders that involve pathologic interactions between the respiratory center and the neuromuscular apparatus. Pulmonary function studies are indicated if changes in lung volumes or respiratory mechanics are suspected.

MANAGEMENT

The fundamental goal in the management of respiratory failure is to facilitate adequate gas exchange to support metabolic function. To that end, management of respiratory failure requires decreasing the resistive load placed on the system, supplementing inspiratory oxygen concentration, supporting the power of the respiratory system to meet gas exchange demand, and treating the underlying illness with definitive therapy.

Support of extrathoracic airway obstruction requires therapy aimed at decreasing upper airway resistance and reversing the underlying disease. Helium/oxygen mixtures are used successfully to reduce the density of inspired air and reduce the frictional resistance of turbulent flow. Nebulized racemic epinephrine is used to relieve symptomatic upper airway edema. Although unproven, it is thought to exert its therapeutic effect by decreasing vasogenic edema of the larynx and subglottic region by vasoconstricting precapillary arterioles in the region.

Noninvasive positive airway pressure can help stent open dynamic obstruction in upper airways from a variety of problems, such as inappropriate pharyngeal reflexes to structural tissue laxity. Noninvasive positive pressure can be delivered via nasal prongs or a form-fitting mask. The fraction of inspired oxygen, inspiratory positive airway pressure, and expiratory positive airway pressure can be titrated to treat hypoxemia and decrease the work of breathing. Continuous positive airway pressure (CPAP) increases the functional residual capacity of the patient and is particularly useful in functional reserve capacity (FRC)-lowering or restrictive lung disease. Maintaining a normal or near-normal FRC can decrease atelectasis, improving $\dot{V}/\dot{Q}$ mismatch, and decrease the work of breathing by shifting tidal breathing to a more compliant lung volume. Biphasic positive airway pressure (BiPAP) works similarly to CPAP, with the addition

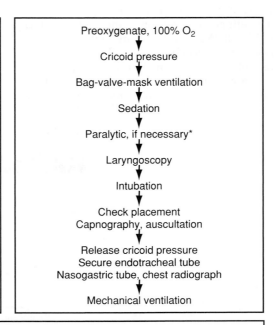

Monitoring
    Heart rate, blood pressure
    Pulse oximetry
Equipment
    Yankauer suction
    Ambu-bag with 15 L oxygen
    Appropriate-sized face mask
    Oral airway
    Laryngoscope
    Endotracheal tube with stylet
Sedation
    Midazolam 0.1 mg/kg, adult dose 2 mg; or
    Morphine 0.1 mg/kg; or
    Ketamine 2 mg/kg
Paralytic*
    Rocuronium 1.2 mg/kg; or
    Vecuronium 0.1 mg/kg; or
    Succinylcholine 2 mg/kg
Support
    Nurses
    Respiratory therapist
    Experienced airway physician

Preoxygenate, 100% O$_2$
↓
Cricoid pressure
↓
Bag-valve-mask ventilation
↓
Sedation
↓
Paralytic, if necessary*
↓
Laryngoscopy
↓
Intubation
↓
Check placement
Capnography, auscultation
↓
Release cricoid pressure
Secure endotracheal tube
Nasogastric tube, chest radiograph
↓
Mechanical ventilation

***Do not** administer unless you are a trained airway physician*

FIGURE 3. Modified rapid sequence intubation.

of phasic variations in the level of positive pressure that correspond to the patient's respiratory cycle. Exhalation is against a set expiratory airway pressure while the patient's own inspiratory effort, when synchronized, is supported by a preset inspiratory airway pressure.

The challenges of noninvasive positive airway pressure include patient compliance, difficulty synchronizing with the patient's respiratory cycle during tachypnea, and the need for continuous close monitoring. Apnea, respiratory pause, or rapid changes in respiratory mechanics can result in serious patient morbidity because there is no fail-safe backup full ventilation capacity with BiPAP or CPAP. BiPAP does have a backup ventilatory rate setting, but the insensitivity of these devices and the presence of mask or prong leaks preclude its use as a reliable backup mechanism. General supportive therapy, such as anti-inflammatory agents, empirical antibiotics, fluids, and nutritional support that addresses the underlying disease, is imperative.

Support of diseases that cause intrathoracic airway obstruction includes the use of anti-inflammatory agents, empirical antibiotics, bronchodilators, and mucolytics. Helium/oxygen mixtures are used to treat lower airway obstruction, although the evidence remains equivocal (Table 3). The proposed mechanism of action is similar to that described with its use in upper airway disease. Some report success in the use of noninvasive positive airway pressure (BiPAP/CPAP) with lower airway obstructive disease. Noninvasive positive airway pressure can decrease expiratory flow velocity, normalizing intraluminal pressure at sites of obstruction and decreasing dynamic collapse at exhalation.

Diseases of the lung and pleura can substantially increase the resistive workload of the respiratory pump. Alveolar fluid, atelectasis, and consolidation impair normal gas exchange and decrease the compliance of the lung. Therefore, tidal ventilation requires greater work and respiratory effort to overcome increased elastic resistance (see Fig. 2). Pleural fluid can decrease pulmonary compliance by not allowing normal lung expansion. Appropriate use of empirical antibiotic therapy, use of chest physiotherapy, and maintaining good pulmonary toilet are mainstays of management. Significant

pleural fluid may warrant a thoracentesis or drainage via chest tube for both diagnostic and therapeutic purposes. CPAP can result in significant symptomatic improvement from diseases that decrease respiratory compliance. Restoration of normal or near-normal FRC by CPAP has the added benefit of decreasing interstitial and lymphatic hydrostatic pressure, resulting in removal of alveolar fluid. Increasing lung volumes to FRC results in decreased work of breathing, allowing for tidal ventilation higher on the pressure–volume curve (see Fig. 2).

Disorders of the respiratory pump can increase resistive work or decrease mechanical function of the respiratory pump to varying degrees. Neuromuscular diseases, such as myasthenia gravis, or the use of medications that result in respiratory muscle weakness can impair the respiratory pump. Diseases such as kyphosis and scoliosis alter the orientation of the thoracic rib cage and can increase resistive load by both increasing airway resistance and decreasing thoracic compliance. Failure of the initiation of the respiratory pump occurs in central apnea and results in hypoventilation. Hypoventilation from diseases of the respiratory pump, if mild, may respond to noninvasive positive-pressure ventilation. Severe neuromuscular weakness or apnea may require intubation and long-term ventilatory support.

Definitive support of the respiratory pump, either for primary failure or inability to match increased resistive work, requires endotracheal intubation and mechanical ventilation. Figure 3 provides a guideline for emergent intubation in the setting of respiratory failure. It is critical, when attempting intubation, to have sufficient monitoring, personnel, and support from an experienced airway physician. Table 4 lists the different modes of ventilation.

Common Pitfalls

Assessment of the severity of respiratory distress and risk of respiratory failure remains the most critical aspect of management. The stigmata of respiratory distress—tachypnea, retractions, flaring, and grunting—should always raise concern. Each is an attempt by the

TABLE 4 Modes of Mechanical Ventilation

Modes	Mandatory			Assisted		
	Trigger	Limit	Cycle	Trigger	Limit	Cycle
VCV	time	flow	volume	patient	flow	volume
PCV	time	pressure	time	patient	pressure	time
SIMV PC	time	pressure	time	patient	pressure	time
SIMV VC	time	flow	volume	patient	flow	volume
PSV	—	—	—	—	—	—
CPAP	—	—	—	—	—	—

CPAP, continuous positive airway pressure; cycle, goal of mechanical breath; limit, limits period and volume of mechanical breath; PCV, pressure control ventilation; SIMV, synchronized intermittent mandatory ventilation; trigger, ventilator triggers mechanical breath; VCV, volume control ventilation.
Modified from Branson RD, Chatburn RL: Technical description and classification of modes of ventilator operation. Respir Care 37:1009–1026, 1992. Reproduced with permission of the American Association for Respiratory Care via Copyright Clearance Center.

respiratory system to compensate for increased resistive work and impaired gas exchange, to support gas exchange. However, each exacts a significant metabolic cost in terms of additional energy expenditure, increased oxygen requirement, and increased carbon dioxide load on an already impaired system. Although these mechanisms provide short-term compensation, if the underlying illness fails to improve and supportive interventions are not made, the progression to respiratory failure is inevitable. The rate of progression to respiratory failure depends on the severity of the acute illness and the patient's respiratory, cardiovascular, and nutritional reserve. Therefore, timely assessment of respiratory failure and intervention is imperative.

SUGGESTED READINGS

1. Lumb AB, Nunn JF: Nunn's Applied Respiratory Physiology, 5th ed. Oxford: Butterworth-Heinemann, 1999. **A comprehensive review of the physiologic principles of the respiratory system in health and disease.**
2. Taussig LM, Landau LI: Pediatric Respiratory Medicine. St. Louis: Mosby, 1999. **An excellent disease-based review of current management principles in pediatric respiratory disease.**
3. West JB: Pulmonary Pathophysiology, 5th ed. Baltimore: Williams and Wilkins, 1998. **Outstanding review of essential physiologic principles of the respiratory system in disease.**
4. West JB: Respiratory Physiology. The Essentials, 6th ed. Baltimore: Williams and Wilkins, 2000. **Outstanding review of essential physiologic principles underlying normal respiratory function.**

Supported			Spontaneous		
Trigger	**Limit**	**Cycle**	**Trigger**	**Limit**	**Cycle**
—	—	—	—	—	—
—	—	—	—	—	—
—	—	—	patient	pressure	pressure
—	—	—	patient	pressure	pressure
—	—	—	—	—	—
—	—	—	patient	pressure	pressure

Anaphylaxis

Erin E. McGintee, Suzanne Beno, and Terri Brown-Whitehorn

KEY CONCEPTS

- Anaphylaxis is a low-incidence disease that can be rapidly fatal if untreated.
- The common causes of anaphylaxis include foods, drugs, hymenoptera stings, latex, allergen immunotherapy, exercise, immunizations, and radiocontrast media.
- Anaphylaxis is largely a clinical diagnosis.
- An elevated serum β-tryptase level, if obtained within 6 hours of the exposure, can support a diagnosis of anaphylaxis.
- Rapid administration of intramuscular epinephrine is first-line therapy for anaphylaxis.
- All patients at risk for a future anaphylactic event should be referred to an allergy specialist for evaluation.
- All patients at risk for anaphylaxis should be prescribed an epinephrine auto-injector, which should be available to them at all times.

Definition

Anaphylaxis is defined as a potentially life-threatening, systemic, immediate hypersensitivity reaction caused by immunoglobulin (Ig) E-mediated release of mediators from mast cells and basophils because of exposure to a substance to which a person has become sensitized. Anaphylactoid reactions are clinically indistinguishable from anaphylaxis, but they are non–IgE-mediated. Patients typically present with cutaneous reactions associated with varying degrees of involvement of the respiratory, cardiovascular, and gastrointestinal systems.

The severity of anaphylaxis can vary greatly, both among patients and within the same patient at different times. Anaphylactic episodes can range from mild and self-limited to fatal. Just because a patient has a mild reaction does not mean subsequent exposures will be mild. Risk factors that may contribute to the severity of an anaphylactic reaction include the offending agent itself, route and constancy of administration of the allergen, and length of time elapsed since the last reaction.

The true incidence of anaphylaxis in the population is difficult to estimate, largely because of under-reporting of reactions by patients. Overall estimates of the risk of anaphylaxis per person in the United States range from less than 1% up to approximately 3%. Fortunately, fatal anaphylaxis is rare, with deaths occurring in approximately 4% of all cases of anaphylaxis. Patients are at higher risk of a severe or fatal anaphylactic reaction if they have a comorbid condition, such as asthma, coronary artery disease, or adrenal insufficiency. Certain medications, such as β-blockers and angiotensin-converting enzyme (ACE) inhibitors, also increase the risk of fatal reaction by disrupting homeostatic mechanisms, making an individual less able to respond to the physiologic changes that occur during an anaphylactic event.

Etiology

By far, the leading cause of anaphylaxis in children is food, accounting for more than half of all cases. Food-induced anaphylaxis occurs in an estimated 1% to 3% of children. Milk, eggs, soy, wheat, peanuts, tree nuts, fish, and shellfish are the most commonly implicated foods in the United States, although virtually any food theoretically could induce anaphylaxis in a susceptible patient. Peanuts, tree nuts, fish, and shellfish are the most likely to induce persistent sensitivity in patients, whereas allergies to most other foods are frequently outgrown.

Another common cause of anaphylaxis in children is drug allergy, with β-lactam antibiotics the most prevalent. Penicillin reactions are responsible for 500 to 1000 deaths per year. Aspirin and nonsteroidal anti-inflammatory drugs can cause anaphylactoid reactions. These reactions tend to be more common in asthmatic patients and are attributable to aberrant metabolism of arachidonic acid. It is thought that inhibition of prostaglandin E, which protects against mast cell degranulation and overproduction of leukotriene C (which enhances degranulation) leads to direct mast cell activation in these individuals.

Allergy to hymenoptera stings is also quite prevalent in both adults and children, affecting anywhere from 0.5% to 5% of the general population. Approximately 40 to 100 deaths per year in the United States are attributed to anaphylaxis caused by hymenoptera venom.

Positive skin testing to latex occurs in approximately 3% of children tested. Latex allergy tends to be even more prevalent in atopic individuals, health care workers, and children with spina bifida. In one study, latex allergy was identified in 67% of children with spina bifida, upward of 17% of health care workers, and 6.5% of patients undergoing multiple surgeries.

Exercise-induced anaphylaxis is becoming increasingly common, although the exact prevalence is unknown. It is most common in patients between 25 and 35 years of age. Exercise-induced anaphylaxis can be food specific, in that anaphylaxis only occurs if the patient has consumed a specific food within 2 to 4 hours of exercise. The skin tests of these patients often show positivity to the food, but they do not react to the food alone in the absence of exercise. Some patients have anaphylaxis with exercise 2 to 4 hours after the consumption of any food.

Other causes of anaphylaxis in children include allergen immunotherapy, immunizations, blood products, and radiocontrast media. Reported cases of anaphylaxis for which no cause can be identified, termed *idiopathic anaphylaxis,* should be considered a diagnosis of exclusion.

Pathophysiology

True anaphylaxis is an IgE-mediated reaction, which requires initial exposure to an antigen. This exposure results in the production of specific IgE antibodies, which are then bound to surface receptors on mast cells. Subsequent exposure to the same antigen results in cross-linking of the mast cell–bound IgE, thus activating the mast cells and triggering the release of the mediators of anaphylaxis, including histamine, leukotrienes, neutral proteases, chemoattractants, and nitric oxide. Together, these mediators lead to vasodilation and increased vascular permeability, bronchoconstriction, and recruitment of inflammatory cells. Anaphylactoid reactions, although clinically identical to anaphylactic reactions, are not IgE-mediated. Anaphylactoid reactions result in the release of mast cell mediators either through complement activation (which leads to mast cell activation) or through direct activation of the mast cell. Causes of anaphylactoid reactions include opiates, radiocontrast media, and blood products.

Clinical Manifestations

Clinical manifestations of anaphylaxis are highly variable. Dermatologic symptoms are the most common manifestations of an allergic reaction, occurring in up to 90% of episodes. Typical findings include urticaria, angioedema, flushing, and warmth. Cardiovascular manifestations include tachycardia and hypotension, although a small subset of patients may exhibit bradycardia. More severe cases progress to cardiovascular collapse. Lower respiratory signs and symptoms include wheezing, cough, chest tightness, and shortness of breath. The lower respiratory tract is involved in 50% to 60% of anaphylactic episodes, and lower respiratory involvement is more common in patients with a history of asthma. Upper airway edema occurs in roughly half of all cases of anaphylaxis and may present with symptoms such as tongue and throat swelling, dysphagia, dysphonia, choking, and stridor. Patients experiencing anaphylaxis may also manifest gastrointestinal symptoms, such as nausea, vomiting, cramping, and diarrhea. Tingling of the mouth and face is commonly an early presenting feature of anaphylaxis, and patients who experience anaphylactic episodes often later report a "feeling of impending doom." Table 1 lists the common clinical manifestations of anaphylaxis and the frequency of symptoms involving each organ system. Because of the variability in presentation, the differential diagnoses of anaphylaxis are quite broad, which underscores the importance of obtaining a careful clinical history when a diagnosis of anaphylaxis is suspected. Box 1 lists the differential diagnoses for anaphylaxis.

The majority of anaphylactic episodes begin within 30 minutes of exposure. The onset of reaction is typically quicker when the allergen is administered parenterally rather than orally. Anaphylaxis may occur as a biphasic reaction with recurrence of equally severe symptoms, typically within 4 hours, but occasionally up to 8 hours after apparent resolution of the initial episode. Biphasic anaphylaxis is reported in up to 20% of cases, although it is seen much less frequently in pediatric patients, with one study reporting an incidence of 6%. Anaphylaxis may also follow a protracted course, in which the cycle

TABLE 1 Common Clinical Manifestations of Anaphylaxis and Frequency of Symptoms

Signs and Symptoms	Frequency
Cutaneous	90%
Urticaria and angioedema	85%–90%
Flushing	45%–55%
Pruritus without rash	2%–5%
Respiratory	40%–60%
Dyspnea, wheeze	45%–50%
Upper airway angioedema	50%–60%
Rhinitis	15%–20%
Dizziness, syncope, hypotension	30%–35%
Abdominal	
Nausea, vomiting, diarrhea, cramping pain	25%–30%
Miscellaneous	
Headache	5%–8%
Substernal pain	4%–6%
Seizure	1%–2%

From the Joint Task Force on Practice Parameters, representing the American Academy of Allergy, Asthma and Immunology; the American College of Allergy, Asthma and Immunology; and the Joint Council of Allergy, Asthma and Immunology: The diagnosis and management of anaphylaxis: An updated practice parameter. J Allergy Clin Immunol 115(3 Suppl.): S483–S523, 2005.

BOX 1 Differential Diagnoses for Anaphylaxis

- Vasodepressor reactions (syncope)
- Systemic mast cell disorders
- Scombroid poisoning
- Anxiety (panic attacks, hyperventilation)
- Status asthmaticus
- Flushing episodes (vancomycin-induced red man syndrome, alcohol, malignancy)
- Hereditary angioedema
- Seizure/stroke
- Pheochromocytoma
- Myocardial infarction
- Other causes of shock

of symptomatic episodes may or may not be interrupted by asymptomatic periods and may persist for days. Both biphasic and protracted anaphylaxis can occur in spite of appropriate therapy, including corticosteroid treatment.

Expert Opinion on Management Issues

ACCEPTED INTERVENTIONS

The diagnosis of anaphylaxis is usually made on the basis of clinical features and an appropriate history of the event. An elevated serum β-tryptase, if obtained within 6 hours of the initial exposure, can support a diagnosis of anaphylaxis in unclear cases. However, the results are not immediately available, so clinical judgment is necessary to initiate therapy. Tryptase is an enzyme released during mast cell degranulation. Tryptase levels peak 60 to 90 minutes after an anaphylactic event and then remain elevated for up to 6 hours. Histamine is also released, but it is more rapidly metabolized and therefore

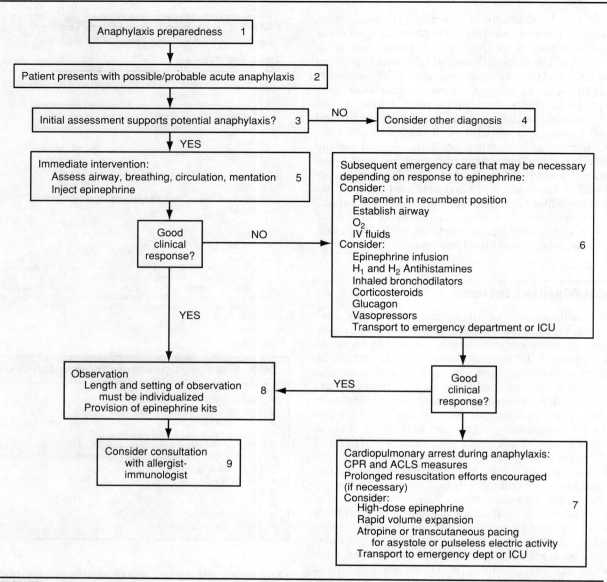

FIGURE 1. Algorithm for the treatment of acute anaphylaxis. ACLS, advanced cardiac life support; CPR, cardiopulmonary resuscitation; ICU, intensive care unit; IV, intravenous. (From the Joint Task Force on Practice Parameters, representing the American Academy of Allergy, Asthma, and Immunology; the American College of Allergy, Asthma, and Immunology; and the Joint Council of Allergy, Asthma, and Immunology: The diagnosis and management of anaphylaxis: An updated practice parameter. J Allergy Clin Immunol 115(3 Suppl):S483–S523, 2005. Copyright 2005. Reprinted with permission from the American Academy of Allergy, Asthma, and Immunology.)

only found in the serum for up to an hour. At times, urinary histamine levels and its metabolites can also be obtained and are useful in supporting a diagnosis of anaphylaxis.

In acute anaphylaxis, as with any type of shock, initial management includes assessment and stabilization of airway, breathing, and circulation. Supplemental oxygen should be administered as necessary. Patients should be placed in the Trendelenburg position whenever possible because the upright position is associated with an increased risk of death anaphylaxis.

The mainstay of pharmacologic therapy for anaphylaxis is epinephrine, a 1:1000 solution, given in a dose of 0.01 mL per kg up to a maximum of 0.5 mL, intramuscularly or subcutaneously. The dose may be repeated every 5 min-

utes as needed for up to three doses. Intramuscular epinephrine injections into the thigh provide more rapid absorption and higher peak plasma levels than either intramuscular or subcutaneous epinephrine injections into the arm. In cases of anaphylaxis, the need for rapid administration of intramuscular epinephrine simply cannot be stressed enough. An intravenous line should be placed as soon as possible, and hypotension not responsive to epinephrine should be treated by rapid fluid resuscitation with either a crystalloid or colloid solution.

Both H_1 and H_2 histamine blockers should be administered parenterally every 6 hours. The exact role for corticosteroids in the management of anaphylaxis is not established, but they are believed to help prevent the late-phase reaction. The data conflict as to whether

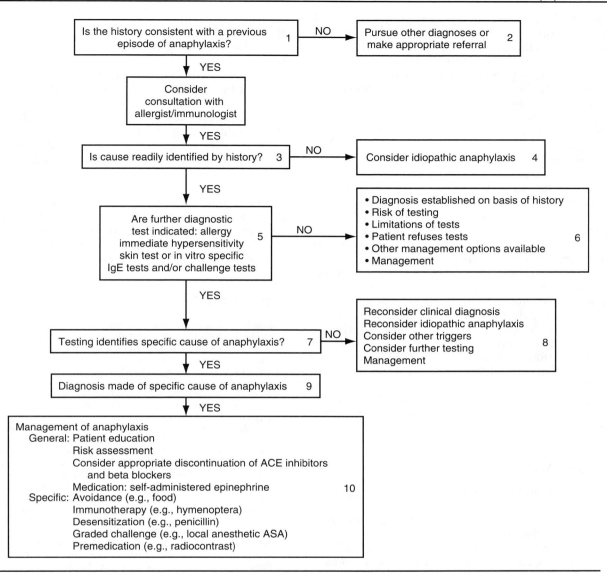

FIGURE 2. Algorithm for the initial evaluation and management of a patient with a history of an episode of anaphylaxis. ACE, angiotensin-converting enzyme. (From the Joint Task Force on Practice Parameters, representing the American Academy of Allergy, Asthma, and Immunology; the American College of Allergy, Asthma, and Immunology; and the Joint Council of Allergy, Asthma, and Immunology: The diagnosis and management of anaphylaxis: An updated practice parameter. J Allergy Clin Immunol 115[3 Suppl]:S483–S523, 2005. Copyright 2005. Reprinted with permission from the American Academy of Allergy, Asthma and Immunology.)

corticosteroids prevent biphasic or protracted anaphylaxis, but nonetheless, they are considered part of standard therapy for anaphylaxis. An inhaled β-agonist such as albuterol may be used for wheezing not responsive to injected epinephrine, but albuterol should be used only as an adjunctive therapy. Intramuscular epinephrine is the first-line pharmacologic therapy for the treatment of wheezing or other respiratory symptoms.

Persistent hypotension may require an infusion of a vasopressor such as dopamine. In patients taking β-blocking drugs who experience anaphylaxis, glucagon is the drug of choice for treating hypotension unresponsive to epinephrine because glucagon has an inotropic effect that is catecholamine independent. In situations of severe laryngospasm or bronchospasm not responsive

to pharmacotherapy, endotracheal intubation may be necessary. Figure 1 illustrates an algorithm for the treatment of acute anaphylaxis.

No standardized observation period is established following resolution of an anaphylactic episode; nor are there any reliable predictors of biphasic or protracted anaphylaxis on the basis of clinical presentation. Most allergists would agree on a minimum of 4 hours of observation following an anaphylactic event, but individual circumstances must be taken into consideration for each patient. If the patient has a history of a biphasic or protracted anaphylactic event, or if there is any question of the patient's ability to return to the hospital in the event of relapsing symptoms, he or she should be admitted overnight for observation. All patients who have experienced an anaphylactic episode, upon discharge from the hospital, should be prescribed an epinephrine auto-injector and instructed on its use. They should also be told that a biphasic reaction is a possibility, and therefore they should remain close to home with immediate access to medical care, should it become necessary. Outpatient follow-up with an allergy specialist should be arranged. Figure 2 illustrates an algorithm for the initial evaluation and management of a patient with a history of anaphylaxis.

In patients with a history of anaphylaxis to hymenoptera, antibiotics, radiocontrast media, or exercise, measures can be taken to prevent or lessen the severity of a future reaction. Immunotherapy with hymenoptera venom protects an estimated 98% of patients with a history of anaphylaxis to venom in the case of a future sting. In cases of antibiotic anaphylaxis, using an alternate drug is optimal, but when this is not possible, antibiotic desensitization can be quite effective. Both the patient and the caregivers should be aware that once the drug is discontinued, the patient must undergo repeat desensitization if the drug is needed on another occasion. In patients with a history of anaphylactoid reaction to radiocontrast media, pretreatment with corticosteroids and a combination of H_1 and H_2 antihistamines, along with the use of low-osmolality nonionic dye, can reduce the incidence of recurrent episodes to approximately 1%. Patients with exercise-induced anaphylaxis can reduce the risk of an episode by avoiding exercise for at least 4 hours after eating.

Common Pitfalls

- Symptoms are underestimated or not recognized as anaphylaxis.
- Administration of intramuscular or subcutaneous epinephrine is delayed.
- Bronchodilator therapy is administered instead of epinephrine to treat lower respiratory symptoms of anaphylaxis.
- Patients are not observed for an appropriate length of time following anaphylactic events.
- Epinephrine auto-injectors are not prescribed following an anaphylactic event, and patients are not trained in the proper use of the device.
- Patients do not fill the prescription of the epinephrine auto-injector, have it available at the appropriate time, or use it in a timely manner.
- Patients are not referred to an allergy specialist.

Referral

A referral to an allergist should be provided following any anaphylactic event. An allergist can perform appropriate allergy testing based on the clinical history.

Communication and Counseling

When treated promptly, most patients recover completely from an anaphylactic event without lasting sequelae.

Patients must understand their risk for future anaphylactic episodes and how to avoid exposures. They need to be trained in using the epinephrine auto-injector and in reading food labels, when appropriate. In cases of hymenoptera allergy, patients should be offered venom immunotherapy. Patients with a history of anaphylaxis to radiocontrast media should be aware of the need for premedication with corticosteroids and antihistamines prior to a radiographic procedure.

In summary, anaphylaxis is a medical emergency that requires prompt identification by the patient and caregiver. Immediate recognition and administration of appropriate medication is key to survival. Although fatalities are rare in pediatrics, they do occur. Knowledge about the risk of a future anaphylactic event, how to avoid it whenever possible, and how to manage the event, should it occur, is of the utmost importance in ensuring a good outcome in patients at risk for anaphylaxis.

SUGGESTED READINGS

1. Lee JM, Greenes DS: Biphasic anaphylactic reactions in pediatrics. Pediatrics 106(4):762–766, 2000. **Describes the incidence of biphasic reactions in pediatric patients, which is considerably less than the incidence reported in adults.**
2. Lieberman P, Kemp SF, Oppenheimer J, et al: The diagnosis and management of anaphylaxis: An updated practice parameter. J Allergy Clin Immunol 115:S483–S523, 2005. **Updated practice parameter on anaphylaxis as issued by the American Academy of Allergy, Asthma, and Immunology, the American College of Allergy, Asthma, and Immunology, and the Joint Council of Allergy, Asthma, and Immunology.**
3. Neugut AI, Ghatak AT, Miller RL: Anaphylaxis in the United States: An investigation into its epidemiology. Arch Intern Med 161:15–21, 2001. **Reviews current medical literature to obtain prevalence data on different types of anaphylaxis in the United States.**
4. Pumphrey RSH: Lessons for management of anaphylaxis from a study of fatal reactions. Clin Exp Allergy 30:1144–1150, 2000. **Underscores the fact that few obvious risk factors for predicting fatal anaphylaxis exist, and therefore careful avoidance of triggers and early and aggressive treatment of episodes once they occur are of the utmost importance in managing anaphylaxis.**
5. Sampson HA: Anaphylaxis and emergency treatment. Pediatrics 111:1601–1608, 2003. **Discusses prevalence, signs and symptoms, diagnosis, and acute and long-term management of food-induced anaphylaxis in the United States.**
6. Sampson HA, Mendelson L, Rosen JP: Fatal and near-fatal anaphylactic reactions to food in children and adolescents. N Engl J Med 327(6):380–384, 1992. **Emphasizes that although children are less likely to have fatalities caused by anaphylaxis, they do occur.**
7. Sampson HA, Munoz-Furlong A, Bock SA, et al: Symposium on the definition and management of anaphylaxis: Summary report. J Allergy Clin Immunol 115:584–591, 2005. **Summary report on the definition and management of anaphylaxis, compiled by leading anaphylaxis experts who represent 12 professional, governmental, and lay organizations.**
8. Simons FER, Roberts JR, Gu X, et al: Epinephrine absorption in children with a history of anaphylaxis. J Allergy Clin Immunol 101(1): 33–37, 1998. **Discusses the ideal site and method of injectable epinephrine delivery in children, as determined by plasma epinephrine concentrations and monitoring of side effects.**
9. Yocum MW, Butterfield JH, Klein JS, et al: Epidemiology of anaphylaxis in Olmsted County: A population-based study. J Allergy Clin Immunol 104(2):452–456, 1999. **Retrospective, population-based cohort study aimed to determine the incidence of anaphylaxis, rate of recurrence, prevalence of atopy, cause of anaphylaxis, rate of specialist referral, hospital admission rate, and fatality rate.**

Head Injury

N. Paul Rosman

KEY CONCEPTS

- With head injuries, always remember to examine the *entire patient*.
- When a head-injured child is in *shock*, the cause is usually outside the head.
- With acute head injuries that are moderate (Glasgow Coma Scale [GCS] 9 to 12) or severe (GCS 3 to 8), the imaging modality of choice is a *cranial CT scan*.
- In medical management of acutely elevated intracranial pressure, *osmolar therapies* (mannitol, hypertonic saline) are the treatments of choice.
- With skull fractures, be mindful of possible *underlying pathologies*.
- With *concussion during contact sports*, recommendations from the American Academy of Neurology (AAN) for withholding such athletes from returning to competition, although reasonable, are not based on scientific study.
- In cerebral contusion or laceration, only *early post-traumatic seizures* (those occurring within 1 week of the injury) can be prevented with anticonvulsants.
- The most important predictor of *neurologic outcome* after head trauma is the severity of the head injury.

Throughout the world, trauma continues to be the leading cause of death and disability. Pediatric head injuries are an important contributor to this morbidity and mortality: In the United States, 2 to 5 million children sustain some degree of head trauma each year. The frequency is greater in children from birth to 5 years of age than in those who are older, and in young children, head injury is the most common neurologic cause of death and disability. Such injuries, twice as frequent in boys as in girls, have many different causes: falls; bicycling, skateboarding, snowboarding, and other recreational activities; competitive sports (e.g., football, ice hockey, and boxing); motor vehicle accidents; hand gun injury; and physical assault, including child abuse. Of these head-injured children, 200,000 are hospitalized; 30,000 suffer permanent disability, including seizures, motor disorders, cognitive impairment, learning difficulties, and behavioral and emotional problems; 5000 of these children die, with 1500 of those deaths from child abuse. Prompt diagnosis, early treatment, and active long-term management, when needed, minimize childhood morbidity and mortality in such cases.

Expert Opinion on Management Issues

DIAGNOSIS

Patient History

It is essential to determine the specific circumstances of the head injury and to identify predisposing factors. Attention should be paid to memory loss, repetitive questioning, confusion, visual disturbance, and symptoms of increased intracranial pressure, such as irritability, altered consciousness, vomiting, headache, and changes in vital signs. The principal mechanisms of head injury are direct contact and acceleration-deceleration. Lesions caused by direct contact with the head include scalp laceration, skull fracture, extradural hematoma, brain contusion, and intracerebral hemorrhage. By contrast, acceleration-deceleration, which results from head movement immediately after the injury (leading to intracranial and intracerebral pressure gradients and to shearing, tensile, and compressive strains) is responsible for cerebral concussion, diffuse axonal injury, and subdural hematoma.

General Physical Examination

Vital signs demand immediate attention and, at times, emergency treatment. Characteristic changes in pulse, blood pressure, and respirations may indicate shock, signaled by decreased blood pressure and increased pulse, or intracranial hypertension, manifested by increased blood pressure, decreased or increased pulse, and slowed or irregular respirations. A fall in blood pressure in a head-injured child is usually caused by an injury in another location, such as intra-abdominal bleeding (e.g., from a ruptured spleen) or bleeding into soft tissues (e.g., surrounding a long-bone fracture). Occasionally, however, hypotension can originate extracranially (e.g., with a large subgaleal hematoma) or intracranially (e.g., from an epidural hematoma).

The entire body should be checked for signs of trauma. Long-bone fractures, which occur in one third of patients with severe head injuries, may be complicated by fat embolism. The neck should be examined with particular care because of possible injury. With suspected neck trauma, the neck should be immobilized with sandbags and adhesive tape or a firm collar. Neck injury is suggested by cervical abrasions, cervical spine tenderness, or meningism. Meningism can also result from subarachnoid bleeding or cerebellar tonsillar herniation. The scalp should be inspected and palpated for areas of tenderness or depression. All scalp lacerations should be probed with a sterile gloved finger in search of a foreign body or an underlying skull fracture. Tension of the anterior fontanelle should be assessed in young infants. Periorbital hemorrhage ("raccoon-eyes" sign), ecchymosis behind the ear (Battle sign), blood behind the eardrum (hemotympanum), and bleeding from the ears or nose should be noted. These signs, along with cerebrospinal fluid (CSF) otorrhea or rhinorrhea, indicate a basilar skull fracture.

Neurologic Examination

The neurologic examination should assess the child's alertness, orientation, and memory. The presence and extent of any retrograde and anterograde (post-traumatic) amnesia should be determined. The latter can be inferred if a head-injured child repeatedly asks the same question. The level of consciousness may range widely. The Glasgow Coma Scale (GCS), with scores ranging from

TABLE 1 Glasgow Coma Scale

Best Motor Response	Score	Best Verbal Response	Score	Eye Opening	Score
Obeys	6	Oriented	5	Spontaneously	4
Localizes pain	5	Confused conversation	4	To speech	3
Withdraws	4	Inappropriate words	3	To pain	2
Flexion to pain	3	Incomprehensible sounds	2	None	1
Extension to pain	2	None	1		
None	1				

3 (worst) to 15 (best), provides a useful and reproducible scoring system for quantifying the level of consciousness and for following a head-injured child's clinical course systematically (Table 1). Although most studies report a correlation between a low GCS score and severe neurologic morbidity and substantial mortality, children with a low GCS score (3 to 5) sometimes do surprisingly well if the head injury is not complicated by a hypoxic-ischemic insult.

Neuro-ophthalmologic evaluation should note pupillary size and reactivity. Small pupils are seen with diencephalic and pontine injuries; a unilateral dilated pupil suggests temporal lobe herniation occurring on the same side. The fundi should be examined carefully, and evidence of retinal and preretinal (subhyaloid) hemorrhages and papilledema should be sought. Abnormalities of ocular gaze and position should be noted. If there is clearly no neck injury, the oculocephalic ("doll's-head") maneuver can be used to assess any apparent limitation of eye movements. Lateral gaze can also be tested in the comatose patient by caloric stimulation. In an alert child, visual acuity, visual fields, and opticokinetic nystagmus should be tested.

The extent of examination of the motor system depends on the child's alertness. The distribution (e.g., hemiparetic, paraparetic) of any muscle weakness, hypotonia, or spasticity should be observed. Abnormal posturing (e.g., decorticate, decerebrate) should be noted. In the responsive child, more detailed motor, coordinative, and sensory testing is possible. Testing for abnormal reflexes (e.g., palmar grasp, suck, root), eliciting deep tendon reflexes, and evaluating the plantar responses complete this portion of the examination.

Investigative Studies

Plain Radiography

The need for radiologic examination of the child with a head injury is dictated by the severity of the head trauma. Enthusiasm for eliminating unnecessary and expensive radiologic examinations in children with minor head trauma is increasing because of the infrequency of abnormalities found. Although some recommend that plain skull radiography be abandoned in favor of cranial CT, which is wise in a severely head-injured child who needs immediate care, many fractures (e.g., linear, basilar, and facial fractures; focal depressions) are visualized better on skull radiographs than with CT. *Severe* head

injuries, with significant loss of consciousness and focal neurologic signs (GCS score 3 to 8), require plain radiographs and further neuroradiologic study in most patients. The initial radiologic examination should include anteroposterior and lateral views of the cervical spine; anteroposterior and inclined anteroposterior (Towne projection), and left and right lateral views of the skull; and at least one lateral view taken with a horizontal beam (cross-table) to demonstrate any air-fluid levels in the cranial cavity or in the paranasal sinuses (indicative of a compound or basal fracture). With extensive head or facial trauma, radiographic views should include a Waters projection of the facial bones and films of the orbits. In *moderate* head trauma, with localizing neurologic signs or a history of loss of consciousness (GCS score 9 to 12), routine skull radiographs alone usually suffice, unless there was an accompanying neck injury. In *mild* head trauma, without focal neurologic signs or loss of consciousness (GCS score 13 to 15), skull and spine films are usually not needed. If a depressed skull fracture is suspected, tangential views should be obtained in addition to standard views.

Cranial Computed Tomography and Magnetic Resonance Imaging

In cases of moderate or severe head trauma and/or in cases with localizing neurologic signs, the most helpful and least invasive imaging modality is cranial CT. A cranial CT scan should probably also be done in anyone who has lost consciousness after a head injury, is amnestic for the injury, or who has signs of a basilar or calvarial fracture. Acute intracranial hemorrhage is usually easily seen on CT without contrast enhancement as a relatively dense mass. After several days, however, extravasated blood, which is semisolid, may appear to have the same density as contiguous brain tissue; thus CT scans taken at that time should be done with and without contrast enhancement. In addition to disclosing the presence of blood within brain parenchyma (as in contusion) or outside the brain (as with subdural and subarachnoid hemorrhage), cranial CT scanning can show brain edema, midline displacements, hydrocephalus, loss of brain tissue, and most skull fractures.

MRI of the brain is assuming an increasing role in the evaluation of head-injured children. Advantages of MRI include safety (no known biologic hazards and no reported side effects); the ability to obtain images in any plane; excellent demonstration of normal and pathologic anatomy; the ability to identify vessels without contrast injection (magnetic resonance angiography); and superior demonstration of the posterior fossa, where bone artifacts interfere with CT imaging. Also, MRI often shows parenchymal abnormalities in head-injured patients in whom no abnormalities are seen on CT. Substantial limitations in using MRI with critically ill patients exist, however, particularly the inability to monitor such patients adequately while they are being imaged. Also, acute intracranial bleeding (i.e., that seen within the first 1 to 3 days after injury) is much easier to see with CT than with MRI (although edema surrounding acute parenchymal hemorrhage is very well seen with MRI). Thus, with acute head injuries, CT is almost always the imaging procedure of choice, whereas MRI is of greatest assistance in evaluating brain lesions that are isodense on CT, such as subacute (3 to 14 days) or chronic (more than 14 days) extra-axial hematomas. In addition, diffuse white matter shearing injuries (diffuse axonal injuries) are seen very well with MRI.

Lumbar Puncture

Lumbar puncture should not be performed in the child with a head injury unless complicating central nervous system (CNS) infection is suspected. Lumbar puncture is usually contraindicated when intracranial pressure is significantly increased, and it is absolutely contraindicated when there is evidence of an intracranial mass.

Subdural Taps

Subdural taps may be indicated as a diagnostic or therapeutic measure, or both. A maximum of 15 mL of fluid is removed from each subdural space, without aspiration. The taps can be repeated within 1 to 2 days.

Other Studies

In selected cases, additional studies may be indicated, including a complete blood cell count; serum liver function tests and an amylase; urinalysis; platelet count and clotting studies; toxicology screening examination on blood, urine, and gastric aspirate; and a skeletal survey for old and recent fractures.

TREATMENT

Home Treatment versus Hospitalization

A head-injured child can usually be managed at home if the head injury was mild, with no more than a brief (several minutes) loss of consciousness, *and* if no significant abnormalities are noted on the physical and neurologic examinations. In addition, close and reliable monitoring of the child's progress at home must be assured; without such assurance, the child should be hospitalized for further management. Hospitalization is also indicated with changing vital signs; seizures; altered mental status, particularly prolonged unconsciousness; persisting memory deficit; focal neurologic signs; depressed or basilar skull fractures; enlarging scalp swellings; persistent severe headache, especially with neck stiffness; recurrent vomiting; unexplained fever; neuroradiologic abnormalities of concern on CT scan or MRI; and an unexplained injury (raising the possibility of child abuse).

General Support

Treatment of the child with head injury must be directed to the entire patient. The head and neck must be stabilized; with suspected neck trauma, a firm cervical collar, or sandbags, or tape and Velcro straps attached to a backboard should be used to immobilize the vertebral column until a spinal injury can be excluded. Life-threatening obstruction of the airway may result from blood, vomiting, secretions, a foreign object, or the tongue. Accessible foreign objects must be removed, with patency of the airway maximized by proper positioning and gentle suctioning. Ventilatory management is assisted by inserting an airway into the oropharynx; if needed, ventilatory support should be provided. If loss of consciousness or some other consequence of the head injury produces airway obstruction or if airway reflexes (e.g., gag, cough) are diminished or absent, orotracheal or nasotracheal intubation is needed. Nasotracheal intubation should not be used if a basilar skull fracture is suspected. One hundred percent oxygen (at 3–10 L/min) should be given by bag and mask or by nasal prongs, with the Pao_2 maintained at 90 to 100 mm Hg.

An intravenous (IV) line should be established and circulatory support provided. Active bleeding should be stopped. With infrequent exceptions, shock is not a sign of head injury in childhood but is caused by an associated injury, such as rupture of an abdominal organ (e.g., liver), by bleeding into extracranial soft tissues (e.g., next to a pelvic fracture), from peritonitis after intestinal perforation, from traumatic pancreatitis, or from an accompanying spinal cord injury ("spinal shock"). In all children with a severe head injury, a central venous line should be placed to monitor central venous pressure and assist in fluid management, and an arterial line should be inserted to monitor arterial blood pressure, assess cerebral perfusion pressure, and facilitate blood gas measurements. Hypovolemia (loss of more than 20% of blood volume) is corrected by IV crystalloid (such as normal saline) or colloid (such as 5% albumin). A slowing in pulse rate may indicate an encouraging response to treatment for circulatory insufficiency, but it can also be a danger signal, reflecting increased intracranial pressure. Circulatory failure is treated with epinephrine or norepinephrine. With cardiac arrest, in addition to ventilation and chest compressions, the child should be treated in accordance with the pediatric advanced life support (PALS) recommendations.

Accompanying injuries, such as those to the scalp, chest, great vessels, abdominal viscera, pelvis, limbs, or spine, may require specific treatment. Chest films to look for rib fractures, pneumothorax, and mediastinal widening should be obtained. With suspected abdominal bleeding or intestinal perforation, abdominal ultrasonography or CT scanning or diagnostic peritoneal lavage should be done. Fractured limbs should be splinted. The stomach should be emptied by nasogastric intubation to prevent

TABLE 2 Clinical Symptoms and Signs of Acutely Raised Intracranial Pressure

In Both Infants and Children	In Infants	In Children
Altered mental state Vomiting Strabismus (cranial nerve VI or III palsies); "setting sun" sign Altered vital signs (increased blood pressure, decreased or increased pulse, decreased or irregular respirations) Signs of herniation	Full fontanelle Separated sutures Macrocrania Papilledema	Headache Papilledema

vomiting, aspiration, and pressure on the diaphragm, which can cause secondary respiratory compromise. The bladder should be catheterized. Fever should be controlled by sponging, antipyretics, or a cooling blanket. If circulatory status is adequate, iso-osmolar fluids should be given at or slightly above normal maintenance. Electrolyte abnormalities and coagulation defects should be corrected. Vital signs should be followed with care. An elevation of systolic blood pressure, a slowing or speeding of the pulse, and slowed or irregular respirations are indicative of increased intracranial pressure. When seizures occur, anticonvulsants should be given.

Post-traumatic Seizures

Early post-traumatic seizures, which occur within the first week after a head injury, develop in approximately 5% of children hospitalized after head trauma. Of these seizures, two thirds occur within the first 24 hours (immediate seizures). Approximately 20% to 30% of patients with early post-traumatic seizures have additional seizures beyond the first week (late post-traumatic seizures). Infants and young children are at greater risk for early post-traumatic seizures than older children and adults. Management of post-traumatic seizures in children is essentially the same as treatment of nontraumatic seizures.

Raised Intracranial Pressure

Intracranial pressure is considered elevated if it measures more than 15 mm Hg in older children or adolescents, greater than 5 mm Hg in children ages 1 to 5 years, or greater than 3 mm Hg in newborns. In acute head trauma, causes of raised intracranial pressure include bleeding into the epidural, subdural, or subarachnoid spaces or into the brain; brain hyperemia causing diffuse brain swelling (days 2 to 3 after injury); brain edema accompanying brain contusion or hematoma (days 3 to 5); acute hydrocephalus from subarachnoid bleeding and impaired resorption of CSF fluid (days 7 to 10); and pseudotumor cerebri. Table 2 shows the clinical symptoms and signs of acutely elevated intracranial pressure.

Supportive Measures

When intracranial pressure is raised, respiratory and circulatory support must be provided. The head should be elevated to 30 degrees above horizontal and stabilized in the midline. Sufficient fluid should be given to maintain a state of isotonic normovolemia. Maintenance of an adequate blood volume is essential to ensure a satisfactory cerebral perfusion pressure to help prevent intracranial hypertension. Sometimes crystalloid, colloid, or vasopressors are required. Under normal circumstances, one should try to maintain serum osmolality between 300 and 320 mOsm/L. Fever should be treated aggressively with antipyretics and a cooling blanket, if needed. Seizures must be stopped with IV anticonvulsants.

Intracranial Pressure Monitoring

Continuous monitoring of intracranial pressure is especially valuable in poorly responsive head-injured patients because they are difficult to follow by clinical parameters alone. Such monitoring is indicated when the Glasgow Coma Scale (GCS; Table 1) is 5 or less, or 8 or less with CT evidence of a mass lesion or brain injury (such as contusion or diffuse cerebral swelling) and in any head-injured child who is unconscious or in shock, who has a deteriorating neurologic examination, or whose cranial CT scan shows distortion or displacement of the brain.

MEDICAL MANAGEMENT

Several medical measures are useful in managing acutely elevated ICP with head trauma. Table 3 summarizes these treatments.

Osmolar Therapies

Two osmolar therapies (mannitol, hypertonic saline) are very useful in the treatment of raised intracranial pressure. Brain capillaries (the site of the blood–brain barrier) are nearly impenetrable to both mannitol and saline. *Mannitol* produces a rapid reduction in intracranial pressure by lowering blood viscosity, which results in reflex cerebral vasoconstriction and a decrease in cerebral blood volume. This effect is transient, lasting less than 75 minutes. The second mechanism by which mannitol reduces intracranial pressure is by an osmotic effect. Mannitol given IV remains in plasma and creates an osmotic gradient, causing water to move from the brain through capillary walls into their lumina, thereby reducing intracranial pressure. This effect develops more slowly, in 15 to 30 minutes, and lasts for 1 to 6 hours. When mannitol is administered repeatedly, fluid and electrolyte imbalances, dehydration, hypotension, and renal

TABLE 3 Medical Management of Acutely Raised Intracranial Pressure in Head Trauma

Agent	Dose	Administration	Onset of Action	Peak Action	Advantages	Side Effects or Limitations
Mannitol	0.25–0.5 g/kg	Every 1–4 hr IV	5–30 min	15–90 min	Prompt action	Fluid-electrolyte imbalances; renal failure; intracranial bleeding; rebound
Hypertonic saline (3%)	0.1–1.0 mL/kg	Every hr IV	10 min	Approximately 3 hr	Prompt action	Renal failure; subarachnoid hemorrhage; rebound
Hyperventilation	Reduce $Paco_2$ to 35–30 mm Hg	Continuous	Seconds to minutes	2–30 min	Very prompt action	Effect may not be sustained; cerebral ischemia
Pentobarbital	Loading: 10–15 mg/kg; infusion: 1–3 mg/kg	Every 1–3 hr IV	1–2 min	Minutes	Prompt action; no rebound	Hypotension; renal failure; need for careful monitoring
Hypothermia	90°F–91°F (32°C–33°C)	Continuous	Approximately 1 hr	2–3 hr	No rebound	Cardiac arrhythmia; coagulopathy; need for careful monitoring

failure may result; thus the serum osmolality should be kept below 320 mOsm per L. Additionally, mannitol can potentiate intracranial bleeding. Mannitol may accumulate in injured brain regions and a reverse osmotic shift may occur, with fluid moving from the circulation to the brain parenchyma, which can exacerbate intracranial hypertension ("rebound"). This effect is most marked when mannitol is in the circulation for extended periods of time, which supports the use of intermittent IV boluses. Effective bolus doses, from 0.25 g/kg to 0.5 g/kg, can be given every 1 to 4 hours.

Resurgence in the use of *hypertonic saline* in the treatment of increased intracranial pressure is noted. The mechanisms of action are the same as with mannitol. A continuous infusion of 3% saline, between 0.1 to 1.0 mL/kg/hour, is given, using the minimum dose needed to maintain intracranial pressure at less than 20 mm Hg. With hypertonic saline, a serum osmolarity of up to 365 mOsm per L can be tolerated, even when given with mannitol. Potential side effects include rebound intracranial hypertension, central pontine myelinolysis, subarachnoid hemorrhage, and renal failure.

Hyperventilation

Hyperventilation can produce a rapid reduction in intracranial pressure. It induces hypocapnia, which leads to vasoconstriction and a reduction in cerebral blood flow, resulting in a decrease in intracranial pressure. Hyperventilation is associated with a risk of iatrogenic cerebral ischemia, however, and there is a move away from the use of aggressive hyperventilation in the management of severe traumatic brain injury. Thus, with hyperventilation, the $Paco_2$ should be lowered to between 35 and 30 mm Hg (below 25 mm Hg, complicating cerebral ischemia may result). Brief aggressive application of hyperventilation can be very effective, however, and in

the setting of acute neurologic deterioration and/or impending herniation, it can be lifesaving. Hyperventilation works quickly, and it does not lead to a secondary increase in intracranial pressure (i.e., rebound). An acute reduction in arterial $Paco_2$ of 5 to 10 mm Hg lowers intracranial pressure by 25% to 30%.

Induced Coma

Induction of coma with *barbiturates* is sometimes helpful in the management of intracranial hypertension after severe head injury where other measures have failed. Pentobarbital is the barbiturate most often used. Barbiturates reduce increased intracranial pressure by reducing cerebral metabolism, and they can do so by as much as 50%. They also reduce intracranial hypertension by causing cerebral vasoconstriction, thereby reducing cerebral blood flow and lowering intracranial pressure. Serum pentobarbital levels sufficient to achieve electrical silence or burst suppression on electroencephalogram (EEG) should be maintained. Such levels are usually 3 to 5 mg/dL. From 10 to 15 mg/kg of pentobarbital is given as a loading dose over 30 minutes, with 1 to 3 mg/kg given every 1 to 3 hours. Advantages of barbiturate coma include rapidity of action and absence of rebound.

Hypothermia

Hypothermia is an additional means of treating increased intracranial pressure. Lowering the body temperature to 86°F (30°C) decreases the cerebral metabolic rate by almost 50%. The target temperature in moderate hypothermia is 90°F to 91°F (32°C to 33°C). The mechanisms of action, advantages, and limitations of hypothermia are very similar to those of barbiturate-induced coma, with a 6% reduction in cerebral blood flow for each degree the temperature is lowered. Hypothermia works more slowly than pentobarbital in reducing intracranial hypertension and is probably never adequate as the sole method of managing increased intracranial pressure.

Drug Therapies

Steroids such as dexamethasone (Decadron) act more slowly than hyperosmolar agents to reduce increased intracranial pressure. Despite their widespread use in managing head injuries, steroids are not effective for that use.

Diuretics reduce brain water and decrease formation of CSF fluid and therefore are used in treating increased intracranial pressure. These agents include acetazolamide (Diamox), furosemide (Lasix), and ethacrynic acid (Edecrin). Diuretics alone are not very effective in rapidly reducing major elevations in intracranial pressure, but they may be effective in chronic treatment when only a moderate reduction in pressure is needed. Acetazolamide probably should not be used in patients with head injuries because its central vasodilator effect may cause intracranial pressure to rise.

SURGICAL MANAGEMENT

On occasion, elevations in intracranial pressure cannot be adequately reversed by specific interventions or by the medical means just discussed. In such a circumstance, surgical management may be indicated, such as aspiration of the subdural spaces, ventricular tap with slow withdrawal of CSF, or decompressive craniotomy.

Clinical Syndromes in Acutely Head-Injured Children

SCALP INJURIES AND SWELLINGS

Contusions and lacerations of the scalp are the most frequent complications of head injury. Lacerations should be cleaned thoroughly and sutured, if necessary. An underlying (depressed) skull fracture should be sought. Antibiotic and tetanus prophylaxis may be needed. In the older child, most scalp swellings following head trauma are caused by subgaleal hematomas, but in infants, particularly newborns, there are additional causes. In the neonate, diffuse scalp swelling with decreased transillumination suggests a subgaleal hematoma; diffuse scalp swelling with increased transillumination indicates a caput succedaneum. If the scalp swelling is focal, particularly in the parietal region, and transillumination is decreased, the newborn very likely has a cephalhematoma (with an underlying skull fracture occurring in 5% to 25% of cases). If the swelling is focal and transillumination is increased, a porencephalic or leptomeningeal cyst with an associated "growing" skull fracture may be present. No treatment is required for subgaleal hematoma, caput succedaneum, or cephalhematoma; in fact, aspiration of fluid from the scalp is contraindicated because of the risk of complicating infection. A leptomeningeal cyst must be treated surgically, however, by removing or replacing the protruding cyst and repairing the dural tear.

SKULL FRACTURES

The six major varieties of skull fractures in childhood are linear, depressed, compound, basal, diastatic, and "growing." *Linear* skull fractures constitute 75% of all pediatric skull fractures; they are most frequent in children younger than 2 years and are most often temporal-parietal. Although these fractures need not be treated, they may overlie serious intracranial pathologic conditions, such as epidural hemorrhage, for which treatment is urgently required. Skull radiographs showing a fracture involving a temporal bone or the sagittal suture should be followed by a CT scan. Linear fractures in the infant or young child should raise the possibility of neglect or inflicted injury, and if such injuries are suspected, long-bone and chest radiographs should be obtained. Linear skull fractures normally heal within 1 to 2 months.

In *depressed* skull fractures, either continuity of the bony calvaria is disrupted or, particularly in the newborn, the skull may simply be indented, causing a "ping-pong" or pond fracture. Focally depressed skull fractures may be missed if one fails to obtain tangential radiographic views of the skull, which usually demonstrate a double density (bone-on-bone) appearance at the fracture site. Although depressed skull fractures are seen best with plain radiographs, many can also be seen on CT, particularly when a bone fragment is displaced. Depressed skull fractures are of particular concern because the underlying brain may be contused or lacerated. Although surgical elevation of depressed fractures is advised if the depression is more than 5 mm deep or if the depressed fragment extends below the inner table of the skull, such elevation appears not to reduce the risk of post-traumatic epilepsy.

A compound or open skull fracture accompanied by a laceration of the scalp extending to the fracture site is of urgent concern because of the danger of complicating infection. Treatment should include meticulous debridement of the wound, search for a foreign body, copious irrigation with a sterile solution before closure, administration of parenteral antibiotics, and, if needed, tetanus prophylaxis. Any depressed fracture fragments should be elevated promptly.

Two main varieties of *basal* fractures are frontobasal and petrous. Only 20% of basal skull fractures can be visualized on standard skull radiographs because of the anatomic complexity of the base of the skull. Although the addition of multiplanar tomography and thin-section cranial CT scanning substantially increase the frequency with which such fractures can be seen radiographically, a firm diagnosis of basal skull fracture frequently depends on the recognition of coexisting signs. These include hemorrhage in the nose, nasopharynx, or middle ear; over the mastoid bone (Battle sign); or around the eyes ("raccoon-eyes" sign). Cranial nerve palsies sometimes occur, most frequently affecting cranial nerves I, VII, and VIII. CSF rhinorrhea and otorrhea, reflecting fractures of the cribriform plate or petrous temporal bone, respectively, are worrisome signs of basal fracture because of the risk of complicating bacterial meningitis. The responsible organism is most often *Streptococcus pneumoniae*, with *Haemophilus influenzae, Streptococcus pyogenes,* and *Neisseria meningitidis* less frequent causative organisms. Results from several studies, including a meta-analysis of more than 1200 patients with basilar skull fracture, indicate that antibiotic prophylaxis does not prevent meningitis. If signs of meningitis are present, empiric coverage against most organisms can be achieved with vancomycin in combination with either ceftriaxone or cefotaxime. Ninety percent of CSF leaks close within 7 to 10 days. Hemorrhage into the cranial sinuses can cause a radiographic appearance simulating sinusitis. Skull films may show intracranial air (pneumocephalus), indicating continuity between a paranasal or mastoid sinus and the inside of the skull.

Diastatic skull fractures are traumatic separations of cranial bones at one or more suture sites. They most frequently affect the lambdoid suture and are seen most often in the first 4 years of life. Diastatic fractures should be monitored closely in children younger than 3 years of age because they can become sites of growing fractures.

Growing skull fractures are caused by herniation of tissue through torn dura (and an accompanying linear or diastatic fracture) into the overlying scalp. These fractures occur most often in the parietal region. The herniating tissue can be solid brain parenchyma or cystic, either a porencephalic cyst (communicating with a lateral ventricle) or a leptomeningeal cyst. Growing skull fractures usually develop within 1 to 6 months of the head injury. They are rare in children older than 3 years. They require surgical repair.

CEREBRAL CONCUSSION

Cerebral concussion is characterized by an alteration in mental state, with confusion and amnesia, with or without loss of consciousness, occurring immediately after a head injury. The force of injury needed to cause a concussion is less than that required to produce a skull fracture, and the causative trauma is usually a blunt impact. Concussion is much more likely to occur when the head moves freely after the impact (acceleration-deceleration) than when the head is firmly in place (compression). Concussion can occur also in the absence of direct head trauma if sufficient whiplash force is applied to the brain. Concussion appears to be caused by an increase in intracranial pressure followed by a temporary shear strain on the upper brain stem. No consistent morphologic abnormalities are found in the concussed brain, but it continues to be debated whether such are present—the absence of proof of pathology is not proof of its absence. Early symptoms of concussion (minutes to hours) include headache, dizziness, lack of awareness of surroundings, nausea, and vomiting. When accompanied by loss of consciousness, concussion is associated with three types of amnesia: a temporary retrograde amnesia (extending back to events predating the head injury by some years); a permanent retrograde amnesia (encompassing the few seconds or minutes that immediately preceded the injury); and a temporary post-traumatic or anterograde amnesia (characterized by impaired ability to form new memories, usually lasting for some hours). Late symptoms of concussion (days to weeks) are many and include headache, lightheadedness, inattention, memory difficulties, fatigability, irritability, photophobia, sonophobia, anxiety, depression, and sleep disturbance.

CONCUSSION AND CONTACT SPORTS

Sports injuries in children 7 to 13 years of age occur in 1 to 2 of every 100 athletic events. One percent of these injuries are concussions, with 300,000 sports-related concussions seen each year in the United States. Grade I concussion is characterized by transient confusion, no loss of consciousness, and clearing of mental status in less than 15 minutes. Grade II concussion is the same as grade I except that the mental status changes last longer than 15 minutes. In grade III concussion, there is a period of unconsciousness.

Based on the severity of the concussion and the sideline evaluation of the concussed athlete (including mental status testing, neurologic tests, provocative exercise tests), recommendations for return to competition are suggested by the American Academy of Neurology. With a grade I concussion, if the player becomes asymptomatic within 15 minutes, he or she may then return to the game. With a grade II concussion, the player should not be permitted to return to competition that day but may return after a full week, if the player is asymptomatic. With a grade III concussion, the player should be withheld from competition for 1 week if the loss of consciousness was brief (lasting seconds) or for 2 weeks if more prolonged (lasting minutes). If the player sustains a second concussion of the same severity, return to competition should be delayed for a minimum of 1 week (grade I), 2 weeks (grade II), or 1 month (grade III).

These recommendations, based on expert opinion, receive only weak endorsement for practice, for many feel that once any serious complication of a head injury can be excluded (e.g., intracranial hemorrhage), a decision to withhold such athletes from participation in competition may be unwarranted. That said, repeated concussions cause cumulative neuropsychological damage, even when the incidents are separated by months or years. Further, the second-impact syndrome, the result of a second relatively minor blow while an affected individual still is symptomatic from a recent mild head injury, can be catastrophic, with permanent disability or death.

POSTCONCUSSIVE SYNDROME

Although the majority of children with concussion recover uneventfully, a few develop a postconcussive syndrome. Symptoms in adolescents, which include headache, dizziness, irritability, and impaired ability to concentrate, are usually relatively mild and self-limited. By contrast, younger children show aggression, disobedience, behavioral regression, inattention, and anxiety that can last from several days to several months and, on occasion, can persist. The pathogenesis of the postconcussion syndrome is unsettled. Organic, environmental, and emotional factors are variously cited.

CEREBRAL CONTUSION AND LACERATION AND POST-TRAUMATIC EPILEPSY

In contusion and laceration, in contrast to concussion, there is a bruising (contusion) or tearing (laceration) of brain. A blunt head injury predisposes to contusion, whereas a penetrating injury or a depressed skull fracture predisposes to laceration. Brain lesions can occur directly beneath the site of impact (coup injury), resulting from forceful impact against the dural septa or irregular bony projections of the skull; lesions can also occur more remotely, beneath the skull, opposite to the site of impact (contrecoup injury). The poles and undersurfaces of the frontal and temporal lobes are especially vulnerable. The diagnosis of contusion or laceration is established clinically by the presence of focal neurologic signs, including seizures, known or presumed to be absent before the head injury. The cranial CT scan or MRI often provides radiologic confirmation.

One complication of special concern in cerebral contusion and laceration is post-traumatic epilepsy (PTE). PTE occurs more often with laceration than with contusion. With a complicating skull fracture, PTE is more likely when the fracture is depressed than when it is linear. When a grade III concussion has also occurred, PTE is more likely when the duration of unconsciousness is more than 1 hour and if the post-traumatic amnesia lasts longer than 24 hours. An EEG is not helpful in predicting the occurrence of PTE in head-injured children.

Approximately 5% of children who are hospitalized following head trauma experience a seizure within the first week after their injury (early PTE). The more severe the head injury, the more likely it is that early PTE will occur. In 20% to 30% of early PTE cases, seizures continue beyond the first week. Another 5% of children who are hospitalized because of head trauma develop seizures more than 1 week after the injury (late PTE). As with early PTE, late PTE is more likely to occur when the head injury was more severe. Of the patients who develop late PTE, seizures eventually stop completely in approximately 50%; approximately 25% continue to have 10 to 15 seizures per year that are usually resistant to treatment, and another 25% have infrequent or rare seizures. Maintenance anticonvulsant drug therapy is clearly indicated in patients with late PTE, and many also prescribe it for children with early PTE.

NONACCIDENTAL HEAD INJURY IN CHILDREN

One quarter of all of head trauma in children less than 2 years of age is nonaccidental; most of these cases are caused by child abuse, with inflicted head injury the most common cause of traumatic death in infancy. Nonaccidental head trauma in young children with accompanying intracranial hemorrhage (subdural, subarachnoid) and ocular hemorrhage (preretinal or subhyaloid; retinal), often with minimal external evidence of trauma, strongly suggests the diagnosis of shaken-infant syndrome. Such injuries are attributable to repetitive whiplash motions of the relatively hyperextensible neck of the young child. Direct trauma is often also inflicted as well, and, in fact, most abused infants have evidence of blunt impact to the head. Thus the term *shaking-impact syndrome* may reflect more accurately than *shaken-infant syndrome* the pathogenesis of these injuries. With nonaccidental head trauma, evidence of external injury is seen in only 40% of infants younger than 1 year but is found in 75% of older infants and children up to 8 years of age.

ACUTE EPIDURAL AND SUBDURAL HEMATOMAS

See the article "Epidural and Subdural Hematoma."

Prognosis in Acute Brain Injuries

Most children hospitalized after concussion, skull fracture, or cerebral contusion recover completely, usually within 1 to several days. A small number of such children develop a postconcussion syndrome or post-traumatic seizures. An even smaller number of these patients sustain severe head injuries with prolonged coma followed by persisting cognitive, behavioral, or motor deficits.

SEVERE HEAD INJURIES AND NEUROLOGIC OUTCOME

The severity of a head injury, as reflected by the GCS, is the most important predictor of outcome. In the absence of accompanying systemic injury, severely head-injured children with a GCS score of 6 to 8 rarely, if ever, die; with a GCS score of 4 or 5, death still is unlikely; but with a GCS score of 3, mortality is between 50% and 100%.

Children with a GCS score of 6 or better have an 80% to 90% chance of recovering independent function with only minimal neurologic disability. With a GCS score of 4 or 5, cognitive, academic, and other neurologic deficits are found in 50% to 60% of children. Children with a GCS of 3 who survive have a high probability of cognitive and other neurologic deficits, usually substantial in degree.

DURATION OF POST-TRAUMATIC COMA AND NEUROLOGIC OUTCOME

Post-traumatic coma injury in the head-injured child lasting less than 24 hours is rarely associated with permanent neurologic or neuropsychological sequelae, except when there is severe focal brain injury. In severely head-injured children 10 years of age or younger, the average length of coma for those returning to normal intelligence is 1.7 weeks; for borderline intelligence, 3 weeks; for mild retardation, 8 weeks; and for severe retardation, 11 weeks. Children older than 10 years usually have longer durations of coma and a similar relationship between duration of coma and cognitive outcome. Such benchmarks notwithstanding, children and adolescents have a greater capacity than adults for recovering from severe head injuries, and they can show improvement in cognitive and social skills for more than 3 years.

NEUROLOGIC OUTCOME IN MILD HEAD INJURIES

Outcome data on neurologic sequelae after mild head injuries vary considerably in different series. Most of these children appear to recover quickly and completely, although later neurologic deficits, often quite subtle, are sometimes found.

AGE AS A FACTOR IN NEUROLOGIC OUTCOME

Many reports show that following head injuries of comparable severity, children usually recover more fully than adults. In head-injured patients with similar GCS scores, a 1-year rate of good outcome was found in 55% of patients 19 years of age or younger but in only 21% of older patients.

SUGGESTED READINGS

1. American Academy of Neurology: Report of the Quality Standards Subcommittee: Practice parameter: The management of concussion in sports (summary statement). Neurology 48:581–585, 1997. **Guidelines for return to competition following cerebral concussion.**
2. Barkovich AJ: Brain and spine injuries in infancy and childhood. In Barkovich AJ (ed): Pediatric Neuroimaging, 3rd ed. Philadelphia: Lippincott Williams & Wilkins, 2000, pp 157–249. **Wonderful images with excellent legends and focused descriptions of accompanying clinical features.**
3. Hauser WA, Pavone A (eds): Posttraumatic epilepsy. Epilepsia 44 (Suppl 10):1–39, 2003. **Most up-to-date summary of this important disorder, highlighting many still unanswered questions.**
4. Haydel MJ, Preston CA, Mills TJ, et al: Indications for computed tomography in patients with minor head injury. N Engl J Med 343:100–105, 2000. **Summarizes clinical features most likely to yield positive CT findings.**
5. Narayan RK, Wilberger JE, Povlishock JT (eds): Neurotrauma, New York: McGraw-Hill, 1996. **Most definitive textbook on head injury and spinal cord injury.**
6. Rosman NP, Oppenheimer EY, O'Connor JF: Emergency management of pediatric head injuries. Emerg Med Clin North Am 1:141–174, 1983. **Discussion of clinical and radiologic evaluation, medical and surgical management, with many accompanying photographs.**
7. Rosman NP: Traumatic brain injury in children. In Swaiman KF, Ashwal S (eds): Pediatric Neurology: Principles Practice, 3rd ed. St. Louis: Mosby, 1999, pp 873–897. **Updating of earlier material, with addition of sections on prognosis, prognostic indicators, and drug trials to minimize neurologic morbidity.**
8. Vinken PJ, Bruyn GW, Klawans HL (eds): Head Injury. Handbook of Clinical Neurology, vol. 57 (RS 13): Amsterdam: Elsevier, 1990. **Broad survey of the most important aspects of head injuries with contributions from a worldwide group of experts.**

Facial and Middle Ear Trauma

Paul R. Krakovitz and Peter J. Koltai

KEY CONCEPTS

■ At birth, the craniofacial ratio is 8:1, with the face located in a recessed position relative to a large skull. By 2 years of age, the cranium has achieved 80% of its mature size. Brain and ocular growth are near completion by 7 years of age, but facial growth continues into the second decade of life. In the adult the craniofacial ratio is 2:1. The consequence of the child's having a higher craniofacial ratio is that the cranium absorbs the majority of the impacting force. This accounts for the higher proportion of pediatric skull fractures compared to facial fractures.

■ Other resilient features of a young child's facial makeup are the thick soft tissue, lack of sinus pneumatization, and elasticity of the bones. The greater proportion of cancellous to cortical bone explains the higher incidence of so-called greenstick fractures in children. The presence of unerupted and mixed dentition in the maxilla and mandible increases the resistance to fracture.

■ Craniofacial bone growth is a complex and incompletely understood process, and even less is known about the effects of trauma on this process. Contemporary thought holds that the genetic program within the enveloping soft tissues and regional growth sites controls facial growth. The nasal septum has received much attention for its role in the downward and outward thrust of the midface. Although it is doubtful that the septum is the only pacemaker of midfacial development, both experimental and clinical data support its role as an important regional growth site.

Following the first month of life, trauma is the number-one cause of pediatric mortality and a major cause of long-term morbidity. Despite these statistics, facial fractures in children are uncommon, with 70% occurring between 13 and 18 years of age.

Motor vehicle accidents are the major cause of serious pediatric facial trauma. Fortunately, less than 1% of traffic accidents result in pediatric facial bone fractures. Other trauma etiologies include childhood play, falls, violence, and sports injuries. Facial fractures, in particular mandible and nasal fractures, can be the result of child abuse.

Nasal fractures in children are the most common facial bones fractured. Mandible fractures are the most common facial fractures in children requiring hospitalization. Complex facial fractures are rare in children. Associated injuries are a common feature of childhood maxillofacial trauma.

Expert Opinion on Management Issues

The first step in evaluating pediatric facial trauma is to follow the basic principles of trauma management. If at all possible, an accurate history should be obtained, with the focus on the mechanism of injury as well as the energy and direction of the impact. An injury that appears inconsistent with the history should raise suspicion of child abuse.

Facial trauma often complicates maintaining a stable airway. Orotracheal intubation is necessary when there is concomitant cranial trauma, severe bleeding associated with midfacial fractures, or oropharyngeal obstruction and posterior retrusion of the mandible. Orotracheal intubation ideally is accomplished after securing the cervical spine.

The secondary survey of the head and neck proceeds in an orderly fashion beginning with the neurologic assessment, evaluation of the neck and cervical spine, inspection of the eyes, otoscopy, rhinoscopy, and, finally, examination and manual palpation of the face and oral cavity.

Computed tomography (CT) has revolutionized the evaluation of pediatric trauma. The gold standard for displaying the mandible is the panoramic view (Panorex). This can be difficult to obtain in a multiply injured or uncooperative child, in which case CT scans should be used. Routine radiograph for isolated pediatric nasal trauma is rarely useful. But when significant flattening or deformity of the nasal dorsum has occurred, both axial and coronal CT should be obtained to determine the integrity of the naso-orbito-ethmoid (NOE) complex.

Practical concepts for the repair of facial fractures in children are based on the known effects of trauma in the growing face as well as on an understanding of the operational mechanics of facial development. The mandible appears generally resistant to abnormalities of growth as a result of trauma, unless there is alteration of its function because of injury in or near the temporomandibular joint. The nose, nasoethmoidal complex, and maxilla are more prone to growth abnormalities as a result of trauma.

Management of complex fractures requires an understanding of both the risks and benefits of rigid fixation. The unresolved question is whether transient stabilization of the facial skeleton results in permanent growth disturbances. We can safely conclude that fixation should be done with caution and be reserved for fractures where the original features are difficult to restore by other means (Box 1).

Mandibular fractures are divided by the subsite (condylar, angle, body, symphyseal, and parasymphyseal) of the injury. Frequently, there are multiple fracture sites. Mandibular fractures that manifest with normal occlusion and mobility can often be treated conservatively with a soft diet and movement exercises. Mandibular fractures that manifest with malocclusion or movement limitation are treated either with 2 to 3 weeks of immobilization (maxillomandibular fixation [MMF] or with open reduction and internal fixation (ORIF).

Midface fractures in children are rare and manifest clinically with severe facial edema, prominent orbital ecchymosis, and malocclusion. Concomitant neurocranial injuries are frequent. Early operative intervention is ideal; however, this might not be possible because of the global medical condition of the child. Significant fracture displacement should be reduced within 10 days.

Zygomaticomalar complex (ZMC) fractures correspond to the maxillary sinus pneumatization and are uncommon prior to 5 years of age. Minimally displaced fractures can be treated conservatively. When simple reduction techniques result in unstable or nonanatomic reduction, ORIF is indicated.

Nasal fractures in young children are rare because of minimal projection but are common in the adolescent. With fractures that significantly displace the nasal skeleton, a high index of suspicion should be maintained for more extensive, but occult, nasoethmoidal and orbital injuries. The initial examination of a child with a suspected nasal fracture is often of limited value with regard to the external deformity because of edema. But immediate intranasal examination is essential to evaluate for septal injury, particularly septal hematoma. Nasal obstruction is the hallmark of septal hematoma and can be observed on anterior rhinoscopy as an obvious purple bulge on one side of the nose. Septal hematoma is a serious complication and should be treated immediately with evacuation.

Injuries to the orbit and nasoethmoidal region can leave children with significant functional and cosmetic defects. The scope of these injuries is related to the magnitude of the impacting force and can vary from relatively minor fractures, such as blowout of the orbital floor, to complex fractures. Associated facial fractures occur in 30% of orbital fractures. Suspected orbital trauma warrants an ophthalmologic evaluation. Periorbital edema and hypoesthesia, ecchymoses, and subconjunctival hemorrhage, diplopia, and mobility reduction are indicative of orbital injury.

Orbital-floor fractures are the most common injuries of the middle component of the orbit. They occur as isolated blowout fractures or in conjunction with zygomaticomalar or Le Fort–type fractures. So-called trapdoor and saucer fractures are the two major types of blowout or orbital-floor fractures seen in the pediatric population. The trapdoor, or white-eyed, fracture is a pure orbital-floor fracture and usually the consequence of low-velocity blunt trauma. The trapdoor fracture can be subtle on presentation and should be suspected when supraduction mobility is limited. Serious ocular injury with blowout fractures occurs in less than 5% of cases.

Fractures of the NOE complex can vary from minimal dislocations to highly comminuted compound fractures. The four-sided NOE fracture is anatomically defined by fractures of the nasofrontal suture, nasal bones, medial orbital rim, and infraorbital rim. Most NOE fractures are best treated with ORIF. Although correction is technically difficult, overcorrection of the NOE fracture is superior aesthetically to undercorrection.

BOX 1 Basic Intervention Tenets for Repair of Pediatric Fractures

- Careful restoration of injured soft tissue
- Close attention to septal injuries with an emphasis on realignment rather than resection
- Reduction of fractures to their stable anatomic locations
- Correct realignment of suture lines
- Minimal periosteal elevation
- Three-dimensional stable fixation of complex fractures
- Use of bone grafts in areas of bone loss

Common Pitfalls

- Reconstruction of pediatric facial fractures requires an understanding of craniofacial development and the consequence of injury on future growth. The patterns of facial fracture differ significantly between children of different ages. Repair of bony injuries is often best accomplished by techniques that may adversely affect craniofacial development. Therefore, a rational approach to treatment must be formulated.

- More severe types of pediatric facial trauma are associated with other concomitant injuries between 30% and 60% of the time. Optimal timing for fracture repair must be tempered with the medical stability of the patient.
- Complications of pediatric fractures include infection, nonunion, malunion, malocclusion, dental injury, and temporomandibular joint dysfunction.
- Prolonged follow-up is mandatory, and orthodontia may be an important adjunct in the long-term management of mandible fractures. Early and persistent movement with an elastic jaw exerciser generally prevents the development of ankylosis and aids in restoring function.

Communication and Counseling

Children sustain severe maxillofacial injuries that require appropriate repair. The primary factor that distinguishes the treatment of pediatric and adult fractures is facial growth. Trauma to the mandible is well compensated, and growth disturbances are uncommon when treated appropriately. Inadequate treatment of upper and midfacial injuries may result in serious alterations of facial growth. CT scanning, craniofacial exposure,

bone grafting, and the advent of resorbable rigid fixation facilitate the ability to reconstruct the most complex three-dimensional disfigurements. Cosmetic deformities, as well as functional impairment in nasal breathing, vision, dental occlusion, and hearing, are all potential long-term sequelae from childhood facial and middle ear trauma (Box 2).

SUGGESTED READINGS

1. Dahlstrom L, Kahnberg KE, Lindahl L: 15 years follow-up on condylar fractures. Int J Oral Maxillofac Surg 18:18–23, 1989. **Study showing long-term effects of condylar fractures.**
2. Enlow DH: Facial Growth, 3rd ed. Philadelphia: WB Saunders, 1990, pp 1–24. **Detailed account of facial development.**
3. Hardt N, Gottsauner A: The treatment of mandibular fractures in children. J Craniomaxillofac Surg 21:214–219, 1993. **Thorough description of treatment options for mandibular fractures.**
4. Hatton MP, Watkins LM, Rubin PA: Orbital fractures in children. Ophthalmic Plast Reconstr Surg 17(3):174–179, 2001. **Complete explanation for treatment of orbital fractures.**
5. Iizuka T, Thoren H, Annino DJ Jr, et al: Midfacial fractures in pediatric patients. Frequency, characteristics, and causes. Arch Otolaryngol Head Neck Surg 121(12):1366–1371, 1995. **Study recounting the etiology of midfacial fractures.**
6. Koltai PJ: Maxillofacial injuries in children. In Smith JD, Bumsted R (eds): Pediatric Facial Plastic Reconstructive Surgery. New York: Raven Press, 1993, pp 283–316. **In-depth discussion of pediatric facial trauma.**
7. McGraw BL, Cole RR: Pediatric maxillofacial trauma. Age-related variations in injury. Arch Otolaryngol Head Neck Surg 116(1):41–45, 1990. **Discussion highlighting the differences in facial trauma between age groups in children.**
8. McGuirt WF, Salisbury PL: Mandibular fractures: Their effect on growth and dentition. Arch Otolaryngo Head Neck Surg 113:257–261, 1987. **Study relating the long-term effects of injury to the mandible.**
9. Scott JH: The analysis of facial growth from fetal life to adulthood. Angle Orthod 33:110–113, 1963. **Comprehensive discussion of facial growth.**
10. Yaremchuk MJ, Fiala TG, Barker F, Ragland R: The effects of rigid fixation on craniofacial growth of rhesus monkeys. Plast Reconstr Surg 93:1–10, 1994. **Animal study demonstrating the effects of manipulating the developing face with ORIF.**

3

BOX 2 Middle Ear Trauma

- Middle ear trauma is frequently the result of either blunt or penetrating injuries.
- Penetrating trauma to the middle ear ranges from minor injuries from such as cotton tip applicators to major gunshot wounds.
- Hot sparks and slag injury can result in tympanic membrane perforation.
- Penetrating trauma to the ear or excessive bleeding should alert the caregiver to potential vascular injury and a radiographic blood flow study should be performed.
- An audiogram should be obtained in anyone suspected of middle ear trauma.
- Patients with dizziness, vertigo, or nystagmus require vestibular studies, such as electroneurography.
- Any otologic injury requires the evaluation of facial nerve function.
- Traumatic penetration of the tympanic membrane in the posterosuperior quadrant has a higher risk of ossicular damage. This observation demands close evaluation for nystagmus because of possible subluxation of the stapes into the vestibule of the labyrinth.
- Trauma to the middle ear can be associated with temporal bone fractures. These injuries are frequently the result of blunt trauma. Associated injuries include facial nerve damage, cerebrospinal fluid (CSF) otorrhea, and damage to the cochlea and vestibular systems. Other common findings include hemotympanum and tympanic membrane perforation. Any finding suggestive of such injuries warrants a temporal bone CT scan.
- Hemotympanum typically resolves with watchful management. Close follow-up is imperative.
- Injuries to the ossicular chain are common and frequently correctable with exploratory surgery.

Stabilizing the Injured Child

Arthur Cooper

KEY CONCEPTS

- Pediatric trauma kills and maims more children than all other diseases combined.
- Pediatric injuries with a demonstrable threat to life are associated with an Injury Severity Score of 10 or higher or a Pediatric Trauma Score of 8 or lower.
- Most pediatric trauma is a disease of airway and breathing, not bleeding and shock.
- Airway opening is crucial because the funnel-shaped upper airway is prone to obstruction.
- Cervical spine stabilization must accompany airway opening to protect the cervical spine.
- Oxygen is the key pharmacologic agent and is given to all patients with pediatric trauma via nonrebreather

KEY CONCEPTS—cont'd

mask in respiratory distress or via bag-valve-mask in respiratory failure or coma.
- Volume resuscitation, when necessary, should be titrated against tissue perfusion.
- Broad-spectrum systemic intravenous antibiotics are indicated for penetrating trauma. Tetanus toxoid is indicated for tetanus-prone wounds unless immunizations are up to date.

Trauma, defined as forceful disruption of bodily homeostasis, comprises those injuries whose severity poses a demonstrable threat to life, which corresponds, in children, to an Injury Severity Score (ISS) of 10 or higher or a Pediatric Trauma Score (PTS) of 8 or lower. It remains the leading cause of death and disability in children worldwide, despite the ample availability of proven measures for injury prevention. The principles of early care for the injured patient are promulgated internationally by the American College of Surgeons Committee on Trauma via their Advanced Trauma Life Support and Trauma Evaluation and Management (TEAM) Programs, which are periodically revised to ensure that treatment guidelines are based on current evidence. Box 1 summarizes the key concepts in pediatric trauma resuscitation.

BOX 1 Key Concepts in Pediatric Trauma Resuscitation

Primary Survey and Resuscitation

Airway/Cervical Spine

- Open: Modified jaw thrust/cervical spine stabilization
- Clear: Excessive secretions suctioned/particulate matter removed
- Support: Oropharyngeal/nasopharyngeal airway
- Establish: Orotracheal intubation for respiratory failure, shock, coma[1]
- Maintain: Primary/secondary confirmation of endotracheal tube placement[2]
- Bypass: Needle cricothyroidotomy for complete upper airway obstruction.

Breathing/Chest Wall

- Ventilation: Chest rise; air entry/effort/rate
- Oxygenation: Central color/pulse oximetry
- Support: Distress, NRB; failure, BVM
- Chest wall: Integrity ensured/lungs expanded
- Tension pneumothorax: Needle decompression, chest tube[3]
- Open pneumothorax: Occlusive dressing, chest tube
- Massive hemothorax: Volume resuscitation, chest tube.

Circulation/External Bleeding

- Bleeding stopped: Direct pressure, clamps avoided
- Shock evaluation: Pulse rate/character, skin temperature/moisture, CRT, LOC[4]
- Blood pressure: Over/undercorrection avoided
- Infant/child: Low normal = 70 + (age × 2) mm Hg
- Adolescent: Low normal = 90 mm Hg
- Volume resuscitation: Possibly lactated Ringer, packed cells
- Infant/child: 20 mL/kg lactated Ringer, possibly repeat × 1–2; 10 mL PRBC
- Adolescent: 1–2 mL, possibly repeat × 1–2, 1–2 U PRBC.

Disability/Mental Status

- Pupils: Symmetry, reaction
- LOC: GCS
  - Track and trend as vital sign
  - Significant change = 2 points
  - Intubate for coma = GCS 8

- Motor: Strength, symmetry
- Abnormality/deterioration: Neurosurgeon called
  - Mild TBI (GCS 14–15): Should be observed, CT considered for history of LOC
  - Moderate TBI (GCS 9–13): Should be admitted, CT obtained, CT repeated in 12–24 h
  - Severe TBI (GCS 3–8): Should be intubated, ventilated, CT obtained, CT repeated in 12–24 h.

Exposure and Environment

- Disrobe: Clothes cut off
- Log roll: Requires four people
- Screening examination: Front and back
- Hypothermia: Patient kept warm.

Adjuncts

- Foley catheter unless contraindicated[5]
- Gastric tube unless contraindicated[6].

Secondary Survey and Reevaluation

History and Physical Examination

- SAMPLE history:
  - **S**ymptoms: "What hurts?"
  - **A**llergies
  - **M**edications
  - **P**ast illnesses
  - **L**ast meal
  - **E**vents/Environment: "What happened?"
- Complete examination:
  - Incorporates ongoing review of primary survey
  - Head to toe; includes neurologic evaluation
  - Inspection, palpation, percussion, auscultation
  - "Tubes and fingers in every orifice".

Adjuncts

- Imaging and laboratory studies:
  - Plain radiographs[7]
  - Special studies.[8]

---

[1]RSI (rapid sequence intubation technique): Preoxygenation; cricoid pressure; etomidate, 0.3 mg/kg; succinylcholine, 1–2 mg/kg.

[2]First degree: Chest rise, air entry. Second degree: Exhaled carbon dioxide (CO_2) detector, esophageal detector device; watch for DOPE (Dislodgement, Obstruction, Pneumothorax, Equipment failure).

[3]Do not wait for confirmatory chest radiograph.

[4]For CRT and LOC, consider obstructive and neurogenic as well as hypovolemic shock. Exclude tension pneumothorax, cardiac tamponade, spinal shock.

[5]Meatal blood, scrotal hematoma, high-riding prostate.

[6]CSF, otorrhea/rhinorrhea, basilar skull fracture, midface instability.

[7]Chest, pelvis, lateral cervical spine; others as indicated.

[8]FAST (Focused Assessment by Sonography in Trauma) and CT as indicated.

BVM, bag-valve-mask ventilation; CRT, capillary refill time; CSF, cerebrospinal fluid; GCS, Glasgow Coma Scale; LOC, level of consciousness; NRB, non-rebreather mask; PRBC, packed red blood cells; TBI, traumatic brain injury.

Expert Opinion on Management Issues

RESUSCITATIVE MEASURES

Major pediatric trauma is a disease of airway and breathing, not bleeding and shock, because most pediatric trauma is blunt trauma involving the head, as demonstrated by data from the National Pediatric Trauma Registry showing that among children who have significant mortality risk (ISS $\geq$10, PTS $\leq$8), the abnormalities in respiratory rate and low Glasgow Coma Scale scores are five times more common (40% vs. 8%) than abnormalities of blood pressure. Thus, in pediatric patients, the main focus of the ABCDEFGs (defined later) of the primary survey is on support of ventilation and oxygenation, rather than on maintenance of perfusion. The primary survey comprises the rapid cardiopulmonary and critical injury assessment that identifies the need for urgent resuscitation and is therefore conducted before the history and physical examination, which thereupon becomes the secondary survey.

Airway opening is crucial because the narrow funnel-shaped larynx is prone to obstruction from soft tissues, abundant secretions, and particulate matter. Obstruction must be fully relieved by airway adjuncts, oropharyngeal suctioning, and foreign body removal while manually stabilizing the cervical spine in a neutral position. *Breathing* assistance with high-concentration supplemental oxygen is also essential, via either nonrebreather (NRB) mask or bag-valve-mask (BVM) device, the choice depending on adequacy of spontaneous respiratory effort. Orotracheal intubation with an uncuffed tube is additionally necessary for the child with an unmaintainable airway or in respiratory failure, as well as for the child in decompensated shock or traumatic coma. Needle cricothyroidotomy is needed for the child with complete upper airway obstruction that cannot be relieved; needle thoracostomy, followed by tube thoracostomy, is required for the child with evidence of tension pneumothorax. *Circulation* support is vitally important for the child with abnormal tissue perfusion, after obtaining vascular access using large-bore cannulas inserted into the antecubital veins bilaterally, or if this cannot be accomplished, via the femoral veins in the older child, or the tibial bone marrow in the infant, using appropriate-sized central lines or intraosseous needles. *Disability*, or neurologic evaluation, follows next. Its purpose is to identify the need for immediate neurosurgical involvement, through pupillary examination, to detect a potential mass lesion, and Glasgow Coma Scale score determination, to document an altered mental status. *Exposure* of the patient to be sure no injuries are missed (taking care to avoid hypothermia because of the child's thin skin and large body surface area) completes the primary survey, and transitions to the secondary survey—the complete history and physical examination—after insertion of a *Foley catheter* and a *gastric tube*, unless these are proscribed by signs of pelvic or craniofacial fracture.

DRUG THERAPY

Supplemental oxygen is the key pharmacologic agent used in pediatric trauma resuscitation because respiratory failure, hemorrhagic shock, and traumatic coma all result in failure of oxygen delivery to end organs. Balanced salt solutions, to promote tissue perfusion, followed by packed red cells as needed, to permit oxygen delivery, are given to hypovolemic trauma patients. There is no contraindication to high-concentration oxygen in the injured child, but volume resuscitation should be titrated against tissue perfusion because overhydration may worsen cerebral edema following traumatic brain injury. Vasopressors have no role in the early care of hypovolemic trauma patients. Phenytoin is used for seizure prophylaxis only during the first week after moderate to severe traumatic brain injuries. Steroids are contraindicated following such injuries. Broad-spectrum intravenous antibiotics are administered following penetrating trauma but not after blunt trauma. Tetanus-prone wounds require tetanus toxoid, with or without tetanus immune globulin, depending on immunization status and degree of contamination.

SURGICAL THERAPY

Although management of blunt visceral trauma in pediatric patients is largely nonoperative, it is not nonsurgical because mature surgical judgment is required to determine whether, or when, surgical intervention may be required. Traumatic brain injury is the most common cause of mortality and morbidity, and it requires aggressive management in a pediatric critical care unit by clinicians who are expert in pediatric neurotrauma, in accordance with nationally recognized guidelines that take into account the far greater incidence of diffuse cerebral injuries in children than adults. Blunt abdominal trauma associated with solid organ disruption can be managed nonoperatively in 98% of kidney injuries, 95% of spleen injuries, and 90% of liver injuries in accordance with nationally recognized guidelines, but management of blunt pancreatic injuries is controversial. In contrast, hollow organ disruption always requires surgical intervention, with the exception of extraperitoneal bladder injuries, for which catheter drainage is indicated.

Skeletal injuries constitute the majority of cases in which surgical intervention is necessary, although for pelvic fractures, interventional radiology may also be used. With few exceptions, hypotensive pediatric trauma patients require immediate operation. Indications for abdominal exploration also include peritoneal irritation, but not peritoneal fluid, unless hemodynamic lability coexists. Penetrating injuries of the head, neck, and abdomen also require surgical intervention, but most intrathoracic injuries, whether blunt or penetrating, require only tube thoracostomy. Resuscitative emergency department thoracotomy has a dismal outcome in childhood. Therefore, it is indicated only for patients with penetrating chest trauma with signs of life at the scene or in the emergency department.

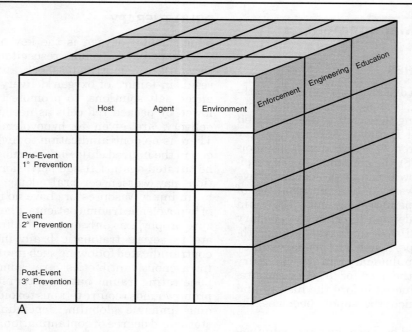

Haddon Factor Phase Matrix

	Occupant (host)	Vehicle (agent)	Highway system (environment)
Pre-crash (pre-event)	Licensing restrictions, Driver education, abiding road laws	Collision avoidance, anti-lock brakes, **crash test dummy based safety design**	Road design, markings and surface **safety standards**
Crash (event)	**Seat belt use, child safety seat use**	**Air bags, restraint design** vehicle size and mass **bumper and crumple zone design**	Collision speed, bullet vehicle mass road side hardware
Post-crash (post-event)	Gender, severity, age, underlying morbidity	Ease of extrication, burn resistant fabrics	EMS system, quality trauma care, traffic management system

B

FIGURE 1. Haddon factor-phase matrix.

PREVENTIVE MEASURES

Injuries are not accidents, but predictable events rooted in a complex web of social, cultural, and economic factors that affect the host, agent, and environment. Yet people respond to established harm reduction strategies applied before, during, and after the injury event as depicted in the Haddon factor-phase matrix, expanded into a cube that demonstrates tactics as well as strategies (Figure 1). Thus, to be effective, injury prevention programs must be based within the community and must function through meaningful collaboration with civic leaders, government agencies, and neighborhood coalitions. Within this environment, they must create successful partnerships between trauma programs and local public health entities to measure and track injury incidence by locality and make specific plans to target high-frequency risks. This requires substantial personal and institutional commitment on the part of trauma professionals and trauma centers, including commitment of necessary resources. Strong physician leadership and effective program coordination are essential for success. The National Safe Kids Campaign (http://www.safekids.org) and the Injury Free Coalition for Kids (http://www.injuryfree.org) have both proved highly effective in reducing the burden of childhood injury. The ABCDEs of injury prevention were recently described:

- *Analyze* injury data through local injury surveillance.
- *Build* neighborhood coalitions that support and empower community leaders.

- *Communicate* the problem by raising local awareness that injuries are a preventable public health problem.
- *Develop* targeted interventions and injury-prevention activities to create safer environments and activities.
- *Evaluate* prevention activities with ongoing injury surveillance.

Common Pitfalls

Preventable deaths following major pediatric trauma result chiefly from failure to support ventilation and oxygenation by recognizing and managing airway obstruction and tension pneumothorax and from failure to maintain organ and tissue perfusion by detection and control of intracranial and intra-abdominal hemorrhage. These tragedies arise mainly from failure to appreciate that major pediatric trauma is mostly a disease of airway and breathing, which results from limited knowledge of developmental anatomy and physiology. Specifically, it is important to recognize that the narrower upper airway is more susceptible to soft tissue obstruction, the mobile mediastinum has a greater propensity to shift under tension, and the pediatric vasculature has a greater ability to constrict in response to hypovolemia, so that a child may be in shock despite normal systolic pressure.

Injured children are also at high risk for respiratory failure, owing to their higher metabolic oxygen requirements yet lower functional residual capacity, as well as their horizontally aligned ribs and poorly developed intercostal muscles (which make small children diaphragmatic breathers). Therefore, signs of respiratory insufficiency must be vigorously reversed. Gastric dilation because of air swallowing, unless decompressed by a nasogastric or orogastric tube, also limits ventilation and oxygenation by compromising diaphragmatic excursion and causing aspiration pneumonitis, and it may mimic or mask intraperitoneal hemorrhage.

Injudicious volume resuscitation is frequently problematic; patients in shock need an effective volume resuscitation including red blood cells (RBCs), but excessive fluids should not be administered to patients with traumatic brain injury.

Unwarranted or inappropriate attempts to practice nonoperative management of solid visceral injuries, although well intentioned, can be fatal in the absence of appropriate resources for tertiary-level pediatric trauma care.

The higher elastin content and horizontal facet joints of the cervical spine can predispose to spinal cord injury without radiographic abnormality (SCIWORA). SCIWORA can be missed on initial physical examination, particularly in comatose patients, necessitating full spinal immobilization until a spinal cord injury is excluded by clinical evaluation and radiologic imaging. Imaging consists at a minimum of anteroposterior, lateral, and open mouth views.

Improper restraint use during motor vehicle crashes can result in diaphragmatic rupture, Chance fractures of the lumbar spine, and proximal intestinal hematoma or perforation.

Communication and Counseling

The case fatality rate following major pediatric trauma is nearly 3%. The complication rates are 23% for injury complications and 11% for treatment complications. Population-based studies demonstrate improved mortality and morbidity for pediatric trauma patients managed in pediatric-capable trauma centers. Functional limitations are present in 90% of major trauma patients at discharge but then decrease significantly unless traumatic brain injury is present, and quality of life is fairly well maintained.

Counseling of parents of injured children is essential. Most express significant guilt about their child's injury, even though they are seldom responsible. Reassurance that is compassionate, yet realistic, is most likely to be regarded as helpful. Family presence during resuscitation should be routinely encouraged, and most regard it as helpful.

SUGGESTED READINGS

1. Aitken ME, Tilford JM, Barrett KW, et al: Health status of children after admission for injury. Pediatrics 110:337–342, 2002. **This study reviews the medium-term effects of pediatric trauma on child health status, concluding that 90% of children surviving major trauma had residual functional deficits at hospital discharge, although only 57% of children had persistent deficits 1 month later, and only 28% of children had persistent deficits 6 months later.**
2. American College of Surgeons Committee on Trauma: Advanced Trauma Life Support for Doctors Student Course Manual, 7th ed. Chicago: American College of Surgeons, 2004. **These consensus-based guidelines are the recognized standard for the early care of the injured patient.**
3. American College of Surgeons Committee on Trauma: National Trauma Data Bank Pediatric Report 2004. Chicago: American College of Surgeons, 2005. **This annual report contains the best information currently available on the epidemiology of childhood trauma.**
4. American College of Surgeons Committee on Trauma: Trauma Evaluation and Management: Early Care of the Injured Patient, 2nd ed. Chicago: American College of Surgeons, 2005. **This brief summary serves as an excellent review of the principles of advanced trauma life support.**
5. Carney NA, Chesnut R, Kochanek PM, et al: Guidelines for the acute medical management of severe traumatic brain injury in infants, children, and adolescents. J Trauma 54:S235–S310, 2003. **These evidence-based guidelines detail the standards, guidelines, and options for optimal care of severe pediatric traumatic brain injury.**
6. Davidson LL, Durkin MS, Kuhn L, et al: The impact of the Safe Kids/Healthy Neighborhoods Injury Prevention Program in Harlem 1988 to 1991. Am J Public Health 84:580–596, 1994. **This report was first to document the steep decline in injury rates that typically result from community-based pediatric injury prevention programs.**
7. DiScala C: National Pediatric Trauma Registry Annual Report. Boston: Tufts University Rehabilitation and Childhood Trauma Research and Training Center, 2002. **This final report of the National Pediatric Trauma Registry remains the greatest single repository of functional outcome data in seriously injured children.**
8. Jurkovich GJ, Pierce B, Pananen L, et al: Giving bad news: The family perspective. J Trauma 48:865–870, 2000. **This study relates what families view as most important when being told of the death of a loved one, concluding that the most important**

features are attitude of the news giver, clarity of the message, privacy, and knowledge and ability to answer questions.

9. Knapp J, Mulligan-Smith D, and the American Academy of Pediatrics Committee on Pediatric Emergency Medicine: Death of a child in the emergency department. Pediatrics 115:1432–1437, 2005. **This report reviews the scientific literature on family presence during resuscitation, concluding that most family members favor having the choice to be present during resuscitation attempts and feel that being present was helpful.**

10. Potoka DA, Schall LC, Gardner MJ, et al: Impact of pediatric trauma centers on mortality in a statewide system. J Trauma 49:237–245, 2000. **This population-based study demonstrates the salutary effect of specialized pediatric trauma care on injury mortality following major injury.**

11. Potoka DA, Schall LC, Ford HR: Improved functional outcome for severely injured children treated at pediatric trauma centers. J Trauma 51:824–834, 2001. **This population-based study demonstrates the salutary effect of pediatric trauma care on functional outcome following major injury.**

12. Pressley JC, Barlow B, Durkin M, et al: A national program for injury prevention in children and adolescents: The Injury Free Coalition for Kids. J Urban Health 82:389–402, 2005. **This report describes the optimal method of community-based injury prevention.**

13. Stylianos S: Evidence based guidelines for resource utilization in children with isolated liver or spleen injury. J Pediatr Surg 35:164–167, 2000. **These evidence-based guidelines describe the optimal management of pediatric liver and spleen injuries.**

14. van der Sluis CK, Kingma J, Eisma WH, ten Duis HJ: Pediatric polytrauma: Short-term and long-term outcomes. J Trauma 43:501–506, 1997. **This study reviews the short- and long-term functional outcomes of pediatric trauma and their perceived effects on quality of life, concluding that although 22% of pediatric patients surviving major trauma had persistent functional deficits 1 year after injury, only half remained physically disabled 9 years after injury, and they enjoyed a quality of life comparable with that of uninjured children.**

Management of Sepsis and Septic Shock

John C. Lin and Joseph A. Carcillo

KEY CONCEPTS

- Sepsis is the second leading cause of death in children in the United States and a dominant cause of death in children worldwide.

- Early recognition of sepsis—defined by tachypnea, tachycardia, and poor feeding—and early treatment with appropriate antibiotics reduce mortality eightfold.

- Early recognition of septic shock, defined by tachycardia plus prolonged capillary refill longer than 2 seconds or hypotension, and early treatment, with fluid resuscitation and stepwise addition of inotropic support, reduce mortality 10-fold.

- Three interventions are required to reverse shock in the first hour: intravenous (IV) fluid boluses (often more than 60 mL/kg of saline or colloid); IV adrenaline (beginning at 0.05 µg/kg/minute titrated to response); and for those with adrenal insufficiency, IV hydrocortisone (from 2 mg/kg bolus plus 24-hour infusion of 2 mg/kg/day, up to 50 mg/kg bolus plus a 24-hour infusion of 50 mg/kg/day).

- When intubation is needed, it should be performed with volume loading (40 mL/kg), induction with atropine (.01 to .02 mg/kg), and ketamine (2 mg/kg), and, if the physician is comfortable, neuromuscular blockade with rocuronium (1 mg/kg). Ketamine can be continued at 2 mg/kg/hour until central access is attained to maintain sedation and analgesia without cardiovascular compromise.

- Staphylococcal septic shock should be treated with supplemental clindamycin to reduce toxin production, and group A streptococcal septic shock should be treated with intravenous immunoglobulin (IVIG) to neutralize toxin.

Sepsis is the second leading cause of death of children, after trauma and accidental injury, costing more than $4 billion per year in the United States. The burden of sepsis is also overwhelming in the developing world, where the leading killers of children are pneumonia, diarrhea, measles, and malaria. Mortality in these children is significantly reduced by giving antibiotics to those with severe forms. Sepsis is defined as tachypnea, tachycardia, and poor feeding in newborns and infants with infection. An eightfold reduction in infant mortality was observed when Indian infants with these signs of sepsis were treated by rural health care workers with 5 days of oral cotrimoxazole and intramuscular (IM) gentamicin (cost: US$5 per day). The leading risk factor for death in children with sepsis is the development of septic shock, which occurs when sepsis is not recognized and not treated early with antibiotics that kill infection. Shock is recognized clinically as tachypnea, tachycardia, poor feeding, and either delayed capillary refill of longer than 2 seconds or hypotension. A 10-fold reduction in meningococcal septic shock mortality was attained in the United Kingdom when physicians at St. Mary's Hospital taught community physicians early recognition of shock and early time-sensitive resuscitation with fluids and inotropes. Similarly, but no less amazingly, in a randomized, controlled trial of four types of fluid resuscitation, physicians in Vietnam showed 100% survival in all four groups when children with stage III and stage IV dengue shock were fluid resuscitated aggressively within the first hour of presentation!

Expert Opinion on Management Issues

More than 90 experts were convened by the American College of Critical Care Medicine and endorsed by the American Heart Association and Pediatric Advanced Life Support Guidelines Committee to draft evidence-based guidelines for the hemodynamic support of term newborn and child septic shock. Two important points are emphasized in this document:

1. Time-sensitive recognition and therapy gives best outcomes; hence all efforts should be made to reverse shock within 1 hour.

2. Best outcomes can be attained when resolution of shock is defined as return to normal capillary refill (1 to 2 seconds), normal heart rate and blood pressure for age, and, in patients with superior vena cava access, a venous oxygen saturation of more than 70%.

Age-specific management guidelines were developed to attain these goals in term newborns, infants, and children (Figs. 1 and 2).

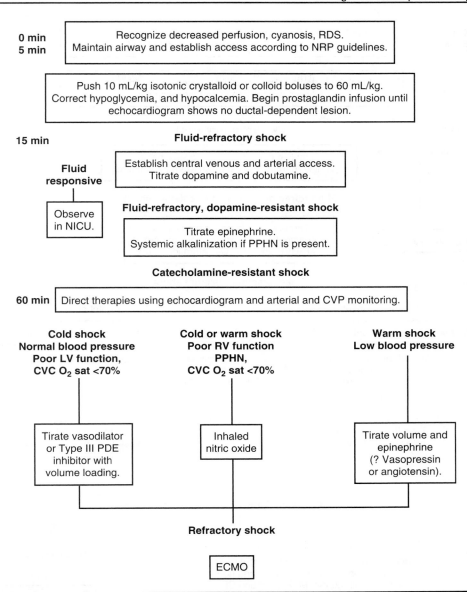

FIGURE 1. Recommendation for stepwise management of hemodynamic support with goals of normal perfusion and perfusion pressure (MAP-CVP), and pre- and postductal oxygen saturation difference of less than 5% in near-term newborns with septic shock. CVC, central venous catheter; CVP, central venous pressure; RDS, respiratory distress syndrome; ECMO, extracorporeal membrane oxygenation; LV, left ventricle; MAP, mean arterial pressure; NICU, newborn intensive care unit; NRP, Neonatal Resuscitation Programme; O2 sat, oxygen saturation; PDE, phosphodiesterase; PPHN, persistent pulmonary hypertension of newborn; RDS, respiratory distress syndrome; RV, right ventricle; sat, saturation.

Term newborns with septic shock commonly have elevated pulmonary blood pressure or persistent pulmonary hypertension of newborn (PPHN). This complicates the shock state with right ventricular failure. Newborns also have the highest resting heart rates (120 to 160 beats per minute [bpm]) and elevated vascular tone. Adults with shock can increase cardiac output by increasing heart rate, for example doubling heart rate from 70 to 140 bpm, but newborns cannot improve cardiac output by doubling heart rate because 240 bpm is supraventricular tachycardia. Infants maintain blood pressure with vasoconstriction, which paradoxically reduces cardiac output by increasing the afterload against which the heart must pump. Newborns who die from septic shock do so

from right ventricular and left ventricular failure. Newborns with shock are fluid resuscitated, given glucose, and placed on inotropic therapy. Inhaled nitric oxide is administered to unload the right ventricle in patients with PPHN, and extracorporeal membrane oxygenation (ECMO) is used for those with refractory shock from right and/or left ventricular failure.

The hemodynamic response of infants and children lies closer to the neonate than the adult. Although 20% show the classic high cardiac output and low systemic vascular resistance state seen in adults, 80% have a low cardiac output with high, normal, or low vascular tone. For operational purposes only, *warm shock* is the term used for high output/low vascular resistance shock, and

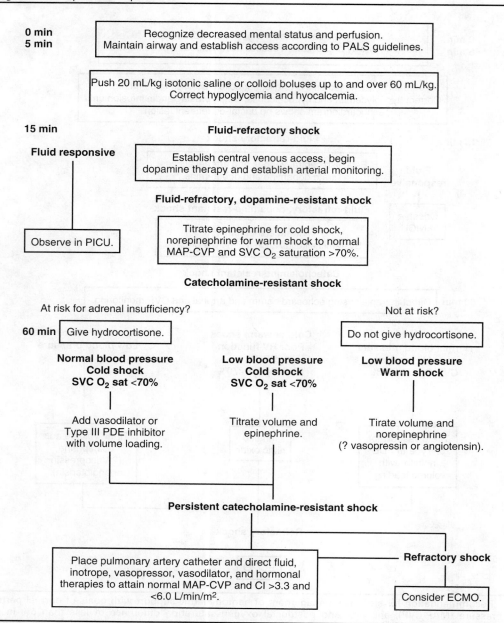

FIGURE 2. Recommendation for stepwise management of hemodynamic support with goals of normal perfusion and perfusion pressure (MAP-CVP) in infants and children with septic shock. Proceed to next step if shock persists. CI, cardiac index; CVP, central venous pressure; ECMO, extracorporeal membrane oxygenation; MAP, mean arterial pressure; O₂ sat, oxygen saturation; PALS, pediatric advanced life support; PDE, phosphodiesterase; PICU, pediatric intensive care unit; SVC, superior vena cava.

cold shock is used to describe low cardiac output shock. Typically, 20 mL/kg boluses are pushed until shock is resolved, rales or hepatomegaly develop, or 60 mL/kg are given in 10 to 15 minutes. If shock persists, inotropes are started (epinephrine for cold shock and norepinephrine for warm shock). Hydrocortisone is administered to those with suspected or proven adrenal insufficiency (defined as known risk factors or a cortisol less than 18 μg/dL in a patient requiring epinephrine or norepinephrine). Vasopressin or angiotensin can be used in those with refractory warm shock, and a type IV phosphodiesterase inhibitor (milrinone, amrinone, pentoxifylline, or enoximone) can be added in those with refractory cold

shock. Norepinephrine can also be added in children with hypotensive refractory cold shock. The pulmonary artery catheter or the pulse-induced contour cardiac output (PiCCO) catheter are used to further direct therapy in these patients, and ECMO can be lifesaving in children with refractory shock despite all other interventions.

ANTIBIOTICS, ANTITOXINS, AND SOURCE CONTROL

Patients cannot survive sepsis and septic shock without killing and removal of infection. Antibiotics should be administered empirically according to local resistance patterns. For example, in some communities there is a 30% incidence of methicillin-resistant *Staphylococcus aureus* (MRSA). Patients with nosocomial infections and those with immunodeficiencies should be treated empirically with antipseudomonal microbial agents and antifungal therapies. Cessation of antibiotics should be considered if organisms are not identified with exhaustive search and C-reactive protein levels remain normal. Antitoxin therapies, including IVIG, steroids, and clindamycin, should be considered in patients with group A streptococcal or staphylococcal septic shock, as should source control. Removal of colonized central lines, dead tissue, and abscesses, and debridement of fasciitis and necrotic wounds are paramount. *Clostridium difficile* colitis should be considered in patients with nosocomial sepsis.

GLYCEMIC CONTROL

Glucose requirements can be attained with administration of D10 solutions at maintenance, and control of hyperglycemia with insulin reduces sepsis mortality and prevents nosocomial sepsis in adults.

ACUTE RESPIRATORY DISTRESS

Surfactant administration improves outcomes in newborns and children with acute respiratory distress syndrome (ARDS). Avoidance of volutrauma and barotraumas is advised even if permissive hypercapnia occurs.

OLIGURIA AND ANURIA

Diuretics can be successfully used in volume-loaded children to reverse oliguria and fluid overload states after resuscitation. The combination of low-dose aminophylline (adenosine antagonist), furosemide (proximal loop inhibitor), and hydrochlorothiazide (distal loop inhibitor) is most effective. Daily continuous renal replacement therapy is used successfully in patients with recalcitrant oliguria.

DISSEMINATED INTRAVASCULAR COAGULATION AND THROMBOCYTOPENIA

Systemic thrombosis occurs in patients who receive late resuscitation. Activated protein C is used in adults and is being studied in children. At present, the anticoagulant proteins protein C, antithrombin III, and ADAM TS13 can be delivered with plasma infusion or in volume-overloaded patients through plasma exchange.

IMMUNE RESTITUTION

The fastest-growing group of children with sepsis is the one with immunodeficiencies. These children cannot survive sepsis unless chemotherapy and immune-suppressant therapies are withdrawn and the immune system restored. Therapies used to restore immune function include granulocyte colony-stimulating factor (G-CSF), granulocyte-macrophage colony-stimulating factor (GM-CSF), and IVIG. Patients with primary immunodeficiencies require specific therapies (e.g., chronic granulomatous disease is treated with white blood cell transfusions and interferon).

Common Pitfalls

- Delayed recognition and/or inadequate resuscitation
- Inadequate antibiotic therapy, antitoxin therapy, or source control
- Failure to provide glucose requirements and maintain euglycemia
- Failure to taper immune suppression and restore immune function.

SUGGESTED READINGS

1. Acute Respiratory Distress Syndrome Network: Ventilation with lesser tidal volume as compared with traditional tidal volume for acute lung injury and acute respiratory distress syndrome. N Engl J Med 342(18):1301–1308, 2000. **Shows that limiting effective tidal volume to 6 to 8 mL/kg reduces mortality in adult ICU patients with acute respiratory distress syndrome.**
2. Bang AT, Bang RA, Baitule SB, et al: Effect of home-based neonatal care and management of sepsis on neonatal mortality: Field trial in rural India. Lancet 354(9194):1955–1961, 1999. **Shows that giving antibiotic to neonates with signs of sepsis reduced all causes of mortality sixfold.**
3. Booy R, Habibi P, Nadel J, et al: Reduction in case fatality rate from meningococcal disease associated with health care delivery. Arch Dis Child 85(5):386–390, 2001. **Shows that delivery of time-sensitive resuscitation in the community hospital with subsequent transfer to the tertiary center reduces mortality for meningococcal septic shock 10-fold.**
4. Carcillo JA: Pediatric septic shock and multiple organ failure. Crit Care Clin 19(3):413–420, 2003. **Provides an in-depth review of pathophysiology and management principles in pediatric septic shock and multiple organ failure.**
5. Carcillo JA, Fields AI, ACCM Task Force: Practice parameters for hemodynamic support of pediatric and neonatal patients in septic shock. Crit Care Med 30(6):1365–1378, 2002. **Provides evidence-based recommendations for hemodynamic support of newborns and children with septic shock.**
6. Nhan NT, Phuong CXT, Kneen R, et al: Acute management of dengue shock syndrome: A randomized double-blind comparison of 4 intravenous fluid regimens in the first hour. Clin Infect Dis 32:204–212, 2001. **Shows that aggressive fluid resuscitation in the first hour in the emergency department achieves 100% survival in children with dengue septic shock.**
7. Schiffel H, Lang SM, Fischer R: Daily hemodialysis and the outcome of acute renal failure. N Engl J Med 346(5):305–316, 2002. **Daily hemodialysis improves outcomes when compared to every other day or greater hemodialysis in adult patients in the intensive care unit (ICU) with acute renal failure.**
8. Van Den Berghe G, Wouters P, Weekers F, et al: Intensive insulin therapy in critically ill patients. N Engl J Med 345(19):1359–1363, 2001. **Shows a twofold reduction in an adult surgical intensive care unit when hyperglycemia is controlled with insulin. All benefits are in prevention and improved survival from sepsis and multiple organ failure.**
9. Watson RS, Carcillo JA, Linde-Zwirble WT, et al: The epidemiology of severe sepsis in the United States. Am J Respir Dis Crit Care Med 167(5):695–701, 2003. **Provides the U.S. epidemiology of newborn and pediatric sepsis.**
10. Yamamoto LG: Emergency airway management: Rapid sequence intubation. In Fleisher GR, Ludwig S (eds): Textbook of Pediatric Emergency Medicine, 4th ed. Philadelphia: Lippincott Williams and Wilkins, 2000, p 74. **Recommends atropine, ketamine, and a neuromuscular blocker as the drugs of choice for rapid sequence intubation in children with severe shock.**

Hypotension in the Neonate

Martin Kluckow and David Osborn

KEY CONCEPTS

- Systemic blood pressure depends on both systemic blood flow (SBF) (or cardiac output) and systemic vascular resistance, and consequently the relationship between blood pressure and blood flow is not constant.
- Some infants, in particular premature infants, have a significant reduction in the SBF on the first day of life that is not always recognized by measuring blood pressure alone.
- Low SBF, with or without hypotension, is associated with significant morbidity.
- Determining whether the infant is likely to have high or low vascular resistance is important in directing treatment of the underlying cause.
- The underlying pathophysiology of cardiovascular compromise in the neonate is variable, and treatment should be tailored to these differences.

Varying clinical scenarios lead to cardiovascular inadequacy in the neonate. Systemic hypotension may be the presenting sign in some of these situations, but not all. The variation in the underlying cause and pathophysiology of cardiovascular compromise means that different therapeutic combinations are important in each case. Hypotension may be associated with low cardiac output, more accurately described as low systemic blood flow (SBF) in the preterm infant. SBF falls dramatically in many extremely premature infants in the first hours of life, and this reduction in flow is usually associated with high vascular resistance. A substantial proportion of these infants initially have normal blood pressure (i.e., they are in compensated shock). Subsequently, approximately 80% of extremely preterm infants who developed low SBF also develop hypotension. Using hypotension to direct cardiovascular interventions, however, results in a considerable delay in support for infants with low SBF and results in some infants with low SBF not being recognized at all. Hypotension may also be associated with normal or even a high SBF, as frequently occurs in the preterm infant with persisting hypotension after the first days of life or term infants with hyperdynamic sepsis. These infants generally have low systemic vascular resistance.

Despite the potential limitations of using systemic blood pressure as the only measure of cardiovascular adequacy, to many clinicians blood pressure is the main clinical information available when making decisions on the need for cardiovascular support. Data regarding the normal physiologic range of systemic blood pressure at various gestational and postnatal ages are readily available. A rule of thumb often used is to maintain the mean blood pressure above the infant's gestational age in weeks, based on reference data from Watkins. Measurement of the systemic blood pressure is best obtained via the invasive route and, when only noninvasive measurement is available, a validated and accurate oscillometric technique should be used.

Documenting the blood pressure invasively or noninvasively and comparing to accepted norms is the current standard for newborn cardiovascular management. However, other ways of assessing the cardiovascular

TABLE 1 Table for Medications Used to Treat Hypotension

Generic Name	Dose, Route, Regimen	Maximum Dose	Dose Formulations
Dopamine	2–15 µg/kg/min IV	20 µg/kg/min	Injection
Dobutamine	2–15 µg/kg/min	20 µg/kg/min	Injection
Adrenaline	0.05–0.1 µg/kg/min	1.0 µg/kg/min	Injection
Milrinone	0.75 µg/kg/min for 3 hr (loading), then 0.2 µg/kg/min	0.75 µg/kg/min	Injection
Hydrocortisone	2–10 mg/kg/day (bid/qid)	2.5 mg/kg/dose	Injection
Dexamethasone	0.25 mg/kg	0.25 mg/kg	Injection

bid, two times per day; CNS, central nervous system; qid, four times per day; SBF, systemic blood flow.

system, such as assessment of cardiac function and measurement of cardiac output using echocardiography, have the potential to improve the management of newborn infants.

Expert Opinion on Management Issues

The appropriate management of hypotension in the neonate differs according to the associated features. The clinician must take into account a number of factors, including the infant's gestational age, postnatal age, other measures of cardiovascular adequacy, such as cardiac output and SBF, if available, and associated pathologic processes. In addition, an understanding of the underlying risk factors for hypotension and low SBF (e.g., immature gestational age or infants with significant ventilatory requirements) is important. An early echocardiogram can assist greatly in the diagnostic process by providing information about the presence, size, and direction of the ductus arteriosus shunt, presence of pulmonary hypertension, assessment of cardiac contractility, adequacy of venous filling, and measurement of cardiac output or SBF.

Prior to instituting treatment for hypotension, potentially reversible causes, such as a measurement error (transducer height in relation to the heart, calibration of the transducer), patent ductus arteriosus, hypovolemia from blood or fluid loss, pneumothorax, use of excessive mean airway pressure, and adrenocortical insufficiency, should be considered and managed appropriately. Available therapeutic options that have a physiologic basis for efficacy and have been subjected to clinical trial include volume loading (crystalloid or colloid), inotropic agents, and hydrocortisone and other steroids. Table 1 provides details of these medications, and Table 2 summarizes an approach to the use of these therapies according to the likely underlying mechanism of cardiovascular compromise.

VOLUME EXPANSION

Hypotension in the preterm infant is rarely associated with hypovolemia unless perinatal blood loss has occurred. Hypovolemia should be suspected where pallor is associated with tachycardia, especially in the setting of peripartum blood loss or a very tight nuchal cord. Infants with sepsis, particularly of later onset, may have significant hypovolemia because of leakage of fluid into tissue spaces and may benefit from volume expansion. Other scenarios associated with hypovolemia include infants with necrotizing enterocolitis or other abdominal surgical conditions and occasional infants with subgaleal hematomas or other intracavity hemorrhage. Evidence does not support routine use of volume expansion in preterm infants on the first day to improve outcome. There appears to be little difference in the effect of crystalloid and colloid solutions in the treatment of systemic hypotension. Crystalloid solutions are preferred because colloid solutions are blood-derived products and more expensive. Colloid solutions should only be used in specific circumstances (e.g., if the infant is thought to be hypovolemic from protein loss).

3

Common Adverse Reactions	Therapeutic Concentrations	Comments
Decreased SBF, tachycardia, tissue necrosis if extravasates	Unknown	Improves blood pressure, may decrease SBF
Tachycardia, arrhythmia, hypotension	Unknown	Less peripheral vasoconstriction
Decreased SBF, tachycardia, tissue necrosis if extravasates	Unknown	Useful in infants not responding to dopamine or dobutamine
Hypotension	150–300 ng/mL	Used in term infants after cardiac surgery; experimental use only in preterm infants
Hyperglycemia, gut perforation, CNS	Unknown	Useful if hypotension unresponsive to inotropes
Hyperglycemia, gut perforation, CNS	Unknown	Useful if hypotension unresponsive to inotropes; one randomized, controlled trial supports use

TABLE 2 Treatment Options According to Underlying Mechanism of Cardiovascular Compromise

Patient Group	Clinical Issues	Cardiovascular Parameters	Suggested Management
Extreme preterm infant	Early low SBF	Normal or low BP Low blood flow/cardiac output Large ductus arteriosus High systemic vascular resistance Poor myocardial contractility	Saline, 10–20 mL/kg Dobutamine, 10–20 µg/kg/min: adjust to blood flow Second line: add dopamine, 5 µg/kg/min; titrate to BP
Preterm infant	Low BP after first 24–48 hours	Normal/high SBF Low systemic vascular resistance	Dopamine, 5 µg/kg/minute titrated to BP
Preterm infant with PDA	Low BP ± PDA signs	Low BP Large PDA, left-to-right shunt	Indomethacin first, then treat SBF/BP
Infant with asphyxia	Myocardial damage, low SBF	Normal or low BP Poor myocardial contractility	Saline, 10–20 mL/kg Dobutamine, 10–20 µg/kg/min: adjust to blood flow Second line: addition of dopamine, 5 µg/kg/min; titration to BP or adrenaline
Infant with suspected sepsis: high output	High output cardiac failure secondary to sepsis	Normal or low BP High SBF Low systemic vascular resistance/capillary leak	Volume replacement (may require more than 20 mL/kg) Dopamine, 5 µg/kg/min titrated to BP Second line: adrenaline, 0.05 µg/kg/min titrated to BP
Infant with suspected sepsis: low output	Sepsis and poor myocardial function	Normal or low BP Normal or low SBF High systemic vascular resistance	Saline, 10–20 mL/kg Dobutamine, 10–20 µg/kg/minute (adjust to blood flow) Second line (low blood flow): Adrenaline, 0.05 µg/kg/min Second line (hypotension): addition of dopamine, 5 µg/kg/min; titration to BP or adrenaline
Infant with mainly respiratory distress: often term	Pulmonary hypertension	Normal or low BP Normal or low SBF High pulmonary vascular resistance	Dobutamine, 10–20 µg/kg/ min (adjust to blood flow) Second line: Adrenaline, 0.05 µg/kg/min Pulmonary vasodilators: nitric oxide
Infant with acute fluid loss (intraventricular/pulmonary hemorrhage)	Acute hypovolemia	Normal or low blood pressure Poor venous filling pressures	Volume replacement (may require more than 20 mL/kg, including blood transfusion) Dopamine, 5 µg/kg/minute titrated to BP Second line: Adrenaline, 0.05 µg/kg/min titrated to BP

BP, blood pressure; PDA, patent ductus arteriosus; SBF, systemic blood flow.

Randomized trials show improvement in blood pressure in hypotensive infants given volume but no change in short- or long-term outcomes. One trial showed dopamine to be more effective than albumin in improving the blood pressure in normotensive infants (mean blood pressure: 29 to 40 mm Hg). Observational studies show a short-term improvement in blood flow after volume expansion.

Because accurate diagnosis of hypovolemia is difficult in the neonate and inotropes are not as effective in the presence of hypovolemia, it is reasonable initially to treat hypotension or low SBF with 10 to 20 mL/kg of normal saline solution administered over 30 minutes. Trials that used a volume load prior to giving a vasodilator inotrope (e.g., dobutamine) report no reflex tachycardia in response to inotrope, suggesting that volume load may ameliorate the reduction in preload that occurs with vasodilation. In an infant requiring positive pressure respiratory support, even if the infant is not hypovolemic, a volume load may increase the central venous pressure sufficiently to improve venous return to the heart. Given the association of excess fluid administration in premature infants and adverse outcomes, including an increased incidence of patent ductus arteriosus, necrotizing enterocolitis, and mortality, excess and inappropriate administration of volume should be avoided.

INOTROPES

Inotropes used in neonates include dopamine, dobutamine, epinephrine, isoprenaline, and milrinone. The mechanisms of action of these vasoactive agents are complex, affected by the developmental maturation of the cardiovascular and autonomic nervous systems, and they usually involve some effect on the peripheral vasculature. Consequently, these agents can alter the relationship between the systemic blood pressure and SBF. If only the blood pressure is monitored, a change in the blood flow may not be appreciated.

Dopamine, a naturally occurring catecholamine, is the most commonly used pressor agent in the treatment of neonates. At lower doses it acts via increasing myocardial contractility, but at higher doses (more than 10 μg/kg/minute), peripheral vasoconstriction and increased afterload play an increasing role in its effect on blood pressure. Dopamine is compared in randomized trials in hypotensive infants to volume expansion, dobutamine, and epinephrine. Dobutamine is a synthetic catecholamine that increases myocardial contractility but also has a peripheral vasodilatory effect. Dobutamine is compared to dopamine in several randomized trials, but, as with dopamine, it has never been subjected to trial against placebo or no treatment in newborns. Systematic review finds that dopamine is better than dobutamine at increasing blood pressure, but to date it has not been better at improving clinical outcomes in hypotensive infants. In contrast, in infants with low SBF on the first day, dobutamine was better at increasing blood flow. Epinephrine is often used in refractory hypotension in neonates. In a single trial comparing low- to moderate-dose dopamine and low-dose epinephrine in hypotensive very-preterm infants on the first day, similar increases were reported in cerebral blood flow and oxygenation as measured by near-infrared spectroscopy. Both inotropes were equally efficacious at increasing blood pressure. No other clinical benefits to either inotrope were reported.

The choice of first-line inotropes depends on the underlying physiologic circumstances. In the setting of hyperdynamic sepsis with a vasodilated periphery, inotropic agents with a vasoconstrictive effect on the peripheral vasculature have the most effect. In the case of a preterm infant in the first day of life with an immature myocardium sensitive to increased afterload, the imposition of an agent that causes peripheral vasoconstriction may further reduce SBF. Dobutamine, which has a vasodilatory effect on the periphery, may be a better choice of inotrope with the goal of improving cardiac output. In infants who remain hypotensive, the addition of dopamine or epinephrine to gently increase vascular resistance, titrated to the minimally acceptable blood pressure, is logical. Table 2 outlines the suggested appropriate use of each of the inotropic agents according to the underlying physiologic circumstances.

Finally, the pulmonary circulation should not be ignored when selecting the most appropriate inotrope. Higher pulmonary vascular resistance is often found in the immature preterm infant with low SBF and in the ventilated term infant with high oxygen requirements (pulmonary hypertension). Pulmonary hypertension can be treated selectively by the use of inhaled nitric oxide. When treating hypotension, dobutamine reduces both systemic and pulmonary vascular resistance and dopamine increases both systemic and pulmonary vascular resistance, especially at higher doses, whereas epinephrine tends to increase systemic more than pulmonary vascular resistance. Although dopamine may decrease right-to-left shunts associated with pulmonary hypertension, it may exacerbate the low cardiac output in those infants with low SBF and poor myocardial function.

STEROIDS

Glucocorticoids affect multiple organ systems, including the cardiovascular system. Recent case reports and clinical trials highlight the usefulness of both dexamethasone and hydrocortisone in increasing blood pressure. The effect is particularly seen in the setting of hypotension unresponsive to standard therapy. Antenatal steroids also seem to have an additional protective effect against hypotension in the preterm infant. The mechanism of action is uncertain but may relate either to treatment of relative adrenal insufficiency or possibly to an effect on adrenal receptor density. Because significant short-term (especially spontaneous intestinal perforation) and long-term side effects are increasingly recognized with the use of glucocorticoids, particularly in the preterm infant, caution is advised in their use in this setting. Table 1 provides information regarding dosage of these agents when treating resistant hypotension.

SUMMARY

Hypotension in the neonate has a range of underlying causes, and proper consideration of these prior to treatment allows for more appropriate treatment (Figure 1). Very little data are available regarding the long-term benefits or harms of many of the cardiovascular interventions used in neonates. The data available highlight the importance of assessing and supporting not only systemic blood pressure but also blood flow to achieve the ultimate aim of maintenance of adequate tissue perfusion and oxygenation. Both hypotension and low SBF are associated with poor long-term neurodevelopmental outcome. Management of these problems is becoming increasingly important as we try to reduce neurodevelopmental complications in term and, in particular, preterm infants.

Common Pitfalls

- Trying to treat all infants with hypotension using the same strategy
- Neglecting the other components of cardiovascular adequacy—the cardiac output, the afterload, and the myocardial contractility
- Failing to treat low SBF or treating hypotension associated with normal SBF because of a lack of physiologic information, such as that provided by echocardiography

Communication and Counseling

The problem of hypotension in the neonate is common and treatment has been available for many years. Preterm infants with hypotension and low SBF are at substantially increased risk of mortality and developmental impairments, with more than 70% of infants with low SBF subsequently dying or developing an impairment. Despite this, the larger area of neonatal hemodynamics is relatively new, and appropriate treatment approaches using all of the new information now available are only

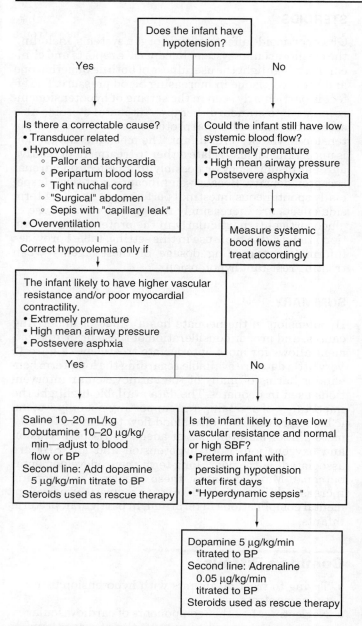

2. Engle WD: Blood pressure in the very low birth weight neonate. Early Hum Dev 62:97–130, 2001. **Authoritative review of the issues surrounding blood pressure in neonates.**
3. Klarr JM, Faix RG, Pryce CJ, Bhatt-Mehta V: Randomized, blind trial of dopamine versus dobutamine for treatment of hypotension in preterm infants with respiratory distress syndrome. J Pediatr 125:117–122, 1994. **Clinical trial addressing the different mechanisms of action of dobutamine and dopamine in the treatment of cardiovascular compromise.**
4. Osborn DA, Evans N: Early volume expansion for prevention of morbidity and mortality in very preterm infants. Cochrane Database Syst Rev 2:CD002055, 2004. **Systematic review of the issues in using volume in preterm infants.**
5. Osborn DA, Evans N: Early volume expansion versus inotrope for prevention of morbidity and mortality in very preterm infants. Cochrane Database Syst Rev 2:CD002056, 2001. **Systematic review of the issues in using volume versus inotropes in preterm infants.**
6. Osborn D, Evans N, Kluckow M: Randomized trial of dobutamine versus dopamine in preterm infants with low systemic blood flow. J Pediatr 140:183–191, 2002. **Clinical trial addressing the different mechanisms of action of dobutamine and dopamine in the treatment of cardiovascular compromise.**
7. Seri I: Circulatory support of the sick preterm infant. Semin Neonatol 6:85–95, 2001. **Excellent review of the physiology and treatment of the circulation in the preterm infant.**
8. Subhedar NV, Shaw NJ: Dopamine versus dobutamine for hypotensive preterm infants. Cochrane Database Syst Rev 3:CD001242, 2003. **Systematic review of the use of the two major inotropes used in the management of hypotension in preterm infants.**

FIGURE 1. Therapeutic algorithm for managing cardiovascular compromise. BP, blood pressure; SBF, systemic blood flow.

Hypertensive Emergencies

Martin A. Nash

KEY CONCEPTS

- Hypertensive encephalopathy requires immediate treatment, usually with an intravenous antihypertensive drug.
- Acute lowering of blood pressure should be modest in degree, sufficient to reestablish cerebral blood flow autoregulation.
- Severe hypertension not associated with encephalopathy or heart failure can be treated initially with oral medication, aiming for complete normalization of blood pressure over days to weeks.
- Hypertension found coincidentally should not be treated initially but referred for prompt investigation and possible eventual therapy.

just beginning to be assessed. As a result, counseling parents about the most appropriate treatment for the infant with hypotension or low SBF is a difficult area and will remain so until further studies into the efficacy and long-term benefits of both existing and newer treatments become available.

SUGGESTED READINGS

1. Bourchier D, Weston PJ: Randomised trial of dopamine compared with hydrocortisone for the treatment of hypotensive very low birthweight infants. Arch Dis Child 76:F174–178, 1997. **Randomized clinical trial demonstrating the potential efficacy of hydrocortisone in the treatment of resistant hypotension.**

Severe acute hypertension is usually separated into the overlapping groups of hypertensive emergencies and hypertensive urgencies. *Hypertensive emergencies* are those patients with severe hypertension associated with manifestations in other organs, whereas those with *hypertensive urgencies* have severe elevations of blood pressure but without secondary involvement of other organs. The organ system most frequently involved is the nervous system, with clinical manifestation of seizures, occasionally hemiplegia or hemiparesis, and, rarely, cortical blindness that is generally transient. Cardiac involvement may manifest with congestive heart failure or acute pulmonary edema. The retinopathy characteristic of malignant hypertension in adults (retinal hemorrhages, exudates, and papilledema) is rare in pediatric patients. As opposed to adults, decreased renal function in children (increased creatinine and blood urea nitrogen [BUN]) is most often the *cause* of the hypertension rather than a secondary effect of the elevated blood pressure.

The distinction between emergencies and urgencies is important in that there are differences in management (discussed later) with emergencies requiring immediate and aggressive therapy to resolve the secondary neurologic or cardiac manifestations. Some patients without secondary organ involvement may be judged imminent emergencies because of an extraordinary elevation of blood pressure, decreased awareness, or tachypnea, and they should be treated as true emergencies. Those patients without such clinical manifestations, judged hypertensive urgencies, require expeditious but more gradual therapy, often with oral, rather than parenteral, medication.

It is difficult to apply an absolute blood pressure level to define hypertensive emergencies and urgencies. Normal, and therefore abnormal, levels of blood pressure vary widely with age and body size. The Fourth Task Force defines stage 2 hypertension as systolic or diastolic blood pressure more than 5 mm greater than the 99th percentile for age and height and suggests that these patients begin evaluation and treatment within 1 week if asymptomatic. Acute rises in blood pressure are less well tolerated and more likely to become symptomatic than more chronic elevations, and they often need earlier intervention despite similar absolute numbers for systolic and diastolic pressures. In general, however, the identification of those children who require emergency or urgent therapy for hypertension does not rest on subtle deviations from published normal values. The extreme elevations of blood pressure are readily recognized as far outside the normal limits.

The most common etiology of severe hypertension in pediatric patients is renal or renovascular. Poststreptococcal acute glomerulonephritis and hemolytic uremic syndrome are the most common causes of de novo acute hypertension. More often, patients present with an exacerbation of known hypertension or with previously unrecognized severe hypertension. This is most associated with the glomerular diseases of focal segmental glomerulosclerosis and membranoproliferative glomerulonephritis, with segmental renal scarring secondary to vesicoureteral reflux and with renal artery stenosis. Children on hemodialysis who have had an injudicious splurge in the intake of salt and water may present with a severe exacerbation of hypertension. Table 1 shows other associated conditions. In adolescents, the possibility of toxic ingestion, especially cocaine, should be considered. Although the use of oral contraceptives is frequently included in lists of causes of severe hypertension, this is rarely the case with the current formulations with lower estrogen content, although they may exacerbate underlying hypertension of another etiology.

Expert Opinion on Management Issues

The aggressiveness of therapy for severe hypertension depends on whether or not there are associated symptoms (seizures, cortical blindness, pulmonary edema). Cerebral blood flow is normally autoregulated over a wide range of blood pressures. With severe hypertension this regulatory range may be exceeded, exposing small arterioles and capillaries to pressures that cause hyperfiltration of fluid into the extravascular space. The occipital areas of the brain are the most vulnerable. On MRI this is recognized as hypointense signals over the occipital lobes on T1-weighted images and hyperintense signals on T2-weighted images. These clinical and MRI findings are called "reversible posterior leukoencephalopathy" because all findings are generally reversible with lowering of blood pressure. The goal of therapy should be to lower blood pressure into the autoregulatory range. One should not attempt initially to lower pressure into the normal range because it may produce cerebral ischemia. There are no established guidelines for the desired rapidity of the decrease, but an approach might be to determine the difference between the observed blood pressure and the 95th percentile for normal children of the same age. An initial lowering of 25% of this difference over several minutes if the child has encephalopathy or over 4 to 6 hours if the child is asymptomatic (except for possible headache and vomiting) is suggested. Another 25% reduction could take place over the subsequent 24 to 36 hours, with the final reduction over the next several days or weeks.

Based on these considerations, initial therapy should be intravenous to permit a controlled lowering of blood pressure, thereby avoiding the risk of cerebral ischemia

---

TABLE 1 Causes of Severe Hypertension Requiring Emergency or Urgent Treatment

Acute Glomerular Diseases
Poststreptococcal glomerulonephritis
Hemolytic uremic syndrome

Renal Artery Stenosis (main or branch arteries)
Previous umbilical artery catheter
Fibromuscular dysplasia
Middle aortic arch syndrome
Neurofibromatosis

Exacerbation of Existing or Previously Unrecognized Hypertension
Focal segmental glomerulosclerosis
Membranoproliferative glomerulonephritis
Reflux nephropathy

Endocrine
Pheochromocytoma

Cardiac
Coarctation of aorta

Miscellaneous
Dialysis patients with excessive volume expansion
Known hypertensive patients unable to retain antihypertensive medication or noncompliant
Toxins: cocaine

TABLE 2 Drugs for Hypertensive Emergencies

Drug	Dose	Route	Onset	Duration	Repeat or Increase Dose
Sodium nitroprusside	0.5–8.0 µg/kg/min	IV	Immediate	Seconds	30–60 min
Labetalol	0.2–1 mg/kg/dose over 2 min *or* 0.4–3.0 mg/kg/h	IV	1–5 min	6–24 hr	10 min
Nifedipine	0.25–0.5 mg/kg/dose; max: 10 mg/dose	PO	5–15 min	2–6 hr	15 min
Nicardipine	0.5–3.0 µg/kg/min	IV	1–3 min	15 min–3 h	15 min
Fenoldopam	0.5–2.0 µg/kg/min	IV	15 min	15–30 min	

IV, intravenous; PO, by mouth.

or hypotension. Table 2 lists the agents most useful in the acute treatment of severe hypertension in children.

- Although in theory intravenous therapy is preferable, in practice, the oral agent nifedipine, a calcium channel blocker, is effective and safe in the acute treatment of severe hypertension in pediatric patients. The cardiac and cerebral side effects observed in some adults occur only rarely in children. The drug can be administered by asking the child to bite and then swallow the capsule or by puncturing the capsule and expressing the contents sublingually. The major absorption takes place in the stomach.
- Sodium nitroprusside leads to the production of nitric oxide and is therefore a direct vasodilator. It is most useful in the intensive care unit (ICU) setting because it requires continuous monitoring of blood pressure and fast adjustment of the rate of infusion to avoid hypotension. The container and lines must be covered with foil to protect the solution from exposure to sunlight. With use beyond 48 to 72 hours, blood levels of thiocyanate and cyanide must be followed.
- Labetalol is a combined α- and β-adrenergic blocker. It can be used acutely in an emergency department or ICU. A relative contraindication is asthma or congestive heart failure.
- Nicardipine, an intravenous calcium blocker, is effective in acute hypertension in children and can be used in the emergency department or ICU.
- Fenoldopam is a dopamine-1 agonist. In addition to arterial dilation with decrease in blood pressure, it increases renal and cerebral blood flow, increases glomerular filtration rate, and improves left ventricular function.

Hypertension found incidentally during a visit for an unrelated reason should not be treated but referred for early evaluation. Premature treatment may complicate the subsequent investigation for etiology. Likewise, hypertension related to pain or to severe anxiety should be treated with analgesics or sedation, not antihypertensive medication.

Seizures alone can cause elevated blood pressure, either real or factitious, because of muscle contraction that normalizes on control of seizures. It is sometimes difficult to distinguish cause from effect.

Common Pitfalls

- Lowering blood pressure too quickly or to levels too low to assure normal cerebral and renal blood flow.
- Not recognizing that in some situations the elevated blood pressure may be secondary to pain or anxiety in which appropriate therapy would be analgesic or anxiolytic drugs and not antihypertensive medications.
- Treating prematurely the child whose elevated blood pressure is found coincidental to another unrelated problem. Later investigation for etiology may be compromised.
- Not arranging appropriate follow-up after the acute episode is treated.

Communication and Counseling

The importance of adequate follow-up for evaluation and possible treatment should be discussed with families and children who have newly discovered hypertension. For children presenting with hypertensive encephalopathy, follow-up neurologic care and imaging studies should be arranged. Those children with acute hypertension because of noncompliance with medication or diet should be counseled on the importance of these areas in the context of their overall care.

SUGGESTED READINGS

1. Adelman RD: Management of hypertensive emergencies. In Portman RJ, Sorof JM, Ingelfinger JR (eds): Pediatric Hypertension. Totowa, NJ: Humana Press, 2004, pp 457–469. **This textbook is a comprehensive up-to-date resource on all aspects of pediatric hypertension.**
2. Cherney D, Straus S: Management of patients with hypertensive urgencies and emergencies: A systematic review of the literature. J Gen Intern Med 17:937–945, 2002. **An evidence-based review of various drug regimens in adults.**
3. National High Blood Pressure Education Program Working Group on High Blood Pressure in Children and Adolescents: The fourth report on the diagnosis, evaluation, and treatment of high blood pressure in children and adolescents. Pediatrics 114(Suppl):555–576, 2004. **The latest report, with tables of normal blood pressures by age and height.**
4. Singhi P, Subramanian C, Jain V, et al: Reversible brain lesions in childhood hypertension. ACTA Paediatr 91:1005–1007, 2002. **A discussion of posterior leukoencephalopathy.**

Disorders of Temperature Control

Todd J. Kilbaugh, Jimmy W. Huh, and Mark A. Helfaer

KEY CONCEPTS

- Both hyperthermia and hypothermia can result in multi-organ system dysfunction.
- Treatment for hyperthermia and hypothermia involves removing the offending agent and diagnosing and treating the underlying disease process while simultaneously providing advanced life support.
- Hyperthermic patients who have attempted strenuous exercise or have been hypotensive are at risk for myoglobinuria and renal failure.
- Hypothermic patients are especially prone to life-threatening ventricular arrhythmias or asystole.
- Chronic (longer than 24 hours) hypothermic patients are at risk for core-temperature afterdrop when they are rewarmed.

The body's core temperature, under normal conditions, remains within plus or minus 1°F (plus or minus 0.6°C), even when the person is exposed to temperatures between 49°F to 140°F (9.4°C to 60°C) in dry air. Balancing the rates of heat production and heat loss is crucial for controlling body temperature. Heat is produced by hormones (thyroxine, growth hormone, testosterone), sympathetic agents (epinephrine, norepinephrine), and muscle contractions caused by shivering. Heat is lost by radiation of infrared heat rays, conduction to air and objects, convection through air currents that surround tissues, and evaporation. Under normal conditions, radiation accounts for 60% of the total heat loss. Conduction and convection to air represents 15% of heat loss, whereas conduction to objects represents a small (3%) portion of heat loss. Evaporative heat loss accounts for 22%. Temperature sensation initially occurs in the preoptic nucleus of the anterior hypothalamus, skin, and deep tissues (spinal cord, abdominal viscera, and the great veins). Temperature sensory signals are then transmitted to the posterior hypothalamus, which controls temperature regulation. Hyperthermia or elevated body temperature causes cutaneous vasodilation, sweating, and decreased heat production (inhibition of shivering). Hypothermia or decreased body temperature results in cutaneous vasoconstriction and increased heat production (by shivering and thyroxine).

Hyperthermia

Hyperthermia occurs when excess heat production or impaired heat dissipation overwhelms the body's thermoregulatory mechanisms. Oxygen (O_2) consumption and carbon dioxide (CO_2) production increase as a result of an increase in metabolic rate and heart rate. Because hyperthermia is usually associated with volume depletion,

central venous pressure or preload is often low. Patients with underlying heart disease may have ischemia, arrhythmias, or congestive heart failure because of hyperthermia. Elevated temperatures can cause seizures in young children, and extreme hyperthermia can produce confusion, delirium, and coma. In addition, hyperthermia can worsen preexisting brain injury. Hematologic abnormalities associated with hyperthermia include leukocytosis, thrombocytosis, hemoconcentration, and disseminated intravascular coagulation. Azotemia and elevated serum levels of muscle enzymes, with associated renal failure and rhabdomyolysis, and elevated serum levels of liver enzymes, with hepatic failure, may occur. Mortality rate tends to increase as temperature increases.

Expert Opinion on Management Issues

Prevention, such as wearing light-colored clothing that allows for heat loss by evaporation and that prevents radiant heat gain, is the first approach to hyperthermia. Exposing a person to heat for several hours per day while doing active play or work (as tolerated) allows the person to develop increased tolerance to heat in 1 to 3 weeks. Children with cystic fibrosis who are at risk for excess salt loss in their sweat do not respond to acclimatization.

The next priority is diagnosis and treatment of the underlying disease while simultaneously providing ABCDE (*a*irway and possibly *a*ntibiotics, *b*reathing, *c*irculation, *d*isability or neurologic and possible *d*extrose, *e*xtracorporeal support if all else fails) and metabolic/hematologic support (Table 1). The patient's clothing should be removed and the skin should be sponged with tepid water to increase heat loss. Environmental temperature should be dropped and bedside fans should be used. Ice packs are placed on the neck, scalp, axillae, and groin, and the patient is placed on a hypothermic mattress. Ice baths are very effective for hyperthermic emergencies, although monitoring and access to the patient may be troublesome. Iced intravenous and body cavity irrigation with cold saline (pleural, peritoneal, gastric, bladder, and rectal) can be used to treat severe hyperthermia. Finally, extracorporeal cooling may be used as a last resort. The body temperature should be continuously monitored to avoid hypothermia. Antipyretics such as acetaminophen and ibuprofen are commonly used. Potential side effects, such as hepatic, hematologic, and renal dysfunction, must be closely monitored. In addition to therapies to decrease body temperature, ongoing support of the cardiovascular and metabolic systems is of paramount importance. Cooled fluids to 39.2°F (4°C) may precipitate arrhythmias. Hydration status should be closely monitored by physical exam, such as capillary refill, vital signs (especially heart rate), electrolytes, hematocrit, urine output, and, if necessary, invasive monitors for central venous pressure and arterial blood pressure. Intravenous boluses of isotonic solution (lactated Ringer solution, 0.9% saline) should be used for volume repletion as needed. In cases of intractable seizures or muscle cramps, hypertonic saline solution (3% saline, 5 mL/kg by intravenous [IV] bolus) may be used.

TABLE 1 Management of Hyperthermia

History and Physical

ABCDE
Underlying disease diagnosed and treated
Vital signs, pulse oximetry, electrocardiogram
Clothing removed, skin moistened, and patient placed in cool
    environment (e.g., fans)

Laboratory Tests

Electrolytes, BUN, creatinine, glucose, Ca, Mg, P
Serum creatinine phosphokinase (CPK)
Urinalysis, including myoglobin
CBC with differential, PT/PTT, fibrinogen
Arterial blood gas
Additional labs, if appropriate

Active Cooling

Ice packs, hypothermic mattresses, ice baths
Iced IV fluids
IV hydration with isotonic or hypertonic (3% saline) solutions
Body cavity irrigation
Possibly antipyretics and inotropic support (e.g., vasodilators)
Avoidance of anticholinergic agents that may inhibit sweating
    (e.g., atropine)
Therapy for myoglobinuria
Euvolemia assured and urine output >1 mL/kg/h maintained
Possibly furosemide (0.5–1 mg/kg IV) and/or mannitol (0.25–1 g/kg IV)
Urine alkalized to pH above 7

ABCDE, *a*irway and possibly *a*ntibiotics, *b*reathing, circulation, *d*isability or neurologic and possible *d*extrose, *e*xtracorporeal support if all else fails; BUN, blood urea nitrogen; Ca, calcium; CBC, complete blood count; IV, intravenous; Mg, magnesium; P, phosphorus; PT, prothrombin time; PTT, partial thromboplastin time.

TABLE 2 Clinical and Laboratory Findings Associated with Malignant Hyperthermia

Clinical Signs	Laboratory Findings
Muscle rigidity despite neuromuscular blockade	Mixed metabolic and respiratory acidosis
Masseter spasm	Increased $Paco_2$
Hypertension	Decreased Pao_2
Hyperthermia	Hyperkalemia
Ventricular arrhythmias	Increased CK
Skin mottling	Myoglobinuria
Tachycardia	Abnormal coagulation tests
Cola-colored urine	Elevated plasma lactate levels
Significantly elevated end-tidal CO_2 despite a marked increase in minute ventilation	

CO_2, carbon dioxide; CK, creatine kinase; $Paco_2$, partial pressure of carbon dioxide, arterial; Pao_2, partial pressure of oxygen, arterial.

Inotropic support may be needed for hemodynamic instability despite fluid administration. Dobutamine and milrinone can provide enhanced myocardial contractility (inotropy) while increasing peripheral vasodilation to promote heat loss. However, these drugs can also cause hypotension. Dopamine may also be administered, when infused at low rates to support myocardial contractility without vasoconstriction. Drugs with α-agonist properties (such as high-dose dopamine, epinephrine, and norepinephrine) are not initially recommended because they prevent heat dissipation by causing vasoconstriction. Anticholinergic agents, such as atropine, that inhibit sweating should also be avoided. However, α-adrenergic agents may be needed when refractory hypotension is present, especially if low systemic vascular resistance from vasodilation is responsible for the hypotension.

Patients who have been hypotensive or have attempted vigorous exercise should be especially monitored for renal failure and myoglobinuria. Urine output, serum electrolytes, especially potassium, calcium, magnesium, and phosphorus, blood urea nitrogen (BUN) and creatinine, serum creatinine phosphokinase (CPK), urinalysis, and urine for myoglobin should be monitored. An elevated CPK and urinalysis that is orthotolidine (Hematest) positive without red blood cells (RBCs) and shows red-gold granular casts is suggestive of rhabdomyolysis. Once the patient's intravascular volume, cardiac output, and arterial blood pressure is restored, rhabdomyolysis should be treated with aggressive hydration to maintain urine output greater than 1 mL/kg/hour, diuresis with furosemide (0.5 to 1 mg/kg IV) and/or mannitol (0.25 to 1 g/kg IV), and alkalinization of the urine with a sodium bicarbonate infusion to keep urine pH above 7.

MALIGNANT HYPERTHERMIA

Malignant hyperthermia (MH) is a potentially fatal hypermetabolic syndrome triggered in susceptible patients exposed to depolarizing muscle relaxants (e.g., succinylcholine) and/or inhaled, volatile, halogenated anesthetic agents (e.g., halothane). The clinical signs of MH are O_2 depletion, excess CO_2 production, and massive heat production. This is followed by myocyte cell death and rhabdomyolysis causing hyperkalemia. Often the presenting sign for MH is not hyperthermia; rather, it is tachycardia, hypertension, increasing minute ventilation in a spontaneously breathing patient, and a rising $Paco_2$ evident by a significant rise in end-tidal CO_2 not associated with hypoventilation. In addition, MH should be strongly considered in a patient exhibiting muscle rigidity or masseter spasm, which according to some experts is pathognomonic for MH. The decision to treat a suspected MH crisis should be made on clinical observations; however, an arterial blood gas with a mixed metabolic and respiratory acidosis in combination with clinical suspicion without any other explanation should initiate treatment (Table 2).

Treatment includes management of hyperthermia as outlined in Table 1 and the administration of Dantrolene, 2.5 mg/kg rapidly, repeated until a decline in end-tidal CO_2. Continued management includes dantrolene, 1 mg/kg every 6 hours for 36 hours, and management of the sequelae of the hypermetabolic state: hyperthermia, metabolic acidosis, hyperkalemia and any associated arrhythmias, and rhabdomyolysis. A nonprofit MH hotline is available 24 hours, staffed by experts, for guidance in diagnosis and treatment of MH: online at www.mhaus.org or 1–800-MH-HYPER.

TABLE 3 Clinical Findings Associated with Heat Exhaustion and Heat Stroke

Heat Exhaustion	Heatstroke
Temp usually <104°F (41°C)	Temperature usually >104°F (41°C)
Orthostatic	Symptoms of heat exhaustion
Sweating, possibly anhydrosis	Hyperdynamic cardiovascular system including tachyarrhythmia
Nausea and vomiting	Central nervous system dysfunction: altered mental status, seizures, coma, and decerebrate posturing
Piloerection	Coagulation disorders
Weakness	Respiratory distress and failure
Tachycardia	Renal insufficiency, hematuria, oliguria, anuria, acute renal failure

HEAT EXHAUSTION AND HEAT STROKE

The pediatric populations at greatest risk for heat exhaustion and heat stroke include neonates and children engaged in physical activity during high ambient temperatures without proper hydration. This is often referred to as exertional heat stroke. Heat exhaustion and heat stroke progress from dehydration and electrolyte losses to the eventual overwhelming failure of the body's thermoregulatory mechanisms by heat stress. Following exposure to heat stress, the clinical signs of heat exhaustion are often nonspecific and resemble a viral illness: fatigue, irritability, nausea, vomiting, muscle cramps, headache, and dizziness (Table 3). Heat stroke includes all the symptoms of heat exhaustion and the critical features of central nervous system (CNS) dysfunction: altered mental status, confusion, hallucinations, and eventually coma. Prevention of exposure to hot environments without air conditioning or proper ventilation (e.g., automobiles) and adequate hydration are keys to avoidance.

FEVER

Exploring the differential of fever is far beyond the scope of this chapter. However, it is important to observe the clinical characteristics of fever to narrow a differential diagnosis. Infectious causes can also trigger a cascade that leads to hypothermia, temperatures less than 97°F (36°C) in overwhelming sepsis. There are noninfectious causes: malignancy, rheumatoid disease, recent immunizations, and so on. Infants younger than 28 days of age and infants younger than 60 days of age with temperatures higher than 100°F (38°C) require careful attention.

SEROTONIN SYNDROME

Serotonin syndrome is a potentially adverse reaction to a serotonin agonist via excessive stimulation of 5-HT (hydroxytryptamine) 1A and 5-HT2 receptors. The syndrome is usually triggered by several mechanisms: administration of a serotonin agonist, enhanced serotonin release (e.g., Ecstasy or cocaine), decreased serotonin reuptake (e.g., tricyclic antidepressants, selective serotonin reuptake inhibitors [SSRIs]), decreased serotonin

metabolism (e.g., monoamine oxidase inhibitor [MAOI]), and excessive administration of serotonin precursors or agonists (e.g., trazodone, L-tryptophan). Clinical features of the serotonin syndrome include cognitive and behavioral changes, autonomic dysfunction, and neuromuscular abnormalities. Autonomic dysfunction manifests as hyperthermia, sweating, dilated pupils, tachycardia, and hemodynamic lability. Cognitive and behavioral changes include confusion, agitation, and coma. Neuromuscular abnormalities often manifest as hyperreflexia, shivering, and ataxia. Diagnosis is clinical, and in children it is important to obtain a complete history from the patient and household members. Therapy is usually supportive, and the condition is usually self-limiting and resolves within 24 to 48 hours. As with all ingestions, treatment should be coordinated with a regional poison center.

NEUROLEPTIC MALIGNANT SYNDROME

Neuroleptic malignant syndrome (NMS) is defined as an idiosyncratic reaction secondary to neuroleptic medications (e.g., haloperidol, fluphenazine, risperidone, promethazine, clozapine, prochlorperazine). NMS presents clinically with hyperthermia, muscle rigidity, altered mental status, and autonomic dysfunction. The onset can be within hours or up to 4 weeks following the initiation or escalation of dosage. Laboratory evidence that may aid in the diagnosis includes elevated CPK, myoglobinemia, elevated transaminases, and a normal lipoprotein (LP). The electroencephalogram (EEG) may be suggestive of nonspecific encephalopathy or normal. Treatment consists of stopping the causative drug and instituting supportive treatment (including treatment of hyperthermia). In addition, dantrolene, 0.5 mg/kg two times per day initially, increased to 0.5 mg/kg two to four times per day, then by increments of 0.5 mg/kg to 3 mg/kg two to four times per day as needed, not to exceed 100 mg four times per day, may be administered to aid in skeletal muscle relaxation. Bromocriptine, a dopamine agonist, is effective in adults to shorten the course of NMS.

MISCELLANEOUS TOXICITY

Hyperthermia is often one of the presenting symptoms of toxic ingestions (either accidental or intentional) of illicit drugs, over-the-counter cold preparations or prescriptions, such as antihistamines (e.g., chlorpheniramine and diphenhydramine), and decongestants (e.g., pseudoephedrine and phenylephrine). Antihistamine toxicity is caused by anticholinergic properties and produces an anticholinergic troxidone that includes hyperthermia, agitation, urinary retention, dilated pupils, and dry, hot, flushed skin. Treatment is usually supportive, and the symptoms typically resolve in 24 to 48 hours.

AUTONOMIC DYSFUNCTION SYNDROME

Autonomic dysfunction syndrome (ADS) is a constellation of clinical findings associated with post–head injury complications: fever, hypertension, tachycardia, tachypnea, extensor posturing, and pupillary dilation. ADS occurs following traumatic brain injury, intracranial tumors, hydrocephalus, subarachnoid hemorrhage, and intracerebral hemorrhage. Any insult that results in injury to the hypothalamus or the cortical and subcortical areas that moderate the hypothalamic activity has the potential to upset a complex, delicate autonomic balance. Hyperthermia is an independent risk for lower Glasgow Coma Scale score and longer pediatric intensive care unit (PICU) stay in head-injured children. It is imperative to consider the possibility of acute infection in this patient population as a differential diagnosis or perhaps a parallel process. Bromocriptine, a dopamine agonist, is effective in treating hyperthermia and diaphoresis associated with ADS.

THYROID STORM

Thyroid storm is a constellation of clinical findings induced by thyrotoxicosis. It is an acute, life-threatening hypermetabolic disorder that manifests acutely with fever, tachycardia, hypertension, widened pulse pressures, diaphoresis, and neurologic abnormalities. Thyroid storm is a rare complication of hyperthyroidism and is frequently precipitated by stress. It is a clinical diagnosis often manifesting with historical features of weight loss, palpitations, chest pain (symptoms of congestive heart failure [CHF]), heat intolerance, anxiety, fatigue, and so on. Therapy may be initiated with β-blockade.

Hypothermia

Hypothermia is defined as a core temperature at or below 95°F (35°C). Esophageal temperature probes are commonly used in intubated patients, although heated air may cause falsely high readings. Bladder and rectal temperatures may lag behind changes in core temperature. Hypothermia increases gas solubility in blood, resulting in a lower partial pressure of CO_2 (Pco_2) and O_2 (Po_2), and a higher pH. However, shivering in response to the cold can increase O_2 consumption and CO_2 production. The oxyhemoglobin-dissociation curve shifts to the left, resulting in decreased O_2 release from hemoglobin at the same Po_2. Respiratory depression because of altered mental status and cold-induced bronchorrhea can result in aspiration and airway obstruction. Increased lactate production from tissue hypoxia and shivering, along with impaired lactate metabolism by the liver, can result in a metabolic acidosis.

There is a transient rise in blood pressure, which then decreases when the temperature continues to fall. Progressive bradycardia contributes to a fall in cardiac output. T wave inversion, prolongation of the PR, QRS, and QT intervals, and the pathognomonic J waves (elevation at the junction of the QRS wave and ST segment) often occur. Atrial fibrillation occurs below 91°F (33°C). Below 82°F (28°C), ventricular fibrillation occurs in adults, whereas infants progress to asystole. Deep tendon reflexes decrease. Pupils become fixed and dilated at temperatures below 86°F (30°C). The electroencephalogram progresses to electrical silence at 68°F (20°C). Hypothermia increases sensitivity to inhalational anesthetics and produces sedation at 91°F (33°C) and narcosis at

86°F (30°C). Coagulopathy often occurs, despite the normal prothrombin and partial thromboplastin time, because these tests are usually done at 99°F (37°C). Platelet number and function is decreased. Disseminated intravascular coagulation may also occur. The initial elevated central blood volume and vasoconstriction causes a diuresis. Severe hypothermia, however, impairs urine production. Gastrointestinal motility decreases and may lead to ileus and constipation. Hepatic/renal drug metabolism and clearance are impaired. Hyperglycemia may result from impaired insulin release. Pancreatitis and/or pancreatic necrosis may occur.

Expert Opinion on Management Issues

Therapy for hypothermia (Table 4) simultaneously includes ABCDE and metabolic/hematologic support. Patients with respiratory depression, altered mental status, and increased secretions should be intubated but as gently as possible to prevent arrhythmias. Heated and humidified air should initially be used in the intubated patient. Blood gas analyzers warm the patient's blood to 99°F (37°C) before measuring pH and the partial pressures of the gas. Using uncorrected arterial blood gas values is called alpha-stat or the ectothermic principle. In hypothermic patients, the "normal" Pco_2 is lower and

---

TABLE 4 Management of Hypothermia

History and Physical

Gentle handling of patient to prevent arrhythmias
ABCDE: cardiopulmonary resuscitation for ventricular fibrillation and asystole
Underlying disease diagnosis and treatment
Vital signs, pulse oximetry, electrocardiogram
Wet or cold clothing removed and patient placed in warm environment

Laboratory Tests

Arterial blood gas analysis corrected for temperature
Electrolytes, BUN, creatinine, Ca, Mg, P
CBC with differential, PT/PTT, fibrinogen
Glucose, amylase/lipase
LFT
Additional labs, if appropriate, such as toxicology screen

Passive Rewarming

≥32°C in patients who are capable of spontaneous thermogenesis

Active Rewarming

<32°C, cardiovascular instability, patients at risk for developing hypothermia
Close monitoring for core-temperature afterdrop
Acute: external and/or core rewarming
Chronic (<90°F [32°C] for over 24 hr): core rewarming
Extracorporeal membrane oxygenation (ECMO)
Availability of rapid deployment

ABCDE, *a*irway and possibly *a*ntibiotics, *b*reathing, *c*irculation, *d*isability or neurologic and possible *d*extrose, *e*xtracorporeal support if all else fails; BUN, blood urea nitrogen; Ca, calcium; CBC, complete blood count; LFT, liver function test; Mg, magnesium; P, phosphorus; PT, prothrombin time; PTT, partial thromboplastin time.

the arterial pH is higher than is encountered at 99°F (37°C). The hypothermic patient should be gently handled to prevent arrhythmias because ventricular fibrillation may occur at temperatures below 82°F (28°C). Closed chest massage should continue until the patient is rewarmed above 86°F (30°C), when electrical defibrillation will be more effective. Drug therapy may be potentially dangerous as a result of decreased hepatic and renal metabolism. As the patient is rewarmed and peripheral vasoconstriction decreases, intravascular volume becomes depleted. Warmed (104°F [40°C]) intravenous isotonic saline (lactated Ringer solution or 0.9% saline) should be administered to avoid worsening hypothermia. If the patient is coagulopathic, fresh-frozen plasma may be administered. Hyperglycemia, which may occur from impaired insulin release, should be observed to avoid hypoglycemia when the patient is rewarmed. However, hypoglycemia should be treated with IV glucose.

Warming of the patient can be done passively (preventing heat loss) or actively (providing heat). For patients with mild hypothermia (90°F [32°C] or more) who are capable of spontaneous thermogenesis, passive rewarming may be adequate. Passive methods begin with removal of cold clothing and covering the patient, including the head, with a blanket in a warm environment. Active rewarming should be used when there is cardiovascular instability and severe hypothermia (less than 90°F [32°C]). Patients who are at risk for developing severe hypothermia (i.e., malnutrition and endocrinopathies) and patients who are unable to thermoregulate spontaneously should also be actively rewarmed. Active rewarming may involve external and core rewarming techniques.

Active *external* rewarming involves the direct exposure of the patient's skin to exogenous heat, such as heating blankets and mattresses and warm packs (to the scalp, neck, axillae, and groin). However, there are concerns regarding core-temperature afterdrop, which is a delayed decrease in core temperature. Chronic (longer than 24 hours) hypothermic patients who are prone to diuresis and third spacing (because of increased capillary permeability) are especially vulnerable to afterdrop. This complication occurs when the warming of the extremities and skin causes peripheral vasodilation and shunting of cold, acidemic, and hyperkalemic blood to the core, resulting in severe hypotension. External rewarming limited to the head and trunk, in conjunction with active core rewarming, may minimize afterdrop.

Active *core* rewarming techniques are less prone to develop afterdrop or life-threatening arrhythmias. These methods are especially important in patients with severe chronic hypothermia (less than 90°F [32°C] for more than 24 hours). Heated humidified air or oxygen by a face mask or an endotracheal tube can prevent respiratory heat loss and can raise the body temperature by 1°C to 2°C per hour. Peritoneal and pleural lavage with heated (104°F [40°C]) sterile isotonic saline solutions may also be effective in active core rewarming. However, the left thoracostomy tube should be avoided to decrease the risk of ventricular fibrillation. Gastric, bladder, and colonic irrigation allows a small surface area available for heat transfer. Complications may include perforation of the viscus and myocardial irritation from gastric tube placement. As a last resort, extracorporeal rewarming by cardiopulmonary bypass or hemodialysis are the most efficient methods for active rewarming. These methods may be considered for patients in refractory cardiac arrest, with severe electrolyte abnormalities, and/or when a body part is frozen.

NEAR DROWNING

Near-drowning accidents are categorized by the temperature of the water in which the submersion takes place: cold-water drowning (temperatures less than 20°F [−7°C]), warm-water drowning (more than 20°F [−7°C]), or very cold-water drowning (less than 5°F [−15°C]). Observational studies and retrospective reviews clearly show that patients arriving to the hospital in cardiopulmonary arrest following submersion in warm water have a very bleak prognosis, and the benefits of resuscitation should be continually reassessed. In patients submerged for less than 1 hour in cold water less than 20°F (−7°C), full resuscitative efforts should be employed. Hypothermic management should continue as outlined here, remembering that hypothermia may exacerbate arrhythmias, acidosis, and hypoxemia secondary to profound bradycardia and vasoconstriction. Extracorporeal membrane oxygenation (ECMO) should also be considered in patients refractory to conventional rewarming techniques. Finally, neuroprotective effects of hypothermia seem to only occur in very cold-water near drowning.

PERIOPERATIVE HYPOTHERMIA

Perioperative hypothermia is common in pediatric surgical patients. Several randomized, controlled trials prove that even mild perioperative hypothermia (95°F to 93°F [35°C to 34°C]) can increase the incidence of wound infections, coagulation disorders, arrhythmias, impaired immune function, and prolonged hospitalization. Therefore, prevention of hypothermia by the anesthesiologist in the operating room is essential with cutaneous warming (e.g., forced warm air, warm-water blankets), warming IV fluids, humidified warm air, and high ambient temperatures in the operating room. Postoperative hypothermia should be evaluated and managed aggressively in high-risk surgical patients admitted to the intensive care unit (ICU), with cutaneous warming (blankets, forced warmed air, overhead warmers).

Common Pitfalls

- When cooling a hyperthermic patient, cooled fluids to 39.2°F (4°C) may precipitate arrhythmias.
- When cooling a hyperthermic patient, dobutamine and milrinone can provide enhanced myocardial contractility (inotropy) while increasing peripheral vasodilation to promote heat loss. However, these drugs can also cause hypotension.
- When warming a hypothermic patient, core-temperature afterdrop can occur, which is a delayed decrease in core temperature.

SUGGESTED READINGS

1. Baum CR: Environmental emergencies. In Fleisher GR, Ludwig S (eds): Textbook of Pediatric Emergency Medicine, 4th ed. Philadelphia: Lippincott Williams & Wilkins, 2000, pp 943–963. **Review of environmental and exertional heat illness and accidental hypothermia.**
2. Danzl DF, Pozos RS: Accidental hypothermia. N Engl J Med 331 (26):1756–1760, 1994. **Provides evaluation and evidence-based rewarming strategies following hypothermia.**
3. Guyton AC, Hall JE: Body temperature, temperature regulation, fever. In Guyton AC, Hall JE (eds): Textbook of Medical Physiology, 9th ed. Philadelphia: WB Saunders, 1996, pp 911–922. **Detailed physiology of thermoregulation.**
4. Kochanek PM, Safar PJ: Therapeutic hypothermia for severe traumatic brain injury. JAMA 289(22):3007–3009, 2003. **Review of evidence-based practice of therapeutic hypothermia and discussion of potential practice parameters.**
5. Lake CL: Extracorporeal circulation circulatory assist devices in the pediatric patient. In Lake CL (ed): Pediatric Cardiac Anesthesia, 3rd ed. Stamford: Conn, Appleton and Lange, 1998, pp 232–252. **Detailed description of hypothermic cardiopulmonary bypass and the brain.**
6. Litman RS: Malignant hyperthermia. In Litman RS (ed): Pediatric Anesthesia: The Requisites in Anesthesiology, 1st ed. Philadelphia: CV Mosby, 2004, pp 174–181. **Review of pathophysiology and evidence-based management strategies for malignant hyperthermia.**
7. Sessler DI: Perioperative heat balance. Anesthesiology 92(2):578–596, 2000. **Reviews the physiology, morbidity, and treatment of perioperative hypothermia.**
8. Simon HB: Hyperthermia. N Engl J Med 329(7):483–487, 1993. **Describes selected hyperthermic disorders and evidence-based management of hyperthermia.**

Orthopedic Trauma

Joshua E. Hyman and Derek W. Moore

KEY CONCEPTS

- Approximately 3.5 million children in the United States go to the emergency department every year to be evaluated for orthopedic trauma.
- Once airway, breathing, and circulation are addressed, a meticulous secondary survey evaluating for musculoskeletal injury should be performed.
- Adequate documentation of the neurovascular examination before and after manipulation is essential.
- If compartment syndrome is suspected because of physical findings, fracture patterns, or a history of crush injury, serial examinations must be performed over 12 to 48 hours.
- A high suspicion for physical abuse and neglect is necessary.
- Elbow injuries are common and prone to complications, so a low threshold for orthopedic consultation should be held.
- The majority of children with displaced tibia fractures need to be admitted for observation of compartment syndrome.

Remarkable gains in pediatric injury control have been made over the last 2 decades. In the United States, pediatric unintentional injury mortality fell by 45.3% between 1979 and 1996, with the largest decreases in children between 5 and 9 years of age. This progress can be attributed to an increasingly scientific approach to injury causation and more effective prevention programs. Despite these enormous gains, trauma remains the leading cause of death among children older than 1 year and exceeds all other causes of death combined. Each year, approximately 20,000 children and teenagers die as a result of injury, and an estimated 22.5 million children go to the emergency department for evaluation. Skeletal trauma accounts for a staggering 10% to 15% of these emergency department visits. To care for this immense patient population effectively, primary care and emergency department physicians need to have a solid understanding of the guidelines for pediatric orthopedic trauma evaluation, treatment, and referral.

Expert Opinion on Management Issues

EVALUATION

Caring for an injured child in an acute setting requires specific pediatric knowledge, meticulous attention to detail, and precise management. Ideally, evaluation should be performed by emergency department physicians specializing in pediatrics or trauma surgeons who are familiar with tenets of modern pediatric trauma care. Once airway, breathing, and circulation are addressed, a meticulous secondary survey evaluating for musculoskeletal injury should be performed. Careful evaluation of every extremity is essential. First, inspect and palpate for gross deformity or tenderness. Then assess carefully for presence of distal pulses and nerve function. Adequate documentation of the neurovascular examination before and after manipulation is essential. Evaluate for compartment syndrome in all extremities even if no gross deformity exists. If a compartment syndrome is suspected because of physical findings, fracture patterns, or a history of crush injury, serial examinations must be performed over 12 to 24 hours. Splint fractured limbs to reduce ongoing hemorrhages. Initial splints should be radiolucent or easily removable so they do not sacrifice the quality of screening radiographs.

A high index of suspicion for abuse is required. Abuse is responsible for a shocking percentage of pediatric injuries. Fractures are the most common presentation of physical abuse behind skin lesions. Spiral fractures, corner fracture, multiple fractures at different stages of healing, fracture patterns inconsistent with the history, unwitnessed fractures, and suspicious skin lesions are all red flags that warrant a complete skeletal survey. Keep in mind, however, that there is no pathognomonic fracture for child abuse.

Radiographs should always include the joint above and below the injury. If the fracture is in a region where ossification is not complete, contralateral radiographs may be useful, especially for pediatric elbow fractures. CT scans are useful for articular fractures that are difficult to delineate on plain radiographs and for complex physeal fractures as seen in the distal tibia.

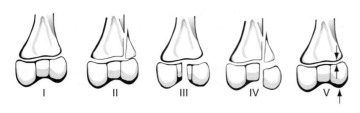

FIGURE 1. The Salter-Harris classification of growth plate injuries. (Adapted from Salter RB: Disorders and Injuries of the Musculoskeletal System, 3rd ed. Baltimore: Williams and Wilkins, 1999.)

The biomechanics surrounding the growth plates differentiate pediatric fracture patterns from adult fractures. A basic understanding of the Salter-Harris classification system is helpful to the diagnosis and treatment of pediatric fractures. In addition, it effectively communicates information regarding the injury to consulting orthopedic surgeons (Fig. 1).

CLAVICLE

The clavicle is one of the most commonly fractured bones in children. These injuries tend to occur in the region of the middle of the clavicle. The majority can be managed with a sling for 2 to 3 weeks. By then there is sufficient healing that the child should be able to support his or her own arm comfortably. The purpose of the sling is for comfort, not to reduce the ends of the fractured bones. These injuries have a tremendous capacity to remodel and reform a nearly normal bone. Surgical intervention is reserved for rare open fractures, severe tenting of the skin, neurovascular compromise, or symptomatic nonunion.

ELBOW

Injuries to the pediatric elbow are extremely common, representing approximately 9% of all fractures in children. Because they can be difficult to diagnose and have the potential for significant complications, they remain a challenge in pediatric orthopedic trauma. A careful neurovascular examination must be performed and documented before and after any manipulation. Initial radiographs should include true anteroposterior and lateral radiographs. Comparison views are occasionally helpful to differentiate normal anatomy from injury. Because the fracture line can be difficult to view on plain radiographs, anterior and posterior fat pad signs on radiographs and the clinical examination play an important role in the diagnosis. Table 1 shows the frequencies of different elbow fractures, peak incidence, and the need for surgery.

Supracondylar Fractures

Representing 41% of elbow injuries and 60% of elbow fractures, supracondylar fractures are common and often require operative treatment. The peak incidence in children is 5 to 8 years of age. Extension-type injuries make up 96% of supracondylar fractures. Neurologic deficits are found in 7% to 15% of supracondylar fractures; thus it is essential to document the neurologic examination before and after manipulation. The anterior interosseous branch of the median nerve is most commonly involved, followed by the radial nerve and ulnar nerve. Most nerve injuries are neurapraxias and do not require treatment. Vascular injury, although less common with an incidence of less than 1%, has higher potential for morbidity. Anterior displacement of the proximal humerus can impinge on or damage the brachial artery. Closed reduction often relieves impingement on the artery and should not be delayed when there are diminished pulses. Prompt orthopedic consultation is critical in this scenario. Management of a pulseless hand that is warm, pink, and has adequate capillary refill is controversial in the orthopedic community, but the trend is toward nonoperative management. Treatment of uncomplicated supracondylar fractures is based on the degree of displacement. Only a completely nondisplaced fracture is amenable to nonoperative treatment in a long arm cast with the elbow at 90 degrees for 2 to 3 weeks. Displaced fractures are treated surgically with closed reduction and percutaneous pinning followed by casting. Postoperatively, the patient is observed for 24 to 48 hours to ensure normal vascular flow and rule out a Volkmann ischemic contracture.

Radial Head Subluxation

More commonly known as nursemaid's elbow, these injuries are most common in children 2 to 5 years of age. The injury is caused by longitudinal traction applied to an extended arm resulting in subluxation of the radial head and interposition of the annular ligament into the radiocapitellar joint. A child with radial head subluxation tends to hold the elbow flexed and the forearm pronated. Pain is localized to the lateral aspect of the elbow. There are no abnormal radiographic findings with this injury.

TABLE 1 Elbow Injury Frequency

Fracture Type	Elbow Injuries (%)	Peak Age	Requires Surgery
Supracondylar fractures	41%	7	Majority
Radial head subluxation	28%	3	Rare
Lateral condylar physeal fractures	11%	6	Majority
Medial epicondylar apophyseal fracture	8%	11	Minority
Radial head and neck fractures	5%	10	Minority
Elbow dislocations	5%	13	Rare
Medial condylar physeal fractures	1%	10	Rare

Reduction is performed by manually supinating the forearm with the elbow in 60 to 90 degrees of flexion. While holding the arm supinated, the elbow is then maximally flexed. During this maneuver, the physician's thumb applies pressure over the radial head. A palpable click is often heard with reduction of the radial head. Immobilization is not necessary, and the child may immediately resume use of the arm. Follow-up is only needed if the child does not resume normal use of the arm in the following weeks. Recurrence occurs in 5% to 39% of cases but generally ceases after 5 years of age.

Lateral Condyle Fractures

Lateral condyle fractures are common, and their outcomes historically are worse than supracondylar fractures. The combination of the fracture's articular nature and diagnostic challenge leads to an unacceptably high incidence of malunion and nonunion. The physical examination lacks the deformity often seen with supracondylar fractures. Swelling and tenderness are usually limited to the lateral side. If the lateral condyle and capitellum have not ossified, radiographic findings can be subtle. Contralateral radiographs are very important. MRI and arthrograms can be helpful as well. To obtain good treatment results, the articular surface must be perfectly reduced. Only when one is confident the fracture is nondisplaced should nonoperative treatment with casting be performed. More often, the fracture is displaced and should be treated by open reduction and percutaneous pinning in the operating room. Intraoperative arthrograms are valuable to delineate the fracture and ensure anatomic reduction. Delay in diagnosis and improper treatment can lead to nonunion or malunion. In these cases, cubitus valgus and tardy ulnar nerve palsy may result. These complications, coupled with the fracture's high prevalence and subtle radiographic findings, should keep lateral condyle fractures on the forefront of the physician's mind when evaluating elbow injuries in children.

Medial Epicondyle Fractures

Medial epicondyle fractures make up approximately 8% of all elbow injuries. They are found in children 10 to 14 years of age. The medial epicondyle serves as the origin of the forearm flexor muscles and the medial collateral ligament. When a valgus force is placed on the elbow while the forearm flexor muscles are contracted, an avulsion of the medial epicondyle may occur. If this force is strong enough, the elbow will dislocate. Fifty percent of medial epicondyle fractures are associated with elbow dislocations. Ulnar nerve dysfunction is found in 10% to 16% of these fractures, so a careful neurovascular examination is critical.

Most medial epicondyle fractures are minimally or nondisplaced and may be treated with immobilization in a posterior molded splint with the elbow flexed to 90 degrees. After 3 to 4 days, the splint is discontinued and active range of motion is begun. A sling can be worn for comfort. For displaced medial epicondyle fractures, treatment is controversial in the orthopedic community. An absolute indication for operative treatment is an incarcerated irreducible fragment in the elbow joint. Controversial indications for surgery include ulnar nerve dysfunction and elbow instability. Operative treatment includes percutaneous pinning or open reduction with screw fixation, depending on the age of the child.

Elbow Dislocations

Elbow dislocations are rare and occur in older children as the result of a fall on a hyperextended elbow. Most dislocations are posterolateral. There is a high association with elbow fractures, especially medial epicondyle fractures. A careful neurovascular examination must be performed because injury to the brachial artery, median nerve, and, less commonly, the ulnar nerve can occur. Reduction should be performed in a timely matter under conscious sedation. The maneuver consists of first reducing medial or lateral displacement, then slowly flexing the elbow while longitudinal traction is applied. Gently pronating and supinating the forearm during this maneuver may aid the reduction. Avoid reduction in hyperextension because it is associated with median nerve entrapment. After reduction, the stability of the elbow should be tested. If it is stable, immobilize it for 1 week and then begin range of motion exercises. If it is unstable, immobilize it in a position of stability for 3 weeks and then begin motion exercises, making sure to avoid full extension until 6 weeks. The need for surgery is rare and is reserved for open dislocations, median nerve entrapment, brachial artery injuries, or treatment of an associated fracture.

Radial Head and Neck Fractures

In children, fractures of the proximal end of the radius typically involve the radial neck and physis. The radial head is rarely involved. Patients typically present with lateral elbow swelling and pain exacerbated by motion, especially supination and pronation. A portion of the radial neck is extra-articular, and therefore effusion and fat pads signs are sometimes absent. A radiograph with the beam directed 40 degrees in the proximal direction, known as the Greenspan view, is helpful to visualize the fracture. Nonoperative treatment is indicated for minimally displaced fractures with less than 30 degrees of angulation. If there is greater than 30 degrees of angulation, closed reduction with or without percutaneous pinning should be performed in the operating room. The indication for open treatment is a fracture that cannot be adequately reduced with closed methods. Open reduction is associated with a greater loss of motion than closed reduction.

FOREARM AND WRIST

Pediatric forearm fractures are very common, composing 45% of all pediatric fractures. Eighty-one percent of these fractures occur in children older than 5 years, with a peak incidence occurring from 10 to 12 years of age in girls and 12 to 14 years of age in boys. Fractures of the diaphysis include both bone fractures and greenstick

TABLE 2 Overview of Forearm and Distal Radius Fractures

Region	Frequency	Type
Diaphysis	20%	Radius and ulna fracture Greenstick fracture
Metaphysis	62%	Displaced distal radius fractures Torus fractures
Distal physis	14%	Salter-Harris I–V
Fracture with dislocation	4%	Monteggia fracture Galeazzi fracture

TABLE 3 Acceptable Angulation in Pediatric Forearm Fractures

Age (yr)	Acceptable Bayoneting	Shaft Acceptable Angulations	Distal Radius/ Ulna Acceptable Angulation
<4	<1 cm	20 degrees	30 degrees
4–10	<1 cm	15 degrees	20 degrees
>10	None	10 degrees	15 degrees

TABLE 4 Femur Fracture Management

Age (yr)	Isolated Injury
Neonate	Splinting for 2–3 wk until united.
1–5	If <1.5 cm of shortening, then immediate spica cast in emergency department under conscious sedation If >1.5 cm shortening, then external fixation, intramedullary flexible nailing, or skeletal traction
6–10	External fixation, flexible nailing or plating, or skeletal traction
10–14	Flexible nailing for stable fractures
>14	Reamed, locked intramedullary nailing using trochanteric entry point if growth center is open

fractures where one cortex is disrupted but one remains intact. Fractures of the metaphysic include "torus" (buckle) fractures and displaced distal radius fractures (e.g., Colles' fracture). Fractures of the distal physis include Salter-Harris fractures I through V. Although rare, compartment syndrome should be carefully ruled out in forearm fractures. In addition to severe swelling, pain out of portion to the injury and pain with passive extension of the fingers are the most sensitive findings to identify a developing compartment syndrome. Table 2 shows a breakdown of different forearm and wrist fractures and their frequency.

The majority of forearm and wrist fractures are treated nonoperatively with closed reduction under conscious sedation followed by casting. The reduction maneuver and accepted angulation is defined on a case-by-case basis depending on the age of the patient, the location of the fracture, and the type of deformity (angulation, rotation, bayoneting). The radius and ulna function as a single rotational unit. Therefore, a final angulation of 10 degrees in the diaphysis can block 20 to 30 degrees of rotation. Rotational deformities do not remodel and are not acceptable. Bayonet apposition, or overlapping, of less than 1 cm does not block rotation and is acceptable in patients younger than 10 years. Acceptable angulations are controversial in the orthopedic community. Table 3 gives commonly accepted angulations in the forearm based on the age of the patient.

Immobilization consists of a long arm cast for 6 to 8 weeks with the possibility of conversion to a short arm cast after 4 weeks, depending on the type of fracture and healing response. One exception is the torus fracture, which may be immobilized in a short arm cast for 2 to 3 weeks. For all forearm fractures, serial radiographs should be taken every 1 to 2 weeks to ensure the reduction

is maintained. Operative treatment is indicated for fractures in which acceptable angulation cannot be obtained through closed reduction, comminuted fractures with segmental bone loss, and open fractures. The most common fractures that require open reduction and internal fixation are bone fractures in a child older than 10 years and articular Salter-Harris fractures (types III through V) of the distal radial physis.

Monteggia fracture is a fracture of the proximal ulna with an associated dislocation of the radial head. Although rare, it is notable because reports show that up to 50% of these fractures are missed in the emergency department. This emphasizes the need for "joint above and joint below" radiographs in all orthopedic injuries. The majority of Monteggia fractures can be treated nonoperatively, especially in younger children. Galeazzi fractures, defined as a fracture of the middle to distal third of the radius with disruption of the distal radioulnar joint, are rare in children.

FEMUR FRACTURES

Femoral shaft fractures represent 1.6% of all fractures in the pediatric population and are the most common fractures requiring hospitalization. The distribution of incidence is bimodal, with the first peak at 2 to 4 years of age and the second at mid-adolescence. During adolescence, a geometric increase in the diameter of the cortex leads to a corresponding increase in bone strength. Therefore fractures in adolescents are caused by high-energy trauma, 90% of which are motor vehicle accidents. In younger children, femur fractures are caused by low-energy injuries. Abuse is responsible for 80% of femur fractures in children not yet walking and 30% in toddlers. The remaining causes for this type of injury primarily are low-energy trauma such as falls. Radiographs must include hip and knee films to rule out associated injuries. Fracture management is directed by the age of the child, the amount of energy causing the fracture, and the presence of additional injuries. Table 4 gives guidelines for treatment based on the age of the child.

TIBIA FRACTURES

Tibia fractures represent the third most common pediatric fracture after femur and forearm fractures. Table 5 lists common causes of tibia fractures. On the forefront

TABLE 5 Causes of Tibia Fractures

Cause	% of Tibia Fractures
Pedestrian vs. motor vehicle accident	50%
Indirect rotational forces	22%
Falls	17%
Motor vehicle accident	11%

of any physician's mind when presented with a tibia fracture should be compartment syndrome. Palpation of the anterior, lateral, and posterior compartments of the leg are essential, and a careful neurovascular examination, including palpation of the dorsalis pedis, should be performed. Compartment syndrome is a clinical diagnosis in children who are alert and oriented. In a child with altered mental status, the examination is unreliable and compartment pressures should be read. Pressures greater than 30 mm Hg or within 30 mm Hg of diastolic blood pressure should receive emergent fasciotomies of all four compartments to avoid neurologic and ischemic sequelae. If compartment syndrome is not present but the child has significant soft tissue damage or swelling, the patient should be admitted overnight for observation and elevation following reduction and casting.

Proximal Tibia Metaphyseal Fractures

Proximal tibia metaphyseal fractures constitute 11% of pediatric tibia fractures and have a peak incidence of 3 to 6 years of age. These fractures are significant for their tendency to develop a valgus deformity. The parents should be counseled about this possibility in advance. If progressive valgus deformity occurs, it may be watched for 12 to 18 months with expectation of spontaneous correction. If correction does not occur, surgical correction with epiphysiodesis or osteotomy may be required. Nondisplaced fractures are treated with a long leg cast in 10 degrees of flexion at the knee. Displaced fractures are reduced under general anesthesia, and a long leg cast is applied in full extension with varus molding to prevent valgus collapse and malunion. Casts are maintained for 6 to 8 weeks with serial radiographs, and weight bearing may be allowed after 2 to 3 weeks. If interposed tissue prevents closed reduction, an open reduction should be performed.

Diaphyseal Fractures of the Tibia

Thirty-nine percent of tibia fractures occur in the diaphysis. Of these, 30% are associated with a fibula fracture. If the fibula is intact, these fractures have a tendency to migrate into varus. If the fibula is involved, they migrate into valgus. The majority of these fractures can be managed nonoperatively with closed reduction under conscious sedation followed by immobilization. Acceptable reduction in children is 50% apposition, less than 1 cm of shortening, and less than 5 to 10 degrees of angulation in the sagittal and coronal planes. Immobilization is performed with a long leg cast with the knee flexed to provide rotational control and prevent weight bearing. Serial

radiographs are performed to monitor for developing deformity. Operative management is indicated in less than 5% of tibia shaft fractures. Indications for surgery include open fractures, complex fractures that cannot be reduced, compartment syndrome, neurovascular injury, and multiple long bone fractures. Methods of fixation include external fixation, plates, or intramedullary rods, depending on the age of the patient and degree of soft tissue injury. Tissue flaps or skin grafts may be required for skin closure. Postoperatively, a long leg cast is applied.

Toddler Fracture

Most toddler fractures occur in children younger than 2.5 years. The classic description of the mechanism is external rotation of the foot with the knee in a fixed position. This creates a torsional force that leads to a spiral fracture of the tibia without involvement of the fibula. Management consists of a long leg cast for 2 to 3 weeks followed by 2 to 3 weeks in a short leg cast. Manipulation is usually not necessary. This is a low-energy injury, and the suspicion for compartment syndrome is less than other tibia fractures, so it is usually not necessary to admit the patient for observation.

Distal Metaphyseal Tibia Fractures

Fractures of the distal third of the tibia compose approximately 50% of pediatric tibial fractures. There is a peak incidence between 2 and 8 years of age. For nondisplaced or minimally displaced fractures, treatment includes reduction under conscious sedation followed by long leg casting. After 3 to 4 weeks, the cast may be converted to a short leg cast. Surgical intervention is reserved for open fractures or complex fractures where stable reduction is not possible by closed means. Usually surgical treatment is performed with closed reduction and percutaneous pinning followed by a long leg cast and serial radiographs. For open fractures, external fixation is the treatment of choice.

ANKLE FRACTURES

Ankle injuries are common, accounting for 25% to 38% of all physeal injuries. An estimated 58% of these injuries occur during athletic participation. Peak incidence is from 8 to 15 years of age. After 16 years of age, adult fracture patterns are seen. On examination, check for proximal fibula tenderness. If tenderness is present, be sure to include tibia-fibula radiographs to rule out a high fibula fracture. Fractures may be isolated to the physis of the fibula or the tibia or they can involve both, depending on the mechanism and amount of energy.

ISOLATED LATERAL MALLEOLUS INJURIES

In children, ligaments are relatively stronger than bones. Therefore bones and growth plates tend to fracture before ligaments tear. Thus ankle sprains are less common in children than adults. More common is a Salter-Harris I fracture of the distal fibula. Because both have negative radiographic findings, the only way to distinguish them is by careful physical examination. With an ankle sprain there should be swelling and tenderness directly over the talofibular ligament, whereas with a distal fibula physis fracture, the tenderness will be over the lateral malleolus growth plate. Treatment of a sprained ankle includes elastic (Ace) bandage, ice, elevation, and weight bearing as tolerated. Treatment for an isolated Salter-Harris I of the distal fibula is a short leg cast with weight bearing as tolerated for 3 to 6 weeks. For a Salter-Harris III or IV fracture of the distal fibula, closed reduction with percutaneous pinning and subsequent casting may be indicated.

ISOLATED DISTAL TIBIA PHYSEAL FRACTURES

Fractures of the distal tibia physis pose a diagnostic challenge and often have a poor prognosis secondary to physeal growth arrest. Axial compression can lead to a Salter-Harris V injury to the physis. Diagnosis is often delayed until premature physeal closure is found with a leg length discrepancy. In the distal tibia, the medial physis fuses first, and for approximately 18 months, the lateral physis remains open while the medial physis is closed. This explains the occurrence of the juvenile Tillaux fractures (lateral Salter-Harris III fracture) and triplane fractures. If either of these fractures is suspected, a CT scan is essential for diagnosis.

Closed reduction and casting is the treatment of choice for Salter-Harris I and II fractures. A long leg cast for 3 weeks followed by a short leg cast for 3 weeks is standard. For Salter-Harris III and IV fractures, Tillaux fractures, and triplane fractures, anatomic reduction is required. If there is less than 2 mm of displacement following closed reduction, treatment is a long leg cast for 4 weeks followed by a short leg cast for 3 weeks. If more than 2 mm of displacement remains, reduction under general anesthesia is followed by percutaneous pinning or open reduction and internal fixation with Kirschner wires or screw fixation. Postoperative casting with a long leg cast for 4 weeks followed by a short leg walking cast for 3 weeks is required.

Common Pitfalls

GENERAL EVALUATION

- Failure to perform and document neurovascular examination before and after manipulation.
- Failure to recognize compartment syndrome.
- Failure to remove splints or use radiolucent material when taking screening radiographs.
- Failure to identify injury caused by physical abuse and neglect.

UPPER EXTREMITY ORTHOPEDIC TRAUMA

- Failure to identify diminished pulses in a supracondylar fracture leading to a delay in orthopedic consult and subsequent compartment syndrome (the Volkmann ischemic contracture).

- Missed diagnosis of lateral condyle fracture leading to elbow deformity or tardy ulna nerve palsy.
- Failure to diagnose a Monteggia fracture.

LOWER EXTREMITY ORTHOPEDIC TRAUMA

- Patient with a minimally displaced tibia fracture is sent home and develops compartment syndrome of the lower leg during the night.
- Failure to diagnose a fracture of the distal tibial physis leads to physis arrest and leg length discrepancy or malunion.

SUGGESTED READINGS

1. Browner BD, Trafton PG, Green NE, et al (eds): Skeletal Trauma in Children, 3rd ed. Philadelphia: Elsevier Science, 2003. **Detailed description of pediatric orthopedic fracture diagnosis and treatment.**
2. Flynn JM, Schwend RM: Management of pediatric femoral shaft fractures. J Am Acad Orthop Surg 12(5):347–359, 2004. **Describes diagnosis and management of pediatric femoral shaft fractures.**
3. Kovall KJ: Handbook of Fractures, 2nd ed. Philadelphia: Lippincott Williams & Wilkins, 2002. **Concise overview of pediatric orthopedic fracture diagnosis and treatment.**
4. Kocher MS, Kasser JR: Orthopaedic aspects of child abuse. J Am Acad Orthop Surg 8:10–20, 2000. **Reviews clinical and radiographic diagnosis of orthopedic child abuse injuries.**
5. Noonan KJ, Price CT: Forearm and distal radius fractures in children. J Am Acad Orthop Surg 6:146–156, 1998. **Review of management and diagnosis of forearm fractures.**
6. Shearman CM, el-Khoury GY: Pitfalls in the radiologic evaluation of extremity trauma: The upper extremity. Am Fam Physician 57 (5):995–1002, 1998. Part II. The lower extremity. Am Fam Physician 57(6): 1314–1322, 1998. **Review of commonly missed radiographic findings in the upper and lower extremities.**

Metabolic Emergencies in the Newborn

Charles P. Venditti and Gerard T. Berry

KEY CONCEPTS

- When a metabolic disorder is suspected, consult a biochemical geneticist immediately for advice about specimen collection and treatment protocols.
- Screening labs should include quantitation of plasma amino acids, urine organic acids, plasma acylcarnitines, blood lactate, and plasma ammonia.
- Vitamin cofactors, such as thiamine, hydroxycobalamin, riboflavin, and biotin, must be available.
- Alternative nitrogen pathway medications and hemodialysis/hemofiltration capability are needed to manage hyperammonemia.
- Critically ill patients should be transferred to a facility that can offer appropriate therapy and monitoring on site.

The inborn errors of carbohydrate, ammonia, amino acid, and organic acid metabolism are associated with acute, life-threatening disease during the newborn period.

BOX 1 Inborn Errors of Carbohydrate Metabolism

- Hereditary galactosemia
- Glycogen storage diseases
- Hereditary fructose intolerance
- Fructose-1,6-bisphosphatase deficiency

BOX 2 Inborn Errors of Ammonia Metabolism

- Carbamoylphosphate synthetase deficiency
- Ornithine transcarbamylase deficiency
- Argininosuccinicaciduria
- Citrullinemia
- Arginase deficiency
- N-acetylglutamate synthetase deficiency
- Transient hyperammonemia of the newborn

BOX 3 Inborn Errors of Amino Acid Metabolism

- Maple syrup urine disease
- Hereditary tyrosinemia type 1
- Nonketotic hyperglycinemia
- Methionine synthetase deficiency
- Phenylketonuria

BOX 4 Inborn Errors of Organic Acid Metabolism

- Methylmalonic acidemia
- Propionic acidemia
- Isovaleric acidemia
- Multiple carboxylase deficiency
- Glutaric acidemia type 1
- Fatty acid oxidation disorders
  - Glutaric acidemia type 2
  - Very-long-chain acyl-CoA dehydrogenase deficiency
  - Medium-chain acyl-CoA dehydrogenase deficiency
  - Short-chain acyl-CoA dehydrogenase deficiency
  - Long-chain 3-hydroxy acyl-CoA dehydrogenase deficiency
  - Carnitine transporter defect
  - Carnitine palmitoyltransferase type I deficiency
  - Carnitine palmitoyltransferase type II deficiency
  - Acylcarnitine translocase deficiency
- Defects in ketone metabolism
  - Ketothiolase deficiency
  - Succinyl-CoA:3-ketoacid-CoA transferase deficiency
  - 3-Hydroxy-3-methylglutaryl-CoA lyase deficiency
- Primary lactic acidoses
- Pyruvate dehydrogenase complex deficiency
- Pyruvate carboxylase deficiency
- Phosphoenolpyruvate carboxykinase deficiency
- Mitochondrial respiratory/electron transport chain defects
  - Barth syndrome
  - Pearson syndrome
- Leigh disease

Although a single biochemical genetic defect may exhibit more than one mode of presentation, this chapter presents the most severe neonatal-onset phenotype for each disorder. Boxes 1 through 4 outline the disorders that constitute each group. The primary lactic acidosis and mitochondrial respiratory chain disorders, as well as the defects in fatty acid oxidation, are included in the section on inborn errors of organic acid metabolism. Selected vignettes are presented and discussed.

Expert Opinion on Management Issues

INBORN ERRORS OF CARBOHYDRATE METABOLISM

Hereditary Galactosemia

Galactose-1-Phosphate-Uridyltransferase Deficiency

The three enzymes of the galactose metabolic pathway responsible for the rapid hepatic conversion of galactose to glucose after ingestion of dietary lactose are galactokinase (GALK), galactose-1-phosphate-uridyltransferase (GALT), and uridine diphosphate galactose-4-epimerase (GALE). All three enzymes are associated with inborn errors of galactose metabolism, but typically references to the disease galactosemia imply GALT deficiency. The clinical syndrome of transferase-deficiency galactosemia has changed since the advent of newborn screening for galactosemia. In the past, a severe multiorgan toxicity syndrome was a much more common occurrence, associated with weeks of unlimited intake of lactose in the proprietary formula or breast milk. However, the disease can be devastating even in the first 1 or 2 weeks of life because of *Escherichia coli* sepsis.

The most common initial clinical sign of GALT deficiency is poor growth; vomiting and poor feeding also occur in most patients. Jaundice may be present in the first few weeks of life and may persist. The jaundice may be caused initially by indirect hyperbilirubinemia and may only later be associated with an elevation of direct bilirubin as well. While consuming lactose in the first 2 to 3 weeks, many infants with galactosemia present with poor feeding, growth impairment, jaundice, and mild irritability or lethargy. With continual ingestion, a multiorgan toxicity syndrome ensues, associated with liver disease that may progress to cirrhosis with portal hypertension, splenomegaly, ascites, renal tubular dysfunction, and sometimes the full-blown renal Fanconi syndrome, with anemia primarily because of decreased red blood cell (RBC) survival, lethargy, and brain edema associated with a bulging fontanelle.

Two clinical phenomena deserve further mention: cataracts and *E. coli* sepsis. Cataracts may be evident in the first few weeks of life, but often they are detected after 2 weeks of age. However, some infants are born with congenital cataracts associated with abnormalities of the embryonal lens; they are central and require slit-lamp examination for documentation. *E. coli* sepsis is the most devastating complication in the newborn period, with the mortality rate exceeding 50%.

After initiation of a lactose-free diet in the newborn period, the problems related to liver and kidney disease, anemia, and brain edema usually disappear, unless severe organ damage has occurred, such as hepatic cirrhosis. Most infants begin to grow and develop at a normal rate. However, we know now that even prospectively treated patients may have long-term complications related to speech defects, delays in language acquisition, learning problems in school, and hypergonadotropic hypogonadism in most of the females. The cause of these so-called dietary-independent complications is unknown. When hereditary galactosemia is initially diagnosed, either through the newborn screening program or because of the recognition of clinical signs, blood galactose levels may be as high as 5 to 20 mmol per L, and the RBC galactose-1-phosphate level is significantly elevated, as are urine galactitol levels. During this phase of severe hypergalactosemia, positive reducing substances are present in the urine.

One of the first abnormalities to be detected—albuminuria—reflects a poorly understood renal glomerular component. This develops within 24 to 48 hours of ingestion of lactose and disappears as quickly after elimination of lactose from the diet. In addition to hyperbilirubinemia, there may be mild to severe elevations of serum alanine transferase (ALT) and aspartate transaminase (AST) levels and various abnormalities related to renal tubular dysfunction, such as hyperchloremic metabolic acidosis, hypophosphatemia, glucosuria, and generalized aminoaciduria. Vitreous hemorrhages can occur in the newborn period. After the patient is started on a lactose-free diet, the RBC galactose-1-phosphate levels in patients with classic galactosemia fall, but they never return to the normal range, remaining mildly elevated for the patient's lifetime. This is also true for the urinary metabolite galactitol and may be related to endogenous galactose production.

The deficiency of the enzyme GALT may be detected in RBCs in patients with most common forms of galactosemia. The newborn screening programs in various states use an enzymatic method, a metabolite method, or both. Liver disease of any cause and congenital hepatic vascular shunts may lead to impaired galactose tolerance and a positive newborn screening test result for galactosemia.

Treatment

- Stop lactose.
- Begin soy-based formula.
- Perform sepsis workup if necessary and administer intravenous (IV) broad-spectrum antibiotics.
- Evaluate for clotting factor abnormalities and administer fresh-frozen plasma (FFP) as necessary.

INBORN ERRORS OF AMMONIA METABOLISM

- Ornithine transcarbamylase (OTC) deficiency
- Argininosuccinate lyase (ASAL) deficiency
- Argininosuccinate synthetase (ASAS) deficiency
- Carbamoylphosphate synthetase I (CPS-I) deficiency

Genetic diseases involving each of the five enzymes of the hepatic mitochondrial urea cycle are described. In the urea cycle, carbamoylphosphate, which carries the nitrogen atom from ammonia, condenses with ornithine to form citrulline in a reaction catalyzed by the enzyme OTC. The most common defect among the inborn errors of the urea cycle is OTC deficiency. Citrulline subsequently interacts with aspartate to form argininosuccinate (ASA), and in the process, another waste nitrogen atom is shuttled into the urea cycle substrate. Arginine is formed from ASA, and arginase, the terminal enzyme in this cycle, converts arginine to urea for urinary excretion while regenerating ornithine to complete the cycle. The first step in this cycle involves the synthesis of carbamoylphosphate, and this reaction, catalyzed by carbamoylphosphate synthetase type I (CPS-I), requires an activator, N-acetylglutamate, which is synthesized from acetyl coenzyme A (CoA) and glutamate via the enzyme N-acetylglutamate synthetase (NAGS). Rare patients may have reduced activity of NAGS.

Each of these enzyme deficiencies is associated with disease in the newborn period. Clinical presentation in the newborn period is similar for all these defects. Almost all the infants are well in the first 12 to 24 hours of life when they begin to manifest poor feeding, vomiting, hyperventilation, lethargy, and coma, usually with seizures. When these diseases are untreated, they are almost always fatal. The treating physicians must consult a local or regional metabolic specialist prior to the initiation of therapy in a patient with hyperammonemia. The treatment requires specific therapy to lower the waste nitrogen burden, including the toxic substance ammonia. An additional clinical finding is increased intracranial pressure. As with maple syrup urine disease (MSUD), the severe encephalopathic and life-threatening features may be related to brain edema. Chronic hepatomegaly is reported in patients with argininosuccinic aciduria, whereas in the other urea cycle disorders, hepatomegaly is evident only during hyperammonemic episodes. Histologic examination of the liver shows modest fatty infiltration and fibrosis. Children with argininosuccinic aciduria may also manifest a specific abnormality of the hair, trichorrhexis nodosa.

The main laboratory finding in the urea cycle enzyme defects (UCEDs) is a plasma ammonia elevation. Plasma ammonia values may vary in different laboratories. In general, however, with automated chemistry testing for ammonia, the normal plasma values in older infants, children, and adults range between 10 and 35 μmol per L. However, the normal plasma ammonia value in newborns may be as high as 110 μmol per L. In patients with newborn-onset UCEDs who are acutely ill, the plasma ammonia levels are often higher than 1000 or 2000 μmol per L. Patients with UCEDs usually do not have metabolic acidosis unless they are in a terminal state with vascular collapse or respiratory failure. Instead, the characteristic acid-base abnormality associated with hyperammonemia is respiratory alkalosis because of the effect of ammonia on the respiratory control centers in the brain stem.

The various UCEDs can usually be distinguished on the basis of the pattern and levels of plasma amino acids. Because citrulline is the product of the CPS-I and OTC reactions and the substrate for argininosuccinate synthetase (ASAS), its value is critical. In newborn-onset CPS-I and OTC deficiencies, plasma citrulline concentrations are zero to trace. With *OTC deficiency*, there is increased urinary orotate excretion secondary to carbamoylphosphate accumulation and pyrimidine synthesis. With *CPS-I deficiency*, carbamoylphosphate production is decreased or absent, and orotate excretion is decreased. Theoretically, a defect in the production of the activator of CPS-I, namely NAGS, resembles a partial CPS-I deficiency. In citrullinemia, the plasma citrulline concentrations are markedly elevated. With argininosuccinic aciduria, plasma citrulline concentration is moderately elevated, in the range of 100 to 300 µmol per L, and it can be readily detected during an analysis of plasma by amino acid column chromatography.

Because the ability of infants with these disorders to excrete waste nitrogen as urea is impaired, therapy initially centered on the reduction of nitrogen intake by decreasing dietary protein and providing essential amino acids or the ketoacid analogues. This approach theoretically permits adequate growth without an excess nitrogen load. Excessive protein leads to hyperammonemia. However, too great a restriction of protein during long-term therapy leads to poor growth. Actually, this approach fails when the patient is in negative nitrogen balance as occurs in the catastrophically ill infant presenting in the first week of life with massive hyperammonemia. For such an infant with hyperammonemia and coma, the mainstay of therapy is dialysis treatment. According to Summar (2001), hemodialysis is preferred because it affords the greatest clearance of ammonia and should be used in conjunction with another continuous hemofiltration method. Although the ammonia clearance of hemofiltration is not as great as hemodialysis, the continuous nature of hemofiltration affords significant ammonia clearance over many hours. Peritoneal dialysis is not recommended for specific UCED therapy in the newborn period because the clearance of ammonia is many times less than hemodialysis.

While the intensive care personnel are waiting for dialysis therapy to be instituted, alternative waste nitrogen therapy using IV sodium benzoate, sodium phenylacetate, and, for patients with ASAS and ASAL deficiencies, arginine hydrochloride should be initiated (Batshaw, MacArthur, Tuchman, 2001). Patients with OTC and CPS-I deficiencies should also receive IV arginine hydrochloride because body arginine pools can begin to deplete as arginine becomes an essential amino acid with a complete block in cycle function. The plasma arginine levels are usually low in all sick newborns with UCED. Unless corrected, arginine deficiency accentuates the hyperammonemia by promoting negative nitrogen balance and, theoretically, by failing to provide its usual stimulation of NAGS. A second role of arginine is to stimulate alternative pathways of waste nitrogen excretion. It does so by promoting synthesis and excretion of citrulline and ASA in citrullinemia and argininosuccinic aciduria, respectively. Argininosuccinate contains waste nitrogen atoms destined for excretion as urea. It has a renal clearance rate equal to the glomerular filtration rate, provided it is continuously synthesized and excreted. Accordingly, ASA should serve as an effective substitute for urea as a waste nitrogen product.

Like ASA, citrulline can be a means to excrete waste nitrogen, but it contains only the one nitrogen atom derived from ammonia, lacking the second nitrogen atom derived from aspartate. Citrulline also has a more limited urinary excretory capacity than ASA. Thus therapy with arginine is less effective for citrullinemia. With citrullinemia and the other urea cycle disorders, arginine therapy is combined with sodium benzoate and sodium phenylacetate, both of which promote excretion of waste nitrogen. Sodium benzoate is conjugated with glycine to form hippurate, which is cleared by the kidney at five times the glomerular filtration rate. Theoretically, 1 mole of waste nitrogen is synthesized and excreted as hippurate for each mole of benzoate ingested. The hippurate synthetic mechanism resides primarily in the hepatic mitochondria and depends on an intact mitochondrial energy system for adenosine triphosphate (ATP) synthesis. The glycine consumed in this reaction can be replaced by either serine or the glycine cleavage pathway. Sodium phenylacetate, as well as sodium phenylbutyrate, which is used for long-term therapy in the absence of sodium benzoate, conjugates with glutamine to form phenylacetylglutamine, which is excreted by the kidney. Sodium phenylbutyrate is converted to phenylacetate in the liver. Glutamine contains two nitrogen atoms, and glycine contains one. Two moles of waste nitrogen are removed for each mole of phenylacetate administered. This acetylation reaction occurs in the kidney and the liver.

The outcome for patients with severe newborn-onset CPS-I and OTC deficiencies is poor. Sometimes, even dialysis therapy cannot rescue severely affected boys with X-linked OTC deficiency in the first few days of life. Prospectively administered alternative pathway therapy in conjunction with administration of high-calorie fluids usually prevents death and severe hyperammonemia in these patients. Even after institution of successful therapy, however, the morbidity and mortality rates are high in such patients. At present, liver transplantation is recommended for patients with CPS and OTC deficiencies who present in the newborn period and have almost no residual enzyme activity. Alternative pathway therapy has led to a 92% 1-year survival rate in newborns who recover from hyperammonemic coma, but most of the survivors are mentally retarded (Msall et al., 1984). There is a significant correlation between the duration of newborn hyperammonemic coma and the developmental quotient (DQ) score at 12 months of age. Four of five reported children in whom duration of coma was 2 days or less had normal IQ scores, whereas all seven children in whom coma lasted 5 days or longer were severely mentally retarded. This fact points to the devastating effects of prolonged newborn hyperammonemic coma and the importance of early diagnosis and treatment. Mutational analysis of DNA is available for most of these disorders. If the lesion in a particular family is known, prenatal diagnosis by means of direct DNA analysis is also feasible. With the exception of OTC deficiency, all the UCEDs are inherited as autosomal recessive traits.

Treatment

- Hemodialysis
- Protein stopped

- Nutritional support (IV glucose and/or infusion of protein-free formula via nasogastric tube)
- IV insulin to correct hyperglycemia (blood glucose [BG] >150 mg %)
- IV arginine
- IV sodium phenylacetate and sodium benzoate
- Carbamoyl glutamate for NAGS deficiency
- Support for brain edema.

TRANSIENT HYPERAMMONEMIA OF THE NEWBORN

Transient hyperammonemia of the newborn (THAN) is a distinct clinical syndrome first identified by Ballard and colleagues in 1978. The disease usually develops in premature infants during the course of treatment for respiratory distress syndrome. The plasma ammonia level may be enormously elevated, as high as that found in any of the patients with the most severe type of UCED. Its onset is usually in the first 24 hours after birth when the infant is undergoing mechanical ventilatory support. Affected babies can manifest all the signs associated with hyperammonemic coma. The diagnosis may be difficult to determine, however, because many of these same infants are receiving sedatives and muscle relaxants to optimize therapy of their life-threatening pulmonary disease. Important clues are the absence of deep tendon reflexes, the absence of the normal newborn reflexes, and the decrease or absence of response to painful stimuli. As with hyperammonemic coma in the UCED patient, this medical emergency requires dialysis therapy.

The cause of THAN is unknown. The plasma amino acid levels are similar to those found in CPS-I or OTC deficiency. Investigators hypothesize that the disorder may be caused by impairment of hepatic mitochondrial energy production or shunting of portal blood away from the liver (such as with a patent ductus venosus). The mortality rate in THAN is high. A patient who can be treated early and aggressively may survive the episode. No evidence indicates that any of the survivors suffer any further episodes of hyperammonemia, nor is there any further evidence of impaired ammonia metabolism. The treatment is identical to that for the urea cycle disorders, with the exception of considering carbamoylglutamate.

INBORN ERRORS OF AMINO ACID METABOLISM

Maple Syrup Urine Disease

Branched-Chain 2-Keto Dehydrogenase Complex Deficiency

MSUD is a rare inborn error of amino acid metabolism. It is inherited as an autosomal recessive trait secondary to a deficiency of the enzyme branched-chain 2-keto dehydrogenase (BCKAD) complex. This enzyme catalyzes the conversion of each of the 3-ketoacid derivatives of the branched-chain amino acids (BCAAs) into their decarboxylated coenzyme metabolites within the mitochondria. The disease occurs in 1 in 200,000 newborn infants worldwide, but in the Mennonite communities in the

United States, the frequency is 1 in 358 because of a founder effect for a point mutation in the E_1 alpha gene.

In most patients, including those from the Mennonite community, the classic form of the disease occurs. It is associated with severe and catastrophic illness in the newborn period and usually results in death without specific medical intervention. The infants typically are well at birth; only after 2 or 3 days of ingestion of breast milk or formula do they begin to manifest poor feeding and spitting up. Lethargy becomes evident; their cry may be shrill and high pitched. There may be hypotonia alternating with hypertonia and opisthotonic posturing. The odor of maple syrup may be detected in the saliva, on the breath, in the urine and feces, and in cerumen obtained from the ear. The infants become more and more obtunded and eventually lapse into a deep coma. The anterior fontanelle may be bulging. Seizures may develop. The life-threatening encephalopathic features may simply be related to brain edema.

Laboratory findings consist of metabolic acidosis. The anion gap may be raised but not necessarily. Ketonuria is almost always present. The plasma ammonia values are not usually elevated. The complete blood count (CBC) is not usually abnormal. The levels of the plasma BCAAs—leucine, isoleucine, and valine—are elevated, with striking elevation in leucine. In the past, almost every newborn infant recognized to have MSUD and in a severely decompensated state received peritoneal dialysis in a tertiary care center. The treatment did not allow for as rapid a rate of reduction in plasma BCAA levels as does hemodialysis or continuous arteriovenous hemofiltration (CAVH).

It is now clear that a nutritional approach works just as well as peritoneal dialysis in newborns with MSUD (Berry et al., 1991). The approach consists of the use of a BCAA-free enteral formula (e.g., nasogastric infusion) or a modified parenteral nutrition therapy for infants as well as older children with acute metabolic decompensation. Insulin therapy usually is also necessary to curtail the effects of catabolic stress. On the basis of the rate of plasma leucine decline, this nutritional therapy appears comparable to peritoneal dialysis when the plasma leucine levels are as high as 25 to 40 mg/dL (normal value, 0.4 to 2.0 mg/dL). Hemodialysis achieves the greatest rate of reduction of the plasma BCAAs and their corresponding branched-chain ketoacids (BCKAs) when the levels of leucine are beyond the range of treatment by nutritional therapy (i.e., 60 mg per dL or more) (Puliyanda et al., 2002). Most patients who are successfully treated by 7 days of age do not have mental retardation. Patients whose diagnosis and therapy are delayed, however, and perhaps even those whose disorder is diagnosed in the first week of life but who have suffered such severe damage because of increased intracranial pressure, often have substantial decreases in DQ or IQ as well as signs compatible with spastic diplegia or quadriplegia.

The mainstay of long-term therapy for patients with MSUD who survive the newborn period is a special formula devoid of the BCAAs. The amount of BCAAs necessary to sustain growth but maintain the plasma, leucine, isoleucine, and valine levels in the normal range is supplied with a regular proprietary formula in limited amounts. In the first week of life, this is approximately 100 mg of leucine per kilogram of body weight daily and 50 mg/kg daily of both isoleucine and valine. The BCAA requirements and thus the rates of use of the BCAAs for protein accretion drop rapidly in the first year of life in conjunction with the decline in growth velocity in young infants. As with phenylketonuria (PKU), the administration of the special amino acid formula must be carefully monitored by means of frequent plasma amino acid quantitations. One of the most common errors made in the treatment of MSUD is the failure to administer adequate amounts of supplemental isoleucine and valine solutions to maintain the normal plasma levels because proprietary formulas alone do not always meet the needs of each growing infant (i.e., adequate amounts of each BCAA are not supplied by a formula alone). Deficiency of BCAAs may result in a severe exfoliative rash and anemia. The rash may mimic that of severe acrodermatitis enteropathica.

As with many of the inborn errors of amino acid, organic acid, and ammonia metabolism, protein administration in the infant whose disease is under previous good control and in metabolic balance with diet therapy must be discontinued during periods of intercurrent infections because catabolism (possibly driven by counterregulatory hormones or cytokines) triggers metabolic decompensation through release of BCKA from skeletal muscle. Metabolic decompensation is further exacerbated by poor nutritional intake. During these times, adequate calories and fluids must be given to prevent the crisis from escalating into a medical emergency.

In selected instances, a molecular diagnosis of MSUD may be undertaken; such a diagnosis is especially useful in targeted populations such as the Mennonites. Rarely, patients have a defect in the E_2 component or, as discussed earlier, in the E_3 component.

Treatment

- Enteral BCAA-free formula via continuous nasogastric tube infusion
- Parenteral BCAA-free modified total parenteral nutrition (TPN) solution via IV if the gastrointestinal (GI) tract is shut down
- Hemodialysis if plasma leucine level is more than 5000 µmol/L
- Intravenous insulin to correct hyperglycemia (BG >150 mg %)
- Isoleucine and/or valine administration to prevent deficiency state
- Support for brain edema.

INBORN ERRORS OF ORGANIC ACID METABOLISM

Defects in the catabolism of the BCAAs are responsible for most of the disorders of organic acid metabolism. Typical examples are methylmalonic, propionic, and isovaleric acidemias. An organic acid is any organic compound that contains a carboxy functional group but no α-amino group as in an amino acid. In this section, we consider the disorders of fatty acid oxidation, ketone

body metabolism, and lactic acid metabolism as well as the more classic inherited defects in organic acid metabolism.

What is true for all these disorders is that the ability to establish a diagnosis depends primarily on the suspicion of the clinician caring for the sick infant. Most of the disorders also require sophisticated testing such as gas chromatography–mass spectrometry (GC-MS) to identify the specific organic compound responsible for the toxic syndrome. In some states and countries, these metabolic errors can be diagnosed by newborn screening using tandem mass spectrometry (MS-MS). As discussed earlier, acidosis and encephalopathy are usually the hallmarks of these syndromes when they manifest in the newborn period.

Methylmalonic Acidemia

L-Methylmalonyl-CoA Mutase Deficiency

Methylmalonic acidemia and propionic acidemia are the most common of the disorders of organic acid metabolism. Although more than one enzyme defect may result in methylmalonic acidemia, all are inherited as autosomal recessive traits. The enzyme most often deficient is L-methylmalonyl-CoA mutase (MCM). This enzyme is present in mitochondria, and it uses adenosylcobalamin as a cofactor. Impaired function may result from either a mutation of the L-methylmalonyl-CoA mutase apoenzyme or deficient availability of the adenosyl form of vitamin B_{12}. The latter may result from impaired cellular metabolism of vitamin B_{12}, including defective activity of the enzyme ATP:Cob(I)alamin adenosyltransferase or mutations in the MMAA gene product. Some patients, but not usually newborn infants with methylmalonic acidemia, are responsive to pharmacologic therapy with vitamin B_{12}. Methylmalonic acidemia, therefore, is one of the important disorders considered a vitamin-responsive inborn error of metabolism. Because of the deficient activity of L-methylmalonyl-CoA mutase, the substrate L-methylmalonyl CoA accumulates in mitochondria and is subsequently hydrolyzed to methylmalonic acid. Methylmalonic acid is capable of diffusing out of cells in which it is being produced, so it may be detected in excess in the blood, cerebrospinal fluid (CSF), and urine of patients with these various forms of the disease. The precursors of L-methylmalonyl CoA are the BCAAs isoleucine and valine, as well as methionine, threonine, thymine, and odd-chain fatty acids.

The many different phenotypes of methylmalonic acidemia range from severe, catastrophic newborn-onset disease in the first days of life to an almost benign form that is detected in adults with partial L-methylmalonyl-CoA mutase deficiency. The phenotypes are the newborn-onset type, the intermediate variety with onset in early and late infancy, the intermittent form with onset usually in late infancy and childhood, and an adult or benign phenotype.

Most patients who present in the newborn period have a severe phenotype. In some of the patients who present in the first week of life with catastrophic illness, even dialysis therapy is not effective, possibly because of a delay in diagnosis and treatment. The most striking presentation is in the second or third day of life. The infant is usually well at birth but then gradually begins to manifest problems with feeding, vomiting, lethargy, temperature regulation, and perhaps seizures. There may be respiratory distress as a manifestation of metabolic acidosis. The liver may be enlarged as a consequence of diffuse steatosis. The important laboratory findings include a metabolic acidosis usually associated with an increased anion gap, ketosis, and hyperammonemia. The elevation of plasma ammonia may be as high as in the severe newborn-onset hyperammonemic syndromes. Because ketonuria is relatively uncommon in newborn infants and diabetes mellitus is so uncommon in the newborn period, the physician caring for newborn infants must always consider an inborn error of organic acid metabolism when confronted with an acutely ill infant with ketosis. Other laboratory findings are thrombocytopenia, leukopenia, and anemia because of effects of the metabolite on the hematopoietic elements in bone marrow. Older patients with methylmalonic acidemia during a crisis suffer acute pancreatitis as well as devastating lesions to the basal ganglia. Plasma amino acid analysis may reveal elevations of several amino acids, such as glycine and alanine. Secondary carnitine deficiency with elevations of carnitine esters is expected. Methylmalonic acid may be detected in urine with GC-MS, and affected infants have increased propionylcarnitine in their newborn blood spots.

The diagnosis can be confirmed with an assay of the activity of L-methylmalonyl-CoA mutase enzyme in cultured skin fibroblasts. In addition, the various other disturbances in vitamin B_{12} metabolism can also be studied by analyzing skin fibroblasts in culture. The treatment of acute disease consists of protein restriction, empirical therapy with vitamin B_{12} (1 mg intramuscularly [IM] per day), IV fluids with 10% glucose and sodium bicarbonate to correct dehydration, electrolyte imbalance and acidosis, high-calorie feeds via a nasogastric tube, and, often, dialysis. The use of carnitine, 25 to 200 mg/kg/day IV or orally, is controversial. The treatment of the chronic state centers on the judicious use of a low-protein diet and administration of alkali to eliminate any acid–base imbalance. Liver transplantation and combined liver-kidney transplantation are used to treat severely affected patients with mixed results. This therapy does not cure the biochemical abnormalities but does prevent recurrence of acute metabolic decompensations, which carry an appreciable mortality risk in such patients.

Treatment

- IV glucose
- IV sodium bicarbonate to correct acidosis
- High-calorie, protein-free formula via nasogastric tube
- Parenteral vitamin B_{12} therapy
- IV L-carnitine
- Enteral metronidazole (Flagyl)
- Support for hematologic cytopenias
- Hemodialysis.

Propionic Acidemia

Propionyl-CoA Carboxylase Deficiency

Propionic acidemia, because of a selective deficiency of propionyl-CoA carboxylase (PCC), is inherited as an autosomal recessive trait and was the first classic defect in organic acid metabolism described in humans. This disorder was originally called *ketotic hyperglycinemia* because of the elevations of plasma glycine in conjunction with ketosis. The precursors of propionyl-CoA include the amino acids isoleucine and valine plus methionine, threonine, the pyrimidine compound thymine, and odd-chain fatty acids. Of the several hundred patients described with this disease, most present in the newborn period with poor feeding, vomiting, lethargy, and hypotonia. Not uncommonly, the patients manifest seizures and hepatomegaly because of steatosis. The metabolic acidosis may be severe with or without an increase in the anion gap. Ketosis is usually but not always present. Patients who survive often manifest choreoathetosis because of persistent damage to the basal ganglia. Episodes of metabolic decompensation characterized by acidosis and ketosis can be precipitated by excessive protein intake or infection. Such episodes may result in permanent neurologic damage. Subsequent findings therefore include developmental delay, seizures, cerebral atrophy, and electroencephalogram (EEG) abnormalities. During the acute attacks, leukopenia, thrombocytopenia, and, less rarely, anemia, probably because of suppression of maturation of bone marrow hematopoietic precursors, may occur.

The diagnosis may be confirmed by GC-MS analysis of urine in an organic acid quantitation. As in methylmalonic acidemia, affected infants have increased propionylcarnitine in their newborn blood spots. The urine has excess concentrations of various propionate metabolites, such as methylcitrate, propionylglycine, 2-methyl-3-hydroxybutyrate, and 2-methylacetoacetate, as well as several other, rarer compounds. The plasma glycine value may be elevated, and during acute attacks, the plasma ammonia value is frequently increased. The enzyme activity of propionyl-CoA carboxylase may be assayed in white blood cells (WBCs) or extracts of cultured skin fibroblasts for definitive diagnosis. Several mutations are identified in the genes that encode the two nonidentical subunits (α and β) of the propionyl-CoA carboxylase enzyme.

Therapy consists of a low-protein diet and adequate calories. As in L-methylmalonyl-CoA mutase deficiency, a secondary carnitine deficiency with elevations of propionylcarnitine can exist. The use of L-carnitine to relieve a deficiency of free carnitine and promote greater urinary excretion of propionylcarnitine to lower mitochondrial propionyl-CoA levels is controversial. This therapy does not result unequivocally in an improvement in the clinical state but should always be given to an ill infant to both maximize propionylcarnitine formation and relieve acute coenzyme A accretion. Because gut bacteria can also contribute to propionate production, antimicrobial therapy with metronidazole is used during an acute attack. In the acutely ill newborn, the immediate treatment consists of elimination of protein administration or total parenteral nutrition, administration of an adequate amount of calories (10% glucose IV and/or administration of a nonprotein formula, such as Mead-Johnson 80056 or Ross Pro-Phree products, via nasogastric tube infusion); administration of alkali to eliminate metabolic acidosis; and platelet transfusion if warranted by thrombocytopenia. Often, because of the severe acidosis and coma, patients need dialysis therapy. It is unclear whether administration of sodium benzoate and sodium phenylacetate, as in the treatment of hyperammonemia associated with UCEDs, is of benefit to the patient with secondary hyperammonemia. Several patients with propionic acidemia have undergone liver transplantation, with mixed success. Most of the patients with severe newborn-onset disease do not survive the first decade of life.

Treatment

- IV glucose
- IV sodium bicarbonate to correct acidosis
- High-calorie, protein-free formula via nasogastric tube
- IV L-carnitine
- Enteral metronidazole (Flagyl)
- Support for hematologic cytopenias
- Hemodialysis.

Isovaleric Acidemia

Isovaleryl-CoA Dehydrogenase Deficiency

Isovaleric acidemia is caused by a selective deficiency of the enzyme isovaleryl-CoA dehydrogenase (IVCD). It is inherited as an autosomal recessive trait. There are two major phenotypes: An acute form manifests as catastrophic disease in the newborn period, and the late-onset type is characterized by chronic intermittent episodes of metabolic decompensation. In the acute form, the infants become extremely sick in the first week of life. There is usually a history of poor feeding, vomiting, lethargy, and, often, seizures. The characteristic sweaty feet or rancid cheese odor because of isovaleric acid (IVA) is noted. Metabolic acidosis, usually with an elevated anion gap and ketosis, is present. There may be secondary hyperammonemia, thrombocytopenia, neutropenia, and sometimes anemia, resulting in pancytopenia. The infants usually lapse into a coma. Dialysis therapy may be necessary. As with other organic acid disorders for which an amino acid determines organic acid production, treatment also consists of protein or total parenteral nutrition restriction, IV fluids with glucose and perhaps sodium bicarbonate, protein-free formula with calories via nasogastric tube, and glycine, 250 mg/kg/day; IV L-carnitine may be beneficial.

Most patients with late-onset isovaleric acidemia are mentally retarded. In contrast, most of the patients with the acute phenotype are not severely retarded, but most do not survive the newborn period, attesting to the severely toxic nature of this organic acid disorder in the newborn period. The diagnosis may be made from measurement of marked elevations of isovalerylglycine in urine. There is usually also increased excretion of 3-hydroxyisovaleric acid. Elevated C5-OH acylcarnitine species are seen and provide the basis for detecting this disorder by newborn screening. The enzyme IVCD can be assayed in extracts of cultured skin fibroblasts. The gene is identified and assigned to human chromosome 15. Various mutations are described.

Treatment

- IV glucose
- IV sodium bicarbonate to correct acidosis
- High-calorie, protein-free formula via nasogastric tube
- IV glycine
- IV L-carnitine
- Support for hematologic cytopenias
- Hemodialysis.

Fatty Acid Oxidation Disorders

Very-Long-Chain Acyl-CoA Dehydrogenase, Medium-Chain Acyl-CoA Dehydrogenase, and Short-Chain Acyl-CoA Dehydrogenase Deficiencies

In general, the defects in fatty acid oxidation are associated with coma, hypoglycemia, liver disease, cardiomyopathy, and skeletal myopathy. All of these defects involve abnormalities in the enzymes that participate in or facilitate the mitochondrial β-oxidation of fatty acids. In general, the pathophysiology associated with these disorders has the potential to put the patient in a life-threatening condition in which there is a state of catabolism and enhanced liberation of free fatty acids by adipose stores.

Patients with very-long-chain acyl-CoA dehydrogenase (VLCAD) deficiency may be ill in the newborn period because of liver disease, with hypoglycemia, cardiomyopathy, and skeletal myopathy. VLCAD deficiency may be fatal; sudden death in early infancy is reported. The most common of these disorders, the medium-chain acyl-CoA dehydrogenase (MCAD) deficiency, is discussed later. The short-chain acyl-CoA dehydrogenase (SCAD) deficiency, previously thought rare prior to the initiation of expanded newborn screening, can feature a severe newborn-onset disease with feeding problems and vomiting, lethargy, and hypotonia in the first week of life in some. Others may have persistent metabolic abnormalities, such as ethylmalonic aciduria and elevated butyrylcarnitine species in the plasma, but they are asymptomatic. The long-chain 3-hydroxy acyl-CoA dehydrogenase (LCHAD) deficiency is associated with acute illness, fasting-induced hypoketosis, hypoglycemia, cardiomegaly, and muscle weakness. Women who are carriers for this disease may also have the acute fatty liver of pregnancy syndrome.

Each deficiency has a characteristic pattern of abnormalities detected on metabolic analysis and acylcarnitine profiles that can allow for newborn screening. Specific dietary regimens are different, but in the newborn period, symptomatic treatment is similar.

The MCAD deficiency is the most common disorder of fatty acid oxidation and has a prevalence of approximately

1 in 15,000 newborns. More than 200 patients are described, and with implementation of expanded newborn screening, many more have been identified. Most patients do not present until late infancy. The typical patient is an older infant who, after an infection, experiences anorexia, vomiting, dehydration, lethargy, and hypoglycemia that may be associated with seizures. Similarly, older patients have features that mimic those of Reye syndrome and can die because of brain edema. Onset of symptoms in the newborn period is rare, but symptoms can occur and must be considered in the setting of severe or unexplained hypoglycemia. Because modern newborn screening methods can diagnose the condition with great sensitivity and specificity, affected patients can now be diagnosed in the newborn period, before a crisis occurs.

In MCAD deficiency, the initial episode is associated with a high mortality rate. The laboratory studies usually show hypoglycemia and an absence of moderate to large ketones in urine that would be expected to accompany hypoglycemia. The plasma ammonia values may be mildly elevated, the liver may be enlarged, and the serum ALT and AST levels may be slightly increased. During an acute episode, urine GC-MS analysis of organic acids characteristically shows increased levels of adipic, suberic, and sebacic acids as well as the unsaturated analogues of these medium-chain dicarboxylic acids. Greater urinary excretion of dicarboxylic acids is common in many of the defects of carnitine or fatty acid metabolism. However, this is not pathognomonic of a disorder of fat metabolism because infants fed medium-chain triglyceride-enriched formulas also manifest dicarboxylic aciduria. Fatty acid analysis of plasma from patients with MCAD deficiency demonstrates increased levels of octanoic and 4-decanedioic acids. Urine also contains glycine conjugates such as suberylglycine and hexanoylglycine. A secondary carnitine deficiency can be present, and the acylcarnitines analyzed by MS-MS have higher concentrations of 4-, 5-, 6-, 8-, and 10-carbon monounsaturated acylcarnitine species. The MCAD enzyme may be assayed in cultured skin fibroblasts.

The MCAD gene has been cloned and sequenced, and several mutations are now identified. The most conspicuous one is *R329E*, a highly prevalent mutation in people of northern European ancestry. The major treatment is to avoid fasting; if an episode occurs with hypoglycemia or encephalopathy, IV administration of glucose and calorie support should be instituted quickly. Because of the possibility of the development of brain edema, obtunded patients may have to be aggressively treated to relieve increased intracranial pressure. Avoidance of free fatty acid mobilization during relative insulin deficiency and catabolic stress and prevention of hypoglycemia are the cornerstones of therapy.

Primary Lactic Acidosis

The term *primary lactic acidosis* (PLA) refers to a group of diseases in which impaired lactate metabolism is caused by a defect in the mitochondrial respiratory or electron transport chain (ETC), the tricarboxylic acid (TCA) (Krebs) cycle, or the accessory components that support mitochondrial function and shuttling of reducing equivalents, or in which there is a primary defect in pyruvate metabolism that secondarily leads to impaired lactate handling. However, a limited number of reports are available on inborn errors of the TCA cycle. Most of the information on PLA focuses on mitochondrial ETC, pyruvate dehydrogenase (PDH) complex, and pyruvate carboxylase (PC) defects.

Some patients present with overwhelming lactic acidosis. In others, lactate may be elevated only in CSF, a "cerebral" lactic acidosis syndrome. Depending on the nature of the enzyme deficiency, lactate and pyruvate as well as alanine can be elevated in blood. The ratio of blood lactate to pyruvate (L/P ratio) can be helpful in distinguishing the different types of inborn errors. For example, the L/P ratio is often normal (10 to 20) in the PDH and PC deficiencies but elevated in an ETC defect.

The most common cause of a primary defect in pyruvate metabolism is PDH complex deficiency. This complex, located in the mitochondria, has several components, the E_1 alpha and E_1 beta subunits, the E_2 subunit, the E_3 subunit, the X-lipoate subunit, and the PDH phosphatase and kinase subunits. Most mutations are reported in the E_1 alpha subunit. Unlike the other components, the E_1 alpha subunit is encoded on the X chromosome. Because of the key importance of the PDH complex in energy metabolism, even partial defects of the complex may be associated with severe CNS disease. In addition, even though the E_1 alpha subunit defect is an X-linked disease, many females are also affected, so it can be considered a dominant mutation. All the other defects are inherited as autosomal recessive disorders.

The several different phenotypes of PDH complex deficiency are based on the severity of the enzyme deficiency. Some patients, but perhaps those without life-threatening acidosis, even have congenital lesions associated with cystic lesions in the cerebral hemisphere; cerebral atrophy; cystic lesions in the basal ganglia; and facial dysmorphism, including features that resemble those of fetal alcohol syndrome, such as a narrowed head, frontal bossing, wide nasal bridge with upturned nose, a long poorly developed philtrum, and flared nostrils. In addition, there may be partial or complete agenesis of the corpus callosum and impaired migration of neurons within the cerebral hemispheres, identified as heterotopic dysplasia on neuropathologic examination of brain tissue. Patients with less severe defects manifest progressive psychomotor retardation including the entity termed *Leigh disease*, or *subacute necrotizing encephalomyelopathy* (SNE), as discussed later, and older male patients with variant lesions may manifest only intermittent ataxia during childhood with a mild or intermittent lactic acidosis. Secondary hyperammonemia may be detected.

No effective treatment is available for any of the defects in PDH complex metabolism that manifest in the newborn period. A response to thiamine megatherapy is reported in a few patients. Metabolic imbalance in the patient with PDH deficiency, as well as in other PLA defects, may be further compromised by high- or selective-carbohydrate feedings. Some success is achieved in reducing lactate accumulation using a ketogenic diet. Dichloroacetate, an inhibitor of the PDH kinase, is being studied as a treatment for several PLAs.

Mitochondrial Respiratory Chain or Electron Transport Chain Defects

Oxidative phosphorylation is the key process performed by the mitochondria of cells. Any inborn error of metabolism that involves the tightly coupled and regulated process of mitochondrial energy metabolism may have profound effects on health and disease because oxidative phosphorylation is the process by which we convert food into energy. The various derivatives of foodstuffs such as pyruvate and fatty acids are converted to carbon dioxide in mitochondria. The energy derived from such controlled chemical combustion is harnessed by allowing the reducing equivalences (in the form of nicotinamide adenine dinucleotide [NADH] or the reduced form of flavin adenine dinucleotide [FADH$_2$], which are derived from such metabolism) to combine with oxygen to form water, and in the process, the synthesis of ATP is coupled to the orderly flow of electrons down the respiratory chain components.

Early Lethal Lactic Acidosis

In an unknown fraction of patients with primary disturbances in mitochondrial oxidative phosphorylation or ETC defects, massive lactic acidosis develops within 24 to 72 hours after birth. Not uncommonly, the condition is untreatable because it is relentless and unresponsive to alkali therapy. Dialysis is a remedy but not a cure. Affected infants often have no obvious organ damage early in the course or evidence of malformations. This statement is also true for infants with the PDH complex deficiency, which is probably a more common cause of overwhelming acidosis in the first week of life. In addition, acidemia per se can easily explain the coma or impaired cardiac contractility that may be encountered. With aggressive therapy, some infants survive. Anecdotal reports also suggest the existence of a transient disease process.

The care of infants with these different forms of severe lactic acidosis almost always brings an ethical and moral dilemma to the forefront for the physicians and nurses of the neonatal intensive care unit (NICU) as well as for the families. To further complicate the issues, enzymatic and molecular analyses usually are not immediately available. The disease in most patients probably remains idiopathic, and no DNA mutation, nuclear or mitochondrial, can be identified. A rigid approach to care is impractical and unwise. Decisions regarding management must be individualized because the mitochondrial dysfunction and resultant pathophysiology may vary among infants.

Common Pitfalls

- Beware of inaccurate results (e.g., plasma ammonia).
- If you consider a metabolic disease, stop protein feeding and provide calorie support while waiting for a consultation.
- Watch for dosing errors.

- Do not fail to institute dialysis therapy in a timely fashion.

Communication and Counseling

In the event of an unknown diagnosis, counseling should be guarded. If a presentation of hyperammonemia is part of the symptom complex, a risk of 50% for an affected male in a future pregnancy should be entertained considering OTC as the diagnosis. All other conditions carry a 25% recurrence risk. The course and symptom complex between affected infants in a sibship is expected to be similar. Achieving a diagnosis is paramount, and a metabolic autopsy may be required in some circumstances to obtain a definitive answer.

SUGGESTED READINGS

1. Batshaw ML, MacArthur RB, Tuchman M: Alternative pathway therapy for urea cycle disorders: Twenty years later. J Pediatr 138 (1 Suppl.):S46–S54, 2001. **Reviews the use of alternative pathway therapy in urea cycle disorders.**
2. Berry GT, Heidenreich R, Kaplan P, et al: Branched-chain amino acid–free parenteral nutrition in the treatment of acute metabolic decompensation in patients with maple syrup urine disease. N Engl J Med 324:175, 1991. **Describes the use of parenteral nutrition to treat MSUD.**
3. Fernandes J, Saudubray J-M, van den Berghe G (eds) Inborn Metabolic Diseases: Diagnosis and Treatment, 3rd ed. New York: Springer-Verlag, 2000. **Clinically focused one-volume reference text.**
4. Msall M, Batshaw ML, Suss R, et al: Neurologic outcome in children with inborn errors of urea synthesis. N Engl J Med 310:1500, 1984. **Original source of neurologic outcome data in urea cycle disorders.**
5. Puliyanda DP, Harmon WE, Peterschmitt MJ, et al: Utility of hemodialysis in maple syrup urine disease. Pediatr Nephrol 17(4):239–242, 2002. **Discusses hemodialysis in MSUD and useful comparison of clearances by different modalities.**
6. Summar M: Current strategies for the management of neonatal urea cycle disorders. J Pediatr 138(1 Suppl.):S30–S39, 2001. **Reviews the acute treatment by dialysis in urea cycle disorders.**
7. Scriver CR, Beaudet AL, Sly WS, et al (eds) The Metabolic and Molecular Bases of Inherited Disease. New York: McGraw-Hill, 2001. **Comprehensive reference textbook in four volumes.**

Rhabdomyolysis

Karen I. Gerber-Vecsey and Wayne R. Waz

KEY CONCEPTS

- The most common causes of rhabdomyolysis are alcohol abuse, crush injury, overexertion, certain medications and toxic substances, infections, and metabolic disturbances. Rhabdomyolysis secondary to hereditary causes, such as metabolic myopathies, is usually triggered by exercise.
- Complications include electrolyte abnormalities, acidosis, compartment syndrome, clotting disorders, hypovolemia, myoglobinuria, and acute renal failure.
- Early recognition and treatment of complications are crucial to successful outcome.

- The major goal of therapeutic efforts is to prevent or delay the onset of acute renal failure. Early volume replacement represents the single most important factor in this prevention. After initial volume expansion, treatment includes a forced mannitol-alkaline diuresis.
- Development of renal failure is related to extent of muscle injury and correlates with the serum creatine kinase (CK) concentration.

Rhabdomyolysis is a clinical and biochemical syndrome that occurs when muscles are stressed by a variety of etiologies resulting in damage to myocytes and significant third-space fluid loss (Table 1). Release of intracellular contents after damage to cell and sarcolemma membranes can lead to myoglobinuria, electrolyte abnormalities, acidosis, clotting disorders, and acute renal failure. A variety of conditions are associated with this potentially life-threatening syndrome. These diverse groups of clinical diseases share a final common pathway in the mechanism of myocyte injury. Through either direct membrane disruption or depletion of cellular energy (adenosine triphosphate), they result in an acute increase in cytosolic and mitochondrial calcium concentrations. This rise in calcium activates a chain of events that ultimately leads to muscle necrosis.

In pediatric patients with evidence of rhabdomyolysis or myoglobinuria, it is important to look for an underlying cause if one is not obvious at initial presentation. Rhabdomyolysis after general anesthesia often unmasks a tendency toward malignant hyperthermia or reveals the presence of muscular dystrophies and metabolic myopathies. Likewise, muscular dystrophies, metabolic myopathies, or other underlying disorders, such as sickle cell trait, are often subsequently diagnosed in children and adolescents who have exertional rhabdomyolysis after exercise. The use of recreational drugs, particularly amphetamine and amphetamine analogues, which are increasingly associated with strenuous physical activity (sports participation, dancing), is emerging as an important cause of rhabdomyolysis in adolescents. Statins and other lipid-lowering drugs may also cause rhabdomyolysis.

Clinical signs and symptoms of rhabdomyolysis can be divided into local, systemic, and urinary. Local symptoms include muscle pain and weakness. On exam, localized bruising and swelling may be apparent. Large muscles of the thighs, calves, and lower back are most often involved. These symptoms are usually self-limiting, resolving in days to weeks. Systemic symptoms are nonspecific and include fever, malaise, nausea or vomiting, oliguria, and central nervous system signs, such as confusion, agitation, and delirium. Urine appears brown or tea colored secondary to myoglobinuria. History and physical exam provide clues to the diagnosis of rhabdomyolysis, which is then confirmed with laboratory studies. Although myoglobin levels are elevated, the most rapid and least expensive screening test for rhabdomyolysis is the serum creatine kinase (CK) level. Typically, the CK level begins to rise at 2 to 12 hours postinjury; it then peaks at 1 to 3 days and declines after 3 to 5 days. Several studies show a correlation between the CK level and the risk of developing acute renal failure. The critical CK level in these studies varies from 5000 to 75,000 U/L. Other important biochemical findings are hyperkalemia, hyperphosphatemia, hypocalcemia, and hyperuricemia. Aldolase, lactate dehydrogenase (LDH), aspartate aminotransferase (AST) or serum glutamic oxaloacetic transaminase (SGOT), and carbonic anhydrase III are frequently elevated. Metabolic acidosis results from the release of phosphate, sulfate, uric acid, and lactic acid from the damaged myocytes. Urinalysis usually demonstrates large blood on dipstick examination, but few, if any, erythrocytes are seen on microscopy. Protein, brown casts, and uric acid crystals are also present. Disseminated intravascular coagulation (DIC) may also develop.

Rhabdomyolysis accounts for 5% to 7% of acute renal failure in the United States, and acute renal failure occurs in approximately 15% of cases. The following three mechanisms contribute to the development of renal failure: decreased renal perfusion, cast formation with tubular obstruction, and direct toxic effects of myoglobin on renal tubules. Decreased renal perfusion develops secondary to hypovolemia from third-space loss and renal vasoconstriction, which occurs in the presence of myoglobin. Vasoconstricting substances released include endothelin and platelet activating factor. Depressed myocardial function from hyperkalemia and hypocalcemia may also contribute. Casts form in the renal tubules when myoglobin binds to Tamm-Horsfall protein and precipitates. The binding is enhanced in acidic conditions. These casts may obstruct urine flow in the tubules. Myoglobin can cause iron-enhanced free radical damage, especially to the proximal tubule.

TABLE 1 Causes of Rhabdomyolysis

Trauma	Crush injury, third-degree burns, electric shock
Excessive muscular activity	Sports/military training, status epilepticus, status asthmaticus
Infections	Bacterial/viral/fungal/parasitic
Inflammatory	Polymyositis, dermatomyositis
Recreational drugs	Alcohol, cocaine, amphetamines, methylenedioxymethamphetamine (MDMA; Ecstasy), heroin
Prescription drugs	Statins, immunosuppressants, antibiotics, narcotic analgesics, salicylates, antidepressants, antipsychotics
Toxins	Snake, hornet, and spider venoms, quail ingestion, hemlock
Ischemia	Vascular injury, compression, sickle cell trait
Metabolic	Electrolyte abnormalities (hypokalemia, hypophosphatemia), diabetic ketoacidosis
Temperature extremes	Malignant hyperthermia, heat stroke, frostbite
Inherited	Enzyme deficiencies of carbohydrate metabolism (e.g., McArdle syndrome) or lipid metabolism (e.g., carnitine palmitoyltransferase deficiency), myopathies

Expert Opinion on Management Issues

For patients presenting in a state that may predispose to rhabdomyolysis, initial management (Table 2) should include monitoring for intravascular volume depletion, cardiac arrhythmias, electrolyte abnormalities, acidosis, progressive renal failure, DIC, and compartment syndrome. If the latter complication develops, surgical intervention for possible fasciotomy may be needed.

The major goal of therapeutic efforts is to prevent or delay the onset of acute renal failure. For crush victims in particular, early intravenous fluids, preferably at the time of extraction/reperfusion, may significantly prevent this complication. After initial volume replacement, therapy most often consists of a mannitol-alkaline diuresis, although this treatment is controversial.

Evidence to support the use of bicarbonate and mannitol is mostly from animal studies. Human studies supporting their use have small sample sizes or flawed design. A study by Homsi and colleagues shows no benefit to administration of mannitol and bicarbonate once adequate saline expansion is provided; although it was a small study of only 24 patients. Brown and colleagues reviewed more than 2000 trauma patients. They found that a serum CK level greater than 5000 U/L is associated with an increased risk of acute renal failure. For patients with CK levels from 5000 to 30,000 U/L, mannitol and

bicarbonate administration did not prevent renal failure. There was some indication that mannitol and bicarbonate treatment for patients with CK levels greater than 30,000 U/L is beneficial. A prospective, controlled, multicenter trial is needed to compare the effectiveness of these medications versus standard crystalloid resuscitation alone.

Successful treatment protocols use the following medications, summarized in Table 3:

- Saline: 1.5 to 2 times maintenance with isotonic saline/5% dextrose. Patients may initially need more fluid, given as boluses of 20 mL/kg of isotonic saline to replace fluid deficits, to maintain central venous pressure, and establish adequate urine output (>3 mL/kg/hour).
- $NaHCO_3$: 25 to 50 mEq/L of intravenous fluid. Sodium bicarbonate provides rapid correction of metabolic acidosis and prevents myoglobin precipitation, which occurs at a lower urine pH, but bicarbonate use can be complicated by metabolic alkalosis, volume overload from excessive administration in oliguric or anuric patients, and exacerbation of hypocalcemia by precipitation of calcium phosphate salts in injured tissues. Urine pH should be kept greater than 6.5.
- Mannitol: 1 g/kg up to 25 g per dose. Because of the risk of hyperosmolar volume overload, mannitol should not be given unless good urine output is established, and it should be stopped if the patient becomes oliguric or anuric. Frequent monitoring of serum electrolytes, osmolarity, and patient volume status is required with its use.
- Furosemide: 2 mg/kg up to 120 mg every 6 to 12 hours or continuous infusion (0.05 mg/kg/hour, with the dose titrated to clinical effect). Some authors express concern regarding the use of furosemide because of the possibility of exacerbating metabolic acidosis, whereas others stress the need to maintain a steady diuresis. No clinical trials have compared management of rhabdomyolysis with and without furosemide, and consideration of its use should depend on the clinical setting.
- Acetazolamide (5 mg/kg per dose) to maintain urine pH greater than 6.5 in patients who have developed metabolic alkalosis from bicarbonate infusions. No studies of its efficacy are published, but no serious side effects are reported when it is used.

In massive disasters (e.g., earthquakes), where adequate intravenous fluids and materials may be unavailable, oral therapy with the following solution may be helpful: Na^+, 80 mEq/L; Cl^-, 50 mEq/L; HCO_3^-, 30 mEq/L; dextrose, 100 mOsm/L. This solution can be prepared by mixing 1 liter of water, 1 teaspoon of sodium chloride, 1 teaspoon of sodium bicarbonate, and 1 tablespoon of sugar. In response to recent earthquake disasters, the international nephrology community and international health organizations, assisted by the rapid communication made available by the Internet, now have the ability to respond quickly with resources and personnel necessary to prevent and treat rhabdomyolysis-associated acute renal failure.

TABLE 2 Monitoring Needs for Patients with Rhabdomyolysis

Electrocardiogram/cardiac monitoring
Blood pressure, central venous pressure
Foley catheter for measurement of urine output
Laboratory monitoring: every 4–6 h: sodium, potassium, chloride, total CO_2 (or HCO_3), glucose, phosphorus, calcium, uric acid, lactate dehydrogenase, aspartate aminotransferase, creatine phosphokinase, complete blood count, prothrombin time, partial thromboplastin time, fibrinogen
Monitoring for compartment syndrome

CO_2, carbon dioxide; HCO_3, bicarbonate.

TABLE 3 Recommended Treatment of Rhabdomyolysis

Saline: 1.5–2 × maintenance with isotonic saline/5% dextrose, fluid boluses of 20 mL/kg of isotonic saline to replace fluid deficits, maintain CVP, and establish UOP >3 mL/kg/h
Mannitol: 1 g/kg up to 25 g
Furosemide: 2 mg/kg up to 120 mg every 6–12 hr or continuous infusion (0.05 mg/kg/h, with dose titrated to clinical effect)
$NaHCO_3$ (25–50 mEq/L of IV fluid): to maintain urine pH >6.5
Acetazolamide (5 mg/kg per dose): to maintain urine pH >6.5 in patients who have developed metabolic alkalosis from bicarbonate infusions

CVP, cell volume pressure; IV, intravenous; UOP, urine output.

In addition to the overall management strategy discussed, several specific problems may also arise, including hyperkalemia, metabolic acidosis, hypocalcemia, and DIC. Management of hyperkalemia should include avoidance of potassium-containing intravenous fluids and may require the use of sodium polystyrene sulfonate (Kayexalate), calcium, glucose and insulin infusions, sodium bicarbonate, and β_2-agonists. Management of metabolic acidosis primarily involves the use of sodium bicarbonate, but in oliguric or anuric patients who are volume overloaded, dialysis may be required. In the absence of hypocalcemic symptoms (tetany, carpopedal spasm, laryngeal stridor, seizures), hypocalcemia should not be treated with calcium supplementation because of the risk of metastatic calcification related to hyperphosphatemia. Metastatic calcification is more likely to occur in patients with combined hyperphosphatemia and normal or increased serum calcium (a product of calcium [mg/dL] × phosphorus [mg/dL] of greater than 70 suggests a greater likelihood of metastatic calcification). Some authors recommend the use of calcium channel blockers, although no trials demonstrating their efficacy are published as yet. DIC, manifested as thrombocytopenia, increases prothrombin and partial thromboplastin times, and consumption of clotting factors, including fibrinogen, may complicate the course of rhabdomyolysis. Although DIC often improves spontaneously with treatment of the underlying cause of rhabdomyolysis, more severe cases may require the use of heparin and newer therapies, including the use of protein C concentrates, antithrombin III, and tissue plasminogen activator.

When measures to prevent acute renal failure are unsuccessful, dialysis is necessary to control the metabolic and fluid perturbations of rhabdomyolysis and myoglobin-induced acute renal failure. Dialysis is necessary when medical management of the following problems is unsuccessful: metabolic acidosis, hyperkalemia, volume overload, oliguria or anuria that is unresponsive to diuretics, and symptomatic uremia. Of the available dialysis modalities, none is particularly effective in removing myoglobin, and a modality should be selected on the basis of the ability to correct metabolic and fluid abnormalities during recovery from the acute injury. Hemodialysis, as well as slow continuous therapies that include CAVH (continuous arteriovenous hemofiltration), CVVH (continuous venovenous hemofiltration), CAVHD (continuous arteriovenous hemodiafiltration), or CVVHD (continuous venovenous hemodiafiltration) are all used with success. However, hemodialysis provides the most effective clearance of potassium and other toxic molecules. The choice of modality may ultimately depend on access to equipment and local expertise, particularly in large disasters. Peritoneal dialysis, although safe and technically simple, may not be effective during the acute phase of rhabdomyolysis.

Future therapies for rhabdomyolysis should attempt to achieve the goals of maintaining adequate renal and peripheral blood flow, speeding the repair of cell and sarcolemmal membranes, and minimizing free radical and myoglobin-induced cell damage. Possible therapies currently under consideration include free radical scavengers, antioxidants such as glutathione and vitamin E,

nitric oxide synthesis inhibitors, the endothelin receptor antagonist bosentan, platelet-activating factor (PAF) receptor blockers, the iron chelator desferrioxamine, and dantrolene.

Common Pitfalls

- Failure to recognize rhabdomyolysis on initial presentation is a potential pitfall that can delay prompt fluid administration and prevention of complications.
- Failure to closely monitor for life-threatening complications, such as hyperkalemia or compartment syndrome, can result in permanent sequelae or death. Hyperkalemia is an early complication, with potassium levels peaking around 12 to 36 hours after injury. Compartment syndrome can occur early or late in the course of the syndrome. Decompressive fasciotomy should be performed if the compartment pressure is greater than 30 mm Hg. Delay of more than 6 hours can lead to irreversible muscle damage.
- It is necessary to monitor patients closely for the development of oliguric renal failure to prevent complications such as congestive heart failure and pulmonary edema.

Communication and Counseling

Prognosis of rhabdomyolysis depends on the underlying cause. In patients who develop acute renal failure, the duration of renal failure requiring dialysis is often 10 to 30 days, with most patients recovering sufficient renal function to discontinue dialysis. Progression to end-stage renal disease is rare. Chronic neuromuscular injury often occurs and may require long-term rehabilitation services.

For patients whose illness is secondary to ethanol, illegal drugs, or prescription medication, counseling should be provided on the discontinuation of the offending substance. Patients should be referred to rehabilitation services when appropriate. Counseling on exercise in moderation and attention to hydration status should be given to patients with hyperthermia/exertional rhabdomyolysis. Families with inherited conditions that predispose to the development of rhabdomyolysis should receive genetic counseling.

SUGGESTED READINGS

1. Baggaley PA: Rhabdomyolysis. Available online at http://members.tripod.com/~baggas/rhabdo.html (retrieved July 2004). **Discusses specific pathogenesis of rhabdomyolysis in several hereditary and acquired causes.**
2. Brown CV, Rhee P, Chan L, et al: Preventing renal failure in patients with rhabdomyolysis: Do bicarbonate and mannitol make a difference? J Trauma 56(6):1191–1196, 2004. **Retrospective study comparing the outcome in trauma patients with rhabdomyolysis who received mannitol and bicarbonate with those who only received saline resuscitation.**
3. Brumback RA, Feeback DL, Leech RW: Rhabdomyolysis in childhood: A primer on normal muscle function and selected metabolic myopathies characterized by disordered energy production. Pediatr

Clin North Am 39(4):821–857, 1992. **Information on basic anatomy and physiology of skeletal muscle and discussion of several metabolic myopathies.**

4. Cheney P: Early management and physiologic changes in crush syndrome. Crit Care Nurs Q 17(2):62–73, 1994. **Discussion of pathophysiologic changes that occur with crush syndrome on a cellular and systemic level.**

5. Craig S: Rhabdomyolysis. Available online at http://www.emedicine.com/emerg/topic508.htm (retrieved July 2004). **Review of causes, clinical presentation, workup, and treatment of rhabdomyolysis.**

6. De Meijer AR, Fikkers BG, de Keijzer MH, et al: Serum creatine kinase as predictor of clinical course in rhabdomyolysis: A 5-year intensive care survey. Intensive Care Med 29(7):1121–1125, 2003. **Study showing that serum CK levels can predict the development of acute renal failure.**

7. Holt SG, Moore KP: Pathogenesis and treatment of renal dysfunction in rhabdomyolysis. intensive Care Med 27(5):803–811, 2001. **Review of pathogenesis and treatment of renal failure because of rhabdomyolysis.**

8. Malinoski DJ, Slater MS, Mullins RJ: Crush injury and rhabdomyolysis. Crit Care Clin 20(1):171–192, 2004. **Pathophysiology and treatment of myoglobinuric renal failure caused by traumatic rhabdomyolysis and crush injuries.**

9. Oda J, Tanaka H, Yoshioka T, et al: Analysis of 372 patients with crush syndrome caused by the Hanshin-Awaji earthquake. J Trauma 42:470–476, 1997. **A retrospective study showing that peak CK levels and the number of injured extremities estimate the severity of crush syndrome.**

10. Sauret JM, Marinides G, Wang GK: Rhabdomyolysis. Am Fam Physician 65:907–912, 2002. **Review of causes, clinical features, and treatment of rhabdomyolysis.**

Epistaxis and Nasal Trauma

Jane M. Lavelle

EPISTAXIS

KEY CONCEPTS

- In most cases, epistaxis is a benign, self-limited condition.
- In the majority of cases, bleeding comes from the anterior septum.
- Conservative therapy with direct pressure followed by application of antibiotic ointment at the site of bleeding treats the majority of patients successfully.
- Patients with a posterior bleeding site may require nasal packing; referral to an otolaryngologist is indicated.
- Patients with severe or recurrent episodes should be evaluated for a coagulation and nasoseptal abnormality.

Epistaxis is a very common, most often self-limited ailment of childhood. It occurs rarely in the first 2 years of life. Approximately 30% of all children 0 to 5 years of age, 56% of those 6 to 10 years of age, and 64% of those 11 to 15 years of age have at least one episode of epistaxis during their lifetime. The richly vascular structure of the nose and nasal septum, in conjunction with the normal frequent occurrence of upper respiratory tract infections, allergy, desiccation, and minor trauma, predispose toddlers and children to epistaxis. In most cases,

---

BOX 1 Causes of Epistaxis
Common
Local inflammation caused by viral/bacterial infection
Allergic rhinitis
Minor trauma
Foreign body
Uncommon
Coagulopathy
Nasal polyps
Juvenile angiofibroma
Telangiectasia
Drugs
Tumors

bleeding results from a normal vessel without any obvious abnormality and is thus called idiopathic epistaxis. Box 1 provides a list of common and uncommon causes of epistaxis. Epistaxis rarely occurs as a manifestation of systemic disease. Severe and/or recurrent epistaxis in children can be associated with coagulopathies, other hematologic disease, nasal septum abnormalities, and tumors. Unlike in adults, hypertension rarely causes epistaxis in children.

Sandoval and colleagues reviewed 178 children who were referred for hematologic evaluation following recurrent epistaxis. One third of this referred population was found to have a coagulopathy; all of them had prolonged partial thromboplastin times (PTTs). Many had a family history of bleeding. The most common disorders included von Willebrand disease (33 of 59) and platelet aggregation disorders (10 of 59). Other studies suggest that 5% to 10% of children with recurrent epistaxis have undiagnosed von Willebrand disease.

The vast majority of children present with bleeding that originates from the Little area located in the anterior septum where a number of arteries anastomose to form the Kiesselbach plexus under the thin mucosa. It is not uncommon to have several episodes over a few days as the mucosa heals. Physical examination reveals unilateral excoriation or scabbing on the medial surface of the anterior septum. Posterior bleeding should be suspected if an anterior site is not identified, if bleeding is poorly controlled by adequate external pressure, or if there is blood in the oropharynx or in both nares. Occasionally, patients may also present with a complaint of hematemesis or melena secondary to swallowed blood.

Evaluation includes a thorough history and physical examination. The vital signs should be reviewed and the site of the bleeding located. If epistaxis is associated with trauma, careful evaluation for nasal fracture and septal hematoma is required. Lack of systemic symptoms, petechiae, abnormal bruising, adenopathy, or hepatosplenomegaly aid in excluding hematologic, oncologic, and infectious etiologies. Children with recurrent and/or severe epistaxis should be evaluated with a complete blood count (CBC), prothrombin time (PT), PTT, and ristocetin cofactor. Referral to a pediatric hematologist and or an otolaryngologist may be indicated for further evaluation.

Expert Opinion on Management Issues

There is no consensus on effectiveness of interventions for epistaxis other than direct pressure. Other available therapies include silver nitrate cautery, application of antibiotic cream, petroleum jelly, nasal saline spray, oxymetazoline, desmopressin, or ε-aminocaproic acid.

ACCEPTED INTERVENTIONS/URGENT INTERVENTIONS

Direct pressure over the nasal alae for 5 to 10 minutes is the mainstay of therapy. In addition, a rolled gauze pad can be placed under the upper lip to compress the labial artery. Topical vasoconstrictors, such as phenylephrine or oxymetazoline, are rarely needed. Silver nitrate sticks can be used to cauterize exposed vessels in the anterior septum if bleeding persists. However, this requires that the bleeding site be visible, easily accessible, and not bleeding briskly. Cautery is painful and causes vessel sclerosis and mucosal thickening, resulting in crusting, which can induce nose picking. It has a high failure rate and can cause atrophy of the nasal septum. A recent prospective study comparing the use of silver nitrate cautery to application of a topical antibiotic ointment demonstrates that cautery does not reduce rebleeding in children with recurrent idiopathic epistaxis.

Parents can use petroleum jelly or topical antibiotic ointment at the site of the septal scab in an attempt to provide lubrication and reduce itching and discomfort, which results in continued trauma. Antibiotic ointment may help reduce any local low-grade mucosal infection and promote healing. A recent prospective study comparing use of an antibiotic ointment to no treatment in children with recurrent idiopathic epistaxis revealed no differences in the rate of repeat episodes of bleeding. Another study comparing application of petroleum jelly to the septum and no treatment showed no impact on the rate of rebleeding in a similar population.

Nasal packing with absorbable oxycellulose material or petroleum jelly gauze is required if bleeding continues or if the site of bleeding cannot be located (posterior bleeding). Oral antibiotics should be administered while the packing is in place to reduce the risk of sinusitis and toxic shock syndrome.

Patients with known intranasal lesions or hematologic disorders benefit from otolaryngology and/or hematology consultation. Cautery should be avoided. Juvenile angiofibroma is a benign angiomatous tumor seen in adolescent boys presenting with nasal obstruction and epistaxis. Hereditary hemorrhagic telangiectasia is an autosomal disorder characterized by abnormal capillaries, which cause recurrent epistaxis.

Children with recurrent epistaxis may require referral to an otolaryngologist for electric cautery of the vessels of the anterior septum under general anesthesia. In refractory cases, a limited septoplasty may be necessary. Children in whom vascular abnormalities or tumor is suspected require MRI/MRA (magnetic resonance imaging/magnetic resonance angiography) to delineate the etiology as well as vascular supply. Therapies include embolization and/or surgical excision.

Common Pitfalls

- Failure to identify the source of bleeding, as well as other unusual causes.
- Failure to perform a careful history and physical exam to exclude systemic causes of coagulopathy.
- Failure to consider the possibility of nasal fracture and septal hematoma in children with trauma-associated epistaxis.
- Routine evaluation of hemoglobin, platelets, and clotting times is not indicated in the vast majority of patients.

Communication and Counseling

Parents and patients should be reassured that epistaxis is a benign, self-limited condition in the vast majority of cases. It is not unusual for children to have another nosebleed as the mucosa heals. If the child experiences recurrent or severe episodes, an evaluation by a pediatric hematologist and/or otolaryngologist may be indicated.

NASAL TRAUMA

KEY CONCEPTS

- Nasal contusions are common in children; nasal fracture/dislocation are rare.
- During the acute evaluation, septal hematomas must be identified and treated.
- Patients with marked deformity, nasal obstruction, uncontrolled epistaxis, and/or cerebrospinal fluid (CSF) rhinorrhea require immediate otolaryngology consultation.
- An otolaryngologist should evaluate patients with significant nasal swelling, periorbital ecchymosis, and/or nasal mucosal laceration 72 hours after injury.
- Optimal timing for surgical reduction is 5 to 7 days following the injury.
- Closed reduction under general anesthesia is the method most commonly used.
- Future surgical nasal reconstruction may be required to correct deformity.

Because of its central, protuberant position, nasal trauma in children occurs very frequently. Falls, play, sports, and occasionally fights account for nasal injury. Abuse should always be considered in the differential diagnosis. Although nasal trauma most often results from lower-energy mechanisms, it is important to focus on assessment and maintenance of the vital life functions in children with more forceful mechanism of injury and in those with multiple injuries.

The nasal cartilages are supported by nasal processes of the frontal bone superiorly and the maxilla inferiorly. Overlying the nasal cartilages is a thin layer of soft tissue, muscle, and mucous glands. In children, the nose is mostly cartilaginous, and thus fractures of the nasal bones rarely occur. As the child grows, nasal bone fractures are more common.

Expert Opinion on Management Issues

ACCEPTED/URGENT INTERVENTIONS

A careful account of the mechanism and timing of injury is important. Serious injuries should be evaluated and treated first. The cervical spine, the orbits, facial bones, maxilla, mandible, and teeth should be examined for injury in children with nasal trauma. In patients with periorbital ecchymosis and intercanthal distance greater than the length of the palpebral fissure, a nasoethmoidal fracture should be suspected. The nose should be palpated for deviation, step-off, tenderness over the proximal nasal skeleton, crepitus, depression, shortening, and subcutaneous emphysema. In the initial evaluation, it may be very difficult to appreciate deviation of the nasal bones/septum following the injury because of the presence of overlying soft tissue swelling. However, deformity and/or significant swelling are usually present with nasal fracture/dislocation. Periorbital ecchymosis, nasal obstruction, mucosal laceration, and epistaxis are highly suggestive of nasal fracture. Internal examination at the time of the injury may be challenging. A nasal speculum, suction, good light source, and use of topical vasoconstrictors, such as oxymetazoline, and anesthetics, such as Xylocaine, are needed. The otolaryngologist may use a rigid nasal endoscope or fiberoptic scope to fully evaluate the nasal septum. The nasal septum should be evaluated for the presence of deviation and/or septal hematoma. A septal hematoma appears as a purplish grape-like swelling on the medial surface of the anterior nasal septum. CSF rhinorrhea is rarely associated with nasal fracture.

The presence of a septal hematoma is an emergency for the otolaryngologist. The collection of blood between the septal mucosa and the cartilaginous septum must be drained to avoid necrosis and/or abscess formation, which results in permanent septal damage and the saddle nose deformity. The hematoma is treated with incision and drainage, followed by careful packing with antibiotic gauze. Systemic antibiotic coverage is also recommended.

Because the nose is mostly cartilage in young children, nasal radiographs are unreliable and can be misleading; thus they are not recommended routinely. If there is associated orbital abnormality, CSF rhinorrhea, malocclusion, or extensive facial swelling, CT scan imaging is indicated to delineate the associated fractures.

Open wounds over the cartilage surface should be gently debrided and carefully repaired to provide complete coverage. An otolaryngologist or a plastic surgeon should evaluate cartilage laceration. The child's tetanus status should be reviewed. The decision to treat with oral antibiotics is individualized.

Because children heal more quickly than adults, therapy should not be delayed. Patients with significant edema can be discharged with scheduled follow-up in 72 hours with an otolaryngologist. Conservative therapy, with head elevation, ice, and analgesia, is recommended. Patients with marked deformity, nasal obstruction, septal hematoma, and/or uncontrolled epistaxis may benefit from immediate evaluation by an otolaryngologist and precise reduction. Fracture reduction is generally done under general anesthesia and includes meticulous septal examination followed by closed reduction. In children, a more conservative surgical approach is taken because of the presence of cartilaginous growth centers. Future nasal reconstruction may be necessary after the skeleton matures. In adolescents, septorhinoplasty may be indicated. Postsurgical treatment includes extranasal and intranasal splints, antibiotics, steroids, and follow-up.

CONTROVERSIAL INTERVENTIONS

The current management strategies for acute nasal fractures result in a high incidence of post-traumatic nasal deformities in published series of adult patients. Differentiating between new and old nasal injury/deformity can be challenging, so photographs are useful. Definitive treatment of nasal fractures should be done within 5 to 7 days following the injury. There is controversy in adult literature regarding closed reduction versus performing septorhinoplasty in achieving the best aesthetic and functional results. In children and adolescents, however, closed reduction under general anesthesia remains the treatment of choice.

Common Pitfalls

- Missing associated injuries by failing to complete a thorough physical examination of the head and neck
- Failure to identify a septal hematoma
- Failure to ensure follow-up with a pediatric otolaryngologist within 72 hours for patients with suspected nasal fracture.

Communication and Counseling

Conservative therapy with head elevation, ice application, and acetaminophen analgesia is the mainstay of therapy. Children with suspected nasal fracture should be evaluated by an otolaryngologist 72 hours after injury. All patients should be counseled regarding the need for further nasal procedures.

SUGGESTED READINGS

1. Burton MJ, Doree CJ: Interventions for recurrent idiopathic epistaxis (nosebleeds) in children. Cochrane Database Syst Rev 1: CD004461. **Reviews and compares the efficacy of application of Vaseline, antiseptic cream, nasal cautery, and no treatment in children with recurrent epistaxis.**
2. Fernandes SV: Nasal fractures: The taming of the shrewd. Laryngoscope 114:587–592, 2004. **Reviews the controversy regarding nasal fracture management with closed reduction versus staged septorhinoplasty in providing optimal outcome in adult patients.**
3. Katsanis E, Lee KH, Hsu E, et al: Prevalence and significance of mild bleeding disorders in children with recurrent epistaxis.

J Pediatr 113:73–76, 1988. **Reviews the types of coagulopathies identified in children referred to a pediatric hematologist for evaluation of recurrent epistaxis.**

4. Kubba H, MacAndie C, Botma M, et al: A prospective, single-blinded, randomized controlled trial of antiseptic cream for recurrent epistaxis in children. Clin Otolaryngol 26:465–468, 2001. **Compares the efficacy of application of antiseptic cream and no treatment in children with recurrent epistaxis.**

5. Loughran S, Spinou E, Clements WA, et al: A prospective, single-blind, randomized controlled trial of petrolatum jelly/Vaseline for recurrent pediatric epistaxis. Clin Otolaryngol 29:266–269, 2004. **Compares the efficacy of application of petroleum jelly and no treatment in children with recurrent epistaxis.**

6. Lusk RP, Muntz HR: Introduction to pediatric rhinology. In Wetmore RF, Muntz HR, McGill TJ, et al (eds): Pediatric Otolaryngology: Principles Practice Pathways. New York: Thieme, 2000, pp 439–452. **Review written by a pediatric otolaryngologist covering nasal anatomy and the etiologies and recommended treatment of children with epistaxis.**

7. Rohrich RJ, Adams WP: Nasal fracture management: Minimizing secondary nasal deformities. Plast Reconstr Surg 106:266–273, 2000. **Reviews the controversy regarding nasal fracture management with closed reduction versus staged septorhinoplasty in providing optimal outcome in adult patients.**

8. Ruddy J, Proops DW, Pearman K, Ruddy H: Interventions for recurrent idiopathic epistaxis in children. Int J Pediatr Otolaryngol 21:139–142, 1991. **Compares the efficacy of application of antiseptic cream and silver nitrate cautery in children with recurrent epistaxis.**

9. Sandoval C, Dong S, Vistainer P, et al: Clinical and laboratory features of 178 children with recurrent epistaxis. Pediatr Hematol Oncol 24:47–49, 2002. **Reviews the types of coagulopathies identified in children referred to a pediatric hematologist for evaluation of recurrent epistaxis.**

10. Senders CR: Pediatric facial trauma. In Wetmore RF, Muntz HR, McGill TJ, et al (eds): Pediatric Otolaryngology: Principles Practice Pathways. New York: Thieme, 2000, pp 497–512. **Chapter written by a pediatric otolaryngologist that reviews presentation of nasal fractures in children and makes recommendations regarding optimal treatment.**

11. Toback S: Nasal septal hematoma in an 11-month-old infant: A case report and review of the literature. Pediatr Emerg Care 19:265–267, 2003. **Discusses epidemiology, presentation, and treatment for children with septal hematoma.**

Acute Poisoning

Diane P. Calello

KEY CONCEPTS

- The pediatrician should be familiar with the drugs for which even one pill can be toxic to a young child.
- Supportive care is the cornerstone of management of all poisoned patients.
- Activated charcoal is the method of choice for initial gastrointestinal (GI) decontamination.
- Further methods to enhance elimination include whole bowel irrigation, multiple-dose charcoal, alkalinization, and extracorporeal removal.
- Antidotes are available for some poisons and should be used in conjunction with supportive care and consultation with the Poison Control Center.
- There is no substitute for prevention.

Poisoning exposures in children younger than 6 years of age represent more than 50% of cases reported to poison

TABLE 1 Drugs Toxic in Small Doses

Agent	Toxicity
Calcium channel antagonists	Hypotension, bradycardia, cardiac arrest
β-receptor antagonists	Hypoglycemia, hypotension, bradycardia
Local anesthetics: benzocaine, dibucaine	Methemoglobinemia, dysrhythmias
Oral hypoglycemics	Hypoglycemia
Diphenoxylate (Lomotil)	CNS and respiratory depression
Camphor	CNS depression, seizures
Cyclic antidepressants	Dysrhythmias, seizures
Methyl salicylate (oil of wintergreen, found in topical preparations)	Salicylate toxicity: acidosis, seizures
Lindane	Seizures

CNS, central nervous system.

control centers each year. Pediatric poisonings follow a bimodal age distribution; toddlers frequently ingest substances in an exploratory fashion, and adolescents are poisoned under conditions of self-harm or intentional abuse. Young children who ingest toxic substances usually fare well, with few fatalities each year because of the small volumes ingested. Adolescents, however, are much more likely to have serious manifestations of poisoning.

The most common poison exposures each year involve analgesics, household cleaning products, cosmetics, sedatives, topical medications, cough and cold preparations, antipsychotics, and antidepressants. Acetaminophen toxicity is the most common, with the potential for fulminant hepatic failure if untreated. Household cleaners may be caustic, leading to respiratory or gastrointestinal (GI) tract burns, or they may have a hydrocarbon base, the ingestion of which can cause pneumonitis.

Of particular note are the exposures that, in seemingly small amounts, can be lethal to a young child. An exploratory gulp in children is estimated at 5 mL, and less than 5 mL of a hydrocarbon or a caustic can have devastating results. One or two pills of either a calcium channel or β-receptor antagonist can cause bradycardia, hypotension, and cardiac arrest. One oral sulfonylurea pill (glipizide, glyburide) can cause refractory hypoglycemia for several days. Table 1 lists some potent poisons for toddlers.

The local poison control center should be contacted for all poisoning cases, which not only helps maintain the national database but also provides the physician with up-to-date information on management and the opportunity to discuss issues with an on-call toxicologist if needed. This is particularly helpful in the critically ill patient and the patient requiring antidotal therapy (see later).

Expert Opinion on Management Issues

GENERAL POISONING MANAGEMENT

As with any emergency department patient, poisoned patients first require basic resuscitation. The majority of poison exposures do not require specific antidotal therapy but need excellent supportive care. This begins with the ABCs (airway, breathing, circulation) and pediatric advanced life support (PALS) modalities but also includes fluid resuscitation, use of pressors, respiratory or ventilatory support, and close monitoring of hemodynamic and metabolic parameters, such as blood glucose.

DECONTAMINATION

Once resuscitation is under way, decontamination, the process by which any retrievable poison is removed from the patient, should be carried out if possible. For patients with ocular or dermal exposure, this involves irrigation and removal from the source (if indicated) with careful attention to prevent exposure of health care providers caring for the patient.

Because ingestion is by far the most common route of poisoning, GI decontamination is often the most important. However, performing GI decontamination in obtunded or vomiting patients is not without risk. Gastric emptying methods such as gastric lavage through a large-bore orogastric tube and induction of emesis have little, if any, benefit when performed beyond 30 minutes after ingestion. Furthermore, because of problems associated with inappropriate use and lack of convincing evidence, syrup of ipecac is no longer recommended for initial decontamination in the home by the American Academy of Pediatrics (AAP) and is only rarely, if ever, used in the hospital setting.

Activated charcoal has emerged as the decontamination method of choice; 1 g/kg of oral or nasogastric activated charcoal, up to 100 g, binds most poisonous compounds. Exceptions include metals (lead, lithium, iron), ethanol, caustics, and many hydrocarbons. Activated charcoal should be given carefully in the case of obtunded or vomiting patients because it is emetogenic and increases the risk of charcoal aspiration pneumonitis. To that end, some patients may require esophageal intubation for airway protection during charcoal administration. Contraindications to charcoal include caustic ingestions because it may worsen esophageal damage without benefit, and hydrocarbon exposures, in which emesis greatly increases the risk of hydrocarbon pneumonitis.

ENHANCED ELIMINATION

Whole bowel irrigation with a polyethylene glycol solution through a naso- or orogastric tube at 500 to 2000 mL per hour can flush additional pills or other substances through the GI tract, inhibiting further absorption and hastening elimination. This procedure is not necessary in all cases but should be considered for ingestions of sustained-release preparations, drug-smuggling packets, potentially lethal substances (calcium channel antagonists, β-receptor antagonists, tricyclic antidepressants, colchicine), drugs expected to form gastric pill bezoars (carbamazepine, enteric-coated aspirin), and those not absorbed by charcoal. Similarly, multiple doses of activated charcoal (MDAC), given 2 hours apart, act in the

GI tract as an absorption column, drawing toxin out of the circulation into the gut for fecal elimination. This may have some benefit in serious ingestions as well but is often complicated by severe constipation. However, due to the potential for electrolyte disturbance, charcoal should be used without sorbitol for repeat doses.

Alkalinization of the serum is employed for substances whose acid–base characteristics require an alkaline milieu to prevent further tissue distribution, and it is used to ameliorate drug-induced cardiac sodium channel blockade. It is therefore useful in poisoning by salicylates, tricyclic antidepressants, type Ia and Ic antidysrhythmics, and a number of other substances. Urinary alkalinization enhances elimination of various compounds, including salicylates, phenobarbital, and methotrexate. The addition of three ampoules of sodium bicarbonate to 1 liter of a 5% dextrose solution, infused at 1.5 times the patient's maintenance fluid requirements, is a good starting point. The desired serum pH is above 7.4; the urine pH should be maintained above 7. Failure to maintain serum potassium at greater than 4 mmol/L may lead to inadequate urinary alkalinization.

Lastly, hemodialysis (circulation of blood volume and removal of a substance over 4 to 8 hours through a semipermeable membrane), hemoperfusion (circulation of blood volume through a charcoal column to absorb toxin), and hemofiltration (continuous slow-rate circulation and removal through a membrane or dialysis circuit) have a definite role in certain poisonings and may be beneficial in others. To be amenable to hemodialysis, a substance must have a low molecular weight, have a low affinity for protein binding, be water soluble, and have a small volume of distribution (reflecting its tendency to stay in the blood rather than distribute to the tissues). Table 2 lists the indications for hemodialysis. Charcoal hemoperfusion is not limited by protein binding and so is useful with severe poisoning from phenobarbital, carbamazepine, and others. Hemofiltration may be of use for larger molecular weight compounds; however, the slow rate of removal is suboptimal in massive acute overdoses.

TABLE 2   Indications for Dialysis*

Definite

- Lithium
- Ethylene glycol
- Methanol
- Salicylates
- Theophylline
- Bromides

Possible

- Ethanol
- Valproic acid
- Refractory metabolic acidosis

---

*The exact serum level at which each toxin should be dialyzed depends on a number of factors, and the decision should be made in conjunction with a nephrologist and the local Poison Center.

TABLE 3 Common Antidotal Therapies

Antidote	Indication	Dosage	Comments
N-Acetylcysteine PO	Acetaminophen	140 mg/kg loading; then 70 mg/kg q4h for 17 doses	Foul smelling; may induce emesis.
N-Acetylcysteine IV	Acetaminophen	150 mg/kg load over 1 h; then 150 mg/kg over 20 h	Rate-related anaphylactoid reactions.
Physostigmine	Anticholinergic delirium	0.02 mg/kg IV over 5 min	Lowers seizure threshold.
Octreotide	Sulfonylureas	1 µg/kg SC q6h	
Digoxin-specific antibody fragments	Digoxin	(Level)(Weight in kg)/100	Use care in patients requiring therapeutic digoxin levels.
Naloxone	Opioids	0.1 mg/kg up to 2 mg	Short (30–60 min) duration of effect.
Fomepizole	Toxic alcohols	15 mg/kg load, then 10 mg/kg q12h (change dose for patients on dialysis)	Safer, easier than ethanol infusion.

IV, intravenous; PO, by mouth; qxh, every x hours; SC, subcutaneous.

ANTIDOTAL TREATMENTS

There are a number of poisoning exposures for which specific antidotal therapy is indicated and supported by recent evidence. In severe anticholinergic delirium, physostigmine may reverse delirium where high doses of benzodiazepines fail. The most significant side effect of physostigmine is lowered seizure threshold, so patients with a seizure predisposition either by medical history or circumstances of ingestion should not receive this therapy. Octreotide reverses hypoglycemia associated with sulfonylurea poisoning. Fomepizole, an alcohol dehydrogenase inhibitor, is safe and effective for patients with ethylene glycol and methanol poisoning, in conjunction with dialysis. Carnitine corrects valproate-induced hyperammonemia and may have a role in encephalopathy after valproic acid overdose. Digoxin-specific antibody fragments can prevent ventricular dysrhythmias in digoxin and plant-derived glycoside (oleander, foxglove) toxicity.

Acetaminophen-induced hepatotoxicity is completely prevented with timely (within 8 hours) administration of N-acetylcysteine. Recent studies find both the intravenous (IV) and oral (PO) preparations effective. IV N-acetylcysteine therapy, however, has a higher incidence of rate-related anaphylactoid reactions, so caution should be used in patients with a strong tendency for bronchospasm. The IV preparation is given over 24 hours, and the PO preparation over 72 hours; however, neither should be discontinued until hepatic transaminitis is resolving and the acetaminophen concentration is below detectable levels.

Table 3 describes some commonly used antidotal therapies with dosage and administration guidelines. Consultation with a local poison control center is strongly encouraged when employing these treatments.

Common Pitfalls

- Failure to recognize that certain drugs ingested in small doses can be highly toxic to a toddler.
- Performing GI decontamination without adequate airway protection.
- Allowing a patient to drink polyethylene glycol for whole bowel irrigation. The rates required to achieve clear rectal effluent in the desired time (4 hours) are nearly impossible to achieve in all but the most determined patients (500 mL/hour for toddlers; 2 L/hour in adults).
- Allowing an agitated patient to thrash in restraints for the purposes of maintaining a physical exam; patients can easily become hyperthermic and unstable, especially if the specific poisoning causes thermodysregulation (e.g., anticholinergics, phenothiazines, serotonin syndrome).
- Failure to maintain serum potassium (>4 mmol/L) when attempting urinary alkalinization.

Preventive Measures

No discussion of pediatric poisonings is complete without emphasis on prevention. Preventive legislation in the United States, such as the Poisoning Prevention Act of 1970, drastically decreased the incidence of and morbidity from poisoning in young children. Still, these exposures continue to occur and are largely preventable. Anticipatory guidance from the pediatrician should include the following:

- All prescription medications should be kept in childproof containers and not transferred to pillboxes or other more accessible vessels.
- Household chemicals should under no circumstances be transferred to containers originally intended for consumption, such as coffee cups or soda cans.
- All hazardous substances should be kept out of reach of children.
- Household visitors introduce additional risk because suitcases and other luggage may contain pills that are easily accessible.
- The Poison Control Center hotline number (1–800–222–1222) should be kept near all phones, should an exposure occur.

3

SUGGESTED READINGS

1. American Academy of Clinical Toxicology, European Association of Poison Centres and Clinical Toxicologists: Position statement: Single-dose activated charcoal. J Toxicol Clin Toxicol 35:721–741, 1997. **Guidelines for the use of charcoal for GI decontamination.**

2. American Academy of Pediatrics: Committee on Injury, Violence, and Poison Prevention. Poison treatment in the home. Pediatrics 112:1182–1185, 2003. **AAP statement recommending the discontinuation of syrup of ipecac use.**

3. McLaughlin SA, Crandall CS, McKinney PE: Octreotide: An antidote for sulfonylurea-induced hypoglycemia. Ann Emerg Med 36:133–138, 2000. **Study demonstrating safety and efficacy of octreotide in sulfonylurea overdoses.**

4. Osterhoudt KC: The toxic toddler: Drugs that can kill in small doses. Contemp Pediatr 3:73, 2000. **List of exposures that in small amounts can cause serious toxicity in young children.**

5. Perry HE, Shannon MW: Efficacy of oral versus intravenous *N*-acetylcysteine in acetaminophen overdose: Results of an open-label clinical trial. J Pediatr 132:149–152, 1998. **Study in pediatrics demonstrating safety and efficacy of IV *N*-acetylcysteine.**

6. Milstein MJ, Bronstein AC, Linden C, et al: Acetaminophen overdose: A 48-hour intravenous *N*-acetylcysteine treatment protocol. Ann Emerg Med 20:1058–1063, 1991. **Study demonstrating efficacy of intravenous *N*-acetylcysteine comparable to oral *N*-acetylcysteine.**

7. Watson WA, Litovitz TL, Klein-Schwartz W, et al: 2003 Annual Report of the American Association of Poison Control Centers Toxic Exposure Surveillance System. Am J Emerg Med 22:335–404, 2004. **Yearly report of national database with poisoning epidemiology and outcomes in the United States.**

Mammalian Bites and Bite-Related Infections

F. Meridith Sonnett, Robert A. Green, and Peter S. Dayan

KEY CONCEPTS

- The largest proportion of mammalian bites are caused by dogs.
- The majority of dog bite fatalities occur in children younger than 10 years.
- The most common cause of morbidity from bites is wound infection.
- Human bites, cat bites, and bites to the hand are at greatest risk for infection.
- Meticulous wound cleansing is essential to potentially prevent wound infection.
- Primary closure of bite wounds is controversial, although potentially disfiguring wounds, such as those that involve the face, can often be sutured.
- Prophylactic antibiotics, targeted toward the most likely pathogens causing infection, should be seriously considered for bites to the hand and bites caused by humans and cats.
- Amoxicillin-clavulanic acid or ampicillin-sulbactam provides excellent single-agent coverage for the most commonly identified pathogens in bite wounds.
- Infected bite wounds generally require inpatient intravenous therapy.
- The need for tetanus, rabies, human immunodeficiency virus (HIV), and hepatitis prophylaxis must be comprehensively reviewed for all bite victims.

An estimated 5 million or more mammalian bites are reported annually in the United States, with nearly half of these occurring in children. This figure undoubtedly underestimates the true incidence because a proportion of victims do not seek medical attention. Approximately 80%, 10%, and 3% of reported mammalian bites are caused by dogs, cats, and humans, respectively. Mammalian bites account for up to 1% of all annual visits to pediatric emergency departments in the United States.

Dog bites are most often caused by a pet belonging to family or friends, whereas cat bites are frequently caused by strays. Although mortality is uncommon, dog attacks result in 15 to 20 deaths annually in the United States, the majority of which occur in children younger than 10 years. As compared to adults, who most often sustain bites to the hands and arms, young children are at increased risk of bites to the head, neck, and face because of their smaller height. Upward of 70% of bites involve the head or neck in young children.

The most common cause of morbidity of mammalian bites is wound infection. In general, bites to the hand and cat and human bites are at a significantly increased risk for infection. Although dog bites account for the majority of bite-related infections, cat and human bites more frequently result in infection. Of patients presenting to medical attention, the literature suggests a 5% to 16% infection risk for dog bites, 50% for cat bites, and 25% to 50% following human bites. The greater relative risk of infection from cat bites is thought to result from the puncture nature of the bite, with deposition of cat oral flora deep into the patient's tissues.

Expert Opinion on Management Issues

Clinicians are generally presented with three main categories of acute issues:

1. Management of a bite wound prior to infection
2. Management of infected wounds
3. Tetanus, rabies, hepatitis, and human immunodeficiency virus (HIV) prophylaxis.

The discussion here is restricted to mammalian bite-wound management resulting from dog, cat, or human bites.

MANAGEMENT OF A BITE WOUND PRIOR TO INFECTION

General Wound Management

Clinicians must perform a complete history for all patients presenting with animal or human bite wounds. The history must include how and when the bite was obtained (provoked or unprovoked attack); the type of offending animal; the immunization status of the animal (rabies vaccination record); and the patient's pertinent medical history, including vaccination and immune status. Bites from stray animals heighten the concern for potential rabies infection because most strays are not immunized.

The most serious of human bites, so-called clenched-fist bites, occur when a closed fist hits the teeth of another person, resulting in a laceration over the metacarpal head (usually the third and/or fourth metacarpals). The majority of these result from an altercation. Patients, unaware these types of injuries are at extremely high risk for infection and consequent compromise in joint function, may fail to disclose how the injury was obtained. Clinicians should have a heightened suspicion for seemingly innocuous disruptions of the skin over the metacarpal bones.

A bite wound must be thoroughly and meticulously examined. Sufficient pain control will be required in young children to perform the examination and to thoroughly cleanse and debride the wound. With bite injuries to a limb, the clinician must perform and document a thorough motor and sensory exam and assess tendon and ligament integrity. Deep facial injuries may involve the facial nerve. After thorough examination of the wound, plain radiographs should be considered if bony fracture, joint penetration, or foreign body is suspected. Surgical consultation may be required if there is tendon, ligament, or nerve injury or if a joint space was violated.

Pain management should include topical analgesia, such as a gel containing lidocaine, epinephrine, and tetracaine (LET gel). Topical anesthetics provide particularly effective analgesia for face and scalp wounds, often negating the need for subcutaneous lidocaine infiltration. Topical anesthesia may also lessen the pain associated with lidocaine infiltration, if needed. Although no perfect oral sedative exists, midazolam provides fairly effective anxiolysis in 60% to 80% of children. Interventions by a child-life specialist may also reduce patient anxiety. Children with extensive bite wounds should not be allowed oral intake in anticipation of requiring parenteral (moderate) sedation and analgesia for examination and repair of wounds. Only credentialed clinicians should administer parenteral sedation.

Thorough wound cleansing is an important measure to prevent bite-related infections. Standard cleansing techniques allow for removal of contaminating bacteria, dried blood, and other debris. Wounds that are superficial and do not extend through the epidermis should be cleansed with standard agents such as normal saline.

For wounds that penetrate through the epidermis, irrigation under pressure is the preferred cleansing technique. The optimal amount of pressure needed to cleanse the wound mechanically is controversial, but it should be enough to clean out debris yet not so forceful as to cause tissue damage. Although fully equipped commercial kits are available, irrigation can be readily accomplished by attaching a 16- to 18-gauge angiocatheter to a 20- to 30-mL syringe filled with normal saline and applying pressurized flow directly into the wound. Clinicians should use a splashguard to protect themselves from contaminated irrigation fluid. Most wounds, unless very extensive and heavily contaminated, are adequately cleansed with 300 to 500 mL of normal saline. For wounds inflicted by animals that potentially harbor rabies, some clinicians recommend cleansing with soap and water after initial irrigation.

Devitalized tissue is generally caused by occlusional bites that crush tissue. Clinicians should debride the minimum amount of tissue to obtain vascularized refined wound edges. Debridement of devitalized tissue is recommended to reduce the risk of infection and promote adequate wound healing.

Much controversy surrounds whether an open bite wound should be sutured. The overriding concern is that suturing bite wounds might increase the risk of infection by creating a closed space in which bacteria can proliferate. Although no randomized clinical trials are available, the following recommendations can be made:

- Consensus suggests that bite wounds to the hand and foot should not be sutured. These should be allowed to drain and subsequently heal by secondary intention if small (<1.5 cm) or by delayed primary closure if larger.
- For sites other than the hand and foot, the literature suggests that primary closure for dog bites does not increase the risk of infection and is therefore a reasonable strategy. However, suturing is not recommended for wounds greater than 8 to 12 hours old, with the exception of facial wounds.
- Although scant supportive literature exists, the authors recommend refraining from suturing cat and human bites unless they are potentially disfiguring.
- Bite wounds to the face can be quite disfiguring and should be sutured by an experienced practitioner. Facial wounds have a lesser tendency to become infected because of the plentiful vascular supply to the face and therefore can be sutured even if the wound is greater than 12 but less then 24 hours old.
- For those wounds selected for closure, clinicians should use a single layer of nonabsorbable sutures. Multiple layer closures should be avoided.

Antibiotic Prophylaxis

Wounds caused by mammalian bites are prone to infection because of the inoculation of the wound with microbiologic flora from the mouth of the offending animal. Although not much literature exists specifically targeting bite wounds, data concerning wounds in general suggest a potential small reduction in infection risk with application of topical antibiotics.

The use of systemic prophylactic antibiotics for the prevention of infection from mammalian bites is controversial, stemming from the relative paucity of randomized clinical trials performed in this area. A Cochrane Collaboration meta-analysis of existing randomized, controlled trials provides the data on which to make recommendations regarding prophylaxis for preventing infections. Recommendations are based on categorizing bites by type of animal and nature of host, type of wound, and site of wound and structures involved (Box 1).

Type of Animal

There are suggestive but very limited data to recommend antibiotic prophylaxis for cat and human bites. The data do not, however, suggest antibiotic efficacy for dog bites as a whole. In six trials included in the Cochrane meta-analysis, there was no significant difference in infection rates between those who did and did not receive antibiotics for dog bites (odds ratio [OR] 0.74, 95% confidence interval [CI] 0.30, 1.85, in the direction favoring prophylaxis).

Type of Wound

Limited data from two randomized clinical trials are suggestive but not do conclusively demonstrate the efficacy of antibiotic prophylaxis for puncture wounds (OR 0.22, 95% CI 0.01, 8.37, in the direction favoring prophylaxis). Data do not support the use of prophylactic antibiotics for lacerations and avulsions as the sole criterion for therapy. Two randomized trials of lacerations caused by mammalian bites showed no statistical difference in infection risk in 129 patients (OR 0.80, 95% CI 0.05, 13.67). Two clinical trials of patients with avulsions noted no difference in the risk of infection with and without antibiotics (OR 1.07, 95% CI 0.11, 10.63).

Site of Wound

Hand wounds are the only site for which prophylactic antibiotics have efficacy in preventing infection. In the Cochrane systematic review, the odds of infection were substantially decreased in patients who received prophylactic antibiotics (OR 0.10, 95% CI 0.01, 0.86).

Box 2 lists the recommended prophylactic antibiotics. Recommendations are based on the organisms likely to cause infection, as discussed later. Prophylactic antibiotics should be administered for 3 to 5 days.

MANAGEMENT OF INFECTED WOUNDS

Wounds should be considered infected if there is pain and swelling at the wound site and/or surrounding erythema, evidence of abscess, purulent drainage, or lymphangitis. Fever may or may not be present. Although some clinicians may use the peripheral white count as a marker for infection, the physical examination is sufficient to make the diagnosis in most cases.

Most dog, cat, and human bite infections are polymicrobial and include both aerobic and anaerobic gram-negative and gram-positive pathogens, with a mean of three to five organisms isolated. Those organisms most commonly causing infection include *Staphylococcus aureus, Pasteurella multocida, Streptococcus* species, *Eikenella corrodens,* and *Corynebacterium, Fusobacterium,* and *Bacteroides. E. corrodens* is most often associated with human bite wounds and rarely isolated from dog or cat oral flora. *P. multocida* is most often associated with cat bites; it is not found in human oral flora. Infection with *Capnocytophaga canimorsus,* found in dog oral flora, is associated with significant morbidity in both healthy and immunocompromised hosts.

Certain manifestations of infection appear associated with specific types of pathogens. Anaerobes are more likely to be recovered from bite-wound abscesses, whereas staphylococci and streptococci species are recovered more often from nonpurulent wounds. Infections from dog bites presenting in less than 24 hours from the time of the bite often involve *P. multocida,* whereas infections that develop more than 24 hours after the bite are frequently caused by staphylococcus and streptococcus species.

An established bite-wound infection requires prompt antibiotic therapy broad enough to cover the expected polymicrobial nature of the infection. Wound cultures should be obtained prior to antibiotic administration to identify the pathogens. Culture results allow for adjustment of therapy as necessary. Incision and drainage may be necessary if a fluctuant abscess is apparent. The clinician may want to consult with a surgeon if the abscess overlies a vital area of function or an area at high risk for significant scarring.

Box 2 and Box 3 detail recommended oral and intravenous antibiotics. Although supportive data are lacking, several authors recommend an initial intravenous dose of antibiotics even in those cases for which the patient will be subsequently discharged home on an oral agent.

BOX 3 Inpatient Intravenous Therapy Recommendations for Infected Canine, Feline, and Human Bite Wounds

First Choice

- Ampicillin/sulbactam (Unasyn): 100–200 mg/kg/day div q6h

Alternative/Penicillin Allergy*

- Trimethoprim (TMP)-sulfamethoxazole (SMX): 8–10 mg/kg/day of TMP div q12 h *plus* clindamycin: 25–40 mg/kg/day div tid or qid
- Cefoxitin[†] (Mefoxin): 80–100 mg/kg/day div q6–8h
- Cefuroxime[†] (Zinacef): 75–150 mg/kg/day div q8h (max 6 g/24 h)

*Other second- and third-generation cephalosporins with anaerobic activity can be used as well.

[†]Caution should be exercised in using cephalosporins in patients with *severe* penicillin allergy.

bid, twice daily; div, divided; q*x*hr, every *x* hours; qid, four times per day; tid, three times per day.

TABLE 1 Tetanus Prophylaxis Recommendations for Human, Dog, and Cat Bites

History of Adsorbed Tetanus Toxoid (Doses)	dT*	Tetanus Immune Globulin
<3 or unknown	Yes	Yes
≥3[†]	No[‡]	No

DTaP, diphtheria, tetanus toxoids, and acellular pertussis; dT, diphtheria-tetanus toxoid.

Adapted from Red Book: American Academy of Pediatrics, 26th ed. Elk Grove Village, Ill: American Academy of Pediatrics, 2003, p 614. Used with permission of the American Academy of Pediatrics.

*DTaP should be administered in children younger than 7 years. If pertussis is contraindicated, dT should be administered.

[†]If only three doses of toxoid have been administered, a fourth dose is recommended.

[‡]Yes, if more than 5 years since last dose.

An antibiotic that combines a penicillin and a β-lactamase inhibitor provides effective intravenous or oral therapy. Clindamycin, dicloxacillin, first-generation cephalosporins (e.g., cephalexin), and erythromycin are not recommended as single-agent antibiotics because *Pasteurella* and *Eikenella* species do not respond well to these organisms in vitro.

Inpatient or outpatient disposition is dictated by the severity and extent of the infection. Patients presenting with signs of sepsis, lymphangitis, lymphadenitis, tenosynovitis, septic arthritis, osteomyelitis, or rapidly progressing cellulitis (developing in less than 24 hours) should be hospitalized for intravenous antibiotic therapy and further supportive management. Consultation with a general, plastic, and/or orthopedic surgeon may be necessary. Admission should also be seriously considered for patients with bites invading the dermis, deep puncture wounds, infections to functionally or cosmetically important areas (e.g., hand or face), and for patients who have been taking oral antibiotics. The duration of intravenous antibiotics and hospitalization is often 10 to 14 days but depends on the nature of the infection, the immunocompetence of the patient, and the rapidity of response to antibiotic therapy and infection resolution. For any patient with an infection who is treated as an outpatient, we recommend an initial dose of intravenous antibiotics followed by oral antibiotics therapy for 10 to 14 days. Clinicians should assure follow-up within 24 to 48 hours to check for wound healing and response to antibiotic therapy.

TETANUS AND RABIES PROPHYLAXIS

Tetanus and rabies prophylaxis must be addressed for all mammalian bite wounds. Bite wounds are all considered tetanus prone, and patients who have received fewer than three primary tetanus immunizations should receive both tetanus immune globulin and tetanus toxoid. For patients who have received only three tetanus toxoid

vaccines, a fourth vaccine is recommended. Table 1 details further recommendations for tetanus prophylaxis.

Infection from the rabies virus results in death in all cases. Rabies postexposure prophylaxis should be considered even with seemingly superficial wounds if the offending animal is at high risk for rabies infection. This includes the following circumstances:

- Animals known to harbor rabies
- A stray animal
- An unprovoked attack
- The inability to capture and observe the offending animal
- Factors endemic to the geographic area.

In humans, the average incubation time of rabies is 4 to 6 weeks, ranging from 5 days to greater than 1 year. Ideally, prophylaxis should begin within 24 hours of exposure. Prophylaxis should be administered even in cases where there is a delay in seeking medical attention. When making the often difficult decision to initiate rabies prophylaxis, the clinician should ideally act in consultation with local health officials. The health department provides information on the risk of rabies for specific geographic areas and for particular animals. Table 2 outlines recommendations for rabies postexposure prophylaxis.

The clinician should also consider hepatitis B and HIV prophylaxis when the biter (perpetrator) is at high risk for having these infections. Some authors recommend administering hepatitis vaccine and hepatitis immune globulin to victims otherwise not immunized for hepatitis B. Bites at greatest risk for HIV transmission include those that draw blood from the victim and are the result of a bite from an individual known to be HIV infected. All reported cases of HIV transmission from a bite have occurred when there was significant break in the victim's skin with mixing of the victim's blood and the biter's saliva. When available, consultation with an infectious disease specialist may help in deciding if prophylaxis is warranted. In the United States, the national postexposure prophylaxis hotline is available for assistance in making difficult management decisions (1–888–448–4911).

TABLE 2 Rabies Postexposure Prophylaxis for Dog and Cat Bites

Evaluation and Disposition of Animal	Postexposure Prophylaxis Recommendations*
Healthy animal captured and confined for 10-day observation period by a veterinarian	Prophylaxis only if animal develops signs of rabies.[†]
Rabid or suspected of being rabid[‡]	Immediate immunization and human rabies immune globulin (HRIG).
Unknown	Consult local public health officials (local health department) for advice.

Adapted from Red Book: American Academy of Pediatrics, 26th ed. Elk Grove Village, Ill: American Academy of Pediatrics, 2003, p 517. Used with permission of the American Academy of Pediatrics.

*If rabies prophylaxis is initiated, 5 total doses (1 mL per dose) of the vaccine must be administered intramuscularly on days 1, 3, 7, 14, and 28. Human rabies immune globulin (HRIG) must also be administered for passive immunization on day 1. The dose of HRIG is 20 IU/kg, with half the dose infiltrated around the site of the wound and the remainder given intramuscularly.

[†]Initiate treatment with HRIG and rabies vaccine at the first sign of rabies in the biting animal. The animal should be euthanized and tested immediately.

[‡]Holding animal for observation is *not* recommended. The animal should be euthanized and tested as soon as possible. If negative, immunization can be discontinued.

Common Pitfalls

- Failure to obtain adequate history or explore the wound thoroughly, resulting in a retained foreign body; undiagnosed bone fracture; nerve, tendon, or ligament injury.
- Underestimating the extent of involvement caused by a puncture wound.
- Failure to recognize that a seemingly innocuous disruption of the skin over the metacarpal bone represents a clenched-fist bite.
- Failure to recognize need for rabies and/or tetanus prophylaxis.
- Use of antibiotics that may be ineffective for infected bite wounds, including erythromycin and first-generation cephalosporins, such as cephalexin.

Communication and Counseling

Clinicians should educate children and caretakers about the behaviors and interactions with dogs and cats that may put the child at increased risk for being bitten. In general, formal, structured educational programs reduce those behaviors in children that put them at increased risk for dog bites. Continued effectiveness requires repeated exposure to the educational intervention.

Adults must be educated on the paramount importance of supervising infants and children in the presence of animals, particularly unfamiliar animals. Children must be taught to avoid contact with stray, unfamiliar, or unrestrained animals. They should be cautioned against provoking animals by attempting to take away food or other items the animal may have in its mouth or playing aggressively with them. Parents and caretakers should be cautioned to make responsible and educated choices when bringing a pet into the home. Pit bulls, Rottweilers, and German shepherds are more aggressive than other dogs and most frequently associated with dog-attack fatalities.

The clinician must be cognizant of the potential for significant psychological trauma, including the development of post-traumatic stress disorder, in children who were attacked by an animal. This can occur in children with minimal wounds as well as in those with disfiguring injuries. Referral for psychological support services should be considered. When treating these injuries in the emergency setting, the availability and expertise from child-life specialists can be critical in reducing the child and caretaker's fears and anxiety.

SUGGESTED READINGS

1. American Academy of Pediatrics: Summaries of infectious diseases. In Pickering LK (ed): Red Book: 2003 Report of the Committee on Infectious Diseases, 26th ed. Elk Grove Village, Ill: American Academy of Pediatrics, 2003, pp 514–520. 611–616. **Summary of the current recommendations of the American Academy of Pediatrics concerning antibiotics and rabies and tetanus prophylaxis for animal bite wounds in infants, children, and adolescents.**
2. McCaig LF: National Hospital Ambulatory Medical Care Survey: 2002 Emergency Department Summary. Advance Data from Vital and Health Statistics. CDC 340:1–36, 2004. **Detailed information on the epidemiology of mammalian bites.**
3. Medeiros I, Saconato H: Antibiotic prophylaxis for mammalian bites. Cochrane Database Syst Rev 2:CD001738, 2001. **Comprehensive review of randomized controlled trials determining the effectiveness of prophylactic antibiotics in preventing bite-wound infections.**
4. Talan DA, Abrahamian FM, Moran GJ, et al: Clinical presentation and bacteriologic analysis of infected human bites in patients presenting to emergency departments. Clin Infect Dis 37:1481–1489, 2005. **Multicenter prospective study delineating bacteriology of infected human-bite wounds and determining the most effective antibiotic therapy.**
5. Talan DA, Citron DM, Abrahamian FM, et al: Bacteriologic analysis of infected dog and cat bites. Emergency Medicine Animal Bite Infection Study. N Engl J Med 340:85–92, 1999. **Prospective study identifying the polymicrobial nature of infected dog and cat bites.**

Venomous Snakebite

Robert L. Norris

KEY CONCEPTS

- Snake venom poisoning is a dynamic process that requires close monitoring for symptoms and signs of progression. Even an apparently mild bite can progress over hours to severe poisoning.
- The cornerstone of management of venomous snakebite is antivenom therapy.

- Antivenom should be started as soon as possible in any patient with symptoms or signs of systemic venom poisoning or with evidence of progressive local findings.
- Any child with an apparent dry bite (nonenvenomation) should be observed for a minimum of 8 hours before discharge to a reliable home environment.
- Antivenom should be started before beginning any infusion of necessary blood products to avoid feeding further fuel to a consumptive coagulopathy.
- Surgical fasciotomy is rarely needed and should only be performed in the face of objectively measured increases in intracompartmental pressures.

Venomous snakes exact a variable toll in terms of human morbidity and mortality around the world. Although no reliable statistics are available on the true extent of the problem, an estimated 2.5 million venomous snakebites occur in the world each year and as many as 125,000 deaths. Children make up a sizable proportion of those bitten. Their natural curiosity, lack of experience, and, particularly with adolescent boys, bravado, all tend to increase the risk. In North America, almost half of all venomous snakebites occur to individuals younger than 20 years of age, and 20% of deaths occur in children. The overall mortality rate for treated snakebite in North America, however, is less than 1%.

The indigenous venomous snakes of North America include the pit vipers (rattlesnakes, cottonmouth water moccasins, and copperheads) and the coral snakes. Approximately 98% of snakebites in North America are caused by pit vipers. Pit viper venoms are complex mixtures of enzymes, low-molecular-weight polypeptides, and other constituents that disrupt cell membranes, create vascular leaks, disrupt the coagulation cascade, and, in some cases, interfere with neuromuscular transmission. Essentially, any organ system can be affected, but the typical pit viper bite results in immediate pain, rapidly progressive swelling, and ecchymosis. Over a period of hours to days, hemorrhagic or serum-filled blebs can develop at the bite site and variable tissue necrosis can occur. Victims of pit viper venom poisoning often develop abnormalities of coagulation tests but usually without any evidence of clinically significant bleeding (see later), although bleeding from any body site can occur.

Coral snake bites are uncommon because of the secretive, fossorial habits of these animals but can occur in children who are prone to picking up the brightly colored (red, yellow, and black) serpents when found. Coral snake venom primarily affects the neuromuscular system and can lead to cranial nerve dysfunction, paralysis, and respiratory arrest.

The clinical course of a venomous snakebite can be quite variable—from so-called dry bites, where no venom is injected, to severe bites that can be fatal. Countless factors are involved in determining the severity of any particular bite. Some of these include the size, species, health, and demeanor of the snake and the size and health of the victim. Because of their smaller size and reduced circulating blood volume to dilute injected venom, children may have a worse outcome in venomous snakebites than adults. Thus any physician faced with treating a child bitten by a venomous snake must be knowledgeable on the subject, alert for findings consistent with toxicity, and aggressive in managing the case.

Expert Opinion on Management Issues

Management begins with ensuring that the victim's airway, breathing, and circulation are intact. Although breathing difficulty is unusual, victims showing signs of respiratory embarrassment, difficulty handling secretions, or signs of cranial nerve dysfunction (particularly following a coral snake bite) should be intubated and placed on mechanical ventilation. At least one intravenous line suitable for volume infusion should be established—two if any hemodynamic instability is evident. Cardiac and pulse oximetry monitoring should be established, and vital signs should be taken and repeated at frequent intervals. Early consultation with an expert in snake venom poisoning is prudent and can be obtained by calling a regional poison control center.

Blood for workup can be drawn while establishing intravenous lines. A sample should be sent early on for blood type and screening. A complete blood count (looking for consumption of platelets or evidence of hemolysis) and a basic metabolic panel (evaluating kidney function) as well as a coagulation screen (prothrombin time, partial thromboplastin time, fibrinogen and fibrin degradation products) are important tests for evidence of systemic venom poisoning. Urine should be checked for evidence of occult blood by bedside testing with each voided specimen.

The child's bitten extremity should be marked with an indelible pen at two or three sites (e.g., just above the bite site and more proximally). Limb circumferences should be checked at these sites every 15 minutes to determine if swelling, and therefore overall venom poisoning, is progressing. Such measurements should continue until the patient is clearly stable. The limb should be kept at about heart level during the initial observation period.

If any systemic poisoning is evident, based on the victim's symptoms, signs, or laboratory abnormalities, or if there is evidence of local venom toxicity that is progressing, antivenom is indicated. Although currently two antivenoms are produced in the United States for management of pit viper bites, the newest, most effective, and safest product is CroFab (Savage Laboratories, Melville, NY). This antivenom is produced in sheep and consists of Fab fragments of the ovine immunoglobulin molecules against the snake venoms with which the sheep are immunized. Although only four different pit viper species are used in production of CroFab, the venoms of all the North American pit vipers are antigenically similar enough to allow use of this product regardless of the species inflicting the bite.

CroFab is administered intravenously at a dose of four to six vials diluted in 250 mL of normal saline, although more diluent can be used if desired (up to 20 to 40 mL/kg body weight to a total of 1 L). The antivenom is packaged in a lyophilized state and requires reconstitution prior to use, a laborious process that can take 20 to 30 minutes. Pit vipers tend to inject similar quantities of venom into children as adults; thus the dose for antivenom is not based on body weight but rather on the quantity of antibodies thought necessary to counter the effects of a typical pit viper's venom delivered in a defensive bite. The antivenom is given over 1 hour, and no preliminary skin testing for potential allergy is necessary or recommended. However, the treating physician must be available during antivenom administration to intervene immediately if the child develops any acute reaction to the product. Although allergic reactions to CroFab appear much less common and less severe than reactions that sometimes occurred to the older equine antivenom, all the supplies needed to treat anaphylaxis (epinephrine, airway equipment, etc.) must be immediately available during antivenom infusion.

Once the initial dose of CroFab is given, the child is watched over the next hour for any evidence of worsening symptoms or signs (including local changes and limb circumferences). If any sign of progression is noted, the starting dose is repeated in like fashion. Such cycles of antivenom followed by observation and reassessment can be repeated until the child is clearly improving. Thereafter, CroFab should be repeated in a dose of two vials intravenously every 6 hours for three more doses. The Fab fragments in CroFab are cleared quickly from the circulation—faster than snake venom components are cleared—and repeat dosing on a schedule helps reduce the risk of recurrence of symptoms, signs, or laboratory abnormalities. Laboratory work that was abnormal initially should be repeated every few hours until stable. Laboratory work that was normal initially should be repeated every 6 to 8 hours for the first 24 hours to ensure stability.

Once antivenom is started (if indicated), the patient's bitten extremity should be elevated above the heart to reduce swelling. The extremity will be more comfortable if placed in a well-padded splint, with cotton between the digits. If there is any concern for a compartment syndrome in a swollen, painful extremity, a surgeon should measure the intracompartmental pressure (ICP). Only if the ICP is elevated above 30 to 40 mm Hg and remains elevated for more than an hour despite antivenom therapy and elevation of the extremity should a fasciotomy be considered. The rate of necessary fasciotomy for pit viper bites in North America is probably less than 1%. Although there is new evidence that fasciotomy might actually increase myonecrosis, fasciotomy still could be required to relieve pressure on vital nerves in the compartment.

If the victim develops blood- or serum-filled blebs at the bite site, these can be debrided 3 to 5 days after admission, as long as coagulopathy has resolved. Alternatively, blebs can be left intact and only debrided if they rupture. Patients who develop laboratory or clinical evidence of coagulopathy during their initial hospitalization are at risk of developing recurrent coagulopathy up to 2 weeks following the bite. Again, this coagulopathy tends to be clinically occult and of unclear clinical importance. But patients should be warned to avoid contact sports and

any elective surgery during the first 3 weeks following the bite and to report any evidence of unusual bleeding.

Delayed serum sickness, once a common occurrence following administration of equine pit viper antivenom, appears much less common with CroFab. Children should be returned to the hospital if they develop hives, fever, myalgias, arthralgias, and so on, at 1 to 2 weeks following treatment with antivenom. Serum sickness is treated with oral steroids (e.g., prednisolone orally at 1 to 2 mg/kg/day) until the symptoms and signs resolve. The steroids are then tapered over 1 to 2 weeks. Symptomatic treatment with diphenhydramine and acetaminophen is also helpful.

Although the mortality rate of snake venom poisoning in North America is very low, the complication rate related to loss of function or tissue in the bitten extremity is higher—as high as 30% following upper extremity bites and 10% following lower extremity bites. Wound care should include conservative debridement of clearly necrotic tissue after coagulation studies have normalized, followed by tissue grafting as necessary. Secondary infections are uncommon, and prophylactic antibiotics are not needed. Tetanus status, however, should be updated as appropriate.

Children who are envenomated should be admitted to a monitored setting for observation and further management. Once stable, and once all necessary antivenom is given, they can be transferred to a floor bed for further wound care.

Management of the rare child clearly bitten by a definitively identified coral snake is challenging and should be guided by someone knowledgeable in these bites. If coral snake antivenom (currently produced in the United States only by Wyeth-Ayerst Laboratories, Philadelphia, Pa.) is available, it should be started regardless of the presence or absence of symptoms or signs of poisoning because once these begin, it is difficult to halt progression of neuromuscular paralysis even with treatment. This antivenom, an equine product, should be administered according to the manufacturer's package insert. The child should be monitored closely in an intensive care unit setting for any evidence that would suggest the need for intubation (development of cranial nerve dysfunction, difficulty handling secretions, etc.). A victim of an apparent dry bite by a coral snake should be admitted for at least 24 hours of observation because of a possible delay in onset of clinical findings with this snake's venom.

Common Pitfalls

- Failure to anticipate progression of severity of venom poisoning, a very dynamic process, could result in underestimating the gravity of the bite and undertreatment.
- Failure to administer antivenom in a timely fashion when it is indicated (i.e., in the face of progressive local findings or any systemic findings) can lead to a worsened clinical outcome.
- Failure to prepare in advance for a possible allergic reaction to antivenom (e.g., having epinephrine and

airway equipment immediately available) delays intervening when and if this occurs, possibly resulting in a worse outcome for the child.

- Failure to document intracompartmental pressures in a patient with potential compartment syndrome could result in either missing a developing rise in pressures or unnecessary surgery if the pressures are normal.
- Failure to observe a child with an apparent dry bite by a pit viper for at least 8 hours could result in premature discharge when, in fact, symptoms and signs requiring antivenom treatment could still arise.

Communication and Counseling

Victims of snake venom poisoning can be discharged from the hospital when they show signs of definite improvement and all laboratory tests are normalized. Ongoing outpatient physical therapy may be arranged as needed. Parents/guardians should be cautioned about possible recurrence of coagulopathy and symptoms of serum sickness.

Children with apparent dry bites should be observed in the emergency department for at least 8 hours. If, after that time, they are still asymptomatic with normal vital signs and all of their laboratory work (both initial and repeat) is normal, they can be discharged home with a reliable adult. The family should be instructed to watch the child closely for 24 hours and to bring the child back immediately if any symptoms or signs of envenomation develop.

Parents should instruct their children at an early age not to pick up or handle any snake without permission, and they should teach their children to be observant for snakes when playing in a likely snake habitat.

SUGGESTED READINGS

1. Banner W: Bites and stings in the pediatric patient. Curr Probl Pediatr 18:9–69, 1988. **A review of the approach to pediatric victims of various bites and stings, including snakes.**
2. Gold BS, Dart RC, Barish RA: Bites of venomous snakes. New Engl J Med 347(5):347–356, 2002. **A comprehensive up-to-date review of snake venom poisoning in the United States.**
3. Lavonas EJ, Gerardo CJ, O'Malley G, et al: Initial experience with Crotalidae polyvalent immune Fab (ovine) antivenom in the treatment of copperhead snakebite. Ann Emerg Med 43(2):200–206, 2004. **An analysis of recent experience with CroFab in patients (including children) bitten by copperheads.**
4. Norris RL: Venom poisoning by North American reptiles. In Campbell JA, Lamar WW (eds): Venomous Reptiles of the Western Hemisphere. Ithaca, NY: Cornell University Press, 2004, pp 683–708. **A comprehensive review of the management of snake venom poisoning in North America, including a species-by-species review of snake venoms and their effects.**
5. Ruha A-M, Curry SC, Beuhler M, et al: Initial postmarketing experience with Crotalidae polyvalent immune Fab for treatment of rattlesnake envenomation. Ann Emerg Med 39(6):609–615, 2002. **An analysis of experience with CroFab in treating patients (including children) bitten by rattlesnakes.**
6. Russell FE: Snake Venom Poisoning. New York: Scholium International, 1983, pp 1–562. **An enjoyable comprehensive review of the problem of snake venom poisoning, including much historical information and information on exotic venomous snakes.**

Burns

Jeffrey Lukish

KEY CONCEPTS

- Focus initial care on primary survey: ABCDE (airway, breathing, circulation, disability, and exposure).
- Determine percentage total body surface area (%TBSA) burn injury using the Lund-Browder chart.
- Establish intravenous fluid resuscitation according to the Parkland formula.
- Determine depth of burn injury using clinical criteria.
- Determine requirement for transfer to a burn center using American Burn Association guidelines for major thermal burns in children.
- Establish pain and anxiety control followed by initial burn wound care.

In 2001 an estimated 99,400 children 14 years of age and younger were treated in hospital emergency rooms for burn-related injuries. Burn injury remains the fifth leading cause of unintentional injury–related death among children in the United States. Nearly all pediatric burns are preventable. Most occur in the home; the kitchen and bathroom are the most dangerous areas. Scalds are the most common type of burn injury in children (50% to 60%), followed by flame (30%), and contact with hot solids (10%). Chemical and electrical burns are relatively rare (less than 5%). There is a distinct gender difference, with boys accounting for approximately two thirds of burns. Flame burns from house fires usually result in severe burn injury and concomitant inhalational injury. Grease-type scald injuries are devastating because they are deeper and involve the hands and face. Child abuse is not an uncommon cause of infant and adolescent burns, accounting for approximately 5% of admissions.

Children 4 years of age and younger are at the greatest risk and have a fire- and burn-related death rate nearly twice that of all children. Young children have a less acute perception of danger, limited ability to respond quickly and properly to a life-threatening fire or burn situation, and increased metabolic demands. They are also less able to tolerate toxic combustion products physically, rendering them more susceptible to fire-related asphyxiation. Additionally, because younger children have thinner skin than adults, their skin burns at lower temperatures and injury occurs more deeply.

The pediatric burn examination is relatively straightforward; however, the severity of injury is often underestimated, resulting in suboptimal initial care. Because of the challenges of initial diagnosis and therapy, pain control, and frequent cleansing to avoid infection, many of these children require inpatient hospital care.

Expert Opinion on Management Issues

Childhood burn injuries should be approached as any major pediatric traumatic injury: primary survey (airway, breathing, circulation, disability, and exposure [ABCDE]) and resuscitation followed by secondary survey and definitive care. But there are unique features of thermal injury in children that need to be considered.

The physician must stop the burning process. Many children are wearing synthetic fabrics that can become adherent and continue to smolder. These must be removed, with care taken to minimize the risk of hypothermia. The child's core temperature is maintained above 95°F to 97°F (35°C to 36°C). Heating of the resuscitation room, overhead bed and radiant warmers, and warmed resuscitation fluids and inhaled gases preserve core body temperature and minimize heat loss.

Pediatric burn airway management is divided into two distinct problems: upper airway obstruction and lower airway damage. Upper airway obstruction occurs in children who are burned on the face and neck with indirect heat injury, causing edema to the posterior pharynx and supraglottic areas. The onset of acute obstruction may be subtle until complete airway closure occurs. A child may have an increased respiratory rate or work of breathing, increase in secretions, or hoarseness. Suspicion of injury or signs of airway obstruction should be managed by endotracheal intubation. Lower airway damage results from inhalation of hot gas, most commonly smoke. Certain signs suggesting inhalational injury should be recognized early because this injury may not become apparent for 24 to 48 hours (Table 1). Findings include dyspnea, rales, rhonchi, and wheezing. Meticulous pulmonary care and judicious fluid management are the cornerstones of therapy. Pulmonary status must be closely monitored because the increased secretions may obstruct the small lumen of the endotracheal tube.

Supporting the circulating blood volume is the next priority. The Advanced Trauma Life Support (ATLS) algorithm now suggests that two attempts be made to place large-bore peripheral intravenous lines (IVs) in the upper extremities. An unburned site is preferable, but if none is available, lines can be placed through burned skin. If percutaneous placement is unsuccessful, an intraosseous (IO) line should be placed in a child less than 6 years of age. If the child is older than 6 years of age, a venous cutdown should be performed at the ankle, or with adequately trained personnel, a percutaneous femoral line should be placed. Fluid resuscitation should begin with normal saline or a lactated Ringer bolus of 20 mL/kg IV.

The single most important step in the evaluation of a burned child is accurate estimation of burn size. This permits appropriate planning of immediate medical management and fluid therapy and dictates the need for

definitive care. Burn size is expressed as percent total body surface area (%TBSA) burned. Several methods are used to determine %TBSA. The region covered by the child's hand is 1% TBSA. The rule of nines, used to calculate adult %TBSA, is not applicable for children. The Lund-Browder chart should be used to calculate %TBSA in children, permitting a more accurate assessment of burn size based on age and involved body part.

Following determination of %TBSA burned, resuscitation can be initiated. The objective of resuscitation is to replace fluid losses through the burned skin and into the third spaces with the minimal amount of fluid required to maintain organ function. Precision with regard to pediatric burn resuscitation is critical; excess fluid is never advantageous. Initial therapy should be instituted according to the Parkland formula (Figure 1). Fluid rates are adjusted half hourly to achieve proper urine volumes.

Depth of burn injury is important in determining the choice of care and the ultimate functional and cosmetic outcome. Partial-thickness burns involve the epidermis and a portion of the dermis. These burns can be superficial, appearing erythematous (first degree) to a deeper injury, appearing mottled with edema and blister formation (second degree). The surface is usually weeping and painfully hypersensitive. Third-degree, or full-thickness, burns appear waxy white or dark and leather-like. The surface is generally dry and, because all dermal elements have been destroyed, is painless.

Immediate cooling of a burn wound with tap water for 30 seconds shortly after the burn provides pain relief and may decrease burn depth. Application beyond this immediate period or the application of ice risks the development of hypothermia and has no role in modern burn management. The burned region is washed with dilute antiseptic soap and water. Moistened gauze is used to remove all loose tissue. Small blisters on the palms or soles may be left intact.

First-degree burns are sunburn and water scald burns. There is little risk for infection and scarring with these burns. Treatment includes cool water compresses, pain medication, and application of emollient creams. Second-degree burns can be expected to heal within 30 days. These burns are seen after significant scald or flash-type burns. Treatment involves wound protection to avoid conversion to full-thickness burns. These are best treated by debridement followed by wound closure with the application of a biologic dressing, such as Transcyte (Smith & Nephew, Largo, Fla) or Biobrane (Bertek Pharmaceuticals, Morgantown, WVa). Full-thickness burns, unless they are very small (<2 cm), require debridement, topical antimicrobials (silver sulfadiazine), and skin grafting.

Optimal care of major thermal burns in children requires a multidisciplinary approach that is best delivered by a burn center (Table 2). Children with these burns should undergo primary survey and initial resuscitation followed by transfer to a regional burn center.

Common Pitfalls

Evaluation of the burned child is similar to any trauma evaluation. Wound care is considered in the secondary

---

TABLE 1 Signs Suggesting Inhalation Injury

History of confinement in a burning building
History of explosion
History of decreased level of consciousness
Carbon deposits around the mouth or in the oropharynx
Inflammatory changes in the oropharynx
Carbonaceous sputum
Singed facial hair

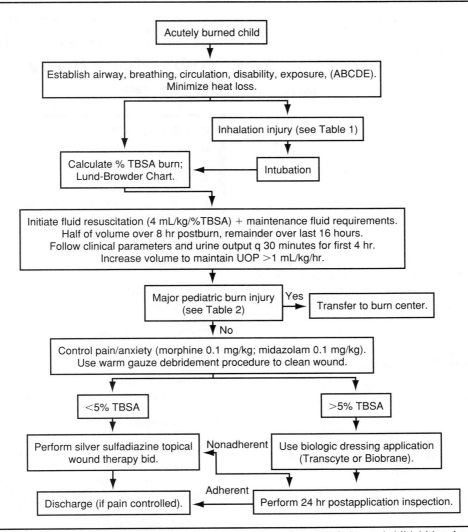

FIGURE 1. The algorithm represents a clinical pathway for the care of an acutely burned child. bid, twice daily; q, every; %TBSA, percentage total body surface area burn.

TABLE 2 American Burn Association Criteria for Major Pediatric Burns
Partial-thickness burns greater than 10% total body surface area (TBSA)
Burns that involve the face, hands, feet, genitalia, perineum, or major joints
Full-thickness (third-degree) burns
Electrical burns, including lightning injury
Chemical burns
Inhalation injury
Burn injury in children with preexisting medical disorders
Burn injury with concomitant trauma
Burned children in hospitals without qualified personnel or equipment
Burns in children who require special social, emotional, or long-term rehabilitative intervention

survey after the ABCs of trauma care. Children younger than 2 years of age; those with preexisting disease (neurologically impaired); and those with burns of the face, hands, feet, or perineum present unique problems of wound management and overall care and should be transferred to a burn center regardless of burn size or depth.

The fluid volume determined by a burn formula is only a starting point of resuscitation. Adequate resuscitation in a child is based on clinical outcome: normal mentation, normal and stable vital signs, and a urine output of 1 mL/kg/hour.

It is often difficult to characterize the depth of the burn injury at presentation. The safest wound management strategy is twice-daily cleaning and topical silver sulfadiazine. Surgical evaluation early after burn injury is essential to determine whether further debridement, biologic dressing, or skin grafting is indicated.

Nonadherence of a biologic dressing indicates that the burn is significantly deeper than the clinical appearance. In these cases, surgical consultation is indicated, and transfer to a regional burn center is warranted because

TABLE 3 Child Abuse: Suspicious Burn Injuries

Multiple burns of the same or different ages
The presence or absence of splash marks
Bilateral symmetry (stocking-and-glove distribution)
Well-demarcated waterlines
Burns on the soles of the feet
Spared burn regions
Associated nonburn trauma (whip marks, bruises, fractures)
Buttocks/genitalia/perineum burns.

many of these injuries require further debridement and grafting.

Child abuse must always be considered when caring for a burned child. This injury pattern is commonly in a child younger than 4 years of age and results from tap water immersion. The incidence of death and further injury is high; therefore, suspicious injuries warrant involvement of a social worker and child protective services (Table 3).

Communication and Counseling

The current pressures and trends in health care financing have created a heightened need for effective and cost-efficient treatment of pediatric burns. Early wound closure of partial-thickness burns in children by an occlusive dressing or an adherent skin substitute increases the rate of healing, decreases pain, improves function, and reduces the length of hospitalization. This form of wound care is a practical alternative to silver sulfadiazine wound care in children and is quickly becoming the standard of care.

Regardless of size or severity, the goals of burn therapy in children are clear: limit pain and anxiety, prevent infection, decrease metabolic demand, promote healing, and minimize disability.

SUGGESTED READINGS

1. Centers for Disease Control and Prevention: Web-Based Injury Statistics Query and Reporting System (WISQARS). Fatal injury reports [Online]. 1999–2000 [cited 2003 February 3]; National Center for Injury Prevention and Control, Centers for Disease Control and Prevention (producer). Available online at http://www.cdc.gov/ncipc/wisqars. **Current epidemiology of pediatric burn injury.**
2. Golianu B, Krane EJ, Galloway KS, Yaster M: Acute pain in children: Pediatric acute pain management. Pediatr Clin North Am 47:1–24, 2000. **Detailed description of pain management.**
3. Lukish JR, Eichelberger MR: Accident victims and their emergency management. In Grosfeld JL, O'Neill JA, Fonkalsrud EW, et al: Pediatric Surgery. Philadelphia: Elsevier (in press). **Detailed description of the primary survey, vascular access, and fluid resuscitation in injured children.**
4. Lukish J, Eichelberger M, Newman K, et al: The use of a bioactive skin substitute decreases length of stay for pediatric burn patients. J Pediatr Surg 36(8):1118–1121, 2001. **A study documenting standard burn wound management and the advantages of biologic dressings in partial-thickness burns in children.**
5. Purdue GF, Hunt JL, Burris AM: Pediatric surgical emergencies, pediatric burn care. Clin Pediatr Emerg Med 3:76–82, 2002. **Detailed description of pediatric burn care.**

Drowning and Near Drowning: Submersion Injury

Katherine Biagas

KEY CONCEPTS

- Submersion injury is one of the leading causes of accident-related childhood mortality and morbidity.
- Two age groups are primarily affected: infants and toddlers and adolescents.
- Injury is primarily hypoxic-ischemic brain injury.
- Additional shock and acute lung injury may be seen.
- Immediate therapy is focused on restoration of oxygenation and circulation at the scene. Rapid transfer to an emergency department and pediatric intensive care facility is needed.
- Therapy is largely limited to good supportive care and avoidance of secondary insults. Repeated assessments of brain function over time can offer some prognosis of functional outcomes.
- Prevention of submersion injuries is a public health goal.

Submersion injuries are the second leading cause of accidental death in childhood. A drowning event is a fatal submersion injury; a near-drowning event is one in which the victim survives, albeit survival may be with important disabilities. In the United States, submersion events account for approximately 1000 deaths and more than 3000 emergency department visits annually for children less than 19 years of age. Despite recent efforts to prevent such events and advances in medical care, outcomes from all but brief submersion events remain, in many cases, quite poor.

Epidemiology

The majority of submersions occur in fresh water, with a large proportion of these occurring in natural bodies of water: rivers, creeks, lakes, and ponds. Submersions also occur frequently in domestic sites—home pools, spas, or bathtubs—and recreational community pools, water parks, and schools. As few as 4% of events occur in salt water, although this incidence is much higher in coastal communities. Three groups of children are at particular risk for submersion injuries: the very young, adolescent males, and nonwhites. Infants 6 to 11 months of age largely drown in home bathtubs. Older infants and young children may drown as result of a fall into a shallow body of water such as a wading pool or spa, as well as in bathtubs. Moreover, infants and toddlers are least likely to be involved in a witnessed drowning event, a condition associated with poorer outcome. In boys 15 to 19 years of age, submersion events are generally related to recreational water activities. The incidence of fatal submersion injuries is higher in African Americans and Hispanics than the general pediatric population (Ibsen and Koch, 2002). Certain medical conditions may predispose children to submersion events. Drowning risk is elevated in children with epilepsy, with most events occurring in bathtubs and pools. Drowning events are reported in patients with long QT syndrome because such patients are prone to ventricular tachyarrhythmias, particularly torsades de pointes, and fibrillation. In fact, swimming may be an arrhythmogenic trigger. The use of alcohol or other intoxicating substances is associated with submersions in older adolescents. Submersion injuries in older children and adolescents may be associated with cervical spine injury.

Pathophysiology

The initial sequence of events in drowning was studied in the 1930s and consists of the following: initial struggle sometimes with a surprise inhalation, suspension of movement and exhalation of a little air frequently followed by swallowing, violent struggle, convulsions with spasmodic respiratory efforts through an open mouth, loss of reflexes, and death. During the initial seconds of submersion, small amounts of fluid are aspirated causing laryngospasm. Victims who are resuscitated at this phase have little water aspiration, but ventilation by rescue breathing may be difficult because of glottic closure. If the victim loses muscle tone, larger quantities of fluid may be aspirated. In addition, a victim may vomit, aspirating gastric contents.

Much is made of possible fluid shifts and electrolyte disturbances in drowning, but important disorders of vascular volume are not often found. Hemodilution and hypervolemia are generally mild. Hypovolemia after salt-water drowning may be seen in severe cases, usually in victims who do not survive. The development of hypothermia is extremely common in drowning victims, resulting from rapid radiant heat losses in tepid water. The presence of hypothermia in most cases should not be interpreted as a "cold water drowning." All submersion victims go through some period of hypoxia. For those with brief episodes, hypoxemia is limited to the duration of apnea and may not be present on initial medical evaluation. However, some patients, even those with relatively short duration hypoxia, develop lung injury with increased permeability of pulmonary capillaries with alveolar fluid leak and dysfunction of surfactant. Aspiration of gastric contents may cause additional caustic injury to airways and alveoli, and neurogenic pulmonary edema may be present. In combination, these processes create the clinical syndromes of acute lung injury (ALI) and acute respiratory distress syndrome (ARDS). The hallmark of cardiovascular dysfunction with submersion injury is shock. The most important sequela of submersion injuries is global hypoxic-ischemic brain injury. The combination of hypoxemia and low flow states results in a host of pathologic processes, including energy failure, lipid peroxidation, production of free radicals, inflammatory responses, and release of excitotoxic neurotransmitters. There is disruption of neuronal and glial functions and cellular architecture. The vascular end zones are particularly vulnerable, and "watershed" infarctions may be appreciated on CT scans. With more extensive hypoxic-ischemic insult, the injury becomes more global and involves more of the cortex.

Expert Opinion on Management Issues

Management at the scene should focus on rapid restoration of oxygenation and spontaneous circulation with basic cardiopulmonary resuscitation (CPR). Emergency medicine services should be summoned as quickly as possible. Bystanders should perform mouth-to-mouth breathing even before the victim is removed from the water. No attempts should be made to drain water from the lungs before initiation of rescue breathing. Once on solid ground, chest compressions should be performed unless the presence of a pulse is established. Cervical spine immobilization should be performed in cases with history of diving or when the mechanism of injury is not known. Advanced life support efforts should be initiated by paramedics.

Definitive management of submersion injuries begins in the emergency department. Advanced life support should focus on establishing adequate oxygenation and ventilation, adequate circulation, and determination of neurologic functioning. Initial neurologic status is approximated using the Glasgow Coma Score (GCS). A more thorough neurologic examination is performed later in the emergency room or upon admission to the hospital. Repeated GCS determinations during the first 12 hours of treatment and repeated neurologic examinations throughout hospitalization are necessary to document changes in function. Definitive warming should be initiated for all but mild hypothermia (95°F to 97°F [35°C to 36°C]). The simplest warming techniques include the use of warmed intravenous fluids, external radiant heat, ventilation with heated gas, and immersion in a warm bath. More aggressive efforts are necessary for moderate hypothermia: warmed peritoneal lavage or dialysis fluids and bladder washes with warm fluids. For severe hypothermia (temperatures less than 82°F [28°C]), passive rewarming can induce "rewarming shock." Peripheral vasodilatation and impaired cardiac output can ensue. The use of cardiopulmonary bypass is advocated for core rewarming in severe hypothermia. Failure of restoration of circulation within 30 minutes of rewarming to 90°F (32°C) or greater suggests that further resuscitation efforts are unlikely to be successful. Given the encouraging data about the neuroprotective effects of mild hypothermia after cardiac arrest, consideration should be given to maintaining a core temperature of 93°F to 95°F (34°C to 35°C); certainly overwarming should be avoided.

Children who do not regain full consciousness in the emergency department should be transferred to a pediatric intensive care facility. There, ongoing efforts should be to treat aggressively any cardiorespiratory dysfunction. An "open lung" strategy should be employed for patients with ALI or ARDS. Usual ventilator settings include limiting ventilator peak pressures to 25 torr, tidal volumes to 6 to 8 mL per kg, and fraction of inspired oxygen to less that 0.60. Liberal use of positive end-expiratory

---

BOX 1 Anticipatory Guidance Concerning Water Safety for Infants and Children Younger Than 5 Years

- Parents and caregivers should be advised never to leave infants and children alone while in bathtubs, pools, or spas or when near standing bodies of water.
- Supervising adults should be within "touch distance" of an infant or young child.
- Home swimming pools should have four-sided fencing that prevents direct access from the home.
- Unless developmentally precocious, children should not be given swimming lessons until after 4 years of age.
- Swimming lessons do not drown-proof any child or adult.
- Parents and caregivers should know basic CPR.
- Flotation devices approved by the U.S. Coast Guard, such as life preservers, should be readily available.
- Air-filled swimming aids, such as "water wings," are not flotation devices and should not be substituted for flotation devices.
- Parents should inquire about exposure to water hazards when children are out of their immediate care, such as in day care.

Policy Statement. Committee on Injury, Violence, and Poison Prevention. Prevention of Drowning in Infants, Children, and Adolescents. AAP Policy 2003:112:437–439. Used with permission of the American Academy of Pediatrics.

BOX 2 Anticipatory Guidance Concerning Water Safety for Children 5 Years and Older and Adolescents

- Children should be taught to swim.
- Children should be taught the principles for safe swimming in pools and in naturally occurring bodies of water, with emphasis on judging conditions under which it is safe to swim.
- Children should never swim alone or be without adult supervision.
- Children should use a personal flotation device, such as a life preserver, when boating or in danger of falling into water.
- Diving into water can cause injury, and the depth of water should be determined before diving.
- Feet-first jumping should be the first entry into a body of water.
- Parents and children need to recognize the drowning risks posed in winter while engaging in activities near frozen or thawing bodies of water.
- Children with seizure disorders should have adult supervision when swimming or bathing.
- Adolescents should be counseled about the dangers of combining consumption of alcohol or other illicit substances with water-related activities.
- Adolescents should learn CPR.

Policy Statement. Committee on Injury, Violence, and Poison Prevention. Prevention of Drowning in Infants, Children, and Adolescents. AAP Policy 2003:112:437–439. Used with permission of the American Academy of Pediatrics.

---

pressure (PEEP) may improve oxygenation dramatically. Permissive hypercapnia, a commonly used lung protective strategy, is contraindicated if intracranial hypertension is suspected. Administration of exogenous surfactant has been used to treat severe ARDS following submersion injury when surfactant washout or dysfunction is suspected (Onarheim and Vik, 2004). Continuous vasoactive infusions may be required to treat myocardial dysfunction and correct abnormal peripheral vascular resistance. Care should concentrate on normalizing blood pressure, organ perfusion, and gas exchange as quickly as possible, and frequent repeated examinations are necessary to detect deterioration in cardiorespiratory functioning.

The other focus of care in the intensive care unit (ICU) should be on restoring cerebral function. Having said this, no definitive treatment exists to reverse the neuronal injury processes previously discussed. Instead, care of the brain is largely supportive. Hypermetabolic states, such as seizures and fevers, should be treated aggressively. Routine electroencephalography should be used to detect subclinical seizures and to titrate antiepileptic therapy. In cases of severe global brain injury, consideration should be given to maintaining mild hypothermia for 24 to 48 hours, as previously discussed. To maintain a hypothermic state, patients may require the use of neuromuscular blocking agents, which interfere with performance of the neurologic examination. Intracranial hypertension is often seen in cases of severe brain injury. However, despite previous enthusiasm for intracranial pressure (ICP) monitoring and treatment, no evidence indicates that such management affects ultimate outcome. Rather, raised ICP is a marker of poor neurologic prognosis.

Preventative Measures. The outcome of a drowning event is determined in the first few minutes of submersion.

Because there is little by way of primary therapy for these injuries, an emphasis on prevention is necessary. Prevention strategies focus on calling attention to the common causes of childhood drowning, specifically bathtub drowning and recreation-related incidents (Wintemute, 1990). Slogans such as "Don't Turn Your Back on Me" alert parents to the proper supervision of infants and toddlers. Other alerts focus on specific events, for example the installation of a home pool. Most pool-related submersions occur within the first 6 months of pool exposure (Thompson and Rivara, 2005). The absence of proper pool fencing may increase the odds of pool-related drowning as much as three- to fivefold (Thompson and Rivara, 2005). Written alerts about drowning risks are generally distributed with the purchase of a new pool.

Additional prevention strategies focus on the family pediatrician. The American Academy of Pediatrics issued a policy statement in 2003 to guide pediatricians in incorporating regular teaching about water safety in their anticipatory guidance to families. Box 1 outlines these guidelines for infants and young children; Box 2 does so for older children.

Common Pitfalls

The development of hypothermia is extremely common in drowning victims. The presence of hypothermia in most cases should not be interpreted as a "cold water drowning." Having said this, there is a definite clinical entity of brain preservation in so-called cold water drowning with good and even normal neurologic outcomes observed despite extensive submersions. Cold water drowning is a misnomer in that the submersion must occur in ice-cold fresh water and is a phenomenon restricted to northern climates and cold weather. Young children are particularly susceptible to rapid cooling of the brain when exposed to icy water because of little subcutaneous fat insulation and a large head-to-body ratio. Moreover, activation of the "diving reflex" with ice-cold water submersion slows metabolism and preserves some perfusion to the heart and brain. The result is rapid brain cooling in the face of residual perfusion and provision of brain substrates. Brain cooling, itself, may be neuroprotective in hypoxic-ischemic injury, and better than expected neurologic outcomes are possible. Numerous reports document dramatic cases of intact neurologic functioning in children who almost drowned in icy water.

Communication and Counseling

Counseling families in the immediate postsubmersion period is difficult because outcome from drowning is related to the extent of cerebral injury, which cannot be reliably determined initially. Poor prognostic signs include an unwitnessed event, prolonged time to resuscitation, the need for CPR at the scene and in the emergency department (Horisberger, Fischer et al., 2002), and prolonged coma. The best independent predictor of survival is submersion time (Quan, Wentz et al., 1990; Suominen, Baillie et al., 2002); however, in many patients these data are not known. In the emergency department, a physical examination remarkable for nonreactive pupils or a GCS of 5 or less predict poor neurologic outcome (Lavelle and Shaw, 1993), but these are not absolute predictors. Specific prognostic scales are similarly less satisfactory in discriminatory function. A reasonable approach therefore is to avoid determining in the field or emergency room which patients should receive initial treatment based on prognostic factors. Rather, the "treat them all approach" applies with aggressive efforts even with an initial lack of heartbeat (Lavelle and Shaw, 1993). The adage "You're not dead until you're warm and dead" applies. Prognosis is deferred until circulation is restored and perfusion optimized. At that time, the patient can be examined more completely. For those patients who do not regain consciousness, efforts are made to determine the likelihood of good neurologic outcome with appropriate counseling of the family as time passes.

SUGGESTED READINGS

1. Horisberger T, Fischer E, Fanconi S: One-year survival and neurological outcome after pediatric cardiopulmonary resuscitation. Intensive Care Med 28(3):365–368, 2002. **This is a retrospective review of the medical records and prospective follow-up of CPR survivors in a tertiary care pediatric university hospital. Predictors of survival were location of resuscitation, CPR during peri- or postoperative care, and duration of resuscitation. Independent determinants of long-term survival of pediatric resuscitation are location of arrest, underlying cause, and duration of CPR.**
2. Ibsen LM, Koch T: Submersion and asphyxial injury. Crit Care Med 30(11 Suppl):S402–S408, 2002. **Discusses the epidemiology, pathophysiology, and treatments applied to near-drowning victims, with an emphasis on the difficulties predicting outcome using current methods.**
3. Lavelle JM, Shaw KN: Near drowning: Is emergency department cardiopulmonary resuscitation or intensive care unit cerebral resuscitation indicated? Crit Care Med 21(3):368–373, 1993. **Retrospective review of hospital records for patient condition on arrival in the emergency department and ICU, treatments, hospital course, and ultimate outcome after a submersion event. No predictor was absolute. Two patients who arrived in the emergency department without vital signs, requiring cardiopulmonary resuscitation and cardiotonic medications, had full neurologic recovery. The results emphasize the need for initial full resuscitation in the emergency department.**
4. Onarheim H, Vik V: Porcine surfactant (Curosurf) for acute respiratory failure after near drowning in 12 year old. Acta Anaesthesiol Scand 48(6):778–781, 2004. **Describes rapid and persistent improvement after one single dose of porcine surfactant (Curosurf), 0.5 mL per kg (−1) (40 mg per kg) intratracheally, for ARDS with severe oxygenation failure 8 hours after freshwater near drowning in a 12-year-old girl.**
5. American Academy of Pediatrics committee on Injury, Violence and Poison Prevention: Prevention of drowning in infants, children, and adolescents. Pediatrics 112(2):437–439, 2003. **Reviews drowning-related death in children. A number of preventative strategies are discussed. Pediatricians play an important role as educators and advocates.**
6. Quan L, Wentz KR, Gore EJ, Copass MK: Outcome and predictors of outcome in pediatric submersion victims receiving prehospital care in King County, Washington. Pediatrics 86(4):586–593, 1990. **Predictors of outcome in pediatric submersion victims were studied. The two more common risk factors were submersion duration greater than 9 minutes (28 patients) and cardiopulmonary resuscitation duration longer than 25 minutes (20 patients). Both factors were ascertained in the prehospital phase of care.**
7. Suominen P, Baillie C, Korpela R, et al: Impact of age, submersion time and water temperature on outcome in near-drowning. Resuscitation 52(3):247–254, 2002. **In this retrospective study of children and adults with near-drowning submersion time was the only independent predictor of survival. Patient age, water temperature, and rectal temperature in the emergency room were not significant predictors of survival.**
8. Thompson DC, Rivara FP: Pool fencing for preventing drowning in children. Cochrane Database Syst Rev (2):CD001047. **The authors conclude that pool fences should have a dynamic and secure gate and should isolate (i.e., four-sided fencing) the pool from the house.**
9. Wintemute GJ: Childhood drowning and near-drowning in the United States. Am J Dis Child 144(6):663–669, 1990. **Reviews epidemiology and neurologic outcomes in children with submersion injury. The authors describe two distinct high-risk groups: children under 5 years of age and boys 15 to 19 years of age. Among survivors, the clinical course is bimodal; intact survival and survival with severe permanent disability are the most likely outcomes. The outcome of an immersion event is determined within a few minutes of the onset of immersion, mandating an emphasis on primary prevention, including requirement for pool fencing, caretaker training in cardiopulmonary resuscitation, and alcohol abuse prevention programs.**

3

Blunt Abdominal Trauma

Steven Stylianos, Barry A. Hicks, and Richard H. Pearl

KEY CONCEPTS

- The standard treatment of hemodynamically stable children with splenic injury is nonoperative, and this concept has now been successfully applied to most blunt injuries of the liver, pancreas, and kidney.
- CT has become the imaging study of choice for the evaluation of injured children because of several advantages. CT is now readily accessible in most health care facilities,

KEY CONCEPTS—cont'd

it is noninvasive, and it is a very accurate method of identifying and qualifying the extent of abdominal injury.

- Application of specific treatment guidelines in children with isolated spleen or liver injury based on injury severity resulted in conformity in patient management, improved use of resources, and validation of guideline safety. Significant reduction of ICU stay, hospital stay, follow-up imaging, and activity restriction was achieved without adverse sequelae.

- Based on alarmingly high rates of operative treatment for blunt spleen injury, adult trauma surgeons caring for injured children must consider the anatomic, immunologic, and physiologic differences between pediatric and adult trauma patients and incorporate these differences into their treatment protocols.

- The need for imaging in the patient with blunt trauma and microscopic hematuria is not as clear cut. The degree of hematuria does not always correlate with the degree of injury.

- Frequent physical exams and vigilance are required for the subset of injuries caused in children with lap belt restraints presenting with visible "seatbelt signs" on physical exam. Multiple studies have documented increased abdominal injuries to both solid and hollow organs with this finding.

- The decision *not* to operate in pediatric trauma is always a surgical decision.

No one could have imagined the influence of James Simpson's publication in 1968 on the successful *nonoperative* treatment of select children presumed to have splenic injury. Initially suggested in the early 1950s at the Hospital for Sick Children in Toronto, Canada, the era of nonoperative management for pediatric spleen injury began remarkably with the report of 12 children treated between 1956 and 1965. Four decades later, the standard treatment of hemodynamically stable children with splenic injury is nonoperative, and this concept is now applied successfully to most blunt injuries of the liver, kidney, and pancreas as well. Surgical restraint is the theme based on an increased awareness of the anatomic patterns and physiologic responses characteristic of injured children. Clinicians in adult trauma care have slowly acknowledged this success and applied many of the principles learned in pediatric trauma to their patients.

Expert Opinion on Management Issues

DIAGNOSTIC MODALITIES

The initial evaluation of the acutely injured child is similar to that of the adult. Radiography of the cervical spine, chest, and pelvis are obtained following the initial survey and evaluation of the ABCs (airway, breathing, circulation). Simple abdominal films offer little in the acute evaluation of the pediatric trauma patient. As imaging modalities have improved, treatment algorithms have changed significantly for children with a suspected intra-abdominal injury. Prompt identification of potentially life-threatening injuries is now possible in the vast majority of children.

Computed Tomography

Computed tomography (CT) is the imaging study of choice for the evaluation of injured children for several reasons. Readily accessible in most health care facilities, CT is a noninvasive, very accurate method of identifying and qualifying the extent of abdominal injury and reduces the incidence of nontherapeutic exploratory laparotomy. Use of intravenous contrast is essential, and dynamic methods of scanning optimize vascular and parenchymal enhancement. A head CT, if indicated, should be performed first without contrast, to avoid concealing a hemorrhagic brain injury. Enteral contrast for enhancement of the gastrointestinal tract is generally not required in the acute trauma setting and can lead to aspiration.

Not all children with potential abdominal injuries are candidates for CT evaluation. Obvious penetrating injury often necessitates immediate operative intervention. The hemodynamically unstable child should not be taken out of an appropriate resuscitation room for a CT. These children may benefit from an alternative diagnostic study, such as focused abdominal sonography for trauma (FAST), laparoscopy, or open operative intervention. The greatest limitation of abdominal CT scanning in trauma is its inability to identify intestinal rupture reliably. A high index of suspicion should exist for the presence of a bowel injury in the child with intraperitoneal fluid and no identifiable solid organ injury on CT scanning.

Ultrasonography

Clinician-performed FAST for the early assessment of the injured child is currently being evaluated to determine its optimal use. This bedside exam may be useful as a rapid screening study, particularly in those patients too unstable to undergo an abdominal CT scan. Early reports find FAST a useful screening tool in children, with a high specificity (95%) but a low sensitivity (33%) in identifying intestinal injury.

Laparoscopy

Multiple studies (principally in adults) demonstrate the utility of laparoscopy in trauma evaluation and in definitive management of related injuries. The extent of operations feasible is directly related to the skill of the surgeon with advanced laparoscopic techniques and the overall stability of the patient. As with elective abdominal surgery, the role of laparoscopy in trauma will increase substantially as training programs and trauma centers redirect their training of residents to this modality and as more pediatric centers report outcome studies for laparoscopic trauma management in children.

TREATMENT OF BLUNT SOLID ORGAN INJURY

Spleen and Liver

The spleen and liver are the organs most commonly injured in blunt abdominal trauma, with each accounting for one third of the injuries. Nonoperative treatment of

TABLE 1 Resource Use and Activity Restriction in 832 Children with Isolated Spleen or Liver Injury

Resource Use and Activity Restriction	CT Grade			
	I (n = 116)	II (n = 341)	III (n = 275)	IV (n = 100)
Admitted to ICU	55.0%	54.3%	72.3%	85.4%
Hospital stay (mean)	4.3 days	5.3 days	7.1 days	7.6 days
Hospital stay (range)	1–7 days	2–9 days	3–9 days	4–10 days
Transfused	1.8%	5.2%	10.1%*	26.6%*
Laparotomy	None	1.0%	2.7%†	12.6%†
Follow-up imaging	34.4%	46.3%	54.1%	51.8%
Activity restriction (mean)	5.1 wk	6.2 wk	7.5 wk	9.2 wk
Activity restriction (range)	2–6 wk	2–8 wk	4–12 wk	6–12 wk

ICU, intensive care unit.
*Grade III vs. grade IV, P <0.014.
†Grade III vs. grade IV, P <0.0001.

TABLE 2 Proposed Guidelines for Resource Use in Children with Isolated Spleen or Liver Injury

Guideline	CT Grade			
	I	II	III	IV
ICU days	None	None	None	1 day
Hospital stay	2 days	3 days	4 days	5 days
Predischarge imaging	None	None	None	None
Postdischarge imaging	None	None	None	None
Activity restriction*	3 wk	4 wk	5 wk	6 wk

ICU, intensive care unit.
*Return to full-contact competitive sports (e.g., football, wrestling, hockey, lacrosse, mountain climbing, etc.) should be at the discretion of the individual pediatric trauma surgeon. The proposed guidelines for return to unrestricted activity include standard age-appropriate activities.

isolated splenic and hepatic injuries in stable children is now standard practice. Although nonoperative treatment of children with isolated blunt spleen or liver injury is universally successful, the management algorithms used by individual pediatric surgeons vary greatly. The American Pediatric Surgical Association (APSA) Trauma Committee analyzed a contemporary multi-institution database of 832 children treated nonoperatively at 32 centers in North America from 1995 to 1997 (Table 1). Consensus guidelines on length of stay in the intensive care unit (ICU), length of hospital stay, use of follow-up imaging, and physical activity restriction for clinically stable children with isolated spleen or liver injuries (grades I through IV) were defined by analysis of this database (Table 2). *Note:* These proposed guidelines assume hemodynamic stability.

The guidelines were then applied prospectively in 312 children with liver or spleen injuries treated nonoperatively at 16 centers from 1998 to 2000. There were no differences in compliance by age, gender, or organ injured. Compared with the previously studied 832 patients, the 312 patients managed prospectively by the proposed guidelines had a significant reduction in ICU stay (P < 0.0001), hospital stay (P < 0.0006), follow-up imaging (P < 0.0001), and interval of physical activity restriction (P < 0.04) within each grade of injury.

From these data we concluded that prospective application of specific treatment guidelines based on injury severity resulted in conformity in patient management, improved use of resources, and validation of guideline safety. Significant reduction of ICU stay, hospital stay, follow-up imaging, and activity restriction was achieved without adverse sequelae when compared to the retrospective database.

Not surprisingly, adult trauma services report excellent survival rates for pediatric trauma patients; however, analysis of treatment for spleen and liver injuries reveals alarmingly high rates of operative treatment. This discrepancy in operative rates emphasizes the importance of disseminating effective guidelines because the majority of seriously injured children are treated outside of dedicated pediatric trauma centers. Adult trauma surgeons caring for injured children must consider the anatomic, immunologic, and physiologic differences between pediatric and adult trauma patients and incorporate these differences into their treatment protocols. The major concerns are related to the potential risks of increased transfusion requirements, missed associated injuries, and increased length of hospital stay. Each of these concerns is without merit.

Pancreas

Injuries to the pancreas occur in less than 10% of children sustaining blunt abdominal trauma. Two centers (Toronto and San Diego) reported their experience with divergent methods of managing blunt traumatic pancreatic injuries. The striking differences in these series are the 100% diagnostic sensitivity of CT scanning in Toronto versus 69% in San Diego and the 44% operative rate in San Diego versus 0% in Toronto. These reports from major pediatric trauma centers clearly conflict. Some favor and document the efficacy and safety of observational care for virtually all pancreatic traumas (including duct disruption), whereas others advocate aggressive surgical management with debridement and/or resections. Because proponents of each treatment plan supply compelling data for these treatment algorithms, individual hospital/surgeon preference will probably determine which treatment plan is selected. But with simple transection of the pancreas at or to the left of the spine, clearly spleen-sparing distal pancreatectomy can accomplish definitive care for this isolated injury with short hospitalization and acceptable morbidity. With this controversy in mind, we favor conservative therapy whenever possible with these features:

- Early spiral CT with oral and IV contrast in all patients who by history, physical examination, or mechanism of injury may have blunt trauma to the pancreas.
- Documentation of injuries and early endoscopic retrograde cholangiopancreatography (ERCP) to provide duct stenting in selected cases.
- Nonoperative management with nothing by mouth (NPO) and total parenteral nutrition (TPN).
- Expectant management of pseudocyst formation.
- Percutaneous drainage for symptomatic, infected, or enlarging pseudocyst.

Kidney

The kidney is the most commonly injured organ in the urogenital system, and children appear to be more susceptible to major renal trauma than adults. Several unique anatomic aspects contribute to this observation, including less cushioning from perirenal fat, weaker abdominal musculature, and a less-well-ossified thoracic cage. The child's kidney also occupies a proportionally larger space in the retroperitoneum than does an adult kidney. In addition, the pediatric kidney may retain fetal lobulations, permitting easier parenchymal disruption. Preexisting or congenital renal abnormalities, such as hydronephrosis, tumors, or abnormal position, may predispose the kidney to trauma despite relatively mild traumatic forces. The frequency of congenital abnormalities in injured kidneys ranges from 1% to 5%. Renal abnormalities, particularly hydronephrotic kidneys, may be first diagnosed after minor blunt abdominal trauma. Most often, these patients present with hematuria following blunt trauma. Others may present with an acute abdomen secondary to intraperitoneal rupture of the hydronephrotic kidney.

Once the patient is resuscitated and life-threatening injuries are addressed, evaluation of the genitourinary system can be undertaken. Following any blunt injury, the presence of hematuria (microscopic or gross), a palpable flank mass, or flank hematomas are indications for urologic evaluation. Most major blunt renal injuries occur in association with other major injuries of the head, chest, and abdomen. Urologic investigations should be undertaken when trauma to the lower chest is associated with rib, thoracic, or lumbar spine fractures. They should also be undertaken in all crush injuries to the abdomen or pelvis when the patient has sustained a severe deceleration injury. Because a renal pedicle injury or ureteropelvic junction disruption may not be associated with one of the classic signs of renal injury, such as hematuria, radiologic evaluation of the urinary tract should always be considered in patients with a mechanism of injury that could potentially injure the upper urinary tract.

Gross hematuria is the most reliable indicator for serious urologic injury. The need for imaging in the patient with blunt trauma and microscopic hematuria is not as clear cut. The degree of hematuria does not always correlate with the degree of injury. Renal vascular pedicle avulsion or acute thrombosis of segmental arteries can occur in the absence of hematuria, whereas mild renal contusions can manifest with gross hematuria. Detection of significant renal injury increased to 8% with significant microhematuria (more than 50 red blood cells per high power field [RBC/HPF]), and 32% in those with gross hematuria after blunt trauma. The presence of multisystem trauma significantly increases the risk for significant renal damage. Therefore, it is reasonable to consider observation with no renal imaging in children with microscopic hematuria of less than 50 RBC/HPF who are stable and without a mechanism of injury that is suspect for renal injury.

Historically, intravenous urography (IVP) was the radiographic imaging study of choice in suspected renal trauma. Sensitivity was as high as 90% in diagnosing renal injury. Unfortunately, IVP misses other intra-abdominal injuries and may miss or understage renal injury in children by 50% compared to CT scans. CT scans are now used almost exclusively as the imaging study of choice for suspected renal trauma in hemodynamically stable adults and children. CT is both sensitive and specific for demonstrating parenchymal laceration and urinary extravasation, delineating segmental parenchymal infarcts, and determining the size and location of the surrounding retroperitoneal hematoma and/or associated intra-abdominal injury. CT also allows for accurate staging of the renal injury.

In most patients, attempts should be made to manage all renal injuries conservatively. Minor renal injuries constitute the majority of blunt renal injuries and usually resolve without incident. The management of major renal parenchymal lacerations, although accounting for only 10% to 15% of all renal trauma patients, is controversial. Surgery is not always mandatory, and many major renal injuries caused by blunt trauma may be managed conservatively. When necessary, the goals of surgical renal exploration are either to treat major renal injuries definitively with preservation of renal parenchyma when possible or to thoroughly evaluate a suspected renal injury. The need for surgical exploration is much higher in patients with penetrating trauma as opposed to blunt trauma.

When conservative management is chosen, supportive care with bed rest, hydration, antibiotics, and serial hemoglobin and blood pressure monitoring is required for uneventful healing. After the gross hematuria resolves, limited activity is allowed for 2 to 4 weeks until microscopic hematuria ceases. Early complications can occur with observation within the first 4 weeks of injury and include delayed bleeding, abscess, sepsis, urinary fistula, urinary extravasation and urinoma, and hypertension.

The greatest risk is delayed hemorrhage occurring within the first 2 weeks of injury, which may be life threatening. Immediate surgical exploration or angiographic embolization is indicated. Angiographic embolization is an alternative to surgery in a hemodynamically stable patient in whom persistent gross hematuria signifies persistent low-grade hemorrhage from the injured kidney. Persistent urinary extravasation is managed successfully by percutaneous drainage. Hypertension in the early post-trauma period is uncommon. Hypertension may develop in the ensuing months and in most instances is treated with medical management.

Common Pitfalls

Frequent physical exams and vigilance are required for the subset of injuries caused in children wearing lap belt restraints while passengers in high-speed automobile crashes. These children present with visible *seat belt signs* on physical examination of the abdomen (Figure 1). Multiple studies document increased abdominal injuries to both solid and hollow organs with this finding. An interesting triad of injuries is noted in patients with a seat belt sign: abdominal wall contusions/herniation, Chance fractures of the lumbar spine, and isolated jejunal/ileal perforations. In a study of 95 patients, all wearing seat belts, who were admitted with abdominal trauma, 60 had a seat belt sign. The proportion of patients with intestinal injuries with and without the seat belt sign were 9 of 60 and 0 of 35, respectively. The more common injuries just described can distract both the patient and trauma team and delay the diagnosis of serious vascular injuries involving the aorta and iliac vessels.

Communication and Counseling

Recent advances in the delivery of trauma and critical care in children have resulted in improved outcome following major injuries. Pediatric surgeons must familiarize themselves with current treatment algorithms for life-threatening abdominal trauma such as "damage control" and the consequences of the abdominal compartment syndrome. Radiologists and endoscopists are making important contributions in the diagnosis and treatment of children with abdominal injury. Clinical experience and published reports addressing specific concerns about the nonoperative treatment of children with solid organ injuries and recent radiologic and endoscopic contributions have made pediatric trauma care increasingly nonoperative. Although the trend is in this direction, the pediatric surgeon should remain the physician of record in the multidisciplinary care of critically injured children. The decision not to operate is always a surgical decision.

SUGGESTED READINGS

1. Abou-Jaoude WA, Suggerman IM, Fallat ME, Casale AJ: Indicators of genitourinary tract injury or anomaly in cases of pediatric blunt trauma. J Pediatr Surg 31:86–89, 1996. **Historically, congenital abnormalities in injured kidneys have been reported in from 1% to 21% of patients. More accurate recent reviews have shown that incidence rates are 1% to 5%.**
2. Acierno SP, Jurkovich GJ, Nathens AB: Is pediatric trauma still a surgical disease? Patterns of emergent operative intervention in the injured child. J Trauma 56:960–966, 2004. **Details high incidence of operative intervention required in pediatric trauma patients supporting the need for a qualified pediatric trauma surgeon.**
3. Canty TG Sr, Weinman D: Management of major pancreatic duct injuries in children. J Trauma 50:1001–1007, 2001. **Report on 18 patients with major pancreatic injuries with distal pancreatectomy performed on 8 patients (44%).**
4. Chandler CF, Lane JS, Waxman KS: Seatbelt sign following blunt trauma is associated with increased incidence of abdominal injury. Am Surgeon 63:885–888, 1997. **Documenting that increased abdominal injuries to both solid and hollow organs occur when the seatbelt sign is present.**
5. Lutz N, Nance ML, Kallan MJ, et al: Incidence and clinical significance of abdominal wall bruising in restrained children involved in motor vehicle crashes. J Pediatr Surg 39:972–979, 2004. **Review of a database created by the State Farm Insurance Company on 147,985 children who were passengers in motor vehicle crashes indicating that those with the seatbelt sign were 232 times more likely to have a significant intra-abdominal injury then those without a bruise.**
6. Mooney DP, Forbes PW: Variation in the management of pediatric splenic injuries in New England. J Trauma 56:328–333, 2004. **Review of the New England Pediatric Trauma Database in the 1990s contrasting the care of 2500 children with spleen injury depending on the training of the surgeon with respect to pediatric trauma.**
7. Morey AF, Bruce JE, McAninch JW: Efficacy of radiographic imaging in pediatric blunt renal trauma. J Urol 156:2014–2018, 1996. **A meta-analysis of all reported series of children with hematuria and suspected renal injury noted that only 2% (11 of 548) of patients with insignificant microscopic hematuria (<50 RBC/HPF) had a significant renal injury.**
8. Patel JC, Tepas JJ: The efficacy of focused abdominal sonography for trauma (FAST) as a screening tool in the assessment of injured children. J Pediatric Surg 34:44–47, discussion 52–54, 1999. **Early reports have found FAST to be a useful screening tool in children, with a high specificity (95%) but a low sensitivity (33%) in identifying intestinal injury.**
9. Shilyansky J, Sen LM, Kreller M, et al: Nonoperative management of pancreatic injuries in children. J Pediatr Surg 33:343–345, 1998. **Report on 28 patients with major pancreatic injuries with no pancreatic resection required.**
10. Stylianos S, and the APSA Trauma Committee: Evidence-based guidelines for resource utilization in children with isolated spleen or liver injury. J Pediatr Surg 35:164–169, 2000. **Multi-institution**

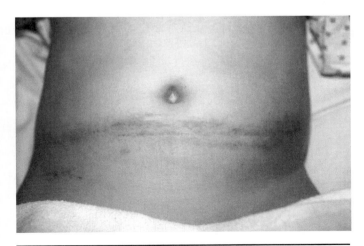

FIGURE 1. Seatbelt sign across lower abdomen.

database of 832 children with isolated liver or spleen injury based on CT grading treated nonoperatively at 32 centers in North America from 1995 to 1997.

11. Stylianos S, and the APSA Trauma Study Group. Prospective validation of evidence-based guidelines for resource utilization in children with isolated spleen or liver injury. J Pediatr Surg 37:453–456, 2002. **Prospective application of consensus guidelines in 312**

children with liver or spleen injuries treated nonoperatively at 16 centers from 1998 to 2000.

12. Tepas JJ, Frykberg ER, Schinco MA, et al: Pediatric trauma is very much a surgical disease. Ann Surg 237:775–781, 2003. **Details high incidence of operative intervention required in pediatric trauma patients supporting the need for a qualified pediatric trauma surgeon.**

Perinatal Care at the Threshold of Viability

Avroy A. Fanaroff

KEY CONCEPTS

- Most deaths occur in developing countries and at home.
- Infant mortality in the United States is 6 to 7 per 1000 live births.
- Mortality is related to race, birth weight, gestational age, gender, place of delivery, and intrauterine growth.
- Survival of infants of low birth weight improved with antenatal corticosteroids and surfactant, but for the past few years it has been static.
- Infants with a birth weight below 1 kg account for approximately 0.4%, and those below 750 g 0.2% of all deliveries, but these infants account for the bulk of the mortality and contribute disproportionately to the morbidity.
- Decisions regarding the limits of viability include medical and technologic issues compounded by moral, ethical, economic, social, religious, and sometimes even judicial issues.

Infant mortality is an important outcome measure of the health services of a population. Of the 130 million infants born every year worldwide, approximately 4 million die in the first 4 weeks of life. A similar number of infants are stillborn. Most neonatal deaths (99%) occur in developing countries; approximately half occur at home. In the United States, where approximately 4 million births are recorded each year, infant mortality hovers around 7 per 1000 live births. For the first time in more than 40 years, the infant mortality rate rose in 2002 to 7.0 deaths per 1000 live births from 6.8 per 1000 in 2001. Whereas the perinatal mortality rates for the past few decades have noticeably declined, the prematurity rate has remained fairly constant. The outlook for infants of extremely low birth weight and low gestational age has also improved remarkably in places where neonatal intensive care is available. Many factors influence neonatal mortality. In addition to race, birth weight, gestational age, gender, place of delivery, and intrauterine growth, there are wide variations in population descriptors, the criteria used for starting or withdrawing treatment, the reported duration of survival, and care.

A major challenge is the optimal management of the mother and infant when delivery takes place at the threshold of viability. When the topic of the limits of viability was addressed in the previous edition of this book, Marilee Allen said, "There are neither easy answers nor straightforward protocols when faced with the question of how aggressively to manage preterm infants born at the lower limit of viability." Despite new knowledge and insight concerning these infants, her comments remain appropriate at this time. Furthermore, given the complexity of the problem, no easy remedies are anticipated in the near future. Medical and technological issues are compounded by moral, ethical, economic, social, religious, and sometimes even judicial issues. The database for sophisticated decision making is insufficient, so health care providers are commonly forced to straddle the decision line of how and when to provide appropriate care, with a chance for a reasonable outcome, however defined, and not merely prolong life and suffering. Lines of communication among all the health care providers must be maintained at all times, and the family must be intimately involved in the decision-making process.

The factors that determine viability and the current neurodevelopmental outcomes of infants of extremely low birth weight are reviewed here to establish a foundation for decision making prior to and at the time of delivery. Although infants with a birth weight less than 1 kg account for approximately 0.4% and those below 750 g for 0.2% of all deliveries, they are responsible for the bulk of the mortality and contribute disproportionately to the morbidity. Because of technological advances, the ability to resuscitate and temporarily support even pre-viable infants is available. These relatively few deliveries tax the resources of any institution and require coordinated effort, skilled professionals, and excellent communication to meet the needs of all the parties involved. The use of resources is excessive with prolonged technology-dependent intensive care after extensive periods of hospitalization.

Expert Opinion on Management Issues

LIMITS OF VIABILITY: FACTORS DETERMINING MORTALITY

Improved survival of infants who are extremely immature and of low birth weight has blurred the definition of viability. Definitions of viability vary and include the ability to sustain independent life, to sustain life with the aid of a ventilator, to survive following intensive care, or to live and to grow and develop normally. The definition of viability will continue to change, so specific birth weight and gestational age numbers should be used only as a guide for decision making. Importantly, the available outcome data pertain to groups, but decisions must be made for individuals. Survival for the lowest gestational ages (currently 23 to 24 weeks) is complicated by very high rates of short- and long-term morbidity. These infants are at greater risk for cerebral palsy, mental retardation, deafness, and blindness. The perinatal team must coordinate all the perinatal information, inform the family and present them with their available options, be aware of their wishes regarding active resuscitation and intervention, and communicate the action plan to all individuals who may attend the delivery.

The prospective parents must be fully informed not only of the national data but also of the local outcome data and the risks and benefits of various interventions. Marked variations are apparent even within regions, depending on the aggression of caregivers regarding resuscitation and supportive care of infants born at the fringe of viability. The family must be informed of the complexities of care required for an extremely premature infant and the potential short- and long-term adverse outcomes. The risks and outlook may change frequently after the birth. Decisions about neonatal management made prior to delivery may be modified by the infant's condition, size, estimated gestational age, and responses to simple or invasive resuscitative measures. Repeated discussions with the families and consistency from the health care providers may facilitate a difficult task. Counseling must be sensitive to cultural and ethnic diversity, and a skilled translator should be available for parents whose primary language differs from the language of the care providers.

The appropriate management of infants born at the limits of viability is a subject of considerable debate. Strongly polarized viewpoints are held with and without supporting data. Reports on the outcomes of these pregnancies relate either to birth weight or gestational age. Whereas birth weight can be measured precisely, this number is not available prior to delivery, and estimates of birth weight may vary substantially from the actual birth weight. Gestational age is not nearly as precise unless an early ultrasound was performed. Ultrasonography may be helpful at the time of delivery when the date of the last menstrual period is uncertain, and it may also identify malformations, severe growth restriction, hydrops fetalis, or other conditions that could change the management plan. Intrapartum ultrasounds should not be used to alter the estimated gestational age, and they are not reliable enough in predicting birth weight when small differences may tilt the scales between what is considered to be a viable or nonviable fetus.

Race is an important determinant of mortality. In the United States in 2002, mortality rates were 5.8 per 1000 for non-Hispanic white infants; 13.9 per 1000 for non-Hispanic black infants, and 5.6 per 1000 for Hispanic births. African American women have many more preterm and very early preterm births, which, in part, explains the doubling of their fetal and infant mortality rates. Although for the total birth cohort, blacks have a higher mortality risk than whites, the reverse is noted at the lower weight group/gestational age distributions.

Birth weight and gestational age are the key factors determining perinatal outcome. Gestational age–specific outcomes depend on the criterion used to assess gestational age. Gestational age traditionally is reported as completed weeks from the last menstrual period, although some round to the closest week. The gestational age is also influenced by further adjustment according to ultrasound measures of fetal age. The postnatal assessment of gestational age, especially at 26 weeks' gestation and less, overestimates fetal age by up to 2 weeks, despite recent modifications in the examination. Gestational age outcomes are reported by the number of completed weeks. The outlook for an infant delivered at 24 1/7 weeks who weighs 550 g is very different from an infant at 24 6/7 weeks who weighs 900 g. Yet both would be considered at a gestational age of 24 weeks. A review of the world literature and our own experience reveals that at 23 weeks' gestation, survival ranges from 2% to 35%. At 24 weeks' gestation, the range is 17% to 62%, and at 25 weeks' gestation, 35% to 85%. Differences in population descriptors, in the initiation and withdrawal of treatment, and the duration of survival considered may account for the wide variations in the reported ranges of survival. Thus, every effort is made at 24 weeks' gestation and earnest decisions after due consultations at 23 weeks.

The birth weight at any given gestational age varies enormously as does the mortality rate. Specific outcomes related to birth weight are influenced by the fact that some reports pertain to birth weights of 500 g and above (e.g., 500 to 599 g), whereas others calculate from 501 g (e.g., 501 to 600 g). Because of a tendency to round off birth weight, such differences may influence survival rates. In 2001–2002, approximately 20% of infants weighing between 401 and 500 g survived their nursery stay, and 55% of infants between 501 and 750 g lived. Survival of infants weighing between 501 and 600 g approximates 40%; 60% of infants at birth weighing between 601 and 700 g and almost 80% of those between 701 and 800 g lived. These numbers continue to change and should be used as guidelines rather than absolute criteria when plans for resuscitation and ongoing intensive care are formulated. Despite the widespread publicity they receive, few with a birth weight below 500 g survive; the majority are females who are small for gestational age. The very poor neurodevelopmental outcomes and debilitating lung and eye morbidity of children less than 500 g birth weight probably reflect the combined effects of prematurity and severe intrauterine growth failure.

Gender is an important determinant of survival, and females have approximately a 20% lower risk of mortality at all immature gestational ages. Decisions regarding active resuscitation and viability thus should take into consideration the combination of projected birth weight, gestational age, and gender, as well as maternal history. Unfortunately, in many instances, the perinatal team is confronted by a patient who will deliver imminently with uncertain dates and has received no prenatal care. Neither birth weight nor gender is known. Perinatal morbidity and mortality are significantly increased in multiple gestations, and the incidence of severe handicap is increased in survivors of multiple gestations, which accounts for 26% of deliveries with birth weight below 1500 g.

Little to no success has been achieved with reducing the incidence of preterm birth, intrauterine growth restriction, and congenital malformations. However, over the past 20 years, the survival for infants of extremely low birth weight (<1500 g) has increased from 74% to 85%. Specific factors responsible for reducing mortality include the introduction of surfactant therapy for respiratory distress syndrome in 1990 and the widespread use of antenatal steroids that followed the National Institutes of Health (NIH) Consensus Conference in 1994. Prior to that time, only 20% of women who delivered infants with a birth weight of 1500 g or less received antenatal corticosteroids. That number now exceeds 80% in most centers in the United States and may be even higher in other parts of the world. Exposure to antenatal corticosteroids appears to be a critical determinant of survival for infants at the borders of viability. Care of infants with birth weights of 750 g or less has become more aggressive, so the rate of cesarean delivery has increased from 17% to 60%, and active resuscitation as evidenced by delivery room intubation has increased from 54% to 74%.

OBSTETRIC MANAGEMENT

No clear-cut guidelines are available regarding the obstetric management of the infants of extremely low birth weight. A cesarean delivery necessitates a vertical uterine incision, with increased risk of maternal morbidity. Furthermore, there is minimal documentation of improved outcome with cesarean delivery for extremely premature infants. Management of the infant should always be humane and compassionate, with provision of warmth and comfort. The Fetus and Newborn Committee, Canadian Pediatric Society, Maternal-Fetal Medicine Committee, and Society of Obstetricians and Gynaecologists of Canada are very specific regarding the management of women with threatened birth of an infant of extremely low gestational age:

Fetuses with a gestational age of less than 22 weeks are not viable and those with an age of 22 weeks rarely viable. Their mothers are not, therefore, candidates for cesarean section, and the newborns should be provided with compassionate care rather than active treatment. The outcomes for infants with a gestational age of 23 and 24 weeks vary greatly. Careful consideration should be given to the limited benefits for the infants and potential harms of cesarean section, as well as the expected results of resuscitation at birth. Cesarean section, when indicated, and any required neonatal treatment are recommended for infants with gestational ages of 25 and 26 completed weeks; most infants of this age will survive. And most survivors will not be severely disabled. Treatment of all infants with a gestational age of 22 to 26 weeks should be tailored to the infant and family and should involve fully informed parents.

Fetus and Newborn Committee,
Canadian Paediatric Society,
Maternal-Fetal Medicine Committee,
Society of Obstetricians and Gynaecologists of Canada

Common Pitfalls

- Available data only provide group data; we deal with individuals.
- Gestational age is not always reliable.
- Families do not always listen carefully or fully comprehend the complex survival data with which they are presented.
- It is nearly impossible to predict the outcome for an individual patient.
- The media over-report the "miracles" and under-report the bad outcomes, leading to unrealistic expectations.

Communication and Counseling

When resuscitation is not performed because of extreme immaturity or other considerations, the family must be carefully supported. They must be allowed access to support personnel, including the hospital staff, clergy, relatives, and close friends. They should be encouraged and permitted to hold, touch, and interact with the infant. The infant should be weighed and measured and the information provided to the mother. The infant should be gently handled and kept warm and comfortable. Ongoing support following the infant's demise is essential. Counseling regarding the mourning process as well as for future pregnancies is mandatory.

In summary, the obstetric and pediatric team, supported by nursing specialists, social workers, and bioethicists, should confer and then counsel the family. Realistic outcomes must be presented, including the risks for moderate or severe disability, mental retardation, cerebral palsy, visual impairment including blindness, hearing loss, and the need for special education. The team must take into consideration the fact that there is no ethical distinction between withholding and withdrawing life-sustaining treatments. Humane care must be provided to all infants including those where life-sustaining interventions are either being withheld or withdrawn. Parents should be encouraged to participate actively in the decision-making process concerning the treatment of their infant. Families should be treated with dignity and compassion at all times. In this manner, a course of action for the delivery and immediate management of the fetus can be established. Continuation of care is based on the condition of the infant with the family fully informed of the condition and plans at all times.

The limits of viability will remain a moving target as long as viability means the ability to survive so that life would be considered worthwhile to the infant or the parents. Hospital neonatal survival rates of infants at the limits of viability are significantly lower with the inclusion of fetal deaths. This information should be considered when providing prognostic advice to families when mothers are in labor at 22 to 25 weeks' gestation.

Early Childhood Outcomes

Advances in perinatal care have led to the survival of increasing numbers of children born at the lower limits of viability. Children with very low birth weight have poorer outcomes relative to normal birth weight term-born controls in neurologic and health status, cognitive and neuropsychological skills, school performance, academic achievement, and behavior. Outcomes are highly variable but related to neonatal medical complications of prematurity and social risk factors. With more survivors, there are both increased numbers who survive intact as well as a greater number of handicapped survivors (Wilson, 2005).

The major morbidities that influence later development include bronchopulmonary dysplasia (BPD), severe brain injury, necrotizing enterocolitis (NEC), nosocomial infections, and retinopathy of prematurity. Additional neonatal factors associated with later outcomes include transient hypothyroxinemia and breast-milk feeding. Morbidity increases with decreasing gestational age and birth weight, and it varies according to demographic and clinical therapeutic practice differences. Fifty percent of survivors of less than 750 g birth weight and the majority at 24 to 25 weeks' gestation have one or more neonatal complications. Many infants are discharged home on oxygen and apnea monitors, and they require rehospitalizations for respiratory complications associated with BPD. Factors predictive of poor neurodevelopmental outcome include low birth weight; male gender; the severity of cerebral ultrasound abnormality, including periventricular leukomalacia (PVL) and persistent ventriculomegaly; BPD; and growth failure. In addition to gross neurologic deficits, including cerebral palsy, hydrocephalus, and hemiplegia, these infants are susceptible to growth failure, deafness, and blindness. Many of the severely disabled children have multiple impairments. Furthermore, many infants who are neurologically intact and appear normal at 18 to 24 months of age have a variety of learning problems at school.

Major neonatal morbidity increases with decreasing gestational age and birth weight. At 23 weeks' gestation, chronic lung disease occurs in 57% to 86% of survivors; at 24 weeks, in 33% to 89%; and at 25 weeks, in 16% to 71% of survivors. The rates of severe cerebral ultrasound abnormality range from 10% to 83% at 23 weeks' gestation, 9% to 64% at 24 weeks, and 7% to 22% at 25 weeks. Of 77 survivors at 23 weeks' gestation, 26 (34%) have severe disability (defined as subnormal cognitive function, cerebral palsy, blindness and/or deafness). At 24 weeks' gestation, the rates of severe neurodevelopmental disability range from 22% to 45%, and at 25 weeks, 12% to 35%. The continuing toll of major neonatal morbidity and neurodevelopmental handicap is of serious concern. Vohr (2005), on the basis of evaluation of a multicenter cohort at 18 to 22 months' corrected age, noted that infants of extremely low birth weight (<1 kg) are at significant risk of neurologic abnormalities, developmental delays, and functional delays. Twenty-five percent of the children had an abnormal neurologic examination; 37% had a Bayley II Mental Developmental Index less than 70; 29% had a Psychomotor Developmental Index less than 70; 9% had vision impairment, and 11% had hearing impairment. Neurologic, developmental, neurosensory, and functional morbidities increased with decreasing birth weight. Factors significantly associated with increased neurodevelopmental morbidity included BPD; grades III and IV intraventricular hemorrhage (IVH); PVL; the use of steroids for BPD and NEC; and male gender. With the expanded use of more sophisticated imaging techniques, many preterm infants with normal ultrasounds are found by MRI to have evidence of white matter injury, including white matter atrophy, periventricular leukomalacia, ventricular dilation, thinning of the corpus callosum, and enlarged subarachnoid space. The correlation between these MRI findings and developmental outcome are ongoing.

Early Childhood Neurodevelopmental Outcomes

The majority of reports of early childhood outcomes consider children severely disabled or impaired if they have either a major neurologic abnormality, such as cerebral palsy; unilateral or bilateral blindness; deafness requiring hearing aids; and/or cognitive functioning less than two standard deviations of the mean (mental development less than 68 or 70). These measures are criticized; however, few measures of functioning and quality of life have been validated during early childhood. Factors affecting the rates of disability include survival selection, the sociodemographic descriptors of the population, varying rates of neonatal complications and resultant chronic disease, whether the age of the child is corrected for preterm birth, and the duration and rates of follow-up. There is also variation in the clinical diagnosis of cerebral palsy and definition of lesser degrees of neurosensory and cognitive dysfunction. Children from lower sociodemographic backgrounds are more commonly lost to follow-up, which may influence outcomes. In general, the rates of disability increase with decreasing gestational age and birth weight, but this varies, possibly because of the poor reliability of determining gestational age and the selected survival of lower risk infants of 23 and 24 weeks' gestation.

In the majority of studies, the rates of subnormal cognitive function are much higher than those of neurosensory impairment. Half or more of the children considered impaired may thus have global developmental delay without cerebral palsy or other neurosensory impairments.

The overall consensus, despite improvements in survival following the introduction of surfactant therapy, is that the rates of neurodevelopmental handicap remained unchanged in the early to mid–1990s. However, increased survival, but deteriorating developmental outcomes for 23 to 25 weeks' gestation infants born during the latter part of the 1990s, is attributed to increased use of postnatal corticosteroids.

Survival of infants of extremely low birth weight and gestational age increased in the early 1990s because of the combined effects of increase in assisted ventilation at delivery, surfactant therapy, and possibly increased use of antenatal steroid therapy. The gestational age of viability, considered to be 23 to 24 weeks' gestation, has not changed, but survival has increased slowly at these limits of viability. Current technology and methods of care appear to have encountered a biologic barrier. The next major breakthrough is awaited. Of major concern is the fact that the already high rates of neonatal morbidity, including BPD, sepsis, and poor growth, have persisted or even increased. High rates of neurodevelopmental handicap during early childhood have also persisted and possibly increased. When these children reach school age, high rates of school failure and learning problems can be anticipated. It is worth noting, too, that most survivors are ambulatory and mainstreamed at school, but 50% to 70% of the children who have normal cognitive scores demonstrate learning disorders.

Families must be made aware that the treatment of the extremely immature and small infant is, to a certain extent, still experimental and fraught with a high mortality and prolonged neonatal morbidity. Although most surviving children eventually lead fairly normal lives, major developmental and learning problems must be anticipated. Because it is not possible to predict how an individual child will later develop, ongoing assessment and support with proactive programs need to be provided from infancy and into the school years.

In sum, the majority of infants born at 22 weeks or less, and with a birth weight of less than 500 g, should receive only comfort care. For those born at 23 weeks, flexibility is recommended with regard to resuscitation, with careful consideration of the views of the family, the pregnancy history, and the condition of the infant at birth, whereas for infants born at 24 weeks and beyond, full resuscitation is warranted.

SUGGESTED READINGS

1. American Academy of Pediatrics Fetus and Newborn Committee, American College of Obstetricians and Gynecologists Committee on Obstetric Practice. Perinatal care at the threshold of viability. Pediatrics 96:974–976, 1995. **The dilemma of defining threshold of viability.**
2. Fetus and Newborn Committee, Canadian Paediatric Society, Maternal-Fetal Medicine Committee, Society of Obstetricians and Gynaecologists of Canada: Management of the woman with threatened birth of an infant of extremely low gestational age. CMAJ 151(5):547–553, 1994. **How the experts define the borders of viability.**
3. Lawn J, Cousens S, Zupan J: 4 million neonatal deaths; When? Where? Why? The Lancet Neonatal Survival, March 2005. Available online at http://www.thelancet.com. **Global approach to perinatal mortality.**
4. MacDorman MF, Martin JA, Mathews TJ, et al: Explaining the 2001–02 infant mortality increase: Data from the linked birth/infant death data set. Mon Vital Stat Rep 24; 53:1–22, 2005. **Provides most recent data on perinatal mortality, neonatal mortality, and related subjects.**
5. Marlow N, Wolke D, Bracewell MA, Samara M: EPICure Study Group: Neurologic and developmental disability at six years of age after extremely preterm birth. N Engl J Med 6; 352:9–19, 2005. **Outstanding follow-up of a national cohort (the EPICure study).**
6. Vohr BR, Allen M: Extreme prematurity—the continuing dilemma. N Engl J Med 352:71–72, 2005. **Editorial discussing outcome at age 6 for infants born at 22–25 weeks of gestation.**
7. Wilson-Costello D, Friedman H, Minich N, et al: Improved survival rates with increased neurodevelopmental disability for extremely low birth weight infants in the 1990s. Pediatrics 115 (4): 997–1003, 2005. **The cost of survival—balancing death and disability.**

Preventing Childhood Injuries

Joel L. Bass

4

KEY CONCEPTS

- Injuries are the leading cause of death in children ages 1 through 19 years and are an important cause of death in the first year of life.
- The most frequently occurring injuries in children include motor vehicle accidents, drowning, fires, poisoning, and falls.
- In addition to causing death, injuries are also a very significant cause of morbidity, resulting in both emergency department visits and hospital admissions.
- Although most injuries are preventable, many children continue to sustain injuries because of factors both within and outside the home.
- Passive interventions that require no parental action are usually the most effective.

Injuries are the leading cause of death in children ages 1 through 19 years and are an important cause of death in the first year of life. The most frequently occurring injuries in children include motor vehicle accidents, drowning, fires, poisoning and falls. In addition to causing death, injuries are also a very significant cause of morbidity resulting in both emergency department visits and hospital admission. Although most injuries are preventable, many children continue to sustain injuries owing to a variety of factors both within and outside of the home.

Conceptually, there are two major models of the childhood injury—epidemiologic and biomechanical. The epidemiologic model is based on host-agent issues that consider the child, the parent, and the environment within the social context as interdependent factors that serve to cause, modify, or prevent an injury. The biomechanical model incorporates dynamic principles that view an injury as resulting from a pathologic energy

TABLE 1 Haddon's Matrix

Stage	Education	Technology	Government Action
Pre-event	Prevent the injury occurrence.		
Event	Reduce the severity of the injury.		
Postevent	Improve the treatment of the injury.		

TABLE 2 Passive Approaches to Injury Prevention (1953–1974)

Approach	Result
Flammable Fabrics Act	Clothing ignition deaths decreased by 71% (males) and 82% (females)
Poison Prevention Packaging Act	Virtual disappearance of salicylate poisoning
Children Can't Fly	50% decrease in falls (New York City)
Child Protection and Toy Safety Act	Substantial decrease in toy injuries
Federal Crib Standard	40% decrease in deaths caused by head entrapment

exchange involving mechanical, thermal, electric, or chemical energy with the child. Both models are useful in understanding how injuries occur and in designing preventive strategies. Haddon's matrix, first described in 1977, provides a useful framework for planning preventive strategies. Haddon proposed a triphasic temporal approach (Table 1) that could be linked to various intervention strategies. The approach provides a logical framework on which preventive programs can be developed.

The role of the physician in injury prevention includes direct communication with individual parents and participating in public education programs. As passive interventions, which require no parental action, are usually the most effective (Table 2), legislative and regulatory advocacy to promote adoption of these strategies are also a critically important physician responsibility.

Expert Opinion on Management Issues

Effective counseling about preventing childhood injuries requires familiarity with a large body of rapidly changing information. A major resource containing expert opinion on childhood injury control is the American Academy of Pediatrics (AAP). As an example, guidelines for appropriate infant and child restraints, which can significantly protect children from motor vehicle passenger injuries, are available from the AAP (Fig. 1). All current AAP policies regarding childhood injuries, and examples of parent teaching materials, can be found on the AAP web site (http://www.aap.org). The AAP publication, "Injury Prevention and Control for Children and Youth," also provides a wealth of information on many important childhood injury-related topics.

Additionally, helpful written and web-based resources are available from government agencies such as the Centers for Disease Control and Prevention (http://www.cdc.gov) and the Consumer Product Safety Commission (http://www.cpsc.gov). A comprehensive web-based directory, the Injury Control Resource Network (http://www.injurycontrol.com/icrin/) maintained by the Center for Injury Research and Control based at the University of Pittsburgh, provides access to up-to-date information from every major public and private source on all relevant injury control issues.

Common Pitfalls

- The primary care physician should not miss opportunities to teach parents about injury prevention.
- The physician should not fail to recognize both socioeconomic and cultural issues that may affect parental compliance with injury prevention messages.
- The physician should provide parents with current information about safety messages. Just as with immunizations, it is essential to frequently review guidelines from professional sources such as the AAP (see Fig. 1).

Visits for minor trauma should be viewed as opportunities to analyze the situation that led to the injury. Although such "teachable moments" can be effective times to review and consolidate injury prevention messages, these should not substitute for an organized educational program incorporated into health supervision visits. A disorganized approach to this problem will lead to significant gaps in potentially beneficial parental practices. In either counseling situation, the physician must provide accurate and current advice to parents to maintain credibility on this issue.

The AAP Children's Safety Research Project was implemented to understand family concerns about safety and what they did to keep children safe. One of their interesting findings was that parents were strongly influenced by their concepts of what a good parent does. Urban parents, who felt that good parents keep an eye on their children, sometimes felt that equipment was unnecessary because they directly supervised their children. In contrast, suburban families, who felt that a good parent uses safety equipment, were more inclined to follow advice about preventive devices.

Communication and Counseling

The pediatrician is in a unique position to counsel parents of young children about injury prevention. Studies show that not only are parents quite anxious about the possibility of their child experiencing an injury, but they also view the pediatrician as an important educational resource. Also, primary care–based counseling sometimes results in educational acquisition, behavioral change, and even injury reduction. The studies of behavioral change—which demonstrate increased use of car seats, seat belts, and smoke detectors—are of particular

Infant and Child Restraints:
Selecting the Appropriate Type

- The safest place in a car for all children is the rear seat.
- Never place a rear-facing infant seat (child under 1 year and 20 lb) in the front seat of a vehicle with a passenger-side air bag.
- In an emergency, if a child (more than 1 year and 20 lb) must ride in the front seat, make sure he or she is properly restrained and then move the vehicle seat as far back as possible, away from the air bag.

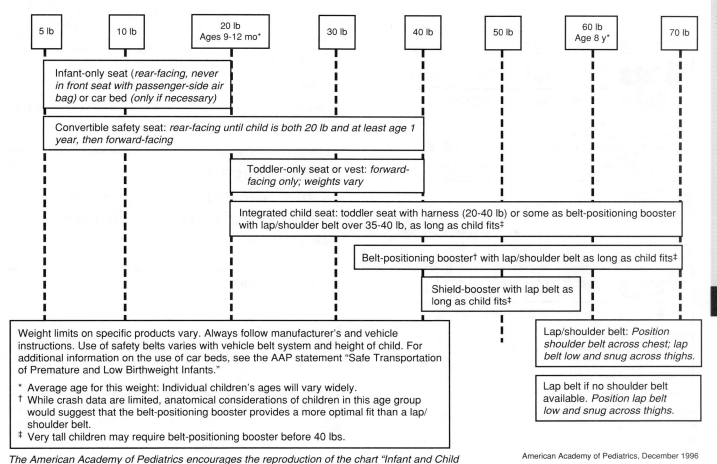

The American Academy of Pediatrics encourages the reproduction of the chart "Infant and Child Restraints: Selecting the Appropriate Type" for noncommercial, educational purposes.

American Academy of Pediatrics, December 1996

FIGURE 1. American Academy of Pediatrics guidelines for infant and child restraints. (AAP Guidelines/AAP TIPP Program. Used with permission of the American Academy of Pediatrics.)

importance because the inherent efficacy of these interventions is quite substantial (Table 3). Both the United States Preventive Services Task Force and the Canadian Task Force on the Periodic Health Examination concluded that the existing evidence supports pediatricians' counseling parents to prevent childhood injuries.

A system for implementing injury prevention counseling in primary care settings, the Injury Prevention Program (TIPP), has been developed by the AAP. The program is based on the AAP policy to provide office-based counseling to prevent injuries and includes both a counseling schedule and a series of age-appropriate information sheets for parents that serve to emphasize and reinforce the most important safety messages at every age. Additionally, TIPP includes the Framingham Safety Surveys, a series of developmentally oriented questionnaires that are designed to meet the specific counseling needs of the caretaker. Each survey is designed as a multiple-choice questionnaire with a physician copy in which "at-risk" responses can be readily identified (Fig. 2). A Physician Counseling Guide, which includes specific injury prevention messages, is also included in the program. Use of TIPP allows the pediatrician to implement a comprehensive program that is updated regularly by the AAP.

Although this discussion has focused on counseling parents of young children, counseling the parents of older children and adolescents and the children and teens themselves is important. The evidence of counseling efficacy has not been demonstrated in these groups. The pediatrician's role, as an advocate who communicates with legislators about injury prevention

TABLE 3 Effective Injury Prevention Methods

Method	Decreased Injuries	Decreased Mortality
Car seats	67%	54%–71%
Seat belts	45%–55%	40%–50%
Smoke detectors	88%	86%

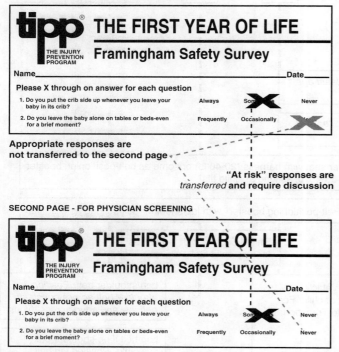

FIRST PAGE - FOR PARENTAL RESPONSES

SECOND PAGE - FOR PHYSICIAN SCREENING

FIGURE 2. Framingham safety surveys. (Reprinted from American Academy of Pediatrics' Injury Prevention Program Guide, 1994. AAP Guidelines/AAP TIPP Program. Used with permission of the American Academy of Pediatrics.)

legislation such as graduated driving licenses and handgun control, is a more important function for these children.

SUGGESTED READINGS

1. Bass JL, Christoffel KK, Widame M, et al: Childhood injury prevention counseling in primary care settings: A critical review of the literature. Pediatrics 92:4, 1993. **A systematic review of the literature concerning the efficacy of primary care–based injury prevention counseling.**
2. Bonnie RJ, Fulco CE, Liverman CT (eds): Reducing the burden of injury: Advancing prevention and treatment. Committee on Injury Prevention and Control, Division of Health Promotion and Disease Prevention, Institute of Medicine, Washington, DC: National Academies Press, 1999. **A high-quality source of information on the public health aspects of injury prevention including a chapter on economic issues.**
3. Committee Injury and Poison Prevention. Injury Prevention and Control for Children and Youth, 3rd ed. Elk Grove Village, Ill: American Academy of Pediatrics, 1997. **Summary of information on childhood injuries and AAP preventive recommendations.**
4. National Committee for Injury Prevention and Control. Injury Prevention. Meeting the Challenge. New York: Oxford University Press, 1989. **Detailed historical perspective on the process of injury prevention.**
5. National Safety Council. Injury Facts, 1999 Edition. Washington, DC: National Safety Council, 1999. **A good source of information on injury statistics (updated annually).**
6. Spady DW, Saunders DL, Schopflocher DP, et al: Patterns of injury in children: A population-based approach. Pediatrics 119:3, 2004. **A recent report on the use of administrative data to identify age-specific patterns of injury.**
7. U.S. Preventive Services Task Force. Guide to Clinical Preventive Services, 2nd ed. Baltimore: Williams & Wilkins, 1996. **Detailed analysis of the effectiveness of clinical preventive services (including injuries) published periodically by the U.S. Preventive Services Task Force.**
8. Wilson MH, Bake SP, Teret SP, et al: Saving Children. A Guide to Injury Prevention. New York: Oxford University Press, 1991. **A detailed survey of the field of childhood injury prevention.**

Adherence to Treatment in Children and Adolescents Living with Chronic Illness

Dorothy Fielding and Alistair J. A. Duff

KEY CONCEPTS

- Partial adherence should be viewed as a normative response in complex treatment regimens for pediatric chronic illness.
- A collaborative, "blame-free" problem-solving approach in multidisciplinary management is crucial.
- A clear standard should be adopted for each adherent behavior within a treatment program.
- Evidence-based psychoeducational, behavioral, and organizational methods should be part of treatment protocols for children with chronic illness.
- Preparing patients and caregivers for relapse in adherent behavior is essential.
- Individual or family intervention with a team psychologist or mental health specialist may be necessary when nonadherence is pervasive, influenced by family conflict, or part of a complex reaction to an illness and treatment.
- Motivational interviewing is a promising new approach for young people for whom avoidant coping or peer group pressures are important barriers to optimal adherence.

The delivery of pediatric health care is in part dependent on the willingness of patients to follow prescribed regimens. No matter how effective treatments are, if parents and children are unable to follow medical instructions adequately, then health care will be compromised.

Engaging parents, children, and young people in treatment plans is a major and essential task for all child health care providers. However, studies have estimated that the nonadherence rates in some chronic conditions are so high that poor adherence should be viewed as a normative response to the demands of treatment and illness. This is a worldwide problem; many countries report adherence rates of around 50% (World Health Organization, 2003). Moreover, recent investigations that employ electronic monitoring to measure adherence suggest that even this estimate is optimistic.

Problems in adherence can lead to serious medical complications. For example, ketoacidosis in children and adolescents with juvenile diabetes, compromised pulmonary function in children with cystic fibrosis, recurrent symptoms in young children with asthma, and length of graft survival in children and adolescents with renal transplants have all been linked to low levels of adherence in some patient groups. Such difficulties in following prescribed regimens have been described as a "cost problem," because the resultant nonadherence leads to increased rates of hospitalization, greater length of hospital stay, and increased health care expenditures. It is, therefore, essential that methods to assess and improve adherence become integral to the treatment process.

Expert Opinion on Management Issues

DEFINITIONS

Traditionally, compliance has been defined as *the extent to which a person's behavior coincides with medical advice*. However, this narrow definition has been criticized, because it implies that patients are the passive recipients of expert advice and can be categorized using a simple dichotomy of "compliant" or "noncompliant." In contrast, current approaches suggest that children, young people, and their families have more active and collaborative roles, working with clinical teams in planning and implementing treatment. Exponents of these recent approaches argue that adherent behavior is better conceptualized on a continuum in which the extremes of "complete adherence" and "nonadherence" are rare. Furthermore, it is now clear that even within disease categories, adherent behaviors are not strongly correlated with one another. For example, children may follow a physician's instructions precisely regarding oral medication regimens but following dietary recommendations may be more problematic.

A further difficulty in defining adherence arises from the fact that in many cases, there are no clear or simple instructions to be followed. Many treatment regimens are complex and require judgments to be made by a parent, child, or adolescent. Additionally, there may be a lack of precise information about what should be considered sufficiently adherent for a particular condition and the prescribed course of therapy.

Current definitions reflect the need to adopt reasonable criteria, developed to suit the specific context of an individual patient's behavior. The World Health Organization now defines adherence as "the extent to which a person's behavior...corresponds with *agreed* recommendations from a health care provider." There is also a much greater acknowledgment that patients and their families should be supported in ways that consider their individual needs and preferences.

FACTORS AFFECTING NONADHERENCE

Poor treatment adherence is associated with a wide range of factors. Such factors can be useful in helping to identify children who are particularly "at risk" for adhering suboptimally and in directing the choice of interventions to assist them and their families (Table 1).

Adherence problems have been found to increase with increasing time from diagnosis in a number of chronic conditions. The longer a child has to maintain a treatment regimen, the more difficult adherence can become. Additionally, adherence problems appear to be greater when a child has greater functional impairment or an additional physical handicap.

Adherence also appears to be poorer with complex and time-consuming regimens (e.g., cystic fibrosis, diabetes, end-stage renal failure) and when treatment offers no perceived immediate benefit (e.g., nebulized therapies in the treatment of cystic fibrosis). Side effects and the palatability of oral medication may also be important factors, because these can also deter young patients from engaging in treatments.

Age is also an important factor. For instance, studies with diabetic patients indicate that adolescents have poorer rates of adherence to daily insulin injections, exercise, diet, and glucose test prescriptions as compared to younger children. Similar findings have been

---

TABLE 1 Factors Influencing Treatment Adherence in Children and Adolescents Living with Chronic Illness

Illness and Treatment	Patient	Family	Social and Material Resources	Health Care Provider
Duration of illness (longer time since diagnosis) Functional impairment and physical handicap Complexity of regimen Treatment side effects	Limited knowledge and/or skills Age and developmental stage (adolescents more nonadherent) Adjustment and coping (anxiety, depression, and avoidant coping style)	Poor problem solving Lack of cohesion Poor communication Large family size	Financial constraints Lack of social support	Poor communication Organization of clinics

Amended from Fielding D, Duff A: Compliance with treatment protocols: Interventions for children with chronic illness. Arch Dis Child 80:196–200, 1999.

noted for children with chronic renal diseases in which adherence to fluid restrictions are important.

Adjustment and coping are also important. Children who have had difficulties in adjusting to diagnosis and those showing high levels of distress or avoidant coping styles are more likely to experience difficulties with their treatment regimens.

Family factors are also important. Children with parents who are more supportive, more flexible, less critical, and good at problem solving have been observed to have fewer problems with adherence, possibly because such parents can supervise and support children through difficult aspects of the regimen without excessive conflict or difficulty.

Finally, good communication by the clinical team, well-organized clinics, and effective training of health care staff have all been noted as essentials in promoting adequate adherence. Determining the extent to which families can cope with complex regimens, responding accordingly, and minimizing the number of lifestyle changes are essential to effective pediatric care.

MEASUREMENT

Adherence rates vary according to the patient sample (age, disease, treatment regimen), the specific behavior being assessed (pill taking, injections, glucose monitoring, inhaler use), the method of measuring adherence (patient diaries, electronic pill dispensers), and the classification system used. Table 2 summarizes the advantages and disadvantages of a number of different methods of measuring adherence.

Methods for measuring adherence over time are increasingly included in pediatric treatment protocols. Continuous and positive feedback about how well children are adhering to their treatment is important in the proactive management of any condition. As far as possible, the chosen method for regular monitoring of adherence should balance practicalities with reliability. Moreover, the measurement of adherence should not be confused with the measurement of health status; each should be assessed separately.

Fundamental to the whole approach of assessing adherence is an open and "blame-free" approach from the multidisciplinary clinical team. Accepting and explaining adherence problems as an inevitable aspect of living with and treating childhood chronic illness is a first step in this process.

INTERVENTIONS

Organizational, educational, and psychotherapeutic strategies have all been used alone or in combination in studies to improve adherence in children with chronic illness. There is now considerable evidence for the effectiveness of these strategies.

Organizational

Organizing and coordinating team responses and shared team values are crucial to facilitating good patient relationships and meaningful attempts to address adherence. Much can be done at a team level to provide the environment for encouraging and supporting adherent behaviors, and organizational changes have been built into many of the programs set up to help children and their families (Table 3).

Psychoeducational Methods

Psychoeducational approaches attempt to improve adherence by promoting knowledge about the condition (e.g., its cause, prognosis, and treatment), and providing training in recognition of factors that adversely affect adherence (e.g., negative emotional reactions to

TABLE 2 Methods of Assessing Treatment Adherence

Method	Advantages	Disadvantages
Biochemical measures (assays, markers, etc.)	Direct correlates of drug consumption Specific measures	Not for long-term use. Expensive, invasive.
Electronic or mechanical monitors	Precise monitoring (date and time) Continuous data over long time periods Eliminates self-report bias	Expensive, possible technical difficulties. Only certain behaviors are measured (pill taking, nebulizer/inhaler use). May still be subject to "faking."
Pill counts	Easy to administer Confirms patient/parent report	Only one aspect of regime covered. Relies on patient/parent to remember to return unused medication.
Standardized questionnaire	Simple, inexpensive Covers all aspects of regimen Identifies barriers to adherence	Subject to reporting and recall bias. Underestimates nonadherence.
24-hour retrospective recall, telephone interview	Improves recall Easy to administer	Requires trained interviewers. Can be time-consuming.
Diary/log	Completed daily, less subject to recall problems, can cover most behaviors	Time-consuming for patient/parent. Data may be complex. Reporting and recall bias still possible.
Physician/health professional ratings	Easy to use Identifies adherent patients	Limited objectivity. May confuse health status with adherence if global ratings used. Overestimates adherence. Does not engage the family.

diagnosis) and techniques improve adherence. Such interventions should also use the substantial body of evidence, now available, on how to construct written leaflets for patients that are easy to read and understand. This includes advice on how materials can be organized and categorized to aid retention (see Table 3).

Psychotherapeutic Approaches

Effective psychotherapeutic approaches are predominantly based on behavioral and cognitive principles. These interventions generally incorporate techniques based on social learning theory and, more recently, work on attitudes, beliefs, and cognitions. The assumption underlying such strategies is that some existing behaviors are difficult to change because they have been established over long periods of time. Accordingly, lasting change involves the breaking down of habitual patterns of behavior and the establishment of new routines. These new behaviors may be quite difficult to develop because they may be accompanied by negative side effects, which can outweigh the more nebulous and longer-term promise of improved health outcomes.

In some cases psychopathology may act as a barrier to treatment adherence (e.g., depression, anxiety, family conflict), and more individualized psychotherapeutic approaches are needed. Clearly, such difficulties impinge on the ability of a patient and/or family to engage with medical teams and treatments. Again, there is good evidence for the effectiveness of psychological therapies for these types of difficulty.

INTERVENTIONS WITH PROMISE

The success of strategies aimed at improving treatment adherence is in part dependent on a child, young person, or parent's motivation and readiness to change. Motivational interviewing is a form of psychological intervention that shows promise in improving rates of adherence. It is also an approach that can be used by all members of the multidisciplinary team.

To date most studies have been concerned with the treatment of substance abuse, and systematic reviews have reported impressive effect sizes; however, studies aimed at evaluating the effectiveness of similar interventions to improve treatment adherence in children

---

TABLE 3 Methods to Improve Adherence

Components	Examples
Organizational	
Shared multidisciplinary team approach to adherence strategies	Shared perspective of "blame-free approach," normalizing non-adherent behaviors providing aids to adherence
Improving accessibility to health care	Outreach clinics, removing barriers to attending, support by telephone
Child-, family-friendly settings	Same health care professional each visit, clinic play facilities
Minimizing treatment negative side effects	Simplifying treatments
	Tailoring treatments to family lifestyle
Psychoeducational	
Information about the illness and treatment.	*How*: leaflets, videos, CDs, slide shows, program handouts.
Description of side effects together with the problems of adhering to complex regimes.	Demonstrations, use of age-appropriate models, behavioral rehearsal.
Recognition of barriers to adherence.	*To whom*: individual children, parents.
The benefits of using long-term consistent strategies to improve adherence.	*Where*: during normal clinic visits, during separate visits to clinics, by separate telephone calls, at home
Relapse prevention training.	*By*: doctors, nurses, therapists, member of psychosocial team
Psychotherapeutic (e.g., behavioral and cognitive interventions)	
Self-monitoring	Parental or child diaries of medication intake
Control over stimuli that evoke patterns of behavior that need to change	Teeth brushing (stimulus) causing drinking (behavior) in children on dialysis
Goal-setting	Level of frequency of glucose monitoring.
Behavioral contracting	Written contract with child, parent, and doctor about the specific behaviors that are required.
Corrective feedback and reinforcement	Avoidance of blame and criticism. Systematic encouragement and rewards for approximations to goals.
Motivational	
Establish and express empathy.	Listen to and understand the patient's perspective.
Provide choice (to change or not).	Respect patient choices, values, and decisions.
Clarify patient's treatment goals.	Facilitate patient's consideration of the advantages
Help to develop discrepancy (between current behavior and patient's own goals).	and disadvantages of behavior change.
Empathize and work with resistance.	Avoid arguing for change. Resistance is not directly opposed. New perspectives are invited but not imposed. Accept that goals of treatment will vary between patients and patients and doctors.
Remove barriers to change.	Patient is encouraged to find own answers and solutions.
Provide frequent and regular feedback.	Positively reinforce any small changes or contemplation of change.
Support the development of patient self-efficacy.	Health professional supports patients' growing sense that they can bring about change.

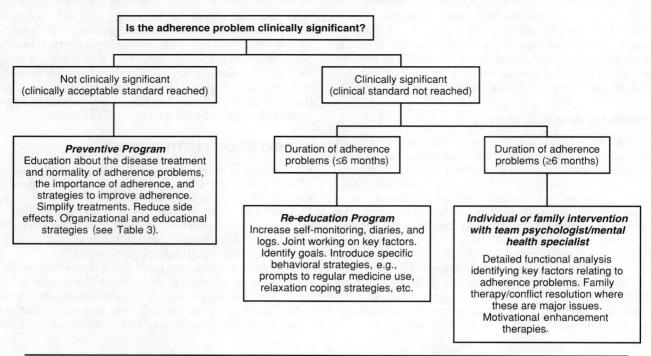

FIGURE 1. Timing of interventions to improve treatment adherence in pediatric chronic conditions.

and young adults with chronic illnesses are beginning to emerge. In helping patients to change their adherence behavior, the emphasis is on a collaborative rather than a coercive approach in which patients' choices, values, and decisions are respected, goals negotiated, and ambivalence openly explored.

The style is client centered and client led and consequently particularly appropriate when working with adolescents and young adults because it draws on their own perceptions, treatment goals, and values at a time when they are establishing an identity as autonomous individuals, separate from their parents and other family members (see Table 3).

Common Pitfalls

Earlier sections have commented on a range of methods and approaches to improve adherence. However, key issues remain concerning how, when, and by whom such methods are delivered. Some psychosocial interventions can be costly and labor intensive and it is essential that they are adopted in the most appropriate ways. It is also important that all members of the multidisciplinary team are engaged in methods to facilitate adherence behaviors. Some researchers in this area have considered adoption of a primary, secondary, and tertiary prevention program to improve adherence. Figure 1 presents this diagrammatically.

Communication and Counseling

Adherence rates can be affected by the quality of the interaction between patient and health care professional and directly correlate with patient/parent satisfaction with their clinic visit.

Families are often unwilling to express their concerns and problems concerning the effects of treatment with their doctor. Furthermore, many studies have now indicated that physicians appear to underestimate the degree of interaction desired by parents in relation to their child's illness. Parents' commitment to treatment recommendations can be strengthened when health care professionals take account of those needs. The ability of health care providers to adapt clinical approaches to consider the needs of parents, child, or adolescent has an important influence both on adherence and the ultimate long-term health of the pediatric patient.

SUGGESTED READINGS

1. Drotar D (ed): Promoting adherence to medical treatment in chronic childhood illness; concepts, methods and interventions, Mahwah, NJ: Lawrence Erlbaum Associates, 2000. **A comprehensive reference book, bringing together chapters from key researchers and clinicians in the field. It is divided into eight sections covering concepts, models, influences on adherence, impact of adherence on health, and interventions to improve adherence.**
2. Fielding D, Duff A: Compliance with treatment protocols: Interventions for children with chronic illness. Arch Dis Child 80: 196–200, 1999. **A brief article summarizing the key findings in this area and citing many of the studies providing the evidence base for this chapter.**
3. Lemanek KL, Kamps J, Chung N: Empirically supported treatments in pediatric psychology: Regimen adherence. J Pediatr Psychol 26:253–275, 2001. **In this article, a set of criteria developed by the American Psychological Association Task Force on Promotion Dissemination of Psychological Procedures (Chambless Criteria, 1995) are applied to eight intervention studies on asthma, 4 on juvenile rheumatoid arthritis, and 11 on type 1 diabetes. Although no**

interventions achieve the highest Chambless rating, several fall within the "effective" category.

4. Ley P: The use and improvement of written communication in mental health care and promotion. Psychol Health Med 3:19–53, 1998. **A useful review of findings from studies investigating the effectiveness of written communications.**

5. Miller WR, Rollnick S (eds): Motivational interviewing. New York/London: Guilford Press, 2002. **This is the second edition of this influential text. It will be most useful for those wanting an in-depth account of motivational interviewing. This set of techniques, which originated in the treatment of adults with substance abuse problems, has more recently been used with adolescents with chronic illnesses.**

6. Rapoff MA: Adherence to pediatric medical regimens. New York: Kluwer/Plenum, 1999. **This book combines a well conceptualized review of the area with practical case examples. It is written in a very accessible style with useful summaries, learning points, and examples of assessment methods and treatment regimes.**

7. World Health Organization: Adherence to long-term therapies: Evidence for action. Geneva: WHO, 2003. **This report gives an up-to-date account of current knowledge in the field for both adults and children with long-term conditions. There are chapters on asthma, cancer, diabetes, epilepsy, human immunodeficiency virus, and acquired immune deficiency syndrome.**

Children of Divorcing Parents

George J. Cohen

KEY CONCEPTS

- Divorce is a process, not an event: the ongoing anger and disagreement between parents, and the actual separation affect children's emotions and behavior.
- Supporting relatives and friends, familiar routines and activities, consistent discipline, and remaining in the same home lead to better outcomes for children.
- Anticipatory guidance and professional counseling help reduce the negative effects of divorce on children and parents.
- Children must be assured that they are not the cause and cannot be the solution to the divorce.
- Custodial and legal issues can be difficult for parents to deal with. Appropriate legal and mental health advice may be helpful.

The marriage rate among women in the United States declined from 100/1000 in the 1920s to 80/1000 in the 1990s, whereas the divorce rate climbed from 10/1000 to 40/1000. Currently half of first marriages and 60% of second marriages end in divorce. Each year 1 million children in the United States are affected by divorce or separation of their parents.

Divorce and separation take their toll on children and parents. The rancor that generally precedes the actual separation can be a factor in children's emotional and behavioral problems before, during, and after the divorce. However, children whose parents do not display antagonism toward each other may be equally at risk, as they may be devastated by the unexpected departure of a parent or the announcement of divorce proceedings.

The age of a child is a factor in the type of response he or she will have to the parents' divorce. In those younger than 3 years old, fearfulness, irritability, crying, and separation anxiety are common, as are sleep problems, aggression, and regression. Four-year-olds and 5-year-olds may blame themselves for the divorce and may become clingy, fear abandonment, and have nightmares, temper tantrums, and increased fantasy activity. School-age children often externalize their behavior with defiance, limit testing, and aggression. School-age children may feel rejected or deceived by a parent, yet they may feel guilty about the divorce and feel they should be punished themselves. Often there is a marked decline in school success. Adolescents may feel loss of self-esteem but attempt premature autonomy to show that the divorce does not affect them even though they are angry, confused, and depressed. School performance is likely to suffer, and antisocial behavior is a frequent reaction. Delinquency is less likely if teenagers are separated from the same-sex parent with whom they have a poor relationship. Girls have been reported to enter puberty earlier and become sexually active earlier after parental separation, but this is less so if there is continuing direct good-quality parental care.

Although most children of divorce function adequately as adults, some show continued anxiety and wariness about interpersonal relationships. Child abuse is observed more frequently in families of divorce and situations with single parenting.

Expert Opinion on Management Issues

Many studies show that continuing the children's normal routines and activities, consistent discipline, ensuring ongoing support from friends and family, and remaining in the family home all help children function more comfortably and capably when their parents separate. A variety of interventions help ameliorate untoward reactions of both children and parents. These include programs that offer parents information on legal issues, community services, or programs that focus on children's needs and improving parental communication. Counseling programs that work with children and families individually or in groups may be helpful. In some cases long-term psychotherapy is needed to help children deal with emotional problems.

A fundamental message that children must hear is that the divorce is not their fault and that they cannot change the situation between their parents. Efforts to assure affected children that each parent loves them and will continue to be a positive part of their lives are crucial.

Common Pitfalls

Although early intervention is ideal, all too often the pediatrician learns of the divorce only when confronted with child behavior problems, the family's financial status declines, or the family moves. Custody and legal issues pose problems as well. Each state or other jurisdiction is likely to have its own laws regarding divorce, and judges may differ in their skills and knowledge of child and family issues. The complexity of different custody arrangements (joint or individual, residential, and legal) may lead to confusion for the parents and unhappiness for all. What is in the "best interest of the child" is often a matter of individual perception for each parent, the judge, and the parents' attorneys. The advice of the pediatrician and a knowledgeable mental health advisor may help the family make a comfortable custody decision.

Parental dating and remarriage may cause potential problems for the child joining a "new" and "blended" family. Parental authority, child discipline, and privileges must be negotiated with all of the stepchildren's needs and comfort in mind.

Communication and Counseling

Communication and counseling are the essence of anticipatory guidance, which includes identifying health risks and offering early intervention and prevention strategies and ongoing management. Part of anticipatory guidance should be inquiry into the functioning, stability, and happiness of the family and its members. If problems are noted, the pediatrician can offer advice to help the child adjust to stressful situations, suggest resources for children and parents, and make appropriate referrals if needed for specialist consultation.

These activities are time-consuming, and realistic reimbursement becomes an issue that can be addressed with proper coding of symptoms and treatments. The *Diagnostic and Statistical Manual for Primary Care (DSM-PC) Child and Adolescent Version* is a resource. Situational diagnosis codes are v61.0 for family divorce, v61.1 for family discord, and v62.8 for domestic violence. Disorder codes can include 309.0 for adjustment disorder with depressed mood, 309.24 for adjustment disorder with anxiety, 309.28 for adjustment disorder with mixed anxiety/depressed mood, 309.3 for adjustment disorder with disturbance of conduct, 311.0 for depressive disorder not otherwise specified (NOS), and 296.12x for major depressive disorder. The code V65.45 is for sadness variation, and v40.3 is for sadness problem. Of course, complete and proper documentation in the child's medical record is essential.

Ideally, the pediatrician is able to remain available to help children and parents deal with issues that may occur as children mature and consider their situation from a new vantage point.

SUGGESTED READINGS

For Pediatricians

1. Braver SL, Ellman IM, Fabricius WV: Relocation of children after divorce and children's best interests: New evidence and legal considerations. J Fam Psychol 17(2):206–219, 2003. **Discusses moves of each parent and effects on their sons and daughters after divorce.**
2. Burns A, Dunlop R: Parental marital quality and family conflict: Longitudinal effects on adolescents from divorcing and non-divorcing families. J Divorce Remarriage 37:57–74, 2002. **Considers adolescents' perceptions of family life and their adjustment 10 years later.**
3. Cohen AJ, Adler N, Kaplan SJ, et al: Interactional effects of marital status and physical abuse on adolescent psychopathology. Child Abuse Negl 26:277–288, 2002. **Child abuse and divorce/separation are associated with attention deficit hyperactivity disorder (ADHD) in teens.**
4. Cohen GJ, Committee on Psychosocial Aspects of Child and Family Health, American Academy of Pediatrics: Helping children and families deal with divorce and separation. Pediatrics 110: 1019–1023, 2002. **Age-oriented approach and role of the pediatrician.**
5. Committee on Psychosocial Aspects of Child and Family Health, American Academy of Pediatrics. The child in court: A subject review. Pediatrics 104:1145–1148, 1999. **Addresses the pediatrician's role in helping children appearing in court.**
6. Ham BD: The effects of divorce on the academic achievement of high school seniors. J Divorce Remarriage 38:167–185, 2003. **Students from intact families performed better in school than those from disrupted families.**
7. McKenzie B, Bacon B: Parent education after separation: Results from a multi-site study on best practices. Can J Commun Ment Health Summer (4 Suppl):73–88, 2002. **Child well-being improved after education program for divorcing parents.**
8. Pruett MK, Williams TY, Insabella G, et al: Family and legal indicators of child adjustment to divorce among families with young children. J Fam Psychol 17:169–180, 2003. **Mediating effect on child outcomes by paternal involvement, attorney involvement, and parent-and-child relationships.**
9. Quinlan RJ: Father absence, parental care, and female reproductive development. Evol Hum Behav 24:376–390, 2003. **Divorce/separation of parents of young girls is associated with girls' early reproductive development.**
10. Videon TM: The effects of parent-adolescent relationships and parental separation on adolescent well-being. J Marriage Fam 64:489–503, 2002. **Child delinquency and depression associated with parental separation and relationship with child.**
11. Wallerstein JS, Blakeslee S: What about the kids? Raising your children before, during and after divorce. New York: Hyperion, 2003. **Age-oriented, practical information regarding behavior, custody, and family adjustment.**
12. Wolchik SA, Sandler IN, Millsap RE, et al: Six-year follow-up of preventive interventions for children of divorce. JAMA 288:1874–1881, 2002. **Intervention programs with mothers or mothers and teens versus controls produce less externalizing problems in teens.**

For Families

1. Adams E, Adams K: On the day his daddy left. Morton Grove, IL: Albert Whitman, 2000. **For elementary school age. Also has a page for adults.**
2. American Academy of Pediatrics. Divorce and Children (brochure). Elk Grove Village, IL: AAP, 1999. **Practical advice for parents.**
3. Bode J, Mack S: For Better, for Worse. New York: Simon & Schuster, 2001. **Interviews with children and parents. For preteens and teens.**
4. Cadier F, Daly M: My Parents Are Getting Divorced. New York: Amulet Books, 2004. **For preteens and teens.**
5. Johnson J, O'Neill C: How Do I Feel About My Stepfamily? Brookfield, CT: Copper Beech Books, 1998. **For fourth grade and older.**
6. Kimball G: How to Survive Your Parents' Divorce: Kids' Advice to Kids. Chico, CA: Equality Press, 1994. **For ages 12 through 18 years.**
7. Rogers F, Judkis J: Let's Talk About It: Divorce. New York: GP Putnam's Sons, 1996. **Mister Rogers talks to elementary-age kids.**
8. Wallerstein JS, Blakeslee S: What About the Kids?: Raising Your Children Before, During and After Divorce. New York: Hyperion, 2003. **Practical, sensitive age-oriented advice for parents about child reactions, counseling, and custody.**

The Child and the Death of a Loved One

Cynthia W. Moore and Paula K. Rauch

KEY CONCEPTS

- A child's understanding of death is informed by his or her phase of development.
- A death is grieved acutely, and the loss is revisited throughout a child's subsequent life.
- Children will benefit from open, age-appropriate communication about death and from a secure environment in which normal routines are maintained.
- Parents should anticipate that children will have a range of feelings and reactions to a death.
- Parents will benefit from education about how to prepare their children for end-of-life rituals.

After the death of a loved one, the pediatrician can provide information about how children commonly react to loss, an understanding of the many ways grief is expressed, and suggestions about when to seek professional help for a grieving child. The sensitive inquiries of a caring pediatrician who appreciates the impact of a loss can do much to allay the anxieties children and their parents experience about the days and weeks ahead.

Expert Opinion on Management Issues

A child's understanding of a death is dependent on his or her developmental level. It is key for clinicians to understand these age-appropriate differences and to convey them to the parents of a bereaved child (Table 1). Under stress it is common for children to regress and behave temporarily in ways that are more typical of an earlier developmental stage. It is helpful to share with parents that regression is a common response to stress and to educate them about the common reactions to loss seen in both current and earlier phases of development that may be expressed by their child.

Although developmental level greatly influences a child's understanding of death, children of all ages have many needs in common after a loss. First, they need to feel safe, secure, and part of the family. This will be facilitated by a timely return to a child's regular routines and schedules and by providing as much normalcy as can be achieved at home.

Children will benefit from being included in the end-of-life rituals but will need to be given information about what to expect and a choice about how to participate. A familiar adult should describe what the child will see and hear at the funeral, detailing the physical and emotional setting ("You'll see a coffin in front, many people crying . . ."), then should discuss with the child whether or not he or she will attend. It can be helpful to have an adult who could, if necessary, leave

part way through the service with a younger child or children. If an older child makes a choice not to attend, some one-on-one talking time with that child about how he or she might feel may be helpful.

In the months following a loss, children need adults around them to model that it's all right to discuss good and bad memories, to talk about what they will miss and not miss about the deceased, and to provide opportunities to remember the deceased over time. They also need to know that they are not alone with their feelings and that caring adults understand what they are experiencing.

CHILDREN'S GRIEF

Although it was questioned in the past whether children are capable of real grief, we have come to recognize that although the form of a child's grief differs from that of an adult, it is just as heartfelt. Even children too young to understand death's finality still have strong emotional reactions to separation from the deceased, expressed in their play and behavior.

Although the most intense distress may subside within a month or two of a loss, losses tend to be reprocessed at each new developmental stage and milestone. Thus, grief is a lifelong process, not something accomplished once and for all in the first year following a death. Contrary to earlier notions that it was protective to help children forget a dead loved one or to remember the person as perfect, parents are currently encouraged to invite their child to remember the deceased person realistically, respecting the person's strengths and flaws. Many children describe having a relationship with a deceased family member in which they either talk to the person for guidance or have the comforting sense that the person is watching over them. Parents may be reassured to know that most children go on to enjoy happy and productive lives following deaths of even parents or siblings.

Much is accomplished in the grief process. First, children come to understand that someone has died, and they gradually accept the reality of the loss and its implications. Then children come to face and bear the pain of the loss. Over time and at different stages of development, a child will re-evaluate his or her relationship with the deceased, work out how to maintain an internal connection to the person, and adjust to an environment in which the person is missing. Simultaneously, the child will gradually invest in new relationships, resume age-appropriate activities, and generally re-engage in life. Children may experience a transient increase in distress around developmental transitions or specific anniversaries and may show behavioral regression at those times.

A child's reaction to a death is influenced by many factors (Box 1). However, it may be useful to review some general principles for children of different ages. Symptoms of grief wax and wane over time, and there are no strict guidelines regarding when behavior should appear nearly normal after a close family member's death. Expected and unexpected triggers may cause a transient return of distress, usually lasting

TABLE 1 How Children Understand Death

Conceptualization of Death	Helpful Adult Responses
Infants	
Sensitive to disruptions in their routine.	Consistent caregivers, routines (feeding, soothing, nighttime)
Pick up on caregivers' distress.	and settings.
Preschoolers (2–6 years)	
Aware of the absence of a loved person.	Patience in repeating over and over that deceased person isn't coming back.
Understand death as prolonged separation, may believe the deceased is alive elsewhere.	Provide concrete descriptions of death (dead person's body doesn't work any more; he can't see, hear, or feel anything; his heart stops pumping and he stops breathing).
Do not appreciate that death is irreversible, and offer "solutions" to death, such as replacing batteries, watering the dead person, or giving him/her more medicine.	Explore the child's understanding of a death and dispel guilt by correcting misconceptions.
Concept of forever is inconceivable, so death is not experienced with the full weight of finality.	Reassure child that nothing they did caused the death.
Lack of causal logic combined with egocentricity facilitates explanations for death that are inaccurately self-centered: may blame selves for a death, or interpret surviving adults' withdrawal as a sign that the child has disappointed adults.	If a parent is withdrawn, explain that the parent is sad, and why, and that the child did not cause the adult's distress.
Think concretely, so euphemisms like "The angels came for him," will create confusion and worry about who may be "taken" next.	Maintain consistent caregivers, preschool attendance, play dates, meal times, and bedtime rituals.
School-Age Children (6–12 years)	
Understand that a dead body cannot come back to life, but may struggle to comprehend discussions about spirituality, such as about a loved one's "being in heaven now."	Understand that the quest for information serves to help them feel more in control of the situation.
Experience a sense of mastery by accumulating information and skills, so may ask very detailed questions that some parents find objectionable (e.g., "Do worms really eat the body?").	Provide clear, accurate information about causes of death.
Understand information about the causes of death and may also ask detailed questions about how someone died.	Elicit and answer questions warmly and openly.
Gaps in their understanding can lead to particular fears, such as the fear that they themselves might "catch" an illness, such as cancer.	Elicit and correct misconceptions about causes of death.
Generally focused on learning and playing by the rules that may lead them to find ways the loss wasn't fair: "Grandpa takes horrible care of himself and he's alive; why did Dad have to die when he took great care of himself?"	Help put guilt and other concerns in perspective.
May experience guilt about things they did or did not do with or for the deceased.	Maintain predictable routines and expectations.
May worry about the health of surviving adults.	
Adolescents	
Understand that death is final, irreversible, and universal.	Allow and encourage discussions with appropriate nonparental adults.
With new abstract reasoning skills may struggle with abstract questions about justice and the meaning of life and suffering.	Respect adolescent's wish for privacy and control over dissemination of information about a loss, as much as seems reasonable.
Egocentrism and emotional immaturity may still cause them to focus on the personal effects of a loss in ways that can feel selfish to surviving adults, for example, being concerned that a funeral could interfere with preparations for the junior prom.	Do not expect adolescents to assume adult responsibilities.
May take on adult worries, e.g., about finances.	
May feel anxious about their own mortality, e.g., susceptibility to a heritable illness.	Watch for evidence of risk-taking behavior or substance abuse in response to the news of a death.
Sensitive about how a loss sets them apart from peers and may feel embarrassed about peers knowing of a death.	
Relationship with deceased may have been complex or conflictual; this may produce guilt, regrets, and resentment that complicate grief.	

hours to days rather than weeks to months. It is common to see noticeable behavioral changes in the first 2 weeks that reflect both the loss and disruptions in the child's life. However, children often return to their usual activities quickly, and parents may worry that they are not dealing with their grief. Parents can be reassured that being active helps children cope. After 2 to 4 weeks, children have generally returned to a fairly typical schedule of activities and will have fewer symptoms of behavioral disruption.

In the weeks and months after a loss of a close family member, children commonly have a wide range of emotional reactions, including sadness, anxiety, anger, and guilt. Sadness and longing may be triggered by the realization that a favorite activity can no longer be enjoyed together or an accomplishment cannot be

---

> ## BOX 1 Factors That May Compromise a Child's Adjustment to a Loss
>
> ### Context of Death
> - Violent death, especially if witnessed by child
> - Suicide
> - Child's or adult's belief that the child influenced or somehow caused the death
> - No opportunity to say good-bye, convey love
>
> ### Child Factors
> - Poor premorbid functioning
> - Ambivalent or very dependent relationship with deceased
>
> ### Family Factors
> - Surviving parent's functioning
> - Inconsistency in caregivers
> - Family secrecy, unwillingness to discuss the loss or answer questions
> - Surviving parent dating within first year of spouse's death
> - Inconsistent discipline
> - Little attention paid to child's feelings and needs
> - Little or no preparation for the funeral
> - Needing to move
> - Diminishment of financial resources

> ## BOX 2 Red Flags
>
> ### In First Weeks after a Loss
> - Self-destructive behavior or expressed desire to die.
> - Guilt about things other than actions taken or not taken by the survivor at the time of the death; belief they are not deserving of having a good life because the other person died.
> - Morbid preoccupation with worthlessness.
> - Marked psychomotor retardation.
> - Prolonged and marked functional impairment.
> - Hallucinatory experiences other than thinking he or she hears the voice of or transiently sees the image of the deceased.
> - Drug or heavy alcohol use.
>
> ### After 1 Month
> - Symptoms of post-traumatic stress disorder: recurrent intrusive recollections or dreams of the death, intense distress at exposure to cues that symbolize the death, avoidance of stimuli related to the death and numbing of general responsiveness, and symptoms of increased arousal (difficulty sleeping, concentrating, exaggerated startle response, irritability).
> - Ongoing worsening difficulties with sleep, appetite, anxiety (e.g., clinging to caretakers, nighttime fears, reluctance to go to school), frequent crying, or aggression or acting out.
> - Failure to re-engage in activities and friendships; difficulties in two or more arenas of functioning (home, school, peers).
>
> ### After 2 Months
> - Persistent signs of depression: sad mood, reduced energy, eating and sleeping disturbances, poor concentration, or a diminished interest in activities previously enjoyed persisting for 2 months or more after loss.
>
> ### After Several Months
> - Infants who are not growing as expected may be experiencing problems attaching to a new caregiver, or have no consistent new caregiver.

shared with the deceased. If a parent died, they often experience anxiety about the well-being of surviving caretakers. School-age children may pester parents about quitting smoking; preschoolers may be extra clingy at separations; adolescents may point out inconsistencies in parents' expectations of them, and the parent's own behavior. Anxiety about children's own safety is also common. Anger may be directed at God, at the deceased person for leaving them, or at other people or forces the child perceives as somehow responsible for the death. Children who have lost a sibling may feel jealous about the attention lavished on the ill child, then may feel guilty about these feelings. School-age children and adolescents may feel guilty about enjoying anything in life without the deceased and about actions taken or not taken, things said or not said, to the deceased.

Children of all ages may be more accident prone and may have less confidence in their ability to effect change or master their environments. Children may have difficulty coping with challenges and are likely to regress to earlier ways of managing frustration.

Some behavioral reactions are more typical of children of certain ages and developmental stages. *Infants* may be particularly fussy and harder to soothe. Their sleep can be disrupted, and they may wake frequently at night. They may be less willing to try new foods. *Preschoolers* may have a hard time settling down at bedtime, complain of bad dreams, lose gains in toileting, show increased clinging or separation difficulties, and handle relationships with peers in ways typical of themselves at an earlier age (e.g., regressing to biting, grabbing). *School-age children* frequently have somatic complaints such as headaches and stomachaches. They may have a hard time falling asleep and may complain of nighttime fears, and they may become picky eaters. At school, they may daydream and have difficulty concentrating. Some experience problems with peers, sometimes increased conflict, and sometimes withdrawal.

Adolescents' intense, adult-like emotions will likely alternate with enjoyment of some usual activities. They may question why the death happened and struggle to understand and place death in a larger context. Some social withdrawal, difficulty concentrating, and difficulty falling asleep or sleeping more than usual are not uncommon.

Because children's grief may manifest at school, it is helpful for parents to inform the school staff of a significant loss. Teachers, guidance counselors, and school nurses can be important sources of support for a child and also provide valuable information to parents about the child's coping, when properly informed. Adolescents may want a say in which teachers are told, and some children may be quite clear that although they want a teacher to know of a loss, they don't ever want the teacher to talk about it. Whenever possible these preferences should be respected.

Common Pitfalls

Some children experience serious emotional or behavioral difficulties after the death of an important person. It can be helpful to schedule a meeting approximately 4 to 6 weeks after a death to identify family members who may be struggling to cope with a loss and require a referral to a mental health clinician. The child should be seen by a counselor if at about 6 weeks after a death his or her symptoms are getting generally worse rather than better or if the grief is interfering significantly with schoolwork or causing withdrawal from friends. Pediatricians need to recognize the symptoms that indicate a child needs professional help in managing his or her grief (Box 2). Even difficulties that are quite common soon after a loss warrant a referral if they do not resolve by about 4 to 6 weeks after the loss.

Communication and Counseling

Parents may find it helpful to remember:

- Grief is a natural, lifelong process that is different for everyone.
- Most children do well in the long run and live happy, productive lives.
- Children are likely to cope with a death in keeping with their style of coping with other challenges.
- It is important to support the child's reinvestment in life and to respect the pace and style of his or her grief.
- Within 6 weeks of a loss, children generally function fairly well in school, with peers, and at home. If problems persist, and particularly if problems occur in two or more arenas, seek professional assessment.
- Children need adults who can help them remember the lost person with stories, pictures, and so on, when the child is ready.
- Anniversaries, holidays, and developmental milestones are likely to be difficult; a temporary increase in symptoms is not uncommon around those times.

SUGGESTED READINGS

Books for Children and Adolescents

1. Brown MW: The Dead Bird. New York: HarperTrophy, 1995. (Ages 3–6). **Simple language and drawings tell the story of a dead bird found in the forest and answer young children's questions about death.**
2. DePaola T: Nana Upstairs, Nana Downstairs. New York: Putnam, 2000. (Ages 4–8). **Tells the story of a young boy's warm relationship with his great-grandmother, and his reaction to her death.**
3. Fitzgerald H: The Grieving Teen: A Guide for Teenagers and their Friends. New York: Fireside, 2000. **Written for adolescents, answers typical questions about an adolescent's experience of grief.**
4. Viorst J: The Tenth Good Thing about Barney. New York: Atheneum, 1971. (Ages 6–10). **Tells the story of the death of an elementary school-age child's beloved cat and discusses feelings stemming from a loss surrounding a death.**

Books for Parents

1. Grollman E: Talking about Death: A Dialogue Between Parent and Child, 3rd ed. Boston: Beacon Press, 1990. **This book is a guide for adults and children to read together; it includes a story, and answers to questions children ask about death.**
2. Trozzi M, Massimini K: Talking with Children about Loss: Words, Strategies, and Wisdom to Help Children Cope with Death, Divorce, and Other Difficult Times. New York: Perigee, 1999. **Explains how to talk with children and adolescents about loss, with discussions about how children interpret death, helping children face funerals, and when to seek professional help.**

Articles for Professionals

1. Baker J, Sedney MA, Gross E: Psychological tasks for bereaved children. Amer J Orthospychiat 62(1):105–116, 1992. **Describes the grieving process in bereaved children.**

The Child with a Serious Ongoing Condition

Ruth E. K. Stein

KEY CONCEPTS

- Certain conditions may have serious implications for a child's development and for family members collectively and individually.
- These conditions challenge the clinician to provide the usual preventive health care and care of intercurrent illnesses, address complications, and deal with comorbidities.
- The goals of care are to maximize the child's development and to normalize the child's functioning to the fullest extent possible within the family and community context.
- Collaboration and communication are essential with family, other caretakers, specialists and consultants, educators, child care providers, and agencies that provide special services to the child and family
- Care must be available, accessible, coordinated, and comprehensive.
- Lines of responsibility should be clear and a plan should be developed in partnership with the family and the team members.
- Transitions, both developmental and institutional, present major challenges that require planning and organization.
- Children with complex conditions should receive thorough periodic re-evaluations.
- As more information becomes available about the genetic risks of conditions, parents and the adolescent should be offered genetic counseling.

A substantial fraction of children have serious ongoing conditions that persist over long periods of their lives. Regardless of their individual diagnoses, these children can be identified because of the presence of a disorder with a biologic, psychologic, or cognitive basis that has lasted or is virtually certain to last for at least one year and produces one or more of the following functional sequelae (or consequences): limitation of function, activities, or social role in comparison with healthy age peers in the general areas of physical, cognitive, emotional, and social growth and development; dependency on medications, special diet, medical technology, assistive device, or personal assistance to compensate for or minimize limitations of function, activities, or social role; or the need for medical care or related services, psychological services, or educational services above the usual for the child's age, or for special ongoing treatments, interventions, or accommodations at home or in school.

These consequences distinguish these children in functional terms from their healthy peers and may also require pediatric practitioners to deal with a range of special issues. These issues also may have a major impact on the child's development and pose real challenges to both family members and health care professionals in caring for the children and their siblings. These children often require complex services of a wide variety, making their care both extremely challenging and rewarding.

Expert Opinion on Management Issues

Children with ongoing conditions are prone to all the usual illnesses and normal developmental issues that their healthy peers experience. Additionally, they may be predisposed to complications or illness as a result of their biologic condition or its treatment. The specific nature of the problems that may develop is likely to vary with the biology of the health condition (e.g., pneumococcal infection in the presence of nephrotic syndrome, gallstones secondary to hemolytic anemia, sepsis secondary to immunosuppression). These special considerations and vulnerabilities, together with the frequent presence of other comorbidities, may make delivery of medical care to children with serious ongoing conditions complex. The clinician must be aware of the range of problems that can arise and be alert to recognize when intervention is indicated.

Because so many of these children require the consultation of subspecialists, primary care clinicians are often in the position of sharing care responsibilities rather than working independently. From the first referral to a subspecialist, concerns and plans must be communicated so that the family experiences a cohesive care package. As the child enters school or early intervention programs, other types of service providers are also likely to be involved. It is desirable to have open communication with other key personnel such as teachers and caretakers, whose greater involvement may facilitate care. Primary practitioners can play an essential role in helping coordinate the issues that arise and helping to ensure good communication between the members of the care team. In many cases they are the physicians who provide a *medical home*. A medical home consists of care that is accessible, family-centered, continuous, comprehensive, coordinated, compassionate, and culturally effective. Whether the medical home is provided by the primary provider or by a subspecialist, primary providers can ensure that the family knows where the medical home is and has ample opportunity to have questions answered and who to ask if problems arise.

The goals of treatment are not only to handle the primary condition and the intercurrent issues but also to maximize the child's development and normalize the child's function to the fullest extent possible within the context of the family and community. This objective requires that clinicians maintain a balanced approach and emphasize the child's strengths and deficits or limitations. It is also important to foster opportunities for increased independence as the child grows up and to ensure the gradual transfer of responsibility from the parents to the child as he or she becomes more independent.

One feature that distinguishes long-term conditions from those that are more acute is the need to know more about what family members think or believe to develop treatment priorities with their input. The large extent to which families assume ongoing responsibility for management of the child's condition on a daily basis requires the practitioner to step out of the prescriptive mode of care. Instead, it is helpful to use a much more collaborative strategy that recognizes the parents and, later, the older child and adolescent as true partners in the care. This approach involves joint planning and participation in decision making, and respecting and supporting values, information, and opinions expressed by family members.

To solve the logistic problems that accompany the challenges of providing home treatment, it is often necessary to discuss details of family life. This may initially be uncomfortable for both practitioners and families and may feel like prying. However, a nonjudgmental exploration of ways to make life easier often identifies key information that can lead to safe modification of the treatment plan. Attention to details contributes to success in implementing and sustaining treatment plans. For example, it is often much easier and more successful to adjust a child's medication schedule to fit in with family routines than it is to expect the family to adhere to a schedule of medications that is incompatible with other family responsibilities.

To maximize adherence to recommended management, it is critical to obtain a realistic sense of the family's understanding and beliefs about the condition and its etiology and prognosis, and their perceptions and preferences about alternative management strategies. Forming a therapeutic alliance involves establishing trust and mutual respect and has important long-term benefits. An essential ingredient in this process is honest and open sharing of information, including uncertainty when the answers to questions are not readily available.

Another area in which the primary care pediatrician can make important contributions is in helping the family anticipate special problems that may arise and in preparing for potential emergency situations and transitions. It terms of preparation for emergencies, it is useful to provide the family with a letter summarizing key medical information, especially when they are traveling or away from their usual source of care. A convenient technique for ensuring that children with serious ongoing conditions are never without access to lifesaving emergency care is the use of a medical alert bracelet that allows easy identification of the child's essential medical information and emergency care needs.

Transitions often present special challenges for children with serious conditions and their families. This is true for developmental transitions, such as school entry, or changing from elementary to middle or high school and for transitions because of systems that have age limits or other special qualifications that require children to change service settings or to apply for new services. In the former case, the strain is often emotional, as these transitions bring to light differences in functioning of children who are healthy and those with serious ongoing conditions. The latter case often involves the hassle of changing and requalifying and all the paperwork that accompanies the transition, along with the stress of beginning new relationships with new service providers.

Families often look to their practitioners for information about local and regional resources for children with special health conditions. These resources include a wide range of services, from suppliers of special equipment to recreational opportunities, financial assistance programs, parent support groups, and information about the school system. Familiarity with these resources helps the family gain access to them.

Over time, many families are able to develop skills to coordinate care and to be effective managers of the many systems with which they must interact. Others may need help with case management. The clinician together with members of the clinician's office staff should enable the child and family to become as independent as they can, but to provide some oversight and a safety net for those who need more assistance.

Common Pitfalls

- Not being honest with family members.
- Failing to clarify who is doing what when there are multiple providers or services involved.
- Omitting routine services such as developmental assessments, screenings, and immunizations.
- Brushing off parental concerns.
- Failing to take the time to explore what is really going on when things don't add up, such as when responses to treatment become mystifying.

Physicians are increasingly trained to expect scientific answers to all medical questions, and although there is much new knowledge to inform the care that we provide to children with serious ongoing health conditions, there is still a great deal of uncertainty. Thus, answers to parents' questions are often elusive, and the pediatrician must be willing to share uncertainty and disclose what he or she does know about the child's condition, its treatment, or its prognosis. The pediatrician will generally find that honesty is appreciated by the family members and that there is much to be accomplished in helping to orchestrate the care among the team members and to ensure that the child is obtaining the full range of needed services, including those the pediatrician is best equipped to provide: developmental assessments, screening, and health care maintenance. Such services are badly needed to avoid duplication or omission of important elements of care, two very common problems in long-term care of children with serious ongoing conditions.

Pediatricians should also remember that when parents raise concerns, it is often because they know their child best and often see signs of a problem before it is evident to others. Finally, every pediatrician who treats children with ongoing health conditions has had the experience of having an unusually frustrating or disappointing response to treatment. Physicians should be alert to the possibility that other factors are interfering with treatment. These may be errors in diagnosis, a complicating medical condition, or difficulties in adherence that range from parental disbelief in the treatments to competing and complicating psychosocial issues. In all these instances it is prudent to spend some time reassessing what is really going on. Often the sooner time is invested in making a differential assessment of all the possible reasons for treatment failure, the more time is saved in the long run. Long-term outcomes will be maximized in these situations only with the proper and comprehensive reassessment of all the possible elements.

Communication and Counseling

Whenever possible, it is helpful to include multiple family members in discussions so that one adult is not left carrying questions and messages back and forth. This goal can be accomplished by planning to sit down, even briefly, with adult caretakers on a periodic basis or around critical events and transitions in the child's development or disease. At these times it is helpful to allow time for questions and to take stock of how the parents and siblings are doing. It is important to assess the needs of all family members because, at times, some may be inappropriately neglected while so much effort is focused on the child who has a serious ongoing health condition. It is also useful to inventory competing family and personal priorities that may affect the care of a child who has a serious ongoing health condition, and healthy siblings.

Having a child with any serious chronic condition has a substantial impact on the family as individuals and as a unit. Typically, parents struggle with the question of why their child has a health condition. They may have considerable guilt about a range of real and imagined things that may have contributed to the child's situation. In some cases they are also concerned about the genetic implications of the child's condition for other children and their offspring. As more is learned about the heritability of many serious ongoing conditions this is becoming an area of increasing interest, but it may lead to increased blame and guilt within the family. Coupled with these emotions is the sense of burden of having to provide special care at home and through the health care system. This care has considerable cost in terms of time, energy, and money and often restricts individual and family options. Among the concerns that families often raise are those relating to the cause of the condition and its prognosis and impact on daily life. It is helpful to families when members of the health care team are available to listen to these concerns, but they should not to feel forced to provide solutions, especially when answers are unclear. Many families find it helpful to find someone who will listen, and most appreciate support and honesty more than guesses. Moreover, statistics, although often requested and helpful to some people, only predict for groups of children, whereas the family cares about the specific outcome for an individual child, which clinicians cannot supply. In the face of uncertainty, continued support and availability of the practitioner may become the mainstays of a relationship.

All these issues intensify the psychological and social implications of treating the conditions and require the practitioner to address a range of issues. The nature of the psychological and social issues is likely to be similar across a range of diverse medical conditions. This similarity can be empowering to pediatric practitioners, because experience with patients having one condition may be helpful and have important implications when dealing with another condition. Although the vast majority of children and families do very well, some experience overwhelming difficulty and require intensive involvement of the pediatric practitioner or other members of the health care team. In such cases, assisting families to successfully cope with a chronic health condition can be an extremely rewarding aspect of practicing pediatrics.

SUGGESTED READINGS

1. Stein REK, Bauman LJ, Westbrook LE, et al: Framework for identifying children who have chronic conditions: The case for a new definition. J Pediatr 122:342–347, 1993. **Discusses the similarities of issues across conditions and the rationale for the noncategorical approach; also is the source of the definition cited in the introduction.**
2. Stein REK: Challenges in long-term care of children. Ambul Pediatr 1:280–288, 2001. **Discusses issues in handling competing priorities in the care of children with serious long-term conditions.**
3. Cooley WC, McAllister JW: Building medical homes: Improvement strategies in primary care for children with special health care needs. Pediatrics 113(5 Suppl):1499–1506, 2004. **Reviews the key roles of pediatricians and the medical home concept.**
4. Stein REK: Chronic physical disorders. Pediatr Rev 13:224–229, 1992. **Summarizes a wide range of issues that affect children with ongoing conditions and their families as well as some of the challenges for health care providers.**
5. American Academy of Pediatrics; American Academy of Family Physicians; American College of Physicians-American Society of Internal Medicine. A consensus statement on health care transitions for young adults with special health care needs. Pediatrics 110:1304–1306, 2002. **Discusses current recommendations for handling adolescents as they move out of the service systems geared toward children.**
6. Perrin JM, Kuhlthau K, Walker DK, et al: Monitoring health care for children with chronic conditions in a managed care environment. Matern Child Health J 1(1):15–23, 1997. **Devoted to a discussion of quality-of-care measures and the challenges of meeting them.**
7. Johnson CP, Kastner TA, Committee/Section on Children with Disabilities: Helping families raise children with special health care needs at home. Pediatrics 115:507–511, 2005. **Discusses many of the day-to-day issues in the lives of families raising a child with an ongoing condition, especially those that affect functioning.**

The Child Cured of Cancer

Jacqueline Casillas and Stephen A. Feig

KEY CONCEPTS

- The National Cancer Institute defines a cancer survivor as follows: "An individual is considered a survivor from the time of diagnosis, through the balance of his or her life. Family members, friends, and caregivers are also impacted by the survivorship experience and are therefore included in this definition."
- A late effect is an outcome that occurs more than 5 years from the time of diagnosis of cancer, as a result of the previous cancer treatment, and may be physical, psychological, or social in nature.
- Key components of long-term follow-up care are risk-based, longitudinal, providing continuity, and employing a multidisciplinary approach.
- Delivery models of care for childhood cancer survivors include specialized late effects clinic-delivered in the pediatric oncology setting (most common) or in transition settings in which specialized adult providers screen for late effects, in the adult oncology setting or in the general primary care setting within the community.

Although childhood cancer is a relatively rare phenomenon, in the United States approximately 12,400 children and adolescents younger than 20 years of age are found to have cancer each year. However, the success of treatment is excellent, and the number of survivors is increasing rapidly. The current overall survival rate for childhood malignancies is estimated to be 78%, which means that approximately 1 per 1000 persons in the general U.S. population is a childhood cancer survivor. Furthermore, pediatric cancer survivorship is a relatively "new" phenomenon; prior to 1970, most children died from their primary cancer diagnosis. Now, owing to multimodal treatment regimens with chemotherapy, radiation therapy, and surgery coupled with aggressive supportive care regimens, survival rates continue to rise. Cure from cancer, however, is not without its complications. Virtually every organ system can be affected by previous cancer therapy. Accordingly, comprehensive long-term follow-up care is essential for this at-risk population.

Expert Opinion on Management Issues

Screening for late effects is essential to ensuring the health and well-being of childhood cancer survivors because at least 44% will experience at least one significant late effect as a result of their previous therapy for childhood cancer. Specific sociodemographic factors are associated with a higher risk for the development of late effects. According to a study by Hudson and associates, these include female gender, lower levels of educational attainment, and low family annual income

TABLE 1 Selected Physical Late Effects and Screening Recommendations

Therapeutic Exposure	Physical Late Effect	Examples of Recommended Screening
Anthracycline antibiotic (e.g., doxorubicin)	Cardiomyopathy	Echocardiogram and electrocardiogram
Epipodophyllotoxins (e.g., etoposide) or alkylating agents (e.g., cyclophosphamide)	Second malignant neoplasm (e.g., acute myelogenous leukemia [AML])	Annual history and physical and complete blood count (CBC)
Antitumor antibiotic (bleomycin) or alkylating agent (busulfan)	Pulmonary fibrosis	Pulmonary function tests
Heavy metal (cisplatin)	Ototoxicity/hearing loss	Brainstem auditory evoked response (BAER) or audiogram
Corticosteroids (prednisone, dexamethasone)	Osteopenia, osteoporosis, and cataracts	Bone density evaluation (e.g., DEXA) and annual eye examination
Blood or serum product transfusion prior	Hepatitis B and C, HIV	Transfusion prior to 1993 (hepatitis C serologies), 1972 (hepatitis B serologies), 1985 (HIV screening)
Cranial/spinal irradiation	Endocrine dysfunction	Monitoring of height/weight/BMI, free T_4, TSH, LH, FSH, estradiol, testosterone
Chest irradiation	Breast cancer in females	Monthly breast self-examination, annual clinical breast examination, mammography

BMI, body mass index; DEXA, dual-energy x-ray absorptiometry (scan); FSH, follicle-stimulating hormone; HIV, human immunodeficiency virus; LH, luteinizing hormone; T_4, thyroxine; TSH, thyroid-stimulating hormone.

(<$20,000/year). Hudson and colleagues observed that relative to survivors of acute lymphoblastic leukemia (ALL), survivors of brain tumors, sarcomas, and bone tumors have significantly higher probability of reporting adverse outcomes in at least one domain of health status. Furthermore, according to a 2003 Institute of Medicine Report entitled *Childhood Cancer Survivorship: Improving Care and Quality of Life,* approximately 25% of survivors will experience a late effect that is severe or life-threatening. Thus, it is essential for a childhood cancer survivor to receive annual, comprehensive long-term follow-up care throughout childhood and adulthood.

The Children's Oncology Group (COG) has developed evidence-based screening recommendations based on *previous therapeutic exposure* that can now be followed for the provision of long-term follow-up care to survivors during childhood, adolescence, and young adult life. Table 1 lists some examples of treatment exposures and associated physical late effects with recommendations for screening that should be completed (as outlined in the COG long-term follow-up guidelines and are available for review at http://www.survivorshipguidelines.org).

Psychological Late Effects

An emerging body of literature in pediatric cancer survivorship research indicates that childhood cancer survivors are, overall, experiencing good psychological health years after completion of their cancer treatment. Various studies demonstrating no difference between survivors with comparison groups, including sibling and general population norms, have assessed the prevalence of major depression, somatic distress, and general psychological functioning as measured by the Symptom Checklist–90 and the Brief Symptom Inventory.

Other studies have demonstrated risk factors for adverse psychological outcomes in small populations of survivors. The risk factors that have been identified include female sex, low socioeconomic status, and exposure to intensive chemotherapy in leukemia and lymphoma survivors. According to Hudson and associates, quoted above, three diagnostic groups (Hodgkin disease, sarcomas, or other bone tumors) are also at increased risk for continued cancer-related anxiety. Importantly, Hudson and colleagues hypothesized that their observations may be because adolescents, the age group with those diagnoses, have a better understanding as compared to younger children about the meaning of their diagnosis and risks of treatment, because adolescence is the period in which abstract thinking develops.

Neurocognitive deficits as a result of cranial irradiation at a young age deserve special attention because these can have a devastating impact on psychosocial outcomes. The two most important risk factors for neurocognitive delay are age at cranial irradiation exposure and total cumulative dose (particularly brain tumor survivors who receive higher total doses). This also includes patients who have had exposure to whole-brain irradiation (ALL survivors). Treatment with cranial irradiation prior to the age of 3 years has been shown to place a survivor at high risk for neuropsychological impairment because the brain is undergoing rapid development during the time of irradiation. However, as childhood cancer survivors continue to be monitored for several years in post-therapy, studies have indicated that there is also risk for intellectual compromise among older children. Exposure to intrathecal chemotherapy such as methotrexate can also place childhood cancer survivors at risk for neurocognitive dysfunction. It is, therefore, imperative to provide regularly scheduled neuropsychological evaluation coupled with appropriate special education and psychosocial support services to maximize academic performance and psychosocial outcomes for all survivors who have had cranial and/or intrathecal chemotherapy.

Common Pitfalls

Given the myriad of late effects for which childhood cancer survivors are at risk, it is essential that their long-term follow-up care be delivered by knowledgeable providers with expertise in risk-based health care so that appropriate follow-up and screening can be tailored to the individual child, adolescent, or young adult. Referral to multidisciplinary long-term follow-up programs for childhood cancer survivors that maintain ongoing communication with the primary care providers is the cornerstone of high-quality care for this at-risk patient population.

Unfortunately, it has been demonstrated that a significant number of survivors are not receiving a general physical examination, a cancer-related visit, or a cancer center visit. According to Oeffinger and associates, factors associated with a lack of access to medical care include no health insurance, male sex, and lack of concern for future health by the survivor. They further showed that the likelihood of patients reporting that a visit is being made as a cancer-related follow-up visit, or of having a general physical examination focused on this issue, decreases significantly as survivors age or as the time from cancer diagnosis increased. This is particularly concerning because it has been shown that childhood cancer survivors have greater than a 10-fold excess risk in overall mortality when compared to the general U.S. population.

Among those survivors whose cause of death was determined, 67.4% died from relapse of primary malignancy and 21.3% from treatment-related mortality. Death rates due to subsequent cancers and other causes increased more rapidly in the time period of 15 to 25 years postdiagnosis as compared to 5 to 15 years postdiagnosis. It is therefore critical that childhood cancer survivors be educated about the importance of lifetime annual long-term follow-up care, including screening for disease recurrence and late effects as a result of therapy.

Communication and Counseling

The most effective method of health education/counseling for late effects for childhood cancer survivors requires further investigation. The childhood cancer experience is unique in that some survivors, given their young age at diagnosis, may not remember the diagnosis and the treatment received with respect to their cancer. For some survivors, parents may not have even talked to them about their history of cancer. Thus, the findings by Kadan-Lottick and associates show that important knowledge deficits about past diagnosis and treatment when childhood cancer survivors are questioned are not surprising. In view of these findings, Kadan-Lottick and colleagues recommended that much of a patient's history alone cannot be trusted to guide medical management for late effects evaluations; instead medical records must be obtained from the treating institutions. It is imperative, therefore, that both the survivor and/or the family and the primary care providers be given a treatment summary in an attempt to optimize screening for the late effects of childhood cancer treatment.

It is an exciting time in the field of pediatric oncology because cure rates are reaching an all-time high and childhood cancer survivorship can now be considered an "epidemic." It is crucial for providers caring for this population to recognize the significant risk for late effects, monitor the childhood cancer survivor longitudinally, and make appropriate referrals to long-term follow-up care programs.

SUGGESTED READINGS

1. Anderson DM, Rennie KM, Ziegler RS, et al: Medical and neurocognitive late effects among survivors of childhood central nervous system tumors. Cancer 92:2709–2719, 2001. **Study of medical and neurocognitive late effects of therapy for childhood central nervous system tumors.**
2. Anderson DM, Rennie KM, Ziegler RS, et al: Medical and neurocognitive late effects among survivors of childhood central nervous system tumors. Cancer 92:2709–2719, 2001. **Late medical and neurocognitive effects.**
3. Duffner PK, Cohen ME: Long-term consequences of CNS treatment for childhood cancer. Part II. Clinical Consequences. Pediatr Neurol 7:237–242, 1991. **A look at the clinical consequences of central nervous system treatment for childhood malignancies.**
4. Elkin T, Phipps S, Mulhern R: Psychological functioning of adolescent and young adult survivors of pediatric malignancy. Med Pediatr Oncol 29:582–588, 1997. **A paper on psychosocial aspects of cancer survival.**
5. Hudson MM, Mertens AC, Yasui Y, et al: Health status of adult long-term survivors of childhood cancer: a report from the Childhood Cancer Survivor Study. JAMA 290(12):1583–1592, 2003. **An important childhood cancer survival study.**
6. National Cancer Institute Office of Cancer Survivorship. Cancer survivorship research. Available online at http://dccps.nci.nih.gov/ocs/about.html. **A useful website.**
7. Kadan-Lottick NS, Robison LL, Gurney JG, et al: Childhood cancer survivors' knowledge about their past diagnosis and treatment: Childhood Cancer Survivor Study. JAMA 287(14):1832–1839, 2002. **Revealing study that not all survivors of childhood cancer know the details or even the diagnosis of a past malignancy.**
8. Landier W, Bhatia S, Eshelman DA, et al: Development of risk-based guidelines for pediatric cancer survivors: The Children's Oncology Group Long-Term Follow-Up Guidelines from the Children's Oncology Group Late Effects Committee and Nursing Discipline. J Clin Oncol 22(24):4979–4990, 2004. **Risk-based guidelines.**
9. Mertens AC, Yasui Y, Neglia JP, et al: Late mortality experience in five-year survivors of childhood and adolescent cancer: The Childhood Cancer Survivor Study. J Clin Oncol 19(13):3163–3172, 2001. **Late mortality in survivors.**
10. Mitby PA, Robison LL, Whitton JA, et al: Utilization of special education services and educational attainment among long-term survivors of childhood cancer: A report from the Childhood Cancer Survivor Study. Cancer 97:1115–1126, 2003. **Educational outcome and utilization from the Childhood Cancer Survivor Study.**
11. Oeffinger KC, Eshelman DA, Tomlinson GE, et al: Programs for adult survivors of childhood cancer. J Clin Oncol 16(8):2864–2867, 1998. **A study about programs and risks.**
12. Oeffinger KC, Hudson MM: Long-term complications following childhood and adolescent cancer: Foundations for providing risk-based health care for survivors. CA Cancer J Clin 54(4):208–236, 2004. **A study of long-term complications and their use in developing risk-based health care.**
13. Oeffinger KC, Mertens AC, Hudson MM, et al: Health care of young adult survivors of childhood cancer: A report from the Childhood Cancer Survivor Study. Ann Fam Med 2(1):61–70,

4

2004. **Health care among young adults who are cancer survivors.**

14. Ries LAG, Smith MA, Gurney JG, et al (eds): Cancer Incidence Survival among Children and Adolescents: United States SEER Program 1975–1995. National Cancer Institute, SEER Program. (NIH Pub. No.99–4649). Bethesda, MD, 1999. **National data from the SEER database and National Cancer Institute.**

15. Ries LAG, Eisner MP, Kosary CL, et al (eds): SEER Cancer Statistics Review, 1973–1999. Bethesda, MD: National Cancer Institute, 2002. **National data from the SEER database and National Cancer Institute.**

16. Teta MJ, Del Po MC, Kasl SV, et al: Psychosocial consequences of childhood and adolescent cancer survival. J Chronic Dis 39:751–759, 1986. **A paper on psychosocial aspects of cancer survival.**

17. Weiner SL, Simone JV, Hewitt M (eds): Childhood cancer survivorship: Improving care quality of life. National Cancer Policy Board, Institute of Medicine and National Research Council. Washington, DC: National Academies Press, 2003, p 32. **Institute of Medicine report outlining a policy agenda for improving health care delivery and follow-up for childhood cancer survivors.**

18. Zebrack BL, Zeltzer LK, Whitton J, et al: Psychological outcomes in long-term survivors of childhood leukemia, Hodgkin's disease, and non-Hodgkin's Lymphoma: A report from the Childhood Cancer Survivor Study. Pediatrics 110:42–52, 2002. **A paper on psychosocial aspects of cancer survival.**

End-of-Life Care for Pediatric Patients

John J. Collins

KEY CONCEPTS

- Pediatric palliative care aims to provide the best possible quality of life by the providing holistic care at every stage of the illness trajectory, irrespective of location of care.
- Caring for a dying child is complex and includes a need to provide care beyond the physical that includes psychosocial, spiritual, and other domains of care.
- The symptom burden of children dying in the hospital is high.
- Anxiety about death is perhaps the central emotional problem of any seriously ill child.
- The majority of children with life-threatening illness have insight into the seriousness of their illness and that worry is a highly prevalent symptom.
- A child's understanding of death evolves as she or he goes through developmental stages.
- The death of a child is recognized as one of the most stressful life events for caregivers. In comparison with other individuals in different relationships to the deceased, parental grief is more intense and longer lasting.
- The grief response of siblings will, in part, depend on their developmental understanding of death.

The landmark World Health Organization (WHO) document, *Cancer Pain Relief and Palliative Care in Children,* details principles of pain management and

principles of palliative care that are universal and applicable to any child dying of cancer, irrespective of location. A further impetus for clinicians to embrace these principles is a study indicating that the memory of the suffering and physical symptoms of a dying child may be retained in the memory of parents and caregivers for many years after the death. This chapter considers palliative care using the child with terminal cancer as an example, but the principles are applicable to children dying of other causes.

Expert Opinion on Management Issues

WHAT IS PEDIATRIC PALLIATIVE CARE?

The pediatric palliative care paradigm concerns holistic care for children with progressive disease in whom death is expected before the adult years. The holistic viewpoint of palliative care encompasses the physical, psychological, social, spiritual, and other domains of care. There is a common mistaken belief that palliative care teams should be consulted only when there is disease progression and resistance to treatment. However, the palliative care paradigm is often applicable to children earlier in their disease trajectories. The aim of pediatric palliative care is to provide the best possible quality of life by providing holistic care at every stage of the illness trajectory, irrespective of location of care.

EVOLUTION OF PEDIATRIC PALLIATIVE CARE PROGRAMS

Pediatric palliative care has lagged behind the development of adult palliative care programs. In part this may be related to the long-held Western belief that death should be hidden, not discussed, and the assumption that a sick child will die in a hospital behind closed curtains. Additionally, until recently, there has been a lack of resources or support for a child to die in any other place but in the hospital. This practice is slowly changing as we come to understand the complexities of caring for a dying child, as we accept the need to provide care beyond the physical to include psychosocial and spiritual, and as more resources are being devoted to this area of medicine.

The evolving paradigm includes the notion of implementing palliative care principles at the earliest possible stage of a child's life-threatening illness and creating an integrated pediatric palliative care system around every child and family to meet their needs. The standard of palliative care in each location should be high and should not be less than that which could be provided in the hospital. As many of the conditions requiring palliative care may last for years, respite care is an integral feature of any pediatric palliative care program.

Despite the existence of treatment options for several conditions of childhood that now may result in long-term survival, there remains a significant risk of dying. Entry into a pediatric palliative care system can be a complex process of decision making because prognostic information about some diseases is scant and the prognosis is guarded. Children can "graduate" from a pediatric palliative program because of survival. For example, with the advent of liver transplantation, but because of the high risk of dying while waiting for a liver transplant, children may enter a palliative care program but, owing to their survival following transplantation, no longer require such care.

TRAJECTORY OF CANCER AS A LIFE-THREATENING ILLNESS IN CHILDHOOD

Prognosis depends on tumor type, risk indicators, and extent of disease (e.g., rhabdomyosarcoma, high white cell count at the diagnosis of acute lymphocytic leukemia, stage 4 disease). Even if remission is achieved, relapse may well herald a worsening prognosis. It is appropriate to include the pediatric palliative care paradigm into the protocols of children who have a poor prognosis at diagnosis.

SYMPTOMS OF CHILDREN AT THE END OF LIFE

There has been an increasing awareness that dying children need better symptom management. Wolfe found that 89% of 103 parents whose children died of cancer in a hospital setting reported that their children experienced "a lot" or "a great deal" of discomfort from at least one symptom in their last month of life. In the children who were treated for specific symptoms, parents considered treatment successful in only 27% of those with pain and in only 16% of those with dyspnea.

In a study by Drake and associates, symptoms and symptom characteristics during the last day of life were determined from interviewing a nurse who cared for a specific dying child during the last 24 hours of life using a symptom-assessment instrument. The dominant disease process was cancer, and the most common location of death was an intensive care unit. The mean duration of the "active phase of dying" was 25.2 hours, and the major physiologic disturbances at this time were respiratory failure and encephalopathy.

The mean ($\pm$SD) number of symptoms dying children reported was 11.1 ± 5.6, and significantly more ($P < 0.02$) symptoms occurred in children dying on the general ward (14.3 ± 6.1) as compared to those dying in intensive care (9.5 ± 4.7). Six symptoms (lack of energy, drowsiness, skin changes, irritability, pain, and edema of the extremities) occurred with a high prevalence (affecting 50% or more of the children) in the last week of life. The level of patient comfort as perceived from the medical notes indicated that the majority of children were "always comfortable" to "usually comfortable" in the last week (64%), day (76.6%), and hour (93.4%) of life. Taken together, these data suggest that the symptom burden of children dying in the hospital is high. Ironically, in Drake's survey, the symptom burden was significantly reduced in the intensive care unit, in which the most aggressive interventions were undertaken.

CHILDREN'S UNDERSTANDING OF DEATH

The paper *Who's Afraid of Death on a Leukemia Ward?* suggests that death anxiety is perhaps the central emotional problem of any seriously ill child. This study made clear that the majority of children with life-threatening illness have insight into the seriousness of their illness and that worry is a highly prevalent symptom. This fear seems to be universal. Children from diverse cultures are able to differentiate a potentially fatal illness from an acute or chronic nonfatal illness.

A child's understanding of death evolves with his or her developmental stage, starting spontaneously in the toddler years. However, when a child's thinking is at a preoperational or concrete stage (according to the developmental stages of Piaget), young children may have misconceptions about what has caused a death. Given their egocentric view of the world, young children may believe that what happens to others is directly related to their own thoughts, wishes, and actions. During ages 5 to 10 years, children gradually absorb the irreversible, universal elements of death and cease to see the dead as continuing to function. Older children can conceptualize the biological, social, and psychological changes that ensue following death.

PARENTS AS CAREGIVERS OF THE DYING CHILD

The Emotional Responses

Many parents experience anger and fear when the terminal phase of their child's illness is reached. The potential responses of parents to the impending death of their dying child include denial, anger, bargaining, depression, and acceptance. In addition to emotional support, the parents may need help in preparing their child and their other children for the death of the sibling. When death draws near, providing information about the way the child may die and how the child's discomfort and pain will be relieved will be helpful to parents.

Supporting Parents

Communicating the diagnosis of a child's life-threatening illness is an important but little-researched area. In general, parents have valued open, sympathetic, direct, and uninterrupted discussion of the diagnosis in private that allowed sufficient time for them to process the bad news and for doctors to repeat and clarify information. Parents dislike evasive or unsympathetic interviews and vividly remember the way the diagnosis was imparted, continuing to be preoccupied with this many years later. Ongoing open communication between health care providers and parents throughout the disease process is an integral part of the therapeutic relationship.

Home Care

There is a progressive trend for dying children to be cared for at home. Recent literature suggests this is a feasible option if families are adequately supported with appropriate expertise. Although the literature examining the experience of parents caring for their dying child at home is limited, evidence suggests the psychological adjustment of parents is better if the dying child is cared for at home rather than in the hospital.

A study conducted in Sydney, Australia, investigated the problems faced by parents caring for their dying child at home. Twenty families participated in this study, which was conducted by interview. The interval between death of the child and interview ranged from 6 months to 41 months. The child's age at death ranged from 4 months to 16 years, and time at home receiving palliative care ranged from 3 days to 184 days (mean, 46 days). The place of death was home for 16 children, 3 died in the hospital, and 1 child, whose home was far from the hospital, died in rented accommodation close to the hospital.

Multiple reasons led to the decision to proceed with the option of home care. The child's own wish to be home, parental perception the child would be happier at home, easier access of family and friends, freedom from the negative aspects of hospital life, less disruption to family life, and ability to cater for the child's food preferences were some of the reasons. Home-based palliative care was perceived as a positive experience for the majority of parents, allowing the participation of the siblings in the care of the child and making it easier to attend to the needs of the siblings. Some parents said home care enabled them to spend more time with their dying child. This enabled the family to be present at the time of death and be able to grieve in an unhurried manner.

All parents volunteered that the most difficult aspect of home care was watching their child's physical decline. Two thirds of parents perceived the night as particularly difficult. Various fears surfaced for many during the period of home care: fear of what would happen at the time of death, fear of not coping, and the child's own fear of death. The nursing responsibility, household duties, care of other siblings, finances, and uncertainty about what procedure to follow at the time of death were other perceived difficulties.

The results of this study imply that services must be comprehensive and include 24-hour support, as the palliative emergencies of pain, discomfort, and distress can occur at any hour. Parents seek education, request group support, and need help in negotiating the hospital system. Health care providers working in the area of pediatric palliative care must be able to stand by families who have fears and experience loneliness and isolation.

Subsequent Psychological Adjustment of the Family

In one study, 24 families who had participated in a home care program for children terminally ill with cancer and 13 families whose children had died in the hospital completed inventories on parent and sibling personality and family functioning 3 months to 29 months after the child's death. Parents of patients who received terminal care in the hospital appeared more anxious, depressed, and defensive and had a greater tendency toward somatic and interpersonal problems compared to parents of patients in the home care program. Siblings of patients who received terminal care in the hospital seemed more emotionally inhibited, withdrawn, and fearful compared to their counterparts in the home care program. Although some group differences in parental personality may have antedated terminal care, these results support parental reports of more adequate family adjustment following participation in a structured home care program. There are currently no comparative data on the psychological adjustment of families following the death of a child in a children's hospice.

Common Pitfalls

- Late referral to a palliative care program is an inappropriate way to prepare a child and his or her family for death.
- Parents will remember unrelieved distress in their dying child for many years to come unless meticulous attention is given to symptom management.
- Failing to communicate with a dying child without recognizing that a child's understanding of death evolves during developmental stages.
- Failing to understand that the death of a child is one of life's most stressful events for caregivers. Strategies must be put into place to care for bereaved parents and siblings.

Communication and Counseling
COMMUNICATING WITH DYING CHILDREN

Communicating with a dying child about death is difficult and is arguably one of the most poignant of life's tasks. Discussion about death remains a taboo subject, and consequently some families and staff overprotect, cover up, evade, or even lie to a dying child in an effort to avoid an unpleasant reality. This may stem from a common fear adults have about what to say should a child directly ask, "Am I going to die?" Nevertheless, open communication with children is generally thought to reduce a child's sense of isolation in the dying process and reduce anxiety.

As a child's understanding of death is developmental in nature it is not necessary for a child to have a mature understanding of death as a necessary outcome of discussions prior to death. The transition from life to death will be easier if fears are allayed, misconceptions corrected, and the sense of isolation reduced.

BEREAVEMENT
Parental Grief

The death of a child has been recognized as one of the most stressful life events that can occur. In comparison with others, who have different relationships to the deceased, the grief of parents is more intense and longer lasting. There is a high incidence (50%) of emotional disturbance in at least one family member after the child's death. A recent study indicated that parental grief appears to remain quite intense for at least 4 years.

The phenomenon of survivor guilt may account for why the resolution of grief is a difficult task for bereaved parents. Thoughts of suicide, self-accusations, inconsolable grief, and social withdrawal are common parental reactions to the loss. Because both parents are simultaneously confronted with the loss, each loses the primary support of the other. It should be emphasized that there may be lack of synchronicity in grieving styles in partners and that this could lead to dissimilar expectations and coping strategies.

Sibling Grief

Three important notions form the basis of our current understanding of sibling grief. First, children do have feelings that need to be validated by adults. Second, children do grieve, although their grief will be contingent on their understanding of death. Third, sibling relationships are important. Many children have at least one sibling with whom they will share a greater part of their life span than with any other person.

Siblings have both acute and long-term responses to a sister or brother's death. The immediate responses have been described as shock and indifference. No matter how prepared one may be for the inevitable death of a loved one, the initial reaction is often one of shock. No degree of anticipatory grief adequately prepares family members for the reality of death. Children are individuals and will respond to this shock in their own way. When children hear bad news or are anxious they often cope by resorting to familiar activities (e.g., playing) as a way of gaining control over a difficult situation. A behavior that may be interpreted as indifference by adults may, in fact, be the way a particular child copes with a stressful event.

Pediatric practice is slowly coming to understand the complexities of caring for a dying child, to accept the need to provide care beyond the physical, including psychosocial and spiritual care, and to allocate more resources to this important area of medicine

SUGGESTED READINGS

1. Binger CM, Ablin AR, Feuerstein RC, et al: Childhood leukemia: emotional impact on patient and family. N Engl J Med 280: 414–418, 1969. **Outlines the emotional impact of caring for a child with cancer.**
2. World Health Organization: Cancer Pain Relief and Palliative Care in Children. Geneva: World Health Organization, 1998. **Landmark WHO document mandating pain relief and palliative care to be incorporated into the care of every child with cancer, irrespective of geographical location.**
3. Chambers EJ, Oakhill A, Cornish LM, et al: Terminal care at home for children with cancer. BMJ 298:937–940, 1989. **Outlines the complexity of caring for a dying child at home.**
4. Collins JJ, Stevens MM, Cousens P: Home care for the dying child. Aust Fam Physician 27(7):1–5, 1998. **Outlines the complexity of caring for a dying child at home.**
5. Davies B: After a child dies: Helping the siblings. In Armstrong-Dailey A, Zarbock Goltzer S (eds): Hospice Care for Children. New York: Oxford University Press, 1993, pp 140–153. **Outlines support need to care for siblings.**
6. Davies B, Eng B: Special issues in bereavement and staff support. In Doyle D, Hanks GWC, MacDonald N (eds): Oxford Textbook of Palliative Medicine. New York: Oxford University Press, 1998. **Outlines bereavement needs of families and staff support required.**
7. Drake R, Frost J, Collins JJ: The symptoms of dying children. J Pain Symptom Manage 27(7):6–10, 2003. **Retrospective study documenting systematically the symptoms of children dying in hospital.**
8. Faulkner KW: Children's understanding of death. In Armstrong-Dailey A, Zarbock Goltzer S (eds): Hospice Care for Children. New York: Oxford University Press, 1993, pp 9–21. **Summary book chapter of a child's understanding of death.**
9. Goldman A: Palliative care for children with cancer. Arch Dis Child 65:641–643, 1990. **Landmark article on this issue.**
10. Hazzard A, Weston J, Gutterres C: After a child's death: factors related to parental bereavement. J Dev Behav Pediatr 13:24–30, 1992. **Outlines the potential emotional sequelae of caring for a dying child.**
11. Heffron WA, Bommelaere K, Masters R: Group discussions with the parents of leukemic children. Pediatrics 52:831–840, 1973. **Paper outlining concerns of parents of children with leukemia.**
12. Kubler-Ross E: On Children and Death. New York: Macmillan, 1983. **Landmark book on this issue.**
13. Mulhearn RK, Lauer ME, Hoffmann RG: Death of a child at home or in hospital. Pediatrics 71:743–747, 1983. **Indicates psychological sequelae in survivors may be less in families who cared for a dying child at home.**
14. Vernick J, Karon M: Who's afraid of death on a leukemia ward? Am J Dis Child 109:393–397, 1965. **Landmark paper demonstrating that death anxiety is one of the central psychological themes of any seriously ill child.**
15. Wolfe J, Grier HE, Klar N, et al: Symptoms and suffering at the end of life in children with cancer. N Engl J Med 342(5):326–333, 2000. **A retrospective study indicating that the memory of pain and suffering in dying children is retained in the memories of parents for many years.**
16. Woolley A, Stein GC, Forrest GC, et al: Imparting the diagnosis of life threatening illness in children. BMJ 298:1623–1626, 1989. **Outlines preferences for parents in the ways bad news is communicated.**

5 Special Problems in the Infant and Neonate

Respiratory Distress Syndrome

Roger F. Soll and Robert H. Pfister

KEY CONCEPTS

- Despite advances in care, respiratory distress syndrome (RDS) remains a significant source of morbidity and mortality.
- Antenatal interventions, specifically the use of antenatal corticosteroids in mothers at risk for delivering prematurely, decrease the risk of RDS and mortality.
- A variety of means of respiratory support are available and effective in treating infants with RDS, including NCPAP (nasal continuous positive airway pressure), conventional mechanical ventilation, and high-frequency ventilation.
- Postnatal treatment with intratracheal surfactant decreases the risk of pneumothorax and mortality. Earlier treatment leads to the best results.

Respiratory distress syndrome (RDS) affects the majority of infants of very low birth weight. In 2002 more than 4000 infants in the United States died from prematurity, and an additional 1000 infants died from factors directly related to RDS. Along with this significant mortality, RDS is associated with a significant morbidity and high cost to society.

A deficiency of pulmonary surfactant and structural immaturity of the lung causes RDS and leads to a cycle of atelectasis, ventilation-perfusion mismatch, hypoventilation, hypoxia, hypercarbia, and pulmonary vasoconstriction.

Mortality caused by RDS has decreased dramatically during the past decades thanks to effective antenatal and postnatal care. These interventions include the regionalization of high-risk maternal and neonatal care, effective use of tocolytic agents, and antenatal administration of corticosteroids to enhance lung maturity. After delivery, a variety of interventions, including improved understanding of neonatal homeostasis, respiratory support (including continuous positive airway pressure [CPAP], conventional mechanical ventilation, and high-frequency ventilation), and surfactant therapy contribute to improved outcome in infants with RDS.

Expert Opinion on Management Issues

ACCEPTED INTERVENTIONS

Antenatal Interventions

Currently available tocolytic therapy does not forestall labor sufficiently to decrease the incidence of premature delivery. But tocolytic therapy may lead to short-term delays that allow a window for therapy with corticosteroid treatment. Antenatal corticosteroids may induce lung structural maturation (increasing gas exchange surface), induce type II cell maturation, and increase surfactant synthesis. Meta-analysis of randomized, controlled trials concludes that antenatal corticosteroid administration prior to an anticipated preterm delivery is associated with a substantial reduction in the incidence of early neonatal death, as well as respiratory distress syndrome, intraventricular hemorrhage, and necrotizing enterocolitis. In follow-up studies, exposure to antenatal corticosteroid therapy does not adversely affect physical growth or psychomotor development.

Dexamethasone and betamethasone are the preferred corticosteroids for antenatal therapy. Treatment with two doses of 12 mg of betamethasone, given intramuscularly 12 hours apart, or four doses of 6 mg of dexamethasone, given intramuscularly 12 hours apart, is effective. Strong evidence exists for neonatal benefits from a complete course of antenatal corticosteroids, starting at 24 hours and lasting up to 7 days after treatment. Data are inadequate to establish the clinical benefit beyond 7 days after antenatal corticosteroid therapy. It is unclear whether and when to give repeat doses of antenatal corticosteroids.

Postnatal Interventions

Respiratory Support

A variety of techniques of respiratory support are improving the outcome of infants with RDS. These range from the least invasive methods of support, such as nasal continuous positive airway pressure (NCPAP), to aggressive support with either conventional mechanical ventilation or high-frequency ventilation.

Nasal CPAP may help maintain functional residual capacity in infants affected with RDS. Studies that examine the variation in outcomes and practice among centers suggest the early use of NCPAP may reduce the incidence of chronic lung disease. In addition, studies using historical controls demonstrate an improved outcome with introduction of the early application of NCPAP. However, few data are available from randomized, controlled trials.

Success in providing assisted ventilation to the newborn was noted in the early 1970s when time-cycled pressure-limited ventilation was introduced. Although not subjected to rigorous trials, the introduction of time-cycled pressure-limited ventilation led to striking decrease in mortality in infants of very low birth weight. Recent technical improvements, including synchronized intermittent mechanical ventilation, are not of great clinical benefit. However, patient-triggered ventilation and other methods of pressure support are widely used in neonatal intensive care. High-frequency ventilation, particularly high-frequency oscillation, has gained widespread use in infants with RDS. Meta-analyses of these trials suggest a decrease in lung injury (decreased oxygen dependency at 36 weeks' adjusted age) but no change in mortality. Concern from initial studies regarding an increased rate of intraventricular hemorrhage (IVH) is not supported in current meta-analyses.

Pulmonary Surfactant

Numerous randomized, controlled trials show that the intratracheal administration of exogenous surfactant preparations is effective in both the prevention and treatment of RDS. Both synthetic and animal-derived (natural) surfactant products have been tested. Meta-analyses of the randomized, controlled trials show that when compared to conventional management without surfactant replacement, surfactant therapy results in a significant decrease in the risk of mortality and pneumothorax. In comparative trials, animal-derived surfactant extracts decrease the risk of pneumothorax and neonatal mortality when compared to the use of currently available non–protein-containing synthetic surfactants. Current studies are under way using protein-containing synthetic surfactants.

Administration of surfactant is tested using two strategies: prophylactic and rescue treatment. In prophylactic therapy, surfactant is administered in the delivery room to infants at high risk for developing RDS (infants less than 30 weeks' gestation), usually within 10 to 15 minutes of birth. In rescue or selective surfactant therapy, surfactant is administered to infants after they develop signs of RDS. Prophylactic administration of surfactant in the delivery room offers the theoretical advantage of replacing surfactant before the onset of respiratory disease, decreasing the need for ventilator support and avoiding secondary barotrauma that may result from even short periods of assisted ventilation. Meta-analysis of the eight randomized, controlled trials that evaluated the benefits of prophylactic surfactant therapy compared to surfactant treatment of infants with established respiratory distress syndrome demonstrates that prophylactic administration of natural surfactant extract leads to a significant reduction in the risk of pneumothorax and

a significant reduction in the risk of neonatal mortality. An analysis of the number needed to treat indicates that prophylactic administration of natural surfactant is an appropriate and cost-effective intervention. It saves one life for every 20 infants receiving treatment. It is unclear whether extremely early therapy (within the first hour of life) is as effective as prophylactic therapy and will allow for greater discrimination regarding the need for treatment.

POTENTIAL INTERVENTIONS

Early Surfactant Administration with Rapid Extubation to Nasal Continuous Positive Airway Pressure

An approach that combines aspects of both early delivery room surfactant administration and early stabilization on NCPAP was tested in Denmark. Infants received intratracheal surfactant and then were rapidly extubated to NCPAP. Trends toward less need for mechanical ventilation and lower mortality were noted in these studies.

Permissive Hypercapnia

The idea of so-called gentle ventilation is universally accepted as a goal of respiratory management. Some investigators advocate ventilation that allows for a slight increase in $Paco_2$ above normal ranges to minimize the need to increase ventilator support and the secondary lung injury that may ensue. However, no randomized, controlled trials demonstrate a benefit to this management strategy.

NO BENEFIT

Early Aggressive Use of Diuretics

Edema of the pulmonary interstitium and alveolar spaces is a significant complicating factor in the pathophysiology of RDS. Prior to the era of surfactant replacement, clinicians observed that a spontaneous diuresis (usually between 36 and 72 hours of age) heralds acute improvement and resolution of RDS. These observations led to several trials of postnatal diuretic therapy early in the course of RDS. Despite the theoretical rationale, the early use of diuretic therapy demonstrates no clinical benefits.

Early Postnatal Steroids

Antenatal steroids are clearly indicated in women at risk for preterm delivery to promote lung maturity, but the use of glucocorticoids in the immediate postnatal period is more problematic. Glucocorticoids are thought to reduce pulmonary inflammation and decrease pulmonary interstitial edema. When used early, glucocorticoids may decrease oxygen dependency at 28 days' and 36 weeks' gestation. However, serious short-term (gastrointestinal perforation, infection, hypertension) and long-term (cerebral palsy, developmental delay, growth retardation) complications preclude use in this fashion to prevent chronic lung disease.

Use of Sedation and Analgesic Agents

The use of sedation and analgesic agents to decrease pain and discomfort in ventilated premature infants is widespread despite the paucity of evidence concerning correct dosing regimens, safety, and efficacy. A trial of morphine in ventilated preterm infants demonstrates a decrease in clinical signs of pain but is associated with a significant increase in adverse outcomes (IVH, periventricular leukomalacia [PVL], and/or death). Review of trials of intravenous midazolam as a sedative in neonates demonstrates that use of intravenous midazolam infusion may prolong hospital stays. Although ventilation asynchrony may cause complications during mechanical ventilation, such as pneumothorax, intraventricular hemorrhage, and barotrauma, the routine use of neuromuscular blockade of ventilated preterm infants cannot be recommended based on current evidence. In fact, oral sucrose, breast milk, and skin-to-skin contact are safe and effective for reducing procedural pain from single painful events in stable, older, nonventilated infants. Although humane and ethical considerations for providing comfort exist, the decision to use sedation or analgesia will likely be guided by expert opinion and personal preference among clinicians. Further research on the effectiveness and safety of sedation in neonates is needed.

Common Pitfalls

- Overzealous support in the delivery room or early in the course of treatment may predispose to chronic lung disease.
- Waiting to administer surfactant treatment while other aspects of general care are pursued (e.g., line placement for monitoring) may delay treatment unnecessarily.
- In infants who do not improve after initial stabilization on appropriate respiratory support and surfactant treatment, pneumothorax, infection, and patent ductus arteriosus should be considered.
- Intensive care is a multidisciplinary effort; the approach to respiratory support that the team is most comfortable with should be used.

Communication and Counseling

- Appropriate communication and counseling begins prior to delivery.
- When counseling parents, it is critical to give an accurate assessment of risks based on gestational age.
- Clinicians must be prepared to resuscitate and treat as early as the time of birth (in the delivery room).
- The risks associated with prematurity and RDS, including pneumothorax, IVH, chronic lung disease, and death, must be understood.
- Effective communication is difficult in the stressful environment of intensive care.

SUGGESTED READINGS

1. Arias E, Macdorman MF, Strobino DM, et al: Annual summary of vital statistics, 2002. Pediatrics 112(6 Pt 1):1215–1230, 2003. **Basic review of causes of death and injury in the United States.**
2. Avery ME: Surfactant deficiency in hyaline membrane disease: The story of discovery. Am J Respir Crit Care Med 161(4 Pt 1):1074–1075, 2000. **The story of the experiments that led to the understanding of the pathophysiology of RDS.**
3. Avery ME, Tooley WH, Keller JB, et al: Is chronic lung disease in low birth weight infants preventable? A survey of eight centers Pediatrics 79(1):26–30, 1987. **Comparison of chronic lung disease at eight centers involved in lung research, noting the center that practiced the least invasive form of respiratory support (NCPAP) had the lowest rate of chronic lung disease.**
4. Effect of corticosteroids for fetal maturation on perinatal outcomes: NIH Consensus Development Panel on the Effect of Corticosteroids for Fetal Maturation on Perinatal Outcomes. JAMA 273(5):413–418, 1995. **Review of the impact of antenatal corticosteroids in women at risk for premature delivery and specific guidelines for use.**
5. Jobe AH: Drug therapy: Pulmonary surfactant therapy. N Engl J Med 328:861–868, 1993. **Review of surfactant replacement therapy.**
6. NICHD. Cochrane neonatal home page. http://www.nichd.nih.gov/cochrane/cochrane.htm. **Access to reviews and meta-analyses of a variety of neonatal interventions.**
7. Verder H, Albertsen P, Ebbesen F, et al: Nasal continuous positive airway pressure and early surfactant therapy for respiratory distress syndrome in newborns of less than 30 weeks' gestation. Pediatrics 103(2):E24, 1999. **Study of use of surfactant replacement therapy and NCPAP.**

5

Persistent Pulmonary Hypertension of the Newborn

Tina A. Leone and Neil N. Finer

KEY CONCEPTS

- Persistent pulmonary hypertension of the newborn (PPHN) most often occurs in the presence of other diseases causing pulmonary pathology.
- The clinical presentation of PPHN includes lability of oxygenation and blood pressure and pre- and postductal oxygenation gradients during the initial presentation.
- The exclusion of cyanotic congenital heart disease is important in the evaluation of the hypoxemic infant.
- Therapy for PPHN should be directed toward the underlying/associated pathophysiology, initiated promptly, and elevated in accordance with the clinical condition of the infant to prevent undesirable outcomes.

Persistent pulmonary hypertension of the newborn (PPHN), a disorder that occurs in approximately 2 per 1000 live births, is associated with a 10% to 20% risk of mortality. An understanding of normal fetal and transitional circulation is essential to understanding the pathophysiology of PPHN. Multiple underlying diseases of primarily pulmonary origin are associated with the onset of PPHN and influence the ultimate outcome.

During fetal life, gas exchange takes place in the placenta, and increased pulmonary vascular resistance results in only approximately 10% to 20% of the total cardiac output providing pulmonary blood flow. The remainder of the fetal cardiac output is shunted through the foramen ovale and the ductus arteriosus to the systemic circulation. After birth, the lungs are expanded, and pulmonary vascular resistance decreases in response to increased oxygen tension and the initiation of breathing, which results in increased pulmonary blood flow. After the transition from fetal to neonatal circulation, the majority of which takes place in the first few minutes of life, the entire cardiac output provides pulmonary blood flow. Blood may flow through the ductus arteriosus and the foramen ovale from the side of higher pressure to the side of lower pressure until those structures close.

The mechanisms involved in regulating pulmonary vascular resistance perinatally are multifactorial. The intrinsically muscular pulmonary arteries in the fetus are compressed by the small fluid-filled lung, decreasing pulmonary blood flow, and the compression is released after birth when the lung fluid is replaced with air. A balance among vasoactive substances in the pulmonary environment enables the fetal pulmonary vessels to exist in a predominantly vasoconstricted state and changes in the balance create a state of predominant vasodilation in the newborn. The predominant vasoconstrictors include endothelin–1 (ET–1), which interacts with ET_A receptors, leukotrienes, and thromboxane A_2, and the predominant vasodilators include endogenous nitric oxide (NO) and the prostaglandin PGI_2, both stimulated by bradykinin. Nitric oxide is released from endothelial cells when endothelial nitric oxide synthase (eNOS) is stimulated. The activity of nitric oxide on smooth muscle cell relaxation is mediated by an interaction of NO with guanylyl cyclase, producing cyclic GMP (guanosine monophosphate). The complex interaction of these vasoactive substances in response to changes in oxygen tension and physical forces within the lungs control the pulmonary vascular resistance in the perinatal period.

When the normal decrease in pulmonary vascular resistance does not occur after birth, PPHN develops. Elevated pulmonary vascular resistance postnatally results in a fetal blood flow pattern in which blood is shunted through the patent ductus arteriosus (PDA) and the patent foramen ovale (PFO). The direction of blood flow is dynamic depending on the relative pressures of the pulmonary and systemic circulations. The hallmark of PPHN is lability of oxygenation and intravascular pressure. Transient increases in pulmonary pressure occur during periods of stress for the infant, resulting in shunting of blood in a right-to-left direction through the foramen ovale and ductus arteriosus, causing systemic hypoxemia. This phenomenon is exacerbated when systemic pressure is low, which occurs commonly in PPHN for several reasons. As pulmonary blood flow is reduced, the pulmonary venous return to the left atrium is also reduced, decreasing preload to the left ventricle. The contractility of the heart may also be compromised by an enlarged right ventricle bowing into the left ventricle. When left ventricular output is reduced, the coronary arteries are poorly perfused, and in the presence of right-to-left shunting at the atrial level, they receive poorly saturated blood, placing the myocardium at risk for injury.

Failure of reduction in pulmonary vascular resistance is influenced by conditions of hypoxia and acidosis. Therefore, PPHN most often occurs in association with pulmonary diseases such as respiratory distress syndrome, meconium aspiration syndrome, pneumonia, and sepsis. Pulmonary hypoplasia, such as occurs in congenital diaphragmatic hernia (CDH) or associated with prolonged oligohydramnios, may also elevate pulmonary vascular resistance in the neonate and cause severe PPHN. Approximately 20% to 25% of cases of PPHN occur in the absence of any other pathology and are known as idiopathic PPHN.

The diagnosis of PPHN is facilitated by recognizing the clinical syndrome of lability of oxygenation and blood pressure associated with the disorder. The main differential diagnosis is cyanotic congenital heart disease (CHD), which causes a fixed hypoxemia. Although generally thought of as a disease of term or near-term infants, PPHN may occur in infants of any gestational age with pulmonary pathology, and it is seen in the very preterm infant with moderate to severe respiratory distress syndrome. A high index of suspicion is necessary when caring for any infant requiring oxygen or ventilation. Early in the course of illness, shunting occurs primarily at the ductal level, creating a pre- and postductal oxygenation difference, with the more saturated blood at the preductal site. As the disease progresses, shunting occurs at the level of the foramen ovale, and the pre- and postductal gradient is lost. Most infants with PPHN have an increase in Po_2 when exposed to 100% oxygen as opposed to infants with cyanotic CHD. Continuous positive airway pressure (CPAP) may or may not improve oxygenation in infants with cyanotic heart disease. A murmur may be heard consistent with tricuspid regurgitation. Chest radiograph findings are usually consistent with the underlying pulmonary pathology and demonstrate decreased pulmonary vascular markings. An echocardiogram can be used to rule out CHD and confirm the clinical diagnosis of PPHN with the typical findings of right-to-left or, most commonly, bidirectional shunting at the PDA and PFO, a dilated right ventricle with a flattened or bowed intact ventricular septum (IVS), and tricuspid regurgitation, which can be used to calculate the actual pulmonary artery pressure. The oxygenation index (OI) ([mean airway pressure × Fio_2 × 100]/Pao_2) may be used as an indication of progression of disease in relation to how much respiratory support is being provided.

Expert Opinion on Management Issues

The overall goals of management are to decrease pulmonary vascular resistance, support the infant with adequate oxygenation until the PPHN resolves, and treat any associated pathology. Such treatments include but are not limited to antibiotics for pneumonia and sepsis, surfactant for primary surfactant deficiency or conditions of surfactant inactivation (e.g., meconium aspiration syndrome), and restoration of adequate ventilation and oxygenation. A stepwise approach to therapy is necessary because of the wide range of severity of illness associated with this condition.

The initial steps in treating an infant with PPHN involve providing adequate oxygen and ventilation to support lung function. The level of oxygenation provided is controversial at this time, but there is general agreement that the oxygen saturation should be maintained at a minimum of 96% to 97%. Keeping the infant calm and avoiding noxious stimuli helps prevent additional elevation in pulmonary artery pressures. This may be accomplished with appropriate analgesia and/or sedation, a quiet environment, and in very severe cases a trial of neuromuscular blockade. Maintenance of adequate tissue perfusion and blood pressure to prevent right-to-left shunting of blood and further clinical deterioration is a critical component of therapy. Blood pressure support may be achieved with volume infusion or pharmacologic therapy, such as with dopamine, dobutamine, milrinone, or other agents. Milrinone may be particularly useful in this circumstance because it is a phosphodiesterase inhibitor and may increase levels of cyclic GMP. Steroids are often used to increase blood pressure and cardiac function and reduce inflammation, but like many other therapies for this condition, they have not been proved efficacious.

The most extensive clinical evidence of benefit exists for the use of inhaled nitric oxide (iNO) for the treatment of PPHN. Inhaled nitric oxide acts specifically as a pulmonary vasodilator because it is administered by inhalation and has an extremely short half-life, preventing systemic effects. In term or near-term infants, iNO improves oxygenation and reduces the need for extracorporeal membrane oxygenation (ECMO). Although the initiation of iNO at an OI of 25 is recommended, we believe it is more appropriate to consider starting iNO at an OI of 10 to 15 to provide maximal benefit and to prevent escalating illness. Other vasodilators used in the past have systemic activity causing hypotension. The ability to provide other medications, such as prostacyclin and phosphodiesterase inhibitors, by inhalation is creating the potential for new therapies. Phosphodiesterase inhibitors, such as sildenafil, prevent the degradation of cyclic GMP, prolonging the vasodilatory effect of nitric oxide. Phosphodiesterases are specific to different tissues, and therefore selective phosphodiesterase inhibitors may be effective in specifically causing pulmonary vasodilation. Current clinical trials are evaluating these therapies, and specific recommendations for their use must await these results.

Significant evidence supports the use of ECMO as a lifesaving rescue therapy for refractory PPHN. ECMO allows the infant time to resolve the increased pulmonary vascular resistance while preventing lung damage from high ventilator pressures. Venovenous ECMO is particularly efficacious in PPHN because it delivers highly oxygenated blood directly to the pulmonary artery, helping reduce the pulmonary artery pressure while avoiding the need to cannulate the carotid artery. Many complications are associated with the use of ECMO, making patient selection for ECMO critical. ECMO is only done in a limited number of centers, and referral to an ECMO center must occur at a time when transport and treatment can be initiated prior to further deterioration. ECMO centers often consider an infant's OI of 40 a criterion for initiating ECMO. Non-ECMO centers should consider transport to an ECMO center when the OI reaches 25, and at a minimum they should consult with their regional center when an infant has an OI of 25 or greater.

CDH, a condition resulting from incomplete formation of the diaphragm and causing herniation of the abdominal contents into the chest, is often associated with severe PPHN. The lungs become compressed by the herniated abdominal contents and are usually hypoplastic, more severely on the side of the hernia, although both lungs are usually affected. A permissive approach to ventilation with the intent to avoid barotrauma improves outcomes. Although no proven benefit is demonstrated from the use of surfactant or iNO in this disorder, some infants may benefit from their use.

Common Pitfalls

Failure to recognize PPHN and provide early intervention may result in more severe clinical disease. Once the infant is stabilized, a slow methodical approach to weaning should be followed. Excessively rapid weaning may result in a more severe state of PPHN, which on occasion can be intractable. Recognizing the destabilizing effects of procedures such as airway suctioning and weighing, these procedures when necessary should be done with a consideration for the prior use of sedation/analgesia. Careful monitoring for disease progression and timely transfer to an appropriate level of care can be lifesaving in this condition. Overall therapy must include appropriate treatment of the underlying pathology.

Communication and Counseling

When discussing PPHN with family members, it is important to explain it is a disease of transition from the fetal to neonatal environment. Conveying an understanding of the labile nature of this condition and the possibility of worsening status prior to improvement is also helpful in counseling parents. Discussion of length of treatment depends mainly on the underlying pathology. Each institution needs to determine when transfer to another institution is appropriate, and this potential situation should be presented to the family. Prior to discharge, discussion should include an overview of outcome for these infants, which includes a risk for some level of neurodevelopmental dysfunction and the risk of frequent respiratory infections in the first few years of life, including the possibility of rehospitalizations.

SUGGESTED READINGS

1. Dukarm RC, Steinhorn RH, Morin FC III: The normal pulmonary vascular transition at birth. In Glick PL, Irish MS, Holm BA (eds): New Insights into the Pathophysiology of Congenital Diaphragmatic Hernia. Clinics in Perinatology. Philadelphia: WB Saunders, 1996, pp 711–726. **Description of transitional circulation.**

5

2. Finer NN, Barrington KJ: Nitric oxide for respiratory failure in infants born at or near term. Cochrane Database Syst Rev 4: CD000399, 2001. **Meta-analysis of the use of nitric oxide for PPHN in term and near-term infants.**

3. Hansell DR: Extracorporeal membrane oxygenation for perinatal and pediatric patients. Respir Care 48:352–362, 2003. **Overview of ECMO.**

4. Heymann MA: Control of the pulmonary circulation in the fetus and during the transitional period to air breathing. Eur J Obstet Gynecol Reprod Biol 84:127–132, 1999. **Review of mechanisms controlling transitional circulation.**

5. Kinsella JP, Shaul PW: Physiology of nitric oxide in the developing lung. In Polin RA, Fox WW, Abman SH (eds): Fetal and Neonatal Physiology, 3rd ed. Philadelphia: WB Saunders, 2004, pp 733–743. **Detailed description of endogenous and inhaled nitric oxide in the fetal and transitional circulation and treatment of PPHN.**

6. Lipkin PH, Davidson D, Spivak L, et al: Neurodevelopmental and medical outcomes of persistent pulmonary hypertension in term newborns treated with nitric oxide. J Pediatr 140:306–310, 2002. **Outcome at 1 year of age of infants treated with iNO.**

7. Neonatal Inhaled Nitric Oxide Study Group: Inhaled nitric oxide in term and near term infants: Neurodevelopmental follow-up of the neonatal inhaled nitric oxide study group (NINOS). J Pediatr 136:611–617, 2000. **Outcome at 2 years of age of infants treated with iNO.**

8. Travadi JN, Patole SK: Phosphodiesterase inhibitors for persistent pulmonary hypertension of the newborn: A review. Pediatr Pulmonol 36:529–535, 2003. **Review of phosphodiesterase inhibitors as therapy for PPHN.**

9. Walsh-Sukys MC, Tyson JE, Wright LL, et al: Persistent pulmonary hypertension of the newborn in the era before nitric oxide: Practice variation and outcomes. Pediatrics 105:14–20, 2000. **Epidemiologic description of PPHN, variation in practice, and outcome.**

10. Weinberger B, Weiss K, Heck DE, et al: Pharmacologic therapy of persistent pulmonary hypertension of the newborn. Pharmacol Ther 89:67–79, 2001. **Overview of pharmacologic therapies available for PPHN.**

Bronchopulmonary Dysplasia in the Neonate

Kristi L. Watterberg and Elizabeth A. Perkett

KEY CONCEPTS

- Bronchopulmonary dysplasia (BPD) is a leading morbidity for infants of extremely low birth weight and a significant risk factor for adverse neurodevelopmental outcomes. Infant development should be carefully monitored.

- Mechanical ventilation almost always precedes the development of BPD; consider techniques to limit or avoid ventilation.

- Early in the disease, hyperoxia may worsen BPD; later, premature withdrawal of oxygen may contribute to growth failure.

- Systemic dexamethasone should not be given routinely for prevention or treatment of BPD.

- Inhaled steroids have no proven benefit in preventing or decreasing the severity of BPD.

- Few respiratory interventions are supported by multi-center long-term studies; supportive care is paramount.
  - Monitor nutrition and growth closely; give more calories if needed.

- Ensure full immunization of infants, including influenza vaccine for family members.
- Avoid infections by good hand washing and limited contact outside family.
- Emphasize the importance of a smoke-free environment.
- Provide adequate oxygen supplementation for growth.

Bronchopulmonary dysplasia (BPD), chronic lung disease following neonatal lung injury, was first described in 1967. It was initially attributed to the injurious effects of oxygen and mechanical ventilation; however, as our patient population has evolved to include ever smaller and more immature infants, our understanding of this disease has also continued to evolve. The pathogenesis of BPD is undoubtedly multifactorial, with many injurious factors—such as chorioamnionitis, mechanical ventilation, and infection—acting on a susceptible, immature host to produce a disease that frustrates the many attempts to prevent and treat it.

Today, perhaps because of improved therapies, BPD occurs infrequently in larger premature infants. However, the disease still affects up to half or more infants of extremely low birth weight (ELBW) (2002 Vermont-Oxford database: 69% of surviving infants 500 to 750 g birth weight; 44% of those 750 to 999 g). Its incidence varies widely from nursery to nursery, perhaps reflecting differing patient populations, variations in management techniques, or both. Because the severity of BPD varies considerably, a new classification is proposed (Table 1).

EARLY INPATIENT MANAGEMENT OF DEVELOPING BRONCHOPULMONARY DYSPLASIA

Expert Opinion on Management Issues

As our understanding of BPD evolves and adverse effects of our therapies come to light, recommendations for therapies to prevent or treat BPD change over time. One striking example of such change is *dexamethasone*, which has been given for extended periods of time to prevent or decrease inflammatory lung injury. Reports of adverse neurologic outcomes from this therapy led the American Academy of Pediatrics to state that "routine use of systemic dexamethasone for the prevention or treatment of chronic lung disease in infants with very low birth weight is not recommended." Many other therapies currently used for BPD have little foundation in evidence-based medicine. From the Cochrane Database systematic reviews, there is insufficient evidence of long-term benefit to recommend diuretics, systemic or inhaled steroids, bronchodilators, or "permissive hypercapnia–minimal ventilation strategies." Vitamin A, which decreased BPD in a multicenter trial, has not gained widespread acceptance, possibly because of the need for many subcutaneous injections and the small perceived benefit (7% increase in survival without BPD).

TABLE 1 Definition of Bronchopulmonary Dysplasia

Treatment with oxygen for at least 28 days *plus*		
Severity of BPD	Infants <32 Weeks' Gestation	Infants ≥32 Weeks' Gestation
Mild	Breathing room air by 36 weeks PMA	Breathing room air by 56 days
Moderate	Need for <30% oxygen by 36 weeks PMA	Need for <30% oxygen at 56 days
Severe	Need for ≥30% oxygen and/or positive pressure at 36 weeks PMA	Need for ≥30% oxygen and/or positive pressure at 56 days

BPD, bronchopulmonary dysplasia; PMA, postmenstrual age.

MECHANICAL VENTILATION

BPD rarely occurs in nonventilated infants; therefore, techniques to avoid mechanical ventilation are worth pursuing, including:

■ Early use of continuous positive airway pressure (CPAP)
■ Accepting moderate hypercapnia on CPAP, rather than intubating to achieve normal Pco_2 values
■ "In-and-out" intubation for surfactant

Such techniques may be useful; however, their benefits and risks in high-risk ELBW patients are yet to be evaluated in multicenter randomized trials.

Oxygen therapy is obviously essential; however, appropriate saturation targets are less clear. A large randomized trial of infants with retinopathy of prematurity (the Supplemental Therapeutic Oxygen for Prethreshold Retinopathy for Prematurity [STOP-ROP] trial) showed that high oxygen saturation targets (96% to 98%) resulted in more BPD. An oxygen saturation range as low as 70% to 90% is suggested by some but has not yet been tested in a multicenter trial with assessment of long-term neurologic outcomes. Currently, a middle-of-the-road approach seems reasonable, targeting oxygen saturations of 85% to 94%. Fluctuations in oxygen saturation should be minimized by limiting interventions and clustering care, by giving additional ventilation before increasing Fio_2 in ventilated infants, and by increasing or decreasing Fio_2 in small increments, remaining at bedside until the situation stabilizes.

BRONCHODILATORS

Because increased lung inflammation may result in increased airway reactivity, both systemic and inhaled bronchodilators are administered to infants with developing BPD. However, the effectiveness of bronchodilators early in the course of the disease is not established, and their routine use is not warranted. If an infant shows evidence of airway hyperreactivity, an inhaled bronchodilator (albuterol) may be tried. Evidence does not support use of a systemic bronchodilator; however, clinicians may occasionally choose to try aminophylline in an unstable patient with bronchospasm.

DIURETICS

Because continuing lung inflammation in BPD can result in increased lung water, diuretic therapy (furosemide, hydrochlorothiazide) is advocated to improve pulmonary compliance and decrease oxygen need; however, the effect of diuretic therapy on long-term respiratory outcome is unclear. Diuretics clearly do cause renal wasting of electrolytes and thus complicate nutritional management. If diuretic therapy is used, electrolytes must be monitored, and dosing should be reduced to every-other-day therapy and discontinued as soon as possible. Evidence does not support a role for the addition of potassium-sparing diuretics to either furosemide or thiazide therapy.

Common Pitfalls

Focusing on the respiratory symptoms of BPD, we can easily overlook the paramount importance of *nutrition* in its management, probably the most important therapy we have, other than oxygen, to support infants with BPD. Illness, fluid restriction, and feeding difficulties can lead to decreased intake, whereas increased work of breathing requires increased calories. This combination puts these infants at extremely high risk for growth failure, additionally impairing lung growth and repair. Therefore, weight, length, and weight-for-length measurements should be closely monitored.

Immunizations are often deferred but should be given on schedule unless the infant is unstable. All infants should receive palivizumab (Synagis) before discharge during the local respiratory syncytial virus (RSV) season.

Communication and Counseling

Plans for care after discharge should be discussed with the family in the nursery and again at the first outpatient visit. Families need to know that the recovery process is slow, compared to the neonatal intensive care unit (NICU) environment. Many BPD infants may be on supplemental oxygen for up to a year, in part because the oxygen is contributing not just to survival but also to

TABLE 2 Medications

Generic Name (Trade Name)	Dose/Route/Regimen	Maximum Dose	Formulations	Common Adverse Reactions	Comments
Albuterol/salbutamol (numerous)	MDI: 1–4 puffs Nebulizer: 1 vial q4–6h	6×/day	MDI: 90 µg/puff Nebulizer: 2.5 mg/3 mL	Tachycardia, tremor	Inhaler must be used with holding chamber.
Budesonide (Pulmicort Respules)	0.25–0.5 mg q12h	0.5 mg bid	0.25, 0.5 mg vials	Thrush, facial irritation; adrenal suppression: rare	Use jet nebulizer, face mask; must rinse mouth after use.
Dexamethasone (Decadron)	For extubation, 0.15 mg/kg q12h × 4; then 0.05 mg/ kg q12h × 6 IV or PO	Unclear: may still be too high a dose	4 mg or 10 mg/mL, preservative-free	Many (e.g., ↑ glucose, hypertension, cardiac hypertrophy, GI irritation, growth impairment)	Because of numerous adverse effects, use short term in infants with previous failure of extubation. Avoid concurrent indomethacin use.
Fluticasone (Flovent MDI)	1–2 puffs q12h	440 µg/day	44, 110, 220 µgMDI	Thrush, facial irritation; adrenal suppression: rare	Must use holding device.
Furosemide (Lasix)	1 mg/kg IV; 1–2 mg/kg PO q12–48h	2 mg/kg IV; 6 mg/kg PO per dose	10 mg/mL (use IV solution: has no alcohol)	↓ Na, ↓ K, dehydration; renal calcifications	Monitor electrolytes.
Hydrochlorothiazide (HydroDIURIL)	1–2 mg/kg PO q12h	2 mg/kg per dose	10 mg/mL	↓ Na, ↓ K, dehydration	Monitor electrolytes; do not confuse with chlorothiazide (Diuril).
Metoclopramide (Reglan)	0.1–0.2 mg/kg PO q6h	0.8 mg/kg/day	1 mg/mL syrup	GI discomfort, sedation; rarely, extrapyramidal symptoms at high doses	Space dosing evenly throughout day, before meals, and at bedtime.
Palivizumab (Synagis)	15 mg/kg IM Monthly	N/A	50-mg, 100-mg vial	Pain/swelling at site	Give during RSV season; recommended for infants <2 years of age with BPD.
Ranitidine (Zantac)	2–5 mg/kg/dose PO q12h	10 mg/kg/day (maximum 300 mg)	15 mg/mL oral solution	Minimal; possible GI changes or discomfort	Oral solution has 7.5% alcohol; for very young infants, use unpreserved IV solution, stable 7 days refrigerated.

BPD, bronchopulmonary dysplasia; GI, gastrointestinal; IM, intramuscular; MDI, metered-dose inhaler; N/A, not applicable; PO, by mouth; q, every; RSV, respiratory syncytial virus.

optimal growth. Additionally, parents should be counseled that BPD is a risk factor for adverse developmental outcomes; therefore, development should be followed closely, with early intervention if indicated.

CONTINUING OUTPATIENT TREATMENT OF ESTABLISHED DISEASE

Expert Opinion on Management Issues

GENERAL GUIDELINES

These infants should be followed monthly for assessment of weight, length, head circumference, respiratory rate, blood pressure, oxygen saturation, and diet history (volume and calories). Ideally, infants should come to the office at a time when they will not be exposed to infectious diseases. Infants with BPD and their entire families should receive influenza vaccine, and infants should continue to receive palivizumab (Synagis) while RSV is active in the community.

NUTRITION

Optimal nutrition is extremely important for infants with BPD, with a goal of approximately 15 to 30 g per day weight gain. The first year of life is a critical period for lung development and growth. Increased calories are frequently required to support normal growth, catch-up growth, and increased work of breathing. These infants generally require a minimum of 140 kcal/kg, and sometimes up to 160 kcal/kg, for growth. The increased volume required to achieve this caloric intake may stress the infant both with increased respiratory and feeding effort, necessitating the use of high-density formulas. Monthly follow-up is usually sufficient to assess growth, but if an infant is not gaining adequate weight, more frequent assessments are needed.

Gastroesophageal reflux (GER) is a frequent complication during the first year of life. The only symptom may be increased respiratory rate, with or without cough, as infants attempt to protect their airway. Infants with increased respiratory rates have the most difficulty protecting their airways and are at risk for microaspiration. Infants with suspected GER should receive frequent small feedings and be kept upright after feedings. Thickening of formula may also be useful. If symptoms persist, antireflux medical therapy is indicated (acid blockers [ranitidine] and prokinetic drugs [metoclopramide]).

ENVIRONMENT

Infants should be in a nonsmoking environment. Environmental temperatures either too hot or too cold can increase caloric needs, so infants should be in a home where extremes of temperature can be avoided. Hand washing by family members is important to avoid transmission of infectious diseases. Contact with large numbers of people should be avoided, again to reduce exposure to pathogens.

OXYGEN

Although guidelines for the use of home oxygen remain unclear, numerous studies document benefits from home oxygen, including improved weight gain, increased dynamic compliance, decreased work of breathing, and decreased pulmonary hypertension. The most common guideline used is oxygen sufficient to maintain saturations higher than 92%, or 94% to 96% in infants with pulmonary hypertension.

RESPIRATORY THERAPY

Although BPD is defined by pulmonary damage, there is no specific therapy for the lungs. Nutrition, appropriate oxygen therapy, and avoidance of infections allow the infant to grow and resolve respiratory symptoms. No evidence indicates that inhaled medications benefit an infant with BPD, unless the infant has reactive airways. If an infant develops wheezing or increased work of breathing, a therapeutic trial of inhaled albuterol can be given. Infants with documented reactive airway disease requiring daily albuterol should be given inhaled steroids. Those with lower systemic absorption are preferred (i.e., fluticasone or budesonide, rather than beclomethasone).

Common Pitfalls

Solids should not be introduced too soon. The caloric density of solids is low, compared to infant formulas. The major source of calories for the first year for most patients should be breast milk or formula. Foods may be introduced for tasting but not for calories.

Improper mixing of formula is a potential problem. Parents should be given written instructions about the proper preparation of high-density formulas.

Premature withdrawal of supplemental oxygen is a potential problem. Infants may require increased oxygen therapy after hospital discharge, perhaps because of increased activity at home. Oxygen saturations at rest may not reflect oxygen needs when the infant is more active. If an infant has decreased saturations when feeding or active or fails to gain weight with adequate caloric intake, a trial of higher supplemental oxygen is warranted.

Nebulized medicines should be carefully administered. The dosage of aerosolized medications cannot be determined when given blow-by. Most inhaled medications can be given by metered-dose inhaler with a mask and spacer. Proper dosing is particularly important for inhaled steroids; if nebulized steroids are used, they must be given with an appropriate mask.

Communication and Counseling

Parents should be made aware that infants with BPD have limited respiratory reserves and can rapidly develop increased respiratory distress with infections. They may require increased oxygen therapy and even hospitalization for a mild viral illness. However, increased respiratory symptoms may also be caused by fluid overload (too large a volume of feedings), temperature (too hot or too cold), and gastroesophageal reflux. The importance of a nonsmoking environment—including wood stove and other sources of smoke, in addition to cigarettes—cannot be overemphasized.

SUGGESTED READINGS

1. AAP policy statement of the Committee on Infectious Diseases and Committee on Fetus and Newborn: Revised indications for the use of palivizumab and respiratory syncytial virus immune globulin intravenous for the prevention of respiratory syncytial virus infections. Pediatrics 112:1442–1446, 2003. **Contains current guidelines for use of palivizumab for premature infants, both with and without BPD, as well as revised recommendations for children with cyanotic congenital heart disease.**
2. Allen J, Zwerdling R, Ehrenkrantz R, et al: for the ad hoc subcommittee of the Assembly on Pediatrics, American Thoracic Society: Statement on the care of the child with chronic lung disease of infancy and childhood. Am J Respir Crit Care Med 168:356–396, 2003. **Exhaustive review of BPD, particularly emphasizing evaluation and continuing management of the infant with established BPD.**
3. Ellsbury DL, Acarregui MJ, McGuinness GA, et al: Controversy surrounding the use of home oxygen for premature infants with bronchopulmonary dysplasia. J Perinatol 24:36–40, 2004. **The authors found a lack of consensus and wide variation in criteria for initiation of home oxygen therapy and oxygen saturation targets. Presents a review of literature regarding effects of oxygen supplementation.**
4. Jobe AH, Bancalari E: Bronchopulmonary dysplasia: NICHD/NHLBI/ORD workshop summary. Am J Respir Crit Care Med 163:1723–1729, 2001. **Review of current understanding of pathogenesis and interventions for developing BPD.**
5. Smith VC, Zupancic JAF, McCormick MC, et al: Rehospitalization in the first year of life among infants with bronchopulmonary dysplasia. J Pediatr 144:799–803, 2004. **Infants with BPD are rehospitalized twice as often as other premature infants.**
6. Vohr BR, Wright LL, Dusick AM, et al: Neurodevelopmental and functional outcomes of extremely low birth weight infants in the NICHD Neonatal Research Network, 1993–1994. Pediatrics 105:1216–1226, 2000. **Large (1151 infants) cohort study of factors affecting outcomes at 18 months of age, showing that BPD is a significant risk factor for increased neurodevelopmental disability.**

Stabilization of the Neonate with Congenital Heart Disease

Robert H. Pass

KEY CONCEPTS

- Clinical assessment of the neonate with suspected congenital heart disease is still the cornerstone on which evaluation and therapy rest.
- Learning to assess the second heart sound accurately is critical in the evaluation of this patient group.
- Presence of a murmur or cyanosis in the first days of life in the absence of lung disease is a highly suspicious finding for important congenital heart disease. In the absence of

echocardiography, the hyperoxia test, in concert with the clinical assessment, is still of great value.
- Prostaglandin E_1 (PGE_1) should not be withheld in an infant with cyanosis and murmur or poor pulses or in the setting of clinical decompensation.
- Careful and accurate echocardiography is critical to the management of this patient group, particularly in the newer era of repair of congenital heart defects in the newborn period.

The approach to identification and management of neonates with congenital heart disease continually changes because of improvements in prenatal identification as well as the growing application of echocardiography in the initial evaluation and assessment of infants with congenital heart problems. Previously, accurate diagnosis of newborns with significant congenital heart disease largely depended on the clinician's expertise in examining a newborn and auscultating the heart. Although both skills are clearly important, their role in the precise anatomic elucidation of heart disease is perhaps less critical in the age of echocardiography and cardiac MRI. Finally, with the ever-growing realization that early neonatal repair of many congenital cardiac anomalies offers significant advantages over palliative surgery, a shift from a purely clinical diagnostic pathway to a combined clinical and biotechnologic approach is now mandatory to provide the cardiac surgeon with pertinent, detailed information. Thus, whereas the stethoscope and clinical exam are still of paramount importance, it would no longer be heretical to frame them as one of many essential diagnostic tools.

Expert Opinion on Management Issues

Once an accurate diagnosis is made, the appropriate approach to stabilizing such an infant with congenital heart disease is fairly straightforward. However, in many centers, the absence of the echocardiogram makes the first appropriate step unclear. After an infant shows appropriate and adequate patterns of breathing, the decision of whether to maintain ductal patency through the use of prostaglandin E_1 (PGE_1) must be made. In general, the use of PGE_1 in the treatment of a patient with presumed congenital heart disease and cyanosis is most likely the correct decision. A recent study, using information theory, assessed which patients were most likely to benefit from PGE_1 before an echocardiogram was obtained. They concluded the following:

- The risk of withholding PGE_1 changed with the patient's clinical condition. Patients in extremis will likely benefit more on average than those who are stable.
- A cyanotic patient with a murmur and a noncyanotic patient with poor pulses likely present good clinical scenarios where PGE_1 is useful and appropriate.
- The presence of cyanosis or abnormal pulses alone are likely good enough reasons to consider starting PGE_1.

TABLE 1 General Principles of Preoperative Treatment or Stabilization

Lesion	Initial/Preintervention General Management
Right-sided obstructive lesions	
TOF	Provide pulmonary blood flow: PGE_1.
TOF/PA	Intubate/sedate for catheterization or surgery if unstable.
PS	
PA/IVS	
Left-sided obstructive lesions	
HLHS	Provide systemic blood flow: PGE_1.
AS: valvar/subvalvar	Intubate/sedate for catheterization or surgery if unstable.
Aortic coarctation	Transcatheter atrial septoplasty for HLHS with restrictive ASD.
Aortic interruption	Raise pulmonary vascular resistance if too much PBF:
	1. Hypoventilation
	2. Ventilate with $Fio_2 = 0.21$
Single ventricles	
Tricuspid atresia	Provide pulmonary blood flow if needed: PGE_1.
Complex heterotaxy disease	Raise pulmonary vascular resistance if too much PBF:
	1. Hypoventilation
	2. Ventilate with $Fio_2 = 0.21$
Single ventricles: miscellaneous	
D-transposition of great arteries	Provide pulmonary blood flow: PGE_1.
	Consider balloon atrial septostomy for restrictive ASD.
Tachyarrhythmias	Pharmacologic management: level of aggressivity predicated on degree of hemodynamic embarrassment.
Bradyarrhythmias	Level of aggressivity predicated on degree of hemodynamic embarrassment. Consider surgical temporary or permanent epicardial pacing wires.

AS, aortic stenosis; ASD, atrial septal defect; HLHS, hypoplastic left heart syndrome; IVS, intact ventricular septum; PA, pulmonary atresia; PBF, pulmonary blood flow; PGE_1, prostaglandin E_1; PS, pulmonary stenosis; TOF, tetralogy of Fallot.

In general for cyanotic congenital heart disease, the decision to start PGE_1 only theoretically harms patients with obstructed pulmonary venous return (and this point is debatable). Finally, it is possible that patients with D-transposition of the great arteries with intact atrial and ventricular septi are not helped by this drug.

Discussion of the appropriate management schemes for all the different congenital lesions is clearly beyond the range of this chapter, but Table 1 reviews some guiding principles for management. In addition, the patient with low cardiac output typically benefits from inotropic support, such as α- and β-adrenergic agonists and phosphodiesterase inhibitors.

Common Pitfalls

- Failure to administer PGE_1 appropriately before echocardiography is available.
- Inappropriate use of PGE_1 in patients with lung or other problems that cause symptoms similar to congenital heart disease.
- Failure of PGE_1 to improve patient clinical status. This may be seen in patients with left-sided obstructive lesions either because of poor ventricular function with low cardiac output or inability of PGE_1 to open the ductus adequately (in rare circumstances) because of obstruction at the atrial septal level. Failure of PGE_1 is also seen in patients with D-transposition of the great arteries (D-TGA) and with intact atrial and ventricular septi requiring urgent balloon atrial septostomy.

- Certain inotropic agents or phosphodiesterase inhibitors may alter pulmonary or systemic vascular resistance to a degree that adversely affects the physiologic balance between the pulmonary and systemic circulations.

SUGGESTED READINGS

1. Castaneda AR, Mayer JE Jr, Jonas RA, et al: The neonate with critical congenital heart disease: repair—A surgical challenge. J Thorac Cardiovasc Surg 98:869–875, 1989. **Excellent early review of neonatal surgery and its potential implications for the cardiologist by the true original proponents of this now accepted approach.**
2. Danford DA, Gutgesell HP, McNamara DG: Application of information theory to decision analysis in potentially prostaglandin-responsive neonates. J Am Coll Cardiol 8:1125–1130, 1986. **An interesting application of information theory in determining the best approach in deciding who might need prostaglandin without the help of an echocardiogram.**
3. Marino BS, Wernovsky G: General principles: Preoperative care. In Chang AC, Hanley FL, Wernovsky G, Wessel DL (eds): Pediatric Cardiac Intensive Care. Philadelphia: Lippincott Williams & Wilkins, 1998, pp 151–162. **Review of general principles for managing children with congenital heart disease prior to repair or palliation.**
4. Nadas AS: Hypoxemia. In Fyler DC (ed): Nadas' Pediatric Cardiology. Philadelphia: Hanley & Belfus, 1992, pp 73–76. **Description of the central problem in many children with congenital heart disease by one of the true pioneers in the field.**
5. Penny DJ, Shekerdemian LS: Management of the neonate with symptomatic congenital heart disease. Arch Dis Child 84:F141–F145, 2001. **General concepts related to assessment and therapy for most common congenital heart lesions in infancy.**
6. Rossi AF: Cardiac diagnostic evaluation. In Chang AC, Hanley FL Wernovsky G, Wessel DL (eds): Pediatric Cardiac Intensive Care. Williams & Wilkins Philadelphia, 1998, pp 37–43. **Outstanding general review of the clinical assessment of children with congenital heart disease.**

Sudden Infant Death Syndrome

Alex Kline and Eric Gibson

KEY CONCEPTS

- Sudden infant death syndrome (SIDS) remains the leading cause of postneonatal mortality in the United States.
- Since initiation of the "Back to Sleep" campaign, the incidence of SIDS has decreased 50%.
- All healthy infants should be placed on their backs to sleep, and parents should be counseled about the risks of smoking.
- Infants born prematurely are at an increased risk for SIDS.
- Home monitors are not proven effective in the prevention of SIDS.

Beckwith defined sudden infant death syndrome (SIDS) as "the sudden unexpected death of an infant less than 1 year of age, with onset of the fatal episode apparently occurring during sleep, that remains unexplained after a thorough investigation, including performance of a complete autopsy and review of the circumstances of death and the clinical history."

SIDS was originally defined in 1969 at the Second International Conference on Causes of Sudden Death in Infants. It was revised in 1989 to exclude infants older than 1 year. It also specified that an examination of the death scene and review of the clinical history should be a part of the investigation. The present definition was delineated in April 2004 when a panel of experts met in San Diego, California, to address many of the controversies and pitfalls in SIDS diagnosis.

SIDS is now classified in the following categories:

- Category 1A: infants older than 21 days and younger than 9 months, with a normal term pregnancy and no circumstances that might explain the death
- Category 1B: cases in which the investigation is not considered complete
- Category 2: cases that meet category 1 criteria but classic criteria are not met, including atypical age ranges or certain circumstances of death or findings at autopsy

A separate category of unclassified sudden infant death includes those cases that do not meet the criteria for categories 1 or 2 and those cases in which an autopsy was not performed.

Despite a dramatic decrease in the incidence of SIDS cases since the American Academy of Pediatrics introduced the "Back to Sleep" campaign in 1992, SIDS remains the leading cause of postneonatal mortality and the second leading cause of infant mortality, after congenital anomalies. Approximately 2500 SIDS deaths occur per year in the United States, with an overall incidence of 0.6 per 1000 live births. This rate is doubled for premature infants, affecting almost 1.5 per 1000 live births. African American infants have a two to five times higher risk of SIDS compared to white infants. This increased risk persists even after implementation of the "Back to Sleep" campaign. A recent educational intervention at the Women, Infants, and Children (WIC) Programs was effective in informing caregivers about the importance of a safe sleep position that appeared to extend to the first 6 months of life when an infant is at highest risk for SIDS. In contrast, Asian Americans and Hispanics have lower SIDS rates when compared to whites.

The typical age distribution at which SIDS occurs is one of its characteristic features. Less than 3% of all SIDS deaths occur in the first month of life. The incidence peaks between 8 and 15 weeks, and 90% of all SIDS deaths occur by 6 months of age.

Certain groups of infants are at an increased risk for SIDS. As stated earlier, premature infants have a twofold increased risk compared with term infants, but the postconceptional age at death is not different between those infants born at term versus those born prematurely. Siblings of SIDS victims also have a slightly higher SIDS risk, with surviving twins having an even higher risk. Twins also have a higher rate of SIDS (1.3 of 1000 live births) than singletons (0.7 of 1000 live births). Infants who have acute life-threatening episodes (ALTEs) also have a slightly higher incidence of SIDS.

The differential diagnosis of an ALTE includes many of the etiologies thought to play a role in SIDS, including gastroesophageal reflux, seizures, infection, and abuse. Contrary to previously held beliefs, infants with a history of apnea of prematurity do not have a higher incidence of SIDS than premature infants who do not have apnea.

Overall SIDS risk factors include prematurity, low birth weight, maternal smoking during and after pregnancy, male gender, low socioeconomic status, limited prenatal care, young maternal age, single parenthood, and multiple gestations. Additional risk factors relate to unsafe sleeping conditions, which include sleeping prone and on the side, use of soft bedding, and sleeping with items such as pillows, comforters, and stuffed animals. Overheating is also an important risk factor. With the dramatic decrease in the rate of prone sleeping, maternal smoking now has emerged as the most important modifiable risk factor for SIDS. Co-sleeping may play a role in SIDS, especially if the parent is a smoker. Recent studies find that infants in child care settings have an increased risk of SIDS, with 15% of all SIDS deaths occurring in a child care setting, much higher than the 8% expected from the U.S. Census Bureau data. The reasons are unknown because infants in child care settings are no more likely to be placed or found prone, and they are more apt to sleep on a safe sleep surface.

Expert Opinion on Management Issues

The etiology of SIDS remains elusive. Although a single cause is unlikely, SIDS is most probably caused by multifactorial mechanisms, which may not be the same for all infants. Many of the initial theories revolved around difficulties with respiration, although problems with the cardiovascular system, as well as infectious and metabolic problems, were also evaluated. The fact that SIDS most often occurs during a predictable time period also raises speculation about possible deficits in the maturation of neural control.

Some form of respiratory failure is a common theme in many theories that attempt to explain SIDS. The infant airway is small and easily occluded at several points by external forces. In addition, failure of protective reflexes, such as coughing, sneezing, and pharyngeal and laryngeal closure, could foster occlusion of the airway and lead to obstruction. Decreased chemoreceptor sensitivity to hypoxia and hypercarbia may cause a failure to initiate respirations in an infant with an immature central nervous system.

Apnea has long been considered, although not proven, to play a central role in the etiology of SIDS, and some believe it is the final common pathway. Premature infants, siblings of infants with SIDS, and infants who experienced an ALTE all have higher rates of apnea than the general population. Infants with apnea have abnormalities in their ventilatory response to hypoxia and hypercarbia, in particular when carbon dioxide is rebreathed. The initial increase in ventilation seen with hypoxia is replaced by apnea and decreased ventilation after several minutes.

Another factor that puts infants at increased risk for SIDS is heat stress. Studies show hypoventilation in infants under conditions of heat stress. Research from Australia and England demonstrates that infants who die from SIDS are often in more heavily heated rooms and more wrapped than controls. In addition, infants with infection have an increased metabolic rate, which could lead to increased thermal stress and its associated effects on respiration.

Infection is also considered a factor in some SIDS cases. Studies show that 60% to 75% of infants with SIDS had signs of viral respiratory infection prior to their death. The similar age distribution of SIDS cases and the age of most severe cases of airway obstruction as evidenced by hospitalization for bronchiolitis is further evidence of a possible link. In addition, the winter peak in SIDS cases also corresponds to the time of year at which most viral respiratory infections occur.

The cardiovascular system, in particular the conduction system of the heart, is also postulated as important in some cases of SIDS. The conduction system became a focus of SIDS research in the 1970s when researchers discovered areas of apoptosis followed by replacement fibrosis in the myocardium of some infants with SIDS. Since then, many have postulated that SIDS may result from fatal cardiac electrical activity. Postmortem studies of the heart and conduction system show histopathologic changes in a variety of areas of the conduction system in infants with SIDS. Conduction abnormalities, particularly related to abnormal autonomic nervous supply to the cardiorespiratory system, continue to be an intriguing area of research.

Many studies examined the role that home monitors might play in the prevention of SIDS. Although monitors may be useful in detecting apneic and bradycardic events in infants, monitors are not effective in the prevention of SIDS or the identification of infants who are at increased risk.

"BACK TO SLEEP"

The first studies showing a link between SIDS and prone sleeping, conducted in Australia and England in the late 1980s, were retrospective. Subsequent prospective studies showed similar results. In 1991, New Zealand began the National Cot Death Prevention Program. Also in 1991, "Back Is Best" campaigns started throughout the United Kingdom. The American Academy of Pediatrics followed suit and in 1992 initiated the "Back to Sleep" campaign, encouraging parents to put all healthy infants to sleep on their sides or back. The incidence of SIDS subsequently dropped from 1.3 per 1000 live births in 1991 to 0.6 per 1000 live births in 1999, a reduction of greater than 50%. Some, but not all, infants with craniofacial or other airway anomalies and infants with severe gastroesophageal reflux may be exceptions to the rule that all infants should be placed to sleep on their backs.

Further modification of the infants' sleeping environment helps prevent SIDS. Parents should be encouraged not to place infants on soft bedding and not to use comforters or other objects such as stuffed toys in the crib. These increase the risk of suffocation.

Maternal smoking during pregnancy and afterward has long been recognized as a risk factor for SIDS. Research shows that exposure to smoke, both in utero and after birth, may be a major factor in as many as 60% of all SIDS deaths. Passive smoke exposure from all household members is also a risk factor for SIDS. Although the exact mechanism is unknown, effects of nicotine on respiratory centers may play a role. Nicotine affects airway chemoreceptors and can thus alter an infant's control of respiration. Other substances of abuse are also proposed risk factors for SIDS but are not substantiated in studies.

Breast-feeding should be encouraged in all situations where no contraindications exist. In addition to the many other benefits of breast-feeding, several studies show decreased SIDS among breast-fed infants.

NEWEST FINDINGS

In late 2004, significant data emerged to support bed sharing as a significant risk for SIDS. Earlier work had suggested this connection. With the dramatic drop in SIDS rates following the "Back to Sleep" campaign, some studies demonstrate that of the remaining cases of SIDS, greater than 50% of infants were in bed with a parent, sibling, or other related individual. As a result, many U.S. cities began programs to encourage infants sleeping by themselves. Some even provided cribs to families who were not able to get one on their own.

Common Pitfalls

■ Failure to counsel parents about the importance of placing their infants to sleep on their backs

5

- Failure to counsel parents about other modifiable risk factors, such as smoking and maintaining a safe sleeping environment
- Failure to recognize infants at higher risk for SIDS
- Failure to advise that all SIDS cases have an autopsy performed as well as a complete review of the circumstances of the death and the clinical history

Communication and Counseling

As stated earlier, parents and anyone caring for infants should be counseled about the importance of placing all healthy infants to sleep on their backs. Many parents are concerned about the possible risk of aspiration, but repeated studies show that infants who sleep supine are not at increased risk of aspiration compared with infants placed prone. All household members should be counseled about the role of smoking in increasing the risk for SIDS. In addition, caregivers should be instructed about safe sleeping environments, including avoidance of excessive blankets, soft mattresses, swaddling, and stuffed toys and animals. African American families in particular should be counseled on the risks of prone sleeping because African American infants have a twofold risk of dying from SIDS, likely related to the increased tendency of caregivers to place infants to sleep in the prone position.

In the event of a SIDS death, immediate attention should be available to the grieving family. Parents should be reassured they are not responsible for the death. Review of current information about SIDS and the fact that its causes are unknown may help the family. Counseling should be arranged for the parents and any siblings, depending on their ages, who may also be experiencing extreme guilt. Referral to support groups may also help the family continue the recovery from their loss.

Parents of SIDS victims continue to be very important in promoting initiatives both for SIDS research and educational programs.

SUGGESTED READINGS

1. Beckwith JB: Defining the sudden infant death syndrome. Arch Pediatr Adolesc Med 157:286–290, 2003. **Discusses the limitations of previous definitions of SIDS and offers an approach for handling cases for both case management and research purposes.**
2. Daley KC: Update on sudden infant death syndrome. Curr Opin Pediatr 16:227–232, 2004. **Reviews the definition, etiology, and risk factors for SIDS and emphasizes ways to target at-risk populations to promote further reduction in SIDS rates.**
3. Getahun D, Demissie K, Shou-En L, Rhoads GG: Sudden infant death syndrome among twin births: United States, 1995–1998. J Perinatol 24:544–551, 2004. **Demonstrates that twins are at higher risk for SIDS than singletons and shows a similar epidemiology of SIDS between twins and singletons.**
4. Krous HF, Beckwith JB, Byard RW, et al: Sudden infant death syndrome and unclassified sudden infant deaths: A definitional and diagnostic approach. Pediatrics 114:234–238, 2004. **Offers a new general definition for SIDS, which is further stratified to facilitate research and consistency in how the term is applied.**
5. Mitchell EA: Sleeping position of infants and the sudden infant death syndrome. Acta Paediatr Suppl 389:26–30, 1993. **Reviews early and evolving evidence for the decrease in SIDS with supine sleep position.**
6. Moon RY, Oden RP, Grady KC: Back to Sleep: An educational intervention with Women, Infants, and Children Program clients. Pediatrics 113:542–547, 2004. **Demonstrates that a short educational session with a small group of parents is effective in changing parental behavior and informing parents about the importance of the infant's sleep position.**

Abdominal Wall Defects and Disorders of the Umbilicus

Robert A. Cowles and Charles J. H. Stolar

KEY CONCEPTS

- Abdominal wall defects are serious life-threatening conditions of the newborn.
- Gastroschisis is associated with intestinal atresia and long-term intestinal dysfunction but not with other genetic or congenital anomalies. Omphalocele is often (50%) associated with other congenital conditions.
- Umbilical hernia is not an emergency, and repair is often delayed until 3 or 4 years of age.
- Developmental abnormalities of the urachus or omphalomesenteric duct can result in umbilical abnormalities that are treated surgically.

The term *abdominal wall defect* describes a wide range of conditions. Gastroschisis and omphalocele are severe and potentially life-threatening abdominal wall defects commonly seen on prenatal studies and often obvious at birth. Less severe abnormalities of the abdominal wall and umbilicus, such as umbilical hernia and abnormalities of the urachus and omphalomesenteric duct, may not be noted in the neonatal period.

Expert Opinion on Management Issues

ABDOMINAL WALL DEFECTS

Gastroschisis

Gastroschisis is an abdominal wall defect most commonly located just to the right of the normal umbilicus. The intra-abdominal structures, most often small bowel, herniate through this defect and are exposed to the amniotic fluid without a covering membrane. The size of the defect is variable, but it is generally smaller than the defect seen in neonates with omphalocele (Table 1). The chronic exposure of the intestine to the contents of the amniotic sac causes it to become inflamed, matted, and foreshortened.

Delivery of children with known gastroschisis, or any abdominal wall defect, should preferably occur at a center with pediatric surgical capability. Expertise in neonatal care and pediatric anesthesia should also be available. After delivery, the neonate should be resuscitated according to usual protocols, with special attention given to fluid resuscitation and respiratory support. With regard to the exposed viscera, the bowel should be kept warm and moist. A so-called bowel bag may be used to cover the lower half of the infant to help prevent massive fluid loss from the bowel and help keep the child warm. The bowel should be propped in a position that prevents kinking of its blood supply during this initial phase. At this point, the newborn should be prepared for surgery with adequate intravenous (IV) access, endotracheal intubation, and nasogastric decompression.

At surgery, the bowel is inspected. Often the bowel cannot be fully evaluated because of the associated serositis. After enlarging the abdominal wall defect for 2 to 3 cm, the bowel should be returned to the abdominal cavity, taking care to avoid the creation of an abdominal compartment syndrome. If full reduction of the eviscerated contents is not possible or appears unwise, a silo is constructed, placed over the exposed viscera, and sutured to the fascial defect. Over the next several days, the contents of the silo can be gradually, manually reduced until a final abdominal wall closure can be performed.

Parenteral nutritional support is of vital importance in newborns with gastroschisis. These children often have a prolonged ileus or an associated intestinal atresia (10% to 15%), making enteral nutrition quite difficult or even impossible for days to weeks. The development of parenteral nutrition strategies has markedly improved the outcome in these children, and thus a central venous catheter becomes an important part of the management strategy. With modern neonatal care and nutritional support, the current survival rate is greater than 90%.

Omphalocele

Omphalocele is a central abdominal wall defect. The abdominal contents herniate through an open umbilical ring. The herniated viscera are covered with a membrane that protects them from the irritating amniotic fluid. Thus the viscera are not matted or inflamed as in gastroschisis. Omphaloceles can range in size from small defects of the umbilical cord to giant omphaloceles that contain a majority of the intra-abdominal organs. Except in cases where the omphalocele appears minor, mothers carrying a fetus with a known omphalocele should be referred to a center with pediatric surgery, pediatric anesthesia, and advanced neonatology capabilities.

After delivery, the treatment of newborns with omphalocele is similar to that for newborns with gastroschisis. The infant should be resuscitated using standard procedures. The omphalocele should be inspected, and if the covering membrane is intact, the omphalocele sac can be covered with dressings. A search for associated anomalies should ensue. In contrast with newborns with gastroschisis, approximately 50% of newborns with omphalocele have serious associated conditions (see Table 1). A thorough physical examination, chest radiograph, and transthoracic echocardiogram are recommended as part of the initial evaluation before surgery. These studies reveal anomalies of the circulatory or respiratory system that may be important prior to administering a general anesthetic. As recommended in

TABLE 1 Features Associated with Omphalocele and Gastroschisis

Feature	Omphalocele	Gastroschisis
Location	Central	Right of umbilicus
Size of defect	Small to large	Small
Sac	Present	Absent
Gastrointestinal abnormalities	Malrotation	Malrotation, prolonged ileus, intestinal atresia, inflamed bowel
Associated anomalies/ syndromes	Common	Rare
Maternal age	Normal	Younger

newborns with gastroschisis, stable IV access, endotracheal intubation, and nasogastric decompression should be routine in preparation for surgery.

The decision to operate on a newborn with omphalocele is less pressing than in gastroschisis. There is time to search for life-threatening anomalies and for physiologic stabilization of the child. In children who are severely premature or have serious comorbid conditions, the surgeon may wait days before considering repair. If surgery within the first several days is considered too risky, some authors advocate treatment of the omphalocele sac with silver sulfadiazine, escharification of the sac, and delayed abdominal wall hernia repair. The operation for omphalocele begins with the careful removal of the omphalocele sac and ligation of the umbilical vessels and structures. If primary closure of a small omphalocele appears possible, the fascia is approximated and the defect closed with interrupted sutures. When the omphalocele is large or when attempts at primary closure are likely to cause an abdominal compartment syndrome, placement of a silo is indicated. This silo is fashioned and sutured to the abdominal fascial defect. The contents of the silo are gradually reduced into the abdominal cavity and a final fascial closure performed. The whole process can take up to 14 days.

Children with omphalocele have fewer intestinal and nutritional complications compared with those with gastroschisis, and they often can be nourished enterally soon after definitive closure of the abdominal wall. The overall survival of children born with omphalocele is 70% to 80%, with a majority of the mortalities attributed to associated structural and genetic abnormalities.

DISORDERS OF THE UMBILICUS

Umbilical Hernia

Umbilical herniae occur when the umbilical ring fails to close. They occur with similar frequency in boys and girls, and the incidence among African American children is significantly higher than in whites. Although no genetic associations are made, umbilical herniae are often seen in children with certain conditions, such as trisomy 21, trisomy 18, and Beckwith-Wiedemann syndrome.

Children often present with a history of an umbilical bulge since birth, which is easily confirmed on the physical examination. The open fascial ring and its limits can be appreciated on palpation of the defect.

Umbilical herniae can close spontaneously depending on the size of the defect. Defects of 0.5 cm or less have a closure rate of 96% over a 6-year period, whereas larger defects close more infrequently. Another important aspect of the clinical behavior of umbilical herniae is that they rarely incarcerate. For these reasons, most surgeons recommend a period of observation until 3 to 4 years of age prior to recommending operative repair.

When the hernia persists or becomes complicated by incarceration, surgical repair is warranted. During surgery, a small periumbilical incision is made, the fascial ring is isolated, and the hernia sac is resected. The fascial defect is closed with interrupted sutures and the skin is reconstructed over the fascial closure. Repair of umbilical hernia is an outpatient procedure, and the results are predictably good.

Umbilical Granuloma

After separation of the umbilical cord, a mass of fragile granulation tissue may form at the site that is often moist and can bleed. Initial treatment involves application of silver nitrate or surgical excision (in the case of a large granuloma). If adequate treatment with silver nitrate is unsuccessful, an umbilical cord polyp should be considered and treated with surgical excision.

Omphalomesenteric Duct Remnants

Omphalomesenteric duct abnormalities comprise a range of defects in closure of the vitelline duct. The most obvious visible abnormality at the umbilicus is the ileoumbilical fistula, where a clear, open communication between the terminal ileum and the umbilicus allows enteric contents to drain from the child's umbilicus (Figure 1). The treatment of an ileoumbilical fistula is surgical. Through an infraumbilical incision, the patent fistulous tract is followed down to its attachment to the ileum. This attachment is divided, the often large vitelline vessel ligated, and the ileum closed as in any other intestinal procedure.

Urachal Remnant

The urachal remnant usually consists of a fibrous cord-like band extending from the umbilicus to the dome of the bladder. As it obliterates, the urachus can remain patent, resulting in a fistula between the bladder and the umbilicus that can be a source of urinary tract infection. Alternatively, a cyst can form along the urachus as it obliterates, resulting in an urachal cyst (Figure 2).

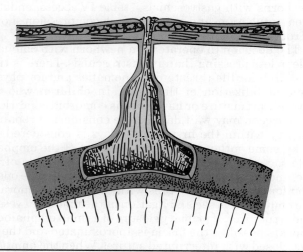

FIGURE 1. Omphalomesenteric duct remnant with umbilical-intestinal fistula. The ileal mucosa extends from the small bowel to the skin of the umbilicus.

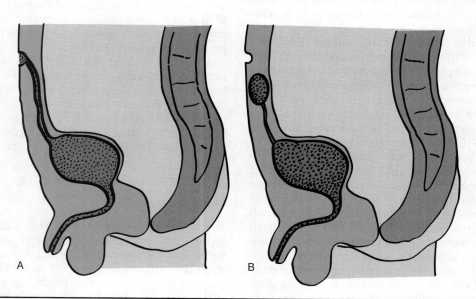

FIGURE 2. Urachal anomalies. *A,* Urachal fistula from bladder to umbilicus. *B,* Urachal cyst.

Urachal fistulas should be excised and ligated surgically to prevent recurrent urinary infections, which can be accomplished through an infraumbilical incision. The fistulous connection can be identified and traced to the bladder. Once excised, the dome of the bladder is closed and the umbilicus repaired.

Urachal cysts can remain asymptomatic and often become apparent because of increasing size or as a result of infection. If an infection or abscess is suspected, the cyst should be drained immediately, and it should be excised once the inflammation resolves. Noninfected urachal cysts are excised electively using an approach similar to the approach already described for a patent urachal fistula.

Common Pitfalls

- Failure to distinguish an omphalocele from gastroschisis. The location of the defect and presence of a sac are key to diagnosis.
- Closure of an abdominal wall defect resulting in abdominal compartment syndrome. Poor venous return, oliguria, and difficulty with mechanical ventilation are the possible outcome.
- Repair of asymptomatic umbilical hernia in the first 2 years of life. The defect may close without surgery. These children also have a higher rate of hernia recurrence.
- Prolonged treatment of umbilical drainage with silver nitrate. If no resolution occurs after two or more treatments, surgical excision may be warranted.

Communication and Counseling

Newborns with abdominal wall defects are challenging, and families require continuous reassurance and support. After prenatal diagnosis, parents are sometimes told that abdominal wall defects carry an unacceptably high mortality. The data do not support this, and, in fact, the overall survival rates are quite encouraging. The acute surgical treatment is often complete by 2 weeks. The long-term consequences of intestinal dysfunction in gastroschisis and associated anomalies in omphalocele determine the long-term outcome. Families should be prepared for certain aspects of their child's care, such as the appearance and reasoning for placement of a silo, because this part of treatment can be frightening.

Umbilical defects are easily treated, and discussions with parents are often not stressful. Almost all of these children are treated as outpatients. The most difficult discussion can be with a parent of a child in the first year of life who has a large umbilical hernia. Parents often see this as an ugly defect and want it repaired whatever the cost. It is important to stress the threefold reasoning behind expectant management of umbilical hernia:

1. The hernia may close on its own, thereby avoiding surgery.
2. If an umbilical hernia is repaired before the child's fascia and abdominal musculature are mature, there is an increased risk of recurrence requiring a second operation.
3. Umbilical hernia, in contrast to inguinal hernia, only rarely incarcerates, making expectant management safe.

SUGGESTED READINGS

1. Abdominal wall defects: In O'Neill JA, Grosfeld JL, Fonkalsrud EW, et al (eds): Principles of Pediatric Surgery, 2nd ed. St. Louis: Mosby, 2004. **An excellent concise overview with illustrative photos.**
2. Beasley SW: Vitellointestinal (omphalomesenteric duct) anomalies. In Spitz L, Coran AG (eds): Rob & Smith's Operative Surgery—Pediatric Surgery. London: Chapman & Hall, 1995. **Excellent description of omphalomesenteric duct anomalies with good illustrations.**
3. Langer JC: Abdominal wall defects. World J Surg 27:117–124, 2003. **Review of the diagnosis and management of the fetus with an abdominal wall defect.**
4. Nuchtern JG, Baxter R, Hatch EI Jr.: Nonoperative initial management versus silo chimney for treatment of giant omphalocele. J Pediatr Surg 30:771–776, 1995. **Description of the nonoperative treatment for giant omphaloceles.**
5. Walker SH: The natural history of umbilical hernia. Surgery 6:29–32, 1967. **Classic reference supporting the expectant management of umbilical hernia based on the natural history.**
6. Wilson RD, Johnson MP: Congenital abdominal wall defects: An update. Fetal Diagn Ther 19:385–398, 2004. **Most recent review of the modern literature from 1985 to 2003.**

Infants of Diabetic Mothers

Karen D. Hendricks-Muñoz

5

KEY CONCEPTS

- Approximately 5% to 10% of all pregnancies are complicated by diabetes.
- Exposure to maternal poor glycemic control during embryogenesis (less than 7 weeks' gestation) is associated with a three- to sixfold increased risk of congenital malformations, especially neural and cardiac defects.
- Fetal exposure to maternal hyperglycemia beyond 20 weeks' gestation stimulates fetal pancreatic insulin release, affecting organ development.
- Elevated maternal hemoglobin A_{1C} levels more than 8.5%, a marker of maternal glucose control, is associated with adverse infant outcomes.
- Clinical signs, dependent on gestational exposure to maternal glucose and fetal insulin production, include organ and growth disturbance such as macrosomia, organomegaly, lung immaturity, and metabolic disturbance.
- Intrauterine growth restriction may occur in infants born to mothers with vascular complications of diabetes.
- Careful intrauterine fetal monitoring (e.g., glucose tolerance test, lung maturity, and fetal growth/well-being assessments) are important to address the potential birth complications of infants born to diabetic mothers (IDMs).
- Management and treatment of the newborn is tailored to the clinical manifestations of the disease.

Diabetes ranks as one of the most common medical diagnoses of pregnancy, with approximately 5% to 10% of all

TABLE 1 Diagnosis of the Infant of the Diabetic Mother: White's Classification of Diabetes in Pregnancy (Modified)

Gestational Diabetes	Abnormal Glucose Tolerance Test, Diet-Maintained Euglycemia; If Diet Alone Insufficient, Insulin Is Required
Class A	Diet alone, any duration or age of onset
Class B	Age of onset: ≥20 yr; duration: <10 yr
Class C	Age of onset: 10–19 yr; duration: 10–19 yr
Class D	Age of onset: <10 yr; duration: >20 yr; background retinopathy or hypertension (not preeclampsia)
Class R	Proliferative retinopathy or vitreous hemorrhage
Class F	Nephropathy, with >500 mg/day proteinuria
Class RF	Criteria for both classes R and F coexist
Class H	Arteriosclerotic heart disease clinically evident
Class T	Prior renal transplantation

Adapted from White P: Classification of obstetric diabetes. Am J Obstet Gynecol 1978;130:228–230.

pregnancies in the United States complicated by some form of the disease. The prevalence of gestational diabetes (glucose intolerance with an onset during pregnancy) ranges from 2.5% to 4% of pregnancies. Prevalence varies by race and ethnicity; rates for African Americans and Hispanics are 2.8% each, and rates for non-Hispanic whites and Asians are 2.4% and 2.6%, respectively. The infant born to a mother whose pregnancy is complicated by diabetes is at increased risk of antenatal disordered growth, perinatal morbidity and mortality, and poor long-term outcome in direct proportion to the control of the maternal glucose state. Those infants born to insulin-dependent mothers with pregestational diabetes or fasting hyperglycemia gestational diabetes have an estimated three- to sixfold increased risk of congenital malformations and higher morbidity as compared to the general newborn population.

The White classification of maternal diabetes groups pregnant diabetic women according to age at onset, duration of disease, and presence of vascular complications (Table 1). The classification is useful in clinical care decisions to identify risk and compare clinical outcomes of mothers and infants. Maternal hemoglobin A_{1C} levels greater than 8.5% are associated with a 22.4% risk of fetal complications and further identify the likelihood of adverse outcomes in infants. Many centers simplify diabetic care management by classifying pregnancy in the diabetic woman as gestational diabetes, type 1 diabetes, or type 2 diabetes, focusing on glycemic control of the mother. Regardless of the classification of diabetes during pregnancy, improvement in the management of the poorly controlled diabetic mother has led to decreased infant mortality and morbidity and supports the need for a specialized approach to care to ensure the delivery of a healthy child.

Effect of Maternal Diabetes on the Fetus

From a developmental standpoint, the fetus of the diabetic pregnancy depends completely on maternal glucose delivery. Maternal glucose, a major substrate for fetal energy metabolism and growth, reaches the fetus by carrier-mediated diffusion until fetal levels approximate 70% to 80% of the maternal plasma glucose concentrations. Fetal hormonal responses, independent of the mother, are mediated by glucose because none of the maternal peptide hormones are transported to the fetus. Hyperglycemia, as a result of maternal diabetes, results in continuous fetal exposure to glucose. When fetal glucose uptake exceeds the requirement of energy production and growth, the excess glucose is stored in the fetus as glycogen and triglycerides.

Although maternal glucose control is attributed to diabetic embryopathy, no single cellular pathogenic mechanism is clearly defined to explain the diverse problems observed in the infant of the diabetic mother (IDM). However, timing of this environmental exposure results in a variety of altered fetal responses (Table 2).

Prior to 20 weeks' gestation, uncontrolled maternal diabetes, with its associated hyperglycemia, affects fetal development, altering growth, oxygenation, iron metabolism, and organ development. Poor glycemic control of the pregnant diabetic mother occurring during the period of embryonic organogenesis, prior to the 7th week of gestation, is associated with a fourfold increase in fetal congenital malformations. Malformations that affect neural plate development are particularly prominent and include caudal regression syndrome, a disorder of agenesis or hypoplasia of the femur in conjunction with lower vertebrae and sacrum agenesis; spina bifida; hydrocephalus; and anencephaly. In addition, cleft palate and cardiac, skeletal, and urogenital malformations are increased. Cardiac malformations may occur at a prevalence rate of up to 15 times greater in the infant of the insulin-dependent diabetic mother. Conotruncal defects, such as truncus arteriosus, tetralogy of Fallot, transposition of the great arteries, and double-outlet right ventricle, have an increased occurrence rate of threefold greater in the IDM.

Beyond 20 weeks' gestation, with continued glucose exposure, the newly formed fetal pancreas responds with hyperinsulinemia progressing to fetal pancreatic islet cell hypertrophy and beta-cell hypersensitivity. However, the continued fetal exposure to hyperglycemia and hyperinsulinemia creates a fetal environment that affects the development of the entire organism. Persistent hyperglycemia and hyperinsulinemia lead to inappropriate parathyroid hormone response, elevated calcitonin, and altered vitamin D metabolism, with associated postnatal infant hypocalcemia and hypomagnesemia. Continued fetal hyperglycemia and hyperinsulinemia increase fetal total body oxygen consumption, leading to fetal hypoxia, elevated erythropoietin secretion, and fetal polycythemia. Increased fetal iron requirements are not met in this scenario, leading to inadequate brain and cardiac

TABLE 2 Pathogenesis of the Infant of the Diabetic

Fetal Hyperglycemia	Fetal Hyperinsulinemia	Fetal Hyperglycemia and Hyperinsulinemia
Congenital anomalies (0–20 wk): caudal regression, cardiac defects	Postnatal, neonatal: Hypoglycemia	Fetal macrosomia/organomegaly: Dystocia/birth asphyxia Cardiomyopathy Transient tachypnea of newborn (TTN)
Decreased growth (0–20 wk)	Stimulate hormones: Growth hormone Erythropoietin	Metabolic demands/fetal hypoxia: Polycythemia Renal vein thrombosis Stroke Iron deficiency
Hyperinsulinemia >20 wk gestation	Immature liver metabolism, hyperbilirubinemia Surfactant deficiency: Inhibit surfactant gene expression	

Adapted from Nold JL, Georgieff MK: Infants of diabetic mothers. Pediatr Clin North Am 2004;51:619–637.

TABLE 3 Complications of the Infant of the Diabetic Mother

Growth	Intrauterine growth restriction (IUGR <5th percentile) Macrosomia/large for gestational age (LGA >95th percentile)
Birth trauma	Shoulder dystocia, birth asphyxia, clavicular fracture, especially macrosomic infants
Metabolic	Hypoglycemia (<50 mg/dL), hypocalcemia (<7 mg/dL), hypomagnesemia (<1.5 mg/dL)
Hematologic	Polycythemia (central hematocrit >65%), hyperbilirubinemia, iron deficiency
Lung immaturity	Respiratory distress syndrome (may have absence of phosphatidylglycerol [PG] with normal L/S [lactase/sucrase] ratio)
Gastrointestinal	Poor feeding, small left colon syndrome, and gut dysmotility syndrome
Cardiac	Cardiac failure: cardiac septal hypertrophy and outflow obstruction
Congenital anomalies	Nervous system defects (caudal regression), cardiac defects, skeletal anomalies, cleft lip

5

iron stores as well as reduced serum ferritin concentrations. Combined with impaired maturation of hepatic enzymes, hyperbilirubinemia is often seen in the IDM. Hyperinsulinemia inhibits type II pulmonary alveolar cell surfactant proteins SPA and SPB gene expression, leading to surfactant deficiency and an increased risk of respiratory distress syndrome (RDS). Fetal growth hormone release is stimulated, resulting in excessive infant growth or macrosomia (birth weight more than the 95th percentile) and associated organomegaly. Macrosomic infants are at increased risk of birth dystocia and birth injury.

In contrast, infants of mothers who have advanced diabetic vascular disease often suffer placental vascular insufficiency and protein malnutrition independent of maternal glycemic control. These infants present with fetal growth restriction, birth weight less than the 5th to 10th percentile for gestational age. Early presentation of placental insufficiency in mothers with severe vascular disease leads to symmetrical growth restriction in the infant, where the body and head are proportionately sized. Later onset, or milder vascular disease, may present with head sparing in these infants. But the chronic deficiency environment of growth restriction leads to an increased risk of infant mortality and delivery room–related morbidity. Following birth, the supply of

maternal glucose is abruptly discontinued. The IDM, whether large for gestational age or intrauterine growth restricted, has inadequate circulating glucagon and catecholamine responses. Continued elevated circulating insulin levels further compound the inability to mobilize glucose to meet energy needs in these infants, leading to hypoglycemia, a major presenting sign.

Expert Opinion on Management Issues

The management of the IDM is tailored to the individual clinical manifestations of the disease (Table 3). Obstetric antenatal assessments of fetal well-being are important to perinatal care and include biophysical profile, lung maturational studies, and fetal ultrasound assessments. Preparation for delivery often involves careful antenatal multidisciplinary communications to infant care providers that include maternal diabetic classification, possible presentation of macrosomia or growth-restricted infants, and additional identified pregnancy complications. At birth, careful physical examination adds to the antenatal history, and expectant management of clinical signs and symptoms is necessary, as outlined in the section on complications of the IDM.

ACCEPTED INTERVENTIONS

Infant growth disturbances of macrosomia or restriction are excellent markers of IDM risk status that identify needed infant interventions. Organomegaly, in the macrosomic IDM, places the infant at risk for organ hemorrhage of the liver, spleen, adrenals, or external genitalia. Potential birth complications include shoulder dystocia, cephalohematoma, facial palsies, clavicular fractures, and brachial plexus injuries, as well as possible birth asphyxia. Hypoglycemia (glucose less than 40 mg/dL), occurring within 1 to 3 hours after birth, is common in up to 50% of IDMs who are macrosomic or growth restricted. Recommended therapy includes timely surveillance of glucose status, early feedings in at-risk infants, and appropriate glucose infusions to maintain glucose homeostasis. In addition, transient hypocalcemia (less than 7 mg/dL), occurring in up to 50% of IDMs, as well as hypomagnesemia (less than 1.5 mg/dL) can occur within the first 72 hours and is most marked in those with associated growth alterations. These metabolic disturbances can also be potentiated by prematurity or asphyxia.

Polycythemia (central hematocrit more than 65%) and hyperbilirubinemia frequently need early assessment and treatment. Cardiorespiratory assessment identifies cardiac functional abnormalities in up to 30% of IDMs. Septal hypertrophy of the heart, a common disorder resulting from glycogen deposition in the cardiac septum, can lead to hypertrophic subaortic stenosis with cardiomyopathy, obstructive left heart failure, and cardiomegaly. When severe, outflow obstruction in hypertrophic subaortic stenosis can be treated with β-blockers and may be exacerbated by hypovolemia and inotropic agents. Early diagnosis and treatment of RDS with surfactant and respiratory support is indicated to respond to poor pulmonary compliance and loss of lung volume but is less common in the growth-restricted infant. Antenatal markers of pulmonary maturity, especially including presence of the phospholipid phosphatidylglycerol (PG) (more than 3%), should be part of expectant care of those infants targeted for early delivery because of maternal complications. Retained fetal lung fluid (transient tachypnea) after cesarean delivery or persistent pulmonary hypertension of the newborn (PPHN) can further complicate the respiratory course in these infants. Furthermore, persistent fetal hyperglycemia is associated with gastrointestinal dysfunction, with feeding intolerance, transient small left colon syndrome, or intestinal dysmotility syndrome.

The long-term health of the IDM depends on the antenatal, fetal, and neonatal course. The IDM is predisposed to develop later diabetes at a rate five to ten times higher than the normal infant. There is an increased risk of later childhood obesity and an increased risk for delayed cognitive development. In the growth-restricted infant, this risk is increased further. A significant correlation exists between second- and third-trimester glucose control and delayed cognitive development that is unexplained by adverse antenatal and perinatal events.

URGENT INTERVENTIONS

Clinical risk assessment for presence of congenital malformations, birth weight discordance, metabolic disturbances, hematocrit value, and cardiorespiratory stability should be made at birth for every IDM to identify need for early treatment. Early care decreases adverse events such as neonatal seizures and lessens the risk of impaired long-term cognitive development. Anticipatory diagnosis of RDS should be determined to provide therapy and lessen lung injury or the risk of development of PPHN in these infants. Polycythemia requires prompt treatment with partial exchange transfusion to avoid potential vascular compromise. IDMs are at risk for vascular thrombosis; thus the decision for placement of umbilical catheters should be made cautiously.

CONTROVERSIAL INTERVENTIONS

Controversy exists related to diagnostic glucose challenge criteria for maternal gestational diabetes. More aggressive testing in high-risk populations seems warranted. Maternal diabetes without other factors is no longer considered an indication for early delivery. Antenatal management of the diabetic pregnant mother, with an infant with discordant growth, requires a coordinated medical approach to care. Communication between obstetric and pediatric providers is paramount to provide appropriate delivery and postnatal management of the infant and mother. Admission to infant special care units, where clinical course assessment and treatment can be anticipated, should be considered in the management of these infants. Although glucose normative values are lacking, most clinicians recommend early screening of at-risk infants and treatment of glucose levels less than 50 mg/dL.

Common Pitfalls

Failure to coordinate an obstetric and pediatric approach to care, as well as identifying the potential multisystem complications of the IDM, is a pitfall. Fetal growth discordance, associated macrosomia or intrauterine growth restriction, can lead to unexpected delivery room complications of birth injury or postnatal metabolic conditions that can lead to asphyxia, seizures, and further neurologic impairment. Lung dysmaturity, if unrecognized, can lead to severe morbidity. Untreated polycythemia can lead to hyperviscosity syndrome, thrombosis, stroke, or necrotizing enterocolitis; undiagnosed hyperbilirubinemia can lead to increased risk of kernicterus.

Communication and Counseling

In the well-controlled pregnant diabetic mother, most infants can have normal gestation and recover without sequelae. Preconceptual and strict glucose control in pregestational or gestational diabetic patients should be part of antenatal counseling to optimize perinatal survival and decrease morbidity. Counseling should include expectations of achieving circulating glucose levels as close to normal as possible, as well as expected delivery room and postnatal specialized care. Tests of fetal well-being, including a nonstress test, biophysical profile, and fetal activity determinations, should be conducted, with the goal of long-term glucose control and delivery of an infant with normal circulating glucose levels to lessen severity of associated morbidity.

SUGGESTED READINGS

1. Kousseff BG: Gestational diabetes mellitus (class A): A human teratogen? Am J Med Genet 83:402–408, 1999. **Reviews the pathogenesis of diabetic embryopathy, contrasting pregestational and gestational diabetic exposure.**
2. Lucas MJ: Medical complications of pregnancy: Diabetes complication pregnancy. Obstet Gynecol Clin North Am 28(3):513–536, 2001. **Identifies the medical complications of the pregnant mother with diabetes.**
3. Nold JL, Georgieff MK: Infants of diabetic mothers. Pediatr Clin North Am 51:619–637, 2004. **Describes the pathophysiology, clinical manifestations, and treatment strategies for the infant of the diabetic mother.**
4. Petry CJ, Hales CN: Long-term effects on offspring of intrauterine exposure to deficits in nutrition. Hum Reprod Update 6(6):578–586, 2000. **Describes pregnancy-related environmental influences and their effects on later life.**
5. Piper JM, Xenakis EM, Langer O: Delayed appearance of pulmonary maturation markers is associated with poor glucose control in diabetic pregnancies. J Matern Fetal Med 7:148–153, 1998. **Details the impact of poor glucose control and lung maturation.**
6. Rowley DL, Danel IA, Berg CJ, Vinicor F: The reproductive years. In Beckles GLA, Thompson-Reid PE (eds): Diabetes and Women's Health across Life Stages. Centers for Disease Control and Prevention. Available online at http://www.cdc.gov/diabetes/pubs/pdf/women.pdf. **Describes the changing ethnic and racial incidence of diabetes in pregnancy.**
7. Sheffield JS, Butler-Koster EL, Casey BM, et al: Maternal diabetes mellitus and infant malformation. Obstet Gynecol 100: 5(Pt 1):925–930, 2002. **Details the rate of infant malformations in the pregestational diabetic mother.**
8. Silverman BL, Rizzo T, Green OC, et al: Long-term prospective evaluation of offspring of diabetic mothers. Diabetes 40(Suppl 2):121–125, 1991. **Identifies the increased risk for development of obesity and diabetes in the infant of the diabetic mother.**
9. Wren C, Birrell G, Hawthorne G: Cardiovascular malformations in infants of diabetic mothers. Heart (British Cardiac Society) 89 (10):1217–1220, 2003. **Describes the prevalence and spectrum of cardiac malformations in the infant of the diabetic mother.**

Hypoglycemia in the Newborn Infant

Eugenia K. Pallotto and Rebecca A. Simmons

KEY CONCEPTS

- The signs and symptoms of neonatal hypoglycemia are often subtle and nonspecific, so closely monitoring the high-risk infant (infant born to diabetic mother [IDM], small for gestational age [SGA], sepsis) is very important.

- Hypoglycemia is defined as a glucose level less than 40 mg/dL the first day of life, less than 50 mg/dL during the first week of life, and less than 60 mg/dL subsequently, regardless of gestational age.
- Whole blood glucose concentrations, such as those measured by Dextrostix, are 10% to 15% lower than plasma glucose concentrations because of the dilutional effect of the red blood cell mass.
- The testing of the sample should not be delayed because it can result in an artificially low value caused by red cell oxidation of glucose.

The fetus is completely dependent on its mother for glucose and other nutrient transfer across the placenta. In the basal nonstressed state, placental transport of glucose meets all of the fetal glucose requirements. The human fetal liver has the enzymatic capacity for gluconeogenesis and glycogenolysis as early as the third month of gestation. However, the absolute levels of gluconeogenic enzymes are far lower than those of adults, and it is unlikely the fetus produces much glucose under normal conditions. The fetus prepares for extrauterine survival by increasing energy stores and developing enzymatic processes for rapid mobilization of stored energy.

Development of carbohydrate homeostasis in the newborn infant results from a balance among hormonal, enzymatic, neural regulation, and substrate availability. The newborn infant must supply its own substrate to meet the energy requirements for maintenance of body temperature, respiration, muscular activity, and regulation of blood glucose. The concentration of glucose in the umbilical venous blood approximates 70% to 80% of that in the mother and is higher than in the umbilical arterial blood. During the first 4 to 6 hours of postnatal life, glucose values fall, stabilizing between 50 and 60 mg/dL. Blood glucose concentration is normally maintained at a relatively constant level by a fine balance between hepatic glucose output and peripheral glucose uptake. Hepatic glucose output depends on adequate glycogen stores, sufficient supplies of endogenous gluconeogenic precursors, a normally functioning hepatic gluconeogenic and glycogenolytic system, and a normal endocrine system for modulating these processes.

At birth, the neonate has glycogen stores that are greater than those in the adult. Because basal glucose use doubles, however, these stores are rapidly depleted and begin to decline within 2 to 3 hours after birth, remain low for several days, and then gradually rise to adult levels. Both serum glucagon and catecholamine levels increase three- to fivefold in response to the cutting of the umbilical cord. Circulating insulin levels usually decrease in the immediate newborn period and remain low for several days. The depressed serum insulin and elevated glucagon and epinephrine levels (along with elevated serum growth hormone levels) at birth favor glycogenolysis, lipolysis, and gluconeogenesis. Changes in various hormone receptors also modulate these processes. Hepatic glucagon receptors increase in number and become functionally linked with cyclic adenosine monophosphate (cAMP) responses. Neonatal

BOX 1 Conditions Associated with Neonatal Hypoglycemia

BOX 1 Conditions Associated with Neonatal Hypoglycemia

Limited Glycogen Supply
- Prematurity
- Perinatal stress
- Glycogen storage disease

Hyperinsulinism
- Infant of a diabetic mother
- Congenital hyperinsulinism
- Beckwith-Wiedemann syndrome
- Maternal drug therapy
- Erythroblastosis fetalis

Diminished Glucose Production
- SGA infant
- Inborn errors of metabolism

Others
- Hypothermia
- Sepsis
- Polycythemia
- Hypothalamic or hypopituitary disorders
- Adrenal insufficiency

SGA, small for gestational age.

BOX 2 Signs and Symptoms of Hypoglycemia

- Apnea
- Bradycardia
- Cyanosis
- Jitteriness
- Lethargy
- Poor feeding
- Seizures
- Tachypnea
- Temperature instability

glucose homeostasis also requires appropriate enzyme maturation and response in the newborn. After birth, glycogen phosphorylase activity is increased and glycogen synthetase activity is decreased, allowing for the rapid depletion of hepatic glycogen. Phosphoenolpyruvate carboxykinase activity, the rate-limiting enzyme for gluconeogenesis, also increases during the immediate postnatal period. Thus hormonal and enzymatic activity in the fetus provide for anabolism and substrate accretion, whereas those in the newborn period provide for the maintenance of glucose homeostasis in response to the abrupt interruption of maternal glucose supply.

The incidence of hypoglycemia is estimated at 1 to 5 per 1000 live births but is higher in at-risk populations. Specifically, reports of the incidence of hypoglycemia in infants with intrauterine growth retardation vary from 15% to 50%. A wide variation in reported incidence is due, in part, by a variety of historical definitions of hypoglycemia in clinical use.

There is no consensus defining a blood glucose level diagnostic of hypoglycemia. Earlier data defining hypoglycemia as a blood glucose level less than 35 mg/dL in term infants and 25 mg/dL in preterm infants were derived from data in fasted infants and probably invalid. In these studies, blood glucose levels below 2 standard deviations (SD) of the mean were considered hypoglycemic, which led to the common misconception that infants of low birth weight and premature infants could tolerate lower plasma glucose levels in comparison to full-term and normally grown infants.

Concerns about the long-term effects of asymptomatic neonatal hypoglycemia, first raised by Pildes, led to efforts to change the definition of hypoglycemia. In newborns, brain metabolism probably accounts for at least 85% to 90% of total glucose consumption, and the newborn brain is not able to use other substrates adequately for its metabolic needs. Therefore, many neonatologists and pediatricians now define hypoglycemia as a glucose level less than 50 mg/dL, regardless of gestational age. Importantly, whole blood glucose concentrations, such as those measured by Dextrostix, are 10% to 15% lower than plasma glucose concentrations because of the dilutional effect of the red blood cell mass. The testing of the sample should not be delayed because it can result in an artificially low value caused by red cell oxidation of glucose.

Many pathophysiologic conditions influence neonatal glucose homeostasis leading to hypoglycemia. Most of these are related to an inadequate production of or increased use of glucose. A lack of glycogen stores and/or decreased gluconeogenesis (intrauterine growth retarded infants, premature infants) leads to inadequate production of glucose. Increased use of glucose is associated with hyperinsulinism (infants of diabetic mothers, congenital hyperinsulinism) or an increased rate of anaerobic glycolysis (septic infants, asphyxiated infants). Each of these categories is associated with several different disease states (Box 1).

Signs and Symptoms

The signs and symptoms of neonatal hypoglycemia are often subtle and nonspecific (Box 2). In fact, some infants with low glucose values are asymptomatic. This difficulty is compounded by the occurrence of symptoms at different blood glucose concentrations that vary from neonate to neonate and the lack of a universal threshold below or above which symptomatology may occur. Thus close monitoring of the high-risk infant (infant born to diabetic mother [IDM], small for gestational age [SGA], sepsis) is crucial. The maternal and perinatal history may yield useful information in helping decide which infants may be at risk for low blood glucose. High-risk situations include the presence of diabetes mellitus, any history of glucose intolerance, maternal use of medications, history of preterm labor, and preeclampsia. Risk factors in the perinatal history include cold stress, asphyxia, trauma, and sepsis. The symptomatic infant may be jittery, lethargic, cyanotic, apneic, bradycardic, and hypotonic. Occasionally an infant seizes or suffers a cardiac arrest.

Expert Opinion on Management Issues

All infants at risk for development of neonatal hypoglycemia should be monitored. Blood glucose values less than 40 mg/dL in the first day of life should be verified and treated. The treatment of hypoglycemia depends on several factors. Infants who are asymptomatic with borderline glucose levels and capable of enteral feeds may receive either formula or 5% dextrose water as initial therapy. Infants with symptomatic hypoglycemia or more severe asymptomatic hypoglycemia should be given intravenous glucose solutions consisting of an initial bolus of 100 mg/kg of 10% dextrose in water solution (1 mL/kg) followed by a continuous infusion of 6 mg/kg/minute of 10% dextrose in water. Infants of diabetic mothers and SGA infants often need to be treated with a constant infusion of glucose. Many of these infants need between 8 and 10 mg/kg/minute of 10% dextrose in water solution to keep the serum glucose values in the normal range. The rate of infusion can be titrated to achieve a normal glucose level. The use of a peripheral vein or an umbilical venous catheter is preferable to the use of an umbilical arterial catheter because the latter is associated with hyperinsulinism secondary to direct pancreatic stimulation. Boluses of glucose should be avoided because rebound hypoglycemia may occur when the hyperresponsive beta cell produces an insulin surge. Neonates needing prolonged glucose therapy or dextrose infusion rates above 12 mg/kg/m^2 should be investigated for refractory causes of hypoglycemia, such as congenital hyperinsulinism and inborn errors of metabolism.

Occasionally infants who were born very prematurely, are severely growth restricted, or had perinatal stress develop prolonged hypoglycemia that can persist for several weeks. Usually these infants can be managed by increasing the caloric density of feeds or by feeding more frequently. Diazoxide therapy can be used if the infant does not tolerate increased calories or frequent feedings. Prior to starting diazoxide, other causes of hypoglycemia must be ruled out, and follow-up with a pediatric endocrinologist is recommended.

Common Pitfalls

Neonatal hypoglycemia is a common problem that is difficult to define, understand, and manage. In the past three decades, many published reports addressed this clinical issue, but confusion still remains regarding both the definition of hypoglycemia and its management. In the neonate, glucose homeostasis is a complex balance between systemic or organ needs and the capability to produce and regulate glucose. It was generally believed prior to the early 1990s that newborns were resistant to the pathophysiologic effects of hypoglycemia observed in older infants and adults because newborns are often asymptomatic at low levels of serum glucose. However, unlike older infants and adults, glucose is the principal substrate of cerebral metabolism in the neonate. The evidence is now clear from human and animal studies that severe, prolonged hypoglycemia leads to acute neurologic injury that can often result in permanent sequelae.

Abnormal sensory-evoked potentials are observed in full-term infants with whole blood glucose values of less than 45 mg/dL in the first 72 hours of life. A majority of these newborns are asymptomatic. In addition, numerous case-control studies of preterm and term infants find an adverse neurodevelopmental outcome in newborns who had plasma glucose values less than 45 mg/dL within the first 72 hours of life. SGA preterm infants who had one or more plasma glucose values of less than 45 mg/dL in the first few days of life also demonstrate abnormal neurodevelopmental outcomes and decreased head growth.

Communication and Counseling

Parents should be counseled that most newborns with mild hypoglycemia have no long-term sequelae. However, those infants who develop symptomatic hypoglycemia are at high risk for abnormal neurodevelopmental outcome and should be followed carefully.

SUGGESTED READINGS

1. Cowett RM: Hypoglycemia and hyperglycemia in the newborn. In Polin RA, Fox WW (eds): Fetal and Neonatal Physiology. Philadelphia: WB Saunders, 1998, p 596. **A thorough review of the pathogenesis of altered glucose homeostasis in the newborn.**
2. Girard J: Gluconeogenesis in late fetal and early neonatal life. Biol Neonate 50:237–258, 1986. **Physiology of glucose metabolism in the fetus and newborn.**
3. Hay WW: Fetal and neonatal glucose homeostasis and their relation to the small for gestational age infant. Semin Perinatol 8:101–116, 1984. **A review of pathophysiology of glucose metabolism in the small-for-gestational-age infant.**
4. Jones RAK, Robertson NRC: Problems of the small for dates baby. Clin Obstet Gynecol 11:499–524, 1984. **A discussion of glucose metabolism in the SGA infant.**
5. Kalhan SC, Saker F: Disorders of carbohydrate metabolism. In Fanaroff A, Martin R (eds): Diseases of the Fetus and Newborn, 6th ed. St. Louis: Mosby, 1997, pp 1439–1462. **A review of carbohydrate metabolism in the fetus and newborn.**
6. Koh TH, Eyre JA, Aynsley-Green A: Neonatal hypoglycemia—the controversy regarding definition. Arch Dis Child 63:1386–1398, 1988. **A discussion of the definition of hypoglycemia in the newborn.**
7. Lucas A, Morley R, Cole TJ: Adverse neurodevelopmental outcome of moderate neonatal hypoglycemia. BMJ 297:1304–1308, 1988. **A discussion of the consequences of neonatal hypoglycemia in relation to neurodevelopmental outcome.**
8. Schwartz R, Gruppuso PA, Pelzold K, et al: Hyperinsulinemia and macrosomia in the fetus of the diabetic mother. Diabetes Care 17:640–648, 1994. **Glucose homeostasis in the infant of the diabetic mother.**
9. Srinivasan G, Pildes RS, Cattamanchi G, et al: Plasma glucose values in normal neonates: A new look. J Pediatr 109:114–177, 1986. **A large clinical study of glucose values in normal newborns.**
10. Stanley CA: Hyperinsulinism in infants and children. Pediatr Clin North Am 44:363–374, 1997. **A review of the causes of congenital hyperinsulinism.**

5

Treatment of Neonatal Hyperbilirubinemia

Ronald L. Poland

KEY CONCEPTS

- Bilirubin is toxic to all cells and can produce irreversible brain damage.
- Prevention of brain damage is the goal of treating hyperbilirubinemia.
- Albumin protects against bilirubin toxicity.
- Sepsis, hemolytic disease, undernutrition, certain drugs, and hypothermia can reduce the bilirubin-binding capacity of albumin.
- Frequent milk feedings (not water supplementation, not intravenous hydration) prevent hyperbilirubinemia by reducing intestinal reabsorption of bilirubin.
- Visual assessment of jaundice is not as reliable as once thought.
- Hour-specific bilirubin concentration is a valuable measure of risk for the development of severe hyperbilirubinemia.
- Phototherapy is used to prevent exchange transfusion, but exchange transfusion is the treatment of choice once laboratory criteria are met or the infant shows signs of bilirubin neurotoxicity.
- Prompt exchange transfusion can reduce the incidence or severity of permanent brain damage in infants showing symptoms of acute bilirubin neurotoxicity.

Managing neonatal hyperbilirubinemia is important for two reasons: High concentrations of bilirubin can cause permanent brain damage and may be a sign of a pathologic condition (e.g., hemolytic disease, gastrointestinal disease, infection). This chapter concentrates on the management of the jaundice itself in term and near-term infants.

Successful management of neonatal jaundice should start with a protocol for prevention and surveillance. Bilirubin is toxic to any cell it might enter. High concentrations affect platelet function and renal function as well as central nervous system functions, but the potential for permanent damage of central neurons is the main reason for surveillance and treatment of hyperbilirubinemia. The main host defense against bilirubin toxicity is serum albumin. Albumin, which circulates in plasma and other extracellular fluid, binds very tightly to bilirubin in a 1:1 molar ratio and prevents bilirubin from entering cells. However, some conditions interfere with the binding of bilirubin to albumin. For example, sepsis, undernourishment, and hypothermia all raise circulating free fatty acid concentrations, and free fatty acids compete for bilirubin-binding sites on albumin. In addition, products of hemolysis and certain drugs, such as sulfonamides, diuretics, and some analgesics, can displace bilirubin from albumin. Bilirubin that is not bound to albumin can penetrate cell membranes, including those in the brain.

The best management strategy is prevention. Obstetricians prevent most instances of Rh isoimmunization (erythroblastosis fetalis) with the use of anti-Rh (D) immune globulin during and right after pregnancies at risk. Because the enterohepatic circulation of bilirubin contributes significantly to the development of jaundice in newborn infants, early and frequent breast or formula feedings (as often as every 2 hours) are effective in reducing bilirubin concentrations. The gastrocolic reflex is the likely mechanism. *Oral supplementation of feedings with water or glucose water is ineffective in decreasing jaundice, as is intravenous supplementation.*

The next best strategy is surveillance. This starts with family history (e.g., previous jaundiced infants, hemolytic diseases) and laboratory investigations during pregnancy (e.g., ABO and Rh groupings as well as a screen for antibodies) and in the newborn period (e.g., Coombs test, blood type, and Rh if mother is untested; screening for hypothyroidism, galactosemia). In addition, every infant should be screened for hyperbilirubinemia. Visual assessment is less reliable than previously thought, so an objective screening test is preferred. Available methods include measurement of skin reflectance (transcutaneous bilirubin assessment) or serum bilirubin concentration. Screening should occur at least once prior to initial hospital discharge and again on initial follow-up, or whenever the infant appears jaundiced. Follow-up visits should be scheduled for 24 to 48 hours after discharge if the initial hospital discharge occurs prior to 72 hours of age. Each bilirubin value should be plotted on an hour-specific nomogram (Fig. 1) to assess the risk of developing significant hyperbilirubinemia. Obtaining two bilirubin concentrations at least 4 hours apart improves the predictive value of the estimates. Hour-specific screening values help the clinician better plan the timing of discharge and of follow-up visits.

If the rate of rise of total bilirubin exceeds 0.5 mg/dL per hour, a hemolytic condition should be assumed. In that case, recheck for isoimmune disease; obtain a blood smear for abnormal red cell morphology and an enzyme analysis for red cell glucose–6-phosphatase deficiency (G6PD). If isoimmune disease is diagnosed, an intravenous globulin infusion (0.5 to 1 g/kg over 2 hours) can reduce the rate of hemolysis. This can be repeated in 12 hours. If jaundice persists beyond 10 days of age, total and direct bilirubin should be measured. If the direct bilirubin is abnormally high, an investigation for cholestasis or hepatocellular injury, including infectious and metabolic causes, should be pursued.

Expert Opinion on Management Issues

Two methods of reducing bilirubin concentration are well accepted. The first is phototherapy, which decreases bilirubin concentration by photoisomerization and photo-oxidation of bilirubin. Both processes detoxify bilirubin and assist in its excretion. Phototherapy does

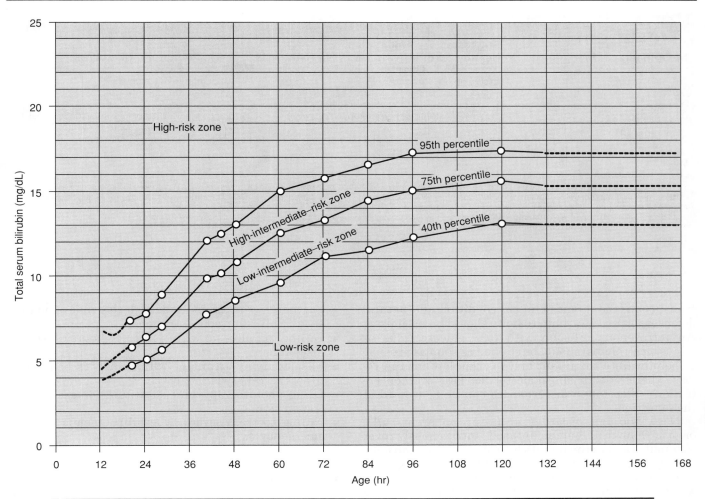

FIGURE 1. Bhutani nomogram. (From Bhutani VK, Johnson L, Sivieri EM: Predictive ability of a predischarge hour-specific serum bilirubin for subsequent significant hyperbilirubinemia in healthy term and near-term newborns. Pediatrics 103:6–14, 1999. Used with permission of the American Academy of Pediatrics.)

BOX 1 **Signs of Acute Bilirubin Neuropathy**
■ Obvious jaundice
■ Poor feeding
■ Irritability, lethargy
■ Opisthotonos, retrocollis
■ Abnormal Moro reflex
■ Apnea, failed BAER (brainstem auditory evoked response)

not prevent bilirubin neuropathy, however, and it is not a substitute for exchange transfusion when exchange transfusion is indicated. It does, however, reduce the number of infants meeting criteria for exchange transfusion.

When infants exhibit acute symptoms of bilirubin toxicity (Box 1), the only appropriate treatment is exchange transfusion as soon as possible. This procedure is done infrequently today and requires a team of caregivers who are proficient in intensive care. Candidates for exchange transfusion should be admitted directly to a facility that can deliver intensive care and has experience with exchange transfusion in newborn infants. Having such infants seen first in emergency facilities leads to delays that can be avoided by arranging direct admission.

When an exchange transfusion is indicated, it is impossible to start immediately. Arranging hospital admission; obtaining laboratory tests, including complete blood count (CBC), electrolytes, and total and direct bilirubin; procuring the appropriate blood product; and confirming the need for the procedure all take time. This time can be put to good use to first document the history and physical examination, in part to determine whether the infant shows any signs of encephalopathy on admission. Then, while preparing to do the exchange

TABLE 1 Guidelines for Management of Hyperbilirubinemia <30 mg/dL Based on Bilirubin-to-Albumin Ratios

Molar Ratio	B/A (mg/g)*	Suggested Treatment Plan Healthy Term or Near Term; No Hemolysis	Sick, Premature, Hemolysis[†]
1.0	9	Exchange transfusion ASAP	Exchange transfusion ASAP
0.9	8	Exchange transfusion if bilirubin not decreasing >1–2 mg/dL in 4 h with phototherapy	Exchange transfusion ASAP
0.8	7	Dietary adjustment, phototherapy	Exchange transfusion if bilirubin not decreasing >1–2 mg/dL in 4 h with phototherapy
0.7	6	Options: dietary change, phototherapy, or just observe	Dietary adjustment, phototherapy
0.6	5		

Note: If jaundiced infant has clinical signs of bilirubin encephalopathy, exchange as soon as possible regardless of ratio. When close to exchange transfusion criteria, phototherapy should be intensive (>25 µW/cm^2 in the 430–390 nm band). Dietary adjustments include milk feedings every 2 hours and, when close to exchange level, switching from breast to formula feeding temporarily.

*Bilirubin (mg/dL) divided by albumin (g/dL) values are rounded to whole numbers. The total serum bilirubin is used for this ratio.

[†]Or is receiving a drug that interferes with bilirubin binding to albumin.

ASAP, as soon as possible.

transfusion, the infant's clinical condition and natural defenses against bilirubin toxicity should be optimized. An intravenous infusion with 10% glucose (plus or minus electrolytes) should be started as soon as possible to help hydrate the infant and to stimulate insulin release, thereby decreasing nonesterified fatty acid concentrations. Electrolyte disturbances can be addressed at the same time.

Next, if no signs of cardiac failure are apparent, 1 g/kg of 5% human albumin infused intravenously over 30 minutes add to the infant's bilirubin-binding capacity. Finally, the blood exchange should be considered an emergency. If obtaining specifically cross-matched blood will cause undue delay, type O, Rh negative cells mixed with AB plasma (reconstituted whole blood) should be used, and the exchange performed sooner rather than later. Clinical signs of kernicterus can be reversed by prompt exchange transfusion.

Table 1 provides a set of guidelines for the treatment of hyperbilirubinemia based on the molar ratio of bilirubin (mg/dL) to albumin (g/dL). It can be used as long as the bilirubin concentration is less than 30 mg/dL (513 µmol/L). Exchange transfusion is the only recommended treatment for bilirubin concentrations higher than that. When an infant's total bilirubin concentration is higher than 15 mg/dL (257 µmol/L), the albumin concentration should be measured. Serial albumin levels are not necessary because the concentration varies little over short periods of time. The ratio of the two values is more closely related to the risk of toxicity than the total bilirubin alone. Until the free or unbound bilirubin concentration is available to clinicians, this ratio is the best measure of risk for bilirubin brain damage.

Common Pitfalls

■ Trusting your eyes rather than measuring bilirubin concentration to gauge risk

■ Discharging an infant in the high-risk zone of hour-specific bilirubin concentration
■ Failing to follow up within 24 to 48 hours of early discharge
■ Misclassifying an infant with hemolysis or other illness as "otherwise healthy"
■ Using phototherapy as a substitute for exchange transfusion
■ Failing to treat severe hyperbilirubinemia as an emergency

Communication and Counseling

Parents should be counseled and given some written information about neonatal jaundice prior to taking their infant home, including the causes of this common condition, how to look for jaundice, and when to contact their health care provider about it. The American Academy of Pediatrics provides a fact sheet for parents online at http://www.aap.org/family/jaundicefaq.htm

SUGGESTED READINGS

1. American Academy of Pediatrics, Subcommittee on Hyperbilirubinemia: Management of hyperbilirubinemia in the newborn infant 35 or more weeks of gestation. Pediatrics 114:297–316, 2004. **Latest comprehensive national guidelines.**
2. Johnson LH, Bhutani VK, Brown AJ: System-based approach to management of neonatal Jaundice and prevention of kernicterus. J Pediatr 140:396–403, 2002. **Ninety documented cases of kernicterus in apparently healthy newborns.**
3. Kaplan M, Hammerman K, Maisels MJ: Bilirubin genetics for the nongeneticist: Hereditary defects of neonatal bilirubin conjugation. Pediatrics 111:886–893, 2003. **Genetic defects combine with other causes of jaundice to produce severe hyperbilirubinemia.**
4. Maisels MJ, Watchko JF: Treatment of jaundice in low birthweight infants. Arch Dis Child Fetal Neonatal Ed 88:F459–F463, 2003. **Provides guidelines for treating premature infants based on literature review and expert opinion.**
5. Shapiro SM: Bilirubin toxicity in the developing nervous system. Pediatr Neurol 29:410–421, 2003. **A review of the pathophysiology of bilirubin neurotoxicity.**

Intracranial Hemorrhage in the Newborn

Jeffrey M. Perlman

KEY CONCEPTS

- Intraventricular hemorrhage (IVH) remains the most common serious neurologic lesion of the newborn period, particularly in the premature infant of less than 1000 g birth weight.
- Most IVH develops in the first 72 hours of postnatal age.
- Outcome is strongly related to the associated white matter involvement (grade IV IVH).
- Posthemorrhagic hydrocephalus complicates up to 50% of severe IVH.
- Antenatal glucocorticoid administration reduces the incidence of severe IVH.
- Postnatal indomethacin is associated with a reduced incidence of severe IVH.

Periventricular-intraventricular hemorrhage (PV-IVH) remains the most common serious neurologic lesion of the neonatal period. Although the overall incidence of PV-IVH is declining, the occurrence of severe IVH remains a significant problem in the infant of very low birth weight (less than 1000 g) (Table 1). The severe form of hemorrhage is associated with both neonatal mortality and long-term neurodevelopmental deficits.

Pathogenesis

Bleeding originates from capillaries within the germinal matrix, a transitional gelatinous region that provides limited support for prominent but immature vessels that course through it. The genesis of the bleeding is likely multifactorial, in part related to intravascular, vascular, and extravascular influences. More specifically, intravascular factors related to perturbations in cerebral blood flow (CBF) are of particular importance. Thus the cerebral circulation of the sick newborn infant appears to be pressure passive (i.e., changes in CBF directly reflect changes in systemic blood pressure). This situation increases the potential for cerebral injury during periods of systemic hypotension or hypertension. Moreover, the peculiar venous drainage of the region (i.e., the draining vessels) take a U-shape course opposite the head of the caudate nucleus, which increases the potential for venous distention and rupture at this most common site of bleeding. The risk for IVH is greater in the intubated infant with respiratory distress syndrome in whom cerebral perturbations are most likely to occur.

Clinical Features

PV-IVH occurs within the first 72 hours of postnatal life in 85% to 90% of cases. In the smallest infants (i.e., less than 750 g birth weight), the onset tends to be early, within the first 24 hours, whereas in the larger premature infant, the onset is later, from 25 to 72 hours. Later onset bleeding may be observed in the sick infant of very low birth weight. Most cases (up to 70%) are clinically occult and only detected by screening cranial ultrasound imaging. Infants with severe IVH frequently exhibit clinical signs, including a bulging fontanel, seizures, a fall in hematocrit, hyperglycemia, metabolic acidosis, and pulmonary hemorrhage.

Cranial Ultrasound Scans

The ultrasound scan (US) is the modality of choice for screening, diagnosing, and grading the severity of IVH. The appropriate times for obtaining screening US are not entirely clear. However, any recommendation regarding screening protocols should take into account the following: Most IVH is clinically occult, severe lesions occur most often in the tiniest of premature infants, and there seems to be a shift toward a delayed presentation of the clinically more significant lesions. Based on these observations, Table 2 indicates a suggested timetable for screening US.

The grading of IVH is important vis-à-vis management and prognosis. When grading a hemorrhage, the amount of ventricular blood, the degree of ventricular dilation, and the size and location of the associated parenchymal involvement must be estimated (Table 3).

Posthemorrhagic Hydrocephalus

A major complication observed in approximately 40% to 50% of severe IVH cases is posthemorrhagic hydrocephalus (PHH). The progression of PHH may be rapid (i.e.,

TABLE 1 Frequency of Severe Intraventricular Hemorrhage (IVH) in Infants of Birth Weight 500–1500 g (1995–1996)

Grade of IVH	501–750 g (*N* = 1002)	751–1000 g (*N* = 1084)	1001–1250 g (*N* = 1053)	1251–1500 g (*N* = 1229)
Grade III IVH	13%	6%	5%	2%
Grade III IVH and IPE	13%	6%	3%	1%
Total IVH	26%	12%	8%	3%

IPE, intraparenchymal echodensity; often referred to as grade IV IVH. Adapted from Hill A, Volpe JJ: Normal pressure hydrocephalus in the newborn. Pediatrics 75:719, 1981.

TABLE 2 Suggested Timing of Screening Cranial Ultrasound Examinations

Birth Weight (g)	Timing of Screening (days)	Projected Finding
<1000	Initial: 3–5 Identify increased PVE	Identify 75%–80% of IVH
	Second: 10–14 Identify early hydrocephalus Identify early cyst formation	Identify 95% cases of IVH
	Third: 28	Identify most or all IVH Assess ventricular size Assess periventricular white matter Identify late lesions
	Fourth: predischarge	
1000–1250	Initial: 3–5	As above
	Second: 28	As above
	Third: predischarge	As above
1250–1500	Initial 3–5	As above
	Second: predischarge	

TABLE 3 Grading of Severity of Periventricular-Intraventricular Hemorrhage (PV-IVH) by Cranial Ultrasound Imaging

Grade 1	Blood confined to the germinal matrix only
Grade 2	Blood filling <50% of the lateral ventricle on sagittal view
Grade 3	Blood filling >50% of the lateral ventricle with distension on sagittal view
Grade 4 IV/IPE	Increased periventricular echogenicity (of greater intensity than the choroid plexus) located in periventricular white matter observed on both coronal and sagittal images

IPE, intraparenchymal echodensity; IVH, intraventricular hemorrhage.

days) or slow. In the former, the obstruction is secondary to an impairment of cerebrospinal fluid (CSF) absorption caused by a particulate clot at the foramen of Monro or the aqueduct of Sylvius and usually associated with an elevation in intracranial pressure. Treatment is usually immediate, via external drainage above the site of obstruction. The more common presentation is a communicating hydrocephalus that slowly evolves over 1 to 4 weeks following the diagnosis of hemorrhage. The hydrocephalus in these cases is secondary to an obliterative arachnoiditis in the posterior fossa distal to the outflow of the fourth ventricle. The usual clinical criteria of evolving hydrocephalus (i.e., full anterior fontanel and rapid head growth) do not appear for days or weeks after ventricular dilation is already present. Possible reasons for this discrepancy include a relative excess of water in the centrum semiovale, a relatively large subarachnoid space, and a paucity of myelination. Thus serial US are necessary to observe the evolution of PHH.

It is also important to understand the natural history in the management of PHH. In the majority of cases, the ventricular dilation is under normal pressure, hence the slow progression. In approximately half the cases, the progression spontaneously ceases, usually within 30 days. In the remaining 50% there is progressive ventriculomegaly and underpressure. Intervention becomes mandatory in this group of patients. A pressure measurement should be obtained when a lumbar puncture or ventricular tap is performed in an infant with hydrocephalus. The ventricular fluid invariably reveals numerous red blood cells, an elevated white blood cell count, an elevated protein, and a low glucose concentration.

Management

The management choices are threefold: close surveillance (for the 50% that resolve spontaneously); temporizing diversion techniques to control ventricular size, such as external ventricular drainage, subgaleal shunt placement, and serial lumbar punctures; and administration of medications that decrease CSF production. For serial lumbar punctures to be effective there has to be communication between the lateral ventricles and the lumbar subarachnoid space, and adequate quantities of CSF have to be removed to induce a decrease in ventricular size (approximately 10 to 15 mL/kg per tap). If this is successful, daily lumbar punctures are then continued for 1 to 3 weeks, with the frequency based on the rapidity with which the ventricles return to a dilated state after the puncture and the degree of that dilation. Several medications are used to decrease CSF production, including isosorbide, glycerol, and acetazolamide. Acetazolamide decreases CSF production by up to 50%. Most neurosurgeons prefer to place a definitive shunt only when the infant has reached a reasonable size (i.e., more than 1500 g).

Expert Opinion on Management Issues

The primary goal in the management of severe IVH is prevention, which would be achieved most effectively by

BOX 1 Suggested Approach to the Management and Prevention of Periventricular-Intraventricular Hemorrhage
<ul><li>Administer antenatal glucocorticoids where possible.</li><li>Identify highest risk infant:<ul><li>Weight less than 1000 g.</li><li>No antenatal steroids.</li><li>Intubated.</li><li>Respiratory distress syndrome.</li><li>Vascular perturbations.</li></ul></li><li>Avoid vascular perturbations:<ul><li>Synchronized mechanical ventilation.</li><li>Sedation.</li><li>Paralysis.</li><li>Avoid systemic hypotension and/or hypertension.</li><li>Use pharmacologic interventions: indomethacin (0.1 mg/kg every 24 hours for three doses, beginning 6 to 12 hours of age).</li></ul></li></ul>
From Shalak L, Perlman JM: Hemorrhagic-ischemic cerebral injury in the preterm infant: Current concepts. Clin Perinatol 29:745, 2002.

TABLE 4 Relationship of Grade of Periventricular-Intraventricular Hemorrhage (PV-IVH) and Outcome

Grade of PV-IVH	Incidence of Definite Neurologic Sequelae
I	10%
II	20%
III	35%
Grade IV/IPE	
Large >1 cm	100%
Localized <1 cm	80%

IPE, intraparenchymal echodensity.

preventing premature birth. Failing that, the antenatal administration of antenatal glucocorticoids prior to delivery (associated with a reduction in severe IVH) should be considered in all cases of preterm labor.

The incidence of severe IVH is also lower in infants born to mothers with pregnancy-induced hypertension. The most effective mode of delivery to prevent IVH remains unclear. Postnatal strategies of prevention should focus on the infant at highest risk for severe IVH. Thus IVH is more common in infants of younger gestational age, lower birth weight, male sex, intubation (the risk for IVH in the nonintubated infant is less than 10%), and with respiratory distress syndrome. For infants with respiratory distress syndrome, the risk for IVH is even greater when there are complications, such as pneumothorax or pulmonary interstitial emphysema, or when there are perturbations in cerebral blood flow or venous return. These vascular perturbations, which in part are related to the infant's own respiratory mechanics, can be minimized with careful ventilator management, including the use of synchronized mechanical ventilation, assist control ventilation, sedation, or, in more difficult cases, with paralysis. Postnatal medications to reduce severe IVH include phenobarbital, vitamin E, and indomethacin. Only indomethacin is associated with a reduction in severe IVH.

Communication and Counseling

Parents need to be educated regarding the outcome following IVH. Long-term motor and cognitive deficits relate to severity of the hemorrhage, and in particular when there is associated parenchymal involvement (Table 4). Moreover, the outcome with parenchymal involvement depends on the size of the echogenicity noted on the US. Thus large lesions (i.e., more than 1 cm in diameter in both the coronal and sagittal plane) invariably are associated with a poor outcome. Such infants commonly exhibit severe motor deficits (spastic quadriplegia) as well as significant cognitive impairment. The outcome for small lesions is less precise. Although the risk for neurodevelopmental deficits is substantial, it is not universal, and, indeed, a normal outcome may occur.

SUGGESTED READINGS

1. Hill A, Volpe JJ: Normal pressure hydrocephalus in the newborn. Pediatrics 75:719, 1981. **Discusses the natural history of hydrocephalus and when to intervene.**
2. Lemons JA, Bauer CR, Oh W, et al: Very low birth weight outcomes of the National Institute of Child Health and Human Development Neonatal Research Network, January 1995 through December 1996. Pediatrics 107:E1, 2001. **Indicates the incidence of IVH in a large cohort of infants of very low birth weight.**
3. Perlman JM, Rollins N: Surveillance protocol for the detection of intracranial abnormalities in premature neonates. Arch Pediatr Adolesc Med 154:822–826, 2000. **Provides information on when to screen for IVH and other neurologic conditions common to the infant of very low birth weight.**
4. Schmidt B, Davis P, Moddemann D, et al: Long-term effects of indomethacin prophylaxis in extremely-low-birth-weight infants. N Engl J Med 344:1966–1972, 2001. **In this study the administration of indomethacin versus placebo reduced the incidence of severe periventricular and intraventricular hemorrhage (9% versus 13% in the placebo group; odds ratio, 0.6; P = 0.02). The rate of survival without neurosensory impairment at 18 months, however, was not altered between groups.**
5. Shalak L, Perlman JM: Hemorrhagic-ischemic cerebral injury in the preterm infant: Current concepts. Clin Perinatol 29:745, 2002. **Review article that covers the most recent literature regarding pathogenesis, treatment strategies, and long-term outcome with IVH and in particular with severe IVH.**
6. Volpe JJ: Periventricular-intraventricular hemorrhage. In Volpe JJ (ed): Neurology of the Newborn, 3rd ed. Philadelphia: WB Saunders, 2001, pp 428–473. **The chapter on IVH reviews pathogenesis, complications including posthemorrhagic hydrocephalus, and treatment strategies.**

Common Pitfalls

- Failure to administer antenatal steroid when a premature birth is suspected
- Failure to follow progression of hemorrhaging with sequential US
- Failure to detect progressive ventricular involvement

Birth Injuries

Philip Roth

KEY CONCEPTS

- Risk factors for the occurrence of birth injuries are highly associated with a complicated labor and delivery process.
- Despite the risk factors, the majority of birth injuries follow uncomplicated births.
- Because many birth injuries coexist in the same patients, meticulous physical assessment and use of radiologic studies are critical.
- For most injuries, expectant management is appropriate and the prognosis for recovery is good.

Birth injuries occur predominantly as a result of mechanical forces experienced during labor and delivery. Although improvements in obstetrical care have resulted in a reduced incidence of birth injuries, they continue to occur in the setting of macrosomia, fetal malpresentation, instrument-assisted deliveries, prolonged labor, and precipitous deliveries. Table 1 outlines the classification of birth injuries according to location and organ/tissue type.

SUPERFICIAL INJURIES

Superficial injuries involve facial structures such as the eyes and nose. Retinal hemorrhages, subconjunctival hemorrhages, and lid edema are rather common and not of significant concern. More significant injuries, such as corneal trauma, lid lacerations, hyphema, and vitreous hemorrhage, occur with the use of forceps and/or fetal scalp electrodes and require the attention of an

TABLE 1 Classification of Birth Injuries

Superficial/Facial
Nasal septal dislocation
Ocular
Head
Intracranial
Extracranial
Caput succedaneum
Cephalohematoma
Subgaleal hemorrhage
Skull fracture
Neuromuscular
Brachial plexus injury
Facial nerve palsy
Laryngeal nerve paralysis
Spinal cord injury
Congenital torticollis
Bone and Soft Tissue Injury
Clavicular fracture
Long bone fracture
Intra-abdominal injury
Liver
Spleen
Adrenals

ophthalmologist. In examining the nose, distinction must be made between simple nasal compression and septal dislocation. The latter involves displacement of the triangular cartilaginous portion of the septum from the vomerine groove, resulting in airway obstruction.

Expert Opinion on Management Issues

Deviation of the nose to one side along with leaning of the nasal columella to the side opposite the dislocation (the Metzenbaum sign) and collapse of the nostrils with pressure on the lip of the nose (Jeppesen and Windfeld test) confirm the diagnosis of septal dislocation. To avoid long-term septal and cosmetic deformities, manual reduction should be performed prior to 3 days of age.

Common Pitfalls

Failure to distinguish septal dislocation from simple nasal compression may result in long-term deformity. If one moves the tip of the nose to the midline, the nostrils appear symmetrical in nasal compression but not with septal dislocation.

HEAD INJURIES

Because intracranial injuries are discussed in the chapter "Intracranial Hemorrhage in the Newborn", this chapter discusses extracranial injuries, which can be classified according to the tissue plane in which they occur (Figure 1). Table 2 summarizes the clinical features distinguishing caput succedaneum, cephalohematoma, and subgaleal hemorrhage. Because caput succedaneum and cephalohematoma are confined to restricted spaces, blood loss is generally not clinically significant. In contrast, the space beneath the galeal aponeurosis, which extends from the orbital ridges to the occiput and laterally to the ears, can accommodate large volumes of blood.

Skull fractures, which primarily involve the parietal bones, result from compression against the maternal

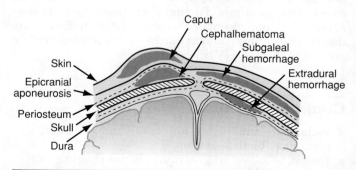

FIGURE 1. Sites of extracranial hemorrhages in the newborn. Schematic diagram of important tissue planes from skin to dura. (Reprinted with permission from Volpe JJ [ed]: Neurology of the Newborn. Philadelphia: WB Saunders, 2001, p 814.)

symphysis or sacral spines or because of application of forceps. Although most fractures are linear, nondepressed, and not associated with intracranial injuries, occasionally inward buckling of the compliant neonatal skull bone results in the so-called Ping-Pong depressed fracture.

Expert Opinion on Management Issues

Initial management should focus on proper identification of the type of extracranial hemorrhage. Caput succedaneum, which appears shortly after birth and does not expand significantly in size, requires no treatment and resolves within days. Although a cephalohematoma may increase in size after birth, the magnitude of blood loss is rarely sufficient to cause significant decreases in hematocrit and blood pressure. Like cephalohematoma, subgaleal hemorrhage may enlarge after birth, but it differs in that blood loss may result in severe anemia and shock. Management should be supportive, with emphasis on volume replacement, transfusion, and correction of any underlying coagulopathy.

Intervention is generally not required for nondepressed fractures. A dural tear occasionally accompanies a linear fracture, resulting in fluid accumulation and formation of a leptomeningeal cyst. In the case of a depressed skull fracture, which generally is clinically detectable, investigation to rule out intracranial injury is required. Surgical intervention is indicated if bone fragments are detected in the cerebrum, neurologic deficits are present, signs of intracranial hypertension are present, or the accumulation of subgaleal cerebrospinal fluid (CSF) is demonstrated.

Common Pitfalls

- Because progression of subgaleal hemorrhage frequently occurs, acute clinical deterioration may occur in patients who initially appear stable.
- Attention must also be given to the appearance of jaundice and hyperbilirubinemia in babies with significant extravascular blood collections, as in cephalohematomas and subgaleal hemorrhages.
- Although skull fractures are associated with 5% to 10% of cephalohematomas, the vast majority are linear and nondepressed and do not require treatment.
- If neurologic symptoms accompany the presence of a cephalohematoma, additional imaging (e.g., CT scan) is required to search for intracranial lesions.

- Although spontaneous elevation of depressed skull fractures is described, the incidence is not known. Therefore, prior to surgical intervention and assuming there are neither bone fragments in the cerebrum nor extradural/subdural blood collections and the patient is neurologically stable, use of digital pressure and/or a breast pump or obstetrical vacuum extractor to elevate the fracture are recommended. Failure of these approaches may be a further indication for surgical elevation. Avoidance of surgical intervention should also be considered in depressions smaller than 2 cm and those that are located over major venous sinuses in neurologically stable infants.

Communication and Counseling

Although caput succedaneum resolves within days, cephalohematoma may be present for weeks. With calcification of a cephalohematoma, swelling may be present for months. In cases of subgaleal hemorrhage, parents should be made aware of its seriousness, with mortality rates of approximately 15% to 20%.

In contrast, parents need to be reassured that, in the vast majority of cases, skull fractures are benign and extensive imaging is not indicated. However, once radiographs are performed and demonstrate fracture(s), follow-up studies should generally be done several months later to document resolution as well as absence of widening of the fracture line, which would indicate a leptomeningeal cyst.

BRACHIAL PLEXUS INJURY

Injury to the brachial plexus occurs when excessive lateral traction is applied at birth, resulting in weakness or paralysis of the muscles innervated by spinal nerves C5-C8 and T1. Table 3 describes the patterns of injury encountered. As with many other birth injuries, brachial plexus injury occurs more frequently in the setting of macrosomia, shoulder dystocia, instrument-assisted deliveries, and abnormal fetal presentation.

Expert Opinion on Management Issues

Ninety percent of infants with brachial plexus injury recover spontaneously. The best outcomes occur in those who begin to recover within 2 to 4 weeks, have an upper

---

TABLE 2 Clinical Features of Major Extracranial Hemorrhages

Hemorrhage Type	Location	Crosses Suture Lines	Large Blood Loss
Caput succedaneum	Subcutaneous	(+)	(−)
Cephalohematoma	Subperiosteal	(−)	(−)
Subgaleal hemorrhage	Subaponeurotic	(+)	(+)

TABLE 3 Brachial Plexus Injury: Clinical Presentations

Type	Frequency (%)	Affected Spinal Nerves	Biceps Reflex	Grasp	Clinical Appearance	Associated Neurologic Findings
Erb palsy (upper)	90	C5, 6, 7	(−)	(+)	"Waiter's tip" position; shoulder adduction/internal rotation; extension of elbow; pronation of forearm; flexion of wrist and fingers	Diaphragmatic paralysis
Klumpke palsy (lower)	<1	C8, T1	(+)	(−)	Weakness of intrinsic hand muscles; weakness of wrist and finger flexors	Horner syndrome
Total	10	C5–8, T1	(−)	(−)	Flaccid	Diaphragmatic paralysis; Horner syndrome

rather than lower or entire plexus injury, and do not have an associated Horner syndrome or diaphragmatic paralysis. At the neuronal level, patients who experience neurapraxia (temporary conduction block secondary to hemorrhage and edema) or axonotmesis (severing of axons with preservation of surrounding elements) have a better prognosis than those who experience neurotmesis (postganglionic disconnection of nerves because of rupture of axons and their surrounding sheaths) or avulsion (preganglionic disconnection from the spinal cord). Initial management consists of immobilization for the first 7 to 10 days to avoid exacerbation of any hemorrhage or edema. At that time, passive range of motion exercises and, according to some experts, splinting of the wrist should be undertaken to avoid development of contractures.

Patients who show no signs of recovery of function by 2 to 3 months should be referred to specialized surgical centers. Neural grafting is generally undertaken between 3 and 6 months if there is no evidence of contractions in the involved muscle groups or detectable antigravity function in the deltoid and biceps muscles. Surgical exploration should also be undertaken in infants with pseudomeningocele, which are cystic lesions resulting from tears in the nerve root sleeves that allow CSF to collect and become encased in fibrotic membranes.

Common Pitfalls

Although risk factors are identified, 40% of brachial plexus injuries occur in patients with no history of shoulder dystocia or other complications of labor and delivery, making it very difficult to anticipate this type of injury. Once brachial plexus injury is diagnosed, systematic evaluation must be undertaken to look for associated abnormalities, including Horner syndrome, diaphragmatic paralysis, bony fractures, especially of the clavicle and humerus, facial nerve palsy, and injury of the cervical spinal cord. Presence of these abnormalities affects both treatment and prognosis.

Communication and Counseling

Because Erb palsy is the most common form of brachial plexus injury and carries the best prognosis, counseling of parents in most cases should be optimistic. For infants who require surgery, discussion should clarify that reinnervation may take months and sequential examinations are the mainstay of follow-up.

FACIAL NERVE PALSY

Facial nerve palsy arises from traumatic compression of the peripheral portion of the nerve as it emerges from the stylomastoid foramen or as it passes over the ramus of the mandible. Although forceps-assisted delivery is a frequently cited risk factor, apposition to the maternal sacral promontory is probably responsible for most cases. In addition, abnormal in utero positioning of the angle of the jaw against the fetal shoulder is responsible for a significant number of cases.

Expert Opinion on Management Issues

Patients with facial nerve palsy display a lower motor neuron pattern of involvement with weakness of both upper and lower facial muscles. The typical infant has flattening of the nasolabial fold, absence of forehead wrinkling, and inability to close the eye on the affected side, along with drawing of the mouth away from that side during crying. Because 90% of patients recover completely, usually within 2 weeks, active intervention is not required. Management should address prevention of corneal injury through installation of artificial tears and in some cases application of tape to keep the eye closed.

Common Pitfalls

In patients with facial nerve palsy, care must be taken not to overlook findings that suggest a nontraumatic etiology, as is the case with the Möbius, Goldenhar, Poland, and DiGeorge syndromes as well as trisomies 13 and 18. In addition, congenital hypoplasia of the depressor anguli oris muscle may be mistaken for facial nerve palsy because of the infant's inability to move the affected side of the mouth laterally and downward during crying.

Communication and Counseling

Prognosis for recovery in traumatic facial nerve palsy is excellent, as already noted.

LARYNGEAL NERVE PARALYSIS

Excessive lateral flexion of the neck may result in compression of the superior branch of the laryngeal nerve against the thyroid cartilage above or of the recurrent branch against the cricoid cartilage below, leading to abnormal swallowing and vocal cord paralysis, respectively. Signs of the latter include stridor, respiratory distress, hoarse cry, and/or recurrent aspiration.

Expert Opinion on Management Issues

Diagnosis of laryngeal nerve paralysis can be made with direct laryngoscopy. While awaiting recovery, small feeding volumes administered through gavage tubes may be necessary. In addition, intubation and possibly tracheostomy may be required to treat respiratory distress, especially in the setting of bilateral vocal cord paralysis.

Common Pitfalls

In the absence of a history of excessive traction, additional studies should be performed to rule out injuries or anomalies of the central nervous system.

Communication and Counseling

Vocal cord paralysis caused by traction injuries has an excellent prognosis for spontaneous recovery, usually within months.

SPINAL CORD INJURIES

Spinal cord injuries, fortunately rare, result from longitudinal traction along with rotation of the spinal cord. The combination of ligamentous laxity, incomplete mineralization of the vertebral bodies, and relatively weak muscles permits the spinal column to stretch beyond the limits of the spinal cord, which may be lacerated, disrupted, or completely transected. Aside from acute hemorrhage and edema, excitotoxic mediators are released and lead to cell death. The gradual occurrence of fibrosis, focal cystic necrosis, and vascular occlusions of the cord contribute to long-term loss of function. Injury is localized primarily to the upper cervical cord following forceps rotation during vertex delivery and to the cervicothoracic cord following vaginal breech delivery accompanied by hyperextension of the head and neck or head entrapment with cephalopelvic disproportion. The three clinical syndromes that may ensue are stillbirth or rapid neonatal death, neonatal respiratory failure, or neonatal hypotonia and weakness. In addition to severe hypotonia, other findings include paucity of movement, absent deep tendon reflexes, and failure to respond to pain below the level of injury.

Expert Opinion on Management Issues

A focus on prevention is essential with cautious management of breech presentations and dysfunctional labor and cesarean delivery in situations involving hyperextension of the head and neck. If spinal injury is suspected clinically, the head, neck, and spine should be immobilized immediately. Intubation and ventilation should be provided to patients with evidence of apnea or poor respiratory effort. Spinal ultrasound or MRI should be provided to confirm the diagnosis as well as to rule out occult dysraphic states or extramedullary masses, which are amenable to surgical decompression. Steroids may have an ameliorating effect if given within 8 hours of injury.

Common Pitfalls

Because hypoxic-ischemic encephalopathy may occur in isolation or concurrently in patients in this clinical setting, diagnosis of spinal cord injury may be delayed. Furthermore, additional evaluation is required to rule out intracranial injury, primary neuromuscular disorders, and congenital abnormalities of the spinal cord.

Communication and Counseling

Prognosis for patients with spinal cord injury is generally poor, especially if they remain dependent on a ventilator for longer than 24 hours. Mortality is close to 50%, and survivors frequently remain ventilator-dependent and have severe neurologic disabilities.

CONGENITAL TORTICOLLIS

The final common pathway for the development of congenital torticollis is thought to be replacement of sternomastoid muscle by fibrotic tissue. Whether the inciting event is the tearing of muscle with resulting hematoma or malposition leading to ischemia and edema, the clinical presentation includes torticollis with mass ("sternomastoid tumor"), torticollis without mass ("muscular torticollis"), or torticollis without a mass or apparent muscle tightness ("postural torticollis").

Expert Opinion on Management Issues

The head of an infant with torticollis is tilted toward and rotated opposite to the side of the lesion. If torticollis is suspected, ultrasound may be performed to rule out abnormalities of the cervical spine. The mainstay of therapy is prolonged active and passive stretching of the neck. With vigorous physiotherapy, surgery is rarely required.

Common Pitfalls

By reducing the limitation to lateral bending and rotation, plagiocephaly (flattening of the skull) can be avoided. Plagiocephaly because of torticollis or simple supine positioning of infants may be treated with cranial remolding orthoses (helmets).

Communication and Counseling

If limitation of motion is less than 10 degrees, the prognosis for complete resolution is virtually 100%. Persistent limitation of motion lasting months and greater than 15 degrees carries a more guarded prognosis and may need to be evaluated for surgical release procedures.

BONE FRACTURES

Although fractures of long bones rarely occur, fracture of the clavicle is probably underreported because of missed diagnosis at birth. Risk factors for clavicular fracture are similar to those for many other birth injuries and include macrosomia, prolonged second stage of labor, shoulder dystocia, and instrument-assisted deliveries. The clinical presentation may vary from no symptoms to decreased movement of the ipsilateral arm. On physical examination, there may be crepitus, palpable bony abnormalities, and/or discoloration over the site of injury. Risk factors for long bone fractures, which primarily involve the femur and humerus, are breech presentation, cesarean delivery, and low birth weight. Like patients with clavicular fractures, these patients present with reduced movement, pain, and crepitus.

Expert Opinion on Management Issues

Because clavicular fractures and humeral fractures clinically resemble and frequently coexist with brachial plexus injury, plain films are essential to make the diagnosis. In cases of asymptomatic or "incomplete" fracture of the clavicle, no treatment is required. However, in "complete" or symptomatic cases, some experts recommend immobilization of the arm for 7 to 10 days by pinning the sleeve of the affected arm to the patient's shirt. Long bone fractures can generally be treated with immobilization and splinting. However, in cases of displaced fractures, closed reduction and casting are required.

Common Pitfalls

- Because of the possible coexistence of humeral fractures, clavicular fractures, and brachial plexus injuries, ruling in one of these entities by no means rules out the others.

- Despite the association with traumatic births, the majority of fractures occur with uncomplicated deliveries, making the occurrence of these injuries highly unpredictable.
- Fractures involving separation of nonossified epiphyses may not be apparent on plain films. In such situations, ultrasound may be helpful, whereas plain films, repeated 7 to 10 days later, show evidence of callus formation.

Communication and Counseling

Long-term sequelae of fractures of either the clavicles or long bones are rare. Although unusual, intrinsic diseases of bone should be considered, especially osteogenesis imperfecta, when the injury seems disproportionate to the clinical history.

INTRA-ABDOMINAL INJURY

Although unusual, injuries to intra-abdominal organs are more likely to occur in the setting of complicated deliveries, prematurity, and conditions associated with hepatosplenomegaly, coagulopathy, and asphyxia. Direct trauma or compression of the chest leading to damage to the surface of organs or tearing of their ligamentous insertions results in rupture or subcapsular hemorrhage of the liver, spleen, or adrenals in order of decreasing frequency. Clinical presentation depends on the degree of blood loss, which is more precipitous in cases of rupture than of subcapsular hematoma.

Expert Opinion on Management Issues

Patients with severe, acute blood loss can be distinguished by the presence of pallor, shock, and abdominal distention and discoloration. Abdominal CT scanning is generally diagnostic but may be difficult to perform in unstable patients. Ultrasound is therefore frequently used because of its diagnostic accuracy and immediate availability at the bedside. Abdominal paracentesis is positive in the setting of hemoperitoneum. Treatment should focus on volume replacement and correction of associated coagulopathy. If the patient is hemodynamically stable and a subcapsular hematoma is present, conservative management is appropriate. However, if rupture of the involved organ has occurred and/or the infant is hemodynamically unstable, surgical exploration is indicated.

Common Pitfalls

Infants with slow clinical progression are more likely to have a subcapsular hematoma. In the event of a sudden rapid deterioration, rupture should be considered and treated as such until proven otherwise. Although significant hemorrhage into any organ may cause hypotension and shock, adrenal hemorrhage is unique in that there may be concurrent deficiency of adrenal steroids, requiring replacement therapy.

Communication and Counseling

Close observation is required to avoid sudden catastrophic deterioration. Rupture of a hepatic subcapsular hematoma or hemoperitoneum is associated with a significant morbidity and mortality.

SUGGESTED READINGS

1. Piatt JH: Birth injuries of the brachial plexus. Pediatr Clin North Am 51:421–440, 2004. **Reviews clinical features, prognosis, and surgical management of brachial plexus injuries.**
2. Rosenberg A: Traumatic birth injury. NeoReviews 4:e270–e276, 2003. **Describes risk factors and common presenting findings of traumatic birth injuries.**
3. Uhing MR: Management of birth injuries. Pediatr Clin North Am 51:1169–1186, 2004. **Describes approach to management of common birth injuries.**
4. Volpe JJ (ed): Neurology of the Newborn, 4th ed. Philadelphia: WB Saunders, 2001, pp 813–838. **Reviews clinical aspects of head and neuromuscular injuries sustained at birth.**

Anemia of Prematurity and When to Transfuse

Helen M. Towers

KEY CONCEPTS

- Preterm infants do not mount adequate erythropoietin response to hypoxia and anemia.
- Iatrogenic losses can exceed blood production.
- Few, if any, clinical signs and symptoms in preterm infants can be related to hemoglobin concentrations.
- Oxygen delivery to the tissues is influenced by many factors other than hemoglobin concentration.
- Reduction of the need for blood transfusions is associated with rigorous transfusion policies and restrictive blood testing.
- Exogenous replacement of erythropoietin has minimally altered transfusion practice in preterm infants.

Anemia of prematurity is a normochromic, normocytic anemia characterized by low hemoglobin levels, decreased reticulocyte production, and low serum erythropoietin levels. First described by Shulman in 1959, it is now a common finding in premature infants and infants of low birth weight (LBW). Approximately 80% of very LBW (VLBW) infants (<1500 g) and 95% of extremely LBW (ELBW) infants (<1000 g) receive at least one red blood cell (RBC) transfusion during their stay in the neonatal intensive care unit (NICU). Controversy continues regarding the relationship of low circulating hemoglobin to commonly seen clinical symptoms in the preterm infant, including apnea, tachycardia, and desaturation. Historically attributed to anemia, it is now

recognized that resolution of these symptoms may be a maturational process, not a hematologic issue. Other symptoms, including failure to thrive and lethargy, are more difficult to interpret in the face of low, sometimes very low hemoglobin concentrations, but little literature supports the use of RBC transfusions. There is also a lack of consensus about the timing and effectiveness of currently available therapeutic modalities, including recombinant human erythropoietin (rHuEPO).

Anemia of prematurity can result from increased blood loss, decreased RBC production and increased RBC destruction, or any combination of these causes.

Increased Blood Loss

Preterm infants lose blood in different situations, some more avoidable than others. Elevating the infant above the level of the placenta may lead to fetal-placenta transfusion of up to 30 mL in a minute. Cord accidents or losses from indwelling lines are known to occur. The most common form of blood depletion in the preterm population is iatrogenic losses secondary to blood sampling. Very tiny infants can lose close to their entire blood volume (approximately 85 mL per kg) within a few days of life, necessitating frequent blood transfusions.

Decreased Blood Cell Production

During embryologic life, red blood cell production occurs in extramedullary sites such as the yolk sac and liver, with production in the bone marrow beginning after the first trimester. By 32 weeks' gestation, RBCs are produced approximately evenly from both the liver and bone marrow. Erythropoietin, one of many erythropoietic growth factors, develops in the liver in cells of monophage/macrophage origin, with production shifting to the peritubular cells of the kidney after term gestation. Interrupting a pregnancy prematurely does not alter these ontological processes. Erythropoietin (EPO) production is thought to be controlled by an oxygen-sensing mechanism in the liver and kidney, and both anemia and hypoxia stimulate mRNA transcription and EPO protein production. The liver is less sensitive than the kidney in response to these stimuli. Because it remains the major source of EPO in the preterm infant, RBC production may be blunted. The kinetics of EPO metabolism in neonates lead to a larger volume of distribution and faster elimination, whether it is given exogenously or produced endogenously, which may lead to alteration in bone marrow stimulation and reduced RBC production.

Increased Red Blood Cell Destruction

The average life span of neonatal RBCs is approximately a half to two thirds that of the adult RBC. This shorter life span is due to the lower levels of intracellular ATP, enzyme activity, and carnitine levels as well as the increased susceptibility to lipid peroxidation and susceptibility of the cell membrane to fragmentation.

Expert Opinion on Management Issues

INDICATIONS TO TRANSFUSE

The acutely ill premature infant on mechanical ventilator support and oxygen therapy with unstable hemodynamic status and requiring frequent blood testing presents little doubt as to the need to maintain circulating hemoglobin. Consensus would suggest transfusion if the hemoglobin falls below 12 g/dL. As this same infant recovers and weans to little or no respiratory support and begins to gain weight, the need for transfusion fades rapidly. Infants who clearly demonstrate a falling hematocrit with poor reticulocytosis, oxygen requirement, and lethargy may require transfusion if the hemoglobin falls below 8 g/dL. The best available evidence on restrictive transfusion practice shows no increase in important neonatal complications, such as intraventricular hemorrhage, necrotizing enterocolitis, chronic lung disease, or sepsis.

RATIONALE FOR NOT TRANSFUSING

RBC transfusion increases oxygen-carrying capacity and ultimately delivery of oxygen to the tissues. But oxygen delivery to the tissues is influenced by type of hemoglobin, the concentration of 2,3-diphosphoglycerate (2,3-DPG), and the cardiopulmonary function of the infant. The normal postnatal maturational effects of switching from fetal hemoglobin to adult hemoglobin (also seen following transfusion) and the normal rise in 2,3-DPG is actually associated with greater tissue oxygen availability even in the face of falling hemoglobin concentrations. Methods of assessing tissue oxygenation in the clinical setting are not currently possible. Surrogate measures, such as the measurement of peripheral fractional oxygen extraction (FOE) by near infrared spectroscopy or the measurement of whole blood lactate levels, can certainly be performed, although neither are reliable indicators of the need for transfusion. Box 1 lists the indications to transfuse RBCs in preterm infants.

WHAT TO TRANSFUSE

Packed RBCs are the most common blood product administered to premature infants. The functional integrity of transfused adult cells depends on storage and age. The anticoagulant preservatives used today, with additives such as Adsol, allow a shelf life up to 42 days and maintain a hematocrit of approximately 60%. Rapid and large-volume transfusions should be performed with blood less than 5 days old in light of the potential for elevated potassium levels in older blood. Gamma irradiation to prevent graft-versus-host disease is usual, and high-efficiency leukodepletion filters are commonly used, the latter without proven benefit. RBC components used in the preterm population should be cytomegalovirus (CMV) negative.

ERYTHROPOIETIN

Multiple studies on the use of rHuEPO show an effective ability to stimulate erythropoiesis; however, overall transfusion rates are not altered much. It appears that implementing restrictive blood sampling and paying attention to transfusion parameters affect the transfusion rate more than supplying exogenous rHuEPO. Other medical supplements used to treat anemia of prematurity include iron, vitamin E, folic acid, and vitamin B_{12}. Table 1 lists the medications used in the treatment of anemia of prematurity.

PREVENTIVE MEASURES

Blood donors for children less than 1 year of age should ideally be repeat donors who have tested negative for all microbiologic markers. The use of dedicated smaller aliquots from a single donor to be used sequentially for an individual infant greatly reduces exposure to multiple donors.

Common Pitfalls

The most common problem associated with anemia of prematurity is identifying the threshold for transfusion. The nadir of anemia prematurity occurs at approximately 4 to 6 weeks of age and resolves at 3 to 4 months. Immature infants who have tachycardia, apnea, and desaturation episodes generally do not require blood transfusions, despite hemoglobin concentrations that can fall to 6 g/dL, and especially if evidence of reticulocytosis is present. Other pitfalls include failure to consider a family's religious beliefs regarding transfusion and failure to consider alternatives to transfusion such as rHuEPO. If transfusion is required, it is suggested that larger volume (20 mL/kg), rather than smaller volume (10 mL/kg), leads to higher rises in hemoglobin and fewer overall transfusions. Box 2 lists the complications of blood transfusions.

Communication and Counseling

The normal course of anemia of prematurity should be explained to parents as soon as it is recognized. Parents are often anxious about potential transfusion complications and the risks and benefits of blood transfusion, and

---

BOX 1   Indications to Transfuse Packed Red Blood Cells in Premature Infants

- Acute blood loss with associated hypovolemic shock.
- Acutely ill preterm infant with Hct less than 35% or Hgb less than 12 g/dL and O_2 requirement.
- Non-acutely ill preterm infant with falling Hct (<20%), Hgb (<6 g/dL), and low reticulocyte count (<1%), with failure to gain weight, requirement for supplemental O_2, and unexplained lethargy.
- Infant with Hct less than 25% if surgery is considered.

Note: Volume to transfuse is 20 mL/kg.
Hct, hematocrit; Hgb, hemoglobin.

TABLE 1 Medications Used in the Treatment of Anemia of Prematurity

Generic Name (Trade Name)	Dosage/Route/ Regimen	Maximum Dose	Dosage Formulations	Common Adverse Reactions	Therapeutic Concentrations	Comments
Epoetin alfa (Epogen)	400–1400 U/kg/wk subcutaneously given every day or every other day	1400 U/kg/wk	Injection	Few reported	Titrated to rise in hemoglobin	Infants require supplemental iron and vitamin E.
Ferrous sulfate	6 mg/kg/day PO based on elemental iron		Syrup, drops, and elixir	GI upset		Interferes with vitamin E absorption.
Folic acid	50 µg/day PO		Tablet, elixir	Caution if used concurrently with phenytoin	>6 µg/mL	May contain benzyl alcohol as preservative.
Vitamin E	25 IU/day PO		Drops		0.5–3.5 mg/dL	May induce vitamin K deficiency.
Vitamin B$_{12}$	0.4 µg PO IM	0.9 µg	Injection, tablets		200–900 pg/mL	

GI, gastrointestinal; IM, intramuscular; PO, by mouth.

BOX 2 Complications of Blood Transfusions

- Infection (cytomegalovirus)
- Immunosuppression
- Alloimmunization to RBC, WBC, and platelet antigens
- Graft-versus-host disease
- Altered erythropoietin response

RBC, red blood cell; WBC, white blood cell.

---

alternative therapies should be explained clearly to allay parental fears. Many institutions require written consent for blood transfusions, which provides an excellent opportunity to discuss this important topic with parents.

SUGGESTED READINGS

1. Alkaly AL, Galvis S, Ferry DA, et al: Hemodynamic changes in anemic premature infants: Are we allowing the hematocrits to fall too low? Pediatrics 112:838–845, 2003. **Study discussing benefits of transfusion practice guided by measures of cardiac function.**
2. Anderson C: Critical hemoglobin thresholds in premature infants. Arch Dis Child Fetal Neonatal Ed 84:F146–F148, 2001. **Discusses relationship of oxygen transport and tissue oxygen delivery to hemoglobin transfusion.**
3. Canadian Paediatric Society: Position statement: Red blood cell transfusions in newborn infants: Revised guidelines. Paediatr Child Health 7(8):553–558, 2002. **Discusses reasons for transfusion in newborn infants and types of blood products used.**
4. Murray NA, Roberts IAG: Neonatal transfusion practice. Arch Dis Child Fetal Neonatal Ed 89:F101–F107, 2004. **Practical review of current transfusion practice in the newborn.**
5. Ringer SA, Richardson DK, Sacher RA, et al: Variations in transfusion practice in neonatal intensive care. Pediatrics 101:194–200, 1998. **A study that highlights discretionary rather than necessary transfusion practice in NICUs.**
6. Widness JA, Lowe LS, Bell EF, et al: Adaptive responses during anemia and its correction in lambs. J Appl Physiol 88:1397–1406, 2000. **Detailed account of metabolic and cardiovascular adaptive responses to anemia.**

5

Hemolytic Disease of the Newborn

Steven Alan Ringer

KEY CONCEPTS

- Hemolytic disease is characterized by immune-mediated hemolysis, anemia, and hyperbilirubinemia, following maternal sensitization to incompatible fetal erythrocytes.
- Major causes include ABO and RhD incompatibility; minor blood groups can be responsible, especially Kell, c, and E.
- Rh disease is more severe and present at birth. ABO disease is more common but less severe and usually develops over the first 24 hours after birth. Among diseases caused by minor antigens, that caused by Kell sensitization may be severe.
- All pregnant women should be tested for ABO and RhD blood types and have a serum screen for isoimmune antibodies.
- Intrauterine monitoring is recommended for cases in which sensitization is identified. Intrauterine transfusion or early delivery may be necessary.
- The goals of therapy in the newborn are to prevent or correct hemodynamic compromise from anemia and neurologic injury from hyperbilirubinemia.

Continued

KEY CONCEPTS—cont'd

- The newborn should be assessed immediately after birth, and the level of bilirubin and hematocrit should be determined.
- Guidelines for the institution of phototherapy are based on hour-specific levels of bilirubin. Hemolytic disease should be treated at lower bilirubin levels than other causes of hyperbilirubinemia.
- Intravenous immunoglobulin (IVIG) is effective in reducing the need for exchange transfusion when used with phototherapy but may not prevent the need for late transfusion.

Hemolytic disease of the newborn is really a group of disorders characterized by isoimmune hemolysis resulting in anemia and hyperbilirubinemia. The destruction of fetal and neonatal erythrocytes is mediated by maternal immunoglobulin (Ig) G antibodies reacting against an antigen on the cell surface, and the released hemoglobin is metabolized to bilirubin. The range of presentation extends from relatively mild, with moderate jaundice associated with only laboratory evidence of hemolysis, to very severe anemia, hyperbilirubinemia, and hydrops fetalis. Severe disease may be life-threatening or it may be associated with serious disability from the complications of hydrops or the toxicity of hyperbilirubinemia.

The process begins when fetal cells enter the maternal circulation via a fetomaternal hemorrhage, which happens in at least 50% of pregnancies and during abortions, even with losses that are so early the pregnancy may not even be recognized. One or more of the fetal cell-surface antigens that determine major and minor blood groups may be foreign to the mother, who produces antibodies against them. Only IgG antibodies cause hemolytic disease because the crystallizable fragment (Fc) component necessary for the uptake and transport of the antibody across the placenta is not present in IgM or IgA. The most common causes of hemolytic disease are anti-A or anti-B antibodies from a type O mother or anti-D antibodies from a mother who is RhD negative.

Hemolytic disease caused by untreated Rh incompatibility (Rh disease) typically has the most severe presentation. The hemolytic anemia often develops during fetal life and is present at birth; the hyperbilirubinemia may be manifest at birth or develop rapidly thereafter. If the fetal anemia is severe, the disease may progress to hydrops, with cardiac failure, skin edema, effusions, and hepatosplenomegaly.

Because the prevalence of the Rh-negative genotype ranges from as high as 21% among European whites to essentially zero among East Asians and Native Americans, the incidence of Rh disease varies among ethnic groups. Once a woman is sensitized by RhD positive cells, the severity of Rh disease does increase in each successive pregnancy in which the fetus is RhD positive. However, for several reasons, only a small percentage of the infants borne by Rh-negative women actually develop hemolytic disease. First, not all Rh-negative women mount a significant antibody response, sometimes because a coexisting A-O or B-O incompatibility causes rapid clearing of fetal cells from the maternal circulation. Second, the disease rarely occurs in first pregnancies because the initial maternal antibody response is an IgM class that does not reach the fetus. Finally, some subsequent infants of sensitized women are themselves Rh negative.

ABO hemolytic disease is generally less severe than Rh disease, and it rarely results in hydrops fetalis or the need for exchange transfusion. In part, the relatively sparse distribution of the A or B antigens on the red cell membrane decreases the rate of hemolysis. As a result, the anemia and hyperbilirubinemia are not usually present right at birth but develop in the first day of life. This disorder is fairly common, although the 3% of pregnancies in which it occurs is still only a small fraction of ABO-incompatible pregnancies. Unlike Rh disease, the severity often fluctuates in pregnancies subsequent to the initial sensitization and does not increase progressively.

Hemolytic disease can theoretically occur when there is an incompatibility of any one of the numerous other blood group antigens, although most of them are weakly antigenic. The majority of these uncommon cases involve the Kell, c, or E antigens, but antibodies against Dombrock, Duffy, Kidd, Lutheran, M, S, and others are reported in isolated cases. Some of the cases involving so-called minor or atypical antigens can be as severe as Rh disease, particularly those involving Kell sensitization.

Expert Opinion on Management Issues

PREVENTION: SCREENING AND PROPHYLAXIS

Because small fetomaternal hemorrhages are common and not preventable, the one preventive measure for hemolytic disease would be to ensure that the fetal erythrocytes have no antigens to which the mother is sensitized. Preimplantation diagnosis of the Rh genotype was investigated as a means of preventing Rh disease, but it is not currently available. It is possible to perform Rh genotyping accurately on fetal cells obtained by amniocentesis or chorionic villus sampling, with nearly 100% sensitivity and specificity, but this generally offers little advantage over other screening methods. In standard practice, the American College of Obstetrics and Gynecology and the American Academy of Pediatrics (AAP) agree that all pregnant women should be tested for both ABO and RhD blood types during gestation, and their serum should be screened for the presence of unusual isoimmune antibodies. This testing identifies the women at risk for possible RhD sensitization, so they may receive prophylactic treatment during gestation with concentrated anti-D immunoglobulin G (RhoGAM). It also identifies those fetuses already at risk for hemolytic disease. These fetuses can then be monitored closely during gestation for signs of anemia or developing hydrops fetalis. It also identifies those mother–infant pairs in whom ABO incompatibility may develop, so they may be assessed more carefully in the newborn period and appropriate therapy started.

MANAGEMENT OF FETAL HEMOLYTIC DISEASE

If Rh sensitization is identified during gestation, the maternal anti-D titer should be measured and followed monthly because rising titers correlate with more severe disease. Although specific quantitative tests are available in research settings, further evaluation of pregnancies in which the anti-D titer is rising is typically done by amniocentesis. The sampled amniotic fluid is tested for optical density at 450 nm (OD_{450}), which measures the bilirubin concentration. Disease severity is estimated by plotting OD_{450} at different gestational ages. Based on the initial work of Liley, such a plot can be divided into zones that reflect disease severity and the risk of the infant's needing an exchange transfusion. Measurements in the lowest zone should be repeated in 2 to 4 weeks, whereas those in the upper zones or crossing zones are an indication for fetal blood sampling or transfusion. These measurements are similarly useful for monitoring the in utero progress of the other causes of hemolytic disease.

When screening reveals isoimmune antibodies of any type, the fetus should also be monitored by ultrasonographic examination. These examinations demonstrate any signs of developing hydrops, and Doppler flow measurements of the velocity of blood in the middle cerebral artery can be performed. These noninvasive measurements are highly sensitive for identifying moderate to severe anemia and have a low false-positive rate.

If severe anemia is detected or the fetus is already developing hydrops fetalis, a decision must be made electively either to deliver the fetus or to treat in utero by transfusion. If the gestational age is close to term, the infant can usually be more effectively treated in a neonatal intensive care unit. The same is true at earlier gestational ages when the mother has already received antenatal corticosteroids. If the gestational age is very premature, especially if moderate or severe hydrops is present, the safer course is often to attempt in utero treatment because survival ex utero may be impossible.

The first therapy is to treat severe anemia (hematocrit less than 30%) by in utero transfusion. The older technique of intraperitoneal transfusion is still used in some cases, but access to the umbilical vein can usually be established using techniques similar to those used in amniocentesis. The fetal blood is then sampled to measure the hematocrit, and a direct transfusion of O negative blood is completed, with a target final hematocrit of 40% to 45%. Repeat monitoring should be done at an interval appropriate to the severity of disease, and repeat transfusions can be given as needed. These transfusions not only correct the anemia, but they also slow the disease progression by blunting the accelerated erythropoiesis that produces new erythrocytes susceptible to immune-mediated destruction.

SCREENING AND TREATMENT OF THE NEWBORN

When a mother's blood type is RhD negative, the infant's blood type should be determined in cord blood, and the unsensitized mother should be given additional RhoGAM to prevent sensitization. The dose should be determined by estimating the amount of fetal blood in the maternal circulation using a Kleihauer-Betke test. In cases of known sensitization against RhD or any other antigen, the infant should be evaluated soon after birth, and the complications of hydrops or respiratory compromise corrected if present. A sample of cord blood should be obtained for the measurement of bilirubin level, and a hematocrit, reticulocyte count, and direct antiglobulin test (Coombs) should be done soon after birth. If the cord bilirubin level is greater than 3 to 4 mg/dL, phototherapy should be started right away. In this instance, or if the laboratory tests confirm significant hemolysis, immunoglobulin therapy should also be given. Repeat bilirubin levels and hematocrit measurements should be done at an interval determined by the level and rate of rise.

In the absence of identified maternal antibodies, it is not helpful to screen infants born to mothers with blood type O, but these infants should be monitored more closely than others for the development of clinical jaundice. If hemolytic disease is suspected, the hematocrit and reticulocyte count should be measured. Even if there is no suspicion of early jaundice, the bilirubin level should be measured before discharge as part of a universal screening program.

PHOTOTHERAPY

The risk of bilirubin-induced neurologic injury is increased when the bilirubin level is high. Although levels up to 20 to 25 mg/dL may be safe for a perfectly healthy term infant, the presence of hemolysis increases the risk at any level. Phototherapy is the mainstay of treatment for rising serum bilirubin levels. The decision of when to begin phototherapy depends on both the level and the infant's age in hours (Figure 1). The trigger levels for exchange transfusion are discussed later.

Phototherapy is the use of visible light at a wavelength of 460 to 470 nm to illuminate as much of the infant's skin surface as possible. The major photoreaction is a structural isomerization of bilirubin that irreversibly converts it to lumirubin, a water-soluble compound excreted in bile and urine. Three factors determine the effectiveness of this therapy:

1. The wavelength of the light needs to be close to the absorption maximum for bilirubin while eliminating as much ultraviolet and infrared light as possible. Commercial units all do this, and the effectiveness of overhead, spotlight, and blanket units are roughly equivalent.
2. Effectiveness is proportional to light intensity, and hemolytic disease frequently requires two or more devices to illuminate the infant.
3. Effectiveness is also proportional to the surface area of irradiated skin, so this should be maximized while ensuring thermal stability. Unless the hemolysis is very brisk, intensive phototherapy (defined as irradiance of $30\,\mu W/cm^2$ illuminating the maximum surface area) should result in a decrease in serum bilirubin in the first 24

hours. When used to treat significant hemolytic disease, phototherapy should not be interrupted for feedings or visiting.

INTRAVENOUS IMMUNOGLOBULIN THERAPY

Intravenous immune globulin (IVIG) is used in an effort to avoid the need for exchange transfusion. In several small studies, mostly focusing on Rh disease, administration of IVIG along with phototherapy significantly reduced the degree of hemolysis and the need for exchange transfusion, and it shortened the duration of the phototherapy. Many studies used 0.5 to 1.0 g/kg/day for 1 or 2 days, but no one has determined the most effective regimen. In clinical practice, the administration of 1.0 g/kg/day for 2 days (in conjunction with phototherapy) is a reasonable approach. Importantly, this therapy does not eliminate the antibodies, and they continue to cause slow hemolysis for several weeks. As a result, most treated infants develop a late anemia and often require a conventional red cell transfusion. IVIG therapy is not associated with many of the complications of exchange transfusion, but it may not reduce the donor exposure to the infant.

EXCHANGE TRANSFUSION

When phototherapy and IVIG therapy are not effective in blunting the rise in bilirubin levels, exchange transfusion may be required. This procedure is now done infrequently and should only be undertaken in centers with adequate experience, equipment, and personnel to en-sure maximum safety. Figure 1 indicates the bilirubin trigger levels for exchange transfusion. These levels presume that intensive phototherapy and IVIG have already been given. No good recommendations for trigger levels in the first 24 hours after birth exist, but the procedure should probably be done if there is a continued rate of rise in bilirubin level of 0.5 mg/dL/hour or more despite intensive phototherapy and IVIG.

Most often the procedure is performed through a single large umbilical venous line, but it may be done using individual venous and arterial lines. The total volume of blood exchanged should be twice the calculated circulating blood volume of 80 mL/kg, done in aliquots of approximately 4 mL/kg, and the procedure should be completed over approximately 90 to 120 minutes. This method exchanges close to 90% of the infant's blood, which should decrease the bilirubin level drawn immediately after the procedure to approximately 50% of the preprocedure level. Serum bilirubin levels may then increase over 2 to 3 hours to approximately two thirds of the pre-exchange level. If the immediate postexchange level is significantly higher than expected, it indicates severe ongoing hemolysis, and another exchange transfusion should be performed.

Common Pitfalls

When hemolytic disease is suspected or identified, vigilance in monitoring and close communication between caregivers is necessary. In the antenatal period, protocols must be followed to ensure that fetal complications are diagnosed early, so decisions about therapy or timing of delivery can be optimized. Antenatal monitoring provides an assessment of severity and postnatal needs, and the careful communication of this information by the obstetrician to the neonatologist or pediatrician ensures that necessary equipment, personnel, and blood are at hand.

The therapies for hyperbilirubinemia and hemolytic disease are not free of complications. Phototherapy increases insensible water losses, and intravenous therapy or feedings must compensate. It also disrupts parent-infant interactions, often interferes with breast-feeding, and requires careful explanation to anxious parents. Exchange transfusion is usually quite safe, but potential complications can be severe, including air embolism, necrotizing enterocolitis, acidosis, hypoglycemia, sepsis, or, rarely, death.

Communication and Counseling

Early antenatal detection of hemolytic disease is now possible, and therapies can be offered during fetal life that may minimize or eliminate many of the problems seen in the newborn. Hydrops fetalis, probably the most severe sequela of hemolytic disease other than bilirubin-induced neurologic injury, can be treated in utero and dramatically improved. In some cases, the evolution of hyperbilirubinemia and anemia after birth occurs rapidly, and caregivers must monitor these patients

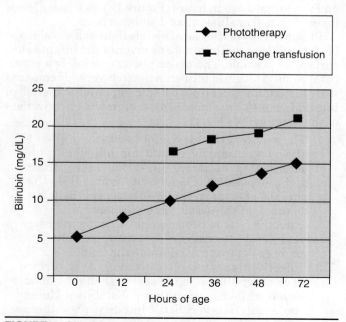

FIGURE 1. Bilirubin levels that should prompt phototherapy and exchange transfusion.

aggressively and begin therapy as early as necessary. This approach most often results in effective treatment and resolution of the disorder. Parents must be as fully informed as possible starting at the time of detection, and obstetric and pediatric caregivers must maintain clear and open communication.

SUGGESTED READINGS

1. Gottstein R, Cooke RW: Systematic review of intravenous immunoglobulin in hemolytic disease of the newborn. Arch Dis Child Fetal Neonatal Ed 88:F6–F10, 2003. **A systematic review of available studies on use of IVIG.**
2. Hsia DYY, Allen FH, Gellis SS, Diamond LK: Erythroblastosis fetalis. VIII: Studies of serum bilirubin in relation to kernicterus. N Engl J Med 247:668–671, 1952. **A hallmark paper with the first description of hemolytic disease and hydrops.**
3. Ip S, Chung M, Kulig J, et al: The American Academy of Pediatrics Subcommittee on Hyperbilirubinemia: An evidence-based review of important issues concerning neonatal hyperbilirubinemia. Pediatrics 114:e130–e153, 2004. **Contains evidence on risks of exchange transfusion.**
4. Palleau S, Le Tourneau C, Jrad I, et al: ABO incompatibility and newborn hemolytic disease: Two cases with major erythroblastosis. Ann Biol Clin (Paris) 62(3):344–348, 2004. **A reminder that ABO disease can be severe.**
5. Subcommittee on Hyperbilirubinemia: Management of hyperbilirubinemia in the newborn infant 35 or more weeks of gestation. Pediatrics 114:297–316, 2004. **Excellent review of hyperbilirubinemia, its screening, and therapy, which sets the current standard.**
6. Van den Veyver IB, Chong SS, Cota J, et al: Single-cell analysis of the RhD blood type for use in preimplantation diagnosis in the prevention of severe hemolytic disease of the newborn. Am J Obstet Gynecol 172:533–540, 1995. **Research on preimplantation diagnosis of the Rh genotype.**
7. Westhoff CM: The Rh blood group system in review: A new face for the next decade. Transfusion 44:1663–1673, 2004. **A complete discussion and description of the blood groups most associated with hemolytic disease of the newborn.**
8. Westhoff CM, Reid ME: Review: The Kell, Duffy, and Kidd blood group systems. Immunohematol 20(1):37–49, 2004. **A complete description of these minor blood groups.**

Apnea of Prematurity

Terry M. Baird, Michael D. Reed, and Richard J. Martin

KEY CONCEPTS

- Apnea of prematurity is almost universal in very preterm infants, although specific etiologies, notably sepsis, must be considered.
- Standard (impedance) respiratory monitoring fails to identify apnea prolonged by obstructed inspiratory efforts.
- Spontaneous episodes of bradycardia and desaturation are almost always the result of apnea or hypoventilation.
- Resolution of apnea in preterm infants is typically complete by 43 to 44 weeks' postconceptional age.

Apnea is a common disorder of prematurity that reflects immature development of respiratory control in these infants. The incidence of apnea increases with lower birth weight and younger gestational age. Almost all infants weighing less than 1000 g exhibit apneic episodes during the early postnatal period. The onset typically occurs during the first week of life or after termination of assisted ventilation. Thereafter, the frequency and duration of apnea decrease as postconceptional age approaches term. Nonetheless, infants with extremely low birth weight may exhibit persistent apnea beyond 40 weeks' postconceptional age, typically with resolution by 44 weeks. It is unclear whether persistence of neonatal apnea is a marker of impaired neurodevelopmental outcome in some high-risk preterm infants.

Physiologic studies of neonatal respiratory control demonstrate decreased ventilatory responses to hypercapnia, hypoxia-induced respiratory depression, and strong respiratory inhibition elicited from laryngeal afferents, all of which may contribute to apnea of prematurity. These phenomena are associated with a greater influence of inhibitory neurotransmitter-mediated pathways during early development. Infants who exhibit apnea of more than 20 seconds' duration or shorter apnea accompanied by bradycardia or oxygen desaturation to less than 80% may require medical intervention. Many of these infants have bradycardia thought to be a result of obstructed or ineffective inspiratory effort. This is a consequence of the upper airway (pharyngeal, laryngeal) closure that accompanies many spontaneous apneas. The respiratory component of these events can be missed because current monitoring technology may fail to trigger an apnea alarm in this setting. An infant can be presumed to have idiopathic apnea of prematurity once other precipitating causes of apnea, including infection, intracranial pathology, metabolic disorders such as hypoglycemia, or impaired oxygen delivery (secondary to hypoxemia or anemia), are ruled out.

Expert Opinion on Management Issues

The pharmacologic agents most widely used for the treatment of apnea of prematurity are the methylxanthines theophylline and caffeine (Table 1). Both agents are very effective and widely used now for nearly 30 years. Caffeine is available in oral and intravenous preparations with doses expressed here as caffeine citrate. A loading dose of 20 mg per kg caffeine is followed by 5 mg per kg caffeine once daily to achieve serum concentrations in

TABLE 1 Methylxanthines for Apnea of Prematurity

Drug	Loading Dose (mg/kg)	Maintenance Dose (mg/kg)
Caffeine (citrate)	20	5
Theophylline	5–6	1–2

the range of 5 to 20 μg per mL, although serum levels are not monitored routinely. For infants who have received theophylline therapy within the past 2 to 3 days, the caffeine-loading dose should be decreased by 25% to 50%, depending on the amount and duration of the previous theophylline therapy. Theophylline is administered as an initial loading dose of 5 to 6 mg per kg, followed by a maintenance dose of 1 to 2 mg per kg every 12 hours. When intravenous administration is needed and intravenous theophylline is not available, aminophylline (theophylline ethylenediamine, 79% theophylline by weight) may be given at doses that are 20% higher.

Serum concentrations of theophylline should be monitored whenever aminophylline or theophylline is used because disposition and the resultant serum concentrations are highly variable. The initial therapeutic theophylline plasma concentration range is 5 to 10 μg per mL. In the absence of achieving desired clinical benefits, higher theophylline plasma concentrations may be necessary for maximal response. In such infants, theophylline dose escalation to achieve plasma theophylline concentrations as high as 15 to 20 μg per mL may be targeted with close patient monitoring for drug-related side effects. The therapeutic effect of theophylline may include the contribution of its caffeine metabolite, which is commonly found in serum at approximately 30% of the concomitant theophylline concentration. For both agents the most commonly observed toxic effects are tachycardia, feeding intolerance, and hyperexcitability. No serious long-term sequelae are reported, although this remains under study.

Presumably, the methylxanthines stimulate central neural output to the respiratory muscles, probably via antagonism of adenosine receptors; however, the precise site of action and modulation of neurotransmitter interactions is not determined. Clinical guidelines for xanthine therapy are not clearly defined and include prophylactic use to decrease need for intubation or ensure successful extubation. Xanthine therapy should be discontinued when clinically significant apnea appears resolved, ideally well prior to discharge. The infant should then be monitored closely for 5 to 7 days to ensure that apneic episodes do not recur. Doxapram, another respiratory stimulant, is proposed for infants in whom xanthines are ineffective but it has not gained broad acceptance. Although reflux of gastric contents to the larynx induces reflex apnea, no clear evidence indicates that treatment of reflux affects the frequency of apnea in most preterm infants.

As an alternative to xanthine therapy, continuous positive airway pressure (CPAP) delivered by nasal prongs at a pressure of 2 to 5 cm H_2O is a safe and effective way to treat apnea of prematurity. CPAP is thought to decrease the frequency of apnea by splinting the upper airway with positive pressure in addition to stabilizing functional residual capacity and oxygenation. Therefore, CPAP may be most effective in infants whose apneic episodes are precipitated or prolonged by pharyngeal obstruction. When prolonged apnea persists in spite of these therapeutic efforts, endotracheal intubation and artificial ventilation should be initiated at minimal ventilator settings to allow for spontaneous ventilatory effort and minimize the risk of barotrauma.

Common Pitfalls

- The use of supplemental oxygen for treatment of episodic desaturation in preterm infants with baseline normoxemia cannot be recommended.
- Pharmacologic management of gastroesophageal reflux is unlikely to affect apnea in preterm infants.
- Home monitoring of cardiorespiratory events in former preterm infants is not a practical means of preventing sudden infant death syndrome (SIDS).

Communication and Counseling

Parents need to be educated that apnea, with accompanying bradycardia and desaturation, although alarming to observe, is a sign of immature respiratory control that resolves spontaneously. Although SIDS is more common in former preterm infants, no evidence indicates that apnea of prematurity is a precursor of SIDS. The prone position should be avoided after discharge to minimize the risk of SIDS.

SUGGESTED READINGS

1. Barrington KJ, Finer N, Dejuan L: Predischarge respiratory recordings in very low birth weight infants. J Pediatr 129:934–940, 1996. **Describes apnea events in preterm infants prior to discharge, resolution of events, and their relationship to apparent life-threatening events (ALTEs).**
2. Brouillette RT, Morrow AS, Weese-Mayer DE, et al: Comparison of respiratory inductive plethysmography and thoracic impedance for apnea monitoring. J Pediatr 111:377–383, 1987. **A comparison of apnea detection by device.**
3. Di Fiore JM, Arko MK, Miller MJ, et al: Cardiorespiratory events in preterm infants referred for apnea monitoring studies. Pediatrics 108:1304–1308, 2001. **Indicates the relationship between breathing pauses, bradycardia, and oxygen desaturation.**
4. Eichenwald EC, Aina A, Stark AR: Apnea frequently persists beyond term gestation in infant delivered at 24 to 28 weeks. Pediatrics 100:354–359, 1997. **A description of apnea resolution in the most premature infants.**
5. Kimball AL, Carlton DP: Gastroesophageal reflux medications in the treatment of apnea in premature infants. J Pediatr 138:355–360, 2001. **Indicates that treatment for gastroesophageal (GE) reflux may not affect the occurrence of apnea episodes.**
6. Miller MJ, Martin RJ: Pathophysiology of apnea of prematurity. In Polin RA, Fox WW, Abman SH (eds): Fetal Neonatal Physiology, 3rd ed. Philadelphia: WB Saunders, 2004, pp 905–918. **A general discussion of the pathophysiology of apnea.**
7. Ramanathan R, Corwin MJ, Hunt CE, et al: Cardiorespiratory events recorded on home monitors: Comparison of healthy infants with those at increased risk for SIDS. JAMA 285:2199–2207, 2001. **The largest study to date of recorded events in the home; addresses the issue of resolution of apnea.**
8. Steer PA, Henderson-Smart DJ: Caffeine versus theophylline for apnea in preterm infants. Cochrane Database Syst Rev 2: CD000273, 2000. **A thorough review comparing the methylxanthines.**
9. Taylor HG, Klein N, Schatschneider C, et al: Predictors of early school age outcomes in very low birth weight children. J Dev Behav Pediatr 19:235–243, 1998. **One of a limited number of studies assessing the possible effect of apnea on long-term neurodevelopmental outcome.**

Neonatal Intestinal Obstruction

William Middlesworth and Angela Kadenhe-Chiweshe

KEY CONCEPTS

- The clinical presentation of intestinal obstruction depends on the degree and the location of the obstruction.
- When intestinal obstruction is complicated by intestinal ischemia, the diagnosis must be established and treated urgently. Bilious emesis is malrotation with midgut volvulus until proven otherwise.
- Protection of the lungs from soilage by gastric secretions is a top priority in the initial management of esophageal atresia and tracheoesophageal fistula.
- Operative correction of pyloric stenosis is not an emergency. Patients should be well hydrated and have normal electrolytes before they are taken to surgery.
- Of babies with congenital duodenal obstruction, one third have Down syndrome and one third have congenital heart disease. Each affects outcome adversely.
- Contrast enema is extremely useful in distinguishing jejunoileal atresia from meconium ileus and Hirschsprung disease. It is also of therapeutic benefit in meconium ileus and meconium plug syndrome.
- Enterocolitis is the most common cause of death in children with Hirschsprung disease. It should be treated aggressively with rectal irrigation and antibiotics. Colostomy is indicated in severe cases.

The causes of intestinal obstruction in the newborn are as varied as the clinical presentation. One of the most common surgical problems encountered in the newborn period, obstruction of the gastrointestinal (GI) tract, may occur at any point throughout its course from esophagus to anorectum. Surgical intervention, either emergently or urgently rendered, almost always serves as definitive therapy. The clinician must therefore be knowledgeable about the etiologies, diagnoses, and therapies for intestinal obstruction and ensure that treatment is instituted in a timely way and not delayed. The morbidity and mortality associated with intestinal obstruction is directly related to timing of diagnosis and intervention, especially when there is vascular as well as luminal occlusion.

It is useful to stratify intestinal obstruction with respect to location, etiology, and degree: proximal versus distal, mechanical versus functional, and partial versus complete. Proximal bowel obstruction does not cause abdominal distention to the degree that distal obstruction does, however vomiting occurs earlier and turns bilious sooner with proximal small bowel obstruction. The failure of relaxation of the bowel characteristic of Hirschsprung disease is an example of a functional cause of obstruction. Duodenal atresia and duodenal web are variants of the same process and demonstrate the difference between complete and partial obstruction.

Prenatal consultation with a pediatric surgeon is important whenever intestinal obstruction is suspected. The surgeon should be an active participant in the initial management of infants with suspected intestinal obstruction because timely surgical intervention is most often required.

Expert Opinion on Management Issues

PRENATAL DIAGNOSIS

Antenatal features of intestinal obstruction vary in specificity. The sonographic double-bubble sign is highly specific for duodenal obstruction (duodenal atresia or web); however, the finding of echogenic bowel may exist absent any ultimate abnormality or may be associated with meconium ileus, intestinal atresia, or chromosomal abnormalities. Polyhydramnios is generally present when there is proximal intestinal obstruction (duodenal or jejunal atresia) but is frequently absent when the obstruction is more distal (anorectal malformation). The presence of a dilated upper esophagus and a small stomach raise suspicion for esophageal atresia, although the sensitivity of sonography is less than 50%. Fetal MRI offers improved detection of the varied forms of intestinal obstruction.

ESOPHAGEAL ATRESIA/ TRACHEOESOPHAGEAL FISTULA

The live-birth incidence of esophageal atresia (EA) is 1:4500 in the United States. The majority of affected infants have an associated tracheoesophageal fistula (TEF). Some studies show a male preponderance, and an associated major anomaly exists more than half the time. Although many variants of EA/TEF are described, three variants comprise more than 95% of cases: atresia with distal fistula (85%); isolated atresia (atresia without fistula, 6%); and isolated fistula (H- or N-type fistula, 6%). Symptoms of EA with TEF are apparent in the immediate postnatal period and include excessive drooling and intolerance of the first feed. Inability to pass a nasogastric (NG) tube beyond the upper esophagus is diagnostic. A plain film of the chest and abdomen shows the NG tube in the dilated proximal esophageal pouch. Presence of air in the GI tract confirms the presence of a TEF; a gasless abdomen establishes the diagnosis of isolated EA.

Initial management of EA with TEF includes continuous aspiration of salivary secretions from the proximal esophageal pouch and elevation of the infant's head and chest. These interventions reduce aspiration risk. Intravenous fluids are provided and supplemental oxygen is administered as required. Positive-pressure ventilation is avoided where possible because it may result in gastric distention with elevation of the diaphragm or even gastric rupture. In addition to chest and abdominal radiographs, renal ultrasound and echocardiogram are performed to determine whether renal or cardiac anomalies exist. The priorities of operative intervention are closure of the fistula and establishment of esophageal continuity. Correction of coexistent congenital heart disease may take priority over esophageal repair. A long gap between the upper and lower esophagus (seen commonly in isolated atresia) may make primary repair impossible. In this case a gastrostomy is performed to administer enteral nutrition, allow for growth of the distal esophagus, and achieve primary repair at a later date. Although both isolated atresia and atresia with distal TEF are repaired by thoracotomy, isolated fistula is approached through a cervical incision.

PYLORIC STENOSIS

Infantile hypertrophic pyloric stenosis is the most common cause of gastric outlet obstruction and the most common condition requiring surgery in the neonatal period. The incidence is 1:400 with a male preponderance of 4:1. Presentation of this disease is at 2 to 6 weeks of age. The cause of the hypertrophy of the circular fibers of the pylorus is not known, although abnormalities in the innervation of the pylorus and local deficiency of nitric oxide synthase are implicated.

The hallmark symptom is progressive nonbilious projectile vomiting after feeding. When diagnosis is delayed, patients can show significant dehydration, weight loss, and characteristic electrolyte abnormalities (hypokalemia, hypochloremia, metabolic alkalosis). Visible gastric peristalsis and a palpable upper abdominal mass are important physical findings. Abdominal ultrasound, the diagnostic study of choice, shows an elongated thickened pylorus and a fluid-filled stomach. Pyloromyotomy, the definitive treatment for pyloric stenosis, is performed only after correction of electrolyte abnormalities and restoration of intravascular volume are demonstrated by adequate urine output. Isotonic crystalloid fluid boluses are generally used for the initial resuscitation and followed by intravenous fluid at 1.5 times the maintenance rate. Whether by laparoscopic or open approach (typically a curved supraumbilical incision), the serosa of the pylorus is incised longitudinally and the incision is bluntly carried down to, but not through, the mucosa. As the muscle layer is gently spread, the mucosa herniates into the myotomy, restoring the lumen. Postoperatively, feeding is resumed with clear liquids and advanced in an incremental fashion to full-strength formula or breast milk.

CONGENITAL DUODENAL OBSTRUCTION

Duodenal atresia, stenosis, or web has an incidence of 1 in 5000 to 10,000 live births, accounting for half of all small bowel atresias. This intrinsic duodenal obstruction occurs early in gestation and is thought to result from a failure of the initially solid alimentary cord to canalize in the fifth to tenth week of gestation. This error of organogenesis occurs at or below the ampulla of Vater in the preponderance of cases, and it may be associated with annular pancreas. Prenatal diagnosis is common. Both prenatal sonogram and postnatal plain films show the characteristic double-bubble sign caused by dilation of the stomach and proximal duodenum. In cases of incomplete obstruction, air may be seen distally in the GI tract, although it is absent in duodenal atresia. Associated anomalies are frequent, with trisomy 21 and congenital heart disease each occurring in a third of cases. The typical clinical presentation is bilious vomiting in the first day of life. Gastric decompression usually yields a large volume of bile-stained fluid; nonbilious aspirate in this setting indicates obstruction proximal to the ampulla of Vater. It is important to differentiate duodenal atresia from malrotation with midgut volvulus, a more urgent problem. Upper GI contrast studies may be helpful in this regard.

The management of duodenal atresia begins with resuscitative measures (GI decompression and intravenous hydration) and a search for coexistent anomalies. Perioperative antibiotics are administered and surgical correction is achieved by duodenoduodenostomy. Care is taken to avoid injury to the ampulla of Vater. Anomalous drainage of the pancreatic and bile ducts into a duodenal web may occur. Postoperatively, gastric decompression is maintained. Duodenal dysmotility may delay institution of oral feeding. Placement of a transanastomotic feeding tube at the time of duodenoduodenostomy may eliminate the need for parenteral nutrition and allow enteral feeding while duodenal peristaltic function improves. Decreasing drainage from the NG tube indicates return of duodenal function. Oral feeds may then be started and gradually increased.

Most patients fare very well from their operation. It is the associated congenital anomalies and prematurity that influence overall morbidity and mortality. In addition to congenital cardiac disease and trisomy 21, anorectal malformations and EA/TEF may coexist and affect outcome adversely. A delay in operative intervention to allow for growth or correction of heart disease is sometimes appropriate.

MALROTATION AND MIDGUT VOLVULUS

Between the fifth and twelfth week of gestation, the human fetus undergoes the normal process of bowel herniation: a 270-degree rotation around the superior mesenteric artery axis, reduction of bowel back into the abdomen, and retroperitoneal fixation. Aberrancy in this process is referred to as *malrotation*. A consequence of malrotation is a narrow mesentery with unfixed bowel, resulting in an elevated risk of midgut volvulus (twisting of the bowel about its mesentery with resultant vascular compromise). This causes obstruction at the level of the duodenum. The risk of midgut volvulus is highest in the newborn period, with approximately 80% of all cases manifesting in the first month of life. Volvulus is a life-threatening condition because the progressive bowel ischemia can lead rapidly to circulatory collapse and death.

The ominous presenting symptom of malrotation with midgut volvulus is bilious emesis. All patients who present with bilious emesis must be evaluated expeditiously with an upper GI series for malrotation. Rightward displacement of the duodenojejunal junction is evidence of malrotation. Duodenal obstruction implies volvulus. Bilious vomiting caused by malrotation (with or without midgut volvulus) is a surgical emergency. Any patient with bilious emesis who presents with signs of bowel compromise—blood per rectum, peritonitis, abdominal wall discoloration, homodynamic instability, acidosis, or thrombocytopenia—should bypass any diagnostic studies and undergo emergency laparotomy.

Upon entering the abdomen, the bowel is detorsed until the mesentery is clearly no longer twisted. The bowel is allowed to recover from the vascular compromise and then is carefully inspected. When the entire bowel is viable, the mesenteric root is broadened, the duodenum is mobilized, filmy peritoneal attachments of the right colon that cross the duodenum are lysed, and appendectomy is performed. The bowel is placed in the abdomen in a "nonrotated" state with the small bowel on the right and the colon on the left. An important operative principle is that a bowel of questionable viability is not resected but rather is reexamined in 24 hours at a second-look operation. This is done to mitigate intestinal loss and reduce the likelihood of intestinal failure. All frankly necrotic bowel is resected. Such decision making depends on the extent of bowel loss, the condition of the remaining bowel, and the condition of the patient.

Postoperatively, bowel function may take up to a week to return, during which time parenteral nutrition should be employed. In unfortunate cases in which patients have undergone massive bowel loss, a lifelong dependency on parenteral nutrition ensues, and such patients should be referred for possible small intestinal transplantation. The potentially devastating consequences to an infant that can result from a delay in surgical treatment underscore the emergent nature of this problem. Intestinal ischemia can be deceptive: An outwardly well-appearing infant may harbor severely compromised bowel.

JEJUNOILEAL ATRESIA

With an incidence of 1 in 1000 to 1 in 5000 live births, jejunoileal atresia is a congenital interruption in the continuity of the small bowel. Although several theories regarding its etiology are proposed, the most widely accepted one holds that in utero injury to mesenteric vasculature causes the atresia (unlike duodenal atresia; see earlier). The atresia may be single or multiple and can occur anywhere along the length of the small intestine. Colonic atresia is rare. A classification was developed based on both the anatomy of the atretic bowel and the associated mesenteric defect. Of note is the so-called apple peel atresia with its precarious blood supply. In this type there is a proximal atresia and a deficient superior mesenteric artery. The bowel distal to the atresia is supplied by a marginal branch of the ileocolic or right colic artery, around which it spirals in a corkscrew fashion. Although associated congenital abnormalities are rare, intestinal atresia is seen with gastroschisis. Prematurity, intrauterine growth restriction, and rotational abnormalities are seen with an increased frequency in apple peel atresia.

Dilated bowel and polyhydramnios on prenatal sonogram should raise the suspicion of jejunoileal atresia. Bilious emesis along with significant abdominal distention is a classic presentation. Plain films may show the dilated bowel and air-fluid levels indicative of obstruction. Gastric decompression is an essential component in initial management as is intravenous fluid resuscitation. Water-soluble contrast enema is very valuable in differentiating atresia from both meconium ileus and Hirschsprung disease because the clinical presentation may be similar.

Once the diagnosis is established, laparotomy is performed to establish intestinal continuity. It is sometimes necessary to resect or taper a segment of massively dilated bowel or to perform multiple anastomoses to salvage as much viable bowel as possible when adequacy of bowel length is uncertain. Patients with jejunoileal atresia and sufficient bowel have an excellent prognosis. Intestinal failure caused by the short bowel syndrome, with its attendant risk of recurrent infection and hepatic failure, is the most significant cause of morbidity and mortality.

MECONIUM DISEASE OF INFANCY

Meconium ileus results from the inspissation of thick, sticky meconium in the distal small bowel. It is a manifestation of cystic fibrosis, an autosomal recessive disease that affects the secretory functions of pulmonary and GI organs. The clinical presentation is that of distal small bowel obstruction: abdominal distention, vomiting, and failure to pass meconium. Meconium ileus may be complicated by distention and necrosis, volvulus of the distal ileum, and perforation. Perforation may be pre- or postnatal. Prenatal perforation is termed *complicated meconium ileus* or *meconium peritonitis*. Meconium ileus has characteristic findings on plain films: a soap bubble or ground-glass appearance of the bowel that represents the inspissated meconium infiltrated with bowel gas. In cases of complicated meconium ileus, extraluminal calcifications can be seen on radiograph. Contrast enemas are both diagnostic and therapeutic because the hyperosmolar contrast agent causes intraluminal fluid shifts, loosening the meconium and evacuating intestinal contents. In complicated meconium ileus where intrauterine perforation has occurred, contrast enema therapy is inadvisable. The approach to such cases is operative and entails exploratory laparotomy and, in some cases, creation of an ileostomy. The outcome of such interventions is good, but these infants must still contend with the long-term pulmonary and GI complications of cystic fibrosis: pneumonia, malabsorption, intestinal dysmotility, and constipation.

Meconium plug syndrome is an obstruction of the distal colon or rectum by a large meconium plug. It is seen in premature infants, those exposed to magnesium, and infants of diabetic mothers. These conditions lead to colonic dysmotility and ileus in an otherwise histologically and functionally normal colon and rectum. A contrast enema is useful to dislodge and help evacuate the meconium plug. The study may demonstrate a small colon distal to the obstructing meconium. This gave rise to the term *small left colon syndrome*. Because meconium plug syndrome is sometimes seen in association with Hirschsprung disease or cystic fibrosis, rectal biopsy and sweat test may be indicated.

HIRSCHSPRUNG DISEASE

Hirschsprung disease (HD) occurs in approximately 1 in 5000 live births and is more common in boys than in girls. It results from the congenital absence of ganglion cells in the distal bowel. This abnormally innervated portion of the colon loses its ability to relax and thus causes obstruction. The bowel proximal to this segment becomes dilated and hypertrophic. The extent of aganglionosis is variable. In 75% of cases, the aganglionic segment extends from the anus to the distal sigmoid colon. The affected segment may extend more proximally, however, to the ileum (total colonic Hirschsprung) or even to the duodenum (total intestinal aganglionosis). Total intestinal aganglionosis is rare, and long-term survival is unusual in this variant.

The majority of cases of HD manifest in term infants in the neonatal period. Delayed passage of meconium until after 24 hours of life is the hallmark sign, accompanied by abdominal distention and vomiting. Initial management must include gastric decompression and intravenous fluid hydration. Patients with HD show a bowel gas pattern on plain film consistent with distal obstruction. A contrast enema is useful in establishing the diagnosis of HD and often shows a transition zone between proximal dilated, normally innervated bowel and distal normal-caliber aganglionic bowel. Although localization of the transition zone is important in planning surgical intervention, rectal biopsy is the gold standard

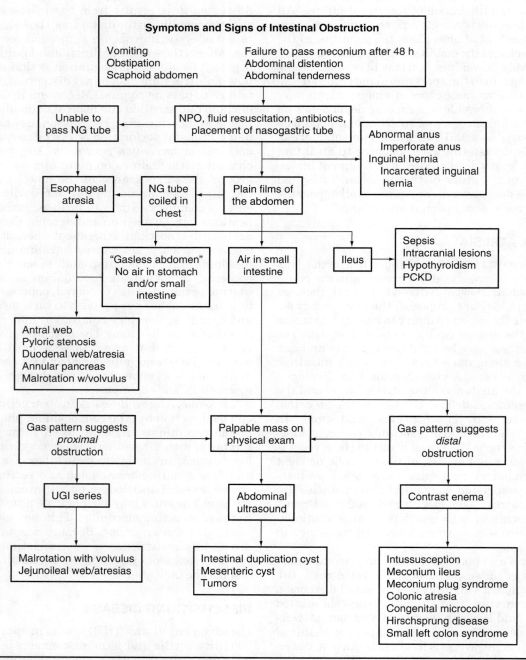

FIGURE 1. Algorithm for management of neonatal intestinal obstruction. NG, nasogastric; NPO, nothing by mouth; PCKD, polycystic kidney disease; UGI, upper gastrointestinal.

confirmatory diagnostic test. A bedside suction biopsy performed at least 2 cm above the dentate line usually yields sufficient tissue to make the diagnosis. Absence of ganglion cells and hypertrophy of nerve fibers in the submucosal and myenteric plexus provide histologic confirmation of the diagnosis of HD.

Surgical therapy for HD has evolved significantly over the past 30 years. Patients were treated historically with a "leveling colostomy" just proximal to the transition zone. Definitive surgery to bring normally innervated colon to the anus was done at a later stage. Currently, when the bowel can be adequately decompressed with enemas, and absent enterocolitis or severe colonic dilation, a single-stage pull-through in the newborn period is often performed. The most significant threat to the health of the patient with HD is enterocolitis. Bacterial overgrowth and bacterial translocation are believed to be part of the pathogenesis, caused by the functional obstruction. Enterocolitis can have a fulminant course, and prompt treatment with rectal irrigation and parenteral antibiotics must be instituted when the diagnosis is suspected. It may occur before or after definitive surgery and is the most common cause of death in affected children. Figure 1 illustrates a logical approach to the workup of intestinal obstruction.

Common Pitfalls

- Positive-pressure ventilation should be avoided preoperatively, when possible, in infants with EA/TEF because gastric distention can result in regurgitation of gastric secretions through the fistula into the lungs or gastric rupture may result.
- The diagnosis of pyloric stenosis is sometimes delayed in a hospitalized patient with a distracting other problem. Forceful nonbilious vomiting at 2 to 6 weeks of age should prompt an abdominal ultrasound.
- The apple peel atresia has a worse prognosis than the other types of jejunoileal atresia with a higher incidence of complications and short bowel syndrome.
- Meconium ileus may be uncomplicated and treated successfully with contrast enema, or it may be complicated by segmental volvulus or perforation. Laparotomy, not contrast enema, is indicated in the setting of perforation.
- Cystic fibrosis and Hirschsprung disease must be suspected in infants with meconium plug.
- Children with both Hirschsprung disease and Down syndrome are especially susceptible to enterocolitis, and they are at increased risk of overwhelming sepsis.

Communication and Counseling

Most causes of intestinal obstruction are amenable to surgical correction if diagnosed promptly. Referral to a pediatric surgeon when there is a prenatal diagnosis of suspected intestinal obstruction allows for a calm discussion of interventions that may occur in the peripartum period. In addition, when the surgeon meets the parents in advance of the delivery, he or she can provide the reassurance of a familiar face in the emotionally charged atmosphere of the delivery room.

Effective communication among obstetricians, neonatologists, and surgeons, of course, is the cornerstone of timely and effective care, and its importance cannot be overstated. Primary caregivers must be well versed in the presenting symptoms of intestinal obstruction and should promptly investigate the etiology with their surgical colleagues. An awareness of those conditions that must be handled with urgency (malrotation, enterocolitis) is essential.

SUGGESTED READINGS

1. Aschcraft KW, Holcomb GW III, Murphy JP: Pediatric Surgery, 4th ed. Philadelphia: Elsevier, 2005. **Succinct, easy-to-read standard text.**
2. Bianchi DW, Crombleholme TM, D'Alton ME: Fetology: Diagnosis Management of the Fetal Patient. New York: McGraw-Hill, 2000. **Comprehensive and detailed text that catalogs virtually all prenatally diagnosed abnormalities; thoroughly referenced and well illustrated.**
3. Hajivassiliou CA: Intestinal obstruction in neonatal/pediatric surgery. Semin Pediatr Surg 12(4):241–253, 2003. **Discusses both common and unusual causes of large and small bowel obstruction, emphasizing the importance of early and expeditious diagnosis and treatment.**
4. Kays DW: Surgical conditions of the neonatal intestinal tract. Clin Perinatol 23(2):353–371, 1996. **Discusses the management of obstructive and nonobstructive surgical diseases of the alimentary tract.**
5. Oldham KT, Colombani PM, Foglia RP, et al: Principles and Practice of Pediatric Surgery. Philadelphia: Lippincott Williams & Wilkins, 2005. **Concise and thorough text that highlights key concepts in the management of surgical disorders of infants and children. Some chapters include a brief historical perspective of the topic under consideration.**

Necrotizing Enterocolitis

Rachel E. Brown and Josef Neu

KEY CONCEPTS

- Necrotizing enterocolitis (NEC) is a disease predominantly of premature infants.
- Infants may present with a variety of signs and symptoms, so monitoring for NEC must be vigilant.
- The pathogenesis of NEC is multifactorial. It involves a triggering event in combination with intestinal immaturity, leading to mucosal disruption, introduction of inflammatory mediators, and finally ischemia, necrosis, and potentially perforation. Genetic predisposition is also likely to play a role, but specific loci are not yet delineated.
- Diagnosis of NEC uses the clinical presentation, including the physical examination (abdominal distention, bloody stools, marked increase in gastric residuals), radiologic findings (pneumatosis intestinalis, portal venous

Continued

Necrotizing enterocolitis (NEC) is one of the most enigmatic diseases in neonatology. Although NEC is the most commonly encountered gastrointestinal emergency in neonates, questions remain regarding its etiology, diagnosis, prevention, treatment, and outcome. As survival rates improve in neonates of low and very low birth weight, the incidence of NEC has increased. NEC affects 3% to 5% of patients in the neonatal intensive care unit (NICU), and only 7% to 10% of these cases involve term infants. Approximately 10% to 50% of neonates with NEC die, leading to an estimated 1000 infant deaths per year. In addition, many infants affected with NEC survive with various sequelae, including feeding intolerance, stricture formation, and short bowel syndrome. The fear of NEC is one of the major factors that discourage neonatologists from using enteral feedings to nourish infants early in their hospital course. Delayed enteral feeding is associated with increased risk of sepsis and cholestasis with prolonged parenteral nutrition.

The pathogenesis of NEC is not clearly understood, but it is well accepted as multifactorial. The major factor contributing to NEC is intestinal immaturity. Immature motility patterns lead to stasis and subsequent bacterial overgrowth. Bacteria then overload the physiochemical protective factors of the mucosal lining, which is adapted to interact with a huge antigenic and microbial load when mature but not during early development. After an initial mucosal disruption occurs, bacterial toxins, such as lipopolysaccharide (LPS), possibly incite an inflammatory response with mediators such as platelet-activating factor (PAF), tissue necrosis factor (TNF), endothelin, leukotriene C_4 (LTC$_4$), thromboxane B_2 (TXB$_2$), oxygen radicals, and interleukin–6 (IL-6). The immature intestine appears exquisitely sensitive to propagation of the inflammatory response, which appears to act through the IκB/NFκB transduction pathway. The inflammatory response then triggers ischemia, apoptosis, and further mucosal disruption, leading to pneumatosis (caused by bacterial fermentation by microorganisms that enter the intestinal lining) as well as coagulation necrosis. If allowed to continue, this situation can lead to perforation, peritonitis, and death. Figure 1 illustrates the predisposing factors for NEC.

As already discussed, the primary risk factor for NEC is prematurity coincident with gut immaturity, but other factors, including aggressive enteral feedings and infections, can contribute to the development of NEC. In addition, there is speculation about a genetic predisposition to the development of NEC. It occasionally occurs in infants who have never been fed, but most frequently NEC occurs in premature infants receiving enteral feedings. Extremely premature infants are at risk for

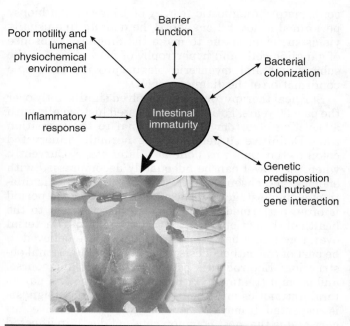

FIGURE 1. Predisposing factors for necrotizing enterocolitis. (From Weiss MD, Williams JL, Ledbetter DJ, et al: Necrotizing enterocolitis. In Polin RA, Yoder MC, Burg FD (eds): Workbook in Practical Neonatology. Philadelphia: WB Saunders, 2001, p 462.)

developing NEC for a protracted period. Their risk for NEC remains high until the postconceptional age of 35 to 36 weeks. The lower gestational age infants (less than 28 weeks) tend to develop NEC later than intermediate gestational age infants or full-term infants. Often these infants encountered minimal problems immediately after birth and were convalescing as "feeders and growers" when they developed NEC. It is unclear why the onset of NEC is later with decreasing gestational age, but it is likely related to intestinal immaturity combined with a changing intestinal microflora and increasing enteral volumes. In addition, if enteral feeds are increased aggressively, the risk for NEC is particularly high. Feedings advanced greater than 20 kcal/kg/day are associated with an increased incidence of NEC. In contrast, studies demonstrate that minimal enteral feedings used to stimulate gastrointestinal (GI) mucosal development are not associated with increased incidence of NEC. Of note, the incidence of NEC is lower in infants fed with breast milk compared to those fed with formula.

Infectious agents are likely to contribute to NEC, but it is unclear whether the presence of these bacteria, commonly found in the intestine, is causative or coincident. Bacteria commonly isolated from infants with NEC include gram-negative rods, most commonly *Klebsiella* species, *Escherichia coli*, *Enterobacter* species, and *Pseudomonas* species. Other microorganisms occasionally associated with NEC are *Clostridium difficile*, *Staphylococcus epidermidis*, coronavirus, and rotavirus. It is possible that overgrowth of commensal microorganisms, in the milieu of an immature mucosa, may provide enough stimuli to trigger this pathogenic cascade.

TABLE 1 Modified Bell's Staging Criteria for Necrotizing Enterocolitis

Stage	Systemic Signs	Intestinal Signs	Radiologic Signs
IA: Suspected NEC	Temperature instability, apnea, bradycardia, lethargy	Increased gastric residuals, mild abdominal distention, emesis, guaiac-positive stool	Normal intestinal dilation, mild ileus
IB: Suspected NEC	Same as above	Bright red rectal blood	Same as above
IIA: Definite NEC; mildly ill	Same as above	Same as above, plus absent bowel sounds, ± abdominal tenderness	Same as above, plus pneumatosis intestinalis
IIB: Definite NEC; moderately ill	Same as above, plus mild metabolic acidosis, mild thrombocytopenia	Same as above, plus definite abdominal tenderness, ± abdominal cellulitis, or right lower quadrant mass	Same as IIA, plus portal venous air, ± ascites
IIIA: Advanced NEC; severely ill; bowel intact	Same as IIB, plus hypotension, bradycardia, severe apnea, combined respiratory and metabolic acidosis, DIC, neutropenia	Same as above, plus signs of peritonitis	Same as IIB, plus definite ascites
IIIB: Advanced NEC; severely ill; bowel perforation	Same as IIIA	Same as IIIA	Same as IIB, plus pneumoperitoneum

DIC, Disseminated intravascular coagulation; NEC, necrotizing enterocolitis.
Adapted from Walsh MC, Kliegman RM: Necrotizing enterocolitis: Treatment based on staging criteria. Pediatr Clin North Am 33:187, 1986.

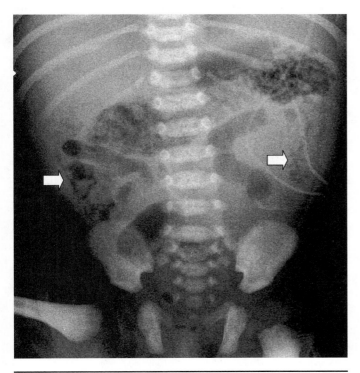

FIGURE 2. Classic findings of necrotizing enterocolitis.

NEC manifests clinically with a myriad of signs and symptoms. These may include increasing oxygen requirement or ventilatory support, increased number of apneas and bradycardias, feeding intolerance, abdominal distention and/or tenderness, occult or frank blood in the stools, sepsis, and shock. These signs and symptoms, together with radiographic findings, form the basis of the modified Bell's staging criteria (Table 1). Initial radiography for NEC is often nonspecific, including dilated bowel loops, bowel wall thickening, and air-fluid levels, but it may also demonstrate a persistently dilated loop. Any fixed, dilated loop should increase suspicion for NEC. Definitive radiographic findings include pneumatosis intestinalis (gas in the bowel wall), portal venous gas, and/or pneumoperitoneum. Figure 2 demonstrates the classic findings of pneumatosis. Serial films, including films taken in the left lateral decubitus position for better evaluation of free air, are necessary if the diagnosis of NEC is suspected.

In an infant with suspected NEC, complete blood counts, metabolic panels, and measurements of lactate can help evaluate the severity of disease. A high or low white blood cell count with a shift toward immature precursors, falling absolute granulocyte count, and thrombocytopenia along with acidosis often indicate increasing severity of NEC.

Because pathologic findings of NEC are obtained through autopsy or through specimens obtained when surgical intervention is necessary, they reflect severe disease. Gross examination reveals predominant involvement of the terminal ileum and proximal colon, but any length of the intestine may be affected. Histologic findings include mucosal edema, hemorrhage, coagulation necrosis, and mucosal ulceration.

Expert Opinion on Management Issues

Therapies for NEC depend on the severity and progression of the disease. Clinical judgment is essential for treatment, but Bell's staging criteria (see Table 1) can be a useful guideline. If there is suspicion of NEC, a rule-out sepsis workup, usually consisting of blood and cerebrospinal fluid (CSF) cultures, antibiotics, bowel decompression, and nothing by mouth (NPO) should be initiated. Close monitoring of the infant's condition dictates the length of antibiotic therapy and NPO and how aggressively the patient is monitored with radiographs and laboratory tests. Initial antimicrobial therapy should include gram-positive and gram-negative coverage. Ampicillin and gentamicin are appropriate choices. If resistant *Staphylococcus epidermidis* is suspected, vancomycin should replace ampicillin. In addition, antimicrobial therapy should be tailored using unit-specific antibiograms. The bowel is decompressed using a large-bore orogastric tube placed to low intermittent suction. If the infant improves or if there is no further progression, reinstitution of enteral feedings at a slightly lower volume than prior to the episode should be considered within 24 to 48 hours.

Once the definitive diagnosis of NEC is established (Bell's stage II or above), the infant should receive a minimum of 7 days of NPO, bowel decompression, and antibiotic therapy. Pediatric surgery should be notified of the infant's diagnosis at this time. Fluids, electrolytes, acid–base status, hematologic parameters, and abdominal exam must be carefully monitored. The infant may have significant third spacing of fluids, resulting in losses of sodium and protein. Potassium and acid–base imbalances may occur, and renal compromise is common. The infant may require intensive respiratory and circulatory support. If acidosis continues with deterioration of platelet and white blood cell counts or if perforation occurs, surgery may be indicated. Surgical options include exploratory laparotomy and/or peritoneal drainage. If perforation occurs or if surgery is necessary, additional antibiotic coverage should include anaerobic coverage with clindamycin or metronidazole. A decision regarding the reinstitution of enteral feedings following stage III (surgical) NEC should be made jointly by the neonatologists and the pediatric surgeons. Feedings will likely be reinstituted at minimal volumes and slowly progressed.

Common Pitfalls

- The presentation of NEC is variable. Subtle signs need to be recognized, but because they are frequently nonspecific, they may lead to measures that are neither preventive nor therapeutic (i.e., prolonged NPO and prolonged antibiotic therapy that may predispose to colonization with resistant microorganisms).
- Some infants, especially of very low birth weight, may develop isolated intestinal perforations, without intestinal necrosis, usually in the first several days of life. Whether these lesions are part of the spectrum of NEC is not known, but they are likely to have a different etiology than the disease that involves actual necrosis.
- Minimal enteral feedings do not increase the risk of NEC. In fact, the lack of enteral feedings is associated with mucosal atrophy, a lack of hormonal output, and prolonged parenteral nutrition with its attendant complications.
- Lack of communication with pediatric surgery may delay surgery and worsen the prognosis for an infant with NEC.

Communication and Counseling

The parents of premature infants must be aware of NEC as a potential cause of morbidity and mortality in their infants. They must be educated about the slow, steady introduction of enteral feedings and the benefits of human breast milk. If their infant develops NEC, parents must be warned of its seriousness. In addition, discussion must involve the potential for surgical intervention and the possible outcomes, including death.

SUGGESTED READINGS

1. Berseth C, Biquera J, Paje V: Prolonged small feeding volumes early in life decreases the incidence of necrotizing enterocolitis in very low birth weight infants. Pediatrics 111:529–534, 2003. **Prospective study comparing minimal versus advancing feeding schedules and incidence of NEC.**
2. Boccia D, Stolfi I, Lana S, et al: Nosocomial necrotizing enterocolitis outbreaks: Epidemiology and control measures. Eur J Pediatr 160:385–391, 2001. **Analysis of previously reported NEC outbreaks and proposed control measures.**
3. Bohnhorst B, Müller S, Dördelmann M, et al: Early feeding after necrotizing enterocolitis in preterm infants. J Pediatr 143:484–487, 2003. **Retrospective study to evaluate recurrence of NEC with early initiation of enteral feedings.**
4. Demestre X, Ginovart G, Figueras-Aloy J, et al: Peritoneal drainage as primary management in necrotizing enterocolitis: A prospective study. J Pediatr Surg 37:1534–1539, 2002. **Prospective study evaluating peritoneal drainage as the first step in treatment of NEC.**
5. Hsueh W, Caplan MS, Qu XW, et al: Neonatal necrotizing enterocolitis: Clinical considerations and pathogenetic concepts. Pediatr Dev Pathol 6:6–23, 2003. **Investigates the contribution of platelet-activating factor (PAF) to the development of necrotizing enterocolitis.**
6. Neu J: Necrotizing enterocolitis: The search for a unifying pathogenic theory leading to prevention. Pediatr Clin North Am 43:409–432, 1996. **A comprehensive review of NEC.**
7. Pierro A, Hall N: Surgical treatment of infants with necrotizing enterocolitis. Semin Neonatol 8:223–232, 2003. **Considers the surgical management options for NEC.**
8. Reber KM, Nankervis CA: Necrotizing enterocolitis: Preventative strategies. Clin Perinatol 31:157–167, 2004. **Examines current and emerging strategies for prevention of NEC.**
9. Safeties D, Squeaky C, Catalos C: Neonatal necrotizing enters colitis: An overview. Curr Opin Pediatr 16:349–355, 2003. **Presents the need for further advances in the treatment of NEC.**

Neonatal Sepsis

Samuel J. Garber and Mary Catherine Harris

KEY CONCEPTS

- A high index of suspicion is required to identify the septic neonate whose initial symptoms may be minimal and nonspecific.
- The premature infant, at higher risk of morbidity and mortality, merits even greater vigilance for prompt diagnosis and treatment.
- Laboratory investigations are useful but may fail to identify the at-risk infant or falsely identify the uninfected infant.
- The role of the lumbar puncture remains controversial.

TABLE 1 Common Pathogens Associated with Early- and Late-Onset Disease in Neonates

Early-Onset Disease	Late-Onset Disease
Group B streptococcus (GBS)	Coagulase-negative staphylococcus (CoNS)
Escherichia coli, other gram-negative species	GBS
Listeria monocytogenes	*E. coli*, other gram-negative species
Staphylococcus aureus	*S. aureus*
Enterobacter species	Enterococci
	Candida

Regardless of gestational age, rule-out sepsis remains one of the most frequent diagnoses encountered in the neonatal intensive care unit. There is the symptomatic newborn for whom a sepsis evaluation is required. Perhaps more common, however, is the asymptomatic newborn with risk factors for sepsis. The older newborn with a hospital-acquired infection requires special consideration.

The incidence of early-onset sepsis (less than 1 week of age) is low (less than 1 to 4 per 1000 births); that of late-onset disease (more than 1 week of age) ranges from less than 1 to 2 per 1000 births. For both, delayed initiation of treatment can result in significant morbidity and mortality. Traditionally, risk factors for early-onset disease include maternal fever higher than 100.4°F (38°C) during labor, rupture of membranes greater than 18 hours, signs of chorioamnionitis, or positive rectovaginal culture for group B streptococcus (GBS). Risk factors for late-onset disease include prematurity, the presence of indwelling central venous catheters, and prolonged duration of mechanical ventilation. Table 1 lists the predominant organisms associated with both early- and late-onset disease.

The advent of the Centers for Disease Control and Prevention (CDC) guidelines aimed at preventing GBS sepsis has resulted in a dramatic decrease in early sepsis but not late-onset disease. These guidelines were revised employing universal screening at 35 to 37 weeks' gestation for all pregnant women along with a risk-based approach for women with unknown GBS status. Concern was raised that a decrease in GBS would be accompanied by an increase in disease caused by other pathogens. Although not observed in term infants thus far, new evidence suggests an increase in ampicillin-resistant gram-negative sepsis in infants of very low birth weight.

Heightened vigilance is required to identify the infected neonate because clinical manifestations may be subtle or nonspecific. A common antenatal finding is fetal tachycardia. Signs of infection in the newborn infant include respiratory distress (e.g., apnea, tachypnea, cyanosis, increased work of breathing), feeding intolerance (e.g., emesis, ileus), seizures, temperature instability, lethargy, and altered glucose regulation.

Expert Opinion on Management Issues

Little controversy surrounds the management of the symptomatic neonate, who requires close monitoring, prompt attainment of vascular access, and initiation of antibiotic treatment. Identifying the asymptomatic at-risk infant prior to the onset of symptoms presents more of a challenge for clinicians.

It is for these asymptomatic infants that laboratory data are used to help determine the need for antibiotics as well as the length of treatment. The ideal laboratory test for diagnosing sepsis should have a high sensitivity (no missed cases) *and* a high negative predictive accuracy (a normal sepsis value is not present). A positive blood culture is considered the gold standard for diagnosis, but the sensitivity of the blood culture is far from perfect because of intrapartum administration of antibiotics, an insufficient volume, or blood sent for culture-intermittent bacteremia in some infected infants.

Emphasis has also been placed on the complete blood count (CBC) with differential as a marker for sepsis. Among the neutrophil indexes (absolute neutrophil count, absolute band count, and immature-to-total (I:T) neutrophil ratio, neutropenia (<1750 per mm^3) has the best specificity but can be observed in association with other conditions (e.g., pregnancy-induced hypertension-related birth asphyxia). An elevation of the white blood cell (WBC) count is nonspecific and much less helpful. In contrast, an I:T neutrophil ratio of 0.2 or more is generally considered a sensitive indicator of neonatal sepsis; however, recent studies using an upper limit of 0.3 suggest this ratio may be less useful than previously thought. Furthermore, there are natural peaks and troughs of neutrophil production, with an expected rise in the WBC count between 4 and 12 hours after birth. Timing of the CBC, source of the blood (e.g., arterial versus venous), and the neonate's activity level, moreover, can affect results. The key issue is that WBC indexes may be normal shortly after birth, failing to identify those at risk, and a healthy neonate may have abnormal WBC values.

Additional laboratory markers are adjuncts to guide decision making. C-reactive protein (CRP) is an acute-phase reactant produced by the liver 6 to 8 hours after an inflammatory stimulus. Levels peak at 24 to 48 hours, with normal values less than 1.5 mg/dL. If blood is drawn shortly after birth, CRP may not be elevated because of the slow rise in the early phases of infection. In addition, maternal fever, prolonged rupture of membranes, fetal distress, and perinatal asphyxia can all trigger an inflammatory response in the absence of sepsis. Delaying measurement of CRP until at least 12 hours of life, with a repeat level 12 to 24 hours later, increases the sensitivity and especially the negative predictive accuracy.

Newer markers of infection, including the cytokines interleukin (IL)–8 and IL–6, are the focus of much investigation. IL–6 stimulates CRP production and rises sharply after an infectious exposure, providing a means for earlier detection. A lack of accepted reference ranges and limited clinical availability prevent widespread use at this time.

ROLE OF THE LUMBAR PUNCTURE AND URINE CULTURE

The role of the lumbar puncture (LP) as part of the sepsis workup remains controversial, especially in the asymptomatic at-risk term neonate in the first week of life. Retrospective studies both support and refute the notion that a lumbar puncture is mandatory. In the past, the LP was considered a routine part of the septic workup before antibiotics were administered. However, in the revised CDC guidelines, the LP is recommended only for the symptomatic infant unless contraindicated by clinical status. There is no question of the need for cerebrospinal fluid (CSF) examination with a positive blood culture or symptomatic infant.

For late-onset disease, the role of the LP is much clearer because the incidence of meningitis increases in the absence of bacteremia. Results of one study suggest as many as a third of infants of very low birth weight with meningitis may have negative blood cultures. With this

in mind, an LP is indicated for all infants evaluated for sepsis after the first week of life.

A word must be said regarding the routine use of urine cultures. In the first 72 hours of life, routine urine cultures are not recommended because of relatively low yield. However, in older infants in whom sepsis is suspected, a urine culture (preferably a catheterized specimen) should always be obtained.

SEPSIS SCREENS

Despite the limitations of laboratory markers, it is commonplace to combine tests as part of a sepsis screen to improve diagnostic accuracy. Figure 1 shows a decision-making algorithm from our institution for both term and preterm infants using point values from the sepsis screen. Overtreatment of neonates is common, but the benefits of early therapy outweigh the risk of antibiotic use.

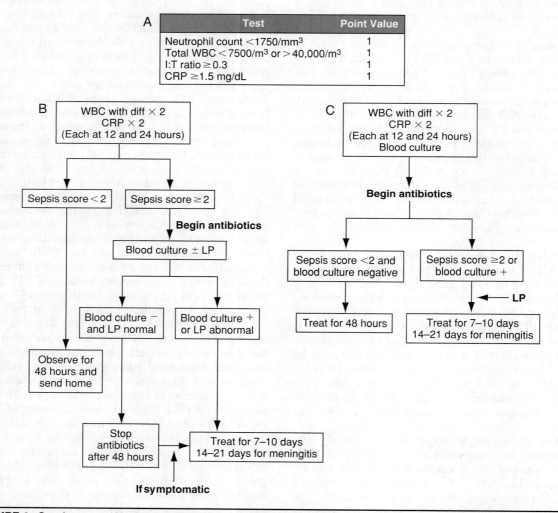

A	Test	Point Value
	Neutrophil count <1750/mm³	1
	Total WBC <7500/m³ or >40,000/m³	1
	I:T ratio ≥0.3	1
	CRP ≥1.5 mg/dL	1

FIGURE 1. Sepsis screen (A) with algorithm to evaluate (B) term (>35 weeks) and (C) preterm asymptomatic infants (<72 hours old) with risk factors (≥1) for sepsis. CRP, C-reactive protein; diff, differential; I:T, immature-to-total neutrophil ratio; LP, lumbar puncture; WBC, white blood cell.

TABLE 2 Dose Recommendations for Commonly Used Antibiotics to Treat Neonatal Sepsis

Antibiotic	Postnatal Age (days)	Gestational Age (wk) or Weight (g)	Dose (mg/kg/dose)	Interval (h)
Ampicillin	<7 days	All weights	50*	12
	7–21 days	All weights	50*	8
Gentamicin[†]	<7 days	<28 wk GA	2.5	24
		28–34 wk GA	2.5	18
		>34 wk GA	2.5	12
	>7 days	1200–2000 g	2.5	12
		>2000 g	2.5	8
Vancomycin[‡]	<7 days	<1000 g	10	24
		1000–2000 g	10	18
		>2000 g	10	12
	7–30 days	<1000 g	10	18
		1000–2000 g	10	12
		>2000 g	10	8
Oxacillin	<7 days	<2000 g	25	12
		>2000 g	25	8
	>7 days	<1200 g	25	12
		1200–2000 g	25	8
		>2000 g	25	6
Cefotaxime	<7 days	All weights	50	12
	7–28 days[§]	<2000 g	50	12
		>2000 g	50	8·
Amphotericin	All ages	All weights	1	24

Adapted from Pharmacy Handbook and Formulary, Children's Hospital of Philadelphia.
*Ampicillin at 100 mg/kg/dose for severe GBS sepsis and meningitis.
[§]Cefotaxime at 45 mg/kg/dose for meningitis.
[†]Goal: gentamicin peak 5–10 mg/dL and trough <2 mg/dL.
[‡]Goal: vancomycin trough 5–12 µg/mL.
GA, gestational age.

CHOICE OF ANTIBIOTIC

Empirical coverage should consider the neonate's age and risk factors as discussed earlier. Ampicillin and an aminoglycoside, most commonly gentamicin, provide broad-spectrum coverage against the common pathogens associated with early-onset disease. Synergy between these two agents exists versus both GBS and *Listeria*. If concern exists for gram-negative infection, particularly meningitis, a third-generation cephalosporin (e.g., cefotaxime) may achieve better central nervous system (CNS) penetration.

Coagulase-negative staphylococcus (CoNS) remains the most common cause of nosocomial infection, although GBS and gram-negative organisms are also common pathogens (see Table 1). Vancomycin typically is the initial choice of therapy for suspected nosocomial disease in combination with an aminoglycoside. However, a reasonable alternative may be to start with oxacillin if the infant is clinically stable because CoNS infections tend to be indolent with low mortality. Aminoglycosides are the preferred agents for gram-negative infection, but coverage should be tailored to individual resistance patterns. In addition, double coverage may be required in the presence of meningitis or highly resistant gram-negative organisms (e.g., *Serratia*, *Klebsiella*, *Citrobacter*). Lastly, amphotericin is the treatment of choice for suspected or proven *Candida* infection.

Table 2 shows dosage recommendations for antibiotics. Once an organism is identified and sensitivities are known, the regimen may be adjusted using the narrowest spectrum agents.

Common Pitfalls

- Failure to identify risk factors in the asymptomatic neonate may delay diagnosis and therapy.
- Signs and symptoms of sepsis can be subtle and nonspecific. The suspicion for sepsis must remain high, with consideration of resistant organisms and broadening of coverage if the infant fails to respond as expected.
- A single set of laboratory markers, especially if drawn too soon after birth, may fail to identify the at-risk asymptomatic infant.

Communication and Counseling

Neonatal sepsis is an uncommon occurrence but one associated with significant morbidity and mortality, particularly if there is a delay in diagnosis and initiation of antibiotic therapy. Signs and symptoms may be subtle and nonspecific, and laboratory data may not identify the septic neonate. Heightened vigilance and appropriate antibiotic therapy with careful monitoring of the clinical status remain the foundation for diagnosis and management of the septic neonate.

SUGGESTED READINGS

1. Escobar GJ, De-kun L, Armstrong MA, et al: Neonatal sepsis workups in infants >2000 grams at birth: A population-based study. Pediatrics 106:256–263, 2000. **Study describing the role of laboratory tests in determining the presence of neonatal infection.**

5

2. Gerdes JS: Diagnosis and management of bacterial infections in the neonate. Pediatr Clin North Am 51:939–959, 2004. **Comprehensive review of early-onset sepsis.**
3. Ottolini MC, Lundgren K, Mirkinson LJ, et al: Utility of complete blood count and blood culture screening to diagnose neonatal sepsis in the asymptomatic at risk newborn. Pediatr Infect Dis J 22:430–434, 2002. **Study describing limited use of blood count and blood culture to detect the septic neonate.**
4. Schrag S, Gorwitz R, Fultz-Butts K, Schuchat A: Prevention of perinatal group B streptococcal disease. Revised guidelines from the CDC. MMWR Recomm Rep 51(RR–11):1–22, 2002. **Revised governmental guidelines for prevention of group B streptococcal sepsis.**
5. Stoll BJ, Hansen N, Fanaroff AA, et al: Changes in pathogens causing early-onset sepsis in very low birth weight infants. N Engl J Med 347:240–247, 2002. **Study showing trends in organisms responsible for early-onset disease since advent of the CDC guidelines.**
6. Stoll BJ, Hansen N, Fanaroff AA, et al: To tap or not to tap: High likelihood of meningitis without sepsis among very low birth weight infants. Pediatrics 113:1181–1186, 2004. **Study showing high incidence of meningitis in infants of very low birth weight with negative blood cultures.**

Hydrops Fetalis

Catherine A. Hansen and David A. Bateman

KEY CONCEPTS

- *Hydrops fetalis* refers to an accumulation of excess extracellular fluid in the fetus. One widely recognized definition requires two or more of the following abnormal fluid collections: generalized skin edema (>5 mm), ascites, pleural effusion, pericardial effusion, or placental thickening (>6 cm). Polyhydramnios accompanies hydrops in up to 75% of cases but is not usually considered a separate criterion.

- The causes of hydrops fetalis are usually classified into one of two groups: immune hydrops, caused by severe fetal anemia secondary to maternal red cell alloimmunization, and nonimmune hydrops, with numerous other causes. Before the introduction of Rh immune globulin (RhoGAM) in 1968, Rh sensitization occurred in approximately 1% of pregnancies and caused more than 80% of the cases of fetal hydrops. Currently, nonimmune hydrops accounts for 90% to 95% of cases.

Immune Hydrops Fetalis

Hydrops caused by red cell alloimmunization is a well-defined disease with an established diagnostic approach and therapy. In immune hydrops, maternal antibodies formed against paternally derived fetal red cell antigens cross the placenta and produce hemolysis and anemia. The most common antigens causing sensitization are the D antigen (Rh disease) and the Kell antigen. Hydrops develops when the hematocrit falls below 15% to 20%. The severity of hemolysis can be estimated from serial changes in the concentration of bilirubin in amniotic fluid (ΔOD450) and the level of anemia ascertained by direct measurement of fetal blood sampled via cordocentesis.

Severe fetal anemia (hematocrit <30%) is considered grounds for intravascular or intraperitoneal transfusion (IVT or IPT). Because IPT is contraindicated in hydrops and has a higher rate of complications, IVT (via the umbilical vein) is the preferred method. Complications of IVT include hemorrhage, umbilical vein compression, and cardiac failure resulting from overtransfusion. High-dose intravenous immunoglobulin (IVIG), administered either antenatally to the mother or to the infant after birth, modifies the severity of fetal hemolytic disease. Exchange transfusion and phototherapy are the mainstays of postnatal therapy.

Hydropic newborns are at high risk for morbidity from severe respiratory distress syndrome, hypoglycemia, hypoproteinemia, perinatal asphyxia, cardiac failure, and a host of problems typically associated with prematurity that are all exacerbated by the hydropic state. In a review of 19 case series that included a total of 175 hydropic fetuses, immune hydrops fetalis carried a mortality of 26%.

Nonimmune Hydrops Fetalis

Nonimmune hydrops fetalis (NIHF) is caused by a variety of diseases that can be difficult to diagnose and often have limited or no treatment options. Overall, NIHF has a much higher mortality rate than immune hydrops, but some causes may resolve spontaneously or respond to intrauterine therapy.

In unselected populations, NIHF occurs in 1 out of 2500 to 3700 pregnancies. The reported incidence in fetuses diagnosed before 20 weeks' gestation is 1 in 1700; this higher incidence reflects the high rate of intrauterine demise prior to the third trimester. The incidence is reported to be as high as 1 in 165 in some tertiary referral centers, presumably because of referral bias.

Antenatal detection of fetal hydrops depends on ultrasonography. Doppler ultrasonographic measurement of systolic and diastolic blood flow velocity in placental and fetal vessels is useful to evaluate fetal blood flow distribution in the presence of altered placental perfusion and hypoxemia. Pulsed and color flow Doppler sonography is used to survey fetal cardiac and vascular anatomy. M-mode sonography is useful in the diagnosis of fetal arrhythmias and for making linear measurements across fetal body cavities and bony structures.

Hydrops fetalis represents a severe complicating feature of numerous diseases that, even without hydrops, usually have substantial mortality. In one series, the overall perinatal mortality for fetuses with NIHF (including spontaneous fetal losses and pregnancy terminations) ranged from 82% to 93%. The overall mortality of lesions considered treatable is approximately 32%. In general, the mortality rate for a specific cause is higher the earlier in pregnancy that hydrops is detected; noted prior to 20 to 24 weeks, hydrops is almost always lethal. A notable exception is hydrops resulting from anemia caused by parvovirus B19 infection. This condition occurs at a median gestational age of 23 weeks and may resolve or respond to intrauterine transfusion.

Routine midtrimester ultrasonographic fetal assessment and the application of aggressive efforts to diagnose and treat fetal hydrops have the potential to drastically alter the context in which hydropic infants present at birth. A report from a tertiary referral center of 83 pregnancies with NIHF is illustrative. The cause of NIHF was identified prenatally in 80% of the cases; one third of these were due to chromosomal and syndromic abnormalities. Nearly all of the chromosomal/syndromic cases were identified prior to 24 weeks' gestation, and termination of pregnancy was elected in nearly all. Altogether, pregnancy was terminated in 38% of NIHF cases; another 20% suffered intrauterine demise. Intrauterine treatment was given in 57% of the pregnancies not terminated. Less than half (43%) of the original cohort of NIHF fetuses survived to delivery. In most of these, hydrops was diagnosed after 24 weeks, with fetal arrhythmias and hydrothorax the two most common causes. The neonatal survival rate of delivered NIHF infants was 69%. This study suggests that when sophisticated antenatal efforts to detect, diagnose, and treat nonimmune hydrops in utero are appropriately applied, the prognosis of newborns who survive to delivery is far from hopeless and often justifies aggressive resuscitation and neonatal intensive care.

ETIOLOGY

Despite the poor overall survival, every effort should be made to determine the etiology of NIHF, either specifically or as part of a general disease category, as early in the pregnancy as possible, for the following reasons:

- Several causes of hydrops are amenable to intervention during the fetal period (e.g., pharmacologic treatment of tachyarrhythmias, drainage of chylothorax). The success of these procedures may diminish as hydrops becomes established and fetal well-being deteriorates.
- Most parents require a period of emotional adjustment before coming to terms with a lethal or severely compromising fetal condition. The earlier a specific diagnosis is made, the broader the set of options available to parents. In severe or lethal conditions, parents may elect to terminate the pregnancy.
- Many specific causes of hydrops are inherited, with implications for future pregnancies.

Expert Opinion on Management Issues

CONDITIONS RESPONSIBLE FOR NONIMMUNE HYDROPS FETALIS

More than 100 different disorders cause nonimmune hydrops. These can be divided into categories, in the manner of several review articles, as follows.

Chromosomal Disorders

Chromosomal disorders are responsible for 10% to 28% of NIHF cases detected throughout the entire pregnancy, but as many as 45% to 78% when NIHF is detected before 20 weeks' gestation. This fact reflects the high rate of fetal loss in chromosomal NIHF. Turner syndrome (45X), trisomy 21, and trisomy 18 are the most common associations. Overall, perinatal survival in chromosomal NIHF is virtually nil, but exceptions are reported (e.g., an infant with trisomy 21 and isolated chylothorax). Turner syndrome associated with hydrops and cystic hygroma is usually lethal.

Cardiovascular Lesions

Cardiovascular lesions account for 13% to 26% of NIHF cases in studies that include the entire pregnancy, but the proportion is only 5% to 7% when hydrops is detected prior to 20 weeks. This category includes structural heart lesions (hypoplastic left heart and endocardial cushion defects are most commonly associated), which have a dismal prognosis; these lesions may manifest with hydrops. However, 30% to 50% of cardiovascular NIHF cases are caused by arrhythmias, with tachyarrhythmias three times more likely than bradyarrhythmias. Tachyarrhythmias often respond to maternal administration of such antiarrhythmic agents as digoxin, verapamil, or flecainide, with possible resort to direct fetal therapy in refractory cases. With treatment, two thirds of infants survive the neonatal period. Because of bradyarrhythmias, NIHF has a much poorer prognosis. In half these cases the bradyarrhythmia is due to fetal heart block caused by transplacental passage of antibodies associated with maternal connective tissue disease. Fetal bradycardia occasionally is the presenting symptom of maternal lupus. Treatments include maternal administration of corticosteroids, inotropic and β-mimetic agents, and intrauterine pacing, all without consistent success.

Syndromic Disorders

Syndromic disorders account for approximately 5% to 10% of NIHF cases in published series. The category includes numerous individually rare entities, nearly all of which carry a poor prognosis for survival. Two large subgroups of the category are the chondrodysplasias, including lethal dwarfing conditions (thanatophoric dwarfism, rhizomelic type Conradi disease, osteogenesis imperfecta, hypophosphatasia, achondrogenesis, and others) and hypomobility syndromes (arthrogryposis, multiple pterygia, Neu-Laxova, Pena-Shokeir, myotonic dystrophy, and others). The pathogenesis of fluid accumulation in these entities is unknown but may be related to decreased fetal movement. Cystic hygroma and Noonan syndrome are also associated with NIHF. A specific diagnosis of the disorder is essential for genetic counseling and involves documentation of fetal limb length, limb deformities, and fractures, as well as postnatal photographs and radiographic, histopathologic, and genetic

TABLE 1 Workup of Nonimmune Hydrops Fetalis that Manifests with Additional Ultrasonographic Findings

Ultrasound Findings	Etiology	Other Investigations (Karyotype Universal)*	Treatment	Prognosis	Comment
Tachyarrhythmia	SVT; atrial flutter	Echocardiography: M-mode, Doppler, 2-D.	Maternal antiarrhythmic agents: digoxin, verapamil, flecainide, etc.	66% postnatal survival with therapy	Not usually associated with structural heart disease (~5%); direct fetal treatment (intravascular, intraperitoneal) with adenosine, amiodarone occasionally successful in refractory cases.
Bradyarrhythmia	Complete AV block; structural lesions	Echocardiography (see above); maternal serum cardiolipin (anti-SS-A, -SS-B antibodies).	Consider maternal corticosteroids, β-mimetics, digoxin; fetal pacing.	Limited survival even with therapy	Complete fetal heart block is usually associated with maternal connective tissue disease; case reports of transplacental β-methasone responsiveness.
Congestive heart failure	Anemia	Fetal cordocentesis: CBC, smear, parvovirus serology/PCR, Hgb electrophoresis; maternal Kleihauer-Betke smear; parental G6PD assay; Doppler echocardiography.	Consider intrauterine transfusion (hematocrit <30%).	Variable	Anemia from parvovirus infection has good prognosis with treatment and sometimes resolves spontaneously; α-thalassemia considered lethal.
	Tumor; AV malformation	US examination for fetal AV malformation, tumor, placental chorioangioma.	Consider fetal surgery for sacrococcygeal teratoma.	Variable	Sacrococcygeal teratoma may present with fetal anemia caused by hemorrhage.
Structural heart disease		Echocardiography.	Usually none.	Usually lethal	Hypoplastic left-heart syndrome most common lesion associated with NIHF.
Cardiac tumors		Echocardiography; family evaluation for tuberous sclerosis.	Usually none.	Poor	Fetal rhabdomyomas may cause tachyarrhythmias; fetal resection of benign tumor reported.
Pulmonary masses and effusions	(Lesions below)	Echocardiography, plus:			Decision for fetal intervention must be individualized; these lesions usually lethal when accompanied by other abnormalities.
	CDH	Assess risk for pulmonary hypoplasia.	Repair; tracheal occlusion.	Poor	Fetal intervention not shown to improve outcome.
	CCAM	Assess for single versus multiple cysts.	Thoracoamniotic shunt; lobectomy.	60% survival with in utero intervention; poor without	20% of lesions regress spontaneously.

Presentation	Diagnosis	Evaluation	Treatment	Outcome	Comments
	BPS	Assess vascular supply to distinguish from CCAM.	Thoracoamniotic shunt.	>90% survival with in utero intervention; poor without.	
	Hydrothorax/ chylothorax	Fetal thoracentesis for fluid chemistry, cytology, cell count.	Thoracoamniotic shunt.	High survival rate for isolated lesion	Poor prognosis for fetuses with Turner, or Down syndromes or cardiac lesions associated with chylothorax; isolated chylothorax may resolve spontaneously.
Twin pregnancy	TTTS	US evaluation of placental structure, fetal discordance, cardiac anatomy, Doppler flow.	Consider blood transfusion to donor via umbilical vein; amniotomy for recipient twin; laser ablations of anastomoses.	Survival 25–50%	Mortality higher in recipient than donor fetus; compromised developmental outcome in 5%–50% of survivors.
Multiple fetal anatomic abnormalities; limb anomalies; arthrogryposis		Studies suggested by family history and by specific pattern of anomalies.	None.	Usually lethal	Labeled "syndromic" if karyotype normal; thorough genetic evaluation; consider termination.
Ascites, hepatosplenomegaly predominate	Possible metabolic, infectious	Amniotic fluid cell culture, viral cultures; maternal serologic/PCR studies for TORCH entities; US evaluation of placenta; detailed maternal family history for metabolic diseases and viral/ toxoplasmosis/drug exposures.	Usually none; penicillin for syphilis; pyrimethamine/ sulfa for toxoplasmosis.	Usually lethal	Ascites may be dominant finding in lysosomal storage disorders. Rule out TORCH infections. Consider termination.
Ascites; abnormal genitourinary anatomy	Prune belly syn, obstructive uropathies, cloacal malformation.	Detailed anatomic survey; Doppler evaluation of renal perfusion.	Usually none; consider vesicoamniotic shunting for distal obstruction.	Usually lethal	Consider termination.

*Karyotype can be performed on fetal samples obtained via chorionic villous sampling, amniocentesis, cordocentesis, or from fetal or placental tissues obtained postmortem.
AV, atrioventricular; BPS, bronchopulmonary sequestration; CBC, complete blood count; CCAM, congenital cystic adenomatoid malformation; CDH, congenital diaphragmatic hernia; G6PD, glucose-6-phosphate dehydrogenase; Hgb, hemoglobin; PCR, polymerase chain reaction; syn, syndrome; SVT, supraventricular tachycardia; TORCH, T (toxoplasmosis), O (parvovirus, adenovirus, other viral etiology), R (rubella), C (cytomegalovirus), H (hepatitis, herpes simplex); TTTS, twin-to-twin transfusion syndrome; US, ultrasound.

studies. The assistance of an experienced clinical geneticist is essential.

Metabolic Disorders

Metabolic disorders account for less than 5% of cases in published series. Lysosomal storage diseases are inherited as an autosomal recessive trait; in the presence of hydrops, fetal or early neonatal mortality is universal. Gaucher disease, GM1 gangliosidosis, sialidosis, mucopolysaccharidosis VII, and I-cell disease are among those most often reported. Hypoproteinemia and venous obstruction by hepatocytes swollen with storage material may be responsible for the hydrops, in which ascites predominates. Lysosomal storage diseases can manifest with characteristic physical, radiographic, and laboratory findings that allow the specific diagnosis to be targeted. Histologic examination of placental tissue can be invaluable in narrowing the list of possible diagnoses.

Thoracic Lesions

The incidence of thoracic lesions ranges from 0% to 15% of NIHF cases (lowest in studies excluding fetuses more than 20 weeks' gestation). Included are chylothorax, congenital diaphragmatic hernia, congenital cystic adenomatoid malformation of the lung, and bronchopulmonary sequestration. All of these lesions have a high mortality rate when accompanied by hydrops, but in utero drainage of pleural effusions in isolated chylothorax and bronchopulmonary sequestration (BPS) and fetal surgery to remove congenital cystic adenomatoid malformation (CCAM) can improve survival. At least two thirds of those with isolated chylothorax and BPS, treated with thoracoamniotic shunt, and CCAM, treated with shunt or lobectomy, survive. Hydropic fetuses less than 32 weeks' gestation with CCAM and BPS are candidates for intrauterine intervention; beyond this gestation, antenatal steroids should be administered if indicated and the mother counseled for delivery and postnatal resection.

Anemia

Anemia occurs in 10% to 20% of NIHF cases. The proportion is greatest among Asian populations that have a high incidence of α-thalassemia. In non-Asians the major causes include parvovirus B19 infection, twin-to-twin transfusion (see later), and chronic fetomaternal hemorrhage. The etiologies of fetal anemia can be divided between those in which compensatory hemopoietic activity is intense and involves extramedullary sites, particularly the liver (e.g., in α-thalassemia and fetomaternal hemorrhage), and those in which erythropoiesis is suppressed (e.g., in congenital parvovirus infection). Fetal congestive heart failure is presumed the main mechanism by which anemia produces hydrops.

Fetal anemia is diagnosed by direct fetal blood sampling (cordocentesis). In addition to hematocrit, red cell indexes, and smear, fetal blood should be tested for α-thalassemia in susceptible individuals, using DNA testing or hemoglobin electrophoresis. Reports correlate the degree of fetal anemia with Doppler ultrasonographic measurement of peak flow velocity of the middle cerebral artery.

Hydrops caused by significant fetal anemia (hematocrit less than 30%) can be treated successfully with intrauterine transfusions. Although transfusion for anemia in congenital parvovirus infection appears indicated (with survival rates approximately 75%), many instances of anemia due to parvovirus infection resolve spontaneously without transfusion. Fetomaternal transfusions may be chronic or acute and massive, leading to sudden demise. The volume of transfused fetal blood in the maternal circulation can be estimated from the proportion of fetal red cells on the maternal Kleihauer-Betke smear.

Infections

Infections account for approximately 5% to 20% of NIHF cases, but the known proportion has increased with the advent of viral polymerase chain reaction (PCR) analysis. In addition to parvovirus B19 infection, responsible for so-called fifth disease in children and adults, NIHF has resulted from fetal infection caused by cytomegalovirus (CMV), *Toxoplasma,* herpesvirus, *Treponema pallidum,* and adenovirus, among others. Individually, each of these diseases makes a small contribution to the overall incidence of NIHF. Aside from congenital syphilis, which caused substantial perinatal mortality in the era before penicillin, there are insufficient data to estimate the mortality rate from hydrops caused by a specific organism. Both syphilis (with penicillin) and toxoplasmosis (with pyrimethamine/sulfa combination) are potentially amenable to maternal treatment during pregnancy. Antenatal serologic testing for syphilis is routine in most places; testing for toxoplasmosis is limited to cases in which maternal infection is suspected or fetal ultrasonographic findings suggest the diagnosis.

Chronic Twin-to-Twin Transfusion Syndrome

Chronic twin-to-twin transfusion syndrome (TTTS) causes 3% to 8% of NIHF cases, with a mortality of 75%. Both the recipient and the donor twin are at risk for fetal or neonatal demise and compromised neurologic outcome. TTTS occurs when large vascular anastomoses in a monochorionic placenta shunt blood from the donor to the recipient twin. Hydrops develops in the recipient twin as a result of progressive volume overload, polycythemia, and congestive heart failure. It develops in the donor twin as the result of severe anemia. IVT may be indicated for the donor twin. Serial removal of fluid from the recipient sac (amnioreduction) and laser ablation of the connecting vessels may improve survival.

Tumors

Tumors are responsible for 1% to 3% of NIHF cases, with poor probability of survival. The mechanism of hydrops varies with tumor type and location. Space-occupying tumors in the thorax (e.g., neuroblastoma) can cause increased central venous pressure; tumors such as sacrococcygeal teratomas and placental chorangiomas can cause high-output cardiac failure because of their high demand for blood flow. Chronic hemorrhage in sacrococcygeal tumors resulting in anemia can also contribute to hydrops. Successful intrauterine removal of sacrococcygeal teratomas is reported.

Genitourinary Abnormalities

Genitourinary abnormalities account for 2% to 3% of NIHF cases, with poor probability of survival. Congenital nephrosis produces low serum protein levels that can lead to hydrops. Prune belly syndrome, other obstructive uropathies, and cloacal malformations are also associated with fetal hydrops, although the mechanism of generalized fluid accumulation is unclear because urinary ascites usually remains localized in the abdomen.

Idiopathic Hydrops

The proportion of hydrops cases ascribed to unknown causes ranges from 5% to 35% in published series and depends on the thoroughness and sophistication of the workup.

Table 1 recategorizes the preceding diagnostic categories according to presenting ultrasonographic features. Table 2 lists investigations appropriate to determining the cause of fetal hydrops. This list is generic and must be tailored to the specific features of the clinical presentation.

POSTNATAL MANAGEMENT OF THE HYDROPIC INFANT

Given appropriate antenatal diagnostic and therapeutic efforts, the hydropic newborn whom the pediatrician encounters at delivery is likely to be one whose diagnosis is known or suspected, has had intrauterine therapy (if indicated), and whose parents have been advised and involved in decision making. In this situation the bulk of pediatric effort involves assembling a team of practitioners (neonatologists, surgeons, pathologists, radiologists, or cardiologists) who can tailor resuscitative efforts to the specific lesion and can perform the diagnostic and therapeutic interventions that are appropriate for the infant's disease. The attention to detail required to organize an effective team must not be underestimated; prewritten protocols that provide detailed instructions about the processing of blood and tissue samples and anticipate other difficulties can be indispensable to the success of the effort.

Most recent published reports on the causes and outcome of NIHF involve cases identified in utero via second-trimester ultrasonographic surveillance and referred to tertiary centers. However, such surveillance is not necessarily routine in low-risk pregnancies, and it is not clear what proportion of the total number of NIHF cases evades prenatal detection and manifests outside of tertiary centers at the time of delivery. The distribution of causes and the survival rates of these infants may differ considerably from those whose hydrops was diagnosed earlier. Table 3 outlines some features generic to the postnatal management of NIHF.

TABLE 2 Investigation of Fetal Hydrops

Maternal and family history:
  Ethnic background
  Consanguinity
  Previously affected infants
  Family history of metabolic or hereditary conditions
  Maternal medical conditions and exposures
  Lupus, anemia, diabetes, infections (especially parvovirus, toxoplasmosis exposure), G6PD deficiency
  Medications that trigger hemolysis or suppress erythropoiesis
Maternal laboratory investigation:
  Complete blood count, indexes, smear
  Hemoglobin electrophoresis
  Blood type and antibody screen
  α-Fetoprotein/triple screen
  Kleihauer-Betke smear
  Serology for syphilis, toxoplasmosis, CMV, parvovirus
  Hemoglobin electrophoresis and immunoassays, DNA analysis for alpha globin gene deletion*
Ultrasound:
  Two- and three-dimensional ultrasound surveys for congenital malformations
  Fetal echocardiography with M-mode and pulsed and color flow Doppler
Limb length measurements
Fetal movement evaluation
Serial scans to monitor fluid accumulation, fetal growth, cardiac status, fetal well-being
Amniocentesis:
  Fetal karyotype*
  Viral culture and PCR for parvovirus, adenovirus, enterovirus
Test for fetal lung maturity
Cell culture for lysosomal storage diseases and other inherited metabolic diseases†
Restriction endonucleases for α-thalassemia*
Fetal blood sampling†:
  Fetal karyotype*
  CBC with reticulocyte count
  Blood type and antibody screen
  Hemoglobin electrophoresis for α-thalassemia
Liver function tests including total protein/albumin
Total IgM
Serology (IgG, IgM), PCR for CMV, toxoplasmosis, parvovirus, adenovirus, enterovirus
Chromatographic analysis of metabolic products related to gene deletions in lysosomal storage diseases, etc.
Postnatal tests†:
  Analysis of fluid (paracentesis, thoracentesis, pericardiocentesis) for cell count, cytology, protein, culture
Tests listed under fetal blood sampling above
Urinalysis
Placental gross and histologic examination; cell culture
Consultation by clinical geneticist
Radiologic studies and skeletal survey†
Complete autopsy if the infant dies
Thorough history provided to pathologist
Photographs
Infant/placental tissue samples frozen for future metabolic studies

---

*Samples for fetal karyotype may be obtained by chorionic villous sampling in first trimester of pregnancy or by amniocentesis or cordocentesis by mid–second trimester.

†As indicated. The extent of this workup should be modified by ethnicity, history, ultrasonographic findings, and positive results of screening tests.

CBC, complete blood count; CMV, cytomegalovirus; G6PD, glucose–6-phosphate dehydrogenase; PCR, polymerase chain reaction.

Common Pitfalls

Obstetric ultrasonography is a sensitive and specific tool for detecting hydrops and many of the associated

TABLE 3 Management of Nonimmune Hydrops Fetalis at Delivery

Timing and route of delivery depends on:
  Diagnosis and available therapeutic interventions
  Fetal well-being
  Progression of disease
  Fetal maturity
Preparation for delivery should include:
  Antenatal steroids if indicated
  Ultrasound assessment of ascites and hydrothorax; possibly intrauterine drainage
  Preparation for resuscitation, umbilical catheterization, and paracentesis or thoracentesis
  Assembly of an experienced resuscitation team
  Assessment for anemia and preparation of blood products for simple or exchange transfusion (O-negative cells crossmatched against maternal serum)
  Formulation of detailed postnatal management plan
  Preparation for processing of diagnostic samples, including blood, effusion fluid, placental specimens, etc.
  Counseling and preparation of parents for a sick newborn
Postnatal management strategies may include:
  Treatment of compromised circulating volume and cardiac output
  Positive-pressure ventilation, drainage of effusions, surfactant, inhaled nitric oxide (iNO)
  Phototherapy; simple transfusions and exchange transfusions
  Peritoneal drainage; appropriate fluid management (usually fluid restriction), diuretics (substantial weight loss anticipated)
  Parenteral nutrition
Ongoing diagnostic efforts, as indicated

anomalies and diseases that produce the condition. However, both false-positive and false-negative diagnosis of hydrops may potentially harm the fetus if conditions amenable to therapy are overlooked or if inappropriate therapy is undertaken. For example, thick subcutaneous fat can mimic subcutaneous edema, and muscles of the abdominal wall sometimes appear very hypoechoic and can resemble ascites. Pulmonary sequestration can be mistaken for cystic adenomatoid malformation unless a careful search is undertaken to establish the arterial blood supply of the sequestered lobe.

At delivery, resuscitation of a hydropic infant may be made more difficult by the presence of cystic hygroma or other lesions involving the neck, airway, or thoracic cavity. Ventilation and cardiac output may be compromised by pulmonary, pericardial, or abdominal effusions that require acute drainage. Consideration should be given to draining these under sonographic guidance prior to delivery; failing this, knowledge of their location, size, and relation to organs like the liver and spleen may help avoid a therapeutic catastrophe. Hyperkalemia and other electrolyte abnormalities usually complicate the early hospital course of an extremely premature hydropic infant. If large volumes of transfused blood are required, use of washed red cells can prevent exacerbation of the potassium overload.

Communication and Counseling

The decision to diagnose or treat fetal hydrops aggressively (for reasons outlined previously) needs to be made with the informed agreement of the parents.

Investigating the cause of hydrops is potentially expensive, procedure intensive, and time consuming, and parents must have a clear understanding of how each step contributes to establishing a diagnosis. But focusing on the importance of identifying treatable lesions may raise unrealistic expectations about the treatability of hydrops in general. Both parents and physicians sometimes overlook the fact that the causes of hydrops are mostly untreatable and fatal, and even those considered treatable have a substantial mortality rate. For some families, the reasons for investigating the causes of hydrops may be outweighed by religious and ethical commitments. These may prohibit some forms of intrauterine testing and therapy, as well as pregnancy termination and autopsy. Physicians must be sympathetic to such commitments. In any case, most causes of hydrops that remain unknown have a relatively low risk of recurrence. Finally, as with any chronic condition that has a generally poor prognosis, communication needs to be consistent, frank, frequent, and repetitive, with full sympathy for the emotional toll that involved families must bear.

SUGGESTED READINGS

1. Bukowski R, Saade GR: Hydrops fetalis. Clin Perinatol 27:1007–1031, 2000. **A thorough review of the obstetric diagnosis and management of nonimmune hydrops.**
2. Gallagher PG (ed): Non-immune hydrops fetalis. Semin Perinatol 19:435–532, 1995. **An entire issue, including nine separate well-researched reviews, on all aspects of the topic.**
3. Koenig JM: Evaluation treatment of erythroblastosis fetalis in the neonate. In Christensen RD (ed): Hematologic Problems of the Neonate. Philadelphia: WB Saunders, 2000, pp 209–238. **A brief, well-written overview of the history and current therapy of alloimmune hydrops.**
4. Machin GA: Hydrops revisited: Literature review of 1,414 cases published in the 1980s. Am J Med Genet 34:366–390, 1989. **The numerous causes of hydrops are divided into 15 categories, with a pathophysiologic discussion of each.**
5. Sohan K, Carroll SG, de la Fuente S, et al: Analysis of outcome in hydrops fetalis in relation to gestational age at diagnosis, cause, and treatment. Acta Obstet Gynecol Scand 80:726–730, 2001. **The outcome, including neonatal survival, of hydrops cases detected before and after 24 weeks' gestation.**

Patent Ductus Arteriosus

Karna Murthy and Jacquelyn R. Evans

KEY CONCEPTS

- Persistence of the ductus arteriosus is associated with an increased risk of a number of adverse sequelae in infants of very low birth weight.
- Clinical exam is neither sensitive nor specific in diagnosing a patent ductus arteriosus (PDA); echocardiography is required for accurate diagnosis.
- The three general approaches to the timing of the PDA closure are prophylactic, presymptomatic, and symptomatic.
- Prophylactic indomethacin use in infants less than 1 kg birth weight is associated with a reduction in severe

intraventricular hemorrhage (IVH), symptomatic PDA, and need for surgical ligation, with no difference in long-term neurodevelopmental outcome.

■ Surgical ligation of a persistent ductus should be strongly considered for premature infants with necrotizing enterocolitis (NEC), gastrointestinal (GI) perforation, or pulmonary hemorrhage (PH).

■ Antenatal indomethacin exposure is associated with an increased risk of a symptomatic PDA and a decreased responsiveness to postnatal indomethacin.

■ A PDA, as well as the therapies used for ductal closure, pose various risks. Decisions on appropriate therapy should be individualized and take into account the infant's gestational and postnatal age, pulmonary status, and other risk factors, as well as the baseline risk of certain complications of prematurity in the unit in which care is provided.

The ductus arteriosus is a normal fetal vascular communication between the main pulmonary artery and the descending aorta. In infants greater than 34 weeks' gestation, the ductus usually closes spontaneously in the first 3 to 4 days after birth. Postnatal ductal persistence remains a common problem in infants born very prematurely and can result in a left-to-right shunt that overloads the pulmonary circulation and causes inadequate perfusion to the brain, gastrointestinal (GI) tract, and kidneys. Patent ductus arteriosus (PDA) is associated with an increased risk of a number of adverse outcomes, including bronchopulmonary dysplasia (BPD), intraventricular hemorrhage (IVH), necrotizing enterocolitis (NEC), pulmonary hemorrhage (PH), and mortality. The incidence of a PDA is inversely related to birth weight and gestational age; approximately one third of infants of very low birth weight (VLBW) and two thirds of infants of extremely low birth weight (ELBW) have a clinically apparent PDA at 72 hours. A hyperdynamic precordium, bounding peripheral pulses, pulmonary edema, continuous murmur, and widened pulse pressures can all be physical findings present in the infant with a hemodynamically significant PDA. In the early stages of ductal persistence, however, none of these findings may be present, and the diagnosis can only be made reliably with echocardiography. Despite many years of research, decisions about when and how to treat the PDA remain controversial.

Expert Opinion on Management Issues

Therapy to close a PDA can be either medical or surgical. The only approved medical therapy in the United States is indomethacin, a potent inhibitor of prostaglandin synthesis. Because indomethacin has major effects on cerebral, mesenteric, and renal hemodynamics, as well as on platelet and neutrophil function, a number of absolute and relative contraindications must be considered prior to its administration (Fig. 1 and Table 1). The efficacy of indomethacin in achieving ductal closure decreases with increasing postnatal age, a gestational age above 34

weeks and below 28 weeks, and antenatal indomethacin exposure. Surgical ligation of the ductus, usually reserved for instances of medical failure, remains the definitive therapy for ductal closure.

The three general approaches to timing of intervention for a PDA are prophylactic, presymptomatic, and symptomatic (Fig. 1 and Fig. 2). Failure of the ductus to close once clinical symptoms of cardiovascular compromise develop (approximately 7 to 10 days postnatally) increases neonatal morbidity in premature infants. Therefore, our approach is to close the PDA prior to the development of any hemodynamic significance. Because the incidence of sequelae from PDAs decreases with increasing gestational age, a strategy for intervention based on gestational age is provided.

Prophylactic indomethacin decreases the incidence of symptomatic PDA, the need for surgical ligation, and severe IVH in ELBW infants, with no increase in the incidence of NEC or PH. Despite these substantial short-term benefits, prophylaxis does not improve long-term neurodevelopmental outcome and exposes many infants who would never develop a symptomatic PDA to the risks of indomethacin.

An alternative to the prophylactic approach is to evaluate all ELBW infants with echocardiography 48 to 96 hours after birth and treat only those with ductal patency. The decision on whether to use a prophylactic approach in these infants may depend on individual circumstances and the unit's background rate of severe IVH, symptomatic PDAs, and surgical ligations, as well as the availability of expert cardiac ultrasound and cardiovascular surgery services. Given their high risk of morbidity and the decreased responsiveness to indomethacin with increasing postnatal age and very low gestational age, ELBW infants more than 10 to 14 days of age should be strongly considered for surgical ligation after a failed first or second course of indomethacin. If NEC or PH has occurred, surgical ligation is preferred. In addition, because a history of antenatal indomethacin use predicts failure of subsequent indomethacin treatment in ELBW infants, some authors advocate that ligation be performed after one course of indomethacin in these infants.

In more mature, mechanically ventilated infants between 1 and 1.5 kg birth weight or 27 to 30 weeks gestation, the ductus often closes spontaneously by 48 to 96 hours of age, at which time surveillance with echocardiography can delineate need for treatment. Infants greater than 1 kg birth weight or 30 weeks' gestation who do not require mechanical ventilation are more likely to have spontaneous PDA closure and are at lower risk of developing complications of prematurity or ductal patency. In these infants a strategy that includes careful clinical surveillance for signs and symptoms of a PDA may be appropriate, with intervention only if clinical deterioration occurs.

Digitalis, diuretics, and inotropic agents are temporizing measures at best and do not enhance ductal closure. However, antenatal steroids and restricted fluid intake in the first days after birth are associated with a lower risk of PDA.

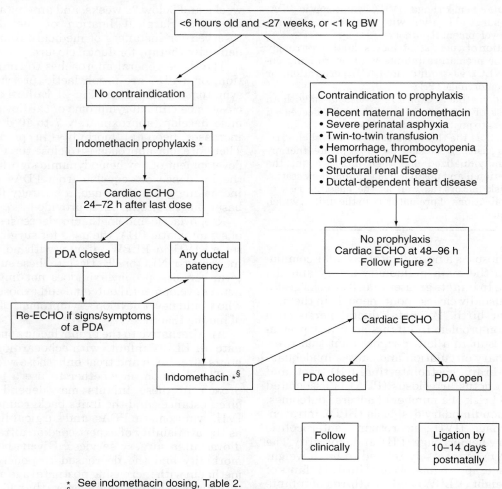

FIGURE 1. Patent ductus arteriosus (PDA) management in infants of extremely low birth weight (ELBW) receiving prophylactic indomethacin. BW, birth weight; ECHO, echocardiography; GI, gastrointestinal; NEC, necrotizing enterocolitis.

TABLE 1 Contraindications to Indomethacin Use

Absolute	Relative
Renal failure	Renal insufficiency
Active hemorrhage	Pulmonary hypertension
NEC/GI perforation	Thrombocytopenia
Ductal-dependent heart disease	Current or recent steroid exposure

GI, gastrointestinal; NEC, necrotizing enterocolitis.

TABLE 2 Dosing and Schedule of Indomethacin

Prophylactic Dosing Regimen (mg/kg/dose)

	<6 h old	T = 24 h	T = 48 h
<1 kg BW or <27 wk	0.1	0.1	0.1

Therapeutic Dosing Regimen (mg/kg/dose)

	T = 0 h	T = 12 h	T = 24–36 h*
<48 h, all weights	0.2	0.1	0.1
2–7 days ≤ 1.25 kg BW	0.2	0.1	0.1
2–7 days >1.25 kg BW	0.2	0.2	0.2
>7 days, all weights	0.2	0.2	0.2

*Most infants should receive the third dose 24 hours after the first dose; infants with renal insufficiency should receive the third dose 36 hours after the first dose.

BW, birth weight; T, time.

Future Directions in Management

Ibuprofen, an alternative prostaglandin inhibitor, was evaluated internationally for the treatment of PDA. Systemic vasoconstriction appears attenuated with ibuprofen as compared with indomethacin; whether this translates to better outcome is not clear. Increasing availability of expert cardiothoracic surgery teams that travel to smaller centers can avoid the problems of transfer and minimize delay in permanent closure of the ductus in those infants not responsive to medical therapy.

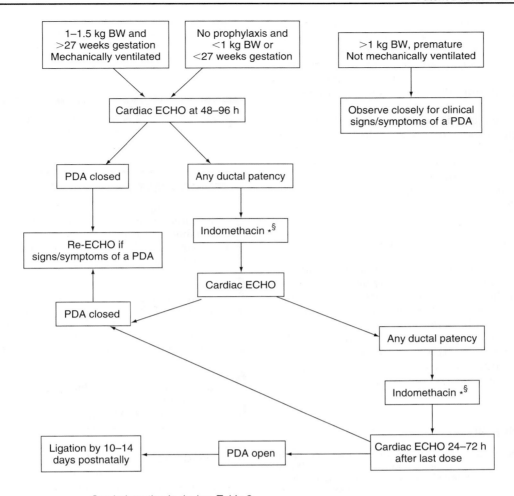

* See indomethacin dosing, Table 2.
§ Consider ligation if PDA with left to right shunting and GI perforation, NEC, or pulmonary hemorrhage.

FIGURE 2. Patent ductus arteriosus (PDA) management for premature infants not receiving prophylactic indomethacin. BW, birth weight; ECHO, echocardiography GI, gastrointestinal.

Thoracoscopic PDA closure, used successfully in older children, is just beginning to be used in premature infants and may reduce some of the complications seen with open thoracotomy closure.

Common Pitfalls

The most common pitfall in treatment of the PDA is delay to permanent closure, thereby substantially increasing the risk of serious sequelae of prematurity. The clinician should be aware that even after documented closure, reopening of the ductus can occur, particularly in association with sepsis or severe pulmonary deterioration. The indomethacin-induced reductions in blood flow in cerebral, renal, and splanchnic circulations raise concern for its use in infants in whom these organ systems are already compromised. Concomitant steroid use may raise the risk of GI perforation. Because indomethacin can impair platelet function, thrombocytopenia should be corrected prior to indomethacin use. The effects on the neonate of *antenatal* indomethacin used for tocolysis are not completely understood. However, in utero exposure to indomethacin is associated in some studies with a decreased postnatal responsiveness to indomethacin and an increased risk of symptomatic PDA, NEC, or focal GI perforation and IVH. Because the vasoconstriction associated with indomethacin is exacerbated with faster infusion rates of medication, the drug should be given as an infusion over 30 to 60 minutes and never by intravenous push.

Metabolism and excretion of many medications are altered during indomethacin treatment. Medications whose clearance depends on renal mechanisms are at particular risk for buildup systemically. Aminoglycoside and vancomycin levels require close attention following indomethacin treatment until renal excretion improves. In addition, careful fluid and electrolyte management is required during the frequent oliguria that follows indomethacin administration, to avoid fluid overload, hyponatremia, and hyperkalemia. Because of its mesenteric vasoconstrictive effects, enteral feedings are contraindicated during indomethacin use, although trophic feedings were used without adverse sequelae in at least one trial.

Surgical ligation is safe when performed by experienced teams. However, mortality, chylothoraces, pneumothoraces, pleural effusions, ligation of adjacent vascular structures, occlusions of bronchial airways, recurrent laryngeal nerve injury, postoperative escalation of cardiopulmonary support, significant hemorrhage, and late thoracic scoliosis are all reported.

Communication and Counseling

Physicians must inform parents that indomethacin therapy has certain risks that are usually acceptable given the potential risks of ductal persistence, and some infants require surgical ligation later despite treatment with indomethacin. Physician counseling prior to ligation should include the routine risks of any surgery but also the specific risks to the structures that surround the PDA in these infants. Most of the surgical complications of ligation occur at a frequency that varies inversely with gestational age.

SUGGESTED READINGS

1. Clyman RI: Recommendations for the postnatal use of indomethacin: An analysis of four separate treatment strategies. J Pediatr 128:601–607, 1996. **Meta-analysis of studies reporting impact of PDA intervention, grouped by treatment strategy.**
2. Cotton RB, Stahlman MT, Bender HW, et al: Randomized trial of early closure of symptomatic ductus arteriosus in small preterm infants. J Pediatr 93:647–651, 1978. **Small trial but only one ever to compare closure of PDA with no closure and no backup treatment.**
3. Evans N: Current controversies in the diagnosis and treatment of patent ductus arteriosus in preterm infants. Adv Neonatal Care 3:168–177, 2003. **Rationale for various treatment strategies reviewed.**
4. Fowlie PW, Davis PG: Prophylactic indomethacin for preterm infants: A systematic review and meta-analysis. Arch Dis Child Fetal Neonatal Ed 88:F464–F466, 2003. **Nineteen trials of indomethacin prophylaxis are reviewed.**
5. Hammerman C, Glaser J, Kaplan M, et al: Indomethacin tocolysis increases postnatal patent ductus arteriosus severity. Pediatrics 102:1202–1203, 1998. **Retrospective review of neonatal impact of prenatal indomethacin exposure.**
6. Knight DB: The treatment of patent ductus arteriosus in preterm infants. A review and overview of randomized trials. Semin Neonatol 6:63–73, 2001. **Review of randomized trials of PDA closure, grouped by postnatal age at intervention.**
7. Koehne PS, Bein G, Alexi-Meskhishvilil V, et al: PDA in VLBW infants: Complications of pharmacological and surgical treatment. J Perinatol Med 29:327–334, 2001. **Higher mortality, lower renal impairment, and no difference in NEC or IVH with surgery versus indomethacin is reported.**
8. Ment LR, Oh W, Ehrenkranz RA, et al: Low-dose indomethacin prevention of intraventricular hemorrhage: A multicenter randomized trial. Pediatrics 93:543–550, 1994. **Prophylactic indomethacin significantly lowered incidence and severity of IVH without significant adverse drug events in infants of less than 1250 g birth weight.**
9. Osborn DA, Evans N, Kluckow M: Effect of early targeted indomethacin on the ductus arteriosus and blood flow to the upper body

and brain in the preterm infant. Arch Dis Child Fetal Neonatal Ed 88:F477–F482, 2003. **Failure of ductal constriction in the first day after birth is associated with subsequent severe IVH.**

Retinopathy of Prematurity

Michael F. Chiang and John T. Flynn

KEY CONCEPTS

- Retinopathy of prematurity (ROP), an abnormal vasoproliferative retinal disease, is a leading cause of childhood blindness throughout the world.
- Major risk factors for ROP include low birth weight, low gestational age, supplemental oxygen exposure, and systemic illness.
- Onset and progression of ROP generally occurs between 31 and 44 weeks' postmenstrual age.
- Because of the narrow time window for diagnosis and treatment, existing guidelines for diagnostic ROP examinations should be followed closely.
- Multiple clinical studies demonstrate that sight-threatening ROP may be treated effectively with laser photocoagulation or cryotherapy.
- Long-term ocular sequelae of severe ROP include retinal detachment, retinal folds, amblyopia, strabismus, glaucoma, high myopia, nystagmus, and retinal scarring.

Retinopathy of prematurity (ROP) is a disease of premature infants characterized by abnormal retinal neovascularization during development. Normal retinal vascularization, which begins at 16 weeks' gestation, is completed by approximately 40 weeks' gestation. For reasons not entirely understood, exposure to the extrauterine environment often disrupts the retinal vascularization process in premature infants, leading to ROP.

Significant risk factors for the development of ROP include low birth weight, low gestational age, supplemental oxygen exposure, systemic illness, white race, and multiple birth status. Specific disease entities correlated with the presence of ROP include respiratory distress syndrome, intracranial hemorrhage, suspected sepsis, and patent ductus arteriosus. The overall incidence of ROP among infants with birth weight less than 1251 g was 65.8% in a major multicenter research study. When it occurs, ROP generally affects both eyes, although the severity may be asymmetrical.

The onset and development of ROP generally occurs between 32 and 44 weeks' postmenstrual age. ROP spontaneously regresses in approximately 90% of cases and is followed by near-normal retinal vascular growth. However, the remaining 10% of cases are characterized by progressively worsening extraretinal neovascularization, which places patients at very high risk for permanent visual impairment secondary to traction retinal detachments and retinal folds that may extend to involve the macula and optic disc (Fig. 1). Overall, ROP is a leading cause of childhood blindness throughout the world, particularly in high- and middle-income countries.

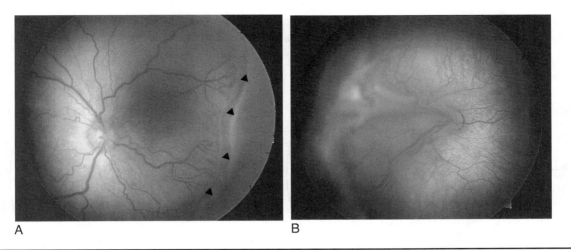

FIGURE 1. *A,* Stage III retinopathy of prematurity (ROP), with mild plus disease. Note area of extraretinal fibrovascular proliferation (*arrows*) at junction of vascular and avascular retina, along with tortuous arteries and dilated veins indicative of plus disease. *B,* Stage IV ROP. Note large retinal detachment, caused by vitreoretinal traction from contraction of extraretinal fibrovascular tissue.

BOX 1 Guidelines for Retinopathy of Prematurity Diagnostic Examination of Premature Infants

- Infants requiring examination
  - Birth weight <1500 g or gestational age ≤ 28 weeks
  - Birth weight 1500 to 2000 g, with unstable clinical course
- Timing of examination
  - Initial exam between 4 and 6 weeks' chronologic age or 31 to 33 weeks' postmenstrual age (whichever is later)
  - Follow-up exams determined by findings at initial exam
- Method of examination
  - Experienced ophthalmologist
  - Dilated examination with binocular indirect ophthalmoscopy

Based on Fierson WM, Palmer EA, Petersen RA, et al: Screening examination of premature infants for retinopathy of prematurity. Pediatrics 108:809–811, 2001.

BOX 2 International Classification of Retinopathy of Prematurity

- **Location:** Three zones, all centered on optic disc.
  - Zone I: Posterior pole. Circle with radius extending from the optic disc to twice the distance from the disc to the center of the macula.
  - Zone II: From edge of zone I to point tangential to nasal ora serrata, and around to area near temporal equator.
  - Zone III: Residual crescent anterior to zone II.
- **Extent:** Specified as clock hours as observer looks at each eye.
- **Severity:** Five stages.
  - Stage I: Demarcation line.
  - Stage II: Ridge.
  - Stage III: Ridge with extraretinal fibrovascular proliferation.
  - Stage IV: Subtotal retinal detachment.
  - Stage V: Total retinal detachment.
- **Plus** disease: Plus (+) qualifier is added when vascular shunting is so marked that veins are enlarged and arteries are tortuous in posterior pole of retina.

Modified from Committee for Classification of Retinopathy of Prematurity: An international classification of retinopathy of prematurity. Arch Ophthalmol 102:1130–1134, 1984.

Additional mechanisms for visual loss in patients with ROP include amblyopia, strabismus, glaucoma, high myopia, nystagmus, and retinal scarring.

Expert Opinion on Management Issues

DIAGNOSIS

The American Academy of Pediatrics, American Academy of Ophthalmology, and American Academy for Pediatric Ophthalmology and Strabismus published a guideline in 2001 proposing requirements for ROP diagnostic examination (Box 1). It states that all infants with birth weight less than 1500 g or with a gestational age of 28 weeks or less should be examined for ROP by an experienced ophthalmologist. Selected infants with birth weight of 1500 to 2000 g should also be examined if they are at high risk because of an unstable clinical course.

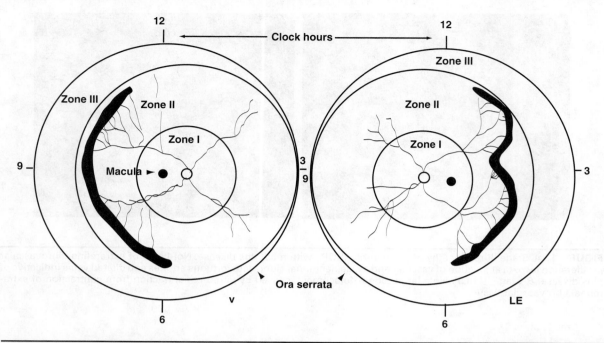

FIGURE 2. Schematic retinal diagram used to describe examination findings according to International Classification of Retinopathy of Prematurity (ICROP) system. Location of disease is described in terms of concentric zones, and extent of disease is described in terms of clock-hour sectors. Pictured image shows five contiguous clock-hour sectors of stage III ROP in zone II of each eye. LE, left eye; RE, right eye.

Initial dilated examination should be performed between 4 and 6 weeks' chronologic age or between 31 and 33 weeks' postmenstrual age, whichever is later. Follow-up examinations are scheduled based on initial findings and intended to observe for disease progression to the point where treatment is required or for spontaneous disease regression followed by normal retinal vascularization. Premature infants must be monitored carefully during pupillary dilation and ocular examination, particularly for episodes of apnea and bradycardia and for signs suggestive of ileus.

The International Classification of Retinopathy of Prematurity (ICROP) is a standardized system for describing the location, extent, and severity of acute ROP (Box 2). *Location* of disease reflects the amount of normal retinal vascularization that occurred before onset of ROP and is delineated by dividing the retina into three zones centered around the optic disc (Fig. 2). ROP in zone I is most severe. *Extent* of disease refers to the number of clock hours affected. In general, involvement of greater retinal circumference reflects more severe ROP. *Severity* is defined by five stages that reflect progressively worsening disease. Stage III is characterized by the development of extraretinal fibrovascular tissue, which has a high risk of causing vitreoretinal traction and eventual retinal detachment (see Fig. 1). *Threshold disease*, the level at which 50% of untreated eyes progress to retinal detachment, is defined by satisfying each of three criteria: presence of stage III ROP in zones I or II; involvement of at least five contiguous clock-hour sectors or at least eight interrupted clock-hour sectors; and presence of plus disease.

TREATMENT

Treatment of ROP is currently based on the results of several major clinical studies. In 1988, the multicenter Cryotherapy for Retinopathy of Prematurity (CRYO-ROP) randomized, controlled trial determined that treatment with cryotherapy to the avascular retina significantly decreases the risk of poor structural or functional visual outcome for infants with threshold ROP. However, long-term follow-up studies involving this cohort of patients found that many of them still develop poor visual outcomes, despite having good structural outcomes after successful treatment.

Laser treatment has largely replaced cryotherapy as the treatment modality of choice for threshold ROP because several clinical studies suggest that laser photocoagulation to the avascular retina is at least as effective as cryotherapy, and laser is less traumatic and more flexible for treating the posterior retina. In 2003, the multicenter Early Treatment for Retinopathy of Prematurity (ETROP) randomized, controlled trial determined that laser photocoagulation significantly decreases the risk of poor structural or functional visual outcome for infants with type 1 prethreshold ROP. This category of ROP was defined as any of the following: zone I, any stage, with plus disease; zone I, stage III, without plus disease; or zone II, stage II or III, with plus disease.

Invasive vitreoretinal surgical procedures may be beneficial for infants with ROP that progresses to stages IV or V despite maximal treatment with laser or cryotherapy. However, outcomes from invasive ocular surgery are variable.

Common Pitfalls

- Because the onset and progression of ROP generally occur between 31 and 44 weeks' postmenstrual age, there is a critical time window for effective diagnosis and treatment.
- For each particular institution, criteria for ROP examination and follow-up should be established by neonatologists, ophthalmologists, and neonatal intensive care unit staff. These criteria should be readily available, and specific personnel should be assigned responsibility for ensuring that all infants meeting criteria are examined.
- If the infant with ROP, or at risk for ROP, is discharged home or transferred to another facility, arrangements for appropriate follow-up ophthalmic examination should be made in advance. If this cannot be done, the infant should not be discharged or transferred.
- If scheduled ocular examinations for infants with acute ROP are missed for any reason, alternative arrangements should be made immediately. The importance of ophthalmic examination for maximizing the likelihood of a favorable outcome must be emphasized to parents verbally and in writing.
- Infants with ROP requiring treatment should receive laser photocoagulation or cryotherapy within 48 to 72 hours. When necessary, arrangements should be made to transfer the infant to a hospital with adequate facilities for treatment and postoperative care.

Communication and Counseling

ROP is an intraocular disease process that cannot be observed without dilated ophthalmoscopy. To help parents understand the disease process and significance of ROP, they should be instructed about the structure and development of the retina, the nature and classification of ROP, and the natural history of ROP. Parents should be updated about progression of disease and, when necessary, provided with information about treatment options as well as possible short-term and long-term outcomes.

Infants of very low birth weight, especially those with severe ROP, require close ophthalmic monitoring throughout childhood because of increased incidence of problems such as retinal detachment, retinal dragging, amblyopia, strabismus, glaucoma, high myopia, and nystagmus. Parents should be given realistic expectations regarding visual prognosis. This is particularly true for infants with severe ROP requiring treatment, given that long-term observational studies demonstrate that many of these infants have poor functional visual outcomes, despite successful treatment with good structural outcomes.

SUGGESTED READINGS

1. Committee for the Classification of Retinopathy of Prematurity: An international classification of retinopathy of prematurity. Arch Ophthalmol 102:1130–1134, 1984. **International consensus statement describing ICROP system for classifying ROP.**
2. Cryotherapy for Retinopathy of Prematurity Cooperative Group: Multicenter trial of cryotherapy for retinopathy of prematurity:

Preliminary results. Arch Ophthalmol 106:471–479, 1988. **Initial results from multicenter randomized controlled CRYO-ROP trial establishing efficacy of cryotherapy for treatment of threshold ROP.**
3. Cryotherapy for Retinopathy of Prematurity Cooperative Group: Multicenter trial of cryotherapy for retinopathy of prematurity: Ophthalmological outcomes at 10 years. Arch Ophthalmol 119:1110–1118, 2001. **Reports long-term data from CRYO-ROP study, indicating long-term value from cryotherapy in treatment of threshold ROP.**
4. Early Treatment for Retinopathy of Prematurity Cooperative Group: Revised indications for the treatment of retinopathy of prematurity: Results of the Early Treatment for Retinopathy of Prematurity randomized trial. Arch Ophthalmol 121:1684–1696, 2003. **Multicenter randomized controlled ETROP trial indicating that earlier treatment of infants with high-risk prethreshold ROP significantly reduces unfavorable structural and functional outcomes.**
5. Fierson WM, Palmer EA, Petersen RA, et al: Screening examination of premature infants for retinopathy of prematurity. Pediatrics 108:809–811, 2001. **Statement from the American Academy of Pediatrics, American Academy of Ophthalmology, and American Association for Pediatric Ophthalmology and Strabismus on guidelines for ROP examination.**
6. Hardy RJ, Palmer EA, Dobson V, et al: Risk analysis of prethreshold retinopathy of prematurity. Arch Ophthalmol 121:1697–1701, 2003. **Describes a computer model, based on data from the CRYO-ROP study, for predicting eyes with prethreshold ROP that have high risk for progressing to unfavorable structural outcome.**
7. McGregor ML, Bremer DL, Cole C, et al: Retinopathy of prematurity outcomes in infants with prethreshold retinopathy of prematurity and oxygen saturation >94% in room air: The high oxygen percentage in retinopathy of prematurity study. Pediatrics 110:540–544, 2002. **Discusses two multicenter randomized controlled trials (HOPE-ROP and STOP-ROP) examining effects of supplemental therapeutic oxygen on the rate of progression from prethreshold to threshold ROP.**
8. Msall ME, Phelps DL, Hardy RJ, et al: Educational and social competencies at 8 years in children with threshold retinopathy of prematurity in the CRYO-ROP multicenter study. Pediatrics 113:790–799, 2004. **Reports long-term data from CRYO-ROP study regarding developmental, social, and educational challenges.**
9. Ng EY, Connolly BP, McNamara JA, et al: A comparison of laser photocoagulation with cryotherapy for threshold retinopathy of prematurity at 10 years: 1. Visual function and structural outcome. Ophthalmology 109:928–935, 2002. **Prospective trial indicating that laser-treated eyes had better structural and functional outcome than cryotherapy-treated eyes.**
10. Reynolds JD, Hardy RJ, Kennedy KA, et al: Lack of efficacy of light reduction in preventing retinopathy of prematurity. N Engl J Med 338:1572–1576, 1998. **Multicenter randomized controlled LIGHT-ROP trial indicating that reduction of light exposure did not lower risk of ROP.**

Circumcision

Helen M. Towers

KEY CONCEPTS

- There is no medical indication for routine circumcision in the newborn.
- Academic societies from Canada, Australia, and Great Britain, as well as the American Academy of Pediatrics (AAP), explicitly do not recommend routine circumcision of the newborn.
- If circumcision is performed, it should be done by experienced personnel with appropriate analgesia.

The history of male circumcision possibly originated in eastern Africa in prebiblical times as a cultural ritual of purification. Religious circumcision for Jews and Muslims was performed for thousands of years, but only in the 19th century did circumcision become a practice governed by the medical community. Cultural, geographic, and socioeconomic influences led to widely disparate views on the subject. The incidence of male circumcision today varies from less than 2% in Scandinavian countries to approximately 64% in the United States, with U.S. numbers trending downward in the past few years. Although the exact frequency is unknown, an estimated 1.2 million males undergo circumcision a year in the United States at a cost of between $150 and $270 million. Ethnicity and race also influence circumcision rates, with whites considerably more likely to be circumcised than blacks or Hispanics (81% vs. 65% or 54%, respectively). Although female circumcision (clitorectomy) occurs predominantly within certain sects of the Muslim community and some African countries, it is now outlawed in many countries and not discussed further here.

Expert Opinion on Management Issues

INDICATIONS

Many indications are presented to support circumcision of the newborn. A common mnemonic is the five M's: Moses, Mohammed, Mother, Money, and Medicine. Ritual circumcision is performed by Jews and Muslims. Maternal education, associated with higher socioeconomic groups, is associated with increased rates of circumcision. Those who perform circumcision clearly benefit financially, and only rarely is there an actual medical reason for it. Phimosis, the inability to retract the foreskin, was commonly presented as a reason to perform circumcision. It is now recognized that separation of the epithelial layers between the glans and the foreskin is incomplete at birth, and the foreskin may not be retractable for at least 5 years in some boys. Minor inflammatory problems occur in both circumcised and uncircumcised males, with meatitis more common in circumcised males and balanitis and inflammation of the foreskin more common in uncircumcised older males.

Hygiene was also suggested as a reason to perform circumcision, but little evidence supports any association between hygiene and penile circumcision. Education regarding the care of the uncircumcised penis should be available to all parents.

It has long been argued that the incidence of urinary tract infection (UTI) is reduced in circumcised males; however, a number of conflicting reports have led to the conclusion there is at best a *potential* benefit in circumcising males for this reason. The rate of UTI in the general population is approximately 1% and approximately 0.2% in circumcised males.

More recent evidence from sub-Saharan Africa suggests an increased risk of female-to-male transmission of human immunodeficiency virus (HIV) in uncircumcised males, although it is a great leap to suggest this as a reason to circumcise males, particularly in countries with a low prevalence of HIV.

PROCEDURE

Circumcision can be performed with a Gomco clamp, a metal cone that fits over the glans and lies between it and the prepuce. The distal foreskin is then removed. A Plastibell is a plastic cone that fits over the glans. The foreskin is stretched over it and a ligature applied at the base. The distal foreskin is then excised. The base of the Plastibell is left in situ and the rest of the cone removed. The plastic base falls off in a few days. A Mogen clamp can also be used, which provides hemostasis by shielding the glans from the scalpel. It is commonly used by mohels, who perform ritual circumcision for those of the Jewish faith.

Pain Control

A subcutaneous circumferential ring of 0.8 mL of 1% lidocaine without epinephrine at the midshaft of the penis can provide adequate analgesia with reduced physiologic stress. A eutectic mixture of local anesthetics (EMLA) cream containing 2.5% lidocaine and 2.5% prilocaine is sometimes used, with 1 to 2 g of cream applied to the distal half of the penis approximately 60 to 90 minutes prior to the procedure. Compared to placebo groups, the pain response appears to be attenuated, but the prolonged time of application and preparation makes this method less likely to be performed correctly and therefore a less effective analgesia in the clinical setting. The use of oral analgesics is inadequate for the procedure itself but can be used with discretion if discomfort appears afterward.

Side Effects

The complication rate of circumcision is between 0.2% and 0.6%. The most common problem is bleeding, seen in approximately 0.1% of cases. Pressure, hemostatic agents, cautery, or sutures are usually sufficient to deal with this infrequent problem. Infection, manifested by redness and purulence, is occasionally seen. Other problems include poor cosmetic result, recurrent phimosis, meatal stenosis, chordee, inclusion cyst, and retained Plastibell devices. It is clearly important that those performing this procedure become proficient and sufficiently skilled to minimize complications.

Ethical Concerns

Importantly, the consent for neonatal circumcision is provided by the parents, not the patient. Given that the majority of circumcisions are nontherapeutic, some practitioners consider the performance of a painful, nonbeneficial procedure unethical.

Common Pitfalls

Common pitfalls in management of circumcision include inadequate explanations or exaggerations to parents regarding the benefits and complications of circumcision. Other areas of concern include inadequate pain control, perhaps secondary to inadequate expertise in performing dorsal penile nerve block (DPNB). Only local anesthetic *without epinephrine* should be used for circumcision. The use of an EMLA as topical anesthetic or oral sucrose solutions is an inadequate analgesic measure for circumcision. If circumcision is performed after the newborn period, general anesthesia should be used. Box 1 shows the absolute contraindications to circumcision in the newborn period.

Communication and Counseling

The importance of discussing both benefits and risks of circumcision with parents should not be underestimated. There is no medical indication for circumcision. An elective, painful procedure, it is performed without apparent benefit to the infant and carries the possibility of harm. However, religious and cultural differences reflect the wide disparity in circumcision rates throughout the world, and sensitivity to these differences should be evident in discussion with parents. All parents of uncircumcised males should be adequately informed of routine hygienic measures that do not involve complete retraction of the foreskin.

SUGGESTED READINGS

1. American Academy of Pediatrics Task Force on Circumcision: Circumcision policy statement. Pediatrics 103(3):686–693, 1999. **Statement that discusses in detail the potential benefits and risks of male circumcision.**
2. Lander J, Brady-Freyer B, Metcalfe JB, et al: Comparison of ring block, dorsal penile nerve block, and topical anesthesia for neonatal circumcision, a randomized controlled trial. JAMA 278(24):2157–2162, 1997. **Study indicating that a block anesthetic should be the analgesia of choice in circumcision.**
3. Taddio A, Goldbach M, Ipp M, et al: Effect of neonatal circumcision on pain responses during vaccination in boys. Lancet 345 (8945):291–292, 1995. **One study that showed increased responsiveness to pain in circumcised males at the time of immunization.**
4. To T, Agha M, Dick PT, Feldman W: Cohort study on circumcision of newborn boys and subsequent risk of urinary-tract infection. Lancet 352(9143):1813–1816, 1998. **Large study evaluating UTIs in circumcised and uncircumcised boys, indicating a small benefit of circumcision of less magnitude than previously described.**

Hearing Loss

Abbey L. Berg

KEY CONCEPTS

- Moderate to significant hearing loss is one of the most common congenital disorders in newborns, occurring in approximately 6 infants per 1000 births. The use of a high-risk register only identifies 40% to 50% of those infants with permanent hearing loss. This impairment can be conductive (dysfunction in the outer and/or middle ear), sensory (dysfunction in the cochlea), neural (dysfunction in the VIII auditory nerve and beyond), or mixed (some combination), and fluctuating, delayed onset, or progressive.
- Permanent congenital hearing loss affects a child's speech/language, literacy, educational, and psychosocial development. Poor communication and literacy abilities can have an impact on earning capacity.
- Hearing loss must be identified early with habilitation implemented as soon as possible because critical periods for language development occur from birth through 5 years of age. To address the need for early identification and habilitation, 38 states and the District of Columbia passed legislation mandating universal newborn hearing screening (UNHS); a standard of care endorsed by the National Institutes of Health (NIH) 1993 Consensus Panel, the American Academy of Pediatrics (AAP, 1999), and the Joint Committee on Infant Hearing (JCIH, 2000). It is recommended that all infants be screened and identified for hearing loss by 3 months of age and receive habilitation and intervention by 6 months of age.

Expert Opinion on Management Issues

ACCEPTED ASSESSMENTS

Only physiologically based methods are acceptable for the screening of newborns: specifically, evoked otoacoustic emissions (EOAEs) and/or auditory brainstem response (ABR), an early evoked potential. Otoacoustic emissions (OAEs), sounds generated by the outer hair cells of the inner ear, are preneural in origin. To observe these responses, an intact outer, middle, and inner ear must be present. To record OAEs, a probe is inserted in the ear canal. The probe stimulates the ear with calibrated click or tonal stimuli and records the responses (sounds) generated by outer hairs in response to the stimuli. These cochlear responses are signal averaged. ABRs are the reflection of averaged electrical activity of the VIII nerve and auditory brainstem pathways that can be detected with scalp electrodes. Synchronous neural firings are required to observe these responses, so they may be absent in infants with neurologic involvement. Note that neither of these physiologic measures tests hearing per se. Hearing involves perception or cortical involvement. These measures assess precortical

TABLE 1 Acceptable Assessments for Measuring Hearing in Infants and Children

Age	Assessment
Newborn screening: two phases	• WBN: OAE first, then ABR • NICU: ABR first, then OAE
Diagnostic assessment: birth–6 mo	• Family history • Immittance (tympanometry and acoustic reflex threshold) using a high-frequency probe tone • OAE • Frequency-specific physiologic measure (i.e., ABR or ASSR); air and bone conduction as appropriate • Behavioral observation of infant's response to sound: warble or frequency-modulated tones and speech • Parental report of emerging communication and auditory behaviors
Diagnostic assessment: 6–36 mo	• Family history • Behavioral response audiometry: VRA for infants 6–24/30 mo; CPA for children 30–36 mo; speech awareness, threshold, and word recognition assessments • Screening of infant's communication milestones • Immittance (tympanometry and acoustic reflex threshold) using low-frequency probe tone • OAE • Frequency-specific physiologic measure (i.e., ABR or ASSR): air and bone conduction as appropriate and for initial evaluation
Diagnostic assessment: special needs children (developmentally delayed)	• Family history • Immittance (tympanometry and acoustic reflex threshold) using a high-frequency probe tone • OAE • Frequency-specific physiologic measures (i.e., ABR or ASSR): air and bone conduction as appropriate • Observation of infant's behavior to tones, preferably by VRA/CPA if possible, as well as responses to speech stimuli • Parental report of emerging communication and auditory behaviors

ABR, auditory brainstem response; ASSR, auditory steady-state response; CPA, conditioned play audiometry; NICU, neonatal intensive care unit; OAE, otoacoustic emission; VRA, visual reinforcement audiometry; WBN, well-infant nursery.

function; however, they correlate well with hearing. Although both of these methods are cost effective, typically within the range of $25 to $40 per infant, an OAE requires less time to administer than an ABR.

A two-phase screening protocol is recommended. Frequently OAEs are administered first, and should the infant be referred, an ABR is administered. This reduces the number of false positives and keeps the referral rate to an acceptable less than 4%; a one-phase screening increases the referral rate to as high as 10%. Research is emerging that screening infants in the neonatal intensive care unit (NICU) initially by ABR and second by OAE better detects those infants at risk for auditory neuropathy/auditory dyssynchrony (AN/AD), a disorder with normal outer hair cell function and abnormal (absent or dyssynchronous) neural function at the level of the VIII nerve. Children diagnosed with AN/AD exhibit a more reduced ability to process auditory information than their behavioral hearing thresholds suggest.

Middle ear status should be assessed using immittance audiometry (tympanometry and acoustic reflex threshold): a high-frequency probe tone for infants younger than 6 months and a low-frequency probe tone for infants older than 7 months. In addition to these physiologic assessments, children 6 months and older should receive a pure-tone behavioral assessment using visual reinforcement audiometry (VRA), a conditioned behavioral technique in which infant responses to a stimulus is shaped. Conditioned play audiometry (CPA) is reliable for children 30 to 36 months of age. Conventional audiometry (i.e., raising hand) can be used for older children (Table 1).

Families need to consult with an otolaryngologist with expertise in childhood hearing loss to determine the etiology of the hearing loss, the presence of related syndromes of the head/neck structures, and related risk indicators. Further, otolaryngologists can determine whether medical and/or surgical interventions are appropriate.

ACCEPTED INTERVENTIONS

Children identified with permanent hearing loss are treated with conventional amplification (i.e., hearing aids) and/or cochlear implants (CIs). CIs, surgically implanted devices, electrically stimulate auditory nerve fibers located in the cochlea and are used when an infant or child cannot benefit from conventional amplification (i.e., hearing aids). The following criteria for infants and children between 12 and 24 months of age must be met for a CI to be approved:

- Bilateral profound deafness
- Minimal benefit from amplification
- Enrollment in early intervention (EI) or a program for children with deafness
- No medical contraindications

Enrollment in a family-centered EI program before 6 months of age is highly recommended to teach and improve auditory communication skill development and

TABLE 2 Prosthetic Treatment for Permanent Hearing Loss

Device	Use
Hearing aids	Amplifies sound
Frequency-modulated (FM) systems: personal or sound field	Improves the signal-to-noise ratio in less than advantageous listening environments (i.e., classrooms, playgrounds); can be beneficial for children who have difficulty processing speech in noise (i.e., children with bilateral hearing loss of any degree, unilateral hearing loss, fluctuating hearing loss, children with auditory processing dysfunction)
Cochlear implants	Amplifies sound for infants and children with severe to profound hearing loss who do not benefit from hearing aids
Other assistive technologies	Includes closed-captioned television, alerting devices, telephone amplifiers, tactile aids

TABLE 3 Indicators for Infants at Risk for Progressive or Delayed-Onset Sensorineural or Conductive Hearing Loss

Indicators

- Parental/caregiver concern regarding hearing, speech, language, or developmental delay
- Family history of permanent childhood hearing loss
- Stigmata associated with a syndrome known to include sensorineural, conductive, or eustachian tube dysfunction
- Postnatal infections associated with sensorineural hearing loss, including bacterial meningitis
- In utero infections, such as cytomegalovirus, herpes, rubella, syphilis, and toxoplasmosis
- Head trauma

- Neonatal indicators: specifically hyperbilirubinemia at serum levels requiring an exchange transfusion, persistent pulmonary hypertension associated with mechanical ventilation, and conditions requiring extracorporeal membrane oxygenation (ECMO)
- Syndromes associated with progressive hearing loss (i.e., neurofibromatosis, Usher's, osteopetrosis)
- Neurodegenerative disorders (i.e., Hunter syndrome, Friedreich ataxia, Charcot-Marie-Tooth disease)
- Recurrent or persistent otitis media with effusion for at least 3 mo

From Joint Committee on Infant Hearing (JCIH), American Academy of Audiology, American Academy of Pediatrics, American Speech-Language-Hearing Association, Directors Speech and Hearing Programs in State Health and Welfare Agencies: Year 2000 position statement: Principles and guidelines for early hearing detection and intervention programs. Pediatrics 106:798–817, 2000.

5

address parental/family concerns. In addition, personal and/or sound-field frequency-modulated (FM) amplification systems, which improve the signal-to-noise ratio in less than advantageous listening environments (e.g., classrooms), can be of extreme benefit to children with all degrees of hearing impairment, unilateral and fluctuating hearing loss, and some forms of auditory processing dysfunction (i.e., difficulty processing speech in noisy environments) (Table 2).

UNACCEPTED INTERVENTIONS

Behavioral observation audiometry (BOA) or any other nonphysiologic measure is unacceptable and not recommended because false-negative results are common.

Common Pitfalls

Timely follow-up of infants referred from newborn hearing screening remains a challenge because there can be long delays between screening, diagnostic evaluation, and amplification. Studies suggest that early identification and habilitation have a positive impact on speech/language and literacy skill development; evidence-based outcome research continues to emerge. A false sense of security may ensue when an infant passes the newborn hearing screen. Hearing loss can occur at any age, and thus surveillance must be ongoing to detect delayed-onset or progressive loss (Table 3).

Fluctuating conductive hearing loss caused by otitis media can affect expressive language abilities as well as school performance. The subtleties of language may be compromised because of the inconsistency of the auditory signal. In addition, unilateral hearing loss is frequently missed in children until they are in school and often is first noticed by the teacher. This type of loss can be problematic for children in compromised listening environments (i.e., classrooms, playgrounds, cafeterias). Children with unilateral hearing loss have a 22% to 35% rate of repeating at least one grade; 12% to 41% receive educational resource services.

CIs are not typically prescribed today for children younger than 12 months; that may change, however, as the Food and Drug Administration (FDA) regulations relax criteria for candidacy. Anesthesia risk to children younger than 12 months must be weighed and balanced with benefits that earlier implantation may provide. In addition, although increases in reported cases of meningitis are reported in children with CIs, prophylactic vaccination and removal of the specific device significantly reduces the risk. Factors that ensure a good CI outcome in children are a source of ongoing research.

Communication and Counseling

Early identification and habilitation of infants and children with permanent hearing loss are essential for improving speech/language and communication skill development outcomes. Professionals need to work in partnership with families. The pediatrician and other primary care physicians make up the infant's medical home and are important in helping develop health care and habilitation for infants identified with hearing loss. Supportive family education, counseling, and guidance needs to be available.

SUGGESTED READINGS

1. Academy of Pediatrics (AAP) Task Force on Newborn and Infant Hearing: Newborn and infant hearing loss: Detection and intervention. Pediatrics 103:527–530, 1999. **AAP position statement endorsing newborn hearing screening.**

2. Cho Lieu JE: Speech-language and educational consequences of unilateral hearing loss in children. Arch Otolaryngol Head Neck Surg 130:524–530, 2004. **Article reviews current literature on the impact of unilateral hearing loss on speech and language development and educational achievement.**

3. Early identification of hearing impairment in infants and young children: National Institutes of Health (NIH) Consensus Statement 11(1):1–24, 1993. **NIH recommendations regarding UNHS, accepted methodologies, interventions, management, surveillance, and educational programs for primary care and caregivers.**

4. Gravel JS, Berg AL, Bradley M, et al: The New York State universal newborn hearing screening project: Effects of screening protocol on inpatient outcome measures. Ear Hear 21:131–140, 2000. **Study describes benefits of two-phase screening protocol.**

5. Gravel JS, Wallace IF: Listening and language at 4 years of age: Effects of early otitis media. J Speech Hear Res 35:588–595, 1993. **Describes language outcomes in a cohort of children with chronic otitis media.**

6. Joint Committee on Infant Hearing (JCIH), American Academy of Audiology, American Academy of Pediatrics, American Speech-Language-Hearing Association, Directors Speech and Hearing Programs in State Health and Welfare Agencies: Year 2000 position statement: Principles and guidelines for early hearing detection and intervention programs. Pediatrics 106:798–817, 2000. **Recommendations from multidiscipline organizations for the identification and management of infants and children with hearing loss.**

7. Keren R, Helfand M, Homer C, et al: Projected cost-effectiveness of statewide universal newborn hearing screening. Pediatrics 110 (5):855–864, 2002. **Increasing the rate of follow-up to diagnostic evaluation after a positive screening test result can potentially increase long-term savings.**

8. Prieve B, Dalzell L, Berg AL, et al: The New York State Demonstration universal newborn hearing screening demonstration project: Outpatient outcome measures. Ear Hear 21:104–117, 2000. **Study describes prevalence of hearing loss in both the well-infant nursery and neonatal intensive care unit and improvement of outcome measures with successive years of program operation.**

9. Thompson DC, McPhillips H, Davis RL, et al: Universal newborn hearing screening: Summary of evidence. JAMA 286(16):2000–2010, 2001. **Comprehensive summary article describing UNHS outcome research.**

10. Yoshinaga-Itano C, Sedey A, Coulter DK, Mehl AL: Language of early and later identified children with hearing loss. Pediatrics 102:1161–1171, 1998. **Study describes increased language abilities of infants identified and receiving habilitation by 6 months of age compared to children identified and receiving habilitation at older ages.**

Special Problems in the Adolescent

Adolescent Gynecology

Jessica A. Kahn, S Jean Emans, Linda M. Kollar and Marc R. Laufer

AMENORRHEA

KEY CONCEPTS

- The differential diagnosis of amenorrhea is extensive, but an underlying condition can usually be identified by a thorough history, physical examination, and selected laboratory studies.
- The average age of menarche is 12.7 years for white girls, 12.2 for Mexican American girls, and 12.1 years for African American girls; 95% of girls have had menarche by age 16.
- Delayed puberty is defined as no secondary sexual characteristics (breast and pubic hair development) by age 13.
- Primary amenorrhea is defined as no spontaneous menses by age 16 years (no menses >4 years after initiation of breast development should also raise concern), and secondary amenorrhea as no menses for 6 months or a length of time equivalent to three previous cycles.

Expert Opinion on Management Issues

Box 1 shows the differential diagnosis of amenorrhea. Box 2 summarizes the history, physical examination, and selected laboratory tests critical in the evaluation of amenorrhea. Treatment for amenorrhea is targeted at the underlying etiology of the problem. For girls who have normal estrogen levels, intermittent oral medroxyprogesterone (e.g., every 1 to 3 months) will yield normal withdrawal flow. For those who are estrogen deficient, estrogen replacement therapy may be instituted using estradiol patches, oral estradiol, conjugated estrogens plus progestin, or hormonal contraceptives (oral contraceptive pill, patch, or ring). Girls who are sexually active should receive hormonal contraceptives. Adequate vitamin D and calcium intake (1300 to 1500 mg per day) and exercise are important adjunctive therapies. Estrogen replacement for girls with anorexia nervosa who are not nutritionally rehabilitated remains controversial. Prolactin-secreting microadenomas are treated with bromocriptine or more recently, cabergoline. Girls with polycystic ovarian syndrome (PCOS) are typically treated with weight loss (if overweight), lifestyle change, hirsutism therapies, combined hormonal medications (such as oral contraceptives), anti-androgens such as spironolactone, and/or insulin-sensitizing agents such as metformin. Patients with congenital anomalies should be referred to an experienced gynecologic surgeon to discuss the options for care. Patients with androgen insensitivity require removal of gonads, hormonal replacement therapy, and counseling about sexuality and fertility issues (see Box 4).

Common Pitfalls

- Failure to obtain an accurate history of sexual activity/risk for pregnancy.
- Failure to assess for eating-disordered behaviors.
- An ultrasound read as "uterine agenesis" in an unestrogenized adolescent girl who in fact has a small prepubertal uterus.
- Not adequately explaining new diagnoses such as vaginal agenesis, PCOS. These diagnoses require multiple visits before the patient can accept/understand the diagnosis.

Communication and Counseling

Adolescents deserve thoughtful office-based counseling with any of the diagnoses listed above. Additionally, print materials and referral to authoritative Internet sites such as www.youngwomenshealth.org will provide teens with the ability to continue learning after their visit.

DYSFUNCTIONAL UTERINE BLEEDING

KEY CONCEPTS

- The normal menstrual cycle occurs every 21 to 35 days and the duration of bleeding is 3 to 7 days, but adolescent cycles are more variable than adult cycles.
- Adolescents frequently have anovulatory cycles in the first 2 years after menarche. Those who have acyclic,

Continued

BOX 1 Differential Diagnoses of Amenorrhea

Hypogonadotropic Hypogonadism

- Hypothalamic tumor (e.g., craniopharyngioma) or history of radiation
- Inadequate gonadotropin-releasing hormone (GnRH) release (Kallmann syndrome)
- Malnutrition secondary to chronic medical conditions (human immunodeficiency virus infection, sickle cell disease, inflammatory bowel disease, celiac disease, chronic renal failure, cystic fibrosis)
- Eating disorder with or without participation in endurance sports
- Stress, depression, psychiatric disorders
- Hyperprolactinemia: pituitary adenoma or drugs/medications (e.g., phenothiazines, haloperidol, metoclopramide, risperidone)
- Hypopituitarism (congenital, head trauma, postpartum necrosis, pituitary infarction, infiltrative disease, radiation)
- Hypothyroidism
- Idiopathic delayed development and menarche

Hypergonadotropic Hypogonadism

- Gonadal dysgenesis and variants: Turner syndrome (45,X), Turner mosaicism, pure gonadal dysgenesis
- Other forms of primary ovarian failure: premature menopause, radiation, chemotherapy, autoimmune oophoritis, resistant ovary, and galactosemia

Ovarian Causes

- Polycystic ovary syndrome
- Gonadal dysgenesis and variants: Turner syndrome (45,X), Turner mosaicism
- Other forms of primary ovarian failure, including premature menopause, radiation, chemotherapy, autoimmune oophoritis
- Ovarian tumor, cyst

Other Endocrine Causes

- Hypothyroidism or hyperthyroidism
- Late-onset congenital adrenal hyperplasia (21-hydroxylase deficiency)
- Addison disease
- Diabetes mellitus
- Cushing syndrome
- Adrenal tumor
- Androgen insensitivity syndrome (AIS)
- 5α-reductase deficiency

Uterine Abnormalities

- Müellerian agenesis (Mayer-Rokitansky-Kuster-Hauser syndrome: absence of the vagina and either absence or severe hypoplasia of the uterus)
- Cervical agenesis or stenosis
- Asherman syndrome (uterine synechiae)

Vaginal and Hymenal Causes

- Müellerian agenesis, transverse vaginal septum
- Imperforate hymen

KEY CONCEPTS—cont'd

prolonged, excessive, and usually painless bleeding may have dysfunctional uterine bleeding (DUB); however, DUB is a diagnosis of exclusion.
- Evaluation of irregular uterine bleeding includes a careful history of the character and timing of bleeding, past menstrual history, history of bleeding disorders in the patient or family members, and history of sexual activity. The physical examination should focus on vital signs (including orthostatics), evidence of androgen excess

or other endocrinologic abnormalities, and signs of a bleeding disorder. A pelvic examination should be performed if it can be done atraumatically.
- Laboratory tests should include a sensitive pregnancy test and a complete blood count. Clotting studies (prothrombin time, partial thromboplastin time, von Willebrand testing, or other platelet function tests) are usually obtained in patients with significant menorrhagia and/or decreased hemoglobin, and a type and cross-matching is done if transfusion is needed. Cervical cultures for gonorrhea and chlamydia should be done if the adolescent is sexually active. Hormonal studies such as thyroid stimulating hormone or tests for polycystic ovary syndrome, a common cause of persistent anovulation, may be indicated.

Expert Opinion on Management Issues

Management of dysfunctional uterine bleeding (DUB) depends upon an accurate diagnosis. Box 3 summarizes the differential diagnosis of abnormal vaginal bleeding. The goals of management in adolescents with DUB are to correct hemodynamic instability, control excessive bleeding, correct anemia, prevent further abnormal bleeding, and provide long-term follow-up. Table 1 summarizes treatment strategies, which depend on the severity of the clinical presentation.

Common Pitfalls

- Not ruling out other disorders, especially pregnancy and infection, as a cause of abnormal vaginal bleeding
- Not interviewing patients confidentially to assess for a history of sexual activity or sexual abuse

Communication and Counseling

The health care provider must be in close contact with adolescents who have moderate to severe DUB during the initial phase of the treatment to ensure that the bleeding is slowing and the patient understands all instructions.

VAGINITIS

KEY CONCEPTS

- Vaginitis involves inflammation and/or infection of the vagina, and common presenting symptoms include vaginal discharge, pruritus, and odor. If the vulva is involved, girls may have vulvar discomfort, a burning sensation, or pruritus.
- Common causes of vaginitis include infectious agents (bacterial vaginosis, candidiasis, and trichomonas), chemical or physical irritants (laundry detergent, soaps, panty liners, chlorine, bubble bath, poor hygiene, tightly fitting clothing), or a foreign body.

BOX 2 History, Physical Examination and Laboratory Studies in Adolescents with Amenorrhea

History

- Growth and pubertal development
- Sexual history, symptoms of pregnancy
- Nutritional status and recent weight loss
- Symptoms of depression
- Recent stresses
- Athletic involvement
- Headaches
- Galactorrhea
- Abdominal pain, diarrhea, blood in stools
- Signs of androgen excess, such as acne and hirsutism
- History of systemic diseases, such as thyroid disease or inflammatory bowel disease
- History of radiation or chemotherapy
- Medications and illicit drug use
- Family history (parental growth and development, mother's and sisters ages of menarche, and gynecologic and endocrinologic disorders)

Physical Examination

- Weight, height, BMI, and blood pressure
- Examination of the thyroid
- Sexual maturity rating of breasts and pubic hair
- Gentle compression of the breasts to identify galactorrhea
- Assessment for any signs of androgen excess, such as acne, hirsutism, or clitoromegaly
- Neurologic examination should assess visual fields, fundi, and ability to smell
- Abdomen: palpate to evaluate for masses
- External genitalia: assess for estrogenization (pale pink vaginal mucosa)
- Assessment of internal pelvic structures (important in primary amenorrhea and normal secondary sexual characteristics)

Laboratory Testing

- Initial tests
  - Urine or serum pregnancy test
  - Complete blood count (CBC)
  - Erythrocyte sedimentation rate (ESR)
  - Thyroid stimulating hormone (TSH) and either free thyroxine (FT_4) or thyroxine (T_4) and thyroxine binding globulin index (TBGI)
  - Follicle stimulating hormone (FSH)
  - Prolactin (PRL)
- Tests if signs of androgen excess
  - Testosterone (and free testosterone), DHEAS, and first morning (8 AM) 17 hydroxyprogesterone; insulin, glucose testing
- Ancillary tests that may be indicated
  - Pelvic ultrasound
  - Assessment of bone density
  - Chemistry panel
  - Karyotype (if elevated FSH)
  - Imaging of central nervous system (e.g., if neurologic abnormalities or elevated prolactin level)

BOX 3 Differential Diagnoses of Abnormal Vaginal Bleeding in the Adolescent

- Pregnancy: implantation bleeding, spontaneous abortion, ectopic pregnancy
- Dysfunctional uterine bleeding
- Infection: cervicitis, pelvic inflammatory disease
- Trauma to the cervix or vagina
- Other gynecologic disorders: cervical hemangioma, uterine anomalies, ovarian cysts or tumors, foreign bodies such as a retained tampon, breakthrough bleeding associated with hormonal contraception
- Hematologic disorders: thrombocytopenia, leukemia, aplastic anemia, von Willebrand disease, other platelet and clotting disorders
- Endocrine disorders: thyroid disease, diabetes mellitus, hyperprolactinemia, polycystic ovary syndrome, ovarian failure
- Systemic diseases
- Medications: anticoagulants, platelet inhibitors, androgens, spironolactone, tricyclic antidepressants, atypical antipsychotics

Expert Opinion on Management Issues

Table 2 gives a summary of diagnostic methods and common treatment options for infectious causes of vaginitis.

Common Pitfalls

- Not recognizing that physiologic leukorrhea (a white, mucoid, asymptomatic vaginal discharge that occurs in girls as puberty begins) is a common cause of vaginal discharge in adolescent girls
- Not taking a confidential history to assess for sexual activity

Communication and Counseling

- Diabetes mellitus, immunocompromise, and excessive moisture in the vulvar area are risk factors for yeast infections; thus, young women with recurrent infections may benefit from treatment of underlying disorders, avoidance of tight-fitting clothing, and so on.
- Adolescents should be advised that douching is a risk factor for bacterial vaginosis.

DYSMENORRHEA AND ENDOMETRIOSIS

KEY CONCEPTS

- All patients with pelvic pain should have a complete history and a general physical examination. Clinicians must rule out a pelvic mass or an anomaly of the reproductive tract. A pelvic examination may be helpful in the patient with pelvic pain but should not be a barrier to or requirement for evaluation. A cotton swab (Q-tip) can be used to

Continued

- Signs and symptoms of cervicitis, vaginitis, and urethritis overlap, so a careful history, physical examination, and directed laboratory studies are important in diagnosis.
- Laboratory evaluation may include saline and potassium hydroxide preparations, an amine or "whiff" test (which evaluates whether or not a drop of 10% potassium hydroxide added to the vaginal sample causes an amine or "fishy" odor), measurement of vaginal pH, and sexually transmitted infection screening in sexually active girls.

TABLE 1 Diagnosis and Management of Dysfunctional Uterine Bleeding

Severity of DUB	Clinical Features	Laboratory Findings	Management Strategies
Mild	Monthly menses lasting >7 days or <21 days for ≥2 months Moderately increased flow	Hemoglobin normal	Menstrual calendar. Oral iron to prevent anemia. NSAIDs during menses to lessen flow.
Moderate	Menses every 7–21 days, often with bleeding lasting >7 days	Hemoglobin normal or mildly decreased	Oral contraceptive pills (OCP) preferred, especially for sexually active adolescents: 0.3 mg norgestrel/30 μg ethinyl estradiol (Lo/Ovral, Low-Ogestrel*) or 0.15 mg levonorgestrel/30 μg ethinyl estradiol (Levlen/Nordette/Levora). OCPs given PO bid for 3–4 days until bleeding stops, then qd to complete 21-day cycle. If the patient does not respond, try taper (see *Severe DUB*).
	Moderate to heavy flow		Medroxyprogesterone acetate (MPA) or norethindrone acetate (NETA) are alternatives (if patient or parent does not desire OCPs or patient has medical contraindication to estrogen). MPA is given 10 mg PO qd for 10 to 14 days each month, started on the day of the visit, the 14th day of the menstrual cycle (e.g., days 14–28) or the first day of each calendar month. NETA 5 mg is used similarly. Continue OCPs (or MPA/NETA) for 3–6 months: if normal cycles do not continue, then restart hormonal treatment. Oral iron to treat/prevent anemia.
Severe	Menses every 7–21 days, often with bleeding lasting >7 days Heavy flow	Hemoglobin decreased, often to <9 g/dL	**Inpatient** Hospitalize if initial hemoglobin <7 g/dL, or if orthostatic with heavy bleeding and hemoglobin <10 g/dL. Consider transfusion *only* if the hemoglobin is very low and patient is hemodynamically unstable. 0.5 mg norgestrel/50 μg ethinyl estradiol (Ovral) or 0.3 mg norgestrel/30 μg ethinyl estradiol (Lo/Ovral) q4h until bleeding stops (usually 4–8 tablets), then qid for 2–4 days, tid for 3 days, and bid for 2 wk. Conjugated estrogens (Premarin) 25 mg IV in patients with acute and severe hemorrhage (rarely needed): q4h for 2–3 doses, and begin 0.3 mg norgestrel/30 μg ethinyl estradiol at the same time (to provide progestin to prevent estrogen withdrawal bleed). If estrogen contraindicated, MPA 10 mg or NETA 5 to 10 mg can be given q4h then qid for 4 days, tid for 3 days, and bid for 2 wk (see *Moderate DUB* for subsequent management). Consider examination under anesthesia, dilation and curettage if bleeding not controlled within 24–36 h. 0.3 mg norgestrel/30 μg ethinyl estradiol (Lo/Ovral) for 3–6 months after interval of 4–7 days from the last OCP. **Outpatient** 0.3 mg norgestrel/30 μg ethinyl estradiol (Lo/Ovral, Low-Ogestrel) or 0.5 mg norgestrel/50 μg ethinyl estradiol (Ovral) PO qid × 2–4 days, tid × 3 days, bid × 2 wk, then continue on cyclic OCP for 3 to 6 months (patients who use 50 μg OCP often can be switched to a 30–35 μg OCP after the first cycle). **All Patients** Antiemetic to prevent nausea on high-dose estrogen therapy and oral iron and folic acid (1 mg/day) to treat anemia.

*Use of brand names does not imply endorsement of a particular product.

bid, twice daily; DUB, dysfunctional uterine bleeding; NSAIDs, nonsteroidal anti-inflammatory drugs; PO, by mouth; qhs, at bedtime; qid, four times a day; q*x*h, every *x* hours; tid, three times a day.

KEY CONCEPTS—cont'd

evaluate the vagina for an obstruction and an ultrasound will evaluate for a pelvic mass.

■ *Primary or physiologic dysmenorrhea* is characterized by pelvic pain on the first day or two of menses; the pain may be related to increases in prostaglandin secretion.

■ *Endometriosis* is a common cause of chronic pelvic pain in adolescents. The most severe symptoms occur typically

just before and during menses, but acyclic pain is also a common presentation. Pain tends to increase with time. In contrast to functional dysmenorrhea, the pain of endometriosis persists and gradually increases despite treatment with oral contraceptives and nonsteroidal anti-inflammatory drugs (NSAIDs). Patients whose symptoms persist or increase on this regimen should be

TABLE 2 Diagnostic Criteria and Treatment of Infectious Causes of Vaginitis in Adolescents

Cause of Vaginitis	Diagnostic Criteria or Methods	Common Treatment Options
Bacterial vaginosis (*Gardnerella vaginalis*, anaerobic microorganisms, mycoplasmas replace normal vaginal flora)	Inspection: homogeneous, adherent white or gray vaginal discharge.* Saline microscopy of vaginal secretions: >20% of epithelial cells are "clue cells,"* positive "whiff" test.* Vaginal pH $\geq$ 4.5* Newer methods: Affirm VP, Fem Exam, PIP Activity Test may be useful.	Metronidazole, 500 mg PO bid for 7 days, *or* Metronidazole gel 0.75% 5 g intravaginally qd for 5 days, *or* Clindamycin cream 2%, 5 g intravaginally qhs for 7 days. Sexual partners are not treated.
Candidiasis (*Candida albicans*, other *Candida* species, and *Torulopsis* species)	Inspection: vulvar erythema, "satellite" lesions, edema, excoriation, white odorless vaginal discharge. Saline microscopy of vaginal secretions (potassium hydroxide may be added): pseudohyphae. Vaginal pH < 4.5	Intravaginal topical azole formulations (Clotrimazole, Miconazole, Terconazole as directed), *or* Fluconazole, 150-mg tablet PO single dose. Sexual partners are not treated.
Trichomoniasis (*Trichomonas vaginalis*)	Inspection: typically frothy, green, malodorous discharge. Saline microscopy of vaginal secretions: active flagellated trichomonads. Vaginal pH > 4.5 Culture, rapid tests may be useful.	Metronidazole, 2 g orally single dose. Sexual partners should be treated.

*Commonly used criteria for diagnosis: 3 or more of these must be present.
bid, twice daily; PO, by mouth; qd, daily; qhs, at bedtime.

referred to a gynecologist for operative laparoscopy to diagnose and surgically treat the possible endometriosis. Most adolescents with endometriosis have normal findings or only mild or moderate tenderness on pelvic examination, without detectable masses or nodularity.

Expert Opinion on Management

DYSMENORRHEA

NSAIDs are usually effective in primary dysmenorrhea, but if the patient does not respond to intensive NSAID therapy (i.e., round-the-clock dosing during the painful portion of the cycle), oral contraceptives may be prescribed (Fig. 1).

ENDOMETRIOSIS

Initial treatment is surgery at the time of diagnosis. All visible lesions of endometriosis should be surgically destroyed, and then medical therapy (e.g., a gonadotropin-releasing hormone agonist) is used to decrease the risk of progression of the disease. All medical regimens are directed toward suppression of ectopic endometrial tissue in the hope of eliminating pain and preventing infertility.

Common Pitfalls

- Not recognizing that endometriosis occurs in adolescents. A delay in diagnosis can cause

persistent pain and possible disease progression and infertility.
- Not recognizing that endometriosis lesions in adolescents may differ in appearance from those in adults. In adolescents, lesions are commonly clear, red, or brown and not the classic "gun powder" color.

Communication and Counseling

Support groups are helpful for adolescents with endometriosis.

PELVIC MASSES

KEY CONCEPTS

- A pelvic mass found on examination or radiologic imaging must be evaluated fully.
- An ovarian tumor, although rare in an adolescent, can occur and is often discovered as an asymptomatic pelvic mass or as a cause of enlarging abdominal girth.
- Severe pain similar to that associated with appendicitis may represent ovarian torsion, torsion or infarction of an ovarian mass, or perforation of a cyst or tumor.
- Pelvic ultrasonography is helpful in the diagnosis of a pelvic mass. Physiologic, developing ovarian follicles reaching a size of 1 to 3 cm are a normal finding, as are small amounts of fluid in the cul-de-sac. MRI is the standard criterion for the evaluation and identification of pelvic anatomy in patients with müllerian anomalies.

6

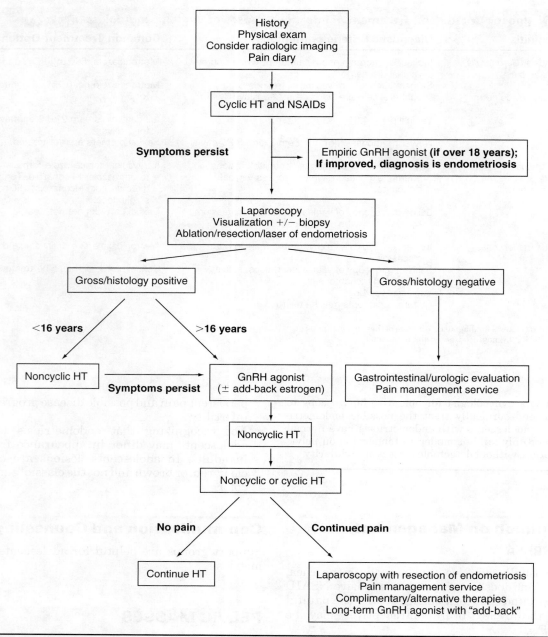

FIGURE 1. Protocol for evaluation and treatment of adolescent pelvic pain and endometriosis. "Add-back," estrogen plus progestin or norethindrone acetate alone; GnRH, gonadotropin-releasing hormone; HT, hormonal therapy (oral contraceptive pills, estrogen/progestin patch, estrogen/progestin vaginal ring, norethindrone acetate, medroxyprogesterone acetate); NSAIDs, nonsteroidal anti-inflammatory drugs; OCPs, oral contraceptive pills. (From Laufer MR, Sanfilippo J, Rose G: Adolescent endometriosis: Diagnosis and treatment approaches. J Pediatr Adolesc Gynecol 16:S3, S3–S11, 2003. Copyright 2003. Reprinted with permission from the North American Society for Pediatric and Adolescent Gynecology.)

Expert Opinion on Management Issues

Table 3 shows the differential diagnoses of pelvic and adnexal masses. If a simple ovarian cyst of less than 6 cm is documented by bimanual examination or ultrasonography in an adolescent, the patient may be followed by serial pelvic examination or ultrasound films until the cyst resolves.

Monophasic oral contraceptive pills are often prescribed to suppress the hypothalamic-pituitary-ovarian axis and prevent the formation of new cysts. Oral contraceptive pills will not shrink an existing cyst. If the cyst has developed on triphasic pills, the patient should be switched to a monophasic pill.

If a cyst is persistent, greater than 6 cm, or causing symptoms, it may be removed laparoscopically, and the fluid and cyst wall should be sent for cytologic-pathologic

TABLE 3 Differential Diagnoses of Pelvic Masses in Adolescents

Location of Mass	Differential Diagnosis
Adnexa/ovary	Ectopic pregnancy, benign ovarian tumors (persistent follicular or corpus luteum cysts of the ovary, mature germ cell tumors), hydrosalpinx, endometriomas, malignant ovarian tumors
Uterus	Pregnancy, uterine anomalies, fibroid
Vagina	Vaginal anomalies, reproductive tract embryonic remnant cysts

study. Attempts should be made to preserve as much ovarian tissue as possible.

Solid or mixed cystic and solid ovarian masses are approached surgically, and a preoperative evaluation is undertaken with the assessment of serum tumor markers to help exclude a malignancy.

Common Pitfalls

- Not including ovarian masses in the differential diagnosis of abdominal or pelvic pain.
- Not evaluating an adolescent with abdominal/pelvic pain and nausea and/or vomiting for possible ovarian/tubal torsion.
- Not attempting to preserve the ovary in cases of ovarian torsion.

ADOLESCENT PREGNANCY OPTIONS COUNSELING

KEY CONCEPTS

- Despite decreases in the prevalence of adolescent pregnancy, the United States has the highest rate of adolescent pregnancy in the industrialized world.
- The goal of pregnancy options counseling is to impart knowledge and facts about all possible options and their implications.
- The environment for the counseling session must be safe for the adolescent to discuss her concerns about the decision.
- The outcome of pregnancy options counseling should be the adolescent's discovery of the right choice for her particular situation.

Expert Opinion on Management Issues

The provider must ensure that rapport has been established and review the parameters of confidentiality. An assurance of unconditional support will allow the adolescent to ask questions and more openly discuss her fears. The provider must provide accurate medical

BOX 4 Questions for Pregnancy Options Counseling

- Have you ever thought about the possibility of pregnancy?
- Have you ever discussed the possibility of pregnancy with anyone?
- What are the positive aspects of pregnancy/abortion/adoption right now for you?
- What are the negative aspects of a pregnancy/abortion/adoption right now for you?
- What do you think it would be like to be a parent?
- Will being a parent change any of your school/career plans?
- What do you think of abortion/adoption?
- What do you think it would be like to have an abortion?
- What do you think it would be like to follow through with an adoption plan?
- Who can you count on to help you?
- Are you safe in your current relationship?
- Has your partner ever hit, slapped, or kicked you?
- Are you safe at home?

information, including gestational age and the relative risks of pregnancy versus abortion, to guide the adolescent in her decision-making process. The current state laws regarding parental consent or notification for abortion or adoption should be shared with the adolescent. The adolescent may need assistance in telling a parent/guardian or trusted adult. The optimal options counseling session is done privately with the adolescent and repeated with whomever she would like to have present: partner, parent/guardian, or other trusted adult. Careful monitoring of the adolescent is required until she has attended her first prenatal appointment or has had an abortion.

Common Pitfalls

- Directive counseling as a result of strong opinions from the provider about the future for the adolescent or potential child.
- Parental ownership of the pregnancy decision.
- Attempting to complete options counseling while the adolescent is in crisis mode and too anxious to concentrate on the decision.

Communication and Counseling

Convey to the adolescent each of the three options: continuing the pregnancy and parenting; continuing the pregnancy and making an adoption plan; or terminating the pregnancy. General questions to consider are included in Box 4. All three of the decisions present challenges for the adolescent. It is particularly important to explore the pregnant adolescent's support systems. More than one meeting may be necessary for the adolescent to make a decision.

SUGGESTED READINGS

1. Braverman PK, Rosenfeld WD (eds): Sexually transmitted infections. Adolesc Med Clin 15:201–421, 2004. **A review of sexually transmitted infections in adolescents; includes discussion of vaginitis.**

2. Emans SJ, Laufer MR, Goldstein DP (eds) Pediatric and Adolescent Gynecology, 4th ed. Philadelphia: : Lippincott-Raven, 1998. **A comprehensive guide to pediatric and adolescent gynecology.**

3. Practice Committee of the American Society for Reproductive Medicine: Current evaluation of amenorrhea. Fertil Steril 82:266–272, 2004. **Guideline for evaluation of amenorrhea in women.**

Sexually Transmitted Diseases in Adolescents

Donald E. Greydanus and Dilip R. Patel

KEY CONCEPTS

- More than half of the nearly 20 million annual sexually transmitted disease (STD) cases occur in sexually active adolescents and young adults, ages 15 to 24 years.
- The most common STDs among youth are infections caused by human papillomavirus, herpes simplex virus, *Chlamydia trachomatis*, *Neisseria gonorrhoeae*, and *Trichomonas vaginalis*.
- Many adolescents are at risk for STDs because of their high coital activity rates, multiple sex partners, substance abuse behavior, immature cervix, difficulties traversing the medical system for comprehensive care, "magical thinking" of adolescents, mistrust of adults, and other factors.
- The 2002 Centers for Disease Control and Prevention Sexually Transmitted Disease Treatment Guidelines are recommended for clinicians.
- Primary prevention of STDs involves proper counseling of youth, immunization for hepatitis A (for males having sex with men and illicit drug users) and hepatitis B (universal), and use of latex condoms for sexually active youth.
- Secondary prevention of STDs involves regular STD screening of all sexually active youth, evaluation for STDs, proper treatment of identified STDs (including asymptomatic infection), and partner notification in the presence of STDs.

There are many types of sexually transmitted diseases (STDs) that can affect youth (Box 1). Many adolescents are at risk for STDs because of their high coital activity rates, multiple sex partners, substance abuse behavior (including use of needles), high risk for other needle injury (tattoos, body piercing, self-mutilation), immature cervix (cervical ectropion), difficulties traversing the medical system for comprehensive care, mistrust of the adult establishment, and "magical thinking" (in which they often feel they are not at risk for consequences of high-risk behavior). Youth at very high risk for the acquisition of STDs include those in jails or detention centers, runaway youth, those engaged in prostitution or other sex-for-survival activity, male homosexual activity, youth who have been abused, mentally retarded youth, and those with a history of STDs. There are several million cases of STDs in youth each year. The most common

---

BOX 1 Sexually Transmitted Agents (Diseases) in Adolescence

- *Chlamydia trachomatis*
- *Neisseria gonorrhoeae*
- Herpes simplex virus (HSV)
- *Trichomonas vaginalis*
- Human papillomavirus (HPV)
- Human immunodeficiency virus (HIV)
- *Treponema pallidum* (syphilis)
- *Molluscum contagiosum*
- Hepatitis A, B, C
- *Haemophilus ducreyi* (chancroid)
- Pediculosis pubis
- Sarcoptes scabiei (scabies)
- Bacterial vaginosis
- *Donovania granulomatis* (granuloma inguinale)
- Behçet disease
- Reiter syndrome
- Others

STDs among youth are infections caused by human papillomavirus, herpes simplex virus, *Chlamydia trachomatis*, *Neisseria gonorrhoeae*, and *Trichomonas vaginalis*. The highest rates of chlamydial and gonococcal infections are in 15- to 19-year-old females.

Expert Opinion on Management Issues

CHLAMYDIA TRACHOMATIS

C. trachomatis bacteria can cause a cervicitis (with vaginal mucosal erythema, hypertrophic cervical erosion, and purulent or mucopurulent cervical discharge), urethritis (with dysuria, urethral discharge), epididymitis, pelvic inflammatory disease (PID), perihepatitis (Fitz-Hugh-Curtis syndrome), and others. All sexually active adolescents should be screened annually (if not more often) for this organism; screening for other STD agents can be done, based on local epidemiologic data. Box 2 reviews *C. trachomatis* cervicitis or urethritis management.

NEISSERIA GONORRHOEAE

N. gonorrhoeae bacteria can cause cervicitis, urethritis, epididymitis, PID, perihepatitis (Fitz-Hugh-Curtis syndrome), disseminated gonococcal infection (including dermatitis, arthritis), and others. Urethral or cervical discharge may be purulent or mucopurulent (mucopurulent cervicitis). The presence of five or more polymorphonuclear leukocytes (PMNs)/1000× magnification defines *urethritis*, whereas *cervicitis* is defined by over 30 PMNs/1000× magnification. Box 2 reviews treatment recommendations for uncomplicated gonococcal urethritis or cervicitis. Infrequently, male urethritis may also be due to *Mycoplasma genitalium* or *Ureaplasma urealyticum*; rarely, it may be caused by *T. vaginalis* or herpes simplex virus (HSV).

BOX 2 Treatment of Cervicitis or Urethritis

***Chlamydia trachomatis* (one of the following)**

- Azithromycin, 1 g orally as one dose
- Doxycycline, 100 mg orally twice a day for 7 days
- Alternative: Ofloxacin, 300 mg orally twice a day for 7 days
- Alternative: Erythromycin base, 500 mg orally four times a day for 7 days
- Alternative: Erythromycin ethylsuccinate (EES), 800 mg orally four times a day for 7 days
- Alternative: Levofloxacin, 500 mg orally once a day for 7 days

***Neisseria gonorrhoeae* (one of the following)**

- Ceftriaxone, 125 mg intramuscularly in one dose
- Cefixime, 400 mg orally in one dose
- Ciprofloxacin, 500 mg orally in one dose
- Ofloxacin, 400 mg orally in one dose
- Levofloxacin, 250 mg orally in one dose
- Alternative: Spectinomycin, 2 g, intramuscularly in one dose
- Alternative: Several others

Herpes Simplex Virus (HSV)

- First episode (one of the following)
    - Acyclovir, 400 mg orally three times a day for 7–10 days
    - Valacyclovir, 1 g orally two times a day for 7–10 days
    - Famciclovir, 250 mg orally three times a day for 7–10 days
- Recurrent episodes (one of the following)
    - Acyclovir, 800 mg orally two times a day, for 7–10 days *or* 400 mg orally three times a day for 5 days *or* 200 mg orally five times a day for 5 days
    - Valacyclovir, 1 g orally once a day for 5 days *or* 500 mg orally twice a day for 3–5 days
    - Famciclovir, 125 mg orally two times a day for 5 days
- Suppressive management
    - Acyclovir, 400 mg orally two times a day, *or*
    - Valacyclovir, 1 g *or* 500 mg orally once a day, *or*
    - Famciclovir, 250 mg orally two times a day

From Workowski KA, Levin WL: Sexually transmitted diseases treatment guidelines: 2002. MMWR Morb Mortal Wkly Rep 51/RR–6:1–79, 2002.

BOX 3 Treatment Options For Pelvic Inflammatory Disease

Oral

- Regimen A
    - Ofloxacin (400 mg orally twice a day for 14 days) *or* levofloxacin (500 mg orally once daily for 14 days)
    - *with or without* metronidazole (500 mg orally twice a day for 14 days)
- Regimen B
    - Ceftriaxone (250 mg intramuscularly in a single dose); *or* cefoxitin (2 g intramuscularly in a single dose) *plus* probenecid (1 g orally concurrently); *or* other third-generation cephalosporin
    - *plus* doxycycline (100 mg orally twice a day for 14 days)
    - *with or without* metronidazole (500 mg orally twice a day for 14 days)

Parenteral

- Regimen A
    - Cefotetan (2 g intravenously every 12 hours) *or* cefoxitin (2 g intravenously every 6 hours)
    - *plus* doxycycline (100 mg orally or intravenously every 12 hours)
- Regimen B
    - Clindamycin (900 mg intravenously every 8 hours) *plus* gentamicin (loading dose 2 mg/kg body weight IV or IM), followed by a maintenance dose (1.5 mg/kg every 8 hours)

From Workowski KA, Levin WL: Sexually transmitted diseases treatment guidelines: 2002. MMWR Morb Mortal Wkly Rep 51/RR–6:1–79, 2002.

6

PELVIC INFLAMMATORY DISEASE

In addition to *C. trachomatis* and *N. gonorrhoeae*, PID, a polymicrobial infection, may involve such agents as *Gardnerella vaginalis*, *M. hominis*, *U. urealyticum*, *Haemophilus influenzae*, coliforms, cytomegalovirus, *Peptostreptococcus*, and other anaerobes. Box 3 lists treatment options for PID, which include various oral and parenteral regimens.

HERPES SIMPLEX VIRUS

Herpes genital infection is usually caused by HSV type 2 (90%) and, less commonly, by HSV type 1 (10%). There are more than 50 million cases, 1 million new cases developing each year. Classic HSV–2 infection in the female usually presents as a cervicitis (often with a mucopurulent discharge) along with vulvar ulcerations. An area of pruritus or hyperesthesia may first develop, followed by small-group vesicles on erythematous bases; these lesions become small, shallow, painful ulcers on the genitals along with inguinal lymphadenopathy. Box 2 reviews herpes genitalis management.

TRICHOMONAS VAGINALIS

T. vaginalis is a unicellular, flagellated protozoan that commonly causes a vaginitis and cervicitis with secondary vulvitis; it produces a profuse, greenish (or gray or yellow-green), frothy ("bubbly") or malodorous discharge. It is intensely pruritic and has a pH of 5.0 to 5.5 or higher. There are 5 million cases each year because of trichomoniasis; many are asymptomatic. "Strawberry marks" (vaginocervical ecchymosis) and swollen vaginal papillae are classic for trichomoniasis. The treatment of choice is metronidazole, 2 g orally as a single dose; an alternative dose of this drug is 500 mg twice a day for 7 days.

BACTERIAL VAGINOSIS

Bacterial vaginosis (BV) is a sexually associated infection caused by an increased growth of anaerobic bacteria, including *G. vaginalis*, Bacteroides species, Mobiluncus and others; *M. hominis* is also found and lactobacilli are reduced. This condition produces a vaginitis in which there is a thin, gray or white, nonpruritic, malodorous ("fishy") vaginal discharge often adhering to vaginal walls. Clinically, the characteristic vaginal discharge, vaginal pH greater than 4.5 (>4.7 on pH paper), positive whiff test, and positive wet mount for clue cells are used for the diagnosis of BV; three of these four criteria make the diagnosis of BV. Box 4 lists the 2002 Centers for Disease Control and Prevention (CDC) recommended treatment of BV.

BOX 4 Management of Bacterial Vaginosis

Preferred (nonpregnant, nonlactating) (one of the following)

- Metronidazole, 500 mg orally, twice daily, for 7 days
- Clindamycin cream (2%), one full applicator (5 g) intravaginally before bedtime for 7 days
- Metronidazole gel (0.75%), one full applicator (5 g) intravaginally two times a day for 5 days

Alternative (nonpregnant, nonlactating) (one of the following)

- Clindamycin, 300 mg orally twice a day for 7 days
- Metronidazole, 2 g orally in a single dose
- Clindamycin ovules, 100 g intravaginally once at bedtime for 3 days

Preferred (pregnant) (one of the following)

- Metronidazole, 250 mg orally, three times a day, for 7 days
- Clindamycin, 300 mg orally, twice a day, for 7 days

From Workowski KA, Levin WL: Sexually transmitted diseases treatment guidelines: 2002. MMWR Morb Mortal Wkly Rep 51/RR–6:1–79, 2002.

BOX 5 Treatment Options for External Genital Warts

Topical Application

- Patient applied
  - Podofilox 0.5% solution or gel
  - Imiquimod 5% cream
- Provider administered
  - Cryotherapy with liquid nitrogen or cryoprobe
  - Podophyllin resin 10% to 25%
  - Trichloroacetic acid (TCA) or bichloracetic acid (BCA) 80% to 90%

Other

- Surgical removal of warts
- Intralesional interferon injection
- Laser surgery

HUMAN PAPILLOMAVIRUS

Human papillomavirus (HPV) accounts for 20 million or more STDs in the United States and are identified with an immunoblot typing system; more than 80 types are now recognized, including some often associated with clinical symptomatology. Most HPV infections are asymptomatic, no warts or condylomas are noted, and the infection is only detected by colposcopy or Pap smear testing. A major concern of HPV infection is the link of some serotypes (16, 18, 31, 33, 35, and others) to cervical neoplasia. The differential diagnosis includes molluscum contagiosum, condyloma lata (syphilis), skin tags (perianal), urethral prolapse, and benign pearly penile papules. Cytology (Pap smear) is the most practical diagnostic tool but has low sensitivity and specificity. Molecular diagnostic modalities include in situ hybridization, dot-blot (commercially available ViraPap/Vira Type), Southern blot, and PCR. The last two are currently used only as research tools. Box 5 lists various measures used to remove the wart-like lesion, although not the viral infection itself.

Common Pitfalls

- Failure to ask adolescents about their possible sexual activity is a potential pitfall.
- Failure to screen for more than one STD can be a problem for some clinicians.
- Adolescents must be afforded the degree of confidentiality that they require to effectively understand and manage high-risk behavior, such as the acquisition of STDs.
- Not all STDs are curable and abstinence is the best message for all adolescents to understand.

Clinicians having the privilege of caring for adolescents should understand the potential problems these patients may have and provide effective management for these conditions. If a clinician is not comfortable with the management of sexual behavior complications of youth, then referral to appropriate experts is recommended. Youth often need to be assured of confidentiality in dealing with such sensitive subjects as sexuality, and clinicians must be prepared to deal with this issue, as allowable by local laws. Failure to accomplish this important clinical goal may result in the adolescent's failing to seek treatment and suffering unnecessary STD complications. Spermicides are no longer considered effective in preventing STD transmission.

It is also important to understand that a sexually active patient may have more than one STD at one time, and thus screening for multiple STDs is important. Local STD patterns can be helpful in guiding this screening process. A negative test for one STD does not mean that other tests will be negative as well. Also, youth and clinicians should understand that some STDs are not curable; for example, treatment does not eradicate HSV or the human papillomavirus. Indeed, abstinence is the best and only sure way to prevent STDs.

Communication and Counseling

Primary prevention of STDs involves proper counseling of youth, immunization for hepatitis A (for males having sex with men and illicit drug users) and hepatitis B (universal), and use of latex condoms for sexually active youth. It is important for clinicians caring for adolescents to ask about the sexual behavior of these youth. Clinicians should educate their patients about the importance of abstinence to prevent STDs (and unwanted pregnancy, as well). Adolescents who are sexually active should consistently and correctly use latex condoms, because many, although not all, STDs can be prevented to a considerable extent by this important practice. *Secondary* prevention of STDs involves regular STD screening of all sexually active youth, evaluation for STDs, proper treatment of identified STDs (including asymptomatic infection), and partner notification in the presence of STDs. Confidentiality is important in the management of adolescents; most state laws allow minors the right to provide their own consent for STD evaluation and management, along with public health requirements for follow-up.

SUGGESTED READINGS

1. Braverman PK, Rosenfeld WD: Sexually transmitted diseases. Adolesc Med Clin 201–428, 2004. **Excellent collection of reviews on STDs in adolescents.**
2. Johnson J: Sexually transmitted diseases in adolescents. In Greydanus DE, Patel DR, Pratt HD (eds): Essential Adolescent Medicine. New York: McGraw-Hill Medical Publishers, 2006, pp 511–542. **Excellent review of important STDs in the adolescent.**
3. Morse SA, Ballard RC, Holmes KK (eds): Atlas of Sexually Transmitted Diseases and AIDS, 3rd ed. New York: Mosby, 2003. **Detailed atlas of STDs.**
4. National Institutes of Allergy and Infectious Diseases: Workshop Summary: Scientific evidence on condom effectiveness for sexually transmitted diseases (STD) prevention 2001. PDF available for download at http://www.niaid.nih.gov/dmid/stds/condomreport.pdf, 2001. **Government document noting the effectiveness of latex condoms.**
5. Workowski KA, Levin WL: Sexually transmitted diseases treatment guidelines: 2002. MMWR Morb Mortal Wkly Rep 1–79, 51/RR–6, 2002. **Standard guidelines for STD treatment from the CDC.**

Adolescent Contraception

David E. Green

KEY CONCEPTS

- Adolescent pregnancy rate in the United States is declining but remains a real health risk and social risk for the adolescent.
- Adolescent contraception must be safe, effective, and reversible.
- Emergency oral contraception is available but underused in the adolescent population.
- Patient education is the cornerstone for preventing unplanned adolescent pregnancy.

The incidence of teen pregnancies in the United States has continued to decline since 1991. In 2003, there were 425,000 teen births, down 5% from 2002. Contraception methods including abstinence have continued to gain acceptance in the adolescent population.

In addition to the increased obstetric complication rate associated with teen pregnancies (preterm birth, pre-eclampsia, operative deliveries, etc.), the long-term social implications continue to be relatively great as well. Sixty-one percent of teen mothers fail to complete high school or take a General Educational Development test (GED) within 2 years of expected high school graduation as compared to 9% of those who did not give birth. Thirty percent of children born to teen mothers are living below the poverty level some 8 to 10 years later. Pregnancy prevention in adolescence is a vital health and social concern.

The goal of adolescent contraception is to provide a safe, effective, and reversible method that is well accepted by the patient. Emergency contraception is available, but many adolescents and clinicians remain unfamiliar with this newer option.

Expert Opinion on Management Issues

Some forms of contraception are not suited for the general adolescent population. Elective sterilization, both male and female, is permanent contraception and therefore not for the average teen. Intrauterine devices are reserved for couples in a long-term, mutually monogamous relationship after at least one birth. The female diaphragm requires fitting, education on proper use, and manipulation of the genitals for insertion; it has up to a 20% failure rate, making it less than ideal for most teens. Male condoms remain the best means for prevention of sexually transmitted diseases (STDs), but they also have an unacceptable failure rate when used as the only means of contraception.

Abstinence is the only 100% effective means of birth control. This remains an individual option that an increasing number of adolescences are choosing. It can be reinforced by practitioners and parents, the educational system, and religious organizations. When adolescents choose to become sexually active, it is imperative that they are knowledgeable about their contraception options if pregnancy is to be avoided.

Hormonal contraception is available in many forms and is the best alternative to abstinence for prevention of adolescent pregnancy. As a category of contraception, hormonal contraceptives are safe, effective, reversible, and well accepted by most users. In addition to the contraceptive effect, many of these products produce beneficial side effects such as decreased menstrual flow and cramping, decreased premenstrual syndrome (PMS) and menstrual migraines, and improved complexion (decreased acne). Serious side effects of these products are rare and the contraceptives are certainly less dangerous to health than pregnancy. Some medicines interfere with efficacy (Box 1).

Medroxyprogesterone acetate, or DMPA (Depo-Provera), is given as a 150-mg injection every 12 weeks beginning with menses. It is 99.9% effective, safe even for the rare adolescents who should not use estrogen products, and reversible (although in rare cases, it may take up to 1 year for normal menses and fertility to return). DMPA is well accepted by most users, although irregular spotting and mild fluid retention may cause some to abandon its use. There are some recent studies that suggest long-term (more than 3 years) DMPA use may induce osteopenia.

Hormonal implant systems (Norplant) are another progesterone-only contraceptive that gained widespread use in recent years. Irregular bleeding and difficulty in removing the implants have resulted in less use by all ages of females.

Oral contraceptives are the most widely used form of reversible birth control in U.S. women. Oral contraceptives contain less than 50 mg of estrogen and one of seven progestins in various combinations. All are equally

---

BOX 1 Medications That May Reduce Efficacy of Hormonal Contraceptives or Oral Contraceptive Pills

Decreased Efficacy of Oral Contraceptive Pills

- Ampicillin
- Carbamazepine
- Felbamate
- Nelfinavir
- Phenobarbital
- Phenytoin
- Primidone
- Rifampin
- Ritonavir
- Tetracyclines
- Topiramate

Decreased Efficacy of DMPA

- Aminoglutethimide

DMPA, medroxyprogesterone acetate (Depo-Provera).

BOX 2 Medical Conditions Precluding Use of Oral Contraceptives in Adolescents

- Pregnancy through 2 weeks postpartum
- History of spontaneous thromboembolic event
- Coronary artery disease
- Congestive heart failure
- Cerebrovascular disease
- Vascular disease associated with:
  - Diabetes
  - Hypertension
  - Systemic lupus erythematosus
- Hypertriglyceridemia
- Antiphospholipid antibodies
- Hepatic adenomas or carcinoma
- Cholestatic jaundice
- Any known or suspected estrogen-dependent neoplasia

---

effective in preventing pregnancy and equally low in side effects such as breakthrough bleeding, nausea, breast tenderness, and so on. Oral contraceptives are begun with menses (on the Sunday after menses begins). Side effects are minimized if the pill is taken about the same time every day. Back-up contraception should be used for the first month and if more than two consecutive pills are missed. If up to two pills are missed, two pills a day are taken until caught up. Decreased menstrual flow (and in some cases amenorrhea) and decreased cramping are to be expected early on, although improved skin complexion (decreased acne) may not be fully realized for up to 6 months.

Because amenorrhea does occur in some users of oral contraceptives, all patients must know that the pill will not abort or otherwise harm an early pregnancy and that it is imperative to begin the next cycle of pills *on time*, even with amenorrhea. Failure to do so is a common cause of "pill failure." The pill should only be stopped when laboratory evidence for pregnancy is positive. Once pills are stopped, normal menses (pre-pill cycles) and fertility resume quickly, usually in less than 90 days. Some medical conditions preclude the use of oral contraceptive pills (Box 2).

Hormonal transdermal patches and vaginal inserts are newer delivery systems for hormonal contraception and evaluation of these products in the adolescent population is lacking. Until such studies are done and show an acceptable failure rate and user compliance, they probably should not be advocated for the average teen.

Emergency oral contraception (EOC) may be particularly suited for the adolescent female. Many first-time and even subsequent episodes of sexual intercourse are unplanned and can result in pregnancy. EOC, if implemented within 72 hours of unprotected intercourse, will decrease the chance of that episode of intercourse resulting in pregnancy by 75%.

Two regimens of EOC are currently available. First, an equivalent of 0.1-mg ethinyl estradiol and 1-mg DL-norgestrel is taken 12 hours apart (two Ovral or four Lo/Ovral tablets orally 12 hours apart). The second regimen is

---

TABLE 1 Adolescent Contraception

Method	Safe	Effective	Reversible	Benefits/Concerns
Abstinence	Yes	Yes	Yes	No STD exposure; unpredictable
DMPA	Yes*	Yes	Yes[†]	Amenorrhea
OCP	Yes*	Yes	Yes	Decreased flow and cramps; decreased acne; interaction with some medications; contraindicated with some medical conditions
Hormonal implants	Probably	Yes	Yes	May require surgical removal and leave scar
Hormonal patches, vaginal inserts	Yes	probably	Yes	Not studied in adolescents
Condoms	Yes	No	Yes	STD prevention; 20% failure rate
Diaphragm	Yes	No	Yes	20% failure rate
IUD	No	Yes	Yes	Reserved for monogamous couple after one child
Male/female sterilization	Yes	Yes	No	Limits lifetime fertility option
EOC	Yes	Yes	Yes	Will decrease pregnancy rate by 75%

---

*Osteopenia may occur in some patients with long-term (>3 yr) use.
[†]Can take up to 12 months to reverse.
DMPA, medroxyprogesterone acetate (Depo-Provera); EOC, emergency oral contraception; IUD, intrauterine device; OCP, oral contraceptive pill; STD, sexually transmitted disease.

taking an equivalent of 0.75-mg levonorgestrel 12 hours apart. Both techniques are equally effective in preventing pregnancy, but the birth control pill regimen, although more readily available, causes more nausea. Use of EOC should prompt the practitioner to discuss better and more effective hormonal contraception with the patient. There are studies suggesting EOC education and treatment packs be given to all women (including adolescents) of reproductive age.

EOC does not abort a pregnancy. If implantation has occurred, the embryo will continue to develop normally. The mechanism of action appears to be rapid alteration of mucus that prevents the sperm from fertilizing the egg. Oral contraceptives taken inadvertently during a viable pregnancy have not been shown to harm the developing fetus.

Elective abortions, medical and surgical, are not contraception and are not included in this discussion. The object here is to prevent unplanned pregnancy and thus not having to deal with an unwanted pregnancy once it has occurred. For an overall synopsis of contraception, see Table 1.

Common Pitfalls

- Failure to educate all adolescents on contraceptive options is a potential pitfall.
- Failure of the adolescent to use the contraceptive method correctly.
- Failure to provide timely EOC and understand its mechanism of action.

Unplanned adolescent pregnancy puts the adolescent and her baby at an increased risk of obstetric complications. Social complications may take generations to overcome. For those adolescents choosing to become sexually active, safe, effective, and reversible methods of preventing unplanned pregnancy are readily available and should routinely be offered by the practitioner.

Communication and Counseling

Because contraception counseling may be awkward in the presence of a parent, attempts should be made to provide this information to the patient alone. Information pamphlets for the adolescent should be placed in private areas of the office, such as the restroom and examination rooms. Helping adolescents understand and accept responsibility for their sexual activity can help avoid undesirable consequences.

SUGGESTED READINGS

1. American College of Obstetricians and Gynecologists: The use of hormonal contraception in women with coexisting medical conditions. ACOG Practice Bulletin 18:674–687, 2000. **A synopsis of medical conditions and medications that affect the various choices of birth control.**
2. Arias E, MacDorman MF, Strobino DM, et al: APGO educational series on women's health issues: Contraception. [monograph]. Annual Summary of Vital Statistics—2002. Pediatrics 112(6): 1215–1230, 2003. **A synopsis of all birth control methods with risks and benefits.**
3. KFF State Health Facts Outline: 50 State Comparisons. Teen Birth Rates, 2002. Available online at http://www.statehealthfacts.org (accessed October 1, 2005.) **Statistical data regarding teen births for 2002.**
4. KFF Fact Sheet. Teen Sexual Activity, January 2003. PDF available online for download at http://www.kff.org/youthhivstds/3040-02.cfm (accessed October 1, 2005.) **Statistical data regarding teen births for 2002.**
5. National Center for Health Statistics: Teen Births, 2002. PDF available online for download at http://www.cdc.gov/nchs/pressroom/03facts/teenbirth.htm (accessed October 1, 2005.) **Statistical data regarding teen births for 2002.**

Issues of Sexual Orientation and Gender Identity

Robert James Bidwell

KEY CONCEPTS

- Homosexuality and bisexuality are part of the spectrum of normal human sexuality.
- Lesbian, gay, bisexual, and transgender adolescents exist within every pediatric practice.
- Lesbian, gay, bisexual, and transgender adolescents have special health needs that are primarily related to growing up in a stigmatizing environment.
- Health providers should provide informed, comprehensive, and supportive health care to lesbian, gay, bisexual, and transgender youth, addressing both medical and psychosocial concerns.

Every pediatric practice has children and youth facing issues of sexual orientation and gender identity. *Sexual orientation* refers to a pattern of affectional and sexual attraction to those of the same or opposite sex. Approximately 3% to 10% of adolescents will recognize that they are lesbian or gay (homosexual) or attracted to both sexes (bisexual). *Gender identity* refers to an inner sense of being female or male. For most individuals, gender identity is congruent with anatomic sex. A small percentage of individuals have a transgender identity in which their gender identity is the opposite of their anatomic sex. They often describe themselves as feeling like they are a male or a female trapped in the body of the opposite sex.

The American Academy of Pediatrics (AAP) has endorsed the position that homosexuality and bisexuality are part of the spectrum of normal sexual development. A lesbian, gay, or bisexual orientation is not chosen and appears to be established by early childhood. Although the classification is controversial, transgenderism (transsexualism) continues to be classified in the American Psychiatric Association's *Diagnostic and Statistical Manual of Mental Disorders, Fourth Edition* (*DSM-IV*) under the rubric "Gender Identity Disorder."

The majority of lesbian, gay, bisexual, and transgender (LGBT) youth are "invisible." This is because most do not fulfill society's stereotypes of what it means to be lesbian, gay, or transgender. Also, when pediatricians address sexuality it is often only in terms of sexual behavior, which is an imprecise indicator of sexual orientation. Perhaps most important, many LGBT youth expect discomfort and disapproval from health providers and therefore are unlikely to reveal their sexual orientation or gender identity even if asked directly.

LGBT adolescents face the same developmental tasks as other teenagers. Nonetheless, their experience is unique because they grow up in an environment that is often unaccepting of LGBT individuals. They are almost completely isolated from accurate information about sexual orientation and gender identity and so they come to accept negative societal beliefs about their sexuality. They lack supportive peer groups, counseling, and visible adult role models. One of their deepest fears is that their sexual identity will become known to their families, friends, and community. The threat of harassment, violence, and rejection is a daily reality for many LGBT adolescents.

Expert Opinion on Management Issues

Like other youth who are isolated, stigmatized, and subjected to violence, many LGBT youth face significant risks to their health. The goal of pediatric management is to facilitate the healthy physical, social, emotional, and sexual development of all LGBT youth. Most of the health risks faced by LGBT youth come from growing up in stigmatizing and hostile environments. For this reason, it is essential that pediatricians be able to provide these adolescents informed, comprehensive, and supportive health care and counseling. This should be in a clinical setting that facilitates open discussion of sexual orientation and gender identity. Because many LGBT youth are "invisible," pediatricians should not presume heterosexuality for any teen. They should recognize the "red flags" of a teenager in distress, including family discord, school problems, substance use, indiscriminate sexual activity, runaway behavior, involvement in the child welfare system, depression, and suicidal ideation. The failure to recognize teens struggling with issues of sexual orientation and gender identity and to address their specific medical and psychosocial needs can result in significant harm. The pediatrician should be able to provide objective information on sexuality, appropriate medical care, supportive counseling, and referral to community resources to all LGBT youth and their families. LGBT adolescents who grow up in an accepting and nurturing environment are at no higher risk of compromised health than other youth.

MEDICAL ISSUES

LGBT adolescents face the same health issues as other teenagers. Like other alienated youth, however, some LGBT adolescents engage in high-risk behaviors that may endanger their physical health. These include substance use, unsafe sexual activity, and suicidal behavior

(see "Sexually Transmitted Diseases in the Adolescent" and "Psychiatric Disorders and Mental Health Disorders in Children and Adolescents"). It should be remembered that sexual activity, heterosexual or homosexual, is an inaccurate indicator of sexual orientation or gender identity. It is likely that only a minority of LGBT youth have engaged in homosexual activity. Many LGBT youth have never been sexually active. Others have been only heterosexually active.

Sexually active LGBT youth, like other adolescents, are at risk for sexually transmitted infections (STIs), pregnancy, and anogenital trauma (see "Adolescent Gynecology" and "Sexually Transmitted Diseases in Adolescents"). In obtaining a sexual history from any adolescent a pediatrician might begin by asking, "Have you ever had sex with another person?" followed in order by the two separate questions, "Have your sexual partners been male (female)?" and "Have any of your partners been female (male)?" Based on responses to these questions, the pediatrician should then ask about specific sexual practices, use of condoms and oral-vaginal barrier protection, contraceptive use, and any history of pregnancy or STIs. Pregnancy and STI screening and Papanicolaou smears should be performed as indicated by an accurate sexual history. Whether a teenager is sexually active or not, it is important to review safer sex practices, STIs, contraception, and pregnancy. The link between substance use and unsafe sexual practices should be emphasized. The provider should also emphasize that abstinence is a healthy option for any teenager.

One of the greatest risks to LGBT adolescents' health is violence from family and peers. The pediatrician should inquire specifically into youths' safety at home, at school, in their dating relationships, and in the community. Depression and suicide are also significant risks and should be discussed with all patients. Transgender youth should receive accurate and nonjudgmental information regarding both hormonal and surgical gender reassignment therapy.

DEVELOPMENTAL AND PSYCHOSOCIAL ISSUES

The developmental and psychosocial issues faced by LGBT adolescents are as important as their medical concerns. It is not the role of the pediatrician to identify every LGBT adolescent. Instead, it is to give all adolescents the message that whatever their sexual orientation or gender identity might be, they are normal and healthy and can look forward to happy and productive lives. This message of acceptance, support, and optimism may be the most important health-enhancing influence a pediatrician has on the life of an LGBT adolescent.

Many adolescents carry negative notions of what it means to be LGBT. The pediatrician should address these misconceptions by giving up-to-date and accurate information on sexual orientation and gender identity. The AAP has developed a brochure titled "Gay, Lesbian, and Bisexual Teens: Facts for Teens and Their Parents," which should be displayed openly in every pediatrician's office. Adolescents' distress about the possibility of being lesbian, gay, or transgender should be explored sympathetically. Nevertheless, LGBT teens should understand that their futures can include loving and committed relationships, parenthood, rewarding careers, and community respect. Visible and respected LGBT role models, including LGBT health providers, can provide invaluable reassurance and hope to LGBT teens and their families.

It is important not to tell an adolescent with homosexual feelings that they are "just going through a phase." Instead, it is more appropriate to say, "I cannot tell you for sure whether you are gay (or lesbian or transgender). Only you can decide this for yourself. But I can give you information and support along the way as you examine your feelings and better understand what they mean for you. As your pediatrician I can tell you that whoever you decide you are in terms of your sexual identity is all right."

It is important to discuss with LGBT youth the realities of growing up in a society not always accepting of their sexual orientation or gender identity. Transgender youth are at highest risk of nonacceptance and violence. Providers should help adolescents address such issues as "coming out" (revealing their sexual identity) and dealing with potential harassment at home, at school, or in the community. "Coming out" too early can be dangerous if a teenager's family and community are unaccepting of who they are. LGBT teens should be introduced to supportive reading materials and web sites and connected to local LGBT teen support groups and supportive counselors. The LGBT adolescent also should know that there is growing societal acceptance of LGBT individuals and that there is no reason that they cannot look forward to a happy, healthy, and fulfilling adulthood.

Parents who learn of their child's LGBT identity often feel anger, guilt, and revulsion. The pediatrician can help heal the rift between parents and an LGBT child by listening to and addressing the parents' specific fears, providing objective information on the spectrum of human sexuality, and connecting families to supportive readings and resources such as local chapters of Parents and Friends of Lesbians and Gays (PFLAG).

Finally, pediatricians have an important advocacy role by educating school and community leaders about normal sexual development and the ethical responsibility to create safe and supportive communities for all LGBT youth. At the same time, pediatricians should inform LGBT students and their parents that they should expect and demand school environments free from harassment and be connected to legal resources if schools do not take this responsibility seriously.

Common Pitfalls

- A major pitfall is the failure to recognize that LGBT adolescents exist in every pediatric practice. In fact, any adolescent may be facing issues of sexual identity.
- It is a mistake to focus only on STDs and safer sex practices when learning an adolescent may be

LGBT. It is just as important to address issues of human sexuality, isolation, diminished self-esteem, and violence.
- Defining same-sex attractions as "only a phase" is misleading and harmful for adolescents discovering their LGBT identities.
- Because of the risk of rejection and violence, parents should be informed of an adolescent's LGBT identity only with the consent of the teen.
- Referring an adolescent to either a secular or religious counselor to change sexual orientation or gender identity is both unethical and dangerous.

Communication and Counseling

One of the most important tasks of pediatricians is to provide LGBT youths and their families informed and supportive care and counseling. Pediatricians should be comfortable in discussing both sexual orientation and gender identity with all adolescent patients. If providers are uncomfortable with or unaccepting of LGBT adolescents, they should refer these youth to colleagues who are able to work with them in a comprehensive, respectful, and supportive manner. Confidentiality should be respected at all times.

Although health providers may have their own issues of concern in working with an individual LGBT youth, they should take time to listen to and address the issues of greatest importance to the individual teen. As LGBT teens grow older, they will face new issues and challenges. It is important that the health provider maintain regular contact with LGBT teens to address these new issues as they arise and provide age-appropriate anticipatory guidance as the teen transitions from childhood to adulthood. Regular contact is especially important because for many LGBT youth the pediatrician may be their only source of objective information and support. This patient-doctor relationship may be literally lifesaving for many LGBT adolescents.

SUGGESTED READINGS

1. Frankowski BL: American Academy of Pediatrics Committee on Adolescence: Sexual orientation and adolescents. Pediatrics 113:1827–1832, 2004. **Clinical report providing guidance for the clinician in rendering pediatric care to LGBT adolescents.**
2. Garofalo R, Harper GW: Not all adolescents are the same: Addressing the unique needs of gay and bisexual male youth. Adolesc Med 14:595–611, 2003. **Review of the developmental, psychosocial, and medical needs of gay and bisexual male youth and how to address them.**
3. Perrin EC: Sexual Orientation in Child and Adolescent Health Care. New York: Kluwer Academic/Plenum Publishers, 2002. **Guidelines on understanding and meeting the health care needs of LGBT youth.**
4. Savin-Williams RC, Cohen KM: Homoerotic development during childhood and adolescence. Child Adolesc Psychiatr Clin N Am 13:529–549, 2004. **Review of research and a reformulated understanding of the development of sexual orientation, sexual behavior, and sexual identity.**
5. Zucker KJ: Gender identity development and issues. Child Adolesc Psychiatr Clin N Am 13:551–568, 2004. **Review of diagnostic, developmental, and behavioral issues, treatment approaches, and ethical concerns related to gender identity disorder.**

Eating Disorders and Obesity

Marsha S. Sturdevant and Bonnie A. Spear

KEY CONCEPTS

- Pediatricians can play a significant role in early detection and medical management of eating disorders and obesity and their coexisting medical morbidities.
- Early recognition of eating disorders and obesity is key to effective treatment.
- Sequential measurement of body mass index is a useful tool in identifying significant changes in weight.
- Medical history screening for purging behaviors such as vomiting, laxative use, or diuretic use during routine health assessments can assist in the early diagnosis of bulimia nervosa.
- Medical comorbidities are common with child and adolescent obesity and include hypertension, obstructive sleep apnea, type 2 diabetes, and hyperlipidemia.
- Laboratory values are often normal in patients exhibiting significant medical malnutrition related to anorexia and bulimia nervosa.
- An interdisciplinary team is considered the standard of treatment for children and adolescents with disordered eating.

Increases in the incidence and prevalence of classic eating disorders—anorexia and bulimia nervosa—have been noted since the 1950s. Over the past decade the prevalence of overweight and obesity in children and adolescents has increased even more significantly and has been accompanied by an emphasis on unhealthy weight loss practices and fad dieting. Along with these increases have come increasing concerns with weight-related issues at younger ages, a growing awareness of disordered eating in males, and increases in the prevalence of disordered eating in minority youth populations.

Underlying psychological issues that coexist with disordered eating include depression, low self-esteem, and family dysfunction. Once problematic eating patterns are established, they can be difficult to change because dysfunctional eating behavior often serves as a coping strategy and becomes habitual.

Early recognition of disordered eating is key to the institution of effective treatment. Pediatricians are often in a position to recognize disordered eating, excessive body image concerns, and weight changes in a timely manner so that early treatment is possible. Unfortunately, physicians often do not recognize or address eating disorders such as anorexia nervosa, bulimia nervosa, or obesity until medical consequences bring young people to their attention. Failure to detect and treat disordered eating at an early stage can result in an increase in severity of the illness, further weight loss in cases of anorexia nervosa, increases in and habituation of purging behavior in bulimia nervosa, or additional weight gain in obesity. Body mass index (BMI), comparing weight to surface area, can be a helpful measurement in tracking weight

and noting early changes. Newly developed growth charts are available for plotting changes in weight, height, and BMI over time and for comparing individual measurements with age-appropriate population norms (http://www.cdc.gov/growthcharts). The purpose of this chapter is to discuss the pediatrician's role in early recognition, medical monitoring, intervention, and case management of adolescents with anorexia nervosa, bulimia nervosa, and obesity.

ANOREXIA NERVOSA AND BULEMIA NERVOSA

Expert Opinion on Management Issues

ACCEPTED INTERVENTIONS FOR ANOREXIA NERVOSA

Several treatment decisions regarding treatment setting and treatment team members follow the initial evaluation of a patient with suspected anorexia nervosa. Anorexia nervosa is a psychiatric condition that leads to significant medical and nutritional compromise. Mental health treatment is the foundation of treatment and should be instituted for all patients in combination with other treatment modalities. Patients who have minimal nutritional and medical issues may be treated in the pediatrician's office in conjunction with a registered dietitian and a mental health practitioner. However, studies demonstrate that over one-half of all children and adolescents with eating disorders not fully meeting all *Diagnostic and Statistical Manual of Mental Disorders, Fourth Edition* (*DSM-IV*) criteria for anorexia or bulimia nervosa still experience significant medical and psychological consequences of these disorders, referred to as *eating disorder not otherwise specified* (EDNOS). Patients with EDNOS require the same careful attention as those who meet the criteria for anorexia nervosa. Rapid weight loss may be associated with physical and psychological compromise similar to marked underweight, even when the patient does not meet the full diagnostic criteria for anorexia nervosa. An interdisciplinary team approach to treatment is generally accepted as the most effective treatment approach, with the team including a physician, nutritionist, nurse, and mental health professional who are each skilled in managing children and adolescents with eating disorders.

In anorexia nervosa, the goals of outpatient treatment are nutritional rehabilitation, weight restoration, cessation of weight reduction behaviors, improvement in eating behaviors, and improvement in psychological and emotional state. Weight restoration alone is not an indicator of full recovery, and forcing weight gain without appropriate psychological support and counseling is not indicated. Cognitive behavioral therapy and interpersonal psychotherapy have been found to be effective in the psychological treatment of anorexia nervosa. Family therapy is also a mainstay in treatment of children and adolescents with eating disorders.

Goal setting for weight restoration generally begins with establishment of a goal weight range at 90% to 100% of median weight for height or, for young adolescents, a BMI of greater than the 10th percentile. In growing children and young adolescents, weight goals must be reevaluated at 4- to 6-month intervals to take linear growth into account. After target goals are set, patients are seen regularly, usually weekly, for physical assessment and nutrition counseling until a steady weight restoration velocity of 0.5 to 2 pounds per week over several weeks has been established. Weekly visits are used to check weight progress, identify ongoing or new barriers to weight restoration, and establish progressive recommendations for physical activity and food intake based on the progress of the previous week. Many patients experience significant medical symptoms during weight restoration and nutritional rehabilitation, including orthostatic lightheadedness, constipation, abdominal pain, and early satiety. These symptoms can be discussed and addressed at weekly surveillance visits.

No psychotropic medication has been Food and Drug Administration (FDA) approved for the treatment of anorexia nervosa. However, many patients are treated with medications for coexisting disorders such as depression, obsessive-compulsive disorder, or generalized anxiety disorders. It is generally prudent to consult a child and adolescent psychiatrist or other clinician with expertise and training in psychopharmacology prior to initiation of psychotropic medication in patients with anorexia nervosa.

ACCEPTED INTERVENTIONS FOR BULIMIA NERVOSA

Medical and nutritional management of patients who binge and purge and are not underweight includes ongoing monitoring for signs and symptoms associated with purging behavior, encouraging regular planned intake of nutritionally balanced meals and snacks with adequate, but not excessive, energy intake, and developing strategies aimed at controlling high-risk situations. Patients are encouraged to initiate steps toward improvement in their eating behavior. For instance, patients need to be encouraged to eat early in the day, at least a small breakfast or mid-morning snack, to avoid the marked hunger and binge eating that may occur at the end of the day. Patients who purge after meals can be encouraged to wait at the table for 15 to 20 minutes after eating. Small, successful changes can be identified and supported by the pediatrician. A registered dietitian working closely with the pediatrician can address specific menu planning and make changes based on the individual patient's progress.

Two serotonin-reuptake inhibitors are approved by the FDA for use in patients with bulimia nervosa, Paxil and Prozac. Only Prozac has FDA approval for use in children and adolescents younger than 18 years of age. Generally it is prudent to seek consultation with a child/adolescent psychiatrist or a physician with specific expertise in psychopharmacology before initiation of psychotropic medications in adolescent patients with bulimia nervosa.

URGENT INTERVENTIONS FOR ANOREXIA NERVOSA AND BULIMIA NERVOSA

The medical and psychiatric complications associated with anorexia nervosa and bulimia nervosa can be potentially life threatening. Medical hospitalization may be required for medical stabilization, initiation of refeeding, and monitoring and management of refeeding syndrome. Medical criteria for hospitalization include weight less than 75% of expected for height, rapid weight loss with associated symptoms and signs of malnutrition, and electrolyte disturbances associated with uncontrollable binging and purging several times each day. Psychiatric hospitalization criteria include suicidal ideation, severe depressive symptoms, or failure of outpatient treatment. However, inpatient psychiatric management is beyond the scope of this chapter; only inpatient medical stabilization will be discussed in this chapter.

At many hospitals, a medical malnutrition protocol is used for nutritional and medical stabilization of patients with anorexia nervosa. The goals of a medical malnutrition protocol are to establish adequate caloric intake, maintain hydration during nutrition rehabilitation, maintain electrolyte balance, maintain medical stability, and block purging behavior. This type of medical protocol is highly structured. Supervisory features include: 1) strict bed rest with bathroom privileges only under nursing supervision, 2) staff supervision whenever food is in the room, 3) removal of containers or vessels in which food or emesis could be hidden, and 4) allowing only the patient to eat in his/her room. Box 1 provides a complete list of the rules for the admission of a medical patient with malnutrition related to anorexia nervosa or bulimia nervosa. Nutritional features of the protocol include an escalating caloric intake beginning at 1200 to 1500 calories per day and rising to a goal of 1800 to 2800 calories per day, as determined by the medical and nutritional status of the patient. After each meal or snack, intake of ordered caloric levels is ensured through replacement for food not eaten via liquid nutritional supplements such as PediaSure or Ensure. These supplements are either drunk by the patient or administered passively through a nasogastric tube if the patient cannot or will not consume the supplement. Every patient is also supplemented with a standard daily multivitamin/mineral tablet.

This protocol provides for a rapid increase in caloric intake, which may lead to symptoms such as lightheadedness, abdominal pain, and constipation, signs such as hypotension, or abnormal laboratory values such as hypoglycemia or hypophosphatemia. Intravenous fluids are administered during the first several days of nutritional rehabilitation to support blood pressure, ameliorate the tendency toward constipation, and replace fluid lost through high urine output. Patient vital signs, including orthostatic pulse and blood pressure changes, are monitored every 4 hours during the first 24 hours of admission, then every 8 hours thereafter. Strict intake and outputs are measured; weights are measured daily in a hospital gown after the morning void and before breakfast. Electrolytes and serum phosphorus are monitored daily during initial escalation of calories. Intravenous fluids

BOX 1 Supervisory Rules for the Inpatient Medical Malnutrition Protocol

Room Inspections

- Nursing staff inspections occur at the beginning and end of each shift.
- No luggage is allowed in the hospital room.
- The room should be free of nonessential items.
- No containers or pitchers are allowed.
- Wastebaskets are kept outside the room, with access under nursing supervision.
- No excess linens are kept in the patient's room.
- Needle and glove boxes are removed from the patient's room and placed outside the door.

No Strenuous Activity

- The patient remains at strict bed rest, with bathroom use under nursing supervision.
- An egg crate mattress is provided for comfort.
- Stretching and range-of-motion exercises are supervised at the bedside by a physical therapist.
- The patient may be up in a chair for meals and a wheelchair for medical tests.

Supervised Bathroom Use

- Patients are allowed 5 minutes per time for voiding or showers.
- Patients use the bathroom only with nursing supervision.
- Patients are allowed one shower daily.

Supervised Consumption of Food and Drink

- All food trays are delivered to the nursing station and checked by the nurse before being served.
- Trays are rechecked after removal from the patient's room.
- All food intake is supervised by nursing staff.
- Nursing staff and the patient keep accurate records of the food eaten.
- Meals may be eaten in bed or up in a chair with a 30-minute time limit for consumption of each feeding.
- After meals and snacks, nursing staff calculates the calorie level of food not eaten and provides liquid supplementation in an equivalent caloric amount.
- Liquid supplement is to be drunk by the patient within 30 minutes; the remaining supplement, if any, is administered via nasogastric tube.
- No food is allowed in the patient's room except during scheduled meals and snacks.
- No access to the bathroom is allowed until 30 minutes after any meal or snack.
- No one except the patient is allowed to eat in the patient's room.

are weaned over several days, with a goal of keeping vital signs relatively unchanged and maintaining blood urea nitrogen of 15 or less.

The medical nutrition rehabilitation protocol is considered complete when the following outcome criteria have been met:

- Adequate caloric intake has been established.
- Symptoms related to the nutritional rehabilitation have been controlled.
- No intravenous fluids have been required for 24 hours.
- The blood urea nitrogen remains 15 or less, with normal serum fasting glucose and stable serum phosphorus.
- Weight is stable off of intravenous fluids.

At completion of the medical nutrition protocol, the inpatient treatment team, which includes psychiatry, medicine, and nutrition, makes recommendations to the patient and family regarding ongoing treatment. Recommendations are based on the combined professional opinions regarding what is the optimal level of treatment required for recovery. Possible recommendations for ongoing treatment include:

- Return to intensive outpatient treatment
- Transfer to an adolescent psychiatry unit for continuation of nutritional rehabilitation and intensification of psychotherapeutic treatment
- Transfer to an eating disorder–specific treatment program
- Transfer to a day treatment program

CONCLUSION

Because of the complicated issues related to eating disorders in adolescents, assessment and ongoing management by an interdisciplinary team is optimal. Medical, nursing, nutritional, and mental health providers should have specific experience in treating eating disorders and expertise in working with adolescents and their families. Within the team, an interested and experienced pediatrician can play important roles in both the inpatient and outpatient treatments of adolescents with eating disorders by providing initial medical assessment, ongoing medical surveillance and case management, and in certain circumstances, initial medical and nutritional stabilization of the patient.

CHILD AND ADOLESCENT OBESITY

Expert Opinion on Management Issues

ASSESSING BODY MASS INDEX

In children and teens, BMI is used to assess underweight, overweight, and risk for overweight (Fig. 1). Children's body fatness changes over the years as they grow. Also, girls and boys differ in their body fatness as they mature. This is why BMI for children, also referred to as BMI-for-age, is gender- and age-specific. The following identifies how to interpret BMI for assessing overweight/obesity (Table 1).

Much of our current understanding of individual/family treatment of pediatric overweight comes from four long-term family-based studies conducted by Epstein. Key findings from Epstein's 10-year follow-up on treatment of overweight and other long-term studies indicate that:

- Child outcomes were improved when both parents and children were targeted for behavior change.
- Increased physical activity was critical to long-term maintenance of weight control in children.
- Youth had more success in maintaining weight loss than parents.

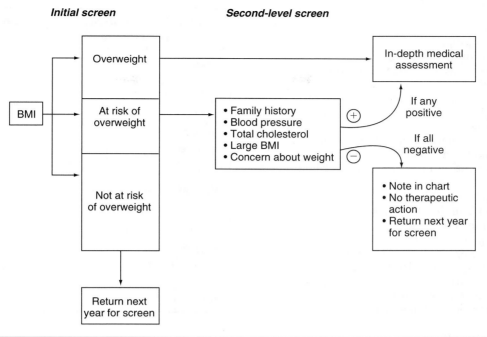

FIGURE 1. Interpretation of body mass index (BMI).

TABLE 1 Interpretation of BMI

Body Mass Index	Interpretation
Greater than 85th but less than 95th percentile	At risk for overweight
Greater than 95th percentile	Overweight

- Longer treatment programs result in greater weight loss.
- The role of parents may be more influential in modifying younger children's behaviors (vs. adolescent behavior).
- Programs using behavior modification (vs. education only) resulted in a greater change in weight status.
- Reducing sedentary activities (rather than increasing structured physical activity) achieved better long-term physical activity levels.
- The caloric intake in most childhood treatment programs ranged from 900 to 1500 kilocalories per day depending on the severity and the presence of medical complications.

Epstein's model shifts the responsibility for habit change from the parent to the child based on the child's developmental capabilities. Although these can be used as a guide, the clinician must evaluate the child's cognitive ability and tailor the program to meet the family/individual's needs. These guidelines include:

- Ages 1 to 5 years—the program must focus on parent management, as parents are the major influences

on child eating and activity. Children of this age are probably not motivated to lose weight.
- Ages 5 to 8—a program in this age group must focus on parent management, but the child must be trained to handle social situations in which food is offered. The child can learn to solicit parental cooperation so that reciprocal reinforcement occurs with the parent or significant adult.
- Ages 8 to 12 years—although children are still responsive to parent management methods, they can take greater responsibility for weight loss. Reading and writing skills are more advanced and children are capable of self-monitoring and goal-setting. Children at this age are more motivated to lose weight to improve athletic performance, look better, and avoid criticism from peers.
- Ages 13 and older—children at this age possess the motivation and capability of managing their program with appropriate support from their parents. Behavior management programs for adolescents must be carefully planned, because conflict can arise when parents are involved as the adolescent is struggling for independence.

ACCEPTED INTERVENTIONS IN CHILD AND ADOLESCENT OBESITY

Interventions that assist in early recognition of overweight/obesity include:

- Plot BMI routinely.
- If there is an increasing BMI percentage, address this before it is greater than 95%.

- Identify children at risk:
  - Parents are overweight.
  - Sibling is overweight.
  - Lower socioeconomic status.
  - Children receive less cognitive stimulation.
- Guidance in nutrition and physical activity
  - Promote consumption of water and milk over juice and soda.
  - Eat as a family.
  - Encourage nonsedentary family activities.
  - Do not use food as a reward.
  - Limit TV/computer/video games to 1 to 2 hours per day.
  - Do not eat in front of the TV.
  - Do not put a TV in the child's room.
- *Family* prevention activities
  - Parents act as role models.
  - Healthy nutrition is practiced at home.
  - Physical activity is practiced at home.
  - Eating out is limited.
  - The family eats meals together.
  - "Special times" do not have to involve food or sedentary activities.
- *School* prevention activities
  - Encourage physical education in grades K through 12.
  - Provide nutritious meals.
  - Control vending machines/encourage healthy vending.
  - Have nutrition and activity education integrated into school curriculum.
- *Community* prevention activities
  - Have safe playgrounds.
  - Provide safe places for bike riding and walking.
  - Promote physical activity outside of school.

STEP APPROACH TO TREATMENT OF OVERWEIGHT CHILDREN

Despite time limitations, the pediatrician can use the steps in Box 2 to begin intervention with the overweight child or adolescent (e.g., for children with BMI greater than the 85th percentile). Many providers have created a prescription pad focusing on improving nutrition and reducing sedentary activities.

CONCLUSION

Obesity is associated with significant health problems in the pediatric age group and is an important early risk factor for much of adult morbidity and mortality. Medical problems are common in obese children and adolescents and can affect cardiovascular health (hypercholesterolemia and dyslipidemia, hypertension), the pulmonary system, the endocrine system (hyperinsulinism, insulin resistance, impaired glucose tolerance, type 2 diabetes mellitus, menstrual irregularity), musculoskeletal system, and mental health (depression, low self-esteem). Pediatricians can play a key role in the prevention and

---

BOX 2 Step Approach to Treatment of Overweight Children

Step 1
- Limit sedentary activities to 1 to 2 hours per day.
- Do not eat in front of TV.
- Eat as a family at least four times a week.
- Limit beverages to milk or water only.

Step 2
- Increase fruit and vegetable servings to 5 to 9 per day.
- Ensure adequate calcium intake (3 to 4 servings per day).
- Increase physical activity.

Step 3*
- Nutrition education.
- Hypocaloric diet.
- Referral to dietitian.

Step 4
- Refer to pediatric weight management program.

*This step might not be done in the doctor's office, because of time and skills needed.

---

treatment of childhood and adolescent obesity through screening, prevention, and initial treatment.

Common Pitfalls

- Laboratory tests can be normal, even in patients with low or high body mass index with significant symptoms. Do not let normal labs lead toward nonintervention in patients with malnutrition or obesity.
- Management with medications for appetite suppression or enhancement should not replace team management and behavioral interventions.
- All members of a management team, whether for anorexia or bulimia nervosa or obesity, need to be skilled in the developmental issues involved in working with children and adolescents.

SUGGESTED READINGS

1. American Academy of Pediatrics: Identifying and treating eating disorders: Policy statement of the AAP. Pediatrics 111(1):204–210, 2003. **Overview of current expert opinion regarding early diagnosis and treatment of disordered eating in children and adolescents.**
2. Epstein LH, Myers MD, Raynor HA, et al: Treatment of pediatric obesity. Pediatrics 101:554–570, 1998. **Provides recommended treatment guidelines based on 10-year longitudinal follow-up.**
3. Glenny AM, O'Meara S, Melville A, et al: The treatment and prevention of obesity: A systematic review of the literature. Int J Obes 21:715–737, 1997. **Reviews the current research of treatment and intervention programs in the area of childhood obesity describing the components of programs that appear to be most effective.**
4. Leiderman SA, Akabas SR, Moore BJ, et al: Preventing childhood obesity: A national conference focusing on pregnancy, infancy, and early childhood factors. Pediatrics 114(4):1139–1173, 2004. **Proceedings of a conference sponsored by Shape-Up America, a nonprofit organization founded by Dr. C. Everett Koop, former surgeon general.**

5. Rome ES, Ammerman S: Medical complications of eating disorders: An update. J Adolesc Health 33(6):418–426, 2003. **Excellent review of current knowledge of medical complications of adolescent anorexia and bulimia nervosa.**

Gynecomastia

David P. Olson and Joseph I. Wolfsdorf

KEY CONCEPTS

- Gynecomastia is common in neonates and adolescents.
- Pubertal gynecomastia is usually a self-limited condition.
- A minority of boys have persistent severe breast enlargement, and they should be thoroughly evaluated.
- No medical therapy has been clearly proven to be efficacious in adolescents with gynecomastia.

Gynecomastia refers to benign proliferation of glandular breast tissue in a male and manifests as a firm or rubbery concentric mass under the areola. In pediatric medicine, it occurs in neonates, rarely in prepubertal children, and in adolescents.

Expert Opinion on Management Issues

INFANCY

In the first few days of life, 60% to 90% of newborn infants have palpable breast tissue caused by transplacental passage of maternal estrogen. Neonatal gynecomastia resolves spontaneously within a few weeks. Neither investigation nor therapy is warranted. Neonatal gynecomastia is occasionally accompanied by galactorrhea (witch's milk). Parents should be advised not to manipulate the baby's breasts in an attempt to discharge the milk as this may lead to infection.

PREPUBERTY

Gynecomastia in a prepubertal boy warrants a thorough exploration of potential estrogen exposures, including creams, lotions, shampoos, contraceptive pills, and contaminated food sources. Identification of the source is often difficult or impossible, because the exposure may have ceased by the time the child presents for evaluation. Precocious sexual development may be associated with gynecomastia; a careful examination of the testes should be performed to stage pubertal development. CT or MRI can be used to search for estrogen-secreting adrenal tumors. Ultrasonography of the testes should be considered to exclude a small, nonpalpable estrogen-secreting testicular tumor. Congenital adrenal hyperplasia (especially 11β-hydroxylase deficiency) and a trophoblastic human chorionic gonadotropin (hCG)-secreting tumor

---

BOX 1 Drugs That Cause Gynecomastia

Hormones
- Estrogens
- Androgens and anabolic steroids
- Human chorionic gonadotropin (hCG)

Antiandrogens and Inhibitors of Androgen Synthesis
- Ketoconazole
- Spironolactone
- Flutamide
- Cyproterone acetate

Psychoactive Medications
- Tricyclic antidepressants
- Diazepam
- Haloperidol
- Risperidone
- Phenothiazines

Recreational or "Street" Drugs
- Marijuana
- Heroin
- Methadone
- Amphetamines
- Alcohol

Cytotoxic Agents
- Vinca alkaloids
- Alkylating agents
- Methotrexate
- Nitrosoureas

Cardiovascular Agents
- Digitoxin
- Calcium channel blockers (diltiazem, nifedipine, verapamil)
- Amiodarone
- Angiotensin-converting enzyme inhibitors
- Methyldopa
- Antimicrobials
  - Isoniazid
  - Ethionamide
  - Ketoconazole
  - Metronidazole
  - Antiretrovirals

Anti-Ulcer Drugs
- Cimetidine
- Ranitidine
- Omeprazole

---

should be ruled out. A rare cause of prepubertal gynecomastia is overexpression of aromatase in extraglandular tissues, which causes increased conversion of androgen to estrogen. Treatment of the underlying disorder will arrest progression of gynecomastia. If the workup is negative, the patient has idiopathic prepubertal gynecomastia that can be expected to resolve within a few years and for which no specific therapy is available. Most cases are idiopathic.

PUBERTY

Sixty percent to 70% of gynecomastia cases occur during puberty. Onset typically occurs at 10 to 12 years of age and is most pronounced between 13 and 14 years of age (at Tanner stages 3 to 4). The breasts are often

TABLE 1 Medical Therapy for Gynecomastia

Drug	Indication and Effect	Comments
Estrogen Modulator		
Tamoxifen citrate	A nonsteroidal antiestrogenic agent that blocks estrogen effect in breast tissue. In uncontrolled trials, most treated individuals with pubertal gynecomastia had ≥50% reduction in breast size. Dose: 10–20 mg PO bid for 3–9 mo.	Low incidence of side effects (nausea and vomiting). Not clear that treatment is more effective than observation alone. Consider a 3-month trial in painful or severe gynecomastia before referring for surgery.
Aromatase Inhibitors		
Testolactone	Synthetic antineoplastic agent that inhibits steroid aromatase activity. Has been used in an uncontrolled trial in a small number of boys with pubertal gynecomastia; 40% decrease in breast size. Dose: 450 mg PO qd for 2–6 mo.	Number of patients who had complete regression was not reported. Not recommended except for rare patients with aromatase excess syndrome.
Anastrozole	A nonsteroidal competitive inhibitor of aromatase enzyme that prevents conversion of androgens to estrogens. Double-blind placebo-controlled trial in pubertal gynecomastia failed to show efficacy. Dose: 1 mg PO qd for 6 mo.	Not recommended except for rare patients with aromatase excess syndrome.

bid, twice daily; PO, orally; qd, every day.

unequal in size and may be slightly tender to palpation. Fat deposition without glandular proliferation (pseudogynecomastia or lipomastia) is common in obese adolescents and must be differentiated from glandular breast tissue. It usually regresses spontaneously within 24 months and does not require intervention. Persistent and severe gynecomastia (diameter of breast tissue >4 cm) infrequently occurs during normal pubertal development. In these cases, pathologic causes of gynecomastia should be ruled out. One should inquire about possible exposure to any of the pharmacologic causes of gynecomastia listed in Box 1. Graves disease, liver disease, and testosterone deficiency syndromes (e.g., Klinefelter syndrome) should be excluded. Serum luteinizing hormone (LH), follicle-stimulating hormone (FSH), and testosterone levels reflect the status of the hypothalamic-pituitary-gonadal axis. Serum estrogen and hCG levels are measured to rule out an estrogen-secreting or an hCG-secreting tumor, respectively.

ACCEPTED INTERVENTIONS

Treatment of gynecomastia is directed at the underlying cause. Specific treatment of endocrinologic disorders associated with gynecomastia should halt progression of breast development but does not always result in satisfactory regression of breast tissue. Surgical breast reduction is indicated when gynecomastia is persistent and severe.

CONTROVERSIAL THERAPIES

Table 1 lists medications that have been used to treat pubertal gynecomastia, but none have been carefully studied in large randomized, controlled clinical trials and their safety and efficacy are not well documented. Testosterone therapy is contraindicated in pubertal gynecomastia because aromatization of exogenous testosterone to estrogen may cause an increase in breast size.

The selective estrogen antagonist tamoxifen has been used to treat pubertal gynecomastia. Some benefit in reducing gynecomastia has been reported; however, its effect may regress after discontinuation. Aromatase inhibitors, which inhibit the conversion of androgens to estrogens, have been used to treat gynecomastia. Testolactone was the first aromatase inhibitor used to treat gynecomastia, but its efficacy is limited. In a recent controlled clinical trial, anastrozole, a newer, more specific aromatase inhibitor, also had little efficacy in pubertal gynecomastia.

Common Pitfalls

- The major pitfall in management is impatience *followed by unnecessary action.*
- Idiopathic gynecomastia in the prepubertal child is a diagnosis of exclusion.

Communication and Counseling

Because gynecomastia is usually transient, the central theme of counseling is reassurance that breast development is a normal variant of physical maturation and can be expected to resolve spontaneously. The potential psychological impact of severe gynecomastia during adolescence, a time when boys are most self-conscious and concerned about their appearance, should not be underestimated. Severe gynecomastia is embarrassing, frequently impairs normal social interactions, and can be emotionally devastating. The psychosocial impact on the affected individual must be evaluated and sensitively addressed.

SUGGESTED READINGS

1. Braunstein GD: Gynecomastia. N Engl J Med 328:490–495, 1993. **Review of gynecomastia in all age groups.**

2. Lazala C, Saenger P: Pubertal gynecomastia. J Pediatr Endocrinol Metab 15(5):553–560, 2002. **Addresses key aspects of pubertal gynecomastia.**

3. Derman O, Danbur NO, Kutluk T: Tamoxifen treatment for pubertal gynecomastia. Int J Adolesc Med Health 15:359–363, 2003. **Use of tamoxifen in the treatment of pubertal gynecomastia.**

4. Braunstein GD: Aromatase and gynecomastia. Endocr Relat Cancer 6:315–324, 1999. **Discusses the role of aromatase in the development of gynecomastia and rationale for aromatase inhibitor use.**

Disorders of Puberty

Rajani Prabhakaran and Madhusmita Misra

The onset of puberty is a complex physiologic event heralded by the activation of the hypothalamic-pituitary-gonadal axis. Very small pulses of gonadotropin-releasing hormone (GnRH) induce elevations of luteinizing hormone (LH) and follicle-stimulating hormone (FSH) throughout childhood. Levels of gonadotropins and the amplitude and frequency of FSH and LH pulses increase slowly but progressively until puberty, when secretion increases, and initial nighttime pulsatility is followed by easily detectable daytime pulsatility. The initial FSH-dominant response to GnRH stimulation progresses to an LH-predominant response.

Age at onset of puberty is approximately 2 years earlier in girls than in boys (average of approximately 9 years in girls and approximately 11 years in boys), and occurs earlier in African American girls than in white girls. Peak height velocity in girls is about 8.3 cm/year and occurs between Tanner stages 2 and 3 (mean age of 11.5 years). In boys, peak height velocity occurs between Tanner stages 3 and 4 (mean age of 13.5 years) and is greater in magnitude (approximately 9.5 cm/year). The 2 additional years of prepubertal height gain in boys and

the greater magnitude of growth velocity contribute to the 10 to 12 cm greater adult height in boys compared with girls. The most visible events occurring at puberty are the pubertal growth spurt and the development of secondary sexual characteristics.

Puberty has two integral components: adrenarche (maturation of the adrenal glands) and gonadarche (maturation of the gonads); events associated with each are described in Figure 1. In girls, gonadarche is heralded by thelarche (onset of breast development); menarche (onset of menses) occurs after approximately 2.4 years of thelarche.

PRECOCIOUS PUBERTY

KEY CONCEPTS

- Puberty is considered precocious if sexual development begins before 8 years in girls (although data from one recent multicentric study suggest that puberty may begin as early as 7 years of age in white girls, and a year earlier in African American girls) or before 9 years in boys.
- In addition to age of onset, a rapid rate of progression of pubertal changes is worrisome.
- Isolated thelarche and adrenarche are usually not associated with bone age advancement or true precocity but require careful follow-up to ensure nonprogression.
- Slow progression of early pubertal changes with commensurate bone age advancement and without compromise of height potential is a variant of normal not requiring treatment.
- Central precocious puberty is isosexual and associated with pubertal secretion of gonadotropins, bone age advancement, and accelerated growth.
- Peripheral precocious puberty results in pubertal progression that is not gonadotropin-driven and is always pathologic; testicular size and symmetry provide clues to etiology of peripheral precocity in boys.

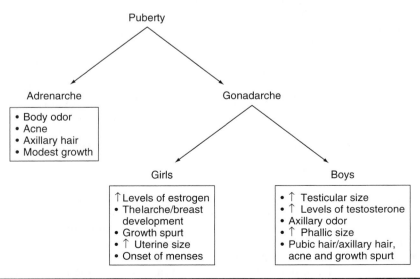

FIGURE 1. Events associated with adrenarche and gonadarche.

BOX 1 Causes of Precocious Puberty

Isosexual Causes

- GnRH-dependent/true/central precocious puberty (CPP)
  - Idiopathic precocious puberty (female-to-male ratio, 10–20:1)
  - CNS disorders (tumors, trauma, infection, hydrocephalus, arachnoid cysts, myelomeningocele, NF1)
  - Associated with early sex steroid exposure (CAH/tumors/McCune-Albright syndrome)
- GnRH independent/peripheral precocious puberty
  - Gonadal causes: granulosa-theca cell tumors, sex-cord stromal tumors, McCune-Albright syndrome, familial male limited precocious puberty
  - Adrenal causes: disorders in steroidogenesis (CAH), adrenal tumors
  - Ectopic causes: hCG secreting tumors (e.g., hepatoblastoma)
- Hypothyroidism
- Exogenous sex hormone exposure (e.g., estrogen- and placenta-containing hair products and creams)
- Incomplete precocious puberty, variants of normal pubertal development
  - Premature thelarche
  - Premature adrenarche
  - Adolescent gynecomastia

Contrasexual Causes

- Virilization in a genetic female (virilizing tumors, exogenous exposure to virilizing hormones, CAH)
- Feminization in a genetic male (estrogen-secreting tumors, exogenous exposure to estrogens, congenital adrenal hyperplasia: 17-hydroxylase, 3β-HSD, 17β-HSD defects)

CAH, congenital adrenal hypoplasia; CNS, central nervous system; GnRH, gonadotropin-releasing hormone; hCG, human chorionic gonadotropin; HSD, hydroxysteroid dehydrogenase; NF1, neurofibromatosis type 1.

BOX 2 Indications for Evaluation of Precocious Puberty

Girls

- All girls <7 years (white) or <6 years (African American) with breast and/or pubic hair development
- All girls >7 years (white) or >6 yrs (African American) with breast development *and*
  - *Rapid progression* (bone age advanced ≥2 years compared with chronological age)
  - *and* predicted adult height ≥2 SD (≥10 cm) below genetic height potential*
  - *CNS-related findings* such as headaches, seizures, focal neurologic deficits; known history of hydrocephalus, arachnoid cysts, CNS infections, tumors, trauma, or NF1
  - *Behavioral issues* where progression of puberty and subsequent attainment of menarche might adversely affect the emotional state of the child or her family

Boys

- Boys with evidence of increased androgen production other than pubic hair development (enlargement of phallus and scrotum, acne, growth spurt) with or without testicular enlargement before 9 years of age

*Genetic height potential in girls (cm) = [(paternal height − 13 cm) + maternal height]/2; genetic height potential in boys (cm) = [(maternal height + 13 cm) + paternal height]/2.
CNS, central nervous system; NF1, neurofibromatosis type 1.

Expert Opinion on Management Issues

Evaluation and management of early puberty depends on the type of precocious puberty and the etiology of the condition (Box 1). When signs of puberty are congruent with the genetic sex of the individual, puberty is *isosexual*. Conversely, when signs are incongruent with the genetic sex of the individual, puberty is termed *contrasexual*. Contrasexual puberty is always pathologic. True precocious puberty results from activation of the hypothalamic-pituitary-gonadal axis, also known as central or gonadotropin-dependent precocious puberty. This may be idiopathic or secondary to central nervous system (CNS) pathology and is always isosexual. Gonadotropin-independent precocious puberty is also called *peripheral precocious puberty*, and it may be isosexual or contrasexual depending on whether the peripheral source of sex steroids is in accordance with the genotype of the individual or not.

Isolated *premature thelarche* refers to breast development in the absence of pubic hair growth or accelerated bone maturation, with a normal predicted height outcome. This is usually seen between birth and 4 years

of age and results from either an aberration in early gonadotropin secretion, with the normal physiological surge of gonadotropins in infancy being larger and longer, or from functional ovarian cysts. FSH levels may be mildly elevated, whereas LH levels are in the prepubertal range. Spontaneous regression is the rule, with normally timed puberty and normal reproductive function. Careful monitoring is necessary to pick up the occasional child who continues to progress into puberty and requires further evaluation.

Isolated *premature adrenarche* refers to predominantly pubic hair development, with mild to moderate acceleration of growth. This is generally seen between 4 and 8 years of age, with gonadarche occurring at the expected time. Evaluation includes a bone age to confirm that skeletal age is not significantly advanced, assessment of levels of dihydroepiandrosterone (DHEAS), androstenedione, and 17-hydroxyprogesterone, and an ACTH stimulation test to pick up mild forms of non-classical congenital adrenal hyperplasia (CAH) if indicated. A greater subsequent risk for hyperinsulinism and polycystic ovarian disease has been described in girls with premature adrenarche.

Evaluation

In addition to age at onset and gender, factors that need to be taken into consideration in evaluation of precocious puberty are rate of progression of sexual development, height potential, presence of pathologic states, and behavior-based factors. Indications for evaluation and referral are described in Box 2; Box 3 describes laboratory and radiologic tests used for evaluation of sexual

BOX 3 Evaluation of Precocious Puberty

History and Physical Examination

- Isosexual or contrasexual
- Complete or incomplete

Laboratory Evaluation

- Serum estradiol, testosterone, LH* and FSH, prolactin, TSH, free T$_4$
- Serum β-hCG (in all boys for hCG-secreting tumors), α-fetoprotein (alternative tumor marker)
- GnRH or GnRH analogue (e.g., leuprolide) stimulation test*
- GnRH stimulation test: 2.5 μg/kg GnRH (maximum 100 μg) given IV with LH and FSH measured at 0 min, 15 min, 30 min, 60 min, 90 min, and 120 min (at least for 1 h); *or* 100 μg GnRH SC with a single sample for LH levels after 40 min
- Leuprolide stimulation test: 500 μg IV or SC with LH and FSH measured at 0, 1, 2 and 3 hours
- Adrenal androgens such as DHEAS, androstenedione, and 8 AM 17-hydroxyprogesterone
- ACTH stimulation test (rule out CAH)

Vaginal Cytology

- Vaginal cytology for maturation index: useful indication of estrogen exposure

Imaging Studies

- Bone age (x-ray left hand and wrist)
- Cranial MRI
- Pelvic sonogram for uterine size (length <35 mm, corpus-to-cervix ratio <1, uterine volume <1.8 mL are prepubertal), presence or absence of endometrial stripe and ovarian cysts and tumors
- CT liver and chest for hCG-producing tumors (e.g., hepatoblastoma), CT adrenals for adrenal tumors
- Skeletal survey for polyostotic fibrous dysplasia if McCune–Albright syndrome suspected

---

*Baseline LH >0.3 IU/L, GnRH stimulated LH >5 IU/mL, leuprolide stimulated LH >6 IU/L suggestive of precocious puberty (third-generation assays for LH measurement).

ACTH, adrenocorticotropic hormone; CT, computed tomography; DHEAS, dihydroepiandrosterone; FSH, follicle-stimulating hormone; GnRH, gonadotropin-releasing hormone; hCG, human chorionic gonadotropin; IV, intravenously; LH, luteinizing hormone; MRI, magnetic resonance imaging; SC, subcutaneously; T$_4$, thyroxine; TSH, thyroid-stimulating hormone.

---

precocity. In boys with precocious puberty, testicular size is an important guide to possible etiology (Fig. 2).

Treatment

Treatment of precocious puberty depends on the etiology, whether it is true/central precocious puberty or GnRH-independent precocious puberty.

GnRH and its agonists are effective in *true/central precocious puberty* and act by downregulating GnRH receptors on gonadotropes, thus suppressing LH and FSH secretion. On cessation of therapy, pubertal responses of gonadotropes to GnRH resume in 3 to 6 months, and menarche usually occurs within 1 year.

The superactive agonist-analogues of GnRH have significantly higher potency, more prolonged duration of action, and less toxicity than natural GnRH. We use depot leuprolide acetate (Lupron Depot) at doses of 0.3 mg/kg every 3 to 4 weeks with excellent results. Adverse effects are few and include local reactions like pain at the injection site and sterile abscesses (seen in approximately 5% with depot preparations). Systemic side effects are unusual. In patients developing sterile abscesses with depot preparations, daily subcutaneous injections of leuprolide acetate (50 μg/kg/day) may be substituted. Inadequate or irregular therapy can worsen final height prognosis because of inadequate suppression of gonadotropins and can even stimulate gonadotropin release. Monitoring is thus important and includes periodic measurement of testosterone levels in boys (should be <20 ng/dL) and estradiol in girls (should be <10 pg/mL), basal gonadotropins (if measured by ultrasensitive assays), GnRH stimulation tests (to determine whether suppression of gonadotropin secretion is adequate), and monitoring of growth, bone age, and secondary sexual characteristics. In girls, serial evaluations of ovarian morphology and uterine size by pelvic sonography may be useful. A deceleration in the rate of growth, regression of secondary sexual characteristics, and slowing in advancement of bone age are reassuring.

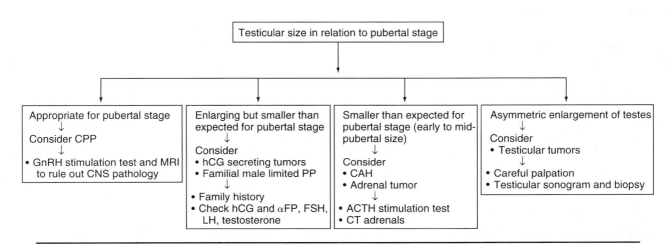

FIGURE 2. Precocious puberty in boys.

Rapid advancement of bone age and suboptimal linear growth after cessation of GnRH analogue therapy often result in an adult height that is less than predicted during therapy. Early institution of therapy is necessary to optimize adult height potential. Simultaneous administration of recombinant human growth hormone in doses of 0.2 to 0.3 mg/kg/week with GnRH analogues has been used to optimize height.

For *GnRH-independent precocious puberty* (such as boys with familial male-limited precocious puberty [FMPP] or girls with McCune-Albright syndrome), GnRH analogues are ineffective in suppressing pubertal progression unless secondary central precocious puberty has supervened. Ketoconazole suppresses gonadal and adrenal synthesis of sex steroids through inhibition of 17-hydroxylase and may be of use. Side effects include mild hepatic injury, reversible renal injury, rash, interstitial pneumonia, and adrenal insufficiency. Testolactone (40mg/kg/day), an aromatase inhibitor, has been successfully used with the antiandrogen spironolactone in boys with FMPP, but resistance to treatment may develop. More potent and specific antiandrogens, such as flutamide and nilutamide, and aromatase inhibitors, such as letrozole, are the latest additions to the therapeutic armamentarium with potentially greater therapeutic efficacy.

Medroxyprogesterone acetate inhibits gonadal steroidogenesis, decreases frequency of menstrual periods and the volume of ovarian cysts, and slows the rate of growth and bone maturation in girls with McCune-Albright syndrome. Unfortunately, some patients escape this effect after 1 to 3 years. Tamoxifen, an anti-estrogen, also reduces bone age advancement, growth rate, and pubertal advancement in McCune-Albright syndrome. Aromatase inhibitors such as letrozole and anastrozole showed initial promise in halting pubertal progression in girls with McCune-Albright syndrome. However, fadrozole, another aromatase inhibitor, was not effective. Other treatment of peripheral precocious puberty includes removal of the etiology (e.g., tumors causing precocity), identification and elimination of exogenous sources of estrogen or androgens, and treatment of congenital adrenal hypoplasia (CAH).

DELAYED PUBERTY

KEY CONCEPTS

- Puberty is considered delayed in girls if thelarche has not occurred by 13 years or if menarche has not occurred by 15 years and breast development is immature.
- Puberty is considered delayed in boys if testicular enlargement (>4 mL) or pubic hair development have not begun by 14 years.
- Absence of menarche by 16 years in the presence of normal breast development in girls is primary amenorrhea.
- Full testicular volume is usually reached within 3.2 ± 1.8 years of onset of puberty, and if progression is unusually slow, pathologic abnormalities may be present.
- Hypogonadotropic hypogonadism (associated with low levels of FSH, LH, and gonadal steroids) includes constitutional delay in growth and puberty, the most common

cause of delayed puberty in boys, but may also be pathologic; associated anosmia suggests Kallmann syndrome.
- A short course of low-dose testosterone may help "jump start" puberty in boys with constitutional delay; treatment is individualized for pathologic causes of hypogonadotropic hypogonadism.
- Hypergonadotropic hypogonadism (associated with elevations in FSH and LH but low levels of gonadal steroids) indicates primary gonadal failure and mandates karyotyping to rule out Turner syndrome in girls and Klinefelter syndrome in boys; elevated gonadotropins are always pathologic.
- Sex steroid replacement is begun in low doses and gradually increased to adult replacement doses to optimize height potential and to mimic endogenous puberty.
- Eugonadotropic causes of pubertal delay include imperforate hymen and vaginal agenesis; levels of gonadotropins and gonadal steroids are normal and surgery may be necessary.

Expert Opinion on Management Issues

EVALUATION

Box 4 lists the causes of pubertal delay. The evaluation of delayed puberty begins with a careful history and examination, including complete nutritional assessment (Box 5). Laboratory evaluation includes assessment of gonadal steroids (testosterone and estradiol), gonadotropins, prolactin, other pituitary hormone deficits, and evaluation for chronic diseases and chronic inflammatory states.

Gonadotropin levels differentiate between hypogonadotropic hypogonadism (hypothalamic or pituitary cause for hypogonadism) and hypergonadotropic hypogonadism (gonadal pathology resulting in elevated gonadotropin levels). The GnRH stimulation test (described in Box 2) unfortunately cannot differentiate between constitutional delay in puberty (the commonest cause of pubertal delay in boys) and idiopathic hypogonadotropic hypogonadism (IHH). However, a family history of constitutional delay with a serial height pattern suggestive of a "late bloomer" points to the former condition. In IHH, but not in constitutional delay, an adrenarchal rise of DHEAS levels is often seen. Following stimulation with GnRH agonists, gonadotropin secretion (especially bioactive gonadotropins) is higher in constitutional delay than in IHH. On the leuprolide stimulation test, a sufficient rise of LH occurs by 180 minutes to permit the discrimination of simple pubertal delay (LH > 6.0 IU/L) from hypogonadotropic hypogonadism (LH < 6.0 IU/L).

Hypergonadotropic patients and all short girls should undergo karyotyping. Turner syndrome is a common cause of short stature in girls, and a 46,XY karyotype in an otherwise healthy phenotypic female suggests complete androgen insensitivity, especially in the absence of pubic and axillary hair. When the karyotype is normal and commensurate with the phenotype, other causes of gonadal failure need to be considered, such as infections, trauma, radiation, chemotherapy, and autoimmune

---

BOX 4 Causes of Pubertal Delay

Hypogonadal Causes

- Hypogonadotropic hypogonadism
  - Constitutional delay in puberty
  - Isolated gonadotropin deficiency: idiopathic hypogonadotropic hypogonadism, Kallman syndrome, mutations in LH and FSH genes
  - Multiple pituitary hormone deficiencies: septo-optic dysplasia, hypothalamic and pituitary tumors, head trauma, radiation, surgery, CNS infections, infiltrative diseases
  - Genetic syndromes: Prader-Willi and Bardet-Biedl
  - Secondary to chronic diseases: undernutrition, anorexia nervosa, intense exercise; gastrointestinal, hepatic, or renal disease; malignancies; chronic infections; iron overload
  - Psychogenic amenorrhea
- Hypergonadotropic hypogonadism in males
  - Klinefelter syndrome
  - Testicular insult: gonadal dysgenesis, anorchia, bilateral cryptorchidism, bilateral orchitis, testicular surgery, radiation, chemotherapy
  - Abnormalities in testosterone synthesis and 5α-reductase deficiency
  - Androgen sensitivity syndromes
  - Noonan syndrome
- Hypergonadotropic hypogonadism in females
  - Turner syndrome
  - Ovarian insults: gonadal dysgenesis, primary or premature ovarian failure (idiopathic, surgical oophorectomy, radiation, chemotherapy, galactosemia)
  - Complete androgen insensitivity

Eugonadal Causes (females)

- Menarche delayed in the presence of breast budding and pubic hair development
- Rokitansky-Meyer-Kuster-Hauser syndrome
- Partial or complete non-canalization of the vagina and imperforate hymen

---

FSH, follicle-stimulating hormone; LH, luteinizing hormone.

BOX 5 Evaluation of Delayed Puberty

History

- Absent versus "stalled" pubertal development
- Cyclic abdominal pain (suggestive of cryptomenorrhea)
- Neurologic symptoms, anosmia, history of head trauma
- General health and nutrition, exercise pattern
- Growth pattern
- Intra- and perinatal history
- Past history of radiation, chemotherapy, or surgery
- Family history of constitutional delay or other causes of pubertal delay
- Use of drugs inducing hyperprolactinemia

Physical Examination

- Standing height, height in relation to weight
- Arm span, upper to lower segment ratio (eunuchoid habitus)
- Thyroid size and consistency
- Secondary sexual characteristics, testicular size and symmetry
- Complete neurologic examination (including tests for anosmia)
- Plotting of serial heights on charts, including pattern for "late maturers"

Laboratory Evaluation

- FSH, LH (hyper- or hypogonadotropic hypogonadism)
- Ultrasensitive estradiol assay, testosterone
- Complete blood count and sedimentation rate (screen for chronic disease)
- GnRH stimulation test in hypogonadotropic hypogonadism
- Thyroid function tests and IGF-1 (if associated slowing of growth is present, to screen for thyroid function and growth hormone deficiency respectively; rule out multiple pituitary hormone deficits)
- Prolactin levels (prolactinomas sometimes manifest as "stalled" puberty)
- Karyotyping (if hypergonadotropic, and in all short girls)

Nutritional Assessment

- Assess nutrition if history and exam suggest nutritional deficiency

Imaging Studies

- Bone age
- Pelvic ultrasound (for uterine and gonadal morphology; also blood-filled and distended uterine cavity and fallopian tubes suggest cryptomenorrhea from vaginal agenesis or imperforate hymen)
- Cranial CT or MRI (to rule out intracranial pathology)
- Consider bone density testing if indicated

CT, computed tomography; FSH, follicle-stiimulating hormone; GnRH, gonadotropin-releasing hormone; IGF, insulin-like growth factor; LH, luteinizing hormone; MRI, magnetic resonance imaging.

---

ovarian failure (in girls). The last is usually a diagnosis of exclusion and mandates investigation for associated autoimmune conditions such as autoimmune thyroiditis and adrenalitis. A low-dose ACTH stimulation test helps rule out primary adrenal failure from autoimmune adrenalitis. Imaging studies are described in Box 5. Bone density testing should be considered in patients who have very delayed puberty and are not taking hormonal replacement.

TREATMENT

Goals of therapy are to (1) induce age-appropriate secondary sexual characteristics, (2) stimulate statural growth by inducing the pubertal growth spurt, (3) optimize psychosocial adjustment, and (4) maximize development of peak bone mass. *Long-term goals* include (1) achievement of fertility, which is easier in patients with hypogonadotropic hypogonadism, and (2) optimal bone mass accrual. Any pathology determined to be responsible for pubertal delay needs to be addressed.

To induce development of secondary sexual characteristics, low doses of gender-appropriate sex steroids are begun at well below the adult replacement dose to avoid compromising adult height. The dose is increased every 6 months such that full replacement dosing is achieved in approximately 2 years. In boys with constitutional delay, a short course of low-dose testosterone (50 mg intramuscularly [IM] every 4 weeks for 4 to 6 months) allows endogenous progression through puberty and may help "jump start" puberty. A role for aromatase inhibitors in increasing testosterone bioavailability and stimulating pubertal progression has been described. Androgens may be required in girls with inadequate pubic hair; however, voice changes and male pattern baldness are side effects. Oral testosterone undecenoate is useful because of its peripheral conversion to dihydrotestosterone, a relatively weak androgen. Anabolic steroids have also been used.

If pubertal delay is a result of chronic illnesses, excessive exercise, or undernutrition, treatment is aimed at correcting the underlying condition. When the underlying cause is hyperprolactinemia, hypothyroidism should be ruled out and a cranial imaging study performed to rule out a prolactinoma. Cabergoline is effective in reducing the size of a prolactinoma and reducing prolactin levels. Adverse effects include headaches, nausea, and postural hypotension, which can be minimized by starting at a low dose (0.25 mg at bedtime given once weekly) and gradually titrating the dose upward to 0.5 mg twice weekly if necessary. Surgery is necessary for an imperforate hymen or in cases of vaginal agenesis.

Common Pitfalls

- Lack of uniformity of gonadotropin assays mandates the gonadotropin stimulation test to diagnose centrally driven precocious or delayed puberty; however, nonavailability of GnRH has resulted in GnRH analogues being used for this test without widely accepted norms.
- Exogenous sources of sex steroids need to be considered when precocious puberty is not gonadotropin driven; however this history can be difficult to elicit.
- Delay in treatment in patients with precocious puberty is associated with poorer height prognosis; thus timely diagnosis and treatment are critical.
- Rapid progression of skeletal maturation after discontinuation of GnRH analogue therapy may result in adult height that falls short of predicted height during therapy.
- Constitutional delay in puberty is a diagnosis of exclusion and can be difficult to differentiate from other causes of hypogonadotropic hypogonadism.
- Failure to recognize other associated endocrine gland failure in children with autoimmune gonadal failure can result in life-threatening situations, particularly if autoimmune adrenalitis is associated.

Communication and Counseling

Communication with the parents and, when possible, the child regarding what constitutes early or delayed puberty, variants of normal, and causes and consequences of early or delayed puberty is critical in management of such patients. Although the majority of children referred to an endocrine clinic for a pubertal disorder have conditions that are variants of normal, recognizing patterns associated with pathology is of paramount importance. Counseling should include a discussion of possible pathology, if applicable, and of height prognosis. Psychosocial issues need to be addressed, especially in children with developmental delays who experience early puberty, in whom the potential for abuse needs to be recognized. When a decision is made not to treat early puberty, parents need to be counseled about pubertal mood swings and the appropriate handling of such situations given the immaturity of the child per chronological age. Reassurance is key in managing children with constitutional delay in puberty, and tips on dealing with peers and societal pressure are invaluable.

SUGGESTED READINGS

1. Eugster EA, Rubin SD, Reiter EO, et al: Tamoxifen treatment for precocious puberty in McCune-Albright syndrome: A multicenter trial. J Pediatr 143:60–66, 2003. **Examines the effects of tamoxifen in slowing pubertal progression in McCune-Albright syndrome.**
2. Herman-Giddens ME, Slora EJ, Wasserman RC, et al: Secondary sexual characteristics and menses in young girls seen in office practice: A study from the Pediatric Research in Office Settings network. Pediatr 99:505–512, 1997. **Examines the ages at which different aspects of puberty begin in boys and girls.**
3. Lee PA: Central precocious puberty: An overview of diagnosis, treatment and outcome. Pediatr Endocrinol 28:901–918, 1999. **Reviews central precocious puberty.**
4. Palmert MR, Malin HV, Boepple PA: Unsustained or slowly progressive puberty in young girls: Initial presentation and long term follow up of 20 untreated patients. J Clin Endocrinol Metab 84:415–423, 1999. **Discusses forms of early puberty that are variants of normal, are not associated with significant bone age advancement, and thus do not require treatment.**
5. Raivio T, Dunkel L, Wickman S, et al: Serum androgen bioactivity in adolescence: A longitudinal study of boys with constitutional delay of puberty. J Clin Endocrinol Metab 89:1188–1192, 2004. **Examines androgen bioactivity in boys with constitutional delay receiving testosterone and an aromatase inhibitor, letrozole versus no treatment, and the effect on pubertal progression.**
6. Roth C, Freiberg C, Zappel H, et al: Effective aromatase inhibition by anastrozole in a patient with gonadotropin-independent precocious puberty in McCune-Albright syndrome. J Pediatr Endocrinol Metab 15(3):945–948, 2002. **Reports the effective use of anastrozole, an aromatase inhibitor in slowing pubertal progression in a patient with McCune-Albright syndrome.**
7. Sedlmeyer IL, Palmert MR: Delayed puberty: Analysis of a large case series from an academic center. J Clin Endocrinol Metab 87:1613–1620, 2002. **Discusses common causes of pubertal delay.**

The Sports Physical

Eric Small

KEY CONCEPTS

- The preparticipation physical evaluation (PPE) is good at picking up musculoskeletal injuries.
- The PPE should be performed 4 to 6 weeks before the sports season.
- One physician in a private setting should perform the entire PPE.
- Certain topics should be briefly touched on in PPE process: sudden death, heat injury, nutritional supplements, concussion, common sports injuries, and weight gain/weight loss.

Each year 15 million children and adolescents have a sports physical or a preparticipation physical evaluation (PPE). There are up to 1500 forms available in various states and schools. Physicians perform them in a variety of ways. Examinations may vary from listening to the heart and lungs to performing a full musculoskeletal examination of multiple joints from head to toe. It is the goal of this chapter to establish a pattern and a process for these evaluations.

One must understand the goals for doing the examinations. The main goal is to ensure the safety and health of athletes during training and competition. Secondary goals include screening for causes of sudden death, screening for conditions that may be exacerbated by sports participation, and allowing for safe and fun participation among athletes.

The exam is divided up into three categories: history, physical, and clearance. This chapter focuses on the process and highlights the salient features of the history, physical, and clearance portions.

Timing of Examination

The examination should be done 4 to 6 weeks prior to the sports season. This means that any pending medical conditions or musculoskeletal injuries can be addressed and resolved or rehabilitated before the start of the season. For example, if an athlete has infectious mononucleosis, 4 to 6 weeks may need to elapse before the spleen returns to normal size and the athlete may safely participate. Another example is an athlete who had anterior cruciate ligament (ALC) reconstruction 5 months earlier. The athlete may be cleared for running and jumping at the time of the examination. The athlete may need another 1 to 3 months before he or she can participate in scrimmages, contact activities, and full competition.

Type of Examination

There are generally two types of examinations that can be performed: individual examination or station examination. The individual examination is definitely preferred as personal health issues such as eating habits, social habits, and family/school functioning can be explored. Ideally, the examination should be done by the student's own personal physician. This physician has the records and has rapport and trust of the patient.

The station examination is one in which multiple examiners examine different parts of the body such as the heart/lung, abdomen, and musculoskeletal systems. There are two variations of the station examination. There may be 6 to 8 different people all examining different body parts or 6 to 8 examiners all doing the entire examination. If more than one examiner is participating, it is preferable to have one examiner do the entire examination as more medical information can be gleaned.

History

It is recommended that the physician use the form included in *The Preparticipation Physical Evaluation*, 3rd edition (see Suggested Readings). I recommend three essential areas to target: cardiac (sudden death or hypertrophic cardiomyopathy), musculoskeletal (sprains, strains, and overuse injuries), and neurologic (concussion, brachial plexus injury). As part of the history it is important to determine whether the young athlete has ligamentous laxity or is tight in the muscles by asking questions, such as, Have you ever dislocated a joint, are you double-jointed, or are you tight in your muscles as compared to your peers?

Expert Opinion on Management Issues

Height, weight, and blood pressure must be taken. A body mass index (BMI) should be calculated to identify athletes who are overweight and obese. The BMI can be used as prevention for diseases and used as a data point for future research.

At a minimum the heart, lung, neurologic systems, and musculoskeletal systems should be examined. When there are positives in the written history or the oral history, these issues should be expanded on in the physical examination. For example, a history of multiple concussions indicates it is physically taxing for the athlete to do maximal push-ups or sit-ups in a time period of 1 minute or to sprint 100 yards. An athlete who has recurrent ankle sprains should be referred to a physical therapist for ankle strengthening, rehabilitation, and supportive bracing.

CLEARANCE

At the conclusion of the PPE one of three choices for clearance status should be assigned: not cleared, not cleared pending further evaluation, or workup required. In the last two categories, it is extremely critical that everyone (physician, school nurse, athletic director, athlete, and athletic trainer) be included in the communication. Regarding the first category, the parent and child should both know why the child was not cleared and what can be done about it.

SUDDEN DEATH

A student dying on the athletic field is a tragedy for all involved: parents, friends, and school staff and personnel. Fortunately these events are rare (perhaps 8 to 12 deaths per year). Important points to cover are family history of sudden death, history of Marfan syndrome, chest pain, and fainting with exercise. Screening electrocardiograms or echocardiograms are not indicated. There are two many false positives and the tests are not cost-effective. If one responds to a family history of sudden death or admits to shortness of breath or chest pain with exercise, then clearance should be withheld until further evaluation by a cardiologist.

HEAT INJURY

Heat injury is an often-overlooked condition that can be prevented. Those participating in multiple bouts of intense exercise throughout the day (two-a-day soccer or football practices), those with a history of heat injury, those on specific medications, and those with specific medical conditions are at risk for heat injury, which includes heat cramps, heat exhaustion, and heat stroke.

MUSCULOSKELETAL CONDITIONS

Anterior Cruciate Ligament

ACL injuries have reached epidemic proportions in adolescents. Since 1993 it has been recognized that females tear their ACL two to eight times more than males, particularly in sports such as soccer and basketball. An injury prevention program, which emphasizes balance and strength, has proven effective.

Stress Fractures

Stress fractures are a result of too much training and not enough time for recovery. An athlete with a history should be counseled on proper training (not to increase training by more than 10% per week) and nutrition. They should be consuming adequate calories for growth and development and physical activity.

Low Back Pain

An athlete with a history of low back pain lasting more than 1 month has a 25% chance of a low-back stress fracture or spondylolysis. When an athlete has a history of low back pain, every effort should be made to determine a diagnosis.

Concussion

Up to 19% of high school football players suffer a concussion at some point during the season. For pediatricians it is not difficult to make a diagnosis. The problem is the return-to-play question. Recent evidence indicates amnesia is a worse prognostic indicator than loss of consciousness.

NUTRITIONAL SUPPLEMENTS

The sports supplement industry is a billion-dollar industry. Children and adolescents look to take sports supplements for a variety of reasons: to gain weight, to lose weight, and to get stronger. Young athletes should be discouraged from using supplements for a variety of reasons: it is unethical, it may place the individual at risk, no short-term and long-term side effects are known, purity of supplements is not guaranteed, and athletes have poor compliance regarding use. It is imperative that

physicians educate young athletes, parents, and coaches about sound nutrition and properly supervised strength and conditioning programs.

CHILDHOOD OBESITY

Childhood obesity has reached epidemic proportions. Overweight and obese athletes present themselves at the sports physical. Unless there is a comorbid finding, the overweight and obese athlete can participate in any sport. In fact, overweight and obese athletes should be encouraged to participate in sports and physical activities.

Common Pitfalls

Having a PPE does not guarantee the student athlete will not suffer from an injury (minor or major). Additionally, the general public and parents wrongfully assume that without a history of chest pain or fainting with exercise and with a normal cardiac physical examination that this guarantees no underlying heart conditions that could result in sudden death.

There are a series of general questions that I believe must be reviewed with each athlete even though the athlete may have previously answered them on the questionnaire. These categories include: asthma, allergies (especially history of anaphylaxis and if the student carries an EpiPen), surgeries, current medication, and recent emergency department visits.

Communication and Counseling

The PPE can serve as a means for reintegrating the child into the health care system. Adolescents are one of the most underserved populations in terms of visits to the health care system. Many adolescents—both male and female—are not happy with their weight. Most want to lose weight and some want to gain weight. This examination is an opportunity to refer these youngsters to appropriate medical specialists, psychologists, and nutritionists. For the overweight child or athlete, suggestions and recommendations can be made for increasing physical activity and improving nutrition.

It is important to be cognizant of the sport the athlete will be participating in. For example, if the youngster is playing football, several questions must be asked. Football players are more likely to suffer from heat injury, concussion, and brachial plexus injuries (burners or stingers). In cross-country runners or track athletes a history of shin pain or stress fractures must be queried. All female athletes, especially those participating in aesthetic sports (dance, gymnastics, figure skating) should be asked about their eating habits, menstrual cycles, and bone health, as these are questions that relate to the female athlete triad (disordered eating, amenorrhea, osteopenia). If a girl demonstrates elements of the female athlete triad, referral should be made to a team of professionals, including the athlete's primary care physician, nutritionist, and psychologist.

In baseball players (especially pitchers and catchers), it is important to ask about elbow and shoulder problems.

The majority of young athletes can safely participate in middle and high school sports. It is our goal as a medical community to assist in their safe participation and promote enjoyment. A concerted effort should be made to reintegrate these young athletes into the health care system by encouraging routine visits to their pediatrician.

SUGGESTED READINGS

1. Arendt E, Dick R: Knee injury patterns among men and women in collegiate basketball and soccer. NCAA data and review of literature. Am J Sports Med 23(6):694–701, 1995. **This reference is the first study to recognize that female athletes suffer noncontact ACL injuries at three times that of male counterparts.**

2. American Academy of Family Physicians, American Academy of Pediatrics, American College of Sports Medicine, American Medical Society for Sports Medicine, American Orthopaedic Society for Sports Medicine, American Osteopathic Academy of Sports Medicine: The Preparticipation Physical Evaluation, 3rd ed. Minneapolis: McGraw-Hill, 2004. **This is the latest edition of the preparticipation evaluation. It is a great reference for those performing the exam and parents.**

3. American Academy of Pediatrics: Medical conditions affecting sports participation. Pediatrics 107:1205–1209, 2001. **This is one of the most frequently quoted articles in sports medicine. It is in table form and gives guidelines whether an athlete can participate with certain medical conditions.**

4. American Academy of Pediatrics Committee on Sports Medicine and Fitness: Use of performance-enhancing substances. Pediatrics 115:1103–1106, 2005. **This policy focuses on sports supplements in general and strongly discourages the use in pediatric patients.**

5. American Academy of Pediatrics Committee on Sports Medicine and Fitness: Climatic heat stress and the exercising child and adolescent. Pediatrics 106:158–159, 2000. **This policy reviews why children are at increased risk for developing heat injury and gives guidelines how to prevent and manage.**

6. American Academy of Pediatrics Committee on Sports Medicine and Fitness: Medical concerns in the female athlete. Pediatrics 106:610–613, 2000. **This policy reviews menstrual abnormalities, energy balance, and bone health in young females.**

7. Maron BJ, McKenna WJ, Danielson GK, et al: American College of Cardiology/European Society of Cardiology clinical expert consensus document on hypertrophic cardiomyopathy: a Report of the American College of Cardiology Foundation Task Force on Clinical expert Consensus Documents and the European Society of Cardiology Committee for Practice Guidelines. J Am Coll Cardiol 42(9):1687–1713, 2003. **This reference discusses the work-up of patients with hypertrophic cardiomyopathy and the level of sports participation.**

8. Maron BJ: Sudden death in young athletes. N Engl J Med 349 (11):1064–1075, 2003. **This reference discusses the common causes of sudden death in the young athlete (hypertrophic cardiomyopathy, viral myocarditis, and total anomalous pulmonary venous return).**

9. National Collegiate Athletic Association: Prevention of heat illness: Sports medicine guidelines. In National Collegiate Athletic Association: NCAA Sports Medicine Handbook 2003–2004, 16th ed. Indianapolis, IN: National Collegiate Athletic Association, 2003, p 22. **This reference reviews risk factors for heat injury and heat injury treatment.**

10. Yeager KK, Agostini R, Nattiv A, Drinkwater B: The female athlete triad: Disordered eating, amenorrhea, osteoporosis. Med Sci Sports Exerc 25(7):775–777, 1993. **This is the first document that outlines the female athlete triad (osteopenia, disordered eating, and amenorrhea) and is a must read for everyone involved with young female athletes.**

Conduct Disorder, Aggression, Violence, and Delinquency in Youth and Adolescents

Eric Jon Sigel

KEY CONCEPTS

- Prevalence of violence, victimization, perpetration, injury, and conduct disorder is high.
- There is a strong biologic and genetic contribution to conduct disorder development.
- The primary care setting is an ideal setting to identify youth at risk.
- Pharmacologic treatment options are proven effective.
- Behavioral interventions can change the trajectory toward violence development.

The spectrum of youth violence is broad and multifactorial, representing an interaction between genetics and environment. Multiple factors contribute to youth violence development, and increasingly pediatricians are being called on to detect, refer, and treat this complicated condition.

Youth are at high risk for violence perpetration, violence victimization, and injury from interpersonal violence. Homicide is the second-leading cause of death in adolescents and young adults, the majority perpetrated by firearms. Overall, 33% of high school students surveyed by the youth risk behavior survey (YRBS) in 2003 were in a physical fight in the last year. Forty percent of males and 25% of females report being in a fight. Injuries from fighting and assault are a significant problem as 4.2% of students who report being injured in a physical fight require medical attention. Grade and gender differences exist: 5% of ninth graders and 3.1% of twelfth graders and 5.7% of males and 2.6% of females report being injured in a physical fight. Ethnically and racially Hispanics and African Americans have a 5.2% and 5.5% rate of injuries compared to 2.9% of whites. Juveniles account for nearly 20% of people arrested for a violent crime. Multiple sequelae associated with delinquency include academic failure, substance use, post-traumatic stress disorder, and other psychological conditions.

Definitions

There is a spectrum of diagnoses that are encountered when addressing youth violence. Oppositional-defiant disorder (ODD) is diagnosed when a pattern of negative, hostile, and defiant behavior lasts more than 6 months and four out of eight criteria are present (Table 1). Two percent to 16% of children and adolescents meet criteria for ODD. Children with ODD may be aggressive but have not become violent.

Conduct disorder (CD) is diagnosed when a repetitive and persistent pattern of behavior in which the basic

TABLE 1 Diagnostic Criteria for 313.81 Oppositional-Defiant Disorder

A. A pattern of negativistic, hostile, and defiant behavior lasting at least 6 months, during which four (or more) of the following are present:*
   1. Often loses temper.
   2. Often argues with adults.
   3. Often actively defies or refuses to comply with adults' requests or rules.
   4. Often deliberately annoys people.
   5. Often blames others for one's own mistakes or misbehavior.
   6. Often touchy or easily annoyed by others.
   7. Often spiteful or vindictive.
B. The disturbance in behavior causes clinically significant impairment in social, academic, or occupational functioning.
C. The behaviors do not occur exclusively during the course of a psychotic or mood disorder.
D. Criteria are not met for conduct disorder, and if the individual is 18 years or older, criteria are not met for antisocial personality disorder.

---

*Consider a criterion met only if the behavior occurs more frequently than is typically observed in individuals of comparable age and developmental level.

From *Diagnostic and Statistical Manual of Mental Disorders*, 4th ed., text revision. Washington, DC: American Psychiatric Association, 1994, pp 93–94. Copyright 2000. Reprinted with permission.

TABLE 2 Diagnostic Criteria for Conduct Disorder

A. A repetitive and persistent pattern of behavior in which the basic rights of others or major age-appropriate societal norms or rules are violated, as manifested by the presence of three (or more) of the following criteria in the past 12 months, with at least one criterion present in the past 6 months:

Aggression to people and animals
   1. Often bullies, threatens, or intimidates others.
   2. Often initiates physical fights.
   3. Has used a weapon that can cause serious physical harm to others (e.g., a bat, brick, broken bottle, knife, gun).
   4. Has been physically cruel to people.
   5. Has been physically cruel to animals.
   6. Has stolen while confronting a victim (e.g., mugging, purse snatching, extortion, armed robbery).
   7. Has forced someone into sexual activity.

Destruction of property
   8. Has deliberately engaged in fire setting with the intention of causing serious damage.
   9. Has deliberately destroyed others' property (other than by fire setting).

Deceitfulness or theft
   10. Has broken into someone else's house, building, or car.
   11. Often lies to obtain goods or favors or to avoid obligations (i.e., "cons" others).
   12. Has stolen items of nontrivial value without confronting a victim (e.g., shoplifting, but without breaking and entering; forgery).

Serious violations of rules
   13. Often stays out at night despite parental prohibitions, beginning before age 13 years.
   14. Has run away from home overnight at least twice while living in parental or parental surrogate home (or once without returning for a lengthy period).
   15. Is often truant from school, beginning before age 13 years.
B. The disturbance in behavior causes clinically significant impairment in social, academic, or occupational functioning.
C. If the individual is 18 years or older, criteria are not met for antisocial personality disorder

Code based on type:
   1. 312.81 Conduct Disorder, Childhood-Onset Type: Onset of at least one criterion characteristic of conduct disorder before 10 years of age.
   2. 312.82 Conduct Disorder, Adolescent-Onset Type: Absence of any criteria characteristic of conduct disorder before 10 years of age.
   3. 312.89 Conduct Disorder, Unspecified Onset: Age at onset is not known.

Specify severity:
   1. Mild: Few if any conduct problems in excess of those required to make the diagnosis and conduct problems cause only minor harm to others.
   2. Moderate: Number of conduct problems and effect on others intermediate between "mild" and "severe."
   3. Severe: Many conduct problems in excess of those required to make the diagnosis or conduct problems cause considerable harm to others.

From Diagnostic and Statistical Manual of Mental Disorders, 4th ed., text revision. Washington, DC: American Psychiatric Association, 2000, pp 90–91. Copyright 2000. Reprinted with permission.

rights of others or major age-appropriate societal norms or rules are violated; major categories include aggression to people and animals, destruction of property, deceitfulness or theft, and serious violation of rules (Table 2). There is a continuum of conduct disorder from mild to moderate to severe. The prevalence of CD is 2% to 8%. Comorbid diagnoses in CD youth are frequent, with substance use and dependence (30% to 80%), attention deficit hyperactivity disorder (ADHD) (30% to 50%), and mood disorders (12% to 20%) being common.

Juvenile delinquency is defined as a minor who has been accused of an offense and adjudicated in a court of law. Delinquent offenses are divided into two groups. Status offenses are those that are illegal only because the perpetrator is a minor (e.g., drinking under age, truancy). Index offenses are illegal acts regardless of age (e.g., burglary, murder). Adolescents account for 13% of all violent crimes, 12% of forcible rapes, 18% of robberies, and 12% of aggravated assaults. Learning disabilities and decreased cognition are found commonly in delinquent youth. Males perpetrate crimes 6 to 13 times more often than females.

Violence occurs once aggressive actions are carried out with the intention (or perceived intention) to physically injure another person, or that lead to emotional or bodily harm to others. Violent behavior can be perpetrated with or without a weapon—hitting, pushing, slapping, grabbing, kicking, hitting with an object, threatening with a weapon, or using a weapon (gun, knife, club). As violent behavior escalates, the consequences become more serious, resulting in emotional trauma, physical injury, or death.

Development of Violence

A detailed discussion of this issue is beyond the scope of this chapter, but a tacit understanding is important for the primary care provider to help recognize and prevent an escalation of behavior. There is strong evidence supporting a genetic influence. Multiple twin studies find that from 50% to 70% of conduct disorder is attributed to genetic influence, and less than 50% of the variance is attributed to environmental factors. Biologically there is a difference between violent CD youth and controls. Several studies find significant underarousal of the autonomic nervous system, with decreased heart rates, electrical skin conductance, and increased heart rate variability. Some data suggest that low levels of serotonin are found in aggressive youth. At the individual level, youth with intellectual deficits, psychiatric disorders (ADHD, depression, psychosis), and traumatic brain injury and those who are victims of sexual or physical abuse are at higher risk. At the family level, poor parenting, lack of a nurturing environment, parental substance abuse, and modeling of violent behavior as a conflict resolution tool contributes to the development of aggressive behavior. At the community level, poverty, lack of community resources, and a general culture of violence can contribute to the promulgation of delinquency.

Expert Opinion on Management Issues

Ideally, primary prevention should be the focus in a primary care setting, beginning with newborn visits. The American Academy of Pediatrics (AAP) has developed a curriculum, Connected Kids, that can help guide primary care practitioners through all phases of childhood, and issues to focus on at different developmental levels. Teaching effective parenting is one key element in changing the trajectory toward conduct disorder. Recognizing parental risk factors such as alcoholism (20% of youth have an alcoholic parent), parental criminality, mental health diagnoses, and attitudes toward punishment and violence are vital, as the primary care practitioner can facilitate treatment and referrals for the parents. It is important for parents to be aware of what their children are exposed to through video games, television, movies, and the Internet. Multiple studies have found correlation between viewing violence and future aggression. Steering parents away from letting youth be exposed to media violence is one factor that may decrease their risk. An additional item to address is presence of a firearm in the home, which is the single most important cause of death in youth: 25% of teenage deaths (homicide, suicide, or accidental) are a result of firearms. There are an almost fivefold greater risk of suicide and threefold greater risk of homicide when a firearm is in the home. Encouraging parents to remove guns from the home, using safety locks, and ensuring safe storage (if guns are kept in the home they should be unloaded and locked away) can set an example for the youth and decrease their risk of injury or death. As children grow up, the focus of primary prevention is on the youth, addressing issues of family relationships, academic performance, peer interaction, and risk taking.

Secondary prevention involves detecting youth at risk for conduct disorder and violence involvement. Recognizing and treating behavioral and emotional issues early is essential. Screening for and treating ADHD and other mental health issues and detecting learning disabilities can help prevent a path toward conduct disorder. Youth

may exhibit oppositional defiant behaviors—referral for further assessment and treatment is important.

Once youth enter adolescence, interviewing them alone about risk and protective factors is essential. The risk behavior syndrome states that if an adolescent is engaging in one risky behavior then there is a significantly increased chance that they are involved in other risky behaviors. The spectrum of risk behavior includes early sexual involvement, lack of condom use, pregnancy or paternity, early age of initiation of substance use (alcohol, marijuana), using tobacco (smoking or chewing) academic difficulties, depression, suicide attempts, questioning sexual orientation, and sexual perpetration. Additional risk behavior that confers specific risk for future violence involvement—perpetration and injury from violence—includes recent fighting, injury from fighting, substance use, poor academic performance, carrying a weapon, gang involvement, and delinquency. Protective factors for future violence involvement include high grade point average, connectedness to parents, high perceived parental expectations for school, connectedness to adults outside the family (for males), and religiosity (females). Teenagers should be counseled about their risk behavior, and linkage between risk behaviors such as violence and substance use should be explored. Treatment of any of the identified problems is essential. Screening youth can be done by the practitioner individually or can be aided by brief screening tools. The Pediatric Symptom Checklist (25 items) or the Strength and Difficulties Questionnaire can be used for general mental health screening that provides sub-scales for depression, aggression, and conduct problems.

As risk factors and behaviors accumulate, the primary care physician may suspect conduct disorder. Diagnosis can be made by using the Diagnostic and Statistical Manual of Mental Disorders, 4th edition (DSM-IV) criteria (Table 3). If the diagnosis is unclear, then referral to a mental health specialist should be made. Because there is significant comorbid diagnosis such as depression, ADHD, psychosis, and bipolar disorder, these also need to be evaluated. A history of traumatic brain injury has been shown to correlate with the development of aggression.

TABLE 3 Violence Assessment and Screening

- When did you last get into a fight?
- How often do you fight?
- Have you ever been injured in a fight?
- Have you used weapons during a fight?
- Do you carry/own a weapon?
- Do you have access to guns?
- Have you committed any illegal acts?
- Have you ever been arrested or on probation?
- How do you solve conflicts?
- How are conflicts solved at home?
- How are you disciplined?
- Have you been the victim of sexual or physical abuse?
- Have you ever forced sex on someone?
- Do you ever think about hurting anyone? Killing anyone? Forcing sex on anyone?
- Are you in a gang? What do you do for the gang? What type of illegal activity does your gang get involved in?
- Do you use alcohol/drugs? What happens to your anger when you are under the influence?

Obtaining information from the school system, probation officers, and employers can be helpful.

Tertiary Prevention Treatment of Conduct Disorder and Violence

PHARMACOLOGIC INTERVENTIONS

If any comorbid diagnoses exist, then treating the specific condition can improve a youth's chances of avoiding violent behavior and delinquency. Several randomized, controlled trials have proved psychoactive medications effective in treating conduct disorder and violent behavior. Two classes of medication are most commonly used: mood stabilizers and atypical antipsychotics. Valproic acid has been evaluated in two randomized, controlled trials, both showing effectiveness in treating conduct disorder. One study compared high-dose to low-dose valproic acid. Fifty-three percent of subjects responded favorably to 1000 mg /day of valproic acid, whereas only 8% responded to the low dose (250 mg). Valproic acid is generally well tolerated and takes 2 to 4 weeks to become effective. Side effects include gastrointestinal distress, diarrhea, sedation, and rash. Valproic acid levels and liver enzymes should be checked every 3 months. Additionally, lithium has proven effective in some studies as well. The use of lithium requires more frequent monitoring and has more significant side effects compared to valproic acid.

The second-generation antipsychotics, such as haloperidol (Haldol), have also been used to treat aggression in conduct disorder patients, although side effects, including extrapyramidal symptoms, have limited its use. The second-generation atypical antipsychotics have fewer side effects and have been used frequently since their development. Risperidone has been studied in several randomized, controlled trials, effectively treating aggression in boys with conduct disorder. The starting dose of risperidone is usually 0.5 mg, titrated up to 3 to 4 mg by 0.5 mg weekly if necessary. Common side effects include sedation, weight gain, and orthostatic hypotension. Newer atypical antipsychotics include ziprasidone and aripoprazole, which have fewer side effects than risperidone but have not been studied.

Clonidine, an α_2-agonist, has been shown to decrease aggression in patients with ADHD, in addition to stimulant medication. Dose ranges from 0.1 to 0.2 mg/day. Side effects include decreased systolic blood pressure, transient sedation, and dizziness.

BEHAVIORAL INTERVENTIONS

Multiple behavioral interventions have been studied in delinquent teenagers and several show promising results. Elliot from the Center for Prevention of Violence has reviewed many intervention programs and highlights Blueprints for Violence Prevention programs that can affect youth. Multisystemic therapy (MST) is a particularly useful intervention that leads to behavioral change. MST is based on social-ecologic theory that views the child and family's school, work, peers, and community as interconnected systems with dynamic and reciprocal influences on the behavior of family members. The goals of MST are to empower parents with the skills and resources needed to rear an adolescent, and to empower adolescents to cope with familial and extrafamilial problems. A therapist works with the family, often in the home, to help improve family dynamics and parents understanding of the youth. The therapist helps the youth at the peer level, helping to decrease involvement with delinquent peers and facilitate involvement with prosocial peer groups through athletics, after-school activities, or church groups. Under the guidance of the therapist, parents are encouraged to work with the school system to promote and monitor the adolescent's academic achievement. At the individual level, interventions target the adolescent's problem-solving skills and social perspective-taking skills. Most communities have MST programs (check the MST web site). Usual length of time for MST is 3 to 5 months.

Another effective treatment modality is family-focused therapy. This intervention targets the family as a functioning system rather than focusing on the identified patient. In randomized, controlled trials, family-focused therapy has been successful at decreasing symptoms of CD and is an option for treatment. Mentoring programs are successful as well, often as a component of multisystem intervention but also independent of other interventions. Youth who do not have a strong role model benefit significantly from a partnership with a caring adult. Recognizing those youth in a primary care setting and referring them to mentoring programs can decrease youth's risk significantly.

Some interventions do not seem to produce the desired effects. Individual psychotherapy, behavior modification, institutional programs (group homes), and boot camps do not appear to change behavior when studied as individual interventions.

Common Pitfalls

Increasingly, primary care practitioners are being called on to address multiple issues that historically fell in the behavioral realm. Significant morbidity and mortality result from mental health issues and require the attention of primary care providers. Primary care providers first need to be open to considering an illness that has such a high prevalence, and although it is challenging, figure out a way to address the issue efficiently and effectively. Primary care providers need to take seriously parents' concerns about their child's behavior, and not attribute behavior to "just being a boy," for example.

Next, the family system needs to be considered in treatment, not just the patient. Addressing parenting styles, and issues such as parental alcoholism, honestly, can have a significant impact on the youth's trajectory toward violence and delinquency. Pharmacologic treatment certainly can help, but it does not address the family dynamic. Determining comorbid diagnosis is challenging but essential to positive outcomes. Treating ADHD in particular, and other mental health problems is important. Poor outcomes may be related to an adolescent's persistent drug use, which may confound the pharmacologic intervention. There is a delicate and challenging balance regarding primary treatment by the primary care provider and referral to psychiatry and other mental health services. One needs to consider the resources of the patient and the community in determining course of treatment. Knowledge of community resources is pivotal.

Communication and Counseling

A key element in treating conduct disorder and aggression is open, honest communication with patients and their families about expectations. If embarking on pharmacologic treatment, parents and patients need to understand risks, benefits, and side effects of the medication. Frequent follow-up is essential, with appointments every 1 to 2 weeks initially as a patient is initiating medication. Contact with the school and mental health counselors is important to help monitor progress and to aid in diagnosis.

If concern is raised at a well-child check without any diagnosis being made, sooner than later follow-up is recommended. The primary care physician should let the parent know that they are available to address these issues. Often parents do not bring up behavioral concerns as they feel it is not in the realm of a busy pediatrician.

If interested, a primary care physician can take on a primary counseling role regarding risk behavior. Discussing anger management techniques, problem-solving skills, and empathy development in a motivational interviewing-type model can be done quickly and efficiently, and has been shown to be effective in decreasing risk.

SUGGESTED READINGS

1. Blueprints for Violence Prevention. Center for the Study and Prevention of Violence, Boulder Colorado. Available at http://www.colorado.edu/cspv/blueprints/ (accessed October 14, 2005). **Summarizes 11 programs that have proven effective in violence prevention for youth. Contains links to programs referenced in the chapter.**
2. Connecting the Dots to Prevent Youth Violence: Training and Outreach Guide for Physicians and other Health Professionals. American Medical Association. PDF available for download from http://www.ama-assn.org/ama1/pub/upload/mm/386/youthviolenceguide.pdf (accessed October 14, 2005). **In-depth discussion of youth violence, and recommendations for primary care practitioners on assessment and treatment in the office setting.**
3. Lorber MF: Psychophysiology of aggression, psychopathy, and conduct problems: A meta-analysis. Psychol Bull 130(4):531–552, 2004. **A meta-analysis of 95 studies that examine biologic factors contributing to aggression and conduct problems, such as low resting heart rate and low electrodermal activity.**
4. Schur SB, Sikich L, Findling RL, et al: Treatment recommendations for the use of antipsychotics for aggressive youth (TRAAY). Part 1. J Am Acad Child Adolesc Psychiatry 42(2):132–144, 2003. **Summarizes specific pharmacologic treatment recommendations for aggressive youth.**
5. Woolfenden SR, Williams K, Peat JK: Family and parenting interventions for conduct disorder and delinquency: A meta-analysis of randomised controlled trials. Arc Dis Child 86(4):251–256, 2002. **A meta-analysis that summarizes family and parenting interventions for juvenile delinquents that reduce time spent in institutions and decrease criminal activity.**

Suicide

Janice Hutchinson and Renée R. Jenkins

KEY CONCEPTS

- Suicide is a major cause of death in children and adolescents.
- Suicidal ideation alone is not uncommon but should be taken seriously when accompanied with a specific plan.
- Children and adolescents with substance abuse problems and other psychiatric disorders are at highest risk for suicide.
- The role of psychotropic drugs in reducing suicide is controversial and unresolved.
- A suicide attempt is a psychiatric emergency and requires a psychiatric assessment.
- Self-administered suicide scales are no substitute for clinical assessment of suicide risk.
- Patient education materials can be useful in alerting parents to signs of children and adolescents in distress and at risk for suicide.

Suicide is the third leading cause of death for 10- to 19-year-olds and the sixth leading cause of death for 5- to 14-year-olds. American Indian and Alaskan Natives have the highest rate of suicide in the 15- to 24-year-old group. Suicide rates rose dramatically for American teens 10 to 19 years old from 1980 to 1995, with rates rising more rapidly among blacks than whites. White students have been significantly more likely than black students to have thought seriously about attempting suicide, but Hispanic students were much more likely than other students to have attempted suicide. Female students are more likely to have thought seriously about suicide, to have made a specific plan to attempt suicide, and to have attempted suicide than male students. Suicidal ideation alone is not uncommon and is not a strong precursor to suicidal behavior. As many as 12% to 25% of older children and adolescents express some form of suicidal ideation. Suicidal ideation accompanied by a specific plan should be taken as a much more serious risk. Prepubertal children may have suicidal thoughts but are not as likely to attempt suicide as are children who have reached puberty. Firearms are used in the majority of youth suicides, although suffocation (hanging) and poisoning follow.

Nearly all studies show a high presence of psychiatric disorders among suicide victims. Mood disorders, substance abuse, and conduct or antisocial and borderline personality disorders are often co-occurring. Substance abuse may be related to 30% to 70% of all suicides and is associated with more lethal methods. Depression seems to be the most common underlying factor whether the person is an adult or a child. The association is high in all forms of the common major affective disorders, approximately 20% of deaths among persons with bipolar disorder and 10% of deaths in persons diagnosed with major depression. Suicide attempts are more likely to occur during depressive or dysphoric mixed-mood states.

Suicide risk is significantly elevated if there is a history of a previous severe depression, prior suicide attempts, and younger age at onset of illness. Other risk factors for suicide include a history of mental disorders, a history of alcohol and substance abuse, a family history of suicide, a family history of child maltreatment, feelings of hopelessness, impulsive or aggressive tendencies, physical illness, easy access to lethal methods, cultural and religious beliefs, local epidemics of suicide, or isolation. Additional factors may include loss (relational, divorce, job, home, legal, financial, etc.), barriers to accessing mental health treatment, and unwillingness to seek help because of stigma attached to mental health and substance abuse disorders or suicidal thoughts. Teenagers may particularly feel the stress of gender-identity issues, self-doubt, and financial and future uncertainties.

Expert Opinion on Management Issues

DRUG THERAPY

Many medications have been developed to treat the affective disorders that frequently underlie suicide (Table 1). Lithium was identified as a prophylactic treatment for depression in 1886. There is growing and consistent research in adults that shows that long-term treatment with lithium results in reduced rates of suicides and attempts. Baldessarini and his group at Harvard have conducted international collaborative studies that show compelling evidence that a long-term maintenance of lithium provides prolonged reduction of suicide risks. Suicide attempts decline by sevenfold. Sharp and/or abrupt discontinuation of lithium results in sharp increases in suicide risks in association with depressive episodes soon after discontinuation. Other mood stabilizers like carbamazepine and valproic acid have not been shown to have antisuicidal effects. Agents such as olanzapine, risperidone, quetiapine, gabapentin, lamotrigine, topiramate, verapamil, nifedipine, and nimodipine that have been used as mood stabilizers have not yet been tested for antisuicide effectiveness. One other medication has been shown to have antisuicidal effects. Clozapine has been effective in patients with chronic psychotic disorders. Clozapine has also been effective in persons with a diagnosis of schizophrenia.

The newest class of antidepressants, selective serotonin reuptake inhibitors (SSRIs) have never been claimed to have direct antisuicide effects. Yet many psychiatric researchers claim that the decline in adolescent suicides in the past decade (1992–2002) is secondary to SSRIs. Teen suicide rates for both males and females declined after the introduction of Prozac in 1988. Some researchers have claimed that SSRIs actually create suicidal ideation, but this is a currently unresolved controversy. In some patients SSRIs behave like the tricyclic antidepressants, causing the "switch" phenomena. Symptoms emerge that are more like the aggressive, impulsive, dangerous behaviors that are exhibited in bipolar mania. Further investigation involving child psychiatry clinicians and researchers is important to clarify behavioral effects of SSRIs.

BEHAVIORAL/PSYCHOLOGICAL THERAPY

Once a person has attempted suicide, others must act immediately to remove endangering devices and secure a zone of safety. A suicide attempt constitutes a psychiatric emergency and requires first medical treatment and stabilization. This should be followed by an immediate psychiatric assessment that includes direct questions regarding the problems associated with the attempt, the circumstances surrounding and prior to the attempt, and ongoing suicidal ideation and plans. Based on the person's responses, the psychiatrist must develop a treatment plan. The first decision is whether to admit the person for inpatient therapy or to release the patient with therapeutic follow-up. An admission is required if the person retains suicidal intent, has a specific plan, is psychotic, has a major psychiatric disorder, has made past attempts, or has a made a violent, near-lethal, or premeditated attempt. Admission should also occur if the person is sad or angry that they have survived the attempt, if there is little or no family and social supports, including housing, if there is inadequate and unavailable timely outpatient follow-up, and if the person remains agitated, has poor judgment, and is uncooperative and unreceptive to help. Medical compromise that includes contributing medical conditions–for example, neurologic, cancer, infections, or toxic life-threatening sequelae of the attempt–may also require admission.

The psychiatrist may discharge that person if the suicidal desire has dissipated and there is no intent or plan, if there is both living and immediate and available social support, and if the person is able to cooperate with the treatment plan for follow-up. Inpatient hospitalization may require initial one-to-one monitoring while antidepressant or antipsychotic medications are introduced as the person is engaged in individual, group, and/or substance abuse treatment. Discharge can occur when the suicidal ideation has stopped and outpatient interventions are available. Outpatient treatment may be more desirable than hospitalization if the person has chronic suicidal ideation and/or self-injury without prior medically serious attempts.

Individual therapy must address the acute stressors, contributing psychiatric and physical diagnoses, and modifiable risk factors. Suicide risk assessment must continue throughout the course of treatment. Treatment of depression and other psychiatric maladies is also important. Frequent appointments, suicide hotline numbers and numbers of treating therapists, and identification of emergency services should be provided. Social service interventions that can assist in vocational training, job and housing stability, and linkages to psychiatric and therapy support are also essential. Enrollment of the person in a day treatment program may provide consistent therapies and medication monitoring and support. Cognitive-behavior therapy (CBT) may be extremely effective in preventing further attempts because it is effective in reducing cognitive distortions, source of depression, and suicidal ideation. CBT may also be useful in addressing the hopelessness that is often a part of suicidal ideation. Multisystemic therapy (MST) has been shown to reduce suicide attempts, especially among African

TABLE 1 Medications for Depression

Generic Name (Trade Name)	Dosage/Route/ Regimen	Maximum Dose	Dosage Formulation	Common Adverse Reactions	Therapeutic Concentrations	Comments
Lithium (influences reuptake of serotonin and/or norepinephrine)						
Lithium (Lithobid, Eskalith, Eskalith CR) Rx	PO: Children: 15–60 mg/kg/day in 3–4 divided doses. Adolescents: 600–1800 mg/day in 3–4 divided doses for regular release or 2 divided doses for sustained release. Initiate at lower dose and adjust based upon levels.	Not to exceed adult doses	Capsule (carbonate): 150, 300, 600 mg. Eskalith: 300 mg; contains benzyl alcohol. Syrup (citrate): 300 mg/5 mL in 5 mL, 10 mL, 480 mL (5 mL≡8 mEq lithium equivalent to 300 mg lithium carbonate); contains alcohol. Tablet (carbonate): 300 mg, extended release (Eskalith CR) 450 mg, slow release (Lithobid) 300 mg.	Concentration related: 1.5–2 mEq/L for GI/tremor; 22.5 mEq/L for confusion/somnolence; >2.5 mEq/L, seizures/death Common: tremor, polyuria, diarrhea, vomiting, drowsiness, muscle weakness, arrhythmia, anorexia, nausea, blurred vision, dry mouth, fatigue	No specific depression range. Draw trough (8–12 hours postdose). Toxic: >1.5 mEq/L.	Renal: Adjust dose if Cl$_{Cr}$ <50 mL/min. Several drug interactions. Avoid altering sodium content of diet, which can alter plasma levels of drug. Syrup may precipitate in feeding tubes.
Selective Serotonin Reuptake Inhibitors (inhibits central nervous system serotonin uptake)						
Fluoxetine (Prozac, Prozac Weekly*) Rx	PO: 8–18 years: 10–20 mg/day, initiate 10 mg/day in lower weight children and increase if needed after 1 wk.	20 mg/day	Capsule: 10, 20, 40 mg. Prozac: 10, 20, 40 mg. Capsule, delayed release (Prozac Weekly*): 90 mg. Oral solution (Prozac): 20 mg/5 mL in 120 mL (contains alcohol and benzoic acid); mint flavor. Tablet: 10, 20 mg. (Prozac): 10 mg, scored.	CNS: insomnia, anxiety, headache, nervousness, somnolence, tremor GI: anorexia, nausea, diarrhea, dry mouth Sexual dysfunction, rash, sweating, weakness	100–800 ng/mL; levels usually not obtained and not well established.	FDA Black Box Warning regarding suicidal ideations in children (2004). Drug interactions: CYP 1A2, 2B6, 2C8/9, 2C19, 2D6, 2E1, and 3A3/4; substrate, 2C9 inducer, 1A2 (high doses), 2B6, 2C8/9, 2C19, 2D6, 3A3/4 inhibitor. May reduce dose in hepatic impairment. Do not use with MAO inhibitors.

*Prozac Weekly not approved in pediatric patients.
Citalopram (Celexa), escitalopram (Lexapro), paroxetine (Paxil, Paxil CR), sertraline (Zoloft) are not FDA-approved for depression in the pediatric patient.
Cl$_{Cr}$, creatinine clearance; CNS, central nervous system; GI, gastrointestinal; MAO, monoamine oxidase; PO, orally; Rx, prescription.

American youth. MST engages a variety mental health professionals, family, and community resources in treatment interventions. Pharmacotherapy and psychosocial interventions together usually constitute the most effective treatment planning.

PREVENTION

The best approach to suicidal ideation and attempts is to prevent them. There must be early recognition of risk factors and referral for early psychiatric assessment, identification, and treatment of mental disorders. Mental, physical, and substance abuse disorders require early and effective treatment planning. Interventions must be available and accessible. Family and community support are critical. It is also important to identify and embrace religious and cultural beliefs that discourage suicide. Parents have to listen carefully to their children and beware of complaints of being a bad person, introduction of verbal hints that they will no longer be a problem, the distribution of prized possessions to family and friends, sudden, unexplained happiness after a depression, and signs of hallucinations and bizarre thinking. Self-administered suicide scales tend to be oversensitive and underspecific and are not to be used in place of a clinical assessment for screening.

Common Pitfalls

Circumstances to avoid in treating suicidal patients include failure to recognize and regard symptoms and signs of suicidality and failure to provide safety and protection to the potentially suicidal person through hospitalization and/or warnings to the person and significant others about signs of deterioration and resources for immediate help. Other events to avoid include failure to prescribe suicidal precautions, that is, one-to-one monitoring in an institutional setting such as a hospital, detention center, or youth home.

Communication and Counseling

Most adolescents who have suicidal thoughts are not at imminent risk of suicide. Suicide attempts are much less common than suicidal ideation. However, children and adolescents who are identified as having suicidal ideation should be further evaluated to determine their risk for attempt. Prior suicide attempt, substance abuse, and the presence of a psychiatric disorder are strong predictors of suicidal behavior. A clinical assessment by a mental health professional is the most appropriate strategy to determine patient management.

SUGGESTED READINGS

1. American Academy of Child and Adolescent Psychiatry: Teen Suicide, Fact Sheet no. 10, August 8, 2004. **Prevention of teen suicides.**
2. American Academy of Child and Adolescent Psychiatry: Practice parameter for the assessment and treatment of children and adolescents with suicidal behavior. J Am Acad Child Adoles Psychiatry 40(7 Suppl):24S–51S, 2001. **Review of literature and recommendations for assessment and treatment.**
3. Centers for Disease Control and Prevention: Teens attempting suicide. MMWR Morb Mortal Wkly Rep 45(No. SS-4): 1–86, 1996. **Epidemiology and demographics of youth suicide.**
4. Centers for Disease Control and Prevention: Methods of suicide among persons aged 10–19 years—United States, 1992–2001. MMWR Morb Mortal Wkly Rep 53(22):471–474, 2004. **Methods and demographics of youth suicides.**
5. Couzin J: Volatile chemistry: Children and antidepressants. Science 305(5683):468–470, 2004. **SSRIs and treatment for suicide.**
6. Huey SJ Jr, Henggeler SW, Rowland MD, et al: Multisystemic therapy effects on attempted suicide by youths presenting psychiatric emergencies. J Am Acad Child Adolesc Psychiatry 43(2):183–190, 2004. **Study found multisystemic therapy superior to emergency hospitalization.**
7. Jacobs J, Brewer M: APA Practice Guideline provides recommendations for assessing and treating patients with suicidal behaviors. Psychiatr Ann 34(5):373–379, 2004. **Treatment of a person's post-suicide attempt.**
8. National Center for Injury Prevention and Control: Suicide: Fact Sheet. Available online at http://www.cdc.gov/ncipc/factsheets/suifacts.htm. **Epidemiology, demographics, and protective factors for suicide.**
9. Roy A: Psychiatric emergencies. In Sadock BJ, Sadock VA, Kaplan HI (eds): Kaplan Sadock's Comprehensive Textbook of Psychiatry, Vol VI. Philadelphia: Lippincott Williams & Wilkins, 2004, pp 1739–1751. **Descriptions of risk factors and management.**
10. Tondo L, Baldessarini R, Jennen J: Lithium and suicide risk in bipolar disorder. Ann N Y Acad Sci 932:24–43, 2001. **Detailed description of use of lithium and other agents in treating suicide.**

Epidural and Subdural Hematomas

Alfred T. Ogden and Neil A. Feldstein

KEY CONCEPTS

- Epidural hematomas (EDHs) are acute by definition and result primarily from arterial bleeding.
- Most EDHs require emergent craniotomy for clot evacuation.
- A diagnosis of EDH should be considered in any patient with a history of impact head trauma.
- EDHs classically manifest with a "lucid interval" of less than 1 to 2 hours; EDHs rarely occur more than 4 hours after injury.
- Prognosis for EDH is excellent if the hematoma is diagnosed and patients are brought to surgery before signs of herniation.
- There is no aspect of the patient's accident history that positively predicts the presence of an asymptomatic EDH.

Epidural hematomas (EDHs) and subdural hematomas (SDH) are common sequelae of pediatric head trauma that require immediate neurosurgical consultation. Both are the result of bleeding inside the skull adjacent to, but not within, brain tissue and are thus termed *extra-axial* hematomas. Epidural hematomas are typically true neurosurgical emergencies in that good outcomes are predicated on the speed with which the hematoma is diagnosed and patients are brought to the operating room. Acute subdural hematomas are often associated with severe underlying traumatic brain injury and edema, such that the benefits of surgical evacuation are questionable in many cases. Although common in middle-age and elderly adults, chronic subdural hematomas are unusual in the pediatric population and generally occur in children with a predisposing neurologic condition. They usually manifest with an indolent course preceded by a remote history of relatively minor trauma.

Expert Opinion on Management Issues

EPIDURAL HEMATOMA

Epidural hematomas (EDHs) typically result from a tear in a meningeal artery during a high-velocity impact injury and therefore are by definition acute hemorrhages. Meningeal arteries lie within the outer layer of dura, can be rather large, and often lie in grooves in the inner table of the calvarium. Growing bone is molded over large meningeal vessels during development. This is particularly true for the largest of these vessels, the middle meningeal, which lies next to the thinnest and most fragile bone in the skull, the temporal bone. Thus, a classic epidural hematoma results from an impact fracture of the temporal bone that shears the adjacent middle meningeal artery.

Clinically, epidural hematomas may manifest with a lucid period following initial injury, followed by rapid neurologic decline. In this scenario, mild brain trauma results in an initial stupor or perhaps a loss of consciousness that resolves over a period of time lasting several seconds to several minutes. The sensorium clears because, at this point, there is no significant damage to or mass effect on the brain. The *intact* state of the patient may lull caregivers into a false sense of security as the epidural space rapidly fills with arterial blood. When a sufficient amount of epidural blood accumulates to produce mass effect on the brain, the patient may develop a hemiparesis. More often, however, the patient experiences headache, nausea, and vomiting followed by a precipitous drop in level of consciousness. The time course of this process is usually 1 to 2 hours. Development of an epidural hematoma more than 4 hours after the initial injury is rare; however, arterial EDHs appearing after negative CT scans have been reported. It should be noted that the absence of a lucid interval in a patient's history does not exclude the possibility of an EDH, as these lesions can occur simultaneously with other brain trauma.

Expedient transportation and diagnosis are probably the most important factors affecting outcome. Diagnosis is made by CT, and MRI is of no additional value in the acute setting. Acute epidural blood is bright on CT and, in contrast to subdural blood, is bilenticular in shape. It can further be distinguished from subdural blood because it does not cross suture lines, where the dura is adherent to the skull. The dilemma in diagnosis and treatment tends to lie not in management choices once the diagnosis is made but rather in the decision of when to image children with "minor" head trauma, particularly when the patient is less than 2 years old. The imaging dilemma has become more accentuated recently as frivolous CT scanning lies at a nexus of criticism from those concerned with economy in medicine and with unnecessary radiation exposure in children. Although aspects of the patient's medical history and the details of the mechanism of injury can be helpful in making the decision to image, no single clinical variable correlates with the presence of an EDH when patients present with a normal neurologic examination. Guidelines for children and infants reflect this uncertainty, although in children younger than 2 years, the presence of an occult lesion is more likely.

With the active input of a neurosurgeon, small asymptomatic epidural hematomas are sometimes treated with observation; however, epidural hematomas are usually surgical lesions. Of all the extra-axial hematomas this is the most pressing operative lesion because the blood source is usually arterial, and these patients are the most salvageable as there is often no underlying brain trauma. Hyperosmolar therapy can and should be administered en route to the operating room, but it is likely of minimal benefit. As with any large intracranial bleed, anemia should be diagnosed and corrected as indicated.

Outcome is predicated on rapid decompression and clot evacuation. Acute blood clots are solid and can only be removed through a wide bony opening (craniotomy). Craniotomy also affords the requisite surgical exposure to identify and cauterize bleeding vessels. This is usually a straightforward operation, and poor outcomes are a result of preexisting underlying brain trauma or a delay to surgery. In cases of isolated epidural hematomas, poor outcomes result from herniation prior to surgery; overall mortality in the CT scan era is around 6%. Short of this extreme, neurologic deficits from epidural hematomas are usually reversible, often within the initial postoperative recovery period.

Blood in the epidural space can be venous in etiology as well. Skull fractures often are associated with bleeding from small emissary veins between the dura and the skull or venous channels within the bone itself. These are usually small and trivial, although a skull fracture associated with any amount of intracranial blood requires a neurosurgical consultation, at least an overnight hospital stay, and serial CT scans.

Epidural blood associated with a skull fracture across suture lines or an abnormal widening of sutures, called *diastasis*, is much more perilous as the bleeding source is potentially from dural sinuses. Dural sinuses are very large V-shaped channels within the dura itself that serve to drain the vast majority of deoxygenated blood from the brain. Sinus blood flow is so great that large sinus tears can result in epidural clots that accumulate at a rate similar to those from meningeal arteries. Smaller tears can produce a clot that gradually becomes symptomatic over the course of a day or two. Thus, a small epidural hematoma in proximity to a sinus associated with a fracture or diastatic suture deserves particular attention. Symptomatic clots of this kind sometimes require surgical decompression, but surgery is complicated by possible exacerbation of sinus injury.

SUBDURAL HEMATOMAS

Subdural hematomas (SDHs) come in acute and chronic varieties. Acute subdurals are viewed in the context of patient presentation and fall into two categories: high-speed accidents and child abuse in infants, the so-called shaken baby syndrome. Acute subdural hematomas occur when the head of a person traveling at high velocity is suddenly decelerated such as in a head-on automobile collision. During such accidents, the brain slides forward in the cranial vault, stretching small bridging veins between the arachnoid and dura matter. In children, these vessels are not under any natural tension and the deceleration force required to tear them is so great that it will almost always shear cortical axons as well, resulting in a devastating pattern of injury called *diffuse axonal injury* (DAI). Because of DAI, patients with acute subdural hematomas are usually comatose from the time of injury and, if so, have a poor prognosis.

Subdural hematomas are diagnosed by CT scan, where they appear bright and concave, following the curve of the skull, and are not bound by suture lines. Sometimes prominent sinuses or prominent venous lakes are confused for SDHs on CT scan. The imperative to remove a subdural clot from trauma patients contrasts with the acute epidural hematoma and must be considered in the setting of the overall prognosis of the patient. Often treatment consists of placement of an intracranial pressure (ICP) monitor to guide medical management of cerebral edema. When medical management fails to control ICP and there is a significant mass effect from a subdural hematoma, decompressive surgery should be performed if the underlying parenchymal injury is deemed to be sufficiently mild to permit a meaningful recovery. MRI can be helpful in assessing the degree of parenchymal injury in such cases.

Acute subdural hematomas in infants are sometimes inflicted by an abusive caregiver (shaken baby syndrome). A CT scan and an ophthalmologic examination should be considered in any infant with neurologic symptoms, whether acute or chronic, and is obviously requisite when abuse is suspected with even the subtlest of neurologic findings. Acute subdural hematomas from shaken baby syndrome are usually thin and diffuse, often entering the subarachnoid space, and rarely require an operation. The imaging characteristics and the ophthalmologic findings predict outcome. Treatment involves medical management of ICP, when present, and the appropriate workup for corroboratory evidence of abuse.

CHRONIC SUBDURAL HEMATOMAS

Chronic subdural hematoma is a diagnosis that is often incorrectly broadened to refer to subdural fluid collections from a variety of etiologies. In adults, subdural hematomas are common and result from small traumatic tears in bridging veins that come under tension during brain atrophy that occurs as part of the normal aging process. Often the trauma is of a trivial nature. Asymptomatic subdural blood leads to an inflammatory response that produces a reactive membrane between the blood and the normal CSF space. Either through recurrent bleeding, an osmotic gradient, or some combination of these, the membrane-enclosed space gradually accumulates fluid over a period of weeks and eventually produces a mass effect on the brain and clinical symptoms.

In infants, the presence of a chronic subdural hematoma again raises the specter of child abuse, as the chronic appearance of the subdural blood on CT scan may be a result of chronic abuse or merely a delay between the event and the patient's medical evaluation. In any event, shaken baby syndrome should be considered along with hydrocephalus and an intracranial mass in any infant with increasing head circumference or other signs of chronically elevated ICP such as a bulging fontanel.

Aside from cases of abuse, chronic subdurals are usually an acquired condition in children, which is to say they are permitted to occur because of some other process that results in an abnormal distance between the dura and the surface of the brain. Neurosurgical patients who have recently received a shunt for hydrocephalus or who have had mass lesions excised fall into this category, as do children with atrophic brains from any cause.

Chronic subdural hematomas manifest with a relatively indolent time course of days to weeks. Infants are likely to present with only irritability and lethargy, whereas older children will complain of headache and fatigue and may demonstrate cognitive symptoms. Hemiparesis occurs as well, although motor findings are more typical in the adult population.

CT scan is the first appropriate diagnostic tool. Chronic subdural hematomas are dark on CT, concave with the curve of the skull, and demonstrate mass effect. They can show mixed signal intensity representing different ages of blood and if so are called "acute-on-chronic." In the absence of an acute component, these lesions are often confused with subdural hygromas, which are benign subdural CSF collections without mass effect, and other benign fluid collections such as postmeningitic effusions.

When symptomatic, chronic subdural hematomas can be evacuated through small openings in the skull—called *burr holes*—as chronic blood clots liquefy with time. Surgery is sometimes delayed in patients with mild symptoms to allow the aging process to proceed and spare the patient a craniotomy. Chronic subdural hematomas are prone to re-accumulate, however, especially when the brain is slow to re-expand into the space created by the clot evacuation. Sometimes chronic subdurals require permanent CSF diversion. Although re-operation is sometimes needed, chronic subdurals generally have excellent outcomes.

Communication and Counseling

Typically, all but the tiniest of epidural hematomas are evacuated, and it is straightforward to advise families that these blood clots need to be removed. If they are not removed, the children and families will often be kept in the hospital, undergoing serial CT scans until the hematoma starts to resolve. In the face of headaches and high anxiety, this can be quite frustrating and, given the risk of acute deterioration and the low risk of surgery, it is generally best to evacuate most epidural hematomas. It can be difficult to counsel families about subdural hematomas because they often are not the primary process causing neurologic symptoms. If the neurosurgeon believes that the hematoma is acting as a significant mass against the brain, then it should be removed. If the symptoms are related to the injury (and its shear effect on the brain and venous drainage), it may not be necessary to evacuate a small subdural hematoma. In either case, with epidural and/or subdural hematomas the choice of observation versus surgery is a balancing act between the likelihood of progression versus the surgical risks of evacuating the blood clot. It is beyond the scope of this chapter to outline an appropriate algorithm that all neurosurgeons would follow, but the important counseling pearl is that it is essential that a neurosurgeon be involved as the primary decision maker in these instances.

SUGGESTED READINGS

1. Committee on Quality Improvement, American Academy of Pediatrics: Commission on Clinical Policies and Research, American Academy of Family Physicians: The management of minor closed head injury in children. Pediatrics 104:1407–1415, 1999. **Guidelines for management of children ages 2 to 18 years old with minor closed head injury.**
2. Bonnier C, Nassogne MC, Saint-Martin C, et al: Neuroimaging of intraparenchymal lesions predicts outcome in shaken baby syndrome. Pediatrics 112:808–814, 2003. **Prognosis of patients with shaken baby syndrome according to CT scan characteristics.**
3. Ersahin Y, Mutluer S, Guzelbag E: Extradural hematoma: Analysis of 146 cases. Childs Nerv Syst 9:96–99, 1993. **A large surgical series of pediatric epidural hematomas.**
4. Kivlin JD: Manifestations of the shaken baby syndrome. Curr Opin Ophthalmol 12:158–163, 2001. **Prognosis of patients with shaken baby syndrome according to ophthalmologic findings.**
5. Ono J, Yamaura A, Kubota M, et al: Outcome prediction in severe head injury: Analyses of clinical prognostic factors. J Clin Neurosci 8:120–123, 2001. **Association between acute subdural hematoma, severe underlying brain injury, and poor prognosis.**
6. Rappaport ZH, Shaked I, Tadmor R: Delayed epidural hematoma demonstrated by computed tomography: Case report. Neurosurgery 10:487–489, 1982. **Case report of an epidural hematoma after an initial negative CT scan.**
7. Schutzman SA, Barnes P, Duhaime AC, et al: Evaluation and management of children younger than two years old with apparently minor head trauma: Proposed guidelines. Pediatrics 107:983–993, 2001. **Proposed guidelines for management of patients under 2 years old with minor head trauma.**
8. Simon B, Letourneau P, Vitorino E, McCall J: Pediatric minor head trauma: Indications for computed tomographic scanning revisited. J Trauma 51:231–237; discussion 237–238, 2001. **Outlines the poor positive predictive value of various clinical factors and the presence of a traumatic intracranial lesion on CT scan.**

7

Diagnosis and Management of Chiari I Malformation

Richard C.E. Anderson and Neil A. Feldstein

KEY CONCEPTS

- In patients with Chiari I malformation, narrowing at the foramen magnum and upper cervical spinal canal leads to brain stem compression, syringohydromyelia (or spinal cord syrinx), cranial nerve dysfunction, and cerebellar dysfunction.
- There is currently no effective medical treatment for patients with Chiari I malformation.
- The goals of surgical treatment are to relieve pressure on the brain stem, restore cerebrospinal fluid flow, and eliminate any pressure differential from the spinal to cranial subarachnoid space that can cause syringohydromyelia.
- Data using intraoperative electrophysiologic monitoring suggest that in pediatric patients, the majority of improvement from surgery occurs after bony decompression and division of the atlanto-occipital membrane rather than after dural opening.
- Surgical results have overall been excellent, but there is some morbidity that can largely be attributed to dural opening or intradural manipulations.

The Chiari I malformation is a congenital anomaly that consists of downward displacement of the cerebellar tonsils through the foramen magnum into the cervical spinal canal (Fig. 1). Although the extent of tonsillar descent is quite variable and is often asymmetric, downward displacement greater than or equal to 5 mm is considered

abnormal. Although the vermis, fourth ventricle, and lower brain stem are typically normal or only minimally deformed in patients with the Chiari I malformation, patients frequently do have other associated anomalies. These anomalies include syringohydromyelia (or spinal cord syrinx), abnormalities of the base of the skull and craniovertebral junction (e.g., small posterior fossa, platybasia, basilar impression, Klippel-Feil deformity, assimilation of the atlas), scoliosis, hydrocephalus, and others (Box 1).

The incidence of Chiari I malformation in the general population is unknown. A recent report of a large pediatric neurosurgical practice revealed that 40% of patients presenting with Chiari I malformation are younger than 5 years of age, 25% are between the ages of 5 and 10 years, and 30% are between 10 and 15 years of age. Prior to MRI, the distribution of Chiari I malformations among the age groups had been the same.

Radiographic criteria for the diagnosis of Chiari I malformation are controversial, because statistically significant differences in tonsillar position with age occur normally. (The cerebellar tonsils ascend with increasing age.) Nevertheless, there is general agreement that reasonable criteria for diagnosis include: (1) herniation of one or both tonsils at least 5 mm below the plane of the foramen magnum or (2) bilateral tonsillar herniation of 3 to 5 mm accompanied by other Chiari I features including syringohydromyelia or abnormalities of the cervicomedullary junction (see Box 1). Acquired tonsillar herniation from an intracranial mass lesion, Dandy-Walker malformation, or hydrocephalus should be ruled out. Despite their less frequent occurrences, the presence of associated craniovertebral anomalies (e.g., assimilation of the atlas, basilar invagination, and fused cervical vertebrae) should be investigated radiographically because

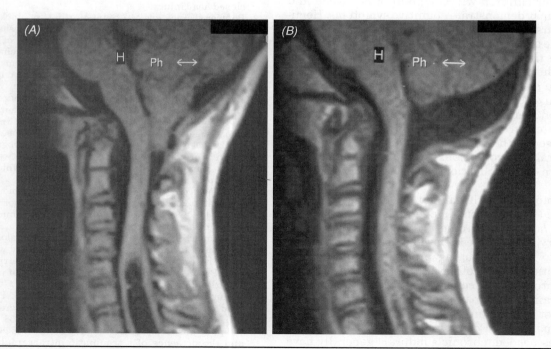

FIGURE 1. Postoperative sagittal T1-weighted MRI at 3 months follow-up (*B*) demonstrates ascension of the cerebellar tonsils and virtual resolution of the syrinx in comparison to a preoperative film (*A*).

BOX 1 Radiographic Evaluation of Chiari I Malformation

Diagnostic Criteria
- Caudal descent of one cerebellar tonsil 5 mm or more below the level of the foramen magnum
- Caudal descent of both cerebellar tonsils 3–5 mm below the level of the foramen magnum if associated with other anatomic abnormalities (e.g., syringohydromyelia or cervicomedullary kinking)
- Pointed or "pegged" appearance of the cerebellar tonsils
- Crowding of the craniocervical subarachnoid space

Associated Anomalies
- Brain: Small posterior fossa volume
- Ventricles: Mild to moderate hydrocephalus (10%–20%)
- Spinal Cord: Syringohydromyelia (50%–75%)
- Skeletal anomalies: Basilar invagination (25%–50%), Klippel-Feil (5%–10%), atlanto-occipital assimilation (1%–5%), scoliosis (30%–50% of those with syringohydromyelia)

BOX 2 Common Presenting Signs and Symptoms of Chiari I Malformation

Brain Stem and Lower Cranial Nerve Dysfunction
- Headache or cervical pain
- Down-beating nystagmus
- Vocal cord paralysis
- Respiratory irregularities
- Facial sensory abnormalities
- Dysarthria
- Palatal or tongue weakness or dysfunction
- Dysphagia
- Recurrent aspiration
- Extraocular movement abnormalities
- Sensorimotor hearing loss
- Vertigo or dizziness
- Hiccups

Spinal Cord Dysfunction (Syringohydromyelia)
- Scoliosis
- Sensory abnormalities
- Dysesthetic pain of trunk and extremities
- Clumsiness, weakness, and atrophy of hands and upper extremities
- Spasticity
- Urinary incontinence

Cerebellar Dysfunction
- Ataxia
- Nystagmus

induced or exacerbated by Valsalva maneuvers such as coughing, laughing, or sneezing. In infants and younger children who are unable to communicate verbally, headaches may manifest with only irritability and crying. Neurologic signs can be divided into three types of presentation: a brain stem syndrome (22%), a spinal cord syndrome (65%), and a cerebellar syndrome (11%) (see Box 2). Specifically, signs include motor and sensory losses, hyperreflexia, hyporeflexia, ataxia, Babinski response, clonus, either vertical or down-beating nystagmus, and respiratory irregularities including sleep apnea. Lower cranial nerve dysfunction can lead to vocal cord paralysis, dysarthria, palatal weakness, tongue atrophy, and recurrent aspiration. Progressive scoliosis is a relatively common manifestation of Chiari I malformation when there is a coexistent spinal cord syrinx. Clinical and radiographic signs that raise the suspicion of an underlying neurologic defect in a patient with scoliosis include a convexity to the left, a single curve, leg or foot asymmetry, vertebral anomalies or other congenital anomalies, and any neurologic deficit.

Expert Opinion on Management Issues

There is no effective nonsurgical treatment for patients with Chiari I malformations. Although the natural history of the disease is not completely known, the benefit of surgery in changing the clinical course of the disease has been documented in many retrospective studies over the last several decades. While the benefit of surgery is clear, major areas of controversy still center on the indications for surgery, the timing of treatment, and the details of the specific operation. Nevertheless, the common goals of management remain the alleviation of presenting symptoms, radiographic reduction of associated syrinx cavities, and arrest or remission of associated scoliosis.

The operative goal of a suboccipital decompression for Chiari I malformation is to enlarge the bony compartment surrounding the craniocervical junction, thereby expanding the space around the brain stem and restoring normal circulation of cerebrospinal fluid. Many different surgical options exist to achieve this objective. They include decompression with or without dural opening, dural opening with or without closing or patching, lysis of adhesions and exploration of the fourth ventricle with or without obex plugging or stenting of the fourth ventricle, resection of the tonsils, various shunting procedures of the syrinx itself, and terminal ventriculostomy. As indicated by surveys of members of the Pediatric Section of the American Association of Neurologic Surgeons in both 1987 and 1998, the majority of pediatric neurosurgeons perform a suboccipital decompression and duraplasty for symptomatic patients with Chiari I malformations.

At the Children's Hospital of New York, our data indicate that the vast majority of improvement in conduction time through the brain stem (as measured by brain stem auditory evoked potentials) occurred after bony decompression and division of the atlanto-occipital membrane.

of their common association with cervical instability. Cine-mode MRI can occasionally be helpful to characterize cerebrospinal fluid flow around the craniocervical junction. When a Chiari I malformation is suspected, it is usually best to be prepared to obtain an MRI of the brain and entire spine in order to exclude other disease processes and investigate any associated abnormalities.

Patients with Chiari I malformation can be asymptomatic, or they may present with a variety of symptoms and signs ranging from mild occasional headaches to severe myelopathy and brain stem compromise (Box 2). The most common presenting symptom is pain (60% to 70%), usually occipital and upper cervical in location, often

We did not see any significant improvement attributable to opening of the dura, suggesting that these patients may not require dural opening and duraplasty for adequate decompression of the brain stem. Accordingly, for the past 2 years we have not routinely opened the dura during surgery, and have seen excellent clinical and radiographic results after bony decompression and division of the atlanto-occipital membrane (without dural opening). A recent report compared the outcomes of suboccipital decompression with and without duraplasty in patients with Chiari I malformations and syringohydromyelia. Although there was no significant difference in symptomatic improvement between the two groups, the postoperative complication rate was 42% in the duraplasty group, compared to 10% in the group without dural opening. At the Children's Hospital of New York, we have not seen any significant operative morbidity in patients after suboccipital decompression without duraplasty.

Common Pitfalls

Surgical complications associated with posterior fossa decompression for the treatment of Chiari I malformation have decreased significantly over time. However, postoperative hemorrhage, infection, new neurologic deficit, subdural hygroma, aseptic meningitis, pseudomeningocele, CSF leak, hydrocephalus, and failure to improve can still occur. Significant morbidity is usually attributable to either opening the dura or performing an intradural procedure.

Progressive neurologic deficits or failure to improve after surgery should alert one to the possibility of craniocervical instability, the presence of ventral brain stem compression, recurrent syringohydromyelia, cerebellar sag, or hydrocephalus. In some cases, regeneration of the foramen magnum with new bone formation has been found to be responsible for delayed recurrence of symptoms after decompression. Stringent selection criteria, thorough knowledge of the disease process, and meticulous operative technique help limit postoperative complications.

Communication and Counseling

Interpretation of surgical outcomes after suboccipital decompression for Chiari I malformation is difficult because of an incomplete understanding of the disease, the different surgical techniques employed, and the absence of any randomized, prospective studies. Overall, results from surgical series are favorable. Symptomatic children with mild neurologic deficits treated early in the course of the disease process have excellent outcomes, with 90% to 95% improving after surgery. Subjective symptoms are more likely to improve than objective neurologic deficits. Patients presenting with symptoms and signs attributable to brain stem compression or cerebellar dysfunction appear to have a better long-term outcome than those presenting with spinal cord dysfunction. A recent study suggested that children younger than 10 years of age with scoliosis less than 40 degrees are more likely to have arrest or resolution of scoliosis after suboccipital decompression than children older than 10 years or with curves greater than 40 degrees.

SUGGESTED READINGS

1. Anderson RCE, Emerson RG, Dowling KC, et al: Attenuation of somatosensory evoked potentials during positioning in a patient undergoing suboccipital craniectomy for Chiari I malformation with syringomyelia. J Child Neurol 16:936–939, 2001. **First report of intraoperative electrophysiological monitoring altering surgical positioning in a child with Chiari I malformation.**
2. Anderson RCE, Emerson RG, Dowling KC, et al: Improvement in BAEPS after suboccipital decompression in patients with Chiari I malformation and syringohydromyelia. J Neurosurg 98:459–464, 2003. **Prospective clinical series demonstrating improvements in intraoperative electrophysiological potentials after bony opening but not after dural opening in patients undergoing suboccipital decompression for Chiari I malformation.**
3. Anderson RCE, Dowling KC, Feldstein NA, et al: Chiari I malformation: potential role for intraoperative electrophysiological monitoring? J Clin Neurophysiol 20(1):65–72, 2003. **Reviews the role of intraoperative electrophysiological monitoring during suboccipital decompression in children with Chiari I malformations.**
4. Brockmeyer DL, Gollogly S, Smith JT: Scoliosis associated with Chiari 1 malformations: the effect of suboccipital decompression on scoliosis curve progression: A preliminary study. Spine 28:2505–2509, 2003. **First detailed retrospective study investigating which patients with Chiari I malformation and scoliosis are most likely to respond to posterior decompression.**
5. Feldstein NA, Choudhri TF: Management of Chiari I malformations with holocord syringohydromyelia. Pediatr Neurosurg 31:143–149, 1999. **Retrospective review of surgical outcomes after suboccipital decompression and duraplasty in patients with Chiari I malformation and large spinal cord syrinxes.**
6. Haroun RI, Guarnieri M, Meadow JJ, et al: Current opinions for the treatment of syringomyelia and Chiari malformations: Survey of the Pediatric Section of the American Association of Neurological Surgeons. Pediatr Neurosurg 33:311–317, 2000. **Results of an international survey of pediatric neurosurgeons investigating patient management, surgical indications, and surgical techniques.**
7. Iskandar BJ, Oakes WJ: Chiari malformations. In Albright AL, Pollack IF, Adelson PD (eds): Principles and Practice of Pediatric Neurosurgery. New York: Thieme, 1999. **Excellent review of the pathophysiology, clinical manifestations, and management of children with Chiari I malformation.**
8. Munshi I, Frim D, Stine-Reyes R, et al: Effects of posterior fossa decompression with and without duraplasty on Chiari malformation–associated hydromyelia. Neurosur 2000, 46:1384–1389; discussion 1389–1390. **Retrospective study that compares surgical outcomes after suboccipital decompression with and without duraplasty for patients with Chiari I malformation and spinal cord syrinx.**
9. Osborn AG: Disorders of neural tube closure. In Osborn AG (ed): Diagnostic Neuroradiology. St. Louis: Mosby, 1994. **Excellent review of the imaging characteristics of patients with Chiari I malformation.**
10. Park JK, Gleason PL, Madsen JR, et al: Presentation and management of Chiari I malformation in children. Pediatr Neurosurg 26:190–196, 1997. **Excellent review of the management of patients with Chiari I malformation at a single institution.**
11. Weprin BE, Oakes WJ: The Chiari malformations and associated syringohydromyelia. In McLone DG (ed): Pediatric Neurosurgery, Surgery of the Developing Nervous System, 4th ed. Philadelphia: WB Saunders, 2001. **Excellent review of the pathophysiology, clinical manifestations, and management of children with Chiari I malformation.**
12. Yundt KD, Park TS, Tantuwaya VS, et al: Posterior fossa decompression without duraplasty in infants and young children for treatment of Chiari malformation and achondroplasia. Pediatr Neurosur 25:221–226, 1996. **Retrospective series providing some early evidence that posterior decompression without duraplasty is sufficient for surgical treatment.**

Abscess in the Central Nervous System

Susan E. Coffin

KEY CONCEPTS

- Obtaining material for culture is important to guide long-term antibiotic therapy.
- Sites of primary infection, such as paranasal sinuses or mastoid air cells, may be a source of culture material to enhance recovery of probable etiologic organisms.
- Anaerobic organisms are commonly associated with brain abscesses that complicate head and neck infections.
- Antibiotics that penetrate the blood–brain barrier are necessary to sterilize infections of the central nervous system.
- Sequential imaging studies are an important tool to determine response to therapy.
- Neurologic sequelae are common after brain abscess, particularly in neonatal patients.

The pathogenesis and microbiology of brain abscess in children is varied. Intracranial abscesses can develop following direct extension of infected paranasal sinuses, middle ear space, or mastoid air cells. Brain abscesses can also occur after hematogenous dissemination, such as bacteremia or septic embolization, and may be associated with bacterial meningitis. Finally, direct inoculation (associated either with a surgical procedure or traumatic injury) can lead to brain abscess. The suspected pathogenesis of infection can help clinicians to choose optimal empiric antibiotic therapy.

The microbiology of intracranial abscess is influenced by patient characteristics and the mechanism of infection. In neonates, most brain abscesses are associated with bacteremia and/or meningitis. The most common pathogens in this age group are gram-negative organisms and group B streptococcus. Among patients with intracranial abscesses associated with otitis media, mastoiditis, sinusitis, or dental infections, *Streptococcus* species are frequently isolated; these infections are frequently polymicrobial, and anaerobic organisms are common when appropriate culture techniques are used. Immunocompromised patients can develop brain abscess with opportunistic pathogens including *Aspergillus* and *Candida* species.

Expert Opinion on Management Issues

The diagnosis of brain abscess is suggested when a child presents with the classic triad of fever, headache, and focal neurologic signs. A CT or MRI scan with contrast can establish the diagnosis while excluding other mass lesions. In young infants with open fontanels, ultrasonography of the head can identify moderate to large abscesses.

Following diagnosis, the acute management of a child with a brain abscess includes empiric antibiotic therapy and, if present, control of elevated intracranial pressure. Upon stabilization, surgical drainage is important for both diagnostic and therapeutic purposes. Aspiration and evacuation of abscess contents provides material for culture and may reduce the burden of organisms. Less frequently, a well-encapsulated lesion can be excised. Because cultures of blood and cerebrospinal fluid are often sterile, it is important to attempt aspiration of the abscess to determine a microbiologic etiology whenever possible. Up to 25% of cultures obtained do not have an organism isolated. If multiple or inaccessible lesions are present, patients can be managed with empirical antibiotic therapy and frequent imaging to evaluate their response to therapy. Finally, culture of fluid aspirated from infected sinuses or mastoids may also provide data to guide antibiotic therapy.

Antibiotic therapy should be guided by susceptibility tests of organisms cultured from the abscess. Initially, empirical therapy should include coverage for organisms associated with meningitis and head and neck infections. Typically, patients are treated with an antistaphylococcal drug (a semisynthetic penicillin or vancomycin based on prevalence of methicillin-resistant *Staphylococcus aureus*) and a third-generation cephalosporin. If the patient has an associated head and neck infection, anaerobic coverage should be added. When a patient develops a brain abscess following a neurosurgical procedure, vancomycin should be included as part of empirical therapy to ensure adequate coverage for coagulase-negative staphylococcus species. Immunocompromised patients should receive antifungal therapy due to the risk of *Candida* or *Aspergillus* infection. When culture and susceptibility data are available, further adjustments of antibiotic therapy can be made. Typically, clinical improvement is assessed by serial examination and repeated imaging. Brain abscesses are usually treated for 4 to 8 weeks depending upon host factors and the response to therapy.

Common Pitfalls

Laboratory testing is often normal in patients with brain abscess. Total leukocyte counts and inflammatory markers are rarely elevated. Lumbar puncture should be avoided because it may precipitate herniation, and analysis of cerebrospinal fluid rarely provides important clinical information.

Selected antibiotics do not penetrate the blood–brain barrier and therefore should not be used to treat patients with brain abscess. For example, clindamycin may be an excellent drug to treat an anaerobic infection of the head and neck; however, it does not penetrate into the CNS space and should not be used to treat a patient with known or suspected anaerobic brain abscess.

Communication and Counseling

Brain abscesses are associated with significant morbidity and mortality. Overall, brain abscesses are associated with a 10% to 14% mortality rate. Factors such as young age, coma at the time of presentation, and multiple abscesses are associated with an increased risk of death. Neurologic sequelae occur in approximately 50% of all children. However, neonatal brain abscesses associated with gram-negative infection can be particularly devastating, with sequelae including hydrocephalus, seizure disorders, and cognitive impairment that can affect up to 70% of survivors.

SUGGESTED READINGS

1. Brook I: Aerobic and anaerobic bacteriology of intracranial abscess. Pediatr Neuro 8:210–214, 1992. **Bacteriology of 39 cases of pediatric intracranial abscesses.**
2. Goodkin HP, Harper MB, Pomeroy SL: Intracerebral abscess in children: Historical trends at Children's Hospital Boston. Pediatrics 113:1765–1770, 2004. **Longitudinal analysis of six decades of pediatric brain abscesses.**
3. Renier D, Flandin C, Hirsch E, Hirsch JF: Brain abscesses in neonates. J Neurosurg 69:877–882, 1988. **Case series of 30 neonates with brain abscess.**
4. Saez-Llorens X, Umana MA, Odio CM, et al: Brain abscess in infants and children. Pediatr Infect Dis J 8:449–458, 1989. **Case series of 101 children with pediatric brain abscess treated in Dallas, Texas, and San Jose, Costa Rica.**
5. Saez-Llorens X: Brain abscess in children. Sem Pediatr Infect Dis 14:108–114, 2003. **Comprehensive review of the microbiology, clinical manifestations, and outcome of pediatric brain abscess.**

Acute and Chronic Immune-Mediated Polyneuropathy

Malcolm Rabie, Howard W. Sander and Yoram Nevo

KEY CONCEPTS

- Management of Guillain-Barré syndrome (GBS) requires expert medical and nursing care. Patients should be referred to centers that have experience in managing this condition.
- Blood pressure and cardiac rhythm in GBS must be monitored for autonomic complications.
- Patients with early cranial nerve involvement may have impending respiratory insufficiency.
- Most children with chronic inflammatory demyelinating polyradiculoneuropathy (CIDP) respond to immunotherapy; however, some children have residual deficits.
- CIDP must be distinguished from hereditary neuropathies by onset, family history, and nerve conduction studies and occasionally by a nerve biopsy.

Acute and Chronic Immune-Mediated Polyneuropathy

This section focuses on the spectrum of Guillain-Barré syndrome (GBS) and chronic inflammatory demyelinating polyradiculoneuropathy in childhood, in which a postulated acquired autoimmune-mediated pathophysiology is directed against the Schwann cell, myelin, axon, or a combination of these components in the spinal roots, plexuses, and peripheral nerves.

GUILLAIN-BARRÉ SYNDROME

The most common cause of acute childhood flaccid paralysis is Guillain-Barré syndrome (GBS), a clinical diagnosis supported by cerebrospinal and electrodiagnostic findings. It affects all ages, races, and sexes, but it is rare in those over the age of 80 years and those younger than 2 years of age. The estimated annual incidence is 0.5 to 1.5 cases per 100,000 population younger than 18 years (adults 0.4 to 4 per 100 000). The clinical features in pediatric cases are similar to those for adults, except that severe sequelae are less common and axonal forms are more frequent in certain populations (Table 1). Maximal neurologic deficit is usually reached within 4 weeks. In half to two thirds of children there is an associated antecedent infection (e.g., *Haemophilus influenzae*, Epstein-Barr, cytomegalovirus, HIV, *Mycoplasma pneumoniae*, *Campylobacter jejuni*), immunization, trauma, toxin, or surgery. The cerebrospinal fluid examination typically reveals a raised protein concentration after several days without cells (albuminocytologic dissociation) and a normal pressure. Ganglioside antibodies offer little diagnostic and prognostic value. In the vast majority of GBS in children in the Western world, nerve conduction studies (NCS) show demyelinating features such as conduction slowing (prolonged distal latencies, slowed conduction velocities, prolonged F-wave minimal latencies, prolonged H-reflex minimal latencies) or conduction block over focal nerve segments. With more advanced disease, there may also be low amplitude compound muscle action potentials. NCS performed early in the course or in mild cases may be non-specific. In Asia, primary axonal variants of GBS (AMAN [acute motor axonal neuropathy], AMSAN [acute motor-sensory axonal neuropathy]) have also been reported.

CHRONIC INFLAMMATORY DEMYELINATING POLYRADICULONEUROPATHY

Chronic inflammatory demyelinating polyradiculoneuropathy (CIDP) is a treatable chronic, predominantly motor neuropathy that manifests with either an acute or insidious onset, with progression of symptoms occurring over a period of at least 2 months. The course may be monophasic, slowly progressive, or relapsing remitting and may result in long-term disability.

The prevalence of CIDP is 1 to 2 cases per 100,000 adults, with onset within the first two decades of life in 20% of patients. Children usually present with gait difficulties, but there may have been preceding sensory symptoms. Antecedent events such as infection and immunization are reported in a third to half of childhood and adult CIDP case reports. The CSF protein concentration is often raised and there are fewer than 5 cells/mm^3 (albuminocytologic dissociation). NCS findings are similar to those described for demyelinating GBS.

TABLE 1 Comparison of Guillain-Barré Syndrome and Main Variants in Children

GBS/Variants	Clinical	Course	Prognosis and Therapy
AIDP/GBS	Clinical: rapid ascending symmetric weakness, CN, ANS, sensory Incidence: main type of GBS in Western countries Pathology: demyelinating Target antigens: unknown (myelin/Schwann cell).	Weeks to months	±90% children and ±75% adults recover. IVIG/PE efficacious.
AMAN	Clinical: ≈AIDP mainly motor (dysautonomia, CN) Incidence: higher in China, Japan, and developing countries Pathology: axonal motor, associated with CJ Target antigens: (motor axolemmal) GM1, GM1b, GD1a, GalNAc-GD1a	≈AIDP; recovery fast, some slow	Good, poorer with CJ+; IVIG/PE efficacy not proven.
AMSAN	Clinical: ≈AIDP, motor-sensory (dysautonomia, CN) Incidence: much less than AMAN Pathology: axonal motor and sensory, associated with CJ+	May be fulminant; very slow recovery	Poorer than AIDP. poorer with CJ+; residual deficits. IVIG/PE efficacy not proven.
Miller Fisher Syndrome	Clinical: external ophthalmoplegia, gait ataxia, areflexia, CSF; albuminocytologic dissociation or normal Target antigen: IgG/M GQ1b	Months	Good (≈mild-moderate AIDP). IVIG/PE probably effective.

≈similar to; AIDP, acute inflammatory demyelinating polyradiculoneuropathy; AMAN, acute motor axonal neuropathy; AMSAN, acute motor-sensory axonal neuropathy; ANS, dysautonomia; CJ+, recent *Campylobacter jejuni* infection; CN, cranial nerve involvement; GBS, Guillain-Barré syndrome.

7

Expert Opinion on Management Issues

GUILLAIN-BARRÉ SYNDROME

With supportive care alone, GBS recovery usually starts within 2 to 4 weeks after the progression of the weakness stops. Most children recover without significant neurologic problems within 3 to 12 months.

Management

The patient's condition may deteriorate rapidly; thus hospitalization and regular monitoring of autonomic and respiratory function is required until maximal disability is reached. Children and adults with rapid disease progression, severe bilateral facial weakness, bulbar/neck/shoulder weakness, or dysautonomia are more likely to require mechanical ventilation.

Indications for intensive care unit (ICU) admission are impending respiratory failure, dysautonomia, complications of the immunotherapy, or later complications (e.g., sepsis, bleeding). Indications for intubation are impending respiratory failure and oropharyngeal paresis (to prevent aspiration) and autonomic complications.

With *impending respiratory failure and oropharyngeal paresis*, respiratory failure is characterized by paradoxical breathing, lethargy, and reduced alertness (hypoxemia until proved otherwise) or hypoxemia diagnosed by pulse oximetry or arterial blood gases. In adults, a vital capacity that has declined to less than 20 mL/kg is also

an indication for intubation and is preferable to avoid emergent intubation. Infants and children with severe respiratory muscle weakness may lack the classic clinical signs of rapid respiratory effort and retractions, having only anxiety and tachycardia.

Autonomic complications include cardiac arrhythmias and hyper- and hypotension. Adynamic ileus and urinary retention must be checked for regularly and treated in this situation.

Early management involves nasogastric tube feeding for significant dysphagia, nutritional support, and positioning the child to avoid pressure palsies and aid pulmonary drainage. Attention for complications such as infections, gastrointestinal hemorrhage/dysfunction, and hyponatremia is necessary. Late management consists of gentle mobilization, physical therapy for early rehabilitation, and, when necessary, speech therapy and occupational therapy.

Specific Treatment

Intravenous human intravenous immunoglobulin (IVIG) and plasmapheresis (PE) are used for treatment. In adults, PE and IVIG significantly reduce the median time to independent walking in untreated patients from 85 days to plus or minus 43 days (PE) and plus or minus 51 days (IVIG); however, the long-term outcome remains unchanged. A similar reduction is reported in several small childhood studies with rapidly progressive weakness. As PE and IVIG have equivalent efficacies, IVIG is preferred in children because PE is invasive. Combined therapy is not thought to be more effective than either alone. Relapse rates in the first few weeks of treatment are similar in both IVIG- and PE-treated groups, and they usually respond to retreatment with the same regimen. CSF filtration, immunoabsorption, or corticosteroids are not recommended in GBS in adults or children.

Contraindications

IVIG is relatively contraindicated where there is hypersensitivity to human immunoglobulin, severe renal disease, or severe cardiovascular disease. Serum immunoglobulin (Ig)A levels should be obtained prior to nonemergent IVIG therapy. In patients with IgA deficiency (prevalence ±1:1000), IgA-poor IVIG or alternative therapies may be used to prevent anaphylaxis. However, the risk of anaphylaxis is not eliminated with the use of IgA-poor preparations. In emergencies, an IgA-poor IVIG preparation may be used until the serum IgA level is available. Avoid PE with marked dysautonomia.

Timing

IVIG or PE should be started promptly, and both are probably effective within 7 days of onset.

Dosage and Administration. Dosing for IVIG and PE is as follows:

- Total dose of IVIG is 2 g/kg given as 1 g/kg/day for 2 days or 0.4 g/kg/day for 5 days given slowly to avoid infusion-related problems.
- In severe childhood GBS, four plasma exchanges over 10 days may be administered. PE is generally not recommended if body weight is less than 10 to 15 kg. Future therapeutic areas under investigation involve modulating cytokine expression, cell adhesion molecules and selective targeting of T cells.

CHRONIC INFLAMMATORY DEMYELINATING POLYRADICULONEUROPATHY

CIDP usually responds to corticosteroids within approximately 2 months; however, there is considerable variability. Treatment should not be withheld if CIDP research diagnostic criteria are not entirely fulfilled, and it should be started as soon as the diagnosis is made. Prior to treatment, baseline strength, reflexes, sensation, and electromyelogram (EMG) and NCS are useful for follow-up. An initial high dose of prednisone or prednisolone, 1 to 2 mg/kg/day orally (maximum of 60–80 mg/day) is recommended for 4 to 6 weeks. Relapses are frequent with rapid tapering; therefore, a slow reduction by 5 mg every 2 weeks is recommended after a clinical response is achieved. Tapering is begun after a significant improvement, but not before 4 to 6 weeks. High-dose pulse corticosteroids may be an alternative approach; however, there may be subsequent deterioration and progressive muscle weakness. PE is an effective temporary adjunctive treatment for chronic progressive and relapsing CIDP; however for the long-term, immunosuppressant drugs are preferred. Both steroids and IVIG are recommended as first-line therapy in children (Table 2). In selected resistant cases or for steroid sparing, azathioprine or cyclosporine may be effective. Other therapies, such as mycophenolate mofetil, have insufficient data. Interferons (INFs) are under investigation in adults, and a few single childhood reports show improvement with IFN-α–2a and IFN-β.

Follow-up and treatment for long-term complications of corticosteroids (hypertension, osteoporosis, diabetes, bleeding, cataract, etc.) is needed. Supplemental calcium and vitamin D, antacids or histamine–2 blocking agents may be considered. Ophthalmologic consultations, monitoring of caloric intake and serum potassium, salt restriction, and bone density evaluation is required. Physical therapy, emotional support, weight reduction,

---

TABLE 2 Therapy in Childhood Chronic Inflammatory Demyelinating Polyneuropathy

Therapy	Advantages	Disadvantages	Dosing
Steroids	Inexpensive and easy to use first-line therapy	Many long-term side effects (e.g., excessive weight gain, hypertension, behavior problems, hyperglycemia, cataracts, gastritis, femoral head aseptic necrosis) Response: weeks to 3–6 mo	PO Prednisolone/prednisone 1–2 mg/kg/day Max dose 60–80 mg
IVIG	Less invasive than PE May be given as outpatient first-line therapy	Expensive. Relapse 1–4 wk S/E: Chills, rash, aseptic meningitis, thrombosis, renal, fluids, anaphylaxis C/I: IgA deficiency, allergy to IVIG, severe renal or cardiac disease	IV 1 g/kg/day for 2 days or 0.4 g/kg/day × 5d Maintenance: 0.4–2 g/kg every 2–4 weeks
PE	Rapid response Temporary adjunctive but may be primary therapy	Expensive. Relapse 2–8 wk Invasive, specialized center, complications (e.g., venous access) Recommended if child's weight >10–15 kg C/I: cardiac, clotting disorder, hypotension	Variable frequency

C/I, relative contraindication; IV, intravenous; IVIG, intravenous human immunoglobulin; PE, plasma exchange; PO, by mouth; S/E, side effects.

ankle-foot orthoses, wrist splints, and a rehabilitation program are important.

Common Pitfalls

GUILLAIN-BARRÉ SYNDROME

- The EMG and CSF protein are often normal in the first week. In some cases, the protein remains normal through the illness.
- Atelectasis and reduced cough reflex may cause earlier respiratory failure.

CHRONIC INFLAMMATORY DEMYELINATING POLYRADICULONEUROPATHY

- Distinguish from hereditary neuropathies by family history, onset, and uniform slowing on nerve conduction studies (as opposed to non-uniform slowing in CIDP).
- In severe or atypical CIDP, nerve histopathology (demyelination and inflammation) may help support the diagnosis.
- Intercurrent infection and immunization may cause a relapse.
- If the CSF white cell count is >10/mm^3, exclude infection such as HIV.

Communication and Counseling

During the recovery from GBS, neurologic deficits including foot drop, hand dysfunction, paresthesias, and ataxia may occur; however, children recover faster than adults and have less residua. Communication, encouragement, and psychological support of children and their families are essential throughout the course of the disease.

In CIDP the prognosis for eventual recovery and long-term remission is less favorable than in GBS and a proportion of patients will suffer neurologic residua.

Family and patient support groups (http://www.guillain-barre.com, http://www.neuropathy.org, and http://www.neuropathy-trust.org) provide useful information about neuropathies.

ACKNOWLEDGEMENT

The authors wish to thank Professor J. Sivan for assistance with the critical care management of children with polyradiculoneuropathies.

SUGGESTED READINGS

1. Burns TM, Dyck PJ, Darras BT, Jones RH, Jr. Chronic inflammatory demyelinating polyradiculoneuropathy. In Jones RH, Jr, De Vivo DC, Darras BT (eds): Neuromuscular Disorders of Infancy, Childhood, and Adolescence, A Clinician's Approach. Boston: Butterworth Heinemann, 2003. **Detailed description of the clinical, pathologic, electrophysiologic and treatment aspects of childhood CIDP.**

2. Connolly AM: Chronic Inflammatory demyelinating polyneuropathy in childhood. Pediatr Neurol 24:177–183, 2001. **A review of childhood CIDP with an overview of therapy from 1980 to 2000.**

3. 88th ENMC International Workshop: Childhood chronic inflammatory demyelinating polyneuropathy (including revised criteria), Naarden, the Netherlands, December 8–10, 2000. Neuromusc Disord 12:195–200, 2002. **Outlines the clinical features, electrophysiology, pathology, therapy, and revised childhood CIDP research diagnostic criteria.**

4. Hughes RA: Management of chronic inflammatory demyelinating polyradiculoneuropathy. Drugs 63:275–287, 2003. **A review of immunotherapy and their adverse effects in adult CIDP.**

5. Nevo Y: Childhood chronic inflammatory demyelinating polyneuropathy. Eur J Paediatr Neurol 2:169–177, 1998. **A detailed review of childhood CIDP.**

6. Nevo Y, Pestronk A, Kornberg AJ, et al: Childhood chronic inflammatory demyelinating neuropathies: Clinical course and long term follow up. Neurology 47:98–102, 1996. **Description of clinical characteristics, treatment and prognosis of CIDP in a group of 13 children.**

7. Report of the Quality Standards Subcommittee of the American Academy of Neurology: Practice parameter: Immunotherapy for Guillain-Barré syndrome. Neurology 61:736–740, 2003. Correspondence and reply in Neurology. 62:1653–1654, 2004. **An evidence-based guide to management of GBS in adults and children.**

8. Sander HW, Hedley-Whyte ET: Case 6–2003: A nine-year-old girl with progressive weakness and areflexia. N Engl J Med 348:735–743, 2003. **CPC discussion of the differential diagnosis and pathology of childhood CIDP.**

9. Sladky JT: Guillain-Barré syndrome in children. J Child Neurol 19:191–200, 2004. **Description of the clinical aspects, pathogenesis and treatment of Guillain-Barré syndrome in children.**

10. The Neuropathy Association Medical Advisory Committee: Guidelines for the Diagnosis and treatment of Chronic Inflammatory Demyelinating Polyneuropathy. J Peripher Nerv Syst 8:281–283, 2003. **A consensus statement designed to allow broader criteria for diagnosing CIDP facilitating access to treatment for patients.**

7

General Concepts in Seizure Management

James J. Riviello, Jr.

KEY CONCEPTS

- Differential diagnosis of seizures: Not all episodes called seizures are epileptic events. Events without an epileptic mechanism are called nonepileptic events or nonepileptic paroxysmal events.
- Classification of seizure type and epilepsy syndrome: Seizure type is determined by the outward clinical manifestations (the signs, or semiology); epilepsy syndrome is classified first by the seizure type and then by various associated findings.
- Etiology of seizures: Seizure etiology is determined by the underlying cause of the seizure—symptomatic, cryptogenic, or idiopathic.
- Management of acute seizure: The airway, breathing, circulation procedures (ABCs) must be adhered to for seizure management. Expert opinion now recommends treatment for a seizure lasting longer than 5 minutes.
- Need for diagnostic studies: An electroencephalogram (EEG) is usually done with other diagnostic studies ordered on an individual basis. These include basic metabolic studies, toxicology studies, lumbar puncture, and

neuroimaging (cranial computed axial tomography [CAT] scan or MRI).
■ Choice of antiepileptic drugs (AEDs): The decision to treat a seizure is usually made when the seizure recurs. Certain AEDs are better for a focal seizure, with or without secondary generalization, and certain AEDs are better for a primary generalized epilepsy, depending on the generalized seizure type: either a generalized tonic–clonic, tonic, myoclonic, or absence seizure.

Seizure management begins with evaluating the presenting event, formulating a differential diagnosis, and selecting the appropriate diagnostic studies. The term *seizure* is not synonymous with *epilepsy*, as it is used for both epileptic and nonepileptic conditions. The International Classification of Epileptic Seizures (ICES), devised by the International League Against Epilepsy (ILAE), is the most commonly used classification system. Classifying epileptic seizure type and epilepsy syndrome guides the diagnostic evaluation, treatment, selection of the appropriate antiepileptic drug (AED), and prognosis. Table 1 summarizes the ILAE definition of specific terms.

The ICES first classifies the seizure type, determined by the actual clinical manifestations, or signs (semiology), and then the epilepsy syndrome (Table 2). The location of seizure onset is important: focal, generalized, or unknown (unclassified). *Focal* indicates a seizure in which the initial clinical manifestations suggest activation of only one part of a cerebral hemisphere. *Generalized* indicates a seizure whose initial clinical manifestations are consistent with more than minimal involvement of both cerebral hemispheres. A generalized tonic–clonic seizure (GTCS) may be primary or secondary, depending on whether or not it has a focal onset. With a focal onset, it is called a secondary GTCS, or secondarily generalized epilepsy, whereas if it is nonfocal, it is called a primary GTCS, or primary generalized epilepsy. Defining the epilepsy syndrome starts with seizure type and then considers associated signs and symptoms typically occurring together: clinical manifestations, age of onset, family history, electroencephalogram (EEG) findings, etiology, and prognosis (benign or malignant).

Seizures may also be classified by etiology and can be identified from either the history or ancillary testing. Symptomatic seizures result from a known or suspected CNS disorder. These are divided into acute symptomatic, resulting from an acute CNS insult, and remote symptomatic, resulting from a past CNS insult. A specific cause is not identified with either cryptogenic or idiopathic seizures. Cryptogenic seizures are presumed symptomatic, because either the neurologic examination or developmental history is abnormal, whereas these are both normal in idiopathic (unprovoked) seizures.

The initial approach depends on whether the event is the acute presentation of a new-onset seizure or the report of a suspicious event or events. When the event is acute, treatment starts with stabilization, following the ABCs (establishment of airway, breathing, and circulation), and then assessing whether the child is acutely ill or has persistent altered awareness. If the seizure

---

TABLE 1 Terms from ILAE Task Force on Classification and Terminology

- Seizure: Sudden clinical event with outward change in neurologic function.
- Ictus: A neurologic event, including stroke, epileptic seizure, or an anoxic event.
- Convulsion: Excessive, abnormal muscle contractions, usually bilateral, that may be sustained or interrupted.
- Epileptic seizure refers to manifestations of epileptic (excessive and/or hypersynchronous), usually self-limited, neuronal activity. Adding the modifier "epileptic" to seizure signifies an epileptic etiology, clearly separating an "epileptic" from a "nonepileptic" seizure.
- Epilepsy refers to:
  - An epileptic disorder: A chronic neurologic condition characterized by recurrent epileptic seizures.
  - Epilepsies: Conditions involving chronic recurrent epileptic seizures.
- Epileptic syndromes: A complex of signs and symptoms that define a unique epilepsy condition.

ILAE, International League Against Epilepsy.

TABLE 2 Features Used to Classify Seizures (A) and Epileptic Syndromes (B)

A: Seizure Type(s):

I. Focal (partial)
   Simple focal
   Complex focal
   Focal with secondary
II. Generalized
   Tonic-clonic
   Absence
   Clonic
   Tonic
   Atonic
   Myoclonic

B: Cluster of Signs and Symptoms Customarily Occurring Together:

III. Unclassified
   Seizure type
   Age of onset
   Etiology
   Anatomy
   Precipitating factors
   Severity: Prognosis, benign, or malignant
   EEG, both ictal and interictal
   Duration of epilepsy
   Associated clinical features
   Chronicity
   Diurnal and circadian cycling

---

continues, an AED must be given to stop it. It is always important to consider the specific causes, especially for a first-time seizure or seizures in infants and younger children, in whom there is a higher incidence of symptomatic seizures. With an acute illness and fever, meningitis and encephalitis must be excluded, especially in the infant, in whom the classic signs of meningitis may not occur. Fever itself may reduce the seizure threshold in infants and young children; these are called benign febrile seizures (management is discussed in a different chapter).

The history is important. Has there been fever, vomiting, diarrhea, or trauma? An important point in considering the need for ancillary testing is whether the child has returned to baseline mental status; persistent altered awareness is more likely with symptomatic seizures. When the child presents after the actual seizure has resolved, often to the pediatrician's office, the history is especially important for determining etiology, whether a prior seizure has occurred, or the need for AED therapy. The physical examination includes both a general and neurologic examination, paying particular attention to signs of increased intracranial pressure, such as papilledema, herniation, or focality. Classification guides the need for additional tests and AED selection. If a benign syndrome is diagnosed, such as absence epilepsy or benign focal epilepsy of childhood, then no testing beyond EEG is needed. AED choice is determined by whether seizures are focal or generalized: certain AEDs are better for focal seizures, whereas other AEDs are better for either generalized seizures or certain epileptic syndromes. Some seizure types or epilepsy syndromes respond favorably to specific AEDs (pharmacologic sensitivity), for example, sodium valproate for juvenile myoclonic epilepsy, whereas others are aggravated by specific AEDs (pharmacologic insensitivity), for example, carbamazepine may aggravate primary generalized epilepsy. However, not every seizure may be classified into a specific syndrome, or the typical syndrome characteristics may not be apparent at the onset.

Recurrent seizures raise different questions. Recurrent seizures in infancy require an evaluation to exclude a specific cause. The evaluation of infantile spasms is covered in another chapter. If the child has not been treated with an AED, this decision may need reconsideration. If the child is on an AED, management questions include: is the AED dose appropriate, should the AED level be checked, and is it the appropriate AED? In general, initial AED dosing is determined by weight and increased in increments over several weeks until either complete seizure control is achieved or side effects occur. At this point, another AED is considered.

Expert Opinion on Management Issues

A prolonged seizure, or status epilepticus (SE), defined as seizure duration greater than 30 minutes, needs AED treatment. Expert opinion recommends lorazepam (LZP), 0.1 mg/kg, for a seizure lasting greater than 5 minutes. In the only childhood study comparing intravenous LZP and diazepam (DZP), the success rate was 70% (19/27) with LZP versus 65% (22/34) with DZP.

Practice parameters using evidence-based medicine have been devised for both the evaluation and treatment of a first unprovoked seizure. The parameter for evaluation recommends a routine EEG, although some experts disagree. Further evaluation, such as laboratory studies, lumbar puncture (LP), and neuroimaging are based on specific clinical circumstances. For a first nonfebrile seizure in a child older than 6 months of age who has

TABLE 3 Conditions with a High Risk for Clinically Significant Findings on Neuroimaging

- Sickle cell disease
- Hemorrhagic disorders
- Cerebral vascular disease
- Malignancy
- HIV infection
- Hydrocephalus
- Travel to area endemic for cysticercosis
- Closed head injury

HIV, human immunodeficiency virus.

returned to baseline, laboratory studies are ordered based on individual clinical circumstances, such as vomiting, diarrhea, dehydration, or history of trauma. Toxicology screening should be considered if there is any question of drug exposure or substance abuse. For the child with the first afebrile seizure, LP is of limited value; LP is considered when there is concern for infection. MRI is the preferred study for neuroimaging, since it is more sensitive than cranial computed axial tomography (CAT) scan. However, if emergent neuroimaging is needed in the emergency department (ED) (new-onset neurologic deficits or persistent altered awareness), this is usually done with CAT scan. In children presenting to the ED with a first nonfebrile seizure, Sharma and colleagues identified two factors associated with clinically significant findings on neuroimaging: predisposing conditions (Table 3), and focal seizures in children younger than 33 months of age. When the child does not return to baseline, all of these studies need consideration.

Freeman suggests the following approach to evaluate a first afebrile seizure:

- Determine if the seizure continues, and address ABCs.
- Obtain history to determine if it was the first seizure; whether there were provoking factors, such as head trauma; and the characteristics of time of day or night, presence of flashing lights, preceding myoclonic jerks, or a focal onset.
- Physical and neurologic examinations.
- Unless special circumstances exist, blood work, LP, and neuroimaging are not needed.

Determining if a seizure continues may not be immediately obvious in all cases, since some seizures may be subtle, with minimal or no obvious manifestations.

Recurrent afebrile seizures in infants need an evaluation, including metabolic studies and neuroimaging. LP is needed to detect certain metabolic disorders: the glucose transporter defect (low glucose), mitochondrial disorders (elevated lactic acid may only occur in CSF), hyperglycinemia, serine deficiency, or folinic acid–responsive seizures).

Evidence-based analyses of AED treatment are sparse in children. For a first unprovoked seizure, the decision to treat or not treat is based on a risk-benefit assessment weighing the risk of recurrence versus the risk of chronic

TABLE 4 Differential Diagnoses of Seizures
• Syncope, pallid infantile syncope, breath-holding attacks
• Cardiac arrhythmias
• Night terrors, somnambulism, parasomnias
• Narcolepsy, cataplexy, hypersomnia
• Hyperekplexia (Startle disease)
• Rage attacks, episodic dyscontrol, panic attacks
• Migraines, especially benign paroxysmal vertigo, acute confusional state
• Basilar artery migraine
• Movement disorders, paroxysmal dystonia, paroxysmal choreoathetosis, tics (especially ocular tics)
• Sandifer syndrome, gastroesophageal reflux, esophageal spasm
• Ocular movements (tics, spasms, nystagmus)
• Infantile masturbation
• Pseudoseizures
• Transient ischemic events

TABLE 5 Choice of Antiepileptic Drugs

Focal/Secondary Generalized	Generalized/Primary Generalized
Phenobarbital	**Generalized Tonic–Clonic Seizure**
Phenytoin	Sodium valproate
Carbamazepine	Felbamate*
Sodium valproate	Lamotrigine
Felbamate*	Topiramate
Gabapentin	Levetiracetam
Lamotrigine	Zonisamide
Topiramate	**Absence Seizure**
Tiagabine	Ethosuximide
Oxcarbazepine	Lamotrigine
Levetiracetam	Clonazepam
Zonisamide	Sodium valproate

*Now used only for refractory epilepsy.

AED therapy. Certain seizure types and epilepsy syndromes (absence epilepsy or infantile spasms) always recur. Ethosuximide, valproate, or lamotrigine are used for absence seizures, but no evidence supports one over another. Ethosuximide is used when absence seizures occur without generalized tonic clonic seizures (GTC), and valproate or lamotrigine is used for absence seizures with GTC seizures.

Common Pitfalls

Correct diagnosis and classification directly affect management. These questions are important:

■ Is the event, or seizure, an epileptic seizure?
■ What is the differential diagnosis? If this is epilepsy, are AEDs needed, and which should be used?
■ What evaluation is needed, if any, and what is the prognosis?

The differential diagnosis of epilepsy in children is extensive (Table 4). The prolonged QT syndrome is an excellent example of asking, "Is the event epilepsy?" Patients typically present with seizures, epilepsy may be diagnosed, and treatment started with an AED rather than an antiarrhythmic, but an electrocardiogram (ECG) is essential for the diagnosis. Pacia and colleagues reviewed the prolonged QT syndrome manifesting as epilepsy: The average age of onset was 4.7 years, yet the time to correct diagnosis ranged from 1 to 28 years. Common symptoms included presyncopal complaints and the feeling of lifelessness prior to the seizures. Remember that clinical manifestations suggest, but do not make, a specific diagnosis; further testing may be needed.

The term *nonepileptic paroxysmal event* (NEPE) is used for recurrent paroxysmal disorders without an epileptic mechanism. NEPEs are common in adults and children, are often called seizures, and mistakenly diagnosed as epilepsy. NEPE occurred in 134 of 833 children monitored recently in an epilepsy unit. EEG does not always differentiate epilepsy from a nonepileptic event. The interictal EEG may be normal in epilepsy, and not all epileptic events have abnormalities detected with surface EEG recordings.

Is the diagnosis epilepsy? The question should be asked in refractory epilepsy. When seizures continue despite appropriate AEDs at appropriate doses (Table 5), the original diagnosis must be suspected. Pseudoseizures, also called psychogenic seizures or psychogenic nonepileptic seizures (NES), may be especially difficult to diagnose and may coexist with epilepsy.

Communication and Counseling

With the initial presentation of seizures, the child is usually presented to the ED or primary care physician's office. Typically, if there is an overt convulsive seizure, or if it persists, presentation is to the ED. If the episode is not obvious, it may be reported later to the primary care physician. Once the initial evaluation is complete, it is important to communicate with the family and address their concerns and fears. Some specific points to discuss: What a seizure is, what activities are allowed, the likelihood of recurrence, and what to do if the seizure recurs. Seizures are very frightening to the child and the family, and many are afraid of dying or fear that the child will die. Death is unlikely from a single seizure, unless prolonged, and even this is unusual. There is a condition called *sudden unexplained death in epilepsy* (SUDEP), but it is rare in children and usually occurs with refractory epilepsy. Parents should also be reassured that brain tumors or strokes rarely present with epilepsy in childhood. Follow-up with the primary care physician is essential, and referral to a child neurologist is reasonable.

Immediate AED treatment is not mandatory for a first epileptic seizure. Many children have a single seizure and never have another. Population-based studies from Nova Scotia show that remission rates and long-term outcome are not affected by AED treatment after a first seizure. Even if treatment is delayed until up to 10 seizures occur, remission rates are unchanged. Families may be appropriately concerned about medication side effects and may be reassured when they realize that delaying treatment is not harmful.

SUGGESTED READINGS

1. Appleton R, Martland T, Phillips B: Drug management for acute tonic-clonic convulsions including convulsive status epilepticus in children. Cochrane Database Syst Rev 2003, CD001905. **Review of published aggregate data; no evidence that lorazepam should replace diazepam as a first-line treatment for status epilepticus.**

2. Blume WT, Luders HO, Mizrahi E, et al: Glossary of descriptive terminology for ictal semiology: Report of the ILAE Task Force on Classification and Terminology. Epilepsia 42:1212–1218, 2001. **Lists all terms used in ictal semiology, including general terms and those describing epileptic seizure semiology.**

3. Camfield C, Camfield P, Gordon K, Dooley J: Does the number of seizures before treatment influence ease of control or remission of childhood epilepsy? Neurology 46:41–44, 1996. **Ten or fewer seizures before treatment does not influence the ultimate control of remission of childhood epilepsy.**

4. Camfield P, Camfield C, Smith S, et al: Long-term outcome is unchanged by antiepileptic drug treatment after a first seizure: A 15 year follow-up from a randomized trial in childhood. Epilepsia 43:662–663, 2002. **These papers show that the subsequent clinical course and remission rates are not affected by treatment of a first seizure, or if AEDs are started before 10 seizures.**

5. Commission on Classification and Terminology of the International League against Epilepsy: Proposal for Revised Classification of Epilepsies and Epileptic Syndromes. Epilepsia 30:389–399, 1989. **The current classification system in use. Gives definitions of focal, generalized, symptomatic, cryptogenic, and idiopathic. Defines and describes the recognized focal epilepsies and epilepsy syndromes.**

6. Freeman JM: Less testing is needed in the emergency room after a first afebrile seizure. Pediatrics 111:194–196, 2003. **Commentary on the need for less testing after a first afebrile seizure.**

7. Gilbert DL, Buncher CR: An EEG should not be obtained routinely after first unprovoked seizure in childhood. Neurology 54:635–641, 2000. **Refutes the recommendation of a routine EEG in the diagnosis of a first childhood seizure.**

8. Hirtz D, Ashwal S, Berg A, et al: Practice Parameter: Evaluating a first nonfebrile seizure in children. Neurology 55:616–623, 2000. **Evidence-based practice parameter for the evaluation of the first afebrile seizure in a child. Routine EEG recommended for the diagnostic evaluation of a first afebrile seizure. Other studies, such as laboratory studies and neuroimaging, are suggested based on specific circumstances.**

9. Hirtz D, Berg A, Bettis D, et al: Practice parameter: Treatment of the child with a first unprovoked seizure. Neurology 60:166–175, 2003. **Evidence-based practice parameter for treatment of the first afebrile seizure in a child.**

10. Hyland K, Arnold LA: Value of lumbar puncture in the diagnosis of genetic metabolic encephalopathies. J Child Neurol 14(Supply 1): S9–S15, 1999. **Reviews the metabolic disorders for which lumbar puncture is essential for diagnosis.**

11. Kotagal P, Costa M, Wyllie E, Wolgamuth B: Paroxysmal nonepileptic events in children and adolescents. Pediatrics 110:e46, 2002. **Excellent review of non-epileptic events.**

12. Lowenstein DH, Bleck T, Macdonald RL: It's time to revise the definition of status epilepticus. Epilepsia 40:120–122, 1999. **Defines both an operational and mechanistic diagnosis for status epilepticus. Suggests a 5 minute duration for treatment because seizures are more likely to stop when treated early.**

13. Pacia SV, Devinsky O, Luciano DJ, Vazquez B: The prolonged QT syndrome presenting as epilepsy: A report of two cases and literature review. Neurology 44:1408–1410, 1994. **Reviews the prolonged QT syndrome, an excellent example of the importance the differential diagnosis of a seizure.**

14. Riviello JJ: Classification of Seizures and Epilepsy. Curr Neurol Neurosci Rep 3:325–331, 2003. **Updates and reviews classification of seizures and epilepsy syndromes. Includes classification of specific situations, neonatal seizures, seizures in infants, and status epilepticus.**

15. Sharma S, Riviello JJ, Harper MB, Baskin MN: The role of emergent neuroimaging in children with new-onset afebrile seizures. Pediatrics 111:1–5, 2003. **Identifies two criteria associated with a high risk of a clinically significant finding on neuroimaging: a predisposing condition and focal seizure in infant less than 33 months of age.**

Acute Ataxia

Claudia A. Chiriboga

KEY CONCEPTS

- Acute ataxia is characterized by broad-based unsteady gait, nystagmus, and dysmetria of sudden onset.
- The most common causes are drug ingestion, acute cerebellar ataxia, and Miller-Fisher variant of Guillain-Barré syndrome.
- Drug ingestion affects mostly toddlers and adolescents.
- Lethargy is usually observed following drug ingestion.
- Urine toxicology should be obtained in all children with acute ataxia.
- Acute cerebellar ataxia (ACA) is usually a monophasic, self-limited disorder.
- Most patients with ACA have viral prodrome.
- Most children with ACA improve within 2 weeks.
- Treatment of ACA is not routinely indicated.
- Opsoclonus-ataxia syndrome (OAS) is characterized by ataxia, altered mentation, opsoclonus and myoclonus.
- Etiology of OAS is paraneoplastic (neuroblastoma) or parainfectious
- OAS patients have a high tendency to relapse during medication taper
- Most children with OAS have neurologic and behavioral sequelae

Ataxia is a relatively common neurologic symptom in children. To identify the causes of ataxia, it is important to distinguish the acuity of symptoms, as etiology differs between acute and chronic ataxia. Acute ataxia is ataxia of short duration (usually less than a week); the affected child is usually normal prior to the onset of ataxia. Chronic ataxias, on the other hand, are long-standing (weeks to months) and more likely to be attributable to brain tumors or neurodegenerative conditions.

Clinically, children with acute ataxia can exhibit a range of symptoms including a broad-based unsteady gait, nystagmus, and dysmetria of sudden onset. Findings, however, are nonspecific regarding etiology. Common causes of acute ataxia include drug ingestion, acute cerebellar ataxia (which includes infectious, parainfectious, and postvaccinal etiologies), and Guillain-Barré syndrome (Miller-Fisher variant). These disorders account for 80% of all cases. Rare cases of ataxia include opsoclonus-ataxia syndrome, encompass cerebellar infarct or hemorrhage, familial periodic ataxia, or a silent cerebellar tumor complicated by an acute hemorrhage. Seizures at times can mimic ataxia, as cases of pseudoataxia are described in which ambulation is affected by

TABLE 1 Evaluation of Acute Ataxia

History

- Family history of recurrent ataxia → suspect familial ataxia.
- Trauma to neck → suspect vertebral dissection (extracranial).
- Viral prodrome → suspect immune-mediated ataxia (OAS, ACA).
- Headache and vomiting → suspect cerebellar hemorrhage.

Examination

- Lethargy → ingestion.
- Absent reflexes → GBS/MFV.
- Isolated ataxia with normal mentation → ACA.
- Ataxia, encephalopathy, myoclonus → OAS.

Laboratory

- Urine toxicology screen (exclude ingestion).
- MRI/CT (exclude posterior fossa tumor or stroke; assess for demyelination).
- Spinal tap.
- Lymphocytic pleocytosis → cerebellitis/ACA.
- Albuminocytologic dissociation → MFV.
- EMG/NC conduction delay, block→ MFV.
- Thoracic and abdominal CT → OAS.
- Urine collection for HVA and VMA.

ACA, acute cerebellar ataxia; EMG/NC, electromyogram/nerve conduction, GBS, Guillain-Barré syndrome; HVA, homovanillic acid; MFV, Miller-Fisher variant; OAS, opsoclonus-ataxia syndrome; VMA, vanillin mandelic acid.

brief, frequent seizures that do not impair awareness but hinder balance.

All children with acute ataxia should have an initial urine drug screening to exclude ingestion. The clinical history should be explored for headaches, vomiting, viral prodromes, sources of ingestion, and neck trauma (diving or cartwheels). Except for mild cases of ataxia that improve rapidly, the ataxic child's evaluation should include an imaging study to exclude a mass lesion or stroke. Brain magnetic resonance imaging (MRI) is the preferred imaging modality because it readily identifies demyelination (cerebellar white matter signal changes) and infarct (as noted on diffusion-weighted images). MRI is also more sensitive in detecting tumors. See Table 1 for evaluation of acute ataxia.

Expert Opinion on Management Issues

DRUG INGESTION

Drug ingestion typically affects the young toddler who may consume alcohol after a house party (morning after syndrome) or medications available in the household. A second peak in intoxication is seen during adolescence. Most substances resulting in ataxia are CNS depressants. Consequently, in addition to ataxia, the intoxicated child usually exhibits lethargy and slurred speech.

Investigation

Efforts should be made to identify the substance ingested via either blood (alcohol) or urine toxicology. The treatment of drug ingestion should be tailored according to the specific agent ingested.

ACUTE CEREBELLAR ATAXIA

Acute cerebellar ataxia is usually a monophasic, self-limited disorder. Rarely does it relapse. The pathogenesis is believed to be immune-mediated secondary to molecular mimicry, where antigenic cross-reactivity between the viral pathogen and brain constituents (e.g., myelin basic protein) during or following a bout of infection results in an immune response that targets the cerebellum. Over 70 percent of cases of acute cerebellar ataxia have a history of a viral prodrome. Varicella has been the most common agent associated with acute cerebellar ataxia. Prior to routine vaccination, varicella was found in about one third of all cases. Other agents implicated include enterovirus, mycoplasma, mumps, Epstein-Barr virus, influenza, and nonspecific viral infections. Approximately 3% of cases of acute cerebellar ataxia are vaccination related, especially with varicella.

Investigation

The need for neuroimaging is often based on the progression of symptoms. Children who improve spontaneously in the setting of a typical presentation of acute cerebellar ataxia or ingestion may not require neuroimaging. However, it is prudent to perform neuroimaging on any child with acute unexplained ataxia. The MRI can show high signal on T2 or fluid attenuated inversion recovery (FLAIR) in the cerebellar white matter, but it often is normal. A spinal tap should also be performed in affected children to determine if cerebellitis is present. Cerebrospinal fluid (CSF) may show a lymphocytic pleocytosis. Polymerase chain reaction (PCR) of the CSF may be used to identify suspected viral pathogens, but results do no alter management. Investigation for neuroblastoma is not indicated for typical cases of acute cerebellar ataxia, since ataxia is rarely a presenting sign of neuroblastoma. Evaluation for neuroblastoma may be considered in severe or relapsing cases.

Management

Acute cerebellar ataxia is largely a monophasic, self-limited disorder that usually does not require intervention (Table 2). Most children improve in 2 weeks regardless of intervention, although at times recovery may lag over 3 weeks. During this period of unsteadiness, children should be protected against falls. Recovery is the rule, with ataxia resolving so quickly that physiotherapy and gait training prove unnecessary. Occasionally children may present with severe ataxia and progressive inability to walk. To hasten recovery in such extreme cases, immune modulatory therapy may be tried. Anecdotal case reports described efficacy with IV methylprednisolone, oral prednisone, or a course of IVIG (2 g/kg over 1 or 2 days). It should be noted, however, that no clinical trial has ever been conducted to determine the efficacy of such treatment. Moreover, there is no consensus of opinion with regard to treatment.

TABLE 2 Therapy for Acute Ataxia

Ingestion

- Supportive care.
- Targeted therapy depending on drug ingested (e.g., activated charcoal, gastric lavage, alkalinization; call poison control).

Acute Cerebellar Ataxia

- Routine treatment is not indicated.
- For extreme cases (no consensus or evidence on treatment efficacy):
  - Brief treatment with steroids (IV methylprednisolone; 10 mg/kg/day × 1–2 days) followed by prednisone 2 mg/kg × 1 week. Do not taper.
  - IVIG (2 g/kg) divided over 1 or 2 days.

Opsoclonus-Ataxia Syndrome (regardless if paraneoplastic or parainfectious)

- ACTH 40 IU/day to 150 IU/m²/day. Gradual taper to lowest dose that does not elicit relapse.
- Prednisone 2–4 mg/kg/day. Gradual taper to lowest dose that does not elicit relapse (0.5 mg/kg qod).
- IVIG (2 g/kg) divided over 1 to 2 days q 4 weeks.

Miller-Fisher Variant of Guillain-Barré

- IVIG 0.4 g/kg/day for 5 days*; alternatively 1 g/kg/day for 2 days.
- Plasma exchange for 3 to 5 days.*

*Drawn from class II evidence from adult trials. Immediate treatment with plasmapheresis after ineffective IVIG is not recommended; plasmapheresis should be delayed at least 2 weeks after IVIG is administered.
IVIG, intravenous immunoglobulins; q, every; qod, every other day.

OPSOCLONUS-ATAXIA SYNDROME

Opsoclonus-ataxia syndrome (OAS) (also known as opsoclonus-myoclonus syndrome, opsoclonus encephalopathy, or Kinsbourne encephalopathy) is characterized by sudden onset of severe neurologic symptoms where, in addition to ataxia, children exhibit a profound encephalopathy (severe changes in mentation, hallucinations or agitation), myoclonus (lightning fast proximal jerks) and opsoclonus (dancing eyes). It occurs in young children usually younger than age 6 years (mean age 20 months). Approximately half of OAS cases are paraneoplastic because of neuroblastoma and the rest are caused by parainfectious disorders. Only about 3% of neuroblastomas manifest with OAS. The presence of OAS confers neuroblastoma with a more benign outcome. Unlike adult paraneoplastic disorders that manifest with OAS (e.g., breast cancer), children rarely present with anti-Ri, anti-Yo or anti-Hu antibodies, especially in low stages of neuroblastoma. Although anti-neuronal antibodies are noted in children with OAS, these are not sufficiently specific to be clinically useful. Children with parainfectious OAS present during or following a viral infection. There is overlap between the viral agents linked with acute cerebellar ataxia and OAS. Mycoplasma, influenza, enterovirus, especially coxsackie B virus, hepatitis A and B, and Epstein-Barr virus have all been implicated in OAS. A few reports describe cerebellar atrophy to occur in children with opsoclonus-ataxia and neuroblastoma several years after onset of OAS.

Management

The mainstay of treatment is immune modulatory therapy. None of the treatment options, however, has been tested in clinical trials. Most reports are anecdotal, some describe case series, and others are retrospective. Historically, some of the larger case series describe adrenocorticotropic hormone (ACTH) (30–40 IU/day) and prednisone (2–4 mg/kg) to be equally effective in improving symptoms. Efficacy rates with these treatments vary from 60% to 100%. Doses are gradually tapered to the smallest dose that does not elicit a relapse. A handful of studies also report benefit from intravenous immunoglobulin (IVIG) (2 g/kg) given over 1 or 2 days. Immune modulatory therapy is usually needed for extended periods, as OAS often relapses during steroid taper. A large retrospective study found equal benefit for the therapies described above and no long-term advantage for any single therapy.

MILLER FISHER VARIANT OF GUILLAIN-BARRÉ SYNDROME

Miller-Fisher variant of Guillain-Barré syndrome (GBS) syndrome is an acquired demyelinating nerve disease that is considered a variant of GBS. The syndrome is characterized by ataxia but is easily distinguished from acute cerebellar ataxia because of the presence of ophthalmoparesis and areflexia, symptoms that point toward a neuropathy. Children often have a viral prodrome. Pain and paresthesias may precede ataxia. The child may also complain of diplopia. Young children may refuse to walk or do so by holding onto walls or furniture. Weakness may also be observed, which on occasion will progress to a flaccid paralysis requiring ventilatory support.

Investigation

The neurologic examination points away from the cerebellum and toward a peripheral disorder. The spinal tap, electromyelogram (EMG), and nerve conditions are the main diagnostic modalities. The spinal tap may be normal in 10% to 20% of children but typically shows albuminocytologic dissociation (i.e., high protein without inflammatory cells). Protein elevation often develops during the second week of symptoms. The EMG is usually diagnostic, but may be normal. As with typical GBS, delayed conduction, absent H reflexes, and conduction block may be observed. In the Miller-Fisher variant, there may be markedly reduced amplitude of the distal sensory apparatus as well as frequent axonal degeneration. The Miller-Fisher variant is associated with a high frequency of anti-GQ–1-b antibodies.

Management

The treatment of Miller-Fisher is identical to the treatment of GBS. Supportive care with attention to respiratory capacity is essential to treatment. Several clinical trials in adults show the efficacy of plasmapheresis (also known as plasma exchange) and IVIG treatment (level B recommendation derived from class II evidence in adults). Plasmapheresis involves separating red blood cells (RBCs) from plasma and returning the RBCs to the patient. Venous access may be problematic, especially in young children. IVIG is preferred to plasmapheresis in children because of its ease of use and because it may improve function more quickly than plasma exchange. Clinical trials have not found that oral steroids are effective treatment of GBS.

Common Pitfalls

- Identification of an ataxia-inducing substance may be hindered by lack of sensitivity or scope of the toxicology measure. History is important in identifying possible drugs in the household.
- Rarely there is a presentation of neuroblastoma with typical acute cerebellar ataxia.
- Acute cerebellar ataxia with a posterior fossa tumor/cerebellar hemorrhage is misdiagnosed.
- Mild symptoms of OAS with acute cerebellar ataxia are misdiagnosed.
- Relapse of OAS symptoms occurs with a too-rapid taper of medication.
- A spinal tap is obtained too early in the course of the Miller-Fisher variant, prior to the development of high CSF protein.
- The sensory symptoms of the Miller-Fisher variant are missed in young children.
- Treatment with plasmapheresis soon (<2 weeks) after IVIG in the Miller-Fisher variant negates the benefit of treatment.

Communication and Counseling

Prognosis for recovery in acute cerebellar ataxia is excellent. As noted, children recover within a few weeks to baseline. In a large series, approximately 20% of children had developmental or behavioral symptoms 4 months after the acute ataxia, yet only 8% of affected children had sustained learning difficulties.

All children with OAS show neurologic and behavioral sequelae. Persistent neurologic deficits include speech delay, cognitive deficits, motor delay, and behavioral problems. Behavioral problems described early in the course of the illness include severe irritability and inconsolability in all; later, oppositional behavior and sleep disorders are noted. Expressive language is more impaired than receptive language, as are fine and gross motor abilities. Older children show lower scores in all areas. Although opsoclonus abates in all children, abnormalities in pursuit eye movements are found on finer testing.

Most children with the Miller-Fisher variant improve over the course of 10 weeks and show no residual symptoms. In children with GBS, however, 23% will show long-term mild muscle weakness that has minimal impact on function. Predictors of long-term muscle weakness are young age and a rapid progression to maximal

weakness. The Miller-Fisher variant may, on rare occasions, relapse.

SUGGESTED READINGS

1. Edmondson JC, Nichter CA, Selman JE, DeVivo DC: Use of intravenous gamma globulin therapy for postinfectious acute cerebellar ataxia/opsoclonus of childhood. Ann Neurol 32:440, 1992. **Small series describing efficacy of IVIG in these conditions.**
2. Hughes RA, Wijdicks EF, Barohn R, et al: Practice parameter: immunotherapy for Guillain-Barré syndrome: Report of the Quality Standards Subcommittee of the American Academy of Neurology. Neurology 61:736–740, 2003. **This is a consensus paper on the accepted treatments for GBS in adults and, by extrapolation, in children.**
3. Kanra G, Ozon A, Vajsar J, et al: Intravenous immunoglobulin treatment in children with Guillain-Barré syndrome. Eur J Paed Neurol 1:7–12, 1997. **Large retrospective study in children with GBS showing benefit of shorter course of IVIG therapy (2 vs. 5 days).**
4. Mitchell WG, Davalos-Gonzalez Y, Brumm VL, et al: Opsoclonus-ataxia caused by childhood neuroblastoma: Developmental and neurologic sequelae. Pediatrics 109:86–98, 2002. **Article of recent vintage describing the neurodevelopmental sequelae among children with neuroblastoma-associated OAS.**
5. Petruzzi JM, DeAlarcon PA: Neuroblastoma-associated opsoclonus-myoclonus treated with intravenously administered immune globulin G. J Pediatr 127:328–329, 1995. **Describes benefit of IVIG with OAS.**
6. Pohl KR, Pritchard J, Wilson J: Neurological sequelae of the dancing eye syndrome. Eur J Pediatr 155:237–244, 1996. **Describes the long-term ocular sequelae of OAS.**
7. Shanbag P, Amirtharaj C, Pathak A: Intravenous immunoglobulins in severe Guillian-Barré syndrome in childhood. Indian J Ped 70:541–543, 2003. **Describes improved outcome of IVIG over plasmapheresis in children.**
8. The Guillain-Barré Syndrome Study Group: Plasmapheresis and acute Guillain-Barré syndrome. Neurology 35:1096–1104, 1985. **Large clinical trial in adults demonstrating efficacy of plasma exchange in the treatment of GBS.**
9. Vajsar J, Fehlings D, Stephens D: Long-term outcome in children with Guillain-Barré syndrome. J Peds 142:305–309, 2003. **Paper describes the motor sequelae of children with GBS.**

Diagnosis and Management of Hydrocephalus

Neil A. Feldstein and Richard C.E. Anderson

KEY CONCEPTS

- Hydrocephalus has a prevalence of approximately 1 in 1000 children.
- While often idiopathic, hydrocephalus can be a result of central nervous system infection or hemorrhage.
- Hydrocephalus can be the presenting sign of tumors, especially posterior fossa tumors.
- It can manifest at variable rates (chronic to acute) based on the degree to which spinal fluid is being normally processed by the body.
- A neurosurgical consultation is required when hydrocephalus is diagnosed or suspected.
- It is currently treated with either shunting or endoscopic third ventriculostomy.

BOX 1 Basic Forms of Hydrocephalus

Overproduction
- Choroid plexus hypertrophy
- Choroid plexus papilloma
- Choroid plexus carcinoma

Communicating (nonobstructive)
- Postinfectious
- Posthemorrhagic

Noncommunicating (obstructive)
- Aqueductal stenosis
- Vein-of-Galen malformation
- Tectal glioma
- Pineal masses or cysts

BOX 2 Signs and Symptoms of Hydrocephalus

Infant
- Enlarged head circumference
- Splitting of cranial sutures
- Bulging fontanelle
- Projectile vomiting
- Irritability

Adolescent
- Headaches
- Delay or loss of developmental milestones
- Papilledema
- Ocular nerve palsies
- Nausea and vomiting

Hydrocephalus is a common condition seen in the pediatric population. It affects roughly one in 1000 live births. Any process that augments the production or inhibits flow or reabsorption of spinal fluid can lead to hydrocephalus.

There are many causes of hydrocephalus. In general, hydrocephalus demonstrates itself as an inability for infants or children to adequately control their cerebrospinal fluid volume. The result is an increase in the ventricle size and subsequent increase in intracranial pressure and potentially neurologic complications and death.

The rarest of the three forms of hydrocephalus is that of overproduction (Box 1). This is caused by either choroid plexus hypertrophy or choroid plexus tumors such as papillomas or carcinomas. Treatment of these lesions may lead to the resolution of the hydrocephalus. The other two forms are communicating (nonobstructive) hydrocephalus and noncommunicating (obstructive) hydrocephalus. They are not always completely separate disease processes, and often the child may have both problems affecting spinal fluid pathways. The more common causes of the noncommunicating form of hydrocephalus are aqueductal stenosis and tectal gliomas. The rare vein-of-Galen malformation, as well as other vascular malformations and cysts that can occur near the posterior aspect of the third ventricle or at the aqueduct of Sylvius, can also lead to noncommunicating hydrocephalus. Hemorrhage and inflammatory processes can also lead to obstruction at this site. Problems with reabsorption, the communicating or nonobstructive form of hydrocephalus, are most commonly seen after infection and hemorrhage in the neonate, as well as during infancy and, less commonly, adolescence.

Approximately 80% to 90% of children born with open neural tube defects either have hydrocephalus at birth or develop it shortly thereafter. A second common association is that of the Dandy-Walker malformation. Fifty to 75% of children with this cystic dilation of the fourth ventricle eventually develop hydrocephalus and require the placement of a ventricular and/or a cysto-peritoneal shunt.

The hallmarks of hydrocephalus (Box 2) are very much dependent on both the age at which it occurs and the speed at which it develops. In the newborn and infancy period, children often present with a rapidly enlarging head size with splitting of the cranial sutures, an enlarged and bulging fontanelle, irritability, nausea, and projectile vomiting. The scalp may also appear quite taut, with distended scalp veins. As the hydrocephalus progresses, infants may become lethargic and develop a forced downward gaze.

As infants approach the end of the first year of life and enter into the toddler stage, the hydrocephalus tends to evolve more slowly; therefore, the symptoms may not be as obvious. In addition to enlarged head circumference and persistence and bulging of the fontanelle, it is possible to detect either delays or loss of acquired developmental milestones. As the children mature, they may be able to express a sense of pain or headaches. Funduscopic examination may reveal papilledema, and there may be evidence of sixth nerve palsies.

Hydrocephalus can also develop in later adolescence. Often the hydrocephalus has gone undiagnosed for years and the children have always been noted to have a large head circumference. At this point, they may be manifesting signs of a subtle neurologic difficulty such as clumsiness and, in some, language or emotional difficulties.

Despite the age at presentation, once the diagnosis is raised, the appropriate actions must be taken swiftly. The diagnostic procedure of choice varies depending on the child's age, as well as the severity of the symptoms. For those presenting with clear signs of raised intracranial pressure, an emergency evaluation must be performed. For those presenting in an asymptomatic fashion, but with a growing head circumference, the evaluation is semi-emergent. While the most informative radiologic test available is an MRI scan, not all children with increasing head circumference require such a study. Many times a simple noninvasive ultrasound of the brain is sufficient to make the diagnosis.

On many occasions, an increase in the child's head circumference is not caused by hydrocephalus but rather by an entity that is known as benign external fluid collections of infancy. This condition (also referred to as *external hydrocephalus*) can be confused with progressive hydrocephalus, which is caused by rapidly increasing head circumference. CT scan, MRI, and ultrasound all demonstrate that the fluid accumulation is outside the ventricular system in the subarachnoid space. The ventricles will be normal or slightly enlarged in size. Curiously, this tends to run in families, and often one or both parents or grandparents will demonstrate mild to moderate macrocephaly. Unlike true hydrocephalus, this is usually a self-limited process that does not require surgical intervention.

Expert Opinion on Management Issues

Regardless of the age of the child, once a diagnosis of hydrocephalus is firmly established, the recommended management is usually surgical (Box 3). Until recently, almost all children treated surgically for hydrocephalus were treated with the insertion of a device known as a *shunt*. These devices are placed into the ventricular system and then, depending on the neurosurgeon's practice, tunneled underneath the skin to be placed into the heart, the chest cavity, or the peritoneal cavity. These three different forms of shunts are thus named ventriculoatrial, ventriculopleural, and ventriculoperitoneal, respectively. The majority of shunts placed in the United States today are of the ventriculoperitoneal type.

In certain instances in the neonate of very low weight, a shunt may be required but the surgeon may feel that the infant is too small to receive a permanent shunt. Rather than performing intermittent ventricular or lumbar taps, the surgeon may choose to place a ventriculosubgaleal shunt. This device shunts the cerebrospinal fluid (CSF) to the potential space underneath the scalp over much of the cranium. The scalp can absorb the CSF to some extent and temporize until the infant is of sufficient weight to receive a more permanent shunt system. On occasion, this technique may lead to arrested hydrocephalus and obviate the need for a permanent shunt system.

In the past two decades, there has been an increase in the use of endoscopic or endoscopic-assisted techniques to treat some forms of hydrocephalus. Specifically, the obstructive forms of hydrocephalus such as aqueductal stenosis can at times be treated without a shunt by performing what is known as an endoscopic third ventriculostomy (ETV). Using an endoscope (with or without a stereotactic guidance system), a small perforation is made in the floor of the third ventricle. This opening allows spinal fluid to flow from the ventricular system into the subarachnoid space, bypassing the obstructed aqueduct. Once in the subarachnoid space, CSF is reabsorbed in the usual fashion and does not require a shunt insertion. This procedure is not usable in children who have problems with reabsorption of spinal fluid. In addition, although there was very early optimism that these procedures would be curative for life, it is now becoming apparent that like ventricular shunt systems, third ventriculostomies can fail over time leading to the symptoms of shunt malfunction. There is still much debate regarding how old a child needs to be in order to be a good candidate for an ETV. Under the age of 1 year, the failure rate of the procedure is upwards of 50%, with increasing failure rates in the younger infant population. In addition, some children without clear evidence of obstructive hydrocephalus may still successfully be treated with an ETV.

Common Pitfalls

- Failure to diagnose hydrocephalus in a timely fashion
- Inaccurate measurement of head circumference
- Failure to recognize that after an ETV, children can present months to years later with acute hydrocephalus that can lead to life-threatening emergencies
- Failure to recognize shunt malfunction or shunt infection

Communication and Counseling

Once a shunt system has been inserted or an ETV performed, the children are monitored by the neurosurgeon with head circumference measurements, neurologic assessments, and follow-up radiologic imaging studies. There is no standard recommendation for frequency of such follow-up studies. These children are most often dependent on their shunts for the rest of their lives, although a small number of them will outgrow the need for their shunt system. It is important for the parents, the pediatrician, the neurosurgeon, and ultimately the child to be aware of the common side effects of the shunt system as well as signs of shunt malfunction and/or shunt infection. When the shunt systems are first placed, infants and children will often be uncomfortable when they are sitting or standing upright as a result of excess flow of spinal fluid through the shunt system. This is usually a self-limited process and will correct itself without the need for shunt revision.

The signs of a shunt malfunction in general are the signs of hydrocephalus. These include headaches, vomiting, and lethargy. In some cases, spinal fluid can be seen to collect under the scalp at the site of the valve or anywhere along the tract of the shunt. Large randomized studies have demonstrated that shunt malfunction occurs in 50% to 60% of children within 5 years of initial shunt placement. The bigger fear, however, is that of shunt infection with the potential risk of meningitis and brain abscess formation. Shunt infections usually occur

---

> **BOX 3 Surgical Treatment of Hydrocephalus**
>
> **Shunting**
> - Ventriculoatrial
> - Ventriculopleural
> - Ventriculoperitoneal (most commonly performed)
> - Ventriculosubgaleal (used in neonates generally to temporize)
>
> **Nonshunting**
> - Endoscopic third ventriculostomy (ETV)
> - Excision of choroid plexus lesions (papilloma, carcinoma, hypertrophy)
> - Excision of obstructive lesions (pineal tumors and cysts, posterior fossa tumors)

in the first weeks to months after shunt placement or shunt revision. Common signs and symptoms include unexplained fevers and redness along the shunt valve or shunt tract, implying irritation or cellulitis. Peritoneal shunt infections may also lead to peritonitis and bowel obstruction. In addition to these findings, the infected shunt often shows signs of malfunction. The shunt infection rate is approximately 5%.

The ultimate outcome for a child with hydrocephalus and appropriate treatment is quite variable. The initial degree of ventricular enlargement in general does not correlate with outcome. Outcome best correlates with the thickness of the cortical mantle several months after the shunt has been functioning. It is not uncommon to see a newborn or infant who has a very thin cortical mantle that, after the child recovers from shunting, re-expands to a normal cortical thickness. The outcome from hydrocephalus does not so much depend on the surgical intervention as it does on the primary cause of the hydrocephalus. If detected early, forms such as aqueductal stenosis in which there is a benign obstruction to spinal fluid flow should do quite well. Conversely, hydrocephalus cases associated with severe forms of meningitis, bilateral grade IV hemorrhage, and trauma are less likely to do well.

Modern shunt systems have been developed to grow with the infant or child. The era of elective shunt revision or lengthening has mostly passed. If the shunt system does not clog or fracture, there is no need to plan for revision. There are no official guidelines on the restrictions of children who have shunt systems. There is probably a slight increase in the risk of intracranial bleeding with significant head trauma. This has led some physicians to recommend that severe contact sports be restricted. The effects on the shunt system resulting from rapid changes in pressure are not known, but at this time, there are no restrictions on air travel.

SUGGESTED READINGS

1. Garton HJ, Piatt JH, Jr. Hydrocephalus. Pediatr Clin North Am 51:305–325, 2004. **Although the article focuses on one of the more common forms of hydrocephalus, posthemorrhagic, it draws attention to the fact that hydrocephalus is not a rare condition and can be expected to be seen in most pediatric practices.**
2. Kestle J, Drake J, Milner R, et al: Long-term follow-up data from the Shunt Design Trial. Pediatr Neurosurg 33:230–236, 2000. **The authors reviewed data from a large, randomized, multicenter (12 centers in America and Europe) shunt trial comparing three different shunt valves. Despite preconceived notions, no single shunt was demonstrated to be superior to another in the initial management of childhood hydrocephalus.**
3. Koch D, Wagner W: Endoscopic third ventriculostomy in infants of less than 1 year of age: Which factors influence the outcome? Childs Nerv Syst 20:405–411, 2004. **Review of the authors' experience of attempting ETV in very young children accounting for age and underlying cause of hydrocephalus. As expected, nonaqueductal stenosis had a higher failure rate.**
4. Rekate HL: Selecting patients for endoscopic third ventriculostomy. Neurosurg Clin N Am 15:39–49, 2004. **The author makes a strong argument that many children with nonaqueductal stenosis–type hydrocephalus may still be good candidates for ETV. In addition, the author addresses the option of converting a child to ETV treatment during times of shunt malfunction or shunt infection rather than replacing the shunt system.**
5. Smith ER, Butler WE, Barker FG II: In-hospital mortality rates after ventriculoperitoneal shunt procedures in the United States, 1998 to 2000: Relation to hospital and surgeon volume of care. J Neurosurg Spine 100:90–97, 2004. **Although the data have to be read and interpreted carefully, the authors demonstrated lower in-hospital mortality rates in shunt procedures performed at high-volume hospitals or by "high-volume" neurosurgeons compared to smaller hospitals or "lower-volume" neurosurgeons.**
6. Tuli S, Tuli J, Drake J, et al: Predictors of death in pediatric patients requiring cerebrospinal fluid shunts. J Neurosurg Spine 100:442–446, 2004. **Ten-year review of morbidity and mortality in shunted children.**

Myelomeningocele

Saadi Ghatan

KEY CONCEPTS

- Myelomeningocele is the most common birth defect affecting the nervous system, occurring with a frequency of 1:1000 live births in the United States.
- Neural tube defects occur because of an error in neurulation, the early formation of the nervous system in the first month of gestation.
- Hydrocephalus, spinal and limb deformities, and bowel/bladder dysfunction are the common medical and surgical issues children with spina bifida face throughout life.
- A multidisciplinary approach in a well-coordinated spina bifida clinic is the most effective management strategy for children with myelomeningocele.
- Early and ongoing neurosurgical, orthopedic, and urologic management is coordinated and overseen by the pediatrician.

Despite advances in the understanding of their pathogenesis and prevention, neural tube defects (NTDs) are among the most common of all congenital malformations and remain the most frequent birth defects that affect the central nervous system (CNS). Myelomeningocele, or *spina bifida aperta*, occurs in 1:1000 live births in the United States and presents a lifelong challenge for patient, parent, and practitioner alike. An error in the fundamental process of neurulation, the early formation of the nervous system during the first month of gestation, results in an open neural tube defect, typically at the caudal extent of the spinal cord. Accompanying disorders include the Chiari II malformation, a constellation of CNS anomalies that include midline and hindbrain abnormalities and hydrocephalus. Systemic manifestations include bowel and bladder dysfunction, and depending upon the level of the NTD, truncal, and lower extremity paralysis and sensory deficits.

Between 20 and 28 days' gestation, embryogenesis moves through a series of steps including neural induction, elevation, and apposition of the neural folds and the fusion of these folds to form an intact midline, and secondary neurulation whereby the most caudal extent of the spinal cord develops from the primordial caudal

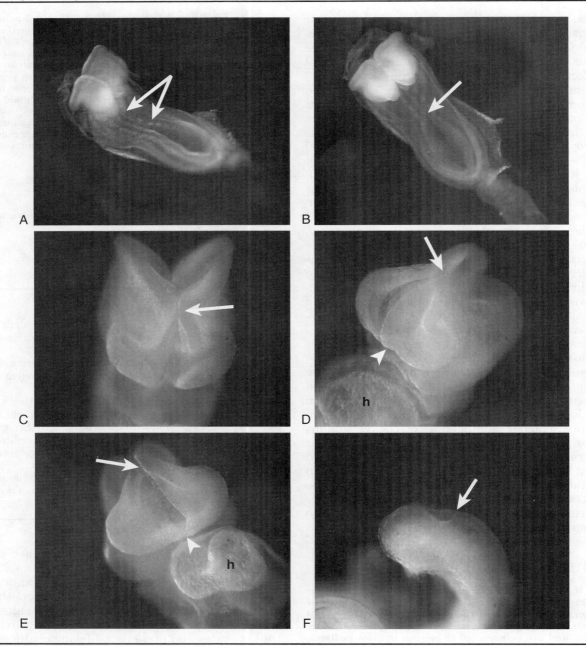

FIGURE 1. Mammalian neural tube closure (**A, B**). Oblique and dorsal images of a 6– to 8–somite pair embryo showing the first site of neural tube closure at the future hindbrain-cervical junction (3 weeks gestation) (*arrows*). **C–E,** Three different views of the head of a 12– to16–somite pair embryo showing the second neural tube closure at the level of the forebrain-midbrain junction (*arrow*), and a third point of closure at the rostral end of the neural tube (*arrowhead*). **F,** The posterior neuropore at the caudal extremity of the neural tube. Closure of the spinal neural tube proceeds from the hindbrain-cervical junction caudally and eventually closes the posterior neuropore at approximately 4 weeks gestation. Arrow indicates the extent of closure in this embryo. **h,** heart.

cell mass. The first closure event occurs at the future mid-brain-hindbrain junction and proceeds both rostrally and caudally as the embryo elongates (Fig. 1). Failure of the hindbrain neuropore to close results in anencephaly or exencephaly, a lethal condition, whereas failure of anterior neuropore closure at the most rostral extent of the embryo is thought to give rise to a nasal dermal sinus tract. When the posterior neuropore fails to close, a

myelomeningocele is created; a dysplastic spinal cord, in which a flattened neural tube and nerve roots are visible, protrudes through a defect in the dura, posterior spinal arches, and soft tissues to the skin surface, covered only by a thin, cystic membrane (Fig. 2).

The pathogenesis for this disorder is multifactorial, but much attention in the past 2 decades has focused on genetic and environmental factors such as maternal

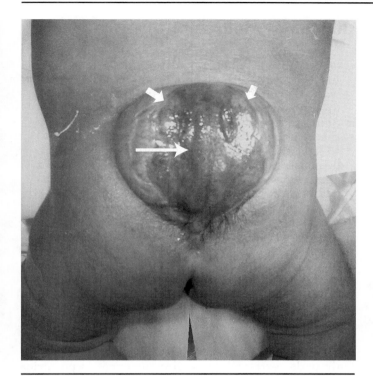

FIGURE 2. Myelomeningocele in a neonate. The neural placode is visible at the surface (*long arrow*) in this lumbosacral myelomeningocele. Abnormal epithelium lines the edges of the cerebrospinal fluid (CSF)-filled cyst (*short arrows*).

diabetes, alcohol exposure, and antiepileptic drugs. Recognition that levels of certain vitamins were abnormally low in mothers carrying fetuses with NTDs led to the widespread use of multivitamins with folate, which has greatly reduced the incidence of the disorder in susceptible populations. Nonetheless, about 30% of myelomeningoceles occur in a familial pattern that is resistant to folate or other vitamin supplementation.

Expert Opinion on Management Issues

A multidisciplinary team in a well-coordinated spina bifida clinic sets the stage for effective, early, and longitudinal management. Pediatrics, neurosurgery, orthopedics, urology, physical and occupational therapy, and social work can communicate and coordinate care to meet the challenges encountered by patient and family alike from infancy through adulthood in this complex patient population.

EARLY INTERVENTIONS

Prenatal recognition is made possible through screening of maternal α-fetoprotein, 2D and 3D ultrasonography, and fetal MRI. Prenatal counseling with a multidisciplinary team that includes obstetrics, pediatrics, and neurosurgery allows for preparation of a birth plan (most children are delivered by elective cesarean

section) and early postnatal closure of the myelomeningocele, ventriculoperitoneal shunting for hydrocephalus, and further postnatal evaluations.

Natural history studies show that expeditious closure of the defect and treatment of hydrocephalus is warranted, unless coexisting anomalies incompatible with long-term survival are identified. Initial assessment after delivery focuses on the neural placode, location, and extent of the defect. Care is taken to avoid trauma to the exposed neural elements, and thus the neonate is kept prone at all times with a sterile, saline-soaked, nonadhesive dressing covering the open defect. Early neurosurgical intervention (within the first 24–48 hours after birth) allows layered closure of the neural tube and soft tissues. Briefly, the neural placode is closed to provide a smaller surface area and prevent retethering (see "Longitudinal Interventions," later), followed by closure of the dura and overlying soft tissues and skin to prevent cerebrospinal fluid (CSF) leak. Excessively large skin defects (>8–10 cm, depending on location and morphology) warrant consultation with plastic surgery for aid in closure of the superficial layers.

Perhaps the most important determinant in preventing CSF leak and ensuring proper wound closure is recognition and treatment of hydrocephalus, which occurs in approximately 90% of children born with myelomeningocele. Hydrocephalus is assessed by fontanelle palpation, head circumference measurement, and cranial ultrasound for baseline values. Shunting, typically ventriculoperitoneal, is not necessary at the time of myelomeningocele closure because CSF decompression occurs during closure of the NTD. A separate procedure for placement of the shunt is preferred by many neurosurgeons to avoid the attendant infectious issues involved in closing a potentially clean-contaminated wound (the myelomeningocele) at the same time that hardware is being placed.

Rarely, severe kyphotic deformity is seen in conjunction with large lumbar myelomeningoceles, and their correction is necessitated at the time of closure. Other orthopedic evaluation is useful to identify lower extremity deformities (club foot) and hip dislocations. Urologic evaluation is critical: renal ultrasonography and a voiding cystourethrogram allow assessment of renal and bladder anomalies, and identification of vesicoureteral reflux in addition to voiding pattern and postvoid residual (PVR).

LONGITUDINAL INTERVENTIONS

The pediatrician maintains well-child care, evaluates urgent issues, and communicates with subspecialists to coordinate effective and comprehensive care. Neurosurgical issues focus on management of hydrocephalus and revolve around diagnosis and management of shunt malfunction. In infants, a bulging fontanelle, excessive head circumference growth, irritability, lethargy, and vomiting might signal shunt malfunction, necessitating evaluation in the form of a shunt series (radiographs of the entire shunt system in anteroposterior and lateral views) and a noncontrast CT scan to assess ventricular volumes. If these symptoms are accompanied by fever, meningismus, or leukocytosis within 6 to 8 weeks of shunt placement or revision, shunt infection must be carefully evaluated. Older children with shunt malfunction present with headaches, lethargy, changes in school performance, or personality change. Most shunts require revision at least once during a 10-year period.

Spinal cord tethering is encountered in a subset of patients, particularly during growth spurts. Scarring of the neural placode to the dura and soft tissues at the closure site manifests as lumbosacral and/or lower extremity pain, spasticity, changes in gait, worsening of bowel/bladder dysfunction, and worsening spinal deformity. Neurosurgical evaluation is necessary and occasionally reoperative cord detethering is necessary to prevent permanent neurologic deterioration. Spinal deformity can often be corrected with cord detethering, but some deformities progress to require bracing or surgical correction.

Longitudinal orthopedic management is necessary to maintain joint alignment, prevent fractures and decubiti, and maximize functional mobility. Bracing and ankle-foot orthoses are employed alone or in combination, depending upon the child's functional level and requirements for hip, trunk, or lower extremity support. Surgery in the form of soft tissue release, tendon transfer, and osteotomy may be necessary in cases of severe deformity.

Long-term urologic evaluation and treatment are critical for the quality of life and life expectancy of the child with myelomeningocele. Lumbosacral spinal cord and nerve root abnormalities lead to bladder and urethral sphincter dysfunction. Management of bladder hypotonia or hypertonia and detrusor and sphincter spasticity is critical in avoiding secondary complications such as recurrent infection, ureteral reflux, hydronephrosis, and renal injury.

Most children require clean intermittent catheterization (CIC) in conjunction with pharmacologic support to reduce bladder contraction or increase outflow resistance. Prophylactic antibiotics may be necessary in the setting of recurrent infections. Finally, advances in surgical techniques have allowed the creation of artificial sphincters and bladder augmentation to assist in cases of severe incontinence and poorly compliant and small-capacity bladders, respectively.

CONTROVERSIAL INTERVENTIONS

In utero closure of myelomeningocele defects has been advocated as a means of protecting the exposed spinal cord during gestation, limiting the incidence of the Chiari II malformation and its attendant problems and reducing the incidence of shunt-dependent hydrocephalus. However, risks to mother and fetus inherent from in-utero surgery, wound dehiscence, epidermoid cysts, and the questionable benefit to neurologic function and hydrocephalus seen in children treated with this method have tempered enthusiasm. Currently, a multicenter randomized, controlled trial of in utero closure, versus standard postnatal management, is being conducted nationally to answer this question.

Common Pitfalls

- In the perinatal period after surgical closure of the defect, the most important determinant in preventing CSF leak and infection and ensuring proper wound healing is recognition and treatment of hydrocephalus.
- Shunt-independent treatment of hydrocephalus in the form of endoscopic third ventriculostomy (ETV) is not indicated in the perinatal period due to demonstrated inefficacy and dangers of attendant anatomic variations with the associated Chiari II malformation.
- Latex allergy is commonly seen in children with myelomeningocele. Avoidance of latex-containing products in the office, hospital, and home setting is imperative.

Emergent manifestations of the Chiari II malformation are also possible; some infants and teenagers present with symptoms and signs of brainstem dysfunction in the form of stridor, dysphagia, vocal cord paralysis, or apnea. Immediate medical and supportive intervention is necessary. Most commonly, hydrocephalus is the inciting factor, and shunt malfunction must be excluded. Only under extremely rare circumstances is posterior fossa decompression necessary to alleviate these potentially life-threatening symptoms.

Communication and Counseling

The pediatrician and specialists must coordinate care in a manner that is safe, convenient, comprehensible, and comprehensive for the child and family. Establishing an efficient strategy for communication between patient and pediatrician and relaying the information to various specialists is critical to the successful management of the many needs of these patients.

SUGGESTED READINGS

1. Copp AJ, Bernfield M: Etiology and pathogenesis of human neural tube defects; insights from mouse models. Curr Opin Pediatr 6:624–631, 1994. **Provides a comprehensive link between laboratory and clinical data.**
2. Copp AJ, Greene ND, Murdoch JN: The genetic basis of mammalian neurulation. Nat Rev Genet 4:784–793, 2003. **Details advances in our understanding of the potential genetic contribution to myelomeningocele.**
3. Karol LA: Orthopedic management in myelomeningocele. Neurosurg Clin N Am 6:259–268, 1995. **An excellent review of orthopedic issues faced by children with myelomeningocele.**
4. Madersbacher H: Neurogenic bladder dysfunction in patients with myelomeningocele. Curr Opin Urol 12:469–472, 2002. **An overview of major urologic problems encountered in children with myelomeningocele.**
5. McLaughlin JF, Shurtleff DB, Lamers JY, et al: Influence of prognosis on decisions regarding the care of newborns with myelodysplasia. N Engl J Med 312:1589–1594, 1985. **Demonstrates the background behind our present management of myelomeningocele.**
6. Tulipan N: Intrauterine closure of myelomeningocele: An update. Neurosurg Focus 16:E2, 2004. **Provides background information on the rationale and early results behind intrauterine surgery for myelomeningocele.**

Cerebral Palsy

Joelle Mast

KEY CONCEPTS

- Cerebral palsy (CP) is a nonprogressive disorder of mobility caused by brain injury early in life.
- Evaluation is based upon history and clinical findings. If etiology is unclear, MRI is recommended over CT because of its greater sensitivity.
- Problems with visual, auditory, speech, language, and oromotor functions are common, and screening for these is recommended.
- An electroencephalogram (EEG) is only recommended if seizures are suspected.
- Testing for coagulopathy should be considered in patients with hemiplegic CP.
- Genetic and metabolic studies are recommended if radiologic studies reveal a structural abnormality or if the clinical picture suggests a genetic or metabolic disorder.
- Treatment of spasticity may include therapy, medication, and surgical management. An interdisciplinary, family-centered approach is suggested with the primary health care provider coordinating a multidisciplinary team.

Cerebral palsy (CP) is a nonprogressive mobility disorder resulting from an abnormality in the brain that occurs early in life. The prevalence of CP is 1.2 to 2.5 per 1000 live births. Etiologies include maternal infection, structural abnormalities, genetic disorders, and other causes of brain injury. Clinical examination is characterized by abnormalities in muscle tone, posture, and deep tendon reflexes. Depending on the nature of the injury, there may be associated neurologic deficits, such as mental retardation, seizures, or movement disorder.

Careful history and physical examination establish the diagnosis. If etiology is not clear, imaging with MRI may be helpful. Structural brain abnormalities are common in children with CP and may provide information about the prognosis. Metabolic and genetic tests should be considered if the clinical or family history suggests such a disorder, or if etiology is not known despite neuroimaging. With hemiplegic CP, workup for a coagulopathy is worth considering. Hearing and vision screening are recommended because of the increased association of vision and hearing deficits in children with CP. An electroencephalogram (EEG) is only recommended if a seizure disorder is suspected.

Expert Opinion on Management Issues

Treatment of cerebral palsy is symptomatic. The goals are to maintain range of motion (ROM), prevent orthopedic complications, and improve the function and quality of life. Children who do not sit by 4 years of age are unlikely to learn how to walk. Nonambulators are at increased risk for hip dislocation, scoliosis, and osteopenia.

The majority of children with CP are hyper- rather than hypotonic. Spasticity interferes with muscle function and causes secondary orthopedic complications. It can be treated with therapy, medication, and surgery. Stretching and ROM are important with all treatments. Physical therapists work on gross motor skills and evaluate assistive devices and other equipment needs. Occupational therapists concentrate on upper extremity function such as feeding, dressing, toileting, bathing, use of adaptive devices, school readiness, and communication systems. Speech therapists focus on language development and oromotor function.

Orthotic devices and adaptive equipment help maintain ROM, improve postural stability, prevent contractures, protect skin from breakdown, aid ambulation, and reduce spasticity. Skeletal alignment, extremely important for upper extremity function, can be improved by seating systems. Various types of splints provide stability and support. A thoracolumbar soft orthosis (TLSO) provides postural alignment and support for the trunk. Ankle-foot orthoses (AFOs) may be used for positioning and standers with appropriate body support provide needed weight bearing. Walkers are useful with disorders of balance. Serial casting can provide stretch to various muscles.

Various medications are useful in reducing muscle tone in combination with therapy. Dantrolene reduces calcium release, thereby decreasing excitation-contraction coupling in skeletal muscle. Dosing is 0.5 mg/kg orally every day, increasing to 2 mg/kg three or four times daily to a maximum dose of 3 mg/kg or 100 mg four times daily. Side effects include sedation, weakness, dizziness, and hepatotoxicity at high doses.

Baclofen is a presynaptic inhibitor activating the γ-aminobutyric acid (GABA)$_b$ receptor. Typical dosing is 10 to 15 mg/day divided every 8 hours, titrating dose every 3 days up to 40 mg in children younger than 8 years or 60 mg in children older than 8 years. Side effects include sedation, nausea, headache, and lowering of seizure threshold. Sudden withdrawal can lead to seizures and hallucinations.

Intrathecal baclofen (ITB) is effective in reducing spasticity, as well as dystonia. Medication is delivered via a pump reservoir. A catheter delivers medication intrathecally. ITB can make hygiene, transfers, and positioning easier in spastic quadriparesis. It is useful in decreasing tone in discrete muscle groups. Complications include infection, catheter dislocation or obstruction, cerebrospinal fluid (CSF) leak, and pump failure.

Diazepam is a benzodiazepine that facilitates the postsynaptic effects of GABA by increasing presynaptic binding. Dosing is 0.12 to 0.8 mg/kg/day orally in divided doses three to four times per day. Side effects include dizziness and sedation.

Tizanidine, another α_2-agonist, acts at central α_2-noradrenergic receptor sites. Postulated actions facilitate glycine, an inhibitory neurotransmitter, and interfere with the release of excitatory amino acids. Dosing begins with 2 to 4 mg orally at bedtime, increasing by 1 mg every 4 to 5 days. Side effects include somnolence, fatigue, dry mouth, orthostatic hypotension, insomnia, nausea, and elevated liver enzymes. Further clinical studies are needed in the pediatric population.

Botulinum toxin (Botox) is used to treat focal dystonias and rigidity in hemiplegic or diplegic spasticity. Botox inhibits release of acetylcholine from the presynaptic site at the muscle nerve junction. The injections last 3 to 5 months; therefore, repeated treatments are necessary. Botox is also used to predict the functional effect of orthopedic surgery such as a tendon release. Botulinum toxin is also used to treat focal dystonias and rigidity in hemiplegic or diplegic spasticity.

If physical therapy and medications fail to adequately treat spasticity, surgical management is a consideration. With selective dorsal rhizotomy (SDR), a percentage of dorsal nerve roots are severed with a resulting decrease in muscle tone. Side effects include postoperative pain, spondylolisthesis, and lumbar lordosis. Good results have been shown to be maintained at 5 years. The relative cost-to-benefit ratio of SDR versus ITB needs further controlled study.

Reduction of spasticity can decrease secondary complications, such as contracture, hip dislocation, and limb length discrepancy. Orthopedic intervention can correct these. Tendon transfers, lengthening, and soft tissue releases can restore balance if contracture is present. Osteotomies alter the shape of bones and improve alignment of limbs. Contractures occur most commonly at the shoulder adductors, elbow flexors, wrist and finger flexors, hip flexors and adductors, knee flexors and ankle plantar flexors. Because of weak dorsiflexors and overactivity of the triceps surae and peroneals relative to the posterior tibials, equinovalgus deformity is common. Asymmetry of the neck or trunk can lead to torticollis and spinal deformation. Scoliosis is most common and severe in nonambulators. Orthoses can retard progression. However, spinal fusion is indicated for curves of more than 40 degree, thoracolumbar curves, and nonambulatory patients.

The goal of surgery is to increase ROM, decrease contracture, and normalize forces on the joint. The orthopedic surgeon must consider all contracted muscles and the role they play in function. Gait analysis may be useful in this regard, as well as in evaluating function postoperatively. It is important to remember that some contracture may be necessary to maintain the strength and stability necessary for a patient to maintain the preoperative level of function.

Oromotor supranuclear bulbar palsy may lead to difficulties with swallowing and articulation and can lead to aspiration pneumonia and drooling. Positioning, medication, and sometimes surgery may be necessary to alleviate these problems. Medications such as trihexyphenidyl hydrochloride, benztropine mesylate, and glycopyrrolate have been helpful with drooling. Side effects include increased activity, irritability, drowsiness, stating, insomnia, dry mouth, vomiting, abdominal pain, and trouble voiding. In some cases surgery is necessary.

The treatments discussed do not change the lesion that caused CP. Although therapy decreases spasticity, ongoing therapy is needed or gains are lost. Adjunctive therapies such as swimming, biking, and riding are helpful adjunctive therapies. Review of the literature shows no scientific evidence to support patterning, neurodevelopmental therapy (NDT), sensory integrative therapy, optometric visual training, and auditory integrative therapy over traditional therapy. Although proponents argue this is a result of poor selection of the outcome variable, prospective controlled studies are needed.

Evaluation of changes in functional independence is the basis for evaluating the efficacy of rehabilitation. The gross motor function measure (GMFM) can be used to assess overall motor function. The Ashworth scale is useful in assessing spasticity. WeeFIM (Functional Independence Measure for Children) and the pediatric evaluation of disability inventory (PEDI) are often used as global measures of activities of daily living.

The American Academy of Pediatrics recommends that pediatricians remain involved with the evaluation of therapy programs for children with disabilities. The pediatrician, as primary care provider, is in an ideal position to oversee the many facets of a child's care and maintain balance in the life of the child and family.

Common Pitfalls

Although CP is described as a static encephalopathy, clinical findings, such as movement disorders or secondary complications, evolve with development. It is important to distinguish the loss of function caused by secondary complications of CP from a misdiagnosis of CP in a child with a progressive disorder. This will become more important as our ability to treat metabolic conditions increases. Glutaric aciduria type I and dopamine-responsive dystonias are two examples of treatable disorders that can present as CP. Some progressive disorders, such as hereditary spastic paraparesis and ataxia telangiectasia, can have such a slow course that also mimics CP.

Failure to inadequately work up the etiology of CP can result in a failure to treat an underlying cause such as a coagulopathy. Although a treatable etiology is rare, determining an etiology is important in order to appropriately counsel parents about prognosis and recurrence risk.

A serious pitfall in the management of spasticity is to treat the sign at the expense of function. Some increased tone may be needed to offset weakness. Some degree of contracture may be useful to maintain the stability necessary for the patient to maintain his level of function.

Perhaps the most common and serious pitfall in the management of CP is basing assessment on an office visit examination and failing to take into account that performance in the real world is often very different from estimates of ability based on a brief examination. A child who can walk a few steps down a hospital corridor may be unable to navigate the long, busy halls of a middle school, for example.

Finally, management of the patient by the book or the practitioner's idea of what is appropriate is another significant pitfall. To maximize success, goals must be tailored to individual patient and family's needs and to function in the real world.

Communication and Counseling

CP is best handled by a multidisciplinary team so that the needs and abilities of the child are put in context. Classification of the child with CP expanded from the clinical to an assessment of functioning in the real world. The International Classification of Functioning, Disability, and Health (ICF) developed by the World Health Organization emphasizes the interaction between health and personal and environmental factors. Similarly, recognition that the family is the central element in a child's life has fostered the development of family-centered care. Family-centered care respects a family's uniqueness and understands that the family is the most important and constant context for a child's development. The relationship between a health care provider and a family is collaborative. Communication is a dialogue between clinician and family. It is important for the clinician to listen to the family, to determine their understanding about their child's condition, their beliefs, and their goals. The clinician helps families acquire the knowledge base and skills necessary to participate with confidence in planning their child's care.

Counseling begins with assessment of the family's needs. It is the duty of the clinician to explain the diagnosis; provide anticipatory guidance; and to help families understand the prognosis over time, answer questions, and explain treatment options. It is, therefore, important for the clinician to be knowledgeable about the professional and therapeutic modalities available. Factors associated with a good prognosis for independent living are attendance at regular school, completion of high school, independence in mobility, ability to travel beyond the home, good hand skills, and living in a small community. Immobility or severe mental retardation decreases life expectancy. Early intervention provides improved interaction between infant and caregiver, support for the parent, and education about how to care for the child at home. As a professional, the clinician has a responsibility to counsel families about the efficacy of treatments based on their scientific merits, to help set functional goals for therapy, to inform parents of the community resources that are available, and to coordinate the care from therapeutic and professional specialists such as pediatric physiatrists, developmental pediatricians, and neurologists. The pediatrician as provider of the medical home for a child is in an ideal position to oversee the many facets of a child's care and to meet the changing needs of the child and family.

SUGGESTED READINGS

1. American Academy of Pediatrics, Committee on Children with Disabilities: The treatment of neurologically impaired children using patterning (RE9919). Pediatrics 104:1149–1151, 1999. **Discusses evidence and lack thereof for this school of therapy for children with disabilities.**
2. Ashwal S, Russman BS, Blasco PA, et al: Practice parameter: Diagnostic assessment of the child with cerebral palsy (CP). Neurology 62:851–863, 2004. **Report of the quality standards subcommittee of the American Academy of Neurology and the Practice Committee of the Child Neurology Society discusses workup of child with suspected CP.**
3. Cooley WC: Providing a primary care medical home for children and youth with cerebral palsy. Pediatrics 114:1106–1113, 2004. **Report of the committee on children with disabilities gives overview of management of children with CP.**
4. Ketelaar M, Vermeer A, Helders PJ: Functional motor abilities of children with cerebral palsy: A systematic literature review of assessment measures. Clin Rehabil 12:369–380, 1998. **Discusses common measures of function used in the pediatric population.**
5. King S, Teplicky R, King G, Rosenbaum P: Family-centered service for children with cerebral palsy and their families: A review of the literature. Sem Ped Neurol 11:78–86, 2004. **Discusses family centered care of children with CP.**
6. Majnemer A, Mazer B: New directions in the outcome evaluation of children with cerebral palsy. Sem Ped Neurol 11:11–17, 2004. **Examines emerging concepts, including new ICF classification by the World Health Organization, in the assessment of outcomes of children with CP.**
7. Michaud LJ: Prescribing therapy services for children with motor disabilities. Pediatrics 115:1836–1838, 2004. **Describes the role of the pediatrician in prescribing physical, occupational, and speech therapy.**
8. Palisano RJ, Snider LM, Orlin MN: Recent advances in physical and occupational therapy for children with cerebral palsy. Sem Ped Neurol 11:66–77, 2004. **Provides a conceptual framework based on family-centered care for reviewing physical and occupational therapy.**
9. Tilton AH: Management of spasticity in children with cerebral palsy. Sem Ped Neurol 11:58–65, 2004. **Reviews therapeutic, medical, and surgical treatment options in CP.**

Movement Disorders

Kent R. Kelley

KEY CONCEPTS

- The major types of movement disorders are athetosis, chorea, dystonia, myoclonus, rigidity, stereotypies, tics, and tremors.
- Movement disorders can be primary or secondary to other diseases (trauma, hypoxia-ischemia, infection/immunologic reaction, drug reaction, metabolic disorders, endocrine disorders and vascular disorders).
- Primary movement disorders can be hereditary or acquired.
- Movement disorders are often associated with neuropsychiatric disorders.

Types of Movement Disorders

Athetosis consists of irregular, slow distal writhing and twisting movements. Athetosis is seen in cerebral palsy, other static encephalopathies, Lesch-Nyhan syndrome, and kernicterus.

Chorea are quick, dancing movements of proximal and distal muscles with irregular unpredictable random jerks. Chorea is seen in infectious and autoimmune encephalopathies such as Sydenham chorea, systemic lupus erythematosus, hyperthyroidism, infectious mononucleosis, pregnancy, reactions to drugs such as anticonvulsants and neuroleptic drugs, closed head injury, carbon monoxide poisoning, hypocalcemia, polycythemia, and Huntington and Wilson diseases.

Dystonia is irregular slow, twisting, sustained movements that may result in abnormal postures and can progress to contractures. Dystonia may be primary-idiopathic (e.g., torsion dystonia) or secondary (Sandifer syndrome, spasmus nutans, reaction to neuroleptic drugs, static encephalopathy, perinatal asphyxia, or familial dystonia).

Myoclonus consists of abrupt, brief, jerk-like contractions of one or more muscles; it is often stimulus sensitive. Myoclonus may arise from multiple levels of the nervous system. Causes include sleep myoclonus, hypoxic-ischemic encephalopathy, uremic encephalopathy, urea cycle defects, side effects of tricyclic therapy, prion disease, hyperthyroidism, opsoclonus-myoclonus, epileptic encephalopathies, mitochondrial and metabolic diseases such as Tay-Sachs disease, Startle disease, sialidosis, and Wilson disease.

Rigidity is resistance to passive movement. It may be sustained (lead-pipe rigidity) or interrupted by tremor (cogwheel rigidity). Rigidity is seen in juvenile Parkinson syndrome, Huntington chorea, and static encephalopathy.

Stereotypies are repetitive, purposeless motions (e.g., body rocking, head rolling) that resemble the voluntary movements often associated with akathisia (sensory and motor restlessness). Stereotypies are seen in autism, Rett syndrome, reactions to neuroleptic drugs, and schizophrenia.

Tics are rapid, sudden, repetitive movements or vocalizations.

Tremors are rhythmic oscillatory movements, both supination-pronation and flexion-extension, seen in a resting state or with activity. Resting tremors are seen in primary juvenile or secondary Parkinson syndrome, and action tremors may be seen in essential (familial) tremor, cerebellar disorders, brainstem tumors, hyperthyroidism, Wilson disease, electrolyte disturbance (e.g., glucose, calcium, magnesium), heavy metal intoxication (e.g., lead, mercury), and multiple sclerosis.

Etiology

Movement disorders may be primary or secondary. Primary movement disorders are hereditary or genetic. Secondary disorders are acquired. Causes of secondary movement disorders include trauma, hypoxia-ischemia, infection/immunologic reaction, drug reaction, metabolic disorders, endocrine disorders, vascular disorders, and unknown etiologies. Laboratory tests are listed in Box 1.

Disorders of movement are characterized by abnormal movements of different types, often with associated neuropsychiatric disorders. The particular movement disorder in itself is rarely etiologically specific. Many movement disorders may be temporarily suppressed, may be incorporated into other voluntary movements, decrease spontaneously during sleep, or increase with stress. Methods of provocative testing include maintenance of posture in extension against gravity,

---

> **BOX 1   Laboratory Testing for Movement Disorders**
>
> - β-Hemolytic streptococcal pharyngeal culture
> - Streptococcal titers (antistreptolysin O titers [ASLO]) and anti-DNase
> - Antinuclear antibody
> - Thyroid function tests
> - Ceruloplasmin
> - Liver function tests
> - Urinary copper
> - Lactate and pyruvate
> - Plasma amino acids
> - Urinary organic acids
> - Urinary vanillylmandelic and homovanillic acids
> - Further metabolic testing as indicated by history and examination

hyperpronation, tongue protrusion, squeezing the examiner's finger, pouring liquid, and drawing a spiral. The diagnosis is made by history and examination that leads to localization and differential diagnosis.

Many movement disorders originate in the basal ganglia (extrapyramidal system). The primary neurotransmitters of the basal ganglia are dopamine, serotonin, and the catecholamines. The basal ganglia are also implicated in disorders of attention, anxiety, obsessions, and compulsions. The disorder may be primary or secondary to developmental, metabolic, traumatic, and infectious etiologies. The etiologies can range from benign to malignant in their effect on the developing nervous system. Testing may include neuroimaging, EEG, and metabolic evaluation. Treatment is directed at the underlying defect and symptoms. In addition, the associated behavioral disorders may require neuropsychological testing, counseling, and treatment of associated symptoms as well as school interventions. The emphasis in this chapter is on the different types of movements, the common syndromes, the treatable syndromes that should not be missed, and symptomatic treatment.

Syndromes

NON-TIC DISORDERS

Benign sleep myoclonus is characterized by rhythmical jerks, both erratic and generalized, that occur only in sleep and may persist weeks to months in the newborn. It may be induced by stimulation and is extinguished by waking the baby.

Sandifer syndrome is characterized by episodes of opisthotonic arching, twisting, and dystonic posturing and is associated with hiatal hernia and gastroesophageal reflux and poor weight gain. Treatment is aimed at the underlying cause.

Self-stimulation involves infants and young children often displaying self-soothing and stimulatory behaviors such as rocking and head banging. Masturbation is more common in girls and is characterized by stiffening, rocking, and flushing. It may be interrupted. It is not associated with a change in consciousness and should be distinguished from infantile seizures.

Shuddering attacks are characterized by a quick shiver in infants 6 to 18 months of age. They commonly occur with presentation of excitatory stimuli and may be associated with a family history of essential tremor.

TIC DISORDERS

Tics are brief, sudden, repetitive, stereotyped, involuntary, and purposeless movements or vocalizations. They most commonly involve muscles of the face, neck, and respiratory tract. They may be increased by anxiety, stress, excitement, and fatigue and are decreased during sleep and relaxation, and during activities involving increased concentration. They can be voluntarily suppressed. At times, a premonitory urge and a sense of release accompany tics.

Motor tics include simple motor functions—eye blinking, eye jerking, face and head twitching, shoulder shrugging, bruxism, abdominal tensing, or shoulder rotation.

Complex tics include throat clearing, sniffing, grunting, barking, snorting, and spitting. Complex vocal tics are classically associated with coprolalia (obscene words), echolalia (repeating another's words), and palilalia (rapidly repeating one's own words). Simple motor tics are common and occur in as many as 10% to 29% of school-aged children. Prevalence of tic disorder is higher in younger children and in males. Transient and chronic tic disorders usually do not have an identifiable cause. However, tics can be found in association with a number of other conditions such as chromosomal abnormalities or developmental syndromes such as autism, pervasive developmental disorder, and Rett syndrome. They can also occur secondary to drugs or infections.

Tourette syndrome was described in 1885 by Georges Gilles de la Tourette as a syndrome of motor tics and vocal tics with behavioral disturbances and a chronic and variable course. The *Diagnostic and Statistical Manual of Mental Disorders*, fourth edition (DSM-IV) criteria for Tourette syndrome requires onset before 18 years of age and persistence of multiple motor and vocal tics over more than 1 year. The tics are frequent, often daily, and there is no period of more than 3 months without tics. The chronic motor and vocal tics must cause significant disturbance in social functioning. Finally, there must be no identifiable medical etiology. Prevalence is reported to be as low as 3 in 10,000 people and as high as 300 in 10,000 people globally. Evaluation includes a detailed developmental, neurologic, and psychiatric history and examination, sometimes an electroencephalogram (EEG), and neuropsychological evaluation for comorbid disorders.

Expert Opinion on Management Issues

TICS AND TOURETTE

For information on Tourette syndrome and tic disorders, see the chapter in Section 22 entitled "Tourette Syndrome."

IATROGENIC MOVEMENT DISORDERS

Acute dystonic reactions may occur within days of initiation of dopamine receptor–blocking drugs. They are characterized by intermittent, involuntary contractions of muscles in the face, neck, trunk, pelvis, and extremities. Oculogyric crises involving conjugate dystonic eye deviation can last minutes to hours. The treatment response is rapid with antihistamines (diphenhydramine 50 mg intravenously [IV]), anticholinergic drugs (benztropine mesylate 1–2 mg intramuscularly [IM]), or benzodiazepines (diazepam 5–7.5 mg IM).

Neuroleptic malignant syndrome is a syndrome of movement (rigidity, tremor, chorea, and dystonia), autonomic dysfunction (fever, hypertension, tachycardia, diaphoresis, irregular respiratory pattern, urinary retention), lapses of consciousness, and rhabdomyolysis with an elevation of creatinine kinase. It occurs within weeks of starting neuroleptics. The adult mortality rate is 20%. Treatment is immediate withdrawal of antipsychotic medication, intravenous hydration and cooling, and dantrolene sodium or bromocriptine. A similar syndrome of overstimulation of serotonin receptors by various serotonergic agents has been described with the beginning of treatment or with overdose.

Tardive dyskinesia is a hyperkinetic disorder of abnormal movements, most commonly involving the face (e.g., lip smacking or pursing, chewing, grimacing, tongue protruding). Tardive dyskinesia occurs during treatment with neuroleptics (e.g., chlorpromazine, haloperidol, metoclopramide) or within 6 months of their discontinuance. This disorder is thought to be secondary to dopaminergic dysfunction of the basal ganglia, because these drugs act as dopamine receptor blockers. Approximately 3 months of continuous or intermittent treatment with neuroleptics is needed before the risk of tardive dyskinesia increases.

HEREDITARY MOVEMENT DISORDERS

Huntington chorea is an autosomal dominant disorder manifested as chorea or rigidity and dementia. It is caused by a CAG trinucleotide repeat on chromosome 4p. The function of the gene product, Huntington, is not known. Genetic testing is available and affected patients typically have more than 30 repeats. The disorder is of paternal origin in more than 70% to 90% of cases. Onset before the age of 20 years is seen in fewer than 10% of cases, and children most often present with rigidity. MRI demonstrates atrophy of the head of the striatum, in particular of the caudate nucleus, and of the frontal cortex. Progression is rapid over years and there is no effective treatment.

Wilson disease (hepatolenticular degeneration) is an autosomal recessive disorder involving copper accumulation in the basal ganglia and liver. Roughly a third of patients present by age 5 years with hepatic involvement, and another third presents after age 8 years with dystonia, rigidity, tremor, dementia, and psychiatric manifestations. Kayser-Fleisher rings (copper clumps in the Descemet membrane) are seen in most children with neurologic involvement. Neuroimaging may show hypodensities of the thalamus and basal ganglia. Markedly decreased levels of ceruloplasmin and low serum copper and high urinary copper are usually seen, but confirmation of the diagnosis may require liver biopsy. Treatment involves chelation of copper with D-penicillamine (up to 0.5–0.75 g per day) in divided doses with gradual increases of dose, because of potential for worsening of symptoms. Pyridoxine 25 mg/kg/day is also recommended because of the antivitamin effect of penicillamine. Side effects include fever, rashes, pyridoxine deficiency, thrombocytopenia, and rarely myasthenic symptoms; alternative treatments are available. Outcome is best in primary hepatic involvement and is more guarded when there is neurologic involvement.

Neuroacanthocytosis, ataxia-telangiectasia, and Lesch-Nyhan syndrome may also produce a hereditary chorea.

SECONDARY MOVEMENT DISORDERS

Chorea

Sydenham chorea (St. Vitus Dance) is a late major manifestation of rheumatic fever caused by group A *Streptococcus* that is characterized by behavioral changes and chorea. Presentation is often subtle and insidious and includes fidgeting, emotional lability, and clumsy movements. Onset is typically after age 3 years and may be asymmetric. Syndemham chorea is somewhat more common in girls. The continuous movements, when fully developed, produce a dancing appearance that makes writing, dressing, and speech very difficult. An electromyogram (EMG) shows bursts of activity. The affected child is hypotonic and has difficulty sustaining contraction. Classically a "milk-maid's" grip is seen (hand grip may alternate between weak and normal). Recovery occurs over months, and there may be later recurrences with intercurrent illness and pregnancy (chorea gravidarum).

Other autoimmune disorders may manifest with chorea and psychiatric manifestations including systemic lupus erythematosus, hyperthyroidism, and encephalitis. Chorea has also been associated with anticonvulsants, anticholinergics, antipsychotics, and birth control pills.

Pediatric autoimmune neuropsychiatric disorders associated with streptococcal infection (PANDAS) is a poststreptococcal neuropsychiatric disorders. It is not clear whether PANDAS constitutes a distinct syndrome or a variation with tics that is expressed more commonly in males. Nosologic considerations aside, treatment strategies are similar to those for Sydenham chorea, but the issue of the need for penicillin prophylaxis has not been adequately addressed.

Treatment of chorea and behavioral abnormalities is symptomatic and commonly includes low-dose haloperidol (0.5–1 mg twice daily) or newer neuroleptics for months as needed followed by gradual discontinuation. Dopamine-blocking agents should be avoided; however, dopamine-depleting drugs such as reserpine have been recommended. Antiepileptic medications, including carbamazepine and valproic acid, are used and avoid the risk of tardive dyskinesia. Penicillin prophylaxis is always indicated because of the risk of rheumatic heart disease in Sydenham chorea.

Myoclonus

Opsoclonus-myoclonus, or dancing eyes–dancing feet as described by Kinsbourne, is also called *infantile polymyoclonus syndrome* or *acute myoclonic encephalopathy of infants*. It is a rare but distinctive movement disorder appearing in children in the first 3 years of life. Opsoclonus is characterized by wild, chaotic, erratic, fluttering, irregular, rapid, conjugate bursts of eye movements (saccadomania). Myoclonus consists of sudden, shock-like muscular twitches of the face, limbs, or trunk. The movements are often intense and may last for months to years with exacerbation by intercurrent infection or decrease of steroids. Affected children are left with motor and speech difficulties, behavioral problems, and mental retardation. The diagnostic workup should include a complete radiologic evaluation and urinary determination for vanillylmandelic and homovanillic acids to detect occult neuroblastoma.

The anatomic site of pathology is thought to be the cerebellum and brain stem and pathophysiology is thought to be autoimmune. Opsoclonus–myoclonus has been associated with viral infection. Neuroblastoma is found in 50% of patients. The management of neuroblastoma is discussed in the chapter "Neuroblastoma" in Section 21.

Chronic symptomatic treatment of opsoclonus-myoclonus is immune modulation with steroids, prednisone 1 mg/kg, or adrenocorticotropic hormone (ACTH). Intravenous gamma globulin (IVIG), plasmapheresis, and chemotherapeutic agents are also used.

Dystonia

Classic torsion dystonia, or dystonia musculorum deformans, comprises a heterogeneous group of disorders mapped to loci referred to as DYT1 to DYT13. Early-onset autosomal-dominant DYT1, located on chromosome 9q34, may be as frequent as 1 per 2000 in the Ashkenazi Jewish population. Presentation commonly occurs after age 5 years with focal, segmental, or generalized dystonia, which often begins with plantar flexion and gait disturbance. There is an extensive list of secondary causes that should be considered, including trauma and drug exposure, but there is no confirmatory laboratory investigation. Dystonic cerebral palsy and childhood-onset Parkinson syndrome should be suspected, and a trial with dopamine is always indicated. The order of preference (per Aicardi) for treatment of dystonia, which is difficult, is:

- Levodopa trial of 25 to 300 mg/day for 1 to 3 months for dopamine-responsive dystonia
- Benzhexol starting at 2 to 4 mg/day increasing by 2.5 mg every 2 weeks up to 30 to 80 mg
- Tetrabenazine 50 to 200 mg/day
- Baclofen 40 to 120 mg/day
- Clonazepam or other benzodiazepine

Dopamine-responsive dystonia (Segawa disease) is a fluctuating dystonia with a diurnal pattern that disappears with sleep and reappears some 30 to 40 minutes after awakening and then increases. There is dramatic response to low-dose levodopa that persists into adulthood. Untreated patients may develop parkinsonism, but even late treatment is effective. It is an autosomal dominant trait with low penetrance and has been mapped to chromosome 14q.

Other Secondary Movement Disorders

Myoclonus may also result from seizures as in the early myoclonic and infantile epileptic encephalopathies (nonketotic hyperglycemia) and in the progressive myoclonic epilepsies, which include Lafora disease, Unverricht-Lundborg disease, and MERRF (myoclonus epilepsy associated with ragged-red fibers). Angelman syndrome manifests with seizures, myoclonus, and ataxia. Evaluation is primarily for the underlying genetic disorder includes chromosomal testing. Treatment is primarily aimed at symptomatic treatment of the epilepsy and rarely with vitamin cofactors.

Disorders of brain iron metabolism with a characteristic "eye-of-the-tiger" sign on MRI have been associated with pantothenate kinase–associated degeneration, hypobetalipoproteinemia, acanthocytosis, retinitis pigmentosa, and poor outcome. Movement disorders are also described with metabolic diseases including gangliosidosis, glutaric aciduria, propionic and methylmalonic acidemias, Leigh syndrome, and other mitochondrial encephalopathies.

PAROXYSMAL MOVEMENT DISORDERS AND CHANNELOPATHIES

Paroxysmal dyskinesias are rare, intermittent, episodic disorders of movement appearing in childhood. They may be sporadic or familial. Classification schemes are evolving, and they have been arranged according to precipitating factors: paroxysmal kinesigenic dyskinesia (PKD), paroxysmal nonkinesigenic dyskinesia (PNKD), paroxysmal exercise-induced dyskinesia (PED), and paroxysmal hypnogenic dyskinesia (PHD).

PKD is primarily idiopathic and is characterized by episodes of dystonic, choreic, or mixed movement disorders that occur up to 20 times per day and last less than 2 minutes; most respond to carbamazepine. PNKD may be idiopathic or secondary; episodes are mainly dystonic and last longer (5–20 minutes) and occur less frequently (daily to monthly). Treatment response is poor, but some patients respond to clonazepam or acetazolamide. PED is predominantly familial, and the episodes are triggered by prolonged exercise, usually walking or running, and can be brief or last for hours. Autosomal-dominant PHD is often responsive to carbamazepine and may be a form of nocturnal frontal lobe epilepsy. Mutations in the gene coding for nicotinic acetylcholine receptors have been found in some families.

Channelopathies are a group of disorders that affect the nervous system in myriad ways. Channels may be voltage-gated and ligand-gated, and disorders are described in both. Phenotypic convergence is seen, and different calcium or potassium channels produce similar syndromes of episodic ataxia. Furthermore, phenotypic divergence is seen with different mutations of the same calcium channel, producing migraine, ataxia, epilepsy, or coma. Channelopathies have also been described in a group of episodic cerebellar ataxias and familial hemiplegic migraine. Familial channelopathies are also described in paroxysmal dyskinesias and in benign neonatal convulsions and autosomal-dominant nocturnal frontal lobe epilepsy. In addition, hypokalemic periodic paralysis, central core disease, and malignant hyperthermia syndrome have been associated with calcium channelopathies.

Hyperekplexia was the first channelopathy identified and involves a mutation in the glycine receptor α_1 in the familial hyperekplexia. This syndrome is characterized by excessive startle and in severe cases, prolonged spasms of grimacing and flexion that can lead to apnea and death. Treatment is symptomatic using benzodiazepines and valproate.

Alternating hemiplegia of childhood is a rare disorder of intermittent, alternating hemiplegia manifesting in early childhood. It is characterized by abnormal eye movements and dystonic episodes, followed by hemiplegia. There may be an autonomic prodrome, and recovery takes hours to days. Children with early onset typically have greater developmental delay and movement disorders. Seizures may occur with the hemiplegia; however, the electrocardiogram (ECG) typically shows only slowing. Flunarizine has been used for treatment and may reduce severity, duration, and frequency of the episodes.

SUGGESTED READINGS

1. Aicardi J: Disease of the Nervous System in Childhood. London: Mac Keith Press, 1998. **This is a beautifully written summation of the extensive experience and erudition of a premier child neurologist. Recommended chapters include "Heredodegenerative Diseases with Diffuse CNS Involvement of the Basal Ganglia" (pp 334–339), which discusses chorea and covers dystonia and its treatment on p. 339. Wilson disease and its treatment is discussed on pages 305–306. Also highly recommended is his collaboration with Emilio Fernandez-Alvarez.**
2. Berg BO: Principles of Child Neurology. New York: McGraw-Hill, 1996. **This volume summarizes the author's extensive clinical experience and teaching in his discussion of the dangers and treatment of neuroleptic malignant syndrome.**
3. Caine ED, McBride MC, Chiverton P, et al: Tourette's syndrome in Monroe County school children. Neurology 38:472–475, 1988. **This is a good epidemiologic study of the prevalence of tics and Tourette in New York state.**
4. Dale RC, Heyman I, Surtess RAH, et al: Dyskinesias and associated psychiatric disorders following streptococcal infections. Arch Dis Child 89:604–610, 2004. **These authors present a well-studied group of children with post-streptococcal movement and psychiatric disorders and fairly discusses the issues surrounding this long-recognized and often poorly understood disorder of Sydenham chorea.**
5. Dale RC: Childhood opsoclonus myoclonus. Lancet Neurol 2:270, 2003. **Dale summarizes the current state of knowledge and treatment in his discussion of opsoclonus-myoclonus.**
6. Fernandez-Alverez E, Aicardi J: Movement Disorders in Children. London: Mac Keith Press, 2001. **Another highly recommended volume by these leading child neurologists.**
7. Holmes GL, Russman BS: Shuddering attacks. Am J Dis Child 140:72–74, 1986. **Holmes and Russman reported on three children with shuddering attacks with V-EEG and characterize it as a benign disorder.**

8. Khalifa N, von Knorring AL: Prevalence of tic disorders and Tourette syndrome in a Swedish school population. Dev Med Child Neurol 45:415–419, 2003. **This is a good epidemiologic study of the prevalence of tics and Tourette in the Swedish population.**

9. Kullmann DM: The neuronal channelopathies. Brain 1256:1177–1195, 2002. **Kullman provides an excellent review of the molecular and cellular mechanisms of the neuronal channelopathies and their various clinical manifestations.**

10. Kurlan R, Como PG, Miller B, et al: The behavioral spectrum of tic disorders: A community-based study. Neurology 59:414–420, 2002. **This volume provides a complement to Caine et al and Khalifa and von Knorring, emphasizing the behavioral spectrum of tic disorders.**

11. Pranzatelli MR, Pedley TA: Differential diagnosis in children. In Dam M, Gram L (eds): Comprehensive Epileptology. New York-Raven Press, 1991, pp 423–447. **Pranzatelli and Pedley provide the clinicians' perspective of the mimickers of infantile seizures and the varied paroxysmal episodes and behaviors of infants and children.**

12. Resnick TJ, Moshe SL, Perotta L, Chambers HJ: Benign neonatal sleep myoclonus: Relationship to sleep states. Arch Neurol 43:266–268, 1986. **Resnick et al reported and characterized the benign disorder of neonatal sleep myoclonus.**

13. Shiang R, Ryan SG, Zhu YZ, et al: Mutations in the alpha 1 subunit of the inhibitory glycine receptor cause the dominant neurologic disorder, hyperekplexia. Nat Genet 5:351–358, 1993. **Shiang et al helped elucidate the point mutations associated with this disorder, which had been clinically described by Gastaut Villeneuve in 1967.**

14. Sutcliffe J: Torsion spasms and abnormal postures in children with hiatal hernia: Sandifer's syndrome. Prog Pediatric Neurol 2:190–197, 1969. **Sutcliffe described and named the disorder of posturing of Sandifer syndrome.**

15. Zeman W, Dyjen P: Dystonia musculorum deformans: Clinical, genetic, and pathoanatomical studies. Psychiatr Neurol Neurochir 70:77–121, 1967. **Zeman and Dyjen described well the clinical entity of dystonia musculorum deformans.**

Degenerative Diseases of the Central Nervous System

Robert H. A. Haslam

KEY CONCEPTS

- The majority of central nervous system (CNS) degenerative disorders are inherited as an autosomal recessive trait.
- Most CNS degenerative disorders have a characteristic age of onset.
- Bone marrow transplantation is effective for some CNS degenerative disorders if accomplished early in the course of the illness.
- Enzyme replacement therapy is a safe and efficacious therapy for Gaucher type 1 disease and Hurler disease.
- Future therapies for CNS degenerative diseases will include enzyme enhancement therapy, stem cell therapy, and the use of attenuated neurotropic viruses.

Central nervous system (CNS) degenerative diseases consist of a diverse group of conditions that are increasing in the pediatric age group as new disorders are identified by genetic and biochemical studies. Most CNS degenerative diseases are the result of a genetic mutation and are diagnosed by a combination of clinical findings, neuroimaging studies, and various biochemical screening tests followed by specific molecular diagnostic testing.

Infants and children may present with a wide range of symptoms and signs varying from lethargy, vomiting, hepatosplenomegaly, convulsions, and coma in the newborn to progressive abnormalities in gait, visual or auditory deficiencies, a change in personality, loss of cognitive function, and deteriorating academic performance in the school-age child. The first and most important step in the delineation of a CNS degenerative disorder is a thorough history and neurologic examination. Many conditions may mimic a degenerative disorder including cerebral palsy, encephalopathy, loss of language skills in a child with autism, the Landau-Kleffner syndrome (a recalcitrant seizure disorder), heavy metal poisoning, toxic levels of anticonvulsant drugs, and drug abuse.

As CNS degenerative diseases consist of a large number of conditions, this chapter focuses on providing a framework for the identification of a degenerative disorder. Whereas most of the conditions discussed in the following sections do not have a specific therapy, their diagnoses are essential for providing appropriate genetic counseling and to offer prenatal diagnosis if available. Table 1 summarizes the mode of inheritance and the genetic defect for each of the diseases. Finally, evidence-based treatment strategies are highlighted in those conditions that are amenable to therapy.

The Sphingolipidoses

Sphingolipidoses are characterized by the accumulation of normal metabolites within the cell that cannot be catabolized because of a deficiency in a specific enzyme or substrate. A recent study found their prevalence as a group to be 1 in 7700 live births. The following provides a brief description of the sphingolipidoses.

GM GANGLIOSIDOSIS

There are three subtypes of GM_1 gangliosidosis, but only two are discussed here. *Infantile GM_1 gangliosidosis* typically manifests at birth with poor feeding, lethargy, and convulsions. The infant has coarse facial features, an enlarged tongue, and hepatosplenomegaly and is unresponsive to sound and visual stimuli. A "cherry-red" spot may be present on examination of the retina. Muscle tone becomes progressively increased. Kyphosis results from "beaking" of the vertebra. In *juvenile GM_1 gangliosidosis*, onset is noted around 1 year of age with progressive ataxia, unsteady gait, generalized convulsions, spasticity, and loss of visual function and with deterioration in cognitive and language function. Dysmorphic facies and hepatosplenomegaly are not present as in the infantile form. Death occurs by 10 years of age.

GM_2 gangliosidosis has four subtypes; only three are discussed here. *Tay-Sachs disease* most commonly occurs in the Ashkenazi Jewish population with a carrier rate of 1/30. Screening programs designed to identify carrier

TABLE 1 Mode of Inheritance and the Genetic Defect for Degenerative Diseases of the CNS

Disease	Inheritance	Gene Location	Enzyme Abnormality
GM$_1$ gangliosidosis	AR	3p14.2	Acid β-galactoside
GM$_2$ gangliosidosis			
Tay-Sachs	AR	15q23-q24	Hexosaminidase A
Sandhoff	AR	15q13	Hexosaminidase A and B
Niemann-Pick (A&B)	AR	11p15.1-p15.4	Acid sphingomyelinase
Krabbe	AR	14q31	Galactocerebroside
Gaucher	AR	1q21-q23	Acid β-glucosidase
MLD	AR	22q13.31qter	Arylsulfatase-A
NLD			
Infantile	AR	1p32	Palmitoyl-protein thioesterase
Late infantile	AR	11p15	Pepinase
Juvenile	AR	16p12	Lysosomal membrane protein
Mucopolysaccharidoses			
Hurler	AR	4p16.3	α-L-Iduronidase
Hunter	XLR	xq28	Iduronate sulfatase
Sanfilippo A	AR	17q25.3	N-sulfatase
Sanfilippo B	AR	17q21	α-N-acetylglucosaminidase
Sanfilippo C	AR	—	Acetyl-CoA α-glucosaminidase
Mitochondrial disorders			
Leigh disease	Maternal transmission (complex V deficiency); autosomal recessive (COX deficiency); X-linked (PDH deficiency)		
MELAS	Maternal inheritance, point mutation at nt 3243 in the tRNA$^{Leu(UUR)}$ gene of mtDNA in majority of patients		
MERRF	Point mutation at nt 8344 of the tRNA^{Lys} gene of mtDNA in majority		
Adrenoleukodystrophy	XLR	xq28	VLCFAs
Peroxisomal (Zellweger)	AR	17q21–22	Abnormality of peroxisome import
Spinocerebellar disorders			
Friedrich ataxia	AR	9q13-q21	Frataxin
Basal ganglia disorders			
Wilson disease	AR	13q14.3	Copper transport
Pelizaeus-Merzbacher	XLR	xq22	Proteolipid protein gene

AR, autosomal recessive; CNS, central nervous system; COX, cyclooxygenase; MELAS, mitochondrial myopathy, encephalopathy, lactic acidosis and stroke-like episodes; MLD, metachromatic leukodystrophy; MERRF, myoclonus epilepsy and ragged red fibers; NLD, neuronal ceroid lipofuscinoses; nt, nucleotide; PDH, pyruvate dehydrogenase complex; VLCFAs, very-long-chain fatty acids; XLR, X-linked recessive.

parents have significantly reduced the prevalence of the disease. Infants are normal at birth but during early infancy demonstrate loss of motor and language skills. Most affected infants have hyperacusis and a "cherry-red" spot. Deterioration occurs rapidly with the onset of generalized convulsions and spasticity. Death usually occurs by 4 to 5 years of age. *Sandhoff disease* shares many features in common with Tay-Sachs disease. The major difference is that infants with Sandhoff disease have splenomegaly. *Juvenile GM$_2$ gangliosidosis* begins in the early school-age child, with progressive difficulties in gait and coordination followed by loss of language and visual skills secondary to optic atrophy. Generalized convulsions are also common and death occurs by the mid-teens.

NIEMANN-PICK DISEASE

Niemann-Pick disease has three subtypes. *Type A* is a uniformly lethal condition that occurs in infants. Although normal appearing at birth, the infant soon develops hepatosplenomegaly associated with loss of developmental milestones including cognitive function. Spasticity becomes a major problem and the child usually succumbs by 2 to 3 years of age. *Type B* is usually detected by the presence of splenomegaly or hepatosplenomegaly. Most individuals are developmentally intact and have normal cognitive function. Some patients ultimately develop a peripheral neuropathy and a few have "cherry-red" spots. Patients with types B and C have marked infiltration of the bone marrow with Niemann-Pick cells. *Type C* patients are normal at birth, although prolonged neonatal jaundice is common. There is a gradual loss of neuromotor and cognitive skills associated with moderate splenomegaly. Death may not occur until mid-adulthood.

KRABBE DISEASE

Krabbe disease (globoid cell leukodystrophy) is characterized by excessive irritability and inconsolable crying, poor feeding, failure to thrive, and fevers of unknown origin beginning during the first few months of life. These infants develop generalized seizures, marked rigidity, unresponsiveness to sound, and loss of visual awareness because of optic atrophy. The child rarely lives beyond 2 years of age. Krabbe disease has been reported in older children and is characterized by progressive optic atrophy and deterioration in ambulation and coordination. MRI using T2-weighted images shows symmetrical zones of high signal intensity in the centrum semiovale.

GAUCHER DISEASE

Gaucher disease has three subtypes. *Type 1* is a disease of adults that results from the accumulation of glycolipid substrates in the reticuloendothelial system causing hepatosplenomegaly, anemia, and bony abnormalities. The condition is most common in Ashkenazi Jews. There are no associated neurologic or cognitive signs. *Type 2* begins during infancy with failure to thrive, hepatosplenomegaly, marked stridor because of involvement of the larynx, and progressive loss of milestones, resulting in death by 2 years of age. *Type 3* is characterized by the onset of neurologic signs during childhood, including the development of dementia and primary muscle disease (type 3a) or an isolated gaze palsy (type 3b).

METACHROMATIC LEUKODYSTROPHY

Metachromatic leukodystrophy (MLD) has six identified subtypes, but only the *late infantile MLD type* is discussed in this chapter. Symptoms of gait disturbances and frequent falls begin prior to the second birthday. Examination reveals hypotonia with absent deep tendon reflexes, difficulty in speaking, and loss of cognitive function. The child is then unable to stand or sit and becomes bedridden. Feeding becomes difficult because of incoordination of swallowing, visual acuity decreases as a consequence of optic atrophy, and death ensues by 4 to 5 years of age secondary to aspiration pneumonia. MRI shows diffuse symmetrical attenuation of the cerebral and cerebellar white matter.

Neuronal Ceroid Lipofuscinosis

Neuronal ceroid lipofuscinosis (NCL) represents the most common CNS degenerative disease in children. The condition results from the deposition of autofluorescent material within neurons. Eight subtypes have been identified. The three most common are infantile, late infantile, and juvenile.

Infantile (Santavuori-Haltia-Hagberg disease): Symptoms begin at approximately 1 year of age with difficult to control myoclonic seizures, loss of developmental milestones, and visual inattentiveness caused by optic atrophy. There is a relentless loss of neuromotor function leading to death by 10 years of age. Significant brain atrophy and hypodensity of the thalamic nuclei is evident by MRI.

Late infantile (Jansky-Bielschowsky disease): Myoclonic seizures begin around 4 years of age in a child with normal development to that point. With the onset of seizures there is a loss of visual awareness caused by optic atrophy and a characteristic brownish pigmentation of the macula, poor coordination, and relentless intellectual decline. The child becomes bedridden a few years later but may

survive for many years. Microscopic examination of a skin biopsy shows inclusions containing curvilinear bodies.

Juvenile (Spielmeyer-Vogt-Sjögren disease): Children with this form of NCL are developmentally normal until early school years. The disease is characterized by progressive visual loss associated with cognitive deterioration. Myoclonic seizures are also present, but characteristically are not as devastating as in the other types of NCL. The retinal changes are similar to those noted in other forms of the disease. CT shows calcification of the outer and inner brain surfaces.

Mucopolysaccharidoses

Mucopolysaccharidoses (MPS) result from the abnormal accumulation of mucopolysaccharides or glycosaminoglycans in lysosomes. At least nine subtypes have been identified. Only the three associated with neurologic involvement are discussed.

Hurler disease: Infants are normal at birth but coarsening of facial features, intellectual deterioration, bony abnormalities including kyphoscoliosis and marked short stature, hepatosplenomegaly, umbilical hernia, and corneal opacities become evident. The disease slowly progresses, causing death by 20 years of age.

Hunter disease: These children develop marked short stature as a result of osseous involvement. They may develop hydrocephalus, cognitive impairment, and sensorineural deafness. The MRI may show ventricular dilation and hypodensity of the surrounding white matter. The life span is variable.

Sanfilippo disease: This disease has its onset in midchildhood with progressive intellectual regression. Generalized convulsions are common. Coarsening of facial features is present but not to the degree of Hurler disease. Death usually occurs by 20 to 30 years.

Mitochondrial Disorders

Mitochondrial diseases are a complex group of conditions caused by mutations of nuclear DNA or mitochondrial DNA. Three disorders are briefly discussed.

Leigh disease: Vomiting, failure to thrive, and seizures may begin in early infancy. Neurologic signs include hypotonia, upper motor neuron signs, optic atrophy, and external ophthalmoplegia. Bilaterally symmetrical hypodense areas of the basal ganglia are evident by MRI or CT.

Mitochondria myopathy, encephalopathy, lactic acidosis, and stroke-like episodes (MELAS): These children present with short stature, psychomotor delay, stroke-like episodes, seizures, headaches, and vomiting. The serum lactate may be elevated, and following the onset of hemiparesis the MRI will show focal lucencies unrelated to the cerebral vasculature. Muscle biopsy often demonstrates ragged red fibers (indicating abnormal mitochondria).

Myoclonus epilepsy and ragged red fibers (MERRF): Progressive myoclonic epilepsy associated with weakness, ataxia, and dysarthria are the hallmarks of MERRF. Neurologic examination is characterized by a myopathy, spasticity, hearing loss, and optic atrophy. The serum lactate is increased in many cases and ragged red fibers are present on examination of a muscle biopsy.

Adrenoleukodystrophy

The incidence of adrenoleukodystrophy (ALD) is approximately 1 in 20,000 boys. The condition begins insidiously during the first decade of life with gait abnormalities and behavioral and cognitive changes. Generalized seizures, increased tone, and pseudobulbar palsy causing difficulty with swallowing dominate the neurologic picture. Approximately half of patients have evidence of abnormal adrenal function manifested by hyperpigmentation of the palmar creases. Very-long-chain fatty acids (VLCFAs) are uniformly elevated with a C26:C22 ratio of 1.6 ± 0.84 in the plasma. MRI shows periventricular demyelination in the posterior regions. Death usually occurs approximately a decade following the onset of symptoms.

Peroxisomal Disorders

Peroxisomal disorders result from a defect in peroxisome transport or an abnormality of a peroxisomal enzyme. *Zellweger* syndrome is the best known peroxisome transport disorder and has typical clinical findings including facial dysmorphism characterized by a high and prominent forehead, hypoplasia of the mid-face, marked hypotonia and weakness at birth, and neonatal seizures. Eye abnormalities include cataracts, corneal clouding, retinal pigmentation, and optic nerve hypoplasia. MRI shows evidence of a migrational disorder with marked pachygyria and associated hypoplasia of the vermis in some cases. Death usually ensues within the first few months of life.

Spinocerebellar Disorders

Friedreich ataxia is a progressive condition that begins with ataxia between 3 to 5 years of age. The ataxia is progressive and is associated with dysarthria, weakness, and skeletal abnormalities, particularly pes cavus and scoliosis. The child becomes nonambulatory around 10 years of age. The neurologic examination is characterized by upper motor neuron signs in the lower extremities and by absent deep tendon reflexes with loss of joint position and vibration sense. Death occurs in the third decade of life secondary to a cardiomyopathy in most cases.

Disorders of the Basal Ganglia

There are several CNS degenerative disorders of the basal ganglia affecting children, including Wilson disease, Hallervorden-Spatz disease, and, rarely, Huntington chorea. *Wilson disease* is a disorder of copper transport and typically begins with a history of hepatitis caused by cirrhosis of the liver during the first 10 years of life. During the second decade of life these children present with a variety of neurologic abnormalities including dystonia, rigidity, tremor, and asterixis.

Behavioral changes and psychiatric disturbances are common and often confound making a correct diagnosis. The finding of a Kayser-Fleischer ring on examination of the eye is pathognomonic. MRI demonstrates hypodensity of the thalamic nuclei and basal ganglia in approximately half of the cases.

Pelizaeus-Merzbacher Disease

Pelizaeus-Merzbacher disease is the result of a genetic defect in myelin formation. These male infants present with marked nystagmus and roving eye movements

TABLE 2 Treatment of CNS Degenerative Diseases

Disease	Treatment Strategy	Reference
Krabbe disease	Bone marrow transplantation—early in course	Krivit et al
Gaucher type 1	Enzyme replacement (miglustat or imiglucerase)	Cox et al
Hurler disease	Enzyme replacement (laronidase)	Wraith et al
	Cord blood transplantation	Staba et al
MLD	Bone marrow transplantation—early in course	Krivit et al
Adrenoleukodystrophy	Hematopoietic cell transplantation—early stage	Peters et al; Mosher et al
Wilson disease	Penicillamine	Loudianos and Gitlin

MLD, metachromatic leukodystrophy.

Cox TM, Aerts JM, Andria G, et al: The role of the iminosugar N-butyldeoxynojirimycin (miglustat) in the management of type 1 (non-neuronopathic) Gaucher disease. J Inherit Metab Dis 26:513–526, 2003.

Krivit W, Peters C, Shapiro EG: Bone marrow transplantation as effective treatment of central nervous system disease in globoid cell leukodystrophy, metachromatic leukodystrophy, adrenoleukodystrophy, mannosidosis, fucosidosis, aspartylglucosaminuria, Hurler, Maroteaux-Lamy, and Sly syndromes, and Gaucher disease type 3. Curr Opin Neurol 12:167–176, 1999.

Loudianos G, Gitlin JD: Wilson disease. Semin Liver Dis 20:353–364, 2000.

Mosher H, Dubey P, Fatemi A: Progress in X-linked adrenoleukodystrophy. Curr Opin Neurol 17:263–269, 2004.

Peters C, Charnas LR, Tan Y, et al: Cerebral X-linked adrenoleukodystrophy: The international hematopoietic cell transplantation experience form 1982 to 1999. Blood 104:881–888, 2004.

Staba SL, Escolar ML, Poe M, et al: Cord-blood transplants from unrelated donors in patients with Hurler's syndrome. N Engl J Med 350:1960–1969, 2004.

Wraith JE, Clarke LA, Beck M, et al: Enzyme replacement therapy for mucopolysaccharidosis 1: A randomized, double-blinded, placebo-controlled, multinational study of recombinant human alpha-L-iduronidase (laronidase). J Pediatr 144:581–588, 2004.

causing head nodding. Hypotonia, developmental delay, and optic atrophy are prominent neurologic findings. MRI T2-weighted images indicate a prominent signal in the white matter of the cerebral hemispheres. The condition is slowly progressive and death occurs by the second or third decade of life.

Miscellaneous CNS Degenerative Disorders

As indicated in the previous section, there are a host of additional CNS degenerative disorders that may occur in children. Some of these include the lipidoses (e.g., sialidosis), Menke disease, multiple sclerosis, Rett syndrome, Alexander disease, and Canavan spongy degeneration. These disorders will not be discussed further in this chapter.

Expert Opinion on Management Issues

The genetic defect is known in many CNS degenerative disorders. It is therefore imperative to establish the diagnosis so that genetic counseling may be discussed and prenatal diagnosis offered as a therapeutic option (see Table 1). Hematopoietic stem cell transplantation has been successful in a number of conditions including Krabbe disease, MLD, adrenoleukodystrophy, Hurler disease, and type 3 Gaucher disease (Table 2). To be effective in preventing progression and prolonging life, transplantation must occur early in the course of the disease. Enzyme replacement has been a safe and effective therapy for the management of type 1 Gaucher disease during the past 10 years. Recently, two studies hold promise for the treatment of Hurler disease including the use of recombinant human α-L-iduronidase (laronidase) and cord blood transplantation. Several novel therapeutic strategies will become available in the future, including enzyme enhancement therapy designed to increase residual function of mutant proteins, additional stem cell therapies, and the use of attenuated neurotropic viruses.

SUGGESTED READINGS

1. Cox TM, Aerts JM, Andria G, et al: The role of the iminosugar N-butyldeoxynojirimycin (miglustat) in the management of type 1 (non-neuronopathic) Gaucher disease. J Inherit Metab Dis 26:513–526, 2003. **An evaluation of miglustat in the treatment of type 1 Gaucher disease.**
2. Krivit W, Peters C, Shapiro EG: Bone marrow transplantation as effective treatment of central nervous system disease in globoid cell leukodystrophy, metachromatic leukodystrophy, adrenoleukodystrophy, mannosidosis, fucosidosis, aspartylglucosaminuria, Hurler, Maroteaux-Lamy, and Sly syndromes, and Gaucher disease type 3. Curr Opin Neurol 12:167–176, 1999. **A review of 400 patients with lysosomal and peroxisomal disorders who underwent hematopoietic stem cell transplantation.**
3. Loudianos G, Gitlin JD: Wilson disease. Semin Liver Dis 20:353–364, 2000. **An excellent review of Wilson disease.**
4. Meikle PJ, Hopwood JL, Clague AE, Carey WF: Prevalence of lysosomal storage disorders. JAMA 181:249–254, 1999. **A summary of all lysosomal storage disorders in Australia from 1980 to 1996.**
5. Mosher H, Dubey P, Fatemi A: Progress in X-linked adrenoleukodystrophy. Curr Opin Neurol 17:263–269, 2004. **Bone marrow transplantation is beneficial in X-linked adrenoleukodystrophy patients with early cerebral involvement.**
6. Peters C, Charnas LR, Tan Y, et al: Cerebral X-linked adrenoleukodystrophy: The international hematopoietic cell transplantation experience form 1982 to 1999. Blood 104:881–888, 2004. **The course of 126 boys with X-linked adrenoleukodystrophy is reported following hematopoietic cell transplantation.**
7. Staba SL, Escolar ML, Poe M, et al: Cord-blood transplants from unrelated donors in patients with Hurler's syndrome. N Engl J Med 350:1960–1969, 2004. **Hematopoietic stem cell transplantation with banked cord blood favorably alters the natural history of Hurler's syndrome.**
8. Wraith JE, Clarke LA, Beck M, et al: Enzyme replacement therapy for mucopolysaccharidosis 1: A randomized, double-blinded, placebo-controlled, multinational study of recombinant human alpha-L-iduronidase (laronidase). J Pediatr 144:581–588, 2004. **Study shows the efficacy of laronidase in the treatment of mucopolysaccharidosis 1.**

Familial Dysautonomia

Felicia B. Axelrod

KEY CONCEPTS

- Familial dysautonomia (FD) is an autosomal recessive disorder that affects neuronal development and survival and results in sensory and autonomic dysfunction.
- DNA diagnosis and general population screening is now possible.
- The disorder is neurologic but other systems are affected and there is considerable variation in expression.
- The disease is progressive but supportive treatments can decrease morbidity and mortality.
- Dysautonomic children have increased risk of febrile and hyponatremic convulsions.
- Gastrostomy and fundoplication prevent aspiration and help maintain adequate nutrition.
- Diazepam is the most effective antiemetic for the dysautonomic crisis, and clonidine is a useful adjunct to control hypertension.
- Artificial tears as well as tear duct or punctal cautery are helpful in increasing baseline moisture.
- Spinal curvature (kyphosis and/or scoliosis) develops in 95% of dysautonomic patients by adolescence.
- Postural hypotension without compensatory tachycardia and episodic hypertension is present in all patients with dysautonomia.

Familial dysautonomia (FD) is one of the hereditary, sensory, and autonomic neuropathies, a group of genetic disorders that affects neuronal development and survival and results in sensory and autonomic dysfunction. Familial dysautonomia is an autosomal recessive disorder especially prevalent in the Ashkenazi Jewish population, where the carrier rate is estimated as 1 in 27. The gene is located on chromosome 9 (9q31), and in 2001, the two Ashkenazi Jewish mutations were identified, permitting DNA diagnosis and general population screening.

A de novo diagnosis, however, is based on the presence of cardinal criteria; that is alacrima, absent fungiform papillae, depressed patellar reflexes, and absent axon flare following intradermal histamine. Further supportive evidence is provided by findings of decreased response to pain and temperature, orthostatic hypotension, and periodic erythematous blotching of the skin.

Although penetrance is complete, there is marked variability in expression of the disease. Signs of the disorder are usually apparent at birth, and neurologic function slowly deteriorates with age so that symptoms and problems will vary with time. Although the newborn is frequently hypotonic and developmental milestones are usually delayed, motor nerve conduction is normal. Thus the motor delays are thought to be caused by central dysfunction, incoordination, and decreased sensory awareness. The sensory issues involve both peripheral and central neuronal tracts. Although dysautonomic children feel internal pain (e.g., stomachache, chest pain), skin and bone pain and temperature sensations are diminished. Burns, pressure sores, and even broken bones may go unnoticed. Central autonomic dysfunction also contributes to high anxiety levels and learning disabilities that are more apparent when the child is stressed physically or emotionally.

Frequent secondary manifestations include feeding difficulties, intractable vomiting, hypotonia, delayed developmental milestones, labile body temperature and blood pressure, absence of overflowing tears and corneal anesthesia, marked diaphoresis with excitement, recurrent aspiration pneumonia, breath-holding episodes, ataxia, and spinal curvature. Although the disease process cannot be arrested, better preventive and supportive treatments have decreased morbidity and mortality. Treatment should be directed toward specific problems, which can vary considerably among patients and at different ages.

Expert Opinion on Management Issues

ACCEPTED INTERVENTIONS

General Neurologic Care

To cope with hypotonia and delayed development, early intervention therapies are recommended. Physical and occupational therapies employing sensory integrative techniques help strengthen muscles in preparation for independent ambulation and reduce pathologic posturing.

Decreased pain and temperature perception requires that children with dysautonomia be taught to protect themselves. If there is any reason to suspect a fracture, a radiograph should be taken. Care must be taken in casting to prevent the development of pressure sores. If possible, complete immobilization should be avoided as children with neurologic problems develop muscle weakness rapidly with disuse. Chest physiotherapy during immobilization and physical therapy after the cast is removed are important.

Dysautonomic children have increased risk of febrile and hyponatremic convulsions. In contrast to the 5% risk for the general population, 32% of dysautonomic children will have at least one febrile seizure. Metabolic seizures, induced by hyponatremia, are more apt to occur during extremely hot weather, when fluid and salt intake have failed to compensate for the excessive sweating manifested by these patients or with prolonged crisis, extreme hypertension, or severe infections.

Gastrointestinal Problems

Oropharyngeal incoordination is an early sign. Poor suck or discoordinated swallow is observed in 60% of infants and is responsible for severe feeding problems that can result in malnutrition or aspiration. Cineradiographic swallowing studies often demonstrate that thin liquids are more apt to be aspirated than softer foods or thickened liquids. If weight gain is inadequate, respiratory problems persist, or the infant has elevated blood urea nitrogen, gastrostomy should be performed. Once bolus gastrostomy feeds start, gastroesophageal reflux (GER) is often apparent. Thus fundoplication is usually performed with gastrostomy. If the swallow is adequate and only GER is identified, medical management with prokinetic agents, H_2-antagonists, thickening of feeds, and positioning can be tried. However, if medical management is not successful, using the criteria of poor weight gain and growth, pneumonia, hematemesis, or apnea, surgical intervention (fundoplication) is recommended.

Recurrent or frequent vomiting can be caused by peripheral, as well as central, autonomic dysfunction. When vomiting is associated with a constellation of systemic symptoms, including hypertension, tachycardia, diffuse sweating, and even personality changes, it is termed the *dysautonomic crisis*. The most common peripheral cause of vomiting is GER. Vomiting as a result of central autonomic dysfunction is noted also in some patients. It can be induced by stress, either physical or emotional. In approximately 40% of dysautonomic patients, the central autonomic dysfunction assumes a pernicious cyclical pattern resulting in daily, weekly, or monthly crises. Cyclical vomiting may represent a type of autonomic seizure activity. In fact, anticonvulsant medications have prevented or decreased crises in some patients.

An acute vomiting or retching episode in a dysautonomic patient, irrespective of the cause, is managed with diazepam, as diazepam appears to be the most effective antiemetic for the dysautonomic crisis (Box 1). Diazepam can be administered orally, intravenously, or rectally at 0.2 mg/kg per dose with a maximum dose of 10 mg. The initial dose of diazepam should be effective in stopping the

7

BOX 1 Drugs for Dysautonomia
■ Clonidine (0.004 mg/kg per dose)
■ Diazepam (0.1–0.2 mg/kg per dose)
■ Fludrocortisone (0.1–0.2 mg/24 h)
■ Omeprazole (20 mg/24 h)
■ Midodrine (0.05–0.1 mg/kg per dose)
■ Ranitidine (2 mg/kg/24 h)

vomiting, normalizing blood pressure, and decreasing agitation. If agitation or hypertension persists, clonidine (0.004 mg/kg/dose) can be given via gastrostomy if the diastolic pressure is greater than 85 mm Hg. Subsequent doses of diazepam and clonidine are repeated at 3-hour intervals until the crisis resolves. Ranitidine (2 mg/kg/24 hours), or Omeprazole (20 mg/24 hours), may be helpful in reducing emesis volume. The crisis usually resolves abruptly, with normalization of personality and return of appetite. A crisis usually can be managed at home, especially if the child has a gastrostomy, which facilitates hydration and giving of medications. Hospitalization is indicated, however, if there is not the expected positive response to medication within 12 hours, if serious infection is suspected because of high fever, if blood or coffee ground material is vomited, if dehydration is suspected, or if there is uncharacteristic behavior, as the latter may be a sign of hyponatremia.

Respiratory Problems

The major cause of recurrent pneumonia is aspiration as a result of either misdirected swallows or GER. Most of the damage to the lung occurs during infancy and early childhood, when oral incoordination is especially poor and the diet is primarily liquid. Therefore lung infections are appreciably decreased with aggressive management of gastrointestinal dysfunction. For those who continue to have misdirected swallows, gastrostomy is indicated and for those who fail medical management of GER, then fundoplication is advised.

Because of the increased risk of aspirating gastric contents, broad-spectrum antibiotics are advised until bacteriologic studies permit specific therapy. The patient's ability to cope with respiratory infections and other causes of hypoxia is compromised because of the decreased chemoreceptor and baroreceptor sensitivity. Hypoxia does not appropriately increase ventilation and can result in systemic hypotension and bradycardia; oxygen desaturation and respiratory acidosis can ensue quickly. Unstable respiratory patterns and apneas during sleep in FD patients are evoked by abnormal interactions between various parameters such as hypoxia, decreased lung volume, and impaired baroreceptor and chemoreceptor control. Increased risk of demise during sleep may be the result of unstable respiratory patterns. All dysautonomic patients must be cautious in settings where the partial pressure of oxygen is decreased, such as at high altitudes or during airplane travel. Diving and underwater swimming are also potential hazards.

Prolonged breath-holding with crying is frequent in the early years. It occurs at least once in 63% of patients. Breath-holding can be severe enough to result in cyanosis, syncope, and decerebrate posturing; it is another example of the patients' insensitivity to hypoxia. Such an episode is frightening but self-limiting and, in our experience, has never been fatal. Electroencephalograms usually are normal or nonspecific, and breath-holding frequency is unaffected by anticonvulsant therapy.

The signs of pneumonia may be subtle. Tachypnea is generally not evident, cough is not consistently present and auscultation may be unrevealing because of decreased chest excursion. Chest physiotherapy, consisting of postural drainage and inhalation, is helpful not only in the acute situation but also as a daily routine for children with residual effects from previous aspirations or infections. In the seriously ill child, blood gases must be monitored. Excessive CO_2 accumulation is not an uncommon problem and it can be severe enough to cause coma and require assisted ventilation.

Fevers

Unexplained fevers were considered characteristic of familial dysautonomia. However it has become apparent that there usually is a reason for the fever, although the etiology may be obscure. Thus a fever lasting more than 24 hours requires a search for a source of infection. In addition to infection, causes can include dehydration, mucus plugs in the bronchi, excessive external temperature, and even stress. Fever is often preceded or accompanied by shaking chills, painful neck and leg muscle spasms, cold extremities, and gastroparesis. Antipyretics and a muscle relaxant often are helpful in reducing the anxiety and muscle spasms associated with hyperpyrexia. Diazepam (0.1 mg/kg/dose) in combination with antipyretic is effective. The child should not be fed orally or by gastrostomy until the chills and the fever subside because of associated decreased gastrointestinal motility.

Ophthalmologic Problems

Lack of overflow emotional tears is a consistent feature of FD and thus remains one of the cardinal clinical criteria for diagnosis. Reflex tearing and baseline eye moisture, however, are variably diminished. Corneal hypoesthesia and decreased blink frequency further predispose the FD eye to corneal complications. Neurotrophic corneal ulcerations occur and may be potentiated by undetected trauma and excessive dryness, especially during acute illnesses as a result of hypertension, fever, and dehydration. Corneal complications have been reduced with the regular use of topical lubricants such as artificial tear solutions. The frequency with which tear solutions are instilled depends on the child's own baseline eye moisture and corneal sensitivity (which regulates the blink frequency) as well as environmental conditions and the child's state of health. Moisture chamber spectacle attachments and goggles can be used to help retain eye moisture and protect the eye from wind and foreign bodies. If an abrasion does occur, the frequency of artificial tear use should increase. Other treatments include use of traditional patching or use of plastic wrap taped to the cheek and forehead, or use of hydrophilic soft contact lenses. Tear duct or punctal cautery is helpful in increasing baseline moisture. Tarsorrhaphy can be done on a temporary basis by use of glue on the lashes. Permanent tarsorrhaphy has been reserved for unresponsive and chronic situations. Corneal transplants have not been successful.

Orthopedic Problems

Spinal curvature (kyphosis and/or scoliosis) develops in 95% of dysautonomic patients by adolescence. Rapid progression can occur at any time. The completion of puberty generally halts the progression of scoliosis, as it does in the idiopathic adolescent form, but puberty is commonly delayed in dysautonomia. Spinal curvature further compromises respiratory function, adding the component of restrictive lung disease to interstitial disease.

Annual examination of the spine allows early diagnosis of scoliosis and permits appropriate institution of brace and exercise therapy. The latter is helpful in correcting or preventing secondary contractures in shoulders and hips. Extreme care is required in fitting the braces as decubiti may develop on the dysautonomic patient's insensitive skin at pressure points. Braces may also inhibit respiratory excursion and exacerbate GER if there is a high epigastric projection. If the brace is not successful in halting progression, or if the patient has a severe curve, spinal fusion is recommended.

Insensitivity to pain can also result in unrecognized fractures. Swelling or mild discomfort with movement may be the only sign of a fracture. Inadvertent trauma to joints also put the dysautonomic patient at increased risk for Charcot joints and aseptic necrosis.

Blood Pressure Lability

Orthostatic change in blood pressure is a cardinal sign of autonomic insufficiency and is present in all patients with dysautonomia. Because of sympathetic denervation, there is no compensatory tachycardia. Clinical manifestations of postural hypotension include episodes of lightheadedness, dizzy spells, blurring of vision, and occasional reports of "weak legs." In rare instances, there may be syncope. Symptoms tend to be worse in the morning, in hot or humid weather, when the bladder is full, before a large bowel movement, after a long car ride, coming out of a movie theater, or with fatigue. Infection, anemia, and dehydration worsen symptoms. Generally, low blood pressure is more troublesome in the adult years and can limit function and mobility. Treatment includes maintenance of hydration and lower extremity exercises to increase muscle tone and promote venous return. Other treatments have included wearing of elastic stockings, extra salt in the diet, and use of fludrocortisone, a mineralocorticoid, and midodrine, an α-agonist. Fludrocortisone 0.1 mg is given in the morning. A second dose is often added at midday. Midodrine is also given in the morning at 0.05 to 0.1 mg/kg/dose and is usually repeated every 4 hours. It should be stopped within 4 hours of bedtime. When the blood pressure is persistently low, then hypoxemia, hypovolemia, severe anemia, or infection should be suspected.

The dysautonomic patient is also susceptible to episodic hypertension. Hypertension is more apt to occur when the patient is supine, or it can occur in response to emotional stress or visceral pain or as part of the crisis constellation. Because blood pressure is so labile, treatment of hypertension should be directed to factors precipitating the hypertension rather than the use of blocking agents. If the hypertension is refractory and is associated with headache or symptoms of crisis, then clonidine or labetalol is indicated.

Anesthesia

Anesthesia for surgical procedures is associated with an increased risk because of blood pressure lability and diminished responsiveness to hypoxia and hypercapnia. Local anesthesia with diazepam as preoperative sedation is preferred whenever possible.

One of the most important factors in reducing risk is maintenance of an adequate circulating volume because vasodilation during anesthesia may be extreme. The patient should be prehydrated the night before surgery with intravenous fluids. Arterial blood pressures and blood gases are monitored throughout surgery via an arterial line. Hypotension should be corrected by decreasing the percentage of gas anesthetic and administering volume expanders. Rarely, pressor agents, such as phenylephrine hydrochloride or dopamine, are required. Postoperative management can be extremely challenging. Gastric secretions tend to be copious during excitatory anesthetic phases. To avoid postoperative aspiration, ranitidine can be given, and the stomach should be kept decompressed. This is facilitated if a gastrostomy is present. Chest physiotherapy decreases mucus plugging and exacerbation of preexisting lung disease. The duration of intubation may need to be extended until the respiratory status stabilizes or there is less reliance on pain medication. Visceral pain is appreciated, and it often causes hypertension, so narcotic pain medication may be required for intra-abdominal or intrathoracic procedures. Ophthalmologic surgery requires minimal pain medication.

CONTROVERSIAL INTERVENTIONS

The FD mutation found on more than 99.5% of FD chromosomes is a single T-to-C change located at base pair (bp) 6 of intron 20 in the *IKBKAP* gene, which encodes the protein IKAP. This mutation causes a splicing alteration that leads to variable skipping of exon 20 in the *IKBKAP* message. The mutation does not cause complete loss of function. Instead, it results in a tissue-specific decrease in splicing efficiency of the *IKBKAP* transcript; cells from patients retain some capacity to produce normal messenger RNA (mRNA) and IKAP protein. The effect of the most common (splicing) mutation varies from tissue to tissue—neuronal tissues seem primarily to express mutant mRNA, somatic tissues express roughly equal levels of normal and mutant mRNA, and FD lymphoblast cell lines primarily express the normal product. It has been speculated that by raising the amount of the normal or wild-type IKAP protein, the progression of the disease will be slowed and that the clinical symptoms of FD may be reduced. Anderson and colleagues state that tocotrienols in cell culture generally increase IKAP levels. They proposed this as a treatment for FD patients and suggest using 50 to 100 mg a day. Only one clinical trial is currently under way but there have been favorable anecdotal reports, especially in regard to increasing baseline eye moisture. Another approach to therapy would be to alter splicing patterns of mammalian mRNA. Two agents appear to have this effect, EGCG (epigallocatechin gallate) and kinetin, a plant cytokinin.

Some patients have started to use the former although neither of these drugs has been tested in clinical trials. Kinetin is not yet approved for study.

Common Pitfalls

- Once bolus gastrostomy feeds start, GER is often apparent. Thus fundoplication is usually performed with gastrostomy.
- Hospitalization should be considered when crisis persists longer than 12 hours, if there is high fever or uncharacteristic behavior, if there is hematemesis, or if dehydration is suspected.
- Hyponatremia can be a serious complication of crisis.
- The febrile child should not be fed orally or by gastrostomy because gastrointestinal motility decreases during stress.
- Extreme care is required in fitting of braces as decubiti may develop on the dysautonomic patient's insensitive skin at pressure points. Braces may also inhibit respiratory excursion and exacerbate GER if there is a high epigastric projection.
- Because blood pressure is so labile, treatment of hypertension should be directed to factors precipitating the hypertension rather than the use of blocking agents.

Communication and Counseling

With greater understanding of the disorder and development of treatment programs, survival statistics have markedly improved and increasing numbers of patients are reaching adulthood. At present, more than 40% of surviving patients are older than 20 years of age. Causes of death are less often related to pulmonary complications, showing that fundoplication and gastrostomy, and treatment of respiratory problems, have been beneficial. For this type of success to occur, a great deal of effort is necessary. The parents must cope with the care of a chronically handicapped child, who may have repeated life-threatening crises, and the physician has to become familiar with the varied manifestations of a multisystem disorder.

SUGGESTED READINGS

1. Anderson SL, Coli R, Daly IW, et al: Familial dysautonomia is caused by mutations of the IKAP gene. Am J Hum Genet 68:753–875, 2001. **Description of the two Ashkenazi Jewish mutations.**
2. Anderson SL, Qiu J, Rubin BY: Tocotrienols induce *IKBKAP* expression: A possible therapy for familial dysautonomia. Biochem Biophys Res Commun 306:303–309, 2003. **Describes in vitro increased transcription of IKAP mRNA in FD-derived cells by tocotrienols and speculates on its use as therapy.**
3. Axelrod FB: Familial dysautonomia. In Mathias CJ, Bannister R (eds): Autonomic Failure, 3rd ed. New York: Oxford University Press, 1999, pp 402–418. **Comprehensive overview of familial dysautonomia.**
4. Axelrod FB, Goldberg JD, Ye XY, et al: Survival in familial dysautonomia: Impact of early intervention. J Pediatr 141:518–523, 2002. **Provides the most current survival statistics and demonstrates improvement in the last 20 years.**
5. Bernardi L, Hilz M, Stemper B, et al: Respiratory and cerebrovascular responses to hypoxia and hypercapnia in familial dysautonomia. Am J Respir Crit Care Med 167:141–149, 2002. **Describes blunted response to hypoxia in FD patients and the subsequent effects on blood pressure and cerebral perfusion.**
6. Maayan Ch, Carley DW, Axelrod FB, et al: Respiratory system stability and abnormal carbon dioxide homeostasis. J Appl Physiol 72:1186–1193, 1992. **Describes abnormal response to hypoxia and hypercapnia during sleep stages.**
7. Slaugenhaupt SA, Blumenfeld A, Gill SP, et al: Tissue-specific expression of a splicing mutation in the *IKBKAP* gene causes familial dysautonomia. Am J Hum Genet 68:598–604, 2001. **Description of the two Ashkenazi Jewish mutations as well as autopsy findings illustrating tissue-specific expression.**
8. Slaugenhaupt SA, Mull J, Leyne M, et al: Rescue of a human mRNA splicing defect by the plant cytokinin kinetin. Hum Mol Genet 13:429–436, 2004. **Describes in vitro correction of missplicing of the FD gene by kinetin and speculates on its use as therapy.**

Neurofibromatosis Type I

Beth A. Leeman and David H. Gutmann

KEY CONCEPTS

- Neurofibromatosis type 1 (NF1) is a neurocutaneous syndrome.
- Autosomal dominant inheritance.
- Inherited tumor predisposition syndrome.
- Wide variety of clinical manifestations, including café-au-lait macules, skinfold freckling, neurofibromas, optic pathway gliomas, Lisch nodules, learning disabilities, scoliosis, tibial bowing, congenital heart defects.
- Clinical diagnosis established by history and physical examination.
- Management involves symptomatic treatment and supportive care.
- Patients benefit from care in multidisciplinary specialized NF clinics.

Neurofibromatosis type 1 (NF1) is the most common genetic disorder involving the nervous system, with an incidence estimated at 1 in 3000. Individuals affected with NF1 may present with pigmentary abnormalities, benign and malignant tumors, learning disabilities, and bony abnormalities, which manifest at different ages (Box 1). The diagnosis of NF1 is established by careful history and physical examination (Box 2).

NF1 is inherited as an autosomal dominant trait; however, nearly 50% of individuals with NF1 represent the first affected individual in their family. Although all patients with NF1 manifest clinical features of the disorder, the specific signs and symptoms may vary greatly between individuals in the same family.

Café-au-lait spots are the most common feature of NF1 and appear as flat, evenly hyperpigmented macules. Freckling, the second most common sign of NF1, occurs in intertriginous, non–sun-exposed regions, such as the

BOX 1 Age-Related Manifestations of Neurofibromatosis Type 1

Birth

- Café-au-lait macules
- Plexiform neurofibromas
- Tibial dysplasia

1–2 Years

- Café-au-lait macules increase in number and size
- Detection of plexiform neurofibromas
- Scoliosis

3–6 Years

- Optic pathway gliomas
- Skinfold freckling
- Learning disabilities, ADHD
- Hypertension
- Migraines
- Lisch nodules
- Precocious puberty
- Enlargement of plexiform neurofibromas

Late Childhood/Preadolescence/Adolescence

- Cutaneous neurofibromas increase in size and number (may herald the onset of puberty)
- Scoliosis
- NF1 vasculopathy, renal artery stenosis with hypertension
- Increasing Lisch nodules

Adulthood

- NF1 vasculopathy, renal artery stenosis with hypertension
- Essential hypertension
- Headaches
- Cutaneous neurofibromas increase in size and number
- MPNSTs

Pregnancy

- NF1 vasculopathy, renal artery stenosis with hypertension
- Cutaneous neurofibromas increase in size and number

Lifelong

- Malignancy
- Cosmetic issues
- Chronic pain

ADHD, attention deficit hyperactivity disorder; MPNSTs, malignant peripheral nerve sheath tumors; NF1, neurofibromatosis type 1.

BOX 2 Diagnostic Criteria for Neurofibromatosis Type 1

Two or more of the following are needed for the diagnosis of NF1:

- Six or more café-au-lait macules, diameter greater than 5 mm if prepubertal, or greater than 15 mm if postpubertal
- Two or more cutaneous neurofibromas *or* one or more plexiform neurofibromas
- Multiple axillary or inguinal freckles
- Optic pathway glioma
- Two or more Lisch nodules
- A distinctive osseous lesion (sphenoid dysplasia, dysplasia, or cortical thinning of long bones) with or without pseudarthrosis
- A first-degree relative with NF1 by the previously listed criteria

NF1, neurofibromatosis type 1.

---

axilla, groin, nape of the neck, areas under the chin and inframammary folds. Lisch nodules are raised, pigmented hamartomas of the iris. They typically do not cause any clinical symptoms.

The most common tumor in NF1 is the benign neurofibroma, which can manifest as a discrete mass involving a single nerve or a more diffuse lesion involving multiple nerves (plexiform neurofibroma). Discrete neurofibromas are benign tumors that may manifest as exophytic, cutaneous growths or subcutaneous masses. These neurofibromas do not commonly cause neurologic compromise and do not undergo malignant transformation. Neurofibromas also commonly grow within the intervertebral foramina as paraspinal masses. They may cause neurologic deficits or pain by compression of associated spinal nerve roots.

Plexiform neurofibromas are typically more diffuse, irregularly shaped lesions. They may grow to affect an entire limb or segment of the body, involving nerve, muscle, vasculature, and overlying skin. With continued growth they may become symptomatic and cause pain, disfigurement or neurologic dysfunction. Complications can include stimulation of neighboring soft tissue or skeletal elements, leading to limb length discrepancy or dysplasia of bone, and hemorrhage into the tumor. In addition, plexiform neurofibromas carry a risk of malignant transformation into malignant peripheral nerve sheath tumors (MPNSTs). These spindle cell sarcomas are particularly aggressive tumors associated with a poor response to treatment, metastasis, and a low 5-year survival rate. Sudden pain, new neurologic symptoms, or rapid growth of a plexiform neurofibroma should alert the patient and physician to the possibility of MPNST development.

Ophthalmologic manifestations of NF1 include low-grade pilocytic optic pathway astrocytomas affecting the optic nerve, chiasm, and hypothalamus in young children. Many of these tumors are asymptomatic. When symptoms do occur, they may include decreased visual acuity, decreased visual fields, color desaturation, and optic atrophy. Involvement of the hypothalamus may lead to endocrine dysfunction or precocious puberty.

Patients with NF1 may have a number of neurologic manifestations, including dural ectasia, seizures, macrocephaly, primary aqueductal stenosis, and migraines. Rarely, cerebrovascular abnormalities may predispose patients with NF1 to cerebral ischemia, infarct, or hemorrhage.

Although frank mental retardation is infrequent, intelligence quotient (IQ) scores are on average 5 to 10 points lower than in the general population. Specific learning disabilities and attention deficit disorder (ADD) are important causes of poor scholastic performance in children with NF1. Some authors have proposed a correlation between the presence of T2 hyperintensities on brain MRI and learning disabilities, although this relationship remains controversial.

Orthopedic issues associated with NF1 include kyphoscoliosis and dysplasia or cortical thinning of long bones. Scoliosis may be idiopathic, or it may be secondary to dysplasias or spinal tumors. Tibial bowing, an anterolateral curvature of the lower leg, may result from dysplasia or cortical thinning. This abnormal thinning may lead to pathologic fractures, and nonunion of the bone fragments may result in "false joint" formation (pseudarthrosis). Dysplasia of the sphenoid bone also occurs in a small number of patients with NF1.

Cardiovascular disease in NF1 manifests as hypertension, vasculopathy, or congenital heart defects. Although elevated blood pressure is most often caused by essential hypertension, other causes may include renal artery stenosis (RAS) resulting from NF1 vasculopathy and pheochromocytomas. Vasculopathy may involve small or large vessels and cause stenosis, occlusion, aneurysm or pseudoaneurysm, rupture, or fistula. Congenital heart disease is common, and a variety of anomalies have been reported, including a high frequency of pulmonary valve stenosis.

Expert Opinion on Management Issues

No definitive medical therapy exists for NF1. The care of patients with NF1 involves anticipatory management, symptomatic treatment, and education (Table 1). Patients benefit from the multidisciplinary team approach found in many specialized NF clinics. Visits should be scheduled on an annual basis in children, or more frequently when indicated.

TABLE 1 Summary of Management Recommendations

Clinical Feature	Management
Cutaneous Manifestations	
Dermal neurofibromas	Surgical removal or laser treatment
Spinal neurofibromas	Surgical removal when appropriate
Plexiform neurofibromas	Surgical removal for enlarging or symptomatic lesions
	Medication trials
MPNSTs	Surgical removal
	Local radiation
	Chemotherapy in selected cases
Ophthalmologic Manifestations	
Optic pathway gliomas	Followed clinically and radiographically if asymptomatic
	Treatment with chemotherapy for symptomatic tumors
Neurologic Manifestations	
Learning disabilities	May require modified educational curriculum
Attention deficit disorder	Stimulant medications (dexamphetamine, methylphenidate)
Orthopedic Manifestations	
Scoliosis	Bracing
	Surgical fusion
Tibial bowing	Bracing

MPNSTs, malignant peripheral nerve sheath tumors.

Café-au-lait macules do not require treatment. Laser therapy has been attempted for cosmetic reasons but often with only transient improvement. Dermal neurofibromas may be surgically removed or treated with laser ablation for cosmetic reasons or functional compromise. Plexiform neurofibromas must be followed clinically, and the patients must be carefully monitored for signs of MPNST formation. Surgical intervention is reserved for those with enlarging or symptomatic lesions. Because of the diffuse, infiltrative nature of the tumor, however, surgical resection is often unsatisfactory. A number of medication trials have been conducted, including use of antihistamines, maturation agents, antiangiogenic drugs, and mast cell stabilizers. Radiation treatment and chemotherapy have not been widely used for neurofibromas.

Development of pain, neurologic dysfunction, or an increase in size of a plexiform neurofibroma should prompt MRI to evaluate for MPNST or hemorrhage. Options for establishing the diagnosis of MPNSTs include fine-needle aspiration (FNA), Tru-Cut biopsy needle, open incisional biopsy, and wide surgical excision. Recent evidence suggests that fluorodeoxyglucose positron emission tomography (FDG-PET) might be useful for discriminating benign from malignant peripheral nerve sheath tumors. Although MPNSTs are typically treated by surgical resection, adjuvant radiation therapy may provide local control and delay recurrence.

In the absence of ophthalmologic or focal neurologic signs or symptoms, baseline testing such as CT, MRI, electroencephalogram (EEG), or visual-evoked potentials is not recommended. Children with NF1 require close follow-up by a pediatric neuro-ophthalmologist familiar with the disorder. If an abnormality is discovered on ophthalmologic or neurologic examination, an MRI with gadolinium should be obtained to detect a possible optic pathway glioma. Asymptomatic optic pathway gliomas without evidence of progression do not necessitate treatment and may be followed with frequent ophthalmologic and MRI examinations. Intervention is reserved for those with symptomatic tumors. Chemotherapy with a combination of carboplatinum and vincristine has been used for these symptomatic gliomas.

Signs of learning disabilities or ADD mandate neuropsychological assessment and individualized education planning. ADD may be treated with stimulants such as dexamphetamine or methylphenidate (Ritalin). Seizures, migraines, and cerebrovascular disease should be treated as they are in the general population.

An orthopedic surgeon familiar with NF1 should be consulted for treatment of bone deformities. In patients with scoliosis, MRI should be performed to identify associated tumors. Scoliosis is treated by bracing or spinal fusion. Tibial bowing should be treated with bracing to prevent fractures.

Hypertension should be treated with antihypertensive medication as in the general population. Pheochromocytomas and renovascular causes of hypertension should be considered in selected cases. Follow-up and treatment of congenital heart defects depends upon the age of the patient and the nature and severity of the defect.

Common Pitfalls

A diagnostic dilemma occurs when children without a family history of NF1 present with only one feature of the disorder. NF1 is still the most likely diagnosis, and the vast majority of such children will develop additional criteria by age 10 years.

Communication and Counseling

Patients and their families should receive counseling regarding the diagnosis of NF1, with special attention to genetic factors, prognosis, psychological issues, and available resources. Family members should be included as important contributors to the patient's care.

SUGGESTED READINGS

1. Ferner RE, Gutmann DH: International consensus statement on malignant peripheral nerve sheath tumors in neurofibromatosis 1. Cancer Res 62:1573–1577, 2002. **Recommendations for treatment of MPNSTs.**
2. Friedman JM, Arbiser J, Epstein JA, et al: Cardiovascular disease in neurofibromatosis 1: Report of the NF1 Cardiovascular Task Force. Genet Med 4:105–111, 2002. **Review of hypertension, vasculopathy, and congenital heart defects in NF1.**
3. Gutmann DH, Aylsworth A, Carey JC, et al: The diagnostic evaluation and multidisciplinary management of neurofibromatosis 1 and neurofibromatosis 2. JAMA 278:51–57, 1997. **Discussion of diagnosis and treatment of NF1 and NF2.**
4. Listernick R, Louis DN, Packer RJ, et al: Optic pathway gliomas in children with neurofibromatosis 1: Consensus statement from the NF1 Optic Pathway Glioma Task Force. Ann Neurol 41:143–149, 1997. **Recommendations for treatment of optic pathway gliomas.**
5. Lynch TM, Gutmann DH: Neurofibromatosis 1. Neurol Clin N Am 841–865, 2002. **A detailed review of NF1.**
6. National Institutes of Health Consensus Development Conference statement: Neurofibromatosis conference statement. Arch Neurol 45:575–578, 1988. **Established the criteria used for diagnosis of NF1.**
7. North KN, Riccardi V, Samango-Sprouse C, et al: Cognitive function and academic performance in neurofibromatosis 1: Consensus statement from the NF1 Cognitive Disorders Task Force. Neurology 48:1121–1127, 1997. **A review of learning disabilities in NF1.**
8. Packer RJ, Gutmann DH, Rubenstein A, et al: Plexiform neurofibromas in NF1: Toward biologic based therapy. Neurology 58:1461–1470, 2002. **Recommendations for treatment of plexiform neurofibromas.**
9. Tedesco MA, Di Salvo G, Natale F, et al: The heart in neurofibromatosis type 1: An echocardiographic study. Am Heart J 143:883–888, 2002. **Study showing high frequency of congenital heart defects and need for screening echocardiography.**

Tuberous Sclerosis Complex

Steven P. Sparagana and E. Steve Roach

KEY CONCEPTS

- Tuberous sclerosis complex (TSC) is a genetic disease, although approximately two thirds of the cases result from a spontaneous mutation.
- TSC affects multiple organ systems with numerous potential medical complications.
- Surveillance screening can help to identify potentially treatable complications and thus help to minimize morbidity.
- The Tuberous Sclerosis Alliance (http://www.tsalliance.org) has up-to-date information for both patients and medical professionals.

Tuberous sclerosis complex (TSC) is a dominantly inherited disorder of cellular differentiation and proliferation with variable clinical manifestations. It can affect not only brain and skin but also the eye, kidney, heart, lungs, and other organs. Mutations of two different genes, *TSC1* (chromosome 9q34) and *TSC2* (chromosome 16p13), can cause TSC. These are tumor suppressor genes, and a mutation in either TSC gene evidently causes nearly identical phenotypes, although subtle gene-specific differences in phenotype are being investigated. TSC may be diagnosed by clinical criteria (Table 1). A DNA test for *TSC1* and *TSC2* mutations is available (Athena Diagnostics, Worcester, Mass). Given the overall complexity of TSC, a comprehensive discussion of all aspects of the diagnosis and treatment of the disease is beyond the scope of this chapter. Two excellent monographs on TSC are listed in the Suggested Readings section.

TABLE 1 Diagnostic Criteria for Tuberous Sclerosis Complex (TSC)*

Major Features

- Facial angiofibromas or forehead plaque
- Nontraumatic ungual or periungual fibroma
- Hypomelanotic macules (three or more)
- Shagreen patch (connective tissue nevus)
- Cortical tuber[†]
- Subependymal nodule
- Subependymal giant cell astrocytoma
- Multiple retinal nodular hamartomas
- Cardiac rhabdomyoma, single or multiple
- Lymphangiomyomatosis[‡]
- Renal angiomyolipoma[‡]

Minor Features

- Multiple, randomly distributed pits in dental enamel
- Hamartomatous rectal polyps[§]
- Bone cysts[¶]
- Cerebral white matter "migration tracts"[†¶]
- Gingival fibromas
- Nonrenal hamartoma[§]
- Retinal achromic patch
- "Confetti" skin lesions
- Multiple renal cysts[§]

*Definite TSC: Either two major features or one major feature plus two minor features.
   Probable TSC: One major plus one minor feature.
   Suspect TSC: Either one major feature or two or more minor features.
   [†]When cerebral cortical dysplasia and cerebral white matter "migration tracts"occur together, they should be counted as one rather than two features of tuberous sclerosis.
   [‡]When both lymphangiomyomatosis and renal angiomyolipomas are present, other features of tuberous sclerosis should be present before a definite diagnosis is assigned.
   [§]Histologic confirmation is suggested.
   [¶]Radiographic confirmation is sufficient.
   Modified from Roach ES, Gomez MR, Northrup H: Tuberous sclerosis complex consensus conference: Revised clinical diagnostic criteria. J Child Neurol 13:624–628, 1998.

Expert Opinion on Management Issues

Epilepsy occurs in 85% of patients with TSC. Although some individuals with TSC and epilepsy have normal intelligence, most have varying degrees of mental retardation. Infantile spasms occur in approximately 50% of children with TSC, often as the first indication of the disease. The most common seizure type overall is complex partial seizure with or without secondary generalized tonic-clonic seizure. Tonic seizures and myoclonic seizures, as well as Lennox-Gastaut syndrome (tonic or atonic seizures, atypical absence seizures, myoclonic seizures, and slow spike-wave complexes on electroencephalogram [EEG]) may also occur in TSC. Epilepsy in individuals with TSC is often difficult to control—only 15% of individuals with TSC have seizure remission long enough to consider discontinuation of antiepileptic drug (AED) therapy.

A catastrophic form of epilepsy called *infantile spasms* (IS) is frequently associated with mental retardation. The American Academy of Neurology and the Child Neurology Society have jointly developed a practice parameter on the medical treatment of IS. Adrenocorticotropic hormone (ACTH) was determined to be "probably effective" for the short-term treatment of IS; however, optimum dosage and duration of treatment with ACTH could not be established based on the evidence. In TSC, vigabatrin was determined to be "possibly effective" for the short-term treatment of IS. Optimum dosage was not determined. Visual field constriction caused by retinal toxicity is a serious potential side effect with vigabatrin treatment. The guideline recommended serial ophthalmologic screening in patients on vigabatrin, although the frequency and type of screening was not clarified. The Food and Drug Administration (FDA) has not licensed vigabatrin for use in the United States, although approval for use in the United States is being sought. There was insufficient evidence to prove that other treatments for IS (valproic acid, benzodiazepines, pyridoxine, and new AEDs) were useful for the treatment of infantile spasms, although these treatments are often attempted prior to ACTH or vigabatrin, or if IS remain uncontrolled.

There are approximately 10 AEDs commonly used to treat complex partial seizures with or without secondary generalized tonic-clonic seizures. The majority of these AEDs have been used as monotherapy agents or in conjunction with each other to treat epilepsy in TSC. No single agent is proven to be superior. As such, AEDs are often selected based upon side effect profile. AEDs are discussed further in the chapter entitled, "General Concepts in Seizure Management."

Individuals with medically refractory epilepsy may be candidates for either a vagus nerve stimulator or resective epilepsy surgery. Video-electroencephalography, cranial MRI, and possibly other specialized neuroimaging studies are usually done prior to the surgical procedures in order to better characterize and determine the site of seizure origin. Comprehensive evaluation by a center specializing in the treatment of epilepsy is useful for children with TSC and medically refractory epilepsy.

SUBEPENDYMAL GIANT CELL ASTROCYTOMA

Subependymal giant cell astrocytomas (SEGAs) occur in approximately 15% of individuals with TSC, and most of those who develop symptoms do so during the first 2 decades of life. SEGAs arise from subependymal nodules, and almost all of them occur in the anterior lateral ventricles. Although SEGAs are not malignant or highly invasive, they can be locally invasive and may also cause symptoms of increased intracranial pressure caused by obstruction of cerebrospinal fluid flow through the foramina of Monro.

SEGAs may remain stable and not require surgical intervention. Criteria for neurosurgical intervention include:

- Obstructive hydrocephalus, with or without symptoms of raised intracranial pressure
- A very large tumor at initial presentation, or if there has been significant growth in tumor size
- A new neurologic deficit or change in neurologic status (e.g., increased seizure frequency), which may be attributable to the tumor.

Surveillance CT or MRI is recommended every 1 to 3 years for children and adolescents with TSC (Table 2).

TABLE 2 Recommended Testing for Individuals Diagnosed with Tuberous Sclerosis Complex

Assessment	Initial Testing	Repeat Testing
Neurodevelopmental testing	At diagnosis and at school entry	As indicated
Ophthalmic examination	At diagnosis	As indicated
Electroencephalography	If seizures occur	As indicated for seizure management
Electrocardiography	At diagnosis	As indicated
Echocardiography	If cardiac symptoms occur	If cardiac dysfunction occurs
Renal ultrasonography	At diagnosis	Every 1 to 3 yr
Chest computed tomography	At adulthood (women only)	If pulmonary dysfunction occurs
Cranial computed tomography*	At diagnosis	Children/adolescents: every 1 to 3 yr
Cranial magnetic resonance imaging*	At diagnosis	Children/adolescents: every 1 to 3 yr

*Either cranial computed tomography or magnetic resonance imaging, but usually not both.
Reprinted from Roach ES, DiMario FJ, Kandt RS, Northrup H: Tuberous Sclerosis Consensus Conference: Recommendations for diagnostic evaluation. National Tuberous Sclerosis Association. J Child Neurol 14:401–407, 1999.

COGNITIVE AND BEHAVIORAL ISSUES

Mental retardation is not included as one of the criteria for the diagnosis of TSC, but it is common, occurring in roughly half of all individuals with TSC. The severity of mental retardation correlates loosely with the number and size (volume) of cortical and subcortical lesions, and the location of the lesions may also play some role. Comorbid behavioral concerns include attention deficit disorder with or without hyperactivity, autism, learning disorders, aggressive behavior, and rarely, frank psychosis. Neurocognitive evaluation is essential for children with TSC, at least by the age of school entry. Ongoing management of psychological and behavioral concerns often requires the full armamentarium of psychopharmacologic agents, as well as the assistance of psychologists and psychiatrists familiar with special-needs children.

RENAL LESIONS

The primary kidney lesions in TSC include angiomyolipomas (AMLs), epithelial cysts, and renal cell carcinoma. AMLs are benign tumors composed of dysmorphic blood vessels, smooth muscle, and fat. They occur in 80% of children with TSC by the age of 11 years. AMLs may grow, and lesions larger than 4 cm in diameter are at greater risk for causing kidney compromise through hemorrhage. Once AMLs reach this size or become symptomatic, endovascular tumor embolism seems to be fairly effective at halting growth and preventing hemorrhage, and in experienced hands it has low morbidity. Surveillance monitoring with renal ultrasonography every 1 to 3 years is recommended (see Table 2).

Small simple cysts or huge and multiple cysts may occur in TSC. Simple cysts usually do not cause dysfunction. Conversely, huge or multiple cysts can result in hypertension and potentially, kidney failure. The *TSC2* gene is adjacent to the gene for polycystic kidney disease (*PKD1*), and individuals with both TSC and severe polycystic kidney disease usually have a contiguous gene syndrome caused by a large deletion.

Renal cell carcinoma occurs in relatively few individuals with TSC. These lesions are characterized by absence of fat on radiographic imaging studies. Although most people with TSC do not develop renal carcinoma, lesions without fat are suspicious enough to warrant biopsy. Renal carcinomas require aggressive management, including nephrectomy.

CARDIAC DYSFUNCTION

Cardiac rhabdomyomata occur in two thirds of children with TSC. These tumors usually involute over the first year or two of life, but surgical intervention may be necessary if hemodynamic dysfunction occurs during infancy. Cardiac arrhythmias may occur later in life.

OPHTHALMIC LESIONS

Retinal findings (retinal hamartomas, pigmentary changes, vascular changes) occur in at least half of individuals with TSC, but in most cases eye lesions do not cause progressive visual loss. Children with large retinal hamartomas or those with macular lesions affecting vision are best followed by a pediatric ophthalmologist.

SKIN

The skin findings of TSC are prominent features of the disease. Many of the skin findings in TSC are cosmetic in nature and are unlikely to require intervention of any sort. However, the facial angiofibromas can become a significant problem. These lesions may occur as early as 1 to 2 years of age and tend to increase significantly at puberty. Treatment of angiofibromas prior to puberty when the angiofibromas are less prominent is recommended. This allows for decreased frequency and intensity of treatments in the long run. Treatment consists of vascular laser therapy, which can be conducted in an outpatient setting by a dermatologist or plastic surgeon. Sedation may be necessary, especially for children with mental retardation or behavior problems. Facial angiofibromas may eventually re-emerge after therapy and retreatment is often necessary.

MOLECULAR DIAGNOSIS

A commercial test for TSC is available. Although genotyping is not necessary to make the clinical diagnosis of TSC in an individual who meets the diagnostic criteria, it is often useful for family planning and counseling or when the diagnosis is uncertain. Positive test results are reliable, but there is a significant false-negative rate (approximately 15%), so mutational testing cannot absolutely exclude the possibility that the individual has TSC.

Common Pitfalls

- Infantile spasms are often mistaken for colic or gastroesophageal reflux disease. It is critical to correctly diagnose IS and commence treatment early.
- Although epilepsy in TSC is sometimes difficult to control, approximately 15% of children with TSC and epilepsy will have seizure remission. Discontinuation of AEDs may be considered after going at least 2 years without seizures.
- In children with TSC and a SEGA, an indication that the SEGA is growing and altering intracranial pressure may be that there is a significant change in seizure profile. One must have a low threshold to consider repeat cranial imaging.
- If it cannot be discerned whether a solid renal lesion has fat in it (i.e., is an AML) with ultrasonography or renal CT scan, the lesion should be biopsied to determine whether it is an AML or whether it might be renal cell carcinoma.
- A negative result on TSC gene mutation testing does not completely rule out TSC.

■ TSC is a protean disease; one should have a low threshold to consult specialists in other disciplines to assist with management of the disease.

Communication and Counseling

While TSC is a complex disease with many potential complications, there is a vast clinical spectrum ranging from those with normal cognition and minimal major organ involvement to those with profound mental retardation and multiple organ involvement. Increasingly, the major medical complications can be effectively treated, and surveillance screening for these treatable complications helps to identify them earlier. TSC research is actively ongoing on both basic science and clinical fronts, with the intent to better understand the nature of the disease and to define the best treatments for it. The Tuberous Sclerosis Alliance (TSA) (http://www.tsalliance.org) is an outstanding resource for families with children affected by TSC, as well as for medical professionals. There are also local groups, called TS Community Alliances, located throughout the United States. Additionally, there are 14 TSC clinics in the United States that specialize in care of children with TSC.

ACKNOWLEDGEMENTS

Treasure Street (Dallas) has kindly supported the care of children in the Tuberous Sclerosis Clinic at Texas Scottish Rite Hospital for Children and has funded many of our clinical research efforts.

SUGGESTED READINGS

1. Curatolo P (ed). Tuberous Sclerosis Complex, From Basic Science to Clinical Phenotypes. London: MacKeith Press, 2003. **Monograph on basic science and clinical features of TSC, including discussion of management of medical complications of the disease.**
2. Ewalt DH, Sheffield E, Sparagana SP, et al: Renal lesion growth in children with tuberous sclerosis complex. J Urol 160:141–145, 1998. **Discusses the profile of angiomyolipomas in children with TSC.**
3. Gómez MR: Tuberous Sclerosis Complex, 3rd ed. New York: Oxford University Press, 1999. **Monograph includes discussion of clinical and molecular features of TSC.**
4. Mackay MT, Weiss SK, Adams-Webber T, et al: Practice parameter: Medical treatment of infantile spasms. Neurology 2004, 62:1668–1681. **Evidence-based analysis of treatment for infantile spasms.**
5. Neumann HH, Schwarzkopf G, Henske EP: Renal angiomyolipomas, cysts, and cancer in tuberous sclerosis complex. Sem Ped Neurol 5:269–275, 1998. **A survey of the kidney lesions found in TSC.**
6. Roach ES, DeMario FJ, Kandt RS, et al: Tuberous sclerosis consensus conference: Recommendations for diagnostic evaluation. J Child Neurol 14:401–407, 1999. **Recommendations for diagnostic testing in individuals newly diagnosed with TSC, and for surveillance monitoring thereafter.**
7. Roach ES, Gómez MR, Northrup H: Tuberous sclerosis complex consensus conference: Revised clinical diagnostic criteria. J Child Neurol 13:624–628, 1998. **Updated clinical diagnostic criteria for TSC.**
8. Torres OA, Roach ES, Delgado MR, et al: Early diagnosis of subependymal giant cell astrocytoma in patients with tuberous sclerosis. J Child Neurol 13:173–177, 1998. **Discusses the rationale for surveillance head imaging, and criteria for surgical intervention.**

Febrile Seizures

Douglas R. Nordli, Jr.

KEY POINTS

■ Simple febrile seizures are the most common form of seizure in children.

■ Complex febrile seizures are either focal, prolonged ($\geq$10 minutes or $\geq$15 minutes), or multiple within the same febrile illness and signify a greater risk of later epilepsy.

■ Susceptibility genes are being discovered, but attendance at day care, prolonged nursery stay, and developmental delay are other important risk factors.

■ Diagnosis is made by exclusion of other causes of symptomatic seizures. Whenever there is a clinical suspicion of meningitis or encephalitis, a lumbar puncture (LP) should be performed.

■ Neuroimaging is reserved for children with complex febrile seizures.

■ EEG has no role in the evaluation of the child with simple febrile seizures.

■ Most children with febrile seizures do not need treatment with anticonvulsant drugs.

■ For children with prolonged febrile seizures, rectal diazepam (0.2–0.5 mg/kg) can be given to abort future prolonged attacks, although it is not formally approved for this use.

■ Counseling is the most important intervention.

The International League Against Epilepsy (ILAE) defines a febrile seizure as a seizure in association with a febrile illness in the absence of a central nervous system (CNS) infection or acute electrolyte imbalance in children older than 1 month of age without prior afebrile seizures. The most common form of seizure in pediatrics, febrile seizures afflict between 3% and 5% of all children in the United States and Europe and 6% to 9% of children in Japan. Most occur in children between the ages of 6 months and 4 years, with a peak incidence at 18 months. The upper age limit is not defined by the ILAE but they are uncommon above age 7 years.

A complex febrile seizure is one that is either focal, prolonged ($\geq$10 minutes or $\geq$15 minutes), or multiple within the same febrile illness. Complex febrile seizures are important to recognize because they connote a greater susceptibility toward development of epilepsy. Risk factors for febrile seizures in general include a family history of febrile seizures in a first- or second-degree relative, attendance at day care, developmental delay, and a prolonged newborn nursery stay of 30 days or more. Rare families have been reported in which members have febrile seizures, epilepsy, or both, and these traits are inherited in an autosomal dominant fashion. This has been termed generalized epilepsy febrile seizures plus (GEFS+). Mutations in the voltage-gated sodium channel β1 subunit gene (*SCN1B*; OMIM link 600235) on 19q13 cause GEFS+ type 1, mutations in the *SCN1A* gene (OMIM link 182389) on 2q24 cause GEFS+ type 2, and mutations in the *GABRG2* gene (OMIM link 137164) on 5q31.1-q33.1 cause GEFS+ type 3. Mutations in the *SCN2A* (OMIM link 182390) gene cause febrile seizures associated with afebrile seizures. The role of such genes in common forms of sporadic febrile seizures remains to be determined.

Expert Opinion on Management Issues

EVALUATION

Depending on the manifestations and the clinician's experience, laboratory tests are not always necessary. Usually, a clinically identifiable infection, such as otitis media, roseola infantum, pharyngitis, or gastroenteritis, is present. Fever after immunization may also trigger a febrile seizure. Any suspicion of meningitis, however, mandates lumbar puncture. Diagnosis is made by excluding other possible causes of the convulsion, such as meningitis, metabolic abnormalities, or structural brain lesions. The 1996 American Academy of Pediatrics (AAP) practice parameter addressed the diagnostic evaluation of a child with a simple febrile seizure between 6 months and 5 years of age and recommended that a lumbar puncture be strongly considered in infants below 12 months. Recall that the typical indicators of meningeal irritation, such as nuchal rigidity and the Brudzinki sign, are not reliable in young infants. If the seizure has focal features or if there are focal neurologic abnormalities, brain imaging is necessary. Electroencephalography (EEG) is not useful because it does not provide information regarding either risk of recurrence of febrile seizures or later development of epilepsy. The role of EEG in patients with complex febrile seizures is not clearly defined.

FEBRILE STATUS EPILEPTICUS

Patients presenting with febrile status epilepticus should be managed according to the protocol for status epilepticus, recognizing that continued therapy beyond the first 24 hours is usually not necessary in most cases. (See "Status Epilepticus" for further details and a table outlining treatment of SE.)

PROPHYLAXIS

In well-designed randomized, controlled clinical trials, both phenobarbital and valproate reduced the risk of a recurrent febrile seizure if regularly administered. However, the vast majority of children with febrile seizures have no long-term consequences and treatment does not alter the risk of developing epilepsy. Adverse drug effects occur in as many as 40% of infants and children treated with phenobarbital, and valproate carries a risk of idiosyncratic fatal hepatotoxicity and pancreatitis. For all of these reasons, most clinicians avoid chronic prophylactic treatment with antiepileptic drugs, even after several isolated convulsions. Indeed, the American Academy of Pediatrics (AAP) recommends no treatment for the child with simple febrile seizures. For children with complex febrile seizures, treatment is also not routinely indicated. Phenytoin and carbamazepine are ineffective.

If treatment is considered, it should be reserved for children with complex febrile seizures who are neurologically abnormal or who have a strong family history

of afebrile seizures. An alternative to chronic drug therapy is intermittent diazepam treatment during febrile illnesses, but the side effects of diazepam militate against its frequent use in this fashion.

Antipyretic treatment for future illnesses provides comfort but does not appreciably reduce the risk of febrile seizures.

Rectal diazepam can be used for prolonged febrile seizures, using the same guidelines as found in "Status Epilepticus" (doses range from 0.2 to 0.5 mg/kg).

Common Pitfalls

- EEGs should not be routinely ordered for children with simple febrile seizures.
- Most patients do not require prophylactic medication, and in most cases treatment may have more adverse effects than benefit.

Communication and Counseling

Approximately one third of children with febrile seizures have more than one attack. Recurrence is highest in infants whose first febrile seizure occurred before the 18 months, who have a family history of febrile seizures, or who have a low peak temperature and duration of fever for less than one hour prior to the seizure (Box 1). When the first seizure is a simple febrile seizure, only 1% of patients have prolonged convulsions later.

The risk of developing epilepsy is increased in children with febrile seizures, but the magnitude of the risk depends on several factors. In children with simple febrile seizures, the risk of epilepsy is 2% to 3%. Higher rates of epilepsy (10%–13%) are seen in children with complex febrile seizures, a short duration of fever before the seizure, three or more febrile seizures, family history of afebrile seizures, and neurologic abnormalities (Box 2). Febrile seizures do not cause mental retardation, poor school achievement, or behavioral problems. Some differences in the outcome of children with febrile seizures are reported. Those with seizures in the first year of life are more likely to require special schooling and those with prolonged convulsions have slightly lower nonverbal intelligence measures. Mortality is not

---

BOX 1 Risk Factors for Recurrent Febrile Seizures

- Family history of febrile seizures
- Age <18 months
- Low peak temperature
- Duration of fever <1 hour prior to seizure

BOX 2 Risk Factors for Epilepsy

- Neurodevelopmental abnormality
- Family history of epilepsy
- Complex febrile seizure
- ≥3 febrile seizures
- Duration of fever <1 hour prior to seizure

increased in children with febrile seizures who are neurologically normal.

Parents are often traumatized by the experience of watching their child have a convulsion. Proper counseling is the most important intervention. Reassurance to dispel any myths the family may have, a review of practical first aid measures, and a special emphasis on the benign prognosis of most children with febrile seizures is particularly appropriate. Parents should be told that epilepsy is neither life threatening nor damaging to the brain. This can be effectively accomplished by counseling at the first emergent visit and repeating the same information at the follow-up visit. The AAP has copies of the guidelines and an information sheet for parents available through their website (http://www.aap.org), and the Epilepsy Foundation provides useful information about febrile seizures that can be downloaded (http://www.epilepsyfoundation.org).

SUGGESTED READINGS

1. American Academy of Pediatrics. Provisional Committee on Quality Improvement, Subcommittee on Febrile Seizures: Practice parameter: The neurodiagnostic evaluation of the child with a first simple febrile seizure. Pediatrics 97:769–772, 1996. **Guidelines for evaluation of children with the first febrile seizure.**
2. Baram TZ, Shinnar S (eds). Febrile Seizures. San Diego: Academic Press, . **An excellent comprehensive resource.**
3. Berg AT, Shinnar S, Shapiro ED, et al: Risk factors for a first febrile seizure: A matched case-control study. Epilepsia 36:334–341, 1995. **Epidemiology of febrile seizures.**
4. Nelson KB, Ellenberg JH: Prognosis in children with febrile seizures. Pediatrics 61:720–727, 1978. **Landmark study of febrile seizures.**
5. Rosman NP, Colton T, Labazzo RNC, et al: A controlled trial of diazepam administered during febrile illnesses to prevent recurrence of febrile seizures. N Engl J Med 329:79–84, 1993. **Use of intermittent diazepam in febrile seizures.**
6. Singh R, Scheffer IE, Crossland K, Berkovic SF: Generalized epilepsy with febrile seizures plus: A common childhood-onset genetic epilepsy syndrome. Ann Neurol 45:75–81, 1999. **Landmark work on the role of channelopathies in common forms of epilepsy and febrile seizures.**
7. Verity CM, Greenwood R, Golding J: Long-term intellectual and behavioral outcomes of children with febrile convulsions. N Engl J Med 338:1723–1728, 1998. **Important reference regarding outcome.**
8. Wallace RH, Wang DW, Singh R, et al: Febrile seizures and generalized epilepsy associated with a mutation in the Na^+-channel beta 1 subunit gene SCN1B. Nat Genet 19:366–370, 1998. **A description of another channelopathy that is important in the group of patients with febrile seizures and epilepsy.**

Infantile Spasms: West Syndrome

Mark S. Scher

KEY CONCEPTS

- West syndrome is an epileptic encephalopathy with onset during infancy.
- It usually manifests in clusters of spasms.
- Consider structural, metabolic, and genetic derangements.

- The classic electroencephalographic pattern of West syndrome is termed *hypsarrhythmia.*
- There are no clear recommendations for treatment.
- Adrenocorticotropic hormone (ACTH) administration is suggested, especially for idiopathic forms.
- Vigabatrin is suggested for spasms in children with tuberous sclerosis.
- Quality-of-life concerns extend into adulthood.

Infantile spasms, or West syndrome, is a devastating age-dependent epileptic encephalopathy. Most children come to medical attention before or around 6 months of age when their parents note sudden recurrent contractures of the head, torso, and/or limbs. As a rule, the younger the age that the child presents, the more atypical the clinical presentation. Initially, parents and even the infant's physician dismiss pathologic movements as exaggerated startle responses or the movements of a colicky child. However, the spontaneous occurrences of these events, their general tendency to recur in clusters of 10 to 20 spasms in a series, and an apparent decrease in the infant's level of interaction during and after the spasms eventually bring this condition to medical attention.

William J. West, a 19th century physician, published in *The Lancet* (1841) a detailed account of his son, who demonstrated rapid spasms in the context of developmental regression. In the mid-20th century, Gibbs introduced the term *West syndrome* to signify infantile spasms, developmental regression, and the characteristic high-voltage chaotic electroencephalographic pattern termed *hypsarrhythmia.* Spasms frequently involve a combination of flexion and extensor movements. Classically, a child will rapidly bow his or her head (salaam), flex at the trunk and hips, and extend the arms forward. Such a posture is maintained for multiple seconds, usually followed by a brief cry. The next spasm occurs within seconds and clusters in the same manner. Clusters consist of 2 to greater than 100 individual spasms just minutes apart. Spasm clusters occur often during the early morning hours, before the child goes to sleep, at nap time, and shortly after feeding. West syndrome is a relatively uncommon type of seizure with an incidence of 0.25 to 0.42 per 1000. Approximately 35% of children evolve into the epileptic syndrome known as Lennox-Gastaut syndrome. Another 23% evolve into partial epilepsy.

Diagnostic Issues

Although the fundamental cause remains unknown, a number of predisposing conditions are recognized. Given the current knowledge concerning the pathophysiologic basis of infantile spasms, a new model is proposed that is based on developmental desynchronization, suggesting that infantile spasms may result from a particular temporal desynchronization of two or more central nervous system developmental processes that result in a specific disturbance of brain function:

- The interaction of developmental processes controlled by primary genes that subserve neuronogenesis, myelination, synaptogenesis, apoptosis, and the development of neurotransmitter systems

- Altered regulatory gene effects, specifically controlled by transcription factors and other modulators
- Environmental factors influencing development including injury, toxicity, and disease processes that interfere with gene expression

The developmental process becomes desynchronized among these processes, maximally at approximately 6 months of age. Modeling of unbalanced maturational patterns has allowed a variety of different anatomic and/or biochemical entities to be considered. Careful scrutiny of structural, metabolic, and genetic derangements have increased the proportion of patients with a definable medical entity to explain these spasms.

Currently, infantile spasms remain idiopathic for approximately 10% to 15% of affected children. Predisposing etiologic factors include cerebral dysgenesis and genetic and metabolic disorders (e.g., tuberous sclerosis and phenylketonuria), intrauterine infections, and hypoxic-ischemic brain injury. At the present time, the consensus is that the diphtheria-pertussis-tetanus (DPT) vaccination is not causally related to the development of infantile spasms. The present use of state-of-the-art neuroimaging (MRI and positron emission tomography [PET]) has greatly enhanced the physician's ability to detect the structural-functional interface for clinical phenotypes associated with forms of infantile spasms.

ELECTROENCEPHALOGRAPHY

The electroencephalogram (EEG) is nearly always abnormal, and it is grossly disorganized if obtained when seizures are well established. Gibbs and Gibbs identified the most characteristic pattern, hypsarrhythmia: irregular slow waves of high voltage occurring asynchronously and randomly over all head regions, intermixed with spikes and polyspikes from multiple independent loci. The etymologic root of *hypsarrhythmia* refers to the high-voltage, mountainous, and disorganized or arrhythmic interictal EEG pattern. Variations of the pattern (modified hypsarrhythmia) are commonly described, such as in very young or older infants, when the EEG is obtained. Like the clinical entity of infantile spasms, the electrographic pattern of hypsarrhythmia is age specific. It is generally less pronounced during slow-wave sleep and may disappear completely during active sleep.

Ictal recordings show various patterns, but the most common accompaniment to a clinical spasm is one or more generalized, high-voltage, slow or sharp-slow waves followed by abrupt voltage attenuation of background activity lasting one to several seconds, termed the *electrodecremental event*. Spasms do not always correlate well with a particular EEG ictal pattern, nor do all spasms have abnormal EEG correlates. However, EEG and clinical improvement usually parallel each other, but they may also become dissociated.

A suggested list of diagnostic studies, listed in Box 1, might be considered for the evaluation of children with infantile spasms.

BOX 1 Suggested Diagnostic Tests to Evaluate the Child

- MRI
- Positron emission tomography
- Electroencephalography, preferably synchronized video-EEG monitoring
- Serum lactate and pyruvate levels
- Serum amino acid analysis
- Urine organic acid analysis
- Cytogenetic analysis (including FISH)
- Lysosomal enzyme analysis
- Tissue sampling for neuropathologic analysis

EEG, electroencephalogram; FISH, fluorescent in situ hybridization

---

Therapeutic Issues—Drug Choices and Pitfalls

The goals of treatment for infantile spasms are straightforward (to control seizures, resolve the hypsarrhythmic pattern on the EEG, and improve neurodevelopment); however, success is difficult to achieve. Although recent practice parameters have been revised for the medical management of children with infantile spasms, there remain a number of controversial issues. Database searches of MEDLINE from 1966 and EMBASE from 1980 have resulted in suggestions for a four-tiered classification scheme that remains controversial. As originally recommended in 1958, adrenocorticotropic hormone (ACTH) is probably the most effective agent for short-term treatment of infantile spasms. However, at this time there is insufficient evidence to recommend the optimum dose and duration for such a treatment. There is also insufficient evidence to determine whether oral corticosteroids are effective. Before the 1990s, phenobarbital, clonazepam, and valproic acid were the best available additional treatment modalities, but response rates were only 30% to 50%. Inasmuch as the natural history of infantile spasms is resolution or evolution into other seizure types, such as the Lennox-Gastaut syndrome, the timing of treatment becomes critical. However, the recent consensus report has no clear recommendation to offer.

In the 1990s, additional antiepileptic medications were approved for use by the Food and Drug Administration (FDA). The FDA subsequently removed vigabatrin because of retinal toxicity in children and adults. Evidence-based medicine suggests that vigabatrin is probably an effective short-term treatment for infantile spasms. If children with tuberous sclerosis are treated with this drug, serial ophthalmologic screening is required.

Other agents have also been evaluated for the treatment of infantile spasms. The consensus report indicates that there is insufficient evidence to recommend other drugs such as valproic acid, benzodiazepines, pyridoxine, and newer antiepileptic drugs or novel therapies for the treatment of infantile spasms.

Finally, the report concludes that insufficient evidence exists to suggest whether any of the antiepileptic medications mentioned above improve long-term outcome and seizure freedom with normal development for children with infantile spasms.

Specific Details of Treatment

Historically, ACTH has been administered at high, low, and very low doses. In a double-blind crossover placebo-controlled trial comparing ACTH (20 IU per day) with prednisone (2 mg/kg/day), no significant difference in response rate was noted, nor any relationship found between the duration of spasms before treatment and outcome. In contrast, a prospective, randomized blinded study comparing high-dose ACTH (150 IU/m^2/day) and prednisone (2 mg/kg/day) in a 2-week course demonstrated the treatment with high-dose ACTH resulted in a response rate of 87% as opposed to a response rate of 29% in the group treated with prednisone.

Historical evidence suggests a mortality rate as high as 5% to 6%, using ACTH. Serious side effects for ACTH include infection, pneumonia, sepsis, dilated cardiomyopathy, severe hypertension, gastrointestinal hemorrhage, and massive weight gain. Cosmetic effects, particularly acne, and behavioral side effects such as irritability can often be severe. Pretreatment evaluation should include a chest x-ray, electrocardiogram, four-extremity blood pressure determination, and an echocardiogram. Infants are commonly placed on a low sodium diet and histamine H_2 blockers to prevent gastric irritation. Close monitoring of blood pressure is essential. Urine should be tested for glucose and stools for occult blood. A clinical response is expected first, followed by normalization of the EEG during sleep. An awake and asleep closed circuit synchronized video and EEG study is useful to monitor the treatment response and timing of the ACTH wean. Return of spasms can be seen in up to one third of infants who may respond to subsequent treatment. Spontaneous remission of spasms occurs by several percentage points each month with a cumulative remission rate at 12 months of 25%.

The use of vigabatrin for the treatment of infantile spasms was first reported in the early 1990s, in France and Italy. Response rates were best in children with tuberous sclerosis (86%). Responses that are more favorable occur in those with cryptogenic etiologies. Less than half of symptomatic infants respond to treatment with vigabatrin, and half of the responders exhibit relapses. In a comparison with ACTH, vigabatrin controlled infantile spasms in 48% of infants compared to 74% treated with ACTH.

A double-blind placebo controlled study of vigabatrin treatment in infants with newly diagnosed infantile spasms showed 78% reduction in spasms versus 26% in a placebo group. Other studies demonstrate notes ranging from 50% for a symptomatic group to look for a cryptogenic group. Common side effects for vigabatrin include somnolence, hypotonia, weight gain, hyperactivity, insomnia, but these effects are usually transient.

Synchronized video EEG recordings during treatment are recommended. As noted above, the FDA has not approved vigabatrin because of the initial concerns regarding retinal toxicity.

Surgical treatment may be considered for a selected group of children with infantile spasms given the improved neuroimaging techniques using MRI and PET. Various forms of brain malformations ranging from focal cortical dysplasia to hemimegalencephaly may be amenable to surgical removal as part of the treatment strategy. This form of treatment is presently retrospective and not supported by evidence-based research. Long-term outcome for this group of children following surgery is unknown.

Communication and Counseling

Families require careful and frequent consultation by the physician regarding the diagnosis, prognosis, and therapeutic options. It should be made clear to the family that infantile spasms is a catastrophic form of epileptic encephalopathy with no approved treatments or clear-cut consensus regarding the best treatment for this syndrome. The guiding principles of treatment are to balance the side effects of the medications with the goal of putting the spasms and EEG pattern of hypsarrhythmia into remission to maximize the infant's developmental outcome. The goals of minimizing seizures and side effects and providing the best possible quality of life remain a high priority. Clinicians must develop appropriate care plans and be aware of the child's changing needs with respect to growth and development. Clinical symptoms involving the catastrophic epilepsies including infantile spasms change over time. Therefore, by understanding the natural history of the child's condition, the physician can ease the transition from childhood to adulthood. Children with catastrophic epilepsy are now reaching adult ages with both medical and nonmedical issues to be considered. Medication side effects, tolerance, and dependence need to be considered. In addition, guardian-caretaker issues, group home applications, and respite care options must be part of the overall strategy to assist the patient and the family. The greatest chance for survival for these patients into adulthood will be possible through multidisciplinary care plans that incorporate resources from health care practitioners, social service professionals, and community agencies.

SUGGESTED READINGS

1. Appleton RE, Peters AC, Mumford JP, et al: Randomised, placebo-controlled study of vigabatrin as first-line treatment of infantile spasms. Epilepsia 40:1627–1633, 1999. **Excellent evidence-based study of drug efficacy using vigabatrin.**
2. Baram TZ, Mitchell WG, Toumay A, et al: High-dose corticotropin (ACTH) versus prednisone for infantile spasms: A prospective, randomized, blinded study. Pediatrics 97:375–379, 1996. **Instructive study comparing two forms of steroid treatment.**
3. Bellman MH: Infantile spasms. In Pedley TA, Meldrum BS (eds): Recent Advances in Epilepsy, vol 1. Edinburgh: Churchill Livingstone, 1983, 113–138. **Good historical review of infantile spasms.**
4. Cowan LD, Hudson LS: The epidemiology and natural history of infantile spasms. J Child Neurol 6:355–364, 1991. **Useful epidemiology review of infantile spasms.**
5. Fejerman N, Cersosimo R, Caraballo R, et al: Vigabatrin as a first-choice drug in the treatment of West syndrome. J Child Neurol 15:161–165, 2000. **Useful comparative study for treatment options for infantile spasms.**

6. Frost JD, Hrachovy RA: Pathogenesis of infantile spasms: A model based on developmental desynchronization. J Clin Neurophysiol 22:25–36, 2005. **Good state-of-science review of the neurobiology of infantile spasms from a developmental perspective.**

7. Gibbs RA, Gibbs EZ: Atlas of Electroencephalography, vol 2: Epilepsy. Cambridge, Mass: Addison Wesley, 1952. **Classic descriptions of the EEG patterns associated with infantile spasms.**

8. Glauser TA: Following catastrophic epilepsy patients from childhood to adulthood. Epilepsia 45(Suppl 5):23–26, 2004. **Realistic expectations of the neurologist's management of intractable epilepsy spanning from childhood to adulthood.**

9. Goodman M, Lamm SH, Bellman MH: Temporal relationship modeling: DTP or DT immunizations and infantile spasms. Vaccine 16:225–231, 1998. **Important study rejecting the association of vaccines and infantile spasms.**

10. Granstrom ML, Gaily E, Liukkonen E: Treatment of infantile spasms: Results of a population based study with vigabatrin as the first drug for spasms. Epilepsia 10:950–957, 1999. **Another demonstrative study of treatment efficacy of vigabatrin.**

11. Hrachovy RA, Frost JD Jr, Kellaway P, et al: Double-blind study of ACTH vs. prednisone therapy in infantile spasms. J Pediatr 103:641–645, 1983. **Earlier but excellent evidence-based study of steroid treatment for infantile spasms.**

12. Hrachovy RA, Glaze DG, Frost JD Jr: A retrospective study of spontaneous remission and long-term outcome in patients with infantile spasms. Epilepsia 32:212–214, 1991. **Important earlier report describing problems with outcome prediction.**

13. Lortie A, Plouin P, Chiron C, et al: Characteristics of epilepsy in focal cortical dysplasia in infancy. Epilepsy Res 51:133–145, 2002. **Representative report of surgical results of patients with infantile spasms.**

14. Mackay MT, Weiss SK, Adams-Webber T, et al: Practice parameter: Medical treatment of infantile spasms: Report of the American Academy of Neurology and the Child Neurology Society. Neurology 62:1668–1681, 2004. **Current guidelines for the medical management of infantile spasms.**

15. Vigevano F, Cilio MR: Vigabatrin versus ACTH as a first-line treatment for infantile spasms: A randomized prospective study. Epilepsia 38:1270–1274, 1997. **Early report comparing vigabatrin and ACTH.**

16. Villeneuve N, Soufflet C, Plouin P, et al: Treatment of infantile spasms with vigabatrin as a first-line therapy and in monotherapy: Apropos of 70 infants. Arch Pediatr 5:731–738, 1998. **Useful study assessing efficacy of vigabatrin.**

Pseudotumor Cerebri Syndrome

Joshua Cappell and Marc C. Patterson

KEY CONCEPTS

- Pseudotumor cerebri (PTC) is diagnosed in the presence of signs, symptoms, or demonstration of high intracranial pressure (ICP) with no identifiable etiology on imaging or cerebrospinal fluid (CSF) examination.
- PTC must be distinguished from cerebral venous sinus thrombosis by magnetic resonance venography.
- Key symptoms are headache, diplopia, blurring, transient visual obscuration, and visual field deficits.
- Acetazolamide is the cornerstone of medical management. In obese patients, weight loss is crucial.

- Surgical procedures are used in severe or progressive visual loss. Options include optic nerve sheath fenestration and lumboperitoneal shunting.
- Treatment decisions are based primarily on serial objective measurements of vision.

The term *pseudotumor cerebri* (PTC) was coined a century ago to describe a syndrome of high intracranial pressure (ICP) without apparent cause. The terms *benign intracranial hypertension* and *idiopathic intracranial hypertension* have also been applied to this entity. PTC is traditionally diagnosed by satisfying the modified Dandy criteria (Box 1): Symptoms or signs of elevated ICP without focal signs, absence of a cerebral mass or hydrocephalus, with cerebrospinal fluid (CSF) that may have elevated pressure but has normal composition. Cerebral venous sinus thrombosis (CVST) should be ruled out by magnetic resonance venography (MRV) before intracranial hypertension is deemed idiopathic. In addition to actual mass lesion and infectious causes of elevated ICP, the differential diagnosis of headaches accompanied by visual obscuration includes vascular or immunologic causes such as carotid dissection, optic neuritis, temporal arteritis, Behçet syndrome, and Susac syndrome. Whereas adult PTC is mainly a disease of young, obese women, in children the sex ratio is nearly even and obesity accounts for fewer cases. Once considered benign, PTC is now recognized as a potential cause of progressive visual impairment in adults and children.

Excluding CVST, the pathophysiology of pseudotumor remains poorly understood. Although sinovenous stenosis may be seen with specialized imaging, this may be a consequence rather than a cause of CSF hypertension. Hypotheses for the association of PTC with obesity range from hormonal effects on CSF dynamics to transmitted intra-abdominal pressure reducing systemic venous return. Rare patients with spinal arteriovenous malformation (AVM) or elevated systemic venous pressure (e.g., caused by atrial septal defect) have presented as PTC. Both PTC and CVST have been associated with vitamin A, tetracycline, and growth, thyroid, or steroid hormone treatments.

BOX 1	**Criteria for Diagnosing Idiopathic Intracranial Hypertension**

- If symptoms are present, they may only reflect those of generalized intracranial hypertension or papilledema.
- If signs are present, they may only reflect those of generalized intracranial hypertension or papilledema.
- Documented elevated intracranial pressure measured in the lateral decubitus position.
- Normal CSF composition.
- No evidence of hydrocephalus, mass, structural, or vascular lesion on MRI or contrast-enhanced CT for typical patients and MRI and MRV for all others.
- No other cause of intracranial hypertension identified.

MRI, magnetic resonance imaging; MRV, magnetic resonance venography.
Adapted from Friedman DI, Jacobson DM: Diagnostic criteria for idiopathic intracranial hypertension. Neurology 59:1492–1495, 2002.

Expert Opinion on Management Issues

ASSESSMENT

Pseudotumor should be suspected in any patient with persistent headache, visual changes, or incidentally discovered papilledema or high ICP. Headache may resemble common migraine, tension headache, retro-orbital pain, chronic daily headaches, or migraine equivalents such as neck pain with torticollis. Pulsatile tinnitus is common. Visual complaints may include blurred vision, transient visual obscuration, diplopia caused by abducens palsy, enlarged blind spot, or constriction of visual fields associated with chronic papilledema.

The physical examination focuses on identifiable etiologies and establishing baseline visual and neurologic function. Follow-up is mandatory and guides management. Ophthalmologic examinations at all visits should include eye movements, pupillary responses, funduscopy, contrast sensitivity, visual acuity, and perimetry. General physical examination should include body mass index, blood pressure, and head circumference and a systematic search for signs of systemic venous hypertension, rheumatologic disease, endocrinopathies, or neurocutaneous syndromes. By definition, the presence of cognitive deficits, weakness, or ataxia excludes PTC. Although by the strict criteria, the only cranial nerve deficits are of II and VI; rarely impairments of III, IV, or VII have been reported in patients who otherwise fit this diagnosis.

Visual-evoked potentials have little added value in this condition and are, therefore, not recommended.

Because there are no reliable clinical features distinguishing CVST from PTC, MRV should be performed in all patients. Hypercoagulability evaluation is performed in patients with CVST. MRI is the preferred modality for excluding intracranial masses and assessing ventricular size, which should not be enlarged, but need not be slit-like. Common MRI findings in PTC include an empty sella turcica and distortion or enhancement of the optic nerves.

CSF pressure should be measured with the patient relaxed in the lateral decubitus position, as tight flexion will elevate the measured ICP. If other positioning is required for radiologic guidance in obese patients, pressure should be measured using the foramen magnum as a reference point. The range of normal CSF pressure is age dependent. In young adults, pressures less than 20 cm H_2O may be considered normal, 20 to 25 cm H_2O as high but of uncertain significance, whereas more than 25 cm H_2O is pathologic.

Patients old enough to cooperate should be provided with printed material in a small font size to read daily as a simple assessment of visual acuity.

ACCEPTED INTERVENTIONS

In the absence of randomized, controlled trials, treatment for PTC is based on expert opinion. The key determinant of decision making is visual function, with deterioration mandating more invasive interventions (Fig. 1). In obese patients, weight loss is the single most important intervention and may be curative. Surgical treatment of PTC is reserved for patients whose vision worsens despite medical therapy with acetazolamide, those who have severely affected vision, or those whose headaches are disabling and unresponsive to medical treatment.

Some patients begin recovering after the first lumbar puncture (LP). It is unclear if this reflects a persistent CSF leak or a change in CSF dynamics interrupting a vicious cycle in the pathophysiology of the disorder. There is no consensus regarding the indications for repeated spinal taps. We recommend repeating the LP only in the event of appreciable worsening of vision despite medical treatment, if a surgical procedure is planned.

Drug Therapy

Acetazolamide (25 mg/kg/day divided into three doses daily up to 250 mg three times per day initially, and a maximum of 30 mg/kg daily divided three times daily up to 500 mg three times daily) is recommended as initial medical management on the basis of standard practice, although its benefit is uncertain (Table 1).

Steroids are believed to provide at least short-term benefit in PTC. However, the potential for weight gain exacerbates the condition, making them undesirable, and they are best avoided.

The weak carbonic anhydrase inhibitor topiramate is currently under investigation for treatment of PTC. Topiramate induces weight loss and may relieve headaches.

Behavioral Therapy

In obese patients, improvement in PTC correlates with weight loss. All obese patients should be counseled on weight loss and referred to a weight reduction program.

Surgical Therapy

Surgical procedures to relieve pressure on the optic nerve provide immediate stabilization or improvement of vision in most cases, but carry a risk of failure that grows over time. Lumboperitoneal shunting reduces CSF pressure but shunt failure requiring revision is common. Optic nerve sheath fenestration (ONSF) halts or even reverses visual loss in most adult patients but there is limited pediatric experience with this procedure. The therapeutic mechanism of ONSF is unclear as visual improvement in the face of persistently high ICP suggests a local effect, but cases of bilateral improvement after unilateral ONSF argue for a broader action. Some patients experience relief from headaches after ONSF, but lumboperitoneal shunting is thought to be more efficacious for relief of intractable headache associated with PTC.

Venous sinus stenting is used to treat PTC, but indications have not been established.

Bariatric surgery can be considered in morbidly obese patients in whom medical management has been unsuccessful. The role of such surgery in children has not been

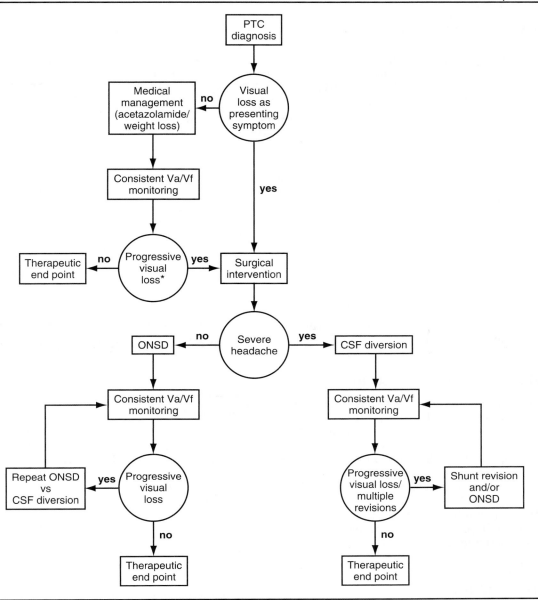

FIGURE 1. Initial management and long-term follow-up of pseudotumor cerebri (PTC) patients. *Visual loss is defined as new onset or progression of a significant visual field defect or loss of greater than two lines on the Snellen visual acuity chart. CSF, cerebrospinal fluid; ONSD, optic nerve sheath decompression; Va, visual acuity; Vf, visual fields. Reproduced with permission from Banta JT, Farris BK: Pseudotumor cerebri and optic nerve sheath decompression. Ophthalmology 107:1907–1912, 2000. Copyright 2000. Reprinted by permission from the American Academy of Ophthalmology.

established. As patients lose weight postoperatively, their CSF pressure normalizes.

Common Pitfalls

- Noncompliance with follow-up can be a major impediment to care, despite the fear of blindness.
- MRI excludes a mass or hydrocephalus but does not exclude sinovenous thrombosis; MRV is essential. Recognition of CVST is important because of the risk of stroke and other vascular complications

of hypercoagulability. Treatments of PTC, such as acetazolamide, are potentially deleterious in CVST.
- Responses to interventions in PTC vary. Even surgical treatment is not definitive as failure is common. Patients on treatment still require close follow-up to detect progression.
- Management of pseudotumor in pregnancy is more challenging because weight loss is contraindicated and acetazolamide is category "C" and should particularly be avoided in the first 20 weeks of gestation. Lumbar puncture may be used in the

TABLE 1 Medications for Pseudotumor Cerebri

Name (Trade Name)	Dosage/Route/ Regimen	Maximum Dose	Formulations	Common Adverse Reactions	Therapeutic Concentrations	Comments
Acetazolamide (Diamox) Rx	PO: target of 25 mg/kg/day, or 300 to 900 mg/m²/day; bid-tid dosing	30 mg/kg/day or 500 mg tid	Tablet: 125, 250 mg Extended release capsule: 500 mg Suspension: 250 mg/5 mL	GI upset, drowsiness, dizziness, photosensitivity	Not established for PTC	Not labeled for PTC
Topiramate (Topamax) Rx	PO: 5–9 mg/kg/day; bid dosing	9 mg/kg/day or 200 mg bid	Sprinkle capsules: 15, 25 mg Tablet: 25, 50, 100, 200 mg	Psychomotor slowing, paresthesiae; risks of acidosis and oligohidrosis	Not established for PTC	Not labeled for PTC

bid, twice daily; PO, orally; PTC, pseudotumor cerebri; Rx, prescription; tid, three times daily.

event of worsening vision. ONSF can be performed in pregnancy, albeit with greater risk.

Communication and Counseling

Patients and parents may be counseled that in most cases pseudotumor is a self-limited disease with resolution over time regardless of treatment. The importance of follow-up with objective measurement of vision must be emphasized owing to the risk of insidious visual loss. Patients who are able to do so should test their vision with appropriate reading material daily until PTC has resolved.

Obese patients should be counseled to lose weight to manage PTC and to improve their overall health. Enrollment in a weight-reduction program may make this easier.

SUGGESTED READINGS

1. Banta JT, Farris BK: Pseudotumor cerebri and optic nerve sheath decompression. Ophthalmology 107:1907–1912, 2000. **Study highlighting the benefits of ONSF.**
2. Brazis PW: Pseudotumor cerebri. Curr Neurol Neurosci Rep 4:111–116, 2004. **A current review that discusses venous outflow obstruction as a cause or effect of PTC.**
3. Farb RI, Vanek I, Scott JN, et al: Idiopathic intracranial hypertension: The prevalence and morphology of sinovenous stenosis. Neurology 60:1418–1424, 2003. **High resolution MRV study supporting sinovenous stenosis as a factor in PTC.**
4. Friedman DI, Jacobson DM: Diagnostic criteria for idiopathic intracranial hypertension. Neurology 59:1492–1495, 2002. **Discussion of addition of radiologic data to Dandy criteria.**
5. Johnson LN, Krohel GB, Madsen RW, et al: The role of weight loss and acetazolamide in the treatment of idiopathic intracranial hypertension (pseudotumor cerebri). Ophthalmology 105:2313–2317, 1998. **Study finding improvement correlated with weight loss.**
6. King JO, Mitchell PJ, Thomson KR, et al: Cerebral venography and manometry in idiopathic intracranial hypertension. Neurology 45:2224–2228, 1995. **Intriguing study suggesting that venous hypertension is effect rather than a cause of high ICP.**
7. Lueck C, McIlwaine G: Interventions for idiopathic intracranial hypertension. Cochrane Database Syst Rev 3:CD003434, 2005. **Analysis of evidence-based medicine in PTC, finding no class I data.**

Cerebrovascular Disease

S. Anne Joseph and Mary L. Zupanc

KEY CONCEPTS

- Strokes can occur in children.
- Rapid diagnosis requires a raised index of suspicion based on the clinical presentation.
- Appropriate diagnostic tests should be ordered based on the type of stroke.
- A thorough search for a cause should be undertaken in all cases.
- Long-term therapy is aimed at preventing stroke recurrence when possible.

Cerebrovascular disease (CVD) or pediatric stroke is being increasingly recognized during childhood. The incidence of CVD during childhood is now estimated at 3.3 per 100,000 population per year. Stroke is defined as the sudden occlusion or rupture of cerebral arteries or veins resulting in focal cerebral damage and focal neurologic deficits (Box 1). Stroke resulting from vascular occlusion takes the form of arterial ischemic stroke, or sinovenous thrombosis. When a cerebral artery or vein is occluded, a bland cerebral infarction results. These bland infarcts can secondarily become hemorrhagic when there is bleeding into the infarcted area. Venous infarctions have a higher propensity to become hemorrhagic.

BOX 1 Types of Stroke

- Bland infarct—arterial or venous thrombosis
- Subarachnoid hemorrhage
- Intraparenchymal hemorrhage

Stroke that results from rupture of a vessel is referred to as *intracranial hemorrhage*. This can take the form of subarachnoid hemorrhage when there is rupture of an aneurysm of the circle of Willis, or intraparenchymal hemorrhage when there is rupture of a vessel that bleeds into the brain tissue.

The ratio of arterial ischemic strokes to sinovenous thrombosis is approximately 3:1. Pediatric intracranial hemorrhage occurs as frequently as ischemic strokes, whereas in adults ischemic strokes are seen three to four times more frequently than intracranial hemorrhage. The overall increased incidence of stroke in children is partially related to survival of previously fatal disorders such as leukemia, congenital heart disease, sickle cell anemia, and tumors. This is also in part because of the availability of more sensitive diagnostic tools such as MRI that improve stroke detection.

Studies of CVD in children are largely descriptive and differ from adult studies. Specifically, the diagnosis of stroke in children is frequently delayed or missed entirely. In addition, developmental differences in the cerebrovascular, neurologic, and coagulation systems result in different etiologies. Very little research has been conducted on the treatment of CVD in children. In addition, by virtue of the different etiologies in pediatric patients, the treatment strategies used for adults with CVD are not broadly applicable.

Etiologies

The etiologies of childhood CVD are very different from those found in adults. The most common etiologies of adult CVD include atherosclerosis, hypertension, atrial fibrillation, and complications of diabetes mellitus. In children, the causes are legion and include acquired or congenital heart disease, coagulation disorders, dehydration, vasculopathies, vasculitis, metabolic disorders, arterial dissection, infection, vascular malformations, and cancer (Box 2). In retrospective case series, 20% to 30% of patients had no identifiable risk factors. Of interest, multiple risk factors for stroke are often present in an individual patient.

CARDIAC DISEASE

Congenital and acquired heart diseases are the most common causes of ischemic stroke in the pediatric

---

BOX 2 Causes of Arterial Ischemic Stroke

- Cardiac disease
- Hemoglobinopathies
- Vasculopathies
- Vasculitis
- Arterial dissection
- Coagulopathies
- Antiphospholipid syndrome
- Pregnancy
- Metabolic disorders

---

population. The overall incidence of stroke from congenital lesions has declined since the 1960s, presumably because of the surgical procedures that can now be performed early in life to repair these lesions. However, complex congenital heart disease remains a risk factor for thromboembolism to the brain directly from the heart or from systemic clots via a right-to-left shunt through an atrial or ventricular septal defect or a patent foramen ovale. Prosthetic heart valves can also be a source of thromboemboli. Congenital cyanotic heart disease with polycythemia and secondary intravascular hyperviscosity is a risk factor for venous clot formation and will be discussed in the section on sinovenous thrombosis. Acquired conditions such as bacterial endocarditis, cardiomyopathy, rheumatic heart disease, and cardiac arrhythmias have also been identified as etiologies of ischemic stroke in children. The mechanism of stroke in these cases is often embolic, with a high risk of recurrence if anticoagulant therapy is not initiated (see the Expert Opinion section).

HEMOGLOBINOPATHIES

Sickle cell anemia is another common etiology of stroke in children. Approximately 25% of all individuals with sickle cell anemia develop cerebrovascular disease. Ischemic strokes can occur in the setting of thrombotic crises. Rarely, aneurysm formation and rupture result in life-threatening subarachnoid hemorrhage. Fortunately, effective treatment is available for patients with this disorder and is anticipated to reduce the morbidity and mortality of CVD in this population. Specifically, blood transfusions can be given in the acute phase to reduce the concentration of the abnormal sickled hemoglobin in blood (see the Expert Opinion section).

VASCULOPATHIES

Moyamoya disease is one of the more common vasculopathies that can produce ischemic stroke. Moyamoya disease is characterized by progressive unilateral or bilateral carotid stenosis with the subsequent development of collateral telangiectatic vessels that bypass the obstruction. *Moyamoya* is the Japanese expression for "something hazy like a puff of smoke drifting in the air," the telltale sign of the telangiectases seen on cerebral angiography. Moyamoya disease can be a primary disorder or can occur in association with other disorders such as Down syndrome, neurofibromatosis, or sickle cell disease. The initial signs and symptoms of Moyamoya disease may be fluctuating transient ischemic attacks, often culminating in persistent and progressive neurologic deficits. Affected individuals have undergone revascularization procedures with good results. However, a study investigating the morbidity and mortality of this disorder failed to show any difference in the outcomes of patients with or without the procedure.

Fibromuscular dysplasia is a noninflammatory arterial wall disorder characterized by alternating areas of stenotic and dilated arterial segments in medium and large vessels. Although it is a disorder that mainly affects women 25 to 45 years of age, it has rarely been reported in children. This disorder of arterial wall dysplasia can affect almost every vascular bed. In the nervous system, it predominantly affects the internal carotid arteries and the vertebral arteries in the neck causing stenosis. In the intracranial vasculature, "berry" aneurysms can be seen in the midsize vessels. Symptoms occur when the lesions are tightly stenotic, causing hypoperfusion; embolize, thrombose, or dissect causing ischemic strokes; or cause an intracranial hemorrhage from aneurysm rupture. The diagnosis is made on angiography with the characteristic involvement of the extracranial neck vessels and often the renal arteries as well.

VASCULITIS

Vasculitis is a relatively rare cause of CVD in children. Vasculitis refers to a heterogenous group of disorders that cause inflammation of the blood vessels. Vasculitis may be secondary to central nervous system (CNS) infections, autoimmune disorders, systemic viral or bacterial infections that have a predilection for inflammation of the cerebral vessels, certain drugs, and isolated primary angiitis of the CNS. Arterial and venous strokes have been described in 5% to 12% of children with meningitis. Pediatric strokes have also been reported in association with systemic infections such as mycoplasma, cat-scratch fever, Rocky Mountain spotted fever, coxsackie B4 and A9, influenza A, human immunodeficiency virus (HIV), parvoviruses B19 and X, and chlamydia.

Transient varicella vasculopathy is now recognized as a distinct clinical entity. Postvaricella angiopathy occurs weeks or months after uncomplicated varicella and results in stenosis of the distal internal carotid or proximal anterior, middle, or posterior cerebral arteries, causing arterial ischemic strokes.

Other causes of vasculitis include systemic lupus erythematosus, rheumatoid arthritis, Behçet disease, and other rheumatologic disorders. CNS vasculitis has been reported with exposure to a variety of drugs including amphetamines, cocaine, and opioids. Recreational drug users are at increased risk for strokes from vasospasm, nonvasculitic occlusion, hemorrhage, and vasculitis.

Primary CNS angiitis is a noninfectious granulomatous cerebral angiitis, unassociated with systemic disease. It exclusively affects the cerebral small and medium-sized leptomeningeal, cortical, and subcortical arteries and to a lesser extent veins and venules. The diagnosis is elusive and is made definitively with leptomeningeal and brain biopsy.

Steroids and other immunosuppressant agents are effective ways to reduce the incidence of stroke from vasculitis.

ARTERIAL DISSECTION

Spontaneous or traumatic injury to the intima of cerebral vessels can result in the accumulation of blood between the layers of the blood vessel and subsequent occlusion of the lumen. Increased awareness of the clinical features and radiographic findings of arterial dissection has resulted in more frequent diagnosis and treatment of this condition.

Traumatic dissection is usually the result of sports injuries or motor vehicle accidents. Carotid occlusion can occur after peritonsillar trauma, such as a fall with a sharp pointed object (e.g., ice-cream stick, toothbrush, and pen). Vertebral or basilar arterial occlusion has been reported after trivial falls involving the neck, as well as after gymnastics, weight lifting, and chiropractic manipulation. Dissection may occur in children who have no underlying risks, or in children with vasculopathy secondary to sickle cell disease, neurofibromatosis, or fibromuscular dysplasia. Spontaneous dissection affects the carotid arteries more frequently than the posterior circulation.

Treatment of cerebral artery dissection in children needs further study. Areas of investigation include angioplasty, stent placement, and pseudoaneurysmal coiling. Vascular occlusion can be performed if the collateral circulation is adequate. However, experience with these procedures in children is very limited. They are also technically difficult and delicate procedures that can result in further disruption of the vessel with the possibility of rupture, hemorrhagic transformation of an ischemic stroke, release of emboli distal to the dissection, or any combination of these sequelae.

COAGULOPATHIES

Coagulopathies can promote thrombosis and increase the risk of ischemic stroke. These disorders are more likely to produce venous thrombosis than arterial thrombosis. Acquired or inherited prothrombotic disorders such as protein C deficiency, protein S deficiency, antithrombin III deficiency, or plasminogen deficiency, as well as factor V Leiden, anticardiolipin antibody, and lupus anticoagulant predispose a child to stroke. These disorders can be hereditary or acquired. If the trait is hereditary and homozygous, the strokes can occur in the neonatal period. Often in children with prothrombotic disorders, thromboembolic events occur in the setting of additional acquired conditions that temporarily increase the risk of thrombus formation such as dehydration. Acquired protein C deficiency can result from liver disease, bone marrow transplantation, sepsis, or disseminated intravascular coagulation. Acquired antithrombin III deficiency can be caused by nephrotic syndrome or protein-losing enteropathy. Both protein C deficiency and antithrombin III deficiency have been associated with L-asparaginase therapy.

ANTIPHOSPHOLIPID SYNDROME

Antiphospholipid antibodies, including lupus anticoagulant and anticardiolipin antibodies, are also associated with CVD. The syndrome is characterized by the presence of these circulating antibodies and diverse systemic clinical manifestations such as thrombosis and recurrent abortions. Antiphospholipid antibodies bind to the phospholipid moieties found on platelets, coagulation factors, and endothelial cells and produce a hypercoagulable state. The etiology of strokes is probably multifactorial and includes an association with valvular disease, cerebral microemboli, thrombosis, and endothelial activation and antibody to brain endothelium. Two forms have been described: the primary syndrome, where there is no evidence of an underlying disease, and the secondary syndrome, which occurs mainly in the setting of systemic lupus erythematosus. Adults are affected more frequently than children are, but case reports of children with these disorders have been described. Furthermore, women with frequent miscarriages should be screened for these antibodies.

BOX 3 Causes of Venous Ischemic Stroke

- Dehydration
- Infection
- Hyperviscous states
- Coagulation disorders
- Pregnancy
- Malignancy

PREGNANCY

Pregnancy and oral contraceptive therapy are also associated with an increased risk of venous and arterial occlusion, probably because of induction of a hypercoagulable state. Pregnancy increases the risk of stroke to approximately 13 times the risk in nonpregnant young women.

METABOLIC DISORDERS

Metabolic disorders such as homocystinuria, Fabry disease, mitochondrial cytopathies, and hyperlipidemia can be associated with childhood stroke. Homocystinuria is a relatively uncommon autosomal-recessive inborn error of methionine metabolism. Several enzymatic defects can produce homocystinuria, the most common one being cystathionine synthetase deficiency. In its classic form, it is associated with skeletal and cutaneous manifestations, ectopic lens, cognitive impairments, epilepsy, and recurrent vascular occlusions. Thromboembolism is the most likely mechanism of stroke. Patients who are heterozygotes for disorders in methionine metabolism may have an increased risk of CVD. Clinical research indicates that individuals with moderately elevated homocystine levels have a significantly increased risk for the early development of CVD. If this research is confirmed, it may be prudent to screen patients for elevated homocystine levels and initiate therapy (e.g., folate supplementation) to reduce their blood levels.

Other metabolic disorders that can result in CVD include mitochondrial encephalomyopathy, lactic acidosis, and stroke-like episodes (MELAS); methylmalonic acidemia; propionic acidemia; isovaleric acidemia; and ornithine transcarbamylase deficiency. The stroke-like episodes are usually preceded by nausea and headache. They occur in a nonvascular distribution and are often transient; the mechanism of action is probably intracellular metabolic failure. Repeated strokes result in progressive neurologic impairment. No effective treatment is available for this disorder.

In Fabry disease, as a result of α-galactosidase deficiency, multiple lacunar strokes occur in affected males during the teenage and early adult years.

Hyperlipidemia can be associated with childhood stroke, and a fasting lipid profile should be performed in any child with idiopathic stroke.

SINUS VENOUS THROMBOSIS

The diagnosis of sinus venous thrombosis (SVT) has increased since the late 1980s, probably because of the use of enhanced radiographic techniques, including MRI, magnetic resonance angiography (MRA), and magnetic resonance venography (MRV). Thrombosis of these vessels results in increased intracranial pressure with subsequent venous infarctions that can transform to hemorrhagic infarctions. The most common sites of venous thrombosis are the sagittal and lateral sinuses. Common systemic conditions that predispose to sinus venous thrombosis include dehydration, inherited or acquired coagulation abnormalities, hypernatremia, localized infections such as mastoiditis and meningitis, malnutrition, congestive heart failure, and cyanotic congenital heart failure with polycythemia (Box 3). Malignancy can also produce sinus occlusion through direct invasion of the sinus by tumor or leukemic cellular occlusion, or by production of a hypercoagulable state. Leukemia is the most common malignancy that causes dural sinus thrombosis. Chemotherapeutic agents such as L-asparaginase can also contribute to producing sinus thrombosis. Occlusion of a major draining cerebral vein results in elevation of cerebral venous pressure, and reduced cerebrospinal fluid reabsorption through the arachnoid granulations. This in turn, leads to raised intracranial pressure and venous infarctions that have a higher propensity to become hemorrhagic when compared to arterial ischemic strokes. The classic triad of lethargy, symptoms, and signs of raised intracranial pressure, and seizures should raise the suspicion of sinus venous thrombosis.

In SVT, there is a greater risk of clot propagation than in arterial thrombosis. Furthermore, recanalization of the vein even days or weeks later can help relieve venous congestion in the affected areas of the cerebrum. As such, the role of antithrombotic treatment in SVT tends to differ from the role of these agents in arterial thrombosis. In superior sagittal sinus thrombosis, bilateral cortical hemorrhagic infarctions are often seen. Deep venous sinus thrombosis of the straight sinus, the internal cerebral veins, or the vein of Galen produces deep hemorrhagic infarctions of the thalami or cerebellum. Treatment includes anticoagulation therapy (see section on Expert Opinion).

HEMATOLOGIC DISORDERS

Thrombocytosis can be seen with Kawasaki disease and it can cause platelet thrombosis with subsequent vessel occlusion. Thrombocytopenia, on the other hand, is more frequently encountered and may be caused by a number of etiologies, including viral illness, sepsis, and medications (e.g., valproate and chemotherapeutic

---

BOX 4 Causes of Intracranial Hemorrhage

- Aneurysm rupture
- Arteriovenous malformation
- Neurocutaneous syndromes
- Tumor
- Radiation effects
- Hypertension
- Drugs

---

agents), or it may be idiopathic. Treatment of this disorder is symptomatic.

Polycythemia can also increase the risk of sinus venous thrombosis, usually by inhibiting venous return. Cyanotic congenital heart disease is one of the most common causes of this hematologic disorder. Dehydration can also produce a relative polycythemia. Treatment is symptomatic, and some degree of fluid resuscitation is usually needed.

Other hematologic disorders that can result in CVD include defects in coagulation, the most common of which is hemophilia A. Intracranial hemorrhage can develop in children with these disorders even after trivial head trauma (Box 4). Effective treatment results in replacement of the missing coagulation factor. Vitamin K deficiency, most commonly found in neonates, can also result in intracranial hemorrhage. A vitamin K–responsive coagulopathy may develop in neonates whose mothers have epilepsy and who are being treated with enzyme-inducing antiepileptic drugs (carbamazepine, phenobarbital, phenytoin, oxcarbazepine, topiramate). They require larger doses of vitamin K at birth. In addition, their mothers should receive vitamin K supplementation during the last trimester of pregnancy.

VASCULAR MALFORMATIONS AND ANEURYSMS

Arteriovenous malformations and other structural vascular lesions are the most common cause of nontraumatic intracranial hemorrhage in children. In one series, they accounted for 42% of cases of nontraumatic hemorrhage in children. Arterial aneurysms are less common than arteriovenous malformations and generally produce subarachnoid hemorrhage. The ruptured aneurysms are managed surgically. Arteriovenous malformations, venous angiomas, capillary telangiectases, and cavernous angiomas usually produce intraparenchymal hemorrhage. Vein of Galen malformations result in altered blood flow in the posterior circulation. In infancy, this malformation is manifested as high-output congestive heart failure. Later in life, the major symptoms are that of cerebral vein thrombosis (i.e., seizures, headache, and signs of increased intracranial pressure). The vascular malformations may be hereditary with familial recurrence, and therapy depends on surgical accessibility of the lesion.

Sturge-Weber syndrome, a neurocutaneous disorder, is characterized by facial hemangiomatosis and ipsilateral intracranial capillary venous hemangioma. These tortuous blood vessels progressively calcify and do not deliver adequate oxygen and other nutrients to the cortex, which often results in focal seizures, progressive hemiparesis, and cognitive decline. In patients with progressive changes, hemispherectomy is curative. Neurofibromatosis can be associated with a vasculopathy, giving rise to aneurysms that can rupture and cause subarachnoid hemorrhage.

TUMOR AND RADIATION EFFECTS

Intracranial tumors can produce intracranial hemorrhage. In one series, 13% of patients with intraparenchymal bleeding were eventually found to have brain tumors. The radiation therapy and chemotherapy used to treat brain tumors can produce occlusive bland infarction or intracranial hemorrhage, probably secondary to a mineralizing microangiopathy.

SYSTEMIC HYPERTENSION

This condition is a relatively rare cause of CVD in children. Some medications can result in hypertension, particularly steroids and adrenocorticotropic hormone (ACTH). ACTH is used in the treatment of infantile spasms and has been reported to cause intracranial hemorrhage, probably because of systemic hypertension (poorly documented).

Radiographic Techniques

Radiographic evaluation of a pediatric patient with CVD has dramatically improved since the late 1980s. Current techniques include MRI, MRA, MRV, MR diffusion-weighted studies, and magnetic resonance spectroscopy (MRS) (Box 5).

State-of-the-art equipment for MRI includes a 1.5-Tesla high-field magnet with echoplanar capability and rapid gradients. Rapid gradients and echoplanar imaging allow faster acquisition without the added risk of movement artifact. Gradient echo imaging is very helpful in detecting blood and blood products found in intraparenchymal hemorrhage. Another technique, diffusion-weighted imaging, is very sensitive in the identification of acute ischemia or infarction. Diffusion-weighted imaging measures the random, brownian movement of water in the brain.

MRA is a newly developed technique that can image the large intracranial veins and arteries without the administration of contrast material. It has proved very helpful in the identification of thromboembolic occlusion of the large vessels.

MR diffusion-weighted images are extremely sensitive in identifying areas of cerebral ischemia within a few hours of onset, even before standard MR images show any changes.

MRS is performed with the same equipment as MRI, except that it measures different metabolites in the brain by using qualitative and quantitative information about hydrogen nuclei in each measured metabolite. For example, MRS can measure lactate in the brain, which is an indicator of anaerobic metabolism and possible ischemia or infarction.

BOX 5 Diagnostic Tests

Confirmation of Stroke and Identification of Vessels Affected

- CT scan
- MRI with diffusion-weight images
- MRA/MRV
- Spinal tap if subarachnoid hemorrhage suspected
- 4-Vessel cerebral angiogram

Tests for Underlying Condition

- Sickle cell disease: complete blood count
- Sepsis: ESR, culture
- Hyperlipidemia: lipid profile
- MELAS: mitochondrial DNA, protein C, protein S
- Prothrombotic states: factor V Leiden, antithrombin III, prothrombin mutation
- Antiphospholipid syndrome: anticardiolipin levels, lupus anticoagulant, β-2 glycoprotein
- Toxins: drug screen
- Homocystinuria: homocystine
- Congenital heart disease: echocardiography
- Valve problems, atrial fibrillation, rheumatic heart disease: electrocardiography

ESR, erythrocyte sedimentation rate; MELAS, myopathy, encephalopathy, lactic acidosis, stroke-like episodes; MRA, magnetic resonance angiography; MRV, magnetic resonance venography.

Although MRA is almost as sensitive as conventional angiogram, conventional four-vessel cerebral angiography remains the gold standard for visualizing vascular changes that are not detected on MRA.

Expert Opinion on Management Issues

The three major barriers to clinical research and evidence-based clinical treatment in children with CVD are delayed or missed diagnosis with missed opportunities for selection of interventions, complex etiologies, and lack of applicability of adult research to children. Treatment of CVD in children is currently aimed at medical stabilization, treating complications of the stroke, management of the underlying cause, and attempting to prevent recurrence or extension of the stroke.

MEDICAL THERAPY

Antiplatelet Therapy

No controlled trials on the use of aspirin or other antiplatelet agents in children with CVD have been performed. However, aspirin is being used with increased frequency in children with ischemic CVD and possible prothrombotic conditions. The suggested dosage to provide an antiplatelet effect is 3 to 5 mg/kg per day. Despite the theoretical risk of Reye syndrome in children taking daily aspirin, not a single case has been reported in the world's literature. The effectiveness of this dosage in children remains unproven.

Antithrombotic Therapy

Heparin

The decision to use heparin is based on one's ability to answer two questions: what is the risk of recurrent emboli or extension of the infarction and what is the risk of inducing hemorrhage with anticoagulation? Heparin should probably be used in children with intracardiac clots, cardiac arrhythmias, arterial dissection, sinus venous thrombosis, coagulation disorders, and other conditions associated with an increased risk of recurrent emboli. Again, no large-scale trials have evaluated the use of heparin in children. The dosage of unfractionated heparin is 20 U/kg per hour for children older than 1 year and 28 U/kg per hour in those younger than 1 year. The targeted activated partial thromboplastin time is 60 to 85 seconds. Drug treatment should be monitored carefully. Adverse effects include hemorrhage and thrombocytopenia. When heparin-induced thrombocytopenia occurs, ancrod or heparinoid are alternative anticoagulants.

Low molecular weight heparins offer general advantages over unfractionated heparin. It is easy to administer subcutaneously twice a day and requires minimal monitoring. Low molecular weight heparins are given to children in doses of 1 mg/kg every 12 hours, or in neonates 1.5 mg/kg every 12 hours. Antifactor Xa levels are monitored aiming for levels of 0.5 to 1 unit/mL in a sample drawn 4 to 6 hours after the subcutaneous dose.

Warfarin

The same decision that results in the use of heparin usually sets the stage for long-term anticoagulation with warfarin. Experience in children with long-term anticoagulation is limited. There has always been the fear that the risk of long-term anticoagulation in active children who may be prone to injuries and falls will outweigh the benefits. This concern appears to be unfounded with respect to the available clinical data. Warfarin is the most effective means of prolonged anticoagulation in children. The dosage is variable. An international normalized ratio (INR) of 2.0 to 3.0 is appropriate for most children taking warfarin; for children with artificial heart valves, the INR should be higher at 2.5 to 3.5.

Acute Treatment of Sinus Venous Thrombosis

Therapy in SVT is aimed at preventing clot propagation and subsequent intracranial hemorrhage, lowering intracranial pressure, and minimizing morbidity such as visual field compromise caused by optic nerve compression. Supportive therapy should also include aggressive treatment of seizures. Medical management in the acute setting, therefore, includes anticoagulation, agents that lower cerebrospinal fluid pressure such as acetazolamide, antiepileptic medications when indicated, aggressive treatment of the underlying cause of the SVT, and continued monitoring for complications of treatment.

Anticoagulation in SVT has been controversial. A randomized, controlled study of heparin therapy for SVT in adults documented the effectiveness of anticoagulation.

A retrospective study of 17 children with SVT in which all but two received anticoagulation therapy showed that anticoagulation did not carry a greater risk of bleeding complications. Another review looked at two small trials involving 79 patients with SVT. This study concluded that anticoagulant treatment in SVT appears to be safe and is associated with an apparent reduction in the risk of death or dependency that did not reach statistical significance. Larger multicenter studies are still needed to study the efficacy of anticoagulation in this condition. In the absence of more information from randomized trials, clinicians will need to base their treatment on the limited information available and on the pathophysiologic basis for morbidity in this condition.

Thrombolytic Agents

The use of thrombolytic agents in children with acute stroke is very limited and not currently recommended. There are numerous reasons, however, for studying these agents in children because the morbidity of stroke in children is more than 50%. However, the diagnosis of stroke in children is often delayed, thereby missing the window of opportunity to use thrombolytic agents such as tissue plasminogen activator (tPA). In adult studies, tPA given within 3 hours of the onset of stroke symptoms can prevent significant morbidity without a heightened risk of bleeding. If early recognition of stroke could be achieved in children, clinical cohort studies using tPA could be performed. In reality, tPA has the potential of becoming a primary treatment in children with ischemic stroke. Certainly, in adults the use of tPA within 3 hours after the onset of stroke can be lifesaving.

Transfusion

Clinical studies have now established that periodic blood transfusion is the single biggest preventive measure in children with sickle cell disease. If the sickle cell hemoglobin in the blood is kept below 30%, recurrent silent strokes can be prevented. Iron toxicity from repeated transfusions remains a problem, but it can be reduced with iron chelation therapy.

SUPPORTIVE MEDICAL CARE

Supportive medical care should include maximizing cerebral perfusion, paying careful attention to fluids and electrolytes, and providing aggressive treatment of conditions that could increase cerebral metabolic needs and further compromise the ischemic penumbra, such as fever, and seizures. Most patients will eventually require rehabilitation. Neurologic rehabilitation should be designed to meet the specific neurologic deficits sustained. In general, they should include therapies aimed at gross motor, fine motor function, swallowing, speech, language, cognition, and behavior. Emotional and psychological support is an important part of the rehabilitation process and must be provided for the patient and the entire family.

SURGICAL INTERVENTIONS

Treatment of aneurysms and vascular malformations are primarily surgical. Aneurysm clipping or coiling of a vascular malformation are surgical procedures that are used in children. Large intraparenchymal hematomas may need to be surgically evacuated. Surgical procedures such as lumbar-peritoneal shunt placement or optic nerve fenestration should be considered in cases of SVT refractory to medical therapy to decrease intracranial pressure and preserve vision. In progressive Moyamoya disease, several bypass procedures have been used. Direct anastomotic procedures from the superficial temporal artery to the middle cerebral artery have been performed in an attempt to improve circulation to the cerebral areas distal to the stenotic blood vessels. Another more indirect procedure is encephaloduroarteriosynangiosis. Several groups have debated the utility of these approaches and have reported varying degrees of success.

PREVENTIVE MEASURES

Minimizing the risk of extension or recurrence of stroke in the acute and chronic phase remains an area of continued debate. Measures to prevent recurrent ischemic stroke include anticoagulation, antiplatelet therapy, as well as education on factors that can increase prothrombotic states such as dehydration, drug abuse, smoking, and certain types of birth control or hormonal therapy. Chronic anticoagulation is indicated currently in a few specific instances such as thromboembolism from atrial fibrillation, or congenital heart disease with right to left shunts or valve abnormalities. The choice of chronic anticoagulation versus antiplatelet therapy is made after careful consideration of risk of stroke recurrence and risk of complications from therapy. Preventive treatment should also include treatment of specific underlying conditions such as exchange transfusions in sickle cell disease, anti-inflammatory or immunosuppressive therapy in vasculitis, and specific therapy of metabolic disorders.

Common Pitfalls

- A low index of suspicion contributes to delayed or missed diagnosis of pediatric strokes.
- CT scan may not show changes in ischemic strokes for at least 24 to 48 hours. CT scans may also not detect small strokes in the posterior fossa, specifically the brainstem. Therefore, a normal CT scan in the acute phase or in specific clinical settings does not preclude a stroke.
- Subarachnoid hemorrhage rarely can be missed on radiographic studies. A high index of suspicion should lead to cerebrospinal fluid analysis specifically looking for red blood cells and xanthochromia. Although fairly sensitive, MRA may not detect a small aneurysm and the gold standard for diagnosis remains conventional angiography.
- Venous sinus thrombosis should be considered with the triad of raised intracranial pressure, lethargy,

and seizures. Funduscopic examination should not be overlooked in these ill children. In the early stages, CT scan and standard MRI may not detect the thrombosis. MRV with specific attention to the veins is highly sensitive in detecting SVT prior to the presence of intraparenchymal hemorrhage or significant cortical ischemia.

■ Vasculitis remains an often elusive diagnosis. Conventional cerebral angiography is useful when abnormal. In the presence of normal cerebral angiography and a clinical picture suggestive of vasculitis, meningeal and brain biopsy remain the definitive diagnostic procedures.

■ Arterial dissection is often detected on MRI studies windowed specifically to detect a dissection. However, if this test is normal, cerebral angiogram remains the definitive diagnostic procedure. In the appropriate clinical setting, dissection should be suspected even when the trauma in question was trivial.

Communication and Counseling

Clear communication with the families as well as with the medical team is crucial in the management of CVD.

The acute period of an ischemic stroke involves progressive edema of the damaged area of the brain that peaks within 3 to 5 days, barring further insult. Potential complications during this phase include either raised intracranial pressure, seizures, intracranial tissue shifts, hemorrhagic conversion spontaneously or secondary to treatment, and recurrent stroke. During the period that the patient is bedridden, there is also increased risk of infection.

During the critical phase of subarachnoid hemorrhage, there is the potential for re-hemorrhage and death, seizures, vasospasm, and raised intracranial pressure.

Arterial dissection either of the carotids or the vertebral system increases the risk of further thromboembolism from the distal edge of the thrombus to the area of the brain supplied by the dissected vessel, placing that entire territory at risk for infarction.

Once the acute phase is over, ultimate functional capacity depends on the size and location of the stroke. Functional improvement in general occurs most rapidly in the first 3 months following the stroke, but continues, albeit at a slower rate for up to 1 to 2 years.

Patients on anticoagulation should be counseled on avoiding contact sports and certain medications that can affect metabolism of the anticoagulant.

Cerebrovascular disorders in children cause significant morbidity. The many different etiologies of CVD in children are distinctly different from those of their adult counterparts. Few treatments of CVD have been established for the pediatric population. The diagnosis is made early when there is a high index of suspicion. In the acute phase, management is geared toward prompt diagnosis utilizing the most appropriate tests, prevention of extension or recurrence, and minimizing damage to the brain. In the chronic phase, attention is focused on rehabilitation and prevention of stroke recurrence. A careful search for underlying etiology should be undertaken in each case.

SUGGESTED READINGS

1. Begelman SM, Olin JW: Fibromuscular dysplasia. Curr Opin Rheumatol 21:41–47, 2000. **A review article on fibromuscular dysplasia, pathologic classification, etiology, and differential diagnosis.**
2. Deveber G, Roach ES, Riela AR, Wiznitzer M: Stroke in children: Recognition, treatment, and future directions. Semin Pediatr Neurol 7:309–317, 2000. **A comprehensive review of pediatric stroke.**
3. De Veber G: Cerebrovascular disease in children. In Swaiman KF, Ashwal S (eds): Pediatric Neurology: Principles Practice. St. Louis: Mosby, 1999, pp 1099–1124. **A comprehensive review on strokes in children, classification, causes, and treatment options.**
4. Einhaupl KM, Villringer A, Meister W, et al: Heparin treatment in venous sinus thrombosis. Lancet 338:597–600, 1991. **A prospective randomized, blinded placebo-controlled study of 20 adult patients with venous sinus thrombosis to assess safety and efficacy of heparin anticoagulation.**
5. Johnson M, Parkerson N, Ward S, de Alarcon P: Pediatric sinovenous thrombosis. J Pediatr Hematol Oncol 25:312–315, 2003. **A retrospective chart review of 17 patients with sinovenous thrombosis to determine if anticoagulation therapy is effective in preventing progression of pediatric sinovenous thrombosis and to determine the safety of anticoagulation in the pediatric population.**
6. Katzav A, Champan J, Shoenfeld Y: CNS dysfunction in the antiphospholipid syndrome. Lupus 12:903–907, 2003. **A review of clinical data obtained from a large series of cases regarding the spectrum of symptoms seen in antiphospholipid syndrome.**
7. Masuhr F, Mehraein S, Einhaupl K: Cerebral venous and sinus thrombosis. J Neurol 251:11–23, 2004. **A teaching review on cerebral sinovenous thrombosis with attention to clinical symptoms, evolution, causes, diagnostic tools, and potential treatments.**
8. Roach ES: Etiology of stroke in children. Semin Pediatr Neurol 7:244–260, 2000. **A review of the causes of stroke in children.**
9. Smith ER, Butler WE, Ogilvy CS: Surgical approaches to vascular anomalies of the child's brain. Curr Opin Neurol 15:165–171, 2002. **An overview of current methods of surgical treatment for pediatric stroke, focusing on indications and use of the surgical approaches.**
10. Stam J, Bruijn S, deVeber G: Anticoagulation for cerebral sinus thrombosis. Stroke 234:1054–1055, 2003. **A review of available evidence regarding the effectiveness and safety of anticoagulant therapy in confirmed cerebral sinus thrombosis.**
11. Younger DS: Vasculitis of the nervous system. Curr Opin Neurol 17:317–336, 2004. **A review of CNS vasculitis including classification, causes, diagnosis, and treatment.**

Reye Syndrome

Lawrence W. Brown

KEY CONCEPTS

■ Reye syndrome is characterized by the combination of liver disease and inflammatory encephalopathy, usually following viral infection in childhood.

■ Infectious, toxic, and metabolic causes (including disorders of fatty acid oxidation and ketogenesis) can mimic Reye syndrome.

Reye syndrome is a systemic mitochondrial disorder associated with viral illness; it is characterized by encephalopathy and hepatic dysfunction in children between 5 and 15 years of age. Although Reye syndrome has been described for more than 40 years, the pathogenesis remains unknown. Incidence peaked in the early 1980s, and it is now a rare disease. Its decline has been attributed to increased public awareness of the possible association of therapeutic salicylate ingestion with prodromal viral illness and the virtual elimination of aspirin in the susceptible population.

Criteria for Reye syndrome (Box 1) include an acute noninflammatory encephalopathy without cerebrospinal fluid (CSF) pleocytosis, characteristic liver histology or markedly elevated serum transaminases or ammonia levels, and no other explanation for the illness. Other possible differential diagnoses include viral hepatitis, acute acetaminophen or chronic salicylate poisoning, viral encephalitis, and inherited disorders of metabolism (Box 2). Varicella infection and nonspecific upper respiratory illness are the most common antecedent illnesses. Vomiting is a consistent feature and usually the first symptom of Reye syndrome; changes in mental status ranging from confusion to delirium to coma define the various stages of the disorder (Table 1). Liver biopsy shows evidence of microvesicular fat and diagnostic mitochondrial alterations on electron microscopy.

The association of Reye syndrome with viral infection has been well established both from epidemiologic and virologic evidence. In addition to varicella as well as influenza A and B, varieties of other viruses have been isolated, including adenovirus, coxsackie, herpes simplex and others. Although some have doubted the importance of viral infection alone in a sporadic disease like Reye syndrome, others have emphasized the variable nature of viral illness and the importance of host genetic factors. Certainly, many viruses are capable of producing overwhelming infection with a wide spectrum of clinical manifestations. Viral infection alone can explain both hepatic disease and brain involvement: Liver function abnormalities are seen in 3% of patients with influenza A and more than 75% of those with varicella. Similarly, many viruses can produce an acute toxic encephalopathy with increased intracranial pressure. Cerebral edema can also develop secondary to fulminant liver failure.

Findings of hyperammonemia, hypoglycemia, and abnormal liver function tests are characteristic. Prolonged prothrombin time and partial thromboplastin time as well as hypoalbuminemia are common, but bilirubin remains normal and jaundice is not part of the syndrome. Acute pancreatitis is an occasional accompaniment. Lumbar puncture findings are benign except for increased opening pressure and hypoglycorrhachia (low cerebrospinal glucose). Electroencephalogram (EEG) shows evidence of a diffuse encephalopathy without epileptiform features. Liver biopsy is diagnostic with panlobular fatty infiltration. Electron microscopy demonstrates mitochondrial abnormalities, peroxisomal swelling and proliferation, and glycogen depletion.

The signs and symptoms of Reye syndrome can vary considerably. It is possible to demonstrate normal cerebral functioning in the presence of otherwise typical recurrent vomiting and hepatic dysfunction following viral illness with demonstration of the pathologic features of Reye syndrome on liver biopsy; this is called stage 0. Stages I and II have increasing confusion, agitation, and lethargy. Coma with increasing intracranial pressure and herniation define stages III and IV. Progression from stage I to stage IV can evolve slowly over several days or appear explosively over hours. Stage V coma is end-stage disease approaching brain death despite evidence of improving blood ammonia and serum liver enzyme activity. Full recovery is expected if the disease never progresses beyond stage III, stage IV carries a poor prognosis, and death or major disability is invariable with stage V. Independent negative indicators include rapid progression through clinical stages, blood ammonia greater than 300 µg/dL, and prothrombin time (PT) more than twice the control levels.

BOX 1 Case Definition of Reye Syndrome

- Acute noninflammatory encephalopathy.
- Microvesicular fatty metamorphosis of the liver confirmed by biopsy or autopsy.
- AST, ALT, or NH_3 greater than three times the upper limit of normal CSF.
- If obtained, must contain less than 9 WBC/mm^3.
- Exclusion of other diagnoses.
- There should be no more reasonable explanation for the neurologic presentation or the hepatic abnormality.

ALT, alanine transaminase; AST, angiotensin sensitivity test; NH_3, ammonia; WBC, white blood cells.

BOX 2 Differential Diagnoses of Reye Syndrome

Infectious Diseases
- Influenza A and B
- Varicella
- Adenovirus
- Coxsackie virus
- Epstein-Barr virus

Metabolic Diseases
- Disorders of fatty acid oxidation and ketogenesis
- Urea cycle disorders
- Disorders of carbohydrate metabolism
- Organic acidurias

Toxic Disorders
- Aflatoxin
- Hypoglycin
- Phenothiazine antiemetics
- Salicylates
- Valproic acid

TABLE 1 Lovejoy Staging of Reye Syndrome

Mental Status	Response to Pain	Other CNS Findings
Lethargy, follows verbal commands	Purposeful	Normal
Stuporous, combative, disoriented, delirious	Purposeful	Hyperventilation, hyperreflexia
Obtunded, comatose	Decorticate	Pupils dilated and reactive
Comatose	Decerebrate	Loss of oculocephalic reflexes, dilated pupils ± hippus
Comatose	Unresponsive	Flaccid, ± seizures, absent brainstem reflexes, Cheyne-Stokes respiration or apnea

CNS, central nervous system.

Expert Opinion on Management Issues

ACCEPTED INTERVENTIONS

Aggressive and supportive treatment in an intensive care setting are essential to maximize survival and minimize neurologic consequences. Even patients in stage I Reye syndrome must be admitted to the hospital; ideally, they should be observed in the PICU or intermediate care unit because rapid deterioration is not uncommon. Efforts are directed at correcting electrolyte abnormalities and maintaining normal blood glucose levels (70 to 110 mg/dL); glucose levels should be checked every 2 to 4 hours.

Patients with stage II to V Reye syndrome need aggressive management in the PICU. Glucose monitoring is even more critical, and they may require hypertonic glucose infusions. Intracranial pressure (ICP) monitoring should be performed to evaluate cerebral perfusion pressure (mean arterial pressure minus mean intracranial pressure). Elevated ICP is the single factor that most directly increases mortality. Standard measures to control elevated ICP include elevating the head in the neutral position, a degree of volume restriction to maintain osmolality in the range of 290 to 320 mOsm, sedatives, paralyzing agents, intubation, hyperventilation to keep Pco_2 25 to 30 mm Hg, control of body temperature within normal range (e.g., cooling blanket), and osmotic diuretics as needed. However, patients have succumbed even if ICP is not apparently elevated.

There are many other general measures that are part of routine PICU care, although some problems are more common in children with stage II to V Reye syndrome. It is important to maintain electrolyte and mineral homeostasis by monitoring sodium, potassium, calcium, phosphorus, creatinine, and BUN (blood urea nitrogen) every 4 hours (in addition to glucose). SIADH (syndrome of inappropriate antidiuretic hormone secretion) and diabetes insipidus are particularly ominous findings sometimes seen in the most severe cases. Hepatic dysfunction predicts the degree of encephalopathy and can produce clotting disorders. It is essential to monitor liver function tests and ammonia levels daily until normal. Prothrombin time and partial thromboplastin time should be initially measured every 8 hours; it may be necessary to reverse coagulation abnormalities with fresh-frozen plasma (FFP) 10 mL/kg intravenously (IV). FFP should be administered for liver biopsy, placement of ICP monitor, or other invasive procedures. Vitamin K (1 mg IV) should be administered every 2 to 3 days. Serum amylase and lipase should be considered because pancreatitis can complicate the disorder. Total parental nutrition is recommended for indolent cases lasting more than 1 week or those complicated by pancreatitis.

Infection must be pursued vigorously with daily blood and urine cultures as well as daily Gram stains of tracheal secretions. Catheter tips should also be routinely cultured. It is critically important to maintain normal systemic arterial blood pressure, central venous pressure, and urinary output using colloids, if necessary, to support volume needs. Adequate cerebral perfusion pressure must be maintained with vasopressors and oxygen carrying capacity with transfusions; these are necessary to ensure oxygen delivery to the brain. Continuous electrocardiographic monitoring can alert caregivers to early signs of dysrhythmia. Virtually all children with moderate disease will require intubation; good pulmonary toilet and chest physiotherapy are standard PICU practices. Gastrointestinal care may include nasogastric suction, gastric pH determination, antacids, and neomycin to decrease ammonia production.

Desperate therapies have been tried over the years, including exchange transfusion, peritoneal dialysis, steroids, carnitine, insulin supplementation with IV fluids (to encourage intracellular uptake of glucose), barbiturate coma, and craniotomies to decompress the massively swollen brain. None of these interventions has compelling evidence, and many have proven to be extremely risky.

Common Pitfalls: Differential Diagnosis

Metabolic conditions that can mimic Reye syndrome include carnitine transport defects (i.e., carnitine palmityl transferase deficiency), disorders of fatty acid oxidation, urea cycle disorders (e.g., ornithine transcarbamylase deficiency), disorders of gluconeogenesis, and organic acidemias. Diagnosis of inborn errors of metabolism may be very difficult to establish and depends on a high index of suspicion plus the availability of laboratory expertise. In the United States and England, surveillance data over the past 20 years have indicated that 12% to 50% of suspected Reye syndrome cases are actually metabolic disorders. Although extremely important to distinguish from idiopathic cases, it remains unlikely that the majority of children with Reye syndrome are presenting with still undefined metabolic diseases.

Toxins need to be considered as a potential cause of Reye syndrome. Jamaican vomiting sickness (from hypoglycin in the ackee fruit) is a known mimicker of idiopathic Reye syndrome. Antiemetics (promethazine and phenothiazine) have been considered to have a possible role, although epidemiologic studies in the 1980s did not support a connection. Valproate hepatotoxicity can also mimic Reye syndrome, although it is unclear whether affected individuals also have an underlying metabolic abnormality brought out by the drug challenge.

Preventive Measures: The Role of Salicylate Elimination

There has been a dramatic decline in the incidence of Reye syndrome since the Centers for Disease Control and Prevention first expressed concerns about salicylates in 1980. This culminated in the 1985 Food and Drug Administration requirement that warning labels against use in children under the age of 12 years be placed on aspirin bottles. There remains controversy, however, because Reye syndrome was already experiencing a decline even before the public awareness campaigns and virtual elimination of aspirin use in children. At the same time, there was better recognition of inherited metabolic disorders as the actual cause of many cases of Reye-like illness. The 1980s saw not only a decline in the frequency of Reye syndrome but also a reduction in the average age of onset from 8 to 3 years. This near elimination in older children without a past history or risk factors of inherited metabolic disease may well represent a population with as yet unidentified metabolic diseases.

There is no doubt that incidence of Reye syndrome has fallen dramatically since peaking in the early 1980s. The reported incidence in the United States fell by 75% between 1986 and 1989, and it remains a rare condition in childhood. It appears that there are several likely possibilities to explain the decline in the incidence of a major pediatric disease: the elimination of routine aspirin use in childhood, the increasing awareness of underlying metabolic disease, and the declining use of phenothiazine antiemetics. Some investigators have suggested that the apparent decline may be explained by the consequence of overdiagnosis of Reye syndrome in the past. A retrospective blind review of 49 individuals with Reye syndrome during 1970 to 1987 by three independent clinicians found certain diagnosis in only one case!

At this point in time, aspirin is no longer used in children except under unusual circumstances. Prolonged administration of high-dose salicylates in children with juvenile rheumatoid arthritis puts them at increased risk for Reye syndrome. It is recommended that these patients be closely monitored for persistent vomiting or changes in mental status, especially during febrile illness. Fortunately, newer effective alternatives are reducing the need for aspirin exposure and thus reducing the risk of this potentially avoidable illness. Folk remedies in immigrant communities and others relying on complementary and alternative medications put children at risk of exposure to aspirin. There are more than 30 over-the-counter products containing aspirin that are still being given to children. Additional preventable cases of Reye syndrome are likely to occur with lapses in professional and public awareness. Influenza and varicella vaccination programs and ongoing educational efforts are critical. Because Reye syndrome is still a potentially fatal disorder, pediatricians and the media should remain vigilant in their attempts to discourage pediatric salicylate usage.

Communication and Counseling

Pediatricians must remember that Reye syndrome remains a serious and potentially fatal threat in childhood. They must be vigilant in avoiding the risks of salicylate administration, since it may be found in over-the-counter and herbal medications. Other infectious, metabolic, or toxic disorders that mimic Reye syndrome must be considered in the presence of coexisting acute hepatic disease and noninflammatory encephalopathy. Reye syndrome had an extremely high mortality when it was first described in the 1960s, but advances in intensive supportive care have reduced mortality from 20% to 10%. Long-term sequelae in survivors can include cognitive impairment, seizures, and motor disability, but most recover completely.

SUGGESTED READINGS

1. Belay ED, Breese JS, Holman RC, et al: Reye's syndrome in the United States from 1981 through 1997. N Engl J Med 340:1377–1382, 1999. **Epidemiology of the decline of Reye syndrome with comprehensive national data from the Centers for Disease Control.**
2. Casteels-VanDaele M, Van Geet C, Wouters C, Eggermon E: Reye syndrome revisited: A descriptive term covering a group of heterogeneous disorders. Eur J Pediatr 159:641–648, 2000. **A comprehensive review of the multiple factors that can predispose to the combination of liver disease and noninflammatory encephalopathy that fulfills criteria for Reye syndrome.**
3. Chow EL, Cherry JD: Reassessing Reye syndrome. Arch Pediatr Adolesc Med 157:1241–1242, 2003. **A cautionary case report that reminds clinicians of the continuing problem of aspirin as a risk factor for Reye syndrome.**
4. Glasgow JTF, Middleton B: Reye syndrome—insights on causation and prognosis. Arch Dis Child 85:351–353, 2001. **New pathophysiologic data that support the epidemiologic evidence linking Reye syndrome with aspirin use during childhood viral illness.**
5. Reye RD, Morgan G, Baral J: Encephalopathy and fatty degeneration of the viscera, a disease entity in childhood. Lancet ii:749–752, 1963. **The original description of the clinical condition and pathology that has withstood the test of time.**

Lead Toxicity

Herbert L. Needleman

KEY CONCEPTS

- Most children with elevated body burdens of lead display few or no symptoms.
- There is no demonstrated threshold for lead toxicity.

- Decreased intelligence quotient (IQ) has been shown in children at levels below 10 µg/dL.
- Any child with recurrent abdominal pain, anemia, growth failure, personality change, irritability, or joint pain should have a blood lead test.
- All children should be screened for lead at 1 and 2 years of age.
- Pica is a dangerous practice.
- Any child with an elevated blood lead level (>10 µg/dL) should have an environmental and a nutritional survey.

The clinical picture of childhood lead poisoning has changed dramatically over the past 20 years. Acute symptomatic lead poisoning, once a common problem, is now a rare event. As a result of the removal of lead from gasoline, blood lead levels around the world have dropped. In 1975, the mean blood lead level in the United States was 15 µg/dL. It is now less than 2 µg/dL. Most pediatric residents will not see a case of acute plumbism during their training; few will encounter the problem in their career. Lead encephalopathy is even rarer. At the same time, epidemiologic studies from around the world of the effects of lead on children demonstrate behavioral and cognitive deficits in the absence of symptoms at levels of blood lead once considered harmless.

The definition of lead toxicity, 60 µg/dL in the 1970s, has been lowered to 10 µg/dL because of careful epidemiology. Studies published since 2000 demonstrate toxic effects below 10 µg/dL. Traditional treatments with chelating agents are ineffective at these levels of lead in blood. As a result, the principal domain of lead toxicity has shifted from the clinic and hospital to the public health arena, where the effect of lead at clinically silent levels on child development remains a major issue. A half million American children show elevated lead levels in the range associated with central nervous system damage.

Expert Opinion on Management Issues

Drug treatment is indicated for children with blood lead levels greater than 40 µg/dL, particularly if they have symptoms. Succimer (dimercaptosuccinic acid) is the agent of choice. It is given orally at 1050 mg/m² for 3 days, and then at 700 mg/m² for 16 days. This usually results in a 40% to 60% decrease in blood lead levels, which slowly begin to rise. A repeat blood lead test should be obtained at 3 to 4 weeks. If the blood lead level at that time is >35 µg/dL, a second course should be given.

If oral succimer is not tolerated, calcium ethylenediaminetetraacetic acid (EDTA) is given by intravenous drip at a dose of 1500 mg/m².

Symptoms or signs of central nervous system involvement (e.g., headache, clumsiness, changes in alertness)

should be harbingers of encephalopathy. These children require urgent treatment. In the rare case of acute encephalopathy, British anti-Lewisite (BAL) therapy is also administered in addition to EDTA or succimer. The dose of BAL is 500 mg/m² intramuscularly divided into six doses.

The central requirement of successful management is early diagnosis, which requires a degree of suspicion that leads to a blood lead test. Pharmacologic therapy is only a small part of the management. An environmental survey to determine and eliminate the source of the lead is essential, along with parental counseling and follow-up.

If neurobehavioral deficits are suspected, children should be evaluated by a neuropsychologist, the nature of the problems identified, and a psychoeducational program instituted. It is important that all siblings be screened for lead.

Common Pitfalls

- The most common error in the management of lead toxicity is the failure to screen asymptomatic children.
- Lead exposure may manifest itself in altered personality, bone pain, anemia, growth failure, headache, or abdominal pain.
- Drug treatment without environmental survey and source control is futile.

Communication and Counseling

Parents of children with elevated lead burdens need information on the potential sources of lead; the dangers of pica, thumb sucking, and nail biting; and the importance of hand washing. All siblings should be tested, and any patient with a high blood lead level (>40 µg/dL) should have a developmental evaluation.

SUGGESTED READING

1. Bellinger DC, Stiles KM, Needleman HL: Low-level lead exposure, intelligence, and academic achievement: A long-term follow-up study. Pediatrics 90:855–861, 1992. **Effects of lead during pregnancy and infancy**
2. Canfield RL, Henderson CR Jr, Cory-Slechta DA, et al: Intellectual impairment in children with blood lead concentrations below 10 micrograms per deciliter. N Engl J Med 348:1517–1526, 2003. **Recent findings of lead effects below current definition of 10 µg/dL.**
3. Grosse SD, Matte TD, Schwartz J, Jackson RJ: Economic gains resulting from the reduction in children's exposure to lead in the United States. Environ Health Perspect 110:563–569, 2002. **Authoritative benefit analysis of the removal of lead from gasoline.**
4. Needleman HL, McFarland C, Ness RB, et al: Bone lead levels in adjudicated delinquents: A case-control study. Neurotox Teratol 24:711–717, 2002. **The association between lead and crime.**
5. Needleman HL: Lead poisoning. Ann Rev Med 55:209–222, 2004. **Review of current literature, history, and treatment.**

7

Respiratory Tract

Disorders of the Larynx

Joseph Haddad, Jr.

KEY CONCEPTS

- The subglottis is the area below the vocal cords; it is the narrowest part of the pediatric airway, and inflammation in this area can cause respiratory distress.
- Stridor, or noisy breathing, results from turbulent airflow related to obstruction. Inspiratory stridor indicates obstruction at or above the larynx. Expiratory stridor indicates tracheal or bronchial obstruction. Biphasic stridor indicates subglottic or high tracheal obstruction.
- Laryngomalacia, or prolapse of supraglottic tissue, is associated with high-pitched stridor developing soon after birth, and it is the most common cause of congenital stridor.
- Flexible bronchoscopy of the upper airway and larynx is easily performed in the office setting and allows a correlation of physical findings with the phase of stridor.
- High-voltage magnified plain films, often using a filter, are routinely employed to evaluate the airway. Fluoroscopy may provide a dynamic view of the airway.
- Bilateral vocal cord paralysis is usually congenital and may be associated with Chiari malformation. Flexible bronchoscopy and MRI are necessary for diagnosis.
- Risk factors for acquired subglottic stenosis include severe prematurity, low birth weight, sepsis, gastroesophageal reflux, and multiple intubations.
- Laryngeal reconstruction using autologous rib or auricular cartilage is routinely performed to correct moderate and severe subglottic stenosis.

The pediatric and adult larynx differ in size, shape, location, and degree of calcification. After a rapid increase in size during the first 6 months of life, there is gradual growth until the adult size is reached in adolescence. The subglottis, the area below the vocal cords and the narrowest part of the airway, is half the diameter of the adult larynx, so a small amount of inflammation in this region severely limits the size of the airway. The infant larynx has a funnel shape, with its narrowest part at the subglottis, which contrasts with the more cylindrical shape of the adult larynx. The epiglottis is omega shaped and more angular in the infant, and the epiglottis and larynx sit higher in the neck compared to the adult larynx. After a relatively rapid descent in the first 4 months of life, the descent is more gradual until the adult position in the lower neck is achieved in adolescence. Gradual calcification of the larynx occurs throughout childhood, with the hyoid ossifying first (2 years of age), followed by the cricoid cartilage. The thyroid cartilage remains cartilaginous until adulthood.

Stridor, or noisy breathing, results from turbulent airflow related to obstruction. Stridor, acute or chronic, may indicate a disorder of the larynx. Respiratory distress often accompanies stridor, with labored breathing, sternal retractions, and cyanosis, which may require emergency management of the airway. A systematic workup for chronic stridor is important, and the initial evaluation should include a history of the problem and characterization of the stridor. Inspiratory stridor indicates obstruction at or above the larynx; expiratory stridor indicates tracheal or bronchial obstruction; and biphasic stridor indicates subglottic or high tracheal obstruction. Greater intensity of the stridor often correlates with more severe obstruction, and higher pitch may differentiate laryngeal from nasal or oropharyngeal obstruction. Quality of voice and cry should be included in the assessment of stridor. A careful history can help identify the etiology of stridor. For instance, acute onset associated with a barking cough and fever suggest croup. High-pitched stridor developing soon after birth, associated with positional changes, suggests laryngomalacia, the most common reason for congenital stridor.

Physical examination includes an evaluation of the entire upper airway, with attention paid to the nose and throat. The quality of the stridor is evaluated, and the infant's position can be manipulated to note if changes occur in the intensity of the stridor. A flexible laryngoscopy is routinely done in the office to achieve a dynamic assessment of the larynx, with the infant or child sitting upright in the parent's lap. Topical lidocaine and decongestant (oxymetazoline) may assist in comfortably passing the scope through the nose. The nasopharynx, pharynx, and larynx can be assessed with this procedure, and the observer can correlate the findings with the phase of audible stridor. The laryngeal examination allows assessment of overall morphology and vocal cord mobility, looking for mass lesions and evidence of congenital abnormalities.

Radiologic assessment can supplement the physical examination. Plain lateral and anteroposterior soft tissue radiographs of the neck can be helpful in evaluating the laryngeal airway. High-kilovoltage magnified plain films, sometimes using a filter to highlight the airway, are routinely employed in both elective and emergency situations. Airway fluoroscopy as an adjunct to plain films allows for an excellent dynamic view of the airway. CT and MRI have limitations in assessing the airway but can give information about soft tissue lesions compressing the larynx or central nervous system, findings that may be affecting the nerve function of the larynx.

Direct laryngoscopy under general anesthesia, often with bronchoscopy to fully evaluate the airway, may be indicated for diagnosis and treatment of certain laryngeal conditions. A wide array of pediatric laryngeal instruments are available with ventilation capabilities and excellent optics, and these allow for management of a large number of laryngeal conditions. Examination of the laryngeal airway under anesthesia affords a visual assessment of all regions of the laryngeal airway and an evaluation of airway size by passage of endotracheal tubes of known diameter.

Expert Opinion on Management Issues

Management of laryngeal disorders is based on diagnosis after evaluation of the patient as just outlined. Disorders can be classified as congenital and acquired and are discussed here by diagnosis.

CONGENITAL ANOMALIES

Laryngomalacia

Laryngomalacia is the most common congenital anomaly of the larynx. It is manifested by prolapse of supraglottic tissue, including the epiglottis and aryepiglottic folds, into the airway during inspiration. The epiglottis may appear narrow and folded. The inspiratory stridor is most pronounced when the child is supine, agitated, or crying. Stridor may lessen when the child is prone because gravity pulls the epiglottis away from the laryngeal inlet. Usually beginning a few weeks after birth, the stridor often clears by 12 to 18 months of age. Severe laryngomalacia can affect feeding, and the infant may fail to thrive. Diagnosis is based on history and physical examination and confirmed by flexible laryngoscopy. Most cases are managed conservatively, and the parents are counseled to monitor breathing carefully during episodes of upper respiratory infection. Severe cases may manifest as failure to thrive with respiratory compromise, and surgical intervention may be indicated. Under general anesthesia, the aryepiglottic folds and redundant arytenoid tissues are divided or excised, using carbon dioxide (CO_2) laser or microlaryngeal scissors. The patient is carefully monitored after extubation, and steroids and humidification are administered. When successful, this procedure may prevent the need for tracheotomy. Gastroesophageal reflux may accompany laryngomalacia and may cause swelling of the larynx and contribute to respiratory compromise.

Vocal Cord Paralysis

After laryngomalacia, vocal cord paralysis is the second most common congenital anomaly of the larynx. Most cases of bilateral vocal cord paralysis (BLVP) are congenital, and many are associated with congenital neurologic conditions, most commonly Chiari malformation, in which there is downward displacement of the brainstem into the foramen magnum with associated vagus nerve compression. Other causes include hydrocephalus, birth trauma, intubation injury, neoplasm, and infections. MRI is done in BLVP and may lead to diagnosis. Infants with BLVP have high-pitched stridor and severe respiratory compromise that worsens with exertion. Voice quality is usually normal. Diagnosis is made by flexible fiberoptic laryngoscopy with the patient awake.

When severe airway compromise is present, the airway is secured with endotracheal intubation. Central neurologic conditions may be surgically corrected and may lead to some recovery of vocal cord function. Tracheotomy often is required for persistent or uncorrectable problems. When vocal cord paralysis does not resolve over time, a surgical procedure may be considered to enlarge the laryngeal airway (vocal cord lateralization or arytenoidectomy) to allow for removal of the tracheotomy tube.

Unilateral vocal cord paralysis (UVP) is often iatrogenic secondary to surgery. The recurrent laryngeal nerve on the left side takes a course around the aorta and is prone to injury during cardiac surgery. Either or both nerves may be injured during tracheal or thyroid surgery. UVP manifests as hoarseness or breathy voice, with a weak cry. Breathing is usually good, but there may be cough and aspiration associated with feedings. When UVP is iatrogenic, nerve function may return after 6 to 9 months. Voice therapy may help with symptoms and improve voice quality.

Laryngeal Web

Congenital laryngeal webs manifest as a weak, hoarse, or muffled cry. When severe, they may cause airway compromise. Most are located in the anterior portion of the glottis and can be visualized on flexible fiberoptic laryngoscopy. However, in an infant, a small web may be obscured by the epiglottis. These small webs are confirmed by direct laryngoscopy under general anesthesia and may be lysed with a scissors or a CO_2 laser. Large or thick webs may require opening the larynx (laryngofissure) and placing a stent, with a keel placed anteriorly to prevent reformation of the web. The presence of subglottic stenosis may necessitate cartilage graft placement as well.

Laryngeal Clefts

Laryngeal clefts are rare lesions that occur in the posterior glottis and manifest with cough, aspiration, and stridor. Diagnosis may be suspected on a barium swallow study and confirmed on direct laryngoscopy by carefully examining and palpating the interarytenoid area. Type 1 is limited to the interarytenoid area above the vocal cords; type 2 extends partially through the cricoid; type 3 extends into the proximal trachea; type 4 extends into the distal airway. Most laryngeal clefts can be repaired to prevent aspiration, through an anterior or lateral pharyngotomy approach, and surgery may require a temporary tracheotomy.

Congenital Subglottic Stenosis

Congenital subglottic stenosis is caused by a malformation of the cricoid cartilage, which has failed to recanalize, with an abnormally small subglottic airway of 4 mm or less. It may manifest with a range of symptoms, from mild recurrent croup to severe stridor. Under direct laryngoscopy, which is necessary to confirm diagnosis, an age-appropriate endotracheal tube cannot be passed. When stenosis is mild, the airway grows with time and surgical intervention is not necessary. More severe cases require tracheotomy to manage the airway and laryngotracheal reconstruction to achieve decannulation.

Subglottic Hemangioma

Hemangiomas are proliferative vascular lesions that affect the skin and other organ systems, and they may occur in the subglottic airway, with symptoms of biphasic stridor or recurrent croup. Approximately half the cases of subglottic hemangiomas are associated with skin lesions. They occur most commonly in the posterior subglottis but when larger can cause circumferential obstruction. A radiograph may demonstrate asymmetric narrowing, and MRI may also demonstrate this lesion, with the diagnosis confirmed by endoscopy. These lesions tend to decrease in size after 1 year of age, but symptomatic children may require intervention. Oral corticosteroid treatment is helpful in some children; surgical treatment by microlaryngoscopy may include laser shrinkage, intralesional steroid injection, or tracheotomy.

Laryngeal Atresia

Laryngeal atresia is a rare condition that results from failure of the larynx to recanalize in week 10 of gestation, with resulting complete or near-complete airway obstruction at birth. Prompt diagnosis and tracheotomy at birth are necessary for the infant to survive. When prenatal ultrasonographic diagnosis is made, an ex utero intrapartum tracheoplasty (EXIT) fetal surgery tracheotomy can be performed. Laryngotracheal reconstruction is performed at a later surgery.

ACQUIRED ABNORMALITIES

Subglottic Stenosis

Acquired subglottic stenosis (SGS) was first recognized in the 1960s when intubation and ventilation were introduced to treat neonates with bronchopulmonary dysplasia. SGS traditionally is seen in premature infants requiring intubation and long-term ventilatory support, and it has become less common in the intervening decades as care of the premature infant has improved. It is less common at institutions where nasal continuous positive airway pressure (CPAP) is administered to avoid intubation. Although the exact etiology of acquired SGS is unclear, possible risk factors include severe prematurity, low birth weight, sepsis, gastroesophageal reflux, and multiple intubations. Tracheotomy may be performed to bypass the stenosis, but it carries significant risks, including mortality.

The surgical treatment of SGS has evolved significantly in the past 30 years. Infants with mild SGS and good pulmonary function are successfully treated with the anterior cricoid split procedure, in which the cricoid and upper tracheal rings are split and an endotracheal tube is left in place nasally for approximately 7 days. More severe cases are treated with laryngotracheal reconstruction using autologous cartilage grafts (taken from the rib or auricle). These grafts may be placed in both anterior and posterior positions to expand the subglottic airway. A variety of techniques may be employed, depending on the severity and location of the narrowing. Stents may be employed, which allow maintenance of a tracheotomy during the healing period, or the tracheotomy can be removed and an endotracheal tube placed for 1 week. Partial cricotracheal resection is performed for severe cases of SGS. In these cases the stenosed segment is removed, and the trachea and larynx are reanastomosed.

Postoperatively, antireflux medications are given, and steroids are used at the time of extubation to minimize swelling and maintain airway patency. A number of measures are taken in an attempt to improve surgical outcomes, and surgical techniques continue to evolve.

SUBGLOTTIC AND LARYNGEAL CYSTS

Short or long intubations can predispose infants and children to the development of subglottic cysts, which arise in this area from the obstruction of mucous gland ducts. These cysts may be single or multiple, and they manifest as biphasic stridor or recurrent croup.

Microlaryngoscopy confirms the diagnosis, and the cysts may be excised by CO_2 laser or marsupialization of the mucosal surface. Close follow-up is necessary because cysts may recur.

Saccular cysts (congenital laryngeal cysts, laryngeal mucocele) occur laterally or anteriorly in the larynx in the region of false vocal cords. They may be congenital or acquired because of inflammation, trauma, or tumors. Symptoms include inspiratory stridor with respiratory distress when cysts are large and a muffled cry. Diagnosis is made on awake flexible laryngoscopy, and cysts are removed surgically with a cup forceps or CO_2 laser. The child is followed carefully for signs of cyst recurrence.

Foreign Bodies

When a large foreign body, such as a chunk of food, obstructs the laryngeal airway, severe airway obstruction occurs that requires emergent action with a Heimlich maneuver. When obstruction is partial, airway distress may be moderate or intermittent, with associated voice change, and the child needs to be taken as soon as possible to the operating room for endoscopic removal of the object because the threat of total obstruction remains. If time permits and the child is not manifesting airway distress, a flexible laryngoscopy and soft tissue film of the neck may indicate type and location of the foreign body. Removal of the foreign body requires close cooperation with the anesthesiologist to maintain the airway, and a bronchoscopy should be done as well to inspect for additional foreign bodies. Undiagnosed small foreign bodies may cause a chronic cough, and a flexible laryngoscopy may be done to inspect for this etiology.

Laryngeal Trauma

Blunt or sharp laryngeal injuries are uncommon in children because of the higher position and softer consistency of the larynx in the neck. When present, these injuries may be life-threatening; symptoms vary from mild hoarseness to severe stridor and respiratory distress. Dysphagia, dyspnea, and hemoptysis may be present, and neck exam may reveal ecchymosis, crepitus, and loss of laryngeal landmarks. Cervical spine injuries are common, and radiographic examination should be obtained. Flexible fiberoptic laryngoscopy is important to examine the larynx for ecchymosis or distortion of the landmarks. CT scan is helpful in evaluating the anatomy. Emergency endoscopy is reserved for severe airway obstruction, with tracheotomy sometimes necessary. When laryngeal fracture is present, appropriate surgical repair can be done after the airway is established. This may be done electively if significant swelling or hematoma is present.

Recurrent Respiratory Papillomatosis

Human papilloma virus (HPV) may lead to the growth of exophytic lesions of the larynx. Usually caused by HPV–6 and HPV–11, this benign tumor is believed transmitted at birth from the genital tract of affected mothers; cases rarely develop in children born via cesarean delivery. Most children present in the first 5 years of life, and although the condition is benign, persistent or recurrent disease can severely impinge on the airway and cause problems with breathing and voice. The standard treatment is surgical excision in the operating room with the CO_2 laser or powered instruments, and as in other laryngeal surgeries, careful

communication is necessary with the anesthesiologist to maintain the airway. Most surgeons try to avoid tracheotomy because some think it can cause spread of disease into the trachea. Recurrences are common, and affected children should be monitored frequently in the office with follow-up flexible laryngoscopies. Because of the chronic nature of recurrent respiratory papillomatosis (RRP), adjuvant treatments are used, including interferon, indole–3-carbinol, intralesional cidofovir, and photodynamic therapy. In most patients with recurrent disease, RRP becomes quiescent during adolescence.

Other Neoplasms

RRP is the most common benign neoplasm of the pediatric larynx. Other neoplasms are quite rare. These include neurogenic tumors, such as neurofibromas, neurilemomas, and granular cell tumors. Neurofibromas may be multiple and associated with other findings, such as café-au-lait spots in Recklinghausen disease. Neurilemomas are typically solitary; granular cell tumors are extremely rare. In most cases, endoscopic removal can be performed to confirm the diagnosis and alleviate symptoms.

Malignancies of the larynx are exceedingly rare in children. Rhabdomyosarcoma is the most common, followed by squamous cell carcinoma. Treatment is multidisciplinary based on stage of disease and may involve radiation therapy, chemotherapy, and surgery.

Common Pitfalls

- Noisy breathing should be carefully evaluated to see if the noise is inspiratory, expiratory, or both because the differential diagnosis changes based on the phase affected.
- Congenital stridor is not always caused by laryngomalacia; flexible laryngoscopy is simple to perform and may demonstrate a treatable lesion.
- Gastroesophageal reflux may accompany stridor and contribute to laryngeal problems.
- Tracheotomy can be a lifesaving procedure, but the presence of a tracheotomy in an infant can pose life-threatening complications.

Communication and Counseling

Laryngomalacia is the most common cause of stridor in infants, and in most cases it is a benign condition that is outgrown during the first year of life. Once the diagnosis is established, parents can be reassured regarding the prognosis, and they are counseled about symptoms that might indicate a worsening of the airway status, such as respiratory distress, cyanosis, and poor feeding. The child should be watched carefully during episodes of upper respiratory tract infection because it may lead to respiratory difficulty. Antibiotics, short courses of steroids, and antireflux medications may all play a role in helping a child recover from an infection.

Some laryngeal conditions require tracheotomy, which can place a burden on the family when the child is discharged to home for care. Discharge should not take place until the family has learned appropriate tracheostomy care, including suctioning of secretions. The parent or caretaker should understand how to change the tracheotomy tube in the event of an emergency obstruction. Care of the skin around the tracheotomy tube is important to prevent infection and breakdown. An oxygen saturation monitor, to alert for emergencies, is commonly recommended for use when the child is asleep. A home-care nurse can play an important role in helping coordinate and monitor outpatient care.

Obstruction of a tracheotomy by a mucus plug can cause sudden death, both in the hospital and at home. Parents and caretakers need to be aware of this potential complication and understand what to do emergently when respiratory distress occurs.

SUGGESTED READINGS

1. Cotton RT, Gray SD, Miller RP: Update of the Cincinnati experience in pediatric laryngotracheal reconstruction. Laryngoscope 99:1111–1116, 1989. **A series of patients treated with laryngotracheal reconstruction for subglottic stenosis and other laryngeal problems.**
2. Holinger LD, Konior RJ: Surgical management of severe laryngomalacia. Laryngoscope 99:136–142, 1989. **An early report on the surgical management of severe laryngomalacia.**
3. Monnier P, Lang F, Savary M: Partial cricotracheal resection for severe pediatric subglottic stenosis. Update of the Lausanne experience. Ann Otol Rhinol Laryngol 107:961–968, 1998. **Work on a new approach, cricotracheal resection, for management of severe subglottic stenosis in children.**
4. Pransky SM, Magit AE, Kearns DB, et al: Intralesional cidofovir for recurrent respiratory papillomatosis in children. Arch Otolaryngol Head Neck Surg 125:1143–1148, 1999. **A report on the use of cidofovir as an adjunct in the treatment of recalcitrant laryngeal papillomas.**

Croup and Epiglottitis

Ian N. Jacobs

KEY CONCEPTS

- Laryngotracheobronchitis (LTB), also known as croup, is usually viral, in contrast to epiglottitis, which is usually bacterial.
- Deglutition and positioning are usually impaired with epiglottitis, but not LTB.
- Radiographs are useful in the diagnosis of both disorders.
- Epiglottitis has become quite rare with the advent of the *Haemophilus influenzae* vaccine.
- Anatomic narrowing of the laryngotracheal airway may predispose to recurrent LTB.
- Epiglottitis may progress rapidly and requires emergent intubation in the operating room.

Upper respiratory infections may affect the larynx, trachea, and bronchi in infants and young children, resulting in severe symptoms. For anatomic reasons, the upper airway in small children is especially vulnerable to infections. The subglottic larynx is only a 5- to 6-mm space in infants compared to 10 to 12 mm in adults, making it susceptible to closed-space infections (Fig. 1). One millimeter of inflammatory mucus effectively reduces the cross-sectional area by 32%.

Both viral and bacterial infections may cause inflammation in the pediatric airway. There have been dramatic changes in recent years in the pattern of pediatric infectious diseases of the upper airway. The *Haemophilus influenzae* vaccination has affected the incidence of bacterial epiglottitis, and newer resistant strains of bacteria have emerged in recent years. Daycare and widespread uses of antimicrobial agents have also had an impact on both laryngotracheobronchitis (LTB) and epiglottitis (Table 1).

Expert Opinion on Management Issues

ACUTE LARYNGOTRACHEOBRONCHITIS

Laryngotracheobronchitis (LTB), also known as croup, is inflammation of the upper trachea and larynx

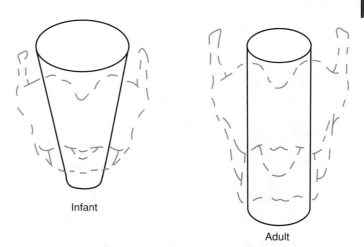

Infant

Adult

FIGURE 1. Comparison of the pediatric to the adult larynx. The infant larynx is funnel shaped with the narrowest portion in the subglottis whereas the adult larynx is narrowest at the glottis. (From Cotton RT: Management and prevention of subglottic stenosis in infants and children. In Bluestone CD, Stool SE, Kenna MA (eds): Pediatric Otolaryngology, 3rd ed. Philadelphia: WB Saunders, 1996, p 1373.)

TABLE 1 Comparison of Croup and Acute Epiglottitis

	Croup	Epiglottitis
Age	Infant	Older toddler or child
Infection	Viral	Bacterial or fungal
Swallow	Normal	Impaired
Cough	Present	Absent
Position	Normal	Abnormal

resulting in varying degrees of airway obstruction. It is usually caused by a viral infection such as parainfluenza type 1 and 2 and respiratory syncytial virus (RSV). LTB can progress rapidly and occurs most often between 1 and 3 years of age. Children typically present with barky seal-like coughs, biphasic stridor, and retractions. A child can progress to near total airway obstruction in a short time.

Diagnosis

The typical clinical picture of a small child with a croupy barking cough, rhinorrhea, stridor, and upper airway symptoms suggests the diagnosis of LTB. Tachypnea and chest retractions may be observed as well. In contrast to epiglottitis, there is usually no drooling, odynophagia, or abnormal positioning. Diagnosis is confirmed by plain films of the neck that show the classic "steeple sign" narrowing for 1 to 2 cm in the subglottic airway (Fig. 2). Other findings include ballooning and overdistention of the hypopharynx.

Flexible fiberoptic laryngoscopy is rarely needed to confirm the diagnosis, but it rules out other pathology including epiglottitis (Fig. 3). Rigid endoscopy in the operating room is generally not advised because instrumentation of the airway may increase the degree of airway obstruction. The differential diagnosis includes epiglottis and bacterial tracheitis.

Treatment

The management of LTB, which is mostly supportive, includes humidification, hydration, steroids, and parental reassurance. Most cases may be treated in the outpatient setting. Children with severe stridor, chest retractions, and respiratory distress should be hospitalized. They can be given intravenous hydration and warm humidity ("croup tent") while on telemetry. Supplemental oxygen may be needed as well. Intensive care unit (ICU) observation is occasionally needed for severe cases.

Although the use of corticosteroids remains controversial for LTB, they may be useful for severe cases because they relieve soft tissue edema and improve airway symptoms. For outpatients with marked stridor, oral prednisone at 1 to 2 mg/kg/day may be helpful. For the hospitalized patient in the ICU, intravenous dexamethasone may be administered at 0.5 to 2 mg/kg/dose every 8 hours.

In the acute situation, nebulized racemic epinephrine may be given to relieve upper airway edema for several hours but may lead to rebound swelling several hours later. Helium and oxygen mixtures, called *heliox*, are occasionally given to lesson the viscosity of airflow and maintain ventilation as the infection subsides. The measures just described may avoid the need for endotracheal tube intubation. Nevertheless, some patients get worse despite all interventions, and intubation is required. The endotracheal tube should be appropriately sized for the age of the child and severity of the LTB. A smaller-than-age-appropriate endotracheal tube should be selected and daily air leaks checked. When leak pressure falls below 25 cm H_2O, extubation should be attempted. Children who fail extubation may require a tracheotomy.

Rarely are direct laryngoscopy and rigid bronchoscopy indicated for long-standing or persistent LTB that fails to resolve within 7 to 10 days or for children with recurrent bouts. When there is acute inflammation, instrumentation of the airway should be avoided, but

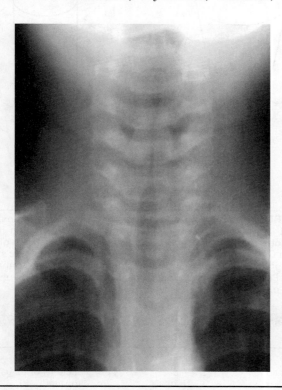

FIGURE 2. AP radiograph revealing a long segment of glottic and subglottic narrowing. Normally the glottic narrow segment is less than 1 cm.

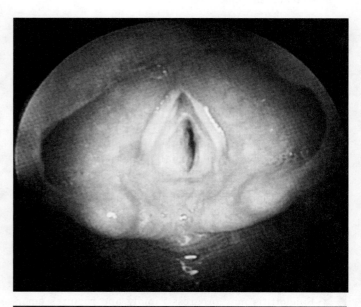

FIGURE 3. Direct endoscopic view revealing glottic and subglottic inflammation with laryngotracheobronchitis.

for various reasons, some cases do not resolve. With recurrent LTB, endoscopy should be deferred until no signs of acute infection remain. In such cases, an underlying airway pathology, such as subglottic stenosis, hemangioma, or cysts (Fig. 4), may be diagnosed and treated to prevent further bouts of croup.

ACUTE EPIGLOTTITIS

Epiglottitis is an acute inflammation of the epiglottis and the supraglottic larynx. It is usually caused by bacterial infection of the airway. The epiglottis may swell and progress rapidly to complete airway obstruction. The most common bacterial organism is *H. influenzae,* but with the advent of the *H. influenzae* vaccine, the incidence of bacterial epiglottitis has declined dramatically in the last 15 years. Nevertheless, it can still occur and may be related to other types of pathogens.

Diagnosis

Typical signs and symptoms of acute epiglottitis include drooling, odynophagia, and "hot potato voice." The child often positions in an extended and upright posture to maximize airflow. The patient often has difficulty handling secretions and pain upon swallowing (odynophagia). Acute epiglottitis may progress to complete airway obstruction in a very short time. Any agitation may provoke complete obstruction.

Diagnosis is made by clinical history and lateral neck radiographs that reveal an enlarged and thickened epiglottis, also known as the "thumbprint sign" (Fig. 5). When there is impending airway obstruction, the diagnosis is confirmed by direct inspection in the operating room (Fig. 6). The patient should be transported under close supervision to the operating room where there are experienced staff and available airway equipment. The patient should undergo a smooth mask induction with spontaneous ventilation until the airway is secured by intubation. Depending on the preference of the staff at the hospital, the patient may be intubated orally or nasally. During the intubation, rigid laryngoscopes, bronchoscopes, and a tracheotomy set should be at hand in the event the airway is lost.

Treatment

Once the diagnosis is made, the airway is secured and the patient is kept intubated for several days. Special care should be taken to avoid accidental extubation. Treatment includes broad-spectrum antibiotics to cover *H. influenzae* and intubation for 48 to 72 hours until epiglottic swelling subsides. Direct inspection at

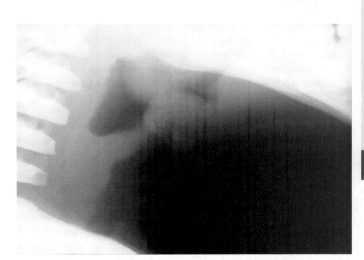

FIGURE 5. Lateral radiograph revealing thumbprint sign with thickened epiglottis.

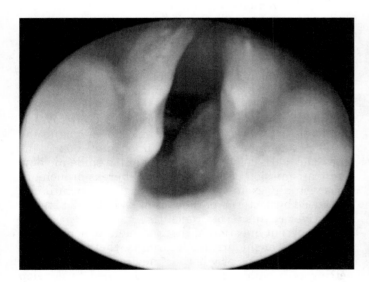

FIGURE 4. Subglottic cysts that predispose to laryngotracheobronchitis.

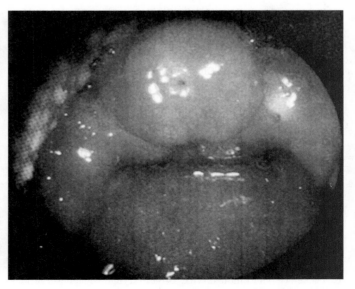

FIGURE 6. Direct endoscopic visualization of epiglottis.

the bedside with an intubation laryngoscope can confirm resolution of the process. As an alternative, an air leak test can be performed at the bedside to assess the airway status prior to extubation; however, direct visualization with a laryngoscope at the bedside is preferable. Extubation is accomplished in the ICU with continued telemetry, respiratory care, and intravenous antibiotics until discharge.

Common Pitfalls

With LTB, failure to understand the significance of recurrent LTB or LTB at an exceedingly young age may indicate an anatomic problem. An infant with persistent LTB symptoms has an anatomic anomaly until proven otherwise. Recognition and treatment of the anomaly help prevent future episodes of LTB.

With the widespread use of the *H. influenzae* vaccine, epiglottitis is now exceedingly rare. Newly trained clinicians may not be familiar with the treatment protocols, which may lead to a failure to recognize and treat epiglottitis properly. New house staff should discuss and review standard protocols of epiglottitis management.

Communication and Counseling

Most cases of epiglottitis and LTB can be easily diagnosed and treated for successful outcomes. It is imperative to understand the clinical features of epiglottitis and LTB because their treatment is quite different. The *H. influenzae* vaccine has made epiglottitis an exceedingly rare disorder. When epiglottitis does occur, one must move rapidly and skillfully toward securing a safe airway in a protected environment where all support is available.

SUGGESTED READINGS

1. Grosz A, Jacobs IN, Cho C, Schears G: Use of helium oxygen mixtures to relieve upper airway obstruction in a pediatric population. Laryngoscope 111:1512–1514, 2001. **A review of how oxygen and helium gas mixtures are used to treat LTB and other airway diseases.**
2. Holinger PH, Kutnick SL, Schild JA, et al: Subglottic stenosis in infants and children. Ann Otol Rhinol Laryngol 85:591–599, 1976. **Review of the anatomy of subglottic stenosis and the effective reduction in the cross-sectional area of the airway with these disease processes.**
3. Hudgins PA, Jacobs IN, Castillo M: Pediatric airway disease. In Som PM, Curtin HD (eds): Head Neck Imaging. Chicago: Mosby, 1996, pp 545–611. **Radiologic description of the infant and child airway with illustrations of radiologic features of LTB and epiglottitis.**
4. Shah RK, Roberson DW, Jones DT: Epiglottitis in the *Haemophilus influenzae* type B vaccine era: Changing trends. Laryngoscope 114(3):557–560, 2004. **The effect of the vaccine on the incidence of epiglottitis.**
5. Spector GJ: Developmental anatomy of the larynx. In Ballenger JJ (ed): Diseases of the Ear, Nose, and Throat, Head and Neck, 13th ed. Philadelphia: Lea and Febiger, 1985. **A review of the embryology and development of the pediatric airway.**
6. Tucker G: The infant larynx: Direct laryngoscopic observations. JAMA 99:1899–1902, 1932. **Original description of the anatomic features of the infant larynx.**

Bronchitis and Bronchiolitis

Julian Lewis Allen

KEY CONCEPTS

- Bronchitis affects the completely cartilaginized conducting airways. Bronchiolitis affects the partially cartilaginized conducting and respiratory bronchioles.
- Bronchiolitis is nearly exclusively viral in origin. Bronchitis, although predominantly viral, can also be caused by bacteria, mycoplasma, chlamydia, and *Bordetella pertussis*.
- Bronchiolitis is transmitted by fomites and direct contact; adherence to strict infection control is an effective means of prevention.
- The relationships among bronchiolitis, bronchitis, and asthma are unclear; management depends on accurate recognition of the underlying role asthma may play. Bronchitis should not be treated with bronchodilators, and asthma exacerbations should not be treated with antibiotics.
- Effective prophylaxis exists for prevention of respiratory syncytial virus (RSV) bronchiolitis. Treatment of established disease is more controversial: Bronchodilators, corticosteroids, epinephrine, and antiviral agents may be effective in some, but by no means all, infants, and they should not be considered routine therapy.

Lower respiratory tract infections (LRIs) include bronchitis, bronchiolitis, and pneumonia; this chapter deals with the first two, and the third is discussed in the article "Pneumonia" in the section on infectious diseases. These are very prevalent conditions; for bronchiolitis alone, nearly all infants are infected by the respiratory syncytial virus (RSV) by 2 years of age; 25% to 40% of these infants develop bronchiolitis, and 1% are hospitalized, with 57% of those hospitalized younger than 6 months of age.

The distinctions among bronchitis, bronchiolitis, and pneumonia are both anatomic and symptomatic. Bronchitis affects the completely cartilaginized conducting airways (generations 0 to 3). Bronchiolitis affects the partially cartilaginized conducting and respiratory bronchioles (generations 4 to 16). The size of the airways affected by bronchiolitis changes with age. In adults, bronchioles are approximately 0.6 mm (more peripheral airways) to 5 mm (more central airways) in diameter. In infants, they can be an order of magnitude smaller. Pneumonia is alveolar in location. Box 1 outlines the pathology, causative agents, epidemiology, and transmission of bronchiolitis. Whereas bronchiolitis is virtually exclusively viral in origin, bronchitis can be caused by bacterial pathogens as well. Box 2 lists the causative organisms of bronchitis.

A recurrent question in the treatment of acute bronchitis and bronchiolitis in children is whether they are de novo conditions or whether they have arisen in the setting of a child who has or is destined to develop asthma. RSV bronchiolitis, for example, is clearly associated with the development of asthma; up to 50% of

BOX 1 Pathophysiology of Bronchiolitis

Pathology

- Infected bronchiolar epithelial cells in airways 75 to 300 μm in diameter resulting in necrosis and sloughing of cells into the airway lumen.
- Partial or complete airway obstruction, increased airways resistance, hypoxemia, and cyanosis.
- Mononuclear cells (lymphocytes and macrophages) infiltrate the peribronchial tissue, leading to airway wall and interstitial edema. Neutrophils are the most common inflammatory cells recovered from bronchoalveolar lavage.
- Regeneration of bronchiolar epithelium may take months and lags behind clinical signs of recovery.

Causative Agents

- Respiratory syncytial virus (RSV) most common cause (50% to 90% of those infants hospitalized).
- Other agents associated: human parainfluenza viruses (type 3 is second most common cause), influenza, adenovirus, human metapneumovirus, *Mycoplasma pneumoniae* (in older children).

Epidemiology

- Occurs from late fall through the winter and early spring in the United States, earlier in the Southeast and throughout the year in some areas (e.g., Florida, Hawaii).
- Infection rate: 68.8 of 100 infants less than 1 year of age; 82.6 of 100 infants during the second year.
- Mortality: primary RSV infection in otherwise healthy children: 3.1 deaths per 100,000 person-years in infants under 1 year of age; approximately 1% to 3% among children with underlying conditions.
- Risk factors for acquisition of RSV infection: birth during the months of April through September; daycare attendance or older siblings in daycare; crowded living conditions; lower socioeconomic status; exposure to environmental cigarette smoke or other air pollutants; lower cord serum RSV antibodies; absence of breast-feeding; multiple births.

Transmission

- Close contact with infected secretions, large particle aerosols, and fomites.
- Self-inoculation of conjunctivae or nose with infected hands.
- Secretions remain infectious on countertops and stethoscopes for up to 6 hours, rubber gloves for 1.5 hours, and on hands or tissue for approximately 30 minutes.
- Viral shedding: up to 21 days after infection but can extend to several weeks or months in immunocompromised patients.

BOX 2 Causative Agents of Bronchitis

- **Viral:** Rhinovirus, RSV, parainfluenza.
- **Bacterial:** *Haemophilus influenzae, Streptococcus pneumoniae, Bordetella pertussis.*
- **Other:** *Mycoplasma pneumoniae, Chlamydia pneumoniae.*
- **Disease specific:** *Pseudomonas aeruginosa* in cystic fibrosis and chronic bronchitis, encapsulated organisms in B cell deficiencies, for example.

BOX 3 Diagnosis of Bronchiolitis

Imaging

- Findings of chest radiography include:
  - Hyperinflation, flattened diaphragms.
  - Peribronchial thickening.
  - Patchy or more extensive atelectasis.
  - Possible collapse of a segment or a lobe.
  - Diffuse interstitial infiltrates commonly seen.

Rapid Viral Identification

- Immunofluorescence (direct or indirect IFA [immune fluorescent antibody]).
- Enzyme immunoassay (EIA). Advantage: rapid results (15–30 min), does not require the presence of a viable virus. Sensitivity ranges from 57% to 97%; specificity: 69% to 100%.

Viral Culture

- Culture of nasopharynx may improve sensitivity in patients with negative rapid respiratory studies.

---

insults. This may explain why the results of studies evaluating asthma therapies (bronchodilators and corticosteroids) for bronchiolitis, without accounting for the presence of underlying asthma, often conflict. Furthermore, guidelines on asthma therapy from the National Institutes emphasize that acute wheezing illnesses should not be treated with antibiotics unless bacterial superinfection (fever, purulent sputum, positive bacterial cultures) is clearly evident. Thus areas of overlap exist between acute LRIs and asthma exacerbations, and distinguishing the two can be difficult.

Distinguishing LRIs diagnostically is largely based on history and physical examination. Homophonous or central wheezing and rhonchi are often heard in bronchitis, whereas heterophonias wheezing is characteristic of bronchiolitis. Rales or crackles may signify an alveolar component but can be heard in bronchiolitis as well. Box 3 outlines the diagnostic studies for infants with suspected bronchiolitis. Insufficient data exist to show that chest radiograph films reliably distinguish between viral and bacterial disease or predict severity of disease. Numerous studies demonstrate that rapid RSV tests have acceptable sensitivity and specificity, but no data show that RSV testing affects clinical outcomes in typical cases of the disease. The exception might be in febrile infants less than 2 months of age, in whom the knowledge of a positive RSV test might obviate the need for further invasive studies to rule out sepsis.

Treatment of bronchitis and bronchiolitis is controversial; a meta-analysis of studies of bronchiolitis showed no effect of such interventions as steroids, bronchodilators, and ribavirin but noted most studies were underpowered to show differences and did not assess such important outcomes as duration and need for hospitalization. A U.S. Agency for Healthcare Research and Quality report in 2004 reviewed results of studies of ribavirin, epinephrine, ipratropium bromide, β_2-agonist bronchodilators, inhaled and oral corticosteroids, and antibiotics; it concluded that strong and

---

infants with bronchiolitis develop subsequent wheezing. Causality is more difficult to determine: RSV may influence the immune system toward the development of a predominantly T-helper (cell) type 2 (Th2) asthmatic phenotype, but infants with inherent airway hyperreactivity are also more likely to wheeze with viral

convincing evidence of effectiveness was not identified for any of the treatments. Several interventions, however, do show some potential for efficacy, as discussed later, and prophylaxis against bronchiolitis with anti-RSV antibodies, as opposed to treatment, shows clear evidence of effectiveness (Box 4). There are currently two preparations, high-titer human RSV intravenous immunoglobulin (RSV-IVIG) and humanized mouse monoclonal antibodies against RSV (palivizumab). Details of RSV prophylaxis are discussed in the article "Respiratory Syncytial Virus" in the section on infectious diseases. Perhaps the most important preventive measure in patients hospitalized for other reasons are contact precautions, careful hand washing, avoidance of contact with infected patients and staff, and use of gowns, gloves, goggles, and perhaps masks.

Expert Opinion on Management Issues

BRONCHIOLITIS

The only accepted interventions for bronchiolitis are supportive. Outpatient measures include adequate fluid intake and maintenance of nasal airway patency with short-term nasal decongestant and suctioning of secretions with a suction bulb. Inpatient measures include careful fluid hydration and supplemental (warmed and humidified) oxygen therapy given to any patient with hypoxemia. There are a number of controversial interventions, described next.

Bronchodilators

Although bronchodilators are frequently used in the management of bronchiolitis, a meta-analysis of 20 randomized, controlled trials of bronchodilator responsiveness showed modest improvement of clinical signs or symptoms in some patients but no improvement in measures of oxygenation, the rate of hospitalization, or duration of hospitalization. In any meta-analysis, inclusion of studies that enrolls people with recurrent wheeze may bias results in favor of bronchodilators. Small benefits must be weighed against the costs of these agents. One study estimated that if 80% of children with bronchiolitis were treated with bronchodilators, the total annual cost of providing inhaled bronchodilator therapy to infants with first-time RSV bronchiolitis in the United States would be $37.5 million.

Although indiscriminate use of bronchodilators in infants with bronchiolitis is not recommended, there is a subset of infants with bronchiolitis who demonstrate significant bronchodilator responsiveness. Recent advances in infant lung function testing may provide more sensitive measurements of changes in airway function and improve our understanding of the role of bronchodilator therapy in infants with bronchiolitis. Until this procedure becomes more widely available, it is reasonable to give all infants with bronchiolitis with significant wheezing a trial of aerosolized β_2-adrenergic treatment to see if symptoms are relieved at all, especially if there is a history of prior wheezing or family history of asthma or atopy. Theophylline should be avoided because it may worsen gastroesophageal reflux. Methylxanthines may have a role in the treatment of apnea if present.

Nebulized Epinephrine

Because of the known pathophysiologic component of airway edema in bronchiolitis (see Box 1), trials of inhaled agents with both α- and β-adrenergic effects were performed (most notably epinephrine). In a meta-analysis comparing aerosolized epinephrine to placebo and albuterol, insufficient evidence supported the use of epinephrine among inpatients. Although epinephrine was found favorable compared with placebo and albuterol for short-term benefits among outpatients, further large multicenter trials are required before routine use among outpatients can be strongly recommended. Racemic epinephrine and L-epinephrine were studied separately and showed beneficial results compared with β-agonists, but there are no specific guidelines regarding the optimal dose and frequency.

Corticosteroids

Unlike patients with asthma, infants with bronchiolitis usually do not exhibit a favorable response to corticosteroids. It is not possible to determine whether some of the favorable effects of systemic corticosteroids in treating bronchiolitis are the result of treating infants experiencing acute asthma episodes, because some studies include infants with a previous history of wheezing. A recent meta-analysis demonstrated a minimal (half-day) reduction of length of stay and duration of symptoms among those infants receiving corticosteroids. If only the studies excluding patients with previous wheezing were analyzed, however, this difference was no longer significant. The greatest effects of corticosteroid use are seen in those infants with the most severe clinical course (i.e., requiring mechanical ventilation). Administration of systemic corticosteroids during the acute phase of bronchiolitis does not prevent wheezing in the subsequent year or the development of asthma in patients by 5 years of age.

Inhaled corticosteroids are also used in the treatment of acute bronchiolitis. No beneficial effects are seen in infants treated with either budesonide alone or budesonide in combination with terbutaline relative to placebo, either in infants less than 12 months of age or in children 12 to 24 months of age. Similarly, no long-term benefits of inhaled corticosteroids in preventing subsequent wheezing or bronchodilator use are shown.

Leukotriene Receptor Antagonists

One study showed that a 1-month course of therapy with montelukast immediately following hospitalization for RSV bronchiolitis is superior to placebo in preventing subsequent pulmonary symptoms during a 2-month follow-up period.

Antibiotics

Antibiotics are not usually indicated except in rare instances of superimposed bacterial infection.

Antiviral Agents (Ribavirin)

Although ribavirin has in vitro antiviral activity against RSV, placebo-controlled trials do not show consistent benefits in duration of hospitalization, duration of intensive care unit stay, or need for mechanical ventilation. In addition, high cost and exposure of health care workers to potential toxic effects from aerosol administration argue against routine use of ribavirin.

BRONCHITIS

Unlike bronchiolitis, bronchitis rarely results in enough ventilation/perfusion mismatch to cause hypoxemia, unless it is associated with asthma; supplemental oxygen is therefore usually not needed, and if it is, it suggests an asthmatic overlay. Similarly, bronchodilators are not effective in either children or adults unless there is underlying airflow obstruction such as in asthma. Nonspecific bronchitis in healthy children does not warrant antibiotic treatment. Antibiotics may be indicated for suspected or proven bacterial infection by the organisms listed in Box 2. Box 5 summarizes the management of both bronchitis and bronchiolitis.

Common Pitfalls

BRONCHIOLITIS

- Hypoxemia may be clinically inapparent; follow pulse oximetry.

> **BOX 5 Management**
>
> **Bronchiolitis**
> - Accepted: oxygen, fluid replacement therapy
> - Controversial: bronchodilators, corticosteroids, epinephrine, ribavirin
>
> **Bronchitis**
> - Accepted: none
> - Controversial: antibiotics, bronchodilators

- Apnea is possible in young infants, especially former preterms.
- Incipient respiratory failure may be present even in presence of normal oxygen saturations; if supplemental oxygen is given; observe closely for signs of respiratory fatigue, and measure blood gases if incipient respiratory failure is suspected.
- Recognize that bronchodilator therapy is controversial but therapeutic trials may be useful in individual infants, especially if underlying airway hyperreactivity is suspected from history.
- RSV-IVIG (intravenous immunoglobulin) (but not palivizumab) is contraindicated in infants with cyanotic congenital heart disease.

BRONCHITIS

- Antibiotics are often not necessary; most bronchitis is self-limited.
- Most cases of recurrent bronchitis are actually unrecognized asthma; a high index of suspicion is needed.

Communication and Counseling

RSV prevention is critical for high-risk infants, and parents and caregivers should be educated about decreasing exposure and transmission of RSV. Measures such as limiting exposure to child-care centers, limiting exposure to other children and adults with respiratory viral infections, hand hygiene, avoiding tobacco smoke exposure, and scheduling RSV prophylaxis vaccinations should all be reviewed. In addition, the relationship between RSV infection and the development of asthma should be discussed. The difference between asthma exacerbations and bronchitis should be emphasized, especially in the context of avoiding antibiotic use for treatment of asthma flares.

SUGGESTED READINGS

Overviews of Bronchiolitis Pathophysiology, Diagnosis, and Treatment

1. Bordley WC, Viswanathan M, King VJ, et al: Diagnosis and testing in bronchiolitis: A systematic review. Arch Pediatr Adolesc Med 158:119–126, 2004. **Examines sensitivity and specificity**

8

of tests for bronchiolitis but concludes that accurate diagnosis does not necessarily alter outcomes.

2. Fitzgerald DA, Kilham HA: Bronchiolitis: Assessment and evidence-based management. Med J Aust 180:399–404, 2004. **Concludes there is no role for nebulized adrenaline, inhaled and systemic corticosteroids, or inhaled bronchodilators in routine management.**

3. King VJ, Viswanathan M, Bordley WC, et al: Pharmacologic treatment of bronchiolitis in infants and children: A systematic review. Arch Pediatr Adolesc Med 158:127–137, 2004. **A review of 54 randomized controlled trials between 1980 and 2002. The efficacy of interventions such as epinephrine, β₂-agonists, corticosteroids, and ribavirin are analyzed.**

4. Martinon-Torres F: Current treatment for acute viral bronchiolitis in infants. Expert Opin Pharmacother 4:1355–1371, 2003. **Emphasizes importance of supportive care including supplemental oxygen and adequate hydration.**

5. Panitch HB: Bronchiolitis in infants. Curr Opin Pediatr 13:256–260, 2001. **A good overview.**

Bronchodilators for Bronchiolitis

1. Kellner JD, Ohlsson A, Gadomski AM, Wang E.E.L.: Bronchodilators for bronchiolitis. Cochrane Database Syst Rev 2:CD001266, 2000. **Some studies show that bronchodilators produce modest improvements in clinical scores, but there are no differences from placebo in measures of oxygenation or rate and duration of hospitalization.**

Epinephrine for Bronchiolitis

1. Hartling L, Wiebe N, Russell K, et al: Epinephrine for bronchiolitis. Cochrane Database Syst Rev 1:CD003123, 2004. **Although insufficient evidence supports the use of epinephrine for inpatients with bronchiolitis, it may be favorable compared to albuterol or placebo in outpatients.**

2. Mull CC, Scarfone RJ, Ferri LR, et al: A randomized trial of nebulized epinephrine vs. albuterol in the emergency department treatment of bronchiolitis. Arch Pediatr Adolesc Med 158:113–118, 2004. **Infants treated with epinephrine were ready for emergency room discharge after 90 minutes, on average 30 minutes sooner than the albuterol-treated group.**

3. Wainwright C, Altamirano L, Cheney M, et al: A multicenter, randomized, double-blind, controlled trial of nebulized epinephrine in infants with acute bronchiolitis. N Engl J Med 349:27–35, 2003. **Found no significant reduction in length of stay in infants treated with nebulized epinephrine compared to placebo.**

Corticosteroids for Bronchiolitis

1. Chao LC, Lin YZ, Wu WF, Huang FY: Efficacy of nebulized budesonide in hospitalized infants and children younger than 24 months with bronchiolitis. Acta Paediatr Taiwan 44:332–335, 2003. **No benefits (alone or in combination with terbutaline) shown in clinical symptoms or hospital length of stay compared to placebo or terbutaline.**

2. Garrison MM, Christakis DA, Harvey E, et al: Systemic corticosteroids in infant bronchiolitis: A meta-analysis. Pediatrics 105(4): E44, 2000. **Demonstrates modest improvement in length of stay (half day) and clinical scores in the steroid-treated groups.**

Leukotriene Receptor Antagonists for Bronchiolitis

1. Bisgaard H: Study group on montelukast and respiratory syncytial virus. A randomized trial of montelukast in respiratory syncytial virus postbronchiolitis. Am J Respir Crit Care Med 167:379–383, 2003. **Demonstrates montelukast superior to placebo in preventing pulmonary symptoms in the 2 months following hospitalization for RSV bronchiolitis.**

Bronchodilators for Bronchitis

1. Smucny J, Flynn C, Becker L, Glazier R: Beta₂-agonists for acute bronchitis. Cochrane Database Syst Rev 1:CD001726, 2004. **No improvement, unless there is concomitant airflow obstruction.**

Bronchiectasis
Robert W. Wilmott

KEY CONCEPTS

- Bronchiectasis is uncommon, except in children with immune deficiency, abnormal mucociliary clearance, or cystic fibrosis (CF).
- In bronchiectasis, the airway wall is damaged permanently, with dilation of the airway and poor drainage of secretions.
- The most common symptom is a chronic, productive cough.
- Physical examination typically shows an area of dullness to percussion, with coarse inspiratory crackles.
- The diagnosis can be confirmed reliably by high-resolution CT of the chest.
- Treatment consists of a regular program of chest physical therapy, and some patients benefit from bronchodilator treatment.
- Acute exacerbations are treated with broad-spectrum antibiotics guided by sputum culture.
- Surgery has a role in patients with localized disease, obstructing foreign bodies or tumors, and massive hemorrhage.

Laennec first described bronchiectasis in 1819 and defined it as the irreversible dilation of one or more bronchi. It results from structural damage to the airway wall that causes irreversible dilation of airways, with resulting pooling of secretions, impaired mucociliary clearance, and an increased risk of recurrent or persistent infection. Bronchiectasis is now a relatively rare pediatric lung disorder, except in children with an inherited or acquired predisposition toward recurrent pulmonary infection (Table 1). It is classified as cystic, cylindrical, or varicose, based on the morphologic abnormalities of the airways. Clinical features of bronchiectasis are given in Table 2. The majority of children with bronchiectasis present before 7 to 8 years of age.

Expert Opinion on Management Issues

MEDICAL THERAPY

Medical treatment focuses on trying to prevent recurrent infections and the development of further affected areas. A mainstay of medical therapy is daily chest physical therapy that can be delivered manually or with mechanical assistance from a high-frequency oscillating vest (e.g., ThAIRavest) or a mechanical percussor.

Antibiotic therapy is guided by regular culture and sensitivity testing of sputum. Acute pulmonary exacerbations should be treated with short-term courses of antibiotics. In children, a broad-spectrum antibiotic such as trimethoprim-sulfamethoxazole or amoxicillin-clavulanate is usually the first choice. In patients known to have colonization with *Pseudomonas aeruginosa*, the best choice is one of the fluoroquinolones, such as ciprofloxacin, which is now regarded as safe for pediatric use. Pediatric case series demonstrate a good safety profile and allay earlier concerns about risks to developing bone and cartilage. Treatment usually lasts for 10 to 14 days or until symptoms resolve. Routine

prophylactic antibiotics have only limited efficacy for preventing infections, although a Cochrane review demonstrated a small clinical effect from long-term antibiotics. Following the successful introduction of high-dose aerosolized tobramycin in cystic fibrosis (CF), a double-blind placebo-controlled study was performed in adults with bronchiectasis and showed a significant effect on sputum colony counts of *P. aeruginosa* but not on pulmonary function.

Although some patients with bronchiectasis complain of wheezing, they tend to have fixed airway obstruction and may respond poorly, or not at all, to bronchodilator therapy. Unfortunately, there are no randomized, long-term controlled trials of either β-agonist or anticholinergic bronchodilators. Some individual patients do seem to receive clinical benefit from bronchodilator therapy, especially those with reversible airway obstruction demonstrated on pulmonary function testing.

Mucolytic therapy seems intuitively attractive for the treatment of bronchiectasis. Hypertonic saline by aerosol is used successfully in CF, asthma, and chronic bronchitis, although it has not been tested in bronchiectasis. Studies on inhaled mannitol powder show encouraging results, and long-term studies are recommended. DNA released by host neutrophils and bacteria is a major component of sputum and contributes significantly to its viscosity. Inhaled dornase alfa (Pulmozyme), which is efficacious in CF, was studied in a moderately large randomized, controlled trial. After 6 months, the 173 patients who received active drug had significantly more pulmonary exacerbations and a significantly reduced forced expiratory volume at 1 second (FEV_1) compared to 176 patients who received placebo. Dornase alfa is therefore an approved therapy for CF, but it should not be used in children with bronchiectasis.

TABLE 1 Causes of Bronchiectasis

- Retained foreign body
- Asthma with mucus plugging
- Chronic sinusitis
- Recurrent aspiration
- Increased susceptibility to infection
    - Cystic fibrosis (CF)
    - Immunoglobulin (Ig) deficiencies (especially IgG and IgA)
    - Complement deficiency
    - Neutrophil defects
    - Immotile cilia syndrome
    - Human immunodeficiency virus (HIV)
- Severe infections in a normal host
    - Measles
    - Pertussis
    - Tuberculosis
    - Adenovirus
- Inflammation
    - Allergic bronchopulmonary aspergillosis complicating CF or asthma
    - α_1-Antitrypsin deficiency
- Congenital
    - Williams-Campbell syndrome (congenital absence of bronchial cartilage)
    - Mounier-Kuhn syndrome (congenital tracheobronchomegaly)
    - Marfan syndrome
    - Yellow nail syndrome (yellow nails, lymphedema, pleural effusion, bronchiectasis)
    - Isolated congenital bronchiectasis

TABLE 2 Clinical Features of Bronchiectasis

Symptoms	Physical Examination	Laboratory
<ul><li>Chronic cough</li><li>Oral fetor</li><li>Chronic production of yellow or green sputum</li><li>Dyspnea or wheezing</li><li>Chest pain</li><li>Hemoptysis: usually streaking; rarely massive (>450 mL)</li><li>Recurrent exacerbations of symptoms, with fever, increased coughing, change in sputum production, wheezing, and malaise</li></ul>	<ul><li>Productive coughing</li><li>Halitosis</li><li>Digital clubbing (less common in recent series)</li><li>Persistent area of consolidation<ul><li>Dullness to percussion</li><li>Coarse crackles on auscultation</li></ul></li></ul>	<ul><li>Chest radiograph<ul><li>Persistent area of consolidation</li><li>Tram-line shadowing</li><li>Nodular cystic shadowing</li></ul></li><li>CT scan<ul><li>Consolidation</li><li>Tram-line shadowing</li><li>Signet ring sign</li></ul></li><li>Pulmonary function tests<ul><li>Assess severity</li><li>Identify reversible airway obstruction</li></ul></li><li>Sweat test</li><li>Serum immunoglobulins</li><li>Sputum culture<ul><li>*Haemophilus influenzae*</li><li>*Streptococcus pneumoniae*</li><li>*Pseudomonas aeruginosa*</li><li>Tuberculosis</li></ul></li><li>Sputum acid-fast bacilli (AFB)</li><li>Ciliary biopsy</li></ul>

The pathogenesis of bronchiectasis has a component of inflammation, and therapeutic approaches may include the use of anti-inflammatory drugs. The most common are inhaled corticosteroids such as beclomethasone and fluticasone. Controlled trials in adults show therapeutic benefit from both treatments, but no comparable data exist for children. Systemic anti-inflammatory treatment with steroidal or nonsteroidal anti-inflammatory compounds have not been extensively studied in bronchiectasis per se, although ibuprofen was studied in children with CF and resulted in a reduction of the rate of decline in FEV_1, with fewer hospital admissions and improved nutritional status.

SURGICAL THERAPY

Surgery has a smaller role in the management of bronchiectasis compared to 50 years ago, but there are well-accepted indications:

- Removal of a foreign body
- Removal of an obstructing tumor
- Resection of an isolated, severely affected part of the lung
- Control of massive hemorrhage
- Removal of bronchiectatic areas suspected of harboring multiresistant organisms, such as *Mycobacterium avium* complex

In the patient with localized bronchiectasis, surgery has a role in reducing symptoms. Before recommending surgery to such a patient, it is important to verify that the disease is localized by performing high-resolution chest CT scans and by ruling out diseases that usually result in diffuse bronchiectasis. Ventilation-perfusion scans may also be useful to characterize the extent of disease.

Bilateral single lung transplant is now the treatment of choice for patients with CF with advanced pulmonary disease when the FEV_1 drops to the predicted 30% to 40%. It has a 5-year survival rate of approximately 50%. Other causes of severe diffuse bronchiectasis are treated by lung transplantation with good results, although separate statistics on outcomes are not available.

PREVENTIVE MEASURES

Serious infections should be prevented with routine childhood immunizations. These are very successful in reducing the prevalence of bronchiectasis in developed countries, although it is still common in the rest of the world. Prompt treatment of lower airway infections and recognition and treatment of atelectasis caused by mucus plugging in asthma, respiratory syncytial virus (RSV) infection, and other such conditions associated with atelectasis prevent the development of bronchiectasis.

Common Pitfalls

Prior to the development of high-resolution chest CT scans, bronchograms were often used to diagnose bronchiectasis or to evaluate a patient for surgery. This technique had a significant complication rate and since the advent of CT is rarely necessary. Sometimes the surgeon requires more detail in children being evaluated for surgical resection. In such cases, selective bronchograms can be performed safely by flexible bronchoscopy using small amounts of contrast medium.

Complications

The systemic blood supply to the lung, the bronchial arterial system, is in close proximity to the airway. Infection in the airway can therefore result in hemoptysis. This is uncommon, except in CF, where it occurs in a significant proportion of patients and can be severe (massive hemoptysis).

Massive hemoptysis is treated by hospitalization with monitoring of vital signs, hemoglobin, and coagulation times. Bleeding may be localized by CT scan or bronchoscopy. Good results are reported with angiography and embolization using coils or polyvinyl alcohol particles; surgery is required if conservative approaches cannot control the bleeding.

Communication and Counseling

Children with bronchiectasis must be evaluated for infection whenever they have an exacerbation of symptoms or intercurrent infections. Bronchiectasis affecting the upper lobes is usually mild because the lobes drain secretions under the influence of gravity. Bronchiectasis is not necessarily progressive unless there is an underlying immune defect. No evidence indicates that an affected segment or lobe acts as a focus of infection that will spread to other lobes and cause progressive bronchiectasis.

SUGGESTED READINGS

1. Barker AF: Bronchiectasis. N Engl J Med 346:1383–1393, 2002. **A comprehensive review of bronchiectasis in adults.**
2. Barker AF, Couch L, Fiel SB, et al: Tobramycin solution for inhalation reduces sputum *Pseudomonas aeruginosa* density in bronchiectasis. Am J Respir Crit Care Med 162:481–485, 2000. **A placebo-controlled, double-blind randomized trial of aerosolized high-dose tobramycin (TOBI) in 74 adult patients with bronchiectasis. There was a significant reduction in the density of P. aeruginosa in sputum after 4 weeks of therapy but no significant change in pulmonary function.**
3. Evans DJ, Bara AI, Greenstone M: Prolonged antibiotics for purulent bronchiectasis. Cochrane Database Syst Rev 2:CD001392, 2002. **Six clinical trials included 302 patients with antibiotics given for 4 weeks to 1 year, which resulted in a small significant clinical effect.**
4. Konstan MW, Byard PJ, Hoppel CL, Davis PB: Effect of high-dose ibuprofen in patients with cystic fibrosis. N Engl J Med 332:848–854, 1995. **Treatment with high-dose ibuprofen therapy over 4 years resulted in a significant reduction in the rate of decline in FEV_1 for patients who were 5 to 12 years of age, with fewer hospitalizations and improved nutritional status.**
5. O'Donnell AE, Barker AF, Ilowite JS, Fick RB: Treatment of idiopathic bronchiectasis with aerosolized recombinant human DNase I. Chest 113:1329–1334, 1998. **A randomized double-blind,**

placebo-controlled trial of dornase alfa in 349 stable adults with bronchiectasis. After 24 weeks there was a greater decline in FEV₁ and an increased number of exacerbations in the actively treated group.

6. Wills P, Greenstone M: Inhaled hyperosmolar agents for bronchiectasis. Cochrane Database Syst Rev 1:CD002996 2002. **Authors comment that dry powder mannitol improves tracheobronchial clearance in bronchiectasis, and further trials of mannitol and hypertonic saline are indicated.**

Asthma

T. Bernard Kinane and Christina V. Scirica

KEY CONCEPTS

- Asthma is the most common pediatric chronic disease in the developed world.
- The pathogenesis of asthma involves genetic, developmental, and environmental factors that lead to airway inflammation, hyperresponsiveness, and obstruction.
- Comprehensive patient education and follow-up is of paramount importance in the management of asthma.
- An important component of asthma therapy is reduction of exposure to common triggers, such as viral infections, tobacco smoke, animal dander, indoor mold, dust mites, and cockroach allergens.
- A stepwise approach to maintenance asthma therapy is recommended:
  - Children with mild intermittent asthma do not require daily controller medications and should receive treatment only in the setting of active symptoms or worsening pulmonary function.
  - Children with persistent asthma require daily preventive anti-inflammatory therapy, of which the first-line choice is generally an inhaled corticosteroid.
  - The daily dose of inhaled corticosteroids is generally increased, and other medications added, in accordance with the severity of asthma.
  - Treatment should be started at higher-level intensity at the beginning to control asthma symptoms and then ramped down once good asthma control is attained.
- All patients with asthma should receive additional therapy in the setting of acute asthma symptoms. Commonly used medications for this purpose are β-agonists, corticosteroids, and anticholinergic agents.

Asthma is the most common pediatric chronic disease in the developed world, affecting nearly 5 million children in the United States. The pathogenesis of asthma involves a complex interaction among genetic, developmental, and environmental influences that lead to airway inflammation, hyperresponsiveness, and airway obstruction.

The diagnosis of asthma is generally made by obtaining a careful history, performing a thorough physical exam, and measuring lung function objectively. Common signs and symptoms of asthma include cough, shortness of breath, and wheezing. Physical

examination is often normal between flares but may reveal high-pitched expiratory wheezing, a prolonged expiratory phase, and accessory muscle use, particularly during acute exacerbations. Although chest radiographs are a relatively insensitive and nonspecific tool for diagnosing asthma, they often reveal hyperinflation and peribronchial cuffing. Spirometry and measurement of peak expiratory flow may be helpful in diagnosing asthma and monitoring response to therapy, as can provocation testing with exercise or methacholine.

The National Asthma Education and Prevention Program of the National Heart, Lung, and Blood Institute (NHLBI) classifies asthma into four categories: mild intermittent, mild persistent, moderate persistent, and severe persistent (Tables 1 and 2). These categories are used to guide the most appropriate choice of therapy for each individual patient.

Expert Opinion on Management Issues

The NHLBI guidelines call for a stepwise approach to therapy in which patients are managed according to the persistence and severity of their symptoms. The guidelines state that children with mild intermittent asthma do not require daily controller medications and should receive treatment only in the setting of active symptoms or worsening pulmonary function. Children with persistent asthma as defined by the guidelines should be prescribed daily preventive anti-inflammatory therapy, of which the first-line choice is generally an inhaled corticosteroid. The daily dose of inhaled corticosteroids is usually increased, and other medications are added in accordance with the severity of asthma. This stepwise approach calls for treatment to be started at higher-level intensity at the beginning of treatment to control asthma symptoms and for the intensity of therapy to be ramped down once good asthma control is attained. In addition to maintenance therapy, all patients with asthma should receive short-acting bronchodilators as needed for acute asthma symptoms. These and other medications used for asthma are each reviewed in turn in subsequent sections (Table 3).

In addition to treatment with medications, patients must be counseled to avoid common triggers, such as tobacco smoke, animal dander, indoor mold, dust mites, and cockroach allergens. Viral infections, including influenza, are also frequent triggers; therefore all patients older than 6 months of age with asthma should receive the influenza vaccine annually. Furthermore, because comorbid conditions such as sinusitis and gastroesophageal reflux disease (GERD) may worsen asthma symptoms, these conditions should be identified and treated if present.

MAINTENANCE THERAPY

Corticosteroids

Inhaled corticosteroids are the mainstay of therapy for persistent asthma. Inhaled corticosteroids reduce

TABLE 1 Stepwise Approach for Managing Asthma in Infants and Young Children (5 Years of Age and Younger): NHLBI Guidelines

Classify Severity and Clinical Features before Treatment or Adequate Control

Severity of Asthma	Daytime Symptoms / Nighttime Symptoms	Medications Required to Maintain Long-Term Control
Step 4: Severe persistent	Continual / Frequent	**Preferred treatments:** ■ High-dose inhaled corticosteroids *and* ■ Long-acting inhaled β_2-agonists *and*, if needed ■ Corticosteroid tablets or syrup long term (2 mg/kg/day; generally do not exceed 60 mg per day). (Make repeat attempts to reduce systemic corticosteroids and maintain control with high-dose inhaled corticosteroids.)
Step 3: Moderate persistent	Daily / >1 night/wk	**Preferred treatments:** ■ Low-dose inhaled corticosteroids and long-acting inhaled β_2-agonists *or* ■ Medium-dose inhaled corticosteroids. **Alternative treatment:** ■ Low-dose inhaled corticosteroids and either leukotriene receptor antagonist or theophylline. If needed (particularly in patients with recurring severe exacerbations): **Preferred treatment:** ■ Medium-dose inhaled corticosteroids and long-acting β_2-agonists. **Alternative treatment:** ■ Medium-dose inhaled corticosteroids and either leukotriene receptor antagonist or theophylline.
Step 2: Mild persistent	>2/wk but <1/day / >2 nights/mo	**Preferred treatment:** ■ Low-dose inhaled corticosteroids (with nebulizer or MDI with holding chamber with or without face mask or DPI). **Alternative treatment (listed alphabetically):** ■ Cromolyn (nebulizer is preferred or MDI with holding chamber) *or* ■ Leukotriene receptor antagonist.
Step 1: Mild intermittent	≤2 days/wk / ≤2 nights/mo	No daily medication needed.

Quick Relief for All Patients:

■ Bronchodilator as needed for symptoms. Intensity of treatment depends on severity of exacerbation.
  Preferred treatment: short-acting inhaled β_2-agonists by nebulizer or face mask and space/holding chamber.
  Alternative treatment: oral β_2-agonists.
■ With viral respiratory infection:
  Bronchodilator q4–6h up to 24 h (longer with physician consult); in general, repeat no more than once q6wk.
  Consider systemic corticosteroid if exacerbation is severe or patient has history of previous severe exacerbations.
■ Use of short-acting β_2-agonists more than two times a week in intermittent asthma (daily, or increasing use in persistent asthma) may indicate the need to initiate (increase) long-term-control therapy.

DPI, dry powder inhaler; MDI, metered-dose inhaler; NHLBI, National Heart, Lung, and Blood Institute; q, every.

Adapted from NHLBI, National Asthma Education and Prevention Program. Expert Panel Report: Guidelines for the Diagnosis and Management of Asthma—Update on Selected Topics. NIH Publication No. 02–5075. Bethesda, Md: U.S. Department of Health and Human Services, 2002.

symptoms of asthma, decrease airways hyperresponsiveness, improve baseline lung function, reduce the use of rescue medications and systemic steroids, and decrease the rate of urgent care visits and hospitalizations for asthma. Inhaled corticosteroids are available as nebulized solutions, metered-dose inhalers (MDIs), and dry powder inhalers. Corticosteroids may effectively be delivered by MDI with spacer to most young children and infants, although some prefer to use nebulizers in this age group.

TABLE 2 Stepwise Approach for Managing Asthma in Adults and Children Older Than 5 Years of Age: NHLBI Guidelines

Severity of Asthma	Classify Severity and Clinical Features before Treatment or Adequate Control		Medications Required to Maintain Long-Term Control
	Daytime Symptoms Nighttime Symptoms	**PEF or FEV$_1$ PEF Variability**	
Step 4: Severe persistent	Continual Frequent	≤60% >30%	**Preferred treatment:** ■ High-dose inhaled corticosteroids *and* ■ Long-acting inhaled β$_2$-agonists *and*, if needed ■ Corticosteroid tablets or syrup long term (2 mg/kg/day; generally do not exceed 60 mg per day). (Make repeat attempts to reduce systemic corticosteroids and maintain control with high-dose inhaled corticosteroids.)
Step 3: Moderate persistent	Daily >1 night/wk	>60%-<80% >30%	**Preferred treatment:** ■ Low- to medium-dose inhaled corticosteroids and long-acting inhaled β$_2$-agonists. **Alternative treatment:** ■ Increase inhaled corticosteroids within medium-dose range *or* ■ Low- to medium-dose inhaled corticosteroids and either leukotriene modifier or theophylline. If needed (particularly in patients with recurring severe exacerbations): **Preferred treatment:** ■ Increase inhaled corticosteroids within medium-dose range and add long-acting inhaled β$_2$-agonists. **Alternative treatment:** ■ Increase inhaled corticosteroids within medium-dose range and add either leukotriene modifier or theophylline.
Step 2: Mild persistent	>2/wk but <1/day >2 nights/mo	≤80% 20%–30%	**Preferred treatment:** ■ Low-dose inhaled corticosteroids. **Alternative treatment** (listed alphabetically): ■ Cromolyn, leukotriene modifier, nedocromil, *or* sustained-release theophylline to serum concentration of 5 to 15 µg/mL. ■ No daily medication needed. ■ Severe exacerbations may occur, separated by long periods of normal lung function and no symptoms. A course of systemic corticosteroids is recommended.
Step 1: Mild intermittent	≤2 days/wk ≤2 nights/mo	≥80% <20%	

Quick Relief for All Patients:

■ Bronchodilator as needed for symptoms. Intensity of treatment depends on severity of exacerbation.
  Preferred treatment: Short-acting inhaled β$_2$-agonists by nebulizer or face mask and space/holding chamber.
  Alternative treatment: Oral β$_2$-agonists.
■ Use of short-acting β$_2$-agonists more than two times a week in intermittent asthma (daily, or increasing use in persistent asthma) may indicate the need to initiate (increase) long-term-control therapy.

FEV$_1$, forced expiratory volume in 1 second; NHLBI, National Heart, Lung, and Blood Institute; PEF, peak expiratory flow.
Adapted from NHLBI, National Asthma Education and Prevention Program. Expert Panel Report: Guidelines for the Diagnosis and Management of Asthma—Update on Selected Topics. NIH Publication No. 02–5075. Bethesda, Md: U.S. Department of Health and Human Services; 2002.

Triamcinolone and flunisolide have the lowest potency of the available corticosteroids; beclomethasone and budesonide are generally classified as intermediate potency. Fluticasone is usually classified as second-generation corticosteroid because it has a greater anti-inflammatory effect while also demonstrating

TABLE 3 Asthma Medications

Medication	Dosage/Route/Regimen	Maximum Dose	Formulation	Common Adverse Reactions	Comments
Corticosteroids (anti-inflammatory; inhibit cytokine production and inflammatory cell activity)					
Triamcinolone (Azmacort) Rx	INH: 6–12 yr: 1–2 puffs tid-qid; ≥12 yr: 2 puffs tid-qid or 2–4 puffs bid.	6–12 yr: 1200 µg/day; ≥12 yr: 1600 µg/day.	Inhaler: 100 µg/actuation	Pharyngitis, cough, xerostomia, oral candidiasis	Not recommended for children <6 yr; rinse mouth thoroughly after use.
Flunisolide (AeroBid, AeroBid-M) Rx	INH: 2 puffs bid.	2000 µg/day.	Inhaler: 250 µg/actuation	Nausea, diarrhea, vomiting, headache	Not recommended for children <6 yr; rinse mouth thoroughly after each use.
Beclomethasone (Qvar) Rx	INH: (1 actuation = 40 µg): 5–11 yr: 1–2 puffs bid; ≥12 yr: 2 puffs tid-qid; INH: (1 actuation = 80 µg):≥6 yr: 2 puffs bid.	5–11 yr: 160 µg/day; ≥12 yr: 640 µg/day.	Inhaler: 40, 80 µg/ actuation	Headache, pharyngitis, rhinitis	Not recommended for children <6 yr; rinse mouth after use.
Budesonide (Pulmicort Respules, Pulmicort Turbuhaler) Rx	NEB: 1–8 yr: 0.25–0.5 mg qd-bid; INH: ≥6 yr: Start at 1 puff bid and increase as needed; adults: 1–4 puffs bid.	NEB: no prior steroids: 0.5 mg/day; prior steroid use: 1 mg/day; INH: no prior steroids: 800 µg/ day; prior steroid use: 1600 µg/day.	NEB: 0.25, 0.5 mg/2 mL; inhaler: 200 µg/actuation	Rhinitis, cough, oral candidiasis	Rinse mouth after use.
Fluticasone (Flovent, Flovent Rotadisk) Rx	MDI: 4–11 yr: 44–110 µg bid; ≥12 yr: 88–880 µg bid; DPI: 4–11 yr: 50–100 µg bid; ≥12 yr: 100–1000 µg bid.	MDI: 4–11 yr: 220 µg/day; ≥12 yr with no prior oral steroid use: 880 µg/day; ≥12 yr with prior oral steroid use: 1760 µg/ day; DPI: 4–11 yr: 200 µg/day; ≥12 yr with no prior oral steroid use: 1000 µg/day; ≥12 yr with prior oral steroid use: 2000 µg/day.	MDI: 44, 110, 220 µg/ actuation; DPI: 50, 100, 250 µg/actuation	Headache, nasal congestion, pharyngitis, oral candidiasis, dysphonia	Rinse mouth after use.
Prednisone (Deltasone, Sterapred) Rx	PO: 1–2 mg/kg/day PO div qd-bid for 5–7 days.	80 mg/day.	Tablet: 1, 2.5, 5, 10, 20, 50 mg; oral suspension: 5 mg/5 mL	Nausea, vomiting, appetite change, mood swings, hyperglycemia	Taper if treatment exceeds 5–7 days.
Prednisolone (Prelone, Orapred, Pediapred) Rx	PO: 1–2 mg/kg/day PO div qd-bid for 5–7 days.	80 mg/day.	Oral suspension: 5, 15 mg/5 mL	Nausea, vomiting, appetite change, mood swings, hyperglycemia	Taper if treatment exceeds 5–7 days.
Methylprednisolone succinate (Solu-Medrol) Rx	IM/IV: 2 mg/kg first dose, then 2 mg/kg/day div q6h.		IV: (sodium succinate) 40, 125, 500, 1000, 2000 mg/vial; IM: (acetate) 20, 40, 80 mg/mL	Nausea, vomiting, appetite change, mood swings, hyperglycemia	

Leukotriene Receptor Antagonists (inhibit LTD_4 and LTE_4 receptors in the leukotriene pathway)

Drug	Dose	Max dose	How supplied	Side effects	Comments
Zafirlukast (Accolate) Rx	PO: 5–11 yr: 10 mg bid; ≥12 yr: 20 mg bid.		Tablet: 10, 20 mg	Headache, dizziness, nausea, diarrhea.	Use with caution in liver disease.
Montelukast (Singulair) Rx	PO: 12–48 mo: 4 mg qhs (granules); 2–5 yr: 4 mg qhs; 6–14 yr: 5 mg chewable qhs; >14 yr: 10 mg qhs.		Granules packet: 4 mg; chewable tablet: 4, 5 mg; tablet: 10 mg	Headache, flulike symptoms, abdominal pain.	Chewable form should not be used in patients with phenylketonuria.

β-Agonists (cause smooth muscle relaxation by activating adenylate cyclase and increasing cAMP)

Drug	Dose	Max dose	How supplied	Side effects	Comments
Albuterol (Ventolin, Proventil, AccuNeb) Rx	NEB: <1yr: 0.05–0.15 mg/kg/dose q4–6h; 1–5yr: 1.25–2.5 mg/dose q4–6h; 5–12 yr: 2.5 mg/dose q4–6h; >12 yr: 2.5–5.0 mg/dose q6h; aerosol MDI: 1–2 puffs q4–6h; Rotacaps: 200–400 µg q4–6h.		NEB: 5 mg/mL; 2.5 mg/3 mL; aerosol MDI: 90 µg/actuation	Tachycardia, tremor, insomnia, nausea, headache.	For acute exacerbations, may give q20min × 3 then q1–4h.
Levalbuterol (Xopenex) Rx	NEB: 6–11 yr: 0.31–0.63 mg q6–8h prn; ≥12 yr: 0.63–1.25 mg q6–8h prn.		NEB: 0.31, 0.63, 1.25 mg/3 mL	Tachycardia, tremor, insomnia, nausea, headache.	Mixing with other NEB not recommended.
Terbutaline (Brethine) Rx	SC: ≤12 yr: 0.005–0.01 mg/kg/dose q15min × 2; >12 yr: 0.25 mg/dose q15 min × 2; IV: 2–10 µg/kg loading dose then 0.1–0.4 µg/kg/min infusion; PO: 6–12 yr: 0.05 mg/kg tid; 12–15 yr: 2.5 mg tid; >15 yr: 2.5–5 mg tid.	SC: ≤12 yr: max 3 doses; >12 yr: 0.5 mg/4 h; PO: 6–12 yr: 0.15 mg/kg/ dose or 5 mg/day; 12–15 yr: 7.5 mg/day; >15 yr: 15 mg/day.	SC/IV injection: 1 mg/mL; Tablet: 2.5, 5 mg	Tachycardia, tremor, insomnia, nausea, headache.	Titrate infusion in increments of 0.1–0.2 µg/kg/min q30min.
Salmeterol (MDI, Serevent Diskus) Rx	MDI: persistent asthma: >4 yr: 2 puffs bid; exercise-induced asthma: >12 yr: 2 puffs 30–60 min before exercise; DPI: persistent asthma: >4 yr: 1 puff bid; exercise-induced asthma: 1 puff 30–60 min before exercise.	2 puffs/day	MDI: 21 µg/actuation; DPI: 50 µg/actuation	Tachycardia, tremor, insomnia, nausea, headache.	Not for acute treatment; onset of action: 10–20 min.
Formoterol (Foradil) Rx	INH: 12 µg q12h.	24 µg/day.	Inhaler: 12 µg/power cap	Tachycardia, tremor, insomnia, nausea, headache.	Not recommended for children <5 yr.

Nonsteroidal Anti-inflammatory Medications (stabilize mast cell membranes and inhibit eosinophil and epithelial cell activation)

Drug	Dose	Max dose	How supplied	Side effects	Comments
Cromolyn (Intal) Rx	INH: children: 1–2 puffs tid-qid; adults: 2–4 puffs tid-qid; NEB: 20 mg q6–8h.		INH: 800 µg/actuation; NEB: 20 mg/2 mL	Rash, cough, bronchospasm, nasal congestion.	Not for acute treatment; use with caution in renal or liver disease
Nedocromil (Tilade) Rx	INH: 2 puffs qid.		INH: 1.75 mg/actuation	Bitter taste, dry mouth, pharyngitis, cough, nausea.	Not recommended for children <6 yr; may reduce dose to bid-tid after improvement

Continued

TABLE 3—cont'd

Medication	Dosage/Route/Regimen	Maximum Dose	Formulation	Common Adverse Reactions	Comments
Anti-IgE Antibodies					
Omalizumab (Xolair) Rx	SC: 150–375 mg q2–4wk dose based on IgE level and weight.	150 µg/injection site; div doses >150 µg.	SC: 150 mg	Injection site reaction, viral infection, headache.	Not recommended for children <12 yr; for aeroallergen-associated asthma
Methylxanthines (cause smooth muscle relaxation by inhibiting phosphodiesterase and possibly by antagonizing adenosine)					
Theophylline (Theo-24, Theolair, Theophylline and 5% Dextrose, Uniphyl) Rx	PO: Loading dose: 1 mg/kg/dose for each 2 mg/L desired change in theophylline level. Maintenance: >1 yr and wt <45 kg: begin at 12–14 mg/kg/day div q4–6h and may gradually increase to 16–20 mg/kg/day div q4–6h; >1 yr and ≥45 kg: begin with 300 mg/day div q6–8h and may gradually increase to 400–600 mg/day.	If >1 yr and <45 kg: max starting dose is 300 mg/day; max total dose 600 mg/d. Goal therapeutic level 10–20 µg/mL.	Immediate-release: capsule/tablet: 100, 125, 200, 250, 300 mg; solution: 80 mg/15 mL; sustained-release: capsule/tablet: 100, 125, 200, 250, 300, 400, 450, 600 mg	Nausea, headache, vomiting, insomnia.	Serum levels should be monitored as drug metabolism varies widely; sustained release forms should not be chewed or crushed.
Anticholinergic Agents (cause bronchodilation by inhibiting muscarinic acetylcholine receptors)					
Ipratropium (Atrovent) Rx	INH: <12 yr: 1–2 puffs tid-qid; ≥12 yr: 2–3 puffs qid; NEB: infants and children: 250 µg q6–8h; >12 yr: 250–500 µg q6–8h.	INH: 12 puffs/day.	INH: 17 µg/spray (HFA) 18 µg/spray; NEB: 500 µg/2.5 mL	Cough, nervousness, nausea, dry mouth.	Contraindicated if soy or peanut allergy and atropine sensitivity; use with caution in narrow-angle glaucoma or urinary obstruction.
Combination Products					
Fluticasone/Salmeterol (Advair Diskus) Rx	INH: 100/50 µg bid. Titrate as deemed appropriate.	500 µg fluticasone + 50 µg salmeterol bid.	MDI: 100, 250, or 500 mg fluticasone + 50 µg salmeterol per actuation	See fluticasone and salmeterol; pharyngitis, cough, oral candidiasis, dysphonia, tremor.	Not approved in children <12 yr; titrate to lowest strength after asthma controlled.

bid, twice daily; cAMP, cyclic adenosine monophosphate; DPI, dry powder inhaler; div, divided; IM, intramuscular; INH, inhalation; IV, intravenous; LTD$_4$, leukotriene D$_4$; LTE$_4$, leukotriene E$_4$; NEB, nebulized solution; PO, by mouth; prn, as needed; q, every; qd, every day; qid, four times per day; qhs, every bedtime; Rx, prescription; tid, three times per day; SC, subcutaneous; wt, weight.

increased first-pass metabolism and therefore less systemic effect. Common local side effects of inhaled corticosteroids, such as candidiasis and dysphonia, may be minimized through proper technique, use of a holding chamber, and rinsing the mouth after administration. When used at doses less than 400 μg per day beclomethasone equivalent, the risk of systemic side effects is minimal. In contrast, high-dose inhaled corticosteroid use is associated with systemic effects, including adrenal suppression, thinning of the skin, delayed growth, and ocular complications.

Leukotriene Modifiers

Leukotriene modifiers include both the leukotriene receptor antagonists such as zafirlukast and montelukast and the leukotriene synthesis inhibitor zileuton. The leukotriene receptor antagonists generally have greater appeal because of their large therapeutic index and easier dosing. Both zafirlukast and montelukast decrease asthma symptoms, reduce the use of short-acting bronchodilators, and improve lung function. The leukotriene receptor antagonists are generally somewhat less effective than inhaled corticosteroids when used as monotherapy, but they have a role when used either in conjunction with inhaled corticosteroids or alone, particularly in patients with allergy-associated asthma. Zileuton has been discontinued for use in the United States because of its many side effects.

β-Agonists

Data suggest that the addition of a long-acting β-agonist to inhaled corticosteroid therapy is more beneficial than doubling the dose of corticosteroids. The bronchodilating effects of these medications last up to 12 hours and therefore are given twice daily. Of note, salmeterol has a greater delay in onset of action than formoterol. Long-acting β-agonists should not be used for treatment of acute asthma symptoms because of the prolonged half-life and delay in onset of action. In patients who experience exercise-induced asthma, short-acting β-agonists are often used prophylactically prior to exercise to prevent bronchospasm; long-acting β-agonists are also effective for this indication. Long-acting β-agonists may also be used for the treatment of allergen-induced asthma, although they only treat symptoms and do not prevent the underlying inflammation associated with this condition.

Nonsteroidal Anti-inflammatory Medications

Cromolyn and nedocromil stabilize mast cells and reduce eosinophil chemotaxis. These medications are less effective than both inhaled corticosteroids and leukotriene modifiers and are therefore now considered alternative treatments for mild to moderate persistent asthma. They improve symptoms in patients with exercise-induced asthma and are particularly useful for this indication, either alone or in conjunction with a short-acting β-agonist. They may also be used to treat allergen-induced asthma or as pretreatment prior to allergen exposure.

Anti-Immunoglobulin E Medications

Omalizumab is an anti-immunoglobulin (Ig) E antibody treatment recently approved for second-line treatment of children 12 years of age and older with moderate to severe allergy-related asthma. A recent study found that those who used omalizumab in addition to inhaled corticosteroids had fewer asthma exacerbations and were able to decrease their corticosteroid dose.

Methylxanthines

Although rarely used in pediatric asthma therapy because of its low therapeutic index, sustained-release theophylline is occasionally helpful as a steroid-sparing medication in patients dependent on oral corticosteroids and for control of nocturnal asthma symptoms. Studies suggest that lower levels than previously thought are effective in reducing symptoms of asthma. However, theophylline levels should nonetheless be monitored routinely, especially during acute illnesses and when patients are given medications that may reduce its clearance.

THERAPY FOR ACUTE ASTHMA EXACERBATIONS

Oxygen

Patients with asthma often develop hypoxemia because of ventilation-perfusion mismatch. The use of bronchodilators may cause pulmonary vasodilation in poorly ventilated areas, exacerbating hypoxemia. Therefore humidified oxygen should be delivered to maintain an oxygen saturation of 92% to 95%.

Short-Acting β-Agonists

Selective short-acting β-agonists are an essential component of treatment for acute asthma symptoms. The most commonly used inhaled β-agonist is albuterol. Levalbuterol consists of only the R-isomer of racemic albuterol and has greater potency than racemic albuterol. Terbutaline is often used for more severe asthma exacerbations, although studies have failed to demonstrate improved effectiveness compared with albuterol. Although initial data suggested that intravenous (IV) administration of β-agonists was more effective than nebulized therapy, recent studies found that IV infusion offers no benefit compared with inhaled β-agonists and is often associated with increased toxicity. MDIs with spacers appear equally as effective as nebulized solutions in nonintubated asthmatics older than 2 years of age but only if used with correct technique. Side effects of frequent or continuous administration of β-agonists are common and include tachycardia, tremor, hypokalemia, and irritability.

Because of the effectiveness and widespread availability of selective β-agonist medications, subcutaneous epinephrine is rarely indicated for the treatment of asthma. It is sometimes used in very severe cases and in situations in which selective β-agonist medications are not readily available.

Anticholinergic Agents

Ipratropium causes additional bronchodilation when used in conjunction with a β-agonist. Its use reduces admissions and improves lung function when given with albuterol to patients in the emergency department. Data on the use of ipratropium in patients admitted for acute asthma exacerbations are mixed, but the benefit appears greatest in patients admitted with severe exacerbations.

Corticosteroids

The data supporting the use of short-duration systemic corticosteroid therapy are unequivocal. Therefore all patients presenting with moderate-to-severe asthma exacerbations should be given systemic steroids for 3 to 5 days, although longer courses may be required for patients with very severe or prolonged exacerbations. As long as patients are able to tolerate and absorb oral medications, orally administered corticosteroids are equally as effective as parenteral methylprednisolone. Although prednisone or prednisolone was historically given at a dose of 2 mg/kg/day, a recent study found the use of 1 mg/kg/day to be equally as effective as 2 mg/kg/day, with fewer behavioral side effects. Data on the effectiveness of inhaled corticosteroids for the treatment of acute asthma exacerbations are inconsistent. Therefore, until further data are available, routine use of inhaled glucocorticoids for acute asthma exacerbations is not recommended.

Magnesium Sulfate

The use of magnesium sulfate in children with asthma remains controversial. If magnesium sulfate is used, magnesium levels should be checked before and half an hour after administration. Blood pressure should be monitored closely because magnesium may be associated with hypotension.

Methylxanthines

Given the narrow therapeutic indices of theophylline and aminophylline, their use is generally not recommended and should be reserved for severe asthma exacerbations refractory to other therapies. If methylxanthines are used, loading and maintenance doses should be carefully calculated and levels monitored to minimize the risk of toxicity.

Heliox

A 70:30 mixture of helium and oxygen, heliox has lower density than room air and reduces airways resistance among patients with both asthma and severe croup. Its use is generally reserved for patients with severe asthma exacerbations. A significant disadvantage of heliox is its low oxygen content, precluding its use in patients requiring supplemental oxygen.

Bicarbonate

The use of bicarbonate to correct respiratory acidosis is controversial and may be associated with side effects such as rebound metabolic alkalosis and blunting of ventilatory drive. It is therefore not recommended.

Mechanical Ventilation

Bronchospasm, hyperinflation, and air trapping often complicate the intubation and mechanical ventilation of patients with asthma. For this reason, intubation should be considered a therapy of last resort. If necessary, controlled intubation with sedatives and paralytic agents is far safer than emergent intubation of patients with asthma. Once the patient is intubated, complications may be minimized by using short inspiratory times with long expiratory times to allow for adequate expiration and minimize air trapping.

Common Pitfalls

One of the major pitfalls in asthma management is underdiagnosis of the disorder, particularly among infants and young children in whom the diagnosis of asthma may be difficult. Similarly, a frequent finding among patients with suboptimal asthma control is poor understanding and inappropriate use of asthma medications. Older children and adolescents whose asthma treatment plan is inadequately supervised by caregivers are at particular risk for suboptimal therapy. Overuse of short-acting β-agonists and poor inhaler technique are common among patients with asthma. Additional pitfalls include failure to recognize and treat early signs and symptoms of acute asthma exacerbations adequately, as well as identification and management of exacerbating conditions, such as GERD or rhinitis. Medical conditions that may mimic asthma include congenital anatomic abnormalities of the airways, allergic rhinitis or sinusitis, vocal cord dysfunction, and GERD. Misdiagnosis of these conditions as asthma may lead to failure of standard asthma therapy.

Communication and Counseling

Education is of paramount importance in the management of pediatric asthma. Patients and their families must be counseled regarding the avoidance of environmental triggers of asthma symptoms, as well as the precise role of each medication prescribed. Patients and their families should be taught to recognize and monitor the signs and symptoms of asthma that indicate the need for medical evaluation and/or modification of therapy. In addition, many practitioners find it useful to provide patients with a written asthma management plan that outlines the daily care plan as well as steps to take during acute exacerbations.

SUGGESTED READINGS

1. Hendeles L, Sherman J: Are inhaled corticosteroids effective for acute exacerbations of asthma in children? J Pediatr 142:26–33, 2003. **Review of studies on the use of inhaled corticosteroids for treatment of acute asthma exacerbations.**
2. Hsu JT: Are inhalers with spacers better than nebulizers for children with asthma? J Fam Pract 53:55–57, 2004. **Brief review of studies comparing the effectiveness of nebulizers with that of MDIs and spacers in children with asthma.**
3. Kayani S, Shannon DC: Adverse behavioral effects of treatment for acute exacerbation of asthma in children: A comparison of two doses of oral steroids. Chest 122:624–628, 2002. **Prospective, randomized, blinded trial of 1 mg/kg/day versus 2 mg/kg/day of prednisone or prednisolone.**
4. Leone FT, Fish JE, Szefler SJ, et al: Systematic review of the evidence regarding potential complications of inhaled corticosteroid use in asthma: Collaboration of American College of Chest Physicians, American Academy of Allergy, Asthma Immunology, and American College of Allergy, Asthma and Immunology. Chest 124:2329–2340, 2003. **Expert panel report on the safety of inhaled corticosteroid use.**
5. Liu AH, Spahn JD, Leung DYM: Childhood asthma. In Behrman RE, Kliegman RM, Jenson HB (eds): Nelson Textbook of Pediatrics, 17th ed. Philadelphia: WB Saunders, 2004, pp 760–774. **Comprehensive review of the pathophysiology, diagnosis, and treatment of childhood asthma.**
6. Milgrom H: Is there a role for treatment of asthma with omalizumab? Arch Dis Child 88:71–74, 2003. **Review of the mechanism of action of omalizumab and early data on its use in asthma.**
7. NHLBI, National Asthma Education and Prevention Program. Expert Panel Report II: Guidelines for the Diagnosis and Management of Asthma. U.S. Department of Health and Human Services: Bethesda, Md, 1991. NIH Publication No. 97–4051. **Original guidelines for the diagnosis and management of asthma published by the National Asthma Education and Prevention Program.**
8. NHLBI, National Asthma Education and Prevention Program. Expert Panel Report: Guidelines for the Diagnosis and Management of Asthma—Update on Selected Topics. U.S. Department of Health and Human Services: Bethesda, Md, 2002. NIH Publication No. 02–5075. **Updated guidelines for the diagnosis and treatment of childhood asthma.**
9. Rodrigo GJ, Rodrigo CR: The role of anticholinergics in acute asthma treatment: An evidence-based evaluation. Chest 121:1977–1987, 2002. **Review of the literature on the use of anticholinergic agents in acute asthma exacerbations.**

Aspiration Syndromes

Michael R. Bye

KEY CONCEPTS

- If an airway foreign body is a possibility, radiographic evaluation is necessary. If there is any question after the radiographs are done, proceed with bronchoscopy. Pharmacotherapy, chest physical therapy, or other maneuvers are not going to help.
- During anticipatory guidance, families must be reminded to keep cleaning fluids and other substances out of the reach of children. Furthermore, storage of such fluids in readily recognizable drinking containers must be discouraged.
- With acute hydrocarbon ingestion, emesis should not be induced. The child should be evaluated for respiratory signs or symptoms.
- Aspiration pneumonitis of gastric contents does not result in an acute infectious process. Concomitant aspiration of oropharyngeal secretions may introduce bacteria, and in those infants, antibiotics may be beneficial. Children hospitalized with aspiration lung disease or those with chronic respiratory symptoms from aspiration and/or reflux should be evaluated and managed aggressively for swallowing dysfunction and/or reflux. These conditions must be treated adequately to avoid subsequent episodes.

Different from all other organ systems in the body, the lung is at a markedly elevated risk of invasion by any one of a number of substances. These may be in a solid, liquid, or gas state. To many of us, it is almost a surprise that such invasion does not happen more frequently. Several times each minute, we all inspire fresh ambient gas. Along with that air comes a number of pollutants, depending on where we live. The opening to the lungs is surrounded by the forces of swallowing. A normal swallow is a very complex maneuver. A small, even transient, glitch in that complex maneuver may result in food entering the airway. The lung itself has good defense mechanisms. The epiglottis and vocal cords serve as mechanical barriers to penetration of extraneous substances into the lungs. The trachea is replete with cough receptors, as are each of the branch points within the tracheobronchial tree. These receptors trigger a cough, which is an exceptional mechanism for removing foreign substances from the airway. When peristalsis is reversed, especially in the patient with altered mental status, some of this material may pass the defense and enter the lungs. Similar mechanisms may occur with simple gastroesophageal reflux. In this case, aspiration may occur on a chronic small-volume basis or on an acute large-volume basis. Similar to the difficulty with swallowing, aspiration of solid foreign bodies into the airway occurs not infrequently in children, especially toddlers. Lastly, the lung is at risk for end-organ involvement in children who ingest hydrocarbons.

This chapter discusses four types of aspiration syndromes. Unfortunately, for some of these entities, the nomenclature is not standardized. For our purposes here, *aspiration pneumonia* is an acute bacterial process in the lung caused by aspiration of bacteria. *Aspiration pneumonitis* is a noninfectious inflammatory disorder of the lungs, caused most commonly by aspiration of stomach contents into the lungs. *Foreign body aspiration* refers to the aspiration of a usually single solid piece of material into the airway. *Hydrocarbon pneumonitis* occurs after a child has ingested any one of a number of hydrocarbons.

Foreign body aspiration is not uncommon in children, occurring most frequently in toddlers. The lack of molar teeth means that food is not chewed adequately, and larger solid particles may be propelled toward the pharynx, with a possible side trip to the larynx and beyond. Toddlers are less careful than some adults about how much is put into the mouth at any given time, resulting in an inability to chew the food adequately. Toddlers are also more likely than most adults to cough, laugh, and run around while chewing. All of these increase the risk of aspiration.

Ingestion of hydrocarbon liquids remains a problem. Those substances that are highly volatile make their way into the airway during swallowing or during emesis. Substances with low viscosity and high volatility readily spread throughout the tracheobronchial tree after passing the larynx.

Aspiration of stomach contents usually results in a noninfectious inflammation of the airway, a sterile aspiration pneumonitis. The lower the pH of the gastric contents and the greater the volume of gastric contents aspirated, the more severe the insult. Thus acute aspiration pneumonitis may result in a wide spectrum of symptoms, from mild cough and wheeze with mild hypoxemia to acute respiratory failure, including the acute respiratory distress syndrome (ARDS).

Aspirated oropharyngeal secretions are more likely to be infected, especially in children with teeth. In such cases, the patient is at risk for developing acute aspiration pneumonia. This may occur in children with swallowing dysfunction, whether they are neurologically intact or neurologically impaired. In addition, children with some neuromuscular disorders develop swallowing dysfunction as their disease progresses.

Finally, any abnormality in the normal defense increases the risk of retained substances, leading to one of the clinical syndromes just described. Laryngomalacia should protect more readily against aspiration of material into the airway. However, it carries an increased incidence of gastroesophageal reflux. Therefore the abnormal larynx is challenged more than the normal larynx, with the potential for increased aspiration. Vocal cord paralysis also decreases the mechanical barriers to aspiration. Children with neuromuscular disease often have decreased cough ability. This less efficient cough is less likely to expel the foreign material, resulting in chronic or acute aspiration syndrome. Children whose cilia do not function normally are also at risk of retaining material that gets further out along the tracheobronchial tree. Anatomic abnormalities of the tracheobronchial tree, such as tracheomalacia, bronchomalacia, or bronchial stenosis, make the cough less efficient by physically blocking some of the material as the child attempts to eliminate it.

Expert Opinion on Management Issues

FOREIGN BODY ASPIRATION

Foreign body aspiration is more common in toddlers, but it can occur at almost any age. Infants may be given inappropriate foods by well-meaning siblings. Without the ability to chew, these young children are at elevated risk for aspiration of the foreign body. Sudden onset of cough with or without unilateral wheeze during or after a meal or after a witnessed choking episode should raise the index of suspicion. But many airway foreign bodies are not detected until days, weeks, or months after the acute ingestion. Thus the index of suspicion should be high in children with cough, unilateral wheeze, or recurrent pneumonia.

The initial approach should be a plain chest radiograph. If the foreign body is opaque, the diagnosis is made. If nothing is seen on the plain film, maneuvers to deflate the lungs during radiography can be helpful, either by obtaining a lateral decubitus film or by creating a forced exhalation by gently squeezing on the abdomen as the radiograph is taken. If local emphysema is seen on any of these films, the index of suspicion for foreign body should be very high. If these films are negative but the index of suspicion is still high, proceeding to bronchoscopy is advisable. Flexible bronchoscopy may be used to detect an otherwise undetectable foreign body. The flexible bronchoscope is able to creep and crawl further out along the tracheobronchial tree than the rigid bronchoscope. However, if any of these studies results in the diagnosis of foreign body aspiration, rigid bronchoscopy should be performed to remove the foreign body. Antibiotics, corticosteroids, and chest physical therapy are either unhelpful or contraindicated.

Once the foreign body is removed, pharmacotherapy may be helpful. If the endoscopist sees significant amount of purulent material or there are white cells and organisms on the Gram stain, antibiotics could be helpful. If significant inflammatory disease in the airway is seen, partially obstructing the airway, systemic corticosteroids may help.

The best prescription for foreign body aspiration is to avoid it. Anticipatory guidance is important in reminding families which foods children should not eat. Avoiding small foods such as nuts, grapes, raisins, hot dogs, sausage, and seeds should be encouraged until the child is 5 years of age and has adequate chewing ability to handle these substances.

HYDROCARBON INGESTION

The best therapy for hydrocarbon ingestion is avoidance. Families must be reminded to keep such substances away from toddlers and young children. Too often, the substances are kept in recognizable food or beverage containers. If a hydrocarbon is ingested, emesis should not be induced. The child should be evaluated in a pediatric emergency department. If the child is normal, with a normal radiograph and normal gas exchange, he or she may be discharged after 6 to 8 hours. If there is any question of respiratory involvement, the child should be kept in the hospital at least overnight. There is no specific therapy in such cases. Corticosteroids are not helpful. Antibiotics are unnecessary, unless bacterial superinfection occurs. If such infection occurs, it is usually several days after the acute episode. Close initial monitoring of the patient, with particular attention to respiratory and central nervous system (CNS) compromise, is critical. Good follow-up for evaluation of pulmonary sequelae is important.

ASPIRATION PNEUMONITIS

Aspiration pneumonitis may occur as a chronic low-level aspiration of acid contents or as a large-volume aspiration. The latter is usually manifest as an acute severe episode of respiratory distress, which may include the development of ARDS. Unfortunately, the most effective therapy in such cases is supportive (i.e., maintenance of adequate oxygenation, ventilation, and fluid status). Studies do not support the routine use of systemic corticosteroids. Because the stomach contents are acid and therefore uninfected, routine antibiotics are not necessary. But the damage to the airways in addition to the ventilatory support equipment may increase the likelihood of a bacterial superinfection. In addition, there may be concomitant aspiration of oropharyngeal flora. One study showed no difference between clindamycin and penicillin. However, both antibiotics would cover anaerobic organisms. Unfortunately, there was no control group in that study to see if the antibiotics are necessary at all. Another study showed no difference between children treated with clindamycin or ticarcillin-clavulanate and less improvement in those treated with ceftriaxone. If the child develops fever and a new infiltrate or the secretions become purulent, antibiotics should be started. Broad-spectrum antibiotics, ideally guided by sputum Gram stain and/or culture and sensitivity, are suggested. Adequate airway clearance, such as chest physical therapy, is often helpful.

Preventing subsequent episodes is critical. Children with reflux should be started on antireflex medications that could include a combination of prokinetic agents, proton pump inhibitors, dietary changes, and perhaps positional changes when asleep. Such children should be followed carefully to ensure the therapy is effective. Chronic lung disease as a result of recurrent aspiration or an acute severe episode requiring hospitalization is an indication for surgical treatment if the medical therapy does not help. If a gastrostomy is performed, the child should undergo a fundoplication. Some infants do well with insertion of a jejunostomy tube. The presence of other cardiopulmonary or neuromuscular diseases should guide the physician toward early aggressive therapy.

ASPIRATION PNEUMONIA

Aspiration of oropharyngeal secretions, alone or in combination with gastric contents, may result in aspiration pneumonia. In such cases, children benefit from antibiotic therapy. The organisms include the usual organisms of the mouth and pharynx, including *Streptococcus pneumoniae, Haemophilus influenzae, Moraxella*, and anaerobes. Antibiotics should be chosen to cover those organisms. Following the acute episode, the child should undergo further evaluation. Swallowing dysfunction should be evaluated by either fluoroscopy or endoscopy. Although swallowing dysfunction is more common in children who are either neurologically impaired or have significant neuromuscular defects, it is also seen in children who are neurologically intact. In the latter cases, speech pathologists or occupational therapists with an interest in feeding problems in children can be helpful in suggesting a diet that is less likely to enter the airway. Children with neurologic or neuromuscular disease should be considered candidates for gastrostomy or jejunostomy feeds, to reduce the likelihood of subsequent severe episodes of aspiration pneumonia or chronic recurrent aspiration syndrome. If a gastrostomy is to be performed, evaluation for reflux must be done. For the child who has reflux and is to undergo a gastrostomy, strong consideration should be given to performing a fundoplication at the same time.

SUGGESTED READINGS

1. Brook I: Treatment of aspiration or tracheostomy-associated pneumonia in neurologically impaired children; effect of antimicrobials effective against anaerobic bacteria. Int J Pediatr Otorhinolaryngol 35:171–177, 1996. **In these two groups of children, aspiration pneumonia was more successfully treated with either ticarcillin/clavulanate or clindamycin than with ceftriaxone.**
2. Bye MR, Mellins RB: Lung injury from hydrocarbon aspiration smoke inhalation. In Chernick V, Boat TF (eds): Kendig's Disorders of the Respiratory Tract in Children, 6th ed. WB Saunders: Philadelphia, 1998, pp 563–572. **A good comprehensive review of the issue of hydrocarbon ingestion.**
3. Jacobson SJ, Griffiths K, Diamond S, et al: A randomized controlled trial of penicillin vs. clindamycin for the treatment of aspiration pneumonia in children. Arch Pediatr Adolesc Med 152:207–208, 1998. **Comparing the two antibiotics, no difference was found, but there was no control group to see if antibiotics are helpful.**
4. Marik PE: Aspiration pneumonitis and aspiration pneumonia. N Engl J Med 344:665–671, 2001. **A thoughtful review helping to differentiate between the two entities.**
5. Morton RE, Wheatley R, Minford J: Respiratory tract infections due to direct and reflux aspiration in children with severe neurodisability. Dev Med Child Neurol 41:329–334, 1999. **Review of lower respiratory tract infections in neurologically impaired children showing they frequently have reflux and direct aspiration.**
6. Rebuck JA, Rasmussen JR, Olsen KM: Clinical aspiration-related practice patterns in the intensive care unit: A physician survey. Crit Care Med 29:2239–2244, 2001. **A survey of members of the Society of Critical Care Medicine to see what they do with patients who have aspirated. Unfortunately, it includes physicians caring for adults and those caring for children, and the age groups are not separated out.**
7. Reid KR, McKenzie FN, Menkis AH, et al: Importance of chronic aspiration in recipients of heart-lung transplants. Lancet 336:206–208, 1990. **Five of eleven adults post–lung transplant had delayed gastric emptying and/or esophageal dysmotility. All five developed bronchiectasis in the transplanted lung, and three of five developed bronchiolitis obliterans.**

Emphysema

Howard B. Panitch

KEY CONCEPTS

- Most cases of what is termed *emphysema* in children are caused by airway inflammation and mucus plugging and are reversible.
- Postinfectious emphysema usually requires no specific therapy unless recurrent infections, respiratory embarrassment from compression of normal lung tissue by the emphysematous lesion, or spontaneous pneumothorax is present. In such situations, surgical excision should be considered.
- Infants with congenital lobar emphysema experiencing respiratory distress or recurrent infections should undergo resection of the emphysematous lobe. There is no consensus regarding the excision of an emphysematous lobe in infants and children with mild symptoms.

BOX 1 Causes of Emphysema in Children

Reversible Emphysema
- Mucus plugging with airway inflammation
  - Asthma
  - Cystic fibrosis
- Retained foreign body

Infectious Emphysema
- Swyer-James-McLeod syndrome/bronchiolitis obliterans
  - Adenovirus
  - Measles virus
  - *Mycoplasma pneumoniae*
  - *Bordetella pertussis*
  - *Mycobacterium tuberculosis*
- Human papilloma virus
- *Legionella pneumophila*

Congenital Lobar Emphysema
- Intrinsic or extrinsic bronchial obstruction with normal or reduced numbers of alveoli
- Polyalveolar lobe

Acquired Lobar Emphysema

Emphysema refers to enlargement of the respiratory airspaces. By strict definition, the condition is permanent and accompanied by destruction of alveolar walls without fibrosis. This condition, a component of chronic obstructive pulmonary disease (COPD), is common in adults and most often associated with tobacco smoking, exposure to environmental toxins like coal dust, or an inherited deficiency of a protease inhibitor (α_1-antitrypsin deficiency). In children, however, destruction of airspaces in concert with their dilation is uncommon, and the term *emphysema* more often is used to describe simple overdistention of airspaces. The most common cause of this type of emphysema in children is partial airway obstruction associated with the retention of endogenous (e.g., mucus plugs in patients with asthma or cystic fibrosis) or exogenous foreign bodies that create a check valve in the airways (Box 1). Intrathoracic airways normally dilate during inspiration, so inspired gas can enter airspaces distal to the partial obstruction. As the intrathoracic airways narrow during exhalation, however, the obstruction becomes complete and traps air distal to it. The overdistention resolves when mucus plugs are dislodged or the foreign body is removed endoscopically.

Infectious Causes

Emphysema with or without tissue destruction can occur after infection. Postinfectious obliterative bronchiolitis can affect a single lobe or the entire lung. The causative agent is usually viral. The most common is adenovirus or measles, but nonviral infections, including *Mycoplasma pneumoniae*, *Bordetella pertussis*, and *Myobacterium tuberculosis,* are also associated. As the bronchiolar lumen scars down, the distal airspaces become overdistended. The long-standing process of bronchiolar obliteration and inflammation causes regional hypoperfusion. The affected lung or lobe becomes hyperlucent compared with the normal lung because of the reduction in blood flow. Although distal airspace enlargement is present, the unilateral hyperlucent lung, or Swyer-James-McLeod lung, usually becomes smaller than the normal lung. Swyer-James-McLeod syndrome is also described after toxic inhalation or chest irradiation.

Human papillomavirus types 6 and 11 cause laryngeal papillomatosis. Symptoms usually do not appear before the second or third year of life, although infection usually occurs at birth. Infection can spread distally to the trachea and bronchi in approximately 5% of patients over the ensuing 4 to 8 years, resulting in cysts, nodules, emphysema, and recurrent pneumonias. Placement of a tracheostomy enhances progression from laryngeal to pulmonary involvement. In patients with altered T-cell immunity, *Legionella pneumophila* can cause bullous emphysema.

Congenital and Acquired Lesions

Single or multiple lobes of the lung can become overdistended because of congenital or acquired lesions. *Infantile* or *congenital lobar emphysema* (CLE) refers to the massive overdistention of one or more lobes of the lung, with compression of surrounding normal lung tissue. Moderate or severe cases occur within days of birth, and 80% to 90% of cases occur within the first 6 months of life. Mild cases can escape detection until adulthood. The emphysema can result from intrinsic airway obstruction secondary to abnormalities or absence of bronchial wall cartilage; a proliferation of bronchial mucosa; extrinsic airway compression by vessels, lymph nodes, masses, or cysts; or an abnormality in alveolar multiplication, resulting in a polyalveolar lobe. In the case of airway compression, alveolar number is normal or reduced, with marked distention of the airspaces. Often, no discernible cause of CLE can be detected. When it occurs, the left upper lobe is most commonly involved, followed by the right middle lobe and right upper lobe. There is a male predominance, and other anomalies (patent ductus arteriosus, vascular sling, and cardiac septal defects) are described in association with CLE.

Acquired lobar emphysema is described in infants who have required extended courses of airway intubation and mechanical ventilation, especially those infants with bronchopulmonary dysplasia. Bronchial stenosis and intraluminal granuloma formation can cause massive overdistention of the lobe subtended by the airway if the obstruction is partial, or lobar atelectasis if the obstruction is complete. Airway mucosal damage from the tip of the endotracheal tube or from aggressive deep suctioning practices are considered the causes of these lesions. When acquired lobar emphysema is present, the lobes of the right lung are most often involved, and lesions are found at the main carina and in the right main bronchus.

Expert Opinion on Management Issues

Treatment of airway obstruction from mucus impaction and airway inflammation should be directed at the underlying cause. Thus use of anti-inflammatory agents and bronchodilators are the treatments of choice for patients with asthma, and antibiotics, anti-inflammatory therapy, airway clearance techniques, and perhaps mucolytics may be appropriate for patients with cystic fibrosis.

When a foreign body is suspected, chest radiography with inspiratory and expiratory films or lateral decubitus views, in younger patients unable to cooperate, can support the diagnosis. One report suggests the simultaneous presence of hyperaeration with ipsilateral atelectasis, or aeration within an area of atelectasis, is highly suggestive of a retained foreign body. Importantly, radiography can never rule out a possible retained foreign body. If the index of suspicion is high enough, airway endoscopy must be performed. The treatment of choice is removal of the foreign body with an open tube (rigid) bronchoscope with the patient under general anesthesia, so the airway can be controlled and ventilation maintained during the procedure.

The radiographic appearance of a Swyer-James-McLeod lung is of a hyperlucent lung that is smaller than the contralateral one. Often, there is a mediastinal shift toward the affected lung. A radionuclide perfusion scan demonstrates patchy or absent perfusion of the affected area. If necessary, a chest CT scan can demonstrate the presence of the main pulmonary artery to rule out agenesis or hypoplasia. Selective bronchography demonstrates a pruned-tree appearance of the airways, with absent alveolarization of the

contrast medium. Most children with hyperlucent lung syndrome require no specific therapy except during intercurrent illnesses. Although some reports of corticosteroid response in patients with obliterative bronchiolitis exist, no controlled trials of this therapy are available. Because the Swyer-James-McLeod lung is the end result of long-standing bronchial obliteration, systemic steroids will likely be ineffective. If bronchiectasis is also present, medical therapy should be directed toward treating the infection and inflammation. In rare cases of recurrent, severe infections, pneumonectomy is performed and results in improved outcome.

Several trials of antiviral, antimetabolite, and α-interferon therapy are reported in patients with pulmonary spread of laryngeal papillomatosis, with disappointing results. Because tracheostomy placement enhances the distal spread of the virus, attempts should be made to avoid the procedure if possible. Similarly, airway instrumentation is also associated with more distal spread and should be performed judiciously.

Congenital lobar emphysema can usually be diagnosed by plain chest radiograph. Findings consist of a hyperlucent lobe and adjacent compression atelectasis. Because other lesions, such as cystic adenomatoid malformation, can resemble CLE, chest CT scan can be used to differentiate CLE from other lesions. Chest CT may also be useful in identifying the bronchial abnormality that causes the emphysematous lobe. If the role of surgical excision is questionable, a perfusion scan can detect whether or not the emphysematous lobe is functional. When CLE manifests early, it is usually because the infant has tachypnea, dyspnea, cyanosis, and respiratory distress. In such situations, excision of the affected lobe is warranted. Excision of the lobe in children with mild symptoms is controversial. Proponents argue that removal of the space-occupying mass allows for compensatory growth of normal lung and without excision, an acute viral illness can result in life-threatening respiratory distress. Pulmonary function measurements in small series of patients who did not undergo excision of the emphysematous lobe, however, did not disclose differences from those of patients who did have the lobe removed.

Any infant who has a history of prolonged mechanical ventilation and develops persistent lobar overinflation should undergo bronchoscopic examination. Endobronchial lesions can be removed by electrocautery or laser resection. If the emphysematous lobe causes respiratory embarrassment, excision of the lobe is warranted.

Common Pitfalls

A normal chest radiograph never rules out the presence of a retained foreign body. A history of choking is absent in up to one third of cases, so the index of suspicion must be high. Although a few reports of excision of a retained foreign body by flexible bronchoscopy are published, by far the safer route is to remove the object through a rigid bronchoscope.

Patients with Swyer-James-McLeod syndrome can experience chronic wheezing, and if bronchiectasis is present, they may also have recurrent episodes of respiratory infections. Evidence of bronchodilator responsiveness should be sought to justify the use of bronchodilators or inhaled corticosteroids.

As mentioned earlier, airway instrumentation and tracheostomy placement promote the spread of papilloma virus into the lower airways. Because of the association with other congenital anomalies, especially cardiovascular lesions, infants with CLE should be fully evaluated before undergoing surgical excision of the emphysematous lobe.

Communication and Counseling

Most children with Swyer-James-McLeod syndrome do well without regular therapy, but they may require antibiotics during intercurrent illnesses. Recurrent or persistent infection may require excision of the affected lung.

Excision of the affected lobe in infants with CLE typically results in resolution of symptoms. Pulmonary function at follow-up may be normal or disclose small airway obstruction. Children treated conservatively without surgical excision undergo radiographic improvement, with a decrease in hyperlucency of the lesion over time. Children whose emphysematous lobes are not removed should refrain from activities occurring at extremes of barometric pressure (e.g., mountain climbing, scuba diving).

SUGGESTED READINGS

1. Fregonese L, Girosi D, Battistini E, et al: Clinical, physiologic, and roentgenographic changes after pneumonectomy in a boy with McLeod-Swyer-James syndrome and bronchiectasis. Pediatr Pulmonol 34:412–416, 2002. **Case report with 9-year follow-up and literature review of Swyer-James-McLeod syndrome in children.**
2. Gervaix A, Beghetti M, Rimensberger P, et al: Bullous emphysema after *Legionella* pneumonia in a two-year-old child. Pediatr Infect Dis J 19:86–87, 2000. **Case report of a girl with chromosome 22q11 deletion syndrome who developed bullous emphysema after acute Legionella infection, with literature review.**
3. Mani H, Suarez E, Stocker JT: The morphologic spectrum of infantile lobar emphysema: A study of 33 cases. Paediatr Respir Rev 5(Suppl. A):S313–S320, 2004. **Review of the clinical presentation and histopathology of congenital lobar emphysema from 33 cases referred to the Armed Forces Institute of Pathology.**
4. Ozcelik U, Gocmen A, Kiper N, et al: Congenital lobar emphysema: Evaluation and long-term follow-up of thirty cases at a single center. Pediatr Pulmonol 35:384–391, 2003. **Clinical presentation, evaluation, and associated anomalies reported in 30 patients who underwent either surgical excision or conservative treatment for congenital lobar emphysema.**
5. Zawadzka-Glos L, Jakubowska A, Chmielik M, et al: Lower airway papillomatosis in children. Int J Pediatr Otorhinolaryngol 67:1117–1121, 2003. **Review of the clinical courses and radiographic and endoscopic findings of four children with lower airway/pulmonary papillomatosis.**

Pneumothorax and Pneumomediastinum

Brigid K. Killelea and Marc S. Arkovitz

KEY CONCEPTS

- The most common presenting symptoms of pneumothorax and pneumomediastinum are ipsilateral chest pain and dyspnea.
- Severe dyspnea should raise suspicion of tension pneumothorax.
- Pneumothorax is usually diagnosed on upright chest radiograph.
- Pneumomediastinum is a symptom of violation of the upper respiratory tract, intrathoracic airways, and/or lung or esophageal parenchyma.
- Pneumomediastinum may be difficult to diagnose, but CT scan is usually diagnostic.

Pneumothorax, the accumulation of air within the pleural space, is relatively uncommon during childhood, but it is a serious condition that requires careful observation and treatment. Tension pneumothorax develops when air accumulates under pressure, causing compression and displacement of mediastinal structures away from the affected side. With involvement of the heart and major vessels, both respiratory function and hemodynamics quickly become compromised, requiring prompt diagnosis and treatment.

Pneumothorax in children has many causes. Primary spontaneous pneumothorax occurs without trauma or underlying lung disease and usually results from rupture of a lung cyst or bleb. Spontaneous pneumothorax, which may run in families, is frequently seen in teenagers, especially tall, thin boys or those with defects of collagen synthesis, such as in the Ehlers-Danlos and Marfan syndromes. Secondary pneumothorax arises as a complication of an underlying lung disorder in the absence of trauma (e.g., pneumonia, empyema, pulmonary abscess, gangrene, infarct, or in association with a foreign body). Finally, iatrogenic causes of pneumothorax include positive pressure mechanical ventilation, thoracentesis, central venous catheter insertion, bronchoscopy, or cardiopulmonary resuscitation.

Pneumomediastinum, also known as mediastinal emphysema, refers to the presence of air or other gas within the mediastinum. The gas that causes pneumomediastinum usually originates from microscopic alveolar rupture in the lungs, but it may come from the upper respiratory tract (e.g., during intubation), intrathoracic airways, or the gastrointestinal tract (usually the result of an esophageal perforation). Additionally, bacterial infection of the visceral pleural space can result in the production of mediastinal gas, and outside air can reach the mediastinum after trauma or surgery. As gas tracks along tissue planes within the thoracic cavity, edema and subcutaneous air ensue. The inflammation of mediastinal structures (usually from an infectious etiology) and its sequelae are referred to as *mediastinitis*, a serious condition that requires immediate treatment.

Expert Opinion on Management Issues

PNEUMOTHORAX

Medical Therapy

Patients who present with spontaneous pneumothorax require supplemental oxygen and intravenous (IV) access. Depending on the initial size of the pneumothorax, patient symptoms, rate of expansion, presence of tension, and concomitant pulmonary pathology, treatment with chest tube thoracostomy may be indicated. If the patient is asymptomatic and the pneumothorax is unilateral and less than 15% to 20% of chest volume, observation alone may be sufficient. Pleural air typically reabsorbs at a rate of 1.25% per day and can be accelerated by the administration of 100% oxygen. Serial chest radiographs should be performed to document decreasing size. CT scan may or may not be indicated at the first episode of a spontaneous pneumothorax. This decision often depends on the treating physician's preference.

Surgical Therapy

For symptomatic, large (greater than 20% of chest volume), or tension pneumothorax, treatment with chest tube insertion and placement to wall suction is indicated. In the event of tension pneumothorax, if a chest tube is not immediately available or the patient's clinical condition deteriorates during preparation for insertion, needle decompression in the midaxillary line at the level of the third or fourth costal interspace should be performed and can be lifesaving. Large persistent air leaks may suggest damage to the airway, lung parenchyma, or pleura and warrant further diagnostic investigation. Appropriate testing begins with CT scan and may include bronchoscopy. In the case of spontaneous pneumothorax, persistent air leaks may result from chronic underlying conditions, such as cystic fibrosis, bronchopulmonary dysplasia, lung cysts, or blebs. Surgical treatment for these conditions may require open resection or video-assisted thoracoscopic surgery (VATS) to remove or repair the affected lung parenchyma.

PNEUMOMEDIASTINUM

Medical Therapy

Treatment of pneumomediastinum requires investigation of the underlying cause with CT scan, esophagoscopy, esophagogram, and/or bronchoscopy. If all investigative efforts fail to reveal a cause, IV antibiotics and close observation are indicated. In the case of

mediastinitis, broad-spectrum IV antibiotics should be initiated immediately.

Surgical Therapy

Surgical treatment is specific to the underlying cause. Subcutaneous air, although unsightly, requires no surgical management, reabsorbs on its own, and in and of itself poses no medical risk. Mediastinitis often requires a surgical drainage procedure of the affected area. In the case of an esophageal perforation, esophageal diversion may be required.

PREVENTIVE MEASURES

The rate of recurrence of spontaneous pneumothorax varies from 20% to 50%, with increased risk after each subsequent event. Patients with recurrent pneumothoraces need a diagnostic workup starting with a CT scan. Most surgeons agree that a recurrence warrants operative exploration and treatment consisting of, but not limited to, thoracoscopy and pleurodesis. If blebs or cysts are identified pre- or intraoperatively, they can be resected thoracoscopically. Pleurodesis is performed by initiating an inflammatory process of the pleura. With subsequent fibrosis and scarring, the pleura becomes adherent to the chest wall, obliterating potential space for recurrent pneumothorax. The preferred method, mechanical pleurodesis, is performed by scraping the pleura. With chemical pleurodesis, agents such as tetracycline derivatives or talc are instilled into the pleural space, causing local inflammation. If pleurodesis is unsuccessful, the patient may require a pleurectomy.

Common Pitfalls

- Failure to recognize tension pneumothorax.
- Incorrect placement of the chest tube or failure to advance the tube until the last hole is intrapleural, which may result in persistent air leak and pneumothorax in the absence of underlying lung disease.
- Injury to the intercostal vessels during insertion and lung perforation.
- Recurrent pneumothorax after tube removal.

Communication and Counseling

Parents of children with Marfan syndrome or other connective tissue disorders should be counseled by a qualified geneticist to help them understand the predisposition to pneumothorax and other symptoms of the disease, as well as treatment options. Most children with pneumothorax treated with tube thoracostomy recover fully. After tube removal, patients can usually be sent home within 24 hours, provided follow-up chest radiograph shows no residual pneumothorax. Although no large long-term follow-up studies document the ideal time for return to play for sports activities, most experts agree that waiting for 3 to 4 weeks after resolution of pneumothorax is sufficient. Parents should be counseled about the risk of recurrence and what symptoms to look for, namely dyspnea, unilateral pleuritic chest pain that radiates to the neck, shoulder, or back, and/or a dry cough. With regard to air travel, a 1- to 2-month delay is recommended.

SUGGESTED READINGS

1. Ashcraft KW, Murphy JP, Sharp RJ, et al (eds): Pediatric Surgery, 3rd ed. Philadelphia: WB Saunders, 2000, pp 195–196. **Discusses the pathophysiology of pneumothorax.**
2. Chalumeau M, Le Clainche L, Sayeg N, et al: Spontaneous pneumomediastinum in children. Pediatr Pulmonol 31(1):67–75, 2001. **A comprehensive review of spontaneous pneumomediastinum, including epidemiology, differential diagnosis, radiographic findings, and treatment.**
3. Marx JA, Hockberger RS, Walls RM (eds): Rosen's Emergency Medicine: Concepts Clinical Practice, 5th ed. St. Louis: Mosby, 2002, pp 276–277. **Discusses pneumothorax and tension pneumothorax with respect to pediatric trauma.**
4. Oldham KT, Colombani PM, Folgia RP (eds): Surgery of Infants and Children: Scientific Principles and Practice. Philadelphia: Lippincott-Raven, 1997, pp 923–924. **Discusses the diagnosis and management of pneumothorax.**
5. O'Neill JA, Grosfeld JL, Fonkalsrud EW, et al (eds): Principles of Pediatric Surgery, 2nd ed. St. Louis: Mosby, 2004, pp 360–361. **Describes pneumothorax and the chest tube insertion procedure for infants and older children.**
6. Ozcan C, McGahren ED, Rodgers BM: Thoracoscopic treatment of spontaneous pneumothorax in children. J Pediatr Surg 38 (10):1459–1464, 2003. **Describes the authors' experience and results with thoracoscopic treatment of spontaneous pneumothorax in 22 children.**
7. Putukian M: Pneumothorax and pneumomediastinum. Clin Sports Med 23(3):443–454, 2004. **Discusses the incidence of pneumothorax and pneumomediastinum during sports, as well as current recommendations for return to play.**

Pleural Effusion, Empyema, and Chylothorax

Samuel M. Alaish and R. Peter Altman

KEY CONCEPTS

- Signs and symptoms of a pleural effusion vary with the etiology. Pneumonia may cause prominent symptoms, such as cough, dyspnea, and fever, whereas malignant effusions may be asymptomatic.
- Signs and symptoms associated with a small- or moderate-sized pleural effusion may be subtle in an infant or small child.
- CT scans of the chest are useful to differentiate fluid from lung parenchyma as the cause of the radiopaque density on a chest radiograph. The presence of necrosis in the lung parenchyma can also be inferred.
- The proper treatment of empyemas is determined by their stage. For stages II and III empyemas, video-assisted thoracoscopic surgery (VATS) reduces the length of hospitalization.

- For persistent chylous leaks, octreotide (a synthetic somatostatin analogue) is a safe and effective treatment that reduces but does not eliminate the need for surgery.
- In the case of an iatrogenic hemothorax following central line insertion, removal of the line may be required in addition to evacuation of the hemothorax.
- Sputum samples are not readily obtained from children because young children cannot coordinate a cough with the pharyngeal movements needed to expectorate sputum. A nasopharyngeal swab, although less accurate, is relatively easy to obtain and can sometimes be helpful.
- Aminoglycosides penetrate poorly into pleural fluid.
- Central venous thrombosis may be the underlying cause for a chylothorax.
- Long-term drainage of chylous fluid may result in depletion of protein and fat stores and cause severe malnutrition and immunodeficiency.

The classification of pleural fluid into transudate or exudate was established according to criteria developed and tested in adults. Unfortunately, these criteria are not as reliable in children. Table 1 lists the commonly accepted criteria, and Table 2 lists the various etiologies for pleural effusions. Box 1 lists the signs and symptoms and Box 2 lists the diagnostic studies.

Pleural effusion in children is most frequently infectious in origin, with congenital heart disease second and malignancy a distant third. The most common bacterial organisms are *Staphylococcus aureus, Streptococcus pneumoniae,* and *Streptococcus pyogenes.* Since the universal use of the pneumococcal vaccine in 2001, methicillin-resistant *S. aureus* infections have increased dramatically. The most common viruses are adenovirus, influenza and parainfluenza, and *Mycoplasma pneumoniae.* Histoplasmosis is one of the few fungal infections seen frequently in otherwise healthy children that can cause an asymptomatic pleural effusion. Children with underlying chronic disease may have other fungal infections, such as nocardia, blastomycosis, or coccidiomycosis. In children with AIDS, *Pneumocystis carinii* is associated with an effusion in 5% of patients. Lymphoma, the most common malignancy associated with a pleural effusion, is nearly always diagnosed prior to the appearance of the effusion.

Any pleural effusion associated with bacterial pneumonia, lung abscess, or bronchiectasis is a parapneumonic effusion. An empyema, by definition, is pus in the pleural space. In patients with uncomplicated parapneumonic effusions treated with antibiotics, pleural fluid and phagocytes are resorbed through subpleural lymphatics, and mesothelial membranes undergo repair. If untreated with antibiotics, the early inflammatory response is insufficient to prevent bacterial spread, and parapneumonic effusions can progress to an empyema through three stages (Box 3). The first stage is called the *exudative* stage, which occurs in the first several days of a parapneumonic effusion. The pleural fluid is free-flowing and characterized by a low white blood cell count and lactate dehydrogenase (LDH) level and normal glucose and pH; early drainage

TABLE 1 Classification of Pleural Effusions

Type of Effusion	Appearance	Protein (g/dL)	LDH (IU/L)	Protein P/S Ratio	LDH P/S Ratio	pH	Glucose (mg/dL)
Transudate	Straw colored	<3	<200	<0.5	<0.6	≥7.3	S
Exudate	Turbid	≥3	>200	≥0.5	≥0.6	≥7.2	S, >40
Empyema	Turbid or purulent	≥3	>1000	≥0.5	≥0.6	<7.2	<40
Chylothorax	Turbid or milky	≥3	S	≥0.5	≥0.6	≥7.4	S

LDH, lactate dehydrogenase; P/S, pleural/serum value; S, serum value.

TABLE 2 Differential Diagnosis of Pleural Effusions

Transudate	Exudate
Congestive heart failure	Infection
Pericardial disease	Neoplasia
Cirrhosis	Hemothorax
Nephrotic syndrome	Esophageal perforation
Peritoneal dialysis	Pancreatitis
Hypothyroidism	Intra-abdominal abscess
Pulmonary arteriovenous malformations	Drug toxicity
Nonimmune hydrops	Collagen vascular disease
Pulmonary embolic disease	
Urinary tract obstruction	
Iatrogenic (may be transudate or hemothorax):	
Central venous catheters	
Ventriculoperitoneal shunts	

BOX 1 Signs and Symptoms

- Cough
- Dyspnea
- Fever
- Orthopnea
- Chest pain
- Abdominal pain
- Vomiting
- Dullness to chest percussion
- Decreased breath sounds
- Pleural rub (in early phase)
- Decreased vocal fremitus (older children)
- Fullness of the intercostal spaces (older children)
- Mediastinal shift away from the affected side (older children)

usually results in rapid improvement. The second stage is termed *fibrinopurulent* and is characterized by more extensive pleural inflammation and increasingly viscous and turbid fluid. The fluid contains many polymorphonuclear leukocytes, bacteria, and cellular debris. As this stage progresses, the pleural fluid pH and glucose levels fall, and the LDH level rises. Fibrinous material coats pleural membranes, creating a framework for preventing lung expansion and forming intrapleural loculations that impede thoracostomy tube drainage. The final stage of empyema formation is termed the *organizing* stage. Patients in this stage have established empyemas with fibrinous pleural peels, intrapleural loculations, and purulent pleural fluid. Decortication is required to cure the patient in this stage.

Hemothorax is rare in children and usually results from either traumatic or iatrogenic causes, such as a complication following central-line placement or thoracentesis. Metastatic neoplasm and vessel erosion by a neoplasm are rare causes.

Congenital chylous effusions are extremely rare. They are usually idiopathic but may be associated with the Down and Noonan syndromes, tracheoesophageal fistula, and polyhydramnios. Although there may be a history of birth trauma, the underlying defect is congenital. There may be complete atresia of the thoracic duct or absence of communication between small peripheral lymphatics and the larger central vessels as a result of hypoplasia. Chylothorax may be secondary to pulmonary lymphangiectasia, which is a difficult problem.

Traumatic damage to the thoracic duct is largely iatrogenic, usually following cardiac, esophageal, or other thoracic surgery; there are also reported cases following central-line placement. Regardless of the etiology, chylothorax is usually right sided because most of the thoracic duct lies within the right hemithorax.

The diagnosis of chylothorax is confirmed by a pleural effusion with a triglyceride level more than 1.1 mmol/L and a cell count more than 1000 cells/μL, with a predominance of lymphocytes (more than 80%). The diagnosis may be confirmed by administration of cream by mouth or via nasogastric tube. This induces a dramatic change in the color and content of the effused fluid, owing to the transport of absorbed fat in the lacteal system. Pseudochylothorax (cholesterol pleurisy) occurs with long-standing fluid in a fibrotic pleura. The fluid has a high content of cholesterol but no triglycerides or chylomicrons. The gross appearance is the same as that of chylothorax.

Expert Opinion on Management Issues

General supportive measures, including supplemental oxygen and analgesia, are given as needed. Specific therapy varies according to the type of effusion.

BOX 2 Diagnostic Studies

- Frontal, lateral, and decubitus chest radiographs
- Blood cultures
- Computed tomography/ultrasonography
- Nasopharyngeal swabs/sputum samples
- Complete blood count with differential (nonspecific but may indicate underlying infection or blood dyscrasia)
- Thoracentesis if etiology of the effusion unexplained or an undetermined infectious process suspected*
- Pleural fluid† sent for the following:
    - Cell count and differential
    - Protein, lactate dehydrogenase (LDH), glucose, and pH
    - Cultures for aerobic and anaerobic bacteria, mycobacteria, fungi, mycoplasma, and, when indicated, viral pathogens.
- Selective studies: cytopathology, cholesterol and triglyceride levels, amylase, rheumatoid factor, antinuclear antibody, and countercurrent immunoelectrophoresis

---

*Thoracostomy tube placement may supersede the need for thoracentesis if the presentation is consistent with empyema.
†The color and turbidity of the fluid may be indicative of the underlying cause. Clear, pale yellow fluid suggests a transudate. Milky fluid is characteristic of a chylous effusion. Bloody pleural fluid is seen with malignancy or following trauma. Purulent fluid is diagnostic of empyema.

TRANSUDATES AND NONPARAPNEUMONIC EXUDATES

For transudates and nonparapneumonic exudates, treatment is directed at the underlying process. When a pleural effusion is caused by fluid overload as in cardiac failure or renal failure, the transudate can often be managed with diuretics and precise fluid management. For malignant effusions, radiation or chemotherapy often result in clearance.

HEMOTHORAX

In the vast majority of hemothorax cases, the most that may be required is evacuation of the hemothorax by placement of a thoracostomy tube and restoration of normal circulating blood volume. If the rate of bleeding continues to exceed 20 mL/kg of body weight, thoracotomy is indicated, although this is rare.

Technological advances in VATS led to its application in the treatment of fibrinopurulent empyemas, and when combined with a mini-thoracotomy, decortication can be performed to treat organized empyemas. The advantages of VATS include decreased morbidity and pain compared to the standard open thoracotomy. Consequently, the traditional thoracotomy incision is now rarely used for this disease.

Many pediatric surgeons now advocate the use of VATS earlier in the treatment protocol at the time of thoracostomy tube placement. Chest tube insertion in the operating room avoids the trauma associated with the procedure in a child who is awake. Furthermore, should the empyema have progressed to a late stage, VATS can immediately be undertaken. This promotes rapid resolution of symptoms, early discharge from the hospital, and early return to normal function, and it avoids the adverse physical, psychological, and

---

BOX 3 Treatment Algorithm for Empyema

Stage I

Thoracostomy tube drainage plus broad-spectrum antibiotics

Stage II

Video-assisted thoracoscopic surgery (VATS) plus broad-spectrum antibiotics (preferred approach) *or* thoracostomy tube drainage plus broad-spectrum antibiotics *plus* fibrinolytic therapy—VATS if this fails

Stage III

VATS plus mini-thoracotomy plus broad-spectrum antibiotics *or* open thoracotomy (rarely necessary) *plus* broad-spectrum antibiotics

---

BOX 4 Treatment Algorithm for Chylothorax

Initial steps:
- Thoracentesis/thoracostomy tube drainage with fluid analysis
- Medium-chain triglyceride (MCT) diet or total parenteral nutrition (TPN)
- Duplex ultrasound to rule out thrombosis causing lymphatic obstruction

If leak is persistent, try:
- Octreotide therapy (1–4 μg/kg/h intravenous infusion or 10–40 μg/kg/day in three divided doses injected subcutaneously)

For persistent leaks despite octreotide therapy, surgery is usually done. Options include:
- Thoracoscopic ligation with or without fibrin glue if leak is visualized
- Pleurodesis by parietal pleurectomy if no leak is seen
- Pleuroperitoneal shunts

Interventional radiology offers a new approach:
- Thoracic duct embolization (experience with this technique is limited)

---

educational sequelae associated with prolonged chest tube drainage in the hospital.

The time of surgery for a persistent chylothorax is not as well defined as the initial therapy (Box 4). Most surgeons do not proceed to surgical treatment until more than 4 weeks of effusion unless the child develops nutritional complications. Patients with high central venous pressures, a thrombosis of the superior vena cava, or a caval-pulmonary anastomosis are exceptions because nonoperative management usually fails. The traditional surgical approach is open thoracic or abdominal ligation of the thoracic duct. The leak may be identified more easily following the administration of cream orally or via a nasogastric tube before or during the operation. Ligation of all tributaries together with the main duct is successful in as many as 90% of patients. Thoracoscopic ligation causes less postoperative pain and morbidity and offers better visualization by means of magnification. Pleurodesis by parietal pleurectomy is advocated for situations in which the leak cannot be identified. Pleuroperitoneal shunts, although not preferable, can be inserted as an alternative to thoracotomy; thoracoscopic assistance allows more accurate positioning. Shunted peritoneal fluid passes into the venous system via the right lymphatic duct. The procedure has a limited success rate, particularly if the right atrial pressure is raised. Disadvantages include shunt occlusion, chest wall discomfort, and inconvenience.

Common Pitfalls

- Contraindications to thoracentesis include an insufficient quantity of fluid, chest wall infection, and uncorrectable coagulopathy. Potential complications include pneumothorax, hemothorax, the introduction of infection into the pleural space, and hepatic, splenic, or renal laceration.
- Fibrinolytic therapy is usually not considered worthwhile in patients with lungs severely trapped by pleural peels because of the inability of these agents to lyse collagen.
- Failure to perform decortication in stage III empyemas may result in a bronchopleural fistula, or the fluid may drain spontaneously through the chest wall. This situation can lead to an overwhelming pneumonia and subsequent death.
- Diagnosis of chylothorax may not be obvious in a fasting patient or a newborn who has never been fed because the fluid is often straw colored rather than milky.

Communication and Counseling

The prognosis of children with transudative effusions is identical to that of the underlying condition. Children with uncomplicated parapneumonic effusions respond well to conservative management with no apparent sequelae. Even children with complicated empyema respond completely to appropriate management and usually attain complete radiographic resolution within 3 months. Long-term follow-up shows that despite marked abnormalities initially, pulmonary function tests return to normal within 18 months.

SUGGESTED READINGS

1. Beghetti M, La Scala G, Belli D, et al: Etiology and management of pediatric chylothorax. J Pediatr 136:653–658, 2000. **Retrospective review of 51 pediatric patients diagnosed with chylothorax over a 12-year period.**
2. Buttiker V, Fanconi S, Burger R: Chylothorax in children. Chest 116:682–687, 1999. **Retrospective review of 39 pediatric patients diagnosed with chylothorax over a 12-year period. Guidelines for diagnosis and management are provided.**
3. Chen LE, Langer JC, Dillon PA, et al: Management of late-stage parapneumonic empyema. J Pediatr Surg 37:371–374, 2002. **Evidence for decreased length of hospitalization in patients treated with VATS.**
4. Cheung Y, Leung MP, Yip M: Octreotide for treatment of postoperative chylothorax. J Pediatr 139:157–159, 2001. **Case report of two infants who developed chylothorax after cardiac surgery and were successfully treated with subcutaneous octreotide.**
5. Cohen G, Hjortdal V, Ricci M, et al: Primary thoracoscopic treatment of empyema in children. J Thorac Cardiovasc Surg 125:79–84, 2003. **Patients undergoing thorascopic drainage and decortication had significantly shorter durations of intravenous antibiotic therapy, chest tube drainage, and hospitalization.**
6. Gates RL, Caniano DA, Hayes JR, et al: Does VATS provide optimal treatment of empyema in children? A systematic review. J Pediatr Surg 39:381–386, 2004. **The most comprehensive review to date of VATS in the treatment of empyema, providing evidence that VATS leads to a shorter hospitalization.**
7. Merry CM, Bufo AJ, Shah RS, et al: Early definitive intervention by thoracoscopy in pediatric empyema. J Pediatr Surg 34:178–181, 1999. **One of the first studies documenting both effective treatment and decreased morbidity following VATS for empyema.**
8. Ozcelik C, Inci I, Nizam O, et al: Intrapleural fibrinolytic treatment of multiloculated postpneumonic pediatric empyemas. Ann Thorac Surg 76:1849–1853, 2003. **Retrospective review of 72 children treated with intrapleural fibrinolytic therapy for empyemas.**
9. Pratap U, Slavik Z, Ofoe V, et al: Octreotide to treat postoperative chylothorax after cardiac operations in children. Ann Thorac Surg 72:1740–1742, 2001. **Evidence for octreotide therapy in the treatment of persistent chylothorax.**
10. Schultz KD, Fan LL, Pinsky J, et al: The changing face of pleural empyemas in children: Epidemiology and management. Pediatrics 113:1735–1740, 2004. **Documents the increasing incidence of S. aureus, particularly methicillin-resistant S. aureus. Evidence for decreased fever duration and length of hospitalization in children who underwent VATS as initial therapy for empyema.**

Diffuse Alveolar Hemorrhage (Pulmonary Hemosiderosis)

Meeghan A. Hart and Dorr G. Dearborn

KEY CONCEPTS

- Diffuse alveolar hemorrhage (DAH) is a rare diagnosis in pediatrics, but it can be life-threatening.
- The initial evaluation of DAH is directed to ruling out secondary causes, which may be more directly treatable.
- DAH may be a manifestation of systemic disease, associated with glomerulonephritis, or idiopathic.
- Aggressive treatment with corticosteroids is associated with better clinical outcome for treatment of idiopathic pulmonary hemosiderosis (IPH).

Diffuse alveolar hemorrhage (DAH), also referred to as pulmonary hemosiderosis, has many underlying causes. It can occur in association with glomerulonephritis, as a manifestation of systemic disease, or as an isolated phenomenon. Box 1 lists the causes of DAH in children. DAH may have an insidious onset. Patients may present with iron deficiency anemia or failure to thrive, or they may present acutely with hemoptysis, cough, wheezing, tachypnea, and even life-threatening respiratory failure. Thus a good understanding of the evaluation and management of the pediatric patient with pulmonary bleeding is vital.

BOX 1   Causes of Diffuse Alveolar Hemorrhage in Children

Isolated
- Idiopathic
- Possibly Heiner syndrome
- Lung prematurity
- Pulmonary capillary hemangiomatosis

Associated with Other Organ Dysfunction
- Pulmonary-renal syndromes
  - Goodpasture syndrome
  - Wegener granulomatosis
  - Microscopic polyangiitis
  - Henoch-Schönlein purpura
- Cardiac disease
  - Congenital heart disease
  - Mitral stenosis
  - Congestive heart failure
  - Pulmonary venous hypertension
- Collagen vascular disease
  - Systemic lupus erythematosus
  - Scleroderma
  - Rheumatoid arthritis
- Celiac disease

Secondary
- Trauma
  - Suffocation
  - Chest injury
- Drugs
  - D-Penicillamine
  - Nitrofurantoin
  - Propylthiouracil
- Necrotizing pneumonia
- Vascular anomalies
- Infarction/emboli
- Neoplasms
- Graft-versus-host disease
- Radiation
- Clotting disorders
- Possibly toxigenic fungi

When diffuse alveolar hemorrhage (DAH) occurs, alveolar macrophages ingest and process hemoglobin from red blood cells, producing hemosiderin, thus the term *pulmonary hemosiderosis*. A definitive diagnosis of DAH is made when these cells are found in bronchoalveolar lavage (BAL) or lung biopsy. BAL is the procedure of choice because it has good sensitivity and specificity for recovery of hemosiderin-laden macrophages and is less invasive than biopsy. Hemosiderin-laden macrophages can be seen within 72 hours of DAH, and their elevated persistence in BAL beyond 5 to 8 weeks after an acute hemorrhage suggests chronic bleeding.

Expert Opinion on Management Issues

DIAGNOSIS

A thorough history and physical exam in addition to laboratory assessment is essential for proper evaluation of the child with DAH. Initial evaluation includes a complete blood count (CBC) to evaluate the severity of anemia and a reticulocyte count to evaluate the chronicity of bleeding. An elevated reticulocyte count may indicate chronic bleeding, although this measure relies on available iron stores. Chest radiographs obtained during an acute event are nonspecific and may be characterized by patchy or diffuse fluffy infiltrates that are usually bilateral, although unilateral infiltrates are sometimes reported. Plain chest radiographic findings may be fleeting if bleeding subsides, but infiltrates noted on a chest CT may persist longer. Aspiration of small amounts of blood (e.g., traumatic intubation) seldom produces alveolar infiltrates. Chronic DAH resulting in pulmonary fibrosis is characterized radiographically by a diffuse reticular pattern.

It is important to obtain bronchoalveolar lavage fluid (BALF) for the assessment of hemosiderin-laden macrophages within 36 to 48 hours of clinical presentation of acute DAH to determine if the bleeding represented an acute or a chronic event. In addition, the fluid can be cultured to rule out infectious etiologies.

Evaluation of renal function and urinalysis should be performed to rule out disorders associated with glomerulonephritis. Although isolated DAH rarely occurs with coagulopathies, the latter must be assessed as a potential contributing factor. Children outside the infancy age range should receive a full rheumatologic evaluation to exclude collagen vascular disease. Other recommendations include an echocardiogram to rule out cardiac disease and a skeletal survey and head CT to rule out accompanying trauma. Suffocation is very difficult to document but usually produces limited bleeding, seldom requiring ventilatory support. A careful history regarding environmental exposures must be obtained.

TREATMENT

Stabilization of the patient with acute DAH is of the utmost importance; ensuring adequate oxygenation, ventilation, and perfusion of the patient. After an expedited and thorough evaluation, treatment with systemic corticosteroids is highly recommended. Doses ranging from 1 to 5 mg/kg/day administered systemically are used in the treatment of acute idiopathic pulmonary hemosiderosis (IPH), with the dose tapered to 1 mg/kg/day by the time of hospital discharge. Even higher doses up to 500 to 1000 mg per day are used with acute severe persistent DAH related to hematopoietic stem cell transplantation. Although the length of steroid treatment after an apparent isolated DAH has not yet been studied systematically, our paradigm is to continue 1 mg/kg/day prednisone for at least 5 to 8 weeks until repeat bronchoscopy with BAL determines if there is continued bleeding, as indicated by the iron index. The iron index is a hemosiderin score of macrophages. One hundred cells are counted and are each scored 0 to 3 for hemosiderin stain, with a maximum index of 300. Continued bleeding is indicated by an iron index of more than 50 of 300. With an iron index

---

BOX 2 Management Algorithm for Diffuse Alveolar Hemorrhage

- Acute alveolar hemorrhage:
  - Supportive care; burst steroids.
  - Diagnostic evaluation.
- Subacute course:
  - Select treatment modality.
  - Environmental: ETS avoidance.
  - Monitor patient for continued bleeding:
  - Daily: asleep RR, stool guaiacs.
  - Monthly: complete blood count (CBC), reticular count, bronchoscopy (5 to 8 weeks): iron index.*
- Chronic course:
  - Select level of treatment based on severity of continued bleeding/recurrence of acute hemorrhage.
  - Repeat bronchoscopy/iron index for guidance every 3 to 6 months if elevated.

*Iron index, hemosiderin scoring of macrophages; count 100 cells, scoring each 0–3 for hemosiderin stain, with maximum index of 300. ETS, environmental tobacco smoke; RR, respiratory rate.

---

of less than 100 of 300, we recommend weaning to every-other-day prednisone and repeating BAL in another 3 to 4 months. Stool guaiac, hemoglobin, reticulocyte count, and sleeping respiratory rate should be monitored, any of which may indicate recurrent or continued bleeding. Bronchoscopy is advised if any of these indicators is positive. Steroids may be further tapered, or even stopped, if subsequent BAL is consistent with resolution of pulmonary bleeding (normal iron index is less than 20 of 300 in infants).

Although most cases of IPH respond to systemic steroids, the addition of hydroxychloroquine (200 mg once or twice daily), azathioprine (1 to 2 mg/kg/day), or cyclophosphamide (1 to 2 mg/kg/day) may be indicated if pulmonary bleeding persists despite compliance with corticosteroid therapy. Although many question the existence of Heiner syndrome, an empirical trial off dairy products in a toddler with persistent DAH may be worthwhile. Termination of apparent environmental exposures is important, including strict avoidance of environmental tobacco smoke regardless of the etiology of DAH, because this is an apparent trigger for subsequent hemorrhage. Box 2 outlines the management algorithm for DAH.

Common Pitfalls

Children who require long courses of high-dose prednisone are at risk for side effects, including immunosuppression, hypertension, glucose instability, and other manifestations of Cushing syndrome. Children treated with long courses of immunosuppressant therapy should receive *Pneumocystis carinii* prophylaxis.

Children with trisomy 21 and congenital heart disease appear to be at high risk for persistent low-grade pulmonary hemosiderosis even following corrective cardiac surgery. This may be caused by continued increased pulmonary venous pressure, even of subtle severity, and/or inherent weakness in their capillary walls.

Communication and Counseling

The outcome for DAH depends on the nature of the underlying diagnosis and its severity. Current studies support the aggressive use of systemic corticosteroids in treating acute and chronic IPH, with significantly better long-term prognosis than previously thought. Children with IPH are at increased risk for recurrent wheezing, which responds to inhaled bronchodilators. Some children experience an isolated episode of bleeding that never reoccurs, whereas others have repetitive episodes of pulmonary bleeding, placing them at risk for the development of pulmonary fibrosis. Parents need to be educated about the risk of recurrent bleeding, the physical signs that may indicate a recurrent episode, and the importance of avoiding tobacco smoke exposure.

SUGGESTED READINGS

1. Boat T: Pulmonary hemorrhage hemoptysis. In Chernick V, Boat T (eds): Kendig's Disorders of the Respiratory Tract in Children, 6th ed. Philadelphia: WB Saunders, 1998, pp 623–633. **The pathophysiology and workup of IPH is discussed.**
2. Dearborn D, Dahms B, Allan T, et al: Clinical profile of 30 infants with acute pulmonary hemorrhage in Cleveland. Pediatrics 110:627–637, 2002. **A summary of the clinical presentations of infants who presented with acute pulmonary hemorrhage in Cleveland between 1993 and 2000.**
3. Godfrey S: Pulmonary hemorrhage/hemoptysis in children. Pediatr Pulmonol 37:476–484, 2004. **Discusses the causes, management, and prognosis of IPH.**
4. Saeed M, Woo M, MacLaughlin E, et al: Prognosis in pediatric idiopathic pulmonary hemosiderosis. Chest 116:721–725, 1999. **Describes the clinical course and mortality of pediatric patients treated with immunosuppressants.**

Cystic Fibrosis

Mark E. Dovey

KEY CONCEPTS

- Cystic fibrosis (CF) is a chronic, multisystem genetic disorder in which pulmonary disease causes the majority of morbidity and mortality.
- CF is usually diagnosed by either perinatal screening or identification of clinical features, followed by confirmation by sweat chloride analysis or identification of two CF mutations.
- Treatment of CF lung disease targets the triad of viscous secretions, endobronchial infection, and airway inflammation.
- Patients with CF benefit from long-term monitoring and treatment by a multidisciplinary team at an accredited CF care center.

Cystic fibrosis (CF) is the most common life-shortening genetic disease in the white population, with an incidence of approximately 1 in 2500 live births. The disease is present but less frequent in other populations, including Hispanic (1 in 9000), African American (1 in 17,000), and Asian (1 in 90,000). CF is an autosomal recessive disease caused by mutations of the cystic fibrosis transmembrane conductance regulator (*CFTR*) gene on chromosome 7. This gene encodes for the CFTR protein, which functions as a cAMP (cyclic adenosine monophosphate)-regulated chloride channel as well as a regulator of other proteins that conduct ions across epithelial cell membranes in the airways, pancreas, biliary tree, intestines, vas deferens, and sweat glands. Absence or dysfunction of the CFTR protein leads to inadequate hydration of secretions and obstruction of ducts with subsequent organ pathology.

The diagnosis of CF is made through observation of clinical features of the disease and demonstration of CFTR dysfunction through sweat chloride analysis, nasal potential difference measurements, and/or presence of two known *CFTR* gene mutations. Box 1 lists the clinical features consistent with a diagnosis of CF. Sweat chloride analysis, or sweat testing, is performed by obtaining sweat from skin after stimulation with pilocarpine iontophoresis. Sweat chloride concentrations more than 60 mEq/L are consistent with the diagnosis of CF. Nasal potential difference (NPD) measurement detects the abnormal bioelectric properties of the nasal epithelium caused by CFTR dysfunction. The test is technically difficult and only available at certain CF care centers. Genetic testing for *CFTR* gene mutations is now widely available for diagnostic use, prenatal screening, and newborn screening in various states and countries. Most clinical laboratories offer testing for a set panel of the most common CF mutations. Because more than 1000 mutations exist, a negative result from a limited panel of mutations cannot rule out the disease definitively. If a patient has clinical features suggestive of cystic fibrosis, a sweat test should be performed.

Expert Opinion on Management Issues

The estimated median survival for individuals with CF in the United States is now into the fourth decade of life. Although the disease affects multiple organs as noted earlier, more than 80% of mortality is attributable to the pulmonary disease. CF pulmonary disease is characterized by the triad of viscous mucus, endobronchial infection, and neutrophilic inflammation of the airways. This combination leads to obstructive lung disease, progressive damage of the airway walls, bronchiectasis, and eventual respiratory failure. The clinical trajectory is usually marked by slowly progressive pulmonary decline punctuated by exacerbations of the disease. Box 2 outlines the clinical features of a CF pulmonary exacerbation. Treatment of CF pulmonary disease consists of careful monitoring of pulmonary health, maintenance therapies to slow disease progression, and intensive therapy for pulmonary exacerbations.

MONITORING PULMONARY HEALTH

Patients with cystic fibrosis should be referred to an accredited CF care center for longitudinal monitoring

---

BOX 1 Clinical Features Consistent with Diagnosis of Cystic Fibrosis

- Chronic sinopulmonary disease manifested by:
  - Persistent colonization/infection with typical CF pathogens including *Staphylococcus aureus*, nontypeable *Haemophilus influenzae*, mucoid and nonmucoid *Pseudomonas aeruginosa*, and *Burkholderia cepacia*
  - Chronic cough and sputum production
  - Persistent chest radiograph abnormalities (e.g., bronchiectasis, atelectasis, infiltrates, hyperinflation)
  - Airway obstruction manifested by wheezing and air trapping
  - Nasal polyps; radiographic or CT abnormalities of the paranasal sinuses
  - Digital clubbing
- Gastrointestinal and nutritional abnormalities including:
  - Intestinal: meconium ileus, distal intestinal obstruction syndrome, rectal prolapse
  - Pancreatic: pancreatic insufficiency, recurrent pancreatitis
  - Hepatic: chronic hepatic disease manifested by clinical or histologic evidence of focal biliary cirrhosis or multilobular cirrhosis
  - Nutritional: failure to thrive (protein-calorie malnutrition), hypoproteinemia, edema, complications secondary to fat-soluble vitamin deficiency
- Salt loss syndromes: acute salt depletion, chronic metabolic alkalosis
- Male urogenital abnormalities resulting in obstructive azoospermia (congenital bilateral absence of the vas deferens [CBAVD])

From Rosenstein BJ, Cutting GR: The diagnosis of cystic fibrosis: A consensus statement. J Pediatr 132:590, 1998.

BOX 2 Clinical Features of a Cystic Fibrosis Pulmonary Exacerbation

Symptoms

- Increased frequency, intensity, and duration of cough
- Increased sputum production
- Change in appearance of sputum
- Feeling of increased chest congestion
- Increased shortness of breath
- Decreased exercise tolerance
- Decreased appetite
- Fatigue

Signs

- Increased respiratory rate
- Use of accessory muscles for breathing
- Intercostal retractions
- Change in chest auscultatory findings (crackles or wheezing)
- Decline of >10% in forced expiratory volume in 1 second (FEV_1) on spirometry
- Fever and leukocytosis
- Weight loss
- New infiltrates on chest radiograph

Adapted from Ramsey BW: Management of pulmonary disease in patients with cystic fibrosis. N Engl J Med 335:181, 1996. Copyright 1996 Massachusetts Medical Society. All rights reserved. Adapted 2006 with permission.

TABLE 1 Maintenance Therapies for Cystic Fibrosis Pulmonary Disease

	Therapy	Mechanism	Dose
Airway clearance	Chest physiotherapy	Mechanically dislodges secretions from airway walls.	qd-tid
	rhDNase (Pulmozyme)	Decreases sputum viscosity by cleaving DNA released from dying neutrophils in airways.	2.5 mg nebulized qd
	Albuterol, and/or Salmeterol	Bronchodilates and enhances mucociliary clearance.	Standard asthma dosing
Antimicrobial	Inhaled tobramycin (TOBI)	Reduces the density of *Pseudomonas* in airways.	300 mg nebulized bid
	Azithromycin (Zithromax)	Uncertain. Has both antibiotic and anti-inflammatory effects in vitro.	250 mg for <40 kg, 500 mg for ≧40 kg, PO tiw
Anti-inflammatory	Ibuprofen (Motrin)	Uncertain. May reduce neutrophil migration into the airways.	20–30 mg/kg (up to 1600 mg maximum) PO bid to achieve serum levels of 50–100 µg/mL

bid, twice daily; PO, by mouth; qd, every day; tiw, three times a week.

and treatment. Such centers provide state-of-the-art disease-focused care with a multidisciplinary team, including subspecialty physicians, nurses, social workers, nutritionists, and respiratory therapists. In the United States, the Cystic Fibrosis Foundation established clinical practice guidelines for CF care at these centers. The guidelines recommend evaluation every 3 months for optimal monitoring and early intervention for disease progression. Each assessment should include a history, physical examination, nutritional assessment, and psychosocial assessment. Lung function testing should be performed, particularly spirometry, because forced expiratory volume at 1 second (FEV_1) is the most commonly used parameter for measuring acute exacerbations, chronic decline, and response to therapy. Respiratory cultures should be obtained from sputum or a deep oropharyngeal swab. *Staphylococcus aureus, Haemophilus influenza,* and *Pseudomonas aeruginosa* are the most common organisms isolated. Chest radiographs should be obtained every year or two, depending on disease severity. Radiograph findings include hyperinflation and bronchial wall thickening in milder disease and evidence of mucus plugging, bronchiectasis, and infiltrates in more advanced disease.

MAINTENANCE PULMONARY THERAPIES

The goals of maintenance pulmonary therapies for CF are to minimize respiratory symptoms and to slow the progression of airway obstruction and injury. Current treatments target the triad of obstruction, infection, and inflammation. Table 1 outlines the established therapies and their mechanisms of action. The treatment regimen for any given patient must be tailored according to disease severity, tolerance, response to medications, and long-term compliance with treatments. To prevent respiratory complications of typical childhood pathogens, CF patients should receive standard pediatric immunizations, including those for *Streptococcus pneumoniae* and *Haemophilus influenza* type b. In addition, an annual influenza vaccine is recommended. Protection from respiratory syncytial virus with palivizumab (Synagis) seems prudent for

young infants with CF; however, definitive studies of its use in this population are not published.

TREATMENT FOR PULMONARY EXACERBATIONS

Patients with cystic fibrosis have intermittent exacerbations of their pulmonary disease marked by the signs and symptoms listed in Box 2. Standard treatment of these flares consists of antibiotic therapy and intensification of the airway clearance regimen. Choice of therapeutic agents depends on the severity of the exacerbation and the species of bacteria infecting the patient's airways. Antibiotic choices should be based on recent respiratory cultures and sensitivities. For mild exacerbations in those patients infected with *S. aureus,* a number of oral antibiotics may be used, including dicloxacillin, cephalexin, amoxicillin-clavulanate, clindamycin, clarithromycin, or azithromycin. Oral agents for *H. influenzae* include amoxicillin-clavulanate, second- and third-generation cephalosporins, clarithromycin, and azithromycin. For patients infected with *P. aeruginosa,* mild exacerbations may be treated with oral ciprofloxacin. Inhaled antibiotics such as tobramycin or colistin may also be used; however, their efficacy in the treatment of exacerbations is not well studied.

For moderate to severe pulmonary exacerbations, intravenous (IV) antibiotics are indicated, and choice of agents should be based on respiratory culture and sensitivities. *P. aeruginosa* infections may be treated with aminoglycosides, β-lactams, or quinolones. A combination of two antibiotics from these three separate classes should be used to provide synergy and slow emergence of resistance. Pharmacokinetics of antibiotics are altered in CF patients by their larger volume of distribution and more rapid renal clearance. As a result, higher doses are required to achieve the desired peak serum concentrations. Table 2 lists the recommended dosing of IV antibiotics for CF patients.

A standard course of therapy for a CF pulmonary exacerbation ranges from 14 to 21 days. In addition to antibiotic therapy, patients should receive two to three sessions of chest physiotherapy per day. Inhaled bronchodilators are often helpful, particularly for

TABLE 2 Intravenous Antibiotic Dosing for Cystic Fibrosis Pulmonary Exacerbations

Prevalent Bacteria	Antibiotic	Pediatric Dose[1,2]	Adult Dose[2]
Staphylococcus aureus	Cefazolin	30 mg/kg IV q8h	1 g IV q8h
	Nafcillin[3]	25–50 mg/kg IV q6h	2 g IV q6h
Methicillin-resistant S. aureus	Vancomycin[4]	15 mg/kg IV q6h	500 mg IV q6h or 1 g IV q12h
Pseudomonas aeruginosa	β-lactam (choose 1):		
	Ceftazidime	50 mg/kg IV q8h	2 g IV q8h
	Ticarcillin[5]	100 mg/kg IV q6h	3 g IV q6h
	Piperacillin	100 mg/kg IV q6h	3 g IV q6h
	Imipenem[6]	15–25 mg/kg IV q6h	500 mg–1 g IV q6h
	Meropenem[6]	40 mg/kg IV q8h	2 g IV q8h
	Aztreonam	50 mg/kg IV q8h	2 g IV q8h
	plus aminoglycoside (choose 1):		
	Tobramycin[7]	3 mg/kg IV q8h	3 mg/kg IV q8h
	Amikacin[8]	5–7.5 mg/kg IV q8h	5–7.5 mg/kg IV q8h
Burkholderia cepacia	Meropenem	40 mg/kg IV q8h	2 g IV q8h
	plus (choose 1):		
	Minocycline	2 mg/kg IV q12h[9]	100 mg IV q12h
	Amikacin[8]	5–7.5 mg/kg IV q8h	5–7.5 mg/kg IV q8h
	Ceftazidime	50 mg/kg IV q8h	2 g IV q8h
	Chloramphenicol[10]	15–20 mg/kg IV q6h	15–20 mg/kg IV q6h
	Trimethoprim/sulfamethoxazole	4–5 mg/kg of trimethoprim component IV q12h	4–5 mg/kg of trimethoprim component IV q12h

Note: Third drug may be added if synergy testing suggests efficacy.

[1]Most doses are expressed as mg per kg of body weight.
[2]The dose given to children should not exceed that for adults.
[3]To minimize phlebitis, nafcillin should be diluted to a concentration of less than 20 mg/mL.
[4]Vancomycin should be infused slowly to avoid histamine release. Serum concentrations should be monitored; the peak concentration ranges from 20 to 40 μg/mL and the trough from 5 to 10 μg/mL.
[5]Ticarcillin may be associated with occasional platelet dysfunction. Its use is limited by concern about the possibility of selection for resistant organisms, such as Stenotrophomonas maltophilia and B. cepacia.
[6]These drugs are for patients with sensitivity to cephalosporin or multidrug-resistant organisms.
[7]Serum concentrations should be monitored; the peak concentration ranges from 8 to 12 μg/mL, and the trough concentration is less than 2 μg/mL.
[8]Serum concentrations should be monitored; the peak concentration ranges from 20 to 30 μg/mL, and the trough concentration is less than 10 μg/mL.
[9]Should not be given to patients younger than 8 years of age.
[10]Serum concentrations should be monitored; the peak concentration ranges from 15 to 25 μg/mL, and the trough from 5 to 15 μg/mL.
IV, intravenous; q, every.
Adapted from Gibson RL, Burns JL, Ramsey BW: Pathophysiology and management of pulmonary infections in cystic fibrosis. Am J Respir Crit Care Med 168:932, 2003. Official Journal of the American Thoracic Society. © American Thoracic Society.

those patients who demonstrate bronchial responsiveness by spirometry. Systemic corticosteroids may be used, although their efficacy in the setting of a CF pulmonary exacerbation is not proven. Nutritional support with a high-calorie diet is essential because CF patients have increased metabolic needs and decreased appetites during exacerbations.

TREATMENT OF EXTRAPULMONARY DISEASE

Because cystic fibrosis is a multisystem disease, extrapulmonary manifestations of the disease, including chronic sinusitis, pancreatic insufficiency, diabetes mellitus, hepatobiliary disease, and intestinal obstruction, must be identified and treated. Addressing gastrointestinal and nutritional issues is particularly important to pulmonary health because studies show a direct correlation between nutritional status and pulmonary function. Because of increased metabolic demands associated with their pulmonary disease, CF patients require 120% to 140% of the recommended daily allowance of calories for age. A calorically dense diet rich in protein and fat is recommended, and nutritional supplements by mouth or via gastrostomy tube may be required to maintain adequate growth and weight gain. Pancreatic insufficiency is treated with pancreatic enzyme supplements and supplementation with fat-soluble vitamins (A, D, E, and K). Chronic malabsorption and abnormal intestinal mucus predispose CF patients to episodes of acute intestinal obstruction in the form of meconium ileus (in neonates), intussusception, or severe obstipation, called distal intestinal obstruction syndrome. Chronic constipation and rectal prolapse may also occur. Progressive pancreatic scarring may impinge on the islets of Langerhans, leading to diabetes and necessitating insulin therapy.

Common Pitfalls

As newborn screening for CF becomes more widespread, clinicians must be mindful that such screening is not 100% sensitive. Diagnostic evaluation should still be pursued in patients presenting with the clinical features of cystic fibrosis.

In children with CF, it may be difficult to distinguish subtle symptoms of CF from common pediatric ailments. Viral upper respiratory infection (URI) symptoms may herald a pulmonary exacerbation, diarrhea may reflect undertreated malabsorption, and constipation may be secondary to intestinal pathology. Even when health issues are identified as unrelated to CF, treatment may be affected by the CF disease process or therapies. Thus ready communication between a CF patient's pediatrician and CF care team is essential.

Treating CF patients with repeated courses of antibiotics often results in the emergence of antibiotic-resistant organisms, such as methicillin-resistant *Staphylococcus aureus*, multiple-drug-resistant *P. aeruginosa*, or *Burkholderia cepacia*. CF patients may also acquire these organisms from contact with other patients, health care workers, or environmental sources. CF-specific infection control guidelines to minimize such transmission were developed and are published. Education of both patients and health care workers is crucial to the success of these infection control practices.

Communication and Counseling

Given the chronic, progressive nature of the disease, effective communication and counseling are essential components of CF care. Over time, patients and families require developmentally appropriate education and advice about their disease in the context of the social, emotional, and spiritual aspects of their lives. Psychosocial support and therapy must match the trajectory of the disease, which is marked by chronic daily symptoms and treatments interrupted by intermittent crises, such as initial diagnosis, pulmonary exacerbations, diagnosis of new complications, and hospitalizations.

Adherence to a recommended treatment regimen, including diet, multiple medications, and physiotherapy, is a major challenge in CF care. To optimize compliance, communication about treatment should include education about the disease process and therapies, discussion of the impact of such therapies on the quality of life, and counseling about strategies to incorporate therapy into daily living. The patient's age, disease severity, family dynamics, and coping abilities must all be factored into such discussions.

As CF patients enter adolescence and adulthood, issues concerning independent living, reproductive health, and planning for the future should be addressed. Patients often need assistance in developing skills for self-care and negotiating the health care system, particularly as they transition from pediatric to adult care facilities. In addition to standard reproductive health education, men and women with CF should receive disease-specific guidance regarding male infertility, pregnancy in the setting of chronic disease, the impact of pulmonary symptoms on sexual function, and the decision to parent in the setting of a life-shortening disease. Finally, as the disease progresses, communication and counseling must encompass decisions about lung transplantation and end-of-life care.

SUGGESTED READINGS

1. Davis PB: Cystic Fibrosis. Pediatr Rev 22:257–264, 2001. **Offers a general overview of cystic fibrosis.**
2. Fuchs HJ, Borowitz DS, Christiansen DH, et al: Effect of aerosolized recombinant human DNAse on exacerbations of respiratory symptoms and on pulmonary function in patients with cystic fibrosis. N Engl J Med 331:637–642, 1994. **Study showing the efficacy of rhDNase for CF pulmonary disease.**
3. Gibson RL, Burns JL, Ramsey BW: Pathophysiology and management of pulmonary infections in cystic fibrosis. Am J Respir Crit Care Med 168:918–951, 2003. **Comprehensive review of CF pulmonary disease process and management.**
4. Hodson ME, Geddes DM (eds): Cystic Fibrosis. New York: Oxford University Press, 2000. **Comprehensive textbook about cystic fibrosis.**
5. Konstan MW, Byard PJ, Hoppel CL, et al: Effect of high-dose ibuprofen in patients with cystic fibrosis. N Engl J Med 332:848–854, 1995. **Study showing the efficacy of chronic anti-inflammatory therapy with ibuprofen in treating CF lung disease.**
6. Ramsey BW, Pepe M, Quan JM, et al: Efficacy and safety of chronic intermittent administration of inhaled tobramycin in patients with cystic fibrosis. N Engl J Med 340:23–30, 1999. **Study showing the efficacy of inhaled tobramycin for chronic Pseudomonas infection in CF.**
7. Ratjen F, Doring G: Cystic fibrosis. Lancet 361:681–689, 2003. **Concise, evidence-based review of CF pathophysiology, diagnosis, and treatment.**
8. Rosenstein BJ, Cutting GR, et al: The diagnosis of cystic fibrosis: A consensus statement. J Pediatr 132:589–595, 1998. **Outlines the diagnostic criteria for cystic fibrosis.**
9. Saiman L, Marshall BC, Mayer-Hamblett N, et al: Azithromycin in patients with cystic fibrosis chronically infected with *Pseudomonas aeruginosa*: A randomized controlled trial. JAMA 290:1749–1756, 2003. **Study showing the efficacy of chronic azithromycin treatment in CF.**
10. Saiman L, Siegel J: Infection control in cystic fibrosis. Clin Microbiol Rev 17:57–71, 2004. **Evidence-based guidelines for infection control practices for CF.**

Pulmonary Sarcoidosis

Hector H. Gutierrez

KEY CONCEPTS

- Sarcoidosis affects the lung in more than 90% of cases. Infants and younger children most frequently present with lymph node, skin, joint, and eye involvement.
- Spontaneous resolution occurs more often in children, although residual morbidity is also significant in a small number of patients.
- Essential diagnostic factors include compatible clinicoradiologic features, histologic proof of noncaseating granuloma, and exclusion of similar diseases.
- Initial evaluation should aim to confirm the diagnosis, assess the extent and severity of involvement, identify stable versus progressive disease, and decide whether therapy is indicated, a decision generally based on symptoms.
- The mainstay of treatment in pediatric patients is systemic corticosteroids. Less-studied second-line therapy includes antimalarial drugs and methotrexate.

Sarcoidosis is a systemic disease of unknown etiology characterized by noncaseating granulomatous inflammation affecting multiple organs. It has a worldwide

TABLE 1 Chest Radiograph Stratification in Sarcoidosis

Stage	Description	Frequency (%)	Rate of Spontaneous Remission (%)
0	Normal	5–10	—
I	Bilateral hilar lymphadenopathy (BHL)	50	60–90
II	BHL and parenchymal infiltrates	25	50–60
III	Parenchymal infiltrates without BHL	15	10–20
IV	Fibrotic lung disease	5–10	0–5

Adapted from Culver DA, Thomassen MJ, Kaburu MS: Pulmonary sarcoidosis: New genetic clues and ongoing treatment controversies. Cleve Clin J Med 71:88–106, 2004, p 95.

distribution and affects people of any age, sex, and race, with a predilection for those younger than 40 years and for some ethnic groups such as African Americans and Scandinavians. The development of granulomas is the result of a chronic immune response to one or more antigenic triggers (including infectious agents such as *Mycobacterium* and *Propionibacterium*) in a genetically susceptible host. This genetic predisposition, possibly residing in polymorphisms involved in immune cell regulation, T cell function, and antigen processing and regulation, appears to influence the development, presentation, and course of the disease.

Sarcoidosis affects both sexes equally. The clinical manifestations are highly variable, ranging from an acute to an insidious chronic onset. The course varies from self-limited single-organ involvement to a more chronic, progressive multisystemic disease. It affects the lungs in more than 90% of patients. As in adults, childhood cases may remain undetected because the disease can take a subclinical, asymptomatic course. The frequency in which the various organs are affected depends on the age of the patient. Common presenting symptoms in children are usually vague and include fever, weight loss, fatigue, cough, chest pain, and dyspnea. A frequent finding in children is enlargement of peripheral lymph nodes, but the most common occurrence in childhood sarcoidosis is an abnormal chest radiograph. Table 1 describes the four radiologic stages of pulmonary sarcoidosis. Most of the pediatric cases (80% to 90%) involve stages I and II. Children with sarcoidosis have the same organ involvement as adults, but infants and young children (9 to 15 years of age) present most frequently with lymph node, skin, joint, and eye involvement (ocular pain and blurred vision in cases of anterior uveitis). Hepatomegaly and/or splenomegaly may occur in up to 40% of patients during the course of the disease.

The pathologic finding of sarcoidosis is usually a non-necrotizing granuloma. However, finding of a granuloma is not pathognomonic of sarcoidosis. In children, peripheral adenopathy allows for biopsy if no cutaneous lesions are present and provides the best chance for confirmatory diagnosis. When biopsy is refused or negative, additional markers may help make the diagnosis. Among these are elevation of serum angiotensin-converting enzyme (ACE), plasma calcium level, and erythrocyte sedimentation rate (ESR). The presence of abnormal lung function also suggests disease. Pulmonary function tests are sensitive, even early in the course. The most common finding is a restrictive pattern in up to 50% of cases. Less frequent is an obstructive pattern (15%). In addition to the previously mentioned radiographic changes, abnormalities found in high-resolution chest CT scan include peribronchial thickening and upper lobe disease. Gallium–67 scans can demonstrate panda and lambda uptake patterns in the face and chest, respectively. Bronchoalveolar lavage (BAL) shows increased lymphocytes and an elevated CD4-to-CD8 ratio. Figure 1 summarizes the approach to diagnosis.

Expert Opinion on Management Issues

The initial evaluation of patients with sarcoidosis aims to confirm the diagnosis, assess the extent and severity of involvement, identify stable versus progressive disease, and judge whether therapy will benefit the patient. Although pulmonary symptoms are the most common reason for treatment, the sole presence of pulmonary disease is only a relative indication for therapy. Adult asymptomatic patients with radiologic stages II or III may not benefit from systemic therapy, but most physicians treat symptomatic pulmonary disease regardless of its staging. Spontaneous remission is expected in approximately two thirds of patients. The few absolute indications for systemic therapy include cardiac or neurologic involvement, hypercalcemia, ocular disease unresponsive to topical therapy, hepatosplenomegaly, sarcoid hepatitis, and marked lymphadenopathy.

The current therapy of choice for symptomatic multisystem involvement is corticosteroids (Table 2), although patients with isolated anterior uveitis can be treated with topical steroids alone. Data suggest that oral steroids should be used in symptomatic patients in stages II and III, with moderate to severe progressive symptoms and radiographic changes. Despite their use, it is unclear whether corticosteroids improve long-term lung function or alter disease progression favorably. There are no randomized, controlled trials defining the optimal dose and duration of corticosteroid therapy, so the treatment must be individualized for each patient. Oral prednisone or prednisolone is usually initiated at 1 mg/kg/day and maintained for 1 to 2

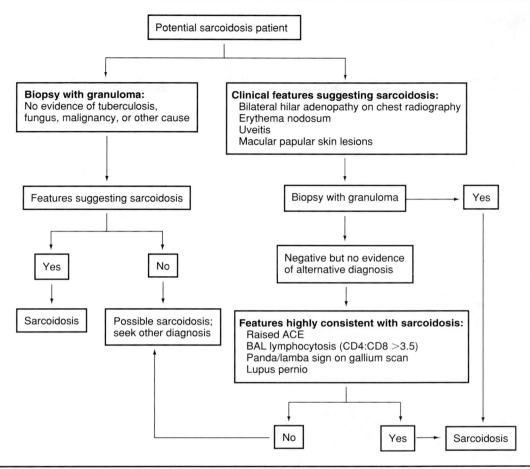

FIGURE 1. Summary approach to diagnosis of sarcoidosis. ACE, angiotensin-converting enzyme; BAL, bronchoalveolar lavage. (From Baughman RP, Lower EE, et al: Sarcoidosis. The Lancet 361:1111–1118, 2003. Copyright 2003. Reprint with permission from Elsevier.)

months. In patients who show significant improvement or resolution of clinical manifestations, prednisone should be slowly tapered over 2 to 3 months to a maintenance dose of 10 to 15 mg/day or to an every-other-day regimen. This maintenance therapy should be continued for a minimum of 6 months for most age groups. After this period, the dose is again tapered (if possible) and maintained until completing 1 full year of corticosteroid use. Patients should be followed after cessation of therapy for possible relapse. In such cases, a reinduction phase may be necessary. Some patients require long-term low-dose therapy to prevent disease. A subset of patients may be unresponsive to therapy or require relatively high doses of corticosteroids to achieve clinical control. This group will require steroid-sparing drugs.

The second line of therapy for sarcoidosis includes cytotoxic agents. Methotrexate (MTX) is frequently used in adults as a steroid-sparing agent in cases of pulmonary, neurologic, cutaneous, and ocular onset. A number of small uncontrolled clinical trials consistently show a benefit for its use as a steroid-sparing agent. Its use in the pediatric age group is limited; however, some success is noted. In one case series, seven children

with biopsy-proven sarcoidosis received a weekly single dose of 10 to 15 mg/m^2 for a minimum of 6 months. This group of children was able to decrease the mean dose of prednisone from 1.3 mg/kg/day to 0.5 mg/kg/day after 3 months of MTX and to 0.2 mg/kg/day after 6 months of MTX use. Adverse effects include liver toxicity, leukopenia, obstructive lung disease, and hypersensitivity pneumonitis. Toxicity of MTX can be minimized by folate supplementation. Blood cell count and liver function should be monitored regularly. The dose is adjusted based on neutropenia, nausea, or other laboratory abnormalities. In adults with sarcoidosis, the drug requires 6 months to become effective, limiting its use in acute disease.

ANTIMALARIAL AGENTS

Antimalarial agents have also been studied for use in pulmonary and cutaneous disease. Ocular toxicity is the major toxicity of this class of drugs. Because of its safer toxicity profile, hydroxychloroquine has been used more frequently. Only small clinical trials (none in children) and case reports demonstrate its efficacy in sarcoidosis.

TABLE 2 Drugs Most Commonly Used in Pediatric Sarcoidosis

Medication Class	Sarcoidosis (Trade Name)	Usual Initial Route/Dose/ Regimen	Maintenance Dose	Dosage Formulations	Adverse Reactions
Anti-inflammatory	Prednisone (Deltasone) Prednisolone (Orapred)	PO: 1–2 mg/kg/day qd or bid, 4–8 wk.	10–15 mg qd to qod; min: 6 mo. See text.	Tablet: 2.5, 5,10, 20, 50 mg; solution: 5 mg/5 mL; solution: 15 mg/5 mL	Weight gain, diabetes, hypertension, osteoporosis, increased risk of infection
Antimicrobial	Hydroxychloroquine (Plaquenil)	PO: 3–5 mg/kg/day, qd or bid. Not to exceed 7 mg/kg/day; max: 400 mg/day.		Tablet: 200 mg	Ocular toxicity, nausea
	Chloroquine (Aralen)	PO: 10 mg base/kg/day qd; max: 300 mg base/day.		Tablet: 250 mg (150 mg base), 500 mg (300 mg base)	Ocular toxicity, nausea
Cytotoxic	Methotrexate (Rheumatrex)	PO, IM, SC: 10–15 mg/m²/wk as a single dose; Cl_{Cr} 61–80 mL/min: decrease dose by 25%; Cl_{Cr} 51–60 mL/min: decrease dose by 33%; Cl_{Cr} 10–50 mL/min: decrease dose by 50%–70%.	10–15 mg/m²/wk, 3–6 mo.	Tablet: 2.5, 5, 7.5, 15 mg; injection: 20 mg/1 g (powder); 25 mg/mL (solution)	Nausea, leukopenia, hepatitis, pneumonitis, pulmonary fibrosis

bid, twice daily; Cl_{Cr}, creatinine clearance; IV, intravenous; PO, by mouth; qd, daily; qod, every other day; SC, subcutaneous.
Adapted from Baughman RP: Pulmonary sarcoidosis. Clin Chest Med 25:521–530, 2004. Dosages adapted from Gedalia A, Molina JF, Ellis GS Jr, et al: Low-dose methotrexate therapy for childhood sarcoidosis. J Pediatr 130:20–25; 1997; Shetty AK, Gedalia A: Sarcoidosis in children. Curr Probl Pediatr 30:145–176, 2000; Taketomo CK, Hodding JH, Kraus DM: Lexi-Comp's Pediatric Dosage Handbook, 11th ed. Hudson, Ohio: Lexi-Comp, 2004.

TABLE 3 Alternative Drugs Used in Adult Sarcoidosis

Medication Class	(Trade Name)	Usual Initial Dose/ Route/Regimen	Maintenance Dose	Dosage Formulations	Adverse Reactions
Cytotoxic	Methotrexate (Rheumatrex)	10 mg once weekly	2.5–15 mg once weekly	Tablet: 2.5, 5, 7.5, 15 mg	Nausea, leukopenia, hepatitis, pneumonitis
	Leflunomide (Arava)	10–20 mg qd	10–20 mg qd	Tablet: 10, 20, 100 mg	Nausea, leukopenia, hepatitis
	Azathioprine (Imuran)	50–100 mg qd	Up to 3 mg/kg qd	Tablet: 25, 50, 75, 100 mg	Nausea, leucopenia
	Cyclophosphamide (Cytoxan)	500–800 mg IV q2wk or 50–100 mg PO qd	1000–2000 mg IV q2–8wk or 50–100 mg PO qd	Tablet: 25, 50 mg Injection: 100, 200, 500 mg; 1, 2 g	Nausea, leukopenia, cystitis, bladder cancer
Cytokine modulators	Thalidomide (Thalomid)	50 mg daily	50–200 mg qd	Capsule: 50, 100, 200 mg	Somnolence, constipation, rash, teratogenicity
	Pentoxifylline (Trental)	400 mg tid	400–1200 mg in divided doses	Tablet: 400 mg	Nausea, diarrhea
	Infliximab (Remicade)	3–5 mg/kg initially and week 2	3–10 mg/kg q4–8wk		Increased rate of infection, anaphylaxis
	Etanercept (Enbrel)	25 mg SC bid	25 mg SC twice a week		Increased rate of infection, local reaction

bid, twice daily; IV, intravenous; PO, by mouth; qd, daily; SC, subcutaneous.
Adapted from Baughman RP: Pulmonary sarcoidosis. Clin Chest Med 25:521–530, 2004.

CONTROVERSIAL INTERVENTIONS

Alternative immunosuppressive agents, such as cyclosporine, azathioprine, chlorambucil, cyclophosphamide, and leflunomide, may be tried in adults (Table 3). Close monitoring for toxicity is necessary, especially regarding bone marrow suppression and gastrointestinal damage. There is only anecdotal use of this group of drugs in children. Cytokine modulators, such as thalidomide, pentoxifylline, infliximab, and etanercept, are used in adult patients with sarcoidosis. At this time, there are not enough data to recommend their use in children, so they should be considered on a case-by-case basis and only on those more severely ill patients not responding to systemic corticosteroids, methotrexate, or antimalarial drugs.

Common Pitfalls

There is no diagnostic test for sarcoidosis. It is a diagnosis of exclusion. A complete history should be performed, including environmental and, if applicable, occupational exposure. Physical examination should look carefully for skin, lung, ocular, neurologic, and cardiac findings. No specific tests are available to help measure disease progression. ACE is not specific for sarcoidosis because it is also elevated in leprosy, tuberculosis, primary biliary cirrhosis, hypersensitivity pneumonitis, α_1-antitrypsin deficiency, histoplasmosis, and so on. ACE is often elevated in active disease and routinely decreases with corticosteroid use in children and adults with sarcoidosis. Its level seems to correlate better with disease activity and effects of therapy in older children with sarcoidosis; in contrast, it is not a useful tool for predicting clinical course and response to treatment interventions in adults.

Communication and Counseling

The acute presentation of sarcoidosis is usually associated with a better prognosis and full recovery. This presentation occurs more commonly in children of Scandinavian origin. African American patients tend to present with the more chronic course that shows a worse long-term morbidity. Sarcoidosis is usually diagnosed in children at 12 to 15 years of age and presents a more favorable prognosis, often with spontaneous resolution. However, residual morbidity may be significant in a small number of patients. Drug therapy is prolonged, usually lasting at least a year.

SUGGESTED READINGS

1. Baughman RP, Lower EE, du Bois RM: Sarcoidosis. Lancet 361:1111–1118, 2003. **Excellent state-of-the-art article that discusses detailed treatment options in adult sarcoidosis.**
2. Baughman RP, Lynch JP: Difficult treatment issues in sarcoidosis. J Intern Med 253:41–45, 2003. **Excellent discussion of management issues in adult sarcoidosis.**
3. Baughman RP: Pulmonary sarcoidosis. Clin Chest Med 25:521–530, 2004. **Updated discussion of adult cases of the pulmonary disease in adults.**
4. Culver DA, Thomassen MJ, Kavuru MS: Pulmonary sarcoidosis: New genetic clues and ongoing treatment controversies. Cleve Clin J Med 71:88–106, 2004. **Good discussion on controversies surrounding etiology, diagnosis, and treatment of sarcoidosis.**
5. Gedalia A, Molina JF, Ellis GSSJr, et al: Low-dose methotrexate therapy for childhood sarcoidosis. J Pediatr 130:25–29, 1997. **Case report of the use of methotrexate in seven pediatric patients.**
6. Hoffmann AL, Milman N, Byg K-E: Childhood sarcoidosis in Denmark 1979–1994: Incidence, clinical features and laboratory results at presentation in 48 children. Acta Paediatr 93:30–36, 2004. **Describes a large series of pediatric cases in the Scandinavian population.**
7. Hunninghake GW, Costabel U, Ando M, et al: ATS/ERS/WASOG statement on sarcoidosis. American Thoracic Society/European Respiratory Society/World Association of Sarcoidosis and Other Granulomatous Disorders. Sarcoidosis Vasc Diffuse Lung Dis 16:149–173, 1999. **Official statement on definitions, diagnostic criteria, and treatment regimens for sarcoidosis.**
8. Pattishall EN, Kendig EL: Sarcoidosis in children. Pediatr Pulmonol 22:195–203, 1996. **Review of pediatric disease.**
9. Shetty AK, Gedalia A: Sarcoidosis in children. Curr Probl Pediatr 30:149–176, 2000. **Comprehensive review of the disease with an extensive list of references.**
10. Wu JJ, Schiff KR: Sarcoidosis. Am Fam Physician 70:312–322, 2004. **Good review of adult sarcoidosis aimed at general practitioners.**

Acute Respiratory Distress Syndrome

Caroline D. Boyd and Andrew T. Costarino, Jr.

8

KEY CONCEPTS

- In acute respiratory distress syndrome (ARDS), disruption of the alveolar-capillary membranes results in noncardiogenic pulmonary edema. ARDS is defined as acute, severe respiratory failure with bilateral opacities on chest radiograph with no clinical evidence of heart failure (pulmonary capillary wedge pressure less than 18 mm Hg).
- The clinical picture of ARDS is the final common pathway of lung injury secondary to numerous etiologies.
- In children, the most common associated conditions with ARDS are shock, sepsis, and acute viral pneumonitis.
- The lung injury in ARDS can be either direct or indirect.
- Estimated mortality rates for ARDS are between 40% and 60%, but death secondary to respiratory failure occurs in less than 20% of cases.
- The only proven intervention to decrease mortality in ARDS is the so-called lung-protective approach of mechanical ventilation. Small tidal volumes (<7 mL/kg) and acceptance of hypercapnia are targeted to avoid overdistention of lung units, thus reducing further alveolar-capillary membrane damage and propagation of the inflammatory cascade.

Acute respiratory distress syndrome (ARDS) is a common cause of hypoxic respiratory failure. It is characterized by diffuse bilateral radiodensities on chest radiograph in the absence of cardiac failure, poorly compliant respiratory mechanics, and hypoxemia. ARDS represents the final common pathway of a wide array of insults leading to alveolar damage and acute respiratory failure. This syndrome usually occurs in the presence of a systemic inflammatory response, leading to the release of inflammatory mediators and damage to capillary beds through the body. Fluid and debris accumulation and atelectasis lead to decreased lung volumes and the disruption of normal gas exchange.

In 1994, the North American–European Consensus Conference (NAECC) on ARDS established a definition of acute lung injury (ALI) and ARDS. ALI and ARDS are on a spectrum of severity. The definition of both entities includes acute onset of respiratory distress symptoms with bilateral opacities on chest radiographs and absent clinical evidence of heart failure (pulmonary artery wedge pressure <18 mm Hg). ALI is distinguished from ARDS exclusively by the severity of oxygenation abnormality. The ratio of arterial oxygen partial pressure to the fraction of inspired oxygen (Pao_2 to Fio_2) is used to quantify the efficiency of oxygenation. If the ratio is less than 200, the patient has ARDS; if greater than 200 but less than 300, the patient is classified as having ALI.

The incidence of ARDS ranges from 1.5 to 75 per 100,000 persons in the general population, depending on the publication referenced. Mortality rates are generally reported between 40% and 60%, with death from respiratory failure occurring less than 20% of the time. It is also possible that mortality rates differ with etiology, and ARDS secondary to a primary pulmonary source has a higher mortality than ARDS secondary to a nonpulmonary source. Studies suggest mortality may be decreasing in patients managed with lung-protective low-lung-volume mechanical ventilation.

Expert Opinion on Management Issues

The three important treatment strategy goals for critically ill children, particularly those with ALI/ARDS, are to control the injury or inflammatory source, to maintain adequate tissue oxygen delivery, and to promote healing. For ALI/ARDS, the specific challenge is to maintain oxygen delivery to tissues while the lung injury induced by mechanical ventilation is minimized.

INITIAL THERAPIES

Oxygen

Patients with ARDS, by definition, are hypoxemic and benefit from oxygen-enriched gas mixtures to boost the Pao_2 and increase the oxygen saturation of hemoglobin (Sao_2). Enriching the inspired gas mixture with oxygen ($Fio_2 > 0.21$) is a simple and usually effective method of raising the partial pressure of oxygen in the arterial blood, thereby increasing the arterial oxygen

saturation of hemoglobin. However, prolonged administration of an oxygen-enriched gas mixture of Fio_2 greater than 0.60 is toxic to the lungs; Fio_2 less than 0.40 is considered safe. Most patients with ARDS require additional therapies to allow adequate tissue oxygenation while receiving Fio_2 in the nontoxic range. Active attempts should be made to decrease the Fio_2 to levels below 0.6 to minimize oxygen toxicity. We recommend tracheal intubation and application of increased mean airway pressure if an Fio_2 greater than 0.6 is required to maintain Pao_2 at 60 mm Hg.

Mean Airway Pressure

Diffuse alveolar collapse is a hallmark of ARDS. The breakdown of the alveolar-capillary barrier secondary to inflammation and surfactant dysfunction allows the formed and nonformed elements of the blood to enter the airspaces. In normal lungs, preacinar arterioles vasoconstrict to shunt blood away from lung regions that are poorly ventilated and hypoxic to the lung regions that have normal oxygen and carbon dioxide gas tensions. In ARDS, this vasomotor response and autoregulation is rendered inadequate because of the large proportion of alveoli affected and modification of the hypoxic pulmonary response caused by inflammation. As a result, regions of the lung, with fluid-filled or collapsed alveoli, are perfused even though they are not ventilated. By counterbalancing the hydrostatic pressure that is collapsing some lung units, an increased mean airway pressure (MAP) can reinflate a portion of the damaged alveoli, allowing a return of ventilation and oxygen delivery to those areas. Although there are noninvasive methods of applying an increased airway pressure, most patients with ARDS require tracheal intubation.

MAP is defined as the average airway pressure throughout one respiratory cycle. It is proportional to the area under the pressure/time curve. When the inspiratory-to-expiratory ratio (I/E ratio) is 1:2 to 1:4, as it is in normal-ratio ventilation, adjustments in positive end-expiratory pressure (PEEP) is most commonly used to increase MAP. Prolongation of the inspiratory time (I time) also increases MAP but has a minimal effect unless the I/E ratio is reversed (inverse-ratio ventilation). Application of inverse-ratio ventilation is uncomfortable for dyspneic patients and often requires they be sedated and/or given neuromuscular blockade. Special ventilatory modalities, such as airway pressure release ventilation, are new strategies to allow patients with ARDS to tolerate reversing the I/E ratio.

The therapy of MAP is targeted to counterbalance the hydrostatic pressure collapsing some lung units; therefore the range of effective MAP is proportional to the vertical dimension of the patient's chest. Thus the effective MAP is generally less in infants and children than in adults. In the pediatric intensive care unit (ICU) population, the MAP in ARDS is usually in the range of 12 to 24 mm Hg. The appropriate MAP must be established at the bedside through therapeutic trial and reevaluated periodically.

LUNG-PROTECTIVE MECHANICAL VENTILATION

Low-Lung Volume

The lung-protective approach to mechanical ventilation includes strategies aimed at preventing overdistention that damages individual lung units and propagates the inflammatory response. Amato and coworkers demonstrated a decreased mortality in ARDS using what they called an "open lung approach." In their study population, they ventilated the control group using traditional tidal volumes (Vts) equal to 12 mL/kg, applied PEEP as necessary to keep Fio_2 less than 0.6, and targeted a $Paco_2$ between 25 and 35. Subjects receiving their open lung approach received a lower Vt (<6 mL/kg), a mechanical ventilation frequency less than 30 breaths per minute, peak inspiratory pressure (PIP) less than 40 cm H_2O, and PEEP adjusted using pulmonary function testing. The I/E ratio was reversed whenever an Fio_2 greater than 0.5 was needed to achieve Pao_2 more than 0.6. They demonstrated that patients treated with the open lung approach had improved Pao_2-to-Fio_2 ratios and static compliance.

In a large multicenter randomized study in adults, decreased mortality was observed when an open lung or low-lung volume approach was used. Low Vt and plateau pressure (Vt of 6 mL/kg and plateau pressure <30 cm H_2O) was compared to traditional ventilation (Vt of 12 mL/kg and plateau pressure <50 cm H_2O). They demonstrated a reduction in mortality rates in the group receiving the open lung approach to ventilation. In the open lung group, fewer patients needed respiratory support at 28 days; there were greater numbers of days free of mechanical ventilation between day 1 and 28 and less nonpulmonary organ failure. This is the only therapy used in ARDS proven to reduce mortality.

Permissive Hypercapnia

A consequence of limiting Vt to 4 to 6 mL per kg (as just described) is that minute ventilation is decreased and the $Paco_2$ rises. Because of the clear benefit of reduced mortality in low-lung volume mechanical ventilation, clinicians must "permit" hypercapnia in treated patients. Permissive hypercapnia has become a target to help track mechanical ventilation adjustments. The goal is to allow the $Paco_2$ to rise as long as the pH remains above 7.15 to 7.2. In fact, clinicians interpret normal $Paco_2$ levels as an indication that their adjustments to reduce mechanical ventilation settings may not be aggressive enough. Any strategy of allowing a respiratory acidosis must be balanced with the overall clinical picture to determine if allowing acidemia is appropriate.

Pressure versus Volume Control

Pressure-control ventilation (PCV) may offer some advantage over volume-control ventilation in patients with ARDS. Volume-control ventilation delivers a preset tidal volume with a constant (square wave) flow pattern, resulting in an airway pressure wave that continuously rises throughout the inspiratory phase. In PCV, the inspiratory pressure is constant with a decelerating inspiratory flow. The pattern of flow in PCV allows for a lower peak airway pressure and a more evenly distributed Vt, thereby minimizing barotrauma to the poorly compliant lungs. The disadvantage of PCV is that breath-to-breath tidal volume may vary, leading to inadequate minute ventilation in the setting of worsening lung compliance. Newer ventilators include modalities in which the inspiratory phase is pressure controlled, but a target tidal volume is set and the ventilator can automatically adjust the pressure up or down as needed to achieve the target Vt. These modes provide a safeguard against unrecognized hypoventilation while also offering most of the advantages of traditional PCV.

HIGH-FREQUENCY OSCILLATORY VENTILATION

High-frequency oscillatory ventilation (HFOV) achieves effective oxygenation by the application of high MAP, low tidal volumes, and the delivery of breaths at a high frequency. In HFOV, both inspiration and expiration are active, that is, controlled by the ventilator. Theoretically, this active expiration results in improved carbon dioxide elimination and reduced gas trapping when compared to other forms of high-frequency ventilation. HFOV is an effective mode of ventilation in patients with ALI and ARDS, using the permissive hypercapnia management strategy. In the short term, HFOV improves oxygenation. There is not enough evidence to conclude whether HFOV reduces mortality or long-term morbidity in patients with ARDS, but some studies demonstrate a trend toward decreased mortality when HFOV is applied.

Airway Pressure Release Ventilation

Airway pressure release ventilation (APRV) is a new mode of ventilation in which a high-level continuous positive airway pressure (CPAP) is briefly terminated each cycle. The short release of high pressure allows improved carbon dioxide clearance. The long high positive pressure to short pressure release ratio allows for maximal alveolar recruitment and improved gas exchange at lower peak airway pressures. The high CPAP is maintained with lower gas flow rates than traditional ventilation. This strategy is designed to allow spontaneous breathing at any phase of the ventilatory cycle, and in some patients it decreases the need for sedation and neuromuscular blockade.

ADJUNCTIVE AND EXPERIMENTAL THERAPIES

Prone Positioning

CT scanning demonstrates atelectasis areas in the posterior lung fields in both healthy and diseased lungs. The quantity of collapsed lung is greater in these regions in patients with ARDS. Both animal and human studies show an improvement in Pao_2 when patients with ARDS are turned from the supine to the prone position. Prone positioning may allow reexpansion of atelectatic regions in the posterior lung fields with subsequent improvement in ventilation/perfusion ($\dot{V} / \dot{Q}$) matching, Although prone positioning provides short-term benefits in patients with ARDS, a reduction in mortality rates has not been demonstrated in studies of this strategy.

Inhaled Nitric Oxide

Inhaled nitric oxide (iNO) may be beneficial in the treatment of ARDS because of its ability to vasodilate pulmonary vasculature selectively. That is, iNO is preferentially delivered to functional lung units, promoting vasodilation of vessels and thereby increasing blood flow to ventilated areas. Inhaled NO does not reach unventilated areas of the lung. Therefore, intrapulmonary shunting decreases, and arterial oxygenation improves. Nitric oxide induces vasodilation by increasing intracellular cyclic guanosine monophosphate levels, which relaxes smooth muscle. Inhaled NO is rapidly inactivated by hemoglobin after it diffuses through the alveolar membrane into the vascular space and therefore offers the benefit of localized selective pulmonary vasodilation with minimal to no systemic vascular effects.

No agreed-upon therapeutic dose of iNO exists. The efficacy of iNO was examined in both adult and pediatric populations with ARDS. Improved oxygenation (Pao_2-to-Fio_2 ratios) were demonstrated in the short term, but no compelling evidence yet supports its use to improve mortality in this disease.

Surfactant

Surfactant is a substance that lines the alveoli, promotes alveolar stability, and decreases surface tension. In the absence of surfactant, surface tension remains constant and small alveoli empty into larger alveoli, leading to collapse of the small alveoli and overdistention of the larger ones.

Inadequate surfactant activity in ARDS leads to decreased pulmonary compliance and alveolar collapse. Pulmonary edema fluid, cell membrane lipids, plasma proteins, and hemoglobin may cause inactivation of surfactant phospholipids.

The beneficial effect of surfactant replacement in premature neonates with hyaline membrane disease prompted the investigation of exogenous surfactant replacement in patients with ARDS. Use of surfactant in patients with ARDS improves oxygenation and respiratory mechanics. Despite improved respiratory mechanics, no improvement in mortality rates is demonstrated.

Extracorporeal Membrane Oxygenation

Extracorporeal membrane oxygenation (ECMO) is a rescue therapy for infants and children suffering from ARDS who fail conventional therapy. ECMO is complex and uses significant hospital resources; the decision to institute it must be made with caution and should be restricted to ARDS patients who are thought to have reversible lung disease. Studies in children with ARDS demonstrate a decreased mortality rate in children treated with ECMO. Contraindications to ECMO include an underlying malignancy, immunocompromised state, and significant neurologic compromise secondary to severe hypoxemia and ischemia.

Partial Liquid Ventilation

Partial liquid ventilation with perfluorocarbon is used experimentally in patients with ARDS. Perfluorocarbons are inert compounds that are nontoxic to the lungs and do not wash out existing surfactant. Liquid perfluorocarbons can dissolve two to three times more oxygen than blood can and reduce surface tension and decrease the production of reactive oxygen species. Multiple animal and human studies of liquid ventilation in ARDS show improvements in oxygenation, ventilation, and compliance. These improvements are attributed to the perfluorocarbon's ability to recruit atelectatic lung regions, improve the end-expiratory lung volume, decrease intrapulmonary shunting, and improve static lung compliance.

Common Pitfalls

- Failure to recognize respiratory insufficiency and impending respiratory failure.
- Failure to institute lung-protective strategies of mechanical ventilation early in a patient's course to minimize morbidity and mortality.
- Failure to treat the underlying cause of disease in patients with ARDS, which results in the continuation of the inflammatory response, worsening respiratory failure, and progression toward multiorgan system failure.

Communication and Counseling

Despite advances in managing patients with ARDS, mortality remains high. Ongoing communication with the patient's family is required to promote understanding and acceptance. Frequent updates and family meetings may be needed. Complications of ARDS and ICU care in general should be anticipated and discussed in advance whenever possible. Social services involvement and contact information of ARDS support organizations should be provided.

SUGGESTED READINGS

1. Amato MB, Barbas CS, Medeiros DM, et al: Effect of a protective-ventilation strategy on mortality in the acute respiratory distress syndrome. N Engl J Med 338(6):347–354, 1998. **Study demonstrating reduction in mortality with lung-protective strategy of mechanical ventilation.**
2. Brower RG, Matthay MA, Morris A, et al: Ventilation with lower tidal volumes as compared with traditional tidal volumes for acute

lung injury and the acute respiratory distress syndrome. N Engl J Med 342(18):1301–1308, 2000. **Study verifying the result of decreased mortality with low tidal volume ventilation in patients with ARDS.**

3. Derdak S, Mehta S, Stewart TE, et al: High-frequency oscillatory ventilation for acute respiratory distress syndrome in adults. Am J Respir and Crit Care Med 166:801–808, 2002. **Randomized controlled trial comparing safety and efficacy of HFOV with conventional ventilation in ARDS.**

4. Dobyns EL, Anas NG, Fortneberry D, et al: Interactive effects of high-frequency oscillatory ventilation and inhaled nitric oxide in acute hypoxemic respiratory failure in pediatrics. Crit Care Med 30(11):2425–2429, 2002. **Study concludes that improved lung recruitment by HFOV enhances the effect of iNO on gas exchange.**

5. Goss CH, Brower RG, Hudson LD, et al: Incidence of acute lung injury in the United States. Crit Care Med 31(6):1607–1611, 2003. **Study estimates the incidence of ALI in the United States as higher than reported previously.**

6. Green TP, Timmons OD, Fackler JC, et al: The impact of extracorporeal membrane oxygenation on survival in pediatric patients with acute respiratory failure. Crit Care Med 24(2):323–329, 1996. **Demonstrates the utility of ECMO as a rescue therapy for ARDS in children.**

7. Howard AE, Courtney-Shapiro C, Kelso LA, et al: Comparison of 3 methods of detecting acute respiratory distress syndrome: Clinical screening, chart review, and diagnostic coding. Am J Crit Care 13 (1):59–64, 2004. **Study suggesting that the incidence of ARDS is underestimated when based on either diagnostic coding or physicians' notes without testing for accuracy of coding.**

8

Congenital Heart Disease

Warren G. Guntheroth

KEY CONCEPTS

- Accurate diagnosis is essential for both the fetus and child. Early diagnosis is particularly important for the fetus, preferably prior to 24 weeks.
- Treatment options range from none required to intensive medical and surgical management. The choice is determined by the severity of the condition and the risks of the interventions.
- When possible, catheter interventions are effective and reasonably safe, but, as with surgery, the experience and skill of the operator determine the success and safety.
- Palliative surgery should be reserved for improving the quality of life; prolonging life should be a secondary consideration.
- Corrective surgery is not justified for some mild conditions, given the risk of surgery.
- Cardiac transplantation is of limited benefit to infants and children in terms of longevity and complications of medical management.
- The medical center and surgeon should be chosen based on the best interests of the child; institutional loyalty should ideally play no part.

Therapy for congenital heart disease (CHD) obviously requires detection and identification of the abnormalities involved, but detection requires considerable expertise and cannot be adequately covered in this volume. An excellent start for practitioners is the book by M.K. Park, *Pediatric Cardiology for Practitioners*.

Treatment may eventually begin in the fetus, but, except for pharmacologic therapy for arrhythmias (see the chapter entitled "Cardiac Dysrrhythmias"), attempts at surgical therapy in utero currently result in inducing labor and a markedly premature neonate with all the complications that accompany that state. Nevertheless, fetal echocardiography is worthwhile to prepare the parents psychologically and to prepare the obstetrical and pediatric team for the occasional urgent problem, such as a ductal-dependent lesion, because the duct may close soon after delivery and will cause the pulmonary blood flow to cease for all practical purposes. It is also necessary to diagnose definitively and before 24 weeks to afford the choice of termination for parents when very serious malformations are present.

Fortunately, most CHD requires no urgent therapy after delivery and, in fact, may never require intervention. But, many diagnoses do ultimately require intervention both to relieve symptoms and to allow a more normal life span. In addition to the natural history of the specific entity, severity of the disorder determines the necessity for intervention, the timing of that intervention, and the type of intervention. In every patient, the risk of the intervention must be weighed relative to the symptoms and the expected limitations of life span and activity that are inherent in the diagnosis. For example, a small ventricular septal defect (VSD) has a 50% chance of spontaneous closure. Most VSDs are asymptomatic, and persons with small VSDs have no proven decrease in longevity; accordingly, the risks of open-heart repair are hard to justify. In contrast, an infant with transposition of the great arteries would have a high probability of dying in the first year if left alone. The risk of the necessary surgery for this lesion is moderate in the hands of an experienced team, and the child's future would likely then be reasonably normal.

Expert Opinion on Management Issues

Therapy considerations include several options, depending on the type of CHD. To begin with, supportive medical management may include simple measures such as oxygen and fluids. Children with congenital cardiac lesions that involve high flow velocities with turbulence should have antibiotic chemoprophylaxis to prevent infective endocarditis as an ongoing need for recurrent procedures such as dental care. Prevention with antibiotics has never been *proven* to be effective, but failure to provide antibiotic coverage can lead to regrets and even litigation if endocarditis occurs. Good dental and oral hygiene have undeniable advantages, and probably are more effective than chemoprophylaxis alone.

PHARMACOLOGIC MANAGEMENT

Pharmacologic management is rarely able to *replace* surgical intervention if the condition is as serious as transposition, but medications may be important in stabilizing the patient so that he or she has a better chance of surviving an operation. In the case of a ductal-dependent lesion such as hypoplastic left heart syndrome, prostaglandins are usually necessary to maintain ductal flow and should be started prior to transportation to a tertiary center. Therefore, parenteral medications should be available even in relatively small hospitals. Closing a ductus arteriosus that remains open as a result of prematurity can frequently be accomplished by administration of indomethacin, but medical therapy does not work for a ductus that represents a congenital defect.

The armamentarium for treating congestive failure has increased a great deal since foxglove was first used, although digoxin is still a good initial choice. Diuretics, drugs to increase cardiac output and lower vascular resistance, and even β-blockers may be helpful (see the chapter titled, "Congestive Heart Failure"). Treatment of pulmonary hypertension because of increased resistance may be required both before and after surgery (see the chapter titled, "Pulmonary Hypertension in Children").

TRANSCATHETER INTERVENTIONS

The initial application was a balloon septostomy to open the foramen ovale more widely in infants with transposition of the great arteries, allowing better mixing of the systemic and pulmonic venous return. Balloon catheters for opening up stenotic pulmonary valves have been successful in the majority of cases. In contrast, opening up a stenotic aortic valve has been less successful and commonly produces regurgitation, and the improvement is less lasting, but it can be lifesaving in critical cases (critical aortic stenosis can lead to sudden cardiac death, whereas aortic regurgitation does not, reflecting the low coronary perfusion pressure in the former). Coarctation of the aorta has been successfully relieved in native coarctation and after partial surgical repairs in which there is residual coarctation. Further catheter-based successes have been achieved by the closure of symptomatic defects or ducts, beginning with devices to close off arterial ducts with one or more coiled filaments (Gianturco coils), a process that generally can safely be accomplished in an outpatient. Just as in surgery, operator experience and skill count in terms of success and safety. So-called clamshell devices delivered to an atrial septal defect by catheters are now accepted by many centers as an effective, safe, and relatively inexpensive means of closing these defects. Similar devices have been used in adults with postinfarction ventricular septal defects, but the risks are arguably excessive for use in infants and children.

Surgical Intervention

Surgical intervention can be palliative or corrective for CHD, if successful. *Palliation* should be reserved for improving the quality of the life of the patient rather than postponing death, unless the prolongation of life is likely to be substantial. The earliest—and still effective—operation is the Blalock-Taussig shunt for cyanotic infants or children whose critical deficiency is inadequate oxygenation secondary to obstructed pulmonary blood flow, as in tetrad of Fallot or tricuspid atresia. In this procedure one of the subclavian arteries is divided, and the end is sutured into the side of one pulmonary artery. Although inefficient, this operation

improves the pulmonary flow and, therefore, the pulmonary venous return to the left heart. This procedure can save lives and greatly improve the quality of life of a markedly cyanotic child. It is still done in early infancy if the size of the pulmonary arteries is too small to allow a complete repair at the time.

Palliation can also be achieved in the patient with tricuspid atresia by bypassing the obstruction and delivering the systemic venous return directly to the pulmonary arteries by means of a bidirectional Glenn procedure (attaching the superior vena cava to the right pulmonary artery, still connected to the main pulmonary artery) or the more complete Fontan procedure (tunneling the inferior vena cava flow through the right atrium to join the Glenn shunt is more effective). The Fontan works only if the pulmonary vascular resistance is low, allowing adequate flow generated by only the systemic venous pressure. The pulmonary venous return in a patient who has had a Fontan procedure permits modest activity and abolishes cyanosis and most of the risk of embolization to the systemic circulation.

Neither the Fontan nor the Blalock-Taussig operation will allow a normal life expectancy. The average survival is only 15 years, although some patients have done well for 25 to 30 years. Although the Blalock-Taussig shunt can be taken down at the time of a complete repair, a Fontan procedure represents a commitment to life with a single ventricle.

Corrective Surgery

Corrective surgery has been possible from the earliest days of safe thoracotomy, enabled by endotracheal anesthesia. The first successful complete correction of CHD was for persistent ductus arteriosus, followed soon after by correction of a coarctation of the aorta. Open-heart surgery had to await the development of extracorporeal circulation, that is, a heart-lung machine. Extracorporeal circulation has allowed the correction of atrial septal defects, ventricular septal defects, endocardial cushion defects (atrioventricular septal defects), tetrad of Fallot, transposition of the great arteries, transposition of the pulmonary veins, truncus arteriosus, and valve replacements of the pulmonic, aortic, and mitral valves. It must be added that these operations are not necessarily curative. In fact, some—particularly valve replacements—will generally require reoperation at intervals of 10 to 15 years.

Transplantation is in some sense the ultimate in surgical correction of CHD, but survival is limited at present to 10 years on average. The life of a child with a cardiac transplant cannot honestly be described as asymptomatic, considering the ravages of rejection and medications intended to retard rejection, which necessarily create a state of immune deficiency. I cannot recommend heart transplantation for an infant, although if the parents are fully informed and choose this option, I would certainly assist them. One advantage of early referral to a transplant service is that the cardiologists in such centers are skillful in managing congestive failure while they wait for a donor heart.

Termination of Pregnancy

Termination of pregnancy is a surgical option when fetal echocardiography has revealed serious CHD with a substantially short life expectancy that can only be palliated. This option requires that a definitive diagnosis is made before 24 weeks of gestation, the age cutoff in most states for abortion. The parents should make the decision to terminate or not after "full disclosure," which should be as free as possible from the physician's own biases or religious beliefs.

Compassionate Care

Compassionate care, preferably at home, is a humane management of some very sick children in whom correction of a severe defect is not feasible. The acceptance of this option requires an unusually mature parent in an era when faith in medical prowess is strong. Nevertheless, it can be a gratifying experience for some parents instead of subjecting their infant to months of futile intensive care.

Common Pitfalls

Almost every medicine or intervention has risks. Even chemoprophylaxis involves a small but definite risk of anaphylactic shock. A surgical mishap or infection may occur in the best of hospitals with the best of surgeons, such as catching an aortic leaflet with the needle sewing a patch on a ventricular septal defect, condemning the patient to severe aortic regurgitation, with all that entails from diastolic overload and ultimate valve replacement.

A primary care physician and cardiologist owe primary allegiance to the patient and not to the patient's hospital or surgeon. There is no doubt that the "occasional surgeon" has a greater mortality and morbidity as compared to a surgeon who does many cases per week in a major cardiac center, with a full team of diagnosticians, intensivists and, particularly, nurses skilled in postoperative management.

Communication and Counseling

Good—and honest—communication is essential in dealing with the parents of a fetus or child with CHD. Reassurance is needed if the situation is realistically not worrisome, but if the outlook is poor, it is our unpleasant task as physicians to explain the situation in as much detail as the parent can accept. It is important to schedule a return visit within a short time to answer questions that will inevitably occur to the parents and family after the first discussion. One should be prepared for some parents to go to websites to check what you have said about a condition, particularly its prognosis. Genetic issues will usually be raised and should be brought up even if the parents don't ask. Generally, CHD has a recurrence rate in a family of 2% to 3%. However, there are the exceptional families in which the rates are much higher, particularly if the same specific anomaly is known to recur in a family.

SUGGESTED READINGS

1. Cetta F, Feldt RH, O'Leary PW, et al: Improved early morbidity and mortality after Fontan operation: The Mayo Clinic experience, 1987 to 1992. J Am Coll Cardiol 28:480–486, 1996. **The 50% survival after a Fontan operation was only 15 years.**
2. Cyr DR, Guntheroth WG, Mack LA: Fetal echocardiography. In Berman M, Craig M, Kawamura D (eds): Obstetrics & Gynecology. Diagnostic Medical Sonography. A Guide to Clinical Practice. Philadelphia: Lippincott, 1990. **Useful for cardiologists, particularly those doing fetal echocardiograms.**
3. Dillard DH, Miller DW: Atlas of Cardiac Surgery. New York: Macmillan, 1983. **Easy to comprehend the abnormal gross anatomy and the steps in surgical correction.**
4. Gill HK, Splitt M, Sharland GK, et al: Patterns of recurrence of congenital heart disease. J Am Coll Cardiol 42:923–929, 2003. **Based on fetal echocardiography, provides frequencies for siblings, maternal, or paternal index cases by severity.**
5. Guntheroth WG: How important are dental procedures in the etiology of infective endocarditis? Am J Cardiol 54:797–801, 1984. **Evidence of causes of endocarditis; probably not the dentist.**
6. Park MK: Pediatric Cardiology for Practitioners. 3rd ed. St. Louis: Mosby. **A well-written and thorough book with enough facts to satisfy even a cardiologist but easy to read and understand.**

Marfan Syndrome

Peter N. Robinson and Yskert von Kodolitsch

9

KEY CONCEPTS

- Marfan syndrome is a relatively common dominantly inherited disorder of connective tissue with prominent manifestations in the skeletal, ocular, and cardiovascular systems.
- Diagnosis of Marfan syndrome depends on recognition of a characteristic combination of manifestations.
- The manifestations of Marfan syndrome are age dependent, with the average age of first diagnosis being around the time of puberty for many clinical features. There is a wide variability both between and among families, and the lack of a specific clinical feature in a child presenting with some manifestations of Marfan syndrome cannot be used to rule out the diagnosis.
- Marfan syndrome is caused by mutations in the gene *FBN1*. Molecular testing, although not routine, may be useful in some circumstances.
- Management revolves around early detection and prevention of serious complications such as aortic dilation and dissection. Regular follow-up by physicians experienced in the care of persons with Marfan syndrome is essential.

Marfan syndrome (MFS) is a dominantly inherited disorder of connective tissue with diverse and age-dependent manifestations primarily involving the skeletal, ocular, and cardiovascular systems. MFS has a frequency of at least 1 in 10,000 people, and approximately 25% to 30% of cases are related to de novo mutations. Timely and correct diagnosis of MFS is essential for providing optimal management and follow-up.

BOX 1   Diagnostic Criteria for Marfan Syndrome*

Skeletal System

A *major criterion* is defined by the presence of at least four of the following:

- Pectus carinatum
- Pectus excavatum severe enough to require surgery
- Reduced upper-to-lower segment ratio (<0.85) or arm span to height ratio (>1.05) (both in absence of severe scoliosis)
- Positive wrist *and* thumb signs
- Reduced extension of the elbows (<170°)
- Medial displacement of the medial malleolus associated with pes planus
- Protrusio acetabuli of any degree (ascertained on radiographs, CT, or MRI)

Involvement of the skeletal system is defined by the presence of two of the preceding features *or* the presence of one of the preceding features and two of the following: pectus excavatum not requiring surgery; joint hypermobility; high arched palate; facial features—at least two of dolichocephaly, malar hypoplasia, enophthalmos, retrognathia, down-slanting palpebral fissures.

Ocular System

A *major criterion* is defined by ectopia lentis of any degree.

Involvement of the ocular system is defined by the presence of at least two of the following:

- Flat cornea
- Increased axial length of the globe (>23.5 mm)
- Hypoplastic ciliary muscle causing decreased miosis

Cardiovascular

A *major criterion* is defined by dissection of the ascending aorta with or without aortic regurgitation and involving at least the sinuses of Valsalva.

Involvement of the cardiovascular system requires the presence of at least one of the following:

- Mitral valve prolapse with or without mitral regurgitation
- Dilatation of the main pulmonary artery, in the absence of valvular or peripheral pulmonic stenosis at younger than 40 years of age
- Calcification of the mitral annulus at younger than 40 years of age
- Dilatation or dissection of the descending thoracic or abdominal aorta at younger than 50 years of age

Pulmonary System

Involvement is defined by either spontaneous pneumothorax or radiographic evidence of apical blebs.

Skin and Integument

Involvement is defined by either striae distensae or a recurrent or incisional hernia.

Dura

A *major criterion* is the presence of lumbosacral dural ectasia.

Family/Genetic History

A *major criterion* is defined by one of the following:

- A first-degree relative who independently meets these criteria
- The presence of a mutation in the *FBN1* gene that is likely to be pathogenic
- The presence of a haplotype around the *FBN1* locus inherited by descent and unequivocally associated with diagnosed Marfan syndrome in the family

*Diagnostic criteria for the Marfan syndrome are also referred to as the *Ghent nosology*. If a first-degree relative is affected by the Marfan syndrome, the person under consideration must have involvement of at least two systems (skeletal, cardiovascular, ocular) and at least one major manifestation (such as ascending aortic aneurysm; ectopia lentis). If no first-degree relative is unequivocally affected by the Marfan syndrome, the propositus must have major manifestations in two systems and involvement of at least one other (skeletal, cardiovascular, ocular).

Expert Opinion on Management Issues

MAKING THE DIAGNOSIS

As in all of medicine, the first step in proper management is to make the proper diagnosis. Although this is relatively straightforward in persons with classic and severe manifestations of MFS, it is often challenging to confirm or exclude the diagnosis of MFS, especially in children with only one or a few features associated with the disorder. The diagnostic criteria for MFS that are in wide use today were developed by a panel of experts in the Belgian city of Ghent, after which they are now often referred as the *Ghent Nosology* (Box 1). This classification gives weight to various clinical features according to their specificity for MFS. For instance, aortic dilation and ectopia lentis are relatively specific for MFS, but many other features often found in persons with MFS, such as scoliosis and pectus excavatum, are also relatively common in the general population. The experience of many centers specializing in MFS is that only half or less of all persons referred with suspected MFS actually do have the condition. Although there are numerous genetic disorders with some degree of overlap with MFS, such as congenital contractural arachnodactyly and familial thoracic aneurysm and dissection, in many cases the clinical question may be whether a person with a "marfanoid" appearance actually has any disorder at all. Persons with homocystinuria may have ectopia lentis and some of the skeletal manifestations of MFS. Although homocystinuria is a rare disorder, it is important to rule it out (by plasma amino-acid analysis in the absence of pyridoxine supplementation) in each patient or family presenting with suspected MFS, because there is effective treatment available for homocystinuria.

Difficulties in making the diagnosis of MFS in children arise primarily from the age-dependent manifestation of most of the clinical features of MFS. Manifestations of the disorder are highly variable, not only between affected families, but also among the affected members within a given family. Thus, a child may be more or less severely affected than other relatives with MFS. Although many of the manifestations associated with MFS, such as scoliosis or aortic root dilation, most often are first diagnosed around the age of puberty, it is important to realize the age of onset is highly variable, ranging from the newborn period to well into adulthood. It is not unusual to see children present at a relatively early age with a single manifestation such as ectopia lentis and then to go on to develop several other clinical features by the time of puberty. Often, the true diagnosis may become apparent only after repeated consultations; when in doubt, close follow-up is essential.

Although *FBN1* mutation analysis is not required to make the diagnosis in straightforward cases, it may occasionally be helpful to carry out molecular diagnosis in children or teenagers who do not (yet) fulfill the clinical criteria. The identification of a characteristic *FBN1* mutation can help identify persons requiring particularly close clinical follow-up. However, the detection rate of *FBN1* mutations is less than 100%, even in persons with classic MFS, and the detection rate is much less in those who do not meet the criteria of the Ghent Nosology. Recently, mutations in the transforming growth factor β receptor II gene (*TGFβR2*) were identified in persons with an MFS-like disorder characterized by prominent aortic, skeletal, and skin/integument anomalies and mild ocular anomalies. It has been debated whether this disorder should be termed "Marfan syndrome," "type 2 Marfan syndrome" or something else. However, *TGFβR2* mutations are probably not common in unselected groups of persons with MFS, and the role of *TGFβR2* mutation screening in clinical practice remains to be defined.

ROUTINE EXAMINATIONS

Optimal care of children with MFS requires a generalist with broad experience in MFS who can refer to specialists as needed and ensure that routine examinations are performed. Several systems require regular assessment throughout childhood and adolescence. The American Academy of Pediatrics (AAP) has published guidelines for health supervision for children with MFS that can be used as a basis for coordinating care of affected children (see Suggested Readings). The following sections offer an overview of the most important management issues for children with MFS.

Cardiovascular Management

Optimal cardiovascular management is the single most important aspect of care for children and adults with MFS. Management generally will include regular monitoring of the heart and aorta and prophylactic treatment with β-blockers, with the primary goal of preventing acute aortic dissection. Insufficiency and other lesions of the mitral valve are also not uncommon and may necessitate surgical repair in some patients.

Although dissection of the aortic root may occur at any time of life (and has even been observed in utero), most persons with MFS do not have severe aortic complications before early adulthood. Many of the cardiovascular complications, such as mitral valve prolapse (MVP), mitral regurgitation, and aortic root dilatation develop in an age-dependent manner and may become more severe with time. It is difficult to predict the exact age of onset of cardiovascular complications in an individual patient, but children with sporadic MFS, with a family history of aortic dissection, or with a younger age at initial diagnosis of MFS have an increased risk of aortic complications. Aortic valve regurgitation is generally an indicator of marked aortic root dilatation.

All children with MFS should undergo yearly echocardiography with assessment of systolic and diastolic left-ventricular function, function of all heart valves, and dimensions of the aorta and pulmonary artery. Presence of mitral valve prolapse should be assessed by recently revised criteria. Aortic root dimensions should be measured in the parasternal long-axis view at all four standard levels by cross-sectional echocardiography, and measurements should be plotted against body surface area using appropriate nomograms. To avoid false-positive diagnosis of aortic root dilatation in MFS, a nomogram for children with tall body size should be consulted. Alternatively, aortic ratios can be calculated as the observed maximum diameter of the aortic root divided by the predicted diameter based on age and body surface area (BSA) of normal individuals. For children younger than 18 years of age, the predicted sinus diameter (cm) is $1.02 + (0.98 \times BSA \text{ [m}^2\text{]})$. For instance, a ratio of 1.3 indicates a 30% enlargement of the aortic root above the mean of normal individuals of the respective age and body surface area. A ratio of 1.18 is the upper 95% confidence limit for a ratio of 1.0. Rapid screening for presence of aortic root dilatation is possible by dividing the diameter of the sinus of Valsalva by the diameter of the aortic annulus; in individuals without aortic annular dilatation a ratio of 1.45 or greater accurately predicts aortic root dilatation.

In general, the risk of acute aortic dissection in MFS increases with increasing diameter of the aortic root. The results of prophylactic aortic root replacement are better than those of surgery following acute aortic dissection, and mortality is significantly less. Therefore, one of the key management issues for MFS is the decision whether surgical repair of the aortic root is indicated for a given patient in any given situation. If possible, surgery should be delayed until adolescence to avoid reintervention for size mismatch of the valve prosthesis caused by growth of the cardiovascular system subsequent to the first intervention. Gillinov and coworkers recommend not delaying mitral valve operations to perform concomitant aortic and mitral valve operations in patients with only mildly or moderately dilated aortic roots. The European task force suggests avoiding routine intervention simply if aortic root dimensions lie outside the upper confidence interval for the normal population but does recommend surgery when dimensions deviate upward from the noted percentile on follow-up echocardiograms. In general, decisions for surgery should be individualized. Ideally, surgery should be performed at centers with experience in treating persons with MFS. Figure 1 summarizes the most frequently recommended criteria for surgical intervention.

Prior to elective vascular surgery, MRI is required for mapping of the entire aorta. Baseline magnetic resonance imaging should be performed within 30 days after elective aortic surgery. Serial postoperative examinations are required at 6-month intervals, which may be extended to yearly intervals when the postoperative course is uneventful and aortic diameters remain stable.

A prospective study by Shores and associates concerning the use of prophylactic β-adrenergic therapy showed that the rate of aortic dilatation was significantly lower, actuarial long-term survival better, and aortic regurgitation, aortic dissection, cardiovascular surgery, and congestive heart failure less frequent in the treatment group as compared to the control group. Retrospective studies have confirmed the effectiveness

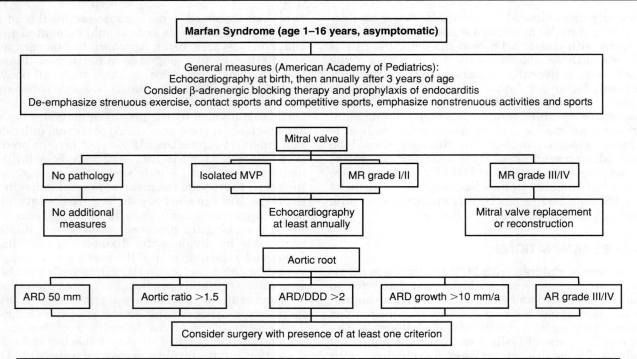

FIGURE 1. Management of cardiovascular manifestations. ARD growth > 10 mm/a: growth of the aortic root diameter by more than 10 mm per year. AR, aortic regurgitation; ARD, aortic root diameter; ARD/DDD, ratio of aortic root diameter divided by the diameter of the distal descending aorta; DDD, diameter of distal descending aorta; MR, mitral valve regurgitation; MVP, mitral valve prolapse.

of β-adrenergic blockade in MFS children. The initial dosage of atenolol or propranolol should be as low as 0.5 to 1.0 mg/kg/day; the dosage of atenolol should then be increased by 12.5 mg to 25 mg per day and propranolol by 20 mg to 40 mg per day until the maximum heart rate remains below 100 beats per minute after moderate exercise such as running up and down 44 steps as rapidly as possible. A study by Rossi-Foulkes and colleagues suggested that if β-blockers are not tolerated, calcium antagonists may also be effective in retarding aortic growth rates. The studies of Shores and associates in 1994 and of Rossi-Foulkes and associates in 1999 suggest that β-adrenergic blockade should be administered to any child with MFS, with calcium antagonists as therapeutic alternatives when β-blockers are not well-tolerated. Medical therapy should be continued after cardiovascular surgery.

Antibiotic prophylaxis is indicated in any patient with MFS when transient bacteriemia is likely to occur. Because MFS patients with heart valve prostheses are at particularly high risk for endocarditis, surgeons recommend broad spectrum intravenous antibiotic prophylaxis for dental, endoscopic, and surgical procedures or with infections of the upper airways or the skin.

Ophthalmologic Management

The most specific ocular manifestation of MFS is ectopia lentis due to progressive elongation of the ciliary zonules. Myopia is often an early manifestation of MFS. Although myopia is very common in the general population, it is a reason for a full ophthalmologic evaluation including cycloplegia, in which even minor degrees of ectopia lentis can be identified. High degrees of myopia up to and exceeding −15 diopters are not uncommon in MFS. Regular ophthalmologic follow-up is indicated to prevent amblyopia. The presence of ectopia lentis should lead to referral to a specialist experienced in the care of persons with MFS and ectopia lentis. In general, a conservative approach with non-surgical visual enhancement is preferable, but reduced visual acuity due to noncorrectable refractive errors, secondary glaucoma, and retinal detachment generally represent indications for surgical lensectomy. It is important to note that about one third of affected persons do not have specific ocular manifestations of MFS.

Orthopedic Management

The skeletal manifestations of MFS include scoliosis, pectus excavatum or carinatum, and joint laxity. Dolichostenomelia (long, slim limbs) can be quantified by measuring the arm span to height ratio (the normal range is less than 1.05), and the ratio of the upper segment to the lower segment (the latter is measured from the symphysis pubis to the floor in a standing position, and the former is calculated by subtracting the lower segment length from the body height; a normal range is above 0.85). Arachnodactyly (long, thin fingers, literally, "spider-fingers") can be quantified by the "wrist sign" (thumb overlaps last joint of little finger when hand is wrapped around opposite wrist) and the "thumb sign" (entire thumbnail projects beyond far side of palm when hand is clenched).

Many of the clinically important problems such as scoliosis and pectus deformities also occur in the general population. It should be noted that the prognosis and indicated form of treatment may be different from those for the general population, and consultation with an orthopedic surgeon with experience with MFS is essential. Approximately two thirds of affected persons will develop scoliosis; scoliosis tends to progress faster than in the general population, tends to respond less well to bracing treatment, and is associated with a higher frequency of postoperative complications. However, in many cases the scoliosis is minor, and only about 10% to 20% of cases require treatment of any kind.

The growth spurt and pubertal skeletal maturation may occur early in MFS, and special growth charts have been developed. These charts should be consulted when predicting adult height. Early endocrinologic consultation is recommended in situations where hormonal treatment to limit adult height is under consideration.

Moderate sporting activity should be encouraged, especially activities such as swimming, cycling, or walking. Contact sports such as karate should be discouraged because of the danger of ectopia lentis. Forms of very strenuous exertion with sudden stops, such as basketball, are not advisable.

Common Pitfalls

- Dismissing the diagnosis of MFS in a child with one or more characteristic manifestations of MFS because the Ghent diagnostic criteria are not fulfilled. Because of the age-dependent nature of many of the manifestations of MFS, repeated follow-up may be needed to make or exclude the diagnosis.
- Excluding the diagnosis of MFS on the grounds of a negative *FBN1* mutation analysis. At present *FBN1* mutation analysis does not detect mutations in all persons with clear MFS; therefore, negative findings do not rule out the diagnosis of MFS.
- Nonreferral. In general, optimal care of persons with MFS is given by centers or specialists with considerable experience treating these individuals.

Communication and Counseling

Improvements in clinical management in the last few decades, such as the use of prophylactic treatment with β-blockers and cardiovascular surgery, have significantly increased life expectancy of people with MFS. Scientific advances including the discovery of mutations in the gene for fibrillin-1 in persons with MFS and novel insights into the molecular pathogenesis of MFS promise to continue to improve quality of life of persons with this disorder. Nevertheless, significant clinical challenges involving diagnosis and choosing the optimal treatment remain. The keys to optimal management include close and careful follow-up of individuals with definite or suspected MFS with early referral to experienced specialists for management of complications.

SUGGESTED READINGS

1. American Academy of Pediatrics Committee on Genetics. Health supervision for children with Marfan syndrome. Pediatrics 98:978–982, 1996. **Guidelines for management of children with Marfan syndrome; available online at http://www.pediatrics.org.**
2. De Paepe AA, Devereux RB, Dietz HC, et al: Revised diagnostic criteria for the Marfan syndrome. Am J Med Genet 62:417–426, 1996. **The Ghent diagnostic criteria.**
3. Erbel R, Alfonso F, Boileau C, et al: Diagnosis and management of aortic dissection. Eur Heart J 22:1642–1681, 2001. **The European task force guidelines for aortic dissection in Marfan syndrome and other disorders.**
4. Freed LA, Levy D, Levine RA, et al: Prevalence and clinical outcome of mitral-valve prolapse. N Engl J Med 341:1–7, 1999. **An interesting study on mitral valve prolapse in the general population with clear descriptions of the diagnostic methods and criteria for mitral valve prolapse.**
5. Gillinov AM, Zehr KJ, Redmond JM, et al: Cardiac operations in children with Marfan's syndrome: Indications and results. Ann Thorac Surg 64:1140–1145, 1997. **An interesting overview of the surgical management of cardiovascular complications of Marfan syndrome in children.**
6. Gott VL, Greene PS, Alejo DE, et al: Replacement of the aortic root in patients with Marfan syndrome. N Engl J Med 340:1307–1313, 1999. **An overview of multicenter results in replacement of the aortic root with a prosthetic graft and valve in patients with Marfan syndrome in order to prevent premature death from rupture of an aneurysm or aortic dissection.**
7. Lipscomb KJ, Clayton-Smith J, Harris R: Evolving phenotype of Marfan's syndrome. Arch Dis Child 76:41–46, 1997. **This article contains information on the average age of onset of many of the manifestations of Marfan syndrome in a study group of 40 children with Marfan syndrome.**
8. Pyeritz RE: The Marfan syndrome. Annu Rev Med 2000; 51:481–510, 2000. **An excellent clinical description of Marfan syndrome.**
9. Robinson PN, Godfrey M (eds): Marfan Syndrome: A primer for clinicians and scientists. Georgetown: Landes Bioscience/Kluwer Academic/Plenum Publishers, 2004. **A comprehensive treatment of the clinical management of persons with Marfan syndrome and basic science aspects of fibrillin and fibrillinopathies.**
10. Roman MJ, Devereux RB, Kramer-Fox R, et al: Two dimensional aortic root dimensions in normal children and adults. Am J Cardiol 64:507–512, 1989. **Nomograms for cross-sectional echocardiography.**
11. Rossi-Foulkes R, Roman MJ, Rosen SE, et al: Phenotypic features and impact of beta blocker or calcium antagonist therapy on aortic lumen size in the Marfan syndrome. Am J Cardiol 83(9):1364–1368, 1999. **A small but interesting study on the effects of β-blocker or calcium antagonist therapy in children and adolescents with Marfan syndrome.**
12. Rozendaal L, Groenink M, Naeff MSJ, et al: Marfan syndrome in children and adolescents: an adjusted nomogram for screening aortic root dilatation. Heart 79:69–72, 1998. **Nomograms useful for children and adolescents with Marfan syndrome.**
13. Shores J, Berger KR, Murphy EA, et al: Progression of aortic dilatation and benefit of long-term β-adrenergic blockade in Marfan's syndrome. N Engl J Med 330:1335–1341, 1994. **The only large-scale prospective study on the use of β-blocker to retard progression of aortic root dilatation in persons with Marfan syndrome.**
14. van Karnebeek CD, Naeff MS, Mulder BJ, et al: Natural history of cardiovascular manifestations in Marfan syndrome. Arch Dis Child 84:129–137, 2001. **A description of the evolution of aortic and mitral valve abnormalities in children with Marfan syndrome.**

Congestive Heart Failure

Joseph D. Kay

KEY CONCEPTS

- Congestive heart failure in children occurs through a variety of distinct mechanisms leading to different physiologic states that require different approaches to therapy.
- Most structural congenital cardiac defects can now be surgically repaired or palliated even during infancy with relatively low mortality and morbidity, precluding the need for prolonged medical therapies.
- Most CHF medical therapies are palliative at best, and none are proved to reduce mortality in children. Any perceived mortality benefit is extrapolated from trials in adults with acquired cardiomyopathies.
- Frequent, repeated clinical assessments are required after initiation of therapies, as responses to therapies vary, and a multistage approach is usually required to ensure adequate growth and development.
- Like all children with chronic medical conditions, adequate nutritional support is critical both preoperatively and chronically to ensure proper wound healing, growth, and development.

Congestive heart failure (CHF) is the physiologic state of increased flow and/or pressure in the pulmonary vasculature, leading to excessive interstitial and alveolar pulmonary fluid referred to as *pulmonary edema.* Children, particularly infants, are very effective in removing this extra alveolar fluid via both lymphatic drainage and increased respiratory rate. Although these adaptations decrease hypoxemia, they also result in an increase in caloric expenditure, which is only compounded by feeding intolerance that occurs, at least in part, because of the inability to coordinate sucking and swallowing in the face of the increased respiratory rate that occurs in this situation. Signs of CHF in children, therefore, differ from those in adults. Rales and lower extremity edema are rarely seen in young children with CHF; more typical signs include tachypnea, tachycardia, hepatomegaly, a hyperactive precordium, poor weight gain, diaphoresis with feeds, and failure to thrive.

The heterogeneous causes of CHF in children preclude simple treatment algorithms. The clinician must identify and understand the physiologic cause and severity of an individual patient's CHF prior to selecting the most appropriate therapy. The treatment approach to a child with moderate to severe valve obstruction is different from that for an infant with an isolated large left-to-right shunt. Additionally, the natural history and treatment options are different for a child with a ventricular septal defect and a child with dilated cardiomyopathy. Box 1 lists common examples of causes of CHF in children. The leading causes of CHF in children from developed countries generally stem from structural congenital heart defects that produce an excessive workload on the myocardium as a result of

pressure or volume overload with or without cyanosis. More prevalent in less-developed countries, but not infrequently seen throughout the world, are cardiomyopathies (both hypertrophic and dilated), which may result from either inherited myopathies (such as the muscular dystrophies or glycogen storage diseases) or from acquired causes (such as infections, toxins, malnutrition, or Kawasaki disease). An increasing cause of CHF over the last few decades is myocardial dysfunction as a sequela from attempted repair or palliation for congenital heart defects.

Expert Opinion on Management Issues

Table 1 lists the more common medical therapies and recommended doses for treating children with CHF. Although there is scant evidence proving that medical treatment for CHF symptoms prior to surgery improves the surgical outcome, most experts agree

---

BOX 1 Causes of Pediatric Congestive Heart Failure

Structural Congenital Heart Defects
- Left-to-right shunts (volume overload)
  - Atrial ventricular canal defect
  - Atrial septal defect (rarely cause CHF)
  - Ventricular septal defect (most common)
  - Patent ductus arteriosus (most common in premature infants)
  - Aortic to pulmonary artery window
  - Truncus arteriosus
- Regurgitant lesions (volume overload)
  - Mitral regurgitation (cleft mitral valve)
  - Aortic regurgitation (bicuspid, aortic root dilation)
  - Tricuspid regurgitation (Ebstein)
  - Pulmonary (absent pulmonary valve syndrome)
- Obstructive lesions (pressure overload)
  - Aortic valvar, subvalvar, or supravalvar stenosis
  - Mitral valvar or supravalvar stenosis
  - Coarctation of the aorta

Cardiomyopathies
- Dilated (myocardial systolic dysfunction)
  - Metabolic (glycogen storage disease, transporter deficiency)
  - Infectious (viral, rheumatic fever, Kawasaki disease)
  - Ischemic (Kawasaki disease, anomalous origin of the left main coronary artery)
  - Congenital (ventricular noncompaction)
  - Arrhythmia induced (tachycardic induced, complete heart block with chronic pacemaker)
- Restrictive (myocardial diastolic dysfunction)
  - Idiopathic
  - Hypertrophic cardiomyopathy (autosomal dominant with variable penetrance)
  - Metabolic (gestational diabetes, glycogen storage disease)

Postoperative Ventricular and or Valvular Dysfunction
- Systemic right ventricle (D-TGA after atrial switch, congenitally corrected transposition)
- Single ventricle
- Postoperative left ventricular systolic dysfunction
- Residual left-to-right shunting
- Residual valvular regurgitation

TABLE 1 Medications for Heart Failure

Drug	Route/Dose	Max Dose	Formulations	Common Adverse Reactions	Comments
Diuretics					
Furosemide (Lasix)	IM/IV: 1–2 mg/kg/dose q6–12h PO: 1–2 mg/kg/dose bid to tid	6 mg/kg/dose 6 mg/kg/dose	IV: 10 mg/mL Oral solution: 10 mg/mL, 40 mg/5 mL Tab: 20, 40, 80 mg	Fluid and electrolyte imbalance (hypokalemia, hypercalciuria, dehydration) hyperuricemia, prerenal azotemia, metabolic alkalosis, ototoxicity, possible renal calcifications in premature infants.	IV dose approximately twice as potent as PO route, therefore adjust dose accordingly when switching from IV to oral.
Ethacrynic acid (Edecrin)	IV: 1 mg/kg/dose PO: 25 mg/dose	IV: not recommended to exceed 1–2 doses per day PO: 2–3 mg/kg/day	IV: 50 mg/vial (diluted in D₅W or NS first) Tab: 25, 50 mg	Fluid and electrolyte imbalance (hypokalemia, hypercalciuria, dehydration) hyperuricemia, prerenal azotemia otoxicity, GI irritation, metabolic alkalosis.	Second line to furosemide in most instances.
Chlorothiazide (Diuril)	IV: Not recommended for infants or children PO: <6 mo, 30 mg/kg/day divided bid Children: 20 mg/kg/day divided bid	<6 mo: 375 mg/day children: 1 g/day	IV: 500 mg/20 mL (mix with 18 mL of sterile water) Oral solution: 250 mg/5mL Tab: 250, 500 mg	Fluid and electrolyte imbalance (hypokalemia, hypercalciuria, hypomagnesemia, hyponatremia, dehydration) hyperuricemia, prerenal azotemia, metabolic alkalosis.	Most effective diuresis when given 1 h prior to loop diuretic.
Metolazone (Zaroxolyn)	IV: not available PO: 2.5 to 10 mg qd-bid	20 mg/day	Tab: 2.5, 5, 10 mg May compound suspension	Fluid and electrolyte imbalance (hypokalemia, hyponatremia, hypochloremia, hypophosphatemia dehydration) hyperuricemia, prerenal azotemia, hemoconcentration, venous thrombosis, GI complaints, ↓ bone marrow suppression, hepatitis, rash.	Most effective when given 30–60 min prior to loop diuretic; causes more profound hypokalemia than other diuretics.
Spironolactone (Aldactone)	IV: not available PO: Children: 1–3 mg/kg/day divided bid-qid	200 mg/day	Tab: 25, 50, 100 mg	Hyperkalemia, gynecomastia, rash. GI upset.	Used commonly in children when moderate to high doses of loop diuretics used to minimize hypokalemia; proven to reduce mortality in adults with CHF.
Inotropic Agents					
Dopamine	IV: 2–20 μg/kg/min, titrated to desired clinical effect	Minimal additive benefit above 20 μg/kg/min	40 mg/mL, 80 mg/mL, and 160 mg/mL; may be mixed with all but alkaline carriers	Tachyarrhythmias; infiltrations may cause local necrosis and should be treated with phentolamine.	Tachyphylaxis may develop because of down regulation of β receptors requiring higher doses. Preferentially through a central venous catheter

TABLE 1—cont'd

Drug	Route/Dose	Max Dose	Formulations	Common Adverse Reactions	Comments
Dobutamine	IV: 2–20 µg/kg/min, titrated to desired clinical effect	Minimal additive benefit above 20 µg/kg/min	12.5 mg/mL; may mix with D_5W or NS	Tachycardia, supraventricular and ventricular arrhythmias.	Tachyphylaxis may develop because of downregulation of β receptors requiring higher doses, preferentially through a central venous catheter.
Milrinone (Primacor)	IV: 50 µg/kg load over 10 minutes, then 0.25–1 µg/kg/min	Questionable added benefit over 1 µg/kg/min	IV: 1 mg/mL	Hypotension, dysrhythmias, hypokalemia, hepatotoxicity, thrombocytopenia.	Effects last 3–5 hours after discontinuation of infusion; dose reduction needed in renal failure.
Epinephrine	0.01–0.2 mg/kg/min	0.2 mg/kg/min		Tachycardia and atrial and ventricular dysrhythmias.	Preferentially through a central venous catheter. Used mainly for postoperative support of stunned myocardium, and with profound shock.
Afterload-Reducing Agents					
Captopril (Capoten)	PO: <2 mo: 0.05–0.1 mg/kg/dose tid >2 mo: 0.1 mg/kg/dose given tid, may double dose to max of 2 mg/kg/dose	6 mg/kg/day	Tab: 12.5, 25, 50, 100 mg	Hypotension, hyperkalemia (particularly when in combination with Aldactone), elevation on Cr, neutropenia, dry cough.	Mild elevations in Cr are not unusual and do not necessarily warrant discontinuation. Contraindicated in renal artery stenosis.
Enalapril (Enalaprilat—IV)	PO: Infants and children: 0.1–0.5 mg/kg/day given bid Adults: 2.5–20 mg bid IV: Infants and children, 0.005–0.01 mg/kg/dose qd-tid Adults: 0.625–1.25 mg/dose q6h	Infants and children: 0.5 mg/kg/day Adults: 40 mg/day	Tab: 2.5, 5, 10, 20 mg May compound suspension IV: 1.25 mg/mL	Hypotension, hyperkalemia (particularly when in combination with Aldactone), elevation on Cr, hypoglycemia, dry cough	Mild elevations in Cr are not unusual and do not necessarily warrant discontinuation. Contraindicated in renal artery stenosis.
Hydralazine (Apresoline)	PO: Infants and children: 0.75–1 mg/kg/day divided q6–12h Adults: 10–50 mg/dose qid IV: Rarely indicated for CHF (may cause profound hypotension)	Infants and children: 25 mg/dose Adults: 75–100 mg/dose	Tab: 10, 25, 50, 100 mg Oral solution: 1.25, 2, 4 mg/mL (needs extemporaneous compounding)	Lupus-like syndrome; hypotension, tachycardia.	Used only for children for whom ACEIs are contraindicated.

Drug	Dosing		How supplied	Adverse effects	Comments
Nitroprusside (Nipride)	IV: 0.5–10 µg/kg/min (Doses > than 6 µg/min not recommended in neonates)		IV: 50 mg/vial	Hypotension, tachycardia, and thyroid suppression.	Thiocyanate levels should be monitored if used >48 hours, in renal failure, and at higher doses.
Nicardipine (Cardene)	IV: 0.5–3 µg/kg/min PO: Not recommended for CHF		IV: 2.5 mg/mL	Hypotension, headache, GI symptoms.	Use with caution in hepatic or renal dysfunction.
Milrinone (Primacor)	IV: 50 µg/kg load over 10 minutes, then 0.25–1 µg/kg/min	Questionable added benefit over 1 µg/kg/min	IV: 1 mg/mL	Hypotension, dysrhythmias, hypokalemia, hepatotoxicity, thrombocytopenia.	Effects last 3–5 hours after discontinuation of infusion; dose reduction needed in renal failure.
β-Adrenergic Blockers					
Propranolol (Inderal)	PO: 1 mg test dose; then 1 mg/kg/day divided tid; increased by 1 mg every 3 days if tolerated IV: Not recommended for treatment for CHF	2 mg/kg/day divided tid	Tab: 10, 20, 40, 60, 80, 90 mg ER caps: 60, 80, 120, 160 mg Solution: 20, 40 mg/5 mL Concentrated solution: 80 mg/mL Susp: 1 mg/mL (needs extemporaneous compounding)	Hypotension, bradycardia, bronchospasm, fatigue, depression, sexual dysfunction.	Not well-studied in children with heart failure to date.
Metoprolol	PO: Start at 0.1 to 0.2 mg/kg/dose given bid; titrated upward to 0.5–1.0 mg/kg/dose IV: Not recommended for CHF	Children: 0.5–2.0 mg/kg/day Adults: 200 mg/day	Tab: 25, 50, 100 mg May compound suspension	Hypotension, bradycardia, bronchospasm, fatigue, depression, sexual dysfunction.	Not well-studied in children with heart failure to date.
Carvedilol (Coreg)	PO: Children: Started at dose of 0.03–0.08 mg/kg/dose given bid; doubled every 2 wk as tolerated Older children and adults: Started with 3.125 mg bid, titrated to goal of 50 mg bid	Children: 0.75 mg/kg/dose Adult: 50 mg/dose	Tab: 3.125, 6.25, 12.5, 25 mg May compound suspension Solution: In study, mixed 3.125-mg tab with 2 mL of water (80% soluble)	Hypotension, bradycardia, bronchospasm, fatigue, depression, sexual dysfunction.	Not well-studied in children with heart failure to date.

ACEI, angiotensin-converting enzyme inhibitors; bid, two times a day; CHF, congestive heart failure; Cr, serum creatinine; D₅W, dextrose 5% in water; ER, extended release; GI, gastrointestinal; IM, intramuscularly; IV, intravenously; NS, normal saline; PO, orally; qd, daily; qid, four times a day; qsh, every x hours; susp, suspension; tid, three times a day.

that optimization of the growth and minimization of pulmonary edema prior to surgery minimizes a child's postoperative convalescent period. Similar principles apply in choosing medical therapies for children with both volume overload states from left-to-right shunts or those with primary myocardial systolic dysfunction. Children with restrictive cardiomyopathies do not tolerate a low preload, and therefore aggressive diuresis should be avoided.

NUTRITIONAL SUPPORT

Because of the combination of decreased caloric intake and the increased caloric expenditure, infants and young children with CHF display poor growth. Unlike adults with CHF, children's oral intake should not be restricted, as maximal caloric intake is vital for growth. Alternatively, the child's caloric intake should be maximized with higher caloric density formulas, typically 22 to 24 kcal per ounce (occasionally higher, if needed), and young children will frequently require up to 125 to 150 kcal/kg/day to maintain near normal growth despite optimal medical therapy. When CHF becomes severe, nasogastric tube placement is often necessary to minimize infants' caloric expenditure and ensure adequate nutrition. Because of hepatic and gastrointestinal distention, children with CHF are also prone to significant gastroesophageal reflux, and additional therapies such as antacids and promotility agents may also be needed.

DIURETICS

Furosemide (Lasix) remains the most common diuretic used in infants and children to relieve pulmonary congestion, and at times may be all that is needed for children with mild CHF. When higher doses are required, significant hypokalemia can develop, prompting many to add spironolactone (Aldactone), a weaker diuretic with potassium-sparing properties. Children with more severe heart failure, however, may develop a tolerance to furosemide because of the development of a hypochloremic metabolic alkalosis. Alternative potent diuretics with slightly different properties have been used with mixed success. Agents that are effective at different sites within the renal tubules and therefore can be used synergistically with furosemide include chlorothiazide (Diuril) and metolazone (Zaroxolyn). When given 30 to 60 minutes prior to furosemide, there is usually a much more brisk diuresis. This combination, however, usually leads to electrolyte abnormalities quickly, requiring more judicious monitoring. Alternatively, ethacrynic acid (Edecrin), a loop diuretic with a slightly different structure than furosemide, is sometimes more effective in children not responding well to furosemide, or it may help the child to have a more brisk diuresis when given in alternating doses with furosemide. Chronic high doses of furosemide can lead to ototoxicity and hypercalciuria, which may eventually deplete the child's calcium stores and can lead to compression fractures.

INOTROPIC AGENTS

Inotropic agents have been used for many years in supporting the failing or overworked myocardium. Digoxin is the oldest agent used to treat both adults and children with CHF and therefore has been studied extensively. Its pharmacokinetics, although complex, have been well studied in children of all ages. Table 2 presents its complex dosing scheme. Echocardiographic and invasive measurements of ventricular function have indicated that digoxin is useful in increasing myocardial contraction. Additionally, it increases vagal tone and thus slows atrioventricular (AV) nodal conduction, which makes it useful for treating some supraventricular arrhythmias. Some specialists also believe that this increased vagal tone and, hence, decreased heart rate seen with digoxin would invariably lead to a decreased myocardial caloric consumption, and potentially to improvement in growth. Little data, however, aside from multiple small case series, exist to support the concept that digoxin leads to improvement of meaningful clinical endpoints in children, such as improved growth or other reproducible improvements in CHF symptoms. Therefore, given the lack of proven efficacy and complex pharmacokinetics, which not infrequently lead to toxicity, digoxin has become a second-line agent after diuretics, usually employed at its lower dose ranges. To avoid toxicity, the practice of

TABLE 2 Digitalis Dosing

Age	Digitalizing Dose*		Maintenance Dose†	
	Oral	IV/IM	Oral	IV/IM
Preterm	30 µg/kg	25 µg/kg	8–10 µg/kg/day divided bid	6–8 µg/kg/day
Term—2 years	65–75 µg/kg	50 µg/kg	8–10 µg/kg/day divided bid	12–15 µg/kg/day
2–10 years	30–40 µg/kg	25 µg/kg	8–10 µg/kg/day	6–8 µg/kg/day
10-adult	1–1.5 mg	0.5–1 mg	125–250 µg/day	100–400 µg/kg/day

*Digitalizing dose—Half the digitalizing dose is given initially, with one fourth the dose given q8h twice. Digitalizing is typically given only when the effect is needed quickly, such as for tachyarrhythmias. It is rarely given for isolated CHF.

†Maintenance dose—Maintenance doses are given to children twice a day because of more rapid metabolism, while older children and adults typically maintain therapeutic doses with once-a-day therapy.

bid, two times daily; IV, intravenously; IM, intramuscularly; q*x*h, every *x* hours.

digitalization is reserved almost exclusively for supraventricular arrhythmias when therapeutic doses are required quickly.

Other inotropes require intravenous (IV) dosing and therefore are used almost exclusively in the intensive care settings. Such agents include milrinone (Primacor), dopamine, epinephrine, and dobutamine. Milrinone is a phosphodiesterase inhibitor that increases cyclic adenosine monophosphate (cAMP) in both myocardial and smooth muscle cells in the pulmonary and systemic vasculature. This agent causes increased myocardial contractility and a drop in both the pulmonary and systemic vascular resistance (PVR and SVR) and has recently been shown to be effective therapy to support the "stunned" myocardium following cardiac surgery in children. Thus, milrinone has become one of the first-line agents for children in the postoperative period. It is also used in children with dilated cardiomyopathies who are not sufficiently stabilized with oral therapies.

Dopamine is a common adrenergic agonist used in children to support the failing myocardium, particularly during periods of hypotension. This agent activates myocardial β_1-adrenergic receptors, thereby increasing myocardial contraction (inotropy). At higher doses, dopamine is useful in increasing blood pressure via its activation of peripheral α_1-adrenergic receptors. Another frequently used adrenergic agent used in the postoperative period is epinephrine, a nonselective α- and β-adrenergic agonist. At lower doses, it increases myocardial contraction, although slightly decreasing SVR, but at moderate to high doses it increases SVR and therefore is useful in supporting blood pressure. One major drawback is that epinephrine has been shown to increase myocardial oxygen consumption and to be arrhythmogenic. Thus, epinephrine is rarely used for extended periods of time outside the postoperative period, unless a child is showing signs of shock unresponsive to other therapies. Dobutamine, a third adrenergic agent, acts primarily by stimulating β_1-adrenergic receptors, thereby increasing myocardial contractility; it also acts via peripheral β_2-adrenergic receptors, thereby decreasing SVR.

These intravenous adrenergic agents are used almost exclusively in the intensive care setting, in neonatal and pediatric intensive care units (ICUs), for short time periods in the postoperative period, to support stunned myocardium, or as a bridge to heart transplant. These three adrenergic-receptor agonists have also been observed to downregulate their own receptors, and tachyphylaxis, therefore, occurs.

Afterload-Reducing Agents

Afterload-reducing agents, such as angiotensin-converting enzyme (ACE) inhibitors and hydralazine, have been shown to be useful in decreasing signs of CHF in small case series in children with either left-to-right shunts or with dilated cardiomyopathies. Studies in adult patients suggest that these agents might also be useful in preventing or delaying adverse myocardial remodeling in children with regurgitant valvular lesions. Although many ACE inhibitors have been studied in adults, only captopril and enalapril have been extensively studied in children with heart failure. However, many animal and human studies indicate that the mechanism for benefit in patients with CHF extends beyond the ability of ACE inhibitors to lower the SVR. ACE inhibitors have been shown to decrease levels of a number of adverse neurohormones, which are elevated in heart failure despite minimal to no effect on blood pressure and SVR.

Hydralazine has been studied in children with CHF and in pediatric hypertension; it is an oral alternative for children with CHF when ACE inhibitors are contraindicated, as with hyperkalemia or pregnancy. However, hydralazine does not have the same degree of beneficial effects on the neurohemal axis as ACEIs and may produce relatively more hypotension. Thus, hydralazine should be considered a second-line therapy.

For children in the intensive care unit, IV therapies with agents that have short half-lives have the advantage in allowing titration of the dose to the desired hemodynamic effects. The most common IV afterload-reducing agents are milrinone (Primacor), nitroprusside (Nipride), and nicardipine (Cardene). Milrinone has become the first-line agent for children with CHF, as mentioned previously, because it both increases myocardial contractility and decreases both the PVR and SVR, with few potential side effects. Nitroprusside has been used effectively for many years in combination with agents such as dobutamine and dopamine, to decrease the SVR, therefore increasing the cardiac output and systemic perfusion. Its major drawback, although rarely seen in clinical practice, is the potential for cyanide toxicity if used in children at high doses for more than 48 hours, owing to its production of thiocyanate. Levels of thiocyanate, therefore, need to be monitored in those instances.

A newer alternative, used more often to control hypertension in the ICU, is IV nicardipine, a short-acting smooth muscle selective calcium channel blocker that causes a dose-dependent drop in SVR without the myocardial depressant effects of other calcium channel blockers. Although nicardipine has the advantage of no toxic metabolic byproducts, its use is somewhat limited by cost and the availability of other effective agents. IV nitroglycerin is another alternative, but its effects are less predictable, and therefore it is infrequently used in children.

β-ADRENERGIC BLOCKERS

Over the last decade, β-adrenergic blockers have been demonstrated to improve mortality and symptoms in adults with ischemic and nonischemic CHF. Recent small case series in children with CHF because of dilated cardiomyopathies, and from left-to-right shunts, have also shown improvement with β-blockers. There are even a few reports of children with severe CHF being removed from the transplant list because of clinical improvement with these agents. To my knowledge, however, the effectiveness of only three β-blockers (propranolol, metoprolol, and carvedilol) has been reported in children with CHF. The use of these agents in children with CHF is still investigational. Thus, β-blockers should be used cautiously, as these agents may lead to cardiovascular collapse in children with marginal cardiac function. Additionally, little is known about how effective these agents would be in more complex congenital heart defects (such as single ventricle), as these patients are more dependent on their ability to increase their heart rate (chronotropic reserve) to maintain adequate cardiac output. Therefore, β-blockers must be started at low doses, with upward titration every 2 to 4 weeks, as tolerated.

MECHANICAL SUPPORT

More recent studies show the value of mechanical support for the failing myocardium in children. Extracorporeal membrane oxygenation (ECMO) has been and remains the most common form of myocardial mechanical support in infants and children. It is effective at supporting a stunned or injured myocardium for short periods of time to either allow recovery or as a bridge to heart transplant. The major disadvantage of ECMO is the high risk of complications associated with the modality, particularly beyond 1 to 2 weeks. Additionally, as opposed to larger adult ventricular assist devices, ECMO is frequently inadequate in decompressing elevated left atrial pressures and mandates an atrial septostomy. Other devices such as intra-aortic balloon pumps may be used for older children, but these devices carry a high risk of vascular complications. More recently, smaller mechanical devices have been developed, such as the Berlin heart (undergoing trials in Europe), and the DeBakey centrifugal pump (recently being studied in a multicenter trial). These smaller devices are hoped to be able to provide safer and longer support as a bridge for transplant.

Communication and Counseling

Most of the medical therapies for CHF in children require close clinical follow-up. In some children, electrolyte testing is advised to ensure improvement in symptoms and growth. Occasionally, infants and young children with left-to-right shunts (e.g., ventricular septal defects) do well enough with therapy consisting of diuretics, digoxin, and occasionally ACE inhibitors, either alone or with adequate nutritional support, to grow and have eventual spontaneous closure of their defects, therefore obviating the need for surgery. Fortunately, however, cardiac surgery has improved dramatically over the last 2 decades so that many congenital defects can be repaired during early childhood with low morbidity and mortality. Medical therapy, however, is still helpful in "optimizing" the child before surgery, reducing operative morbidity. Nonetheless, despite optimal medical, surgical, and nutritional therapies, some children continue to worsen and either die suddenly or require cardiac

transplantation. Future prospective clinical trials that evaluate both medical and mechanical therapy are critical to ensure safety and efficacy of therapies for an increasing population of children with heart failure.

SUGGESTED READINGS

1. Connolly D, Rutkowski M, Auslender M, et al: The New York University Pediatric Heart Failure Index: A new method of quantifying chronic heart failure severity in children. J Pediatr 138 (5):644–648, 2001. **Discusses a new tool developed to objectively quantify severity of heart failure in children, which will aid researchers in assessing meaningful clinical effects of therapy.**
2. Fiser WP, Yetman A, Gunselman RJ, et al: Pediatric arteriovenous extracorporeal membrane oxygenation (ECMO) as a bridge to cardiac transplantation. J Heart Lung Transplant 22(7):770–777, 2003. **Review of the largest pediatric cardiac ECMO service in the United States and references for newer pediatric cardiac mechanical support.**
3. Hetzer R, Loebe M, Potapov EV, et al: Circulatory support with pneumatic paracorporeal ventricular assist device in infants and children. Ann Thorac Surg 66:1498–1506, 1998. **A discussion of the Berlin heart and the first 29 children in whom it was implanted.**
4. Kay JD, Colan SD, Graham TP: Congestive heart failure in pediatric patients. Am Heart J 142(5):923–927, 2001. **Reviews evidence-based medical therapies for pediatric CHF, and discusses needed studies.**
5. Schwartz SM, Duffy JY, Pearl JM, et al: Cellular and molecular aspects of myocardial dysfunction. Crit Care Med 20(10 Suppl): S214–S219, 2001. **Scientific review of the cellular processes involved with heart failure to help understand effects of treatment.**
6. Shaddy RE: Optimizing treatment for chronic congestive heart failure in children. Crit Care Med 20(10 Suppl):S237–S240, 2001. **Excellent review on the state of what is known about chronic medical therapy from the author on most of the published data.**
7. Tabbutt S: Heart failure in pediatric septic shock: Utilizing inotropic support. Crit Care Med 20(10 Suppl):S231–S236, 2001. **Excellent review of up-to-date inotropic therapy for noncongenital heart disease.**
8. Wessel DL: Managing low cardiac output syndrome after congenital heart surgery. Crit Care Med 20(10 Suppl):S220–S230, 2001. **Excellent review of medical and mechanical support used in the postoperative period.**

Myocarditis and Pericarditis

Steven D. Colan

KEY CONCEPTS

- Myocarditis is an inflammatory process within the myocardium associated with cardiac dysfunction.
- Myocarditis is one of many causes of dilated cardiomyopathy, but the two are not synonymous.
- Of the many infectious forms of myocarditis, coxsackie B and adenovirus appear to be the dominant agents.
- At present, endomyocardial biopsy remains the only definitive approach to diagnosis.
- The primary management issues relate to therapy for dilated cardiomyopathy and congestive heart failure.

- Most centers administer immunoglobulin to patients with suspected acute myocarditis.
- Although autoimmunity is believed to be an important aspect of the pathogenesis, the utility of immunosuppressive therapy remains inconclusive.

Myocarditis and pericarditis are inflammatory diseases of the heart muscle and pericardium, respectively. Although myocarditis and dilated cardiomyopathy (DCM) are frequently discussed as if they are the same disorder, DCM is, in fact, a more general disorder characterized by dilatation and diminished function of the left ventricle. Myocarditis is one of many causes of DCM, but most instances of DCM remain idiopathic. Although it has been speculated previously that myocarditis accounts for most instances of chronic DCM, it is now clear that a large proportion is due to familial forms of DCM. The exact relationship between myocarditis and DCM remains uncertain, but a large body of human and animal data has led to the concept of a disease characterized by three sequential phases. The first phase is characterized by an initial myocardial insult that is believed to be a viral infection in the majority of cases. Usually clinically silent, the disease is rarely diagnosed during this phase. The onset of the second phase manifests as progressive myocardial damage because of autoimmunity triggered by the initial injury. Overt congestive heart failure is more common during this second phase, and the inflammatory process is more overt. However, evidence of persistent viral infection is unusual. Despite resolution of the inflammatory process, the third phase with the typical clinical picture of chronic DCM may follow. Clearly, the diagnostic and therapeutic implications of each of these phases are quite different.

The disease is, of course, more complex than this paradigm might suggest, with the various phases frequently overlapping. Some patients experience fulminant myocarditis; some have evidence of latent or persistent viral infection, and some have multiple episodes of recurrent inflammation. The viruses that have been most commonly associated with acute lymphocytic myocarditis are coxsackie B and adenovirus, but, in fact, a large number of viruses have been reported, including most enteroviruses, cytomegalovirus, respiratory syncytial virus, herpes simplex, influenza, human immunodeficiency virus, parvovirus, hepatitis C, varicella, rubella, and the Epstein-Barr virus. However, identification of a virus does not establish a causal relationship to the inflammatory process, particularly because most of the general population have been exposed to these agents. In fact, identification of virus in the myocardium of patients dying from myocarditis is rare. Nevertheless, the existing body of animal and human data is sufficiently compelling to justify the pursuit of diagnostic and therapeutic strategies based on the understanding of an initial infectious insult that triggers an autoimmune disorder and may eventually be followed by end-stage DCM.

Clinical features of myocarditis are variable, including congestive heart failure, chest pain, arrhythmias, syncope, and sudden death. Subclinical or asymptomatic forms are not uncommon, hampering early diagnosis. Although there may be a history of a flu-like illness, this is rarely helpful in diagnosis, and cardiac manifestations often appear well after resolution of the initial symptoms. Although unusual, presentation with circulatory collapse or sudden death is more common in childhood.

Echocardiography is generally the modality used to confirm the presence of ventricular dilatation and dysfunction typical of DCM, but the diagnosis of myocarditis remains problematic. Despite the development of alternative diagnostic modalities, endomyocardial biopsy remains the only method to confirm the presence of an inflammatory process in the myocardium. Measurement of cardiac enzymes is not helpful because they are rarely elevated. Elevation of cardiac troponin I, a marker of myocyte necrosis, is noted in only one third of patients with myocarditis on biopsy. Viral culture is rarely helpful, and serology is not helpful in early management. Several newer methods have been reported to aid in diagnosis of myocarditis, including the presence of contrast enhancement on magnetic resonance imaging and antimyosin scintigraphic imaging, but their role is at present undefined. Ultimately, endomyocardial biopsy remains the final arbiter of the presence of myocardial inflammation. Even this is a less-than-perfect tool, as the process is often focal and can be missed on spot sampling. The availability of polymerase chain reaction methods to amplify small amounts of viral genome has considerably enhanced our ability to identify the presence of virus in the myocardium. Although at present the relevance of this information to a particular patient is uncertain, the overall implications for the disease process are quite important.

Pericarditis is a similarly enigmatic disorder that is largely presumed to be caused by either a viral infection or the immunologic response it incites, but proof is lacking, and 90% of cases remain idiopathic. The clinical presentation of acute pericarditis (friction rub, characteristic pain, and ECG findings) may occasionally be associated with tamponade. Echocardiography is useful to establish the presence of excess pericardial fluid and to help quantify the magnitude of the hemodynamic impact. In the absence of tamponade or predisposing disorders, further testing is not useful. Relapses are not uncommon and are highly specific for idiopathic pericarditis. Pericardial tamponade is significantly more common in patients with purulent, tuberculous, or neoplastic pericarditis, justifying further testing to exclude these possibilities.

Expert Opinion on Management Issues

Treatment of DCM and congestive heart failure is similar regardless of cause, as discussed elsewhere in this volume. There is some evidence that myocarditis predisposes to digoxin toxicity, and, therefore, digoxin should be used with caution and rapid loading should be avoided during the acute phase.

INTRAVENOUS IMMUNOGLOBULIN

Treatment with intravenous immunoglobulin (IVIG) was initially proposed as a means to suppress the immune response in myocarditis, regardless of cause, and to lead to more rapid viral clearance in viral myocarditis. A retrospective analysis of IVIG use in children with myocarditis demonstrated improved 1-year survival and recovery of left ventricular function with IVIG therapy, although improved survival did not achieve statistical significance in the small cohort. Animal studies and preliminary studies in adults were similarly promising, although a single randomized study in adults failed to demonstrate a treatment effect. Nevertheless, based on animal studies indicating that IVIG is more effective during the acute phase, the belief that the therapy may be more effective in children, the lack of other more effective specific therapy, and the very low adverse event rate, IVIG continues to be used by most centers in children suspected of being in the acute phase of myocarditis. Doses employed have been based on the Kawasaki experience (2 g/kg administered over 6 to 12 hours). Potential benefits of retreatment are unknown.

IMMUNOSUPPRESSIVE THERAPY

The large body of animal and human data suggesting a role for autoimmunity during the intermediate stage of myocarditis has led to attempts to reduce or eliminate this response. A double-blind, randomized trial of immunosuppressant therapy for 6 months (prednisone with either azathioprine or cyclosporine) in 111 adult patients with histopathologic diagnosis of acute myocarditis (the Myocarditis Treatment Trial) demonstrated no benefit from treatment. The results of this study have been widely interpreted as showing that immunosuppressive therapy must strike a fine balance between preventing the immune-mediated clearance of virus and permitting an excess response with associated autoimmune damage. Duration of therapy, timing of therapy relative to disease stage, specifics of the inciting virus, and potential activation of latent virus are other factors that may have contributed to the absence of benefit in this trial. Of seven other controlled trials of immunosuppressive therapy in adults with myocarditis, only one found a statistically significant reduction in myocardial inflammation and improvement in cardiac function. The evidence concerning efficacy of immunosuppressive therapy in children is similarly inconclusive, with several uncontrolled series suggesting a benefit. The distinction between use of IVIG and immunosuppression is the much higher risk associated with the latter. Overall, despite the evidence for autoimmunity in mediating the cardiac injury in myocarditis, the currently available data do not support the routine use of immunosuppressive therapy in children with myocarditis.

ANTIVIRAL THERAPY

Preliminary results in children with suspected viral myocarditis using pleconaril, a drug that binds to coxsackie B virus and prevents cell entry, have been favorable. Other agents such as monoclonal antibody against coxsackie B virus and ribavirin have shown efficacy in animal studies. Vaccines effective in preventing adenovirus and coxsackie B virus would prevent the majority of viral myocarditis in children. At present, specific antiviral therapy is only available for human immunodeficiency virus (HIV) and cytomegalovirus (CMV).

PERICARDITIS

For patients with a defined etiology of pericarditis, such as purulent tuberculous or neoplastic pericarditis, therapy is dictated by the underlying disorder. The goal of therapy for acute idiopathic pericarditis is symptomatic relief and intervention for pericardial tamponade. Pain and fever can generally be controlled with aspirin or other nonsteroidal anti-inflammatory drugs alone or in combination. Although aspirin is generally the first choice, indomethacin and ibuprofen are more effective in severe cases. Controversy exists regarding whether to employ steroids in patients who are refractory. Corticosteroids quickly control pain and generally lead to resolution of the pericardial pain. However, there are reports indicating that corticosteroid use increases the risk of relapsing pericarditis, presumably because of their deleterious impact on viral clearance. Once given, withdrawal of steroids is a difficult and prolonged process. It is preferable for patients to endure incomplete symptom control for a period of time to attempt avoidance of steroids. When used, prednisone should be rapidly weaned from initial doses of 1 mg/kg/day down to 0.1 to 0.2 mg/kg/day, in which the risk of symptom recurrence escalates. Further withdrawal is then a difficult and prolonged process of gradual reduction over months, with frequent setbacks.

Common Pitfalls

- The clinical findings are often subclinical, delaying diagnosis until flagrant cardiac compromise is present.
- Cardiac imaging, usually with echocardiography, is a reliable and noninvasive method to document the presence of cardiac dysfunction and should not be delayed if there is any suspicion of the diagnosis.
- The yield from endomyocardial biopsy is highest in the early stages of the disease process. Restricting this investigation to those who do not demonstrate early recovery markedly reduces the diagnostic yield.

Communication and Counseling

The outcome from myocarditis during childhood has generally been relatively equally divided among full recovery, chronic dysfunction with potential for eventual deterioration, and early progression to transplant or death. The ability to predict outcome at the time of presentation is quite limited and therefore early discussion of the possible outcomes including transplantation must be undertaken. Outcome in milder forms or subacute presentation is less well defined, partly because of difficulties in establishing the diagnosis. A risk for arrhythmias and sudden death has been noted in association with active inflammation, and therefore patients are advised to limit activity and to cease sports participation during the early disease phase. For those who fully recover and wish to resume sports activity, at least 6 months to a year from the time of functional recovery may be required for the remodeling process to complete, but there is essentially no information available to provide guidance regarding how long their activities should be restricted.

SUGGESTED READINGS

1. Mason JW: Myocarditis and dilated cardiomyopathy: An inflammatory link. Cardiovasc Res 15; 60(1):5–10, 2003. **Review of evidence relating myocarditis and autoimmunity.**
2. Calabrese F, Thiene G: Myocarditis and inflammatory cardiomyopathy: microbiological and molecular biological aspects. Cardiovasc Res 15; 60(1):11–25, 2003. **Comprehensive review of the data on infectious causes and proposed pathophysiology.**
3. Liu PP, Mason JW: Advances in the understanding of myocarditis. Circulation 28; 104(9):1076–1082, 2001. **General review of diagnosis and etiology of myocarditis.**
4. Wheeler DS, Kooy NW: A formidable challenge: The diagnosis and treatment of viral myocarditis in children. Crit Care Clin 19(3):365–391, 2003. **Review of myocarditis particularly emphasizing the issues that arise in children.**
5. Calabrese F, Rigo E, Milanesi O, et al: Molecular diagnosis of myocarditis and dilated cardiomyopathy in children: Clinicopathologic features and prognostic implications. Diagn Mol Pathol 11(4):212–221, 2002. **Review of current methodology for the diagnosis of myocarditis.**
6. Martin MER, Moya-Mur JL, Casanova M, et al: Role of noninvasive antimyosin imaging in infants and children with clinically suspected myocarditis. J Nucl Med 45(3):429–437, 2004. **Potential utility of antimyosin imaging for detecting biopsy-proven myocarditis.**
7. Burch M: Immune suppressive treatment in paediatric myocarditis: Still awaiting the evidence. Heart 90(10):1103–1104, 2004. **Editorial summarizing the current available data concerning efficacy of immunosuppressive therapy for myocarditis.**
8. Gagliardi MG, Bevilacqua M, Bassano C, et al: Long term follow up of children with myocarditis treated by immunosuppression and of children with dilated cardiomyopathy. Heart 90(10):1167–1171, 2004. **Recent study reporting improved outcome in children with myocarditis treated with immunosuppressive therapy.**
9. Mahrholdt H, Goedecke C, Wagner A, et al: Cardiovascular magnetic resonance assessment of human myocarditis—A comparison to histology and molecular pathology. Circulation 109 (10):1250–1258, 2004. **Study examining the ability of MRI to predict biopsy-proven myocarditis.**
10. Soler-Soler J, Sagrista-Sauleda J, Permanyer-Miralda G: Relapsing pericarditis. Heart 90(11):1364–1368, 2004. **Review of the data concerning treatment of acute and relapsing pericarditis.**

Infective Endocarditis

Samuel R. Dominguez and Robert S. Daum

KEY CONCEPTS

- Although infective endocarditis is relatively rare in children, the incidence has increased in recent years, particularly in children with underlying congenital heart defects and hospitalized newborn infants.
- Obtaining multiple blood cultures is the single most important laboratory procedure in a patient with suspected infective endocarditis.
- Initial, empirical therapy should be guided by the clinical circumstances of the patient and knowledge of the usual pathogens causing infective endocarditis. Continuing therapy should be guided by the identity of the isolated organism and antimicrobial susceptibility testing.
- A prolonged course (usually 4 to 6 weeks) of parenteral antimicrobial therapy, preferably with bactericidal agents, is required for the treatment of infective endocarditis.
- Infective endocarditis prophylaxis should be guided by a patient's underlying cardiac condition and the relative risk of developing bacteremia from the proposed procedure.

Infective endocarditis (IE) is part of a continuum of intravascular infectious syndromes, including infective arteritis and suppurative phlebitis, that have closely related clinical features and management strategies. IE occurs when microorganisms adhere to the endothelial surface of the heart. Intact endothelium is generally a poor stimulator of blood coagulation and is weakly receptive to bacterial attachment. Damaged endothelium, however, is a potent inducer of thrombogenesis and provides a site to which bacteria can adhere and eventually form infective vegetation. In general, cardiac lesions that involve high-velocity, turbulent jets of flow and/or the presence of foreign material are associated with the highest risk of developing IE.

IE remains relatively rare in children and accounts for approximately 1 in 1280 pediatric admissions per year. Although reported rates vary considerably, the frequency of IE among children appears to have increased in recent years. Previously, IE was classified as acute or subacute, based on disease progression, but this terminology has been replaced as a better understanding of the clinical setting in which the disease occurs has taken place. The vast majority of children who develop IE have underlying cardiac disease. Rheumatic fever has ceased to be the primary underlying cause of IE in children, and the majority of children today with IE have had corrective or palliative surgery for congenital heart defects (CHD). IE also occurs as a complication in the management of children with chronic diseases. In particular, long-term venous and arterial catheterization increases the risk of bacteremia, and mechanical injury to the atria can result from trauma induced by a central venous catheter.

BOX 1 Major and Minor Clinical Criteria Used in the Modified Duke Criteria for the Diagnosis of Infective Endocarditis

Major Criteria

Positive blood culture for IE
- Typical microorganisms from two separate blood cultures
  - Viridans streptococci (including nutritional variant strains), *Streptococcus bovis*, or HACEK group or
  - Community-acquired *Staphylococcus aureus* or enterococci, in the absence of a primary focus, or
- Microorganism consistent with IE from persistently positive blood cultures defined as
  - ≥2 positive blood cultures drawn >12 h apart, or
  - All 3 or a majority of 4 or more separate blood cultures, with the first and last drawn at least 1 h apart, or
  - A single positive blood culture for *Coxiella burnetii* or anti–phase 1 IgG antibody titer >1:800

Evidence of endocardial involvement
- Positive echocardiogram for IE defined as
  - Oscillating intracardiac mass, on valve or supporting structures, or in the path of regurgitant jets, or on implanted materials, in the absence of an alternative anatomic explanation, or
  - Abscess, or
  - New partial dehiscence or prosthetic valve, or
- New valvular regurgitation (worsening or changing of preexisting murmur not sufficient)

Minor Criteria

Predisposition: predisposing heart condition or IV drug use
Fever ≥100.4°F (38.0°C)
Vascular phenomena
- Major arterial emboli
- Septic pulmonary infarcts
- Mycotic aneurysm
- Intracranial hemorrhage
- Conjunctival hemorrhages
- Janeway lesions
Immunologic phenomena
- Osler nodes
- Roth spots
- Glomerulonephritis
- Rheumatoid factor
Microbiologic evidence
- Positive blood culture not meeting major criterion, or
- Serologic evidence of active infection with organisms consistent with IE

HACEK, *Haemophilus aphrophilus, Actinobacillus actinomycetem-comitans, Cardiobacterium hominis, Eikenella corrodens,* and *Kingella kingae*; IE, infective endocarditis.
From Li JS, Sexton DJ, Mick N, et al: Proposed modifications to the Duke criteria for the diagnosis of IE. Clin Infect Dis 30:633–638, 2000.

BOX 2 Modified Duke Criteria for Diagnosis of Infective Endocarditis

Definite IE

Pathologic criteria
- Microorganisms demonstrated
  - By culture or histology in a vegetation, or
  - In a vegetation that has embolized, or
  - In an intracardiac abscess, or
- Lesions—vegetation or intracardiac abscess present, confirmed by histology sowing active IE
- Clinical criteria as defined in Box 1
  - 2 major criteria, or
  - 1 major criterion and 3 minor criteria, or
  - 5 minor criteria

Possible IE

- 1 major criterion and 1 minor criterion, or
- 3 minor criteria

Rejected IE

- Firm alternative diagnosis for manifestation of endocarditis, or
- Resolution of manifestations, with antibiotic therapy ≤ 4 days, or
- No pathologic evidence of IE at surgery or autopsy, after antibiotic therapy for ≤ 4 days

IE, infective endocarditis.
From Li JS, Sexton DJ, Mick N, et al: Proposed modifications to the Duke criteria for the diagnosis of IE. Clin Infect Dis 30:633–638, 2000.

---

weight loss, arthralgias, myalgias, rigors, and diaphoresis. As in adults, the clinical findings relate to hemodynamic compromise caused by local infection (e.g., valvitis resulting in regurgitation), peripheral embolization (e.g., renal abnormalities, infarcts), or immunologic responses. Extracardiac manifestations of IE classically seen in adults (e.g., Osler nodes, Janeway lesions, Roth spots, or splenomegaly) are rare in children. The presentation of IE in neonates is often indistinguishable from septicemia or congestive heart failure due to other causes.

The most important diagnostic procedure in a patient suspected of having IE remains the blood culture. The bacteremia associated with IE is usually low-grade and continuous; therefore, it is not necessary to obtain cultures at any particular phase of the fever cycle. It is important to obtain adequate volumes of blood (1–3 mL in infants and young children and 5–7 mL in older children), and cultures should be drawn from indwelling catheters and venipuncture sites prepared with careful aseptic technique. If a patient is clinically stable, at least three blood cultures should be obtained 1 to several hours apart prior to the start of antimicrobial therapy. The microbiology laboratory should be notified that IE is suspected so that cultures will be incubated for at least 2 weeks.

Echocardiography is widely used in the evaluation of children with suspected IE. Transthoracic echocardiography (TTE) in children yields excellent images and has a higher reported sensitivity for detecting vegetations than in the adult population. For these reasons, transesophageal echocardiography (TEE) is usually not required in children and should be considered for

---

These phenomena appear to be the cause of the increased incidence of IE in hospitalized newborn infants. Rarely, IE can occur in the background of a normal heart. These infections arise from *Staphylococcus aureus* bacteremia and primarily involve the aortic or mitral valve.

The diagnosis of endocarditis remains primarily clinical. The most recent modified Duke criteria (Boxes 1 and 2) describe diagnostic criteria based on combinations of major and minor criteria and classify cases as definite endocarditis, possible endocarditis, or rejected cases. The presentation of IE generally is indolent, with prolonged fever and a variety of nonspecific systemic complaints, including fatigue, weakness,

cases in which transthoracic windows are inadequate (lesions involving the aortic valve) or in situations in which technical considerations make TEE images difficult to obtain.

About half of all cases of IE in children are still caused by *Streptococcus viridans* and *Staphylococcus aureus*. The latter is the most common cause of native valve IE. Over the past few years, there has been an increase in the cases of IE due to other organisms, particularly, enterococci, fungi, and so-called HACEK organisms (*Haemophilus aphrophilus, Actinobacillus actinomycetemcomitans, Cardiobacterium hominis, Eikenella corrodens*, and *Kingella kingae*). IE caused by fungi and HACEK species is particularly common in neonates and immunocompromised children. Fungal endocarditis is a severe disease with a poor prognosis found most commonly in neonates requiring extensive intravenous support with hyperalimentation and indwelling catheters. Fungal endocarditis is usually caused by *Candida* species, although IE caused by *Aspergillus* species has been reported. Clinical endocarditis without a positive blood culture is termed *culture-negative endocarditis* and accounts for about 10% to 20% of cases of IE. The most common cause of culture-negative IE is recent or current antibiotic use or infections caused by an organism that grows slowly *in vitro*. Other rare causes of culture-negative IE include *Coxiella burnetii* (Q fever) and *Brucella, Legionella, Bartonella*, and *Chlamydia* species.

Expert Opinion on Management Issues

IE is almost universally fatal if untreated, and it continues to cause substantial morbidity and mortality despite modern antimicrobial and surgical treatments. IE remains a disease in which complete eradication of the organism is required. A prolonged course of therapy (usually 4 to 6 weeks) is necessary for several reasons. The involved organisms embedded in the fibrin-platelet matrix of the vegetation are relatively protected from phagocytes and other host defenses; bacterial division and metabolism rates are low in the vegetation and only a small percentage of the organisms are exposed and susceptible to the effects of antibiotics at any one time. Furthermore, bactericidal rather than bacteriostatic antibiotics should be chosen whenever possible as they have been associated with fewer treatment failures and relapses.

INITIAL THERAPY

Initial therapy is usually empirical and depends on the clinical circumstances and knowledge of the usual pathogens. For community-acquired IE, the most likely causative organisms are *S. viridans, S. aureus*, and the HACEK bacilli. Thus, the usual initial regimen is a β-lactamase–resistant penicillin (nafcillin or oxacillin) plus an aminoglycoside (usually gentamicin). In a milieu with a high incidence of methicillin-resistant *S. aureus* (MRSA) or in patients who have been recently hospitalized, vancomycin should be substituted for the β-lactamase–resistant penicillin. Similarly, in patients who have recently had cardiac surgery, the most common causative organisms are staphylococci, both *S. aureus* and coagulase-negative species. Therefore, the initial regimen should consist of vancomycin and an aminoglycoside. Once the causative organism has been identified, antimicrobial susceptibility testing should be performed and these results should be used to tailor the specific antimicrobial therapy.

SPECIFIC THERAPY (Table 1)

Streptococcal Endocarditis

Treatment of streptococcal endocarditis is dependent on the antimicrobial susceptibility of the organism and the clinical course of the patient. For native-valve endocarditis caused by penicillin-susceptible streptococci (minimum inhibitory concentration [MIC] of <0.1 μg per mL) a 4-week course of parenteral crystalline penicillin G (200,000 U/kg/day) divided into six daily doses has been shown to achieve very high cure rates. In adults, therapy with ceftriaxone has been shown to be equally effective, but no data regarding the use of ceftriaxone in the treatment of IE in children has been published. Despite this limited experience, ceftriaxone (100 mg/kg/day intravenously [IV] or intramuscularly [IM]) may prove to be equally effective in children and has the advantage of potentially allowing for earlier outpatient management. Vancomycin (30 mg/kg/day IV every 12 hours) can be used in patients allergic to penicillin.

Organisms with intermediate susceptibility to penicillin (0.1 μg per mL < MIC <0.5 μg per mL) should be treated with a 4- to 6-week course of penicillin or ceftriaxone and combined with gentamicin for at least the first 2 weeks. Patients with IE caused by nutritionally variant viridans streptococci (*Abiotrophia* species) or highly resistant streptococci (MIC >0.5 μg per mL) always require combination therapy and should be treated in a similar fashion to IE caused by enterococci (see the later section, "Endococcal Endocarditis").

Short-course treatment of IE with a 2-week course of penicillin, ampicillin, or ceftriaxone combined with gentamicin has become increasingly popular in adults and has been shown to have bacteriologic cure rates of up to 98%. In this context, once-daily dosing of the gentamicin has been increasingly used among adult patients. Experience in children regarding both of these regimens, however, is very limited. Short-course treatment should be limited to organisms that are highly susceptible. Patients with chronic endocarditis (>3 months of symptoms), prosthetic valves, hemodynamic compromise at presentation, evidence of emboli, or vegetations greater than 10 mm are probably not candidates for short-course therapy. These patients should be treated with a 4- to 6-week course of penicillin combined with at least an initial 2-week course of aminoglycoside therapy.

Streptococcus pneumoniae is a rare but serious cause of IE, with high morbidity and mortality. Because of its infrequency and the emergence of multidrug-resistant

TABLE 1 Antimicrobial Therapy for Infective Endocarditis in Children

Agent	Dose	Max Dose	Frequency	Route	Duration	Comments
Empiric Therapy						
Community-acquired (low incidence of MRSA)						
Nafcillin or oxacillin *and*	200 mg/kg/day	12 g/day	q4–6h	IV	4–6 wk	
Gentamicin	3 mg/kg/d		q8–24h	IV	4–6 wk	Monitor serum levels.
Community-acquired (high incidence of MRSA)						
Vancomycin *and*	40 mg/kg/day	1 g/day	q6h	IV	4–6 wk	Monitor serum levels.
Gentamicin	3 mg/kg/day		q8–24h	IV	4–6 wk	Monitor serum levels.
Recent hospitalization or cardiac surgery						
Treated same as community-acquired MRSA						
Streptococcal Endocarditis						
*Native-valve and penicillin-susceptible (MIC ≤ 0.1 µg/mL)**						
Penicillin G *or*	200,000 U/kg/day	24 million U/day	q4–6h	IV	4 wk	
Ceftriaxone ±	100 mg/kg/day	4 g/day	q24h	IV	4 wk	
Gentamicin	3 mg/kg/day		q8–24h	IV	2 wk	Monitor serum levels.
Intermediate sensitivity to penicillin (0.1 µg/mL < MIC < 0.5 µg/mL) or prosthetic material						
Penicillin G *or*	200,000 U/kg/day	24 million U/day	q4–6h	IV	4–6 wk	
Ceftriaxone *and*	100 mg/kg/day	4 g/day	q24h	IV	4–6 wk	
Gentamicin	3 mg/kg/day		q8–24h	IV	2 wk	
Penicillin-resistant (MIC > 0.5 mg/mL)						
Penicillin G *or*	300,000 U/kg/day	24 million U/day	q4–6h	IV	6 wk	
Ampicillin *or*	300 mg/kg/day	12 g/day	q4h	IV	6 wk	
Vancomycin *and*	40 mg/kg/day	2 g/day	q6–12h	IV	6 wk	Monitor serum levels.
Gentamicin	3 mg/kg/day	240 mg/day	q8–24h	IV	6 wk	Monitor serum levels.
Streptococcus pneumonia						
Treat same as penicillin-resistant (MIC > 0.5 mg/mL).						
Staphylococcal Endocarditis						
Methicillin- susceptible (MSSA)						
Nafcillin *or*	200 mg/kg/day	12 g/d	q4–6h	IV	6 wk	
Oxacillin ±	200 mg/kg/day					
Gentamicin	3 mg/kg/day	240 mg/day	q8–24h	IV	6 wk	Monitor serum levels.
Methicillin-resistant (MRSA)						
Vancomycin *and*	40 mg/kg/day	2 g/day	q6–12h	IV	≥ 6 wk	Monitor serum levels.
Rifampin *and*	20 mg/kg/day	900 mg/day	q12h	PO	≥ 6 wk	
Gentamicin	3 mg/kg/day	240 mg/day	q8–24h	IV	2 wk	Monitor serum levels.
Enterococcal Endocarditis						
Treat same as penicillin-resistant (MIC > 0.5 mg/mL).						
Gram-Negative Endocarditis						
HACEK, native-valve						
Ceftriaxone	100 mg/kg/day	4 g/day	q24h	IV	≥ 4 wk	Use susceptibility patterns.
Other gram-negative bacilli or prosthetic material						
Use antimicrobial susceptibility patterns in consultation with ID specialist.						
Fungal Endocarditis						
Amphotericin B ±	1 mg/kg/day	1.5 mg/kg/day	q24h	IV		
5-flucytosine	100–150 mg/kg/day		q6h	PO		Monitor serum levels.

HACEK, *Haemophilus aphrophilus*, *Actinobacillus actinomycetemcomitans*, *Cardiobacterium hominis*, *Eikenella corrodens*, and *Kingella kingae*; ID, infectious diseases; IE, infective endocarditis; IV, intravenous; MIC, minimum inhibitory concentration; q*x*h, every *x* hours; PO, orally.
*May be candidates for "short-course" therapy (see text).

pneumococci, optimal therapy for *S. pneumoniae* IE is not established, and treatment should be conducted in consultation with an infectious diseases specialist. Some experts have suggested initial empirical treatment with a third-generation cephalosporin and vancomycin pending susceptibility testing results. Pneumococcal IE should be treated for a minimum of 6 weeks with intravenous antibiotics.

Staphylococcal Endocarditis

The great majority of staphylococci are resistant to penicillin. Therefore, methicillin-susceptible *S. aureus* (MSSA) should be treated with a β-lactamase–resistant penicillin (nafcillin or oxacillin 200 mg/kg/day in four divided doses) for a minimum of 6 weeks. Some experts advocate the addition of gentamicin for the first 3 to 5 days of therapy, but the benefit of this combination regimen has not been proven. In penicillin-allergic patients, first-generation cephalosporin and vancomycin are acceptable alternatives.

Increasing rates of MRSA, both hospital- and community-acquired, have posed new problems for the management of IE because some drugs traditionally used to treat MRSA infections are not effective in the treatment of endocarditis. Patients with native-valve MRSA endocarditis should be treated with vancomycin for a minimum of 6 weeks. MRSA endocarditis on a prosthetic valve or other cardiac prosthetic material is associated with a high mortality rate and has been shown to be an independent risk factor for death. The majority of these patients will require a combined medical-surgical approach with replacement of the valve in addition to antibiotic therapy. Some studies suggest that vancomycin combined with rifampin and gentamicin provides the best therapy. In this instance, gentamicin can be discontinued after 2 weeks, and vancomycin and rifampin continued for a minimum of 6 weeks. Rifampin when used alone selects for resistance and therefore should not be used in this fashion. Importantly, alternative newer drugs such as Synercid and linezolid have been relatively ineffective in the treatment of MRSA endocarditis, as have older regimens such as clindamycin or trimethoprim-sulfamethoxazole. The efficacy of daptomycin in the treatment of endocarditis is under investigation in adults.

Enterococcal Endocarditis

Fortunately, *Enterococcus* species are rare causes of endocarditis in children. Treatment is difficult because of the relative resistance of enterococci to penicillin and ampicillin and their variable resistance to vancomycin and the aminoglycosides. Enterococci are uniformly resistant to cephalosporins. Additionally, the emergence of high-level resistance to vancomycin and ampicillin in some species has further complicated treatment choices. Combination therapy with agents that have synergistic action is required to obtain bactericidal levels of antibiotics. Penicillin G, ampicillin (300 mg/kg/day divided every 4 hours) or vancomycin (for β-lactamase–producing strains) can all be used in combination with gentamicin, preferably for a 6-week course of therapy.

Gram-Negative Endocarditis

Gram-negative bacillary endocarditis is usually caused by the HACEK group of fastidious organisms, with *K. kingae* and *H. parainfluenzae* being the most common. Most children with HACEK endocarditis have underlying cardiac abnormalities. The HACEK group of organisms often makes β-lactamase and is resistant to penicillins. Susceptibility testing should be performed on all isolates. Pending susceptibility testing, initial empirical therapy with a third-generation cephalosporin is suggested. Uncomplicated, native-valve HACEK endocarditis should be treated for at least 4 weeks. To date, no cases of relapse have been reported following 4 weeks of appropriate therapy. Other gram-negative bacteria are rare causes of IE in children. Treatment of such cases must be guided by identification of the organisms and susceptibility testing. Most infectious diseases specialists would recommend treatment with an extended-spectrum penicillin or a cephalosporin together with an aminoglycoside for a minimum of 6 weeks of therapy.

Fungal Endocarditis

With the exception of neonates, surgical intervention is usually needed in conjunction with medical therapy in patients with fungal endocarditis. Amphotericin B remains the mainstay of medical therapy for children with fungal endocarditis. Some experts recommend the addition of 5-flucytosine to amphotericin B at a dose of 100 to 150 mg/kg/day given every 6 hours for endocarditis caused by *Candida* strains susceptible to 5-flucytosine. Experience with azole antifungals such as fluconazole is too limited to recommend their use in acute fungal endocarditis. However, their therapeutic niche may be for long-term therapy after an initial course of amphotericin B. Additional data are needed before this approach can be routinely recommended. Caspofungin, a new echinocandin antifungal, has been anecdotally used to treat a handful of children with endocarditis.

Culture-Negative Endocarditis

Patients believed to have culture-negative IE should generally be treated in a similar fashion to the initial empirical regimens outlined earlier. Particular attention should be paid to the patient's epidemiologic setting in determining therapy, and ongoing therapy should be based on the patient's initial response.

OUTPATIENT THERAPY

Cost and convenience considerations have made outpatient treatment of endocarditis increasingly attractive. Additionally, the emergence of single daily dose therapies, such as ceftriaxone, has added to their popularity. Experience in children, however, is very limited and should be considered only for the most favorable clinical situations. Most experts favor a minimum of 2 weeks of inpatient therapy, the time frame when most complications occur and the time with the greatest need for clinical and laboratory monitoring.

SURGICAL TREATMENT

The role of surgery in the treatment of endocarditis must be individualized. Indications for surgery in a patient with IE include refractory cardiac failure, hemodynamic compromise by valvular obstruction, perivalvular or periannular extension of infection, prosthetic valve dehiscence, ruptured chordae tendineae, papillary muscle, or ventricular septum, "significant embolic events," new-onset conduction disturbances, most cases of fungal endocarditis, and persistent bacteremia despite appropriate antibiotic therapy. In a symptomatic patient, surgery should not be delayed solely because a full course of medical therapy has not been completed or because the patient is still bacteremic.

PREVENTION

The logic surrounding the use of prophylactic antibiotics for the prevention of IE is intuitively appealing. Because bacteremia is a prerequisite for the development of IE, prevention or treatment of the bacteremia should reduce the risk of acquiring IE. Certain invasive procedures are known to cause bacteremia with organisms that cause IE. Therefore, pretreatment with antibiotics prior to these procedures should theoretically decrease the risk of infection. These arguments have made antibiotic prophylaxis the standard of care in most developed countries, despite the lack of evidence concerning its effectiveness.

Certain underlying cardiac conditions are associated with a greater risk of developing IE and with higher rates of morbidity and mortality from IE. These conditions have been stratified by the American Heart Association into high-, moderate-, or negligible-risk categories, based on these associations (Box 3). Prophylaxis is recommended for those conditions in the high- and moderate-risk group. Individuals in the negligible-risk category are presumed to have no greater risk than the general population of developing IE and so prophylaxis is not recommended. Similarly, different procedures are associated with a variable risk of developing bacteremia and IE. Table 2 lists common invasive procedures for which prophylaxis is and is not recommended.

Isolates belonging to the *S. viridans* group (α-hemolytic streptococcus) are the most common pathogens isolated after procedures above the diaphragm. Therefore, for these procedures, amoxicillin is the recommended prophylaxis. Clindamycin is recommended for patients allergic to amoxicillin. Gastrointestinal and genitourinary procedures are most commonly associated with enterococcal endocarditis. Gram-negative bacteremia may result from these procedures, but rarely is complicated by endocarditis. Therefore, for most patients amoxicillin or ampicillin is adequate prophylaxis. Because of their synergistic effect against enterococci, combination parenteral prophylaxis with ampicillin and gentamicin is recommended for high-risk patients. Table 3 presents a summary of prophylactic regimens recommendations listed by procedure and risk category.

Common Pitfalls

- IE should be considered in the differential diagnosis of any child with a fever and a new murmur.
- IE, especially caused by fungi, should be considered in the differential diagnosis of hospitalized infants with congestive heart failure or sepsis, particularly in the presence of indwelling intravenous catheters.
- In a stable patient, antimicrobial therapy should be delayed until multiple blood cultures can be drawn.
- Failure to recognize the importance of MRSA, both hospital- and community-acquired, as a possible cause of IE may lead to treatment failure with "traditional" empirical therapy regimens. In situations in which MRSA is a possible etiology, vancomycin (not a β-lactamase–resistant penicillin) combined with gentamicin should be the initial therapy.
- When indicated, surgical intervention for the treatment of IE should not be delayed, even if a patient has not received a full trial of medical therapy and/or the patient is still bacteremic.

Communication and Counseling

It is important to communicate to colleagues, patients, and families that the incidence of IE has increased in recent years, particularly in children who have undergone surgery for congenital heart disease and in sick infants in the neonatal intensive care unit requiring the use of indwelling intravenous catheters. Although a relatively rare disease, IE remains a serious illness

TABLE 2 Common Invasive Procedures and Antibiotic Prophylaxis

Endocarditis Prophylaxis Recommended	Endocarditis Prophylaxis Not Recommended
Dental Procedures	
Dental extractions	Restorative dentistry
Periodontal procedures	Local anesthetic injections (not intraligamentary)
Dental implant placement and reimplantation of avulsed teeth	Placement of rubber dams
Root canal instrumentation	Postoperative suture removal
Prophylactic cleaning of teeth or implants where bleeding is anticipated	Placement of removable prosthodontic or orthodontic appliances
	Taking of oral impressions
	Fluoride treatments
	Taking of oral radiographs
	Orthodontic appliance adjustment
	Shedding of primary teeth
Oral and Respiratory Procedures	
Tonsillectomy and/or adenoidectomy	Endotracheal intubation
Surgical operations that involve respiratory mucosa	Bronchoscopy with a flexible bronchoscope*
Bronchoscopy with a rigid bronchoscope	
Gastrointestinal and Genitourinary Tract Procedures	
Sclerotherapy for esophageal varices	Transesophageal echocardiography*
Esophageal stricture dilation	Endoscopy with or without biopsy*
ERCP	Vaginal delivery*
Biliary tract surgery	Cesarean section
Surgical operations that involve intestinal mucosa	Circumcision
Prostatic surgery	In uninfected tissues:
Cystoscopy	Urethral catheterization
Urethral dilation	Uterine dilation and curettage
	Therapeutic abortion
	Insertion or removal of intrauterine devices
Other	
None	Cardiac catheterization, including balloon angioplasty
	Implanted cardiac pacemakers, implanted defibrillators, coronary stents
	Incision or biopsy of surgically scrubbed skin

*Prophylaxis is optional for high-risk patients.
ERCP, endoscopic retrograde cholangiopancreatography.
From Dajani AS, Taubert KA, Wilson W, et al: Prevention of bacterial endocarditis: Recommendations by the American Heart Association. JAMA 277:1794–1801, 1997.

TABLE 3 Prophylactic Regimens for Procedures Associated with Endocarditis

Situation	Agent	Regimen
Dental, Oral, Respiratory Tract, or Esophageal Procedures		
Standard general prophylaxis	Amoxicillin	50 mg/kg PO 1 h before procedure
Unable to take oral medication	Ampicillin	50 mg/kg IM/IV 30 min before procedure
Allergic to penicillin	Clindamycin *or*	20 mg/kg PO 1 h before procedure
	Cephalexin *or*	50 mg/kg PO 1 h before procedure
	Cefadroxil *or*	50 mg/kg PO 1 h before procedure
	Azithromycin	15 mg/kg PO 1 h before procedure
Allergic to penicillin and unable	Clindamycin *or*	20 mg/kg IV within 30 min of procedure
To take oral medication	Cefazolin	25 mg/kg IM/IV within 30 min of procedure
Gastrointestinal and Genitourinary Procedures		
High-risk patients	Ampicillin *plus*	30 min before procedure: 50 mg/kg IM/IV
	Gentamicin	6 h after procedure: 25 mg/kg IM/IV
	Vancomycin *plus*	30 min before procedure: 1.5 mg/kg IM/IV
High-risk and allergic to penicillin	Gentamicin	30 min before procedure: 20 mg/kg IV
	Ampicillin *or*	30 min before procedure: 1.5 mg/kg IV
Moderate risk	Amoxicillin	50 mg/kg IV/IM 30 min before procedure
	Vancomycin	50 mg/kg PO 1 h before procedure
Moderate risk and allergic to penicillin		20 mg/kg IV 30 min before procedure

IM, intramuscularly; IV, intravenously; PO, orally.
From Dajani AS, Taubert KA, Wilson W, et al: Prevention of bacterial endocarditis: Recommendations by the American Heart Association. JAMA 277:1794–1801, 1997.

with significant morbidity and mortality. In the sickest children, a combined therapeutic approach in consultation with pediatric cardiothoracic surgeons, intensivists, and infectious disease specialists is often required.

SUGGESTED READINGS

1. Baddour LM, Wilson WR, Bayer AS, et al: Infective endocarditis: Diagnosis, antimicrobial therapy, and management of complications. Circulation 111:e394–e433, 2005. **Discussion of treatment of infective endocarditis (IE) in adults.**
2. Brook MM: Pediatric bacterial endocarditis. Pediatr Clin NA 46:275–287, 1999. **Review of IE in children.**
3. Choi M, Mailman TL: Pneumococcal endocarditis in infants and children. Pediatr Infect Dis J 23:166–171, 2004. **Review of pneumococcal endocarditis in children.**
4. Dajani AS, Taubert KA, Wilson W, et al: Prevention of bacterial endocarditis: Recommendations by the American Heart Association. JAMA 277:1794–1801, 1997. **Presentation of AHA recommendations for prophylaxis against IE.**
5. Eleftherios M, Claderwood SB: Medical progress: Infective endocarditis in adults. N Engl J Med 34:1318–1330, 2001. **Review of IE in adults.**
6. Feder HM, Roberts JC, Salazar JC, et al: HACEK endocarditis in infants and children: Two cases and a literature review. Pediatr Infect Dis J 22:557–562, 2003. **Review of HACEK endocarditis in children.**
7. Ferrieri P, Gewitz MH, Gerber MA, et al: Unique features of infective endocarditis in childhood. Circulation 105:2115–2127, 2002. **Review of IE in children.**
8. Fowler VG, Miro JM, Hoen B, et al: *Staphylococcus aureus* endocarditis: A consequence of medical progress. JAMA 293:3012–3021, 2005. **Review of the global epidemiology of *S. aureus* IE.**
9. Hoen B: Special issues in the management of infective endocarditis caused by Gram-positive cocci. Infect Dis Clin NA 16:437–452, 2002. **Review of treatment of IE caused by Gram-positive cocci.**
10. Milazzo AS, Li JS: Bacterial endocarditis in infants and children. Pediatr Infect Dis J 20:799–801, 2001. **Review of IE in children and summary of modified Duke criteria for diagnosis of IE.**
11. Moreillon P, Que YA, Bayer AS: Pathogenesis of streptococcal and staphylococcal endocarditis. Infect Dis Clin NA 16:297–318, 2002. **Review of pathogenesis of IE.**
12. Olaison L, Pettersson G: Current best practices and guidelines: Indications for surgical intervention in infective endocarditis. Infect Dis Clin NA 16:453–475, 2002. **Discussion of surgical treatments for IE.**
13. Petti CA, Fowler VG: Staphylococcus aureus bacteremia and endocarditis. Infect Dis Clin NA 16:413–435, 2002. **Review of IE caused by *S. aureus*.**
14. Pierrotti LC, Baddour LM: Fungal endocarditis, 1995–2000. Chest 122:302–310, 2002. **Review of fungal endocarditis.**

Acute Rheumatic Fever

Thomas W. Young and William B. Strong

KEY CONCEPTS

- Acute rheumatic fever is an auto-immune inflammatory disease that follows group A streptococcal pharyngitis.
- Prompt and adequate antibiotic treatment of group A streptococcal pharyngitis prevents acute rheumatic fever.
- Diagnosis of acute rheumatic fever is highly probable if there is evidence of antecedent group A streptococcal pharyngitis along with either two major or one major plus two minor Jones Criteria.
- A migratory arthritis of the large joints is the most common manifestation of acute rheumatic fever.
- Carditis is the only manifestation causing significant long-term morbidity.
- Initial therapy for acute rheumatic fever consists of eradicating group A streptococci from the pharynx, bed rest, and aspirin. Prednisone is added for severe carditis.
- Secondary prevention of group A streptococcal pharyngitis with antibiotic prophylaxis is important.
- Penicillin is the antibiotic of choice for both primary and secondary prevention.

Acute rheumatic fever (ARF) is a postinfectious auto-immune inflammatory disease that follows group A streptococcal pharyngitis and affects the heart, brain, joints, blood vessels, and subcutaneous tissue. Although acute rheumatic fever is the most common cause of acquired heart disease in children and young adults in developing nations, it has become much less common in the United States over the past several decades. Nevertheless, localized outbreaks in the United States still occur.

The peak age of onset is between 5 and 15 years of age, with equal distribution in males and females. The latency period between group A streptococcal pharyngitis and the development of ARF is between 1 to 5 weeks (average 2 to 3 weeks). ARF does not (with very rare exception) follow group A streptococcal skin infections. Development of ARF after group A streptococcal pharyngitis depends on both host and organism characteristics. There is a strong genetic predisposition to developing ARF. The marked decline in the incidence of ARF in the developed world can be attributed in part to improved economic standards with decreased crowding and improved access to medical care. More virulent forms of group A streptococci associated with ARF are characterized by specific M protein types and a more "mucoid" capsule.

Expert Opinion on Management Issues

JONES CRITERIA

There is no specific diagnostic test for ARF. Diagnosis is clinical and is based on the Jones criteria, last revised in 1992. The revised Jones criteria apply only to initial attacks of ARF and consist of major and minor criteria.

Major Criteria

Carditis is the only manifestation of ARF that is potentially life-threatening and capable of causing chronic disease. Approximately half of patients with ARF are affected. When pancarditis is present, endocarditis and resultant valvulitis is the most important contributor to acute congestive heart failure (CHF). Myocarditis and pericarditis can contribute to cardiac dysfunction.

The mitral valve is most commonly affected, with the aortic valve a distant second. Valvular insufficiency is present acutely (although stenosis develops years later in some patients). The physical examination is used to diagnose carditis. The apical, holosystolic murmur of mitral insufficiency and the blowing, early diastolic murmur of aortic incompetence are classic. Resting tachycardia (out of proportion to any fever) suggests carditis. Controversy exists over the role of echocardiography, which often detects inaudible insufficiency. Currently, echocardiographic findings are *not* part of the Jones criteria.

Arthritis is the most common manifestation of ARF, occurring in approximately 75% of patients. Classically, an asymmetric migratory arthritis of the large joints (knees, ankles, elbows, and wrists) is present. Each joint tends to be affected for a few days to a week. Arthritis rarely lasts beyond 4 weeks in ARF and is usually responsive to salicylate therapy. Arthritis of longer duration or with poor responsiveness to aspirin suggests another diagnosis.

Sydenham chorea is seen in approximately 5% to 15% of ARF cases. It often starts with emotional lability and progresses to involuntary purposeless movements. After puberty, chorea is much more common in female patients. It often appears 1 to 6 months after group A streptococcal pharyngitis. Although chorea usually resolves after a few weeks, more protracted courses may be seen. Sydenham chorea is associated with a higher rate of chronic heart disease and is seen in approximately 5% to 15% of ARF cases.

Erythema marginatum, an erythematous, macular, nonpruritic rash with serpiginous borders that spread outward with central clearing, is seen in less than 5% of patients. It is seen on the trunk, buttocks, and proximal limbs and does not involve the face.

Subcutaneous nodules are also seen in fewer than 5% of patients and are associated with active carditis. These small, freely mobile nodules are found on extensor surfaces (especially the occiput, over the vertebral spines, and on the elbows, knees, and wrists).

Epistaxis, anemia, and acute abdominal pain are often seen in ARF. They are not, however, part of the diagnostic criteria.

Minor Criteria

The minor Jones criteria are much less specific for ARF. Arthralgia and fever are the clinical minor criteria. Elevated acute phase reactants (erythrocyte sedimentation rate and C-reactive protein) are usually seen in ARF. Although exceptions are seen, normal values suggest another diagnosis. A prolonged PR interval is often seen on EKG and is another minor criterion. It does not represent carditis and does not correlate to the development of chronic heart disease.

In the presence of supporting evidence of antecedent group A streptococcal pharyngitis, a high probability of ARF is supported by the presence of either two major criteria or one major and two minor criteria. A positive throat culture or group A streptococcal rapid antigen test is supportive but is often negative by the time ARF manifests. Both culture and rapid antigen tests do not distinguish between chronic pharyngeal carriers (who do not mount an antibody response) and those with active group A streptococcal pharyngitis. Streptococcal antibody tests are sent to confirm recent group A streptococcal infection. An elevated antistreptolysin O (ASO) titer is seen in approximately 80% of ARF patients. If ASO titer is normal, titers for anti-DNase B or other group A streptococcal specific antibodies should be obtained. Repeat testing 2 weeks later looking for a fourfold rise in titers, which would support the diagnosis, may be necessary in questionable cases.

TREATMENT

Primary prevention of ARF is accomplished by treating group A streptococcal pharyngitis within 10 days of onset. Penicillin remains the treatment of choice, except in allergic patients (Table 1). The intramuscular route ensures adherence, although allergic reactions are more common than with oral dosing. In allergic patients, erythromycin is used although culture sensitivities must by obtained because of a small incidence of erythromycin-resistant group A streptococcal pharyngitis. Azithromycin and some oral cephalosporins are also sometimes used.

Even if there is no evidence of current pharyngitis (including negative cultures), the first step in treating ARF is *eradicating group A streptococcal pharyngitis* from the throat (after adequate cultures are performed), as discussed previously. It is often helpful to delay anti-inflammatory medications until a clear diagnosis is made. Careful observation is necessary during the first 3 weeks, when carditis is most likely to develop. Chest radiograph, EKG, and echocardiography are indicated.

TABLE 1 Treatment of Group A Streptococcal Pharyngitis—Primary Prevention of Acute Rheumatic Fever

Drug	Dosage	Alternative Dosage
Benzathine penicillin G Rx	IM 600,000 U once for patients ≤27 kg 1,200,000 U once for patients >27 kg	
Phenoxymethylpenicillin (penicillin V) Rx	PO Children: 40 mg/kg divided tid Adults: 500 mg bid-tid	Children: 250 mg/dose Adults: 500 mg/dose
Erythromycin estolate Rx	PO 20–40 mg/kg divided bid-qid	1 g/day
Erythromycin ethylsuccinate Rx	PO 40 mg/kg divided bid-qid	1 g/day

bid, two times daily; PO, orally; tid, three times daily.

Anti-inflammatory drugs (aspirin and steroids) do not reduce the incidence of chronic heart disease but can provide symptomatic relief. Arthritis and fever respond dramatically to aspirin (75 to 100 mg/kg divided 4 times daily). This dose is usually given for 2 weeks and then gradually tapered over 4 to 6 weeks. Treatment of carditis is more controversial. Mild or moderate carditis may be treated with aspirin as well (usually for 4 to 8 weeks and then tapered over another 4 weeks depending on clinical response). Severe carditis with CHF is treated with steroids, which appear to help acute morbidity and mortality. Prednisone (2 mg/kg/day orally) is given for 2 weeks and then gradually tapered over 3 to 4 weeks. Approximately a week prior to ending the taper, aspirin at a therapeutic dose is started for another 3 to 4 weeks to prevent rebound of symptoms. Persistent carditis may necessitate much longer courses of steroids. Digoxin, once felt to be contraindicated in ARF, can be used safely if careful monitoring for toxicity is performed. Diuretics and afterload reduction may also be needed acutely.

Bed rest has historically been a mainstay of therapy. Many physicians still keep patients without carditis on bed rest until fever and other symptoms have resolved and acute phase reactants have started to improve (usually 2 to 3 weeks). Development of carditis after this point is uncommon. As the severity of carditis worsens, the duration of bed rest increases.

Chorea is treated with bed rest in a quiet place. In the absence of other manifestations, anti-inflammatory medications are not needed. Phenobarbital, diazepam, haloperidol, and valproic acid have been helpful in more severe cases.

ARF has a high recurrence rate. Asymptomatic infection can trigger a recurrence. The risk of significant residual heart disease increases with each episode of ARF. Secondary prevention of group A streptococcal pharyngitis is, therefore, mandatory and is one of the major reasons for a decrease in the incidence of chronic rheumatic heart disease in the developed world. Table 2 gives recommended doses for secondary prevention. Intramuscular benzathine penicillin *every 4 weeks* (not monthly) is the preferred route to ensure compliance. In high-risk patients, injections can be given every 3 weeks. Duration of prophylaxis is controversial and is summarized in Table 3. Recurrence risk decreases with patient age and with the interval since the last attack of ARF. Importantly, individuals with a higher risk of exposure to group A streptococci (e.g., patients with small children, schoolteachers, and health care workers) should receive a longer duration of prophylaxis.

Common Pitfalls

Because of the lack of a true standard criterion diagnostic test, the potential for over- and underdiagnosis is substantial. Overdiagnosis may be caused by improperly labeling arthralgias as arthritis or benign flow murmurs as carditis. The differential diagnosis is vast and includes juvenile rheumatoid arthritis, systemic lupus erythematosus and other connective tissue diseases, gonococcal arthritis, infective endocarditis, acute leukemia and other malignancies, viral carditis, viral hepatitis, Lyme disease, *Yersinia enterocolitis*, sickle cell anemia, serum sickness, and many other conditions. Therefore, evidence of antecedent group A streptococcal infection is very important. However, a significant minority of school-age children are chronic pharyngeal carriers of group A streptococcus, so many patients without ARF will have a positive throat culture or rapid antigen test.

Underdiagnosis also occurs. Isolated chorea often appears after a latency period of several months with normal acute phase reactants and no evidence of a preceding group A streptococcal infection. Subclinical carditis may also present in the absence of other manifestations. A high index of suspicion is necessary (especially in areas with a high incidence of ARF), as secondary prevention with prophylactic antibiotics may prevent further morbidity. Up to 25% of patients reported no memory of a sore throat prior to their diagnosis of ARF. The Jones criteria pertain only to initial attacks of ARF. A much higher index of suspicion is needed in those patients with a prior history of ARF.

Communication and Counseling

Primary prevention of ARF is essential. Once the diagnosis of group A streptococcal pharyngitis is made, patient adherence to the prescribed antibiotic and appropriate follow-up is very important. Ensuring

---

TABLE 2 Secondary Prevention of Acute Rheumatic Fever

Drug	Dosage
Benzathine penicillin G Rx	IM: 1,200,000 U q3–4wk
Penicillin V	PO: 250 mg bid
Sulfadiazine	PO: 500 mg qd for patients ≤27 kg, 1000 mg qd for patients >27 kg
Erythromycin	PO: 250 mg bid

bid, two times daily; PO, orally; qd, daily; q*x*wk, every *x* weeks; tid, three times daily.

TABLE 3 Duration of Secondary Acute Rheumatic Fever Prophylaxis

Type of Rheumatic Fever	Duration
Rheumatic fever without carditis	5 years after last ARF episode and at least until 21 years old
Rheumatic fever with carditis and no residual heart disease	10 years and well into adulthood
Rheumatic fever with residual heart disease	10 or more years and at least until 40 years old (often lifelong)

ARF, acute rheumatic fever.

adherence to regimens for secondary prevention is more difficult. It should be stressed, especially to the adolescent patient, that chronic prophylaxis is not to make them "feel better" but, instead, to prevent recurrent ARF and worsening of their heart disease. For patients with residual heart disease, additional bacterial endocarditis prophylaxis is required prior to dental surgery or certain procedures that involve the gastrointestinal, genitourinary, or respiratory tracts, because chronic ARF prophylaxis may lead to the proliferation of antibiotic-resistant organisms. Household members of a patient with a history of ARF should be evaluated promptly and treated appropriately if pharyngitis develops.

SUGGESTED READINGS

1. Cilliers AM, Manyemba J, Saloojee H: Anti-inflammatory treatment for carditis in acute rheumatic fever. Cochrane Database Syst Rev (2):CD003176, 2003. **Indicates how steroids offer no advantage over aspirin in preventing chronic rheumatic heart disease.**
2. Dajani AS, Elia A, Bierman FZ, et al: Guidelines for the diagnosis of rheumatic fever: Jones criteria updated 1992. JAMA 268:2069–2073, 1991. **Discusses the revised Jones criteria including exceptions.**
3. Dajani A, Taubert K, Ferrieri P, et al: Treatment of acute streptococcal pharyngitis and prevention of rheumatic fever: A statement for health professionals. Pediatrics 96:758–764, 1995. **Reviews guidelines for primary and secondary ARF prevention.**
4. DiSciascio F, Taranta A: Rheumatic fever in children. Am Heart J 99(5):635–658, 1980. **An excellent review of the clinical presentation of ARF.**
5. Ferrieri P, Baddour L, Bolger A, et al: Proceedings of the Jones Criteria Workshop. Circulation 106(19):2521–2523, 2002. **Reviews the revised Jones criteria and the role of echocardiography in diagnosis.**
6. Ortiz EE: Acute rheumatic fever. In Anderson RH, Baker EJ, McCartney FJ, et al (eds): Paediatric Cardiology, 2nd ed. London: Churchill Livingstone, 2001. **An excellent, exhaustive review of ARF.**
7. Stollerman GH: Rheumatic fever in the 21st century. Clin Infect Dis 33(6):806–814, 2001. **Discusses the pathogenesis of ARF.**

Kawasaki Disease

Jane W. Newburger, William G. Harmon, and Steven E. Lipshultz

KEY CONCEPTS

- Coronary artery aneurysms, or ectasia, develop in approximately 15% to 25% of untreated children with Kawasaki disease (KD); treatment with intravenous immunoglobulin (IVIG) in the acute phase reduces this risk to less than 5%.
- Treatment with high-dose IVIG is recommended for children with at least 4 days of fever and four of five classic clinical criteria. Those with fewer clinical criteria should be treated if coronary abnormalities are noted by echocardiogram. Patients with suspected Kawasaki disease should be treated with IVIG (2 g/kg) and aspirin within 10 days of onset to prevent coronary

aneurysms. A new algorithm from the American Heart Association Committee on Rheumatic Fever, Endocarditis, and Kawasaki Disease (see Fig. 1) may help clinicians to decide which children with suspected Kawasaki disease should undergo echocardiography and/or receive IVIG treatment.
- The best treatment for patients with persistent or recurrent fever after initial IVIG infusion is unknown. IVIG retreatment is usually administered to such patients because of its dose-response effect. Other therapies include treatment with corticosteroids, tumor necrosis factor-α antagonists, plasma exchange, and, in patients developing coronary enlargement, abciximab.
- Regression to normal arterial lumen diameter occurs in approximately one half of aneurysms over the first 2 years after illness onset, but histologic and functional abnormalities remain. Patients with persistent aneurysms are at risk for coronary artery thrombosis, stenosis, and occlusion.
- Long-term management of patients with Kawasaki disease should be tailored to the degree of coronary involvement and may involve long-term anticoagulation. The risk level for a given patient with coronary arterial involvement may evolve over time because of changes in coronary artery morphology.

Kawasaki disease (KD) is an acute vasculitis of infancy and childhood that causes coronary artery aneurysms in approximately 20% of untreated children. Although its incidence is highest in children of Japanese ancestry, it occurs throughout the world in children in all racial groups. In the United States, where approximately 4000 cases are treated annually, KD is the leading cause of acquired heart disease. Despite intensive efforts over the past three decades, the cause of KD remains unknown. Clinical features and differential diagnosis of KD are listed in Boxes 1 and 2. In the absence of full criteria, KD can be diagnosed when coronary abnormalities are present. A significant proportion of children with coronary aneurysms have incomplete KD, that is, not meeting the classic epidemiologic case definition. Incomplete KD is more common in young infants, who are at the highest risk of developing coronary abnormalities. Because complications of KD can be grave and its treatment is safe and effective, new, broader criteria for treatment of suspected KD have been developed (Fig. 1).

Diagnosis

The clinical diagnosis of KD is generally based on extracardiac manifestations. Criteria are widely published and include fever (usually >39°C [102.2°F] and often >40°C [104°F]) of 5 days' duration and the presence of at least four of the five principle features of the syndrome (see Box 1). Such findings are nonspecific, so diseases with similar manifestations need to be excluded (see Box 2).

Children with KD are almost always irritable; joint pain, abdominal pain, and diarrhea may also be present. Aseptic meningitis has been described. Common laboratory findings include an elevated erythrocyte

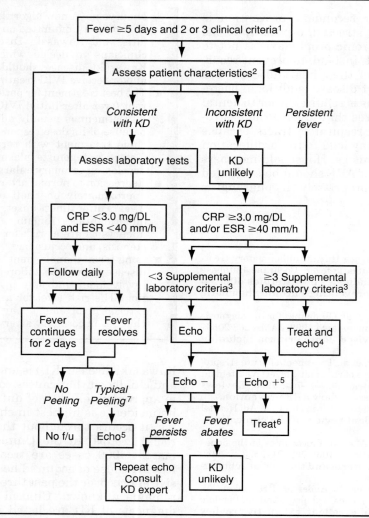

FIGURE 1. Evaluation of suspected incomplete Kawasaki disease (KD). In the absence of a gold standard for diagnosis, this algorithm cannot be evidence-based but rather represents the informed opinion of a committee of experts. Consultation with an expert should be sought any time that assistance is needed. CRP, C-reactive protein; ESR, erythrocyte sedimentation rate; f/u, follow-up.

[1]Infants older than 6 months of age on day greater than 7 of fever without other explanation should undergo laboratory testing and, if evidence of systemic inflammation, an echocardiogram, even if they have no clinical criteria.

[2]Box 1 lists patient characteristics suggesting Kawasaki disease (KD). Characteristics suggesting a disease *other* than KD include exudative conjunctivitis, exudative pharyngitis, discrete intraoral lesions, bullous or vesicular rash, or generalized adenopathy. Consider alternative diagnoses (see Box 2).

[3]Additional laboratory criteria include albumin less than 3.0 g/dL, anemia for age, elevation of alanine aminotransferase (ALT), platelets after 7 days equivalent to 450,000/mm^3, white blood cell count greater than 15,000/mm^3, and urine equivalent to 10 white blood cells per high-power field.

[4]Can treat before performing echocardiogram.

[5]Echocardiogram is considered positive for purposes of this algorithm if any of the following three conditions are met: (1) Z score of left anterior descending (LAD) or right coronary artery (RCA) is >2.5; (2) coronary arteries meet Japanese Ministry of Health criteria for aneurysms; or (3) at least three other suggestive features exist, including perivascular brightness, lack of tapering, decreased left ventricular function, mitral regurgitation, pericardial effusion, or Z scores in LAD or RCA of 2 to 2.5.

[6]If echo is positive, treatment should be given to children who are within 10 days of onset of fever, and to those beyond day 10 who have clinical and laboratory signs (CRP, ESR) of ongoing inflammation.

[7]Typical peeling begins under the nail bed of the fingers and then toes.

From Newburger JW, Takahashi M, Gerber MA, et al: Diagnosis, treatment, and long-term management of Kawasaki Disease: A statement for health professionals from the Committee on Rheumatic Fever, Endocarditis, and Kawasaki Disease, Council on Cardiovascular Disease in the Young, American Heart Association. Pediatrics 114:1708–1733, Dec. 2004. Used with permission of the American Academy of Pediatrics.

sedimentation rate (ESR) or C-reactive protein (CRP), leukocytosis, sterile pyuria, and hypoalbuminemia. Less commonly, gallbladder hydrops, hepatitis, and arthritis are seen. A variety of immunoregulatory changes have been described, including decreased circulating suppressor CD8+ T lymphocytes, increased serum proinflammatory cytokine concentrations, and increased activated B-lymphocyte and monocyte activity. Recent work has documented an immunoglobulin (Ig) A immune response in concert with CD8-positive T-cell infiltration in tissues of children with KD. Similar findings are found in association with known

BOX 1 Clinical and Laboratory Features of Kawasaki Disease

Epidemiologic Case Definition (Classic Clinical Criteria)*

- Fever persisting at least 5 days[†]
- Presence of at least four of the following principal features:
  - Acute changes in extremities: erythema of palms and soles, edema of hands and feet
  - Subacute changes in extremities: periungual peeling of fingers and toes in second and third week
  - Polymorphous exanthem
  - Bilateral bulbar conjunctival injection without exudate
  - Changes in the lips and oral cavity: Erythema and cracking of lips, strawberry tongue, diffuse injection of oral and pharyngeal mucosae.
  - Cervical lymphadenopathy (>1.5 cm in diameter), usually unilateral
- Exclusion of other diseases with similar findings (see Box 2)

Other Clinical and Laboratory Findings

- Cardiovascular findings
  - Congestive heart failure, myocarditis, pericarditis, or valvular regurgitation.
  - Coronary artery abnormalities
  - Aneurysms of medium-sized noncoronary arteries
  - Raynaud phenomenon
  - Peripheral gangrene
- Musculoskeletal system
  - Arthritis, arthralgia
- Gastrointestinal tract
  - Diarrhea, vomiting, abdominal pain
  - Hepatic dysfunction
  - Hydrops of the gallbladder
- Central nervous system
  - Extreme irritability
  - Aseptic meningitis
  - Sensorineural hearing loss
- Genitourinary system
  - Urethritis/meatitis
- Other Findings
  - Erythema and induration at Bacille Calmette-Guérin (BCG) inoculation site
  - Anterior uveitis (mild)
  - Desquamating rash in groin

Laboratory Findings in Acute KD

- Leukocytosis with neutrophilia and immature forms
- Elevated erythrocyte sedimentation rate
- Elevated C-reactive protein
- Anemia
- Abnormal plasma lipids
- Hypoalbuminemia
- Hyponatremia
- Thrombocytosis after first week[‡]
- Sterile pyuria
- Elevated serum transaminases
- Elevated serum gamma glutamyl transpeptidase
- Pleocytosis of cerebrospinal fluid
- Leukocytosis in synovial fluid

*Patients with fever for at least 5 days and fewer than four principal criteria can be diagnosed as having Kawasaki disease (KD) when coronary artery abnormalities are detected by two dimensional echocardiography or angiography.
[†]In the presence of four or more principal criteria, the diagnosis of KD can be made on day 4 of illness. Experienced clinicians who have treated many KD patients may establish the diagnosis before day 4.
[‡]Some infants present with thrombocytopenia and disseminated intravascular coagulation.
From Newburger JW, Takahashi M, Gerber MA, et al: Diagnosis, treatment, and long-term management of Kawasaki Disease: A statement for health professionals from the Committee on Rheumatic Fever, Endocarditis, and Kawasaki Disease, Council on Cardiovascular Disease in the Young, American Heart Association. Pediatrics 114:1708–1733, Dec. 2004. Used with permission of the American Academy of Pediatrics.

BOX 2 Differential Diagnoses

- Viral infections including measles, adenovirus, enterovirus, and Epstein-Barr virus
- Scarlet fever
- Staphylococcal scalded skin syndrome
- Toxic shock syndrome
- Bacterial cervical lymphadenitis
- Drug hypersensitivity reactions
- Stevens-Johnson syndrome
- Juvenile rheumatoid arthritis
- Rocky Mountain spotted fever
- Leptospirosis
- Mercury hypersensitivity reaction (acrodynia)

From Newburger JW, Takahashi M, Gerber MA, et al: Diagnosis, treatment, and long-term management of Kawasaki Disease: A statement for health professionals from the Committee on Rheumatic Fever, Endocarditis, and Kawasaki Disease, Council on Cardiovascular Disease in the Young, American Heart Association. Pediatrics 114:1708–1733, Dec. 2004. Used with permission of the American Academy of Pediatrics.

respiratory viral infections, perhaps supporting an infectious cause with a yet-to-be-isolated virus.

The course of KD can be divided into three clinical phases: acute febrile, subacute, and convalescent. The *acute febrile phase* in the absence of intravenous immunoglobulin (IVIG) treatment usually lasts 1 to 2 weeks and is associated with conjunctivitis, oral and extremity changes, adenopathy, and rash. Irritability also begins at this time. If present, myocarditis and hepatic abnormalities occur at this point.

The *subacute phase* typically encompasses weeks 2 through 4, during which time children are afebrile but may have persistent irritability, conjunctivitis, and abnormalities of skin and oral mucosa. Desquamation of the digits develops during this phase, as does the characteristically elevated platelet count (which frequently reaches 1,000,000 cells/mm^3).

The *convalescent phase* begins with resolution of clinical symptoms and physical findings, usually at week 4, and continues until inflammatory indicators return to normal. Myointimal proliferation and scarring of involved vessels progress during this phase. Most clinicians monitor the sedimentation rate as a marker of ongoing inflammation; it usually returns to normal, marking the end of the convalescent phase 6 to 8 weeks after the onset of symptoms.

Expert Opinion on Management Issues

ACCEPTED INTERVENTIONS

Standard therapy in the acute phase consists of IVIG and aspirin (Box 3). Treatment with IVIG has been proven effective in multiple randomized therapeutic trials to lower the incidence of coronary artery aneurysms when administered in the acute phase of the disease. Patients should be treated with IVIG, 2 g/kg in a single infusion. Because children with acute KD often have decreased left ventricular function and IVIG constitutes a significant volume load, IVIG should be administered over 8 to 12 hours, and sometimes longer in children with overt congestive heart failure or severe

9

BOX 3 General Approach to Treatment

Acute Phase

- IVIG (all patients): 2 g/kg single dose over 12 h.
- Aspirin (all patients): 80 to 100 mg/kg/day divided every 6 h (some advocate a lower dose of 30 mg/kg/day divided every 12 h) for 2 weeks, or until afebrile for 48 h.
- Incomplete response to IVIG: Repeat 2 g/kg single dose. With resistant cases beyond the second dose of IVIG, consider additional IVIG administration, corticosteroids, or other anti-inflammatory agents now under study.

Convalescent Phase

- Aspirin (all patients): 3 to 5 mg/kg single daily dose for 2 months. Discontinue after echocardiographic documentation of normal coronary vasculature.
- Warfarin: In combination with aspirin in children with giant aneurysms (in general, goal INR of 2.0 to 3.0).

Chronic Treatment (Patients with Aneurysms or Stenoses)

- Aspirin: Continue 3 to 5 mg/kg daily dose.
- Warfarin: Used with multiple or giant aneurysms, severe stenosis or history of thrombosis.
- Dipyridamole: Substitute for aspirin after varicella and influenza exposure.

Treatment of Coronary Acute Thrombosis/Chronic Stenosis

- Thrombolytic therapy: Prompt intravenous t-PA (alteplase, reteplase) and IV heparin for acute coronary revascularization.
- Percutaneous coronary interventions (PCI): Percutaneous coronary angioplasty, stent placement or rotational ablation may be effective in some patients. PCI are preferred for the treatment of acute and chronic coronary occlusion in adults.
- Surgical revascularization: Arterial grafts (e.g., internal mammary) are preferred to venous grafts.

INR, international normalized ratio; IVIG, intravenous immunoglobulin.

From Newburger JW, Takahashi M, Gerber MA, et al: Diagnosis, treatment, and long-term management of Kawasaki Disease: A statement for health professionals from the Committee on Rheumatic Fever, Endocarditis, and Kawasaki Disease, Council on Cardiovascular Disease in the Young, American Heart Association. Pediatrics 114:1708–1733, Dec. 2004. Used with permission of the American Academy of Pediatrics.

left ventricular dysfunction. By convention, day 1 of KD is considered to be the first day on which fever is noted. Treatment with IVIG should be administered no later than day 10 and ideally by day 7 of illness. Treatment before day 5 does not lower the risk of coronary aneurysms, but may increase the need for IVIG retreatment. IVIG should also be administered to patients presenting after day 10 if they are still febrile or if they have aneurysms and ongoing inflammation, as evidenced by elevated ESR or CRP. Adverse effects of IVIG include anaphylaxis, hypotension, rigors, headache, and hemolytic anemia. To reduce allergic reactions, intravenous (IV) diphenhydramine, 1 mg/kg, to a maximum of 50 mg, is often administered prior to IVIG infusion. Measles and varicella immunizations should be deferred for 11 months after IVIG treatment. However, if the risk of exposure is considered to be high, these vaccines may be given earlier; in such cases, if the serologic response is inadequate, the child should be re-immunized at least 11 months after IVIG administration.

At least 10% of children with KD fail to respond to initial IVIG therapy, as defined by persistent or recrudescent fever 36 hours or more after completion of the initial IVIG infusion. These children are at greater risk of developing coronary aneurysms. Because studies have shown a dose-response effect of IVIG, most experts recommend retreatment with IVIG, 2 g/kg, for children with persistent or recrudescent fever without other explanation occurring at least 36 hours after completion of initial IVIG.

Aspirin has long been used for treatment of KD for its anti-inflammatory (80 to 100 mg/kg/day in four doses) and antiplatelet (3 mg/kg/day as a single dose) effects, but has never been shown to reduce the prevalence of coronary aneurysms. High-dose aspirin is administered at initial presentation. The aspirin dose usually is reduced after the patient has been afebrile for 48 to 72 hours. Some experts administer high-dose aspirin until the fourteenth day of illness and at least 48 to 72 hours after cessation of fever, whichever is longer.

Low-dose aspirin is continued for 6 weeks in patients without coronary abnormalities and indefinitely for those with coronary abnormalities. Reye syndrome, which has been associated with aspirin use in patients with influenza and varicella, has been reported in children taking high-dose aspirin for KD. The risk of Reye syndrome in children on low-dose aspirin is unknown. Children on chronic aspirin therapy should receive an annual influenza vaccine. Additionally, when such children have a febrile illness that could be consistent with influenza, aspirin should be temporarily withheld and another antiplatelet agent, such as dipyridamole or clopidogrel, substituted. Because ibuprofen antagonizes the irreversible platelet inhibition induced by aspirin, its use should be avoided in children with coronary aneurysms on low-dose aspirin.

The duration of aspirin administration and the need for other antithrombotic therapies are determined by coronary artery status (Tables 1 and 2). Children with giant coronary artery aneurysms, defined as having a maximum diameter of at least 8 mm, are at especially high risk for coronary thrombosis. There have been no randomized trials of optimal antithrombotic management in such children. However, the consensus of experts is that children with giant aneurysms should be treated with low-dose aspirin and warfarin, maintaining the international normalized ratio at 2.0 to 2.5.

CONTROVERSIAL INTERVENTIONS

Controlled data are lacking for treatment of the child who fails to respond to IVIG. Therapies that have been used with success in reducing systemic inflammation include repeated doses of IVIG (see above), corticosteroids; tumor necrosis factor (TNF)-α inhibitors (e.g., pentoxyphylline, infliximab), plasma exchange, and, for those developing coronary artery aneurysms, abciximab. Although cytotoxic agents, such as cyclophosphamide and methotrexate, have been used in severe KD, the risks of these agents exceed the benefits for the vast majority of KD patients.

TABLE 1 Antiplatelet, Anticoagulant, and Thrombolytic Medications

Medication	Route	Dosage
Aspirin	PO	Antiplatelet dose: 3–5 mg/kg qd.
Clopidogrel	PO	1 mg/kg/day,* to maximum (adult dose) of 75 mg/day.
Dipyridamole	PO	2–6 mg/kg/day in 3 divided doses.†
Unfractionated heparin	IV	Load: 50 U/kg. Infusion: 20 U/kg/h. Adjust dose to achieve desired therapeutic level; usually plasma heparin level = 0.35–0.7 in terms of antifactor Xa activity or activated partial thromboplastin time (aPTT) of 60 to 85 seconds.
Low-molecular-weight heparin (enoxaparin)	SC	Infants <22 mo: Treatment: 3 mg/kg/day, divided q12h. Prophylaxis: 1.5 mg/kg/day, divided q12h. Children >2 mo: Treatment: 2 mg/kg/day, divided q12h. Prophylaxis: 1 mg/kg/day, divided q12h. Adjust dose to achieve desired therapeutic level, usually antifactor Xa = 0.5–1.0 U/mL.
Abciximab	IV	Bolus: 0.25 mg/kg. Infusion: 0.125 µg/kg/min for 12 h.
Streptokinase	IV	Bolus: 1000–4000 U/kg over 30 min. Infusion: 1000–1500 U/kg/h.
Tissue plasminogen activator	IV	Bolus: 1.25 mg/kg. Infusion: 0.1–0.5 mg/kg/h for 6 h, then reassess.
Warfarin	PO	0.1 mg/kg/day, given qd (range 0.05–0.34 mg/kg/day—adjust dose to achieve desired INR, usually 2.0–2.5).

*No published studies with children.
†Clopidogrel is preferred to dipyridamole based on studies in adults.
INR, international normalized ratio; IV, intravenously; PO, orally; qd, daily; qxhr, every x hours; SC, subcutaneously.
From Newburger JW, Takahashi M, Gerber MA, et al: Diagnosis, treatment, and long-term management of Kawasaki Disease: A statement for health professionals from the Committee on Rheumatic Fever, Endocarditis, and Kawasaki Disease, Council on Cardiovascular Disease in the Young, American Heart Association. Pediatrics 114:1708–1733, Dec. 2004. Used with permission of the American Academy of Pediatrics.

LONG-TERM MANAGEMENT

The long-term management of children with KD has been stratified according to their relative risk of coronary ischemia; Table 2 summarizes recommendations with respect to medical therapy, physical activity, frequency of clinical follow-up and diagnostic testing, and indications for cardiac catheterization and coronary angiography.

URGENT INTERVENTIONS

The development of coronary thrombosis constitutes the leading cause of death in children with KD. Children with either echocardiographic evidence of coronary thrombosis or with signs and symptoms of myocardial infarction should be treated in an intensive care unit. A variety of treatment regimens may be used, generally in combination with aspirin and heparin (see Box 3). These include:

- Thrombolytic therapy, such as tissue plasminogen activator (tPA)
- Reduced-dose thrombolytic therapy in combination with administration of a glycoprotein IIb/IIIa inhibitor, such as abciximab
- Mechanical restoration of coronary blood flow

Decisions about intervention in individual patients should be made in concert with experienced adult interventional cardiologists and cardiac surgeons.

Common Pitfalls

- Elevated ESR, CRP, or both is nearly universal in KD, but uncommon in viral illnesses.
- A viral illness is more likely than KD if platelet count, ESR, and CRP are normal after the seventh day of illness. Additionally, a viral etiology is suggested by low white blood count, lymphocyte predominance, and low platelet count in the absence of disseminated intravascular coagulation.
- Young infants with KD often have fever without many other classic criteria and are at high risk for coronary artery aneurysms. Echocardiography should be performed on any infant younger than age 6 months with unexplained fever of more than 7 days' duration and laboratory evidence of systemic inflammation.
- Children with KD may present with a unilateral enlarged cervical lymph node and fever. Because such children routinely receive antibiotics, subsequent development of a rash and mucosal inflammation is often mistaken for a drug reaction.
- The presence of sterile pyuria in KD patients may be confused with a urinary tract infection.
- Evidence of aseptic meningitis, with a predominance of mononuclear cells and normal protein and glucose levels, is found in half of children with KD who undergo lumbar puncture, causing the misdiagnosis of partially treated meningitis.

Communication and Counseling

For children with coronary aneurysms and their families, the physician should review the natural history of coronary involvement. Approximately half of coronary artery aneurysms, usually those that are smaller in maximum dimension, regress to normal lumen diameter through myointimal proliferation, reducing the risk of clinical symptoms or events in childhood; however, long-term structural and functional abnormalities of the arterial wall persist. Large or

TABLE 2 Risk Stratification

Risk Level	Pharmacologic Therapy	Physical Activity	Follow-up and Diagnostic Testing	Invasive Testing
I. No coronary artery changes at any stage of illness	None beyond initial 6–8 wk.	No restrictions beyond initial 6–8 wk.	Cardiovascular risk assessment and counseling at 5-yr intervals	None recommended.
II. Transient coronary artery ectasia that disappears within initial 6–8 wk	None beyond initial 6–8 wk.	No restrictions beyond initial 6–8 wk.	Cardiovascular risk assessment and counseling at 3- to 5-yr intervals	None recommended.
III. One small to medium single coronary artery aneurysm per major coronary artery	Low-dose aspirin (3 to 5 mg/kg aspirin per day), at least until aneurysm regression is documented.	For patients in first decade of life, no restriction beyond initial 6–8 wk. For second decade, physical activity guided by stress testing with evaluation of myocardial perfusion every other year. Contact or high-impact sports discouraged for patients on antiplatelet agents.	Annual cardiology follow-up with echocardiogram and ECG, combined with cardiovascular risk assessment and counseling Stress testing with evaluation of myocardial perfusion every other year	Angiography, if noninvasive test suggests ischemia.
IV. One or more large or giant coronary artery aneurysms, or multiple or complex aneurysms in same coronary artery, without obstruction	Long-term antiplatelet therapy and warfarin (target INR 2.0–2.5) or LMW heparin (target: antifactor Xa level 0.5–1.0 units/mL) should be combined in giant aneurysms.	Contact or high-impact sports should be avoided because of the risk of bleeding. Other physical activity recommendations guided by outcome of stress testing with evaluation of myocardial perfusion.	Biannual follow-up with echocardiogram + ECG Annual stress test with evaluation of myocardial perfusion	Initial angiography at 6–12 mo or sooner if clinical indications. Repeated angiography if noninvasive test, clinical or laboratory findings suggest ischemia. Elective repeated angiography under some circumstances.
V. Coronary artery obstruction	Long-term low-dose aspirin. Warfarin or LMW heparin if giant aneurysm persists. Use of β-blockers should be considered to reduce myocardial oxygen consumption.	Contact or high-impact sports, isometrics, and weight training should be avoided because of the risk of bleeding. Other physical activity recommendations guided by outcome of stress testing or myocardial perfusion scan.	Biannual follow-up with echocardiogram and ECG Annual stress test with evaluation of myocardial perfusion	Angiography is recommended to address therapeutic options.

INR, international normalized ratio; LMW, low molecular weight.

From Newburger JW, Takahashi M, Gerber MA, et al: Diagnosis, treatment, and long-term management of Kawasaki Disease: A statement for health professionals from the Committee on Rheumatic Fever, Endocarditis, and Kawasaki Disease, Council on Cardiovascular Disease in the Young, American Heart Association. Pediatrics 114:1708–1733, Dec. 2004. Used with permission of the American Academy of Pediatrics.

giant coronary aneurysms rarely return to normal dimension, and they are associated with a long-term risk of coronary artery stenosis and thrombosis. The signs and symptoms of angina or myocardial infarction should be reviewed, so that children can be brought to prompt medical attention. Patients on long-term antithrombotic therapy, particularly those on warfarin and aspirin, are at risk for bleeding if they participate in collision or high-impact sports. Although patients who never had any coronary abnormalities by echocardiography in any stage of illness have not shown early coronary heart disease with greater than 20 years of careful cardiology follow-up, research studies have shown endothelial dysfunction, increased arterial stiffness, and reduced coronary flow reserve in this population, suggesting a need for long-term follow-up with measurement of a lipid profile, encouragement of exercise, and preventive cardiology counseling.

SUGGESTED READINGS

1. Burns JC, Glode MP: Kawasaki syndrome. Lancet 364:533–544, 2004. **A historical review and recent update of the entire topic.**
2. Cheung YF, Yung TC, Tam SC, et al: Novel and traditional cardiovascular risk factors in children after Kawasaki disease: Implications for premature atherosclerosis. J Am Coll Cardiol 43 (1):120–124, 2004. **Patients with KD, including those who never had coronary artery abnormalities, have an adverse risk profile, including increased arterial stiffness.**
3. Council on Cardiovascular Disease in the Young, Committee on Rheumatic Fever, Endocarditis and Kawasaki Disease, American Heart Association. Diagnostic Guidelines for Kawasaki Disease.

Circulation 0(103):335–336, 2001. **Brief document with photographs of classic physical exam, echocardiographic, and angiographic findings.**

4. Dhillon R, Clarkson P, Donald AE, et al: Endothelial dysfunction late after Kawasaki disease. Circulation 94:2103–2106, 1996. **Demonstrates abnormal endothelial function in children who never had coronary aneurysms.**

5. Holman RC, Curns AT, Belay ED, et al: Kawasaki syndrome hospitalizations in the United States, 1997 and 2000. Pediatr 112(3 Pt 1):495–501, 2003. **Epidemiology of Kawasaki disease in the United States based on administrative hospital discharge data.**

6. Kato H, Sugimura T, Akagi T, et al: Long-term consequences of Kawasaki disease: A 10- to 21-year follow-up study of 594 patients. Circulation 94:1379–1385, 1996. **Natural history of Kawasaki disease.**

7. Muta H, Ishii M, Egami K, et al: Early intravenous gamma-globulin treatment for Kawasaki disease: The nationwide surveys in Japan. J Pediatr 144(4):496–499, 2004. **This study suggested no additional benefit to early (prior to day 5) treatment with IVIG. Early treatment was associated with greater recurrent fever and IVIG retreatment.**

8. Newburger JW, Takahashi M, Gerber MA, et al: AHA Scientific Statement. Revised guidelines for diagnosis, treatment, and long-term management of Kawasaki disease. Circulation 110 (17):2747–2771, 2004. **Scientific statement including most recent guidelines for diagnosis, treatment in the acute phase of the disease, and long-term management.**

9. Oates-Whitehead RM, Baumer JH, Haines L, et al: Intravenous immunoglobulin for the treatment of Kawasaki disease in children. Cochrane Database Syst Rev 4:CD004001, 2003. **Meta-analysis supporting immunoglobulin treatment of Kawasaki disease.**

10. Sundel RP, Baker AL, Fulton DR, et al: Corticosteroids in the initial treatment of Kawasaki disease: Report of a randomized trial. J Pediatr 142(6):611–616, 2003. **Single center randomized trial that suggested that treatment with IV methyl-prednisolone, 30 mg/kg, prior to IVIG shortens duration of fever and hospitalization.**

11. Suzuki A, Miyagawa-Tomita S, Komatsu K, et al: Active remodeling of the coronary arterial lesions in the late phase of Kawasaki disease: Immunohistochemical study. Circulation 101(25):2935–2941, 2000. **Excellent study on the histology of coronary artery aneurysms.**

12. Tsuda E, Kamiya T, Ono Y, et al: Incidence of stenotic lesions predicted by acute phase changes in coronary arterial diameter during Kawasaki disease. Pediatr Cardiol 26(1):73–79, 2005. **Demonstrates that the incidence of coronary artery stenosis in patients with aneurysms increases with duration from disease onset.**

13. Tsuda E, Kamiya T, Kimura K, et al: Coronary artery dilatation exceeding 4.0 mm during acute Kawasaki disease predicts a high probability of subsequent late intima-medial thickening. Pediatr Cardiol 23(1):9–14, 2002. **Demonstrates a significant correlation between initial coronary diameter and intima-medial thickness by intravascular ultrasound.**

Pulmonary Hypertension in Children

Catherine L. Dent

KEY CONCEPTS

- Pulmonary hypertension can occur without an identifiable cause (primary pulmonary hypertension) or, more commonly, may be related to a coexisting disease (secondary pulmonary hypertension).

- Because primary pulmonary hypertension is a diagnosis of exclusion, appropriate evaluation must be performed to exclude all other known causes.

- The goal of medical therapy is to slow or halt the progression of disease, improve quality of life, and increase survival.

- The pulmonary endothelium is an important source of mediators that contribute to the vasomotor tone. Endothelial dysfunction may lead to release of vasoproliferative substances and vasoconstrictors that result in remodeling, obstruction, and obliteration of the pulmonary vasculature.

- Traditional therapy has been directed at reversing vasoconstriction, slowing proliferation, and preventing thrombosis.

- Novel therapies under active investigation include prostacyclin analogues, inhaled nitric oxide delivery systems, phosphodiesterase–5 inhibitors, and endothelin–1 receptor antagonists.

Although pulmonary hypertension remains an incurable disease, recent insights into the pathophysiologic mechanism of the disease have led to the introduction of novel therapies that have resulted in significant symptomatic improvement and longer life expectancy for many patients.

Pulmonary hypertension is defined as an increase in pulmonary arterial pressure above the normal value for age. A mean pulmonary arterial pressure greater than 25 mm Hg at rest or greater than 30 mm Hg with exercise has been considered abnormal in adults. These values are typically applied to pediatric patients as well. Pulmonary hypertension can occur without an identifiable underlying cause (primary pulmonary hypertension [PPH]) or, more commonly, may be related to a coexisting disease or condition, such as congenital heart disease or lung disease (secondary pulmonary hypertension).

Because multiple pathologic conditions may lead to elevated pulmonary arterial pressure, pulmonary hypertension is a manifestation of disease rather than a disease itself. Consequently, treatment plans must be directed primarily at the underlying disease, if at all possible (Table 1). An understanding of the mechanisms that lead to increased pulmonary arterial pressure may help guide diagnosis and determine subsequent therapy. Pulmonary arterial pressure is determined by three factors in accordance with a simple equation:

$$P_{PA} = P_{LA} + Q_P \times R_{PV}$$

where P_{PA} is pulmonary arterial pressure, P_{LA} is the blood pressure in the left atrium (or that opposing pulmonary venous return), Q_P is the blood flow circulating through the pulmonary vascular bed (the entire cardiac output under normal conditions), and R_{PV} is the resistance imposed by this bed to the passage of blood.

Thus, pulmonary hypertension may result from elevated left atrial pressure (or pulmonary venous obstruction), increased pulmonary blood flow, or high pulmonary vascular resistance (Box 1). These three

9

TABLE 1 Treatment of Pulmonary Hypertension

Generic Name (Trade Name)	Dosage/Route/Regimen	Maximum Dose	Dosage Formulation	Common Adverse Reactions	Comments
Prostanoids (Activate adenylate cyclase, increasing cAMP leading to decrease in intracellular calcium and vasodilation)					
Epoprostenol (Flolan)	IV continuous: Start 2 ng/kg/min, ↑ q15min until dose-limiting effects, then ↑ q2wk (to 20–40 ng/kg/min for most patients)	50 ng/kg/min (higher doses have been reported)	IV susp: 0.5 mg vial reconstituted to 3000 ng/mL 5000 ng/mL 10,000 ng/mL 15,000 ng/mL	Sepsis, jaw pain, headache, rash, flushing, leg pain, diarrhea, chest pain, nausea, anxiety, hypotension	Tachyphylaxis: Must ↑ dose. Stable long-term IV access needed. Abrupt withdrawal can cause severe/fatal PHTN. Administer as continuous infusion via portable infusion pump. Patients have been safely transitioned from epoprostenol to treprostinil.
Treprostinil (Remodulin)	SC continuous: Start 1.25 ng/kg/min, ↑ weekly by 1.25 ng/kg/min to effect	40 ng/kg/min (higher doses have been reported)	SC susp: 1 mg/mL 2.5 mg/mL 5 mg/mL 10 mg/mL	Infusion site pain, headache, diarrhea, jaw pain, nausea, rash	
Beraprost (investigational)	Oral : 80 µg qid, ↑ by 80 µg/week as tolerated	480 µg qid	Tablet: 80 µg	Headache, flushing, jaw pain, diarrhea	
Iloprost	Inhaled aerosol: 2.5–5 µg (0.2 µg/kg) over 10–15 min 6–9 times daily	30 µg/day	Inhaled aerosol	Cough, headache, flushing	Has not been studied in children under 18 years of age.
Digoxin (Increases myocardial contractility by inhibition of sodium and potassium across myocardial membrane leading to calcium influx)					
Digoxin (Lanoxin)	Loading dose: (Give half dose initially, followed by one fourth of dose in each of subsequent doses at 6- to 12-h intervals) PO: 1 mo–2 yr: 35–60 µg/kg; 2–5 yr: 30–40 µg/kg; 5–10 yr: 20–35 µg/kg; >10 yr 10–15 µg/kg Adult: 0.75–1.5 mg IV: 1 mo–2 yr: 30–50 µg/kg; 2–5 yr: 25–35 µg/kg; 5–10 yr: 15–30 µg/kg; >10 yr: 8–12 µg/kg Adult: 0.5–1 mg Daily maintenance dose (divided into 2 daily doses if <10 yr, once daily if >10 yr): PO: 1 mo–2 yr: 10–15 µg/kg; 2–5 yr:	0.5 mg/day. Cl$_{Cr}$ 10–50 mL/min: Give 25%–75% of normal daily dose at usual intervals or administer normal dose q36h. Cl$_{Cr}$ <10 mL/min: Give 10%–25% of normal daily dose at usual intervals or give normal dose q48h	Elixir: 50 µg/mL Capsule: 50 µg, 100 µg, 200 µg Tablet: 125 µg, 250 µg, 500 µg Injection: 100 µg/mL 250 µg/mL	Sinus bradycardia, AV block, atrial or nodal ectopic beats, ventricular arrhythmias, drowsiness, fatigue, headache, dizziness, nausea, abdominal pain, diarrhea, blurred vision, halos, yellow or green vision, photophobia	Therapeutic range: 0.8–2 ng/mL; toxicity associated with levels >2 ng/mL. Decreased serum potassium may increase toxicity. Assess renal function in order to adjust dose. Obtain serum concentration 8–12 h after a dose.

Drug	Pediatric Dose	Adult Dose	How Supplied	Side Effects	Comments
	7.5–10 µg/kg; 5–10 yr: 5–10 µg/kg; >10 yr: 2.5–5 µg/kg Adult: 0.125–0.5 mg IV: 1 mo–2 yr: 7.5–12 µg/kg; 2–5 yr: 6–9 µg/kg; 5–10 yr: 4–8 µg/kg; >10 yr: 2–3 µg/kg. Adult: 0.1–0.4 mg				

Diuretics (Inhibit sodium resorption in loop of Henle or distal renal tubule)

Drug	Pediatric Dose	Adult Dose	How Supplied	Side Effects	Comments
Furosemide (Lasix)	PO: 1–6 mg/kg/day divided q6–12h IV: 1–2 mg/kg/dose q6–12h Continuous IV infusion: Bolus 0.1 mg/kg then 0.05 mg/kg/h, titrate to effect	PO: Up to 600 mg has been reported IV: 80 mg q6h Continuous infusion: 0.4 mg/kg/h	Oral soln: 10 mg/mL, 40 mg/5 mL Tablet: 20 mg, 40 mg, 80 mg IV soln: 10 mg/mL	Hypokalemia, hyponatremia, hypomagnesemia, alkalosis, photosensitivity, anemia, ototoxicity, hypotension, nephrocalcinosis	Loop diuretic (acts primarily in ascending loop of Henle).
Chlorothiazide (Diuril)	PO: 20 mg/kg/day in 2 divided doses IV: 4 mg/kg/day divided in 1–2 doses	PO: 1 g/day IV: 20 mg/kg/day	Oral susp: 250 mg/5 mL Tablet: 250 mg, 500 mg Injection: Powder 500 mg	Hypokalemia, hypotension, alkalosis, rash, photosensitivity	Thiazide diuretic (acts primarily in distal renal tubule).

Calcium Channel Blockers (Inhibit calcium from entering channels in smooth muscle, resulting in vasodilation)

Drug	Pediatric Dose	Adult Dose	How Supplied	Side Effects	Comments
Nifedipine (Procardia, Procardia XL, Adalat CC, Nifedical XL)	PO: (immediate release product) 0.5–2 mg/kg/day in 3–4 divided doses	180 mg/day	Capsule: 10 mg, 20 mg Tablet, extended release: 30 mg, 60 mg, 90 mg	Flushing, hypotension, tachycardia, dizziness, nausea, elevated liver enzymes, blurred vision	10 mg capsule ≡ 0.34 mL. 20 mg capsule ≡ 0.45 mL.

Inhaled Nitric Oxide (Increases cGMP activation leading to vasodilation)

Drug	Pediatric Dose	Adult Dose	How Supplied	Side Effects	Comments
Nitric oxide (INOmax)	Inhaled: 5–40 ppm	80 ppm	Inhaled gas	Hypotension, atelectasis, methemoglobin production, impaired platelet aggregation	Administered via endotracheal tube. Alternate routes are under investigation. Monitor methemoglobin levels. Abrupt withdrawal may cause severe rebound PHTN.

Phosphodiesterase-5 Inhibitors (Inhibit action of PDE-5, prolonging cGMP activity and vasodilation)

Drug	Pediatric Dose	Adult Dose	How Supplied	Side Effects	Comments
Sildenafil (Viagra)	Oral: Adult: 50 mg q8h Pediatric (investigational): 0.25–2 mg/kg q6h	100 mg q8h	Tablet: 25 mg, 50 mg, 100 mg	Headache, flushing, nausea, diarrhea, blurry vision, nasal congestion hypotension	

TABLE 1 Treatment of Pulmonary Hypertension—cont'd

Generic Name (Trade Name)	Dosage/Route/ Regimen	Maximum Dose	Dosage Formulation	Common Adverse Reactions	Comments
Endothelin–1 Receptor Antagonists (Block receptors of endothelin–1, a potent vasoconstrictor and smooth muscle mitogen)					
Bosentan (Tracleer)	Oral: 62.5 mg bid, ↑ to 125 mg bid after 4 wk Investigational pediatric dose: <10 kg: 15.625 mg qd × 4 wk, then ↑ to 15.625 mg bid; 10–20 kg: 31.25 mg qd × 4 wk, then ↑ to 31.25 mg bid; 20–40 kg: 31.25 mg bid × 4 wk, then ↑ to 62.5 mg bid; >40 kg: 62.5 mg bid × 4 wk, then ↑ to 125 mg bid)	125 mg bid	Tablet: 62.5 mg, 125 mg	Hepatocellular injury, anemia, headache, flushing, fetal deformities	Monitor liver transaminases monthly. Avoid pregnancy; nonspecific ET–1 receptor antagonist
Sitaxsentan (investigational)	Oral: 100–300 mg daily	300 mg daily	Tablet: 100 mg	Hepatocellular injury, peripheral edema, nausea, dizziness, nasal congestion	Monitor liver transaminases monthly. Specific ET–1 receptor antagonist

↑, increase; AV, atrioventricular; bid, two times daily; cGMP, cyclic guanosine monophosphate; Cl$_{Cr}$, creatinine clearance; ET–1, endothelin–1; IV, intravenously; PDE, phosphodiesterase; PHTN, pulmonary hypertension; PO, orally; ppm, parts per million; qd, daily; qid, four times daily; q×h, every x hours; SC, subcutaneous; soln, solution; susp, suspension.

possibilities, alone or in combination, must be considered in any patient who is found to have abnormally high pulmonary arterial pressure.

PPH is a diagnosis of exclusion. Therefore, appropriate evaluation must be performed to exclude all other causes of pulmonary hypertension. In addition to a careful history and physical examination, diagnostic evaluation may include chest radiography, echocardiography, pulmonary function tests, sleep study, cardiac catheterization, ventilation-perfusion scan, assessment of exercise capacity, and lung biopsy. Appropriate laboratory studies to exclude collagen vascular disease, disorders of coagulation, and infection may also be indicated.

BOX 1 Causes of Pulmonary Hypertension

Increased Pulmonary Blood Flow

Congenital heart lesions with left-to-right shunts: atrial septal defect, ventricular septal defect, complete atrioventricular canal defects, patent ductus arteriosus, truncus arteriosus, aortopulmonary connections

Obstruction to Pulmonary Venous Return

- Pulmonary venous obstruction: veno-occlusive disease, anomalous pulmonary venous return, pulmonary vein stenosis
- Elevated left atrial pressure: mitral stenosis, mitral insufficiency, cor triatriatum, atrial myxoma or thrombus
- Elevated left ventricular end-diastolic pressure: left ventricular failure/cardiomyopathy, left ventricular outflow tract obstruction (aortic stenosis, interrupted aortic arch, coarctation), aortic insufficiency, systemic hypertension, coronary artery disease (anomalous origin of the left coronary artery, Kawasaki disease, transplant coronary vasculopathy)

Increased Resistance of Pulmonary Vasculature

- Pulmonary vascular disease
  - Idiopathic/ PPH
  - Thromboembolic disease: indwelling central lines, ventriculoatrial/ventriculovenous shunts, hypercoagulable states, sickle cell disease, parasitic infection, malignancy, foreign body (talc), sepsis
  - Vasculitis: autoimmune diseases, chemotherapy
  - Collagen vascular disease: scleroderma, systemic lupus erythematosus, mixed connective tissue disease, rheumatoid arthritis, sarcoidosis
  - Peripheral branch pulmonary artery stenosis
  - Drug induced: appetite suppressants (fenfluramine, aminorex), herbs (monocrotalaria), chemicals (toxic rapeseed oil, paraquat)
  - Maldevelopment of pulmonary circulation: meconium aspiration syndrome, persistent pulmonary hypertension of the newborn
  - Maladaptation to extrauterine life: persistent pulmonary hypertension of the newborn
- Pulmonary parenchymal disease
  - Obstructive pulmonary disease: cystic fibrosis, bronchopulmonary dysplasia
  - Restrictive pulmonary disease: sarcoidosis, diffuse interstitial fibrosis, scoliosis
  - Acute lung injury: acute respiratory distress syndrome, pneumonia/pneumonitis
  - Underdeveloped pulmonary parenchymal/arterial bed: congenital diaphragmatic hernia, lung hypoplasia, oligohydramnios
  - Other forms of hypoxic vasoconstriction: high-altitude vasoconstriction, hypoventilation syndromes (sleep disorders, obesity, neuromuscular disease, upper airway obstruction)

Expert Opinion on Management Issues

GENERAL MEASURES

In general, patients with pulmonary hypertension should avoid circumstances that may exacerbate their condition. Most children are allowed to dictate their own level of activity but should avoid strenuous exercise or exertion that induces symptoms. Travel to high altitudes should be avoided because alveolar hypoxia is a potent stimulus for pulmonary vasoconstriction. Pregnancy is usually not advised, because it has been shown to be associated with significant maternal and fetal morbidity and mortality. Oral contraceptives are contraindicated.

Digoxin has been used in patients with pulmonary hypertension to augment right ventricular contractility and improve cardiac output, although its effects may be limited. Digoxin may also counteract the negative inotropic effects of calcium channel blocker therapy (see Table 1). Diuretics are used to relieve symptoms of right heart failure, such as hepatic congestion, ascites, and edema. However, patients on concomitant digoxin and diuretic therapy must be monitored closely to prevent diuretic-induced hypokalemia, which increases the risks of digoxin toxicity. Avoidance of excessive diuresis is important because cardiac output in patients with pulmonary hypertension may be highly dependent on preload. Vasodilator therapy in the setting of intravascular volume depletion from diuresis may also lead to significant hypotension (see Table 1).

Patients with pulmonary hypertension are at risk for the development of thrombosis in pulmonary vessels as a result of intimal proliferation and decreased flow through the vascular bed. Therapy with oral anticoagulants, such as warfarin, has been shown to prolong survival in adult patients with PPH. Less is known about this therapy in children or in other forms of pulmonary hypertension. The use of agents such as low-molecular-weight heparin has been reported but in numbers insufficient to make recommendations for children with pulmonary hypertension.

PRIMARY PULMONARY HYPERTENSION

The pulmonary vasculature of most patients with PPH has a variable combination of vasoconstriction, intimal and medial proliferation, and thrombosis. Until recently, little was known (and less could be done) about the last two mechanisms. Therefore, amelioration of pulmonary vasoconstriction has been the main focus of attention for both researchers and clinicians for many years.

Vasodilator administration is the mainstay of therapy, the main goal of which is aimed at shifting the balance of vasodilatory and vasoconstrictive influences toward vasodilation to achieve diminished right ventricular afterload, improved cardiac output, and symptomatic relief. For a vasodilator to function as such, however, the pulmonary vessels must be in a state of reversible constriction, a situation that is only present relatively early in the disease process. The reversibility of the vasoconstriction is often tested by administering a potent and short-acting vasodilator, such as oxygen or nitric oxide (NO), during cardiac catheterization. The response of the vasculature to vasodilators has allowed identification of potential responders to longer-acting agents such as calcium channel blockers, which can be given orally. Pulmonary vasodilation during inhaled NO is an excellent predictor of the efficacy of other vasodilators. Because serious side effects (prolonged hypotension, shock, or severe vomiting) can develop after administration of oral calcium blockers in approximately 40% of adult patients who do not have a decrease in pulmonary vascular resistance after administration of inhaled NO, the detection of nonresponders seems just as important.

Calcium Channel Blockers

Patients who have a clinical response to short-term vasodilators are usually prescribed calcium channel blockers (nifedipine). The beneficial effects of calcium channel blockers on pulmonary vascular resistance were first reported in the 1980s. The benefit, however, is not universal. Only 30% of patients with PPH experience significant improvement in pulmonary vascular resistance/blood flow with vasodilators, a finding that may relate to the absence of pulmonary vasoconstriction in many of these patients (see Table 1).

Nitric Oxide

Because of its pulmonary selectivity, NO has many characteristics of an ideal pulmonary vasodilator. It is produced from L-arginine in vascular endothelial cells and acts in a paracrine fashion to raise cyclic 3',5'-guanosine monophosphate (cGMP) levels in neighboring vascular smooth muscle cells. The final result is smooth muscle relaxation. When given exogenously by inhalation, NO diffuses into the intravascular space and is rapidly inactivated by binding to hemoglobin, preventing systemic effects. However, because of its short half-life, it must be inhaled continuously, making its administration more difficult. The use of chronic NO therapy via alternate delivery systems such as pulsed nasal cannula delivery is under active investigation. Detrimental effects from NO inhalation appear to be uncommon, although little is known about the effects of long-term use. Short-term concerns have included inactivation of alveolar surfactant production, methemoglobin production, and inhibition of platelet aggregation. Because prolonged administration of NO suppresses NO synthase activity, abrupt withdrawal of therapy is sometimes complicated by rebound pulmonary hypertension and decreased cardiac output (see Table 1).

Antagonists of cGMP-Specific Phosphodiesterase

There is mounting evidence that it is possible to augment the vasodilatory effects of NO on pulmonary vessels. Increases in cGMP-specific phosphodiesterase (PDE_5), the enzyme responsible for cGMP degradation, have been reported in animal models of pulmonary hypertension. Because increased cGMP inactivation may limit the potency and duration of NO therapy, PDE_5 antagonists may have a role in the management of severe pulmonary hypertension. Sildenafil, one such antagonist, has been found to enhance the response to inhaled NO in some patients and has been used to abolish rebound increases in pulmonary arterial pressure after reductions in NO doses in children with pulmonary hypertension after correction of congenital heart disease. As chronic therapy, oral sildenafil has been shown to improve exercise tolerance and cardiac index in adults with PPH and has been shown to augment the pulmonary vasodilatory effects of prostanoids when used as part of combination therapy. It has also shown promise in several secondary forms of pulmonary hypertension, such as human immunodeficiency virus (HIV)-related disease and pulmonary hypertension related to interstitial lung disease. Pediatric trials are ongoing. Phosphodiesterase inhibitors also appear to have antiproliferative effects on vascular smooth muscle cells, which may be beneficial to patients with intimal and smooth muscle hyperplasia (see Table 1).

Prostacyclin (epoprostenol), a metabolite of arachidonic acid, acts as a strong pulmonary and systemic vasodilator, inhibits platelet aggregation, and under some circumstances may prevent smooth muscle proliferation. After binding to a cell surface receptor, prostacyclin activates intracellular adenylate cyclase, which in turn catalyzes production of cyclic adenosine monophosphate (cAMP), causing a decrease in intracellular calcium levels and vasodilation. Prostacyclin may also stimulate the release of endogenous NO. Initially applied to assess short-term pulmonary vascular responsiveness in patients with pulmonary hypertension, it has become an important component of the long-term management of patients with severe pulmonary vascular disease, often delaying the need for lung transplantation. Symptomatic relief and prolonged survival have been reported in adults and children with PPH treated with continuous infusion of prostacyclin. Because similar improvements have been observed after long-term therapy in patients whose pulmonary vascular resistance did not decrease after a test dose of prostacyclin in the catheterization laboratory, it is reasonable to think that the benefits of prostacyclin extend beyond its immediate vasodilating effects. Prostacyclin can be delivered in various forms, although the greatest experience is with continuous intravenous infusion, which has significant drawbacks, including the need for long-term intravenous access and the risk of sepsis. In addition to frequent side effects (headache, jaw pain, hypotension, nausea), tachyphylaxis to prostacyclin occurs, necessitating escalation of dose to maintain a therapeutic response. Additionally, acute interruption or withdrawal of prostacyclin can lead to fatal rebound pulmonary hypertension. More stable analogues of prostacyclin with alternative routes of administration (such as oral beraprost, inhaled iloprost, and subcutaneous treprostinil) hold particular attraction for pediatric patients and are under active investigation.

Endothelin Antagonists

Concentrations of endothelin–1 (ET–1), a potent vaso-constrictor and vascular smooth mitogen, have been found to be elevated in the plasma and lung tissue of patients with severe pulmonary hypertension and in children with congenital heart disease. Two distinct receptors (ET_A and ET_B) mediate the activity of endothelin in the endothelium and vascular smooth muscle cells. Activation of ET_A receptors mediates vasoconstriction and proliferation of smooth muscle, although ET_B receptors are believed to be principally involved in clearance of circulating ET–1. Studies have suggested that ET–1 is a key agent in the pathophysiology of pulmonary hypertension, and the development of ET–1 receptor antagonists has been an active area of research. Bosentan, a nonselective ET–1 receptor antagonist, has been demonstrated to lower pulmonary artery pressure and resistance in adults with pulmonary hypertension and in children with pulmonary hypertension related to congenital heart disease. In theory, selective ET_A receptor antagonists, such as sitaxsentan, may be even more beneficial, by blocking the vasoconstrictor effects of ET_A while maintaining the clearance effects of ET_B. Studies in pediatric patients are in progress (see Table 1).

SECONDARY PULMONARY HYPERTENSION

Congenital Heart Disease

Patients with cardiac lesions causing increased pulmonary blood flow and/or increased pulmonary artery pressures are at risk for developing progressive obstructive changes in the pulmonary vasculature. The treatment of these lesions, by surgical or transcatheter techniques, is aimed at attenuating or abolishing symptoms and preventing the development of irreversible pulmonary vascular disease (Eisenmenger syndrome). The incidence of pulmonary hypertension and the rate of disease progression vary based on the specific lesion and individual patient characteristics (such as the presence of Down syndrome). Patients with significant flow through a systemic-to-pulmonary communication generally undergo complete repair within the first year of life, often in early infancy. Occasionally, when it is necessary to delay definitive repair, a pulmonary artery band is placed to decrease pulmonary overcirculation. With a smaller systemic-to-pulmonary shunt, such as through an atrial septal defect or patent ductus arteriosus, surgical repair is often delayed until early childhood, because the risk of pulmonary hypertension prior to that period is small. Lesions associated with pulmonary venous obstruction are repaired in infancy if amenable to surgical correction.

The management of patients with congenital heart disease and elevated pulmonary vascular resistance later in life can be particularly challenging. Both histologic analysis, obtained from lung biopsy, and pulmonary hemodynamic evaluation have been used to determine if the lesion is considered inoperable, because established pulmonary vascular disease will cause unacceptably high operative risk or will continue to progress despite corrective surgery. As noted earlier, assessing the reactivity of pulmonary vasculature to vasodilators such as inhaled NO or intravenous prostacyclin may also help identify those patients with increased pulmonary vascular resistance arising from smooth muscle hyperreactivity.

Therapy for patients with irreversible pulmonary vascular disease is limited. Prostacyclin has been shown to improve hemodynamic variables in some patients with congenital heart disease and pulmonary hypertension and may provide symptomatic relief and improved exercise tolerance. Treatment with bosentan, an ET–1 receptor antagonist, and/or sildenafil, a PDE_5 inhibitor, hold particular appeal because they may be dosed orally, but studies in this population are ongoing. General measures, such as oxygen, platelet inhibitors/anticoagulants, diuretics, and digoxin may also be beneficial. Long-term outlook, however, remains poor, with lung or heart-lung transplantation often the only hope for survival in these patients.

Pulmonary Disease

Therapy for patients with pulmonary hypertension associated with structural or functional lung disease is directed at the underlying disease. Treatments that decrease hypoxic or hypercarbic contribution to vasoconstriction, such as oxygen or bronchodilators, may be useful. Vasodilator therapy should theoretically decrease right ventricular afterload and improve function, although, in patients with lung disease, such therapy may also override hypoxic pulmonary vasoconstriction, thereby exacerbating ventilation-perfusion mismatch. Inhaled NO has been used in hypoxemic respiratory failure with variable effects. It may be particularly beneficial in patients with intrapulmonary shunting, but it may also worsen hypoxemia by reversing hypoxic pulmonary vasoconstriction. The use of vasodilators in this setting, therefore, may be limited.

Atrial Septostomy

Patients with refractory symptoms of heart failure and low cardiac output, such as recurrent syncope, may benefit from creation of an atrial level communication. Studies of pediatric patients with severe symptomatic PPH demonstrate improved cardiac output and longer survival following atrial septostomy. Atrial septostomy may, therefore, be beneficial as a bridge to lung transplantation, allowing for improved length and quality of life. The procedure, however, is not without risk, with an estimated 5% to 10% risk of mortality, and should be reserved only for patients without other therapeutic options.

PULMONARY TRANSPLANTATION

Before prostacyclin became available, the lack of a long-term therapy left lung or heart–lung transplantation as the only option for survival of patients with severe pulmonary hypertension. In the largest lung transplant centers, transplantation is offered after maximal therapeutic efforts have been attempted (including administration of vasodilators and supplemental oxygen) and when the estimated 2-year survival is less than 50%. Late referral and long waiting time for suitable organs have limited pretransplant survival. Additionally, long-term complications such as organ rejection, bronchiolitis obliterans, and post-transplant lymphoproliferative disease are common. Recent data from the International Society for Heart and Lung Transplantation indicate an overall survival in children of 70% at 1 year and 60% at 2 years. Continued advancements in the understanding of immunosuppression and its relationship to these complications may also improve long-term survival.

Common Pitfalls

The diagnosis of pulmonary hypertension (particularly PPH) is often delayed until later stages, because symptoms are often nonspecific and the physical findings subtle. When the diagnosis of pulmonary hypertension is made, or if it is suspected, a thorough evaluation for secondary causes should be undertaken. Additionally, because pulmonary hypertension is relatively uncommon in pediatrics, and new therapies are under active investigation, early consultation with (and potential referral to) a center with experience in the management of these patients is encouraged.

Communication and Counseling

Despite the frustrating lack of specific therapies for the vascular wall proliferation predominant in the severe forms of pulmonary hypertension, the outlook for children with pulmonary vascular disease has improved considerably in the past few years. The combination of short-term therapies, such as NO, with long-term administration of oral vasodilators or intravenous prostacyclin has lengthened survival, in some cases halting the disease progression and in others making the wait for lung transplantation possible. Improved understanding of the molecular mechanisms has led to development of new therapies, such as ET–1 receptor antagonists and PDE_5 inhibitors. Nevertheless, the prognosis for these patients is guarded and families need to be counseled in regard to the expected outcome and limited experience of many of these therapies in the pediatric population.

SUGGESTED READINGS

1. Atz AM, Wessel DL: Sildenafil ameliorates the effects of inhaled nitric oxide withdrawal. Anesthesiology 91:307–310, 1999. **A study of sildenafil in three postoperative congenital heart patients with rebound pulmonary hypertension after withdrawal of inhaled NO.**
2. Badesch DB, McLaughlin VV, Delcroix M, et al: Prostanoid therapy for pulmonary arterial hypertension. J Am Coll Cardiol 43:56S–61S, 2004. **A review of the pharmacology, mechanisms of action, routes of administration, and study results of prostanoid therapy for pulmonary hypertension.**
3. Barst RJ, McGoon M, Torbicki A, et al: Diagnosis and differential assessment of pulmonary arterial hypertension. J Am Coll Cardiol 43:40S–47S, 2004. **A review of the diagnosis, classification, and evaluation of pulmonary hypertension.**
4. Channick RN, Sitbon O, Barst RJ, et al: Endothelin receptor antagonists in pulmonary arterial hypertension. J Am Coll Cardiol 43:62S–67S, 2004. **A review of the molecular biology of endothelin, its role in the pathogenesis and progression of pulmonary vascular disease, and the results of studies using endothelin receptor antagonists in the treatment of pulmonary hypertension.**
5. Galie N, Seeger W, Naeije R, et al: Comparative analysis of clinical trials and evidence-based treatment algorithm in pulmonary arterial hypertension. J Am Coll Cardiol 43:81S–88S, 2004. **Evidence based review of trials in pulmonary arterial hypertension and recommended treatment algorithm based on level of evidence.**
6. Ghofrani HA, Pepke-Zaba J, Barbera JA: Nitric oxide pathway and phosphodiesterase inhibitors in pulmonary arterial hypertension. J Am Coll Cardiol 43:68S–72S, 2004. **A review of the mechanism of action of NO and the experimental and clinical application of phosphodiesterase inhibitors in the treatment of pulmonary hypertension**
7. Humbert M, Morrell NW, Archer SL, et al: Cellular and molecular pathobiology of pulmonary arterial hypertension. J Am Coll Cardiol 43:13S–24S, 2004. **A review of the complex pathobiology of pulmonary hypertension, the development of pulmonary vascular remodeling and the role of the endothelium in disease development.**
8. Klepetko W, Mayer E, Sandoval J, et al: Interventional and surgical modalities of treatment for pulmonary arterial hypertension. J Am Coll Cardiol 43:73S–80S, 2004. **A review of the available interventional and surgical therapies for pulmonary hypertension, including atrial septostomy, pulmonary endarterectomy, and lung transplantation.**
9. Rich S, Kaufmann E, Levy PS: The effect of high doses of calcium-channel blockers on survival in primary pulmonary hypertension. N Engl J Med 327:76–81, 1992. **A study of 64 patients with PPH and the effects of treatment with calcium channel blockers.**
10. Rondelet B, Kerbaul R, Motte S, et al: Bosentan for the prevention of overcirculation-induced experimental pulmonary arterial hypertension. Circulation 107:1329–1335, 2003. **An animal study demonstrating the effectiveness of an endothelin receptor antagonist in the treatment of overcirculation-induced pulmonary hypertension.**

Systemic Hypertension and the Child at Risk for Cardiovascular Disease

Mark Mitsnefes

KEY CONCEPTS

- Blood pressure levels in children have risen over last two decades owing to the high prevalence of obesity.
- Essential hypertension is most frequently encountered in adolescents and is increasing in frequency in young children.
- Children with hypertension develop target-organ damage such as left ventricular hypertrophy. Children with hypertension and target-organ damage may be at risk for increased cardiovascular morbidity and mortality as they become young adults.
- Blood pressure control can be achieved in children with hypertension through a combination of lifestyle modification and therapy with antihypertensive agents.
- The goal of treatment is to prevent development of target-organ damage by maintaining the blood pressure below the 90th percentile for age and size.

Elevated blood pressure (BP) has been recognized as an important health issue in the pediatric population over the past two decades. Recent data indicate that average BP levels have risen substantially since 1988 among American children. Obesity and other lifestyle factors such as physical inactivity and a diet that includes a lot of high calorie, high salt intake, particularly in fast food, are considered responsible. Hypertension in children is now viewed as a significant risk factor for the development of adult cardiovascular disease. The approach to the evaluation and treatment of hypertension has been recently reviewed in the Fourth Report on High Blood Pressure in Children and Adolescents. This report provides updated normative data for BP for healthy children ages 1 to 17 years according to age, sex, and height, and it presents BP levels for age for 50th, 90th, 95th, and 99th percentiles. The report defines *normal blood pressure* as systolic and diastolic values less than the 90th percentile for age, sex, and height. *Prehypertension* is defined as an average systolic and/or diastolic blood pressure between the 90th and 95th percentiles or BP that exceeds 120/80 mm Hg, even if below the 90th percentile. *Stage 1 hypertension* is defined as an average systolic and/or diastolic BP between the 95th and 99th percentile + 5 mm Hg. *Stage 2 hypertension* is defined as a persistent BP above the 99th percentile + 5 mm Hg.

The causes of elevated BP in children are multiple and described elsewhere. Generally, hypertension can be classified as primary, or essential, with no identified cause; and secondary, with an identified cause. The prevalence of secondary hypertension is inversely related to the child's age. Thus, hypertension in infants and preschool children is almost exclusively secondary and rarely essential. It is also clear that secondary hypertension is generally severe, whereas essential hypertension is usually marked by mild or moderate elevations in BP. Renal and renovascular causes of secondary hypertension such as renal artery thrombosis, renal artery stenosis, congenital renal malformations, polycystic kidney disease, and coarctation of the aorta are the most common causes of hypertension in children up to 6 years of age. In children 6 to 10 years old, renal parenchymal and renovascular disease are the most frequent causes. With age, the prevalence of essential hypertension increases and becomes the leading cause of elevated blood pressure after 10 years of age. The pathophysiology of essential hypertension is not well understood, but it most likely involves a combination of genetic, environmental, and lifestyle factors. Obesity is now emerging as the most frequent cause of essential hypertension in pediatric patients, often manifesting during early childhood.

Expert Opinion on Management Issues

Factors to be considered initially in a child with elevated BP include age, rapidity of onset, and severity of the hypertension, symptoms attributable to hypertension, evidence of target-organ damage, and family history.

Figure 1 presents the diagnostic approach to elevated BP and has been recently updated by the Fourth Report on High Blood Pressure in Children and Adolescents. The primary goal of the evaluation should be to identify potentially correctable conditions producing hypertension. For older, overweight children with a family history of hypertension and who have mild-to-moderate elevation of BP and no indications from the history and physical examination of a secondary cause, few diagnostic tests are required. It is important to confirm hypertension by two to three measurements over a 1-month period. Children with stage 1 or stage 2 hypertension (BP above the 95th percentile) should have a urinalysis, urine culture, complete blood count (CBC), and measurements of serum creatinine and serum electrolytes. If one of these screening studies is abnormal, a renal ultrasound should be performed. In obese children, a fasting lipid profile should be performed to evaluate the levels of plasma triglycerides and low-density lipoprotein (LDL) cholesterol. Evidence for target-organ damage (TOD) manifesting as left-ventricular hypertrophy (LVH) and retinal abnormalities should be sought in children with chronic elevation of BP.

Recently, ambulatory blood pressure monitoring (ABPM) has emerged as a technology that overcomes some limitations of casual office BP measurements. By accomplishing multiple measurements over a 24-hour period in the patient's normal environment during both awake and sleep periods, ABPM can identify or rule out transient "white coat" hypertension due to stress or anxiety. ABPM allows mean 24-hour and mean daytime and night-time systolic and diastolic BPs to be compared against gender- and height-specific 95th percentiles derived from normative pediatric ABPM data. Another ABPM measurement is the calculated BP load, defined as the percentage of blood pressure readings that exceed the 95th percentile for age of the given patient. Finally, ABPM can determine the percent decline in BP with sleep. Normally, BP decreases at least 10% (a phenomenon called *dipping*) during the night; if the decline is less than 10%, the pattern is called *non-dipping*. In adults, non-dipping has been associated with hypertensive end-organ damage.

The pediatrician must recognize hypertensive urgencies and emergencies. Hypertensive emergencies appear as hypertensive encephalopathy, which is manifested by severe headache, vomiting, seizures, ataxia, stupor, and visual disturbances. Treatment should be initiated immediately with the aim of rapidly decreasing the BP with intravenous medications. In infants, severe hypertension can manifest with symptoms of congestive heart failure such as irritability, respiratory distress, and failure to thrive.

The goal of treatment is to reduce BP to a level below the 90th percentile. Specific recommendations for treatment of elevated BP depend on the patient's clinical situation. The initial therapy of the mild elevations of BP seen with essential hypertension without target-organ damage consists of nonpharmacological intervention in the form of lifestyle modification. This includes weight reduction, regular physical activity, and dietary modification with low caloric intake and

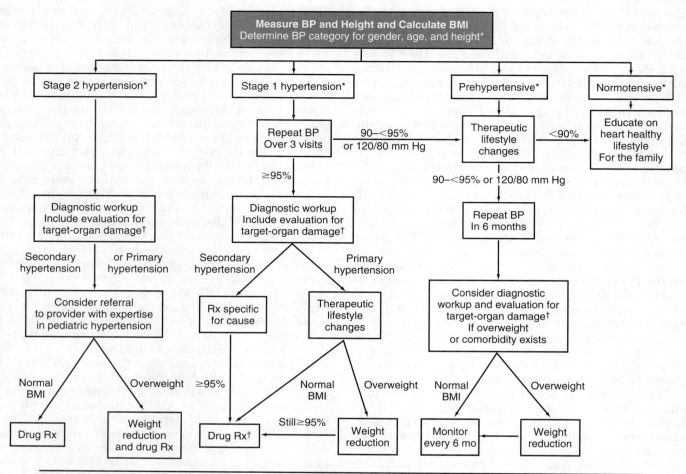

FIGURE 1. Management algorithm of elevated BP in children and adolescents. BMI, body mass index; BP, blood pressure; Rx, prescription.
*Diet modification and physical activity.
†Especially if younger than 10 years old, very high BP, little or no family history, diabetes, or other risk factors.
(From National High Blood Pressure in Children and Adolescents. The Fourth Report on the Diagnosis, Evaluation, and Treatment of High Blood Pressure in Children and Adolescents. Pediatrics 114:555–576, 2004. Copyright © 2004 by the AAP. Used with permission of the American Academy of Pediatrics.)

salt restriction for children with obesity-related hypertension. Weight loss in overweight adolescents generally lowers BP and ameliorates cardiovascular risk factors such as dyslipidemia and insulin resistance. Family-based intervention is vital in achieving BP control in overweight children, because it is the family eating pattern that usually contributes. Sedentary activities including TV, video, and computer games should be allowed for no more than 2 hours per day. Children should spend at least 30 to 60 minutes each day in physical activities. Diet should be changed to a daily sodium intake that should approximate 1.2 g per day for 4- to 8-year-old children and 1.5 g per day for older children. This amount is significantly lower than the current usual sodium intake in the typical American family. Data from DASH (Dietary Approaches to Stop Hypertension) study in adults demonstrate that a high intake of vegetables, fruits, fibers, and low-fat dairy products leads to improvement in BP even in the absence of weight reduction. A similar study in

children and adolescents is currently being conducted by the American Heart Association. Consultation with a nutritionist can provide guidelines and specific recommendations for individualizing the dietary plan. The combination of weight loss, dietary modification, decreased sedentary activity, and improved physical fitness has been shown to significantly reduce BP in children with essential hypertension.

Children with symptomatic essential hypertension, secondary hypertension, hypertension with diabetes, and those who have evidence of target-organ damage (LVH) or failed nonpharmacologic intervention require pharmacologic therapy. Most important in choosing a drug is its safety and efficacy for the given child. The 1997 Food and Drug Administration Modernization Act (FDAMA) and the 2002 Best Pharmaceuticals for Children Act has led to a significant increase in the number of antihypertensive drugs being studied in children. Table 1 summarizes the classification, preparations, and dosages of most commonly used oral

TABLE 1 Antihypertensive Drugs for Outpatient Management of Hypertension in Children 1 to 17 Years Old

Drug	Dose*	Dosing Interval	Evidence[†]	Comments[‡]
ACE Inhibitors				
Benazepril[§]	Init: 0.2 mg/kg/day up to 10 mg/day Max: 0.6 mg/kg/day up to 40 mg/day	qd	RCT	All ACE inhibitors are contraindicated in pregnancy; females of childbearing age should use reliable contraception.
Captopril	Init: 0.3–0.5 mg/kg/dose Max: 6 mg/kg/day	tid	RCT, CS	Check serum potassium and creatinine periodically to monitor for hyperkalemia and azotemia.
Enalapril[§]	Init: 0.08 mg/kg/day up to 5 mg/day Max: 0.6 mg/kg/day up to 40 mg/day	qd-bid	RCT	Cough and angioedema are reportedly less common with newer members of this class than with captopril.
Fosinopril[§]	Children >50 kg: Init: 5–10 mg/day Max: 40 mg/day	qd	RCT	Benazepril, enalapril, and lisinopril labels contain information on preparation of a suspension; captopril may also be compounded into a suspension.
Lisinopril[§]	Init: 0.07 mg/kg/day up to 5 mg/day Max: 0.6 mg/kg/day up to 40 mg/day	qd	RCT	FDA approval for ACE inhibitors with pediatric labeling is limited to children ≥6 yr of age and to children with creatinine clearance ≥30 mL/min/1.73 m^2.
Quinapril	Init: 5–10 mg/day Max: 80 mg/day	qd	RCT, EO	
Angiotensin-Receptor Blockers				
Irbesartan[§]	6–12 yr: 75–150 mg/day ≥13 yr: 150–300 mg/day	qd	CS	All ARBs are contraindicated in pregnancy; females of childbearing age should use reliable contraception.
Losartan[§]	Init: 0.7 mg/kg/day up to 50 mg/day Max: 1.4 mg/kg/day up to 100 mg/day	qd	RCT	Check serum potassium, creatinine periodically to monitor for hyperkalemia and azotemia. Losartan label contains information on preparation of suspension. FDA approval for ARBs is limited to children ≥6 yr of age and to children with creatinine clearance ≥30 mL/min/1.73m^2.
α- and β-Blocker				
Labetalol	Init: 1–3 mg/kg/day Max: 10–12 mg/kg/day up to 12 mg/day	bid	CS, EO	Asthma and overt heart failure are contraindications. Heart rate is dose limiting. May impair athletic performance. Should not be used in insulin-dependent diabetics.
β-Blockers				
Atenolol	Init: 0.5–1 mg/kg/day Max: 2 mg/kg/day up to 100 mg/day	qd-bid	CS	Noncardioselective agents (propranolol) are contraindicated in asthma and heart failure. Heart rate is dose limiting.
Bisoprolol/HCTZ	Init: 2.5/6.25 mg/kg/day Max: 10/6.25 mg/kg/day	qd	RCT	May impair athletic performance. Should not be used in insulin-dependent diabetics.
Metoprolol	Init: 1–2 mg/kg/day Max: 6 mg/kg/day up to 200 mg/day	bid	CS	A sustained-release formulation of propranolol is available that is dosed once daily.
Propranolol[§]	Init: 1–2 mg/kg/day Max: 4 mg/kg/day up to 640 mg/day	bid-tid	RCT, EO	
Calcium Channel Blockers				
Amlodipine[§]	Children 6–17 yrs: 2.5–5 mg once daily	qd	RCT	Amlodipine and isradipine can be compounded into stable extemporaneous suspensions.
Felodipine	Init: 2.5 mg/day Max: 10 mg/day	qd	RCT, EO	Felodipine and extended-release nifedipine tablets must be swallowed whole.
Isradipine	Init: 0.15–0.2 mg/kg/day Max: 0.8 mg/kg/day up to 20 mg/day	tid-qid	CS, EO	Isradipine is available in both immediate-release and sustained-release formulations; sustained-release form is dosed qd or bid.
Nifedipine extended release	Init: 0.25–0.5 mg/kg/day Max: 3 mg/kg/day up to 120 mg/day	qd-bid	CS, EO	May cause tachycardia.
Central α-Agonist				
Clonidine[§]	Children ≥12 yr Init: 0.2 mg/day Max: 2.4 mg/day	bid	EO	May cause dry mouth and/or sedation. Transdermal preparation is also available. Sudden cessation of therapy can lead to severe rebound hypertension.

TABLE 1 Antihypertensive Drugs for Outpatient Management of Hypertension in Children 1 to 17 Years Old—cont'd

Drug	Dose*	Dosing Interval	Evidence[†]	Comments[‡]
Diuretics				
Amiloride	Init: 0.4–0.625 mg/kg/day Max: 20 mg/day	qd	EO	All patients treated with diuretics should have electrolytes monitored shortly after initiating therapy and periodically thereafter.
Chlorthalidone	Init: 0.3 mg/kg/day Max: 2 mg/kg/day up to 50 mg/day	qd	EO	Useful as add-on therapy in patients being treated with drugs from other drug classes.
Furosemide	Init: 0.5–2.0 mg/kg/day Max: 6 mg/kg/day	qd-bid	EO	Potassium-sparing diuretics (spironolactone, triamterene, amiloride) may cause severe hyperkalemia, especially if given with ACE inhibitors or ARBs.
HCTZ[§]	Init: 1 mg/kg/day Max: 3 mg/kg/day up to 50 mg/day	qd	EO	Furosemide is labeled only for treatment of edema but may be useful as add-on therapy in children with resistant hypertension, particularly in children with renal disease.
Spironolactone	Init: 1 mg/kg/day Max: 3.3 mg/kg/day up to 100 mg/day	qd-bid	EO	Chlorthalidone may precipitate azotemia in patients with renal diseases and should be used with caution in those with severe renal impairment.
Triamterene	Init: 1–2 mg/kg/day Max: 3–4 mg/kg/day up to 300 mg/day	bid	EO	
Peripheral α-Antagonists				
Doxazosin	Init: 1 mg/day Max: 4 mg/day	qd	EO	May cause hypotension and syncope, especially after first dose.
Prazosin	Init: 0.05–0.1 mg/kg/day Max: 0.4 mg/kg/day	tid	EO	
Terazosin	Init: 1 mg/day Max: 20 mg/day	qd	EO	
Vasodilators				
Hydralazine[§]	Init: 0.75–1 mg/kg/day Max: 7.5 mg/kg/day up to 200 mg/day	qid	EO	Tachycardia and fluid retention are common side effects. Hydralazine can cause a lupus-like syndrome in slow acetylators.
Minoxidil[§]	Children <12 yr: Init: 0.2 mg/kg/day Max: 50 mg/day Children ≥12yr: Init: 5 mg/day Max: 100 mg/day	qd-tid	CS, EO	Prolonged use of minoxidil can cause hypertrichosis. Minoxidil is usually reserved for patients with hypertension resistant to multiple drugs.

Note: This table includes drugs with prior pediatric experience or recently completed clinical trials.
*Includes drugs with prior pediatric experience or recently completed clinical trials.
[†]The maximum recommended adult dose should not be exceeded in routine clinical practice.
[‡]Level of evidence upon which dosing recommendations are based. CS indicates case series; EO, expert opinion; RCT, randomized controlled trial.
[§]FDA-approved pediatric labeling information is available. Recommended doses for agents with FDA-approved pediatric labels are the doses contained in the approved labels. Even when pediatric labeling information is not available, the FDA-approved label should be consulted for additional safety information.
ACE, angiotensin-converting enzyme; ARB, angiotensin-receptor blocker; CS, case series; EO, expert opinion; init, initial; max, maximum; RCT, randomized, controlled trial.
From National High Blood Pressure in Children and Adolescents. The Fourth Report on the Diagnosis, Evaluation, and Treatment of High Blood Pressure in Children and Adolescents. Pediatrics 114:555–576, 2004. Copyright © 2004 by the AAP. Used with permission of the American Academy of Pediatrics.

antihypertensive drugs. The initial drug choice is based on the mechanism and severity of the hypertension, the patient's demographics, compliance issues, previous history of side effects, the presence of other medical problems, and concomitant drug therapy. In adults, JNC–7 (Joint National Committee on BP) recommends thiazide diuretics as the first line of therapy based on their efficacy, good tolerability, and low cost. In children, angiotensin-converting enzyme (ACE) inhibitors and calcium channel blockers (CCBs) are the most common antihypertensive medications prescribed currently across all pediatric ages. The wide use of these medications is based on their effectiveness and relatively low rate of side effects. ACE inhibitors or angiotensin-receptor blockers are preferable in children with diabetes, microalbuminuria, or chronic kidney disease. CCB or β-blockers are frequently used in children with migraine headaches. Drug therapy usually starts with a low dose of a single agent. The dose is titrated until BP goals are achieved. If adequate BP control is not achieved with a single agent, a second agent should be added.

In the case of hypertensive emergencies, the goal of the therapy is the lowering of BP by one third within first 8 hours after initiation of the treatment and normalization of BP within next 24 to 48 hours. Too rapid reduction of BP may be dangerous, especially in patients with increased intracranial pressure.

TABLE 2 Antihypertensive Drugs for Management of Severe Hypertension in Children 1 to 17 Years Old

Drug	Class	Doses*	Route	Comments
Most Useful†				
Esmolol	β-Blocker	100–500 µg/kg/min	IV infusion	Very short acting; constant infusion preferred. May cause profound bradycardia. Produced modest reductions in BP in a pediatric clinical trial.
Hydralazine	Vasodilator	0.2–0.6 mg/kg/dose	IV, IM	Should be given every 4 h when given IV bolus. Recommended dose is lower than FDA label.
Labetalol	α- and β-Blocker	Bolus: 0.2–1.0 mg/kg/dose up to 40 mg/dose Infusion: 0.25–3.0 mg/kg/h	IV bolus or infusion	Asthma and overt heart failure are relative contraindications.
Nicardipine	Calcium channel blocker	1–3 µg/kg/min	IV infusion	May cause reflex tachycardia.
Sodium nitroprusside	Vasodilator	0.53–10 µg/kg/min	IV infusion	Monitor cyanide levels with prolonged (>72 h) use or in renal failure; or coadminister with sodium thiosulfate.
Occasionally Useful‡				
Clonidine	Central α-agonist	0.05–0.1 mg/dose; may be repeated up to 0.8 mg/dose	PO	Side effects include dry mouth and sedation.
Enalaprilat	ACE inhibitor	0.05–0.1 mg/kg/dose up to 1.25 mg/dose	IV bolus	May cause prolonged hypotension and acute renal failure, especially in neonates.
Fenoldopam	Dopamine receptor agonist	0.02–0.8 µg/kg/min	IV infusion	Produced modest reductions in BP in a pediatric clinical trial in patients ≤12 years old.
Isradipine	Calcium channel blocker	0.05–0.1 mg/kg/dose	PO	Stable suspension can be compounded.
Minoxidil	Vasodilator	0.1–0.2 mg/kg/dose	PO	Most potent oral vasodilator, long acting.

*All dosing recommendations are based on expert opinion or case series data except as otherwise noted.
†Useful for hypertensive emergencies and some hypertensive urgencies.
‡Useful for hypertensive urgencies and some hypertensive emergencies.
ACE, angiotensin-converting enzyme; BP, blood pressure; FDA, Food and Drug Administration; IM, intramuscular; IV, intravenous; PO, by mouth.
From National High Blood Pressure in Children and Adolescents. The Fourth Report on the Diagnosis, Evaluation, and Treatment of High Blood Pressure in Children and Adolescents. Pediatrics 114:555–576, 2004. Copyright © 2004 by the AAP. Used with permission of the American Academy of Pediatrics.

Table 2 demonstrates medications available to treat hypertensive emergencies.

Common Pitfalls

- Failure to recognize and treat hypertension during childhood may lead to a higher risk of myocardial infarction, stroke, peripheral vascular disease, and end-stage renal disease in adulthood.
- Failure to recognize and treat LVH, a marker of prolonged hypertension and independent risk factor for increased cardiovascular disease morbidity and mortality in adults, may lead to increased morbidity.
- The epidemic of obesity in children and difficulties in weight control constitute a significant problem in the managing of elevated BP in children.
- Nonadherence to therapy, particularly in adolescents, is another obstacle in achieving control of hypertension.
- Failure to recognize and treat hypertensive emergencies is potentially dangerous and can lead to irreversible morbidity.

Communication and Counseling

Children with hypertension need careful follow-up. In general, children with mild essential hypertension can be managed by their primary physicians, with an emphasis on nonpharmacologic intervention. If in 6 months BP is not controlled, drug therapy should be started. Referral to an expert in BP evaluation and control in children is advisable at this point. After initiation of pharmacologic treatment, the patient needs to be seen by the pediatrician at 2-week intervals to adjust the dose of medication until BP control is adequate. After 6 months of normal BP, the dose of medication may be tapered down during a 1- to 6-month period of follow-up until off therapy (called the step-down approach). The patient must then be followed carefully for another 6 months and annually to ensure that the BP remains normal. In case of no response to a 1-month trial of antihypertensive therapy, referral to the specialist is essential. Parents should be educated about the long-term consequences of hypertension and obesity, the different options available for treatment, and the safety and efficacy of antihypertensive medications.

SUGGESTED READINGS

1. Lurbe E, Sorof JM, Daniels SR: Clinical and research aspects of ambulatory blood pressure monitoring in children. J Pediatr 144:7–16, 2004. **The most comprehensive review of different aspects of ABPM in children.**
2. Muntner P, He J, Cutler JA, et al: Trends in blood pressure among children and adolescents. JAMA 291:2107–2113, 2004. **Indicates increase in BP among U.S. children over the last decade and describes the role of obesity in elevation of BP.**
3. National High Blood Pressure Education Program Working Group on High Blood Pressure in Children and Adolescents. The Fourth Report on the Diagnosis, Evaluation, and Treatment of High Blood Pressure in Children and Adolescents. Pediatrics 114:555–576, 2004. **Provides new definition of hypertension in children; BP standards based on gender, age, and height; and practical guidelines in management of hypertension in children.**
4. Portman R, Sorof J, Ingelfinger J (eds). Pediatric Hypertension, Totowa, NJ: Humana Press, 2004. **The most up-to-date textbook covering physiology of BP regulation, BP measurement issues, pathophysiological mechanisms, causes, diagnostic approach, and management of elevated BP in children.**
5. Sacks FM, Svetkey LP, Vollmer WM, et al: Effects on blood pressure of reduced dietary sodium and the Dietary Approaches to Stop Hypertension (DASH) diet. DASH-Sodium Collaborative Research Group. N Engl J Med 344:3–10, 2001. **Indicates how a diet of low salt and lots of fruits and vegetables decreases BP in adults.**

Innocent Murmurs

Jon F. Lucas and J. Philip Saul

KEY CONCEPTS

- Innocent murmurs are common, occurring at some point in time in more than half of children between the ages of 2 and 10 years.
- Innocent murmurs can often be differentiated from pathologic murmurs by physical examination alone.
- Murmurs should be evaluated by a pediatric cardiologist in these situations:
  - In a neonate older than 2 days of age
  - In a patient with other signs or symptoms of cardiovascular disease
  - Associated with a thrill, click, or gallop
  - Purely diastolic

Murmurs are common in the pediatric age group, occurring at some point in time in over half of children between the ages of 2 and 10 years. Further, many of these murmurs may be as loud as III or IV/VI, even though they do not reflect underlying cardiac pathology, or are *innocent*. Consequently, primary care physicians are frequently faced with having to decide if a murmur heard during a physical examination is pathologic, requiring evaluation by a pediatric cardiologist, or is innocent. Given the prevalence of innocent murmurs in children, it is important that primary care physicians treating children be able to differentiate these common innocent murmurs from the pathologic, based on their characteristics and simple physical examination maneuvers.

Although innocent murmurs are caused by blood flow in the heart, most pediatric cardiologists, and the American Heart Association (AHA), use the term *innocent*, rather than *functional* or *flow*, to differentiate these murmurs from those caused by flow across an abnormal cardiac structure. Blood flowing through the heart always makes noise. In fact, when a microphone is placed on the tip of a catheter inside the heart, sounds are heard in subjects of any age. These sounds can be heard from the chest surface more commonly in children, simply because the heart is often closer to the stethoscope, because of patient size and a relatively thin chest wall, particularly in 2- to 10-year-olds. The difference between these normal sounds and pathologic sounds is that innocent murmurs typically emanate from either a single cardiac structure, such as a valve leaflet vibrating at a characteristic frequency, or relatively low velocity blood flow, which generates low-frequency eddy currents and turbulence. Alternatively, pathologic murmurs always come from pressure gradients, which generate high-velocity blood flow and a broad mixture of high-frequency eddies. Thus, there is a difference in sound quality between innocent and pathologic murmurs. Innocent murmurs are lower frequency (<200 Hz), often consist of a single frequency (making them sound vibratory), and are usually of lower amplitude ($<$III-IV/VI) (Table 1). Pathologic murmurs are higher frequency (400–1500 Hz), never consist of a single frequency but are always a broad mix of frequencies, making them sound harsh, and are usually higher in amplitude ($\geq$III-IV/VI). Both innocent and pathologic murmurs may be systolic ejection or continuous, but pure diastolic murmurs may always be considered pathologic. Although these rules are not fixed, especially for amplitude, they work very well as guidelines.

Expert Opinion on Management Issues

When a murmur is noted on physical examination, a number of steps can be taken to assist in classifying the murmur as innocent or potentially pathologic. Careful and systematic auscultation of the heart should be performed to determine the location, loudness, sound quality, timing, and radiation of the murmur. The presence or absence of splitting of the second heart sound and any clicks, rubs, or gallops should also be noted. The heart should be auscultated with the patient in different positions, preferably lying supine and

TABLE 1 Characteristics of Innocent and Pathologic Murmurs

Innocent	Pathologic
Lower frequency, <200 Hz	Higher frequency, 400–1500 Hz
Single frequency, vibratory	Broad frequency content, harsh
Lower amplitude, <3/6	Higher amplitude, ≥3/6
Changes with position	Not positional
Changes with physiological state	Less change with physiological state

standing. If the patient is able to cooperate, having him or her perform specific maneuvers to accentuate or extinguish a murmur, such as a Valsalva, may be quite helpful. The most common innocent murmurs in children are Still's murmur, peripheral pulmonary stenosis, pulmonary outflow murmur, and venous hum.

STILL'S MURMUR

Still's murmur is the most common in the pediatric age group. It can be heard at any age, but is typically first heard at around 3 to 5 years of age and often disappears in late adolescence. The characteristic sound of Still's murmur is a low-pitched musical humming or buzzing mid-systolic sound that consists of a single low-frequency tone. Because of its narrow frequency range, the sound quality of Still's murmur is quite distinct from a pathologic murmur. The murmur is most commonly best heard along the left mid to upper sternal border or apex and may radiate to the neck. Classically, the murmur is heard when the patient is supine, and will decrease in intensity or disappear when the patient stands. A Valsalva maneuver will usually extinguish the murmur. Still's murmur can be accentuated by fever, anxiety, exercise, or any other cause of increased cardiac output. Although the precise origin of Still's murmur may vary, most probably originate from a pulmonary or aortic valve leaflet, or an atrioventricular valve chorda that vibrates at a characteristic low frequency as the blood rushes by it, much the way a mast stay vibrates in the wind on a sailboat. Although they are not all so classic, many murmurs fall into the Still's category.

PERIPHERAL PULMONARY STENOSIS

The murmur of peripheral pulmonary stenosis (PPS) is caused by mild turbulence in the branch pulmonary arteries. In fetal life, the ductus arteriosus and foramen ovale shunt blood away from the developing pulmonary vascular bed. Thus, these vessels form with less than a full cardiac output flowing through them, and as a result, they are relatively small compared to the normal postnatal blood flow. It is this mismatch of blood flow and vessel size in the first few months of life that generates turbulence and leads to the murmur of PPS. The murmur is mid-systolic, usually grade I or II, and has a gentle blowing quality. It does not typically change with patient position. The murmur can be heard over the precordium, but because it is generated in the pulmonary arteries, it is typically louder in the axillae or back. It is often louder in one axilla than the other. Once the pulmonary vascular bed matures, the turbulence resolves and the murmur of PPS disappears, typically by 9 months of age. If the murmur persists past 9 months, true pulmonary artery or pulmonary valve stenosis must be suspected.

PULMONARY OUTFLOW MURMUR

The pulmonary valve flow murmur is a grade I or II, high-frequency, blowing systolic ejection murmur heard over the pulmonary valve area when the patient is supine. This murmur sounds very similar to the pulmonary outflow murmur caused by an atrial septal defect. However, a patient with an atrial septal defect should have a fixed, widely split second heart sound and may have a diastolic flow rumble. Neither of these findings will be present in a patient with an innocent pulmonary outflow murmur. The cause of this murmur is not clear, but is presumed to arise from flow across a normal pulmonary valve. This murmur occurs in school-age children and young adults. An innocent pulmonary outflow murmur is also commonly heard in pregnant women, as in other conditions in which cardiac output is increased. A pulmonary outflow murmur will become less prominent and often disappear when the patient sits upright or stands.

VENOUS HUM

A venous hum is a continuous murmur heard at the clavicles or base of the neck when the patient is sitting or standing. The murmur can be quite loud, up to grade III, and is vibratory or blowing in quality. It can be unilateral or bilateral. When the patient is sitting or standing, the neck veins collapse, and the blood flow can become turbulent. The phenomenon is similar to the behavior of a partially occluded straw being lifted from a glass or a rubber tube draining a tank. A venous hum murmur can be extinguished by a number of methods. If the patient lies down, passively increasing the volume of blood in the neck veins, or turns his or her head to the side from which the murmur is heard, temporarily obstructing flow in the neck veins, the murmur will disappear. Light pressure over the neck veins on the side of the murmur will also extinguish the venous hum.

Common Pitfalls

The most common pitfall in evaluating cardiac murmurs is not allowing enough time to perform a complete cardiac examination. Innocent murmurs are distinguished from pathologic murmurs not only by their sound quality but also by their response to changes in patient positioning and maneuvers such as a Valsalva or exercise.

When to Refer to a Cardiovascular Specialist for Evaluation

If a murmur cannot clearly be labeled innocent based on characteristics such as its sound quality, intensity, location and response to posture or physiologic state, then referral to the pediatric cardiovascular specialist is probably indicated. Other indications for referral are any purely diastolic murmur, the additional presence of clicks or gallops, or any other signs or symptoms of cardiovascular disease, such as shortness of breath or decreased exercise tolerance. Additionally, any murmur in a newborn that does not resolve spontaneously by day 2 of life should prompt a consultation prior to or at the time of hospital discharge. Most murmurs in infants younger than 2 months of age probably need evaluation as well.

Although not always necessary, the best single test for determining whether a structural defect is the basis for the murmur is a complete pediatric echocardiogram, performed and interpreted by people specifically trained and experienced with the diagnosis of congenital heart disease. The necessity of a pediatric cardiac specialist comes from a number of differences in the pediatric and adult echo exams, including the views used, use of color Doppler to identify septal defects, identification and examination of all four pulmonary veins, and use of the suprasternal notch view to examine the aortic arch and great arteries. The diagnoses behind pathologic murmurs are obviously quite varied, and each has its own set of tests and therapies, but a full discussion is beyond the scope of this chapter.

Communication and Counseling

Very few lay people understand that murmurs are a common finding in children and do not usually indicate structural heart disease. Thus, once a murmur is identified as innocent, it is vital that the parents and the patient be counseled regarding the lack of any health implications. Specifically, they need to know that the child's heart is normal, that activities need not be restricted, and that antibiotics are not necessary before certain procedures in order to prevent bacterial endocarditis. Further, neither additional diagnostic tests nor future follow-up evaluations are indicated.

There are also a number of patient handouts available that explain innocent murmurs, which can be quite helpful for parents. If the parents are not made to understand that their child's murmur does not signify any abnormality of the heart, the child may be needlessly prevented from participating in athletics, restricted from other activities, or undergo additional diagnostic tests during visits to other physicians. Parents should also be advised that the murmur may be intermittent or transient, even persisting into adulthood. Similarly, it is important to inform the parents that there are situations, such as fever, anemia, or anxiety that can make the murmur louder and more likely to be heard. Parents who understand these points are better prepared to deal with questions that arise when their child is seen by a new physician, such as in an emergency department or dentist's office.

Murmurs will be a frequent finding during the well child pediatric examination and perhaps more frequent during the evaluation of an acute illness, but most of these murmurs are innocent. Understanding the variety of causes of innocent murmurs should help identify them as such. However, referral to the pediatric cardiac specialist is appropriate in newborns and small infants, when the findings are not entirely consistent with an innocent murmur, or when there are other reasons to suspect heart disease.

SUGGESTED READINGS

1. Biancaniello T: Innocent murmurs: A parent's guide. Circulation 109:e162–e163, 2004. **Describes innocent murmurs and their evaluation to parents in understandable terms.**
2. McConnell ME, Adkins SB 3rd, Hannon DW: Heart murmurs in pediatric patients: When do you refer? Am Fam Physician 60(2):558–565, 1999. **Discusses the evaluation of a child with a murmur and includes a parent handout.**
3. Pelech AN: The cardiac murmur: When to refer. Pediatr Clin NA 45(1):107–12, 1998. **Describes common cardiac murmurs and their classification.**
4. Poddar B, Basu S: Approach to a child with a heart murmur. Indian J Pediatr 71(1):63–66, 2004. **Provides a more detailed discussion of the evaluation of a child with a new murmur.**
5. Wiles HB, Saul JP: Pediatric cardiac auscultation. J S C Med Assoc 95(10):375–378, 1999. **Reviews cardiac auscultation and the characteristics of pathologic and innocent murmurs.**

Cardiac Dysrhythmias

Christopher L. Case

KEY CONCEPTS

- The cornerstone of effective therapy for a specific pediatric dysrhythmia first involves obtaining an accurate diagnosis.
- More harm can be done by assuming a pathologic dysrhythmia exists solely on the basis of the clinical history and thus adopting a specific therapy that is either ineffective or unnecessary.
- It is most important to attempt to record and diagnose the dysrhythmia (via surface electrocardiography, Holter monitor, event recorder, electrophysiology study, or a combination of these modalities) before initiating therapy.
- Documenting the diagnosis before treatment is the foundation of accurate therapy for pediatric dysrhythmia.

In the *emergency* treatment of a pediatric rhythm disturbance, it is best to "think simple." If a child is suspected of having pathologic bradycardia or tachycardia causing hemodynamic compromise (loss of consciousness or no recordable blood pressure), it is sometimes proper to institute emergency therapy before recording and obtaining a specific diagnosis. In the presence of bradycardia causing hemodynamic collapse, simple principles of cardiopulmonary resuscitation (airway, breathing, circulation) are used effectively to treat most situations. In the event a pathologic tachycardia causes significant hemodynamic compromise (regardless of its origin), cardioversion or defibrillation is indicated.

General practitioners are diagnosing dysrhythmias in children with greater frequency. This increase in diagnosis reflects a greater awareness by health-care providers of the existence of pediatric rhythm disturbances, as well as technological advances that make high-fidelity recordings of such dysrhythmias possible, even in the youngest of children. Once a pediatric dysrhythmia is diagnosed, a wide range of treatment strategies are available, including nonintervention, pharmacologic therapy, device implantation, and surgical/catheter ablation treatments. This chapter discusses the principles of therapeutics for commonly encountered pediatric rhythm disturbances.

Expert Opinion on Management Issues

The American Heart Association's principles of emergency management of pediatric dysrhythmias should be reviewed periodically by all health care providers. In an emergency situation, the dysrhythmia should be classified simply as "slow" or "fast." Undue time and effort spent refining the specific diagnosis of a compromising tachycardia or bradycardia may jeopardize a child's recovery from the event.

The decision to intervene and treat a pediatric dysrhythmia chronically depends somewhat on the assessment of associated myocardial structure and function. In general, in a child with an abnormal heart, seemingly trivial dysrhythmias such as premature beats may have prognostic significance different from that of an identical rhythm disturbance in a child with a normal heart. Conversely, asymptomatic pathologic sustained tachycardias may sometimes be monitored without treatment in certain pediatric scenarios in which the underlying cardiac structure and function are optimal. Assessing the importance of a specific dysrhythmia in terms of the underlying cardiac structure or function may be important in defining the risk of sudden cardiac death (SCD) associated with the dysrhythmia. Although rhythm disturbances causing SCD in the pediatric population are rare, the clinical context (similar to its adult counterpart) may involve a rhythm disturbance in a child with an associated abnormality in cardiac structure or function.

Because the potential for SCD in most children with dysrhythmias is low, treatment is frequently instituted to avoid bothersome symptoms. In older children, dysrhythmia symptoms are reported in familiar terms, such as palpitations, dizziness, racing heart, and so forth. In younger children, particularly infants, symptoms may be harder to elicit or may be expressed in more obtuse terms (e.g., "chest pains"). Because a younger child may not always be reliable in reporting symptoms, prophylactic treatment of certain rhythm disturbances is sometimes instituted to avoid the consequences of a prolonged, unrecognized, sustained arrhythmia that could result in significant morbidity. Conversely, in an older child, symptoms of dysrhythmias are more reliably reported, so treatment on an as-needed basis may be an effective alternative.

Two different treatment modalities may be used for dysrhythmias. The traditional treatment option involves antiarrhythmic medications. Drugs can be taken every day to avoid dysrhythmia symptoms or can be taken as needed when symptoms occur. Very few antiarrhythmic agents are officially formulated for pediatric use. Only a small number of well-controlled studies outline the effective use of specific antiarrhythmic agents in children. In certain cases, antiarrhythmic agents manufactured only in tablets or capsules have to be modified by pharmacies to a suspension form for use in children. Powerful antiarrhythmic agents such as amiodarone, flecainide, sotalol, and procainamide are examples of such drugs. Thus advanced pharmacologic treatment of childhood dysrhythmias can be quite challenging.

Since 1990, nonpharmacologic treatment options have revolutionized the approach to the treatment of rhythm disturbances in adults and children. In the 1970s and 1980s, open heart surgical ablation procedures that "cured" tachycardias were reserved for severe, life-threatening cases. In the 1990s, the venue for dysrhythmia ablation procedures changed from the operating room to the catheterization laboratory. A variety of tachycardias that previously needed daily antiarrhythmic therapy can now be eliminated by radiofrequency catheter ablation procedures performed in the catheterization laboratory. These procedures were first performed on adult patients and then applied to the pediatric population. Common dysrhythmias such as supraventricular tachycardia (SVT) secondary to an accessory bypass tract can be "cured" with a 90% to 95% success rate and a low (less than 1%) complication rate in the context of a 24-hour hospital admission. Initially, in the early 1990s, the indication for these procedures in children involved dysrhythmias with excessive symptoms or life-threatening potential. Throughout the 1990s, as experience with this modality in children increased, indications for catheter ablation changed so patient/parental choice became the most common reason for performing a pediatric catheter ablation. Many parents elect to have their child's dysrhythmia addressed with this procedure when confronted with the alternative of chronic long-term antiarrhythmic medication therapy.

The use of other nonpharmacologic therapies, such as implantation of pacemakers and defibrillators, has increased in the pediatric population. Implantation of such devices is usually reserved for the control of pediatric dysrhythmias with life-threatening consequences, such as advanced atrioventricular (AV) block (pacemakers) and ventricular tachycardia (VT)/ventricular fibrillation (defibrillators). Once again, most of these implantable devices were designed originally to treat adult disease processes. Their application in pediatric patients sometimes involves unique technical and programming adaptations.

The other consideration in the treatment of pediatric dysrhythmia is the prescription of a proper activity profile commensurate with the child's rhythm disturbance. For a well-controlled dysrhythmia in a child with normal heart structure, the goal is to prescribe unlimited activity, including participation in competitive sports. Dysrhythmias exacerbated by exercise and with associated symptoms generally require some activity restrictions. Such restrictions may be as mild as allowing the child to "rest at will" during the physical activity. However, rhythm disturbances that are sustained and exacerbated by physical activity need "control" before prescription of unlimited physical activity. Also, even minor asymptomatic dysrhythmias (e.g., premature ventricular contractions) in patients with cardiac structure or function abnormalities may require activity restriction because of the concern for SCD. In addition, certain rhythm disturbances that have life-threatening consequences, even though they occur rarely (e.g., the long QT syndrome), require some limitation of physical activities (competitive sports). For children and their parents, these physical limitations are sometimes the most stringent and obtrusive portion of the dysrhythmia treatment plan. Chronic treatment options for commonly encountered pediatric dysrhythmias are reviewed next.

SUPRAVENTRICULAR TACHYCARDIA

SVT is the most common sustained dysrhythmia encountered in children. More than 95% of cases of SVT encountered in younger children are re-entrant in nature, usually secondary to an accessory AV connection. If this accessory connection is manifested on the surface electrocardiogram during sinus rhythm, the condition is termed Wolff-Parkinson-White (WPW) syndrome. Children with WPW syndrome have a small risk for malignant arrhythmias and SCD as a result of rapid antegrade conduction across their accessory connection. In children with accessory connection re-entrant tachycardia (with or without WPW syndrome), the most common circuit for their SVT is antegrade down the AV node with retrograde conduction up the accessory connection. This tachycardia circuit is responsible for most of the paroxysmal events of SVT seen in the majority of children (orthodromic SVT). Acute termination of this SVT can be accomplished with vagal maneuvers (Valsalva) or intravenous adenosine (starting dose, 50 to 100 mcg per kg by rapid intravenous push). In very rare cases, with hemodynamic collapse, re-entrant SVT needs to be cardioverted (1 J/kg). Intravenous verapamil (0.15 mg per kg over a period of 15 to 20 minutes) may also be used to terminate SVT acutely, but its use in children is frequently complicated by hypotension, and it is now supplanted by adenosine. Intravenous verapamil is associated with hemodynamic collapse in infants, so it should be avoided in this population and cautiously used in older children.

If SVT is successfully terminated acutely, prophylactic treatment with a chronic oral antiarrhythmic agent can be chosen to prevent recurrences. If no clear preexcitation is apparent on the surface electrocardiogram, oral digoxin is the drug of choice (10 mcg/kg/day divided twice a day). If WPW syndrome is manifestly present, oral β-blockers are frequently used (propranolol, 2 to 6 mg/kg/day divided three or four times daily, or atenolol, 25 to 50 mg per day in older children weighing more than 25 kg). If WPW syndrome is present and the child has syncope or hemodynamic collapse, catheter ablation of the accessory connection is the treatment of choice. For children with frequent recurrences of orthodromic SVT despite therapy with digoxin, propranolol, or both, catheter ablation is a reasonable therapy, especially if the child is older than 5 years, because natural history studies indicate that SVT could become a chronic problem.

If SVT is initially encountered in a preadolescent or adolescent, the tachycardia circuit is commonly secondary to AV node re-entry tachycardia (AVNRT). This tachycardia is commonly responsible for SVT in the adult population and often first seen in young teenagers. Treatment principles (acutely and chronically) are similar to those for SVT caused by an accessory AV connection. The sudden death potential of AVNRT is small. Many patients choose a catheter ablation procedure for chronic treatment of AVNRT because of its high efficacy and low complication rate.

On rare occasions, SVT in children is recalcitrant to termination with adenosine or verapamil or to cardioversion (or to both modalities). This situation usually necessitates admission to the intensive care unit, intravenous invasive blood pressure monitoring, and the use of powerful intravenous antiarrhythmic agents for termination of the tachycardia (procainamide or amiodarone). After conversion, catheter ablation of the SVT can be considered in view of the recalcitrant nature of the acute rhythm disturbance. If catheter ablation is not feasible, the use of digoxin, propranolol, or more powerful antiarrhythmic agents (e.g., sotalol, amiodarone, flecainide, procainamide) should be considered. The use of antiarrhythmic medications beyond digoxin or propranolol invokes issues of proarrhythmia, which usually necessitates monitoring of the initiation of therapy in a controlled hospital setting.

SVT encountered in infancy deserves special mention. Natural history studies indicate that infantile SVT caused by an accessory connection has a good chance (60% to 70%) of resolving by the age of 1 year. Medications used to control SVT in this age group can frequently be discontinued at 1 year of age without recurrence of SVT. Although SVT in infancy may resolve, many infants with SVT initially have significant symptoms of congestive heart failure and, on occasion, shock with poor cardiac function. This situation arises because SVT in infancy may have subtle symptoms; the infant can be in incessant SVT for days or weeks, and the ultimate manifestation can be dramatic. Thus control of SVT in infancy by medications must be rigorously verified so a repeat scenario is avoided.

Finally, certain rarer SVTs from arrhythmia mechanisms confined to the atria (atrial flutter, atrial ectopic tachycardias [AETs]) can occur in children. Atrial flutter usually occurs at birth or during early infancy. Once the arrhythmia is terminated (cardioversion or spontaneously), the need for chronic treatment (digoxin or propranolol) beyond 1 year of age is rare. AET is an incessant tachycardia in children that is difficult to treat with antiarrhythmic agents. It is frequently manifested as a cardiomyopathy because of its incessant nature. Treatment of AET may involve the use of β-blockers, class I or III antiarrhythmic agents, or catheter ablation. Success rates for catheter ablation of AET are lower than with re-entrant SVTs because of a high recurrence rate and the possibility of multiple foci causing the AET.

VENTRICULAR TACHYCARDIA

VT is a rare but important dysrhythmia in the pediatric population because of the implication involving SCD. In reality, most VTs encountered in children are associated with normal cardiac structure and function; treatment strategies in this scenario usually involve mitigating bothersome symptoms rather than attempting to decrease the incidence of SCD. In contrast, when ventricular arrhythmias are encountered in children with heart disease (postoperative congenital heart disease, cardiomyopathies), treatment is primarily directed at preventing SCD. In most pediatric cardiac disease entities associated with VTs, no pharmacologic or nonpharmacologic therapies are rigorously proved to decrease the incidence of SCD. Also, with the issues of proarrhythmia magnified in children with structural heart disease, more consideration is being given to defibrillator implantation rather than antiarrhythmic therapy to mitigate the risk of SCD caused by ventricular arrhythmias in this patient population. These trends, however, are based on extrapolation of data involving adult SCD caused by VT secondary to coronary artery disease.

Experience is growing with the use of implantable defibrillators in various pediatric cardiac disease states in which SCD secondary to VT is a reality. Such diseases include hypertrophic cardiomyopathy, dilated cardiomyopathy, postoperative congenital heart disease, and the long QT syndrome. The decision to use these devices is sometimes clear cut when an older child has recorded ventricular arrhythmias with a witnessed aborted SCD episode. The decision becomes murkier when implantation is considered for younger children whose initial VT and SCD episode is not well documented but whose cardiac structure or function is abnormal and nonsustained VT is present after the event.

Acute treatment of VT is guided by the clinical context. If the child has hemodynamic collapse, cardioversion or defibrillation (or both) is the treatment of choice. In an emergency situation in which a sustained, hemodynamically stable VT is encountered, intravenous antiarrhythmics can also be used. Lidocaine, procainamide, and amiodarone can be given intravenously to help terminate ventricular irritability. Intravenous use of these medications may have various unwanted deleterious electrophysiologic effects, so the ability to cardiovert, defibrillate, or pace for bradycardia should be available.

Chronic treatment of ventricular arrhythmias involves the use of medications, catheter ablation, defibrillator placement, or a combination of these modalities. Antiarrhythmic medication is generally used to treat sustained VTs in children with normal heart structure. Two types of sustained VT are commonly encountered in children with normal hearts. One emanates from the right ventricular outflow tract; this VT can be exercise sensitive and may respond to β-blocker therapy. The other VT encountered in children with normal cardiac structure entails a re-entry circuit involving the Purkinje network of the posterior fascicle in the left ventricle (posterior fascicular VT). This tachycardia can be terminated acutely with intravenous verapamil and can be prevented with chronic oral verapamil therapy. In children with normal hearts, both these tachycardias may also be cured with catheter ablation, which is a reasonable alternative to chronic drug therapy.

Chronic treatment of VTs in children with abnormal cardiac structure and function usually involves the use of therapies that can prevent SCD. In the past, ventricular arrhythmias encountered in such disease states as dilated cardiomyopathy, hypertrophic cardiomyopathy, and postoperative congenital heart disease were treated with antiarrhythmic medications such as procainamide, flecainide, sotalol, and amiodarone. However, concern about the lack of efficacy and the proarrhythmic potential of these medications made chronic pharmacologic therapy a less attractive alternative for these conditions. The use of device therapy (defibrillation implantation) to prevent SCD in the pediatric population has increased. However, these devices are not always pediatric friendly, and their use in the pediatric population has a unique set of problems.

Two pediatric disease states in which ventricular arrhythmias are common deserve special mention. The first is the long QT syndrome, a genetic condition in which disorders of either sodium or potassium myocardial ionic channels cause repolarization abnormalities and the propensity for malignant ventricular arrhythmias (torsades de pointes). SCD is a frequent outcome in this condition. The initial treatment of long QT syndrome involves the use of a β-blocker (propranolol) and activity restriction. Second-line therapy includes the use of mexiletine (class I antiarrhythmic agent), cardiac sympathectomy, or defibrillator implantation.

VT occurring in infancy is another unique arrhythmia. Similar to SVT, when VT is encountered in infancy, it may be characterized by symptoms of cardiogenic shock as a result of its incessant, unrecognized nature. The substrate underlying ventricular arrhythmias in infancy is usually hamartomatous lesions (plaques) on the ventricular myocardium that exhibit abnormal automaticity and cause ventricular irritability. These hamartomas usually resolve by 5 years of age, and the VT subsides. Until they resolve, these VTs in infancy may require very powerful class I or III antiarrhythmic agents alone or in combination to avoid severe symptoms. On occasion, for medically recalcitrant infantile VT, ablation (either surgical or catheter) therapy is needed to avoid severe mobility or mortality. However, despite the severe initial symptoms, most children with this condition become free of tachycardia without the necessity of any therapy by 4 to 5 years of age.

Finally, the use of catheter ablation techniques to cure VTs in children is increasing. With special three-dimensional mapping systems, more and more complex re-entrant VTs are amenable to cure with catheter ablation techniques. Success rates, however, are lower than those with pediatric SVTs and, depending on the mechanism of the VT, range from 33% to 90%.

PREMATURE BEATS

Premature beats from the atrium, ventricle, or AV junction are encountered frequently in children. If the child has a normal heart and the beats are not exacerbated by exercise, treatment is not usually indicated. If the premature beats cause intolerable symptoms (palpitations), they can sometimes be suppressed with β-blocker therapy.

Premature beats (especially from the ventricle), when encountered in children with abnormal cardiac structure, function, or both, may be of concern because of issues involving prevention of SCD. Although these beats may not require any specific treatment, re-examination of the underlying cardiac substrate may be necessary. A new onset of cardiac ectopy sometimes indicates a cardiac substrate that is changing for the worse. In addition, some restriction of activity in children with cardiac structural disease and new-onset ectopy may at times be warranted.

BRADYCARDIA

Bradyarrhythmias encountered in children that are significant enough to need treatment are extremely rare. If significant sinus bradycardia is encountered in a child with a normal heart, most likely the cause of this arrhythmia is not cardiac. A workup of noncardiac reasons for bradycardia is imperative and includes ruling out apnea, intracranial pathology, endocrine abnormalities, and other systemic diseases. Because the only reliable cardiac treatment of chronic, hemodynamically significant sinus bradycardia is permanent cardiac pacing, searching for other causes of the bradycardia is crucial.

Bradycardia secondary to a high-grade or complete AV block is encountered in children with normal myocardial structure and function (congenital complete AV valve block) and in children who have undergone correction of a congenital heart lesion (surgical AV block). Treatment of both these conditions is permanent cardiac pacing. Pacemakers can be implanted via the epicardial or transvenous route. As pacemaker systems become more miniaturized, the transverse approach is becoming more feasible in younger children. Indications for pacemaker insertion in children with bradyarrhythmias are outlined in the American College of Cardiology/American Heart Association guidelines.

Common Pitfalls

- Not understanding the specific dysrhythmia and its natural history.
- Expending undue time and effort refining the specific diagnosis of a compromising tachycardia or bradycardia, which may jeopardize a child's recovery from the event.
- Failing to realize that in a child with an abnormal heart, seemingly trivial dysrhythmias such as premature beats may have prognostic significance different from that of an identical rhythm disturbance in a child with a normal heart.

Communication and Counseling

It is important to explain to the family that dysrhythmias are being diagnosed more often in children than was the case in past eras. Oral and written explanations both about the dysrhythmia and any therapy should be provided.

In conclusion, as more dysrhythmias are diagnosed in the pediatric age group, the variety of treatment options for these problems is increasing. Both pharmacologic and nonpharmacologic treatment options are available to the practitioner. Proper choice involves knowledge of the specific dysrhythmia, the natural history of the rhythm disturbance, the efficacy of the therapy, and the side-effect profile of the indicated therapy.

SUGGESTED READINGS

1. Bader RS, Goldberg L, Sahn DJ: Risk of sudden cardiac death in young athletes: Which screening strategies are appropriate? Pediatr Clin North Am 51(5):1421–1441, 2004. **Screening assessment.**
2. Cava JR, Danduran MJ, Fedderly RT, Sayger PL: Exercise recommendations and risk factors for sudden cardiac death. Pediatr Clin North Am 51(5):1401–1420, 2004. **Exercise recommendations.**
3. Garson A Jr, Smith RT Jr, Moak JP, et al: Incessant ventricular tachycardia in infants: Myocardial hamartomas and surgical cure. J Am Coll Cardiol 10:619–626, 1987. **This paper reports a series of 21 cases of ventricular tachycardia in young children.**
4. Kugler JD, Danford DA, Houston K, Felix G: Radiofrequency catheter ablation for paroxysmal supraventricular tachycardia in children and adolescents without structural heart disease. Pediatric EP Society, Radiofrequency Catheter Ablation Registry. Am J Cardiol 80:1438–1443, 1997. **Report from the Pediatric Radiofrequency Catheter Ablation Registry.**
5. Kugler JD, Danford DA, Houston KA, Felix G: Pediatric Radiofrequency Ablation Registry of the Pediatric Electrophysiology Society: Pediatric radiofrequency catheter ablation registry success, fluoroscopy time, and complication rate for supraventricular tachycardia: Comparison of early and recent eras. J Cardiovasc Electrophysiol 13(4):336–341, 2002. **Updated report from the Pediatric Radiofrequency Catheter Ablation Registry.**
6. Link MS, Hill SL, Cliff DL, et al: Comparison of frequency of complications of implantable cardioverter-defibrillators in children versus adults. Am J Cardiol 83:263–266, A5–6, 1999. **Eleven pediatric patients are compared to 308 adult patients receiving implantable cardioverter-defibrillators.**
7. Maron BJ: Sudden death in young athletes. N Engl J Med 349(11):1064–1075, 2003. **Overview of factors causing sudden death in young athletes.**
8. Samson RA, Berg RA, Bingham R: Pediatric Advanced Life Support Task Force, International Liaison Committee on Resuscitation for the American Heart Association; European Resuscitation Council: Use of automated external defibrillators for children: An update—an advisory statement from the Pediatric Advanced Life Support Task Force, International Liaison Committee on Resuscitation. Pediatrics 112(1 Pt 1):163–168, 2003. **Recommendations from the Pediatric Advanced Life Support Task Force.**
9. Silka MJ: Implantable cardioverter-defibrillators in children. A perspective on current and future uses. J Electrocardiol 29(Suppl):223–225, 1996. **Review on implantable cardioverter-defibrillators in children.**
10. Van Hare GF, Javitz H, Carmelli D, et al: Pediatric Electrophysiology Society: Prospective assessment after pediatric cardiac ablation: Demographics, medical profiles, and initial outcomes. J Cardiovasc Electrophysiol 15(7):759–770, 2004. **Update on prospective assessment.**

Intestinal Malformations

Martin H. Ulshen

KEY CONCEPTS

- Many intestinal malformations manifest with symptoms at birth; however, some may first become symptomatic at any time in life (e.g., small bowel malrotation or Meckel diverticulum).
- Intestinal malformations that become symptomatic generally require surgical correction.
- Anomalies associated with compromised blood flow to the bowel (e.g., midgut volvulus) are surgical emergencies.
- Normal rotation of the cecum to the right lower quadrant does not rule out malrotation of the small bowel.
- Duplications may manifest with obstructive symptoms or with gastrointestinal bleeding because of the presence of ectopic gastric mucosa.
- Meckel diverticulum may manifest with symptoms of diverticulitis (similar to appendicitis), lower gastrointestinal bleeding (ectopic gastric mucosa), or obstructive symptoms (volvulus or intussusception). The majority remain asymptomatic.
- Improved prognosis of small bowel atresias has resulted from the use of parenteral nutrition.

The human gut undergoes a highly complex and coordinated sequence of embryologic development involving a combination of invagination, elongation, budding, dilation, rotation, and regionalization of function. A failure in any one of these processes results in intestinal malformations, which are among the most common congenital defects. These malformations may be sporadic, but some are clearly inherited or form part of recognized syndromes. The pathogenesis of intestinal malformations is poorly understood. Cell signaling between epithelial and mesenchymal layers appears central to coordination of embryonic development of the gut. Recent studies indicate that mutations in genes of cell signaling (the Hedgehog family of cell signals) are likely to be etiologic in at least some intestinal malformations.

Babies with intestinal malformations may have obvious defects, such as gastroschisis with an abdominal wall defect and herniation of the bowel, signs of intestinal obstruction (abdominal distention, bilious vomiting, obstipation), hemodynamic compromise (shock), sepsis, or a combination of these conditions. Certain minor defects may become symptomatic in later life or be detected as incidental findings. A careful examination for potential associated defects, such as cardiac defects in infants with trisomy 21, must be carried out as well.

Expert Opinion on Management Issues

Definitive management of intestinal malformations is nearly always surgical, either elective in many instances or emergent in some cases. Early recognition and diagnosis of not only the defect but also the clinical state of the child are vital. The first responsibility of the medical staff is resuscitation and stabilization of the child. Recognition that there is an intestinal malformation and further characterization are important in determining the urgency of surgery (e.g., the need for emergent surgery for malrotation with midgut volvulus). Intravenous fluids, institution of nothing by mouth (NPO) status, drainage of intestinal contents by passage of a nasogastric tube, and careful monitoring should be the initial management of almost all children with symptomatic intestinal malformations. Sepsis must always be considered in an ill baby or child, appropriate microbiologic cultures taken, and antibiotic therapy commenced. Intestinal perforation or intraoperative spillage of contents may occur, so administration of broad-spectrum antibiotics effective against sepsis from gut organisms is common during the perioperative period. Postoperative care involves close monitoring of fluid status and vital signs and maintenance of the various drains and vascular lines. Recommencement of feeding depends on the operative procedure undertaken, healing, and clinical signs of recovery of bowel function.

INTRAVENOUS FLUIDS/ELECTROLYTES

Although patients are kept on NPO status, the minimal requirement is to provide maintenance intravenous fluid with glucose and electrolytes. Poor intake before diagnosis and increased loss into the gut may result in dehydration or hypovolemia requiring rehydration as well. For a child who is hypovolemic (in shock), establishing normovolemia to maintain perfusion to vital organs is the first priority. Boluses or infusion of normal saline or lactated Ringer solution are very effective, although, at times, colloid may be necessary. Loss of gastric secretions (e.g., nasogastric suction) should be quantitated and replaced every 4 to 6 hours with one-half normal saline. Although gastric secretions are low in potassium concentration, additional potassium may be necessary with gastric fluid losses. Careful monitoring of serum electrolytes, fluid balance (including urine output), blood sugar, and acid–base status should be carried out to guide replacement.

NOTHING BY MOUTH

In symptomatic children, initial management includes NPO status. In esophageal atresia, NPO status prevents compromise of the airway given the inability to swallow and association with tracheoesophageal fistula. It limits stress on compromised bowel, encourages decompression of distended bowel, and reduces the risk of aspiration if general anesthesia is imminent. Furthermore, it reduces not only the distress of vomiting but also the excessive loss of fluids and electrolytes induced by recurrent emesis.

DRAINAGE OF INTESTINAL LUMINAL CONTENTS

Certain defects prevent passage of a nasogastric tube, which itself can be diagnostic of conditions such as esophageal atresia. Otherwise, a large-bore nasogastric or orogastric tube (size 10 or 12 F, if possible) should be passed into the stomach and either aspirated regularly or kept on free drainage with or without suction. Such treatment helps empty and decompress the bowel.

SPECIFIC INTESTINAL MALFORMATIONS

Atresia and Stenosis

Atresia refers either to complete obstruction of the gut by a membrane or a fibrous band or to complete separation of adjacent sections. Stenosis refers to incomplete obstruction caused by intrinsic narrowing of the internal lumen of the gut. These abnormalities can occur in several portions of the gastrointestinal tract.

Esophageal Atresia

Esophageal atresia occurs in approximately 1 in 3500 live births and has a possible slight male preponderance. Associated anomalies occur in 50% to 70% of patients and most commonly include the following:

- Tracheoesophageal fistula (the basis of various classifications of associations)
- Vertebral (and rib), anal, cardiac (and vascular), tracheal, esophageal, renal, and limb anomalies (VATER or VACTERL association)
- Coloboma, heart, choanal atresia, mental retardation, genital, and ear anomalies (CHARGE association)
- Duodenal atresia and intestinal malrotation.

Given their inability to swallow, affected babies tend to "froth" saliva from their mouths and have episodes of coughing, choking, and cyanosis, especially with feeding. Similar symptoms may occur with laryngotracheoesophageal cleft. The priority is to maintain the airway and prevent aspiration by removing secretions from the mouth, pharynx, and upper part of the esophagus by regular or continuous suctioning and, in some cases, by endotracheal intubation. Abdominal distention may be marked if ventilation is instituted and a tracheoesophageal fistula is present. The baby should be nursed prone and tilted head-up to minimize reflux of gastric contents into the airway.

Surgery involves division of the fistula with primary anastomosis of the proximal and distal ends of the esophagus unless the gap between the two ends is too large. In that case, division of the fistula or its occlusion with a balloon is carried out in isolation, with the formation of a feeding gastrostomy and either a cervical esophagostomy (spit fistula) or regular suctioning to maintain a clear airway. Elongation of the upper pouch together with hypertrophy of the lower pouch during the first 2 to 3 months may allow subsequent anastomosis. Colon or stomach tissue may be used later in the first year to bridge the esophageal gap. In the absence of early complications of an anastomotic leak, fistula recurrence, or stricture formation, oral feeding is commenced within the first week. Gastroesophageal reflux, recurrent chest infections, and dysphagia are common postoperatively and related to dysmotility, incompetent lower esophageal sphincter, or stricture formation. Tracheomalacia is common as well. Overall survival rates are between 70% and 85%, and they approach 100% in babies weighing more than 1500 g without other life-threatening congenital anomalies and in good preoperative condition.

Esophageal Stenosis

Esophageal stenosis occurs in 1 in 25,000 to 50,000 live births, and associated anomalies include esophageal atresia, tracheoesophageal fistula, duodenal atresia, anorectal anomalies, and Down syndrome.

The causes of esophageal stenosis include the presence of ectopic tracheobronchial remnants, a membranous diaphragm, or fibromuscular stenosis. Dysphagia, especially with solid food, vomiting, dribbling of saliva, respiratory distress, and failure to thrive are common findings.

Tracheobronchial remnants are resected, and both an end-to-end esophageal anastomosis and an antireflux procedure are carried out. Surgical resection or repeat endoscopic dilation is used in managing fibromuscular stenosis and membranous diaphragms. Laser treatment has been used for membranous diaphragm as well.

Pyloric Atresia

The incidence of pyloric atresia is low (less than 1% of cases of intestinal atresia). It may be associated with multiple atresias of the small and large bowel or with epidermolysis bullosa lethalis. Persistent nonbilious vomiting occurs from birth. When associated with multiple atresias of the small and large bowel or with epidermolysis bullosa lethalis, the outcome is usually fatal.

If the defect is a thin membrane, excision along with pyloroplasty is the treatment of choice. More complex atresias may require resection and formation of a gastroduodenostomy, pyloroplasty or, less commonly, a gastrojejunostomy. The stomach is kept decompressed after surgery and enteral nutrition commenced in the first week in the absence of complications.

Gastric Antral Diaphragm or Web

The incidence of a gastric antral diaphragm or web is less than 1 in 100,000. The gastric antrum (or pylorus) may be completely or partially obstructed by a circumferential membrane consisting of redundant mucosa and submucosa. Children may have failure to thrive and recurrent nonbilious vomiting from birth or may first present later in life.

Diagnosis is made by contrast radiographs; however, a diaphragm may be missed or falsely diagnosed and endoscopic evaluation is occasionally necessary. Surgical excision is the treatment of choice. Endoscopic transection of the web, balloon dilation, and laser ablation are newer therapies. Complications are minimal, and other bowel atresias should be excluded.

Duodenal Atresia and Stenosis

The duodenum is a common site for atresia or stenosis (occurring in approximately 1 in 10,000 to 30,000 live births). Most occur distal to the ampulla. Associated anomalies may include Down syndrome (up to 40%); esophageal atresia; midgut malrotation; annular pancreas; anorectal, cardiac, and genitourinary defects; and intrauterine growth retardation.

Children with this anomaly may have signs of obstruction, an increased incidence of jaundice, and a classic "double bubble" sign on radiography. Pyloric stenosis results in partial obstruction.

At surgery, the entire duodenum is visualized by mobilizing the right colon. Such mobilization allows identification of the obstruction and exclusion of associated malrotation. A side-to-side or end-to-side duodenoduodenostomy or duodenojejunostomy is carried out. Resection of any obstructing membranes is likely to damage the bile or pancreatic duct and is therefore usually avoided. The presence of other small bowel atresias is excluded at surgery. Survival rates are above 90% in the absence of chromosomal or cardiac defects. Long-term follow-up is needed to monitor the development of complications such as ulceration and duodenal stasis (megaduodenum). The latter may be the result of obstruction at the anastomosis or a duodenal motility disorder. Surgical correction of the obstruction and/or tapering may be necessary.

Jejunal and Ileal Atresia

Jejunal or ileal atresia occurs in 1 in 300 to 5000 live births (higher in certain familial cases), with no sex preponderance. Associated anomalies may include Down syndrome, gastroschisis, malrotation, or cystic fibrosis.

Jejunal atresia and ileal atresia are thought to be the result of ischemic necrosis caused by a focal mesenteric vascular accident, which may be initiated by a variety of events including volvulus and intussusception. Multiple atresias are seen in 6% to 21% of cases. Microcolon may accompany ileal atresias. Signs and symptoms of intestinal obstruction result and may be associated with significant proximal small bowel dilation and perforation.

Surgical repair involves end-to-end anastomosis with the distal section. Multiple atresias may be repaired in this way with attention to preserving final intestinal length, although dense clusters may best be treated by resection of the entire affected bowel. Tapering of dilated proximal bowel may be necessary.

Long-term total parenteral nutrition is likely to be needed if significant resection has occurred, at least until the remaining bowel undergoes compensatory adaptation. At present, the survival rate is approximately 90%, and the prognosis depends on the length and location of residual bowel and availability of total parenteral nutrition. The association with gastroschisis worsens the prognosis.

Colonic Atresia

The incidence of colonic atresia is 1 in 40,000 live births, and associated anomalies may include Hirschsprung disease, small bowel atresia, and gastroschisis. Colonic atresia commonly involves obstruction of the lumen with a membrane or disconnected blind ends to the right of the splenic flexure. It produces signs of progressive distal intestinal obstruction.

Before surgery, multiple atresias and Hirschsprung disease must be excluded. Usually, a staged procedure is carried out with resection of the dilated colon and formation of a colostomy and mucous fistula, subsequently followed by anastomosis. This technique is preferred to primary anastomosis, which carries a higher complication rate. The prognosis depends on associated anomalies and the extent of intestinal involvement, especially small-bowel involvement.

Anorectal Malformations

Anorectal malformations are a complex group of malformations of rectum and anus. They range from anal stenosis to complete agenesis of anus and rectum. Low anomalies are usually treated in the newborn period and generally do well. Anterior displacement of the anus often appears later and only rarely requires surgical correction. Anal stenosis is managed with dilations. An anal membrane is treated by perforation.

High anomalies are much more complex and difficult to manage. Current approaches include posterior sagittal anorectoplasty and laparoscopically assisted anorectal pull-through. Incontinence is the major complication of repair of high anomalies, occurring in at least 25% of cases. Incontinence can be the result of constipation with overflow or anatomic abnormalities of pelvic muscle with poor control. Management is complex, including treatment of constipation with fiber, stool softeners, laxatives, and enemas, as indicated. If the problem is related to abnormalities of musculature and innervation of the distal colon, forming more solid stool with loperamide and then emptying the distal colon with suppositories and enemas may be effective. In children who are unable to retain or do not respond to standard enemas, the regular use of continence enemas or antegrade enemas through a cecostomy or appendicostomy may be necessary.

Duplications and Cysts

Duplications are cystic or tubular malformations of the gut. They may be multiple and often communicate with and share the blood supply of the adjacent gut. Usually, they are composed of intestinal or even ectopic gastric mucosa, submucosa, and smooth muscle coats. The diagnosis may be delayed until enlargement causes compression of adjacent structures, or it may be made after volvulus, intussusception, or investigation of gastrointestinal hemorrhage or perforation. All duplications should be surgically excised to prevent complications.

Esophageal Duplication Cysts

Esophageal duplication cysts typically present as respiratory distress in neonates or dysphagia in older children. They are identified on chest radiograph and delineated by chest CT or MRI. These cysts generally arise in the esophageal wall adjacent to the carina; they share esophageal muscle and contain respiratory epithelium or cartilage. Excision is the preferred method of treatment but may be difficult if the esophagus and duplication share a common wall, in which case stripping off the mucosa with partial resection of the cyst may produce a better result.

Gastric Duplication

Gastric duplication accounts for 4% of gastrointestinal duplications. Associated anomalies may include pancreatic duct abnormalities. This type of duplication may occur in a variety of sites, including duplication in association with the esophagus and pancreas. Enlargement of the cysts can be manifested as obstruction of gastric emptying or compression of adjacent structures. Ulceration, bleeding, or inflammation within the cyst results in either local complications, overt gastrointestinal hemorrhage, or perforation with peritonitis or fistula formation.

Excision of the duplication with minimal loss of adjacent normal stomach is usually possible. In complete or tubular duplications, the normal stomach can be preserved by stripping the mucosal lining, along with variable excision of the cyst. Resection of aberrant or ectopic pancreatic tissue may also be required.

Intestinal Duplications

Cystic duplications tend to involve short segments of the bowel; tubular types occasionally involve the entire intestine. Despite sharing a common wall and blood supply, the mucosa is separate and frequently contains ectopic gastric mucosa. This condition can lead to ulceration, bleeding, inflammation, and perforation within the cyst or adjacent intestine. Complications such as volvulus or intussusception are more common. Rectal duplication cysts can enlarge significantly and obstruct the gut or urinary tract. Malignant change can occur after many years, especially in a rectal duplication cyst.

Cystic duplications can usually be totally excised. Excision of duplications is complicated, however, by their occurrence on the mesenteric border, as opposed to Meckel diverticula, which are normally antimesenteric. Excision of adjacent attached bowel with primary end-to-end anastomosis of the residual intestine is usually necessary. If excessive bowel resection or damage to key structures such as the pancreas or bile duct is to be avoided, mucosa within the duplication should be excised or stripped to remove any ectopic tissue likely to cause problems and the seromuscular layer left in situ. Cystic rectal duplications should be managed by excision because of the long-term risk of malignancy.

Abnormal Rotation and Fixation

The entire gut assumes its normal postnatal position within the abdominal cavity after a carefully sequenced process of physiologic herniation of midgut out of the abdominal cavity in the sixth week of embryonic life. This process is followed by elongation, counterclockwise rotation around the superior mesenteric artery, return into the abdomen in week 10, and fixation of the duodenum and ascending colon to the posterior abdominal wall. Volvulus and obstruction may occur when such rotation and fixation are incomplete or abnormal (malrotation) and can lead to ischemia and infarction of the bowel. Total nonrotation results in the duodenojejunal loop on the right and cecocolic loop on the left side of the abdomen. Symptoms and signs at initial evaluation vary from those of acute obstruction or compromise (e.g., volvulus) to vague chronic gastrointestinal symptoms.

Gastric Volvulus

Gastric volvulus is caused by abnormal rotation of one part of the stomach around another. Most cases have associated abnormal fixation of the stomach at the esophageal junction. Vomiting and acute abdominal pain are typical symptoms, with hemodynamic shock if the diagnosis is delayed. It is a surgical emergency occurring most commonly in the first few months of life. At surgery, the volvulus is reduced and viability of the stomach is assessed. If viable, it is fixed by gastropexy to the abdominal wall or a gastrostomy is fashioned. Repair of any associated defects such as hiatal hernia is necessary. Successful laparoscopic surgery has been reported.

Malrotation and Midgut Volvulus

Malrotation with midgut volvulus occurs in 1 in 6000 live births and is slightly more common in boys.

Associated anomalies may include congenital diaphragmatic hernia, omphalocele, gastroschisis, mesenteric cysts, Hirschsprung disease, intussusception, and intestinal atresia.

Malrotation presents most commonly in the neonatal period. Plain films of the abdomen may be diagnostic, but a limited upper gastrointestinal contrast radiograph series may be necessary. The presence of the cecum in the right lower quadrant does not rule out midgut volvulus secondary to malrotation. Urgency in resuscitation, diagnosis, and treatment is vital to preserve and salvage compromised ischemic bowel. Long-term mortality after loss of the midgut is on the order of 50%. In malrotation, peritoneal (Ladd) bands extending from the cecum to the right upper quadrant may obstruct the duodenum. Furthermore, it often results in a narrow vascular pedicle at the base of the mesentery that is centered around the superior mesenteric artery and vein. Intestinal volvulus with rotation around this narrow pedicle can result in necrosis of the entire midgut and obstruction of the lymphatics with chylous ascites. Clinically, the child has intestinal obstruction that often leads to cardiovascular collapse if treatment is delayed.

During surgery the bowel is fully exposed and carefully examined. It is then normally untwisted by counterclockwise rotation, and any Ladd bands are divided. The mesentery is broadened and an attempt is made to straighten the duodenum and place the intestine in a more normal orientation. The appendix is removed. Ischemic bowel may need a period of observation before abdominal closure, whereas severe ischemia or nonviability of bowel requires resection and anastomosis. The prognosis in the absence of compromised bowel is excellent. Given the increased risk of complications, incidental or asymptomatic malrotation is increasingly managed by elective open abdominal exploration and Ladd procedure.

Abdominal Wall Defects

Ultrasonography has enabled prenatal diagnosis of abdominal wall defects and should allow delivery at a specialized center. These defects occur in approximately 4 per 10,000 pregnancies.

Gastroschisis

Gastroschisis is a small defect in the abdominal wall, lateral and usually to the right of the umbilical cord, that allows a variable amount of intestine and other abdominal organs to herniate out. The bowel is malrotated, not fixed, and uncovered (compare with omphalocele). It is typically inflamed, matted, and shortened. The bowel is covered with a thick "peel," which regresses over 2 to 4 weeks after repair. Intestinal atresia occurs in 5% to 25% of infants with gastroschisis, but it may be difficult to identify initially because of the peel. Associated anomalies are otherwise uncommon.

Neonatal care has significantly improved the survival of children with gastroschisis. At birth, normal resuscitation is undertaken, followed by protection of the exposed bowel with a sterile cover (warm sterile saline wraps or a plastic bowel bag). Given the exposed length of intestine and viscera, adequate fluid replacement and prevention of excessive heat loss are key management strategies. During surgery, the bowel is kept decompressed. The intestine is exposed to check for viability and atresia. The defect is usually enlarged slightly and the abdominal cavity manually stretched before attempting primary reduction of the bowel back into the abdominal cavity and closure.

On occasion, the elevation in abdominal pressure generated by the reduction leads to a number of complications, including decreased cardiac function from compression of caval flow, pulmonary embarrassment from elevated diaphragms, renal failure, decreased limb perfusion, and bowel ischemia itself. If the bowel cannot be fully reduced initially, a prosthetic silo is constructed, allowing gradual reduction of bowel into the abdominal cavity. Atresias are repaired either by resection and anastomosis, which is often difficult with edematous matted bowel, or by staged repair with enterostomy.

Loss of intestinal length in utero, resection, or prolonged ileus can result in short bowel syndrome, which diminishes the otherwise generally good prognosis of uncomplicated gastroschisis repair. Intestinal dysmotility is a common complication of gastroschisis as well. The overall outcome of gastroschisis is largely dependent on the extent of short bowel and the effect of dysmotility on implementation of enteral feedings. Gastroesophageal reflux is common.

Omphalocele

An omphalocele is a central umbilical ring defect through which abdominal contents herniate. In contrast to gastroschisis, a membrane composed of peritoneum and amnion covers the herniated viscera. Defects range from small umbilical cord hernias to the presence of the entire intestine and liver in the sac secondary to huge abdominal wall defects. Rupture of the contents out of the sac can occur.

Omphaloceles are commonly associated with chromosomal abnormalities (trisomy 13, 18, and 21) and with cardiac, musculoskeletal, gastrointestinal, and genitourinary anomalies. It has been associated with Beckwith-Wiedemann syndrome, neural tube defects, and the pentalogy of Cantrell (omphalocele, short sternum, defect of the diaphragm and pericardium, and intracardiac anomaly).

Management is similar to that of gastroschisis. Initial gastric decompression is important to prevent visceral distention. Because the herniated contents are usually covered, heat and fluid loss is less of a problem but a prime consideration nonetheless. Associated anomalies are common and may need to be addressed early. The omphalocele is covered with a protective layer until surgery. Primary reduction with fascial and skin closure, after excising the sac, is usually feasible for small or moderate defects. Careful placement of the viscera back into the abdominal cavity is necessary given the abnormal rotation and fixation of the bowel. Large omphaloceles can be repaired by staged closure with a Silastic silo and frequent manual reductions. Alternatively, giant omphaloceles can be treated with topical agents such as 0.25% merbromin or silver nitrate to encourage epithelialization of the sac, by the application of external pressure with wraps, or by both techniques. Once skin has grown over the sac or reduction has taken place (or both), definitive closure can be carried out.

Complications associated with an increase in intra-abdominal pressure should be monitored. Prolonged ileus is not common, and the prognosis of small and moderate defects is generally excellent in the absence of significant associated anomalies. Mortality is primarily the result of associated anomalies. The incidence of gastroesophageal reflux is increased, and ventral hernias may recur and require additional surgery.

Microgastria

Microgastria is very rare. This condition is nearly always associated with other congenital anomalies, most commonly in the gastrointestinal tract, but also heart, respiratory system, skeleton, kidneys, and central nervous system.

Failure to thrive and gastroesophageal reflux are the most serious problems that an affected infant may have. Aspiration pneumonia secondary to gastroesophageal reflux may occur as well. Surgery is usually attempted only if a feeding strategy of frequent small-volume, high-calorie feeding fails to achieve adequate growth or if symptoms of reflux are prominent. Nasojejunal alimentation and jejunostomy feeding are other options. The aim of surgery is to increase the capacity of the stomach and prevent dilation of the esophagus as a compensatory reservoir. This objective can be achieved by attaching a jejunal pouch to the stomach and forming a distal Roux-en-Y jejunojejunostomy.

Meckel Diverticulum and Other Umbilical Cord Anomalies

In the human embryo, the omphalomesenteric duct connects the yolk sac to the distal small bowel. This duct normally disappears by week 6 of embryonic life. A Meckel diverticulum is a remnant of this duct extending from the distal ileum. Approximately half of these have ectopic mucosa, mainly gastric.

Meckel diverticulum occurs in 1% to 4% of the general population, with a 2:1 male-to-female ratio. These diverticula are usually present on the antimesenteric border of the small intestine. If they contain heterotopic pancreatic tissue or gastric mucosa as opposed to intestinal mucosa, ulceration, bleeding, or perforation can occur with associated symptoms. The bleeding is rectal and typically brisk. Volvulus, intussusception, and prolapse can lead to intestinal obstruction. Carcinoid tumors have been reported. Associated anomalies may include omphalocele, esophageal atresia, and imperforate anus.

A Meckel diverticulum is most commonly detected by ^{99m}Tc pertechnetate uptake (technetium scan). Sensitivity of this scan for detection of ectopic gastric mucosa is about 85% to 95%. The scan is enhanced by pretreatment with an H_2 blocker, such as ranitidine. An inflamed Meckel diverticulum may be identified by ultrasound.

Treatment is by resection of the diverticulum. Broad-based diverticula may require a wedge excision and closure of the bowel. The prognosis is excellent. Resection of an incidentally detected Meckel diverticulum is controversial.

Other Omphalomesenteric Duct Abnormalities

If the entire omphalomesenteric duct remains patent, it continues to form an open communication between the intestinal tract and umbilicus and may discharge gas or feces or permit prolapse of bowel. Obliteration of the duct to form a fibrous cord can act as an axis for volvulus or herniation. Mucosa-lined omphalomesenteric cysts can develop within these cords and enlarge or cause local complications akin to a Meckel diverticulum. Management is by exploration, identification, and excision of the defects.

Aganglionosis (Hirschsprung Disease)

Aganglionosis is thought to result from failure of neuronal migration and ganglia formation to varying extents of the distal end of the bowel. The condition is characterized histologically by an absence of ganglion cells within the submucous and myenteric plexuses extending proximally for a varying distance from the rectum. Consequently, the affected bowel is dysmotile, and symptoms and signs of obstruction, severe constipation, or sepsis result. Management is outlined in the following section.

Meconium Ileus

Approximately 15% of babies with cystic fibrosis (incidence, 1 in 2500 live births) have meconium ileus, which results from the presence of thick viscid inspissated meconium within the intestinal lumen. The viscid meconium results in distal small bowel or colonic obstruction and should be differentiated from a meconium plug or Hirschsprung disease. Simple meconium ileus results from distal small bowel obstruction with proximal dilation and a narrowed empty colon (often referred to as microcolon) and may be complicated by intestinal volvulus, atresia, necrosis, perforation, meconium peritonitis, and pseudocyst formation. This condition is discussed in the section on cystic fibrosis.

Uncomplicated meconium ileus can be treated with hyperosmolar or hydrostatic enemas, such as diatrizoate meglumine (Gastrografin), which appear to free the meconium from the bowel wall, draw in and retain water within the intestinal lumen, and reduce the viscidity of the meconium. The fluid is introduced per rectum with a catheter and, under fluoroscopic guidance, pushed cautiously through the colon and refluxed into the distal end of the small bowel. Meconium is often passed soon after. The patient must be kept well hydrated throughout the procedure. Repeat enemas or the use of saline enemas with acetylcysteine may be needed and have been used with good success.

At least 50% of uncomplicated cases of meconium ileus will have a favorable response. The remaining babies and those with complicated meconium ileus require surgery. In uncomplicated cases, a laparotomy is performed, affected bowel identified, and an enterostomy made in the dilated meconium-filled proximal portion of the bowel, into which a catheter is passed to enable the instillation of *N*-acetylcysteine. Once this agent has taken effect, the less viscid meconium should be able to be milked into the colon and hopefully passed. Some *N*-acetylcysteine is left in situ and the enterostomy closed. If this procedure is not effective, a T tube is inserted for irrigation. Resection and formation of an ileostomy is performed much less commonly than in the past. Resection of cyst or atretic bowel may be required.

Common Pitfalls

- In initial evaluation for a bowel obstruction, an upright radiograph of the abdomen should be included with plain films.
- If an infant or child has possible bowel obstruction, it is best to be cautious and maintain NPO status until the proper radiographic studies are completed. If symptomatic, nasogastric drainage should be considered.
- In a child with acute abdominal pain and obstructive symptoms, a malrotation with midgut volvulus must be considered. This is a surgical emergency and surgical consultation should be sought immediately.
- A normal barium enema does not rule out malrotation of the small bowel. If the diagnosis is suspected and not apparent on plain films, an upper gastrointestinal contrast radiograph series should be performed.

Communication and Counseling

Intestinal malformations generally require surgical correction. This is best performed by a surgeon experienced in the management of infants and children. Most children with intestinal malformations will do well after surgery. The outcome for intestinal atresia is related to the extent of bowel involved, location, and associated conditions (e.g., gastroschisis). If intestinal resection is extensive, duration of recovery is shorter after jejunal than ileal resection and prolonged with gastroschisis. Repair of high anorectal anomalies and Hirschsprung disease may require ongoing postoperative management for constipation and incontinence.

SUGGESTED READINGS

1. Andorsky DJ, Lund DP, Lillehei CW, et al: Nutritional and other postoperative management of neonates with short bowel syndrome correlates with clinical outcomes. J Pediatr 139:27–33, 2001. **Early enteral feeding correlates with shorter duration of parenteral nutrition and reduction in cholestasis. Early restoration of intestinal continuity correlates with decreased cholestasis as well.**
2. Pena A, Hong A: Advances in the management of anorectal malformations. Am J Surg 180:370–376, 2000. **Follow-up of more than 1000 children treated for anorectal malformations with analysis of long-term outcome.**
3. Pena A, Levitt MA, Hong A, et al: Surgical management of cloacal malformations: A review of 339 patients. J Pediatr Surg 39:470–479, 2004. **Recent review of management of the severe anorectal malformations associated with cloacal malformations.**
4. Ramalho-Santos M, Melton DA, McMahon AP: Hedgehog signals regulate multiple aspects of gastrointestinal development. Development 127:2763–2772, 2000. **The pathogenesis of congenital anomalies of the gastrointestinal tract is poorly understood. Recent advances have been made in understanding the regulatory role of cell signaling during embryonic development of the gut and, therefore, the potential role of mutations of cell signaling genes in intestinal malformations.**
5. Stringer MD, Oldham KT, Mouriquand PDE, et al (eds) Pediatric Surgery and Urology: Long-Term Outcomes. Philadelphia: WB Saunders, 1998. **Discussion of intestinal malformations with emphasis on long-term outcomes.**
6. Warner BW: Pediatric surgery. In Townsend CM, Evers BM, Beauchamp RD (eds): Sabiston Textbook of Surgery, 17th ed. Philadelphia: Elsevier Saunders, 2004. **General surgery textbook with excellent pediatric surgery section.**
7. Walker WA, Goulet O, Kleinman RE, et al (eds) Pediatric Gastrointestinal Disease, 4th ed. Hamilton, Ontario, Canada: BC Decker, 2004. **This is an outstanding textbook of pediatric gastroenterology, which covers intestinal malformations in depth.**
8. Oldham KT, Colombani PM, Foglia RP, Skinner MA (eds): Principles and Practice of Pediatric Surgery. Philadelphia: Lippincott Williams & Wilkins. **This textbook of pediatric surgery has excellent sections on intestinal malformations and their management.**

10

Hirschsprung Disease

Jon A. Vanderhoof and Rosemary J. Young

KEY CONCEPTS

- Hirschsprung disease is a relatively uncommon cause of chronic constipation, especially outside of infancy.
- Toddlers and children with fecal retention, stool withholding, and chronic fecal soiling rarely have Hirschsprung disease.
- Hirschsprung disease always begins distally; therefore, the distal rectum is always involved. However, the length of the aganglionic segment varies significantly from patient to patient.
- Absence of myenteric parasympathetic nerve ganglia results in absence of peristalsis in the aganglionic segment and dilated colon to the involved area.
- Because parasympathetic nerves also supply the detrusor muscle of the bladder, Hirschsprung disease may also be associated with defects in bladder function.

Hirschsprung disease, or congenital aganglionic megacolon, first described in 1888, is one of the rare causes of chronic constipation beginning in infancy. Incidence is estimated at 1 in 5000 live births, with a somewhat higher occurrence in Asians. Males predominate in short segment disease and a familial association for total colonic Hirschsprung disease has been observed. There is an association between Hirschsprung disease and other congenital anomalies including Down syndrome and central nervous system disorders. Genetic studies suggest that total intestinal aganglionosis is associated with identified gene mutations involving two signaling pathways, the RET receptor and the endothelin-B receptor, accounting for about half of the cases.

Hirschsprung disease is caused by absence or agenesis of myenteric parasympathetic nerve ganglia in the colon. This results in impeded transmission of peristaltic waves and failure of relaxation of the internal anal sphincter, resulting in obstructed passage of fecal material. The disorder typically manifests during the neonatal period with the late passage of meconium and constipation from birth. If meconium is not passed within the first 48 hours, the likelihood of the child's having Hirschsprung disease is markedly increased. The clinical presentation in later infancy is dependent on the length of the aganglionic segment involved. Box 1 reviews the clinical manifestations of Hirschsprung disease. The disease most commonly affects the rectosigmoid colon, but it always begins distally and ascends to varying degrees proximally. In rare instances, the disease may involve the entire colon and even part or all of the small intestine, particularly in familial cases of Hirschsprung disease.

In addition to chronic constipation, children with Hirschsprung disease may present with enterocolitis. Delayed defecation results in proximal dilation of the colon, with ischemia and bacterial invasion, resulting in severe enterocolitis, a manifestation of the disease that requires immediate medical and surgical intervention and carries with it a high risk of mortality.

Expert Opinion on Management Issues

DIAGNOSIS

Hirschsprung disease is usually a neonatal condition. In rare instances, the disease may be diagnosed later. Although clinicians commonly think Hirschsprung disease is a cause of chronic constipation, outside of the neonatal period it is relatively rare. It is, therefore, important to establish definitively when the constipation began. Most parents will state that the child has always been constipated but, after careful questioning, one can usually establish that the bowel habits very early in life in non-Hirschsprung children were relatively normal. Toddlers or older children who soil their pants rarely have Hirschsprung disease. The typical patient with Hirschsprung disease has small ribbon- or pencil-like stools that are difficult to pass, with no soiling.

Other entities may be in the differential diagnosis. The child with functional fecal retention, by far the most common cause of chronic constipation in toddlers and older children, typically have encopresis and occasionally pass very large bowel movements which not infrequently plug up the toilet. Cow's milk protein allergy has recently been identified as a cause of chronic constipation. Affected children typically present as toddlers but may also present as older children. A variant of this disorder appears to occur in infancy as well.

Stool frequency in breast-fed infants is highly variable. Some breast-fed babies defecate as infrequently as every 5 to 7 days. In these infants, stools are mushy, passed without difficulty, and often quite voluminous. The children grow well, exhibit no discomfort except occasionally on the day of defecation, and are otherwise normal. In this clinical setting in the breast-fed infant, evaluation for Hirschsprung disease is usually unnecessary.

Hirschsprung disease should be considered in a differential diagnosis of the newborn infant with failure to pass meconium within the first 48 hours of life or chronic constipation beginning in early infancy. Other anorectal anomalies such as imperforate anus, anterior displaced anus, and anal stenosis should also be considered. Metabolic causes of constipation, such as hypothyroidism or hypercalcemia, should be considered in the differential diagnosis. Occasionally, infants with allergic proctitis may present with constipation rather than diarrhea. A trial of an extensively hydrolyzed infant formula may be helpful in making this distinction between cow's milk protein intolerance and Hirschsprung disease. More proximal causes of obstruction, such as meconium ileus (usually indicative of cystic fibrosis), should also be included in the differential diagnosis. Additionally, neonatal small left colon

---

BOX 1 Clinical Manifestations of Hirschsprung Disease

■ Delayed meconium passage (>48 hr).
■ Small, ribbon-like or pencil-like stools.
■ Tight anal tone, digital exam reveals no stool in the rectal vault and a "spurt" of stool upon removal of the finger.
■ Poor growth, vomiting, and abdominal distention if extensive aganglionosis.
■ Diarrhea and bloody stools if enterocolitis is present.

syndrome, characterized by a markedly reduced diameter of the descending colon and rectosigmoid, which gradually normalizes with time, should be excluded.

An unprepped barium enema examination will usually exclude the possibilities of other anatomic disorders. In the infant older than 1 month of age, this is probably the first diagnostic study to consider. Older infants with Hirschsprung disease not uncommonly have radiographic studies interpreted as normal during the neonatal period unless the studies are examined by an experienced pediatric radiologist. Frequently, during the first few weeks of life, the only abnormalities seen are "saw-tooth" contractions of the rectosigmoid. The classic transition zone with proximal dilation of the colon usually develops later in life.

If the diagnosis of Hirschsprung disease is suspected, a rectal suction biopsy can be easily performed at a site 2 cm proximal to the dentate line with a rectal suction biopsy apparatus. In the hands of an experienced pediatric gastroenterologist or pediatric surgeon, adequate samples can usually be obtained. Care must be taken to ensure that the biopsies are deep enough to contain sufficient submucosal tissue for histologic examination. Too superficial a biopsy is a common error that may result in a specimen that is interpreted as abnormal or not containing ganglion cells, when in fact, the sample is simply inadequate. Rectal biopsies must be carefully oriented and sectioned serially so that the entire tissue may be examined for the presence of ganglion cells. Normally, only a very few of the serial cuts will show the presence of these cells. The ganglion cells in neonates are often somewhat immature and difficult to recognize unless the specimen is examined by an experienced pediatric pathologist. Cholinesterase staining may be used to make the examination of the tissue a bit easier but, again in inexperienced hands, may result in erroneous interpretation. In our laboratory, hematoxylin and eosin (H & E) staining of the tissue with serial sectioning has been a reliable method of making the diagnosis.

The disorder can also be diagnosed by performing anorectal manometry. A balloon is inflated in the rectum as the pressure of the internal and external anal sphincters is continuously monitored, either with a pressure transducer or perfused catheter. Inflation of the balloon in the rectum in a normal patient will result in relaxation of the internal anal sphincter followed by contraction of the external anal sphincter. In the patient with Hirschsprung disease, the internal anal sphincter does not relax with distention of the rectum. Again, the technique requires an experienced practitioner to be a reliable means of excluding the diagnosis.

TREATMENT

In an otherwise well child with the common form of short segment Hirschsprung disease, a one-stage pull-through operation in the newborn period is the procedure of choice, provided that the child can be kept adequately decompressed for the first few (7 to 10) days of life. A one-stage pull-through in experienced hands is simple, has excellent results, and is typically the standard of care in most institutions. There are several pull-through techniques including the Rehbein, Swenson, Soave, and Duhamel procedures. A staged pull-through is required only for very long segment involvement or if there are other complicating issues. If a staged procedure is performed, a colostomy is placed above the aganglionic segment, which can be identified histologically by frozen sections at the time of surgery. At a later date, a pull-through operation can be performed and the ostomy closed once function has been restored.

Laparoscopic mobilization with transanal anastomosis (thus avoiding abdominal incision) is being adopted by experienced pediatric laparoscopists in selected cases. For short-segment Hirschsprung disease, recent literature suggests that experienced pediatric surgeons have success with a completely transanal procedure. In all cases the external sphincter is left intact, and with removal of the entire aganglionic colon a reasonably normal defecation pattern is usually established. Chronic soiling or persistent constipation is often present, even long after rehabilitation from surgery. In most cases there is no way of restoring an effective internal anal sphincter, so the defecation mechanism is anatomically abnormal and the function achieved is highly variable. Consequently, some children may require long-term laxation; others may need occasional suppositories, although others may require antidiarrheal medications, anal dilations, or combinations of all of these.

Hirschsprung enterocolitis is a particularly difficult situation. In this instance, the infant will develop colonic dilation and bloody diarrhea. In some instances, a catheter may be inserted through the aganglionic segment more proximally and the colon may be lavaged until a colostomy can be performed. In other instances, an emergency colostomy is indicated. Enterocolitis can also occur after surgery due primarily to anal stenosis. Often medical management with antibiotics and anti-inflammatory medications are useful at this time.

Common Pitfalls

- Failure to consider the possibility of Hirschsprung disease in the child with severe enterocolitis and bloody diarrhea. Hirschsprung disease should always be considered immediately in such infants.
- In the early neonatal period, the barium enema is an unreliable means of making the diagnosis. Outside of the neonatal period, a transition zone can usually be identified.
- Barium enema studies, when performed for constipation, should be performed unprepped. Occasionally, radiologists will state in the report that they cannot exclude the possibility of ultra-short segment Hirschsprung disease. Such a report does not necessarily mean they suspect Hirschsprung disease; the radiologist is just stating that the examination cannot completely exclude it. In the absence of a dilated colon with a transition zone, it is quite unlikely that the patient would have

Hirschsprung disease. However, an adequate biopsy or an anorectal motility study would be required to definitely establish a diagnosis.

Communication and Counseling

It is very important to counsel parents prior to surgery that the outcome is highly variable and that the child will probably never achieve totally normal colonic function. It also may be advisable to consider genetic counseling in families with a history of Hirschsprung disease and in those at risk for a child with congenital anomalies such as Down syndrome.

SUGGESTED READINGS

1. Badner JA, Sieber WK, Garver KL, Chakravarti A: A genetic study of Hirschsprung disease. Am J Hum Genet 46(3):568–580, 1990. **A study demonstrating that aganglionosis beyond the sigmoid colon has dominant gene penetrance, whereas if aganglionosis is below the sigmoid colon, the cause is multifactorial or due to a recessive gene.**
2. Berman CZ: Roentgenographic manifestations of congenital megacolon (Hirschsprung disease) in early infancy. Pediatrics 18(2):227–238, 1956. **Classic paper on radiographic appearance.**
3. Bonnard A, de Lagausie P, Leclair MD, et al: Definitive treatment of extended Hirschsprung's disease or total colonic form. Surg Endosc 15(11):1301–1304, 2001. **This paper concludes that the laparoscopic procedure is safe and feasible.**
4. Classic Articles in Colonic and Rectal Surgery. Constipation in the newborn as a result of dilation and hypertrophy of the colon: Harald Hirschsprung, Jahrbuch fur Kinderheilkunde, 1888. Dis Colon Rectum 24(5):408–410, 1981. **Classic paper on the initial description of Hirschsprung disease.**
5. Di Lorenzo C, Colletti RB, Lehman HP, et al: Functional gastrointestinal disorders, gastroesophageal reflux and neurogastroenterology: Working Group report of the second World Congress of Pediatric Gastroenterology, Hepatology, and Nutrition. J Pediatr Gastroenterol Nutr 39(Suppl 2):S616-S625, 2004. **A review of the differential diagnostic features for children with intestinal motility problems.**
6. Elhalaby EA, Teitelbaum DH, Coran AG, Heidelberger KA: Enterocolitis associated with Hirschsprung's disease: A clinical-radiological characterization based on 168 patients. J Pediatr Surg 30(1):76–83, 1995. **This study suggests that it is important to identify whether histopathologic mucosal changes exist in Hirschsprung disease even in the absence of overt symptoms as it affects treatment plans.**
7. Lal DR, Nichol PF, Harms BA, et al: Ileo-anal S-pouch reconstruction in patients with total colonic aganglionosis after failed pull-through procedure. J Pediatr Surg 39(7):e7-e9, 2004. **These authors present a new surgical approach to patients with Hirschsprung disease and previous poor surgical repair.**
8. Langer JC, Durrant AC, de laTorre L, et al: One-stage transanal Soave pullthrough for Hirschsprung disease: a multicenter experience with 141 children. Ann Surg 238(4):569–583; discussion 583–585, 2003. **These authors review the surgical findings of a large group of children undergoing the Soave pull-through procedure for Hirschsprung disease.**
9. Lewis NA, Levitt MA, Zallen GS, et al: Diagnosing Hirschsprung's disease: Increasing the odds of a positive rectal biopsy result. J Pediatr Surg 38(3):412–416, 2003. **This paper demonstrates that key features in the patient's history and examination can predict with great accuracy the diagnosis of Hirschsprung disease versus idiopathic constipation.**
10. Nakao M, Suita S, Taguchi T, et al: Fourteen-year experience of acetylcholinesterase staining for rectal mucosal biopsy in neonatal Hirschsprung disease. J Pediatr Surg 36(9):1357–1363, 2001. **This paper describees the low sensitivity and high specificity of acetylcholinesterase staining for Hirschsprung disease.**
11. Proctor ML, Traubici J, Langer JC, et al: Correlation between radiographic transition zone and level of aganglionosis in Hirschsprung's disease: Implications for surgical approach. J Pediatr Surg 38(5):775–778, 2003. **This paper describes a 90% correlation between the presnce of a radiographic transition zone and aganglionosis and suggests caution to be used when planning a one-stage pull-through.**
12. Soave F: Hirschsprung's disease. Technique and results of Soave's operation. Br J Surg 53(12):1023–1027, 1966. **The initial description of the Soave operation for Hirschsprung disease.**
13. Solari V, Ennis S, Yoneda A, et al: Mutation analysis of the RET gene in total intestinal aganglionosis by wave DNA fragment analysis system. J Pediatr Surg 38(3):497–501, 2003. **Paper on the RET gene and its involvement in Hirschsprung disease.**
14. Swenson O: Congenital megacolon (Hirschsprung's disease); follow-up on eighty-two patients treated surgically. Pediatrics 8(4):542–547, 1951. **Follow-up on surgical experience.**
15. Walker W, Goulet O, Kleinman RE, et al: Hirschprung disease. In Imseis E, Garipey CE (eds): Pediatric Gastrointestinal Disease, 4th ed, vol I. Hamilton, Ontario, Canada: BC Decker, 2004, pp 1031–1043. **A review chapter on the pediatric gastroenterologist's current understanding of the disease.**

Gastroesophageal Reflux

Lynnette J. Mazur and Holly D. Smith

KEY CONCEPTS

- In infants, feeding history should include the amount and frequency (overfeeding/overeating), types of formula, food, and positioning. The pattern of vomiting (frequency, amount, and its association with pain or forcefulness) should be assessed. Warning signs include bilious vomiting and hematemesis.
- In older children, a detailed history of pain character, location, exacerbating and ameliorating factors, and its association with meals or food intake should be obtained.
- The past medical history of infants and young children should include birth history and surgical interventions.
- The family history should include gastrointestinal problems and metabolic or allergic illness in parents or siblings.
- The physical examination should include the height and weight percentiles for all ages.
- Diagnostic tests that are important for assessing gastroesophageal reflux (GER):
  - Upper gastrointestinal series—Useful to evaluate anatomical abnormalities such as pyloric stenosis, malrotation, annular pancreas, hiatal hernia, and esophageal stricture. It is neither sufficiently sensitive nor specific to diagnose GER disease (GERD).
  - Esophageal pH monitoring—Considered the standard criterion for assessing GER.
  - The reflux index, the percentage of time that the pH is less than 4, is the most sensitive parameter. Unable to detect nonacidic GER.
  - Multiple intraluminal electrical impedance—A pH-independent technique based on the registration of gastrointestinal motility. Useful for evaluating GER-related symptoms that are not associated with acidic

reflux. Detects the height of the refluxate in the esophagus.

- Endoscopy and biopsy—Detects the consequences of GER such as esophagitis, strictures, and Barrett esophagus. It is not useful for detecting early disease.
- Scintigraphy—Detects aspiration of gastric contents.
- For infants with uncomplicated GER, no tests are necessary. Parental education and reassurance are usually all that are needed. Thickening of formula and a 1- to 2-week trial of a hypoallergenic formula may be considered.
- For infants with GERD, the differential diagnosis includes food hypersensitivity, intestinal obstruction, metabolic disorders, neurologic disorders, or a urinary tract infection. It may be necessary to obtain a complete blood count, electrolytes, and other appropriate diagnostic tests. A modified barium swallow to assess swallowing, an upper gastrointestinal series, and esophageal pH monitoring may also be helpful. Additional treatments such as lifestyle changes, medications, or surgery are needed to minimize morbidity.

Gastroesophageal reflux (GER) is the retrograde passage of gastric contents into the esophagus. GER disease (GERD) includes symptoms or complications of GER such as abdominal or substernal pain, apnea, dysphagia, esophagitis, failure to thrive, other respiratory disorders, and/or vomiting. Population-based surveys indicate that although regurgitation occurs in up to two thirds of all infants younger than 6 months of age at least once per day, less than 5% have symptoms beyond 1 year of age. The fact that few parents intervene when GER occurs is evidence that it is a normal physiologic event—only 8% change formulas, 2% thicken the feedings, 1% terminate breastfeeding, and fewer than 1% use medication. A good history and physical examination are sufficient to permit health care providers to diagnose GER reliably, and to recognize most complications and initiate management in most infants with GER and older children with epigastric pain and heartburn.

Expert Opinion on Management Issues

For infants, thickened formula improves observable GER (Fig. 1). Thickening slows gastric emptying time and maintains a neutral pH in the stomach for a longer period of time, making the refluxate less injurious to the esophageal mucosa. One teaspoon of rice cereal added to 1 ounce of formula results in a caloric density of about 25 kcal per ounce. Studies that use subjective outcomes (parental report or reflux diary) report improved GER, decreased crying, and awake time in most children. When objective esophageal pH monitoring (EpHM) is used, the results are less convincing; only a few of the parameters show improvement.

Milk composition also influences the occurrence of GER. Human milk is associated with the fastest emptying time and lessens GER. Formula and cow's milk are associated with much slower emptying times and generally worsen GER. Because cow's milk protein

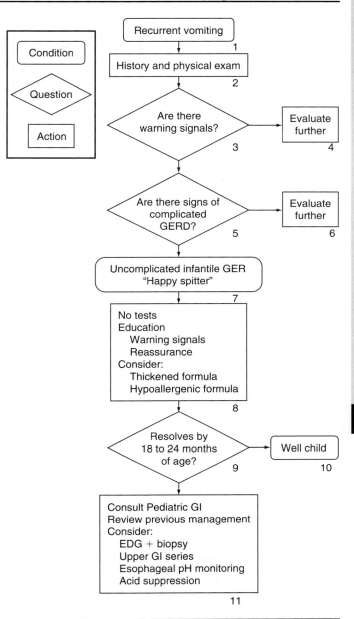

FIGURE 1. Management of an infant with uncomplicated gastroesophageal reflux (GER) disease ("happy spitter"). EGD, esophagogastroduodenoscopy; GI, gastrointestinal.

allergy may mimic the symptoms of GER, a time-limited trial of a hypoallergenic formula may be used.

It is well-known that the prone position is the best position for the alleviation of GER. However, because the prone sleep position is associated with a higher rate of the sudden infant death syndrome (SIDS), the risk of death should be considered when placing children on their stomachs to decrease GER. Other studies show that elevation of the head is not worth the trouble and that infant seats increase GER. In older children there is likely benefit to a left side positioning (Fig. 2).

Lifestyle changes are often recommended therapy for GER in adults. These include avoidance of alcohol, caffeine, and chocolate; limiting fat intake; weight loss; and cessation of smoking. Because most studies

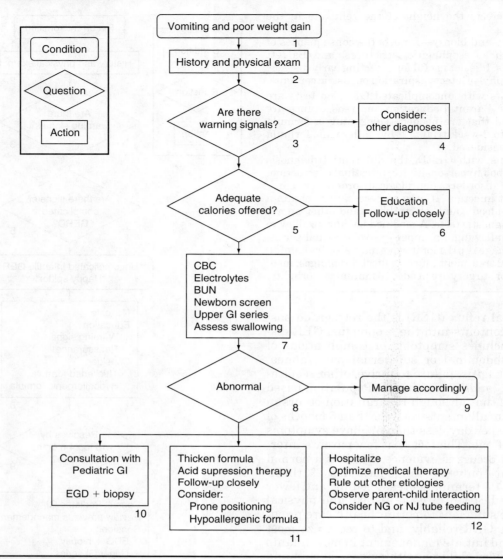

FIGURE 2. Management of an infant with vomiting and poor weight gain. BUN, blood urea nitrogen; CBC, complete blood count; EGD, esophagogastroduodenoscopy; GI, gastrointestinal; NG, nasogastric; NJ, nasojejunal.

of lifestyle changes have been performed in adults, their applicability to children and adolescents remains indeterminate (Fig. 3). Thus, whether lifestyle changes have an additive benefit in young patients receiving pharmacologic therapy is unproven. However, based on the available evidence, it is best to recommend against alcohol, caffeine, and tobacco use, which most likely worsen GER and are otherwise generally contraindicated. Weight loss may help and is recommended if that is an issue.

PHARMACOTHERAPY OF GASTROESOPHAGEAL REFLUX

Pharmacologic agents include acid suppressants and prokinetic agents. The H_2-receptor antagonists cimetidine, ranitidine, famotidine, and/or nizatidine have traditionally been the first-line acid suppressants. Studies on H_2-receptor antagonists suggest that these agents are more effective than antacids but less effective than proton pump inhibitors (PPIs). Additionally, tolerance develops over time, and increasing doses are required to achieve continued benefit.

Prokinetic agents such as bethanecol, domperidone, and metoclopramide improve both clinical and EpHM parameters. However, they are no more effective than antacids. Adverse effects such as bronchospasm, diarrhea, irritability, and tremor (bethanecol); tardive dyskinesia (rigidity and oculogyric crisis) and potentially irreversible parkinsonian reactions (metoclopramide) limit their usefulness in children. A more recent prokinetic agent, cisapride, is no longer recommended because of its association with prolongation of the QT_c or JT_c, malignant ventricular arrhythmias, and sudden death.

PPIs inhibit acid secretion by inhibiting the enzyme responsible for the final step in the secretion of hydrochloric acid by the gastric parietal cell (the acid pump).

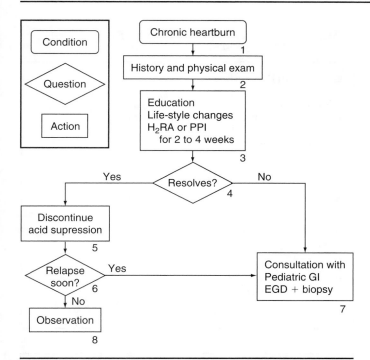

FIGURE 3. Management of a child or adolescent with chronic heartburn. EGD, esophagogastroduodenoscopy; GI, gastrointestinal; H_2RA, histamine–2 receptor antagonist; PPI, proton pump inhibitor.

Acid secretion is inhibited until more enzyme is synthesized, which accounts for its long duration of action (more than 24 hours). Comparison studies with H_2-receptor antagonists show that both agents are effective in decreasing clinical symptoms, improving the histological degree of esophagitis, and reducing esophageal acid exposure; however, PPIs are more effective.

Common Pitfalls

■ Overuse of diagnostic laboratory and imaging techniques in GER results in unnecessary costs and radiation.
■ Overtreatment of GER results in unnecessary costs and side effects of medications, formula changes, and undue parental anxiety.
■ Undertreatment of GERD may lead to asthma, Barrett intestinal metaplasia of the esophagus, chronic aspiration, esophagitis, growth failure, and strictures.
■ It is risky to use pharmacologic agents with no proven benefit in children yet have the risk of side effects.

Communication and Counseling

■ In infants with GER, encourage breastfeeding. Thickened formula can be suggested for symptomatic relief.
■ H_2-recepor antagonists and PPIs but not other medications have been shown to be safe and

effective for the treatment of GERD and its complications in infants and children.

SUGGESTED READINGS

1. Nelson SP, Chen EH, Syniar GM, et al: Prevalence of symptoms of gastroesophageal reflux during infancy: a pediatric practice-based survey. Arch Pediatr Adolesc Med 151:569–572. **Population-based study on the prevalence of gastroesophageal reflux in the real world of private practice pediatrics.**
2. Nelson SP, Chen EH, Syniar GM, et al: One-year follow-up of symptoms of gastroesophageal reflux during infancy. Pediatrics 102:6/e67, 1998. **Follow-up of the authors' previous study.**
3. Rudolph C, Mazur LJ, Liptak GS, et al: Guidelines for evaluation and treatment of gastroesophageal reflux in infants and children: Recommendations of the North American Society for Pediatric Gastroenterology and Nutrition. J Pediatr Gastroenterol Nutr 32:S1-S31, 2001. **A systematic review of the literature and evidence-based guidelines for the diagnosis and treatment of gastroesophageal reflux in infants and children.**
4. Wenzl TG: Evaluation of gastroesophageal reflux events in children using multichannel intraluminal electrical impedance. Am J Med 115(3A):161S–165S, 2003. **A review of a new diagnostic test for GER with comparison to the intraesophageal pH monitoring (EpHM).**

Gastritis and Peptic Ulcer Disease

Michael A. Manfredi and Esther Jacobowitz Israel

10

KEY CONCEPTS

■ Primary peptic ulcer disease is very rare in children younger than 10 years, and most cases in this age group are related to secondary causes.
■ Most children with symptoms of dyspepsia do not have peptic ulcer disease or gastritis. They more likely have nonulcer dyspepsia.
■ Clinical symptoms of peptic disease are poor predictors of actual pathology. Therefore, upper gastrointestinal endoscopy with mucosal biopsy is the investigation of choice for the diagnosis of gastritis and peptic ulcer disease.
■ Minimally invasive tests such as the urea breath test and stool monoclonal antibody test show promise as diagnostic tests for ***Helicobacter pylori*** in children, although further clinical studies are necessary to establish their efficacy.
■ Proton pump inhibitors, when compared to other treatments, including H_2 antagonists, are the most effective medication in healing peptic ulcer disease.

The term *peptic disease* includes both gastritis and peptic ulcer disease, closely related entities that exist on a continuous disease spectrum. Gastritis is thought to be a precursor event leading to ulcer disease. The prevalence of peptic ulcer disease in the adult population is estimated at 5% to 10% but is not well characterized in children. A study from Toronto estimated that 1 in 2500 pediatric hospital admissions was secondary to gastric or duodenal ulcers. The incidence of gastritis without ulcer disease in children is also not well defined.

Peptic ulcer disease occurs when there is an imbalance in the stomach between the so-called aggressive factors, such as hydrochloric acid, pepsin, nonsteroidal anti-inflammatory drugs (NSAIDs), bile acids, stress, smoking, *Helicobacter pylori*, and the so-called protective factors, such as mucus, bicarbonate, mucosal blood flow, prostaglandins, and the mucosal hydrophobic layer.

Gastritis and peptic ulcer disease can be divided into primary and secondary, based on etiology. Most cases of primary gastritis and duodenal ulcers are related to a gastric infection with the gram-negative spiral organism *H. pylori*. Primary peptic ulcer disease is rare in children younger than 10 years, and most cases in this age group are related to secondary causes. The prevalence of primary peptic ulcer disease increases during adolescence.

Approximately 50% of the world population is infected with *H. pylori*. The prevalence varies widely by age, country, ethnic background, and socioeconomic status. *H. pylori* is most commonly acquired during childhood, with up to 70% of children in developing countries infected by 15 years of age. In the United States, the overall prevalence of *H. pylori* infection is low; only 10% of children are infected at 10 years of age. Transmission is believed to occur by fecal–oral, gastric–oral, and oral–oral routes, with increasing evidence that contaminated water is a potential source of transmission.

Secondary gastritis and peptic ulcer disease generally occur as a result of a stressor that disrupts the normal homeostasis of the stomach. These stressors can cause erosive and/or hemorrhagic damage to the gastrointestinal mucosa or nonerosive damage. Box 1 lists some of the causes of secondary gastritis and peptic ulcer disease.

Gastritis is defined as inflammation of the gastric mucosa. A common misconception is that gastritis is diagnosed clinically when in fact it is a histologic diagnosis. Peptic ulcers are defined as deep mucosal lesions that disrupt the muscularis mucosa of the stomach or duodenum. More than 90% of duodenal ulcers are found within the duodenal bulb. *H. pylori* is found in the antral mucosa of almost 90% of children with duodenal ulcer disease, although only 15% of people colonized with *H. pylori* ever develop ulcers. Gastric ulcers, however, are more commonly associated with secondary peptic disease.

Clinical Presentation

The clinical presentation of peptic disease in children varies with age. Box 2 lists signs and symptoms associated with peptic disease. Children older than 10 years usually describe symptoms of dyspepsia, similar to adults. Dyspepsia is defined as abdominal pain or fullness in the upper abdomen, usually in the epigastric area. Young children usually are unable to localize

---

BOX 1   Causes of Secondary Peptic Disease in Children

Erosive and Hemorrhagic*
- Stress (shock, acidosis, sepsis, hypoxemia, burns, major surgery, multiorgan system failure, head injury)
- Trauma (from forceful retching and vomiting)
- Aspirin and nonsteroidal anti-inflammatory drugs
- Other drugs (antibiotics, steroids)
- Alcohol
- Bile
- Henoch-Schönlein purpura
- Exercise-induced
- Radiation.

Nonerosive Gastritis
- Allergic gastritis
- Inflammatory bowel disease
- Celiac disease
- Graft-versus-host disease
- Menetrier disease
- Pernicious anemia.

*There may be some overlap in these two groups.

BOX 2   Signs and Symptoms of Peptic Disease

- Abdominal pain—epigastric in older children and periumbilical in young children
- Recurrent vomiting
- Hematemesis
- Pain awakening the child at night
- Chronic nausea
- Anorexia
- Early satiety
- Irritability with eating in young children
- Weight loss
- Melena stools
- Guaiac-positive stools
- Anemia.

---

abdominal pain. They are more likely to present with periumbilical abdominal pain and symptoms of anorexia, vomiting, and irritability associated with meals. Pain severe enough to awaken a child from sleep is also suggestive of peptic disease. Gastrointestinal tract bleeding, either hematemesis or occult blood in the stool, may be the presenting symptom in some children. Most children with symptoms of dyspepsia do not actually have peptic ulcer disease or gastritis, hence the term *nonulcer dyspepsia*. Box 3 lists the differential diagnoses of dyspepsia. Figure 1 presents an algorithm for the evaluation of epigastric abdominal pain.

Expert Opinion on Management Issues

DIAGNOSIS OF GASTRITIS AND PEPTIC ULCER DISEASE

Clinical symptoms of peptic disease are poor predictors of actual disease. Laboratory findings, such as a low hematocrit, low albumin, or elevated erythrocyte sedimentation rate (ESR) may serve as red flags for systemic disease. Barium studies of the upper gastrointestinal tract may fail to identify duodenal ulceration in up to 86% of children, and gastritis is very poorly defined on radiographic contrast studies. Therefore, upper gastrointestinal endoscopy with mucosal biopsy is the investigation of choice for the diagnosis of gastritis and peptic ulcer disease. Endoscopy may also be therapeutic if an active bleeding ulcer is found. Histologic assessment of mucosal biopsy samples is the gold standard for diagnosing infection with the *H. pylori* organism.

DIAGNOSIS OF *HELICOBACTER PYLORI*

Testing for *H. pylori* infection in children is a controversial topic. Abdominal pain in children is a common complaint; however, studies indicate that *H. pylori* is

> **BOX 3 Differential Diagnoses of Dyspepsia**
>
> - Peptic ulcer disease
> - Gastroesophageal reflux disease (GERD)
> - Cholelithiasis
> - Cholecystitis
> - Pancreatitis
> - Lactose intolerance
> - Hypercalcemia or hyperkalemia
> - Medication induced
> - Parasite infection
> - Inflammatory bowel disease
> - Functional.

seldom the cause of these symptoms. In addition, treatment of children who have nonulcer gastritis associated with *H. pylori* has no proven benefit for relief of abdominal pain. Because of the potential overuse of *H. pylori* treatment in children, an international consensus conference held in 2000 published statements specifically focused on the approach to *H. pylori* infection in children and adolescents. The following conclusions were reached by this conference:

- Screening of children with dyspeptic symptoms for *H. pylori* infection with noninvasive tests is neither indicated nor recommended.
- Screening for *H. pylori* infection in individuals without symptoms is not indicated.
- Children should be evaluated for *H. pylori* infection only when organic disease is suggested by their constellation of signs and symptoms; thus the goal of diagnostic evaluations should be to determine the cause of presenting clinical symptoms and not the presence of *H. pylori* infection.

Minimally invasive methods used in the diagnosis of *H. pylori* infection include serology, urea breath test, and stool antigen testing.

Serology

Infection with *H. pylori* provokes a specific serum immunoglobulin (Ig) G response and takes a while to develop. Serologic tests to detect the presence of *H. pylori* in blood and saliva have both a low sensitivity and specificity in children younger than 12 years of age. Thus the validity of looking at serology in younger

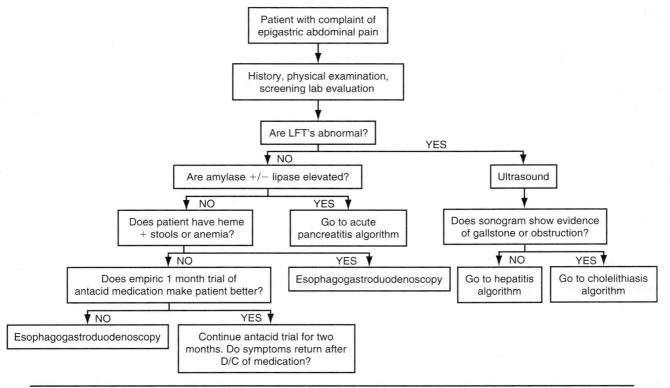

FIGURE 1. Algorithm for evaluating epigastric abdominal pain.

children is questionable, and standardized serologic levels in children are not set. In addition, immunoglobulin (Ig) G levels may remain elevated for years after resolution of the bacteria; therefore a positive test does not imply active disease but rather exposure. No data support treatment of a positive antibody titer. A negative *H. pylori* antibody titer does not exclude the possibility of *H. pylori* infection.

Urea Breath Tests

The ^{13}C urea breath test is a safe and noninvasive method for the diagnosis of *H. pylori* infection. If *H. pylori* is present in the stomach, breakdown of the labeled urea by *H. pylori* urease results in production of labeled carbon dioxide, which is measured in the expired air. This test is 100% sensitive and 92% specific for the diagnosis of *H. pylori* infection in older children. In young children the false-positive rate may be high because of retention of air in the mouth, which also contains urease-producing organisms. The North American Society for Pediatric Gastroenterology, Hepatology, and Nutrition (NASPGHN) does not currently recommend the urea breath test for the diagnosis and treatment of *H. pylori* in children because a positive result does not necessarily denote ulcer disease, and it is not clear that *H. pylori* gastritis needs to be treated in every individual. However, many practitioners, particularly in nonendemic areas, treat a positive breath test rather than follow the guidelines, which suggest performing an endoscopy to identify ulcer disease.

The urea breath test is an excellent tool for assessing treatment success in children. The breath test should be carried out at least 1 month after treatment completion to document resolution of the infection.

Stool Antigen Enzyme Immunoassay

H. pylori antigens in the stool can be detected with immunoassays using monoclonal antibodies. The initial studies in children show a sensitivity of 98% and a specificity of 99% with a positive predictive value of 98%. This test needs further investigation in children younger than 2 years and for evaluation of eradication of the bacteria after treatment. However, this test appears to be a promising diagnostic tool in children. Once again, the presence of *H. pylori* in the stool does not denote ulcer disease, and therefore guidelines do not suggest therapy just on the basis of its presence in stool.

TREATMENT

Disease Associated with *Helicobacter pylori*

Box 4 lists the indications for *H. pylori* treatment for children with proven infection. The treatment of children colonized with *H. pylori* without peptic ulcer disease is a controversial topic. NASPGHN currently does not recommend treatment for *H. pylori colonization*. However, practitioners frequently stray from the guidelines and treat *H. pylori* even in the absence of

---

> **BOX 4 Guidelines for Treatment of Children with Proven *Helicobacter pylori* Infection**
>
> **Definitive Indications for Treatment**
> - Peptic ulcer disease
> - Mucosa-associated lymphoid tissue (MALT) lymphoma
> - Atrophic gastritis with intestinal metaplasia
> - Iron-deficiency anemia unexplained by other causes
>
> **Consider Treatment (because there is insufficient evidence to support or withhold treatment)**
> - Gastritis without ulcer disease
> - First-degree relative with gastric cancer
>
> **Currently Not Indicated**
> - Recurrent abdominal pain symptoms without peptic disease
> - Asymptomatic colonization with *H. pylori*
> - Cancer prevention without family history

> **BOX 5 First-Line Treatment for *Helicobacter pylori****
>
> Each regimen should be administered twice daily for 10 to 14 days:
> - PPI (1–2 mg/kg/day) + amoxicillin (50 mg/kg/day) + clarithromycin (15 mg/kg/day)
> - PPI (1–2 mg/kg/day) + amoxicillin (50 mg/kg/day) + metronidazole (20 mg/kg/day)
> - PPI (1–2 mg/kg/day) + metronidazole (20 mg/kg/day) + clarithromycin (15 mg/kg/day)
>
> ---
> *Based on North American Society for Pediatric Gastroenterology, Hepatology, and Nutrition Recommendations.
> PPI, proton pump inhibitor.

---

ulcer disease. NASPGHN leaves certain clinical settings such as *H. pylori* gastritis and colonization with a family history of gastric cancer up to the discretion of the clinician because there is insufficient evidence to take a position on these two topics.

Box 5 lists the current treatment regimens recommended by the North American Society for Pediatric Gastroenterology and Nutrition. All medications in the regimens should be administered twice daily for 10 to 14 days. Eradication of the infection results in resolution of the gastritis and long-term healing of ulcer disease. The incidence of *H. pylori* resistance to metronidazole and clarithromycin is increasing, and new regimens are being developed.

Non–*Helicobacter pylori* Gastritis and Ulcer Disease

The treatment of non–*H. pylori* peptic disease consists of treating or removing the underlying trigger causing the disease. A high level of acid in the stomach is almost never the underlying cause of peptic disease; however, suppression of acid levels is useful in treating the symptoms as well as healing the mucosa in peptic disease. Treatment with an acid suppression medication for 4 weeks heals ulcers. Different classes of medications are available to treat peptic disease. Table 1 lists recommended doses for each medication.

TABLE 1 Medications for Treating Peptic Ulcer Disease

Medication	Pediatric Dose	Adult Dose
Antacids		
Aluminum/magnesium hydroxide	0.5 mL/kg/dose q3–6h given 1 h after meals and at bedtime	15–45 mL/dose q3–6h, given 1 hr after meals and at bedtime
H₂ Receptor Antagonists		
Cimetidine	Infants: 10–20 mg/kg/day PO/IV div q6h Children: 20–40 mg/kg/day PO/IV div q6h	300 mg PO/IV q6h
Famotidine	Children: 1–2 mg/kg/day PO/IV div q8–12h	20–40 mg/day PO/IV div qd-bid
Ranitidine	Children 2–6 mg/kg/day PO div q8h-q12h 3–4 mg/kg/day IV div q6–8h	150 mg PO bid 50 mg IV q6–8h
Nizatidine	Infants from 6 mo of age to children: 5–10 mg/kg/day div bid	150 mg PO bid
Proton Pump Inhibitors		
Omeprazole	0.5–1.5 mg/kg/day PO div qd-bid Recommended starting dose: 1 mg/kg/day PO QD (10 mg for children 10–20 kg and 20 mg for >20 kg)	10–20 mg PO qd-bid
Lansoprazole	1–2 mg/kg/day PO div qd-bid Recommended starting dose: 1 mg/kg/day PO qd (15 mg for children 15–29 kg) and 30 mg for those >30 kg)	15–30 mg PO qd-bid
Cytoprotective Agent		
Sucralfate	40–80 mg/kg/day div qid	1 g PO qid

bid, twice daily; div, divided; IV, intravenously; PO, by mouth; q*x*h, every *x* hours; qd, every day; qid, four times per day.

10

Antacids

Antacids can be beneficial for symptomatic relief of gastritis and peptic ulcer disease; however, their role in healing is limited. Antacids may also be associated with adverse side effects. Magnesium-based antacids can cause diarrhea, whereas the use of aluminum-containing antacids may result in constipation, hypophosphatemia, and hypocalcemia. Aluminum-containing antacids should not be used in infants and children with impaired renal function. Antacids given concurrently with proton pump inhibitors (PPIs) may lower their efficacy. PPIs should be administered 1 hour before or 2 hours after an antacid.

Prostaglandin Analogues

Misoprostol, a synthetic prostaglandin, acts on the gastric mucosa to increase blood flow and bicarbonate secretion. It also markedly increases the production of mucus. This medication therefore increases the protective factors for the gastric mucosa. It is effective in preventing peptic disease related to use of NSAIDs and aspirin. Misoprostol must not be given to patients who are pregnant, however, because it may lead to miscarriage. The drug often causes diarrhea, which is difficult to manage, thus limiting its use.

Coating and Binding Agents

Sucralfate is a sulfated disaccharide aluminum salt, which splits into negatively charged aluminum and other component particles when ingested. These particles become attracted to the injured mucosa with an affinity six to eight times that for normal epithelium. The particles coat damaged gastric or duodenal mucosa, insulating it and protecting it from further damage to allow the natural healing process to occur. Sucralfate is indicated in the treatment of gastric and duodenal ulcers. Sucralfate can interfere with the absorption of PPIs and lower their efficacy if both are administered concurrently. PPIs should be administered 1 hour before or 3 hours after sucralfate.

H₂ Receptor Antagonists

H₂ receptor antagonists offer a safe method of healing peptic ulcers. These agents can be very effective in the acute treatment of gastritis and peptic ulcers and provide rapid symptomatic relief. H₂ receptor antagonists have no antibacterial effect and do not heal chronic gastritis associated with *H. pylori*. These medications may be associated with rare adverse reactions, including gynecomastia, reversible liver disease, and confusion. These agents can also be used intravenously, which is particularly helpful in patients who present in acute situations where enteral intake is being withheld.

Proton Pump Inhibitors

PPIs inhibit the gastric acid pump (hydrogen/potassium exchanging adenosine triphosphatase [H^+,K^+-ATPase]). They are the most potent inhibitors of gastric acid secretion available. In adult studies, PPIs are the most effective medication in healing peptic ulcer disease. PPIs are effective in preventing peptic disease related to NSAIDs and aspirin. The two most studied

PPIs in children are omeprazole and lansoprazole. PPIs are now available in both liquid and capsule form. In addition, lansoprazole is now available in a fast-dissolving tablet administered sublingually. The PPIs pantoprazole and lansoprazole are available in intravenous form; however, there are no current recommended pediatric dosages.

PPIs are well tolerated. Uncommon side effects include headache, diarrhea, abdominal pain, and nausea, but they are generally self-limited. Bacterial overgrowth in the stomach and small intestine by oral and colonic flora is reported, and the inhibition of gastric acid secretion raises concerns regarding vitamin B_{12} malabsorption and iron deficiency anemia. Patients on prolonged PPI therapy should have their vitamin B_{12} and iron levels checked.

Common Pitfalls

- Gastritis and ulcer disease are commonly over-diagnosed based on clinical symptoms when, in fact, they are both a tissue diagnosis.
- Patients with abdominal pain should have their stool evaluated for occult blood because that raises the suspicion for the presence of true gastritis or peptic ulcer disease.
- The diagnosis and treatment of H. pylori infection based on blood serology tests regardless of symptoms or family history is neither indicated nor recommended.
- Close follow-up is needed to make sure children are compliant with taking triple therapy for H. pylori eradication. Lack of compliance with H. pylori therapy may lead to drug resistance. The urea breath test can be used to monitor efficacy of treatment.

Communication And Counseling

Peptic disease is uncommon in children and can be treated effectively with medication. Epigastric abdominal pain, however, is a very common complaint in children. Figure 1 provides an algorithm for the evaluation and management of the patient with epigastric abdominal pain. Children with symptoms consistent with peptic disease may benefit from a trial of an H_2 antagonist or PPI for 2 to 4 weeks. A lack of improvement on the medication or the inability to wean the medication is an indication for referral to a specialist. Patients with a history of hematemesis, melena, occult blood in the stool, anemia, and/or weight loss should be referred sooner for an endoscopic evaluation.

SELECTED READINGS

1. Dohil R, Hassall E: Gastritis: Other causes. In Walker WA, Goulet O, Kleinman RE, et al (eds): Pediatric Gastrointestinal Disease. St. Louis: Mosby, 2004, pp 513–534. **In-depth review of the pathophysiology of non–H. pylori peptic disease.**
2. Gibbons TE, Gold BD: The use of proton pump inhibitors in children: A comprehensive review. Paediatr Drugs 5(1):25–40, 2003. **Review of the pharmacology of proton pump inhibitors as well as a review of the literature regarding the efficacy of these drugs in children.**
3. Gold BD, Colletti RB, Abbott M, et al: *Helicobacter pylori* infection in children: Recommendations for diagnosis and treatment. J Pediatr Gastroenterol Nutr 31:490–497, 2000. **The NASPGHAN position statement regarding diagnosis and treatment of H. pylori.**
4. Rowland M, Bourke B, Drumm B: Gastritis: *Helicobacter pylori* and peptic ulcer disease. In Walker WA, Goulet O, Kleinman RE, et al (eds): Pediatric Gastrointestinal Disease. St. Louis: Mosby, 2004, pp 491–512. **In-depth review of the pathophysiology of H. pylori disease.**
5. Sherman PM: Appropriate strategies for testing and treating *Helicobacter pylori* in children: When and how? Am J Med 117(Suppl 5A):30S–35S, 2004. **Review of the detection, treatment, and clinical implications of H. pylori.**

Malabsorption

*James P. Keating**

KEY CONCEPTS

- Specific nutrient deficiencies may provide clues to the location of gastrointestinal involvement in a given disease because various nutrients are absorbed in different parts of the intestinal tract. Iron, calcium, and water-soluble vitamins are absorbed in the proximal portion of the small bowel. Fats, sugars, and amino acids are absorbed primarily in the jejunum and ileum. Vitamin B_{12} and bile salts are absorbed in the distal part of the ileum; the colon is responsible for efficiently absorbing water and electrolytes as well as short-chain fatty acids.
- Treatment of malabsorption ideally should be directed at eliminating the underlying condition. In the case of celiac disease, elimination of gluten in the diet results in complete restoration of intestinal function and resolution of malabsorption. In other conditions, modification or supplementation of the diet to compensate for malabsorption must continue indefinitely. Patients with pancreatic insufficiency from cystic fibrosis require pancreatic enzyme and fat-soluble vitamin supplementation for life.
- The best scheme for discussing the treatment of malabsorption is one in which each class of nutrient—carbohydrate, fat, and protein—is addressed separately.

The list of noninfectious disorders that can cause diarrhea is both extensive and varied (Box 1). Those causing malabsorption often have a tremendous impact because of their propensity to contribute to malnutrition. Malabsorption, defined as an inability to absorb a substance across the intestinal barrier, can result from incomplete digestion of food in the intestinal lumen, failure to absorb the products of digestion across the intestinal epithelium, or failure of transport of absorbed nutrients into the portal venous blood or

*Portions of this chapter are taken from the discussion on this topic in the last edition, written by Jenifer Lightdale, MD, and Alan M. Leichtner, MD.

BOX 1 Etiologies of Malabsorptive and Noninfectious Diarrhea

- Human immunodeficiency virus infection
- Postinfectious
  - Carbohydrate malabsorption
  - Malnutrition
  - Bacterial overgrowth
- Dietary
  - Excessive fluid intake
  - Inadequate fat intake
  - Milk protein hypersensitivity
  - Soy protein hypersensitivity
  - Sorbitol intolerance
  - Malnutrition
- Toddler's diarrhea
- Carbohydrate malabsorption
  - Congenital disaccharidase deficiency
  - Lactase nonpersistence
  - Secondary disaccharidase deficiency
  - Monosaccharide malabsorption
- Immune defects
  - Agammaglobulinemia
  - Isolated immunoglobulin (Ig) A deficiency
  - Combined immunodeficiency
  - Human immunodeficiency virus infection
- Autoimmune enteropathy
- Endocrine
  - Hyperthyroidism
  - Adrenal insufficiency
  - Hypoparathyroidism
  - Menses related
  - Hormone-secreting tumors
  - Diabetes mellitus
- Electrolyte transport defects
- Exercise associated
- Celiac disease
- Intestinal lymphangiectasia
- Eosinophilic gastroenteropathy
- Enterokinase deficiency
- Microvillus inclusion disease
- Pancreatic insufficiency
  - Cystic fibrosis
  - Shwachman-Diamond syndrome
  - Chronic pancreatitis
- Liver disease
- Vascular lesions
- Anatomic lesions
  - Hirschsprung disease
  - Malrotation
  - Partial small bowel obstruction
  - Short-bowel syndrome
  - Blind loop syndrome
- Inflammatory bowel disease
  - Ulcerative colitis
  - Crohn disease
- Antibiotic-associated diarrhea
- Toxic diarrhea
- Irritable bowel syndrome

BOX 2 Presentations of Celiac Disease

- Asymptomatic slow growth
- Constipation
- Iron-deficiency anemia
- Hypertransaminemia
- Depression/fatigue
- Pathologic fracture
- Recurrent intussusception
- Dermatitis herpetiformis

BOX 3 Conditions that May Cause a False-Positive Sweat Test

- Heterozygote for cystic fibrosis
- Addison disease
- Glycogen-storage disease 1
- Lysosomal storage diseases
- Localized hyperhidrosis (e.g., ectodermal dysplasia)
- Malnutrition
- Hypo- and hyperthyroidism
- Adult age

Expert Opinion on Management Issues

We now recognize an incidence of CD of 1 in 100 persons with a broad range of clinical presentations (Box 2). Screening is best done serologically using the tissue transglutaminase (tTG) antibody or the endomysial antibody (EMA), and diagnosis is established by biopsy of the small intestinal mucosa. The only available treatment is a lifelong gluten-free diet (GFD). Several groups of the very young are at special risk: children with first-degree relatives who have CD, children with Down syndrome (10% have CD), and children with diabetes mellitus (8% have CD). Surveys of children with Down syndrome indicate that most of them with CD are growing normally before diagnosis; bloating is a common but nonspecific symptom. Some experts suggest screening all children with Down syndrome and diabetes mellitus; but others, noting the difficulty of following a gluten-free diet, prefer to test only those with symptoms that might be alleviated if CD is detected. Given the burdensome aspect of the GFD and the need to maintain it for life, confirming the diagnosis by biopsy before initiating this restrictive diet is strongly recommended.

CF occurs in 1 in 4000 births. In an increasing number of states, all infants are screened for CF in the newborn period, employing some combination of serum trypsinogen, sweat chloride, and genetic testing. The Gibson-Cooke gravimetric pilocarpine electrophoresis sweat test remains the most important diagnostic study, although some affected persons are shown to have the genotype but have a negative sweat test. There are also people with elevated sweat tests who do not have CF (Box 3).

Prematurity and neonatal necrotizing enterocolitis (NNEC) with massive bowel resection results in

lymphatics. The clinical manifestations of malabsorption may be profound and include poor growth and weight loss or be more limited to the sequelae of depletion of specific micronutrients, such as vitamin B_{12} deficiency.

The cause of malabsorption in children is usually cystic fibrosis (CF), celiac disease (CD), or one of a variety of rare anatomic or infectious metabolic problems.

BOX 4 Other Causes of Malabsorption

Anatomic Causes of Malabsorption

- Congenital short (<60 cm) bowel or short bowel after surgery for malrotation
- Chronic volvulus with lymphatic or venous obstruction, also often associated with malrotation
- Stenosis and bacterial overgrowth, sometimes following repair of duodenal or ileal stenosis
- Gastrocolic fistula, often associated with prior abdominal surgery
- Bowel resection

Infections Caused by Malabsorption

- Giardiasis
- Postenteritis enteropathy
- Hepatic or intestinal capillariasis caused by *Capillaria philippinensis* (Philippines)

Metabolic Causes of Malabsorption

- Abetalipoproteinemia
- Vitamin B_{12} malabsorption (five varieties)
- Congenital chloride diarrhea
- Congenital sodium diarrhea
- Congenital bile salt malabsorption
- Hypoparathyroidism

Metabolic/Genetic Causes of Malabsorption

- Exocrine pancreatic deficiency
- Enterokinase deficiency
- Pancreatic resection (e.g., nesidioblastosis)
- Progressive familial intrahepatic cholestasis (PFIC)

malabsorption of all nutrients. These infants often receive parenteral nutrition over extended periods, even years. They sometimes develop a progressive liver injury that may lead to hepatic failure or cirrhosis that may result in death or liver transplantation. Enteral feeding, when tolerated, is usually with a chemically defined lactose-free formula. The mechanism of the liver disease remains unclear and is probably multifactorial, and the repeated infections such infants suffer play a prominent role. Some infants reach a point at which they can survive without intravenous feeding but require frequent feeding of lactose-free diet and selective supplementation. They are frequently in a precarious state, requiring intravenous supplementation during intercurrent viral illnesses. However, they often adapt over several years and can ultimately tolerate a normal or near-normal diet.

An upper gastrointestinal (GI) series with small bowel follow-through is a major part of the diagnostic strategy in pediatric malabsorption. The anatomic causes of malabsorption (Box 4) are usually identified by an experienced pediatric radiologist, often after similar studies were interpreted as normal. The progression of the contrast through the small bowel, especially the first 60 cm, must be directly observed by the radiologist, repositioning the child as needed to ascertain the position of the ligament of Treitz. Similar care in examining the lower small bowel is important to identify rare lesions causing chronic stasis and bacterial overgrowth.

Giardiasis can cause chronic malabsorption in immunocompetent as well as immunologically compromised children. Fecal *Giardia* antigen tests are much more sensitive than the traditional microscopic examination of the stool for ova and parasites. Treatment with metronidazole is recommended, although retreatment is often needed, and newer agents may prove more effective.

CARBOHYDRATE MALABSORPTION

Although newborns, especially if premature, may have difficulty with the initial steps in starch digestion, most cases of carbohydrate malabsorption in humans stem from an inability to hydrolyze disaccharides such as lactose, sucrose, and maltose. Disaccharide malabsorption can result from primary deficiencies of specific enzymes. However, more commonly, carbohydrate malabsorption in young children results from secondary disaccharidase deficiency. Infectious, allergic, inflammatory, toxic, and mechanical disorders can all damage the brush border of epithelial cells, the location where disaccharidases act on substrate. Rotavirus and *Giardia lamblia* are notable infectious causes of carbohydrate malabsorption.

Postinfectious diarrhea, or the persistence of diarrhea or weight loss for more than 7 days after the identification of gastroenteritis, commonly results from secondary disaccharidase deficiency. Among the disaccharidases affected, lactase is often the first to be depleted and the last to recover. The second most frequent deficiency is that of sucrase-isomaltase, whereas glucoamylase deficiency is seen only in the most severe mucosal injuries. Simply put, the degree of mucosal injury affects the severity of the disaccharidase deficiency and the subsequent symptoms of carbohydrate malabsorption, termed *carbohydrate intolerance*. In all cases, unabsorbed carbohydrate is fermented by enteric flora into short-chain fatty acids and other osmotically active molecules that induce secretion of electrolytes and fluid into the bowel lumen. Although the colon may scavenge some short-chain fatty acids, the result is a net loss of calories in the stool.

The clinical features of patients with carbohydrate intolerance can vary from slightly loose stools to explosive watery diarrhea, abdominal distention, and failure to thrive. In infants with mild symptoms resulting from viral gastroenteritis, no change in feeding is required. More severe cases may require a lactose-free formula or a formula with carbohydrate in the form of glucose polymers derived from rice or corn. In the most severe cases, treatment should focus on rehydration and nutritional supplementation, with avoidance of specific carbohydrates. It is imperative to avoid protracted periods of nutrient starvation, which often prolong mucosal injury and exacerbate secondary pancreatic dysfunction. In the most severe cases, elemental diets or parenteral nutrition should be used.

One highly prevalent primary enzyme deficiency is adult-type genetically determined lactase nonpersistence, which, despite its name, may occur as early as

3 years of age. In school-age children, lactase nonpersistence can occasionally even be manifested as isolated abdominal pain. Congenital lactase deficiency is extremely rare and must be distinguished from cow's milk protein allergy, which is the most common etiology of milk intolerance in infancy. Both entities can cause diarrhea and failure to gain weight, and many infants with milk protein allergy undoubtedly also have a secondary lactase deficiency that may be responsible for many of their symptoms.

In its simplest form, treatment of lactase deficiency in older children involves a lactose-restricted diet. Such a diet can be achieved by decreasing the intake of dairy products or substituting commercially available products already treated to decrease their lactose content. Both 70% and 100% lactose-free milk can be purchased. An alternative is for the patient to take enzyme supplements before ingesting diary products. In addition, older and younger patients with lactose intolerance often tolerate yogurt with active cultures, which may be used to augment clinical nutrition, decrease diarrhea, and improve weight gain. Finally, the use of probiotics such as lactobacillus GG may be found in the future to be instrumental in the treatment of older children with lactase deficiency, but such probiotics are not currently recommended routinely.

Human immunodeficiency virus (HIV) infection is directly linked to lactose and carbohydrate malabsorption in children who previously were noted to have growth deficiency of unknown etiology. Interestingly, in this population, symptoms of carbohydrate malabsorption may not be apparent. Therefore, a high index of clinical suspicion for lactose intolerance is necessary in children with HIV infection and malnutrition; such children should receive empirical therapies, including lactose-restricted diets.

Although congenital sucrase-isomaltase deficiency is present at birth, it does not become clinically apparent until the infant is introduced to fruits and fruit juices at approximately 6 months of age, and diarrhea and poor growth subsequently develop. In older children, sucrose-isomaltase deficiency may masquerade as irritable bowel syndrome. Restriction of sucrose lessens the symptoms initially, although increasing age is also associated with diminished symptoms, presumably as colonic bacterial flora and function adapt. An enzyme preparation that can hydrolyze sucrose is now available by prescription.

Consumption of fruit juices in large amounts is also associated with poor carbohydrate absorption in children without sucrase-isomaltase deficiency, usually secondary to the fructose or sorbitol present in many children's foods and soft drinks. The ensuing osmotic diarrhea may account for some cases of toddler's diarrhea and appears in children 6 months to 2 years of age. Affected children can have up to 10 loose stools a day, but they generally maintain normal growth and development. Treatment requires avoidance of the offending foods or beverages. Both pear juice and apple juice, in particular, contain high ratios of fructose to glucose and high amounts of sorbitol.

FAT MALABSORPTION

Because of the hydrophobic nature of dietary fat, digestion and absorption are complicated processes that depend not only on pancreatic lipase and its cofactor colipase but also on bile salts, which emulsify lipid droplets. The process of digestion and absorption of fats ultimately requires their hydrolysis to fatty acids and monoglycerides that are capable of diffusing through the cellular membrane. Fat malabsorption can occur secondary to any disorder that affects pancreatic function or the enterohepatic circulation of bile salts. Disorders that compromise the mucosal absorptive surface or the delivery system that re-esterifies fat and packages it into chylomicrons for export into the lymph can also cause steatorrhea.

Medium-chain triglycerides (MCTs) are digested and absorbed differently from long-chain triglycerides (LCTs) and are important in the management of children with fat malabsorption. MCTs have a lower molecular weight and are more water soluble, which in turn facilitates the action of pancreatic lipase. Thus MCTs are hydrolyzed faster and more completely than LCTs. Furthermore, even in the absence of pancreatic lipase or bile salts, a large fraction of MCTs can be absorbed as triacylglycerol and directly enter the portal venous blood rather than the lymphatics.

Patients with steatorrhea also malabsorb the fat-soluble vitamins A, D, E, and K and may have symptoms of deficiency. All children with significant fat malabsorption should be provided fat-soluble vitamin supplementation, and levels should be monitored carefully to ensure adequate treatment.

Primary pancreatic dysfunction, such as that seen in CF, recurrent pancreatitis, or Shwachman-Diamond syndrome, can lead to massive fat malabsorption and steatorrhea. These diseases can be effectively treated with pancreatic enzyme replacement therapy—optimally, lipase, 5000 IU/kg/day, preferably not exceeding 10,000 IU/kg/day. A reasonable starting dose is 1000 IU/kg/meal in children younger than 4 years and 500 IU/kg/meal in older children. The efficacy of enzyme replacement can be enhanced by enteric coating and by the use of acid blockade medications, such as H_2 antagonists or proton pump inhibitors, to optimize intraluminal pH. Excessive doses of pancreatic enzymes are associated with fibrosing colonopathy, which can result in intestinal obstruction.

Disrupted micelle function may occur as a result of an insufficient concentration of bile acids. It may result from cholestatic liver disease or ileal disease because the ileum is the site of absorption of bile acids. One example of secondarily interrupted enterohepatic circulation that can be manifested as significant steatorrhea is bacterial overgrowth, which may result from structural abnormalities such a blind intestinal loop or loss of the ileocecal valve, dysmotility, or impaired host defenses. The excess bacteria deconjugate bile acids, thereby making them less effective in forming micelles. Treatment of the underlying condition is optimal, but antibiotic therapy is often required.

PROTEIN MALABSORPTION

Although pancreatic enzymes are critical for the initial digestion of proteins, a variety of routes exist for terminal hydrolysis of peptides and their transport into the intestinal epithelial cell. Protein malabsorption rarely occurs as an isolated disorder. Rather, pancreatic insufficiency or small intestinal mucosal injury secondary to a variety of diseases, including CD and Crohn disease, is usually the culprit. Identification of the underlying disorder is therefore mandatory to treat the protein malabsorption effectively. More common than protein malabsorption is protein-losing enteropathy, which is caused by exudation across a damaged intestinal barrier or lymphatic obstruction. Loss of endogenous protein can be profound and result in hypoalbuminemia and edema.

Protein loss is frequently noted in patients with a disrupted intestinal lymphatic system, especially those with increased portal venous pressure or obstruction. Primary intestinal lymphangiectasia is characterized by diffuse or localized ectasia of the enteric lymphatics, often in association with lymphatic abnormalities elsewhere. Patients with intestinal lymphangiectasia often have excessive loss of protein into the gut or into the peritoneal cavity and, consequently, they have edema, growth failure, and a variety of GI symptoms, including steatorrhea. The mainstay of therapy for this disorder is a low-fat, high-protein diet supplemented with MCT, calcium, and fat-soluble vitamins, as needed. Antiplasmin therapy and octreotide are somewhat effective in cases of intestinal lymphangiectasia, although these treatments are still experimental.

Furthermore, patients with cardiac disease and congestive heart failure are at risk for protein loss from increased lymphatic pressure and subsequent secondary intestinal lymphangiectasia. Patients who have undergone the Fontan procedure are particularly at risk for this sequence of events; protein loss in the stool may be profound. Therapy for these patients again focuses on identification and treatment of the underlying disorder, as well as restriction of LCT and supplementation with MCT. Furthermore, corticosteroids and heparin may have a role in the treatment of protein-losing enteropathy after a Fontan procedure. Both therapies may target the inflammatory processes that contribute to lymphatic obstruction after cardiac surgery.

Common Pitfalls

- Failure to do a systematic evaluation. In all cases of diarrhea, empirical trials of antidiarrheal agents should be attempted only in patients with nonspecific, noninfectious disorders who have had a systematic evaluation for all possible infectious or inflammatory etiologies.
- Failure to recognize the potential for complications in severe diseases. Toxic megacolon may develop in patients with severe colitis or bacterial dysentery if gut transit time is decreased with antidiarrheal agents. Thus candidates for symptomatic treatment of diarrhea must be carefully selected.
- Failure to select and follow patients for whom enteral feeding or central hyperalimentation will be required.

Communication and Counseling

Malabsorption leads to troublesome symptoms. During diagnosis and therapy, it is important to work with the affected child and family to achieve nutritional stabilization and to normalize daily life as much as possible.

SUGGESTED READINGS

1. Fasano A: Clinical presentation of celiac disease in the pediatric population. Gastroenterology 128(4 Suppl 1):S68–S73, 2005. **Useful review article on clinical presentation of CD.**
2. Keating JP: Chronic diarrhea. Pediatr Rev 26(1):5–14, 2005. **Review of chronic diarrhea.**
3. Kokkonen J, Holm K, Karttunen TJ, Maki M: Enhanced local immune response in children with prolonged gastrointestinal symptoms. Acta Paediatr 93(12):1601–1607, 2004. **Discusses immune response in children with GI symptoms.**
4. Lowichik A, Book L: Pediatric celiac disease: Clinicopathologic and genetic aspects. Pediatr Dev Pathol 6(6):470–483, 2003. **Summarizes the epidemiology, clinical manifestations, genetics, pathogenesis, and serologic and histologic findings of CD.**
5. Schmitz J: Maldigestion malabsorption. In Walker WA, During PR, Hamilton JR, et al (eds): Pediatric Gastrointestinal Disease: Pathophysiology, Diagnosis and Management, 3rd ed. Hamilton, Ontario, Canada: BC Decker, 2000, pp 46–59. **Useful review.**
6. Ushijima K, Riby JE, Kretchmer N: Carbohydrate malabsorption. Pediatr Clin North Am 42:899–915, 1995. **Article on carbohydrate malabsorptione.**

Intussusception

James P. Keating

KEY CONCEPTS

- Intussusception is a condition with low incidence but potential for high morbidity and mortality.
- Early recognition requires a high index of suspicion.
- Bowel obstruction is a late event and should not be a criterion for pursuing contrast studies.
- Pneumatic reduction, hydraulic reduction, and operative reduction are all effective therapies; the choice of which one to use depends on the availability of skilled practitioners.

Rarely, when the symptoms are nonspecific, minor, or entirely absent, a child with intussusception dies from shock early in the course of the condition. However, the diagnosis is usually suspected by a primary care clinician and is confirmed and treated by a pediatric radiologist or pediatric surgeon with complete recovery.

TABLE 1 Nonclassical Intussusception in Childhood

Condition	Comment
Nodular lymphoid hyperplasia (NLH)	This is probably the lead point in the classic presentation, but NLH can be the result of immunodeficiency disease and may occur later in childhood.
Cystic fibrosis	Thickening of the ileocolonic wall and/or adherent feces provide a lead point.
Celiac disease	Intussusception may be recurrent.
Inverted Meckel diverticulum	These ileoileal intussusceptions are difficult to diagnose before bowel obstruction occurs. Meckel scan may be negative.
Midgut malrotation and intussusception (Waugh syndrome)	3.1% of infants developed intussusception after the Ladd procedure.
Polyposis and cutaneous pigmentation (Peutz-Jeghers syndrome)	The hamartomatous polyps in this dominantly inherited condition causes small bowel intussusception <5 yr of age.
Small-bowel tumor	Include lipoma, lymphosarcoma, American Burkitt, and non-Burkitt lymphoma.
Ectopic gastric mucosa in ileum	Meckel scan can be positive.
Escherichia coli O157H7 and *Yersinia*	These two causes of acute colitis have caused intussusception.
Henoch-Schönlein purpura (HSP)	Fixed intussusception is, happily, rare (<1%). Intense abdominal pain is common in HSP without fixed intussusception.
Hemangioma	May require capsule endoscopy and or laparoscopy to diagnose.
Post-transplant lymphoproliferative disease	Diagnosis is complicated by the underlying disease and opportunistic infections of the bowels.

Although there are a number of possible approaches to treatment, the critical step in achieving a good outcome is early recognition.

Consequently, the details of the clinical presentation and pitfalls that delay the decision to refer the child for evaluation for intussusception are emphasized below. This is information the clinician must retain and review periodically to maintain a high index of suspicion about the diagnosis, because actual encounters with intussusception are rare, given an incidence of 1 in 800 to 1 in 1600 persons. Even a hospital-based specialist (e.g., pediatric radiologist, pediatric surgeon) may see fewer than 5 children with intussusception in any given year.

Who Is at Risk?

The majority of affected infants are healthy, well-grown children with no prior illness or chronic conditions. The inciting lead point is presumably an area of lymphoid hyperplasia in the ileum.

There is a smaller number of children who develop intussusception in the setting of preexisting systemic illness and whose symptoms may vary from most seen in the classical, common form of the condition because of the specific underlying disease and the age of the patient (Table 1).

Classical Ileocecal Intussusception of Childhood

AGE

Eighty percent of those affected are younger than 2 years of age, and the peak incidence is among 4- to 9-month-old infants. Intussusception can occur at any age from the intrauterine period to the teen years, but the further the affected child is from late in the first year of life, the more likely there will be atypical etiologies and presentations. In premature infants, the diagnosis is often delayed, and neonatal necrotizing enterocolitis (NNE) is the most common misdiagnosis.

SYMPTOMS AND SIGNS

Pain is apparent in 90% of patients. However, because infants are unable to describe their symptoms, this important history should be sought by the clinician, who often must elicit it from the parents or caregivers. Episodes of fretting, crying, and flexion at the hips that interrupt sleep, play, and other activities and during which consolation is ineffective may be volunteered by the parent but often will not be apparent until a probing question is asked. Between spasms, the infant may appear entirely well.

Vomiting occurs in 90% of patients, owing to reflex from the stretched mesentery and, late in the course, intestinal obstruction. Early in the course, small-bowel obstruction is absent, and the examiner should not expect to find distention or dilated bowel loops.

Bloody stools occur in 20% of patients. The frequency of blood in bowel movements increases in proportion to the duration of symptoms; 20% of children who have had symptoms for more than 6 hours have visible blood in the stool. A mixture of partially changed blood and mucous yields the "red currant jelly" stool, but frank blood and streaks are more common. At times, the first appearance of blood is on the gloved finger of the examiner.

Mass is felt either by abdominal palpation or on rectal exam in 25% of patients and visibly protrudes from the anus in a few. If the gloved finger can be passed into the rectum alongside a mass protruding from the anus, that mass is likely to be an intussusception, not a rectal prolapse, for which it has been commonly mistaken.

Altered consciousness may be the first and only symptom. This "knocked out" presentation of intussusception was described by Holowach and Thurston from our hospital, a confusing onset that has been confirmed by others. The infant may be flaccid and fail to respond to verbal and noxious stimuli. Children with this presentation are commonly referred for evaluation to neurologists, emergency physicians, or neurosurgeons. Evaluation often includes cerebrospinal fluid examinations, drug screens, brain imaging studies, and skeletal surveys (looking for evidence of shaken baby syndrome). The mechanism of this dramatic alteration in consciousness is unknown.

DURATION OF SYMPTOMS

Intussusception is diagnosed in 80% of children in the first 24 hours after onset of symptoms and in 90% within the first 48 hours, but 10% have symptoms for a longer period, even for a week or more (Table 2). A long duration of symptoms does not, in itself, preclude successful radiographic reduction. The only contraindication to an effort to reduce the intussusception in the radiology suite is shock or peritonitis.

OTHER LESS FREQUENT SYMPTOMS

Symptoms other than the cardinal ones are encountered in patients of all age groups: high fever, 3%; diarrhea, 6%; and constipation, 1%.

DIAGNOSIS AND TREATMENT

Survey films permit a definite diagnosis in only approximately 15% of patients. Additional imaging modalities are used increasingly in the diagnosis of intussusception. Ultrasonography may reveal a so-called doughnut or target sign and is highly sensitive and specific in experienced hands. The inner ring is produced by the intussusceptum and the outer by the intussucipiens. When imaged in a longitudinal plane, a "pseudokidney sign" may be evident. CT and MRI diagnosis are performed more commonly in adults, and little information is available about sensitivity and specificity in children.

When no abnormalities are seen, the clinician must proceed to a contrast study of the colon and ileum. The rate of successful intussusception reduction after air or liquid enema ranges from 50% to 90%; rates in most children's hospitals range from 70% to 85%.

TABLE 2 Duration of Symptoms Prior to Diagnosis

Hours	No.	%
0–6	114	40.1
6–12	49	17
12–24	53	18
24–28	36	13
>48	32	11

From Gierup J, Jorulf H, Livaditis A: Management of intussusception in infants and children: a survey based on 288 consecutive cases. Pediatrics 50:535–546, 1972.

Expert Opinion on Management Issues

Hydrostatic reduction employing barium, water-soluble contrast material, or saline, alternatively, pneumatic reduction are the primary methods of reduction employed in U.S. children's hospitals. An excellent description of this procedure can be found in a "How I Do It" article by an experienced pediatric radiologist, William H. McAlister (see Suggested Readings).

If hydrostatic or pneumatic reduction is successful, observation in the hospital or at home detects recurrence in 10% of cases. Subsequent radiologic reduction is usually successful.

Primary operative reduction is seldom elected in children's hospital settings but may be preferred in community hospitals if radiologists experienced in reduction enema are not available in a timely fashion. Operative reduction or resection is carried out if the intussusception cannot be reduced by enema or if peritonitis, shock, or perforation is present.

Common Pitfalls

- Failing to elicit from the parent the cyclic or intermittent character of the pain.
- Overrelying on a normal abdominal film and failure to proceed with contrast enema.
- Expecting to find all three cardinal features (pain, vomiting, and blood) before proceeding with investigation for intussusception. Vomiting is absent in 45%, rectal bleeding is absent in 90%, and the intussusception is painless in 13%. All three are present in only 3% to 20%.
- Failing to proceed with investigations immediately when you suspect intussusception. Delay reduces the likelihood of successful reduction and increases the likelihood of necrosis and complications.
- Misidentifying the nontender abdominal mass as liver or feces.
- Misidentifying the intussusception protruding from the anus as rectal prolapse.
- Misdiagnosing dysentery. Diarrhea occurs in 7.5% and cyclic intense pain often occurs in dysentery. In one series, delay from this occurred in seven infants, three of whom died.
- Misdiagnosing encephalitis, meningitis, shaken baby syndrome, or ingestion of medication when intussusception manifests with a limp, flaccid infant who does not respond to verbal and noxious stimuli.

Communication and Counseling

It is important to let parents know that recurrence occurs in 10% of children after successful reduction and repeat treatment is generally effective.

SUGGESTED READINGS

1. Byard RW, Simpson A: Sudden death and intussusception in infancy and childhood: Autopsy considerations. Med Sci Law 41:41–45, 2001. **Describes early deaths with few or no symptoms.**

2. Byrne AT, Geoghegan T, Govender P, et al: The imaging of intussusception. Clin Radiol 60:39–46, 2005. **Information on imaging.**

3. Erir SH, Stephens CA, Minor A: The painless intussusception. J Ped Surg 11:563, 1976. **Reminder that even the most common presenting symptom may be absent in some children.**

4. Gierup J, Jorulf H, Livaditis A: Management of intussusception in infants and children: Survey based on 288 consecutive cases. Pediatrics 50:535–546, 1972. **A thoughtful analysis of the presenting symptoms by age and duration of symptoms.**

5. Hernandez JA: Plain film findings in intussusception. Emerg Radiol 10:323, 2004. **The classic triad of an intracolonic mass, obstruction, and paucity of gas in the right lower quadrant occurred in only 1 patient (1%). Plain films of the abdomen were diagnostic of intussusception in only 29% of cases. A completely normal gas pattern was seen in one-quarter of our patients. Most patients with suspected intussusception will require further imaging, either by ultrasound or contrast enema.**

6. Holowach TJ, Thurston DL, McCoy EL: Acute intussusception; analysis of 116 cases at St. Louis Children's Hospital. Arch Surgery 67:68–79, 1953. **Described a study in which many infants with intussusception presented with predominant neurologic symptoms.**

7. McAlister WH: How I do it. Intussusception: Even Hippocrates did not standardize his technique of enema reduction. Radiology 206:595–598, 1998. **Available source of details concerning currently employed methods of reducing ileocecal intussusception.**

8. Ng'walali PM, Yonemitsu K, Tsunenari S: Fetal intussusception in infancy: An experience in forensic autopsy. Legal Med (Tokyo) 5:181–184, 2003. **Describes early deaths with few or no symptoms.**

9. Ravitch MM: Intussusception in Infants and Children. Springfield, IL: Charles C. Thomas, 1959, pp 1–119. **A classic monograph on the topic written by Baltimore surgeon at the time nonoperative reduction was becoming the primary therapy. Full of pictures and wisdom.**

Inflammatory Bowel Disease

John F. Thompson and Erick Hernandez

KEY CONCEPTS

- Pediatric inflammatory bowel disease (IBD), Crohn disease, and ulcerative colitis occur with a variety of clinical presentations, reflecting both the location of the disease activity in the gastrointestinal tract and the type of disease activity in Crohn disease, that is, inflammatory, fistulizing, and stricturing.

- Special issues in children with IBD are growth failure, delayed sexual and psychosocial development, and adherence to therapy.

- Treatment in pediatric IBD involves induction of remission and then maintenance of remission with the least toxic effective therapy.

- Medications to induce remission in ulcerative colitis depend on severity of presentation; 5-aminosalicylic acid (5-ASA)-containing medications and possibly corticosteroids are used for mild to moderate disease and parenteral corticosteroids for severe disease.

- Maintenance of remission in ulcerative colitis is achieved by 5-ASA medications and, if necessary, immunomodulatory medications such as azathioprine or 6-mercaptopurine.

- Induction of remission in Crohn disease is achieved not only with medications but also with enteral nutritional therapy.

- Maintenance of remission in Crohn disease is achieved by a variety of approaches including 5-ASA medications, immunomodulatory medications, and/or anti–tumor necrosis factor agents.

Pediatric inflammatory bowel disease (IBD) includes both ulcerative colitis (UC) and Crohn disease. These conditions share some similarities in that both are chronic idiopathic inflammatory conditions of the gastrointestinal tract. However, marked differences between these conditions exist as well, and therefore, each is considered separately in this chapter. There are estimated to be 1 million people afflicted with IBD in the United States and up to 30% of cases are diagnosed in childhood. IBD is a relatively common and serious public health problem for children in the United States, as evidenced by prevalence of Crohn disease and UC, which were 4.5 and 2.2 per 100,000, respectively, in a recent study of children with newly diagnosed IBD in Wisconsin.

UC is characterized by diffuse inflammation of the colonic mucosa involving the rectum and extending proximately to affect varying lengths of the colon. In children afflicted with UC, the entire colon is usually involved (pancolitis). Symptoms are typical of colitis of any etiology and include diarrhea, often with gross blood and mucus, cramps, urgency, and tenesmus. A history of nocturnal stools is a useful marker of disease activity. Patients with moderate-to-severe disease have signs and symptoms that include anemia, hypoalbuminemia, fever, tachycardia, and severe cramps. Colonoscopy reveals varying degrees of inflammation, including loss of vascular markings, erythema, diffuse ulcerations, exudate, and friability. UC may manifest with acute onset, which is difficult to distinguish from infectious colitis. Similar symptoms, and the pathologic features of crypt abscess and cryptitis, are present in both forms of colitis. Infectious etiologies should be excluded in children presenting with acute-onset colitis. Most infectious causes are self-limited, and therefore, colitis persisting more than 1 month is more likely UC.

Pediatric Crohn disease is characterized by transmural inflammation involving any part of the gastrointestinal tract from the mouth to the anus. Crohn disease occurs as isolated lesions in the small bowel (38% of cases), in both small bowel and colon (38%), and as isolated colonic lesions (20%). Perianal disease is seen in 11% to 18% of children with Crohn disease. Upper intestinal tract disease is often diagnosed by endoscopic and histologic involvement but less often by upper intestinal symptoms. Crohn disease manifests in three forms—inflammatory, stricturing, and fistulizing—and any or all of these may be present in an individual patient. There is some evidence that children who have family members with Crohn disease will present with features similar to those in the afflicted relative.

Symptoms of Crohn disease will reflect the location, form, and severity of involvement. Children with left-sided colonic inflammation will have symptoms of colitis similar to UC. Those with ileal disease and/or right-sided colitis may present with abdominal pain and/or diarrhea. However, symptoms of Crohn disease involving the small bowel and right colon may be very subtle for years and may manifest solely with poor appetite with resulting growth failure because of inadequate caloric intake and increased metabolic rate. Fistulizing disease may be the only presentation, with symptoms such as recurrent perianal abscesses, fistulae, or fissures. Any child who has recurrent perianal fissure or abscess should be evaluated for Crohn disease. Stricturing disease will result in symptoms of partial bowel obstruction in either the small intestine or colon.

Expert Opinion on Management Issues

ULCERATIVE COLITIS

Induction of Remission in Ulcerative Colitis

Mild to moderate disease activity in UC is treated with a 5-aminosalicylic acid (5-ASA) preparation. Table 1 lists a number of these. The first 5-ASA preparation used in UC was sulfasalazine, which is sulfapyridine linked to 5-ASA. 5-ASA is released in the colon by colonic bacterial degradation. Sulfasalazine has been shown to be effective in the treatment of mild to moderate UC, but the side effects of the sulfapyridine moiety are often problematic and include headache and gastrointestinal (GI) distress and occasionally leukocytopenia or severe allergic reactions. The newer 5-ASA preparations (e.g., containing mesalamine) are devoid of the sulfapyridine moiety, thereby eliminating these side effects. These agents use different strategies to deliver mesalamine into the colonic lumen. All mesalamine preparations have been shown to be effective in the treatment of mild to moderate UC. Topical therapy using mesalamine as suppository or enema is useful in patients who have left-sided colitis or proctitis. Topical therapy may also be used as an adjunct to oral mesalamine, because oral mesalamine does not usually reach the sigmoid colon or rectum.

Moderate to severe UC requires corticosteroids to induce remission, as the severity of the symptoms warrants immediate attention. Patients have anemia, hypoalbuminemia, fever, and cramps. Life-threatening complications of severe, fulminant UC associated with significant mortality include perforation and toxic megacolon. Prednisone or methylprednisolone (Solu-Medrol), 1 mg/kg/day, will achieve remission in approximately 80% of children with fulminant UC within 7 to 14 days. Antibiotics such as metronidazole have been used as adjunct therapy for UC, but there are no controlled trials studying the efficacy of antibiotics in this setting.

Failure of induction of remission in 7 to 14 days of systemic corticosteroids in fulminant UC indicates treatment failure. Three therapeutic options are then considered. First, emergency total colectomy and ileostomy with preservation of the rectum with a Hartmann pouch results in rapid resolution of this life-threatening condition. Patients are often discharged from the hospital within as short a time as 3 to 5 days after surgery. Patients subsequently undergo ileoanal pull with a J-pouch within 2 to 4 months. Following this strategy, patients have an average of 4 to 6 loose stools per day and most are satisfied with the outcome. Problems with this surgical approach include incontinence, pouchitis (inflammation and/or infection of the J-pouch) and decreased fertility in females. Also, 2% to 5% of patients who undergo this procedure are subsequently found to have Crohn disease that manifested initially as pancolitis. Finally, patients with acute-onset disease are often not psychologically ready for this life-altering procedure.

A second treatment option in fulminant, steroid-refractory colitis is the use of cyclosporin or tacrolimus, which have been very effective in controlled trials in corticosteroid-resistant severe UC. Frequently, remission is achieved as rapidly as 48 hours after initiating these calcineurin inhibitors. However, the toxicity of these medications prohibits their long-term use in UC. Furthermore, some experiences suggest that most children and adults who needed cyclosporine to induce remission required colectomy within 12 months. Therefore, calcineurin inhibitors are now used as a bridge to either maintenance treatment with a less toxic immunomodulatory agent such as 6-mercaptopurine (6-MP) or azathioprine (AZA) or for stabilization prior to referral for subsequent surgery.

Finally, some recent studies in children with fulminant colitis have reported excellent response to infliximab, a humanized mouse monoclonal anti–tumor necrosis factor antibody that has been used in patients with steroid-resistant fulminant UC. However, not all reports in adults have been favorable. At present, there are no controlled trials in children, but open-label pediatric trials appear to have more favorable results as compared to adult studies, particularly in patients with new-onset fulminant colitis. If clinical remission is achieved with infliximab, the decision about transition to another immunomodulatory agent, continuing long-term infliximab, or performing colectomy must be addressed. Currently, there are no published data or recommendations to guide these decisions. Infliximab is infused intravenously and must be administered in a controlled setting with close monitoring. Infliximab is immunogenic and may result in severe life-threatening infusion reactions including shortness of breath, cyanosis, and hypotension (Fig. 1).

Maintenance of Remission in Ulcerative Colitis

Many controlled trials support the use of 5-ASA medications to decrease the likelihood of relapse in UC. Most of these studies are in adults, but the experience in pediatric patients would support this approach as well. Studies have demonstrated a dose response with 5-ASA medications that favors the use of the newer mesalamine medications rather than sulfasalazine, because higher doses of 5-ASA are tolerated with these newer medications. There appear to be no substantial differences in clinical response with the different 5-ASA preparations. A small number of patients may be sensitive to 5-ASA and experience worsening colitis symptoms with these preparations, which should not be confused with worsening disease activity. Immunomodulatory agents, 6-MP/AZA, have been demonstrated to be effective as maintenance therapy in those patients who fail to sustain remission with 5-ASA preparations and do not wish to undergo colectomy.

CROHN DISEASE

Induction of Remission in Crohn Disease

Therapy for Crohn disease is targeted to induce remission of symptoms. Because Crohn disease produces a variety of clinical problems, therapy is individualized to the patient's particular disease profile. This clinical complexity, along with the high placebo response rate in clinical trials, presents unique problems in the clinical management of these patients and the analysis of evidence-based medicine. The induction of remission in inflammatory Crohn disease has been demonstrated to be achieved by all of the following: elemental diet therapy, aminosalicylates, corticosteroids, immunomodulatory drugs, and infliximab.

Exclusive nutritional therapy, with either elemental or polymeric diets, has achieved remission in up to 80% of children with Crohn disease. This excellent response rate is primarily seen in new-onset inflammatory disease of the small intestine. Most children relapse after introduction of normal diet, although relapse rates may be lower and time to relapse may be prolonged with this initial therapeutic approach. Importantly, this approach usually requires the introduction of nocturnal nasogastric tube feeding or gastrostomy. Because of to the discomfort of tube feeding, elemental nutritional therapy has not been well accepted in the United States but has been more successfully employed in Europe.

Mesalamine is indicated for the treatment of mild-to-moderate Crohn disease. Table 1 notes the varied mesalamine release times for each preparation into the intestinal lumen, in which the drug exerts its topical anti-inflammatory effects. The specific preparation used depends on the location of Crohn disease activity in the gastrointestinal tract. Both Asacol and Pentasa have been demonstrated to be effective in the treatment of patients with active Crohn ileocolitis and colitis. As with UC, studies have demonstrated that higher doses increase the likelihood of achieving remission. Pentasa has also been shown to be effective in ileitis, likely because of its more proximal release in the small intestine as compared to Asacol. Colazal, Dipentum, and sulfasalazine would not be used in jejunoileal disease, because 5-ASA in these preparations is primarily

released in the colon. The response rate to mesalamine in mild to moderate Crohn disease is 40% to 50%.

Corticosteroids are highly effective in inducing remission in Crohn disease, but the toxicity of corticosteroids is problematic. In children, glucocorticoid side effects include psychological effects, cushingoid features, acne, and bone loss. Children with Crohn disease often have decreased bone density, which is exacerbated by corticosteroids. Patients treated with corticosteroids frequently become steroid-dependent; furthermore, corticosteroids are not useful for maintenance treatment. Budesonide is a corticosteroid with extensive first-pass liver metabolism, resulting in low systemic bioavailability. Entocort is formulated to release budesonide into the lumen of the ileum and right colon and, in a dose of 9 mg/day, has been demonstrated in both children and adults to treat mild-to-moderate Crohn ileocolitis as effectively as 40 mg/day of prednisone. It is not indicated for the treatment of Crohn colitis or fistulizing disease, nor is it indicated for maintenance therapy (Fig. 2).

Maintenance Therapy in Crohn disease

Children who have achieved remission with mesalamine should continue this medication as maintenance therapy. It is less clear if mesalamine is effective in patients who have required corticosteroids to induce remission, and there are some data in adults suggesting that corticosteroid treatment may reduce the likelihood of sustained remission with mesalamine. As already stated, corticosteroids are not indicated for the maintenance of remission in Crohn disease. Antibiotics, particularly metronidazole and ciprofloxacin, have been demonstrated to be useful adjuncts in the short term treatment of Crohn disease but are not useful as maintenance therapy because of drug toxicity, lack of efficacy, and development of drug-resistant bacteria.

If mesalamine is ineffective and patients are steroid-dependent, immunomodulatory therapy is indicated. 6-Mercaptopurine and its prodrug azathioprine have been demonstrated to be effective in the maintenance of remission of Crohn disease, including fistulizing disease. 6-MP/AZA is metabolized by thiopurine methyltransferase (TPMT) to the active component 6-thioguanine (6-TG). Homozygous deficiency of TPMT, present in 0.3% of the population, may result is severe bone marrow depression. Optimizing 6-TG blood levels into a therapeutic but nontoxic range is useful in patients who do not respond to standard recommended doses. In patients intolerant of 6-MP/AZA, methotrexate (MTX) has been demonstrated to be an effective maintenance treatment of Crohn disease.

With the discovery that tumor necrosis factor (TNF) is present in high concentrations in the mucosa of patients with active Crohn disease, new therapeutic approaches have been developed to inhibit TNF activity in patients with Crohn disease. Infliximab has been demonstrated to be highly effective in the treatment of both children and adults with moderate-to-severe Crohn disease who had been unresponsive to the

TABLE 1 Drugs for Treating Crohn Disease and Ulcerative Colitis

Generic Name (Trade Name)	Dosage/Route/Regimen	Maximum Dose	Dosage Formulation	Adverse Reactions	Site of Action/ Indication
Aminosalicylates (Modulates arachidonic acid metabolism by the inhibition of lipoxygenase pathway, in particular leukotriene B_4 production, resulting in decreased neutrophil chemotaxis.)					
Sulfasalazine (Azulfidine)	PO: 50–75 mg/kg/day in tid dosing	2–4 g/day	Tablet: 500 mg Oral susp: 250mg/5 ml	Nausea, myalgias, headache, fever, rash, pancreatitis, interstitial nephritis, decreased folic acid absorption	Colonic release
Mesalamine (Asacol)	PO: 50–100 mg/kg/day tid dosing	2.4–4.8 g/day	Tablet: 400 mg	Fever, rash, pancreatitis, interstitial nephritis, alopecia	Terminal ileum and right colon release
Mesalamine (Pentasa)	PO: 50–75 mg/kg/day in tid dosing	4 g/day	Tablet: 250 mg	Fever, rash, pancreatitis, arthralgia, interstitial nephritis, alopecia	Jejunum and colonic release
Colazal (Balsalazide disodium)	PO: 50–100 mg/kg/day tid dosing	6.75 g/day	Capsule 750 mg	Fever, interstitial nephritis, headache, abdominal pain, diarrhea	Colitis
Olsalazine (Dipentum)	PO: 50–75 mg/kg/day (tid)	500 mg bid	Tablet: 250 mg	Fever, rash, pancreatitis, arthralgia, interstitial nephritis, alopecia	Colonic release
5-ASA (Rowasa)	Enema PR: 1–4 g/day Suppository PR: 500 mg/day or bid	4 g/day or bid 1000 mg hs	Enema: 4 g Suppository: 500, 1000 mg	Diarrhea, worsening colitis, fever, rash, pancreatitis, arthralgia, interstitial nephritis	Distal colitis
Antibiotics (Diminish the luminal concentration of intestinal bacteria that may alter the abnormal cellular-mediated immune response.)					
Metronidazole (Flagyl)	PO: 15–20 mg/kg/day (tid)	250–500 mg tid	Tablet: 250, 500 mg Susp: 100 mg/5 mL	Nausea, emesis, headache, epigastric pain, peripheral neuropathy	Colitis and perianal disease
Ciprofloxacin	PO: 20–30 mg/kg/day IV: 10–20 mg/kg/day	PO: 1.0–1.5 g/day IV: 800 mg/day	Tablet: 100, 250, 500, 750 mg Oral susp: 250, 500 mg/5 mL	Nausea, emesis, diarrhea, cartilage damage in animal studies	Colitis and perianal disease
Probiotics (Compete for bacterial-epithelial binding sites, and produce antimicrobial metabolites.)					
Lactobacillus casei strain GG (Culturelle)	PO: 1–2 cap/day	1–2 cap/day	Capsule: 10 billion live cells/capsule	Abdominal pain, nausea, emesis, and diarrhea.	Crohn colitis and ileitis
VSL #3	PO: 6 g/day	PO: 6 g/day	5×10^{11} per g of viable lyophilized bacteria	Abdominal pain, nausea, emesis, and diarrhea	Pouchitis

Corticosteroids (Decrease the release of several inflammatory mediators and inhibit cell-mediated response.)

Drug	Dose		Preparation	Toxicity	Indication
Prednisone	PO: 1 mg/kg/day	20 mg bid	Tablet: 1, 2.5, 5, 10, 20 mg; Oral susp: 1 mg/mL	Fluid retention, hypertension, cataracts, osteopenia, myopathy, mood disorders, weight gain, abdominal striae	Upper gastrointestinal tract, small intestine, colonic disease
Hydrocortisone (Cortenema)	PR: One enema/day	One enema bid	100 mg/60 mL		Distal colitis
Hydrocortisone acetate (suppository)	PR: One suppository bid	One suppository tid	25 mg suppository		Proctitis

Azathioprine or 6 Mercaptopurine (6-MP) (Purine analogues that interfere with protein synthesis and nucleic acid metabolism modifying the immune response. Azathioprine is a prodrug of 6-MP, after absorption (88%) is rapidly converted to 6-MP.)

Drug	Dose	Preparation	Toxicity	Indication
Azathioprine	PO: 2–2.5 mg/kg/day	Tablet: 50 mg; Oral susp: 2, 50 mg/mL	Leukopenia, pancreatitis, elevation of aminotransferase, gastrointestinal intolerance	Corticosteroid-resistant or -dependent patients
6-MP (Purinethol)	PO: 1.5 mg/kg/day	Tablet: 50 mg		

Methotrexate (Folate-inhibitor that impairs DNA synthesis; it also results in the induction of T-cell apoptosis.)

Drug	Dose	Preparation	Toxicity	Indication
Methotrexate	IM or SC: 15 mg/m^2 weekly	Injection: 25 mg/mL	Nausea, anorexia, diarrhea, headache, fatigue, pancytopenia, interstitial pneumonitis, hepatotoxicity	Corticosteroid-resistant or -dependent Crohn patients

Cyclosporine (Inhibits calcineurin, suppressing the cell-mediated immunity.)

Drug	Dose	Preparation	Toxicity	Indication
Cyclosporine	IV: 5–6 mg/kg	Injection: 50 mg/mL	Hepatotoxicity, hypertension, nephrotoxicity, hypomagnesemia, hyperkalemia, hirsutism, leukopenia, gingival hyperplasia	Medically refractory severe ulcerative colitis

Infliximab (Is a chimeric IgG4 monoclonal antibody of tumor necrosis factor-α (TNF-α), which is a potent inflammatory cytokine.). Inhibits TNF-α,

Drug	Dose	Preparation	Toxicity	Indication
Infliximab (Remicade)	IV: 5–10 mg/kg/dose	IV: 100 mg/20 mL injection	Hypersensitive reactions, nausea, headache, opportunistic infections	Medically refractory severe ulcerative colitis and Crohn disease

Note: This is not an exhaustive table, and certain agents mentioned in the text are not included in this table. Newer immunomodulatory agents for which experience is quite limited are not included. Not all of the above drugs are specifically approved for use in children.

bid, two times daily; hs, at bedtime; IM, intramuscularly; IV, intravenously; PO, orally; PR, rectally; SC, subcutaneously; tid, three times daily.

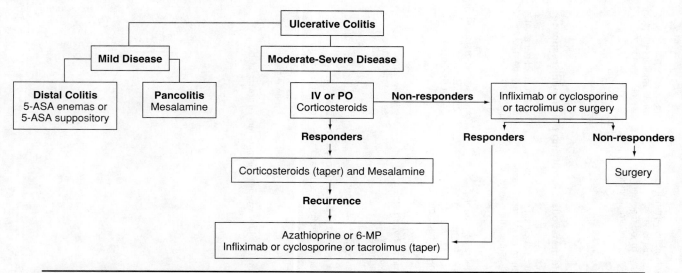

FIGURE 1. Management of pediatric ulcerative colitis. 5-ASA, 5-aminosalicylic acid; IV, intravenous; 6-MP, 6-mercaptopurine; PO, by mouth.

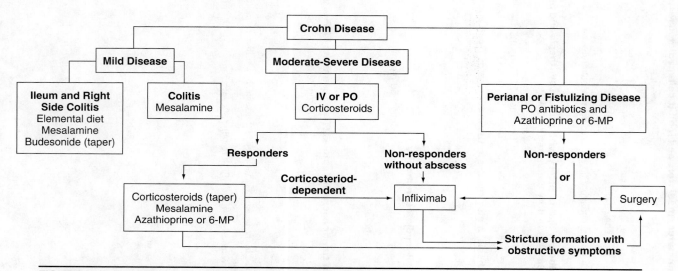

FIGURE 2. Management of pediatric Crohn disease. IV, intravenous; 6-MP, 6-mercaptopurine; PO, by mouth.

conventional therapies. The necessary caution needed with its use is mentioned above. Initially, infliximab is given at 0, 2, and 6 weeks and then every 8 to 12 weeks. Antibodies to infliximab result in higher likelihood of infusion reactions and diminished response to the medication. Concomitant treatment with an immunomodulatory agent may decrease the incidence of anti-infliximab antibody formation and therefore enhance long-term efficacy. Infliximab is an immunosuppressant, and close monitoring for infectious complications is required. Prior to initiating treatment, patients must be assessed for tuberculosis and abscesses, either intra-abdominal or perianal, any of which would preclude infliximab use. A major concern of the prolonged use of infliximab is the development of lymphoma, although at present, it is unclear if infliximab increases the already increased risk of patients with Crohn disease to develop lymphoma.

Special Considerations

Fistulizing disease in patients with Crohn disease may manifest with indolent draining perianal fistulae, which are usually nonproblematic and do not require aggressive therapy. Metronidazole and 6MP/AZA are effective treatments for these fistulae, provided that metronidazole is not prescribed for prolonged periods of time. Perianal fistulae occasionally develop into perianal abscesses when they do not spontaneously drain, and then surgical intervention and/or ciprofloxacin are recommended. Enteric fistulae may develop between adjacent loops of colon or small intestine; enterovesicular, enterovaginal, or enterocutaneous fistulae may also occur. These fistulae are more problematic and usually require surgical intervention, although infliximab may play a role in the treatment of these problems. Intra-abdominal abscesses from enteric fistulae are common and need to be drained and treated aggressively with systemic antibiotics. Infliximab appears to be highly effective in the treatment of complex fistulous disease but is contraindicated in active abscesses.

Some patients have the tendency to develop either small or large bowel strictures, which manifest with partial or complete obstruction. Rectal strictures may manifest with obstipation. Strictures are fibrotic and therefore are not amenable to anti-inflammatory treatment. Balloon dilation performed endoscopically is indicated for colonic or rectal strictures. Surgical stricturoplasty rather than resection should be employed for small intestinal strictures to preserve functional bowel, if possible.

Common Pitfalls

- In fulminant colitis, failure to proceed to alternative therapy after prolonged treatment failure with corticosteroids.
- Inappropriate prolonged or repeated use of corticosteroids in steroid-resistant UC or Crohn disease due to failure to proceed to immunomodulatory medications such as 6-MP/AZA.
- Prolonged medical therapy employing toxic agents when surgical intervention is indicated.

Communication and Counseling

Pediatric IBD is a chronic condition, but it is compatible with a normal life expectancy and normal lifestyle. However, children and their families will need to be vigilant about careful medical follow-up, subtle changes in symptoms, and compliance with the medical regimen. Parents need to be aware of the potential for nonadherence to therapy as the patient reaches the early teens. Families will need to accept the anticipated ups and downs of a chronic illness. Both parents and patient must be knowledgeable regarding the immediate and potential toxicities of the child's chronic medical regimen. Attention and sensitivity should be directed toward the psychosocial development of children and adolescents with IBD as they deal with the potential embarrassment and privacy issues that result from chronic bowel dysfunction.

SUGGESTED READINGS

1. Chang JC, Cohen RD: Medical management of severe ulcerative colitis. Gastroenterol Clin North Am 33(2):235–250, 2004. **Review of current therapy for fulminant colitis.**
2. de Ridder L, Escher JC, Bouquet J, et al: Infliximab therapy in 30 patients with refractory pediatric Crohn disease with and without fistulas in the Netherlands. J Pediatr Gastroenterol Nutr 39:46–52, 2004. **Reports of experience of treatment of Crohn disease in pediatric population.**
3. Escher JC, Taminian JA, Nieuwenhuis EE, et al: Treatment of inflammatory bowel disease in childhood: Best available evidence. Inflamm Bowel Dis 9(1):34–58, 2003. **Review of evidenced-based medicine for pediatric IBD.**
4. Kim SC, Ferry GD: Inflammatory bowel disease in pediatric and adolescent patients: Clinical, therapeutic, and psychosocial considerations. Gastroenterology 126:1550–1560, 2004. **Discussion of unique clinical aspects of pediatric IBD.**
5. Lichtenstein GR, Hanauer SB, Present DH, et al: Crohn's is not a 6-week disease. Lifelong management of mild to moderate Crohn's disease. Inflamm Bowel Dis 10(2):S2–S10, 2004. **Review of literature to support current guidelines of therapy.**
6. Mamula P, Markowitz JE, Cohen LJ, et al: Infliximab in Pediatric Ulcerative Colitis: Two-year follow-up. J Pediatr Gastroenterol Nutr 38:298–301, 2004. **Single-center, open-label experience of infliximab for ulcerative colitis (UC).**
7. Mamula P, Markowitz JE, Baldassano RN: Inflammatory bowel disease in early childhood and adolescence: Special considerations. Gastroenterol Clin North Am 32(3):967–995, 2003. **Review of clinical aspects of pediatric IBD.**

Peritonitis

Melissa S. Camp and Dorry L. Segev

KEY CONCEPTS

- Spontaneous bacterial peritonitis is caused by the infection of preexisting ascites with a single pathogen.
- Secondary peritonitis is caused by multiple pathogens released from a perforated viscus.
- Antibiotics are the primary therapy for spontaneous bacterial peritonitis.
- Management of secondary peritonitis includes surgical intervention in addition to antibiotics.
- Special cases include meconium peritonitis, fungal peritonitis, and peritonitis associated with peritoneal dialysis catheters and ventriculoperitoneal shunts.

Peritonitis is an infection within the peritoneal cavity. Peritonitis can be divided into two major categories: primary or spontaneous bacterial peritonitis, and secondary or polymicrobial peritonitis. The causes and treatments differ, so it is important to distinguish between the two.

Spontaneous bacterial peritonitis develops as a result of infection of preexisting ascites, usually by a single pathogen. The source of infection is thought to be from a transient bacteremia or from translocation of a bowel pathogen. Spontaneous bacterial peritonitis occurs with equal frequency in males and females. Symptoms may include fever, abdominal pain, vomiting, or diarrhea. Physical examination is usually significant for abdominal tenderness and hypoactive or absent bowel sounds. Patients may exhibit rapid shallow breathing, as peritoneal irritation leads to worsening of abdominal pain with deep inspiration. Hypotension and tachycardia may also be present as a result of intra-abdominal fluid shifts.

Secondary peritonitis, in contrast, is caused by a perforated viscus. The most common cause of secondary peritonitis in children is a perforated appendix; Box 1 lists other causes. Bacterial spillage from a perforated viscus is most often polymicrobial in nature. Children with secondary peritonitis can present with fever, abdominal pain, nausea, and vomiting. Abdominal tenderness, with guarding and percussion

---

BOX 1 Causes of Secondary Peritonitis

- Appendiceal perforation
- Strangulated hernia
- Rupture of Meckel diverticulum
- Bowel atresia
- Hirschsprung disease
- Midgut volvulus
- Intussusception
- Hemolytic-uremic syndrome
- Peptic ulcer disease
- Inflammatory bowel disease
- Necrotizing cholecystitis
- Necrotizing enterocolitis
- Typhilitis
- Trauma
- *Neisseria gonorrhea* or *Chlamydia* through the fallopian tubes
- Ventriculoperitoneal shunt
- Peritoneal dialysis catheter

BOX 2 Paracentesis Findings Suggestive of Peritonitis

- A white blood cell (WBC) count >250/mm³ or polymorphonuclear leukocyte (PMN) count >50% PMNs
- a pH >7.35 or arterial-ascitic fluid pH gradient >0.1
- Protein >1 g/dL, glucose >50 mg/dL
- High lactate
- Positive Gram stain or culture

---

tenderness, can be elicited on physical examination, although these peritoneal signs may be more difficult to elicit in neonates and infants. Leukocytosis is common. Upright chest or abdominal films with free air under the diaphragm are classic for a perforated viscus.

Expert Opinion on Management Issues

Management and treatment of children with peritonitis depends on the etiology. For both spontaneous bacterial peritonitis and polymicrobial peritonitis, intensive monitoring is important. Significant morbidity can result from large volume fluid shifts, and mortality rates from peritonitis can be as high as 2%.

SPONTANEOUS BACTERIAL PERITONITIS

One of the initial steps in evaluating a child with preexisting ascites and a suspicion of spontaneous bacterial peritonitis should be diagnostic paracentesis. Patients with chronic liver disease may be coagulopathic, and such patients should be tested for the presence of a coagulopathy, which, if present, should be corrected prior to attempting paracentesis. Paracentesis findings that are consistent with peritonitis include high white blood cell (WBC) count, low pH, high protein, low glucose, high lactate, and positive Gram stain or culture (Box 2). Culture of peritoneal fluid in spontaneous bacterial peritonitis typically results in the growth of a single pathogen. The most frequently isolated pathogens are pneumococcus, group A *Streptococcus*, enterococcus, staphylococcus, and gram-negative rods such as *Escherichia coli* and *Klebsiella*.

A 2-week course of antibiotics is often sufficient for treatment of spontaneous bacterial peritonitis. Empirical therapy should be started initially, with broad-spectrum coverage of gram-positive cocci and gram-negative bacilli. Recommended antibiotic regimens include an aminoglycoside together with either a cephalosporin (cefotaxime or ceftriaxone) or a β-lactam/lactamase inhibitor (ampicillin-sulbactam or ticarcillin-clavulanic acid). Vancomycin is an alternative for patients with penicillin allergy. Imipenem is another possibility for initial empirical coverage, as it covers both gram-positive and gram-negative organisms. Regardless of the initial antibiotics chosen for empirical coverage, antibiotic therapy needs to be narrowed and tailored based on the culture and sensitivity results. If fevers persist despite appropriately tailored therapy, a repeat paracentesis should be performed.

SECONDARY PERITONITIS

Perforated viscus leads to secondary peritonitis, usually from multiple pathogens. Management consists of fluid resuscitation, antibiotics, and surgical consultation. Aggressive fluid resuscitation should begin immediately, as rapid fluid shifts can lead to hypotension followed by hypoperfusion, acidosis, and profound shock. Isotonic fluids should be started with an intravenous bolus of 20 mL/kg and continued until adequate urine output is achieved. Intensive monitoring with central venous and arterial lines is essential for children who are persistently hypotensive despite aggressive fluid resuscitation.

Antibiotics with broad-spectrum coverage should also be initiated for secondary peritonitis. Antibiotics do not treat the underlying disease but instead provide coverage against bacteremia and sepsis. The spectrum of empirical coverage should include gram-positive cocci, gram-negative bacilli and β-lactamase–producing anaerobes. The most common pathogens include enterococci, *E. coli*, *Klebsiella*, and *Bacteroides*. Recommended antibiotic combinations include ampicillin, an aminoglycoside and metronidazole, or an aminoglycoside plus ticarcillin-clavulanic acid. Blood cultures should be drawn, and peritoneal fluid cultures should also be sent intra-operatively to help tailor antibiotic therapy.

A surgical consult should be obtained without delay, as patients with a perforated viscus will most likely require surgical intervention. Aggressive fluid resuscitation and antibiotics should be started preoperatively, and the timing of surgery will depend on the condition of the patient. Hypotension on induction of anesthesia can be a major problem if the patient is not appropriately resuscitated preoperatively.

Surgery may not be required if localized peritonitis develops from a perforated viscus that has been contained within an abscess. Abscess formation can occur not uncommonly in response to a perforated appendix or in association with Crohn disease. A percutaneously placed catheter can be used to drain the abscess, and the fluid should be cultured to guide antibiotic therapy. For abscesses that develop in response to a perforated appendix, interval appendectomy should be performed after percutaneous drainage and a full course of antibiotics (6 to 8 weeks).

Common Pitfalls

- Presumptive diagnosis of spontaneous bacterial peritonitis and resulting failure to recognize a perforated viscus in a patient with preexisting ascites
- Failure to appropriately resuscitate a patient with fluid and antibiotics before surgical management
- Any delay in surgical referral

It is important to keep in mind that although patients with preexisting ascites are at greatest risk for primary or spontaneous bacterial peritonitis, the possibility of secondary peritonitis cannot be excluded in this group of patients. If the workup for presumed spontaneous bacterial peritonitis reveals free air within the peritoneum or culture of peritoneal fluid grows multiple pathogens rather than a single pathogen, a secondary source may be the cause. Patients with preexisting ascites can also develop any of the causes of secondary peritonitis listed in Box 1. Early recognition and diagnosis is important, because secondary peritonitis most often requires prompt surgical intervention.

Special cases of peritonitis include those associated with indwelling pieces of hardware, such as peritoneal dialysis catheters, and nonbacterial causes of peritonitis such as meconium and fungal pathogens.

Peritoneal Dialysis Catheter Peritonitis

Patients undergoing peritoneal dialysis (PD) are at risk for developing peritonitis. Symptoms of peritonitis in a PD patient include cloudy dialysis fluid, abdominal pain and tenderness, fever, diarrhea, nausea, and vomiting. Dialysis fluid containing more than 100 WBC per mm^3, more than half of which are polymorphonuclear leukocytes, is diagnostic. Empirical antibiotic therapy should be initiated with vancomycin and gentamicin, and then antibiotics can be tailored based on culture and sensitivity results. Gram-positive and gram-negative organisms are cultured with equal frequency, and fungal pathogens can also be responsible. Cultures may also be negative, but empirical antibiotics should be continued in these situations if the patient is improving clinically. In general, a 2-week course of antibiotics is sufficient to treat bacterial peritonitis in a PD patient, and antibiotics can be administered in the dialysis fluid. Removal of the PD catheter should be considered in cases in which bacterial peritonitis is recurrent despite appropriate antibiotic therapy, or if cultures are growing fungal or mycobacterial pathogens.

Long-term peritoneal dialysis is also a risk factor for developing sclerosing encapsulating peritonitis. The incidence is 6% in patients who have been on peritoneal dialysis for more than 5 years and 12% in patients who have been on peritoneal dialysis for more than 8 years. CT will reveal peritoneal calcifications, and the diagnosis is confirmed by peritoneal biopsy. Once the diagnosis is biopsy proven, PD should be discontinued.

Ventriculoperitoneal Shunt Peritonitis

Patients with indwelling ventriculoperitoneal (VP) shunts are at risk for bacterial peritonitis in association with shunt infection. Symptoms include abdominal pain, tenderness, nausea, and vomiting. Neurologic symptoms are generally not present with shunt infection but will be present in cases of shunt malfunction. A CT scan may show a fluid collection consistent with infected cerebrospinal fluid (CSF) or may reveal another etiology of peritonitis. For example, VP shunt catheters can cause intestinal perforation leading to peritonitis. Peritonitis caused by infected VP shunts or by intestinal perforation secondary to VP shunts requires surgical removal of the VP shunt and placement of a temporary ventricular drain. Broad-spectrum antibiotic therapy with antibiotics such as vancomycin and gentamicin should be initiated, and antibiotic therapy can be tailored based on culture results from the CSF. A new VP shunt should not be inserted until at least 1 week after negative cerebrospinal fluid cultures are obtained.

MECONIUM PERITONITIS

Spillage of meconium into the peritoneal cavity prior to birth can cause peritonitis in neonates. A distal obstruction in the gastrointestinal (GI) tract, such as intestinal atresia or stenosis, meconium ileus, in utero intussusception, hernia, or gastroschisis can lead to the meconium spillage. Mortality can be as high as 20%. Ultrasound can detect meconium peritonitis prior to birth with the presence of calcifications scattered throughout the peritoneal cavity, but symptoms and signs present after birth include massive abdominal distention, and abdominal wall erythema and edema.

Meconium peritonitis can be differentiated into three types: fibroadhesive, cystic, and generalized. Fibroadhesive peritonitis develops when the perforation is localized and sealed off by adhesions and calcifications in response to a chemical reaction to the meconium. If the perforation is not completely sealed off, a pseudocyst of liquefied meconium can develop, and this is classified as cystic peritonitis. Generalized peritonitis develops when a perforation occurs late and meconium is spread throughout the peritoneal cavity. Exploratory laparotomy to determine the viability of the involved bowel is the operative intervention indicated in patients who present with symptoms of meconium peritonitis. Severely compromised bowel should be resected. A primary anastomosis may be possible if gross abdominal infection is not present, but a temporary stoma is often indicated.

FUNGAL PERITONITIS

Infection of the peritoneal cavity by fungi can occur in patients who have had multiple episodes of bacterial peritonitis, especially for patients with indwelling peritoneal catheters. Treatment for fungal peritonitis should be initiated with a loading dose of intravenous fluconazole followed by intraperitoneal fluconazole. Amphotericin B should be considered in severely ill patients with fungal peritonitis.

Communication and Counseling

Peritonitis can have significant morbidity, and mortality rates are as high as 2%. Early and accurate diagnosis of the underlying etiology of peritonitis is essential to ensure appropriate therapy. Complications that can develop even with appropriate therapy include intra-abdominal abscesses, recurrent bacterial peritonitis in spontaneous bacterial peritonitis, need for bowel resection and/or stoma in peritonitis caused by a perforated viscus, postoperative wound infection, shock, and acute respiratory distress syndrome.

SUGGESTED READINGS

1. Araki Y, Hataya H, Tanaka Y, et al: Long-term peritoneal dialysis is a risk factor of sclerosing encapsulating peritonitis for children. Perit Dial Int 20(4):445–451, 2000. **Study showing how peritoneal dialysis for more than 5 years increases risk of developing peritoneal sclerosis.**
2. Bhuva M, Ganger D, Jensen D: Spontaneous bacterial peritonitis: An update on evaluation, management and prevention. Am J Med 97(2):169–175, 1994. **Review of diagnosis, treatment, and prevention of spontaneous bacterial peritonitis.**
3. Brook I: Microbiology and management of intra-abdominal infections in children. Pediatr Int 45(2):123–129, 2003. **Discussion of the most common bacteria responsible for causing secondary peritonitis, and the treatment of the secondary peritonitis.**
4. Furth SL, Donaldson LA, Sullivan EK, et al: Peritoneal dialysis catheter infections and peritonitis in children: A report of the North American Pediatric Renal Transplant Cooperative Study. Pediatr Nephrol 15(3–4):179–182, 2000. **Study looking at risk factors for developing peritonitis and peritoneal catheter related infections in children receiving peritoneal dialysis.**
5. Gorensek MJ, Lebel MH, Nelson JD: Peritonitis in children with nephrotic syndrome. Pediatrics 81(6):849–856, 1988. **Discussion of the clinical presentation of peritonitis and the most common pathogens responsible for causing peritonitis**
6. Grosfeld JL, Molinari F, Chaet M, et al: Gastrointestinal perforation and peritonitis in infants and children: Experience with 179 cases over 10 years. Surgery 120(4):650–656, 1996. **Discusses the causes of and mortality associated with peritonitis in premature infants and children.**
7. Haecker FM, Berger D, Schumacher U, et al: Peritonitis in childhood: Aspects of pathogenesis and therapy. Pediatr Surg Int 16 (3):182–188, 2000. **Study showing resolution of systemic infection despite persistence of bacteria and endotoxin in peritoneal fluid following operative intervention for perforated appendicitis.**
8. Schaefer F: Management of peritonitis in children receiving chronic peritoneal dialysis. Paediatr Drugs 5(5):315–325, 2003. **Review of risk factors and treatment of peritonitis in children receiving peritoneal dialysis.**
9. Warady BA, Schaefer F, Holloway M, et al: Consensus guidelines for the treatment of peritonitis in pediatric patients receiving peritoneal dialysis. Perit Dial Int 20(6):610–624, 2000. **Practice guidelines for treating peritonitis associated with peritoneal dialysis in children.**
10. Weber TR, Keller MA, Bower RJ, et al: Is delayed operative treatment worth the trouble with perforated appendicitis in children? Am J Surg 186(6):685–689, 2003. **Study comparing immediate appendectomy versus intravenous antibiotics, percutaneous drainage of abscess, and delayed appendectomy in children with perforated appendicitis.**

Pancreatic Diseases

Steven L. Werlin

KEY CONCEPTS

- Acute pancreatitis is typically diagnosed by elevation of the serum lipase or amylase greater than three times normal in the appropriate clinical setting.
- Most cases of acute pancreatitis in children are mild and self-limited.
- Treatment of mild acute pancreatitis consists of intravenous fluids and analgesia.
- A nasogastric tube is required only in the presence of unremitting vomiting.
- Feeding can be resumed when vomiting and pain have resolved; it is not necessary to wait until the amylase and lipase have normalized.
- Pseudocysts commonly follow acute pancreatitis, but most resolve spontaneously.
- Chronic pancreatitis is rare in children.
- A vigorous search for an underlying etiology should be made in all cases of acute recurrent or chronic pancreatitis.
- The most common cause of pancreatic insufficiency in children is cystic fibrosis.

ACUTE PANCREATITIS

Acute pancreatitis is the most common pancreatic disorder in children. Blunt abdominal injury (including child abuse), mumps, other viral illnesses, biliary tract stones, multisystem diseases, biliary tract anomalies, and drugs account for most known causes.

The child with acute pancreatitis has steady, epigastric abdominal pain, persistent vomiting, and fever and often assumes an antalgic position with hips and knees flexed, while sitting upright or lying on the side. The child may be very uncomfortable and irritable and appears acutely ill. The abdomen may be distended and quite tender; a mass may be palpable. The pain increases in intensity for 24 to 48 hours, during which time vomiting may increase and the patient may require hospitalization for dehydration and fluid and electrolyte therapy. The prognosis for the acute, uncomplicated case is excellent.

Acute hemorrhagic pancreatitis, the most severe form of acute pancreatitis, is rare in children. In this life-threatening condition, the patient is acutely ill with severe nausea, vomiting, and abdominal pain. Shock, high fever, jaundice, ascites, hypocalcemia, and pleural effusions may occur. A bluish discoloration may be seen around the umbilicus (Cullen sign) or in the flanks (Grey Turner sign). The pancreas is necrotic and may be transformed into an inflammatory, hemorrhagic mass. The high mortality rate (25%) is related to the development of the systemic inflammatory response syndrome, consisting of shock, renal failure, adult respiratory distress syndrome, disseminated intravascular coagulation, massive gastrointestinal bleeding, and systemic or intra-abdominal infection.

Expert Opinion on Management Issues

DIAGNOSIS

Acute pancreatitis is usually diagnosed by measurement of serum amylase and lipase activities. The serum amylase concentration is typically elevated for up to 4 days. A variety of other conditions may also cause hyperamylasemia without pancreatitis. Elevation of the serum level of salivary amylase may mislead the clinician in a child with abdominal pain. Because the serum amylase is normal in 10% to 15% of patients, the serum lipase, which is more specific than amylase for acute inflammatory pancreatic disease, should be determined. The author now routinely measures only the serum level of lipase in patients with suspected pancreatitis. If the lipase is normal and pancreatitis is strongly suspected the serum amylase is then measured. The serum lipase typically remains elevated 8 to 14 days longer than the serum amylase. Serum lipase may also be elevated in nonpancreatic diseases.

Other laboratory abnormalities that may be present in acute pancreatitis include hemoconcentration, coagulopathy, leukocytosis, hyperglycemia, glucosuria, and hypocalcemia. Elevated γ-glutamyl transpeptidase (GGT) and hyperbilirubinemia suggest biliary obstruction, most commonly because of stones.

ACCEPTED INTERVENTIONS

Most cases of pancreatitis in children are relatively mild and require only maintenance intravenous fluids, analgesia (acetaminophen with codeine), fasting for 1 to 2 days, and possibly a brief period of nasogastric suction. The response to treatment is usually complete over 2 to 4 days. Refeeding may commence after the serum lipase or amylase has peaked and clinical symptoms have resolved. It is not necessary to wait until the enzyme levels are normal to initiate refeeding (Box 1).

FLUID MANAGEMENT

In the patient with more severe pancreatitis, the aims of medical management are restoration of metabolic homeostasis, relief of pain, and removal of the

BOX 1 Management and Treatment of Acute Pancreatitis

- Correction of fluid deficit
- Correction of electrolyte and mineral abnormalities: Na^+, Ca^{++}, Mg^{++}
- Correction of hyperglycemia
- Analgesia for pain control
- Nutrition, with enteral feeding being the route preferred
- Drainage of nonresolving or symptomatic pseudocysts

precipitating cause if possible. These patients are best managed in the intensive care unit by a team including the gastroenterologist, pediatric surgeon, and intensivist. Hypovolemia, when present, must be urgently corrected. Once fluid resuscitation is completed with saline, blood, albumin, and fresh-frozen plasma, intravenous infusions are adjusted for maintenance plus replacement of ongoing fluid and electrolyte losses. Care must be taken to avoid fluid overload. Asymptomatic hypocalcemia is treated by the addition of calcium, 10 to 20 mEq per L, to the intravenous fluids. Seizures and tetany are treated with 10% calcium gluconate (0.1 to 0.2 g/kg) by slow intravenous infusion. Hyperglycemia is treated by adjustment of the glucose infusion rate.

IMAGING

Imaging studies are not required in the case of mild self-limited pancreatitis. When jaundice is present an ultrasound should be performed to evaluate for the presence of biliary lithiasis. In severe or nonresolving pancreatitis a CT scan is generally done. In recurrent pancreatitis, imaging of the biliary ductal system with magnetic resonance cholangiopancreatography (MRCP) or endoscopic retrograde cholangiopancreatography (ERCP) is recommended. All patients should have an ultrasound done 2 to 4 weeks following resolution of the acute illness to evaluate for the development of a pseudocyst.

PAIN RELIEF

Nasogastric suction relieves nausea and vomiting in symptomatic patients but does not shorten the duration of illness and therefore is of no benefit in the mildly ill patient. Adequate analgesia must be administered. Either morphine or meperidine in standard doses may be given as needed. Acetaminophen with codeine or ketorolac may be used for less severe pain.

NUTRITION

The patient should be fasted until nausea and vomiting have resolved and the serum lipase or amylase have peaked. Serum lipase may remain elevated for up to a week after normalization of the serum amylase and therefore cannot be used as a marker for refeeding. If symptoms recur after refeeding, the patient should be fasted again.

OTHER THERAPY

If fasting is necessary for longer than 5 days, nutritional support should be provided. When tolerated, jejunal tube feeding of an elemental diet is preferred over parenteral nutrition. The routine use of antibiotics is of no benefit during the acute phase of mild pancreatitis unless secondary infection is present, but is effective in the prevention of infection in cases of severe pancreatitis. Octreotide (synthetic cyclic somatostatin) does not decrease the duration of illness in severe pancreatitis. Octreotide may be helpful in the treatment of pancreatic pseudocysts and pancreatic fistulas.

SURGERY AND ENDOSCOPIC RETROGRADE CHOLANGIOPANCREATOGRAPHY

Although surgical therapy for acute pancreatitis is infrequently required in children, the treatment of severe acute pancreatitis may involve surgical drainage of necrotic material or abscesses. Endoscopic retrograde cholangiopancreatography (ERCP) is of benefit when pancreatitis is caused by anatomic abnormalities, such as strictures or stones.

PROGNOSIS

Prognostic factors have not been defined for children.

Common Pitfalls

Prolonged use of nasogastric suctioning and delay in refeeding until laboratory abnormalities are completely corrected may lead to unnecessary extended hospitalization. Parenteral nutrition should be reserved for the patient who does not tolerate gastric or jejunal feeding. Because pain can be a major problem, adequate analgesia should be given.

Communication and Counseling

The parents can be informed that acute pancreatitis is a self-limited condition lasting 4 to 5 days. Complete resolution is expected. A pseudocyst may develop 3 to 6 weeks following the acute episode.

Pancreatic Pseudocyst

Pancreatic pseudocysts, sacs delineated by a fibrous wall in the lesser peritoneal sac, are an uncommon sequela to acute or chronic pancreatitis. They may enlarge or extend in almost any direction, thereby producing a wide variety of symptoms. A pseudocyst is suggested when an episode of pancreatitis fails to resolve or when a mass develops after an episode of pancreatitis. Clinical features usually include pain, nausea, and vomiting. A palpable mass is present in 50% of patients and jaundice in 10%. Other findings may include ascites and pleural effusions.

Diagnosis

The most useful diagnostic techniques are ultrasonography, CT scanning, MRCP, and ERCP. Because of its ease, availability, and reliability, ultrasonography should be done first. Sequential studies using ultrasonography have shown that most small pseudocysts resolve spontaneously. The patient with acute pancreatitis should undergo an ultrasound evaluation 2 to 4 weeks after resolution of the acute episode for evaluation of possible pseudocyst formation.

Expert Opinion on Management Issues

Percutaneous and endoscopic drainage of pseudocysts are now the standard of care. The drainage procedure of choice depends on the anatomic location of the lesion and on local expertise. When surgical drainage is required, the pseudocyst must be allowed to mature for 4 to 6 weeks before surgery. Percutaneous and endoscopic drainage may be attempted earlier. ERCP or MRCP should precede surgical treatment to help the surgeon plan the approach and define anatomic abnormalities. It has been our experience that MRCP is not as sensitive as ERCP.

Common Pitfalls

- When surgical drainage is required, the pseudocyst must be allowed to mature for 4 to 6 weeks before surgery. Percutaneous and endoscopic drainage may be attempted earlier.
- ERCP or MRCP should precede surgical treatment to help the surgeon plan the approach and define anatomic abnormalities.
- MRCP is not as sensitive as ERCP in our experience.

Communication and Counseling

Small pseudocysts typically resolve without drainage. There is a low recurrence rate. Infections are uncommon, except when the pseudocyst is associated with severe pancreatitis.

CHRONIC PANCREATITIS

Chronic and recurrent acute pancreatitis in children may be caused by post-traumatic or congenital anomalies of the pancreatic or biliary ductal systems or, less commonly, by cystic fibrosis, abnormalities in the trypsinogen gene (hereditary pancreatitis) or the serine protease inhibitor, Kazal type 1 gene. Hereditary pancreatitis is transmitted as an autosomal dominant trait with incomplete penetrance and variable expressivity. Symptoms frequently begin in the first decade but are usually mild at the onset. Although spontaneous recovery from each attack occurs in 4 to 7 days, episodes become progressively more severe. Hereditary pancreatitis is diagnosed by the presence of the disease in successive generations of a family.

Other conditions associated with chronic relapsing pancreatitis and recurrent acute pancreatitis are hyperlipidemia (types I, IV, and V), hyperparathyroidism, and ascariasis. Although it has been thought that most cases of recurrent pancreatitis in childhood are idiopathic, congenital anomalies of the ductal systems (e.g., pancreas divisum) are probably more common than previously recognized.

Diagnosis

A thorough diagnostic evaluation of every child with more than one episode of pancreatitis, even if mild, is indicated. Serum lipid, calcium, and phosphorus levels are determined. Stools are evaluated for *Ascaris*, and a sweat test is performed. Plain abdominal films are evaluated for the presence of pancreatic calcifications. Abdominal ultrasound or CT scanning is performed to detect the presence of a pseudocyst or stones. ERCP or MRCP should be performed as part of the evaluation of any child with idiopathic, nonresolving, or recurrent pancreatitis and before surgery. Imaging may detect a previously undiagnosed anatomic defect that may be amenable to endoscopic or surgical therapy. Genetic testing for mutations in the trypsinogen and serine protease inhibitor, Kazal type 1 genes must be considered.

Expert Opinion on Management Issues

Metabolic abnormalities such as hyperglycemia and hyperlipidemia should be treated. Pain is treated with analgesics, narcotic or non-narcotic, sufficient for pain relief. A pain service with psychiatric or psychological support is helpful. Abdominal pain may be at least partially relieved by the administration of pancreatic enzymes before meals to induce feedback inhibition of pancreatic secretion. High-dose antioxidants have been shown to reduce the number of painful episodes in adults with chronic pancreatitis. School attendance is encouraged.

Endoscopic treatments include sphincterotomy, stone extraction, and insertion of pancreatic or biliary endoprostheses. Endoscopic therapy allows for successful nonsurgical management of conditions previously requiring surgical intervention.

Common Pitfalls

Failure to search for anatomic and metabolic disorders will lead to recurrent episodes of pancreatitis. Chronic pain because of inadequate analgesia is a major cause of a low quality of life and school absence.

Communication and Counseling

Psychological counseling is beneficial in patients with chronic pain. Genetic counseling is important when any of the hereditary forms of pancreatitis are diagnosed.

PANCREATIC INSUFFICIENCY

In children, exocrine pancreatic insufficiency occurs in cystic fibrosis, in chronic pancreatitis, in the Shwachman-Diamond syndrome, and following massive pancreatic resection for tumor. Isolated deficiencies of lipase and trypsin have been described but are extremely rare. Deficiency of enterokinase, a brush border enzyme required for activation of trypsinogen to trypsin, also leads to malabsorption.

Diagnosis

The diagnosis of pancreatic insufficiency is made by 72-hour fecal fat collection with calculation of the coefficient of absorption in a patient with a normal small bowel biopsy. Complete characterization of pancreatic function can only be made by stimulation with secretin and cholecystokinin and collection of pancreatic fluid. Tests such as fecal elastase and stool staining for lipid droplets may be used for screening but not for diagnostic purposes.

Expert Opinion on Management Issues

The keys to successful therapy are a skilled dietician and the appropriate choice of replacement enzyme therapy. Treatment of exocrine pancreatic insufficiency by oral replacement would seem to be rather simple; however, in practice, creatorrhea can usually be corrected, but steatorrhea is difficult to correct completely because of variability of lipase activity in different commercial preparations, inadequate dosage, incorrect timing of doses, lipase inactivation by gastric acid, and digestion of lipase in the enzyme preparation by chymotrypsin. At present, the enteric-coated products, Pancrease, Creon, Ultrase, and Pancrecarb are those most widely used in the United States.

The dosage of pancreatic replacement for children depends on the amount of food eaten and, therefore, can be established only by trial and error. Because these products contain excess protease compared with lipase, the dosage is estimated from the lipase requirement of 500 to 1500 IU/kg/meal. An adequate dose is one that is followed by the return of the stools to normal fat content, size, color, and odor. Enzyme replacement should be given at the beginning of and with the meal. Enzyme must also be given with snacks.

If adequate fat absorption cannot be realized, gastric acid neutralization with a histamine, receptor-blocking agent, or a proton pump inhibitor is used to prevent gastric acid enzyme inactivation and improve delivery of lipase into the intestine. The coating of enteric-coated preparations also protects lipase from acid inactivation. Complete correction of fat malabsorption may not always be possible.

Common Pitfalls

Untoward effects of pancreatic enzyme replacement therapy include allergic reactions, increased uric acid levels, and nephrolithiasis. Increased dosage of lipase beyond 2500 IU/kg per meal and use of high-potency enzyme preparations do not improve absorption but do increase the risk of fibrosing colonopathy in cystic fibrosis patients.

Supplemental fat-soluble vitamins may be needed to prevent deficiency because of malabsorption. If malabsorption is severe, supplemental tube feedings may be necessary to maintain adequate growth. Because of the introduction of percutaneous endoscopic gastrostomy (PEG), many patients now choose a PEG rather than nasogastric feedings.

Communication and Counseling

A patient who develops pancreatic insufficiency will be required to take replacement therapy for life.

SUGGESTED READINGS

1. Fox VL, Werlin SL, Heyman MB: A medical position statement: The North American Society for Pediatric Gastroenterology and Nutrition. Endoscopic retrograde cholangiopancreatography in children. J Pediatr Gastro Nutr 30:335–342, 2000. **Review of the indications, contraindications, and findings of pediatric endoscopic retrograde cholangiopancreatography.**
2. Werlin SL, Kugathasan S, Frautschy BC: Pancreatitis in children. J Pediatr Gastro Nutr 37:591, 2003. **Recent review of pancreatitis at a large pediatric center.**
3. United Kingdom guidelines for the management of acute pancreatitis. Gut 42(Suppl 2):S1-S13, 1998. **British guidelines for the treatment of acute pancreatitis in adults.**
4. Proesmans M, De Boeck K: Omeprazole, a proton pump inhibitor, improves residual steatorrhea in cystic fibrosis patients treated with high dose pancreatic enzymes. Eur J Pediatr 162:760, 2003. **Demonstrates improvement in fat absorption when omeprazole is added to pancreatic enzyme treatment in cystic fibrosis. The same principle is valid in non cystic fibrosis pancreatic insufficiency.**

Conjugated and Unconjugated Hyperbilirubinemia and Disorders of the Biliary Tree

Wallace A. Gleason, Jr.

KEY CONCEPTS

- Prolonged conjugated hyperbilirubinemia (cholestasis) in a young infant demands explanation because of the possibility that it is due to biliary atresia, a potentially fatal disease that requires surgical intervention by 2 months of age to achieve a successful result.
- The distinction between biliary obstruction and hepatocellular inflammation is the most important responsibility of physicians who encounter infants and children with cholestasis early in the course of the disease.

- Supportive care of infants and children with cholestasis is important in minimizing the nutritional and metabolic consequences of the illness.
- Identification and verification of the diagnosis of Gilbert disease is important to prevent future diagnostic or therapeutic misadventures.

Hyperbilirubinemia is an elevation of the serum bilirubin beyond the normal level of 1 mg/dL. It implies disordered bilirubin metabolism or excretion or production of bilirubin in excess of the capacity of the liver to metabolize and excrete it. Levels of bilirubin above 5 mg/dL usually result in jaundice (icterus), a yellow discoloration most visible in the sclerae and skin. Bilirubin is produced in the reticuloendothelial system from heme and is transported to the liver bound to albumin. Hepatocyte uptake of poorly soluble bilirubin is followed by conjugation with glucuronic acid by glucuronyl transferase to produce soluble bilirubin diglucuronide, which is then excreted via the bile canaliculus to the bile duct system and, ultimately, the intestine.

Most laboratories report serum bilirubin levels as direct and total. The direct fraction, so called because its increased solubility allows a faster reaction with the color reagent, is the conjugated fraction, usually 0.1 mg per dL. Unconjugated bilirubin is the difference between the total and direct bilirubin values. Unconjugated hyperbilirubinemia implies either ineffective conjugation because of impaired bilirubin transport, uptake, or glucuronyl transferase activity, or excess bilirubin production because of hemolysis. Conjugated hyperbilirubinemia results from inability to excrete the conjugated bilirubin into the bile canaliculus and is also known as cholestasis. In most situations causing conjugated hyperbilirubinemia, the level of conjugated fraction is one half to two thirds of the total bilirubin level.

HYPERBILIRUBINEMIA

Unconjugated Hyperbilirubinemia

Unconjugated hyperbilirubinemia occurs mostly in the neonatal period and is discussed in the chapter "The Treatment of Neonatal Hyperbilirubinemia." Gilbert syndrome is the most common cause of recurrent indirect hyperbilirubinemia in children and adolescents. Typically, mild jaundice, with serum bilirubin between 3 and 10 mg/dL, will be noted in an adolescent during another illness, most frequently viral respiratory illnesses. Most patients have no symptoms, although some complain of abdominal pain. The diagnosis is established by an elevated bilirubin in the presence of a normal conjugated bilirubin and normal transaminases, excluding viral hepatitis. This relatively common disorder results from an abnormality in glucuronyl transferase activity. Treatment is unnecessary, and the patient and family are best served by educating them about the disorder to prevent future diagnostic or therapeutic misadventures.

Crigler-Najjar syndrome is a substantially less common autosomal recessive disorder causing unconjugated hyperbilirubinemia manifesting in the neonatal period. Type 1 results from a complete absence of glucuronyl transferase and causes severe hyperbilirubinemia in the newborn, requiring repeat exchange transfusions and prolonged phototherapy. Medical therapy is unsatisfactory, and most of these patients require liver transplantation. Type 2 Crigler-Najjar syndrome is a partial deficiency resulting in less dramatic elevations. Treatment with phenobarbital induces glucuronyl transferase activity, reducing bilirubin levels.

Conjugated Hyperbilirubinemia

Conjugated hyperbilirubinemia in infants (neonatal cholestasis) requires prompt consideration of a wide variety of infectious, metabolic, and anatomic disorders to identify infants who may benefit from timely intervention to correct atresia of the extrahepatic bile ducts. Bacterial infection, including sepsis and urinary tract infection, in young infants can cause cholestasis. Medical therapy involves identification of the infection and antibiotic treatment of the responsible organism. The syndrome of congenital infection classically manifests with failure to thrive, cholestasis, hepatosplenomegaly, thrombocytopenia, and petechiae and is caused by intrauterine infection with cytomegalovirus, herpes simplex, rubella, or toxoplasmosis. Treatment of infants with active cytomegalovirus infection with ganciclovir, an antiviral agent, is controversial. Acyclovir treatment is recommended for infants with active herpes simplex infection, and treatment with pyrimethamine, sulfadiazine, and leucovorin is recommended for infants with active toxoplasma infection. Prednisolone is added if there is evidence of severe central nervous system infection (cerebrospinal fluid [CSF] protein >1 g/dL) or active chorioretinitis. No effective treatment is available for congenital rubella. Congenital syphilis is another bacterial infection that causes neonatal cholestasis and requires penicillin therapy (Box 1).

α_1-Antitrypsin deficiency results from a homozygous mutation resulting in accumulation of an abnormally folded enzyme in the hepatocytes causing progressive cirrhosis. Second only to biliary atresia as a cause of chronic liver disease leading to liver transplantation in children, this disorder frequently manifests with neonatal cholestasis and hepatomegaly. Cholestasis usually resolves, but progressive hepatic dysfunction usually causes cirrhosis by age 5 to 12 years. Liver transplantation, which restores circulating levels of α_1-antitrypsin to normal, is the only successful treatment. Children with cystic fibrosis also may present with transient neonatal cholestasis, with later development of chronic pulmonary disease and pancreatic insufficiency. The neonatal cholestasis requires no treatment and is of little clinical significance except that it may lead to early diagnosis of the underlying disease.

BOX 1 Cholestasis in Infants and Children

Neonatal Cholestasis
- Infectious
  - Bacterial infection
  - Congenital infection (cytomegalovirus, rubella, herpes simplex, toxoplasmosis)
  - Congenital syphilis
- Hereditary and metabolic
  - α_1-Antitrypsin deficiency
  - Cystic fibrosis
  - Galactosemia
  - Hereditary fructose intolerance
  - Hypothyroidism
  - Panhypopituitarism
  - Paucity of intrahepatic bile ducts (Alagille syndrome, arteriohepatic dysplasia)
  - Tyrosinemia
- Anatomic biliary obstruction
  - Biliary atresia
- Other
  - Idiopathic neonatal hepatitis syndrome
  - Multifactorial intrahepatic cholestasis (TPN cholestasis)
  - Inspissated bile syndrome

Cholestasis: Older Infants and Children
- Infectious
  - Viral hepatitis
- Hereditary and metabolic
  - α_1-Antitrypsin deficiency
  - Progressive familial intrahepatic cholestasis
- Anatomic biliary obstruction
  - Choledochal cyst
  - Cholelithiasis
  - Sclerosing cholangitis

TPN, total parenteral nutrition.

Metabolic causes of neonatal cholestasis include galactosemia and hereditary fructose intolerance. In the former, due to absence of galactose-1-phosphate uridylyl transferase, inability to metabolize galactose leads to elevated blood levels of galactose, the basis of some state screening tests for this disorder, which is excreted in the urine and is detected as a reducing sugar. Lactose, the most common dietary carbohydrate in young infants, is hydrolyzed to glucose and galactose; thus a positive test for urinary reducing sugar in a jaundiced infant taking a lactose-containing formula should be followed by prompt elimination of lactose from the diet and measurement of the level of the defective enzyme, which is expressed in red blood cells. The latter disease results from congenital deficiency of fructose-1-phosphate aldolase and manifests when sucrose is introduced into the diet later in infancy or in infants fed sucrose-containing formulas. Treatment involves excluding sucrose from the diet.

Hypothyroidism and hypopituitarism manifest with neonatal cholestasis. They share the dependence of the development of pathways of hepatic bilirubin metabolism on thyroid hormone. Cortisol deficiency also impairs the development of liver function. The diagnosis is made by measuring levels of thyroid hormone and cortisol in blood. Treatment consists of hormone replacement.

Paucity of intrahepatic bile ducts, also known as *Alagille syndrome*, is a disorder in which cholestasis is caused by decreased numbers of intrahepatic bile ducts. It is associated with vascular anomalies, most commonly peripheral pulmonic stenosis, bone abnormalities, most commonly butterfly vertebrae, and eye abnormalities, most commonly posterior embryotoxon. Because of the associated anomalies, it is frequently referred to as *arteriohepatic dysplasia*. Treatment is largely supportive and liver transplantation has been successful.

Tyrosinemia type 1 results from congenital deficiency of the enzyme fumarylacetoacetate hydrolase and is characterized by cholestatic liver disease. Coagulopathy is common, and older infants and children frequently develop rickets. There is an increased incidence of hepatoma in untreated patients. Elevations in blood tyrosine, methionine, and homocysteine reflect accumulation of substrates of the missing enzyme. Elevations in serum α-fetoprotein are consistent with giant-cell transformation in the liver, a nonspecific feature of neonatal cholestasis. The diagnosis depends on demonstration of increased urinary excretion of succinyl acetone, an upstream metabolite responsible for the liver and renal toxicity resulting in cholestasis and the renal Fanconi syndrome. Treatment with the herbicide 2-(2-nitro-4-trifluro-methybenzoyl)-1,3-cyclohexanedione (NTBC) and dietary tyrosine restriction are helpful, but liver transplantation is required to cure the disease.

Biliary atresia is the most important cause of neonatal cholestasis because it causes progressive biliary cirrhosis, which will prove fatal if not recognized early and treated promptly. Identification of the gallbladder by ultrasound after a 6-hour fast makes the diagnosis unlikely; however, a choledochal cyst, a feature of some types of biliary atresia, may be mistaken for a contracted gallbladder. Inability to identify a gallbladder should be followed by a radionuclide hepatobiliary scan after 5 days of pretreatment with phenobarbital to demonstrate excretion of the radionuclide into the duodenum and patency of the extrahepatic bile ducts. If both of these fail to rule out biliary atresia, surgical exploration of the right upper quadrant, operative cholangiography, and, in the event that biliary atresia is found, hepatic portoenterostomy should be undertaken. Although this operation is frequently unsuccessful in reestablishing bile flow, the rate of success is greater if done at younger than 2 months of age. Unsuccessful portoenterostomy usually requires liver transplantation and is the most common indication for liver transplantation in children.

Idiopathic neonatal hepatitis syndrome is an as yet poorly characterized group of disorders causing neonatal cholestasis for which no other cause can be found. Most of these infants are well and anicteric at 1 year of age, but death can occur from liver failure as early as 6 months of age. Treatment is supportive.

Multifactorial intrahepatic cholestasis occurs in premature infants. Although parenteral nutrition is the most prominent cause, analogy to postoperative jaundice in adults suggests that drugs, hypotension, sepsis (systemic or intraperitoneal), anesthesia, and prolonged fasting, all complications of care for premature infants not causing cholestasis individually, contribute to cholestasis as a late complication of prematurity. Treatment is supportive.

The inspissated bile syndrome is neonatal cholestasis appearing during brisk episodes of hemolysis. Typically hemolysis, either autoimmune or extravascular, results in unconjugated hyperbilirubinemia. At or just beyond the peak total bilirubin, the direct fraction begins to rise, and both then decline to normal. This transient, benign cholestasis probably results from saturation of transport and excretory mechanisms because of an increased bilirubin load and immature liver function.

Expert Opinion on Management Issues

Supportive treatment seeks to minimize the nutritional and systemic repercussions of chronic cholestasis.

Medium chain triglycerides are absorbed directly into the portal venous system and do not require emulsification by bile acids in the duodenum, the rate limiting step in the intestinal absorption of long-chain fatty acids. Growth failure because of fat malabsorption is a common consequence of cholestatic liver disease. A formula such as Pregestimil, in which most of the fat is medium-chain triglycerides, improves weight gain in infants with cholestatic liver disease.

Ursodeoxycholic acid is an exogenous bile acid that is less toxic to the hepatocyte than some endogenous bile acids. The inflammatory response to retained bile acids is reduced by replacing the relatively more toxic endogenous bile acids with a less toxic bile acid. Additionally, it is a hydrocholeretic agent, that is, it increases the volume of bile flow. The dose is 10 to 20 mg/kg/day.

Phenobarbital induces hepatic microsomal enzymes and speeds the conjugation and excretion of bilirubin. Although this will decrease the serum bilirubin, concern over the developmental effects of prolonged phenobarbital treatment in view of the lack of serious repercussions of hyperbilirubinemia lessen the enthusiasm for its use. The dose is 5 mg/kg/day.

Fat-soluble vitamins are absorbed poorly in infants with cholestasis. Deficiencies of vitamins A, D, E, and K should be suspected if cholestasis lasts 6 months or longer. This is done by measuring the blood levels of vitamin A, 25-hydroxy vitamin D, the circulating form of vitamin D that best represents vitamin D status and vitamin E. Vitamin K sufficiency is estimated using the prothrombin time. Supplementation uses water-soluble preparations of the fat-soluble vitamins individually, or by a preparation combining them.

Rifampicin is effective in treating pruritus due to bile acid retention in cholestatic illnesses. The dose is 10 mg/kg/day. Other agents that have been used to manage pruritus include anion exchange resins (Cholestyramine, Colestipol). The dose is 0.25 to 0.5 g/kg/day. These agents are less effective and can cause hyperchloremic acidosis in small infants. Concerns about intestinal obstruction because of inspissation of the resin and interference with the absorption of other drugs have limited their use.

DISORDERS OF THE HEPATOBILIARY TREE

Most children presenting with jaundice have viral hepatitis (see chapter entitled "Viral Hepatitis"), but jaundice is occasionally caused by biliary obstruction, and the distinction between them early in the course of the illness is crucial. Hepatitis is characterized by hepatocellular inflammation indicated by substantial elevations in transaminases with only modest elevation of alkaline phosphatase. In contrast, biliary obstruction typically causes a two- to threefold elevation of alkaline phosphatase with only a modest elevation of transaminases. The elevation of alkaline phosphatase results from bile ductular proliferation, the histological correlate of biliary obstruction. Other enzymes more specific to the biliary epithelium—γ-glutamyl transpeptidase (GGT) and 5′-nucleotidase—are also elevated, and measuring them is useful in confirming the biliary origin of the alkaline phosphatase.

Cholelithiasis may manifest with right upper quadrant pain and tenderness, jaundice, or both. The pain is frequently intensified by the stimulation of gallbladder contraction by fat intake. In young children, most gallstones are pigment stones. Cholesterol stones occur more commonly in older children and adolescents. Ultrasonography of the abdomen is an effective diagnostic technique. Treatment by cholecystectomy prevents recurrences.

Choledochal cysts are cystic malformations of the extrahepatic biliary ducts that are in the spectrum of abnormalities seen in biliary atresia. Patients not detected in infancy usually present before 10 years of age with abdominal pain or an abdominal mass. Treatment is surgical resection to deal with current symptoms and to prevent complications such as cholangitis and cholangiocarcinoma.

Sclerosing cholangitis is a rare disorder manifesting with right upper quadrant pain and intermittent jaundice seen most commonly in children with inflammatory bowel disease and Langerhans cell histiocytosis. The diagnosis can be established by cholangiography. Treatment involves achieving remission of the underlying disease. Ursodeoxycholic acid is also useful in treatment.

Common Pitfalls

Many chemical profiles available in newborn nurseries include only a total bilirubin, because the usual purpose for its measurement is to confirm unconjugated hyperbilirubinemia and direct its management. Failure to measure the conjugated bilirubin in an infant with persistent jaundice may lead to delay in diagnosis and management of cholestasis.

Early discharge from the normal newborn nursery and infrequent follow-up of jaundiced infants may lead to delay in appreciating that what appears to be prolonged jaundice may be cholestasis, requiring diagnostic evaluation.

SUGGESTED READINGS

1. Balistreri WF: Intrahepatic cholestasis. J Pediatr Gastroenterol Nutr 35(Suppl 1):S17-S23, 2002. **A review of the pathophysiology of cholestasis.**
2. Btaiche IF, Khalidi N: Parenteral nutrition-associated liver complications in children. Pharmacotherapy 22:188–211, 2002. **A recent review of drug treatment of TPN cholestasis.**
3. Davenport M, Betali P, D'Antiga L, et al: The spectrum of surgical jaundice in infancy. J Pediatr Surg 38:1471–1479, 2003. **A large series of patients referred to pediatric surgeons for surgical management of cholestasis.**
4. Faust TW, Reddy KR: Postoperative jaundice. Clin Liver Dis 8:151–166, 2004. **A discussion of the multiple factors that, acting together, contribute to cholestasis in the postoperative patient. Although the discussion focuses on adults, the discussion of mechanisms is pertinent to the causes of cholestasis seen commonly in growing premature infants.**
5. Haber BA, Russo P: Biliary atresia. Gastroenterol Clin North Am 32:891–911, 2003. **A recent review of the current understanding of the cause, diagnostic evaluation and management of biliary atresia.**
6. Kahn E: Biliary atresia revisited. Pediatr Dev Pathol 7:109–124, 2004. **A recent review focusing on the different types of biliary atresia from a pathologist's point of view.**
7. Kamath BM, Piccoli DA: Heritable disorders of the bile ducts. Gastroenterol Clin North Am 32:857–875, 2003. **A broader view of bile duct disorders with an extensive discussion of the Alagille syndrome.**
8. Karpen SJ: Update on the etiologies and management of neonatal cholestasis. Clin Perinatol 29:159–180, 2002. **An anatomical approach to the differential diagnosis and evaluation of cholestasis in the neonate.**
9. Krawinkel MB: Parenteral nutrition-associated cholestasis—what do we know, what can we do? Eur J Pediatr Surg 14:230–234, 2004. **A recent review of the pathogenesis, prevention and treatment of TPN cholestasis.**
10. Paumgartner G, Beuers U: Mechanisms of action and therapeutic efficacy of ursodeoxycholic acid in cholestatic liver disease. Clin Liver Dis 8:67–81, 2004. **A discussion of the pharmacology of ursodeoxycholic acid in cholestasis.**

Cirrhosis and Portal Hypertension

Manoochehr Karjoo, Philip G. Holtzapple, N. John Cavuto, and Ronald E. Kleinman

CIRRHOSIS

KEY CONCEPTS

- Cirrhosis is a chronic liver disease characterized by architectural changes of the liver associated with collagen accumulation, widespread fibrosis, and regenerative nodule formation. These changes are irreversible and can alter hepatic hemodynamics, nutrition, protein synthesis, and drug metabolism.
- The most common causes of cirrhosis in children include metabolic and genetic diseases such as galactosemia, fructosemia, tyrosinemia, cystic fibrosis, α_1-antitrypsin

10

Expert Opinion on Management Issues

NUTRITIONAL SUPPORT

Most patients with cirrhosis have evidence of significant malnutrition manifested by signs of protein-calorie malnutrition, steatorrhea, fat-soluble vitamin deficiency, and mineral deficiency. Long-term nutritional management with appropriate diet regimens is directed toward promoting growth and development, as well as preventing potential bleeding and ascites. Patients with advanced liver disease may have high fecal fat loss. Their steatorrhea is due to insufficient intraluminal long-chain triglyceride lipolysis secondary to decreased bile acid secretion. In such patients, medium-chain triglycerides that do not require bile salt solubilization before absorption can provide needed calories.

Fat-soluble vitamin supplementation may eliminate significant morbidity in cirrhosis. Vitamin A supplementation (10,000 to 15,000 IU/day) prevents xerophthalmia, night blindness, and thickened skin. Vitamin D supplementation (5000 to 8000 IU/day) or as 25-hydroxycholecalciferol (3 to 5 μg/kg/day) should also be provided to prevent metabolic bone disease, including rickets, and pathologic fractures. In patients with kidney disease, 1,25-hydroxycholecalciferol, 0.25 μg/day, should be considered. Vitamin E deficiency results in areflexia, ophthalmoplegia, cerebellar ataxia, peripheral neuropathy, and posterior column dysfunction. A large dose (up to 50 to 400 IU/day, usually with 150 IU/kg/day as oral α-tocopherol A) may be required. If a patient fails to respond to a large dose of vitamin E orally, intramuscular DL-α-tocopherol (50 mg/day) could be considered. Vitamin K supplementation in an oral water-soluble form may be started at a dosage of 2.5 to 5 mg every other day and increased up to 5 mg/day. Some patients with coagulopathy and bleeding unresponsive to oral therapy may require intramuscular injections of vitamin K. Correction of coagulopathy may still be impaired as a result of a markedly diminished platelet count and inadequate hepatic reserve. The patient's serum calcium, phosphorus, and magnesium levels should be measured and supplemented as needed.

ASCITES

Treatment of ascites starts with a low-sodium diet of 1 to 2 mEq/kg/day (or 250 to 500 mg/day) and fluid restriction to 1000 mL/m^2/day. It is not usually necessary to restrict fluid intake in patients with adequate renal output (urine output more than 500 mL/m^2/day). Diuresis occurs spontaneously in approximately 25% of patients with sodium restriction alone. If this regimen is not sufficient, the aldosterone antagonist spironolactone, 3 to 5 mg/kg/day in three or four divided doses, can be started. The half-life of spironolactone is 12 hours. Approximately 50% of patients undergo diuresis with this dose. For the rest, the dose may be increased up to 10 to 12 mg/kg/day 72 hours after initial therapy. Patients unresponsive to this regimen may require hydrochlorothiazide, 2 to 3 mg/kg/day, or furosemide, 1 to 2 mg/kg every other day up to twice daily. Serum sodium, potassium, urea, and creatine and urinary sodium and potassium should be measured regularly as long as the patient is receiving diuretics. While taking diuretics, patients are prone to prerenal azotemia, hypokalemia, hyponatremia, hypotension, metabolic alkalosis, hepatic encephalopathy, and hepatorenal syndrome. Patients with ascites significant enough to compromise respiratory status may respond to salt-poor albumin infusion, 0.5 to 1.0 g/kg/dose, with close medical supervision, often followed by or given with diuretic. Slow diuresis decreases the potential for renal failure. Therapeutic paracentesis with a slow albumin infusion equal in volume to that removed in the paracentesis also decreases the chance of hepatorenal syndrome. Only a few studies have examined therapeutic paracentesis in children, but it is a relatively safe and effective treatment in adults. Complications of paracentesis include intravascular protein and volume loss, renal failure, and infection.

Ascites is a poor prognostic sign in patients with chronic liver disease. No evidence indicates that treatment of ascites alters the natural history of the underlying disease. The transjugular intrahepatic portosystemic stent shunt is an effective treatment of refractory ascites and hepatorenal syndrome and has a positive effect on nutritional status in adult patients and has been used in children as well.

ENCEPHALOPATHY

Precipitating factors leading to hepatic encephalopathy or coma include gastrointestinal (GI) bleeding, a large dietary protein load, infection, azotemia, vomiting, diarrhea, paracentesis, and severe constipation. Metabolic and electrolyte causes include hypokalemia, hyponatremia, hypomagnesemia, and hypocalcemia; metabolic alkalosis may also contribute. The use of drugs such as diuretics or sedatives can precipitate encephalopathy. A comatose patient should be evaluated for any of these precipitating conditions. Cultures of blood, ascitic fluid, and urine should be obtained. A nasogastric tube should be inserted and gastric lavage performed to investigate for upper GI bleeding. Patients should initially have no protein intake to reduce ammonia production. A nonabsorbable antibiotic, such as oral neomycin, 100 mg/kg/day, should be started. Lactulose, a nonabsorbable sugar, produces short-chain fatty acids in the colon, which leads to a drop in pH and thereby reduces ammonia reabsorption. For patients with end-stage liver disease and recurring hepatic encephalopathy, liver transplantation should be considered.

INFECTIONS

Bacterial peritonitis may occur as a consequence of contamination of the ascitic fluid with pneumococci, *Escherichia coli*, and other enteric organisms. Patients experience a sudden onset of fever, anorexia, diarrhea, abdominal pain, distention, chills, and leukocytosis. Asymptomatic peritonitis is seen in a few patients. If peritonitis is suspected, a diagnostic peritoneal tap should be performed. A combination of ampicillin and gentamicin should be started in asymptomatic patients if the polymorphonuclear leukocyte count is greater than $500/mm^3$ in peritoneal fluid or less than $250/mm^3$ with signs of peritonitis. Antibiotic therapy should be started before sensitivity is known.

LIVER TRANSPLANTATION

Liver transplantation should be considered in patients with cirrhosis in whom end-stage liver disease develops (see the section on liver transplantation).

PORTAL HYPERTENSION

KEY CONCEPTS

- Portal hypertension occurs when blood flow in the portal vein is impeded. It may develop secondary to intrahepatic or extrahepatic pathology, and distinguishing between these two has both clinical and therapeutic implications.
- Cirrhosis acquired as a result of progressive inflammation from disorders that occur in infancy and childhood, such as biliary atresia, chronic viral hepatitis, α_1-antitrypsin deficiency, and tyrosinemia, may produce intrahepatic portal hypertension. Extrahepatic portal hypertension may be a result of either prehepatic (e.g., cavernous transformation of the portal vein, portal vein thrombosis, splenic vein thrombosis) or posthepatic (e.g., Budd-Chiari syndrome) vascular obstruction.
- Portal hypertension may be clinically manifested in various ways. The most common initial sign is upper GI bleeding from ruptured esophagogastric varices. Isolated splenomegaly in the absence of other signs and symptoms may be the initial finding in up to 25% of children. Splenomegaly may be accompanied by evidence of anemia, neutropenia, or thrombocytopenia if hypersplenism is present. Less common initial manifestations include ascites and bleeding hemorrhoids.
- The signs and symptoms noted often follow the development of portosystemic collateral channels. Blood is diverted from the high-pressure portal venous system to the lower-pressure systemic circulation. Collateral flow through the gastric veins results in esophagogastric varices; increased flow through the rectal veins contributes to the development of hemorrhoids. Caput medusae results from dilation of the epigastric vessels in the abdominal wall.

Expert Opinion on Management Issues

DIAGNOSTIC EVALUATION

Ultrasonography is the most helpful diagnostic test for assessing portal hypertension and may aid in distinguishing intrahepatic from extrahepatic causes. Cavernous transformation of the portal vein may be a congenital lesion. Alternatively, portal vein thrombosis, the most common cause of extrahepatic portal hypertension, may result in cavernous transformation of the portal vein. Cavernous transformation is apparent when a normal portal vein cannot be identified and, instead, tortuous collateral vessels are present in the area of the porta hepatis. Cirrhosis does not lead to cavernous transformation of the portal vein, but it is often a cause of portal hypertension. Sonography can identify cirrhosis by the presence of regenerating nodules, which are discrete islands of hepatic parenchyma with a thin border of fibrous and fatty connective tissue of increased echogenicity. Cirrhotic hepatic parenchyma itself may display increased echogenicity due to fatty deposition. Finally, sonography may be able to identify the various portosystemic channels that have developed secondary to portal hypertension.

Doppler ultrasonography is useful in determining the presence and direction of portal vein flow and in delineating the hepatic arteries and veins. It may also be used to assess patency of portocaval shunts surgically placed to relieve portal hypertension. In Budd-Chiari syndrome, slow or absent flow in the hepatic veins may be detected. However, the most reliable technique to demonstrate hepatic vein obstruction is transjugular hepatic venography.

CT scanning may demonstrate abnormalities consistent with portal hypertension, such as ascites, the development of collateral circulation with varices, and liver parenchymal changes. However, it does not usually provide as much information as Doppler ultrasound. Magnetic resonance angiography is increasingly used to image the portal and hepatic vasculature. Angiography aids in evaluation of the vascular anatomy for potential shunting procedures. It also helps assess the distribution of collateral vessels, the dynamics of portal flow, and the site of portal venous obstruction, if any. Direct injection angiography may also be used as an interventional technique to open a narrowed or obstructed vascular channel.

TREATMENT

Therapy for portal hypertension and GI bleeding depends on the clinical situation. Much of the management of portal hypertension in children is based on extrapolation from studies conducted in adults. Few well-controlled, randomized, double-blind trials in children have compared the efficacy of the various therapeutic options. Efforts primarily center on prevention and control of variceal bleeding, although bleeding from ulcers and hypertensive gastropathy also occur in pediatric patients with portal hypertension. Treatment strategies may be based on prevention of the first variceal bleeding episode, management of acute variceal bleeding, and management of recurrent variceal bleeding. Splenomegaly, with or without hypersplenism, rarely requires intervention. Bleeding from thrombocytopenia or infection secondary to neutropenia is a rare event in children with hypersplenism. Splenic embolization in lieu of splenectomy has been successfully used to treat these conditions. Ascites and encephalopathy are other potential complications of portal hypertension. Ascites may become so pronounced that it leads to respiratory compromise. Encephalopathy, which may be precipitated by GI bleeding, should be considered in any patient with portal hypertension and altered mental status. Management of these complications of liver disease is discussed in another chapter.

Factors that place a patient at increased risk for variceal bleeding include large varices, the presence of red "whale" marking on the varix, and marked deterioration in liver function. These risk factors are validated only in studies of adult subjects. Nevertheless, when portal hypertension is discovered before an episode of variceal bleeding, one must consider the risk-benefit ratio of the various therapeutic options versus no intervention. β-Blocking agents reduce portal pressure by constricting the splanchnic circulation and decreasing cardiac output. Treatment with the nonselective β-blocker propranolol for prevention of bleeding in adult patients with varices is strongly recommended because it reduces the risk of bleeding and may improve survival. Studies in children suggest that propranolol should be considered for pediatric patients as well. Extreme caution must be used in patients with cardiac disease, asthma, or diabetes. Blood pressure instability with the use of propranolol is a concern in children because it reduces cardiac output. In younger children, cardiac output depends more on heart rate. Propranolol may prevent the

expected increase in heart rate during an acute variceal bleeding episode and place a child at greater risk for hypovolemic shock. The usual pediatric dosage range is from 2 to 4 mg/kg/day in two equally divided doses. The dose is titrated upward until a 20% reduction in resting heart rate is obtained. Variceal banding may reduce morbidity from esophageal varices in patients who have not bled but are awaiting a liver transplant. But for most patients, this procedure offers no benefit when administered before the first episode of variceal bleeding. Shunt surgery is also not indicated for prophylaxis of variceal bleeding.

MANAGEMENT OF BLEEDING

If a child with portal hypertension has GI bleeding, the initial intervention should be directed toward cardiopulmonary stabilization of the patient. Priority is placed on determining whether the patient is hemodynamically stable. The extent of the blood loss must then be evaluated. Vital signs are closely monitored, including initial assessment for orthostasis. Intravenous access is obtained with the placement of two large-bore catheters, and isotonic solutions such as normal saline or lactated Ringer's solution are infused. Blood is sent for a complete blood count including platelet count, prothrombin time, partial thromboplastin time, electrolytes, glucose, urea nitrogen, and creatine, and for typing and cross-matching.

A nasogastric tube should be placed and the stomach contents aspirated. Gastric lavage with room-temperature or slightly warmed saline is performed to remove old blood and to assess whether the patient is actively bleeding. Blood and platelet transfusions may be required, as well as correction of coagulopathy with fresh-frozen plasma. Although a child with cirrhosis may have a coagulopathy that predisposes to GI bleeding and poses complications for treatment, a child with extrahepatic portal hypertension often has normal liver function without compromised hemostasis. Intravenous H_2 antagonists are often administered in an effort to reduce acid production and offer cytoprotection, although their efficacy in stopping or decreasing GI bleeding is not proven.

Treatment options for acute variceal hemorrhage include pharmacologic management, therapeutic endoscopic intervention, and surgery. Pharmacologic management is used to stabilize the patient by slowing or stopping the bleeding. If the bleeding is from varices in the esophagus or from a visible vessel in an ulcer, therapeutic endoscopy or surgery can then be performed. Drug therapy is the principal treatment for bleeding from severe gastritis or varices located in the stomach or small intestine.

Vasopressin, a drug long used to control acute variceal bleeding, acts by constricting the splanchnic circulation, thereby decreasing portal pressure. Adverse effects are often seen, including oliguria, myocardial ischemia, and cerebrovascular accidents. In adults, there is no advantage to infusion of vasopressin selectively into the superior mesenteric artery to minimize its systemic effects. Intravenous infusion in children of

0.1 to 0.2 U/m^2/minute should be administered. If bleeding continues, the dose may be titrated up to 0.5 U/m^2/minute. After no bleeding has occurred for 12 hours, the infusion may be tapered over the next 24 to 48 hours. Close monitoring for hypertension, oliguria, and hyponatremia is indicated. Vasopressin should be used with caution in patients with seizure disorders, asthma, or vascular, cardiac, or renal disease.

Somatostatin, an endogenous peptide found in the GI tract and hypothalamus, is used in the pharmacologic management of acute GI bleeding. Somatostatin decreases both portal pressure and collateral blood flow. It is currently used in the form of octreotide, a longer-acting synthetic analogue. Octreotide is as efficacious as vasopressin in controlling GI bleeding but does not have the deleterious systemic effects of vasopressin. In the setting of acute GI hemorrhage, we begin with an initial bolus of 1 µg/kg, followed by a continuous infusion at 1 µg/kg/hour. Octreotide may also be dosed intravenously or subcutaneously every 8 hours. After GI bleeding is controlled, doses of 1 to 2 µg/kg three times daily may be used. Serum glucose must be monitored because octreotide is associated with both hyperglycemia and hypoglycemia; these side effects are usually related to the duration of therapy. GI complications include inhibition of gallbladder activity, cramping, and bloating.

The use of a Sengstaken-Blakemore tube to provide balloon tamponade of esophageal or high gastric varices may be considered in patients in whom pharmacologic management has failed and emergency sclerotherapy is not considered safe because of the rapidity of bleeding. Although bleeding is often controlled initially, rebleeding within 24 hours occurs in up to 50% of patients after deflation of the balloon. Balloon tamponade is also associated with potentially fatal complications, including aspiration pneumonia resulting from an inability to drain secretions from the body of the esophagus, large esophageal ulcers or esophageal perforation from pressure-induced injury, and airway obstruction from the balloon itself. The Sengstaken-Blakemore tube should be inserted only by a physician skilled in its placement and with the patient in an intensive care facility. An endotracheal tube must be placed for protection of the airway. Once the tube is passed into the stomach, the gastric balloon is distended with 50 to 100 mL of air and the tube is pulled back until resistance is noted at the gastroesophageal junction. A chest radiograph is then taken to ensure proper placement. Additional air may be infused (up to 150 mL in the pediatric balloon, 250 mL in the adult balloon), and the tube is then pulled taut and taped to a supporting structure outside the body.

Endoscopy often plays a major role in the diagnosis and treatment of acute GI bleeding secondary to portal hypertension. It should not be performed until the patient is hemodynamically stable. Gastric lavage can be performed before endoscopy to afford the best opportunity to visualize the GI mucosa. Endoscopy is useful to determine the cause of the bleeding and, in some cases of variceal bleeding or bleeding from an ulcer, as a means to intervene and stop the bleeding.

The therapeutic course depends on the cause of the portal hypertension. Children with portal vein thrombosis and variceal bleeding at an early age usually undergo sclerotherapy or banding. Those in whom the condition is diagnosed later in childhood or adolescence may be candidates for shunt surgery or variceal obliteration. Children with advanced cirrhosis and a coagulopathy rarely benefit long term from a surgical shunting procedure and usually undergo variceal obliteration or placement of a transcutaneous intrahepatic portosystemic shunt (TIPS), often in anticipation of liver transplantation.

Band Ligation

The technique used in banding is as follows: An "O" ring is inserted within a hooding device placed on the end of the endoscope. The varix to be ligated is invaginated into the hood by suction, and the O ring is released to strangulate the varix. Within a week, the polyp created by the band sloughs off and a shallow ulcer is left. Repeat sessions are indicated until the varices are obliterated.

Surgical Shunts

Surgically created portosystemic shunts are considered, if medical and endoscopic management techniques are unsuccessful in preventing rebleeding and liver transplantation is not an option. If liver transplantation is a consideration, every attempt should be made to avoid a portosystemic shunt because this procedure alters the anatomy and makes future liver transplantation more difficult. However, previous shunt surgery is not an absolute contraindication to liver transplantation. Surgical options include end-to-side and side-to-side portacaval shunts, proximal and distal splenorenal shunts, and cavomesenteric shunts. The most effective procedure to prevent recurrent bleeding is the portacaval shunt, which provides the largest caliber anastomosis. It is generally agreed that shunts constructed from veins larger than 1.0 cm in diameter have a higher long-term patency rate. The distal splenorenal shunt (Warren) was conceived to minimize the reduction in portal blood flow to the liver and decrease the incidence of subsequent encephalopathy. Whereas the proximal splenorenal shunt (Linton) involves ligation of all of the veins feeding the varices as well as splenectomy, the short gastric veins are kept intact during the distal splenorenal shunt procedure and a splenectomy is not required. In adult patients, the incidence of postoperative encephalopathy was lower in several studies with the Warren shunt but survival did not increase. Furthermore, the Warren shunt may be associated with a higher failure rate.

Portosystemic shunts are more difficult to construct in small infants. Pharmacologic and obliterative endoscopic therapy for control of variceal bleeding may be used until the child becomes large enough to be a candidate for shunt surgery. Shunts are more effective in patients with extrahepatic portal hypertension than in those with cirrhosis because liver function is usually normal and a coagulopathy is not present. However, adequate venous channels may not be available to construct such a shunt, as is the case in some patients with cavernous transformation of the portal vein. If shunting is not an option and bleeding cannot be controlled, one may consider transesophageal ligation of varices, transabdominal ligation of varices with gastric devascularization, or the Sugiura procedure, which involves esophageal transection, splenectomy, and devascularization of the lower part of the esophagus and stomach.

Percutaneous Transjugular Shunts

TIPS is being used increasingly in the short-term management of portal hypertension. The procedure involves percutaneous creation of an intrahepatic shunt between the hepatic and portal veins. It is usually performed by interventional radiologists in a relatively brief procedure that lasts from 1 to 3 hours. Patency of the portal vein is first assessed by Doppler ultrasound or by arterial portography if ultrasound visualization is inadequate. An angiographic catheter is then placed in the right internal jugular vein and manipulated into the right hepatic vein. A needle inserted through the catheter then punctures the hepatic vein approximately 2 cm beyond the junction of the hepatic vein and the inferior vena cava and is advanced under fluoroscopic guidance through the hepatic parenchyma into the portal vein. A catheter is placed in the tract created by the needle, and the mean pressure gradient from the portal vein to the inferior vena cava is determined. The tract is then expanded by inflation of a balloon catheter along the length of the tract, and metallic stents are placed to maintain patency of the tract. Before discharge, repeat Doppler ultrasound is performed to confirm patency of the shunt.

TIPS does not interfere with subsequent liver transplantation and is used in patients at high risk for bleeding while awaiting liver transplantation. It is often considered in patients in whom bleeding episodes were not effectively controlled by medical or endoscopic therapy. Complications include portal-systemic encephalopathy, which occurs in 20% of adult patients, transient worsening of liver function, and stenosis or occlusion of the shunt. Shunt insufficiency from stenosis or occlusion over a 6- to 12-month period is reported in 15% to 60% of patients; therefore, TIPS should be considered a temporizing measure. Stenosis may occur secondary to pseudointimal hyperplasia in the stent itself or where the hepatic vein and stent meet.

Ultimately, liver transplantation is the only option for patients with end-stage liver disease and significant unremitting complications of portal hypertension. The possibility of liver transplantation must always be considered when making therapeutic decisions concerning the management of portal hypertension.

Communication and Counseling

As with other chronic problems, both cirrhosis and portal hypertension evolve over time. A close collaboration between the child/family and the treating team are essential to assure adherence, understanding, and trust. Patients with both cirrhosis and portal hypertension should optimally be followed by a team specializing in pediatric liver disease. Many issues can be anticipated, and having an ongoing arrangement with a multidisciplinary team can be most useful.

SUGGESTED READINGS

1. Cabre E, Gassull MA: Nutritional and metabolic issues in cirrhosis and liver transplantation. Curr Opin Clin Nutr Metab Care 3:345–354, 2000. **Discusses cirrhosis and liver transplantation.**
2. Efrati O, Barak A, Modan-Moses D, et al: Liver cirrhosis and portal hypertension in cystic fibrosis. Eur J Gastroenterol Hepatol 15(10):1073–1078, 2003. **Reviews liver disease in CF.**
3. Goncalves ME, Carsos SR, Maksoud JG: Prophylactic sclerotherapy in children with esophageal varices: Long-term results of a controlled prospective randomized trial. J Pediatr Surg 35:401–405, 2000. **As noted, prospective, randomized controlled trial.**
4. Henderson JM, Nagle A, Curtas S, et al: Surgical shunts and TIPS for variceal decompression in the 1990s. Surgery 128:540–547, 2000. **Review of surgical shunts in the 1990s.**
5. Karrer FM, Narkewicz MR: Esophageal varices: Current management in children. Semin Pediatr Surg 8:193–201, 1999. **Reviews esophageal varices in children.**
6. Moustafellos E, Illueca M, Remotti HE, et al: Objective ranking of fibrosis in standard histologic sections of human neonatal liver: Applicability to α_1-antitrypsin deficiency. J Pediatr Gastroenterol Nutr 30:503–508, 2000. **Pathology evaluation of neonatal liver biopsy.**
7. Shilyansky J, Roberts EA, Superina RA: Distal splenorenal shunts for the treatment of severe thrombocytopenia from portal hypertension in children. J Gastrointest Surg 3:167–172, 1999. **Discusses end-stage liver disease.**
8. Sucy FJ, Shneider BL: Neonatal jaundice cholestasis. In Kaplowitz N (ed): Liver and Biliary Diseases. Baltimore: Williams & Wilkins, 1992, pp 442–455. **Classic discussion of neonatal jaundice and cholestasis.**
9. Zetterman RK: Cirrhosis of the liver. In Sherlock S (ed): Diseases of the Liver Biliary System. St. Louis: Mosby, 1992, pp 447–466. **Classic chapter in classic text.**
10. Zetterman RK: Complications of cirrhosis. In Sherlock S (ed): Diseases of the Liver and Biliary System. St. Louis: Mosby, 1992, pp 467–488. **Classic chapter in classic text.**

Acute and Chronic Hepatitis
Daniel S. Kamin and Ronald E. Kleinman

KEY CONCEPTS

- Aside from jaundice, the signs and symptoms of acute hepatitis are nonspecific or subclinical.
- Acute hepatitis generally resolves without sequelae.
- Fulminant hepatitis with liver failure is uncommon but potentially fatal.
- Hepatitis B is a vaccine-preventable infection.
- Serious side effects and modest efficacy characterize the current medical treatment of chronic hepatitis B and hepatitis C viral infections, and generally limit its application to those with active inflammation and fibrosis.

TABLE 1 Most Common Etiologies of Acute and Chronic Hepatitis by Age

Infancy	School-Age	Adolescence
Acute Hepatitis		
Congenital Infections (e.g., herpes simplex virus, rubella)	Hepatitis A Mononucleosis (Epstein-Barr virus)	Recreational drugs/toxins Medications Wilson disease
Systemic viral diseases (e.g., adenovirus)	Medications/toxins	Hepatitis A Hepatitis B

Genetic and metabolic conditions
    Tyrosinemia
    Galactosemia
Hereditary fructose intolerance		

Chronic Hepatitis		

Genetic and metabolic conditions
    α_1-antitrypsin deficiency
    Cystic fibrosis
    Storage diseases
	Celiac disease
	Autoimmune hepatitis
		Wilson disease
		Cystic fibrosis hereditary
		Hemochromatosis
		Autoimmune hepatitis
		Nonalcoholic steatohepatitis
		Hepatitis C

The presentation of hepatitis in childhood ranges from subclinical inflammation to fulminant, life-threatening liver failure. Acute infectious hepatitis generally resolves in 2 to 6 weeks. Chronic hepatitis is said to exist when the inflammatory process persists for more than 6 months. Viral infections are the most common cause of both acute and chronic hepatitis. Other common causes of acute and chronic hepatitis include toxins, drugs, and autoimmune disease. The most common causes of the hepatitis may vary with age (Table 1).

The physical examination of older children with acute hepatitis often reveals only jaundice and slight hepatomegaly with right upper quadrant tenderness. Young children may only have findings suggesting an acute flu-like illness. A spleen tip can be felt in 5% to 25% of well-hydrated patients. If changes in mental status or asterixis are present, liver failure and a fulminant course may be imminent. The biochemical findings characteristic of acute hepatitis include elevated levels of aminotransferases, often to more than 8 times normal. Alkaline phosphatase, γ-glutamyl transferase, and lactate dehydrogenase are minimally elevated. Direct hyperbilirubinemia of varying degree is also often present.

Acute Viral Hepatitis

Although many viral infections can cause acute hepatitis, hepatitis A virus (HAV) and hepatitis E virus (HEV) infections account for the majority of epidemic viral hepatitis worldwide (Table 2). Both infections are typically acquired from contaminated water or food. Outbreaks of HAV may occur in child care centers or institutions from improper handling of human waste; contaminated drinking water is the most common cause of community-wide outbreaks of HEV in developing countries.

HAV and HEV infections manifest themselves differently in children as compared to adults. Children are apt to have clinically silent or nonspecific symptoms, and adults more often develop a flu-like prodrome, an icteric stage during which jaundice, nausea, pruritus, and cholestasis predominate, followed by a convalescent stage during which signs and symptoms gradually resolve over 1 to 2 months. Most infected individuals recover uneventfully, although rarely hepatic failure and death may occur. Risk factors for a fulminant course include pregnancy, concomitant hepatitis C virus (HCV) or human immunodeficiency virus (HIV) infection, and age older than 65 years.

Hepatitis B virus (HBV) infection can also cause an acute hepatitis. As with HAV, infection is more likely to be subclinical in infants and young children. HBV is most often acquired by parenteral or sexual transmission and can be vertically transmitted to the developing fetus by an infected mother. The course of acute infections acquired during childhood is similar to that of HAV, although approximately 5% of acutely infected persons will develop chronic infection.

Other viruses that may cause hepatitis include Epstein-Barr virus (EBV), cytomegalovirus, adenovirus, coxsackie B viruses, human herpesvirus 6, and measles, mumps, and rubella viruses. Some severe cases of acute hepatitis are also associated with systemic viral infections (adenovirus), although others may be subclinical and/or a minor component of the infection (mononucleosis from EBV). Viral infection is suspected to be the cause of the majority of cases of unexplained fulminant hepatitis.

Acute Nonviral Hepatitis

Drugs, toxins, and systemic illness (e.g., sepsis) account for the majority of nonviral acute hepatitis in children. Drugs that have most commonly been associated with hepatitis include nonsteroidal anti-inflammatory medications, antiepileptic agents such as phenytoin and valproic acid, and antimicrobials such

TABLE 2 Summary of Most Common Viral Hepatitides

	Viral Structure	Reservoir	Transmission	Incubation	Clinical	Diagnosis	Chronicity	Treatment	Prevention
HAV	Nonenveloped RNA	Children	Fecal-oral Person-to-person likely	2–4 wk	Most children are asymptomatic. Most adults have classic hepatitis. Occasionally fulminant.	Anti-HAV in serum: IgM (recent infection). IgG (past infection).	Almost always resolves in 3–6 mo. Occasionally relapsing.	No specific therapy.	HAV vaccine if >2 yr of age in high-prevalence communities. *Immunoprophylaxis: 0.02 mL/kg IM within 2 wk of exposure.
HBV	Enveloped DNA	None	Blood-blood Sexual Vertical	7–28 days	Acute: classic hepatitis Fulminant rare. Children more often anicteric. Children more often develop a characteristic papular rash in association with hepatitis B. Chronic: Often asymptomatic. Extrahepatic manifestations 10–20% (e.g. polyarteritis nodosa, glomerulonephritis).	Multiple serologic markers: HBsAg: HBV infection. IgM anti-HBc: early acute infection. HBeAg: active viral replication. Anti-HBe: recovery. HBV-DNA: quantitative viral replicative load.	1%–5% adults. 90% neonates. 20%–50% 1- to 5-yr-olds.	Chronic active hepatitis: Lamivudine Interferon-α	Hepatitis B vaccine. Hepatitis B Immunoglobulin (postexposure prophylaxis).

Virus	Structure		Transmission	Incubation	Clinical Features	Diagnosis	Outcome	Treatment	Prevention
HCV	Enveloped RNA, 6 major genotypes	None	Blood-blood	14–180 days (average 45)	Children most often asymptomatic. 25% adults may have nonspecific acute illness. Chronic infection usually asymptomatic in adults. Up to 38% of adults may have extrahepatic manifestation: Porphyria cutanea tarda Thyroiditis Glomerulonephritis	Anti-HCV antibodies indicative of infection >2 months ago, chronic infection, or past infection. Serum RT-PCR of HCV RNA.	50%–80% develop chronic infection: Adults one third develop cirrhosis after 20 yr of infection. Pediatric infection may be less severe.	Chronic active hepatitis >3 yr of age both agents: Interferon-α 2a. Ribavirin.	Screening blood products. Needle-exchange programs. Vaccine under development.
HDV	Enveloped (HBV provided) RNA	None	Blood-blood Mucosal exposure	Superinfection: 2–8 wk Coinfection: similar to HBV infection	Coinfection: indistinguishable from HBV infection. Superinfection: acute icteric hepatitis, may be severe.	Anti-HDV (only useful if can document rising titers). RT-PCR mostly research tool.	Chronic infection more likely with superinfection vs. HBV coinfection.	High-dose interferon-α for 12 mo. Other antiviral agents not effective.	Prevention and treatment of HB infection.
HEV	Nonenveloped RNA	Unclear	Fecal-oral Rarely person-to-person	3–8 wk	Classic hepatitis. Milder in children. 3rd trimester more severe.	IgM and IgG anti-HEV in serum. HEV RNA in stool.	Acute illness 1–4 wk No chronic phase	No specific therapies. γ-immunoglobulin to exposed pregnant women.	Unclear if antibodies protective. Vaccine in development. Clean water.

*Homosexual men, injection drug users, frequent blood product recipients, high risk occupational exposure, child care center attendees. HAV, hepatitis A virus; HBV, hepatitis B virus; HBc, hepatitis B core antigen; HBe, hepatitis B e antigen; HBs, hepatitis B surface antigen; HCV, hepatitis C virus; IgG, immunoglobulin G; IgM, immunoglobulin M; IM, intramuscularly; RT-PCR, reverse transcriptase polymerase chain reaction.

as isoniazid, nitrofurantoin, and tetracycline. The prognosis of drug-related hepatitis is excellent when the inciting agent is discontinued.

Chronic Viral Hepatitis

HBV and HCV cause the majority of cases of chronic viral hepatitis (see Table 2). Three hundred million people worldwide are chronically infected with HBV, although HCV is the most common cause of chronic liver disease in the United States. Both chronic infections may progress to cirrhosis and liver failure. HCV-related end-stage liver disease is the most frequent indication for liver transplantation in adults. The risk for hepatocellular carcinoma is markedly increased in those chronically infected with HBV and HCV.

Children primarily acquire chronic HBV infection when infection occurs at birth (vertical transmission). Approximately 90% of vertically infected infants will develop chronic infection, whereas approximately 5% of infections acquired during childhood or adult years become chronic. In contrast, chronic infection is likely in the majority of individuals with HCV. Both infections are associated with autoimmune-related extrahepatic diseases (see Table 2).

Expert Opinion on Management Issues

ACUTE VIRAL HEPATITIS

Antiviral medications are not effective against HAV or HEV. Nonimmune individuals should receive immunoglobulin if exposed to persons with acute HAV infection. HAV vaccination is highly effective at preventing infection and is currently recommended for certain high-risk groups (see Table 2). Clean water and universal precautions will prevent the majority of HEV infections.

CHRONIC VIRAL HEPATITIS

Health maintenance for those with chronic viral hepatitis includes periodic ultrasound examinations of the liver and determination of serum transaminases, quantitation of viral replication and immunologic response, and immunization of individuals and family members for HAV and HBV.

Antiviral therapy for chronic HBV in children includes monotherapy with interferon, lamivudine, or adefovir and for HCV, combination therapy with ribavirin and interferon. Significant side effects, the requirement for parenteral administration of interferon, and the modest efficacy of these treatments has limited the therapy to those with ongoing liver injury. Perinatal immunoprophylaxis with HBV vaccine and immunoglobulin has dramatically reduced the incidence of vertical transmission of HBV. HBV immunization is also highly effective at preventing HBV infection in children and adults. No vaccine is yet available to protect against HCV infection

Common Pitfalls

- Failure to appreciate that viral gastroenteritis and acute viral hepatitis may be clinically indistinguishable in children.
- Accepting a diagnosis of HBV or HCV infection without reviewing the specific serologic/virologic evidence.
- Diagnosing acute HAV infection without regard for contact immunoprophylaxis.
- Eliciting medication/toxin exposure history although overlooking use of herbal or alternative medications, including teas, elixirs, and vitamins.
- Lack of recognition that in acute hepatitis a downward trend in serum transaminases in the context of a rising international normalized ratio (prothrombin time) can indicate impending liver failure.
- Failure to consider alternative causes of abnormal transaminases when viral hepatitis serologies are positive.
- Failure to appreciate that an underlying condition is present in otherwise healthy children with mild but persistently abnormal serum transaminase activities.
- Failure to appreciate that muscle inflammation or degeneration may also cause elevation in serum transaminases.

WHEN SHOULD YOU REFER A PATIENT TO A SPECIALIST?

- When hepatitis is associated with signs and symptoms of liver failure or progression to liver failure (coagulopathy, mental status changes).
- When a patient has chronic hepatitis. All patients with chronic hepatitis should be referred to a specialist.

SUGGESTED READINGS

1. Casiraghi MA, De Paschale M, Romano L, et al: Long-term outcome (35 years) of hepatitis C after acquisition of infection through mini transfusions of blood given at birth. Hepatology 39(1):90–96, 2004. **This small but well-designed study suggests that early hepatitis C virus infection has a relatively benign natural history.**
2. Craig AS, Schaffner W: Prevention of hepatitis A with the hepatitis A vaccine. N Engl J Med 350(5):476–481, 2004. **A comprehensive review of the rationale behind and practice of hepatitis A infection prevention.**
3. Ganem D, Prince AM: Hepatitis B virus infection—natural history and clinical consequences. N Engl J Med 350(11):1118–1129, 2004. **A concise but thorough explanation of hepatitis B virus biology and host immune response, with clinical- and treatment-related correlates.**
4. Jonas MM, Mizerski J, Badia IB: Clinical trial of lamivudine in children with chronic hepatitis B. N Engl J Med 346(22):1706–1713, 2002. **A major multicenter, randomized, double-blind, placebo-controlled trial demonstrating efficacy of lamivudine for treatment of hepatitis B virus infection in children.**
5. Keeffe EB, Dieterich DT, Han SH, et al: A treatment algorithm for the management of chronic hepatitis B virus infection in the United States. Clin Gastroenterol Hepatol 2(2):87–106, 2004. **An evidence-based authoritative guide to treatment of chronic hepatitis B virus infection.**

6. Lee WM: Drug-induced hepatotoxicity. N Engl J Med 349(5):474–485, 2003. **Excellent resource that intelligently considers the pathophysiology and clinical repercussions of drug-induced liver injury.**

Viral Hepatitis

David L. Suskind and Karen F. Murray

KEY CONCEPTS

- Children with chronic viral hepatitis are usually asymptomatic and may still have clinically significant liver damage from their infection.
- There are currently approved therapies for children with chronic hepatitis B virus (HBV) or hepatitis C virus (HCV).
- The decision to treat a patient should be made after consideration of the objective evidence of ongoing liver damage and in the context of the risks and benefits of therapy in that individual.
- Children with chronic HBV or HCV should be vaccinated for hepatitis A if not immune.
- The drugs used to treat HBV and HCV have significant potential toxicities and hence must be monitored by someone who has experience using these medications to treat children.

Viral hepatitis has a large impact on the health of children worldwide. Although hepatitis A is the leading cause of acute hepatitis, hepatitis B (HBV) and C (HCV) result in chronic hepatitis with the potential for the development of cirrhosis, end-stage liver disease, and hepatocellular carcinoma.

Worldwide, it is estimated that chronic HBV affects more than 350 million persons. In the United States, an estimated 1 million persons are chronically infected with HBV and 300,000 new infections occur each year, 10% of which are in children. Adoptees from high-prevalence countries account for many of the infected children, but other risk factors include parenteral drug use or blood exposure, sexual contact, perinatal exposure from an infected mother, and horizontal transmission from household nonsexual contacts. After exposure, the chance of becoming chronically infected is inversely proportional to the age at infection—90% to 95% of neonates, 80% of children, and 30% of adolescents become persistently infected. Most children remain asymptomatic, and 1% will spontaneously clear the infection in the first decade of life. In those who remain infected, however, histologic progression may occur, with up to 20% of these individuals progressing to cirrhosis over one to two decades, with the potential for end-stage liver disease and hepatocellular carcinoma.

HCV has an epidemiology similar to that of HBV. Worldwide, more than 300 million persons are chronically infected with HCV. In the United States, 3.5 million residents are chronically infected with 150,000

new infections occurring yearly. The U.S. pediatric population has a seroprevalence for HCV of 0.4%. The risk factors for HCV acquisition are similar to those for HBV, although the perinatal transmission is under 6% and the horizontal transmission is thought to be negligible. Regardless of the age at infection, however, 85% of those exposed will become chronically infected, with the vast majority again remaining asymptomatic. In chronically infected persons, the rate of progressive liver disease is similar to that of HBV, with progression to cirrhosis over decades in some individuals.

For both HBV and HCV the rationale for treatment in the pediatric age group is to halt the progression of the liver disease, and hence prevent the potential for advanced liver injury, failure, and the development of hepatocellular carcinoma. Additionally, the potential to live a viral-free life has profound positive social and psychological implications.

HEPATITIS B

Expert Opinion on Management Issues

Since the advent of routine hepatitis B vaccination and health education regarding hepatitis B modes of transmission, the incidence of acute hepatitis B has decreased by more than 70% in the United States. Health education and vaccination through the primary care provider continue to be strong forces in the prevention of chronic HBV. Infants born to mothers with chronic hepatitis B infection require hepatitis B vaccination and hepatitis B immunoglobulin (HBIG). This prevents transmission of virus in 95% of infants.

Patients with chronic elevation of serum alanine aminotransferase (ALT) are potential candidates for treatment, given the ongoing hepatic inflammation that is reflected in ALT elevation. A liver biopsy is the only way to accurately assess the degree of ongoing liver damage, inflammation, and fibrosis, as ALT levels and serologies do not sufficiently reflect the severity of liver damage. Once HBV hepatitis with persistent elevation of ALT is verified, HBV DNA levels are known, and liver histology, if available, is reviewed, the risks of therapy can be weighed against the potential benefit of viral clearance to determine the best course of action for the given child. As most children are asymptomatic and have been chronically infected at the time of diagnosis, methodical consideration of the need for and timing of therapy can usually be afforded.

APPROVED THERAPIES

The U.S. Food and Drug Administration (FDA) has approved two medications for use in children with chronic hepatitis B, interferon-alfa–2b and lamivudine (Table 1).

Interferon, a cytokine, works by upregulating a person's immune response to HBV. In adult studies,

TABLE 1 Therapy for the Treatment of Chronic Hepatitis B Virus in Children

Generic Name (Trade name)	Dosage/Route/ Regimen	Dosage Formulations	Therapeutic Concentrations	Common Adverse Reactions
Interferon alfa-2b (Intron A*)	3 MIU/m^2 SC tiw for 1 wk, with dose escalation to 6 MIU/m^2 (maximum dose 10 MIU) tiw for 24 wk	Injection: 3 MIU/mL	3 MIU/mL	Fever, myalgias, nausea, vomiting, anorexia, weight loss, diarrhea, depression, thrombocytopenia, neutropenia
Lamivudine (Epivir-HBV†)	3 mg/kg body weight/day (maximum dose 100 mg) PO for 52 wk	Tablet: 100 mg Solution: 5 mg/mL	100 mg/tablet 10 mg/mL	

*Schering.
†GlaxoSmithKline.
MIU, million international units; PO, orally; SC, subcutaneous; tiw, three times per week.

approximately one third of patients seroconverted to a hepatitis B e antigen (HBeAg) negative state, with a corresponding loss of detectable HBV DNA and a normalization of serum transaminases. Additionally, approximately 8% of interferon-treated adults lost hepatitis B surface antigen (HBsAg). Sokal and colleagues performed the largest randomized, controlled trial in children and found similar results. Twenty-six percent of children became HBeAg negative and 10% lost HBsAg. Factors that correlated with a positive response to interferon therapy included stable or decreasing HBV DNA levels, low baseline HBV DNA level, medication dosage, and female gender. The approved dosage of interferon-alfa–2b is 6 million units (MIU)/m^2 injected subcutaneously three times weekly for 24 weeks.

Lamivudine is FDA-approved for use in children 2 to 17 years of age with chronic HBV. The clear advantage that lamivudine has over interferon for the treatment of children is its oral administration and its availability in both tablet and liquid form. As a pyrimidine nucleoside analogue, lamivudine inhibits the reverse transcriptase activity of HBV. In adult trials, seroconversion of HBeAg occurs in 32% and there is transaminase improvement in 41% of patients. Because it works by suppressing replication, few studies show seroconversion from the HBsAg status. In the largest pediatric study, lamivudine, at a dose of 3 mg/kg body weight/day (maximum dose 100 mg) for 52 weeks, showed seroconversion from HBeAg-positive, normalization of serum transaminases, and suppression of HBV DNA in 23% of children.

Vaccination for hepatitis A virus is recommended for any child at least 2 years of age with chronic HBV.

FUTURE THERAPIES FOR PEDIATRIC PATIENTS

Adefovir dipivoxil, a nucleoside analogue of adenosine monophosphate, inhibits HBV DNA polymerase. In adult studies it has been shown to improve histology in 53% to 63% of patients without emergence of resistant HBV mutations after 1 year. Longer duration studies have shown a small number of resistant mutations occurring. Pediatric studies are currently under way.

Common Pitfalls

The most common side affects of interferon include flulike symptoms in 80% of patients, which include fever, myalgias, headache, fatigue, rigors, arthralgia, nausea, vomiting, abdominal pain, anorexia, weight loss, and diarrhea. Depression can result or become potentiated by interferon; consequently, a history of major depression is a relative contraindication for its use. Local injection site reaction with erythema and swelling is common, and the development of neutropenia and thrombocytopenia must be monitored. Although most of these adverse affects are reversible with reduction of or discontinuation of interferon, some more-recently realized neurologic and ophthalmologic effects may not be. Reduction of vision, retinopathies, retinal vascular thrombosis, and optic neuritis have been induced by or aggravated by interferons. Because of the potential neurologic and ophthalmologic toxicities, treatment of children younger than 2 years of age with interferon is not recommended.

Lamivudine's side-effect profile is similar to that of placebo. It has been associated with the development of pancreatitis, however. Additionally, with prolonged administration there is increasing risk of developing a lamivudine-resistant strain of virus, most commonly a strain containing a point mutation termed the *YMDD mutation.*

HEPATITIS C

Expert Opinion on Management Issues

Determining the need for treatment of children with HCV requires a liver biopsy to assess accurately the degree of ongoing liver damage, inflammation,

TABLE 2 Therapy for the Treatment of Chronic Hepatitis C Virus in Children

Generic Name (Trade name)	Dosage/Route/Regimen	Dosage Formulations	Therapeutic Concentrations	Common Adverse Reactions
Interferon alfa-2b (Intron A*)	3 MIU/m² SC tiw for 1 yr	Injection: 3 MIU/mL	3 MIU/mL	Fever, myalgias, nausea, vomiting, anorexia, weight loss, diarrhea, depression, thrombocytopenia, neutropenia
Ribavirin (Rebetol*) (Rebetron,* combination therapy)	200 mg PO bid for 25–36 kg, or 15 mg/kg/day divided bid for 1 yr	Capsule/tablet: 200 mg Solution: 40 mg/mL	200 mg/capsule 40 mg/mL	Hemolytic anemia, teratogen

*Schering
bid, twice a day; MIU, million international units; PO, orally; SC, subcutaneous; tiw, three times a week.

and fibrosis, as serum ALT levels and the HCV RNA level do not accurately reflect the degree of liver damage. Knowledge of the patient's HCV genotype and HCV RNA level can, however, provide valuable information regarding the likelihood of viral clearance with treatment. Once the liver histology, HCV genotype, and HCV RNA levels are available, weighing the risks of therapy against the potential benefit of viral clearance can be done with the patient and their family to determine the best course of action for that child. As most children are asymptomatic and have been chronically infected at the time of diagnosis, methodical consideration of the need for and timing of therapy can usually be afforded.

APPROVED THERAPIES

The only approved therapy for children is the combination of interferon with ribavirin, approved for children older than the age of 3 years (Table 2). Interferon monotherapy was shown to normalize the ALT and reduce the serum HCV RNA to below detectable levels in up to 40% to 50% of adults by the end of 1 year of treatment; however, most of the patients relapsed, leaving the sustained response (6 months after the completion of therapy) around 8% to 35%. Small pediatric trials revealed better but similar results. Ribavirin, a guanosine analogue that inhibits the in vitro replication of RNA viruses, was shown to nicely reduce elevated ALT levels during therapy, but did not, alone, impact the viral load. In combination, however, interferon plus ribavirin results in a sustained response in adults of 30% to 40%. A pediatric trial by Kelly and associates showed comparable results. Combination therapy with interferon-alfa-2b at the recommended doses (3 MIU/m² three times per week on Monday, Wednesday, Friday) subcutaneously and 15 mg/kg/day orally of ribavirin was used for 1 year. The 6-month sustained result was 45%.

Standard of care is currently the use of interferon-α plus ribavirin for 1 year in all subjects treated for chronic HCV. Growing experience in adults would suggest, however, that 6 months of therapy may only be needed in those subjects fortunate enough to have genotypes 2 or 3, rather than 1.

Vaccination for hepatitis A virus is recommended for any child of at least 2 years of age with chronic HCV.

FUTURE THERAPIES FOR PEDIATRIC PATIENTS

The current standard and most recently approved treatment for adults (18 years and older) with chronic HCV is pegylated-interferon-α (PEG-IFN) plus ribavirin. The addition of polyethylene glycol to the molecule of interferon-α results in sustained absorption, decreased systemic clearance, and increased serum half-life, resulting in superior pharmacokinetics and pharmacodynamics. PEG-IFN is delivered once weekly. Initial trials in adults using PEG-IFN plus ribavirin has shown 6-month sustained response rates of between 50% and 60% for all patients treated, and even better response rates in patients with genotypes other than 1.

Pediatric trials are currently evaluating the safety and efficacy of PEG-IFN in children.

Common Pitfalls

The side affects of interferon are the same as those seen during the treatment of HBV with this medication. When the interferon is combined with ribavirin, however, the symptoms are frequently more prominent than with interferon alone. Ribavirin itself can cause hemolytic anemia that is reversible with decrease or cessation of the medication. More concerning is the potency with which ribavirin is both a mutagen and teratogen. Females of childbearing potential must be counseled strongly about the importance of practicing effective birth control, and the manufacturer recommends using two forms of birth control during and for 6 months after discontinuing ribavirin.

Despite the improving efficacy of medications for HCV, many subjects treated will either not respond to treatment or will relapse after therapy is discontinued. Decisions about retreatment versus continued observation must be individualized and based on the prior medications used, the response to those medications, and what new therapies might be available to that patient.

Communication and Counseling

Most children with chronic HBV or HCV are asymptomatic; consequently, diagnosis is made only with a high index of suspicion. Once the determination is made through laboratory testing and/or histological evaluation (required for HCV, should be considered for HBV) that there is ongoing liver damage, therapies are available and should be considered for these infections. The ultimate decision, however, should be made in conjunction with the family and/or patient considering the degree and progression of liver damage, the likelihood of viral clearance with available therapy, and the risks of therapy versus no therapy in a given patient.

SUGGESTED READINGS

1. Comanor L, Minor J, Conjeevaram HS, et al: Statistical models for predicting response to interferon-alpha and spontaneous seroconversion in children with chronic hepatitis B. J Viral Hepat 7(2):144–152, 2000. **Illustrates patient characteristics predicting response to interferon therapy in children.**
2. Dienstag JL, Schiff ER, Wright TL, et al: Lamivudine as initial treatment for chronic hepatitis B in the United States. N Engl J Med 341(17):1256–1263, 1999. **Landmark study using lamivudine for the treatment of hepatitis B in adults.**
3. Jonas MM, Kelley DA, Mizerski J, et al: Clinical trial of lamivudine in children with chronic hepatitis B. N Engl J Med 346 (22):1706–1713, 2002. **Landmark study using lamivudine for hepatitis B in children.**
4. Kelly DA, Bunn SK, Apelian D, et al: Safety, efficacy and pharmacokinetics of interferon alpha-2b plus ribavirin in children with chronic hepatitis C. Hepatology 34(4):680, 2001. **Landmark study using interferon for hepatitis C in children.**
5. Lee WM: Hepatitis B virus infection. N Engl J Med 337(24):1733–1745, 1997. **Review of hepatitis B infection.**
6. Sokal EM, Conjeevaram HS, Roberts EA, et al: Interferon alfa therapy for chronic hepatitis B in children: A multinational randomized controlled trial. Gastroenterology 114(5):988–995, 1998. **Landmark study using interferon with ribavirin for hepatitis B in children.**
7. Wong DK, Cheung AM, O'Rourke K, et al: Effect of alpha-interferon treatment in patients with hepatitis B e antigen-positive chronic hepatitis B. A meta-analysis. Ann Intern Med 119(4):312–323, 1993. **Meta-analysis examining the efficacy of interferon treatment for hepatitis B in children.**
8. Zeuzem S, Feinman SV, Rasenack J, et al: Peginterferon alfa-2a in patients with chronic hepatitis C. N Engl J Med 343:1666–1672, 2000. **Study examining the efficacy of pegylated interferon for hepatitis C treatment in adults.**

Foreign Bodies in the Gastrointestinal Tract

Christa M. H. Zehle and Lewis R. First

KEY CONCEPTS

- An ingested foreign object accompanied by respiratory symptoms is a medical emergency.
- Sharp-pointed objects and batteries lodged in the esophagus require immediate removal.
- A chest x-ray should be obtained in all suspected cases of foreign body aspiration or ingestion to distinguish objects in the gastrointestinal tract from those in the upper airway.
- Ingested coins in the gastrointestinal tract are *enface* in the anterior-posterior view and on edge in the lateral view; coins in the trachea are seen *on edge* in the anterior-posterior view.
- Deviation of the trachea will be in the direction of the obstruction.
- An object should be removed if it remains in the esophagus for more than 24 hours.

Children are at increased risk for ingestion, aspiration, or insertion of foreign bodies into the gastrointestinal (GI) tract. Although the majority of these objects (80%–90%) pass spontaneously, those foreign bodies that remain lodged in the GI tract may lead to serious consequences and are a significant cause of morbidity and mortality. Approximately 10% to 20% of foreign body ingestion will require nonoperative intervention and less than 1% will require surgery.

The majority of foreign body ingestion (80%) occurs in the pediatric population, with a peak age of 6 months to 3 years. The increased risk of ingestion among children is a result of their young age, easy distractibility, tendency to hold objects near or in their mouths, and exposure to foods or playthings inappropriate for their age.

Various materials can become lodged in the GI tract. In pediatrics, these include the less common food impaction and true foreign bodies. True foreign bodies include blunt objects, sharp objects, or disc batteries. Coins are the most common esophageal foreign body (60% to 88%) in children. However, sharp objects account for 10% of foreign bodies ingested and are responsible for the majority of GI complications. These complications include perforation of the GI tract (15% to 35%), which most often occurs at the ileocecal valve. Bones are the most common sharp foreign bodies that children ingest. Button or disc batteries can be harmful because they contain acid or alkali that can lead to liquefaction necrosis and/or perforation. Impaction of food in the esophagus usually occurs secondary to a congenital anomaly, for example, esophageal strictures, achalasia, esophageal spasm, or motor disorder. Impaction of food in the esophagus may also occur following surgical repair of the GI tract.

A foreign body should be suspected if there is an acute onset of choking, coughing, or wheezing or if there is a poorly defined, chronic respiratory complaint. However, both respiratory and GI findings can be present with a GI foreign body aspiration. Respiratory symptoms can occur days or months after the episode and may include coughing, wheezing, stridor, tachypnea, retractions, rales, and decreased/absent breath sounds (only 40% of the time). These symptoms occur usually as a result of tracheal compression from the foreign body. GI symptoms may include vomiting, drooling, dysphagia, and chest or epigastric pain. The physical examination may not be helpful in many cases, but one should evaluate for respiratory distress, risk of aspiration, and evidence of luminal obstruction or perforation.

Locating a GI foreign body is the most important objective in management. Objects often pass spontaneously except for those in the upper or middle esophagus. The most common sites are those of normal esophageal narrowing, which include the cricopharyngeal muscle and thoracic inlet area, the aortic arch, and the gastroesophageal junction. The thoracic inlet is the most common site for esophageal coin lodgment (63%).

Expert Opinion on Management Issue

The management of foreign bodies in the GI tract depends on the patient's age and clinical condition; the object's size, shape, and classification; and the anatomic location of the object.

Initially, one must distinguish foreign bodies in the GI tract from those in the upper airway. A chest and abdominal x-ray is indicated in all cases of suspected foreign body ingestion. An anterior-posterior view of the chest will show an esophageal radiopaque foreign body en face (coronal view), whereas a tracheal object will appear in the sagittal AP plane. If the object is thought to be radiolucent, a thin barium esophagogram should be used to outline the object. A barium swallow, upper GI series, or endoscopy may also be used.

Management varies based on the type of object ingested.

Blunt Object

Coins above the stomach can often be removed using foreign body forceps, a snare, or a retrieval net. Foley catheters under fluoroscopic guidance have a low complication rate; however, they do not allow for control of the object, airway protection, or assessment of the esophagus or esophageal pathology. If a blunt object has passed into the stomach, conservative outpatient management is appropriate, because there is a 98% chance that it will pass spontaneously. Most objects pass within 4 to 6 days; however, some may take up to 4 weeks. Weekly repeat abdominal films should be obtained and objects that remain in the stomach for more than 4 weeks should be endoscopically removed. Surgical removal is indicated if the object remains in the same location for more than a week.

Sharp Object

Sharp objects have a significantly higher complication rate of approximately 35%. These objects should be removed by rigid or flexible endoscopy. If the object has passed into the stomach or duodenum, it should be removed endoscopically if this can be done safely. If endoscopic removal is not possible, daily radiographs should be obtained, and surgical removal is indicated if the object fails to progress for 3 consecutive days.

Batteries

Batteries can be harmful and require immediate removal if lodged in the esophagus, because liquefaction necrosis and/or perforation can occur. Occasionally, the battery can be pushed safely into the stomach. Batteries located in the stomach often pass through the remaining GI tract without consequence and do not need to be retrieved unless there are concerning clinical signs or symptoms. Radiographs should be obtained every 3 to 4 days to monitor the object. GI lavage may be of some benefit; however, emetics and cathartics have little effect.

Food Impaction

Management of food impaction should not be delayed beyond 24 hours. Endoscopy is used to verify and locate the site of impaction and to assist in removal of the food bolus. Occasionally, the bolus can be pushed into the stomach without complications.

Upper esophageal foreign bodies should be removed promptly, as esophageal pressure necrosis can develop and may cause perforation. However, objects located in the middle or lower two thirds of the esophagus can be observed, and a repeat film should be obtained within 12 to 24 hours. If an object remains in the esophagus more than 24 hours, it should be removed.

Endoscopic removal is most common and is usually done using a rigid esophagoscope. This allows for the use of a variety of types and sizes of extraction instruments and for excellent viewing of the esophagus after removal. The success rate for this type of removal is approximately 100%. Other methods of removal include using one of various instruments such as Magill forceps and an overtube, which helps to protect the esophagus; the Foley catheter extraction method; pushing the foreign body into the stomach using esophageal bougienage; the penny pincher technique, which involves insertion of a fluoroscopically guided device that consists of a grasping endoscopic forceps covered by a soft rubber catheter (the procedure is done without anesthesia or sedation); and observation/temporization. There is not significant data supporting one method over another, and removal of the object often depends on the preference and skill of the health care provider.

Common Pitfalls

One of the challenges of managing suspected foreign body ingestions is how to approach the asymptomatic child. Review of the literature suggests that foreign objects should not remain in the esophagus longer than 24 hours. Therefore, it is suggested that children with a simple presentation of an esophageal object, such as a coin, who are asymptomatic and have no history of esophageal disease, can be observed for 12 to 24 hours after the initial radiograph is taken. This period of observation can be followed by a repeat film to assess the location of the foreign body prior to undertaking an invasive procedure to remove the object.

Medications have not proven to be very effective in the management of GI foreign bodies. Glucagon, the most promising pharmacologic agent, has been shown to be effective in adults, but other studies have not found it to be effective in children. In adults, glucagon is considered helpful in dislodging food impacted in the distal esophagus. The mechanism of action of glucagon in this situation is to decrease lower esophageal sphincter pressure and smooth muscle spasm. It is contraindicated in the presence of a pheochromocytoma, insulinoma, or allergy to glucagon. Other pharmacologic agents that have not proven to be helpful are neutralizing solutions, laxatives, and charcoal. Medications that are no longer recommended include papain, an enzymatic digestive agent, because it carries a risk of digestion of the esophageal wall leading to perforation, hypernatremia, or erosion. Ipecac, used to induce vomiting, is contraindicated because of an increased risk of aspiration.

Communication and Counseling

The best therapeutic approach to foreign bodies in the GI tract is to advocate prevention. A child's aspiration or ingestion risk can be reduced significantly through anticipatory guidance. Parents and caretakers need to be educated about the potential dangers of small parts and objects, including button batteries. Better child-proof battery compartments and a clearly written package warning regarding possible toddler ingestion of such batteries will hopefully reduce the incidence of related injuries. It is also valuable for health care providers to emphasize the importance of proper child supervision and safety-proofing the home so that small, possibly ingestible objects are out of reach of small children.

SUGGESTED READINGS

1. Cerri RB, Liacouras CA: Evaluation and management of foreign bodies in the upper gastrointestinal tract. Pediatr Case Rev 3:150–156, 2003. **A case-based review summarizing the evaluation and approach to managing foreign bodies in the gastrointestinal tract.**
2. Eisen GM, Baron TH, Dominitis JA, et al: Guidelines for management of ingested foreign bodies. Gastrointest Endosc 55:802–806, 2002. **A critical review of available data and expert consensus on the management of foreign body ingestion.**
3. McGahren ED: Esophageal foreign bodies. Pediatr Rev 20:129–133, 1999. **A review of evaluating and treating esophageal foreign body ingestion.**
4. Miller RS, Willging JP, Rutter MJ, et al: Chronic esophageal foreign bodies in pediatric patients: A retrospective review. Int J Pediatr Otorhinolaryngol 68:265–272, 2005. **A retrospective study evaluating chronic esophageal foreign bodies in children.**

Nephrology and Genitourinary Tract

Hernias and Hydroceles

Jay J. Schnitzer

KEY CONCEPTS

- Hernias and hydroceles are common.
- Congenital hernias are indirect; direct hernias are always acquired.
- On occasion, hernias can be life-threatening because of incarceration or strangulation.
- Prompt diagnosis and management are mandatory.

Inguinal hernias and hydroceles are two of the most common congenital problems that pediatric surgeons encounter. If not dealt with expeditiously, hernias in particular can be organ- or life-threatening by incarceration or strangulation. Prompt diagnosis and management are mandatory.

Embryology and Pathogenesis

As Galen wrote in AD 176, "The duct descending to the testicle is a small offshoot (processus vaginalis peritonei) of the greater peritoneal sac in the lower abdomen." The *processus vaginalis*, which is a precursor of both the indirect pediatric inguinal hernia and hydrocele, appears in the developing fetus at 3 months' gestation when the testis begins its descent from a retroperitoneal position and follows the gubernaculum to its final position in the scrotum by 8 months' gestation. Normally, the segment of the processus vaginalis enveloping the testis persists as the tunica vaginalis, whereas the remainder of the processus involutes to remove any communication between the peritoneal cavity and the scrotum postnatally (Fig. 1A). If, however, the processus remains patent, an indirect inguinal hernia, a hydrocele, or both become possible. The pattern and degree of patency determine the inguinal anomaly (see Fig. 1B to E). Proximal patency with obliteration of the distal end of the processus produces an inguinal hernia (see Fig. 1B). Complete patency produces a scrotal hernia (see Fig. 1C). An isolated persistent section of the processus vaginalis adjacent to the spermatic cord that may have a tiny connection to the peritoneal cavity produces a hydrocele of the spermatic cord (see Fig. 1D). A persistent narrow opening at the internal ring associated with the distal sac that allows fluid from the peritoneal cavity into this sac produces a communicating hydrocele (see Fig. 1E). Fluid trapped within an isolated tunica vaginalis with an obliterated processus proximally results in an isolated scrotal hydrocele, which resolves spontaneously with time.

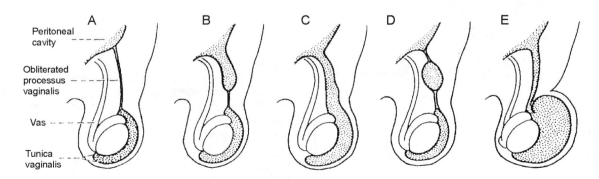

FIGURE 1. Types of inguinal hernia and hydrocele. *A,* Normal anatomy. *B,* Inguinal hernia. *C,* Scrotal hernia. *D,* Hydrocele of the cord. *E,* Communicating hydrocele. (From Lloyd DA, Rintala RJ: Inguinal hernia. In O'Neill JA Jr, Rowe MI, Grosfeld JL, et al. (eds): Pediatric Surgery. St. Louis: Mosby, 1998, p 1072.)

Expert Opinion on Management Issues

INGUINAL HERNIA

Incidence

By definition, a *congenital* inguinal hernia is indirect, and therefore anatomically lateral to the epigastric vessels. Although the exact incidence of indirect inguinal hernia in infants and children is unknown, the reported incidence from several studies ranges from 1% to 5% with an 8:1 to 10:1 male-to-female ratio. Sixty percent of hernias occur on the right side. Premature infants are at increased risk for inguinal hernia, with an incidence of 7% to 30% in boys and 2% in girls. Moreover, the associated risk of incarceration is greater than 60% in this population, so that repair in these infants is recommended before discharge home from the neonatal intensive care unit. Box 1 presents other conditions associated with an increased risk of congenital inguinal hernia.

Direct inguinal hernias are acquired, result from a defect in the transversalis fascia, and are anatomically medial to the epigastric vessels. Direct hernias are rare in children; a third of cases of direct inguinal hernia occur after operative repair of an indirect inguinal hernia. Treatment is operative strengthening of the inguinal floor by suturing transversalis fascia or conjoined tendon to the Cooper ligament. Recurrence is rare in children. *Femoral* hernias result from a defect inferior to the inguinal ligament. They are extremely rare in children and occur two times more frequently in girls than boys. Treatment is operative repair.

Diagnosis

The diagnosis of an inguinal hernia is made on the basis of the history and physical examination. Frequently a parent reports the presence of a groin bulge, particularly after the infant has strained or cried, that often resolves during the night while the infant is sleeping. The differential diagnoses of an inguinal or scrotal swelling include inguinal hernia, hydrocele, retractile testis, undescended testis, varicocele, torsion of the testis, torsion of the appendix testis or epididymis, epididymo-orchitis, trauma, lymphadenitis, and tumor (Box 2). On physical examination, a mass can often be appreciated by inspection as a bulge or a smooth lump in the inguinal region extending from the level of the internal inguinal ring and possibly proceeding past the pubic tubercle and into the scrotum. Increased intra-abdominal pressure may enlarge the mass. In an older child, these findings may be elicited by inducing laughing, coughing, encouraging a Valsalva maneuver, or having the child inflate a balloon, preferably while the child is standing. An infant can be permitted to cry or struggle against gentle restraint. If the mass cannot be appreciated, palpation of a thickened spermatic cord as it crosses the pubic tubercle, the so-called silk-glove sign, is a reliable indicator. Palpation is performed with a single finger placed over and parallel to the cord structures above the canal and lightly rubbing from side to side. In addition, the position of the testicle must be determined and documented because an undescended testicle may manifest as a mass in the groin. Radiographic studies are unnecessary.

On occasion, an inguinal hernia is incarcerated; that is, it cannot be reduced. This condition is a surgical emergency because the vascular supply to the hernia sac contents is in jeopardy. If the incarceration persists, strangulation can occur with infarction of the intestine, gonad, fallopian tube, or omentum.

Inguinal hernias do not heal spontaneously and must be surgically repaired because of the ever-present risk of incarceration. In general, surgical consultation should be obtained at the time of diagnosis and repair performed very soon afterward. Nearly 70% of incarcerated hernias occur within the first year of life.

Surgical Repair in Boys

For most infants and children, the operation can be safely performed electively as an outpatient procedure under general anesthesia with general endotracheal intubation in young children and a mask or laryngeal mask airway for older children. A short transverse

---

BOX 1 Conditions Associated with Increased Risk of Inguinal Hernia

- Abdominal wall defects (gastroschisis, omphalocele)
- Ambiguous genitalia
- Chylous ascites
- Congenital dislocation of the hip
- Connective tissue disorders (Ehlers-Danlos syndrome, Marfan syndrome)
- Continuous ambulatory peritoneal dialysis (CAPD)
- Cryptorchid testis
- Cystic fibrosis
- Exstrophy of the bladder; cloaca
- Hydrops
- Hypospadias; epispadias
- Liver disease with ascites
- Low birth weight
- Meconium peritonitis
- Mucopolysaccharidosis (Hunter syndrome, Hurler syndrome)
- Positive family history
- Prematurity
- Ventriculoperitoneal (VP) shunt

BOX 2 Differential Diagnoses of Pediatric Inguinal or Scrotal Swelling

- Inguinal hernia
- Hydrocele
- Retractile testis
- Undescended testis
- Varicocele
- Torsion of the testis
- Torsion of the appendix testis or epididymis
- Epididymo-orchitis
- Trauma
- Lymphadenitis
- Tumor

incision is made in the groin skin crease. Scarpa's fascia is sharply divided, and the external oblique fascia "roof" of the inguinal canal is opened down to the level of the external ring. Cremasteric muscle fibers are gently dissected free from the cord. The hernia sac is identified, carefully separated from the vas and vessels, and ligated at the level of the internal ring. The testicle is returned to the scrotum, and the wound is closed in layers with a subcuticular skin closure. A long-acting local anesthetic (bupivacaine) is often injected into the wound before closure, and the wound is dressed with a water-resistant dressing such as Tegaderm, OpSite, or collodion. Postoperative analgesia is supplemented with acetaminophen for infants and small children, and codeine may be added for the older child. The wound is kept dry for 48 hours postoperatively, and strenuous activities are avoided for the first week. Some scrotal swelling may be evident postoperatively, but it resolves spontaneously.

Surgical Repair in Girls

The repair in girls is very similar to that of the boys in terms of high ligation of the sac. However, in 21% of the cases, the fallopian tube, or on occasion the ovary or the uterus, is attached to the wall of the hernia sac and forms a sliding hernia. Care must be taken to avoid injury to these structures. Although it was previously believed that an incarcerated ovary did not require urgent surgical exploration, in contrast to the situation in a boy, vascular compromise is now reported more commonly. Thus girls with incarcerated hernias need to be treated expeditiously if the incarcerated structures cannot be successfully reduced. At surgery, the hernia sac is opened, the round ligament divided, the sac ligated at the level of the internal ring, and the internal ring closed.

Patients with testicular feminization (a form of male pseudohermaphroditism resulting from complete androgen insensitivity) may present with an inguinal hernia and a prolapsed gonad. These patients have a 46, XY karyotype and no müllerian structures. Vaginoscopy should be performed at the time of inguinal hernia repair that demonstrates a short or blind-ending vagina with no cervix. Postoperative evaluation should include a karyotypic analysis and pelvic ultrasonography.

The Incarcerated Hernia

The small intestine, cecum, ovary or fallopian tube, or appendix may slide to the hernia sac and become incarcerated. As mentioned earlier, urgent surgical consultation and reduction are required and accomplished with sedation in the Trendelenburg position. If spontaneous reduction does not occur within a short interval, the surgeon should attempt gentle manual reduction. If reduction is successful, the child should be admitted to the hospital, and the hernia repaired the next day. If reduction is not possible, the child requires emergent surgical exploration and repair under general anesthesia. If a strangulated infarcted segment of intestine is discovered at surgery, resection and primary anastomosis are possible and safe through the same groin incision.

Contralateral Exploration

Routine contralateral exploration for unilateral inguinal hernia remains controversial. Children younger than 2 years have a higher incidence of a contralaterally patent processus vaginalis. One approach is routine exploration of both sides of the groin in children younger than 2 years, in older children with a left-sided hernia, in all girls younger than 5 years, and in children with ventriculoperitoneal (VP) shunts, chronic ambulatory peritoneal dialysis catheters, and ascites. Another approach is to inspect the contralateral side for the presence of a patent processus vaginalis with laparoscopy via the opened hernia sac at the time of surgery. Some pediatric surgeons prefer to operate on the affected side only. Bilateral exploration should be considered for any of the conditions listed in Box 1.

Special Considerations

Perioperative antibiotics are recommended for children with foreign bodies (VP shunt, central venous line, peritoneal dialysis catheter), congenital heart disease, prematurity, and incarceration. In addition, preterm infants with a combined gestational age of less than 50 to 60 weeks should be monitored postoperatively overnight for apnea/bradycardia. During high ligation of the congenital inguinal hernia, careful inspection of the neck of the sac at the time of transfixion is mandatory to avoid injury to the fallopian tube, appendix, or bladder when a sliding hernia is encountered. In cystic fibrosis, abnormalities of the vas deferens are found in 100% of patients, as opposed to an incidence of less than 1% in the general population. Therefore, failure to identify the vas deferens at surgery should lead to subsequent or additional evaluation for cystic fibrosis. If the sweat test is normal, evaluation of the upper urinary tract to rule out renal dysgenesis is recommended.

HYDROCELES

Hydroceles are caused by fluid accumulating in a persistent segment of the processus vaginalis, usually the tunica vaginalis, with or without communication via the peritoneal cavity. Unlike hernias, the risk of incarceration or strangulation is minimal. Furthermore, most hydroceles resolve spontaneously during the first year of life. If a hydrocele persists beyond 1 year of age, it is assumed to be in conjunction with a hernia, and surgery is recommended. The diagnosis of a hydrocele is made by physical examination. A hydrocele is manifested as a groin or scrotal bulge, similar to a hernia, but is soft, fluctuant, and nonreducible. Even the most experienced clinicians sometimes find it difficult to distinguish an acute hydrocele of the cord from an incarcerated hernia. Transillumination may be of some benefit, but an infant's small intestine is transilluminated nearly as efficiently as peritoneal fluid.

Thus percutaneous needle aspiration never has a role in the diagnosis or treatment of pediatric hydroceles.

In older children, scrotal hydroceles may appear after trauma, in conjunction with inflammatory illnesses, or with neoplasm. The operation for hydrocele is high ligation of the processus vaginalis, as for inguinal hernia. No attempt is made to remove the distal sac, which is opened widely. Abdominoscrotal hydroceles are rare and managed by surgical resection. Hydroceles in females are rare but do occur as accumulations surrounding the round ligament in the canal of Nuck. They are treated by excision and high ligation of the processus vaginalis.

UMBILICAL HERNIAS

An umbilical hernia results from the failure of closure of the fascial ring through which the umbilical cord protrudes at birth. The overall incidence varies from 10% to 80% and is influenced by age, race, low birth weight, and associated anomalies (e.g., trisomy 21, cretinism, mucopolysaccharidoses, and Beckwith-Wiedemann syndrome). Most umbilical hernias remain asymptomatic and resolve by 4 years of age. Only those that are very large, symptomatic, incarcerated, or persistent beyond 4 years of age are repaired operatively. The operation is performed under general anesthesia via a semicircular incision in the inferior umbilical skin crease. The edges of the fascial defect should be mobilized and closed in a transverse direction with interrupted sutures. The skin is closed with fine absorbable subcuticular sutures. A pressure dressing is applied for 48 hours to minimize the risk of wound hematoma or seroma, which are the most common postoperative complications. Wound infection and recurrence are rare complications.

Common Pitfalls

- The complication rate after inguinal hernia repair in children by a skilled surgeon should be very low; most series report rates from 1.7% to 8%.
- The wound infection rate is between 1% and 2%, and recurrence rates are less than 1%.
- Testicular atrophy following hernia repair is rare but may be more common following emergency surgery for incarcerated hernia.
- Infections are usually managed with opening of the incision and drainage, followed by dressing changes and antibiotics.
- Scrotal swelling and fluid collections (residual hydrocele) almost always resolve spontaneously.
- Injury to the vas should be exceedingly rare when the procedure is performed by an experienced surgeon.

Communication and Counseling

Parents should be advised and educated about an inguinal hernia at the time it is diagnosed. Surgery should be recommended, and in particular parents should be cautioned that there are no other acceptable therapeutic options. Complication risks should be carefully described as part of the informed consent process. An isolated scrotal hydrocele may be managed expectantly, but communicating hydroceles require operation. Because expected outcomes are uniformly excellent, an optimistic tone is appropriate.

SELECTED READINGS

1. Gross RE: Inguinal hernia hydrocele. In Gross RE (ed): The Surgery of Infancy and Childhood. Philadelphia: WB Saunders, 1953, pp 449–466. **Historical text with good descriptions.**
2. Kapur P, Caty MG, Glick PL: Pediatric hernias and hydroceles. Pediatr Clin North Am 45:773–789, 1998. **Review article.**
3. Lloyd DA, Rintala RJ: Inguinal hernia. In O'Neill JS Jr, Rowe MI, Grosfeld JL, et al (eds): Pediatric Surgery. St. Louis: Mosby, 1998, pp 1071–1086. **A more recent text than Gross.**
4. Potts WJ, Riker WL, Lewis JE: The treatment of inguinal hernia in infants and children. Ann Surg 132(3):566–576, 1950. **Historical review.**
5. Rowe MI, Copelson LW, Clatworthy HW: The patent processus vaginalis and the inguinal hernia. J Pediatr Surg 4:102–107, 1969. **Discussion of patent processus vaginalis and inguinal hernia.**
6. Shoog SJ, Conlin MJ: Pediatric hernias and hydroceles. Urol Clin North Am 22(1):119–130, 1995. **Review from the pediatric urology perspective.**
7. Skinner MA, Grosfeld JL: Inguinal and umbilical hernia repair in infants and children. Surg Clin North Am 73(3):439–449, 1993. **Technique of repair.**
8. Weber TR, Tracy TF Jr: Groin hernias and hydroceles. In Ashcraft KW, Holder TM (eds): Pediatric Surgery, 2nd ed. Philadelphia: WB Saunders, 1993, pp 562–570. **Discussion of groin hernias and hydroceles.**

Renal Hypoplasia and Dysplasia

V. Matti Vehaskari

KEY CONCEPTS

- Most cases of renal hypoplasia and dysplasia appear to be sporadic, isolated urinary tract abnormalities but can be associated with syndromes.
- Other associated urinary tract abnormalities such as vesicoureteral reflux and obstruction are frequently present.
- Oligohydramnios may predict severe renal impairment and pulmonary hypoplasia.
- Prognosis in less severe cases is highly variable and, as a rule, favorable when only one kidney is affected.
- Water and electrolyte wasting is common in infants with bilateral involvement.
- Routine nephrectomy of a dysplastic kidney is not indicated.

Hypoplasia refers to a small kidney with a decreased number of nephrons but without anomalous differentiated tissue. The cause is believed to be insufficient branching of the ureteric bud, which induces nephron formation. A dysplastic kidney is the result of abnormal differentiation and may be caused by urinary tract obstruction early during kidney development. The size of the dysplastic kidney is variable, and cysts may be present. A distinction between a small dysplastic kidney and a hypoplastic kidney is often not possible by clinical means. The spectrum of renal hypoplasia/dysplasia ranges from clinically insignificant morphologic deviations to conditions incompatible with postnatal life. If one normal kidney is present, morbidity and long-term impact on life is usually small. Most cases of renal hypoplasia/dysplasia appear to be sporadic and isolated, but affected families, some with a Mendelian inheritance pattern, have been described. Additionally, hundreds of syndromes and chromosomal abnormalities are associated with renal hypoplasia/dysplasia; the reader is referred to available texts and websites for detailed listings. Table 1 lists some of the more common syndromes.

Renal hypoplasia is present in approximately 1 in 400 live births. Two different types of renal hypoplasia are recognized; *oligonephronic hypoplasia (oligomeganephronia)* and *simple hypoplasia*. The former is a rare condition that is always bilateral, characterized by a greatly reduced number of nephrons that are strikingly enlarged. It invariably leads to chronic renal failure, as a rule after a period of progressive azotemia lasting

several years up to a decade or more. Simple hypoplasia may be unilateral or bilateral and of varying severity.

The true incidence of renal dysplasia is unknown. Most cases are unilateral, and males are affected more often than females. At one end of the spectrum is the multicystic dysplastic kidney (MCDK) with large cysts, no recognizable kidney architecture, and no or minimal function at birth; the incidence of MCDK is estimated to be approximately 1 in 4000 live births. At the other end is a normal-size kidney with apparent good function and minimal dysplastic features.

Box 1 shows the presenting signs and symptoms of renal hypoplasia/dysplasia, which vary depending on the age of presentation. Other urinary tract abnormalities are commonly present. For instance, contralateral vesicoureteral reflux (VUR) is present in 15% to 30% of children with MCDK, and contralateral or ipsilateral VUR occurs in most cases of simple hypoplasia. Bilateral dysplasia in boys is most commonly associated with lower urinary tract obstruction due to posterior urethral valves.

Expert Opinion on Management Issues

PRENATAL MANAGEMENT

Prenatal diagnosis of isolated renal hypoplasia or dysplasia requires only counseling before birth, emphasizing good prognosis in unilateral cases. Opinion-based consensus is that antenatal surgical intervention for urinary tract obstruction is not indicated if bilateral hypoplasia or dysplasia is present. If additional malformations are detected, input from an expert in genetics and genetic counseling should be sought.

TABLE 1 Syndromes Associated with Hypoplasia and Dysplasia

Syndrome	Hypoplasia	Dysplasia	Malignancy Risk
Alagille		+	
Bardet-Biedl		+	
Beckwith-Wiedemann		+	+
Branchio-oto-renal	+	+	
Caudal regression	+		
CHARGE association	+	+	
Cornelia de Lange	+	+	+
Infant of diabetic mother	+	+	
DiGeorge/Velocardiofacial	+		
Fetal alcohol	+	+	
Frazier	+		
Goldenhar	+	+	
Hemihyperplasia		+	+
Kallmann	+		
MURCS association		+	
Noonan		+	
Prune belly		+	
Congenital rubella		+	
Tuberous sclerosis		+	+
VATER association	+	+	
von Hippel-Lindau		+	
Williams	+		
Zellweger		+	

CHARGE, colobomas, heart anomalies, choanal atresia, retardation, genitourinary anomalies, and ear anomalies; MURCS, müllerian hypoplasia/aplasia, renal agenesis, and cervicothoracic somite dysplasia; VATER, vertebral defects, anal atresia, tracheoesophageal fistula, renal dysplasia.

BOX 1 Presenting Signs and Symptoms in Renal Hypoplasia/Dysplasia

- Prenatal
  - Hydronephrotic, cystic, small, or missing kidney(s) on ultrasound
  - Oligohydramnios because of fetal anuria or oliguria
  - Recognizable syndrome known to be associated with renal hypoplasia/dysplasia
- Neonatal
  - Recognizable syndrome associated with renal hypoplasia/dysplasia
  - Oliguria or anuria
  - Rising creatinine
  - Problems with fluid and electrolyte balance
  - Respiratory distress because of pulmonary hypoplasia
  - Palpable abdominal mass
  - Incidental finding on imaging study
- After neonatal period
  - Palpable abdominal mass
  - UTI associated with obstruction or vesicoureteral reflux
  - Recurrent dehydration because of renal concentrating defect
  - Signs and symptoms of chronic renal failure
  - Incidental finding on imaging study

UTI, urinary tract infection.

MANAGEMENT AT BIRTH

Babies with bilateral involvement may require treatment for pulmonary hypoplasia and renal problems immediately after birth. If present, lower urinary tract obstruction such as that caused by posterior urethral valves should be relieved as soon as feasible, keeping in mind that massive postobstructive diuresis may ensue, requiring large volumes of intravenous fluids. Because babies with bilateral hypoplastic/dysplastic kidneys commonly have a renal concentrating defect, adequate hydration should be ensured. Inappropriate restriction of fluid intake may worsen renal failure. Supplementation with extra water and electrolytes may become necessary. Prolonged oliguria combined with progressively rising serum creatinine levels constitutes a poor prognostic sign.

In the most severely affected cases, the question of dialysis may arise within days after birth. The decision should be individualized for each patient based on both medical and nonmedical factors. Newborns who remain ventilator dependent because of pulmonary hypoplasia are generally not good candidates for chronic dialysis. Renal transplantation is not usually feasible until a weight of 7 to 10 kg has been achieved.

Because of the frequent association of hypoplasia and dysplasia with VUR and other abnormalities that may predispose the infant to pyelonephritis and further renal damage, most experts recommend obtaining a voiding cystourethrogram during the first weeks of life and antibiotic prophylaxis if high-grade reflux is present. However, this approach has not been proved to improve renal prognosis.

MANAGEMENT AFTER THE NEONATAL PERIOD

Apparent isolated unilateral hypoplasia/dysplasia requires observation only, keeping in mind that subtle contralateral abnormalities may have escaped detection yet may affect long-term renal prognosis. Periodic urine protein or microalbumin determination and imaging by ultrasound suffice in most cases. Routine surgical removal of a unilateral MCDK is no longer recommended. The risk of malignancy and hypertension is minimal, and most MCDKs exhibit partial or total involution during the first years of life. If a poorly functioning hypoplastic/dysplastic kidney with VUR is the cause of recurring pyelonephritic episodes or hypertension, nephrectomy may be considered after a radionuclide scan has demonstrated that the functional contribution of that kidney is insignificant. If the affected kidney contributes 15% or more to total renal function, most specialists would repair the reflux rather than carry out a nephrectomy.

Once renal function has stabilized, varying degrees of fixed fluid and electrolyte losses are often present because of impaired tubular function and may require supplementation, especially in infants. Metabolic acidosis should be corrected with the administration of citrate or bicarbonate. Sodium deficit is difficult to assess; the only sign may be poor weight gain because of subtle volume contraction. In such cases, a trial of sodium supplementation with an extra 1 to 2 mEq/kg/day of sodium is warranted. With progression of renal impairment, standard treatments of chronic renal failure should be instituted as necessary.

Renal dysplasia/hypoplasia is occasionally first diagnosed only in later childhood. The ultimate prognosis varies from eventual end-stage renal disease to virtually no extra morbidity, determined by the extent of the original defect (deficit in number of functioning nephrons) and by any later insults such as episodes of pyelonephritis or hypertension.

Certain genetic conditions (see Table 1) predispose dysplastic kidneys to malignant transformation and therefore, children with these conditions require vigilant monitoring.

Common Pitfalls

- Caution should be exercised in predicting long-term outcome during the neonatal period, because initial imaging and laboratory tests may be misleading. Laboratory values measuring renal function immediately after birth reflect maternal renal status and are not informative about renal function of the newborn.
- Presence of renal dysplasia is difficult to rule out in hydronephrosis due to urinary tract obstruction; favorable long-term prognosis should not be automatically assumed after successful correction of obstruction.
- It is important to recognize when renal hypoplasia/dysplasia is part of a known syndrome or genetic abnormality. If extrarenal manifestations are present, genetic consultation and/or online search to obtain more information should be done. This is particularly important in conditions with high risk of malignancy.
- Failure to recognize extensive fluid and electrolyte losses in an infant may lead to chronic acidosis, volume contraction, and failure to thrive.

Communication and Counseling

The etiology of hypoplasia/dysplasia is unknown in most cases; an effort should be made to alleviate any guilt the parents may feel. In isolated simple hypoplasia or dysplasia without family history the risk of recurrence in future pregnancies is slightly above the background risk. The recurrence risk is higher in many syndromic/genetic conditions.

The commitment to chronic dialysis in a newborn should be made only after careful consideration of the baby's associated medical problems, the social situation, and the family's cultural and religious background. Although most parents want "everything done" for their baby, an attempt to paint a realistic picture should be made, including high morbidity and mortality and risk of long-term consequences of caring for a baby with end-stage renal disease, including possible developmental delay. If it is the family's wish, most centers do not consider withholding dialysis from a newborn unethical, especially if other major medical problems are present.

SUGGESTED READINGS

1. Aubertin G, Cripps S, Coleman G, et al: Prenatal diagnosis of apparently isolated unilateral multicystic kidney: Implications for counseling and management. Prenat Diagn 22:388–394, 2002. **Unilateral MCDK was associated with other urinary tract or genital abnormalities in 33% of cases and with nonrenal abnormalities in 16% of cases. Family history of renal anomalies was reported in 20% of cases.**

2. Atiyeh B, Husmann D, Baum M: Contralateral renal abnormalities in multicystic-dysplastic kidney disease. J Pediatr 121:65–67, 1992. **Associated urinary tract abnormalities were present on the opposite side in 39% of children with unilateral MCDK, most commonly (18%) vesicoureteral reflux (VUR).**

3. Hiraoka M, Hori C, Tsukuhara H, et al: Congenitally small kidneys with reflux as a common cause of nephropathy in boys. Kidney Int 52:874–877, 1998. **This screening study of apparently healthy infants showed an incidence of a small kidney of approximately 1 in 400. All were associated with ipsilateral reflux and more than half with contralateral reflux.**

4. Herndon CD, Ferrer FA, Freedman A, et al: Consensus on the prenatal management of antenatally detected urological abnormalities. J Urol 164:1052–1056, 2000. **Survey of members of the Society for Fetal Urology shows that consensus for surgical intervention for obstruction exists only for cases with oligohydramnios and no evidence of renal dysplasia.**

5. Ismaili K, Schurmans T, Wissig KM, et al: Early prognostic factors of infants with chronic renal failure caused by renal dysplasia. Pediatr Nephrol 16:260–264, 2001. **Shows that estimated creatinine clearance at 6 months is a good predictor of long-term outcome; a value below 15 mL/min/1.73 m^2 is associated with high risk of end-stage renal disease and other complications.**

6. Kuwertz-Broeking E, Brinkmann OA, von Lengerke HJ, et al: Unilateral multicystic dysplastic kidney: Experience in children. BJU Int 93:388–392, 2004. **Follow-up of 97 children with unilateral MCDK showed complete involution in 25% and partial involution in 60%. Abnormalities of contralateral kidney were present in 20%. No malignancies were observed.**

7. Perez LM, Naidu SI, Joseph DB: Outcome and cost analysis of operative versus nonoperative management of neonatal multicystic dysplastic kidneys. J Urol 160:1207–1211, 1998. **No tumor or significant hypertension developed in 49 patients with MCDK, consistent with other reports with only minimally increased risk of Wilms tumor (less than 0.1%) in MCDK.**

8. Roth KS, Carter WH, Chan JC: Obstructive nephropathy in children: Long-term progression after relief of posterior urethral valve. Pediatrics 107:1004–1010, 2001. **During a mean follow-up for 11.3 years, 7 of 10 boys with posterior urethral valves eventually developed end-stage renal disease despite initial successful relief of obstruction, suggesting that presence of dysplasia was an important factor.**

Obstructive Uropathy

Robert L. Chevalier

KEY CONCEPTS

- Congenital obstructive uropathy occurs in 1 in 1000 live births.
- The most common site of obstruction is the ureteropelvic junction, usually unilateral, but increased incidence of abnormalities of contralateral kidney.
- Ureterovesical junction obstruction is less common.
- Posterior urethral valve (PUV) is least common, but prognosis is less favorable.

- Prenatal ultrasound (16 to 20 weeks' gestation) permits early detection of hydronephrosis or bladder dilation.
- Oligohydramnios is an ominous sign, associated with severe bilateral renal impairment and pulmonary hypoplasia.
- Postnatal ultrasound should be performed if prenatal hydronephrosis is suspected; calyceal dilation suggests significant obstruction or reflux.
- Voiding cystourethrography can rule out vesicoureteral reflux and PUV.
- Diuretic renography can determine location and severity of obstruction.
- Two components of long-term outcome are severity of fetal renal maldevelopment and progression of tubulointerstitial disease.

Obstructive uropathy occurs in 1 in 1000 live births and accounts for 23% of chronic renal insufficiency in children. Nearly 7% of neonatal deaths occur in infants with major renal or urinary tract anomalies.

Congenital Versus Acquired

Urinary tract obstruction can be congenital or acquired. Hydronephrosis is the most commonly identified congenital anomaly detected by prenatal ultrasound, and patients with other organ system anomalies should undergo renal sonography to rule out hydronephrosis. The majority of cases of obstructive uropathy in the fetus, infant, and child are due to maldevelopment of the urinary tract, which can result in stenosis of the ureter at the ureteropelvic junction (UPJ), the ureterovesical junction (UVJ), or urethral obstruction because of posterior urethral valves (PUVs) or bladder abnormalities. Acquired urinary tract obstruction can result from tumor, stones, infection (such as fungus ball), or injury to the spinal cord (Table 1).

UPJ obstruction is the most common identifiable cause of congenital hydronephrosis detected prenatally, with an incidence of 1 in 1500. Although generally unilateral, UPJ obstruction has been reported bilaterally in as many as 40% of affected infants. The etiology of the lesion is unknown; it appears to be caused both by intrinsic alterations in the ureter leading to stenosis and by extrinsic compression of the ureter by crossing vessels. UVJ obstruction may result from intrinsic abnormalities of the ureter or from compression of the ureter by a thickened bladder wall. PUVs are abnormal membranous folds in the posterior urethra of affected boys, with an incidence of approximately 1 in 5000. Although less common than UPJ obstruction, impairment of both kidneys and the early fetal onset of this lesion lead to a far more serious prognosis.

Diagnosis

PRENATAL DIAGNOSIS

At present, the most common mode of initial detection of congenital obstructive uropathy is prenatal ultrasonography between 16 and 20 weeks' gestation.

TABLE 1 Evaluation of Upper and Lower Urinary Tract Obstruction

Imaging Study	Upper Tract (UPJ)	Lower Tract (PUV)
Fetal ultrasound	Hydronephrosis, renal pelvic diameter?	↑ Renal echogenicity, hydronephrosis, bladder dilatation?
Postnatal ultrasound (patient well hydrated)	Calyceal dilatation?	Bladder thickening + trabeculation?
Voiding cystourethrography	Vesicoureteral reflux?	Reflux, valves?
Diuretic renography (bladder catheterized)	Decreased uptake or delayed renal clearance on one or both sides?	
Urine stream	Normal	Normal or decreased

PUV, posterior urethral valve; UPJ, ureteropelvic junction.

Interpretation of the fetal sonogram requires an understanding of fetal renal physiology. One of the challenges inherent in fetal ultrasonography is the limitation of resolution—it is difficult to visualize the fetal kidneys prior to 16 weeks' gestation. By this time, many congenital forms of lower urinary tract obstruction are established and poorly reversible. Increased renal echogenicity suggests renal dysplasia (regardless of pelvic dilation). Except for severe obstruction, it is difficult to detect fetal hydronephrosis before the twenty-third week of gestation. Moreover, by the third trimester, the fetus is normally in a state of relative diuresis, such that mild pathologic dilation of the renal pelvis may be difficult to distinguish from normal.

POSTNATAL DIAGNOSIS

The postnatal diagnosis of urinary tract obstruction can be suspected in the infant with an abdominal mass, or the child with flank pain, incontinence, gross hematuria, febrile urinary tract infection, or nephrolithiasis. Renal ultrasound remains the best screening study for suspected obstructive uropathy in the postnatal period, but excretory urography may be of additional benefit to guide surgical intervention in the child with acute flank pain. Voiding cystourethrography is important to rule out vesicoureteral reflux and bladder outlet obstruction, whereas diuretic renography can reveal functional obstruction and its location.

Obstruction

DEFINITION

At present, there is no single reliable prognostic measure of urinary tract obstruction. The outcomes that matter most are progressive renal damage and decreasing renal function. The definition should therefore include the concept that obstruction is a condition that, if uncorrected, will limit the functional potential of a developing kidney. The benefits of avoiding surgical intervention must be balanced against the risks of ongoing obstruction in the face of renal maturation (that continues for at least the first 2 years of life).

CONSEQUENCES OF OBSTRUCTION ON THE DEVELOPING KIDNEY

A number of experimental studies show that urinary tract obstruction can have global effects on the developing kidney. These include delayed maturation of the microvasculature and nephrons, a reduction in the number of nephrons, and progressive tubular atrophy and interstitial fibrosis. There is an increase in renal vascular resistance that is largely mediated by activation of the endogenous renin-angiotensin system.

CLINICAL CONSEQUENCES OF OBSTRUCTION

Severe bilateral obstruction in utero can result in oligohydramnios and the Potter sequence, with pulmonary hypoplasia. Delayed consequences of chronic hydronephrosis include the signs of tubulointerstitial injury, such as urinary sodium wasting, impaired urinary concentration, and impaired distal urinary acidification with hyperkalemia (type 4 renal tubular acidosis).

Expert Opinion on Management Issues

TIMING OF OBSTRUCTION RELIEF IN URETEROPELVIC JUNCTION OBSTRUCTION

There are currently two opposing camps in the management of infants and children with unilateral UPJ obstruction. The first group believes that early surgical intervention for significant UPJ obstruction affords the patient the best long-term renal function and optimizes growth of the obstructed kidney. The second group considers that most cases of UPJ obstruction do not require pyeloplasty but that patients should be closely followed with sequential ultrasound and diuretic renography to monitor for signs of deterioration. As stated previously, there remains no consensus regarding a useful clinical definition of significant urinary tract obstruction. Overall, for infants managed with observation alone, approximately 25% eventually require surgical intervention. The benefits of avoiding an operation must be balanced with the risk of further nephron loss during the period of observation and the individual compliance of the patient's family in adhering to a schedule of serial radiologic studies to monitor the status of the hydronephrotic kidney. Most pediatric urologists agree that for mild dilation of the renal pelvis without calyceal dilation, surgical intervention will be rarely required. There is an urgent need for biomarkers of the severity of obstruction and appropriately controlled clinical trials of the various management options.

Despite the difficulties in correlating fetal renal pelvic volume with outcome, it is generally agreed that in the last trimester, an anteroposterior renal pelvic diameter greater than 10 mm suggests the presence of hydronephrosis, and diameter between 5 and 10 mm in the second trimester suggests ultrasound should be repeated in the third trimester. All fetuses with suspected hydronephrosis should have renal sonography repeated postnatally, ideally after several days of age, and again at 6 to 12 months of age if there is any doubt regarding the status of the pelvis. The studies should be done with the infant in a state of adequate hydration, as volume contraction may mask a potentially significant obstruction.

If renal pelvic dilation is present (and certainly if there is calyceal dilation), a diuretic renal scan should be obtained to measure the location and degree of functional obstruction, and a voiding cystourethrogram to rule out vesicoureteral reflux. If bladder outlet obstruction is suspected (dilated bladder or thickened bladder wall), voiding cystourethrography should be performed promptly after birth, so that catheter drainage can reveal the potential renal function before deciding on ablation of valves or urinary tract diversion. Infants with documented hydronephrosis should be treated with prophylactic antibiotics pending further evaluation or treatment (generally oral amoxicillin at 10 mg/kg/day).

PRENATAL INTERVENTION FOR POSTERIOR URETHRAL VALVES

Because most of the damage to the developing kidney and urinary tract resulting from PUV begins in fetal life, attempts have been made to relieve the obstruction prenatally. In highly selected patients, a catheter may be inserted in the fetal bladder to drain the urine to the amniotic space. In addition to reducing hydrostatic pressure in the collecting system of the developing kidney, this increases the amniotic fluid volume and permits normal pulmonary development (which is impaired in the presence of oligohydramnios). To be considered for such intervention, there must be unequivocal evidence of oligohydramnios and no other organ anomalies or karyotype anomaly, and the parents must recognize the experimental nature of the procedure. Less than 1% of fetuses with suspected hydronephrosis will become candidates for prenatal surgical intervention.

PROGNOSTIC FACTORS FOR PROGRESSION

In patients with PUV managed postnatally, oligohydramnios, prematurity, megacystis, or postnatal glomerular filtration rate (GFR) less than 20 mL/min have been associated with a poor outcome. A majority of patients diagnosed with PUV in fetal or neonatal life develop renal insufficiency by 10 years of age.

Common Pitfalls

- *Evaluation of the contralateral kidney in patients with UPJ obstruction*: In patients with unilateral UPJ obstruction, it is important to evaluate the status of the contralateral kidney with a voiding cystourethrogram. There is an increased incidence of vesicoureteral reflux and other anomalies of the contralateral kidney.

- *Interpretation of ultrasound, scan*: It is important that infants undergoing renal ultrasonography be adequately hydrated at the time of study, as volume contraction may mask an underlying lesion that is revealed only with high urine flow. Diuretic renography (furosemide and MAG3 or DTPA) should generally be performed in infants older than 1 month, to allow for maturation of renal concentrating ability. To allow adequate interpretation of the results, it is important that a catheter be placed in the bladder for the entire procedure.

- *Interpretation of fetal urine electrolytes*: Aspiration of urine from the fetal bladder has been used as an index of the prognosis for fetal renal functional outcome. Thus, fetal urine sodium concentration less than 100 mEq/L, chloride less than 90 mEq/L, or osmolality less than 210 mOsm/kg have been associated with a favorable outcome. Unfortunately, the correlation between these criteria and renal functional outcome has been variable, and more reliable biomarkers of renal impairment are desperately needed.

- *Interpretation of the infant's urine stream*: Severe posterior urethral valves may cause enough resistance to urine flow to reduce the infant's urine stream with micturition. However, compensatory thickening of the bladder wall in fetal life may overcome the resistance, and a normal-appearing urine stream is no guarantee of the absence of bladder outlet obstruction.

- *Long-term follow-up*: The developing kidney has a capacity to compensate for the loss of nephrons through adaptive growth and hyperfiltration of remaining nephrons. Thus, measures of total renal function such as plasma creatinine or nuclide scans do not account for pathologic changes that may not become evident for many years. All children with obstructive nephropathy (whether or not undergoing surgery) should have periodic measurement of blood pressure, plasma creatinine concentration, urinalysis, and renal sonography. Nonsteroidal anti-inflammatory drugs should be avoided or their dose carefully monitored. In the transition from pediatrician to internist, such follow-up should be continued throughout adulthood.

Communication and Counseling

PRENATAL REASSURANCE

There is a very high prevalence of the identification of suspected neonatal hydronephrosis of 0.5% to 1% of pregnancies. It is important to assuage the anxiety of the parents (who fear the implications of possible impairment of a baby's vital organ) by explaining the clinical significance of this finding. Fewer than 20% of fetuses will have UPJ obstruction or vesicoureteral reflux on further evaluation, and less than 50% of these require surgical intervention. For patients without obstruction or reflux, fewer than 10% have moderate or severe pelviectasis after two years' follow-up. The probability of an infant having a clinically significant postnatal abnormality is proportional to the severity of prenatal hydronephrosis. If the prenatal renal pelvic diameter exceeds 20 mm, the probability is greater than 90%, whereas if the diameter is less than 10 mm, the probability is less than 5%.

LONG-TERM FOLLOW-UP

Historically, infants with UPJ obstruction requiring pyeloplasty who had satisfactory postoperative imaging have not subsequently received close follow-up. It is likely that some of these patients will eventually develop proteinuria, hypertension, or chronic renal insufficiency. Of greater concern, many if not most boys diagnosed in fetal or neonatal life with posterior urethral valves develop renal insufficiency by 10 years of age. The parents of the child with obstructive uropathy should understand that there are at least two components to the long-term outcome. The first comprises the renal maldevelopment and dysfunction that result from urinary tract obstruction in fetal life. Most of these changes are irreversible and could not have been avoided. The second includes the factors that lead to progression of renal fibrosis, tubular atrophy, and renal insufficiency. These latter factors can be minimized if the patient and parents understand the rationale for monitoring blood pressure, proteinuria, and renal status, even in the absence of symptoms.

SUGGESTED READINGS

1. Chevalier RL, Roth JA: Obstructive uropathy. In Avner ED, Harmon WE, Niaudet P (eds): Pediatric Nephrology, 5th ed. Philadelphia: Lippincott Williams & Wilkins, 2004, pp 1049–1076. **A detailed overview of the current basic science and clinical management of congenital obstructive uropathy.**
2. Corteville JE, Gray DL, Crane JP: Congenital hydronephrosis: Correlation of fetal ultrasonographic findings with infant outcome. Am J Obstet Gynecol 165:384–388, 1991. **Correlates mean 20-month outcome with fetal pelvic diameter.**
3. Holmes N, Harrison MR, Baskin LS: Fetal surgery for posterior urethral valves: Long-term postnatal outcomes. Pediatrics 108:36–42, 2001. **Demonstrates the overall poor long-term outcome for infants undergoing fetal surgery for posterior urethral valves.**
4. Palmer LS, Maizels M, Cartwright PC, et al: Surgery versus observation for managing obstructive grade 3 to 4 unilateral hydronephrosis: A report from the society for fetal urology. J Urol 159:222–228, 1998. **Describes a controlled prospective study of observation versus pyeloplasty for infants with significant unilateral ureteropelvic junction obstruction, showing the benefits of surgical intervention.**
5. Roth KS, Carter WH Jr, Chan JCM: Obstructive nephropathy in children: Long-term progression after relief of posterior urethral valve. Pediatrics 107:1004–1010, 2001. **Shows that despite surgical correction of posterior urethral valves, 70% developed end-stage renal disease over mean follow-up of only 11 years.**
6. Ulman I, Jayanthi VR, Koff SA: The long-term followup of newborns with severe unilateral hydronephrosis initially treated nonoperatively. J Urol 164:1101–1105, 2000. **Describes mean 78-month follow-up of infants with unilateral ureteropelvic junction obstruction managed with initial observation.**

Enuresis and Voiding Dysfunction

Manju M. Chandra

KEY CONCEPTS

- Nocturnal enuresis (NE) and diurnal urge syndrome are noted in approximately 20% of elementary school children and represent a maturational delay in bladder control in most.
- The treatment of a child with NE should be directed at the contributing mechanisms: polyuria, overactive bladder, and difficult sleep arousal. Difficult arousal from sleep is more prevalent in children with primary as compared to secondary onset of NE and in monosymptomatic NE as compared to NE associated with diurnal voiding symptoms. Although 90% of children with primary monosymptomatic NE have difficulty in sleep arousal as a major pathogenic cause, only 16% of those with secondary onset of NE and associated diurnal voiding symptoms do.
- Diurnal urge syndrome coexists with NE in 50% of the affected boys and 75% of the affected girls.
- History of overactive bladder and stool retention should be repeatedly sought in children with monosymptomatic NE who do not respond to treatment.
- The parents of 40% of children with diurnal urinary urgency, urge incontinence, and urine or stool withholding do not bring these symptoms to the physician's attention, because they ascribe them to the child's laziness and "waiting till the last minute." These problems can be uncovered on detailed interrogation with leading questions, finding evidence of urinary incontinence on perineal examination, or on observing the child's voiding pattern in the office setting.
- The index of suspicion for associated undisclosed diurnal voiding symptoms should be higher in children with NE who manifest the following: psychosocial and learning problems, urinary tract infections after 3 years of age, nocturia more than twice a month, more than one occurrence of wetting at night, easy sleep arousal, secondary onset of NE, stool withholding, or a family history of urinary tract infection and diurnal voiding symptoms during childhood.
- Although children with monosymptomatic NE are not at risk for medical sequelae, those with associated diurnal urge syndrome and discoordinated voiding are at risk for recurrent urinary tract infections, vesicoureteral reflux, renal damage, and stool retention.

A child is labeled as having voiding dysfunction when his or her voiding pattern deviates from what is expected for a child of that age. The common forms of voiding dysfunction in children include diurnal urge syndrome related to overactive bladder, nocturnal enuresis (NE), and infrequent bladder emptying.

Enuresis results when the bladder is able to fill to its functional capacity and contract reflexively. Although diurnal enuresis and NE are normal in infants, a series of maturational processes—hormonal, neural, and structural—result in urinary continence by 5 years of age in most children. These maturational processes result in cortical inhibition of reflex detrusor (bladder muscle) contractions, conscious sensation of bladder fullness, increase in functional bladder capacity, decrease in nocturnal urine volume, and improvement in arousal from sleep in response to bladder fullness or an impending detrusor contraction. Maturational delays or pathologic alterations in one or more of these processes can result in persistence of infantile pattern of voiding (primary enuresis) or secondary onset of NE and/or diurnal urge syndrome.

Expert Opinion on Management Issues

DIURNAL URGE SYNDROME

Urinary frequency, urgency, and urge incontinence in children are generally related to an overactive bladder, that is, a bladder prone to reflex detrusor contractions that are not inhibited by the cerebral cortex. The response to sudden detrusor contractions may be varied in different children and at different times. It may include mad rush to the toilet, total urge incontinence, and sudden tightening of the pelvic floor muscles to postpone voiding and minimize urine leakage. The contraction of the pelvic floor reflexively inhibits a detrusor contraction. Hence, children with overactive bladder frequently use this maneuver to abort or prevent unwanted reflex detrusor contractions.

Children who repeatedly use pelvic withholding maneuvers to obstruct the urine flow put themselves at risk for urinary tract infections (UTI), acquisition or persistence of vesicoureteral reflux , renal damage, and stool retention. Because stool retention predisposes to uninhibited detrusor contractions, a vicious cycle may be initiated that may negatively affect the child socially and psychologically.

Management of Diurnal Urge Syndrome

The treatment of overactive bladder is aimed at preventing uninhibited detrusor contractions and correcting discoordinated pelvic floor tightening maneuvers. An underlying neurogenic or structural cause of voiding dysfunction should be ruled out in all children by obtaining a detailed history of voiding pattern and performing a directed physical examination. Renal and bladder ultrasonography and a voiding cystogram are indicated in those children with UTI and severe voiding dysfunction. Polyuria related to diabetes mellitus or urinary concentrating defect can be excluded by documenting absence of glucosuria and urine specific gravity (SG) of 1.016 or higher in a random urine or in urine collected after fluid deprivation.

Behavioral and Motivational Therapy

The child is taught bladder control by following a regimen of frequent voluntary voids timed before the bladder fills to its functional capacity and manifests reflex contractions. These timed voids help break the cycle of frequent uninhibited detrusor contractions and train the bladder to respond to the brain's commands instead of the child having to respond to the unwanted detrusor contractions. I give an analogy of training the bladder to training a puppy dog; the dog has to follow the master's instructions and not the other way around.

The child is asked to maintain a voiding pattern chart (Fig. 1) to focus his or her attention on the problem just as the schoolteacher provides homework to reinforce the lessons taught. It helps to have all caregivers be involved in motivating and reminding the child in the task of bladder training, with daily checks of the voiding pattern chart. Positive feedback should be provided to the child for efforts and improvement to reinforce the behavior. The voiding interval is gradually increased to every 3.5 to 4 hours if the child can hold urine comfortably for 2 hours without urgency or pelvic withholding maneuvers (Box 1).

About a third of children with diurnal urge syndrome manifest clinically relevant behavioral problems, either an outwardly directed visible behavior such as conduct disorder and attention deficit hyperactivity disorder (ADHD) or internalizing or emotional disorder like social anxiety, sibling rivalry, and depressive disorder. The child's voiding problems may also elicit punitive behavior from the parents, which often appears connected with parental psychosocial problems. Addressing the accompanying psychological or medical problems is as important in managing these children; for example, treating ADHD, if present, will help the child focus better in overcoming his/her voiding problem.

Pharmacologic Therapy of Overactive Bladder

Anticholinergic agents are extremely useful as an adjunct to behavioral treatment. These agents increase the threshold for uninhibited detrusor contractions and decrease their amplitude and frequency. With use of anticholinergic agents, a balance between efficacy and tolerability should be considered, because systemic side effects related to blockade of cholinergic receptors at sites other than the detrusor muscle preclude use of high doses needed to combat detrusor overactivity. The older anticholinergic agents include propantheline (Pro-Banthine 15-mg tablet), hyoscyamine sulfate (Cystospaz, 0.15-mg tablet; Levsin, 0.125 mg orally [PO] or sublingual tablets; Levsin Elixir, 0.125 mg/5 mL; Levsin extended-release tablets, 0.375 mg). The newer agents (Table 1) are more specific for M3-type muscarinic receptors in the bladder. Some have direct

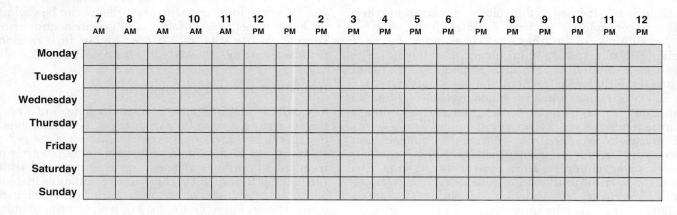

	7 AM	8 AM	9 AM	10 AM	11 AM	12 PM	1 PM	2 PM	3 PM	4 PM	5 PM	6 PM	7 PM	8 PM	9 PM	10 PM	11 PM	12 PM
Monday																		
Tuesday																			
Wednesday																			
Thursday																			
Friday																			
Saturday																			
Sunday																			

Write in one of the following letters as it applies for the appropriate hour:

A - If you leak urine or have an accident   U - If you have an urge   V - When you void at will   B - BM

FIGURE 1. Voiding pattern chart.

BOX 1   Treatment Regimen for Children with Diurnal Urge Syndrome

- Discuss the brain's inhibitory and facilitatory control over the bladder, and how the patient can become the "boss" of the bladder and discipline its behavior.
- Create an every-two-hours voiding schedule, with written record of planned voids (V), urgent voids (U), and accidents (A) in the voiding pattern chart (see Fig. 1).
- Send a note to teachers and other caregivers to allow the child to visit the toilet without having to wait for permission.
- Consider adding an anticholinergic drug; dose titration as per response.
- Increase the voiding interval gradually to every 4 hours if the child can hold urine comfortably for 2 hours.
- Schedule follow-up visits at least every 2 weeks with positive reinforcement for improvement in voiding pattern and for child's efforts.
- Treat associated constipation/stool retention.
- Continue medications for 2 to 3 weeks after normal daytime voiding pattern is achieved, and then gradually taper off, or titrate to the lowest dose required to maintain a normal voiding pattern.

antispasmodic activity on the detrusor muscle as well and have slow-release formulations. Whichever anticholinergic medication is used, the dose should be increased to the maximum tolerable dose if there is not sufficient improvement in voiding symptoms despite motivated efforts on the part of the child.

Treatment of Constipation/Stool Retention

Treatment of associated constipation/stool retention includes patient education about the biologic basis of the problem and institution of dietary modification, laxatives, and gentle persuasion to attempt one or two bowel movements per day with the goal of keeping the rectum empty. Several effective regimens are available (see chapter entitled "Constipation"). I have recently had significant success with the use of the osmotic laxative polyethylene glycol 3350 (MiraLax powder).

Pelvic Floor Relaxation Training

Children with incomplete bladder and rectal emptying because of inadequate pelvic floor relaxation and those with hesitancy of urination and/or bowel elimination will benefit from efforts directed to teach pelvic floor relaxation using slow and deep breathing. Biofeedback training is provided with visual or audio demonstration of the child's pelvic floor electromyelogram activity obtained with sticky patch electrodes placed around the anus. This can also be done by having the child perceive and observe in a mirror the movement of the pelvic floor while using the pelvic withholding maneuver. The child then tries to achieve the opposite, that is, pelvic floor relaxation and descent by relaxing himself/herself.

Controversial Interventions for Overactive Bladder

For children with severe problems related to overactive bladder resistant to standard therapy, other interventions have included periodic intravesical instillation of capsaicin or resiniferatoxin (neurotoxins that desensitize the C-fiber afferent neurons), and electrical stimulation of sacral nerve roots. Injection of botulinum toxin in the detrusor muscle has also been tried. These treatments are unproven.

MONOSYMPTOMATIC NOCTURNAL ENURESIS

Evaluation and treatment of a child whose only complaint is bedwetting should be directed at discovering the predominant pathophysiologic mechanism(s) operative in that particular child, for example, nocturnal polyuria, overactive bladder, difficult sleep arousal, or obstructive breathing. All children with NE should be evaluated for additional diurnal voiding dysfunction and should be labeled as having monosymptomatic NE

TABLE 1 Commonly Used Anticholinergic Agents for Overactive Bladder

Generic Name (Trade Name)	Dosage Formulation	Adult Dosage Regimen	Max Daily Dose	Comments Regarding Pediatric Dosage
Oxybutynin chloride (Ditropan)	Tablet 5 mg; syrup 5 mg/5 mL	5 mg PO bid or tid	30 mg	0.2 mg/kg/dose, max starting dose 5 mg.
Oxybutynin extended release (Ditropan XL)	5-, 10-,15-mg tablets	Start with 5 mg PO qd	30 mg	Start with 5 mg in children >25 kg if they can swallow the tablets.*
Oxybutynin transdermal system (Oxytrol)	3.9 mg/day	2 skin patches/wk	3.9 mg	For children >25 kg, apply to dry, intact skin with reapplication to same site within 7 days; may cause application site rash and burning.*
Tolterodine tartrate (Detrol)	1-, 2-mg tablets	2 mg PO bid; reduce dose if side effects	6 mg	In children 15 to 25 kg, 1 mg bid; >25 kg, 2 mg bid.
Tolterodine long-acting (Detrol LA)	2 mg, 4 mg	4 mg PO qd; reduce dose if side effects	6 mg	In children 15 to 25 kg, 2 mg LA qd; >25 kg, 4 mg LA qd.*

Mechanism of action of anticholinergic agents—Decrease the frequency and amplitude of uninhibited detrusor contractions.
Common adverse reactions—Dry mouth, dry skin, flushed face, blurred vision, drowsiness, risk of heat prostration in high environmental temperature.
Contraindications—Structural obstruction of the urinary tract, gastrointestinal obstruction, risk for narrow angle glaucoma.
Newer agents with no personal experience by author—trospium chloride (Sanctura) 20-mg tablets, darifenacin (Enablex) extended release 7.5-mg and 15-mg tablets, solifenacin (Vesicare) 5-mg and 10-mg tablets.
* Dosage, efficacy, and safety have not been established in children.
bid, two times daily; PO, orally; qd, daily; tid, three times daily.

BOX 2 Treatment Regimen for Monosymptomatic Nocturnal Enuresis

- Limit fluids to 8 ounces at supper 3 to 3.5 hours prior to bedtime; no fluids thereafter.
- Empty the bladder before sleeping.
- Make a bedtime "resolution" to stay dry.
- Discuss mode of action of drugs/moisture alarm and drug side effects; dispense drug/alarm.
- Advise that medication/alarm is the "coach" and the child is the "player."
- Advise that positive internal and external biofeedback signals help hasten central nervous system control of the bladder.
- Keep a calendar of dry and wet nights.
- Encourage child's participation in cleaning up personal and bed clothes.
- Schedule follow-up visits or phone calls at least every 2 weeks, with positive reinforcement for dry nights and efforts.
- Continue use of alarm until 28 consecutive dry nights are achieved, then stop; use medications as directed.
- If bedwetting returns on tapering or discontinuation of medication or alarm, restart nightly medication/alarm.
- If not dry every night, despite motivation and efforts, substitute or add other drug or alarm and rule out undisclosed diurnal voiding problems.

Many modalities for the treatment of bedwetting are available. The common ones include motivational and behavioral approaches, use of a moisture alarm, and drug therapy with either vasopressin analogues or tricyclic antidepressants. Each form of therapy has variable success rates. The best results are obtained when several elements to achieve success are combined in a treatment program. For example, fluid restriction prior to bedtime, bedtime resolution to stay dry, a diary of wet and dry nights, positive external biofeedback (encouragement and reward system), and use of an alarm system and/or appropriate drugs (Box 2 and Table 2).

Behavioral and Motivational Therapy

The child is educated in lay language about the biologic basis for the NE and that bedwetting can be eliminated by behavioral conditioning. If the bladder is kept from emptying itself during sleep for a certain length of time, it may continue with the new pattern. The child is encouraged to help train the bladder in the manner outlined in Box 2 and Table 2. The role of the medication or alarm is compared to that of "coach," with the child being the "player." The child is encouraged to follow the "rules of the game" and return to the physician/health care person for "practice sessions" every 2 weeks, during which performance, motivation, and effort are reviewed and reinforced. The "player," not the "coach," is praised for good results. The child's pivotal role in learning bladder control is emphasized. A telephone conversation with the child may be used in place of a clinic visit.

A minimum period of 4 weeks of consecutive dryness should be achieved before any therapy is discontinued to decrease the chance of relapse.

only when diurnal voiding problems are ruled out with a careful history. In some children with associated diurnal voiding problems, the NE may resolve once the daytime habits are normalized. Specific treatment of obstructed breathing may help cure the NE in others.

Monosymptomatic NE has no adverse medical consequences. However, it is a treatable condition, and treatment does offer psychosocial benefits and improved self-image. Therefore, I recommend treatment in children with persistent monosymptomatic NE beyond 5 years of age if it is stressful to the child and the family.

TABLE 2 Medications for Treatment of Monosymptomatic Nocturnal Enuresis

Generic Name (Trade Name)	Dosage Formulation	Dosage Regimen	Comments
Desmopressin acetate (DDAVP)	Nasal spray pump: 10 µg/0.1mL spray	1 spray (10 µg) per nostril qhs, increasing to 40 µg	Can cause nasal irritation; risk of water intoxication (headache, seizures) hence, restrict fluids 3 h before the dose.
	Tablets: 0.1 mg, 0.2 mg	0.2 mg PO qhs, increasing up to 0.6 mg	Risk of water intoxication.
Imipramine hydrochloride (Tofranil)	Tablets: 10 mg, 25 mg, 50 mg; Tofranil PM capsule 75, 100, 125, 150 mg	1.5–2 mg/kg 2 h before bedtime, not to exceed 2.5 mg/kg or 75 mg maximum	Can cause sleep disturbance, mood alteration, decreased appetite, risk of cardiac arrhythmia with overdose.

Mechanism of Action:
Desmopressin—Decreased urine volume, possible effect on sleep arousal through its action as a central nervous system neurotransmitter
Imipramine—Anticholinergic effect on bladder, increased resistance of bladder outlet, possible central inhibition of micturition reflex, possible effect on sleep arousal by central noradrenergic facilitation
PO, orally; qhs, at bedtime.

Specific Therapy for Monosymptomatic Nocturnal Enuresis

The choice between using an alarm or drug therapy should be made after determining whether the child's predominant problem is polyuria, overactive bladder, or difficult sleep arousal. Assessment of polyuria can be made by the amount of wetness. Nocturnal bladder capacity can be gauged by the number of wetting episodes per night, time of occurrence of wetting in relation to the previous void, and by determining the child's daytime functional bladder capacity. Sleep arousal can be assessed by use of a standardized questionnaire (Chandra, et al.), frequency of nocturia, and the child's awakening after wetting to change clothes. The parents' willingness to awaken their child at night when the bedwetting alarm goes off and parental acceptance of potential drug side effects for a benign condition will often guide the choice of treatment.

Bedwetting moisture alarms have been highly successful in curing bedwetting when used as directed. Because many children with NE are deep sleepers with a high threshold of sleep arousal and are unlikely to awaken with the sound of the alarm, one family member has to wake the child as soon as the alarm goes off and escort him or her to the toilet to finish voiding. This method requires motivation on the part of the child and substantial parental commitment. It is reported to work best in children with high frequency of wet nights and smaller than average bladder capacity for age during the day. The alarm use should be continued until 28 consecutive dry nights are achieved. Overconditioning by increasing fluid intake before bedtime for another 2 weeks before stopping alarm treatment decreases the chance of relapse. Dryness is achieved by sleeping through the night with a full bladder in two thirds and by awakening to void in a third of children.

Recently, vibratory moisture alarms and miniaturized ultrasound bladder volume controlled alarm devices have also been introduced.

Desmopressin (DDAVP) can achieve dryness in some patients with the very first dose. It is most effective in those with low frequency of wet nights, only one wet episode per night and large amount of wetness per night suggestive of nocturnal polyuria. If the patient improves, DDAVP treatment should be continued for 2 to 3 months and then tapered over 2 to 4 weeks. If a child relapses, DDAVP can be restarted. DDAVP treatment is not very good at providing long-term cure, but the drug can be very useful in patients who have a need for immediate and short-term relief for sleep-overs or camp-outs or to prevent aggression in caregivers who cannot cope with the child's bedwetting.

DDAVP therapy can result in water intoxication if the fluid intake is not curtailed. Hence, patients should limit the fluid intake 3.5 hours prior to the bedtime dose of DDAVP.

Imipramine is a better alternative to alarm treatment in children with frequent wet nights and difficult sleep arousal whose parents do not wish to be bothered at night by the child's moisture alarm. Imipramine may lead to dryness from the first dose or may take a few weeks. I prescribe imipramine 2 hours before bedtime until 21 consecutive dry nights are achieved and then continue the drug on an every-other-night basis for 2 weeks. If the patient stays dry, the medication is stopped, although the behavioral therapy is continued for another 4 weeks. In my experience imipramine is more effective than DDAVP in achieving long-term cure.

Imipramine can induce serious cardiac arrhythmias with overdosage or when used in concert with other antipsychotic agents. Thus, children need to be screened for cardiac abnormalities before use, and the family should be cautioned about not exceeding the prescribed dose. The child is encouraged to ask for the medication, although a parent takes charge dispensing it.

Controversial Interventions

Acupuncture and hypnotherapy may also have a place in the management of monosymptomatic NE. However, available reports are anecdotal and uncontrolled.

INFREQUENT BLADDER EMPTYING (BLADDER INERTIA)

Approximately 7% of elementary school children void fewer than three times in 24 hours and/or hold urine for more than 12 hours overnight. These children have larger-than-average bladder capacity and do not manifest urinary frequency, urgency, or pelvic withholding maneuvers. They can be considered to have bladder inertia, that is, a tendency opposite to that of overactive bladder. The pattern of infrequent voiding starts in infancy in some children, although others acquire this habit once they are confronted with public bathrooms.

Children with bladder inertia are at risk for urinary infections because of infrequent washout of bacteria, and those with overstretched bladders, for incomplete bladder emptying. These children do not develop urinary frequency or urgency in response to a UTI but instead present with dysuria, back pain, lower abdominal pain, or fever. Infrequent bowel emptying because of colonic inertia often co-exists with bladder inertia. However, stool retention and leakage because of pelvic withholding maneuvers is distinctly rare in this group.

Treatment

Children who void infrequently need to be trained to reset their voiding pattern by emptying their bladders more frequently, for example, 5 to 6 times a day. These children are often quite stubborn and require gentle coaxing along with a reward incentive. In those with co-existent colonic inertia, more frequent bowel emptying can be facilitated with the use of laxatives.

There is a small group of infrequent voiders whose detrusor contractions are suppressed because of high basal pelvic floor tone. Their pelvic floor spasticity is often a sequel of repeated conditioned pelvic tightening maneuvers related to overactive bladder. This group of children should be treated like those with diurnal urge syndrome.

Common Pitfalls

- Awakening the child at night at a time convenient to the parents is often helpful in achieving some dry nights but does not condition the bladder for long-term cure. Its failure cannot be equated to potential failure of moisture alarm therapy, because the awakening of the child with the alarm is temporally related to the stimulus of a full bladder and a detrusor contraction.
- Many families discontinue moisture alarm use after a few days because of continued bedwetting. The child, however, may have manifested improvement in bladder capacity and sleep arousal in the form of less wetness per episode and occurrence of wetting later in the sleep.
- Parents of children with NE and diurnal urge incontinence of only a few drops of urine often consider the latter problem inconsequential; they are often not initially willing to accept anticholinergic therapy and frequent timed voiding during the day to fix the child's nighttime wetting.
- When advising children with diurnal urge syndrome to void every 2 hours, it should be made clear that 2 hours is the minimum time interval for voiding, and that they can void more often if they wish.
- When toilet training children, emphasize optimal posture during voiding and defecation. Humans have squatted to void for thousands of years. The present one-size-fits-all toilet does not allow foot support for children. The resultant inadequate pelvic floor relaxation interferes with normal bladder and bowel emptying. Children should be provided with small potties or with a footstool when using the regular toilet to obtain foot support.

Communication and Counseling

The rate and rapidity of response to treatment of diurnal urge syndrome and monosymptomatic NE is correlated with the child's motivation and effort and parental encouragement and support. Although the spontaneous cure rate for NE is 15% annually, an estimated 3% of untreated children with bedwetting will continue to have bedwetting as adults. Hence, an attempt should be made to cure this annoying problem in all. Children who have had symptoms of overactive bladder during childhood have a higher prevalence of symptoms related to overactive bladder during their adulthood. Hence, learning the approach to discipline the bladder during childhood is also likely to serve them well in their adult years.

SUGGESTED READINGS

1. Chandra M: Voiding and its disorders in children. In Trachtman H, Gauthier B (eds): Pediatric Nephrology. Amsterdam: Harwood Academic Publishers, 1998, pp 217–229. **Overview of normal voiding mechanism, steps in maturation of voluntary voiding control, and classification of voiding disorders.**
2. Chandra M, Saharia R, Hill V, et al: Prevalence of diurnal voiding symptoms and difficult arousal from sleep in children with nocturnal enuresis. J Urol 172:311–316, 2004. **This study reports presence of diurnal voiding problems in two thirds of nocturnal enuretics and lists clinical features, which should alert the physician to look for undisclosed diurnal voiding problems.**
3. Hjalmas K, Arnold T, Bower W, et al: Nocturnal enuresis: An international evidence based management strategy. J Urol 171:2545–2561, 2004. **Update on pathophysiology and management of NE with input from experts from around the globe.**
4. Kawauchi A, Yamao Y, Nakanishi H, et al: Relationships among nocturnal urinary volume, bladder capacity, and nocturia with and without water load in nonenuretic children. Urology 59:433–437, 2002. **This study demonstrated decreased nocturnal functional bladder capacity as a cause of NE.**
5. Koff S, Wagner T, Jayanthi V: The relationship among dysfunctional elimination syndromes, primary vesicoureteric reflux and urinary tract infections in children. J Urol 160:1019–1022, 1998. **Report of close association between functional constipation and functional problems of the lower urinary tract.**

6. Kruse S, Hellstrom AL, Hjalmas K: Daytime bladder dysfunction in therapy-resistant nocturnal enuresis. A pilot study in urotherapy. Scand J Urol Nephrol 33:49, 1999. **This study suggests that a frequent voiding schedule during the day can help patients with NE who have failed previous treatments.**

7. Loening-Baucke V: Urinary incontinence and urinary tract infection and their resolution with treatment of chronic constipation in childhood. Pediatrics 100:228, 1997. **Report demonstrating improvement of urinary problems with correction of constipation.**

8. Mellon MW, McGrath ML: Empirically supported treatments in pediatric psychology: Nocturnal enuresis. J Pediatr Psychol 25:193, 2000. **Report of behavioral modification approach to the management of NE.**

9. Neveus T, Lackgren G, Tuvemo T, et al: Enuresis—background and treatment. Scand J Urol Nephrol (Suppl) 206: 1, 2000. **Overview of pathogenesis and treatment of NE.**

10. Watanabe H, Kawauchi A, Kitamori T, et al: Treatment system for nocturnal enuresis according to an original classification system. Eur Urol 25:43, 1994. **Authors describe three types of NE based on simultaneous sleep electroencephalogram and urodynamic studies in children.**

- In girls with grades I to III vesicoureteral reflux and normal initial ultrasound, there is no need for follow-up ultrasound in those free of recurrent upper tract infections.
- A follow-up voiding cystourethrogram should be done after 2 years in children with low-grade reflux and every 3 years in those with medium-high grade reflux.
- Renal and perirenal abscesses can manifest at times with normal urine findings. The best diagnostic tool is computed tomography. Most abscesses will respond to 10 to 14 days of parenteral antibiotic therapy with a third-generation cephalosporin, at times augmented by aminoglycosides or anti-staphylococcal agents, followed by oral therapy to complete 3 to 4 weeks of treatment. Surgical intervention is rarely needed.
- Correction of voiding dysfunction and constipation has an important role in protecting the upper tract from infectious and noninfectious damage.

Urinary Tract Infection and Perinephric/Intranephric Abscess

Uri S. Alon

KEY CONCEPTS

- Symptoms in infancy are nonspecific.
- Uncircumcised boys are at higher risk for urinary tract infection (UTI).
- Treatment of neonatal UTI is the same as for neonatal septicemia.
- Beyond early infancy, acute UTI in the nontoxic child can be empirically treated first with oral third-generation cephalosporins, if tolerated. In others, parenteral administration is indicated.
- The yield of routine urinary tract ultrasound in a child with acute UTI and normal prenatal ultrasound is minimal. Therefore, ultrasound in these children can be reserved for complicated cases.
- Cortical imaging studies during the acute infection have limited value but can assist in differentiating between lower tract and upper tract infection. The clinical importance of a small scar detected only by cortical imaging studies in follow-up studies is as yet unknown.
- Thirty percent to 35% of children with pyelonephritis have vesicoureteral reflux.
- A voiding cystourethrogram or a nuclear cystogram can be done either shortly after diagnosis or a few weeks later, in all young children and select older ones, provided the infection has been treated.
- In children younger than the age of 4 years with all grades of reflux and in older children with medium-high grade reflux, prophylactic antimicrobial treatment is indicated.
- Siblings of a child with vesicoureteral reflux have a 30% chance of having vesicoureteral reflux. Family counseling and imaging studies are based on the siblings' ages.

Urinary tract infection (UTI) occurs in children of all ages. During infancy, the male-to-female ratio is approximately 1:1, but in older age groups UTI becomes more prevalent in girls. Uncircumcised male infants are at higher risk for infection. Symptomatology varies with age. Symptoms are nonspecific in infancy and include irritability, fever, vomiting, poor feeding, diarrhea, failure to thrive, and jaundice. In older children symptoms depend on the location of the infection, namely whether it is in the upper or lower urinary tract. Pyelonephritis is characterized by fever, nausea, vomiting, chills, and abdominal and flank pain, whereas cystitis generally manifests with high urinary frequency, urgency, dysuria, hematuria, lower abdominal pain, foul-smelling urine, daytime and nighttime accidents in a child previously fully continent, and either no or low-grade temperature. In many patients with pyelonephritis an element of bladder infection exists as well.

The most common causative organism is *Escherichia coli*, followed by *Klebsiella*, *Enterobacter*, and *Enterococcus* species. Other bacteria are often associated with previous surgery, instrumentation, and anatomic and functional abnormalities of the urinary tract, or they occur in patients receiving antimicrobial prophylaxis. Yeast infections occur in immunocompromised patients and during or after treatment with antibiotics. Rarely, a viral etiology can be the cause of hemorrhagic cystitis, especially in boys. UTI is suspected when a dipstick detects white blood cells (WBCs), and nitrites, either alone or in combination, and urine microscopy demonstrates WBCs and bacteria. However, the definitive diagnosis should always be based on urine culture and colony count. The use of a urine bag in infants is appropriate to rule out an infection, but the presence of bacteria in a urine bag specimen requires an additional urine culture obtained by another method to establish diagnosis. Therefore, in the child in whom urgent antimicrobial treatment is indicated, urine culture should be obtained by methods other than a "bagged urine."

Expert Opinion on Management Issues

During the first 2 months of life UTIs should be treated according to the same guidelines as for septicemia, which is part of the clinical picture in many cases. During later infancy and early childhood all infections should be regarded as upper UTIs and treated with antibiotics for a period of 10 to 14 days (Table 1). In well-hydrated, nontoxic-appearing children, oral treatment, if tolerated, seems to be as effective as parenteral treatment. Otherwise, treatment should start as parenteral therapy and should be switched to oral medications once the child's condition improves. In most children temperature normalizes within 48 to 96 hours.

Until recently, recommendations for imaging studies in a child with a UTI included renal ultrasound and VCUG. However, recent studies have shown that in institutions in which prenatal ultrasound is done routinely, renal ultrasound has very minimal, if any, yield in modifying the treatment of the child with a UTI and history of normal prenatal ultrasound. This is because the vast majority of congenital obstructive uropathies are now diagnosed by prenatal ultrasound, as are some of the cases of high-grade vesicoureteral reflux (VUR). Therefore, in a child with a history of normal prenatal ultrasound it is reasonable to conduct renal ultrasound only if there is evidence of renal failure or inadequate response to antimicrobial therapy. Cortical scintigraphy studies are not routinely required but can assist in the differential diagnosis between lower and upper tract infection. The clinical relevance of small scars detected only by scintigraphy has not been yet proved; therefore, follow-up studies are not indicated. It is recommended to conduct a VCUG in all boys with UTI, girls younger than 4 years of age with first febrile UTI, and older girls with recurrent upper tract infections.

In most young children with VUR, management includes long-term prophylaxis with antimicrobial agents to minimize the risk of acquiring an infection (Table 2). In most cases, trimethoprim alone or in combination with sulfamethoxazole and nitrofurantoin are the agents of choice after age 2 months given as a single evening dose. Before that age a cephalosporin preparation should be used. In a minority of patients, surgical correction or endoscopic injection of dextranomer/hyaluronic acid copolymer is required. It seems very likely that with increasing experience with the latter procedure, more cases of VUR will be corrected by this same-day procedure.

In a girl with reflux grades I to III and with initial normal renal ultrasound, follow-up ultrasounds are of minimal yield and are not routinely needed. Based on the rate of spontaneous resolution of VUR, follow-up imaging studies of the lower urinary tract have to be conducted every 2 years in those with VUR grades I and II, and in children diagnosed younger than 2 years of age with unilateral grade III VUR. In all others, follow-up studies should be done only every 3 years. This minimizes exposure to this invasive procedure and its associated irradiation.

There seems to be no justification for routine periodic urine cultures in the asymptomatic child. However, a high index of suspicion for possible breakthrough infections should be maintained. In such a case an evaluation for possible urologic intervention is required, especially in the child with recurrent infections, evidence of parenchymal damage, noncompliance, and older age.

Lower UTIs occur mostly in school-age and adolescent girls. A course of 7 to 10 days of oral therapy is adequate (see Table 1). In some cases of recurrent infections, prophylactic antibiotics for a period of 6 to 12 months should be tried (see Table 2). In stubborn cases, rotating antibiotics using three agents,

TABLE 1 Antimicrobial Agents for Treatment of Urinary Tract Infection

Antimicrobial Agent	Daily Dosage and Intervals
IV	
Ampicillin*	100 mg/kg divided q8h
Gentamicin	<1 mo old, 3 mg/kg q24h
	>1 mo old, 5 mg/kg divided q8–12h
Third-generation cephalosporins	
Cefotaxime	150 mg/kg divided q6–8h
Ceftazidime	150 mg/kg divided q6–8h
Ceftriaxone	75 mg/kg divided q12–24h (also IM)
Oral	
Amoxicillin*	20–40 mg/kg, divided q8h
Amoxicillin–clavulanic acid	30–40 mg/kg amoxicillin divided q8–12h
Cefixime	8 mg/kg, divided q12–24h
Cefpodoxime	10 mg/kg, divided q12h
Cephalexin	25–50 mg/kg, divided q6h
Ciprofloxacin†	20–30 mg/kg divided q12h
Loracarbef	15–20 mg/kg, divided q12h
Nitrofurantoin‡	5–7 mg/kg, divided q6–8h
Sulfisoxazole§	120–150 mg/kg, divided q4–6h
Trimethoprim/ sulfamethoxazole§	6–12 mg/kg TMP, 30–60 mg/kg SMX, divided q12h

*Many *Escherichia coli* strains are resistant to Ampicillin/Amoxicillin. These antimicrobials can be used to treat gram-positive cocci or after results of the antibiogram are known.
†To be used in otherwise resistant organisms (mainly Pseudomonas).
‡Because of poor tissue penetration, some prefer not to use nitrofurantoin for acute upper tract infections.
§Should not be used for infants <2 months; poorly metabolized.
IM, intramuscularly; IV, intravenously; q*x*h, every *x* hours; SMX, sulfamethoxazole; TMP, trimethoprim.

TABLE 2 Antimicrobial Agents for Prevention of Recurrent Infections

Agent	Daily Dose
Nitrofurantoin	1–2 mg/kg
Trimethoprim/sulfamethoxazole*	1–2 mg/kg TMP, 5–10 mg/kg SMX
Trimethoprim	1–2 mg/kg
Cephalexin†	15 mg/kg divided q12h

*Should not be used for infants <2 months; poorly metabolized.
†For use in infants younger than 2 months of age.
q*x*h, every *x* hours; SMX, sulfamethoxazole; TMP, trimethoprim.

each given for 1 week, or a combination of two daily prophylactic antibiotics can alleviate the problem. It is recommended to give the protective antibiotics at bedtime. It is of crucial importance to correct constipation and abnormal voiding patterns.

RENAL ABSCESS

Most renal abscesses occur at the corticomedullary junction and are secondary to an ascending infection; that is, they have the same etiology of pyelonephritis and are mainly caused by gram-negative bacilli (*E. coli*, *Klebsiella*, *Proteus*). Renal cortical abscesses are usually the result of hematogenous spread and are most commonly caused by *Staphylococcus aureus*. Perinephric abscess may be caused by hematogenous spread or as an extension of intrarenal abscess. The etiologic agents are gram-positive cocci or gram-negative bacilli and at times a mixture of organisms including yeast.

The symptomatology of perinephric and intrarenal abscess is similar to that of acute pyelonephritis, and abscess should be suspected in a patient who fails to respond to 4 to 5 days of antimicrobial therapy. Urinalysis shows findings similar to those of pyelonephritis but may be normal, especially in the case of cortical abscess. Renal sonogram and, even more so, CT are the imaging studies of choice to establish diagnosis.

In general, an intravenous (IV) third-generation cephalosporin or a combination of nafcillin plus gentamicin can be used as initial treatment. Naturally, if an organism is isolated and its susceptibilities are known, the antimicrobial treatment should be appropriately adjusted. Based on the patient's response, 10 to 14 days of IV treatment is needed followed by oral treatment to complete 4 weeks of therapy. In case of failure of the antimicrobial therapy to eradicate the infection, surgical intervention is indicated.

Common Pitfalls

- Failure to obtain a urine culture in a sterile fashion before starting antimicrobial therapy.
- Failure to adjust the antimicrobial therapy based on the causing organism's susceptibilities.
- Failure to appropriately address voiding dysfunction and constipation.
- Performance of invasive radiologic studies more frequently than required, thus exposing the child to potential trauma and irradiation.
- Because of a high rate of resistance to ampicillin among *E. coli* strains, ampicillin should not be used to empirically treat gram-negative infections or as long-term prophylaxis.
- Ruling out renal abscesses based on normal urinalysis and negative urine culture.

Communication and Counseling

Because approximately 30% of children who are siblings of the propositus with VUR may have VUR themselves, it is recommended to conduct a VCUG in siblings younger than 1 year of age. Between ages 1 and 5 years a normal renal ultrasound will generally exclude the need for VCUG, and after age 5 years a thorough medical history ruling out UTIs will suffice.

Parents need to be educated about the symptoms of UTI and the need to approach a health care facility as soon as possible when the child develops symptoms, to allow immediate evaluation and treatment.

SUGGESTED READINGS

1. Elder JS, Peters CA, Arant BS, et al: Pediatric vesicoureteral reflux guidelines panel summary report on the management of primary vesicoureteral reflux in children. J Urol 157:1846–1851, 1997. **Provides indications for medical versus surgical treatment of VUR and the rate of spontaneous resolution of VUR over time.**
2. Hoberman A, Wald ER, Hickey RW, et al: Oral versus initial intravenous therapy for urinary tract infections in young febrile children. Pediatrics 104:79–86, 1999. **Demonstrates the ability to successfully treat orally infants older than the age of 2 months with febrile UTI.**
3. Hoberman A, Charron M, Hickey RW, et al: Imaging studies after a first febrile urinary tract infection in young children. N Engl J Med 348:195–202, 2003. **Demonstrates the lack of influence of urinary tract ultrasound on management of children with newly diagnosed UTI.**
4. Kirsch AJ, Perez-Brayfield MR, Scherz HC: Minimally invasive treatment of vesicoureteral reflux and endoscopic injection of dextranomer/hyaluronic acid copolymer: The Children's Hospitals of Atlanta experience. J Urol 170:211–215, 2003. **Details the endoscopic procedure to correct VUR.**
5. Koff SA, Wagner TT, Jayanthi VR: The relationship among dysfunctional elimination syndromes, primary vesicoureteral reflux and urinary tract infections in children. J Urol 160:1019–1022, 1998. **Indicates the importance of successful treatment of dysfunctional elimination in the management of the child with UTI and VUR.**
6. Lowe LH, Patel MN, Gatti JM, et al: Utility of follow-up renal sonography in children with vesicoureteral reflux and normal initial sonogram. Pediatr 113:548–550, 2004. **Normal initial sonogram excludes the need for follow-up sonogram in girls with VUR grades I to III.**
7. Thompson M, Simon SD, Sharma V, Alon US: Timing of follow-up voiding cystourethrogram in children with primary vesicoureteral reflux: Development and application of a clinical algorithm. Pediatrics 115:426–434, 2005. **Follow-up VCUG is recommended every 2 years in children with low-grade VUR and every 3 years in those with medium-high grade reflux.**
8. Zamir G, Sakran W, Horowitz Y, et al: Urinary tract infection: is there a need for routine renal ultrasonography? Arch Dis Child 89:466–468, 2004. **Routine urinary tract ultrasound in children with newly diagnosed UTI seldom contributes to their management.**

Hemolytic Uremic Syndrome

Sharon Phillips Andreoli

KEY CONCEPTS

- Hemolytic uremic syndrome (HUS) is the most common form of acute renal failure in children.
- Diarrhea-associated HUS (D+ HUS) is the most common cause of this syndrome of microangiopathic hemolytic anemia, thrombocytopenia, and renal parenchymal disease.

- The major therapy is supportive, including acute dialysis and nutritional support.
- Long-term sequelae are common, and children who had full-blown HUS must be followed indefinitely.

The hemolytic uremic syndrome (HUS) is a common cause of acute renal failure in children and leads to significant morbidity and 2% to 5% mortality during the acute phase of the disease. In addition, some children with HUS develop late complications, including proteinuria, hypertension, and renal insufficiency, several years after the acute phase of the illness. The classic clinical features of HUS include the triad of microangiopathic hemolytic anemia, thrombocytopenia, and acute renal failure. However, epidemiologic studies in outbreaks of hemorrhagic colitis and diarrhea-positive HUS clearly show that some patients develop hemolytic anemia and/or thrombocytopenia with little evidence of renal involvement, and other children develop substantial renal disease with a normal platelet count and/or minimal hemolysis. HUS is classified as the epidemic diarrhea-positive HUS (typical, D+ HUS) or diarrhea-negative HUS (atypical, D− HUS) (Box 1). Atypical HUS may be familial and associated with mutations in factor H or associated with medications such as cyclosporine or birth control pills. D+ HUS, the focus of this chapter, is much more common than atypical HUS.

D+ HUS is strongly associated with infection with Shiga toxin–producing *Escherichia coli* that results in hemorrhagic colitis. In the past, the most common vector for transmission of Shiga toxin–producing *E. coli* was undercooked hamburger, but apple juice, radish sprouts, sausages, and other food sources are implicated in the spread of Shiga toxin–producing *E. coli* infections. Person-to-person contact is also an important mode of transmission of Shiga toxin–producing *E. coli* infections. In the United States and Europe, the O157:H7 *E. coli* serotype is the most common Shiga toxin–producing organism involved, but in other areas of the world non-O157:H7 strains are emerging as important pathogens. Two Shiga toxins (also called verotoxins, verocytotoxins (VTs), or Shiga-like toxins

(SLTs) are produced by *E. coli,* including Shiga toxin-1 and Shiga toxin-2. *E. coli* O157:H7 strains isolated from patients with HUS usually produce both ST-1 and ST-2 or only ST-2. Strains that produce only ST-1 are unusual. Once a person is infected with Shiga toxin–producing *E. coli,* the percentage of patients who progress to HUS ranges from approximately 5% to 15%. In children younger than 5 years of age, the attack rate of hemolytic anemia or HUS is 12.9% compared to an attack rate of 6.8% and 8% for children 5 to 9.9 years of age and older than 10 years, respectively. In addition, children with a white blood cell count greater than 13,000 per mm^3 during the initial 3 days of illness with Shiga toxin–producing *E. coli* infection had a sevenfold increase in the risk of developing HUS as compared to age-matched children with a white blood cell count less than 13,000 per mm^3. When HUS develops, the affected child usually appears pale and lethargic at the time the diarrhea is subsiding. Irritability is very common, and some children may also develop petechiae due to the thrombocytopenia. HUS is diagnosed with a triad of findings of microangiopathic (nonimmune) hemolytic anemia, thrombocytopenia, and renal disease (hematuria, proteinuria with or without azotemia) following a gastrointestinal illness that frequently includes bloody diarrhea.

Expert Opinion on Management Issues

The majority of children with HUS develop some degree of renal insufficiency, and approximately two thirds of children with HUS require dialytic therapy. Approximately a third have milder renal involvement without the need for dialysis. Thus the management of HUS encompasses the usual management of children with acute renal failure with additional management issues specific to HUS.

MANAGEMENT OF ACUTE RENAL FAILURE

General management of acute renal failure includes appropriate fluid and electrolyte management, antihypertensive therapy if the child demonstrates hypertension, and initiation of renal replacement therapy when appropriate. The Suggested Readings offer specific detailed management of the child with acute renal failure. This section highlights emergent management of hyperkalemia and hypertension, which can be life-threatening when severe.

Therapy of hyperkalemia is indicated if cardiac conduction abnormalities are noted or if the potassium level is greater than 6 to 7 mEq per L. Table 1 summarizes the therapy of hyperkalemia. Sodium bicarbonate (0.5 to 1.0 mEq/kg/dose) transfers potassium into cells, but this therapy may precipitate seizures and tetany if the serum calcium level is low, resulting in a decreased ionized calcium level. Intravenous glucose and insulin also transfer potassium from the extracellular to the intracellular compartment. Intravenous calcium gluconate increases the threshold

---

BOX 1 Classification of the Hemolytic Uremic Syndrome in Children

- Diarrhea-positive (typical) hemolytic uremic syndrome (D+ HUS)
  - Shiga toxin–producing *E. coli* infection
  - Shiga toxin–producing *Shigella dysenteriae* infection
- Diarrhea-negative (atypical) hemolytic uremic syndrome (D− HUS)
  - Genetic HUS
  - Factor H abnormalities
  - Von Willebrand factor abnormalities
  - Drug-induced HUS
  - Infectious HUS
  - Human immunodeficiency virus (HIV) infection
  - Streptococcus pneumonia–associated HUS
  - Post–bone marrow transplant
  - Associated with systemic lupus erythematosus

TABLE 1 Treatment of Hyperkalemia

Agent	Mechanism	Dose	Onset	Complications
Sodium bicarbonate	Shifts K^+ into cells	0.5–1 mEq/kg IV over 10–30 min	15–30 min	Hypernatremia, change in ionized calcium
Calcium gluconate (10%)	Stabilizes membrane potential	0.5–1 mL/kg IV (10%) over 5–15 min	Immediate	Bradycardia, arrhythmias, hypercalcemia
Glucose and insulin	Stimulates cellular uptake of K^+	Glucose: 0.5 g/kg; insulin: 0.1 U/kg IV over 30 min	30–120 min	Hypoglycemia
β-Agonists (albuterol)	Stimulates cellular uptake of K^+	5- to 10-mg nebulizer (adult dose)	30 min	Tachycardia, hypertension
Sodium polystyrene sulfonate (Kayexalate)	Exchanges Na^+ for K^+ across the colonic mucosa	1 g/kg PO or PR in sorbitol	30–60 min	Hypernatremia, constipation

IV, intravenous, K, potassium; Na, sodium; PO, by mouth; PR, by rectum.

potential of the excitable myocardial cells and counteracts the depolarizing effect of the hyperkalemia. The β-agonist albuterol given as a nebulizer acutely lowers the serum potassium level by stimulating intracellular uptake of potassium. Each of the preceding are temporizing measures and do not remove potassium from the body. Kayexalate given orally, per nasogastric tube or per rectum, exchanges sodium for potassium in the gastrointestinal tract and results in potassium removal. Complications of Kayexalate therapy include possible hypernatremia, sodium retention, and constipation. Depending on the degree of hyperkalemia and the need for correction of other metabolic derangements in acute renal failure, hyperkalemia frequently requires the initiation of dialysis or hemofiltration.

Hypertension in acute renal failure is commonly related to volume overload and/or to alterations in vascular tone. If hypertension is related to volume overload, appropriate fluid removal with dialysis or hemofiltration is necessary if the patient has not responded to diuretic therapy. Depending on the degree of blood pressure elevation and the etiology of the hypertension, antihypertensive therapy may also be indicated. The choice of antihypertensive therapy depends on the degree of blood pressure elevation and the presence of central nervous system (CNS) symptoms of hypertension. For the child with acute renal failure who has severe hypertension and/or is encephalopathic, intravenous therapy with sodium nitroprusside (beginning dose, 0.5 to 1.0 µg/kg/minute), labetalol (0.5 to 3.0 mg/kg/hour), or intravenous nicardipine (1 to 3 µg/kg/min) is indicated to lower the blood pressure acutely. Intravenous hydralazine or sublingual nifedipine can be used for less severe hypertension.

Acidosis, calcium, and phosphorus balance, sodium balance, and nutritional support are other aspects of acute renal failure in children with HUS that require specific attention. Continued oligoanuria with an increasing blood urea nitrogen (BUN) and creatinine and significant electrolyte abnormalities suggests the child is likely to require renal replacement therapy and consultation with a pediatric nephrologist is appropriate.

MANAGEMENT ISSUES SPECIFIC TO ACUTE RENAL FAILURE ASSOCIATED WITH HUS

Issues specific to HUS include management of the hematologic complication of HUS, monitoring for extrarenal involvement in HUS, avoiding antidiarrheal drugs, and possibly avoiding antibiotic therapy. Management of the hematologic complications of HUS, including hemolytic anemia and thrombocytopenia, should involve frequent laboratory studies to include hemoglobin and hematocrit determination on a frequent schedule because children may become quite anemic due to rapid hemolysis. In addition, jaundice, characterized by an increase in indirect bilirubin, may develop as a result of the hemolytic process. Transfusion with packed red blood cells is needed when the hemoglobin is falling rapidly and/or when the hemoglobin reaches 7 to 8 g/dL. Children should be transfused with packed red blood cells over a 2- to 4-hour interval with diuretic therapy as indicated if there is evidence of volume overload. Careful monitoring of blood pressure, urine output, and respiratory status are important to assure that the child does not develop pulmonary edema.

Thrombocytopenia can be profound, and it is tempting to transfuse platelets in the thrombocytopenic child, but platelet transfusions are usually limited to the child in need of a surgical procedure or the child with active bleeding. The rationale for limited platelet transfusions is that platelet transfusions can add further "fuel to the fire" of microthrombi formation, which is thought to result in organ damage. Because microthrombi form during the course of HUS in multiple organs including the kidney, CNS, colon, pancreas, skeletal muscle, myocardium, and other organs, accelerated deposition of microthrombi may occur following platelet transfusions and promote tissue injury. The intravascular volume of the child needs to be considered when a transfusion is indicated because many children with acute renal failure caused by HUS are oliguric and at risk for fluid overload and pulmonary edema. As described earlier, in red blood cell transfusion, attention to fluid status, blood pressure, and respiratory status is important to avoid pulmonary edema.

The kidney and the gastrointestinal tract are the organs most commonly affected in HUS, but other organs are also affected in a substantial number of children. CNS involvement may be manifested as irritability, seizures, obtundation, and/or coma. In some patients, pancreatitis with or without glucose intolerance develops during the acute phase of the disease, and skeletal and myocardial involvement may also be present. It is very important to evaluate the presence and extent of extrarenal involvement because these extrarenal complications of HUS are what contribute to the disease's mortality. Children do not die of renal failure, provided that dialysis is available when needed, but they do die of multiorgan disease that can occur during the course of HUS. In children with HUS, the physical examination and appropriate laboratory studies are needed to monitor for the development of extrarenal manifestations. Neurologic examination screens (for CNS involvement) and radiographic imaging are needed in patients with symptoms including combativeness, irritability, seizures, and decreased level of consciousness. In addition to monitoring the level of renal function, hemoglobin, hematocrit, and platelet count as described earlier, amylase, lipase, glucose, and liver function studies should be performed during the acute phase of the disease.

In children with hemorrhagic colitis caused by Shiga toxin–producing E. coli infection, the use of antimotility agents is associated with a greater risk for the development of HUS. Thus antidiarrheal agents are usually avoided in children with HUS because it is thought they contribute to retention of Shiga toxin within the colon that could enhance absorption of the toxin. The use of antibiotics is also associated with the development of HUS in children with Shiga toxin–producing E. coli hemorrhagic colitis in some studies but not all studies. In vitro studies show that some antibiotics promote production and release of Shiga toxin from E. coli. Currently there is not a consensus on the use of antibiotic therapy in children with hemorrhagic colitis or HUS; however, antibiotics are not usually prescribed in children with HUS until there are specific indications for antibiotic therapy.

Technical advances in dialysis therapy and improved care of the critically ill child has resulted in a significant reduction of mortality caused by acute HUS, so chronic complications in long-term survivors are becoming more apparent. A few children never recover renal function and require long-term renal replacement therapy; those who recover are at risk for the late development of renal disease including the development of proteinuria, hypertension, and possible renal insufficiency several years after the acute episode of HUS. Thus, children who have apparently recovered from HUS need long-term follow-up including a yearly urinalysis and random urine for protein creatinine ratio to evaluate for proteinuria, a blood pressure determination, and a serum creatinine and BUN determination to evaluate renal function.

CONTROVERSIAL INTERVENTIONS IN HUS

Some investigators propose a role of plasmapheresis and/or plasma exchange in typical D+ HUS. Although clearly indicated in some children with atypical HUS (diarrhea negative), a role for plasmapheresis and/or plasma exchange is not proven to be beneficial and may be potentially detrimental in children with D+ HUS.

Common Pitfalls

- Continued hydration of the child who has established renal failure
- Transfusion of platelets when not clinically indicated
- Transfusion of red blood cells without attention to fluid status
- Administration of antimotility agents
- Possibly the administration of antibiotics without clinical indications

Communication and Counseling

Several well-publicized outbreaks of hemorrhagic colitis and HUS have highlighted the morbidity and mortality of HUS associated with Shiga toxin–producing E. coli infections. An outbreak in the western United States associated with consumption of hamburgers resulted in several cases of severe HUS with a high incidence of extrarenal complications. Other well-publicized outbreaks are associated with consumption of apple juice or visiting a petting zoo or state fair. Thus the parents of a child with a diagnosis of "E. coli infection" are likely to have preconceived concepts of severe disease and death. It is important to emphasize to parents that the evolution of hemorrhagic colitis associated with Shiga toxin–producing E. coli occurs in approximately 10% of cases, and if a child develops HUS, the majority recover renal function and do not have residual renal damage. However, long-term follow-up is indicated in all children with HUS because of the potential late complications, including proteinuria, hypertension, and renal insufficiency that can occur several years after the acute episode of HUS.

SUGGESTED READINGS

1. Andreoli SP: Pancreatic involvement in the hemolytic uremic syndrome. In: Kaplan BS, Trompeter R, Moak J (eds): The Hemolytic Uremic Syndrome: Thrombotic Thrombocytopenia Purpura. New York: Marcel Dekker, 1992, pp 131–141. **Discusses pancreatic involvement in HUS.**
2. Andreoli SP: The pathophysiology of the hemolytic uremic syndrome. Curr Opin Nephrol Hypertens 8:459–464, 1999. **Review of the pathophysiology of HUS.**
3. Andreoli SP: Acute and chronic renal failure in children. In Gearhart JP, Rink RC, Mouriquand PDE (eds): Pediatric Urology. Philadelphia: WB Saunders, 2001, pp 777–789. **Review of the management of acute renal failure in children.**
4. Andreoli SP: Acute renal failure: Clinical evaluation management: In Avner ED, Harmon WE, Niaudet P (eds): Pediatric Nephrology, 5th ed. Baltimore: Lippincott Williams and Wilkins, 2004, pp 1233–1254. **Discusses pancreatic involvement in HUS.**

5. Andreoli SP, Bergstein JM: Development of insulin dependent diabetes mellitus during the hemolytic uremic syndrome. J Pediatr 100:541–545, 1982. **Discusses pancreatic involvement in HUS.**
6. Boyce TG, Swerdlow DL, Griffin PM: Escherichia coli O157:H7 and the hemolytic-uremic syndrome. N Engl J Med 33:364–368, 1995. **Review of epidemiology of HUS.**
7. Brandt JR, Fouser LS, Watkins SL, et al: Escherichia coli O157: H7–associated hemolytic-uremic syndrome after ingestion of contaminated hamburgers. J Pediatr 125:519–526, 1994. **Describes one of the largest recent outbreaks.**
8. Cody SH, Glynn K, Farrar JA, et al: An outbreak of Escherichia coli O157:H7 infection from unpasteurized commercial apple juice. Ann Intern Med 130:202–209, 1999. **Describes an epidemic of HUS.**
9. Repetto HA: Epidemic hemolytic uremic syndrome in children. Kidney Int 52:1708–1719, 1997.
10. Rizzoni G, Claris A, Edefonti A, et al: Plasma infusion for hemolytic uremic syndrome in children: Results of a multicenter controlled trial. J Pediatr 112:284–290, 1988. **Study about plasma infusion.**
11. Rowe PC, Orbine E, Wells GA, et al: Risk of hemolytic uremic syndrome after sporadic Escherichia coli O157:H7 infection: Results of a Canadian collaborative study. J Pediatr 132:777–782, 1998. **Discusses risk of developing HUS with E. coli O157:H7 infection.**
12. Safdar N, Said A, Gangnon RE, Maki DG: Risk of hemolytic uremic syndrome after antibiotic treatment of Escherichia coli O157:H7 enteritis: A meta-analysis. JAMA 288:996–1001, 2002. **Article with data about whether risk of developing HUS changes after antibiotic therapy.**
13. Siegler RL, Milligan MK, Burningham TH, et al: Long-term outcome and prognostic indicators in the hemolytic uremic syndrome. J Pediatr 118:195–200, 1991. **Long-term data.**
14. Spizzirri FD, Rahman RC, Bibiloni H, et al: Childhood hemolytic uremic syndrome in Argentina: Long-term follow-up and prognostic features. Pediatr Nephrol 11:156–160, 1997. **Long-term follow-up from a geographic area with high incidence.**
15. Su C, Brandt LJ: Escherichia coli O157:H7 infection in humans. Ann Intern Med 123:698–714, 1995. **Summary of the role of this strain of E. coli in HUS.**
16. Wong CS, Jelacic S, Habeeb RL, et al: The risk of hemolytic uremic syndrome after antibiotic treatment of Escherichia coli O157:H7 infections. New Engl J Med 342:1930–1936, 2000. **Article with data about whether risk of developing HUS changes after antibiotic therapy.**

Nephrolithiasis

Amy Eldridge Bobrowski and Craig B. Langman

KEY CONCEPTS

- The most commonly formed stones in children and adults are composed of calcium salts and are, therefore, radiopaque.
- Normal excretion levels of lithogenic or lithoprotective substances are provided in Table 1.
- Hypercalciuria is the most common cause of calcium-based nephrolithiasis.
- Familial idiopathic hypercalciuria (FIH) is its most common subset and is inherited in an autosomal dominant fashion but with incomplete penetrance.
- Several genetic forms of hypercalciuria are also important causes of stones.
- Urinary tract infections with urease-producing organisms such as *Proteus* species, *Providencia* species, *Klebsiella* species, *Pseudomonas* species, and various

Enterococci species are associated with struvite stones (magnesium ammonium phosphate or carbonate apatite).
- Hyperuricosuria is a rarer cause of stones or hematuria in children compared to those composed of calcium salts.
- Hyperoxaluria may be primary or secondary, and lead to stone disease in either circumstance.
- Cystinuria, an autosomal recessive disease of disordered dibasic amino acid transported in the kidney and gastrointestinal tract, is present in 3% to 10% of children with kidney stones.
- Hypocitraturia is another contributory cause of nephrolithiasis, as citrate is needed to form a soluble calcium salt, preventing calcium oxalate stone formation.
- Stones are common in patients with cystic fibrosis who are undergoing therapeutic use of protease inhibitors or a ketogenic diet and who have had bladder augmentation with defunctionalized intestinal segments.

Nephrolithiasis (kidney stones) occurs when urinary crystals aggregate together with a protein matrix within the urinary tract. Stones come to clinical attention, generally, from obstruction of urinary flow, from stone movement, or from irritation locally at the site of the stone. In children, kidney stones affect males and females equally. They are responsible for from 1 in 1000 to 1 in 7600 pediatric hospital admissions, and are most common in white children. Kidney stones reflect a deviation from the balance between stone-promoting and -inhibiting factors, in favor of the former. In general, higher urinary pH (except in struvite stones, which form in alkaline urine), higher urine volume and dilution, higher urinary citrate, and free flow of urine serve as natural inhibitors of stone formation.

Urinary tract stones may manifest with abdominal, flank, or pelvic pain in about 50% of children with nephrolithiasis, less often than occurs in adults with stones. Gross or microscopic hematuria (occurring in 33% to 90% of affected children) and urinary tract infections (UTIs) are additional common presenting signs in younger patients. Stone disease can be difficult to treat and is often recurrent, and a complete evaluation is one key to success for its eradication.

Calcium-Containing Stones

Sodium salts compose the most commonly formed stones in children and adults, and are, therefore, radiopaque. Table 1 provides information on normal

TABLE 1 Normative Data for Excretion of Selected Lithogenic Substances and Stone Inhibitors

Substance	Reference Range
Calcium	≤ 4 mg/kg/day for children ≥ 2 yr of age
Citrate	≥ 0.4 mg/m^2 BSA/day
Oxalate	≤ 0.5 mmol/m^2/day
Uric acid	Varies with age, up to a maximum of 750 mg/day in adolescence

BSA, body surface area.

excretion levels of lithogenic or lithoprotective substances. Hypercalciuria is the most common cause of calcium-based nephrolithiasis. Familial idiopathic hypercalciuria (FIH), inherited in an autosomal dominant fashion but with incomplete penetrance, is most common. The pathophysiology of FIH is ill-defined in children, and may occur from excessive action of 1,25-dihydroxy-vitamin D in increasing dietary calcium absorption in the gastrointestinal (GI) tract, or from a primary kidney tubular reduction in calcium resorption, or from elements of both processes in an individual patient.

Less common than FIH are several genetic forms of hypercalciuria (listed in Table 2):

- Dent disease (X-linked recessive nephrolithiasis with renal failure, linked to mutations in the *CLCN5* gene that transduces a voltage-gated chloride channel in the kidney)
- Bartter syndrome (nephrolithiasis and/or nephrocalcinosis with one of a series of mutations of genes in the thick ascending limb of the loop of Henle, including *NKCC2* that transduces the Na-K-2Cl transporter, *ROMK* for the K channel, or *CLCNKB* for the chloride channel)
- Distal renal tubular acidosis (growth retardation, metabolic acidosis, nephrocalcinosis, and reduced urinary citrate, associated with deafness in a hereditary disease, with a mutation in the *ATP6B1* gene transducing a vacuolar H^+-ATPase)
- Pseudohypoaldosteronism type II (hypertension, hyperkalemia, and metabolic acidosis linked with mutations in WNK kinases in the distal nephron)
- Hypomagnesemia-hypercalciuria
- Iatrogenic (e.g., loop diuretics, prednisone, adrenocorticotropic hormones)

TABLE 2 Hypercalciuric Conditions Associated with Kidney Stones

Associated with Hypercalcemia	Associated with Normal Serum Calcium
Primary hyperparathyroidism	Familial idiopathic hypercalciuria
Sarcoidosis	Mutations in the kidney chloride channel gene *CLCN5*
Idiopathic infantile hypercalcemia	Familial hypomagnesemia with hypercalciuria and nephrocalcinosis (*PLCN–1* mutation for tight junction protein paracellin–1)
Immobilization	Immobilization
Bartter syndrome	Prematurity, often associated with furosemide therapy
Seibert syndrome	Distal renal tubular acidosis
Thyrotoxicosis	Type I glycogen storage disease
	X-linked hypophosphatemic rickets
	Ketogenic diet
	Activating mutation of the extracellular calcium-sensing gene (generally associated with hypocalcemia)
	Medullary sponge disease
	Inflammatory diseases (e.g., JRA)
	Corticosteroid therapy

JRA, juvenile rheumatoid arthritis.

Infection Stones

Urinary tract infections (UTIs) with urease-producing organisms such as *Proteus* species, *Providencia* species, *Klebsiella* species, *Pseudomonas* species, and various *Enterococci* species are associated with struvite stones (magnesium ammonium phosphate or carbonate apatite). These stones tend to branch out as they enlarge, forming a radiographic staghorn appearance through the kidney-collecting systems.

Uric Acid Stones

Hyperuricosuria is a rarer cause of stones or hematuria in children as compared to those composed of calcium salts. It can occur from causes of hyperuricemia that are secondary to other processes or, more rarely, as a primary abnormality in uric acid metabolism. Some secondary causes include excessive purine intake, gout, intense hemolysis, myeloproliferative disorders, and/or their treatment with irradiation or cytotoxic therapy, and cyanotic congenital heart disease. Lesch-Nyhan syndrome and type I glycogen storage disease are also associated with increased urate production and secondary hyperuricosuria. Increased urate excretion from proximal tubular defects or chronic metabolic acidosis may produce hyperuricosuria. Xanthine kidney stones are formed in an autosomal recessive disorder of mutations in the gene for xanthine dehydrogenase, alone or with an aldehyde oxidase gene mutation. In this condition, uric acid cannot be formed from xanthine precursors and the result may be urinary obstruction.

Hyperoxaluria

Hyperoxaluria (Table 3) may be primary or secondary and leads to stone disease in either circumstance. Secondary causes include enteric oxaluria resulting from increased colon absorption secondary to small bowel malabsorption of fatty and bile acids that increase colonic permeability to oxalate, or more rarely, pyridoxine deficiency (a cofactor in oxalate metabolism), excessive intake of oxalate precursors such as with massive quantities of ascorbic acid or small ingestions of less than 10 mL of ethylene glycol.

Primary causes of hyperoxaluria include the diseases of primary hyperoxaluria type I (PH–1), which is caused by mutations in the alanine glyoxylate aminotransferase gene that transduces the enzyme alanine glyoxylate aminotransferase, and leads to metabolic overproduction of oxalate. The most common mutation (Gly170Arg), coupled with a minor allele polymorphism (P11L), results in the mistargeting of the enzyme from the liver peroxisome into the liver mitochondria. This leads to an inability to metabolize glyoxylate into alanine, and thus shunts glyoxylate to oxalate by other metabolic pathways, instead. Other alanine glyoxylate aminotransferase gene mutations may produce intracellular protein aggregation of alanine glyoxylate aminotransferase, and consequent loss

TABLE 3 Causes of Hyperoxaluria

Primary Overproduction of Oxalate	Secondary Overproduction of Oxalate	Enteric Overabsorption
Primary hyperoxaluria	Ethylene glycol poisoning	Increased serum bile acids
Alanine glyoxylate aminotransferase mutation: I	Vitamin C excess	Inflammatory bowel disease
GR/HPR mutation: II	Pyridoxine deficiency	Dietary oxalate excess
Atypical (gene mutation unknown)		Dietary calcium deficiency
		Small-bowel resection

GR/HPR, glyoxylate/hydroxypyruvate reductase.

of enzyme activity, or prevent vitamin B_6 cofactor binding, needed for optimal alanine glyoxylate aminotransferase activity.

Primary hyperoxaluria type 2 is caused by a mutation in the glyoxylate reductase-hydroxypyruvate reductase gene, and generally has a milder course than that seen in patients with PH–1. *Oxalosis* is a term used to describe the clinical situation in which primary hyperoxaluria leads to calcium oxalate precipitation in multiple organs and joints, impairing renal function secondary to tubulointerstitial nephropathy, in addition to formation of kidney stones. Unfortunately, approximately 30% of patients at any age from childhood through adult life, with primary hyperoxaluria, are diagnosed only after presenting with end-stage kidney disease from oxalosis.

Cystinuria

Cystinuria is present in 3% to 10% of children with kidney stones and is an autosomal recessive disease of disordered dibasic amino acid transport in the kidney and gastrointestinal tract. Affected children have elevated urinary ornithine, arginine, and lysine urinary excretions in addition to cystine, as these amino acids share common transporter mechanisms. Distinct mutations in one of several cystine transport proteins have been demonstrated, but they do not correlate with differences in stone formation rates or recurrence rates or segregate with patient gender.

Hypocitraturia

Hypocitraturia is another contributory cause of nephrolithiasis, as citrate is needed to form a soluble calcium salt, preventing calcium oxalate stone formation. It is seen most commonly in renal tubular acidosis and in a small subset of children with familial idiopathic hypercalciuria.

Systemic Diseases and Stones

Additional clinical situations wherein kidney stones may occur include patients with cystic fibrosis (hyperoxaluria, hypercalciuria, hypocitraturia, and absence of an oxalate-degrading bacterium, *Oxalobacter formigenes*),

in patients undergoing therapeutic use of protease inhibitors (especially indinavir, a poorly soluble drug with a high urine excretion favoring crystallization in the urine), in patients undergoing therapeutic use of a ketogenic diet (hypercalciuria, hypocitraturia), and in patients after bladder augmentation with defunctionalized intestinal segments (struvite stones).

Expert Opinion on Management Issues

DIAGNOSIS

A detailed history and physical should guide evaluation of kidney stones. Family history should focus on members with kidney stones, gout, arthritis, or chronic kidney disease. The presence of a concomitant UTI must be sought, but not accepted as the cause of the stone, and patients should be advised to submit any passed stones or stone fragments for analysis. The structure of stones may be elucidated by polarization microscopy or x-ray diffraction, but not by simple chemical composition studies.

Useful imaging studies may include plain abdominal x-ray films, ultrasonography, and helical CT. Conventional abdominal radiographs may reveal radiopaque but not radiolucent stones, although ultrasound of the urinary tract may demonstrate both radiolucent and radiopaque stones, in addition to the presence of urinary obstruction or nephrocalcinosis. Ultrasound has largely taken the place of intravenous pyelography (IVP) as an initial study for detecting stones, secondary to concerns about radiation and contrast exposure with the latter procedure. Noncontrast helical CT has been found to have high sensitivity and specificity in identifying even small stones without requiring intravenous contrast administration. It may precisely localize stones, and detect obstruction and hydronephrosis.

More than 80% of children with stones have a metabolic problem that is discoverable and generally amenable to therapy. Diagnostic urinary and blood tests for stone evaluation should be obtained although the patient is having a routine activity schedule and diet, and if possible, is free of concurrent UTI. At least two 24-hour urine collections should be performed, and our practice is to wait at least 2 weeks after any acute stone event so that the patient is on his or her usual diet and activity. These collections can assess urinary volume as a reflection of fluid intake, creatinine excretion for completeness of the 24-hour collection (minimum, 10 to 15 mg/kg/day in children older than 2 years; 6 to 9 mg/kg/day younger than 2 years), and measurement of levels of lithogenic substances such as calcium, oxalate, uric acid, and cystine. The collections can evaluate the urine for decreased stone inhibitor levels such as citrate and magnesium. In the blood, levels of uric acid, potassium, calcium, phosphorus, creatinine, bicarbonate (total CO_2), (and biointact parathyroid hormone levels in the blood if hypercalcemia is present) should be obtained as well at the end of the urinary collections.

Consultation with an expert in pediatric stone disorders is encouraged if questions arise about the results of these diagnostic studies.

MEDICAL TREATMENT

See Table 4 for commonly used pharmacologic agents in the care of nephrolithiasis in children.

For all types of stones, increased fluid intake is beneficial, through provision of an increase in urinary volume and urinary dilution, and perhaps by inducing stone particle motion through the urinary tract. All of these factors are nonspecific but act to inhibit stone formation slightly.

Hypercalciuria

Hypercalciuria may be treated with a low-sodium diet, thiazide diuretics, and adequate potassium intake. Thiazide therapy (e.g., hydrochlorothiazide 1 mg/kg/day, maximum of 25 mg per day) in FIH significantly decreases urinary calcium excretion and rate of stone formation in adults, as shown in a study of 175 affected patients by Ohkawa and associates in 1992. A 1998 study by Reusz and colleagues also showed a decrease in urinary calcium excretion with thiazide treatment in 18 children with FIH. In a different population, with hypercalciuria from immobilization, Bentur, Alon, and Berant studied a population of 42 chronically bedridden children in 1987, of whom 18 were hypercalciuric and had a higher rate of fractures. A 3-week course of hydrochlorothiazide plus amiloride in those patients reduced the mean urinary calcium-to-creatinine ratio by 57.7%, although the investigators did not correlate these values with the gold standard of 24-hour urinary data. Dietary calcium intake should not be limited. Citrate therapy (e.g., potassium citrate 2 mmol/kg once daily) is also appropriate in cases of documented hypocitraturia.

Struvite

Struvite stones are treated by prevention of urinary infections, with the possible addition of a urease inhibitor such as acetohydroxamic acid (AHA). AHA has been shown to interfere with the molecular growth of crystals in vitro and also to have clinical benefit in studies of adults with infection-induced urinary calculi. Data in children are lacking.

Hyperuricosuria

Hyperuricosuria may be treated with dietary sodium limitation, oral bicarbonate, or citrate supplementation, or addition of allopurinol if increased uric acid production and hyperuricemia are present.

Hyperoxaluria

All patients with suspected primary hyperoxaluria should be given a therapeutic course of vitamin B_6 (pyridoxine), and urinary oxalate levels used to monitor success or to suggest the need for dose escalation. For patients with reduced kidney function, intensive dialysis followed by liver/kidney transplant can be curative, as a new liver replaces the enzymatic defect in PH–1. Pretransplant hemodialysis for 5 to 6 times per week, and perhaps with additional nightly peritoneal dialysis, is needed to lessen the systemic oxalate burden and prevent recurrence of disease in the transplant kidney. Prompt referral to a pediatric center with expertise in this disorder is suggested (consult the web site of the Hyperoxaluria and Oxalosis Foundation, www.ohf.org, for up-to-date information about these disorders).

Secondary hyperoxaluria that results from enteric hyperoxaluria may be treated with a low-sodium/low-fat diet, high fluid intake, dietary calcium intake at the upper end of the daily recommended intake (DRI), and with limitation of oxalate-containing foods (nuts, pepper, chocolate, rhubarb, spinach [see www.ohf.org for a more complete listing of foodstuffs and oxalate content]), and possible supplementation with magnesium, phosphorus, and citrate salts. The addition of oral calcium leads to a complex salt with the excess oxalate that is present in the gastrointestinal tract, thereby limiting its absorption.

Cystinuria

Cystine stone disease is treated with fluids (minimum of 3 L/1.73m^2/day) and provision of alkali salts, such as citrate. A soluble disulfide thiol, tiopronin, may also be used by someone skilled in pediatric stone disease. This drug may cause allergic side effects such as serum sickness and may reduce smell and taste secondary to zinc depletion. Angiotensin-converting enzyme (ACE) inhibition with captopril therapy has been found beneficial in some patients with cystinuria resistant to alkalinization and fluid therapy alone, and perhaps with less bothersome side effects. Captopril, however, is not as effective as thiol-compound therapy.

SURGICAL TREATMENT/PROCEDURES

Medical therapy alone cannot remove existing stones, although in adults, calcium-channel antagonists or β-adrenergic receptor blockers have been advocated.

TABLE 4 Commonly Used Drugs in the Treatment of Nephrolithiasis

Drug Name	Dosage/Route*	Maximum Dose*	Dosage Formulations	Common Adverse Reactions	Indication
Hydrochlorothiazide (HydroDIURIL)	PO: 1 mg/kg/day every 12–24 hours	50 mg/day 25 mg/day	Oral solution: 50 mg/mL Tablet: 25, 50 mg	Hypokalemia, gastrointestinal distress, photosensitivity, low blood pressure	Hypercalciuria, hyperoxaluria
Chlorthalidone (Thalitone) Chlorothiazide (Diuril)	PO: 20 mg/kg/day in 1–2 doses	500 mg/day	Tablet: 15, 25, 50, 100 mg Oral solution: 250 mg/5 mL Tablet: 250, 500 mg		
Potassium citrate	PO: 5–30 mL in 3–6 ounces water after meals and qhs	30 mL after meals and qhs	Oral solution: 2 mEq/mL K 2 mEq/mL bicarbonate equivalent	Hyperkalemia, diarrhea, metabolic acidosis	Hypocitraturia, hypercalciuria, hyperuricosuria, cystinuria, hyperoxaluria
Pyridoxine (vitamin B₆)	PO: 25–200 mg/day, once daily (titrated to effect with urine oxalate levels)	200 mg/day	Tablet: 25, 50 mg	Nausea, sensory neuropathy, seizure, low folic acid, high AST	Primary hyperoxaluria
Acetohydroxamic acid (Lithostat)†	PO: 10 mg/kg/day divided 3–4 times/day	250 mg 4 times/day	Tablet: 250 mg	Nausea, rash, headache	Struvite stones (urease inhibitor)
Allopurinol (Zyloprim)	PO: 10 mg/kg/day in 2–3 divided doses	800 mg/day	Tablet: 100, 300 mg Oral solution: May be made from tablets	Gastrointestinal irritation, rash, drowsiness	Hyperuricosuria*
Tiopronin (Thiola)	Pediatric: PO: 15 mg/kg/day divided tid Adult PO: 800–1000 mg/day	1000 mg/day	Tablet: 100 mg	Nausea, diarrhea	Cystinuria
Captopril (Capoten)‡	0.1 mg/kg/dose, 2–4 times per day (may be titrated upward)	1 mg/kg/day or 200 mg/day	Tablet: 12.5, 25, 50 Oral solution: 1 mg/mL may be prepared	Low BP, rash, angioedema, hyperK, cough	Cystinuria

*Doses are our recommendations. Physician's Desk Reference dosing may differ.
†Pediatric experience has not been reported.
‡Limited efficacy in cystinuria.
AST, aspartate aminotransferase; PO, orally; tid, three times daily; qhs, at bedtime.

These are not recommended for children with kidney stones at this time.

For large (>1.5 cm) or symptomatic stones, extracorporeal shock wave lithotripsy (ESWL) may be used to fragment stones that may then pass spontaneously or be removed endoscopically. The majority of simple renal calculi (<2 to 3 cm in size, normal kidney anatomy), especially in the upper tract (pelvis, proximal ureter), can be treated successfully with ESWL. The paste-like consistency of cystine stones, however, makes them resistant to ESWL. Success rates for stone dissolution and passage with ESWL range from 80% to 90% in recent reports, and the previous concerns for possible renal damage or hypertension resulting from ESWL in children seem unfounded, as any effects are mild and transient, if present at all. A study by Vlajkovic and associates of 84 children undergoing ESWL looked at glomerular filtration rate (GFR) by kidney scintigraphy before, immediately following, 3 months after, and more than 12 months after treatment. The average immediate post-ESWL GFR decreased to 107 mL per minute from the pretreatment level of 118 mL per minute, but it increased to 121 mL per minute at 3 months and 131 mL per minute at the end of the observation period. ESWL treatment for children with acute obstruction was actually associated with an immediate increase in GFR. Recommendations regarding ESWL are not clear, however, for patients with a solitary kidney or impaired kidney function (chronic kidney disease), and should be referred to a specialist in pediatric stone disorders.

Renal calculi may also be removed by rigid or flexible endoscopy through the urethra or by percutaneous means. Percutaneous nephrolithotomy has a higher stone-free rate and lower retreatment rate than ESWL but is limited in use to stones greater than 2 to 3 cm in size, or in complex renal calculi including staghorn, or in those stones made of materials resistant to ESWL, or when increased patient morbidity may occur with ESWL. Open surgical lithotomy can be done if other techniques fail. Endoscopic laser fragmentation of stones has been used in adults, but its role in children has not yet been established.

Common Pitfalls

- Failure to evaluate the cause of kidney stones in children appropriately, therefore delaying diagnosis and optimal treatment. Because more than one metabolic disturbance may often coexist, an incomplete set of diagnostics may overlook potentially treatable causes of stones.
- Failure to recognize obstruction. With certain forms of nephrolithiasis, complications such as obstruction, renal insufficiency, or infection may occur. Obstruction is a medical emergency, with signs and symptoms including those of acute kidney failure and pain, dysuria, and hesitancy. Early suspicion, diagnosis, and treatment of acute obstruction through consultation with a

specialist in surgical management of kidney stones are critical to avoid morbidity and kidney damage.
- Failure to monitor postobstructive diuresis. Once obstruction is relieved, one should monitor and address the potential for a postobstructive diuresis, to avoid extracellular fluid volume depletion and blood electrolyte abnormalities.

Communication and Counseling

After initial diagnosis and initiation of therapy for kidney stones, there are long-term issues that need to be addressed. An important issue for some patients is that of bone mineral density (BMD) in FIH. A study by Garcia-Nieto of 40 girls with idiopathic hypercalciuria (IH) and their premenopausal mothers showed that bone density lumbar spine Z scores were significantly lower in these patients compared to controls. Of the subjects, 42.5% of the girls and 47.5% of their mothers had lumbar BMD Z scores less than −1. Others have shown that thiazide treatment, in addition to decreasing urinary calcium excretion, can also improve BMD scores in children. Average Z score improved from −1.3 to −0.22 over 1 year of treatment with hydrochlorothiazide and potassium citrate in one study of 18 children by Reusz and associates.

Prognosis for nephrolithiasis depends on type of stones and adherence to therapy. Nephrolithiasis in children, irrespective of cause, generally recurs without treatment. Cystine stones have a recurrence rate of 0.64 per patient year, and obstruction may impair kidney function. Primary hyperoxaluria type I is a progressive disease, often leading to progressive loss of kidney function even with optimal compliance to medical therapy, unless vitamin B_6 responsiveness is established. Kidney stones from hyperuricosuria may continue to occur with or without symptoms despite treatment. Pediatric nephrolithiasis should be referred to an appropriate subspecialist interested in the disorder under most circumstances.

SUGGESTED READINGS

1. Bentur L, Alon U, Berant M: Hypercalciuria in chronically institutionalized bedridden children: Frequency, predictive factors and response to treatment with thiazides. Int. J Pediatr Nephrol 8(1):29–34, 1987. **Demonstrates improvement in urine calcium/creatinine ratios with thiazide treatment in hypercalciuric children. However, these ratios were not correlated with 24-hour urine excretion of calcium, which remains the gold standard in assessing success of medical therapy for hypercalciuria.**
2. Chow G, Streem S: Medical treatment of cystinuria: Results of contemporary clinical practice. J Urol 156(5):1576–1578, 1996. **Shows the effectiveness of D-penicillamine and α-mercaptopropionylglycine (thiols) over hydration and alkalinization alone in decreasing rate of stone formation in a group of patients with cystinuria. Captopril did not clearly add any clinical benefit.**
3. Coe FL, Parks JH: Nephrolithiasis. In Favus MJ (ed): Primer on the Metabolic Bone Diseases and Disorders of Mineral Metabolism. Washington, DC: American Society for Bone and Mineral Research, 2003. **Overview of types of nephrolithiasis and treatment in adults.**

4. Garcia-Nieto V, Navarro JF, Monge M, et al: Bone mineral density in girls and their mothers with idiopathic hypercalciuria. Nephron Clin Pract 94(4):c81–c82, 2003. **Describes high prevalence of osteopenia (lumbar spine BMD Z scores less than −1) in girls and their premenopausal mothers with idiopathic hypercalciuria (IH).**

5. Gillespie R, Stapleton FB: Nephrolithiasis in children. Pediatr Rev 25(4):131–138, 2004. **Review of diagnosis and treatment of kidney stones in children.**

6. Griffith DP, Gleeson MJ, Lee H, et al: Randomized double-blind trial of Lithostat (acetohydroxamic acid) in the palliative treatment of infection-induced urinary calculi. Eur Urol 20 (3):243–247, 1991. **Demonstrates significantly less stone growth with the use of Lithostat versus placebo in a group of adults with chronic urinary infections and stones.**

7. Hoppe B, Leumann E: Diagnostic and therapeutic strategies in hyperoxaluria: A plea for early intervention. Nephol Dial Transplant 19(1):39–42, 2004. **Reviews current methods in diagnosis and options for optimal treatment for primary hyperoxaluria.**

8. Kim S, Kuo R, Paterson R, et al: Urologic aspects of nephrolithiasis management. In Favus MJ (ed): Primer on the Metabolic Bone Diseases and Disorders of Mineral Metabolism. Washington, DC: American Society for Bone and Mineral Research, 2003, pp 522–526. **Outlines surgical interventions for different stone types.**

9. Langman CB: The molecular basis of kidney stones. Curr Opin in Pediatr 16:188–193, 2004. **Reviews current and ongoing development of the understanding of molecular mechanisms behind formation of various stone types.**

10. Langman CB: Nephrolithiasis. In Green T, Franklin W, Tanz R (eds): Pediatrics: Just the Facts. New York: McGraw Hill, 2005, pp 449–451. **Brief overview of key points in nephrolithiasis diagnosis in children.**

11. Ohkawa M, Tokunaga S, Nakashima T, et al: Thiazide treatment for calcium urolithiasis in patients with idiopathic hypercalciuria. Br J Urol 69(6):571–576, 1992. **Randomized, controlled trial showing benefits of thiazides in urinary calcium excretion and rate of stone formation in adults.**

12. Reusz GS, Dobos M, Vasarhelyi B, et al: Sodium transport and bone mineral density in hypercalciuria with thiazide treatment. Pediatr Nephrol 12(1):30–34, 1998. **Demonstrates an increase in Na/K ATPase activity, decrease in urinary calcium to creatinine ratio, and increase in BMD Z -score with thiazide treatment for IH in children.**

13. Vlajkovic M, Lavkovic A, Radovanovic M, et al: Long-term functional outcome of kidneys in children with urolithiasis after ESWL treatment. Eur J Pediatr Surg 12(2):118–123, 2002. **Evaluates short-term (immediate to 3 months) and long-term (12 to 67 months) changes in kidney function after extracorporeal shock wave lithotripsy (ESWL) in a group of children treated for urolithiasis.**

Hematuria and Proteinuria

Rene G. VanDeVoorde III and John J. Bissler

KEY CONCEPTS

- Understanding the detection methodology of urinary protein and blood facilitates result interpretation.
- Patients with isolated proteinuria or hematuria can be approached in a stepwise fashion.
- Persistent hematuria in the absence of proteinuria may be a benign process.
- Persistent nonorthostatic proteinuria with or without hematuria requires prompt evaluation with likely referral.

Isolated hematuria or proteinuria is common in asymptomatic children and is often detected serendipitously by screening urinalysis. Such isolated urinary abnormalities often can be benign, and an in-depth understanding of the diagnostic possibilities is necessary to avoid needless, expensive, and possibly invasive studies. An understanding of renal physiology, disease prevalence, and urinalysis methods greatly aid in the evaluation of the urinary abnormality and helps discern benign from pathologic conditions.

Expert Opinion on Management Issues

PROTEINURIA

Transient proteinuria is reasonably common. Vehaskari and Rapola noted that 10% of Finnish schoolchildren had proteinuria in one of four urinalyses; however, only 2.5% had proteinuria in two of the four urinalyses. A very low rate of protein excretion, comprised primarily of Tamm-Horsfall protein, also called uromodulin, is normal but is below the level of detection using the usual methods. This protein excretion is developmentally regulated. Newborns, with their immature renal function, have increased "physiologic proteinuria."

Understanding the renal handling of protein helps to distinguish benign proteinuria from that accompanying disease. The glomerulus filters plasma water and dissolved solutes into Bowman space. Slit pores limit the passage of proteins into the filtrate, retaining larger molecules but allowing molecules less than 4.5 to 5.0 nm in radius to pass. Additionally, the negatively charged basement membrane proteoglycans repel negatively charged proteins, regardless of size. This charge interaction is why albumin is not filtered in large amounts into the urine under normal circumstances even though it has a small molecular radius (3.6 nm). The proximal tubule also reduces protein excretion by reabsorption of filtered proteins. Perturbations in the glomerular architecture by immune-mediated injury, removal of the net negative charge of the glomerular basement membrane, or renal tubule damage result in increased protein excretion. Less commonly, hyperfiltration or marked increase in serum protein levels can also lead to proteinuria. When there is a loss of overall renal function or an increase in glomerular capillary pressure, each functioning nephron begins to hyperfilter, resulting in increased protein delivery to the tubule. In conditions such as myeloma (increased immunoglobulins), rhabdomyolysis (release of myoglobin), and pancreatitis (increase in amylase), the relevant serum protein is increased, so that more protein must be handled by the tubule. In both hyperfiltration and hyperproteinemia, the filtered load of protein is increased beyond tubular reabsorptive capacity, and proteinuria results.

DETECTION OF PROTEINURIA

The identification of urinary protein may be clinically significant, but the finding must be interpreted with an

TABLE 1 Factors Leading to False-Positive and False-Negative Dipstick Results for Proteinuria

False-Positive	False-Negative
Pyuria	Dilute urine
Bacteriuria	Nonalbumin proteins
Urine pH >7.0	
Antiseptic contamination	
Direct stream of urine (effects on pH buffer)	
Prolonged immersion (effects on pH buffer)	

understanding of the detection methods. A standard urinalysis most often includes a urine dipstick read by an automated analyzer to increase accuracy. The reagent pad for protein contains tetrabromophenol blue and a buffer. In acidic pH ranges, the tetrabromophenol blue reacts with specific amino acid side groups resulting in a colorimetric change from yellow to varying shades of green, depending on the amount of protein present. The amino acid composition of the protein influences the reaction; albumin produces a robust reaction. The dipstick reaction is fallible and can give both false positive and negative results (Table 1).

The dipstick is a screening tool, and most laboratories perform a confirmatory test using a turbidimetric method. Urine turbidity, caused by protein denaturation with an acid such as sulfosalicylic acid, is proportional to the urinary protein concentration. This test will better expose certain proteins that may not be detected as well by dipstick; however, radiographic contrast or penicillin analogues in the urine may lead to falsely positive turbidimetric results.

Both the dipstick and turbidimetric methods are semiquantitative at best. The 24-hour urine collection for protein excretion is the preferred method of quantitation. Protein excretion rates less than 4 mg/m^2/hour are normal, 4 to 40 mg/m^2/hour are abnormal, and more than 40 mg/m^2/hour are considered to be in the nephrotic range. The protein-to-creatinine ratio ($U_{Pr/Cr}$) from a random urine sample correlates well with 24-hour urine protein excretion in adults and children, obviating the need to collect a timed urine sample from a child, which can be impractical. For children older than 2 years, a $U_{Pr/Cr}$ less than 0.2 is considered normal, although for children from 6 to 24 months a value of less than 0.5 is normal. Regardless of age, a $U_{Pr/Cr}$ greater than 1.5 or 2.0 indicates nephrotic range proteinuria (2 g/m^2/day). The relationship between total daily urine protein excretion and $U_{Pr/Cr}$ is expressed by the following equation:

$$\text{Total Urine Protein (g/m}^2\text{/day)} = 0.63 \times (U_{Pr/Cr})$$

Because the urinary creatinine concentration depends on the patient's muscle mass, $U_{Pr/Cr}$ may be inaccurate in children with severe nutritional deficiency, significantly altered muscle mass, or renal insufficiency. Using the first morning void for such analysis limits any possible orthostatic synergism.

HISTORY AND PHYSICAL EXAMINATION

History and physical examination can guide further investigation of proteinuria. A history of gross hematuria, polyuria manifesting as nocturia associated with thirst, oliguria, and edema make proteinuria more concerning. Additional complaints may include headaches from hypertension, fatigability from either anemia or increased effort to move edematous limbs, and abdominal pain from edema and possible compromise of intestinal perfusion. Important family history features include kidney diseases such as polycystic kidney disease, Dent disease, focal segmental glomerulosclerosis, or end-stage renal disease. Past and concomitant medical history of medication usage, such as antibiotics, may also be revealing. It is important to ascertain the presence of systemic conditions, such as human immunodeficiency virus (HIV) or systemic lupus erythematosus (SLE) that may be associated with proteinuria.

Physical findings, including vital signs, height, and weight also aid in determining the significance of the proteinuria. Tachycardia may reflect intravascular volume contraction, and hypertension may reflect renal injury or impairment. Edema, associated with a weight change, may be evident in the extremities, sacrum, scrotum, or labia. Periorbital edema and conjunctival pallor may offer insight into serum albumin levels and anemia, respectively. Hypertension (>90th percentile for height by age), edema, ill appearance, or other significant findings such as the child being small for age indicate an immediate need for a complete evaluation including measurement of renal function and serum proteins.

EVALUATION

Figure 1 outlines the approach to the patient with proteinuria aided by a stepwise evaluation. Asymptomatic patients may have transient or persistent proteinuria. Transient proteinuria (left side of Fig. 1), defined as resolving within 2 weeks, is usually minor and can be associated with fever, exercise, seizures, dehydration, extreme cold exposure, and recent administration of epinephrine. Proteinuria associated with fever often occurs at the onset of the temperature elevation and resolves by the 10th day. Exercise-induced proteinuria correlates with the duration and severity of the exercise and abates within 48 hours. A repeat urinalysis should be done 2 weeks after the initial discovery to confirm the resolution of proteinuria.

Approximately 60% of asymptomatic school-age children with proteinuria that appears persistent have orthostatic proteinuria. Screening for this benign condition is performed by comparing the protein content of the first morning void (obtained immediately after the child arises) with that of a urine sample obtained in the afternoon or evening. A first morning void should have a normal amount of protein ($U_{Pr/Cr}$ less than 0.2, or routine urinalysis with trace or less) as compared to a random void checked later in the day. Long-term studies in adults with orthostatic proteinuria have shown

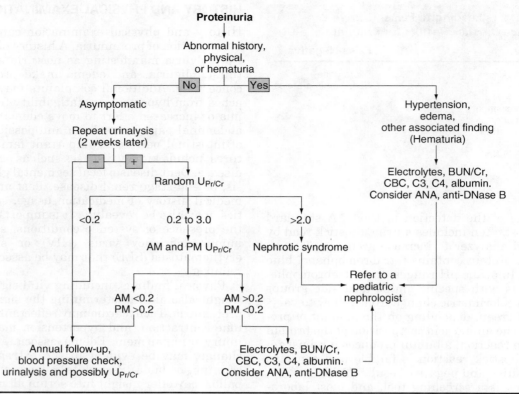

FIGURE 1. Flow diagram for proteinuria. ANA, antinuclear antibodies; BUN, blood urea nitrogen; C3, complement protein 3; C4, complement protein 4; CBC, complete blood count; Cr, creatinine; $U_{Pr/Cr}$, urinary protein-to-creatinine ratio.

TABLE 2 Factors Leading To False-Positive and False-Negative Dipstick Results for Blood

False-Positive	False-Negative
Hemoglobinuria (from hemolysis)	Ascorbic acid
Myoglobinuria (from rhabdomyolysis)	Other antioxidants
Heavily infected urine (bacterial peroxidase)	
Iron sorbitol	
Iodine-containing cleaners	

that orthostatic proteinuria is generally benign and requires no medical intervention. Asymptomatic patients with persistent nonorthostatic proteinuria require referral to a pediatric nephrologist. A renal biopsy may be diagnostic and guide therapy.

HEMATURIA

The vast majority of children who have hematuria are asymptomatic. Prevalence of hematuria in children ranges from 1% to 4%, the majority having asymptomatic microscopic hematuria. The frequency of children with gross hematuria is estimated to be 0.13%. Gross hematuria may be red or brown, depending on whether the pigment is native heme or acid-denatured hematin, respectively. The blood may originate from any of several sources: the renal vasculature as with

trauma, the glomerulus as with glomerulonephritis, the renal tubules as with interstitial nephritis, or the urothelial lining of the urinary tract as with a urinary tract infection.

DETECTION OF HEMATURIA

A dipstick detection of blood may be clinically significant, but as with proteinuria, the result must be interpreted with an understanding of the different detection methods. The urine dipstick pad for blood detects iron, not red blood cells (RBCs). The pad is coated with organic peroxide (diisopropyl benzene dihydroperoxide or orthotolidine peroxide) and a color indicator such as tetramethylbenzidine. The heme iron catalyzes the breakdown of the peroxide, releasing oxygen radicals that oxidize the indicator, resulting in the color change. Urine dipsticks are able to detect one to five RBCs per high power field. Contaminating agents with peroxidase-like activity may cause false-positive results. Table 2 lists potential causes of false-positive results.

Microscopy of urine sediment is required when blood is detected in the urine and may help determine the source of the RBCs. The appearance of gross hematuria in the absence of RBCs is a strong clue for myoglobinuria or hemoglobinuria. Box 1 lists the causes of dark urine that can be mistaken for gross hematuria. RBC casts or small, misshapen erythrocytes suggest glomerular bleeding. Phase-contrast microscopy is useful in detecting glomerular bleeding based on red cell morphology, but may not be available in most laboratories. Leukocytes indicate inflammation and are seen with urinary tract infections or interstitial nephritis. Crystals may be indicative of crystalluria, with bleeding from microtrauma to the lower urinary tract.

HISTORY AND PHYSICAL EXAMINATION

Once hematuria is confirmed, historical details may prove to be invaluable. Hematuria from trauma, exercise or immunoglobulin A (IgA) nephropathy usually occurs concurrently with the inciting event although the hematuria associated with onset of poststreptococcal glomerulonephritis (PSGN) is delayed by 7 to 21 days following infection. Dysuria, urgency, or frequency suggests bladder irritation, possibly a consequence of viral or bacterial urinary tract infection. Colicky flank or back pain suggests nephrolithiasis. Rash may support a vasculitic diagnosis, such as Henoch-Schönlein purpura (HSP) or SLE.

A past medical history of sickle cell disease or trait, congenital heart disease (CHD), or neonatal intensive care unit admission can help direct further evaluation. Patients with CHD may develop endocarditis with ensuing immune complex-mediated glomerulonephritis. Neonates with a history of umbilical catheterization have an increased risk of thrombosis. History of medication use, such as chemotherapeutic agents, antibiotics, nonsteroidal anti-inflammatory drugs (NSAIDs), and diuretics, is helpful. Inquiries into the family history should include questions regarding kidney disease, renal failure, and nephrolithiasis, but one should also search for history of hearing loss (Alport syndrome), hemoglobinopathies (sickle cell, especially trait), coagulopathies (hemophilia), and unexplained hematuria (benign familial hematuria).

Physical examination can also provide clues to the etiology and seriousness of the hematuria. The presence of hypertension, rales, new heart murmurs, abdominal pain, or masses are all significant findings. Costovertebral angle tenderness and flank pain may indicate pyelonephritis, renal inflammation and swelling, or obstruction. The periurethral area should be examined for trauma. Rashes (including purpura), edema, or arthritis are helpful clues and may implicate vasculitic, infectious, or autoimmune processes.

EVALUATION

Isolated microscopic hematuria often is asymptomatic and can be evaluated in a stepwise manner (Fig. 2). Gross hematuria also should be approached in an organized manner (Fig. 3). Hypercalciuria, which accounts for 30% of all isolated hematuria, has the highest incidence in the southeastern United States and may be associated with complaints of vague back or abdominal pain and occasionally gross hematuria. Calcium-containing crystals are hypothesized to irritate the renal tubules and urinary tract, resulting in bleeding and discomfort. Although the observation of crystals in the urine may be suggestive of hypercalciuria, their absence is not helpful. A convenient method to detect hypercalciuria is to measure the urinary concentration of calcium and standardize it by dividing by the urinary creatinine concentration, expressed as the calcium-to-creatinine ratio ($U_{Ca/Cr}$). A $U_{Ca/Cr}$ ratio greater than 0.2 is indicative of hypercalciuria in children beyond infancy. Treatment includes increasing fluid intake and restriction of dietary sodium. Dietary calcium restriction is not helpful, although thiazide diuretics may be used to reduce the calcium excretion. Benign familial hematuria, also called thin basement membrane disease, is an autosomal dominant disorder associated with collagen gene mutations resulting in a thinned lamina densa in the glomerular basement membrane. Affected patients may have microscopic or gross hematuria and the urinary erythrocytes may be slightly dysmorphic. Checking for hematuria in first-degree relatives greatly assists in diagnosis.

Many diseases present with hematuria, but IgA nephropathy, Alport syndrome, and sickle cell disease deserve mention. IgA nephropathy accounts for up to 15% of all persistent, isolated hematuria and is associated with episodes of gross hematuria concurrent with illnesses. Patients are usually normotensive and can lack or have varying amounts of proteinuria. Laboratory evaluation most often reveals normal renal function and C3 concentration. Patients with suspected IgA nephropathy should be referred to a pediatric nephrologist for consideration of a renal biopsy. Twenty-five percent of children with IgA nephropathy develop chronic renal insufficiency. Negative prognosticators include proteinuria, hypertension, older age at onset, and crescentic glomerulonephritis on biopsy. Corticosteroids, vitamin E, and fish oil have all demonstrated efficacy in various studies.

Alport syndrome comprises a collection of genetic disorders of type IV collagen that affects the basement membrane. Classic Alport syndrome is an X-linked disorder that can have an associated high-tone sensorineural deafness and ocular defects. Very early in life patients may present with microscopic hematuria. Later patients will develop proteinuria and occasionally gross hematuria. In the X-linked variety, males progress faster than females, and linkage studies indicate that an autosomal dominant form is unlikely. Approximately 15% of patients with Alport syndrome have mutations in the type IV collagen genes located on chromosome 2 and exhibit autosomal recessive

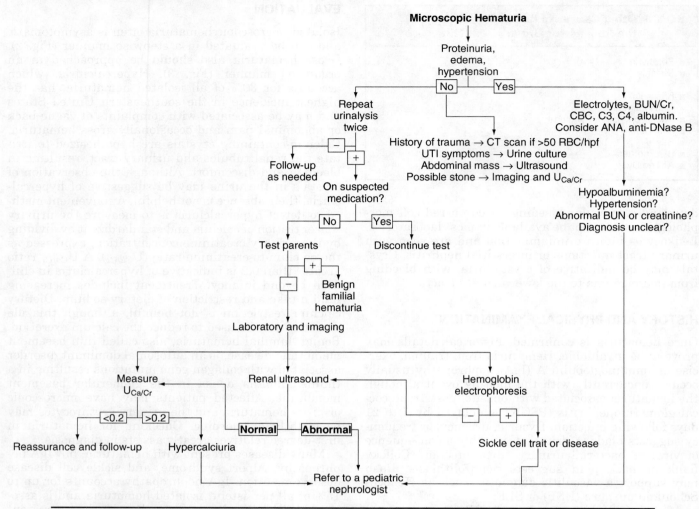

FIGURE 2. Flow diagram for microscopic hematuria. ANA, antinuclear antibodies; BUN, blood urea nitrogen; C3, complement protein 3; C4, complement protein 4; CBC, complete blood count; Cr, creatinine; hpf, high-power field; RBC, red blood cells; $U_{Ca/Cr}$, urinary calcium-to-creatinine ratio; UTI, urinary tract infection.

inheritance. Alport syndrome has no cure, and affected males usually develop renal failure. However, renoprotective agents such as angiotensin-converting enzyme (ACE) inhibitors may delay the onset of renal dysfunction.

Other studies used for evaluation of hematuria include hemoglobin electrophoresis, urine culture, and renal ultrasound. Sickle cell trait causes a greater number of patients with hematuria when compared to sickle cell disease, but this is related to the difference in prevalence. Patients with microhematuria rarely have positive urine cultures. However, an infectious etiology can be found in up to 25% of patients with gross hematuria. A urine culture therefore is recommended for patients with gross hematuria and in children younger than 6 years of age with hematuria. Bladder tumors are rare in children and often manifest with voiding difficulties, negating a need for cystoscopic evaluation of isolated hematuria except in rare cases. Renal ultrasound may be valuable for surveying both renal and bladder wall anatomy. Hemorrhagic cystitis, often

viral in etiology, can cause transient gross hematuria, usually associated with bladder symptoms.

Common Pitfalls

The presence of hematuria with proteinuria should elicit a high degree of suspicion of intrinsic renal parenchymal disease. Microscopic amounts of blood in the urine do not, per se, produce a positive test for protein, but gross hematuria can be associated with as much as 2+ reaction for protein on the dipstick. Therefore, the ominous combination of proteinuria and hematuria can only fully be evaluated after the gross hematuria has subsided. Without a mechanism to assure appropriate follow-up, the occasional patient with intrinsic renal disease will be missed and may suffer otherwise avoidable renal damage. Assuming proteinuria is from gross hematuria without further evaluation can be a missed opportunity for early intervention in an intrinsic renal disease.

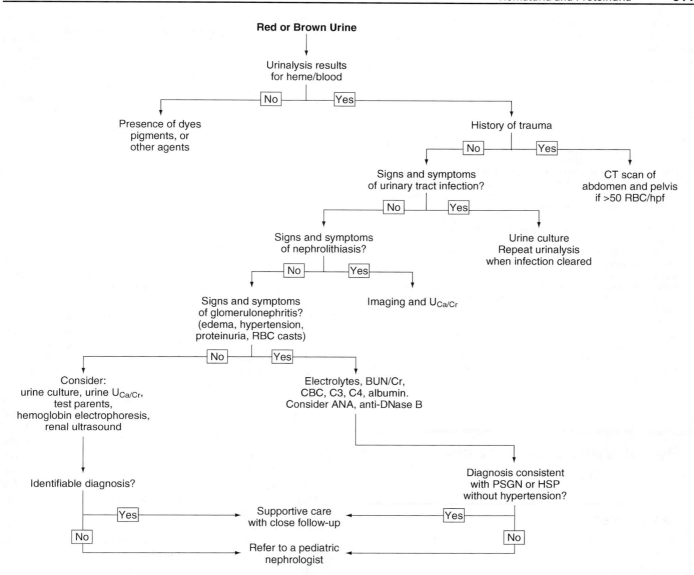

FIGURE 3. Flow diagram for gross hematuria. ANA, antinuclear antibodies; BUN, blood urea nitrogen; C3, complement protein 3; C4, complement protein 4; CBC, complete blood count; Cr, creatinine; hpf, high-power field; HSP, Henoch-Schönlein purpura; PSGN, poststreptococcal glomerulonephritis; RBC, red blood cells; $U_{Ca/Cr}$, urinary calcium-to-creatinine ratio.

Infections severe enough to cause hematuria and proteinuria produce symptoms of bladder irritation. However, the symptoms may not be recognized in children younger than 6 years old, and a urine culture is recommended in all children of this age group with gross hematuria. Laboratory evaluation for patients with both hematuria and proteinuria includes a complete blood count (CBC), blood urea nitrogen (BUN), serum creatinine, complement levels (C3 and C4), serum albumin concentration, and possibly an antistreptolysin O or streptozyme titer. Renal ultrasound should also be considered for evaluation of renal anatomy and size. Persistence of hematuria and proteinuria, accompanying physical examination findings, or abnormalities on initial evaluation can be indicative of an underlying glomerulonephritis (see chapter entitled

"Treatment of Glomerulonephritis"), renal tubular injury (see the chapter entitled "Renal Tubulopathies"), or cystic disease (see chapter entitled "Chronic Kidney Disease"). Therefore, most merit referral to a pediatric nephrologist for further evaluation and treatment.

Communication and Counseling

Hematuria and proteinuria can conjure up fears of renal failure, cancer, and fatality for children and parents. Explaining the prevalence of these findings and the rationale behind the stepwise testing helps diffuse uneasiness and allows the families to realize that there are a variety of diagnostic possibilities. For patients who prove to have more significant findings and require subspecialty referral, an explanation of the abnormal findings reinforces the need for follow-up and assures the family that their primary care physician has communicated with the nephrologist, facilitating patient care.

SUGGESTED READINGS

1. Abitbol C, Zilleruelo G, Freundlich M, et al: Quantitation of proteinuria with urinary protein/creatinine ratios and random testing with dipsticks in nephrotic children. J Pediatr 116:243–247, 1990. **Use of urinary protein-to-creatinine ratios in children.**
2. Diven SC, Travis LB: A practical primary care approach to hematuria in children. Pediatr Nephrol 14:65–72, 2000. **Good insights into the workup of hematuria.**
3. Ettenger RB: The evaluation of the child with proteinuria. Pediatr Ann 23:486–494, 1994. **Guidelines on referral and renal biopsy.**
4. Fitzwater DS, Wyatt RJ: Hematuria. Pediatr Rev 15:102–108, 1994. **History, physical, and laboratory findings that occur with hematuria.**
5. Leung AK, Robson WL: Evaluating the child with proteinuria. J R Soc Health 120:16–22, 2000. **Different etiologies of proteinuria.**
6. Patel HP, Bissler JJ: Hematuria in children. Pediatr Clin North Am 48:1519–1537, 2001. **Review of hematuria with an algorithmic approach.**
7. Vehaskari VM, Rapola J: Isolated proteinuria: Analysis of a school-age population. J Pediatr 101:661–668, 1982. **Incidence of hematuria.**

Renal Vein Thrombosis

Kevin V. Lemley

KEY CONCEPTS

- Renal vein thrombosis (RVT) occurs most commonly in stressed neonates (e.g., premature, infants of diabetic mothers).
- The risk of RVT is increased (in neonates, patients with nephrotic syndrome, etc.) in the presence of genetic thrombophilia.
- Standard therapy involves correction of the acute cause of the thrombosis (dehydration, polycythemia) and, in selected cases, the use of heparin to prevent clot extension or thrombolytic agents to dissolve clots.
- The prognosis if RVT is variable. Decreased renal function and hypertension are long-term sequelae in a minority of patients, necessitating continuing follow-up.

Renal vein thrombosis (RVT) in children is seen most commonly in neonates (with an incidence of approximately 2 per 100,000 live births). Most neonatal cases (more than 80%) occur in infants born to diabetic or preeclamptic mothers or who undergo stresses such as prematurity, infection, perinatal asphyxia or shock, or polycythemia (because of dehydration, congenital adrenal hyperplasia, or congenital heart disease). Males are affected more commonly than females (1.5 to 2:1). RVT usually develops during the first few days of life but may even occur in utero, as indicated by the presence of

BOX 1 Factors Contributing to a Hypercoagulable State

- Genetic thrombophilia (protein C, protein S, antithrombin (AT) deficiencies; polymorphisms leading to increased circulating levels of factors VII, VIII, IX, XI, and von Willebrand factor; factor V Leiden [R506Q]; prothrombin G20210A; MTHFR [5,10-methylene-tetrahydrofolate reductase] C667T; lipoprotein (a); homocystinuria [caused by CBS] mutation)
- Nephrotic syndrome (decreased AT, increased fibrinogen, increased platelet aggregation, hemoconcentration, renal vein compression)
- Antiphospholipid antibodies (lupus anticoagulant, anticardiolipin antibodies)

a flank mass at birth or calcification of the renal thrombus in a newborn. Adrenal hemorrhage is a not infrequent concomitant finding in RVT. In approximately half of neonatal cases of RVT, a predisposing thrombophilia, such as resistance to protein C, is found on investigation. Unilateral RVT is more common in the left renal vein as compared to the right; bilateral RVT is less common, accounting for 21% to 28% of cases. Unlike renal artery thrombosis, RVT is not commonly associated with a central venous catheter in the neonate.

Other settings in which RVT occurs in children include the nephrotic syndrome, particularly congenital nephrotic syndrome, minimal change disease, and focal segmental glomerular sclerosis (FSGS); lupus nephritis, particularly with the nephrotic syndrome; antiphospholipid syndrome (APS); burns; and kidney transplantation. RVT is usually multifactorial in origin—for example, the nephrotic syndrome plus dehydration (e.g., from furosemide therapy); polycythemia and the presence of genetic forms of thrombophilia (Box 1). Compression of the renal veins by tense ascites may contribute to increased RVT risk in the nephrotic state.

The classical clinical presentation of RVT includes increased renal size (flank mass in neonate), gross or microscopic hematuria, acidosis, oliguria or acute renal failure, anemia with erythrocyte fragments on smear, and thrombocytopenia. Hypertension may be found at presentation (8% to 22%). Extension of clot into the inferior vena cava (IVC) is not uncommon (25%), but other associated venous thromboses are rare, as is pulmonary embolus. In sick, high-risk infants, a high index of suspicion for RVT is necessary, as the classic findings are only variably present early in the course. Oliguria, macroscopic hematuria, and thrombocytopenia continue for a median duration of approximately 5 to 7 days. In older children, presentation may be more insidious, with flank pain or lower extremity swelling. Renal function is often better preserved in older children, because of more effective venous collateralization.

Diagnosis may be confirmed with renal ultrasound, which demonstrates increased renal size and a loss of corticomedullary differentiation. Occasionally, a thrombus may be visualized in the renal vein(s) or inferior vena cava (IVC). Doppler sonography shows elevated resistive indices and a lack of typical venous blood flow. Poor ultrasound imaging (especially in neonates) may rarely require the use of alternative imaging modalities such as magnetic resonance angiography (MRA). In older children, Doppler sonography may reveal venous flow, because of the presence of venous collaterals, so that MRA may also be indicated in this setting. Contrast CT should be avoided. Renal scintigraphy (dimercaptosuccinic acid [DMSA]), mercaptoacetyltriglycine [MAG3]) will show poor tracer uptake and decreased excretory function. The utility of adjunctive, confirmatory testing for markers of endogenous fibrinolysis (D-dimers) or clotting factor activation (prothrombin fragment 1 + 2) has not been established.

Expert Opinion on Management Issues

GENERAL MANAGEMENT

Treatable inciting conditions such as polycythemia, dehydration, and hypotension should be corrected. After the RVT has stabilized, a diagnostic workup should be undertaken for genetic thrombophilia, given its high prevalence in the setting of pediatric RVT (see Box 1). Specific factor replacement (such as activated protein C concentrate in protein C deficiency) is not effective.

CONSERVATIVE MANAGEMENT

A conservative approach is appropriate in the setting of unilateral RVT (not complicated by renal failure or extension of clot into the IVC). No anticoagulation is given and close monitoring of the patient is undertaken with frequent serial sonograms looking for clot extension. Remove any central venous catheter in the inferior vena cava if the patient's clinical condition allows. Treat hypertension (Table 1). Severe hypertension may require continuous intravenous infusions (nicardipine); less severe hypertension may respond to isradipine (orally [PO]) or hydralazine (intravenously [IV]) or labetalol (IV). In case of acute renal failure, renal replacement therapy may be necessary.

There is no compelling evidence for the effectiveness of thrombectomy as compared to conservative or medical management, especially in neonates. Thrombosis uniformly extends from the intrarenal veins, so clot cannot be completely removed surgically. Acute nephrectomy also is usually not indicated even in the setting of complete vascular occlusion.

ANTICOAGULATION AND/OR THROMBOLYTIC THERAPY

There have been no controlled trials of either anticoagulation with heparin or thrombolytic therapy (with urokinase, streptokinase or recombinant tissue plasminogen activator [t-PA]). Several anecdotal reports and a few larger, uncontrolled case series suggest that either heparin infusion or thrombolytic therapy may increase the clearance of thrombus and improve long-term outcome. For an RVT extending into the IVC or for bilateral RVT especially with indications of impending renal failure, options include heparin (for prevention of extension during spontaneous fibrinolysis) or heparin plus the addition of t-PA, urokinase, or streptokinase. In neonates, heparin is given as a 50 to 100 U/kg bolus infusion followed by a continuous infusion at 15 to 25 U/kg/hour (to achieve an activated partial thromboplastin time [aPTT] 1.5 to 2 times normal). Lower doses may suffice for older children. Therapy continues for 7 to 10 days, assuming an adequate response. Low-molecular-weight (LMW) heparin (enoxaparin) is an alternative to continuous infusion of unfractionated heparin (see Table 1), especially if heparin-induced thrombocytopenia develops. Clearance of LMW heparin (but not unfractionated heparin) decreases with renal insufficiency. Dosage adjustment may be needed. Consultation with a pediatric hematologist should be sought, if an anticoagulation regimen is to be used.

Thrombolytic therapy may be indicated if heparin infusion does not result in clot stabilization. Thrombolytic therapy is generally contraindicated in postsurgical settings, severe asphyxia, or prematurity less than 32 weeks gestational age, because of an increased risk of significant bleeding. Streptokinase (Streptase) has been infused for periods from 6 hours to 3 days. Urokinase (Abbokinase) has been infused from 10 hours to 4 days. The latter is once again available in the United States. Intra-arterial administration of thrombolytics may be more effective than systemic or selective venous administration, but evidence for this is anecdotal and the procedure is much more invasive than systemic administration. Use of thrombolytics should probably be reserved for severe cases (bilateral RVT with renal failure, kidney transplant) because of attendant risks of bleeding.

Recombinant t-PA may be preferred to streptokinase because of its lower incidence of antigenic reactions and anaphylaxis. Generally, only anecdotal reports of treatment with urokinase, streptokinase, and t-PA have been published. Hemorrhagic rupture of a kidney and fatal cerebral hemorrhage have been reported after t-PA therapy. Combined urokinase plus heparin therapy has been found to be reasonably safe and effective in nonrenal deep vein thrombosis in children. There is no consensus regarding whether low-dose heparin therapy should be continued during thrombolytic therapy (to prevent reformation of clot during fibrinolysis) or restarted immediately following it. The risks of thrombolytic therapy are increased in the settings of thrombocytopenia, low fibrinogen, and low clotting factor levels. Consult a pediatric hematologist before initiating thrombolytic therapy.

LONG-TERM ANTICOAGULATION

Long-term anticoagulation after acute treatment of RVT may be indicated in some cases. There is a risk of cutaneous necrosis with warfarin therapy in patients with protein C or protein S deficiency. Doses are adjusted

TABLE 1 Drugs in the Treatment of Renal Vein Thrombosi

Generic Name (Trade Name)	Dosage/Route/ Regimen	Maximum Dose	Dosage Formulations
Heparin	50–100 U/kg IV bolus, then 15–25 U/kg/h and increased by 5 U/kg/h q4h as needed		Preservative-free: 10, 100, 1000 U/mL
Enoxaparin (Lovenox)	Treatment: 1–1.5 mg/kg SC bid Prophylaxis: 0.50–0.75 mg/kg SC bid	2 mg/kg/dose	30 mg/0.3 mL 40 mg/0.4 mL 60 mg/0.6 mL 80 mg/0.8 mL 100 mg/1 mL
t-PA, Alteplase (Activase)	0.1 mg/kg IV bolus 0.1–0.9 mg/kg/h for 6 h		Lyophilized powder: 2, 50, 100 mg
Urokinase (Abbokinase)	4400 U/kg IV over 10 minutes; then 4400 U/kg/h for 6–12 h		Injection: 250,000 IU
Streptokinase (Streptase)	2000 IU/kg IV bolus; 1000–2000 IU/kg IV maintenance for 6–12 h		Powder for injection: 250,000; 750,000 and 1,500,000 IU.
Warfarin sodium (Coumadin)	0.1–0.2 mg/kg/day for first 2 days, then decreased to 0.05–0,1 mg/kg qd and titrate to INR 2–3		Tablets: 1, 2, 2.5, 3, 4, 5, 6, 7.5, 10 mg.
Nicardipine (Cardene)	0.5–2 µg/kg/h	5 µg/kg/h	Injection: 2.5 mg/mL (10 mL)
Hydralazine (Apresoline)	0.1–0.4 mg/kg/ dose q4–6h	5 mg/kg/day	
Labetalol (Normodyne, Trandate)	0.4–1 mg/kg/h IV 0.25–1 mg/kg IV over 10–20 min, repeated if needed	3 mg/kg/h	Injection: 5 mg/mL. Tablets: 100, 200, 300 mg.
Isradipine (DynaCirc)	0.05–0.15 mg/ kg/dose q8h	20 mg/day	Tablets: 2.5, 5 mg Suspension can be made.

aPTT, activated partial thromboplastin time; bid, two times daily; INR, international normalized ratio; IV, intravenously; PT, prothrombin time; qd, daily; qxh, every x hours; SC, subcutaneously.

Common Adverse Reactions	Therapeutic Concentrations	Comments
Heparin-induced thrombocytopenia in 1%–3% (after 5–10 days of Rx) Hemorrhage Increased liver enzymes	Target aPTT of 1.5–2 times normal. Check aPTT q4–6h during therapy.	
Hemorrhage Increased liver enzymes	Treatment: target anti-Xa 0.5–1.0 U/mL. Prophylaxis: target anti-Xa 0.1–0.4 U/mL.	Heparin-induced thrombocytopenia less common than with unfractionated heparin. Decrease dose for creatinine clearance <30 mL/min.
Hypotension Fever Hemorrhage Allergic reaction	Measure fibrinogen before and 2 h after infusion; correct to >1 g/L.	Use together with heparin is associated with higher bleeding risk.
Hemorrhage Embolism	May prolong treatment (up to 72 h) depending on response.	Check fibrinogen level, PT, aPTT periodically with therapy.
Allergic reactions (urticaria, anaphylaxis, delayed hypersensitivity) Hemorrhage		Check fibrinogen level, PT, aPTT periodically with therapy.
Hemorrhage Hepatotoxicity Skin necrosis	Overlap therapy 4–5 days with heparin.	Interactions with many drugs, foods.
Hypotension AV block Allergic reaction		Relatively rapid onset of action; offset delayed—increase rates slowly. Do not use with high degree AV block, sick sinus syndrome.
Hypotension Edema Lupus-like syndrome	Dose must be adjusted for renal failure.	Slow and fast acetylators react differently.
Hypotension AV block Bradycardia Bronchospasm	Consider nicardipine as continuous infusion therapy.	Contraindicated in severe bradycardia or bronchospasm.
Hypotension Tachycardia Headache Increased liver enzymes	May be given q6h if needed.	Advanced heart block. Sinus bradycardia. Heart failure.

to achieve a target international normalized ratio (INR) of 2 to 3. The duration of oral therapy is 3 to 6 months. LMW heparin represents an alternative long-term treatment option. Recurrent thromboembolism is uncommon (<5%) in children with a history of RVT and seems to occur mostly in children with genetic thrombophilia.

Persistent, treatment-refractory hypertension in the setting of a nonfunctional kidney (shrinking determined by sonography, low function on DMSA or MAG3 examination) may lead to consideration of uninephrectomy, although hypertension is usually a temporary situation. Long-term hypertension associated with atrophy and proteinuria would warrant consideration of a cautious, graded introduction of angiotensin-converting enzyme inhibition (or angiotensin-receptor blockade) for its renoprotective effects.

Common Pitfalls

Anticoagulation and thrombolytic therapy may place sick neonates (especially premature neonates) at risk for intraventricular hemorrhage and other significant bleeding complications in a setting in which conservative therapy is often associated with acceptable short-term outcomes. The risks of aggressive thrombolysis must be weighed against the risks involved in the management of renal failure in a neonate.

Communication and Counseling

Acute survival reflects the underlying etiology and overall clinical setting. Atrophy of involved kidneys is common, even in cases of relatively early reperfusion. Many patients recover all or most of normal renal function (even with atrophy of affected kidneys) at least over the intermediate term. Renal prognosis varies according to whether the RVT is unilateral or bilateral, the completeness of the obstruction to blood flow, and extent of recanalization and collateral formation. The incidence of persistent (medication-requiring) hypertension and/or decreased renal function is approximately 20% to 30%. A fraction of children (2% to 27%) with bilateral RVT will progress to kidney failure after a median follow-up of approximately 4 years. If the IVC is also occluded by thrombosis, subsequent renal transplantation may be difficult. Long-term, close follow-up is necessary in all children who have had a RVT.

SUGGESTED READINGS

1. Brun P, Beaufils F, Pillion G, et al: Thrombosis of the renal veins in the newborn: Treatment and long term prognosis. Ann Pediatr (Paris) 40:75–80, 1993. **A large but uncontrolled experience in 39 neonates suggesting a long-term functional benefit to urokinase therapy.**
2. Kosch A, Kuwertz-Bröking E, Heller C, et al: Renal venous thrombosis in neonates: Prothrombotic risk factors and long-term follow-up. Blood 104:1356–1360, 2004. **A case-control study showing several genetic pro-thrombotic factors increase the risk of renal vein thrombosis (RVT). Based on 59 neonates with renal vein thrombosis and 188 healthy neonates.**
3. Kuhle S, Massicotte P, Chan A, et al: A case series of 72 neonates with renal vein thrombosis. Data from the 1-800-NO-CLOTS registry. Thromb Haemost 92:729–733, 2004. **A large series in which presenting characteristics of neonates with RVT are well-described. Limited reports on follow-up (5/72).**
4. Nowak-Göttl U, Auberger K, Halimeh S, et al: Thrombolysis in newborns and infants. Thromb Haemost 82(Suppl):112–116, 1999. **A review of thrombolytic therapy with reports of a few small series of RVT.**
5. Zigman A, Yazbeck S, Emil S, et al: Renal vein thrombosis: A 10-year review. Ped Surg 35:1540–1542, 2000. **A good review of cases coming for surgical consultation over 10 years in Montreal.**

Treatment of Glomerulonephritis

Diego H. Aviles

KEY CONCEPTS

- Patients with postinfectious glomerulonephritis can present with oliguric renal failure. Early supportive therapies may prevent complications related to volume overload.
- As many as 30% of patients with immunoglobulin A nephropathy can develop renal insufficiency. There is no proven specific therapy for this condition.
- The use of immunosuppressive agents should be considered in patients with membranous nephropathy with risk factors for progression.
- Hepatitis C infection is responsible for a significant number of cases of membranoproliferative glomerulonephritis.
- Treatment of chronic systemic lupus erythematosus nephritis with newer agents such as mycophenolate mofetil appears promising.

Glomerulonephritis (GN) refers to a group of conditions characterized by the presence of inflammation of the glomerular capillaries with clinical signs and symptoms of acute nephritis. These include hematuria, proteinuria, and decreased renal function sometimes associated with hypertension, fluid retention, and edema. GN can occur as a primary disease or as a manifestation of another primary disease process. This chapter discusses the treatment options for the most common diseases that lead to GN in children. When available, treatment recommendations will be evidence-based. Most cases of GN manifest acutely with hypertension, hematuria, proteinuria, and, in most cases, decreased renal function (Table 1). Postinfectious GN is a typical example. Other types of GN that can manifest acutely include Henoch-Schönlein purpura (HSP), systemic lupus erythematosus (SLE) nephritis, and rapidly progressive glomerulonephritis. Other etiologies for GN may present insidiously with only mild symptoms. Examples of this latter group include immunoglobulin A (IgA) nephropathy and membranoproliferative glomerulonephritis (MPGN).

TABLE 1 Suggested Serologic Studies and Interpretation in Patients with Suspected Glomerulonephritis

Serologic Test	Interpretation
Antibodies against Streptococci	Positive results indicate streptococcal infection in the previous 3 months.
Antinuclear antibodies	If positive, should be confirmed with antibodies against double-stranded DNA.
Anti-GBM	If elevated, it is diagnostic of anti-GBM nephritis.
ANCA	If high, confirms with assays for myeloperoxidase and proteinase 3.
	Could be seen in patients with microscopic polyarteritis or Wegener granulomatosis.
Hepatitis C antibody	If positive, suggests previous exposure.
	Confirm with hepatitis C PCR.
Complement	Decreased C3 and CH50 suggest postinfectious GN, MPGN, or SLE.

ANCA, antineutrophil cytoplasmic antibody; DNA, deoxyribonucleic acid; GBM, glomerular basement membrane; GN, glomerulonephritis; MPGN, membranoproliferative glomerulonephritis; PCR, polymerase chain reaction; SLE, systemic lupus erythematosus.

TABLE 2 Therapy in Different Forms of Glomerulonephritis

Disorder	Prognosis	Treatment
Postinfectious GN	Usually complete remission	Supportive therapy.
IgA nephropathy	30% progress to ESRD	Consider if there is hypertension, proteinuria, or impaired renal function.
Membranous GN	Variable	See section in text.
MPGN	ESRD if unresponsive to treatment	Alternate-day prednisone.
		Cytotoxic agents for severe disease.
RPGN	High risk for progression	IV methylprednisolone.
		Plasmapheresis, cytotoxic medications.
SLE	High risk for progression	Diffuse proliferative, cyclophosphamide/steroids; MMF after cyclophosphamide.
		Focal proliferative or membranous, oral prednisone.

ESRD, end-stage renal disease; GN, glomerulonephritis; IV, intravenous; MMF, mycophenolate mofetil; MPGN, membranoproliferative glomerulonephritis; RPGN, rapidly progressive glomerulonephritis; SLE, systemic lupus erythematosus.

11

Expert Opinion on Management Issues

POSTINFECTIOUS GLOMERULONEPHRITIS

Postinfectious GN is a common cause of acute GN in children. It can be preceded by many infections, but it is most commonly associated with group A β-hemolytic streptococcal infection. Most affected patients present with mild symptoms but some may develop renal failure with volume overload, hypertension, encephalopathy, and congestive heart failure. In the absence of renal failure, only supportive therapy with diuretics and antihypertensive medications is indicated (Table 2). The vast majority of children with postinfectious GN recover normal renal function. Hematuria may persist for years after the initial presentation.

Rarely children with postinfectious GN present with rapidly progressive glomerulonephritis with crescents. Although steroid-pulsed therapy has been used for these children, there are no data confirming a positive effect in postinfectious GN.

IMMUNOGLOBULIN A NEPHROPATHY

The most common cause of glomerulonephritis in developed countries is IgA nephropathy. In 40% to 50% of the patients, the disorder initially appears with an abrupt onset of gross hematuria 24 to 48 hours after an upper respiratory or gastrointestinal (GI) viral infection. Edema and hypertension are less common than

in patients with poststreptococcal glomerulonephritis. Patients may present with persistent microscopic hematuria. Acute renal failure, usually reversible, is occasionally seen with episodes of gross hematuria. However, some patients with IgA nephropathy present with a rapidly progressive course and have crescents on renal biopsy. There is no specific diagnostic test other than biopsy, although high levels of IgA-fibronectin complexes have been reported. A renal biopsy may be helpful, especially in the presence of decreased renal function with proteinuria. Specific treatment options for IgA nephropathy are unproven, although a number of trials are promising. Prophylactic antibiotics and tonsillectomy appear to reduce the episodes of gross hematuria in some reports, but the effect on the progression of renal failure is questionable. Immunosuppressive therapy with glucocorticoids and azathioprine has shown promise in uncontrolled pediatric trials. There is no evidence in controlled and prospective studies that immunosuppressive agents improve the long-term outcome for children with IgA nephropathy. However, plasma exchange combined with immunosuppressive agents might be beneficial in patients with rapidly progressive IgA nephropathy (see Table 2).

MEMBRANOUS NEPHROPATHY

Membranous GN may be primary or secondary to a systemic disease or infection. This condition has been associated with hepatitis B and C infections. Most patients present with heavy proteinuria or overt nephrotic syndrome. There is variability in the progression of the disease. A third of the patients enter remission without therapy, another third have persistent proteinuria without renal scarring, and a third may progress to renal failure over 5 to 15 years.

The evaluation of treatment options for this condition has been hampered by its natural history, because so many of those affected remit without therapy. Treatment with immunosuppressive agents should be reserved for patients who have risk factors for progression of renal impairment such as particularly heavy proteinuria, elevated serum creatinine, or evidence or interstitial fibrosis on renal biopsy (see Table 2). In patients with primary membranous nephropathy, a trial with alternate-day prednisone should be considered. The combination of steroids and alkylating agents should be considered for patients with risk factors for progression. Studies in adults show a decrease in the risk of progression among patients treated with alkylating agents. Alternative therapy in treatment failures includes cyclosporine and mycophenolate mofetil. Because patients with membranous GN and heavy proteinuria have an increased risk for thrombosis, the use of low-dose aspirin may be reasonable.

MEMBRANOPROLIFERATIVE GLOMERULONEPHRITIS

Idiopathic MPGN includes three histological variants. All show increased glomerular cellularity with thickening of the glomerular capillary walls and, often, low serum complement (C3) levels (see Table 1).

Types 1 and 3 have subendothelial deposits of immunoglobulin and C3. Patients with type 2 MPGN have evidence of dense intramembranous deposits on renal biopsy. Type 1 disease usually responds to prednisone administered on alternative days for 6 to 12 months followed by a slow taper once remission is achieved on therapy (see Table 2). Types 2 and 3 are treated with alternate-day steroids, but achieving response is less likely as compared to patients with type 1 MPGN. If no benefit is seen, conservative treatment (control of hypertension with medications that should include angiotensin-converting enzyme [ACE] inhibitors to decrease proteinuria) should be implemented. In patients with MPGN who progress to renal failure, transplantation is associated with recurrence in up to 30% of the allografts. MPGN in association with systemic disease (secondary MPGN) is unusual in children. This may occur with infections (hepatitis B and C), cryoglobulinemia, and lymphoma (see Table 1).

RAPIDLY PROGRESSIVE GLOMERULONEPHRITIS

Rapidly progressive glomerulonephritis (RPGN) is defined as glomerulonephritis that is accompanied by rapid and profound loss of renal function. Early renal biopsy is important in such patients, who will have crescents in more than 50% of their glomeruli on biopsy.

The renal biopsy findings permit classification of idiopathic RPGN into antiglomerular basement membrane disease (GBM), immune complex disease and pauci-immune GN.

Anti-GBM antibody disease should be treated initially with intravenous infusions of methylprednisolone. Plasmapheresis to remove the circulating antibody should be initiated early in the course. Long-term use of alkylating agents (cyclophosphamide initially followed by azathioprine or mycophenolate mofetil [MMF]) is necessary to suppress antibody production (see Table 2). If treated early, up to 70% of affected patients generally recover enough renal function to avoid dialysis. However, long-term outcome is unclear.

SYSTEMIC LUPUS ERYTHEMATOSUS NEPHRITIS

Patients with systemic lupus erythematosus (SLE) may present with significant renal involvement. High-dose steroids and intravenous cyclophosphamide have been reported to control lupus nephritis patients with diffuse proliferative nephritis effectively. Cyclophosphamide administered at monthly intervals for 6 to 9 months and then tapered to every 3 months over 2 years is one approach (see Table 2). Alternatively, cyclophosphamide is given for the first 6 months, after which patients are switched to azathioprine. Initial intravenous steroids are followed with oral prednisone. The dose of prednisone is tapered depending on the disease activity. A recent study indicated that MMF is effective in children with SLE nephritis once the disease is treated initially with IV cyclophosphamide (see Table 2). Approximately 75% of the children treated with MMF have functioning kidneys when reviewed at a point 5 years after onset.

In contrast, previous studies indicated that only 25% to 30% of children had functioning kidneys after 5 years.

Common Pitfalls

- Failure to recognize postinfectious GN can lead to life-threatening complications. Excessive fluids in the presence of oliguria can lead to congestive heart failure with volume overload.
- A diagnostic renal biopsy is crucial in the management of RPGN. Delay in the diagnosis may lead to end-stage renal disease. Most children with SLE have renal involvement. Failure to recognize this potential complication could lead to irreversible renal injury.
- Failure to recognize adverse effects related to the use of immunosuppressive agents could lead to life-threatening complications

Communication and Counseling

Only a small percentage of patients with postinfectious GN require hospitalization. As soon as the blood pressure is well controlled and diuresis has begun, children can be followed as outpatients. A low sodium diet might be indicated in the acute phase. However, prolonged dietary restrictions are not indicated.

Patients receiving immunosuppressive therapy should be educated about early signs of infection. Patients receiving high-dose prednisone should be monitored for the development of diabetes and peptic ulcer disease. The adverse effects of immunosuppressive therapy should be discussed with the family. This should include the risk for infertility and malignancies.

SUGGESTED READINGS

1. Cameron JS: Membranous nephropathy in childhood and its treatment. Pediatr Nephrol 4(2):193–198, 1990. **This article reviews the treatment options for children with membranous nephropathy.**
2. Chan Tm, Li FK, Tang CS, et al: Efficacy of mycophenolate mofetil (MMF) in patients with diffuse proliferative lupus nephritis. Hong Kong-Guangzhou Nephrology Study Group. N Engl J Med 343:1156–1162, 2000. **This study compares the safety and effectiveness of a regimen consisting of MMF and prednisolone versus prednisolone and cyclophosphamide for 6 months followed by prednisolone and azathioprine for 6 months. No significant differences were noted at 1 year.**
3. Johnston F, Carapetis J, Patel MS, et al: Evaluating the use of penicillin to control outbreaks of acute post streptococcal glomerulonephritis. Pediatr Infect Dis J 18(4):327–332, 1999. **This study supports the use of benzathine penicillin G to prevent new cases of acute poststreptococcal glomerulonephritis (GN).**
4. Kasahara T, Hayakawa H, Okubo S, et al: Prognosis of acute post streptococcal glomerulonephritis (APSNS) is excellent in children, when adequately diagnosed. Pediatr Int 43(4):364–367, 2001. **The long-term prognosis of children with postinfectious GN is excellent with adequate diagnosis and treatment.**
5. McEnery PT, McAdams AJ, West CD: Membranoproliferative glomerulonephritis: improved survival with alternate day prednisone therapy. Clin Nephrol 13(3):117–124, 1980. **This study shows that alternate-day prednisone significantly improves the long-term survival of children with MPGN.**
6. Wyatt R, Hogg R: Evidence based assessment of treatment options for children with IgA nephropathies. Pediatr Nephrol 16:156–167, 2001. **This article looks for evidence-based evidence for current treatment of IgA nephropathy. The authors conclude that there is no convincing evidence to support the use of ACE inhibitors, tonsillectomy, or fish oil in the treatment of IgA nephropathy.**

The Nephrotic Syndrome

James C. M. Chan and John W. Foreman

KEY CONCEPTS

- Nephrotic syndrome consists of massive proteinuria, with hypoalbuminemia, hypercholesterolemia, and edema as pathophysiological consequences.
- The most common form of this syndrome in children is primary idiopathic nephrotic syndrome.
- Standard therapy involves bringing about remission, usually with glucocorticoids in idiopathic nephrotic syndrome.

- In steroid-dependent minimal lesions nephrotic syndrome, as well as in other forms of nephrotic syndrome, other medications may be used, often immunosuppressive medications.
- Careful attention to salt and fluid intake during episodes is important.
- Focal segmental glomerulosclerosis may progress to renal failure.

The reported annual incidence of nephrotic syndrome is two to seven new cases per 100,000 children younger than 18 years of age, with an estimated prevalence rate of 16 cases per 100,000, making it a major pediatric disease. The primary abnormality is a loss of glomerular membrane selectivity resulting in the massive proteinuria, with hypoalbuminemia, hypercholesterolemia, and edema as pathophysiological consequences. This chapter covers the management and counseling of patients with primary idiopathic nephrotic syndromes, focusing on the minimal-change nephrotic syndrome (MCNS) and the focal segmental glomerulosclerosis (FSGS).

Nephrotic Syndrome

The *sine qua non* of the diagnosis of nephrotic syndrome is a urinary protein loss of 50 mg/kg/24 hours or spot urine of more than 2 mg protein per mg creatinine (Table 1). The age of onset of the disease is helpful in differentiating the types of nephrotic syndrome. Most patients with MCNS present before 5 years of age, whereas most cases of FSGS occur in older children.

A biopsy of MCNS has normal-appearing glomeruli on light microscopy. On electron microscopy, there is diffuse epithelial cell foot process effacement and lipid droplets in the cytoplasm of the visceral epithelial cell. The characteristic feature of FSGS is the segmental sclerosis of the glomerular tuft on light microscopy. Immunofluorescence demonstrates the presence of immunoglobulin (Ig) M in the segmentally sclerotic portion of the glomerulus. Electron microscopy shows vacuoles in visceral epithelial cells and focal foot process effacement. Although the majority of childhood nephrotic syndrome is either idiopathic MCNS or idiopathic FSGS, it is still important to recognize that FSGS can, in rare instances, be secondary, associated with obesity, unilateral renal agenesis, glycogen storage disease, postinfectious glomerulonephritis, obstructive uropathy, lupus nephropathy, sickle cell disease, Alport syndrome, and other renal diseases.

In an uncomplicated case of nephrotic syndrome, the proteinuria clears within a few weeks in response to orally administered corticosteroids and renal function is normal; in such children the diagnosis is presumed to be MCNS. If there is no significant proteinuria between relapses and the relapses continue to respond promptly to corticosteroids, the likelihood of this diagnosis is strengthened. If the child is younger than 10 years of age at the initial presentation, renal biopsy need not be considered at this point. In children older than age

TABLE 1 Diagnosis of Nephrotic Syndrome in Childhood

Clinical Diagnostic Criteria	Laboratory Diagnostic Criteria
Generalized edema, ascites, anasarca, because of massive proteinuria Age of onset: 70% MCNS < 5 years of age 50% FSGS ≥ 6 years of age Congenital nephrotic syndrome <12 months of age	**Primary Findings** Proteinuria (>50 mg/kg per day or >2 mg protein per mg creatinine) Hypoalbuminia (≤2 g/dL) Hypercholesterolemia (>200 mg/dL [5.17 mmol/L]) **Secondary Findings** Hypocalcemia (<9 mg/dL [2.25 mmol/L]) Hyperkalemia (>5 mEq/L [5 mmol/L]) Hypernatremia (<136 mEq/L [136 mmol/L]) Hypercoagulability (decreased partial thromboplastin time)

FSGS, focal segmental glomerulosclerosis; MCNS, minimal-change nephrotic syndrome.

TABLE 2 Drug Doses in Treating Nephrotic Syndrome

Medication	Dosage/Route/Regimen	Comments
Steroidal Agents		
Prednisone	2 mg/kg/day orally (maximum, 80 mg/day)	Daily for 6 wk, followed by alternate-day dosing for 6 wk. This 12-wk regimen is more effective than an 8-wk regimen in reducing relapse. Adverse effects: growth retardation, cataracts, osteoporosis.
Methylprednisolone sodium succinate	30 mg/kg/wk intravenously, combined with prednisone 2 mg/kg on alternate days for variable duration according to underlying diseases	In partial steroid-resistant cases, this relatively high-dose regimen may aid in moderating development of FSGS.
Nonsteroidal Agents		
Cyclophosphamide	2 mg/kg/day for 8 wk, prednisone 60 mg/m^2 on alternate days	May induce steroid sensitivity in later relapses. Adverse effects: sterility, bone marrow depression, sepsis, alopecia. To avoid hemorrhagic cystitis, administer medication early in the day and encourage oral fluid intake.
Chlorambucil	0.2 mg/kg/day for 8–12 wk	Same as for cyclophosphamide. Adverse effects as for cyclophosphamide; risk of bone marrow depression may be higher.
Cyclosporine	5 mg/kg/day to maximum 20 mg/kg per day for up to 4 yr	Effectively maintains remission, but relapses occur on discontinuation. Adverse effect: nephrotoxicity.
Levamisole	2.5 mg/kg/day during remissions	May help to maintain remission in steroid-dependent nephritic syndrome.
Angiotensin-converting enzyme Inhibitors	Varies with medication	Renoprotective by reducing glomerular hyperfiltration. Adverse effects: hypotension, cough.
Mizoribine	2 to 5 mg/kg/day for 24 wk	Reduces relapsing nephrotic syndrome. Blocks purine biosynthesis, Inhibits mitogen-stimulated T- and B-cell proliferation. Adverse effect: hyperuricemia.
Mycophenolate mofetil	25 mg/kg/day in 2 divided doses for up to 1 yr	Effective in conjunction with prednisone to control diffuse proliferative lupus nephropathy. Primary adverse effects are gastrointestinal. Generally well tolerated.
Tacrolimus	0.1 mg/kg divided into 2 doses	This macrolide immunosuppressant inhibits CD4 helper cell. Case series with inadequate follow-up period for valid generalization. Randomized controlled clinical trial pending.

FSGS, focal segmental glomerulosclerosis.

10 years, the increasing risk of different histologic diagnosis pushes most pediatric nephrologists to do a kidney biopsy for histologic diagnosis. Should there be poor or no response to steroid treatment (defined as steroid-resistance disease), biopsy should be considered as soon as the patient is medically stable.

Expert Opinion on Management Issues

The International Study of Kidney Disease in Children (ISKDC) showed that most children with MCNS responded to oral corticosteroid therapy initially. The recommended prednisone dose is 2 mg/kg/day, with maximal dose of 80 mg per day (Table 2). The daily dose should be maintained for 4 to 6 weeks. Before starting corticosteroids, a tuberculin skin test should be placed and read. The Arbeitsgemeinschaft für Pädiatrische Nephrologie, a collaborative pediatric nephrology study group in Germany, recommended that the daily dose be kept constant for 6 weeks followed by an alternate-day schedule for an additional 6 weeks (see Table 2). For 98% of children who have an initial onset of MCNS, proteinuria will resolve with prednisone. However, on long-term follow-up, only 60% remain

TABLE 3 Complications of Nephrotic Syndrome in Childhood

Complication	Incidence	Comments
Cellulitis and sepsis	No data	Predisposed to often serious infections caused by immunosuppressive medications, impaired opsonization from renal wastings of factor B, defective T-cell functions. IgG antibody loss in urine, edema, and ascites.
Peritonitis	2%–5%	Pneumococcal vaccination recommended for frequent relapsers; prophylactic varicella zoster immune globulin. During remissions, varicella vaccine.
Thrombosis	13%	Risk factors: dehydration, immobilization, corticosteroid use. Low molecular weight heparin needs to be considered with in-dwelling catheters.
Hyperlipidemia	No data	HMG-CoA-reductase used in adults; adequate data in children lacking.
Miscellaneous	No data	Growth retardation and bone disease from chronic use of corticosteroids; toxicity of cytotoxic medications; hypothyroidism secondary to renal wasting of iodinated proteins. Acute kidney failure from injudicious diuretic use or bilateral renal vein thrombosis.

Ig, immunoglobulin; HMG-CoA, reductase, β-hydroxy–β-methylglutaryl coenzyme A.

either proteinuria-free or have as few as one or two relapses over a 10-year period following initial presentation. The remainder will fall into two categories called steroid-resistant or frequently relapsing nephrotic syndrome. A patient having more than two relapses in any 6-month period is considered to have frequently relapsing nephrotic syndrome. The Southwest Pediatric Nephrology Group (SWPNG) in the United States showed that a relatively longer initial course of corticosteroids provided better prognosis for patients who experienced frequent relapses.

Table 2 lists medications for patients with steroid-resistant or frequently relapsing nephrotic syndrome. The usual choices are cyclophosphamide and chlorambucil, each of which can be used to achieve a remission or to render the steroid-resistant child more steroid-responsive. Either may be used over 6 to 8 weeks, in conjunction with alternate-day prednisone. But more than 50% of patients experience a relapse, usually within 2 years. Cyclosporine can induce remission, but relapse usually occurs on drug discontinuation, unlike the course following chlorambucil and cyclophosphamide. However, the toxicities of cyclophosphamide and chlorambucil have led many pediatric nephrologists to pursue the use of cyclosporine without first trying the two former agents.

The British Association for Paediatric Nephrology showed that levamisole reduced the frequency of relapses in frequently relapsing nephrotic children. Other ongoing studies are examining the efficacy of mizoribine, mycophenolate mofetil, tacrolimus, and angiotensin-converting enzyme (ACE) inhibitors (see Table 2).

Communication and Counseling

One of the important aspects of managing children with idiopathic nephrotic syndrome, especially MCNS, is teaching the family how to test the urine for protein with a dipstick. It is best to use a dipstick that only measures protein to avoid undue concern about other aspects of the urine, such as pH, specific gravity, and so on. By performing frequent urine tests, the family can detect the recurrence of proteinuria that occurs with relapses before the appearance of edema, facilitating early initiation of therapy.

Families also should be counseled about the probable occurrence of relapses. However, the long-term outcome is quite good with children with idiopathic nephrotic syndrome, especially minimal-change disease, even with many relapses. The mortality of children with minimal-change disease is currently less than 5%. When a fatality occurs, the cause is most often infection or thrombotic complications (Table 3). The majority of children with MCNS will eventually stop relapsing, although usually after some years of intermittent episodes, often in puberty or early adulthood. If there are no relapses after 5 years without medication, the likelihood of a future relapse is virtually nil. Additionally, families of nephrotic children should be counseled on having the child avoid salt, especially during relapses. They should be advised to seek medical attention for fever, significant abdominal pain, or signs and symptoms of thrombosis. Because pneumococcus and varicella pose significant risks to nephrotic patients, parents should be counseled to get their children immunized against these pathogens.

Focal Segmental Glomerulosclerosis

The second most common cause of idiopathic nephrotic syndrome in children is FSGS. Previously, FSGS was thought to account for less than 10% of children with idiopathic nephrotic syndrome, but more recent studies suggest that the prevalence of this disease is now higher, accounting for as many as 40% of children with idiopathic nephrotic syndrome. This epidemiology is especially true for African American children with idiopathic nephrotic syndrome. The diagnosis of FSGS can only be made definitively with a renal biopsy. Therefore, a fraction of children with FSGS who respond to steroids will be missed because they would not usually undergo a biopsy.

Patients with FSGS usually present with nephrotic syndrome, although some patients have only asymptomatic proteinuria. Individual patients with FSGS cannot be clinically distinguished from those with MCNS, except that FSGS patients as a group have a higher incidence of concomitant hematuria, hypertension, and progression to renal failure. They also have a much greater incidence of steroid resistance.

Expert Opinion on Management Issues

Steroids with and without Cytotoxic Drugs

Only approximately 20% to 30% of children with FSGS will respond to a 4-week course of 2 mg/kg/day of prednisone. The lack of a clinical response to steroids thus brings 70% to 80% of children with FSGS to attention, and many are biopsied because they have failed to respond to glucocorticoids. Combining cyclophosphamide with prednisone appears to add no further benefit. A prolonged oral course of steroids for 4 to 8 months, in combination with cyclophosphamide or azathioprine, had a 44% response rate in children and 39% in adults in one study. Mendoza and colleagues, in an uncontrolled trial using a prolonged course of high-dose (30 mg/kg) intravenous methylprednisolone in combination with alternate-day oral prednisone and in some cases with 8 to 12 weeks of cyclophosphamide or chlorambucil, achieved a complete remission rate of 50% (Table 4). However, the patients involved had serious side effects including cataracts, seizures, hypertension, aseptic necrosis of the hip, and infections. Several subsequent smaller studies of intravenous methylprednisolone have reported similar response rates. However, not all have been so sanguine about this approach.

Calcineurin Inhibitors

In a number of uncontrolled studies, cyclosporine has been observed to be highly effective in patients who were initially steroid-responsive; remission rates as high as 80% have been reported. In a controlled trial of cyclosporine (6mg/kg/day) for 6 months in 25 children with steroid-resistant FSGS, all cyclosporine-treated patients had a significant reduction in proteinuria (by 70%), although those who received placebo had

no change. Thirty-three percent of the treated group had a complete remission and 67% had a partial remission. There was no difference in the decline in glomerular filtration rate between the two groups. A retrospective study of African American children with FSGS treated with cyclosporine for a mean period of 27 months had 24% rate of end-stage renal disease (ESRD) as compared to an historical control group who had an ESRD rate of 78% after 8 years. However, 50% of children with nephrotic syndrome treated with cyclosporine for up to 5 years had progression of tubulointerstitial fibrosis in one study.

Only limited data are available concerning the use of tacrolimus in children with FSGS, and no controlled trials have been published. Proteinuria decreased by 50% in the few children with FSGS treated with tacrolimus, and some experienced a complete remission.

Mycophenolate Mofetil

The use of mycophenolate mofetil (MMF) has been reported in only a few children with FSGS, and there are no controlled trials concerning its use. MMF is attractive, because it is an immunosuppressive medication free of nephrotoxicity and adverse renal hemodynamic effects. MMF was effective in reducing the proteinuria in most of the children.

Angiotensin-Converting Enzyme Inhibitors and Angiotensin Receptor Blockers

Angiotensin-converting enzyme (ACE) inhibitors have been successfully used in children with steroid-resistant FSGS to reduce proteinuria. They have been shown to slow the decline in renal function in adults with FSGS, but these studies have not been done in children. Similarly, angiotensin receptor blockers (ARB) have been shown to reduce proteinuria, but only a few children have been studied.

Common Pitfalls

The diagnosis of FSGS can only be made with a renal biopsy. Some patients with FSGS will initially respond to oral steroids and appear to have minimal-change disease only to develop steroid resistance and be found to have FSGS later. Some caution should be exercised in counseling a family about the prognosis of idiopathic nephrotic syndrome until the patient has shown that the nephrotic syndrome remains steroid-responsive for several years.

Although intravenous steroids and calcineurin inhibitors have been effective in some patients in inducing a complete or partial remission, most of these patients have relapsed when the treatment course has been stopped. Many patients continue to lose renal function over time despite improvement in their proteinuria and symptoms with treatment.

All of the agents used to treat nephrotic syndrome have significant side effects. High-dose steroids have

TABLE 4 Mendoza IV Methylprednisolone* Protocol	
Week	**Interval**
Weeks 1 & 2	3 times/week
Weeks 3–10	Weekly
Weeks 11–18	Every other week
Weeks 19–54	Monthly
Weeks 54–80	Every other month

*30 mg/kg to maximum dose of 1 g.
Adapted from Lieberman KV, Tejani A: A randomized double-blind placebo-controlled trial of cyclosporine in steroid-resistant idiopathic focal segmental glomerulosclerosis in children. J Am Soc Nephrol 7:56–63, 1996.

been associated with aseptic necrosis of the hip, in addition to obesity, hypertension, hyperglycemia, and other side effects associated with steroids. Both cyclosporine and tacrolimus have been associated with renal interstitial fibrosis. Cyclosporine is more likely than tacrolimus to cause gingival hyperplasia and hirsutism, although tacrolimus is more likely to cause diabetes. Both cyclophosphamide and chlorambucil are toxic to the gonads and increase the risk of cancer. Cyclophosphamide can cause hemorrhagic cystitis and chlorambucil seizures. All of these agents increase the risk of a serious infection.

Communication and Counseling

The optimal therapy for children with steroid-resistant FSGS has not been clearly demonstrated. Most experts would treat with an ACE inhibitor, an ARB, or a combination of the two to reduce the proteinuria, potentially slow the decline in renal function, and treat the hypertension that often accompanies FSGS. Additionally, they would use either high-dose intravenous methylprednisolone or a calcineurin inhibitor. Parents and patients with FSGS should be counseled about the likelihood of renal failure with time and the possibility of recurrence in the transplanted kidney.

SUGGESTED READINGS

1. Benchimol C: Focal and segmental glomerulosclerosis: Pathogenesis and treatment. Curr Opinion Ped 15:171–180, 2003. **Review of focal segmental glomerulosclerosis.**
2. British Association for Paediatric Nephrology. Levamisole for corticosteroid dependent nephrotic syndrome in childhood. Lancet 337:1555–1557, 1991. **Paper that suggests that levamisole might be a therapy for steroid-dependent nephrotic syndrome.**
3. Eddy AA: Nephrotic syndrome in childhood. Lancet 362:629–639, 2003. **Detailed review of the subject.**
4. Ehrich JH, Brodehl J: Long versus standard prednisone therapy for initial treatment of idiopathic nephrotic syndrome in children: Arbeitsgemeinschaft für Pädiatrische Nephrologie. Eur J Pediatr, 152:357–61, 1993. **Signal paper that established some issues about length of steroid therapy.**
5. Garin EH, Orak JK, Hiott KL, Sutherland SE: Cyclosporine therapy for steroid resistant nephrotic syndrome. A controlled study. Am J Dis Child 142:985–988, 1988. **Controlled trial on cyclosporine in children with nephrotic syndrome.**
6. Gellermann J, Querfeld U: Frequently relapsing nephrotic syndrome: Treatment with mycophenolate mofetil. Pediatr Nephrol 19:101–104, 2004. **Paper suggesting that mycophenolate mofetil may be useful in frequent relapsers.**
7. Gulati S, Sharma AP, Sharma RK, et al: Do current recommendations for kidney biopsy in nephrotic syndrome need modifications? Pediatr Nephrol 17:404–408, 2002. **Discussion of issues around biopsy in childhood nephrotic syndrome.**
8. Honda M: Nephrotic syndrome mizoribine in children. Ped Int 2002;44:210–216, 2002. **Paper suggesting that mizoribine might have a role in nephrotic syndrome.**
9. International Study of Kidney Disease in Children. Nephrotic syndrome in children: Prediction of histopathology from clinical and laboratory characteristics at time of diagnosis. Kidney Int 13:159–65, 1978. **Landmark paper that established characteristics of childhood nephrotic syndrome.**
10. International Study of Kidney Disease in Children. The primary nephrotic syndrome in children. Identification of patients with minimal change nephrotic syndrome from initial response to prednisone. J Pediatr 1981;98:561–564, 1981. **Another landmark paper from the International Study of Kidney Disease in Children (ISKDC) about childhood nephrotic syndrome.**
11. Lama G, Luongo I, Piscitelli A, Salsano ME: Enalapril: Antiproteinuric effect in children with nephrotic syndrome. Clin Nephrol 53(6):432–436, 2000. **One of several papers showing that angiotensin-converting enzyme inhibitors may be useful in nephrotic syndrome.**
12. Lande MB, Gullion C, Hogg RJ, et al: Long versus standard initial steroid therapy for children with the nephrotic syndrome. A report from the Southwest Pediatric Nephrology Study Group. Pediatr Nephrol 18:342–346, 2003. **Signal paper that established some issues about length of steroid therapy.**
13. Lieberman KV, Tejani A: A randomized double-blind placebo-controlled trial of cyclosporine in steroid-resistant idiopathic focal segmental glomerulosclerosis in children. J Am Soc Nephrol 7:56–63, 1996. **A randomized, controlled, double-blind trial of cyclosporine in FSGS.**
14. Loeffler K, Gowrishankar M, Yiu V: Tacrolimus therapy in pediatric patients with treatment-resistant nephrotic syndrome. Pediatr Nephrol 19:281–287, 2004. **Paper suggesting that tacrolimus might be useful in nephrotic syndrome.**
15. Mendoza SA, Reznik VM, Griswold WR, et al: Treatment of steroid resistant focal segmental glomerulosclerosis with pulse methylprednisolone and alkylating agents. Pediatr Nephrol 4:303–307, 1990. **Paper that presented the pulse methylprednisolone approach to treating FSGS.**
16. Pei Y, Cattran D, Delmore T, et al: Evidence suggesting undertreatment in adults with idiopathic focal segmental glomerulosclerosis. Regional glomerulonephritis registry study. Amer J Med 82:938–944, 1987. **Paper discusses longer therapy in both adults in children.**
17. Prasad N, Gulati S, Sharma RK, et al: Pulse cyclophosphamide therapy in steroid-dependent nephrotic syndrome. Pediatr Nephrol 19:494–498, 2004. **Recent paper about use of pulses of cyclophosphamide.**
18. Roth KS, Amaker BH, Chan JCM: Nephrotic syndrome: Pathogenesis and management. Pediatr Rev 23:237–248, 2002. **Accessible review.**
19. Srivastava T, Simon SD, Alon US: High incidence of focal segmental glomerulo-sclerosis in nephrotic syndrome in childhood. Pediatr Nephrol 13:13–18, 1999. **Paper describing changing incidence in FSGS.**
20. Vester U, Kranz B, Zimmermann S, et al: Cyclophosphamide in steroid-sensitive nephrotic syndrome: outcome and outlook. Pediatr Nephrol 18:661–664, 2003. **Recent paper on the use of cyclophosphamide.**

11

Renal Tubulopathies

Alex R. Constantinescu

KEY CONCEPTS

- Suspect renal tubular disorders in children with electrolyte disorders or acidemia.
- Suspect renal tubular disorders in children with failure to thrive.
- Suspect renal tubular disorders in children with rickets or metabolic bone disease.
- Treat based on the specific disorder.

The composition of the urine is determined by the function of transporter and channel proteins residing on the urinary and blood membrane domains of renal tubular epithelial cells, mediating reabsorptive and secretory processes, based on homeostatic needs. As a result, the proximal tubule normally reabsorbs more than 70% of the filtered load of sodium (Na), water, glucose, phosphate, amino acids, and other electrolytes and solutes. The loop of Henle is involved in the concentration and dilution of the tubular fluid. Distal nephron segments, including the distal convoluted tubule and the mineralocorticoid-sensitive collecting duct, contribute to the final renal regulation of salt, water, and acid–base balance.

The group of disorders that have in common the abnormal function of these membrane proteins are described by the term *renal tubulopathies*, implying lack of reabsorption, secretion, or both of ions or solutes. Inadequate reabsorption leads to "spilling" of a particular substance into the urine (e.g., glucose or renal glucosuria). Absence of tubular secretion results in retention of that substance, sometimes to life-threatening levels (e.g., severe hyperkalemia). Tubulopathies can be primary (genetic) or secondary (because of toxins, drugs, or as part of a systemic illness). In the last 15 years, most renal tubular transporters have been characterized at molecular and functional levels, along with their encoding genes and disease-causing mutations, and we currently have a better understanding of their role in the pathophysiology of various tubulopathies than about their interactions and regulation. This chapter briefly reviews the presentation and pathophysiology of the most common primary proximal and distal tubulopathies (Box 1), with emphasis on key concepts and specific therapeutic strategies, most evidence-based.

BOX 1 Renal Tubulopathies
Primary
Proximal
■ Proximal RTA
■ Fanconi syndrome
■ Renal hypophosphatemic rickets
■ Aminoacidurias
■ Glucosuria
Distal
■ Bartter syndrome
■ Gitelman syndrome
■ Hypercalciuria
■ Distal RTA
■ Nephrogenic diabetes insipidus
■ Pseudohypoaldosteronism
Secondary
■ Drug-induced
■ Sickle cell disease
■ Obstruction
■ Immune-mediated disease
■ Amyloid
■ Myeloma and monoclonal gammopathy
RTA, renal tubular acidosis.

Proximal Renal Tubular Disorders
PROXIMAL RENAL TUBULAR ACIDOSIS

KEY CONCEPTS

■ Suspect proximal renal tubular acidosis when hyperchloremic normal anion-gap metabolic acidosis is noted, in absence of diarrhea, urinary diversion, or acetazolamide therapy.

■ Confirm with venous blood gas revealing metabolic acidosis with acidic urine pH, rising above 6.5 at values of serum bicarbonate (HCO_3^-) concentration below normal for age.

■ Evaluate for possible associated causes, such as cystinosis.

■ Treatment consists of correction of the acidosis with alkali.

Urinary acidification is achieved by two major processes: reabsorption of bicarbonate (HCO_3^-) and secretion of protons (H^+). The inability to reabsorb the filtered HCO_3^- completely leads to proximal renal tubular acidosis (pRTA, also called type II RTA), whereas a limited capacity for H^+ secretion leads to distal renal tubular acidosis (dRTA, also called type I RTA). Both types of RTA are characterized by a hyperchloremic, normal anion-gap metabolic acidosis. At times, it is difficult to diagnose the defect and its location, because of significant overlap (i.e., transient HCO_3^- wasting in dRTA). An abnormal Na^+/H^+ exchanger, Na^+/HCO_3^- cotransporter, and carbonic anhydrase isoforms have been implicated in etiology of pRTA, which can occur as an isolated disorder, or as part of Fanconi syndrome. New evidence points toward a role for a potassium (K^+) channel called TASK2 in proximal tubule HCO_3^- transport (features of isolated pRTA are noted in knockout mouse models).

Three categories of isolated pRTA have been identified:

1. Autosomal-dominant pRTA (caused by mutations in *SLC9A3*, a gene encoding one of the five plasma membrane Na^+/H^+ exchangers, called *NHE3*).
2. Autosomal-recessive pRTA with ocular abnormalities (caused by mutations in the kidney type Na^+/HCO_3^- cotransporter [kNBC1] gene, *SLC4A4*).
3. Sporadic isolated pRTA. Mutations in carbonic anhydrase II gene lead to osteopetrosis, RTA (pRTA, dRTA, or both), cerebral calcification, and mental retardation.

Expert Opinion on Management Issues

Limited proximal tubular $NaHCO_3$ reabsorption results in polyuria, with subsequent volume depletion and hypokalemia. Patients usually present with growth retardation in infancy or early childhood, failure to thrive, metabolic acidosis without apparent cause (sepsis, diarrhea, or uretero-sigmoidostomy). To confirm the metabolic acidosis, a venous blood gas simultaneous with a urine pH should be obtained. The next step in management involves establishing whether the pRTA is isolated or is part of a complex tubulopathy (e.g., Fanconi syndrome).

The goal of therapy is to provide adequate alkali to restore the normal serum tCO_2 concentration, correct the associated metabolic abnormalities, and promote weight gain and normal growth. This can be achieved by the administration of sodium bicarbonate, or sodium or potassium citrate (Table 1). Polycitra is preferred over Bicitra for patients with hypokalemia, whereas Bicitra is preferred in patients with hyperkalemia. The therapeutic dose varies and can be as high as 5 to 10 mEq/kg/day. It is prudent to initiate treatment with a lower dose and titrate as appropriate.

Common Pitfalls

Reliance on routine biochemical testing for diagnostic evaluation results in overdiagnosis of RTA. Evaluation for RTA should not be performed during an acute illness. Instead, acid–base balance should be evaluated after recovery from an acute gastrointestinal or other illness.

Many children do not find the necessary medication palatable. Palatability can be improved by chilling the solution at $39.2°F$ $(4°C)$. Additionally, caution must be exercised in patients with renal dysfunction, who may not tolerate a supplemental potassium (K^+) load. Frequent monitoring is required, because other electrolyte abnormalities can occur.

Communication and Counseling

Autosomal-dominant and autosomal-recessive pRTA are usually permanent tubular defects, requiring lifelong alkali therapy. In contrast, sporadic isolated pRTA is transient, and alkali therapy may be discontinued after several years, without reappearance of symptoms.

DISTAL RENAL TUBULAR ACIDOSIS

> **KEY CONCEPTS**
>
> - Suspect distal renal tubular acidosis in patients with failure to thrive, urinary tract anomalies, or kidney stones.
> - Confirm the diagnosis with venous blood gas (metabolic acidosis) and elevated urine pH.
> - Evaluate citrate and calcium excretion, and other organ involvement.
> - Treat the cause, and initiate early alkali therapy.

Distal tubule cells actively extrude hydrogen ion (H^+) into the urine, creating a steep pH gradient between the urine and blood. Autosomal-dominant and autosomal-recessive forms of dRTA are caused by mutations in ion transporters of the acid-secreting Type A intercalated cell of the renal collecting duct. These include the anion exchanger (AE), Cl^-/HCO_3^- exchanger of the basolateral membrane, and at least two subunits of the apical membrane vacuolar $(v)H^+$-ATPase. (Although this is a distal disorder, it is discussed here, so that the reader will have both major forms of RTA to read together.)

Expert Opinion on Management Issues

Patients with dRTA, like those with pRTA, present with failure to thrive, polyuria, and episodes of dehydration. Distal RTA is characterized by the same normal anion gap metabolic acidosis, with normal or low serum K. However, it can be distinguished from the pRTA by the persistent urine pH above 6.5 to 7, even at low serum bicarbonate levels. Additionally, it is associated with hypercalciuria and hypocitraturia, predisposing these patients to nephrocalcinosis and kidney stone formation.

Evaluation of patients suspected of having dRTA should include urinary calcium-to-creatinine ratio (normal <0.2 in older children and adults, <0.6 in infants) and citrate-to-creatinine ratio (normal >0.2). Patients with dRTA require less alkali (1 to 2 mEq/kg/24 hours as bicarbonate or citrate) to buffer the endogenous acid production, than do those with pRTA.

Common Pitfalls

It is important to evaluate the patient for possible urinary malformations or parenchymal abnormalities that can be associated with dRTA (i.e., obstructive uropathy, renal dysplasia). Once alkali therapy is initiated, frequent monitoring of the acid–base balance is important for dose adjustment, to allow optimal growth, and to prevent urolithiasis.

Communication and Counseling

Patients and families need to be made aware of drug interactions and complications of therapy. Once informed about the fact that restoration of normal acid–base balance generally allows patients to grow, normalizes bone mineralization, and minimizes stone formation, patients do tend to have a better compliance with therapy.

Some patients with dRTA have associated high-frequency hearing loss, and it is important to screen affected children.

TABLE 1 Replacement Therapies

Generic Name (Trade Name)	Dosage/Route/Regimen	Maximum Dose	Dosage Formulation	Common Adverse Reactions	Therapeutic Concentrations	Comments
Sodium bicarbonate (NaHCO$_3$)	2–5 mEq HCO$_3$ equivalent/kg/day, PO, in 3–4 divided doses in pRTA, and 1–2 mEq HCO$_3$ equivalent/kg/day, PO, in 3–4 divided doses in dRTA	10 mEq HCO$_3$ equivalent/kg/day.	650 mg tablets, or made as oral solution.	Fluid retention, hypertension, flatulence.	NaHCO$_3$ (1 g = 12 mEq Na and 12 mEq HCO$_3$)	
Citrate (Bicitra, Polycitra, Polycitra-K)		Same as above.	In mEq, Bicitra = 1 Na, 1 citrate; Polycitra = 1 Na, 1 K, 2 citrate; Polycitra K = 2 K, 2 citrate	Citrate preparations can act as laxatives.		Oral liquid preparations should be diluted in water or fruit juice, prior to administration.
Potassium (KCl, or K gluconate)	1–4 mEq/kg/day, PO, q6-12h	4 mEq/kg/day.		GI irritation, ulcerations.	Avoid in patients with renal insufficiency.	
Sodium (NaCl, NaHCO$_3$)	2–8 mEq/kg/day, PO, tid-qid dosing	Titrate to effect.	Oral solutions or tablets	Edema, hypertension.		
Phospha (NeutraPhos, NeutraPhos K)	30–90 mg PO 4/kg/day, PO, tid dosing	Titrate to effect.		Nausea, diarrhea, abdominal pain, tetany, hyperphosphatemia, hyperkalemia, hypocalcemia.	One packet = 250 mg PO4, 7 mEq Na, 7 mEq K	Monitor calcium and phosphate levels to titrate dose.
Magnesium	5–10 mg Mg oxide salt/kg/day, PO (as supplement), or 65–130 Mg oxide salt/kg/day, PO, q6h (in hypomagnesemia)	Titrate to effect and depending on tolerability.	Mg oxide 400 mg	Diarrhea.	1 tablet = 241 mg elemental Mg	Monitor magnesium levels.
Calcium (calcium carbonate, gluconate, acetate)	Neonate: 50–150 mg elemental Ca/kg/day, PO/IV, q4-6h Child: 20–65 mg elemental calcium/kg/day, PO/IV, q4-6h	1 g per day in neonates, 4 g per day in children with normal renal function.	Calcium carbonate suspension, 1250 mg/L or tablets of 500 or 650 mg per tablet	Constipation, hypercalcemia, hypercalciuria, hypophosphatemia.	1 g = 20 mEq or 400 mg elemental calcium	Monitor calcium and phosphate levels.
Vitamin D analogues	Rocaltrol—0.01–0.05 µg/kg/day; DHT—0.05–0.1 mg/24 hr in neonates, and 0.5–1.5 mg/24 hr in children	Titrate to effect.	Rocaltrol 0.25 or 0.5 µg capsules DHT–capsule: 0.125 mg Solution: 0.2mg/mL (concentrate, 20% alcohol) Tablet: 0.125, 0.2, 0.4 mg	Weakness, headaches, vomiting, constipation, hypotonia, polyuria, polydipsia, metastatic calcifications.		Monitor serum calcium and phosphorus.

DHT, dihydrotachysterol; dRTA, distal renal tubular acidosis; GI, gastrointestinal; IV, intravenously; Mg, magnesium; PO, orally; pRTA, proximal renal tubular acidosis; RTA, renal tubular acidosis; qid, four times a day; tid, three times a day.

FANCONI SYNDROME

> ## KEY CONCEPTS
>
> - Suspect Fanconi syndrome in patients with failure to thrive.
> - Confirm by the presence of generalized proximal tubulopathy.
> - Evaluate for primary or secondary causes (Box 2).
> - Treatment depends on the cause.

Fanconi syndrome is a relatively rare tubulopathy characterized by a *generalized* dysregulation of proximal tubule reabsorption. Patients with this disorder exhibit urinary losses of sodium and water, bicarbonate, phosphate, glucose, amino acids, potassium, calcium, and low molecular weight proteins. They usually present with failure to thrive, polyuria and volume depletion, metabolic acidosis (resulting from pRTA), hypokalemia, hypercalciuria, glucosuria, and generalized aminoaciduria. Hypophosphatemic rickets is common as well.

Expert Opinion on Management Issues

The most common primary cause of Fanconi syndrome is *cystinosis*, an autosomal-recessive lysosomal storage disorder, caused by mutations in the gene for cystinosis (*CTNS*) (with regional differences). The gene encoding cystinosin (a protein involved in the transport of cystine out of the lysosomes) is located on chromosome 17. Accumulation of cystine in the proximal tubular cell lysosomes causes significant impairment in these cell transport functions. The clinical manifestations include renal tubular Fanconi syndrome in the first year of life, in addition to growth retardation, hypothyroidism, photophobia, progressive deterioration in renal function by 10 years of age (less with therapy), and late complications such as myopathy, pancreatic insufficiency, and retinal blindness.

A similar accumulation of a toxic metabolite prevails in hereditary fructose intolerance (fructose–6-phosphate), galactosemia (galactose), Wilson disease (copper), and glycogen storage disease (glycogen metabolites). Proximal tubulopathy is the most common presentation of mitochondrial cytopathies, which result from deranged oxidative phosphorylation and cell energy production. A similar mechanism can be postulated in drug (chronic ifosfamide nephrotoxicity) or heavy metal toxicities. Fanconi syndrome may also arise in the context of immune-mediated disorders, involving antibodies directed against proximal tubular antigens.

Treatment of the biochemical abnormalities characteristic of Fanconi syndrome is targeted at replacing the substrates lost in urine. Table 1 provides dosing guidelines. Specific treatments are available for some of the underlying causes of the syndrome. For instance, in cystinosis, therapy with cysteamine (1.3 g/m^2/day, orally, divided in four doses) lowers the cell content of cystine and forestalls many complications. Cysteamine eye drops prevent accumulation of cysteine in the cornea as well. Angiotensin-converting enzyme (ACE) inhibitor therapy diminishes albuminuria in patients with cystinosis and might be used in these patients to slow the progression of renal insufficiency attributed to proteinuria. Growth velocity rate must be monitored, and growth hormone therapy should be initiated early, to achieve catch-up growth.

The specific treatment for fructose intolerance and galactosemia consists of dietary modifications.

BOX 2 Causes of Fanconi Syndrome
Primary
- Cystinosis
- Lowe syndrome
- Hereditary fructose intolerance
- Galactosemia
- Wilson disease
- Glycogen storage disease
- Idiopathic (familial or sporadic)
- Mitochondrial myopathies
Secondary
- Immune-mediated tubulopathies
- Drug toxicity
- Heavy metals toxicity
- Hydrocarbon toxicity
- Hyperparathyroidism
- Vitamin D deficiency
- Multiple myeloma
- Amyloidosis

Common Pitfalls

The success of therapy in a child with renal Fanconi syndrome is based on adequate adherence of the patient with the medications, and monitoring metabolic parameters. Failure to monitor frequently results in unexpected morbidity caused by electrolyte imbalances, and early diagnosis and intervention are essential. It is clear that in cystinosis, the earlier and more consistently cysteamine is administered, the better the outcome.

Communication and Counseling

Despite good compliance, some patients with cystinosis progress to end-stage renal disease (ESRD), although most do well after renal transplantation. However, the extrarenal manifestations (ocular, thyroid, gastrointestinal, and short stature) require continuing therapy even after renal transplant.

RENAL HYPOPHOSPHATEMIC RICKETS

KEY CONCEPTS

- Suspect renal hypophosphatemic rickets in patients with bone deformities and short stature associated with hypophosphatemia.
- Confirm by low tubular reabsorption of phosphate (1-fractional excretion of phosphate, <85%).
- Evaluate possibility of associated abnormalities (hyperparathyroidism [HPTH], hypercalcemia, growth rate, etc.).
- Treatment includes phosphate supplementation, vitamin D, and growth hormone.

Hypophosphatemic rickets comprises a group of disorders characterized by phosphaturia, hypophosphatemia, vitamin D resistance, and rachitic bone changes. There is evidence for a hormone/enzyme/extracellular matrix pathway involved in renal phosphate handling, and research is under way to better understand phosphate homeostasis and mineralization, allowing for improvement in the diagnosis and treatment of hypo- and hyperphosphatemic disorders.

Expert Opinion on Management Issues

The most common of these disorders is X-linked hypophosphatemic rickets. Typically, patients with this disorder have normal vitamin D levels, normal parathyroid hormone levels, and normal serum calcium. Untreated older children and adults present with short stature, dental alterations, and bone deformities including bowed legs and hip and back disorders.

Patients with this disorder were found to have mutations in the *PHEX* gene (phosphate-regulating gene with homologies to endopeptidases on the X chromosome). Its product inhibits phosphatonin, a hormone that under normal conditions stimulates renal phosphate reabsorption via NaP$_i$ cotransporter (located at the apical membrane of the proximal tubule). Phosphatonin also inhibits the activity of renal 24-hydroxylase, thereby decreasing the degradation of 1,25-dihydroxy-vitamin D. Based on this mechanism, a PHEX mutation leads to inhibition of phosphate reabsorption, renal phosphate wasting, and increased clearance of 1,25-dihydroxy vitamin D. Autosomal-dominant hypophosphatemic rickets (ADHR) is caused by gain of function mutations in the gene encoding for the fibroblast growth factor 23 (FGF-23). The mutated cleavage site leads to higher concentration of FGF-23, causing phosphaturia and hypophosphatemia, high vitamin D levels, normal or low parathyroid hormone (PTH), high serum calcium, and hypercalciuria. Phenotypically, ADHR is not significantly different than the X-linked hypophosphatemic rickets (XLHR).

Phosphate supplementation is the key, limited by the appearance of diarrhea and tertiary hyperparathyroidism (HPTH; caused by prolonged very high-dose oral inorganic phosphate [P$_i$] treatment). Hypertension, noted in few treated XLH children, is closely associated with HPTH. Emphasis should therefore be placed on prevention of HPTH as a complication of XLH treatment, and close monitoring for hypertension in those who do develop it.

Common Pitfalls

Oral intake of phosphate can diminish the intestinal calcium absorption, and it is not uncommon for these patients to require calcium supplementation and vitamin D. However, it is important to recognize nephrocalcinosis early, because it can complicate the disease course with hyposthenuria, urolithiasis, and chronic renal insufficiency, with no improvement in final adult height.

Communication and Counseling

Patients must be made aware of the potential complications of therapy, the need for frequent monitoring, and the benefits of therapy with growth hormone (dose of 0.05 mg/kg, daily subcutaneous injections). However, one has to monitor the potential exaggeration of disproportionate truncal growth in prepubertal patients.

AMINOACIDURIAS

KEY CONCEPTS

- Suspect aminoacidurias in failure to thrive, kidney stones, or when a tubulopathy was already diagnosed.
- Diagnose with reverse-phase high-performance liquid chromatography (RP-HPLC) method (age-related reference intervals available), or by stone composition or cystine excretion.
- Evaluate for additional tubulopathies.
- Treatment depends on cause.

Essentially all amino acids (95%) filtered by the glomerulus are reabsorbed via Na-dependent specific transporters in the proximal tubule. Inappropriate urinary losses of amino acids are because of defects in isolated (cystinuria and methioninuria) or charge-specific group (neutral, acidic, or basic) amino acid transporters.

The genes encoding some of these transporters have been identified, improving our understanding of the molecular aspects of renal amino-acid transport. The *SLC7* gene family is divided into two subgroups, the cationic amino acid transporters (the CAT family, SLC7A1-4) and the glycoprotein-associated amino acid transporters (the gpaAT family, SLC7A5-11), also called light chains or catalytic chains of the hetero(di)meric amino acid transporters (HATs). The associated glycoproteins (heavy chains) form the SLC3 family. Members of the CAT family transport essentially cationic amino acids by facilitated diffusion with differential trans-stimulation by intracellular substrates. The HATs are, in contrast, quite diverse in terms of substrate selectivity and function (mostly) as obligatory exchangers. Their selectivity includes large neutral amino acids (system L), small neutral amino acids (Ala-, Ser-, Cys-preferring), negatively charged amino acid [system x(c)(-)], and cationic amino acids plus neutral amino acids [system y(+)L and b(0,+)-like]. Cotransport of Na^+ is observed only for the y(+)L transporters when they carry neutral amino acids. Mutations in b(0,+)-like and y(+)L transporters lead to the hereditary diseases cystinuria and lysinuric protein intolerance (LPI), respectively.

Expert Opinion on Management Issues

Cystinuria, the most common aminoaciduria (incidence approximately 1:7,000 live births), is an autosomal-recessive disorder, which can occur as a result of an isolated defect, or as part of a defect in the transport of all four dibasic amino acids (cystine, lysine, arginine, and ornithine). The human gene for this transporter resides on chromosome 2, and most cystinuric patients have mutations in four exons of both *SLC3A1* and *SLC7A9* genes. The patients are prone to cystine stone formation, because of the insolubility of cystine in aqueous solutions.

Presentation is usually in the second or third decade of life, with renal colic, urinary tract infection, or urinary obstruction, although children with fully recessive (Type I/I) cystinuria have a high risk of stone formation in the first decade of life. The cystine stones represent approximately 8% of all renal stones in children. Examination of the first morning urine allows the identification of characteristic hexagonal cystine crystals, and confirmation is made by quantitating cystine excretion.

The treatment goal is to reduce urinary cystine concentration or increase its solubility. To dilute urinary cystine, patients must drink large amounts of fluids to maintain cystine concentration below 250 mg/L. Reduction of cystine secretion is not yet feasible. To increase its solubility, urine should be alkalinized (pH > 7.5) by oral administration of citrate or sodium bicarbonate (see Table 1). Reduction in dietary methionine, an essential amino acid precursor of cystine, is impractical. If patients continue to form stones, despite conservative management, drug therapy with agents containing free sulfhydryl groups remains an option. These agents, which form thiosulfide bonds with cystine, thereby increasing its solubility, include D-penicillamine and tiopronin. However, their use is associated with a high degree of toxicity: patients develop nephrotic syndrome, pancytopenia, rash, and arthralgia. Patients on D-penicillamine require supplementation of pyridoxine. A low-sodium diet is a helpful adjuvant to the agents described above. Captopril has a free sulfhydryl group; however, its use did not prove to be effective.

Common Pitfalls

Unfortunately, only a small percentage of patients with cystinuria are able to achieve and maintain the goal of decreasing cystine below the saturation concentration, and it appears that those with better insight into their own disease have a better compliance. Greater physician vigilance in complicated stone formers is required to achieve successful prophylactic management, and the cystine crystal volume, in addition to urine pH and specific gravity, was suggested to monitor the compliance and efficacy of therapy (cystine crystal volume $[V_{cys}] > 3000$ micro^3/mm^3 being the threshold risk value). Attention must be paid to the possibility of rebound aciduria (seen with poor compliance to treatment), and increased risk of calcium oxalate stones.

Communication and Counseling

Patients with symptomatic or obstructing stones may require lithotripsy or surgical therapy. Emphasis should be placed on preservation of renal function. However, contemporary medical prophylaxis may be ineffective, and repeated surgical interventions, infections, and obstructions can lead to renal insufficiency. For those with ESRD, renal transplant can be a successful alternative.

GRACILE (*g*rowth *r*etardation, *a*minoaciduria, *c*holestasis, *i*ron overload, *l*actic acidosis, *e*arly death) syndrome is transmitted in autosomal-recessive fashion. Prenatal diagnosis is available for families with these children. Aminoaciduria involving many amino acids is common for patients with different traumatic injuries, and is correlated with a reduction of the total serum calcium concentration (reasons not yet clear).

RENAL GLUCOSURIA

> **KEY CONCEPTS**
> - Suspect renal glucosuria when glucosuria is found incidentally.
> - Confirm when glucosuria is associated with normal serum glucose.
> - Evaluate for associated tubular transport abnormalities.
> - Reassure family of good long-term outcome of isolated glucosuria, without therapy.

Glucose transport in the proximal convoluted tubule and intestine is mediated by Na-dependent glucose transporters, located at the luminal membrane (SGLT1 and SGLT2), and Na-independent ones (GLUT1 and GLUT2), located at the basolateral membrane of these cells. Primary renal glucosuria is a benign condition in which serum glucose level is normal.

Expert Opinion on Management Issues

Renal glucosuria can be isolated (because of mutations in the genes encoding for SGLT transporters), part of Fanconi syndrome, associated with hypercalciuria, or associated with selective aminoaciduria (arginine, carnosine, and taurine). Additionally, cases were described in which renal glucosuria was transient, as seen in patients with acute pyelonephritis, or briefly after initiation of ACE inhibitor therapy for renovascular hypertension.

Mutations in the gene encoding for SGLT1 cause the rare glucose-galactose malabsorption syndrome (mild renal glucosuria, explosive diarrhea following ingestion of sugar or milk, failure to thrive, episodes of dehydration).

Mutations in the *SLC5A2* gene, encoding for the SGLT2, have been identified as responsible for renal glucosuria (both homo- and heterozygous states). These mutations cause a more severe degree of glucosuria, patients being identified by isolated glucosuria at a routine urinalysis, or during an acute illness. They have no history of polyuria, polydipsia, or weight loss, as seen in diabetes mellitus; the fasting serum glucose and oral glucose tolerance tests are normal.

Common Pitfalls

It is important to explore associated tubular defects, such as phosphaturia and aminoaciduria, because these may have developmental implications.

Communication and Counseling

Isolated renal glucosuria requires no treatment, and the long-term prognosis of these patients is excellent.

Distal Renal Tubular Disorders

BARTTER AND GITELMAN SYNDROMES

KEY CONCEPTS

- Suspect Bartter or Gitelman syndrome when hypokalemic metabolic alkalosis is noted.
- Confirm with elevated urinary chloride, sodium, and potassium losses.
- Differentiate between types based on urinary calcium and magnesium excretion.
- Treat according to type and biochemical abnormality.
- Monitor fluid intake, kidney function, development of nephrocalcinosis, and growth rate.

Sodium chloride is reabsorbed in the thick ascending limb of Henle (TALH), by a bumetanide-sensitive sodium-potassium-chloride cotransporter 2 (NKCC2), which is present on the luminal membrane. Net movement of sodium across the epithelium requires recycling of potassium out of the tubular cell into the lumen through the rat outer medulla potassium channel (ROMK), and transport of chloride across a basolateral chloride channel, ClC-Kb. Neonatal Bartter syndrome is caused by mutations in the genes encoding NKCC2 or ROMK, whereas classic Bartter syndrome is caused by mutations of ClC-Kb. Bartter syndrome associated with autosomal-dominant hypocalcemia is linked to mutations of calcium-sensing receptor (CASR). Abnormal activation of ClC-Kb caused by a mutated protein (barttin) can lead to a more severe form of neonatal Bartter syndrome, associated with sensorineural deafness. Gitelman syndrome can be caused by class I (complete) mutations in the thiazide-sensitive sodium chloride (NaCl) cotransporter (located on the apical membrane of distal convoluted tubule cells), some being population-specific, or partially retarded NaCl cotransporter mutants (class II mutations).

Expert Opinion on Management Issues

These two syndromes are rare but well-characterized monogenic disorders associated with mutations of major sodium transport pathways in the distal nephron. Biochemically, patients with either disorder exhibit hypokalemic, hypochloremic metabolic alkalosis. The two syndromes can be distinguished by different rates of calcium and magnesium excretion (Table 2).

In Bartter syndrome, defective sodium chloride absorption in the TALH leads to salt wasting, volume contraction, and activation of renin-angiotensin-aldosterone axis. High circulating levels of aldosterone increase H^+ and K^+ secretion, leading to hypokalemic alkalosis and biochemical features similar to chronic furosemide treatment. Volume contraction and elevated levels of angiotensin II, vasopressin, and kinins stimulate production of prostaglandins, further impairing the tubular sodium reabsorption. Calcium excretion is increased because of the loss of Na-dependent, voltage-driven calcium absorption in the TALH. Neonatal Bartter syndrome can manifest with features of pseudohypoaldosteronism and has to be considered in its differential diagnosis. Careful attention should be paid to patients who develop signs of azotemia, because a small proportion of these patients progress to chronic renal insufficiency.

Patients with Gitelman syndrome present with intravascular volume contraction, hypokalemia, and hyperaldosteronism-induced alkalosis. Because calcium absorption is not affected in Gitelman syndrome, there is hypocalciuria. In contrast, sodium-driven magnesium reabsorption is impaired, leading to hypomagnesemia, and subsequent neuromuscular irritability.

TABLE 2 Differences between Bartter and Gitelman Syndromes

	Age at Diagnosis	Failure to Thrive	Calcium Excretion	Magnesium Excretion	Transporter Mutations
Bartter syndrome	Early	+	Nl–↑	N1	Na-K-2Cl; ROMK; ClC-Kb; CASR in thick ascending limb
Gitelman syndrome	Later	−	↓	↑	Thiazide-sensitive NaCl in distal convoluted tubule

CASR, calcium-sensing receptor; NaCl, sodium chloride; Na-K-2Cl, sodium-potassium–2 chloride; ROMK, rat outer medulla potassium channel.

Prevention of dehydration and replacement of urinary electrolyte losses (see Table 1 for doses of supplements) constitute the mainstay of therapy in Bartter syndrome. Repeated episodes of dehydration in addition to hypokalemic nephropathy have been implicated in the chronic renal failure seen in some of these patients.

Additional approaches have been used, such as:

- Reduction of the urine flow rate by decreasing the glomerular filtration rate (GFR) with indomethacin (1 to 2 mg/kg/24 hours, up to a maximum of 150 to 200 mg/24 hours). Gastrointestinal (GI) side effects consist of GI bleeding, nausea, and vomiting. Decreased platelet aggregation and irritability are also noted.
- Recent studies suggest the use of cyclooxygenase 2 (COX-2) inhibitors (e.g., rofecoxib) to achieve a similar reduction in GFR.
- Further potassium losses may be prevented by addition of amiloride (starting dose 0.1 to 0.3 mg/kg/24 hours, to a maximum dose of 10 mg/day).
- Aldosterone production and its end-organ effects may be decreased with ACE inhibitors. Both captopril (neonate 0.05 mg/kg/dose, to a maximum dose of 0.1 mg/kg/24 hours; infants 0.15 to 0.3 mg/kg/dose, to a maximum dose of 6 mg/kg/24 hours; children 0.3 to 0.5 mg/kg/24 hours) and enalapril (infants and children 0.1 mg/kg/24 hours, to a maximum dose of 0.5 mg/kg/24 hours; adolescents, maximum dose of 40 mg/24 hours). Side effects include hypotension, rash, cough, reduced renal function, and hyperkalemia (not a problem with Bartter syndrome).

Nutritional support, monitoring of growth, metabolic homeostasis, development of nephrocalcinosis, and decline in renal function are the most important aspects in the care of children with Bartter syndrome. In cases of hypomagnesemia, magnesium supplementation has to be considered. No clear evidence exists in the literature, related to magnesium supplementation in cases with normal serum magnesium, although some patients have reported improvement of symptoms.

Therapy for Gitelman syndrome relies on potassium supplementation and curtailing potassium secretion (low sodium intake, or amiloride to prevent sodium absorption which in turn can augment potassium secretion).

Common Pitfalls

Frequent monitoring and detection of side effects of therapy are important, improving the outcome and delaying or even preventing renal insufficiency. Growth rate has to be monitored, and if suboptimal, bone mineral density may be decreased (angiotensin II may be responsible for lowering the uptake of calcium into bone). A recent description of a patient with Gitelman syndrome who, after developing a chronic nephropathy leading to ESRD underwent kidney transplantation, with postoperative course characterized by sustained hyporesponsiveness to the pressor action of angiotensin II and norepinephrine, highlights the importance and the need for careful control of the hemodynamic status of patients with this tubular disorder.

Communication and Counseling

Despite optimal treatment of the metabolic disorder, growth delay can be seen, especially in patients with Gitelman syndrome. Growth hormone therapy has been tried in a few patients with Bartter syndrome, without encouraging results. Increasing the dose of indomethacin (to 4 mg/kg/day) has helped a few children with Gitelman syndrome, providing that the GI complications are minimal.

HYPERCALCIURIA

KEY CONCEPTS

- Suspect hypercalciuria in children with hematuria or kidney stones.
- Confirm by spot urine calcium-to-creatinine ratio or 24-hour calcium excretion.
- Evaluate for additional tubulopathies associated with hypercalciuria, and citrate excretion.
- Treatment goal is to minimize stone formation and alleviate voiding symptoms.

Hypercalciuria is defined as a daily excretion of calcium above 4 mg per kg, a spot urinary calcium-to-creatinine ratio of greater than 0.2 (infants having higher normal values), and is associated with microscopic hematuria in approximately 50% of the patients. In children, the most common etiology of urolithiasis is hypercalciuria, and recent studies indicate that 45% of patients with urolithiasis have an inherited form of the disease. Mutations in the gene encoding the chloride channel (*ClCN5*) have been found in families with Dent disease, a disorder characterized by low molecular weight proteinuria, hypercalciuria, nephrocalcinosis, nephrolithiasis, renal failure, X-linked recessive nephrolithiasis, and XLHR. Hypercalciuria can occur in patients with other tubulopathies, such as dRTA.

Expert Opinion on Management Issues

Therapy for hypercalciuria is directed at reducing the calcium excretion and crystal formation. Calcium intake should be maintained at the recommended daily allowance (RDA) for age, but not lower (to avoid osteopenia). The mainstay of therapy is ensuring high fluid intake and brisk urine output. If patients remain symptomatic despite adequate fluid intake, they may benefit from administration of thiazide diuretics (hydrochlorothiazide 1 to 2 mg/kg/day, or chlorothiazide 10 to 20 mg/kg/day) to enhance calcium absorption in the distal tubule. Side effects of prolonged thiazide therapy include hyperlipidemia and hypokalemia (prevented by potassium supplementation). Amiloride (0.1–0.3 mg/kg/day) has hypocalciuric effects, without causing hypokalemia, and can be an adjuvant to thiazide therapy. Hypercalciuria seen in dRTA can improve after alkali therapy. Patients who develop hypercalciuria as a result of calcium supplementation, such as those with hypoparathyroidism or pseudohypoparathyroidism, need to be monitored for development of nephrocalcinosis and/or kidney stones. On few occasions, calcium stones are found in association with hyperuricosuria, hypomagnesemia, and hyperoxaluria. Bone mineral density is lower in about one third to one fourth of patients with hypercalciuria, and needs to be evaluated in those with bone pain and/or slow growth velocity rate.

Common Pitfalls

Some pitfalls in management include the omission of salt restriction, along with inadequate fluid intake. Citrate excretion has to be evaluated in every patient with kidney stones, because citrate is an inhibitor of crystallization, and, unrecognized, can increase the risk of stone formation. Once on thiazide therapy, lipid profile and K homeostasis need to be monitored at regular intervals.

Communication and Counseling

Compliance with diet, fluid intake, and medical therapy is an effective way of preventing stone formation.

Despite these measures, some patients still form stones, and have to be instructed about associated symptoms and possible interventions in those instances (see chapter entitled "Nephrolithiasis").

NEPHROGENIC DIABETES INSIPIDUS

KEY CONCEPTS

- Suspect nephrogenic diabetes insipidus in patients with episodes of hypernatremic dehydration and failure to thrive.
- Confirm by hyposthenuria, elevated water clearance, and elevated antidiuretic hormone levels.
- Evaluate for genetic mutations.
- Treat to prevent episodes of dehydration and promote adequate growth and development.

Water reabsorption in the distal nephron requires binding of vasopressin (antidiuretic hormone [ADH]) to its receptor, thereby stimulating insertion of water channels (aquaporin-2 [AQP2]) into the urinary membrane. There have been significant advances recently in the understanding of the molecular causes of nephrogenic diabetes insipidus (NDI). The resistance of the collecting duct to the action of ADH in this disorder results from abnormalities in several of the intricate steps that mediate the increase in principal cell hydraulic conductivity in response to the hormone.

X-linked NDI is an autosomal-recessive disorder caused by an abnormal ADH-receptor 2 gene (AVPR2). Males are affected the most in this type of NDI. The non-X-linked NDI is caused by mutations in the gene encoding for the AQP2 water channel. The transmission of this abnormal gene can be autosomal-recessive or dominant. Recent studies reveal that the mutant genes are responsible for impaired trafficking of the channels to the cell membrane, rendering the tubule water impermeable.

Expert Opinion on Management Issues

Regardless of the gene defect, patients with NDI have in common a large daily urinary volume (up to 20 liters). Frequent episodes of dehydration, failure to thrive, and a prenatal history of polyhydramnios are some of the presenting signs. Large volumes of urine cause hydronephrosis and atonic bladder, and hypernatremic dehydration can be the initial presentation.

The two major goals of therapy in NDI are to prevent episodes of hypernatremic dehydration and to reduce the urine output. The first goal can be achieved by providing free access to water. The second goal may be successfully achieved by the administration of:

- Thiazide diuretics, which, by leading to a state of intravascular depletion, promote absorption of water and sodium in the proximal renal tubule (hydrochlorothiazide 1 to 2 mg/kg/day, or chlorothiazide 10 to 20 mg/kg/day).

- Amiloride (0.1 to 0.3 mg/kg/day), which blocks sodium absorption and promotes an initial natriuresis/diuresis followed by increased proximal water reabsorption, has been used alone or, more successfully, in combination with thiazides.
- Indomethacin, a prostaglandin inhibitor, decreases the glomerular filtration rate. The dose used is 1–2 mg/kg/24h, up to a maximum of 150–200 mg/24h. Frequent monitoring of renal function is mandatory.
- COX-2 inhibitors (effects similar to indomethacin) in combination with thiazides.

Recent studies are aimed at pharmacologic rescue of V2 vasopressin receptors, encoded by X-linked NDI, with pharmacologic chaperones.

Common Pitfalls

Therapy is associated with side effects, which include electrolyte abnormalities, renal dysfunction, and dyslipidemia. Therefore, lack of monitoring constitutes a pitfall.

Communication and Counseling

Adequate communication has to exist among caretaker, physician, and school to avoid frequent episodes of dehydration, maintain normal fluid balance, and prevent low self-esteem associated with poor growth. Prenatal diagnosis in families with NDI can provide means of early intervention, which may prevent complications.

PSEUDOHYPOALDOSTERONISM

KEY CONCEPTS

- Suspect pseudohypoaldosteronism in patients with failure to thrive and dehydration who exhibit hyperkalemia and in newborns with hyponatremia and hyperkalemia who do not respond to exogenous mineralocorticoids.
- Confirm a state of hypoaldosteronism, with elevated renin and aldosterone levels.
- Evaluate for urinary tract abnormalities.
- Treat aggressively with sodium supplementation and correction of hyperkalemia.

Pseudohypoaldosteronism (PHA) type I is a rare genetic disorder, typically appearing soon after birth with failure to thrive, vomiting, and dehydration. Although the characteristic renal salt wasting, hypotension, and hyperkalemia with hyperchloremic metabolic acidosis (normal anion gap) resemble a state of hypoaldosteronism, patients have elevated circulating levels of plasma renin and aldosterone. Thus, it represents a state of end-organ resistance to aldosterone. Two modes of transmission are known:

1. Autosomal-dominant transmission (sporadic, milder, caused by a mutation in the gene encoding for the mineralocorticoid receptor to which aldosterone binds) (type Ia).
2. Autosomal-recessive transmission (more severe, caused by an abnormal epithelial sodium channel) ("loss-of-function mutation," type Ib).

Expert Opinion on Management Issues

Type I PHA may be transient in children with vesicoureteral reflux or obstructive uropathy.

In some cases, the electrolyte abnormalities improve with age. Treatment of type I PHA (both subtypes) is similar and includes sodium chloride supplementation. If hyperkalemia is present, Kayexalate needs to be administered (1 g/kg/dose, every 6 hours, orally [PO] or rectally [PR]) or dialysis can be performed to reduce total body K^+ load.

Type II PHA, also known as Gordon syndrome, is a rare autosomal-dominant form of volume-dependent, low-renin hypertension characterized by hyperkalemia and hyperchloremic acidosis. The high serum renin and hypertension distinguish it from type I, and both hypertension and metabolic abnormalities are corrected with low-dose thiazide diuretics.

Common Pitfalls

Infants with hyperkalemia, hyponatremia, or hyperchloremic metabolic acidosis require a renal and bladder ultrasound to rule out structural abnormalities, because correction of the anatomic abnormality may suffice, or reduce the length of time therapy is needed.

Communication and Counseling

Early detection and therapy can lead to adequate growth, and compliance with therapy is essential. Parents should be alerted to the potential side effects of therapy, and the importance of bringing to the attention of the physician any sign of dehydration, failure to thrive, or febrile illness. Genetic testing may be available in selected groups of patients.

SUGGESTED READINGS

1. Brame LA, White KE, Econs MJ: Renal phosphate wasting disorders: Clinical features and pathogenesis. Semin Nephrol 24:39–47, 2004. **In-depth review of phosphaturic states.**
2. Gahl WA: Early oral cysteamine therapy for nephropathic cystinosis. Eur J Pediatr 162(Suppl 1):S38–S41, 2003. **Review of cystinosis and results of early intervention.**
3. Haffner D, Nissel R, Wuhl E, et al: Effects of growth hormone treatment on body proportions and final height among small children with X-linked hypophosphatemic rickets. Pediatrics 113(6):e593–e596, 2004. **Indicates the benefits of growth hormone in these children.**
4. Pietrow PK, Auge BK, Weizer AZ, et al: Durability of the medical management of cystinuria. J Urol 169(1):68–70, 2003. **Pitfalls in management of cystinuric patients.**

5. Reilly RF, Ellison DH: Mammalian distal tubule: Physiology, pathophysiology, and molecular anatomy. Physiol Rev 80:277–313, 2000. **Discussion of Bartter and Gitelman syndromes, hypercalciuria, and distal renal tubular acidosis (RTA).**

6. Sayer JA, Pearce SH: Diagnosis and clinical biochemistry of inherited tubulopathies. Ann Clin Biochem 38:459–470, 2001. **Discussion of diagnosis and molecular mechanisms, facilitating appropriate management.**

7. Tekin A, Tekgul S, Atsu N, et al: Cystine calculi in children: The results of a metabolic evaluation and response to medical therapy. J Urol 165(6 Pt 2):2328–2330, 2001. **Associated hypocitraturia in cystinuric patients.**

8. Vaibich MH, Fujimura MD, Koch VH: Bartter syndrome: Benefits and side effects of long-term treatment. Pediatr Nephrol 19:858–863, 2004. **Frequent monitoring is essential and allows treatment changes that patients may benefit from.**

9. Zelikovic I: Aminoaciduria glycosuria. In Avner E, Harmon W, Niaudet P (eds): Pediatric Nephrology, 5th ed. Philadelphia: Lippincott, Williams & Wilkins, 2004. **In-depth review of pathogenesis, clinical presentation, and therapy.**

Acute Renal Failure

Gaurav Kapur and Tej K. Mattoo

KEY CONCEPTS

- Acute renal failure is a multifactorial process and a single mechanism cannot always explain the pathogenesis.
- Dehydration and nephrotoxins are responsible for most cases of prerenal and intrinsic acute renal failure, respectively.
- Identification of the underlying cause and its elimination are essential to eliminate further damage and to promote recovery of the kidneys from the acute insult.
- Renal failure causes retention of nitrogenous waste; inability to maintain fluid and electrolyte homeostasis may cause life-threatening complications.
- Supportive therapy, which may include renal replacement therapy such as dialysis, is the cornerstone of management of acute renal failure.

Acute renal failure (ARF) is defined as a sudden decrease in the function of previously normal kidneys that results in the retention of nitrogenous wastes in the body, and often leads to fluid and electrolyte problems. ARF may be nonoliguric, in which case the urine output remains normal, or oliguric, defined as urine output of less than 400 mL/day in older children, and less than 1 mL/kg/hour in newborns and infants. ARF is traditionally divided into prerenal, intrinsic, and postrenal types. Prerenal failure occurs when tubular and glomerular function is intact but renal clearance is limited by factors compromising renal perfusion, as may occur with severe hypotension. In intrinsic acute renal failure there is a primary reduction in glomerular and/or tubular function as may occur in acute glomerulonephritis or acute tubular necrosis (ATN), respectively. Postrenal ARF is because of obstruction in urine flow as may occur in patients with obstructive uropathy. Postrenal ARF is more common in infancy as

compared to later childhood, owing to congenital obstructive uropathies.

Diagnosis of ARF starts with a good history that should focus on factors that might cause volume depletion such as vomiting, diarrhea, hemorrhage, congestive heart failure, septic shock, excessive sweating, burns, and renal salt wasting (diabetic ketoacidosis); exposure to nephrotoxic drugs including radiocontrast agents; poor urinary stream (suggestive of posterior urethral valves); and a decrease in urine output. Distinguishing acute from chronic renal failure can be difficult but is essential for appropriate management. A history of chronic symptoms of fatigue, anorexia, nausea, polyuria, nocturia, polydipsia, anemia, and growth failure indicate chronic renal failure. Presence of fever, skin rash, and joint pains raises the possibility of vasculitis such as systemic lupus erythematosus (SLE) and Henoch-Schönlein purpura (HSP). A history of dyspnea and pulmonary hemorrhage may be caused by Goodpasture syndrome, Wegener granulomatosis, Churg-Strauss vasculitis, or pulmonary edema because of volume overload from oliguria/anuria. Abrupt anuria may occur in acute obstruction, severe acute glomerulonephritis, or a sudden vascular catastrophe such as renal vascular thrombosis or embolus. Painless gross hematuria in the setting of ARF suggests acute glomerulonephritis, whereas painful gross hematuria suggests obstruction by blood clots, necrotic renal papilla, or renal stones. Hemoglobinuria and myoglobinuria also cause hematuria and renal failure, and should be suspected in patients with hemolytic disorders and after vigorous exercise, respectively. On physical examination, the clinical signs that are helpful in making a diagnosis include presence of hypertension, signs of fluid overload, pitting edema, skin rashes, joint swelling/tenderness, birthmarks, cardiac murmur, palpable kidneys, and distended bladder. Table 1 gives investigations that help in the diagnosis of ARF.

Expert Opinion on Management Issues

The basis for the management of patients with ARF is the reversal of underlying etiology and, if possible, prevention of further renal injury together with appropriate supportive care until renal recovery occurs (Box 1). Nephrotoxic drugs should be discontinued whenever possible, and the dosages of all drugs with renal excretion should be adjusted for a glomerular filtration rate (GFR) of less than 10 mL/min/1.73m^2.

FLUID THERAPY

In patients with dehydration, restoration of normal renal perfusion is the single most important therapy for the prevention and the treatment of prerenal failure. The volume of fluid replacement depends on the severity of dehydration, and daily clinical assessment of circulatory volume status. It may be necessary to

TABLE 1 Etiology and Diagnosis of Acute Renal Failure

Prerenal	Tubular Necrosis	Glomerulonephritis	Tubulointerstitial Nephritis	Postrenal
	Intrinsic/Renal Failure			
Common causes				
GI losses in vomiting diarrhea, GI drainage	Ischemic-hypoxic insults	Postinfectious GN	Drug-induced	PUV
Renal losses in DI, adrenal insufficiency, diuresis	Nephrotoxicity from drugs such as cisplatin, aminoglycosides, NSAID, IV contrast	MPGN	Infections	Hinman syndrome
Insensible losses in burns	Toxins as in metals, methanol, myoglobin/ hemoglobin	SLE	Idiopathic	Ureteral obstruction:
Hemorrhage		HSP		Intraureteral as in crystals, stones, clots, tumor
Third space loss in sepsis, heart failure, NS, liver failure	Tumor lysis	ANCA + GN		Extraureteral in tumor, peritoneal fibrosis.
		Vascular lesions: HUS, renal artery/venous thrombosis, cortical necrosis		
Urinary findings and laboratory indices				
Urine output: oliguria	Oliguria/nonoliguria	Usually oliguria	Usually nonoliguric	Variable
Urinalysis: usually normal or minor changes	Granular and epithelial casts, epithelial cells, pigmenturia	Hematuria, RBC casts, proteinuria	Pyuria, WBC casts, eosinophiluria	Unremarkable
Fractional excretion of sodium (FeNa)				
<1% Newborn <2.5%	>2% 2.5%–3.0%	<1%	>2%	Variable
Urine osmolality				
>400 mOsm Newborn >350 mOsm	<350 mOsm <300 mOsm	>400–500 mOsm	<350 mOsm	Variable
Urine sodium				
<10 mEq/L Newborn <20–30 mEq/L	>30–40 mEq/L >30–40 mEq/L	<10 mEq/L	>30–40 mEq/L	Variable
Imaging studies				
Ultrasound: normal	Normal or increased echogenicity, loss of corticomedullary differentiation.	Nephromegaly, loss of corticomedullary differentiation	Nephromegaly, increased echogenicity	Diagnostic, dilated pelvis, ureter and/ or bladder depending on the level of obstruction.
Miscellaneous				
		ASO titer, C3, C4, dsDNA, ANCA, ANA	Eosinophilia	

ANCA, antineutrophilic cytoplasmic antibody; ANA, antinuclear antibody; ASO, antistreptolysin O titer; CHF, congestive heart failure, DI, diabetes insipidus; dsDNA, double-stranded DNA; GN, glomerulonephritis; IV, intravenous; MPGN, membranoproliferative glomerulonephritis; NS, nephrotic syndrome; NSAID, nonsteroidal anti-inflammatory drugs; PUV, posterior urethral valves; RBC, red blood cell; SLE, systemic lupus nephritis; WBC, white blood cell.

Modified from Andreoli SP: Clinical evaluation and management. In Avner ED, Harmon WE, Niaudet P (eds): Pediatric Nephrology. Baltimore: Lippincott, Williams & Wilkins, 2004, pp 1233–1251.

place an indwelling bladder catheter to monitor the urine output. Initial resuscitation may require intravenous bolus of 20 mL/kg of body weight of normal saline. Once intravascular circulatory volume is restored, challenge with a loop diuretic, such as furosemide 1 to 5 mg/kg/dose, depending on renal function, may help increase urine output. Subsequent management includes a daily review of fluid input and output records, daily weight monitoring, and clinical assessment for hydration status. To maintain circulatory volume balance, it is best to replace insensible fluid losses at a rate of 300 to 500 mL/m^2/day plus urine output and any other losses such as through drainage tubes. Patients considered euvolemic should receive full urine replacement, whereas patients who are volume-overloaded with pulmonary congestion should receive none or a fraction of daily urine replacement, based on clinical judgment.

ELECTROLYTE HOMEOSTASIS

Patients with ARF are at risk of developing serious and life-threatening hyperkalemia. Potassium should be

---

BOX 1   Guidelines for Management of Acute Renal Failure

Intravenous fluid

- Volume depleted: Restore volume (most important initial step), then prescribe as for euvolemia (initially with isotonic saline).
- Severe hemorrhage: Consider transfusion.
- Euvolemic (fluid intake equal urine output plus 300–500 mL/m^2/day): Replace urine with 0.45 normal saline.
- Overloaded (fluid intake < urine output): Try loop diuretic. Do not replace urine if patient is oligoanuric. Use partial replacement (one third or two thirds depending on clinical status and urine output).
- Fluid challenge: Depending on clinical judgment, a fluid challenge of 10–20 mL/kg may be tried in a patient with oligoanuria and no obvious signs of dehydration. This can be followed by high-dose loop diuretic such as furosemide at 1–5 mL/kg/dose. The rationale for the fluid challenge is that prerenal ARF is reversible by volume depletion.

Is the patient receiving medication?

- No: Check any medications subsequently prescribed for toxicity and adjust doses.
- Yes: Stop nephrotic drugs. Check drug levels and consider dialysis for dialyzable drugs with clinical features of drug intoxication. Adjust medication doses for GFR <10 mL/min/m^2.

Is the patient hyperkalemic?

- No: Restrict potassium intake in diet and IV fluids.
- Yes: Look for source of potassium. If dietary causes excluded, rule out endogenous sources such as acidosis, hemolysis, rhabdomyolysis, ischemic tissue injury, or myonecrosis.

Indications for dialysis

- Fluid overload with pulmonary edema.
- Uremia with encephalopathy, pericarditis.
- Metabolic derangements resistant to conservative management—hyperkalemia, acidosis, and hyperphosphatemia
- Drug intoxications with dialyzable toxins.
- Inadequate nutrition caused by fluid restriction.

Is the nutrition adequate?

- No: Assess need for parenteral or enteral nutrition and calorically rich formulas when fluid restricted.
- Yes: Reassess periodically.

GFR, glomerular filtration rate; IV, intravenous.
Modified from Hutchison F: Management of acute renal failure. In Greenberg A (ed): Primer on Kidney Diseases. San Diego: Academic Press, 2001, pp 275–282. Copyright 2001. Reprinted with permission from Elsevier.

---

restricted in intravenous fluids and medications, low-potassium diet should be instituted, and its blood level monitored carefully. A child with significant hyperkalemia (K >6.5–7 mEq/L) may experience cardiac arrhythmias and sudden death. Electrocardiogram (ECG) should be obtained to look for peaked T waves, prolongation of the PR interval, and widening of QRS complexes. Intravenous calcium gluconate stabilizes the myocardium against hyperkalemia and should be used first. Serum potassium can then be lowered by intravenous administration of sodium bicarbonate, glucose and insulin, or nebulization therapy with albuterol (Table 2). In a patient with no pressing cardiac concern, resin of sodium polystyrene sulfonate (Kayexalate) helps to bind potassium and results in significant stool potassium losses. A dose of 1 g/kg usually results in a fall in serum potassium by 1 mEq/L over a few hours. Intractable hyperkalemia is an indication for expeditious initiation of renal replacement therapy.

Metabolic acidosis should be corrected if the plasma bicarbonate concentration falls below 16 mEqL or the arterial pH is less than 7.20. Sodium bicarbonate is administered to correct metabolic acidosis. The dose can be estimated from the formula:

$$\text{Bicarbonate dose} = 0.3 \times \text{body weight(kg)} \times \text{base deficit(mEq/L)}$$

An alternative approach is to give bicarbonate empirically in a dose of 1 to 2 mEq/kg. Rapid correction by bolus infusion should be done carefully because of the risk of hypertension, fluid overload, and intracranial hemorrhage, particularly in infants.

Hypo- and hypernatremia may occur in ARF. Hyponatremia is more common and occurs usually secondary to an excess of free water because of excessive administration of intravenous fluids, use of hypotonic saline solutions, parenteral antibiotics in 5% dextrose, and enteral and parenteral feeding solutions. Insensible water loss from burn injury is iso-osmotic whereas diarrhea and perspiration increase the requirements for free water.

Decreased renal phosphorus clearance in ARF may result in hyperphosphatemia and concomitant hypocalcemia. Dietary restriction of phosphorus, should be initiated, and agents that bind ingested phosphate, such as calcium acetate and carbonate, should be prescribed with meals. Hypocalcemia frequently complicates ARF, but clinically significant hypocalcemia is rare, as is hypomagnesemia. In cases of significant hypocalcemia, ionized calcium should be monitored and patients should receive intravenous calcium. In patients with severe hypocalcemia and acidosis, care must be taken to replete the calcium stores before acidosis is treated because alkalization can precipitate hypocalcemic tetany.

TABLE 2 Drugs Used in the Management of Hyperkalemia

Medication	Dosing Information	Route	Onset	Mechanism of Action	Complications
Calcium gluconate (10%)	0.5–1 mL/kg over 5–20 min	IV	Immediate	Stabilizes cardiac membrane	Bradyarrhythmia, tissue necrosis when infused subcutaneous
Sodium bicarbonate	0.5–1 mEq/kg over 10–30 min	IV (flush catheter if giving after calcium)	15–30 min	Intracellular shift of K^+	Hypernatremia, alkalosis hypocalcemic tetany
Insulin and glucose	0.1 U/kg 0.5 g/kg	IV IV	30–60 min	Intracellular shift of K^+	Hypoglycemia
Albuterol (0.5%)	0.01–0.05 mL/kg	Nebulized in saline	30 min	Intracellular shift of K^+	Tachycardia, arrhythmia, hypertension
Sodium polystyrene sulfonate (resin) (Kayexalate)	1 g/kg	PO or PR in sorbitol	30–60 min	Exchange of Na^+ for K^+ across gut mucosa	Hypernatremia, diarrhea, long-term constipation

IV, intravenously; PO, orally; PR, rectally.

HYPERTENSION

Hypertension in ARF is commonly related to circulatory volume overload and/or to alterations in vascular tone. The degree of blood pressure elevation, the presence of hypertensive encephalopathy and associated conditions, and the cause of renal failure guide the choice of antihypertensive therapy. Drugs used in the treatment of hypertensive emergency (acute hypertension associated with end-organ damage) include nitroglycerin (starting dose 0.25 to 5 µg/kg/min), sodium nitroprusside (starting dose 0.5 to 1.0 µg/kg/min), labetalol (0.5 to 3.0 mg/kg/hr), nicardipine (0.5 to 5 µg/kg/min), diazoxide (1 to 3mg/kg/dose), or esmolol (25 to 100 µg/kg/min). Serum sodium thiocyanate, a metabolic product that is excreted by the kidneys, should be monitored when using sodium nitroprusside. Apart from the drugs used in the treatment of hypertensive emergency, intravenous enalaprilat (0.005 to 0.01 mg/kg/day), an angiotensin-converting enzyme (ACE) inhibitor, can be used in hypertensive emergency (acute hypertension with no associated end-organ damage). However, it should be used cautiously as it can exacerbate renal ischemia and worsen renal failure. If the hypertension is related to volume overload, fluid removal with dialysis is recommended if the patient does not respond to diuretic therapy.

ANEMIA

Anemia in ARF may result from repeated phlebotomy, decreased production of erythropoietin, uremic bone marrow suppression, hemolytic uremic syndrome (HUS)/thrombotic thrombocytopenic purpura (TTP), and occult or frank bleeding. This can be treated by packed red blood cell (RBC) transfusions, which may aggravate hyperkalemia and may presensitize a child who may be left with residual renal failure. A recent review of literature revealed that in intensive care patients, administration of recombinant erythropoietin helped reduce the frequency of blood transfusions but did not improve the clinical outcome of the patients. One should keep in mind that a child left with chronic renal insufficiency may ultimately need a renal transplant. Therefore, to prevent sensitization, leukofiltered and washed RBC should be used for transfusion.

NUTRITIONAL MANAGEMENT

Nutritional support is essential for infants with ARF and should consist of a minimum of 50 kcal/kg/day. Infants who are able to take enteral feedings should be given a formula that has a low renal solute load and low phosphate content. Fluid restriction makes it difficult to meet the caloric needs of an oliguric infant. Consideration in these cases should be given to the use of calorie enriched formula or ultrafiltration by renal replacement therapy. Most affected infants are critically ill and require parenteral nutrition. Such infants should receive amino acids up to a maximum of 1.5 g/kg/day and intravenous lipid solution up to a maximum of 2 g/day. The concentration of glucose and solutes such as sodium, potassium, calcium, and phosphorus depend on the infant's weight, serum electrolyte concentrations, the severity of the renal failure, and whether or not the patient is on dialysis.

RENAL REPLACEMENT THERAPY

Common indications for acute dialysis include circulatory volume overload, persistent hyperkalemia, severe metabolic acidosis, uremia, and ARF caused by a dialyzable toxin. A comprehensive evaluation is needed to determine the patient's clinical condition and the possible need for ultrafiltration or solute clearance by dialysis. Accordingly, the patient is started on appropriate mode of dialysis that may include hemofiltration, peritoneal dialysis, or hemodialysis.

Common Pitfalls

A review of the literature on ARF highlights the confusion in terminology and wide disparity in the definition of terms used. In a recent consensus conference on ARF, few studies used the same definition of ARF. Also, the diagnosis of ARF hinges on serial analysis of blood urea nitrogen (BUN) and serum creatinine, which are relatively insensitive markers of renal function.

A variety of agents have been tested for their ability to attenuate injury or hasten recovery in ischemic or nephrotoxic ARF. These include "renal-dose" dopamine, calcium channel blockers, and natriuretic peptides. However, none is consistently shown to be of benefit, and they are not routinely used for treatment of patients with ARF.

There is no consensus among nephrologists regarding when to begin dialysis and how frequently to perform dialysis in patients with ARF. Because there are few available studies at present comparing the outcomes achieved by different dialysis modalities, the choice of modality is empirically guided by the underlying illness and the advantages and disadvantages of different modalities that are available locally. Also, it remains to be determined whether early and frequent dialysis with certain biocompatible membranes will increase survival. Further studies are also needed to better define the costs involved with specific dialysis modalities.

Communication and Counseling

Children with acute tubular necrosis and acute interstitial nephritis usually recover completely and are at low risk for any potential long-term complications. Children who have substantial loss of nephrons as in rapidly progressive glomerulonephritis, HUS, or cortical necrosis are at risk of residual renal damage with potential long-term complications. Parents need to be educated about the importance of follow-up, including a need for regular blood pressure checks, renal function monitoring, and urinalysis. For those with significant residual renal damage, which may manifest with persistent hypertension, proteinuria, abnormal urine sediment, and/or elevated serum BUN and creatinine levels, the clinical implications of chronic renal failure need to be discussed with the patient and the parent.

SUGGESTED READINGS

1. Andreoli SP: Clinical evaluation management. In Avner ED, Harmon WE, Niaudet P (eds): Pediatric Nephrology. Baltimore: Lippincott Williams & Wilkins, 2004, pp 1233–1251. **Discusses the etiology, differential diagnosis, and management of ARF.**
2. Bellomo R, Ronco C, Kellum JA, et al: Acute renal failure—definition, outcome measures, animal models, fluid therapy and information technology needs: The Second International Consensus Conference of the Acute Dialysis Quality Initiative (ADQI) Group. Crit Care 8(4):R204–R212, 2004. **Consensus conference discussing definitions and outcomes of ARF.**
3. Flynn JT: Choice of dialysis modality for management of pediatric acute renal failure. Pediatr Nephrol 17:61–69, 2002. **Discusses various dialysis modalities and provides practical guidelines regarding modality selection to the physician involved in management of ARF.**
4. Hutchison F: Management of acute renal failure. In Greenberg A (ed): Primer on Kidney Diseases. San Diego: Academic Press, 2001, pp 275–282. **Reviews the management of acute renal failure.**
5. Thadani R, Pascual M, Bonventre JV: Acute renal failure. New Engl J Med 334(22):1448–1460, 1996. **Comprehensive review on ARF.**

Chronic Kidney Disease

Frederick J. Kaskel and Brook Belay

KEY CONCEPTS

- Early detection and appropriate management of chronic kidney disease, with the use of estimates of glomerular filtration rate, can help prevent or ameliorate morbidity and mortality.
- Children at risk for chronic kidney disease who have normal glomerular filtration rates should be monitored so that early detection of chronic kidney disease can occur and preventive management can be instituted.
- At each stage of chronic kidney disease careful attention must be made to manage all complications, adjust dosages of medications as indicated for renal failure, treat underlying conditions, and prevent further deterioration in kidney function.
- Proteinuria can be detected and should be aggressively controlled.
- Comorbidities including hypertension, hyperlipidemia, evidence of cardiovascular dysfunction, and delayed growth or neurocognitive development are warranted.
- The guidelines developed by the National High Blood Pressure Education Program Working Group need to be used by practitioners for greatest efficacy.

Chronic kidney disease (CKD) is defined as renal failure from structural or functional causes that persists for more than three months or a glomerular filtration rate (GFR) less than 60 mL/min/1.73 m^2 for 3 or more consecutive months. CKD can be classified according to the degree of impairment in GFR. The National Kidney Foundation (NKF) has defined standards for the definition of CKD and guidelines for management. National databases have demonstrated that there is a growing incidence and prevalence of pediatric CKD. The high morbidity and mortality and costs associated with the care of CKD warrant efforts at prevention and early management.

The etiology of CKD in children includes congenital anomalies, anoxic insults, and various nephropathies. CKD generally progresses through stages of increasing renal dysfunction and ultimately to the development of complete renal failure, or end-stage renal disease (ESRD). The treatment and management of CKD in children varies with each stage and focuses on correcting anemia, abnormalities in calcium and phosphorus

TABLE 1 Classification of Chronic Kidney Disease*

Stage	GFR (mL/min/1.73m²)	Description	Action Plan†
1	≥90 with CKD risk factors ≥90	At increased risk Kidney damage w/normal or increased GFR	Evaluation for CKD and risk reduction Treat primary and comorbid conditions; slow progression and reduce comorbidity risk.
2	60–89	Kidney damage w/mild reduction in GFR	Estimate rate of progression.
3	30–59	Moderate GFR reduction	Evaluate and treat complications.
4	15–29	Severe GFR reduction	Prepare for renal replacement therapy (e.g., fistula creation).
5	<15	Kidney failure (ESRD)	Renal replacement therapy.

*This table demonstrates the cutoffs for the five stages of chronic kidney disease as defined by the NKF K/DOQI guidelines. Each stage is accompanied by a specific action plan.

†Stages 2 to 5 include action plans from preceding stages.

CKD, chronic kidney disease; ESRD, end-stage renal disease; GFR, glomerular filtration rate; NKF, National Kidney Foundation.

Adapted from the National Kidney Foundation's K/DOQI Guideline Learning System. National Kidney Foundation: K/DOQI clinical practice guidelines for chronic kidney disease: Evaluation, classification, and stratification. Am J Kidney Dis 39(Suppl 1):S1–S266, 2002.

TABLE 2 Risk Factors for Chronic Kidney Disease in Children with Normal GFRs*

Hypertension
Diabetes (types 1 and 2)
Ethnicity: African American, Native American, Hispanic American
Family history of renal disease or dialysis
Family history of polycystic kidney disease
Small for gestational age/low birth weight
History of hypoxic renal injury
History of acute renal failure
Renal dysplasia/hypoplasia
Urologic disorders (especially obstructive uropathies)
Vesicoureteral reflux
Nephrotic or nephritic syndrome
History of hemolytic uremic syndrome
History of Henoch-Schönlein purpura
Systemic lupus erythematosus

*This table lists common conditions that would be considered placing a child with a normal GFR at risk for the development of CKD.

CKD, chronic kidney disease; GFR, glomerular filtration rate.

Adapted from the National Kidney Foundation's K/DOQI Guideline Learning System. National Kidney Foundation: K/DOQI clinical practice guidelines for chronic kidney disease: Evaluation, classification, and stratification. Am J Kidney Dis 39(Suppl 1):S1–S266, 2002.

metabolism, acidosis, bone disease, and on optimizing growth. Aggressive management should begin very early in the course of CKD and increase in intensity with each stage.

The precursors of adulthood comorbidities begin during childhood in a child with CKD and should be managed accordingly. Known cardiovascular and neurocognitive comorbidities are increasingly recognized as beginning early in the disease course. Recent research has focused on identifying early risk factors or markers for these comorbidities.

Expert Opinion on Management Issues

CLASSIFICATION OF CHRONIC KIDNEY DISEASE

The NKF classification of CKD is divided by GFR into five different stages as shown in Table 1. The GFR can be readily estimated using age-appropriate formulas. Each stage in the NKF plan is accompanied by a specific action plan that focuses on the treatment and management and prevention of comorbidities (lipid abnormalities, hypertension, cardiovascular, and neurocognitive disease), improvement of nutrition and growth, the adjustment of medications, and the preservation of renal function where possible. It has been determined that adequate nutrition and growth are positive prognostic factors indicating lesser morbidity and longer survival. By the time a patient reaches stages 1 to 2, referral to a nephrologist should have been completed. Adequate nutrition and growth often mean nutrient and caloric supplementation and growth hormone therapy, respectively. Children who pass CKD stages 3 to 4 often go on to require renal replacement therapy (RRT). At this time, planning for RRT would necessitate patient and family counseling and perhaps placement of a dialysis catheter or an arteriovenous fistula.

Children with CKD should also have routine monitoring of vaccination status and should receive the influenza virus vaccine each year. It is important to complete immunizations prior to end-stage disease, at which point immunosuppression necessary for transplantation may render immunization more difficult.

Children with normal GFRs who are at risk for CKD (Table 2) include those with a family history of low birth weight, polycystic kidney disease, renal dysplasia/hypoplasia, urologic disorders, and so on. Particular ethnic groups, for example Pima Indians and African Americans, are also at risk for CKD. Children in these groups should be identified so that they may receive preventive management.

PROTEINURIA

Persistent proteinuria (i.e., proteinuria that is not postural or orthostatic in nature) is an early predictor of CKD and often marks a poor prognosis. Proteinuria leads to fibrosis and is probably an independent mediator of renal injury. Glomerular proteinuria is defined as the excretion of albumin into the urine. An increased amount of albumin in the urine that is not detected by standard urine dipsticks is termed microalbuminuria. Microalbuminuria is a sensitive predictor of CKD in patients with diabetes mellitus. Proteinuria encompasses the secretion of glomerular albumin and low molecular weight tubular proteinuria. Measurements of protein forms should be standardized to the amount of creatinine present in the urine. Normal urine protein-to-creatinine ratios on random ("spot") urine tests are less than 0.2 in children older than 2 years old and less than 0.5 in children ages 6 to 24 months old.

Angiotensin-converting enzyme (ACE) inhibitors, along with angiotensin receptor blockers (ARBs), are commonly used to reduce proteinuria. The mechanism of this action is unclear, but these agents have a renoprotective effect via reduction of proteinuria. Table 3 lists commonly used ACE inhibitors, ARBs, and their pediatric doses (for children ages 1 to 17 years) for therapy of chronic hypertension. The doses for renoprotection in children with CKD are not defined, but it is wise to start with a low dose, following the serum potassium level.

CARDIOVASCULAR DISEASE

Cardiovascular disease remains the major cause of death among children with CKD. Hypertension, a major component of cardiovascular disease, is highly prevalent among children with CKD and is often secondary to renal disease. Hypertension is defined in childhood as blood pressures greater than the 95th percentile for age, gender, and height. The National Heart, Lung, and Blood Institute (NHLBI) Fourth Report on the Diagnosis, Evaluation, and Treatment of High Blood Pressure in Children and Adolescents discloses revised guidelines for normal blood pressure (BP) values based on age and height percentile. This report also summarizes the best clinical practices for diagnosis and evaluation of prehypertension and stages 1 and 2 hypertension and their consequences.

Large-scale prospective studies clearly indicate that hypertension is an independent risk factor for the continued progression of CKD and cardiovascular disease. As such, hypertension should be aggressively controlled. It should be noted that even high-normal blood pressures in adulthood confers an increased relative risk for cardiovascular morbidity and mortality. The risks associated with high-normal blood pressure in children are unknown.

Table 3 lists dosages for the commonly used ACEIs and ARBs. Interestingly, there is some evidence that ACEIs may have the additional benefit of remodeling the cardiovascular system in the setting of established renal disease. Other commonly used medications for chronic blood pressure control include calcium channel blockers, β-blockers, diuretics, and centrally acting agents. Table 4 lists dosages of other commonly used antihypertensive agents for children ages 1 to 17 years. The chapter on hypertension considers the treatment of acute hypertensive urgencies and emergencies.

Frequently, children with CKD have abnormal lipid levels. These abnormalities are generally controlled successfully with the use of β-hydroxy-β-methylglutaryl-coenzyme A (HMG-CoA) reductase inhibitors, or statins. Prospective studies indicate that dyslipidemias are risk factors for morbidity and mortality and that treatment

TABLE 3 Commonly Used Angiotensin-Converting Enzyme Inhibitors and Angiotensin Receptor Blockers

Drug	Dosage
ACE inhibitors	
Enalapril	0.08 mg/kg/dose qd-bid (maximum of 0.6 mg/kg/day, up to 40 mg/day)
Lisinopril	0.07 mg/kg/dose qd (maximum of 0.6 mg/kg/day, up to 40 mg/day)
Captopril	0.3 mg/kg/dose tid (maximum of 6 mg/kg/day)
Angiotensin receptor blockers	
Losartan	0.7 mg/kg/dose qd (maximum of 1.4 mg/kg/day, up to 100 mg/day)

ACE, angiotensin-converting enzyme; bid, two times daily; qd, every day; tid, three times daily.

Adapted from the National High Blood Pressure Education Program Working Group on High Blood Pressure in Children and Adolescents. The fourth report on the diagnosis, evaluation, and treatment of high blood pressure in children and adolescents. Pediatrics 114(Suppl 2):555–576, 2004.

TABLE 4 Other Commonly Used Antihypertensive Agents and Their Dosages

Drug	Dosage
Calcium channel blockers	
Amlodipine	2.5–5 mg qd (children 6–17 years)
Isradipine	0.15–0.2 mg/kg/day tid-qid (maximum: 0.8 mg/kg/day up to 20 mg/day)
β-Blockers	
Propanolol	1–2 mg/kg/day bid-tid (maximum 4mg/kg/day up to 200 mg/day)
Metoprolol	1–2 mg/kg/day bid (maximum 6mg/kg/day up to 640 mg/day)
Atenolol	0.5–1 mg/kg/day qd-bid (maximum 2mg/kg/day up to 100 mg/day)
Diuretics	
Hydrochlorothiazide	1 mg/kg/day qd (maximum 3mg/kg/day up to 50 mg/day)
Furosemide	0.5–2 mg/kg/day bid-qid (maximum 6mg/kg/day)
Central agents	
Clonidine	0.2 mg/day bid (children >12 years; maximum 2.4 mg/day); transdermal patch available and is changed once a week

bid, two times daily; qd, daily; tid, three times daily.

Adapted from the National High Blood Pressure Education Program Working Group on High Blood Pressure in Children and Adolescents. The fourth report on the diagnosis, evaluation, and treatment of high blood pressure in children and adolescents. Pediatrics 114(Suppl 2): 555–576, 2004.

with statins reduces this risk. Furthermore, the statins appear to have an anti-inflammatory effect independent of their lipid-reduction effect that may also reduce the lifetime risk of cardiovascular morbidity and mortality. However, these medications may have clinically important side effects and administering them is probably best managed by practitioners comfortable with these drugs. The increasing recognition and diagnosis of type 2 diabetes mellitus, obesity, and the metabolic syndrome are particularly worrisome because they serve as additional comorbidities that may initiate, aggravate, and accelerate renal disease. Therefore, evidence for any of these conditions should be actively sought and preventive therapy instituted.

Recent studies indicate that people with chronic kidney disease may have ongoing evidence of cardiovascular damage in the absence of clinical signs. This evidence comes in the form of surrogate measures—elevated cardiac troponins, apolipoproteins, and β-natriuretic peptide. However, most studies about this issue were conducted in adult hemodialysis patients. The implications, relevance, and predictive (or "tracking") ability of measuring these markers in pediatric CKD patients remain uninvestigated. However, it is likely that children with CKD have early, ongoing cardiovascular damage that may be detected by these methods and, thus, preventively managed. The contribution of carnitine deficiency to cardiovascular disease in these children is under study.

BONE DISEASE AND CALCIUM AND PHOSPHORUS METABOLISM

Calcium and phosphorus metabolism are dysregulated in CKD. These children have hypocalcemia from reduced intestinal absorption, poor nutrition, and reduced renal-activated vitamin D. Hyperphosphatemia results from reduced renal excretion of phosphate. Consequently, treatment follows a multipronged approach. Children with CKD are instructed to reduce their phosphorus intake and to take phosphate binders with their meals—often in the form of calcium-carbonate. These calcium binders must be taken with meals to ensure phosphate binding. Untoward hypocalcemia can be controlled with calcium supplements in between meals. If the renal disease progresses and the GFR continues to decline, then therapy with activated vitamin D can be instituted. Caution is taken not to treat with vitamin D if the calcium X phosphorus products are elevated. Elevated calcium X phosphorus products are associated with an increased risk of calcium and phosphorus deposition in tissues. This can result in painful tissue necrosis, or even calciphylaxis. Interestingly, specialized imaging studies have demonstrated that calcium deposition begins in coronary vessels early on in adolescence in these patients. Such deposition may accelerate cardiovascular disease.

As the GFR declines, the acidosis of renal failure leads to leaching of minerals from bone despite the best efforts at calcium and phosphorus control. Along with the chronic exposure to steroids that some of these children receive, this serves to accelerate the development of bone disease or renal osteodystrophy. Monitoring of parathormone (PTH) levels in addition to electrolytes is helpful in guiding therapy. Bone scans, or even bone biopsies are helpful as well.

ANEMIA

The kidney generates erythropoietin, and with renal failure the levels of this hormone gradually decline and lead to anemia. The anemia of renal failure is complicated by iron deficiency, partly because of poor nutrition. The negative effects of uremia on erythropoiesis are unclear, but clearly present. As a child passes through the stages of CKD, careful attention should be paid to supplement with iron and erythropoietin as indicated. Iron supplementation can be administered orally, whereas erythropoietin must be given subcutaneously or intravenously. Children on hemodialysis can receive these medications intravenously while they are being dialyzed. The optimal hemoglobin target in CKD patients is unclear, but most practitioners aim for hemoglobin levels of 11 to 12 mg per dL in CKD patients. Studies have indicated that lower hemoglobin levels are associated with increased morbidity and mortality and cardiovascular disease. Elevated hemoglobin levels have also been associated with some morbidity. Specifically, "overshooting" with erythropoietin therapy has been associated with hypertension and seizures.

Common Pitfalls

- Our knowledge of the attendant comorbidities in CKD and their management has increased greatly; however, preventive and diagnostic strategies have not yet been optimized.
- Although novel markers for CKD are being evaluated, the predictive ability of these markers and the appropriate therapeutic interventions based on their presence have not yet been identified.
- Awareness of the fact that CKD progresses in stages and that it is necessary to refer early and to control nutritional intake to enhance metabolic balance and growth needs to be disseminated more efficiently among primary care practitioners.

Communication and Counseling

Children with CKD and their families should be carefully informed at every stage about the severity of the illness and the risk of progression of renal failure and risk for other comorbidities. It is especially important to establish a rapport between patient, family, and provider as the disease and comorbidities progress. It should be noted that early in the course of CKD, patients and their families might not appreciate the seriousness of their condition because they otherwise "feel well." Appropriate communication at these times can be immensely helpful in the prevention process. Patients with genetic diagnoses should be counseled, when appropriate, about screening other family members and the chances of "passing the condition along" to their children.

SUGGESTED READINGS

1. Foley RN, Parfrey PS, Harnett JK, et al: Impact of hypertension on cardiomyopathy, morbidity and mortality in end-stage renal disease. Kidney Int 49:1379–1385, 1996. **Provides an estimation of the effect of hypertension in modifying cardiac disease, and overall morbidity and mortality, in ESRD patients.**
2. Goodman WG, Goldin J, Kuizon BD, et al: Coronary artery calcification in young adults with end-stage renal disease who are undergoing dialysis. N Engl J Med 342:1478–1483, 2000. **A widely cited study demonstrating the early presence of coronary artery calcifications by electron-beam CT in dialysis patients, including young adults.**
3. Kannel WB, Stampfer MJ, Castelli WP, et al: The prognostic significance of proteinuria. Am Heart J 108:1347–1352, 1984. **A classic reference on the prognostic significance of proteinuria.**
4. Lipshultz SE, Somers MJK, Lipsitz SR, et al: Serum cardiac troponin and subclinical cardiac status in pediatric chronic renal failure. Pediatrics 112(1):79–86, 2003. **Perhaps the first analysis of the association of renal disease with elevated serum cardiac troponins (a marker of cardiovascular disease) in pediatrics.**
5. Luepker RV, Jacobs DR, Prineas RJ, et al: Secular trends of blood pressure body size in a multi-ethnic adolescent population: 1986–1996. J Pediatrics 134:668–674, 1999. **Population survey demonstrating the epidemic of overweight status and elevated blood pressures in adolescents.**
6. Matsumoto Y, Sato M, Ohashi H, et al: Effects of L-carnitine supplementation on cardiac morbidity in hemodialyzed patients. Am J Nephrol 20:201–207, 2000. **Elegant study demonstrating the improvement in cardiovascular status after L-carnitine supplementation.**
7. National High Blood Pressure Education Program Working Group on High Blood Pressure in Children and Adolescents. The fourth report on the diagnosis, evaluation, and treatment of high blood pressure in children and adolescents. Pediatrics 114 (Suppl 2):555–576, 2004. **A comprehensive expert panel report on hypertension and elevated blood pressures (including prehypertension) in pediatrics spanning diagnosis, evaluation, and treatment.**
8. National Kidney Foundation K/DOQI Pediatric Workgroup Clinical Practice Guidelines. Available at http://www.kidney.org/professionals/kdoqi/guidelines.cfm. **Provides recommended guidelines by the NKF K/DOQI group on management of renal disease in children.**
9. Parekh RS, Carroll CE, Wolfe RA: Cardiovascular mortality in children and young adults with end-stage kidney disease. J Pediatr 141:191–197, 2002. **Provides retrospective database analysis of cardiovascular mortality in pediatric ESRD patients.**
10. Sinha R, Fischer G, Teague B, et al: Prevalence of impaired glucose tolerance among chidden and adolescents with marked obesity. N Engl J Med 346:802–810, 2002. **Demonstrates a high prevalence of altered glucose metabolism in obese pediatric patients.**
11. U.S. Renal Data System: USRD 2003 Annual Data Report. National Institutes of Diabetes and Digestive and Kidney Diseases. Bethesda, Md: National Institutes of Health, 2003. Available from http://www.usrds.org. **Comprehensive data source on the incidence, prevalence, complications, morbidity, and mortality of renal disease in the United States. Text and slides available for download.**
12. Vasan RS, Larson MG, Leip EP, et al: Impact of high-normal blood pressure on the risk of cardiovascular disease. N Engl J Med 345:1291–1297, 2001. **A report of the Framingham Study group implicating high-normal blood pressures to be associated with elevated cardiovascular disease risk.**

Managing End-Stage Renal Disease

Mark R. Benfield

KEY CONCEPTS

- End-stage renal disease (ESRD) is defined as a point where conservative medical therapies are inadequate to correct metabolic abnormalities and dialysis or transplantation is required.
- Careful planning prior to the need for dialysis or transplantation improves long-term outcomes.
- Transplantation is the treatment of choice for children with ESRD.
- With modern immunosuppression, rejection is an uncommon event.
- Infections are now the most common cause of hospitalization.

As children develop worsening kidney function, metabolic abnormalities accumulate, making medical management increasingly less effective. Problems related to clearance of uremic toxins, acid–base imbalance, electrolyte abnormalities, renal osteodystrophy, volume control, growth, and nutrition require the more effective renal replacement therapies of dialysis and transplantation. It is important to plan in advance for the needs of these patients prior to reaching end-stage renal disease (ESRD) (approximate glomerular filtration rate [GFR] of 10 to 20 mL/min/1.73 m^2). This planning should allow time for important decisions about dialysis and transplantation, time to investigate potential living or deceased donor organ sources for transplantation, and, when possible, time to permit pre-emptive transplantation (transplantation prior to the need for dialysis). In many medical and social situations, pre-emptive transplantation is not possible. In these situations it is important to determine the best mode of dialysis (hemodialysis versus peritoneal dialysis) and to establish dialysis access well in advance of the need for dialysis initiation. Both chronic kidney disease and dialysis are associated with abnormalities in growth and neurocognitive development. These abnormalities are significantly improved with renal transplantation, and some urgency should be used in moving children with marked and advancing chronic kidney disease to renal replacement therapy and renal transplantation. After renal transplantation, children can generally participate in all phases of life.

Expert Opinion on Management Issues

TRANSPLANT EVALUATION

As children approach the need for renal transplantation, it is important to thoroughly investigate any potential abnormalities that would adversely affect the

BOX 1 Transplant Evaluation

- Determine primary kidney disease accurately.
- Determine need for native nephrectomy.
- Ensure that the function of the urinary tract is known and optimized.
- Perform a careful medical screen for other medical problems.
- Screen for exposure and response to immunizations and viral infections.
- Determine potential of living donor organ source.

subsequent transplantation (Box 1). The transplant evaluation should include accurate determination of the primary disease that led to renal failure. The most common causes of kidney failure in children involve congenital abnormalities of the urinary tract and kidneys, especially obstructive uropathies, renal hypoplasia, and dysplasia. Urinary tract abnormalities often continue to contribute to adverse outcomes after transplantation. Thus it is essential to work closely and carefully with a pediatric urologist to evaluate and optimize bladder function prior to transplantation. Further, many children with urinary tract abnormalities have a history of recurrent urinary tract infections and pyelonephritis. A native nephrectomy may well be required to minimize continued infections after transplantation.

The next most common causes of renal failure in children are acquired forms of glomerulonephritis; the most common of these is focal segmental glomerulosclerosis (FSGS). Many patients with FSGS continue to have significant proteinuria and nephrotic syndrome even with ESRD and while on dialysis. The edema, nutritional deficits, hyperlipidemia, and hypercoagulable state common to nephrotic syndrome can contribute to allograft thrombosis, and many experts suggest that pretransplant nephrectomy and dialysis be performed to allow for restoration of normal hydration, nutrition, and coagulation prior to transplantation. Unfortunately, FSGS recurs in 40% to 60% of affected patients after transplantation, and this primary diagnosis is associated with much-shortened allograft survival.

Immunizations to prevent common childhood diseases are a vital component of pediatric care. In the transplant patient, defining the immunization and viral exposure status clearly guides further pre- and post-transplantation care. Given the variable response to immunizations and the risk associated with live virus vaccines in immunocompromised patients, every effort should be made to complete the immunizations in the child with chronic kidney disease (CKD) *prior* to transplantation. Viruses in the herpesvirus family cause significant disease after transplantation (e.g., varicella-zoster virus [VZV], herpes simplex virus [HSV], cytomegalovirus [CMV], Epstein-Barr virus [EBV]). Both the patient and donor should be screened for serologic evidence of exposure to these viruses to guide both observation and care after transplantation.

Finally, it is important to investigate potential donor organ sources. In children, the majority of donors are family members (living related donor [LRD]), most often a parent. For the safety of the donor, these family members undergo a thorough evaluation and must be absolutely healthy to be eligible for donation. Living unrelated donation is also possible, and this avenue can also be explored. Unfortunately, the numbers of patients awaiting transplantation are growing at an exponential rate while the numbers of deceased donor organs available for transplantation have stayed fairly constant over the past 20 years. Thus the length of time spent waiting for a deceased donor organ has increased markedly, now 1 to 3 years.

IMMUNOSUPPRESSION

In the early days of transplantation the choices of immunosuppressive drugs were few, and most patients were treated similarly. But the last decade has witnessed an explosion of new immunosuppressive medications (Table 1). Induction therapy was conceived as a means to reduce the number and function of immunologically active cells at the time of transplantation. This was thought to cause an immune modulation that would reduce subsequent rejection and prolong allograft function. Induction agents include antibodies directed at either the T cell receptor or IL–2 receptor. Early registry data suggested that patients who received induction therapy, in fact, had a lower risk of rejection and allograft loss. However, few prospective randomized studies demonstrate long-term improvement in transplantation outcome with the use of induction agents directed at the T cell receptor. Antibodies directed toward the IL–2 receptor show promise in decreasing acute rejection in controlled trials in adults, and their introduction is temporally associated with a marked decrease in the rejection rate in children. Both T-cell receptor and IL–2 receptor antibodies are still commonly used, especially in patients at increased risk for rejection and allograft loss.

Success in renal transplantation was initially made possible by the use of azathioprine (Imuran) and corticosteroids. These remain a mainstay of immunosuppressive therapy. However, numerous choices and combinations are available today, including corticosteroids, antiproliferative drugs (azathioprine, mycophenolate mofetil, sirolimus), and calcineurin inhibitors (cyclosporin, tacrolimus). The large number of choices and combinations, lack of data to demonstrate comparative efficacy, and inability to accurately measure level of immunosuppression make individual decisions regarding immunosuppression exceptionally difficult. However, most patients receive corticosteroids, a calcineurin inhibitor, and an antiproliferative medication long term.

Because of success in transplantation outcomes and increasing incidence of immunosuppression-associated complications, current trends are toward immunosuppression minimization. Multiple trials in adult and pediatric transplantation now demonstrate the possibility of steroid withdrawal, and pilot studies suggest the possibility of complete steroid avoidance. In adult transplantation, many groups report some success with

11

TABLE 1 Kidney Transplantation

Generic Name (Trade Name)	Dosage/Route/ Regimen	Maximum Dose	Dosage Formulations	Common Adverse Reactions	Therapeutic Concentrations
Induction Agents: Polyclonal					
Anti-thymocyte globulin (Thymoglobulin)	1.5 mg/kg/day IV 7–14 days			Fever, chills, leukopenia	Peripheral CD3 counts <25 cells/mm^3
Lymphocyte immune globulin (ATGAM)	10–30 mg/kg/day IV 14–21 days			Fever, chills, leukopenia	None
Induction Agents: Monoclonal					
Muromonab-CD3 (Orthoclone OKT3)	2.5 mg IV for <35 kg 5 mg IV for >35 kg			Cytokine release syndrome	Peripheral CD3 counts <25 cells/mm^3
Basiliximab (Simulect)	10 mg IV for <35 kg 20 mg IV for >35 kg 2 doses: days 0 and 4			Rare	None
Daclizumab (Zenapax)	1 mg/kg 5 doses: days 0, 14, 28, 42, 56			Rare	None
Maintenance Agents					
Corticosteroids					
Prednisone	0.1–2 mg/kg/day PO qd	80 mg/day	Tablets: 1, 5, 10, 20, 50 mg		None
Antiproliferative agents					
Azathioprine (Imuran)	2 mg/kg/day PO qd		Tablets: 25, 50, 100 mg		None
Mycophenolate mofetil (CellCept)	600–1200 mg/m^2/ day PO bid	3000 mg/day	Tablets: 250, 500 mg Oral suspension: 200 mg/mL	GI side effects	Trough AUC 35–60
Sirolimus (Rapamune)	6 mg/m^2/day PO qd		Tablets: 1, 2 mg Oral solution: 1 mg/mL	Hyperlipidemia, thrombocytopenia	10–20 μg/mL
Calcineurin inhibitors					
Cyclosporine A (Sandimmune, Neoral, Gengraf)	10–15 mg/kg/day PO bid		Gel caps: 25, 100 mg Oral solution: 100 mg/mL	Hirsutism, gingival hyperplasia	150–450 μg/mL
Tacrolimus (Prograf)	0.1–0.2 mg/kg/day PO bid		Capsules: 0.5, 1, 5 mg		5–12 μg/mL

AUC, area under the curve; bid, twice daily; GI, gastrointestinal; IV, intravenous; PO, by mouth; qd, every day.

withdrawal or avoidance of calcineurin inhibitors to avoid nephrotoxicity. Although immunologic tolerance has been achieved for many years in preclinical animal studies, this goal remains elusive in humans.

OUTCOME

With improvements in histocompatibility leukocyte antigen (HLA) matching, surgical techniques and care, and immunosuppression, outcomes have improved remarkably in pediatric transplantation over the past 10 to 20 years. Early in the history of transplantation, hyperacute and accelerated rejection were the most severe obstacles to transplantation. With better understanding of preformed HLA antibodies, improved HLA typing and cross-matching, and most recently flow cytometric cross-matching, these forms of rejection have all but disappeared. Over more recent history,

acute cellular rejection was the major obstacle to successful transplantation. In the mid-1980s, 60% to 70% of transplant recipients experienced at least one rejection episode. With improved immunosuppression and monitoring, acute rejection is now reported to occur in only 20% to 25% of patients, and it is no longer the most common cause of allograft failure. Thus it is important to evaluate other causes of allograft dysfunction and confirm the diagnosis of rejection with an allograft biopsy prior to treatment with increased immunosuppression (Box 2).

Similarly, short- and long-term allograft survival has remarkably improved. One-year allograft survival is now 95% for living donor (LD) and 92% for deceased donor (DD) recipients. Long-term allograft survival rates are equally improved: 5-year survival is 84% for LD and 76% for DD recipients; 10-year survival is 75% for LD and 60% for DD recipients.

BOX 2 Approach to Worsening Renal Allograft Function

- Ensure adequate hydration.
  - Push fluids PO/IV 2500–3000 mL/m²/day (so long as renal function supports the fluid load).
- Rule out infections of the allograft.
  - Order clean catch/catheterized urine culture.
  - Screen for evidence of CMV/EBV/BK virus.
- Screen for drug toxicity.
  - Ensure appropriate levels of cyclosporine, tacrolimus, and/or sirolimus.
- Screen for obstruction of urine flow.
  - Conduct allograft ultrasound.
- If none of the above, rule out rejection.
  - Perform diagnostic kidney biopsy.

BK, polyoma virus; CMV, cytomegalovirus; EBV, Epstein-Barr virus; IV, intravenous; PO, by mouth.

Most important, after transplantation children quickly return to a near-normal life. Most children return to school within 1 to 2 months after transplantation. These children need few restrictions in activity or exposures during school, participate in all but collision sports, and can complete normal education, and many are able to have normal families.

Common Pitfalls

The challenge of transplantation always is to provide enough immunosuppression to prevent rejection while allowing sufficient host immune responses to prevent infection and tumors. Over the past years, the most common cause of hospitalization after transplantation has changed from diagnosis and treatment of rejection to diagnosis and treatment of infections. This is secondary to increases in both bacterial and viral infections. The most common bacterial infections are those of the urinary tract; the most common viral infections are those in the herpesvirus family. The majority of children have never experienced these viral infections, but the majority of adult donors have and still harbor these viruses. This sets up a situation in which patients experience their initial infection while significantly immunosuppressed and are at much increased risk of morbidity and mortality. The most serious of these is infection with EBV. When infected with EBV, transplant patients experience a spectrum of disease including asymptomatic viremia, classic mononucleosis syndrome, a lymphoma-like illness (post-transplant lymphoproliferative disease), and frank lymphoma. Care of these patients should include screening of donor and recipient prior to transplantation and vaccination when possible (VZV vaccine), use of antiviral agents to prevent clinical infection early after transplantation (ganciclovir for CMV and VZV), increased awareness and surveillance for infection after transplantation, and decreased immunosuppression with evidence of disease.

Both because of pretransplant disease and treatments and adverse events associated with immu-

nosuppressive medications after transplantation, children are at increased risk for cardiovascular morbidity. Hypertension and hyperlipidemia are common after transplantation and almost certainly increase long-term cardiovascular risks. Finally, many transplant patients continue to have some chronic renal insufficiency and abnormalities in calcium/phosphorus balance, contributing to growth failure. Studies demonstrate that these patients have improved growth with no change in allograft function or rejection when treated with alternate-day steroids. Further, multicenter trials in Europe and the United States showed that growth hormone therapy is both safe and effective in the treatment of this growth failure.

Communication and Counseling

The care and follow-up of a child with ESRD is arduous, requiring much support and education of the child and family. Each of the facets of care described earlier necessitate evaluation, therapy, and monitoring. The optimal approach is via a multidisciplinary team with the necessary expertise and resources to provide support for this effort. Education and careful explanations are necessary both to make life as normal as possible for the child and family and also to ensure adherence to complex medical regimens.

In the past 20 years, remarkable progress has been made in the outcomes of children undergoing renal transplantation. In the early days of pediatric transplantation, we learned by trial and error, extrapolation from experience in adult transplantation, and anecdotal uncontrolled single-center reports. Today, children receive improved care during chronic kidney disease, more often receive pre-emptive transplantation, and are the recipients of improved surgical techniques and care, tissue typing, and HLA matching. Through collaborative efforts of pediatric transplant programs, data registries, and multicenter randomized trials, we are now beginning to have evidence-based medicine to guide approaches to immunosuppressive medications. During this time children have moved from a group with the worst short- and long-term outcomes after transplantation to a group with the best outcomes.

SUGGESTED READINGS

1. Benfield MR: Current status of kidney transplant: Update 2003. Pediatr Clin North Am 60(6):1301–1334, 2003. **Recent review of pediatric renal transplants.**
2. Green M: Management of Epstein-Barr virus-induced post-transplant lymphoproliferative disease in recipients of solid organ transplantation. Am J Transplant 1(2):103–108, 2001. **Discussion of post-transplant lymphoproliferative disease (PTLD).**
3. Groothoff JW: Long-term outcomes of children with end-stage renal disease. Pediatr Nephrol 20(7):849–853, 2005. **Report on long-term outcomes.**
4. Harmon WE, McDonald RA, Reyes JD, et al: Pediatric transplantation, 1994–2003. Am J Transplant 5(4 Pt 2):887–903, 2005. **Survey of pediatric transplantation over a decade.**
5. Hirsch HH, Knowles W, Dickenmann M, et al: Prospective study of polyomavirus type BK replication and nephropathy in

renal-transplant recipients. N Engl J Med 347:488–496, 2002. **Information about polyomavirus in renal transplants.**

6. Neu AM, Ho PL, McDonald RA, Warady BA: Chronic dialysis in children adolescents. The 2001 NAPRTCS Annual Report. Pediatr Nephrol 17(8):656–663, 2002. **Report about dialysis in children.**

7. Seikaly MG, Salhab N, Browne R: Patterns and time of initiation of dialysis in U.S. children. Pediatr Nephrol 20(7):982–988, 2005. **Article from United States Renal Data System (USRDS) demonstrating that dialysis disparities exist in the United States for children.**

8. Smith JM, Nemeth TL, McDonald RA: Current immunosuppressive agents: Efficacy, side effects, and utilization. Pediatr Clin North Am 60(6):1283–1300, 2003. **Review that discusses immunosuppressive agents used in renal transplant.**

Dialytic Therapies

Gina-Marie Barletta and Timothy E. Bunchman

KEY CONCEPTS

- The three types of dialysis are peritoneal dialysis, hemodialysis, and hemofiltration.
- The choice of dialysis depends on why dialysis is required and, for renal disease, whether the patient has acute or chronic renal failure.
- Dialysis is best performed by persons and in centers with experience in dialyzing children.
- Because end-stage renal disease (ESRD) affects multiple organ systems, close attention to nutrition, metabolic issues, growth and development, and general well-being is important.

Dialysis in pediatric patients is used for the management of either acute or chronic renal failure. This chapter offers a brief overview of current perspectives in dialytic therapy for the management of acute and chronic renal failure in infants and children, providing a broad summary of dialytic therapy options and focusing on a few important features that should be considered in patients treated with such therapies.

Expert Opinion on Management Issues

ACUTE DIALYSIS

The indication for acute dialysis in pediatrics is broad and includes acute renal failure (ARF), inborn errors of metabolism, multiorgan dysfunction syndrome (MODS), and intoxications. The overall objective for initiating dialysis is fluid removal and/or solute clearance or, in the case of inborn error of metabolism and intoxication, clearance of a specific metabolite or toxin. The different modalities for acute dialytic therapy include hemodialysis (HD), peritoneal dialysis (PD), and hemofiltration (HF). The latter is further divided into continuous venovenous hemofiltration (CVVH), continuous venovenous hemofiltration with dialysis (CVVHD), and continuous venovenous hemodiafiltration (CVVHDF). In choosing the specific mode of renal replacement therapy (RRT), the particular needs and complexity of the intended patient, as well as specific hemodynamic factors, must be considered. For patients who require rapid clearance (e.g., hyperammonemia, hyperkalemia), a highly efficient form of RRT such as HD is most suitable. For patients requiring less rapid and more continuous clearance, options such as HF or PD are more appropriate.

Hemodialysis is the preferred RRT modality for intoxications and hyperkalemia, but it is difficult to institute in hemodynamically unstable patients. In general, prescriptions for HD consist of a dialysis flow rate of 500 to 800 mL per minute and a blood flow rate between 2 and 8 mL/kg/minute. Prescriptions for the components of the dialysate bath, which include the concentration of bicarbonate, sodium, potassium, calcium, and phosphorous, are determined by the particular needs of the patient. For example, to avoid electrolyte complications related to excessive electrolyte loss during nonacute renal failure indications for HD, such as inborn error of metabolism or intoxications, additional phosphorous or potassium supplementation in the dialysate bath should be considered.

HD is initially preferred over HF for intoxications or inborn errors of metabolism; PD should not be used in such cases. In patients with intoxications or hyperkalemia, HD is more efficient because of the high dialysate flow rate as compared to HF and PD. However, in patients with hemodynamic compromise, HF is preferred over HD because of its gentle nature.

In patients undergoing HD for inborn errors of metabolism, medications that may rescue the patients from their disorder are often cleared as well and therefore may require higher or more frequent dosing schedules. Patients who are at risk for rebound effects from their intoxications (e.g., lithium, vancomycin) or are in situations in which compounds continue to be produced, as in inborn errors of metabolism (e.g., hyperammonemia), may require initial clearance of high levels with acute HD and then transition to HF for continued removal. HD clears toxins/metabolites initially from the vascular space but not from the tissue in these patients. Therefore, once vascular levels are lowered, after initial treatment with acute HD, the reequilibration of the toxin/metabolite from the tissue to the vascular space occurs over time. By transitioning from HD to HF, this rebound phenomenon may potentially be prevented and thereby prevent ongoing intoxication of the drug or metabolite.

The duration of a given HD session is based on adequate clearance of solute and toxins as well as the hemodynamic complexity of the patient. Classically, three to four HD treatments clear approximately three quarters of the solute (e.g., urea) over that period of time, with the highest solute clearance occurring over the first 1 to 2 hours of HD therapy. Ultrafiltration requirements, however, should be extended over a longer period of time to maintain hemodynamic stability.

TABLE 1 Suggested Size and Selection of Vascular Access for Hemodialysis and Hemofiltration

Patient Size	Catheter Size and Source	Site of Insertion
Neonate	Single-lumen 5F (Cook)	Femoral artery or vein
	Dual-lumen 7.0F (Cook/Medcomp)	Internal/external: jugular, subclavian, or femoral vein
3–6 kg	Dual-lumen 7.0F (Cook/Medcomp)	Internal/external: jugular, subclavian, or femoral vein
	Triple-lumen 7.0F (Medcomp)	Internal/external: jugular, subclavian, or femoral vein
6–30 kg	Dual-lumen 8.0F (Kendall, Arrow)	Internal/external: jugular, subclavian, or femoral vein
>15 kg	Dual-lumen 9.0F (Medcomp)	Internal/external: jugular, subclavian, or femoral vein
>30 kg	Dual-lumen 10.0F (Arrow, Kendall)	Internal/external: jugular, subclavian, or femoral vein
>30 kg	Triple-lumen 12.5F (Arrow, Kendall)	Internal/external: jugular, subclavian, or femoral vein

From http://www.pcrrt.com, with permission granted by Timothy E. Bunchman, MD.

Access for Hemodialysis and Hemofiltration

Both HD and HF require short large-caliber venous access (Table 1) to be placed preferably in either the internal jugular or femoral vein and, less desirably, in the subclavian vein. To provide adequate solute clearance, target blood flow rate should be maintained at 2 to 8 mL/kg/minute. In general, access recirculation, a major problem in patients receiving chronic dialysis treatment, is less of an issue in patients requiring acute HD therapy or in patients maintained on HF.

DIALYSIS FOR ACUTE RENAL FAILURE

Newer data for acute renal failure demonstrate that early intervention with HF may be beneficial for both patient survival rate as well as overall decreased intensive care unit costs because it enables more rapid weaning of ventilatory supportive therapy, given the improved volume status of patients it confers.

Hemofiltration

Hemofiltration in the form of CVVH, CVVHD, or CVVHDF is now the standard of care for patients with ARF as a complication of MODS. This treatment modality provides a major advantage by providing continuous removal of solute as well as slow and steady ultrafiltration. This is particularly important in hemodynamically unstable patients in whom rapid fluid shifts may cause significant compromise. Prescriptions for HF vary but are generally based on a blood flow rate of 2 to 8 mL/kg/minute and a convective or diffusive clearance rate of roughly 2000 to 3000 mL/1.73 m²/hour of solute clearance. This is equated to 35 to 45 mL/kg/hour based on data by Ronco and colleagues (2000).

Vascular access for HF is similar to that for HD (see Table 1), and anticoagulation can vary from heparin anticoagulation to the more novel and reliable citrate anticoagulation that has now become the standard of care throughout many programs.

Temperature control can be easily maintained by a newer generation of machines that allow for thermic variation at the bedside as well as for ultrafiltration control with improved accuracy—within 5% of targeted fluid removal rates.

One of the main advantages of HF is that it is *continuous* and therefore permits maximization of nutritional support with total parenteral nutrition (TPN), medication therapy, fresh-frozen plasma (FFP), as well as the other blood components, which may also be administered continuously, depending on the particular needs of the patient. The disadvantage of HF is that because it is continuous, it can interfere with non–intensive care unit (ICU) interventions, such as CT scans/radiographic/surgical procedures. Historically, discontinuation of therapy was necessary during such procedures. However, it is now clear that therapy may be continuously administered intraoperatively or during such procedures in the non-ICU setting.

Dialysis solutions are a major issue in hemofiltration. The first standardized solution approved by the U.S. Food and Drug Administration (FDA) for dialysis was Hemofiltration Solution (Baxter Health Care, Deerfield, IL), which is a lactate-based solution. However, when lactate-based solutions are used for continuous renal replacement therapy (CRRT), measurable plasma levels of lactate can be observed, which makes it difficult to distinguish whether elevated serum lactate levels are caused by the dialysate solution or the development of lactic acidosis in the patient. Barenbrock and colleagues (2000) showed that bicarbonate-based solutions are associated with less hemodynamic compromise as well as improvement in overall patient survival. Many pediatric programs use customized solutions produced in hospital pharmacies for replacement or dialysis fluid. Although customized solutions are produced based on the individual needs of a patient, they tend to be quite expensive and at significant risk for compounding errors, resulting in untoward side effects and even death. Industry-produced standardized solutions, such as Normocarb (Dialysis Inc., Richmond Hills, Ontario, Canada) and PrismaSate (Gambro Healthcare, Lakewood, CO), are now considered standard of care for bicarbonate-based industry-produced solutions. Both of these standardized solutions are approved for dialysate, and data show that Normocarb may also be used as a replacement solution. In addition, these solutions can be used with citrate or heparin anticoagulation for ease of implementation of HF at bedside.

Individual ultrafiltration rate should be based on the hemodynamic status of the patient. Of particular importance is appropriate maintenance of colloid oncotic pressure to promote adequate intravascular volume to allow for fluid removal without inducing hemodynamic instability. To accomplish this, patient serum albumin levels should be maintained at or greater than 3 g per L and adequate hematocrit levels should be sustained to help ensure proper hemodynamic function.

Clinically important hemodynamic instability can occur secondary to reactions to the filtering membrane, as reported with the AN–69 membrane when primed with blood bank blood (low pH). Another major issue is that when the hemofiltration lines are in immediate proximity to infusions such as vasoactive agents, the drugs may be removed and levels will fall. Therefore, very close observation at bedside is required for at least the first 5 to 10 minutes of initiating therapy with HF, optimally longer. Complications for all the continuous dialytic modalities include hemodynamic compromise, clearance of drugs that are used for treatment of the patient, clearance of vasoactive agents, as well as risk of infection caused by catheter placement. In addition, protein and amino acid loss occurs across the HF membrane, which can negatively impact nutrition. Therefore, an increase in the amount of amino acid delivery either by total parenteral or enteral nutrition is necessary to avoid the substantial losses that occur with these modalities.

Peritoneal Dialysis

Many programs still continue to use PD for treatment of patients with ARF. However, PD should not be used to treat inborn errors of metabolism or intoxications because this modality is far less efficient in solute removal as compared to other available dialytic modalities.

Access for PD can be established for either acute or chronic use. The advantage of the acute access is that it can be placed easily at bedside, and therapy can be instituted immediately. Chronic access is also easily placed but requires surgical intervention with omentectomy. Access is established in the pelvic region because of the lower volume of omentum, which can impede the flow of dialysate into or out of the patient, and to avoid puncturing the bowels, liver, and spleen.

Solutions for PD are often produced commercially: lactate based in North America and bicarbonate based in Europe. In addition, dialysate for PD is often made by the hospital pharmacy, classically as a bicarbonate-based solution. However, as with any customized/individualized pharmacy-produced solution, it carries the risk for pharmacy compounding errors.

The physiologic needs of the patient determine the specific choice of solution. For example, if the patient does not have lactic acidosis and is not hemodynamically comprised, a lactate-based solution is reasonable. If the patient is hemodynamically comprised or has a worsening lactic acidosis, alternative solutions, such as pharmacy-made solutions or, outside of North America, standardized industry-made bicarbonate-based solutions, are more appropriate.

Industry-made solutions are often mildly low in sodium and do not contain phosphorous. Potassium can easily be added to these solutions; however, phosphorus should not be added because of its precipitation with the calcium that is already present within the standardized solutions.

The prescription for PD is based on the requirements of the individual patient. Ultrafiltration is best obtained by frequent passes with a short dwell time and using higher concentration/osmolar (glucose) Dianeal. Solute clearance is best achieved by implementing a longer dwell time to allow for improved exchange across the peritoneal membrane.

Complications of PD include leakage at the catheter exit site, impairment of respiratory efforts, pleural effusions because of leakage of dianeal from the peritoneal cavity into the pleural space, and peritonitis. These complications are well described in the literature, and all are identifiable and treatable with early intervention.

CHRONIC DIALYSIS

Often the decision for instituting chronic HD or PD is based on a number of considerations: the distance the patient lives from the nearest pediatric dialysis center, the overall compliance of the family, the size of the patient, as well as the expertise of the individual pediatric nephrology program. Both of these RRT modalities are effective in pediatric patients and should generally be considered only as a bridge to transplantation.

Hemodialysis

HD for chronic dialysis is considered the standard of care in many programs. Chronic HD typically is used in children weighing more than 10 kg, in patients who live close to a pediatric HD center, and in children with families who are considered less responsible to perform PD at home. The choice of HD machinery is based on contracts between institutions and companies, but all have the common benefit of control of ultrafiltration, flexibility in dialysate flow rates, constant temperature control, as well as variable extracorporeal circuit volumes. In general, extracorporeal circuit volumes should not exceed 10% of the patient's calculated blood volume. It is preferable to have as small a proportion of the child's blood volume in the extracorporeal circuit as possible; therefore, if the circuit clots, less blood loss is likely to occur over time.

Blood flow rate during HD is determined by the type of access. Patients with fistulas have different flow rates, recirculation rates, and flow resistance compared to patients with central venous HD catheters. Overall clearance is determined by the blood flow rate, amount of recirculation, and the duration of dialysate exposure. Dialyzer clearance of urea is calculated by Kt/V (where K is the clearance coefficient of the dialyzer, t is the time on dialysis, and V is the volume of distribution of urea); the higher the Kt/V, the better the clearance. Blood flow rates classically are in the range of 2 to 8 mL/kg/minute with the acquired clearance to get a Kt/V on a weekly basis of greater than 1.2. In general, a higher Kt/V results in a higher survival rate, improved nutrition, and improved quality of life compared to lower Kt/V. The dialysate flow rate should run between 500 and 800 mL per minute. Classically, for high-flux dialysis membranes, the dialysate should be maintained at a higher flow rate, approaching 800 mL per minute. This higher flow results in a higher solute clearance, particularly for clearance of so-called middle molecules. Phosphorus clearance should also be improved with these higher dialysate flow rates, although these data in pediatrics are speculative.

Filtration rates by most dialysis machines are within 100 to 300 mL of natural filtration rates per hour. For a standard dialysate rate of 500 mL per minute, most machines have an obligate ultrafiltration rate of 100 mL per hour, yet when the dialysate flow rate is increased up to 800 mL per minute, the natural/obligate ultrafiltration rate may go up to 300 mL per hour. These volumes are in addition to the programmed net ultrafiltration prescribed. Understanding there is an obligatory volume removed is important to avoid excessive ultrafiltration, which can occur if this is not factored into the ultrafiltration needs of the patient during therapy.

Access for HD includes a fistula, a Gortex graft, or an external dual-lumen central HD line. The particular type of HD access is often determined by the predicted/proposed length of therapy. Many programs use HD as a short bridge to transplant. In such cases, the use of a cuffed HD catheter for several months until the time of transplant surgery is reasonable as a short-term bridge. In patients that are cadaveric listed or those patients that have no immediate options for transplantation, longer term access, such as a fistula, should be considered. Overall, fistulas result in longer access survival, better KT/V, and fewer hospitalizations when compared to the other access options. Gortex grafts and extracorporeal HD catheters have an increased risk of clotting, with an increased risk of infection because the presence of a foreign body. However, most infections can be treated with the use of systemic antibiotics without having to remove the Gortex graft or the external catheter. In HD patients who are malnourished, treatment of infected lines is much more problematic because such patients have an overall poor immune response to infection. Therefore, the nutritional status of any patients with recurrent infections should be assessed so appropriate dietary supplementation can be implemented. In addition, many programs now use a combination of heparin with vancomycin or ciprofloxacin to lock HD catheters and thus decrease the potential risk of infections. Data have yet to demonstrate whether this is truly beneficial, yet local standard of care suggests that this works, at least in some patients.

Stable temperature control of dialysis fluid with HD is easily obtained. Most machines have the flexibility of thermic control, from 95°F (35°C) to 98.6 °F (39°C). This is particularly important for treatment of infants who have an increased proportion of heat loss across the extracorporeal circuit, as well as increased heat loss through their skin. Therefore, a higher temperature setting on the machine may be necessary to offset increased heat loss through the extracorporeal circuit.

Peritoneal Dialysis

The choice of PD for chronic renal failure is reasonable in patients with families who are compliant, have no adequate vascular access, and/or who live a long distance from a pediatric dialysis center. In addition, PD is often preferable to treat smaller patients, particularly infants, because vascular access is often difficult and proportionally higher extracorporeal circuit blood volume requirements render chronic HD unfeasible.

Access for PD is achieved using a cuffed catheter, preferably with a so-called swan-necked end. The tip of the catheter should sit in the pelvis, with the curl/swan-neck configuration of the peritoneal dialysis catheter pointing down. At the time of placement of the peritoneal dialysis catheter, an omentectomy is recommended to decrease the risk of inflow/outflow obstruction that often occurs with peritoneal dialysis. It is preferable to have a peritoneal dialysis catheter placed 3 to 6 weeks prior to initiating therapy, to allow time for adequate healing and to avoid any complications of early intervention, such as leakage around the exit site. Many programs recommend these catheters be flushed routinely until they are used regularly. Other programs place these catheters and do not flush them during the 3 to 6 weeks before routine use. Therefore, flushing of the catheter is really based on local determination. Data to date do not demonstrate that one approach is superior to the other.

Perioperative antibiotics are often administered for peritoneal dialysis catheter placement by many programs. Administration of such antibiotics has yet to demonstrate any significant benefit. If perioperative antibiotics are used, it is preferable to treat for a short course (1 to 2 days) of therapy in order avoid complications such as fungal growth.

Many patients treated with PD, particularly infants, require gastrostomy feeding tubes to maximize nutritional support. Simultaneous placement of a gastrostomy tube and a PD catheter may result in a higher incidence of complications and peritoneal infections. Therefore, it is preferable that gastrostomy tubes be placed and used months before PD catheter placement. In those patients who do have simultaneous PD catheter and gastrostomy tube placement or in those patients who have a gastrostomy tube placed *after* PD catheter placement, care should be taken to avoid the possibility of a percutaneous feeding tube puncturing the peritoneum. If the peritoneum is overstretched and the feeding tube is then placed by a percutaneous method, the risk of puncturing the peritoneum is high, with a great risk of causing gastric contents to empty into the peritoneal cavity. This is associated with a higher incidence of fungal peritonitis in the patient.

Once the peritoneal dialysis catheter is in place and matures, so to speak, the peritoneal dialysis prescription should be individually determined. Classically, the particular peritoneal dialysis solution consists of a lactate-based commercial solution. In Europe, bicarbonate-based solutions are now available and clearly preferable to lactate-based solutions. The choice of lactate versus bicarbonate depends on local availability.

The rationale behind the production of lactate-based solutions is because of PD solution bag technology. The older forms of peritoneal bags have a high occurrence of bicarbonate leakage through the membrane. New bag technology in Europe has minimized this and allows for bicarbonate-based solutions to be used for PD.

PD solutions contain an osmolar solution using dextrose to influence ultrafiltration. The standard PD solution options include 1.5% Dianeal, 2.5% Dianeal, and 4.25% Dianeal based on the percentage of dextrose contained in the solution. Some of the newer forms of peritoneal dialysate solutions contain nondextrose polymers that result in similar ultrafiltration, with less glucose and carbohydrate exposure for the patient. In theory, less obesity and less excess weight gain should occur in patients prescribed such solutions. Adult studies prove this to be effective, yet pediatric studies are still in progress to determine the benefit of dextrose- versus nondextrose-containing polymers for ultrafiltration rates as well as overall weight gain/ nutrition.

The volume of peritoneal dialysis is classically begun at 10 mL per kg and then gradually increased over a period of time to a goal of roughly 40 to 50 mL/kg/pass for an average of 8 to 10 passes per 24-hour period. The determination of adequacy of peritoneal dialysis is based on the KT/V. The desired KT/V should exceed 2 on a weekly basis. The KT/V is determined by the volume of dialysate exposure per 24-hour period, the total duration of time, as well as the permeability of the membrane. The permeability of the membrane should be determined by the use of a peritoneal equilibration test (PET) to assess membrane adequacy. Some patients are high convectors of solute, and some patients are high absorbers of glucose. Therefore a PET helps determine the optimal length of time the solution should dwell in the abdomen to achieve adequate solute clearance. In patients who have had several episodes of peritonitis and/or multiple prior abdominal surgeries, the peritoneal membrane may be compromised, resulting in poor solute clearance.

Hyperosmolar solutions, such as the 4.25% dextrose Dianeal, result in improved ultrafiltration rates. However, chronic use of higher concentration dianeal is associated with an increased incidence of membrane sclerosing with resultant thickened and fibrosed peritoneum. Thus a compromise of ultrafiltration rates and fluid intake may be necessary in those children who require PD for a longer period of time to avoid peritoneal membrane sclerosing. In patients who have a fair amount of membrane irritation or fibrin production, the use of heparin at 250 to 500 U per L may be necessary to avoid fibrin formation with subsequent clogging of the PD catheter. In general, intraperitoneal heparin does not induce systemic heparinization, so there should not be any contraindication for instilling heparin into peritoneal fluid in those patients at risk for bleeding complications.

PD may be performed by an automated PD system, such as continuous cycling peritoneal dialysis (CCPD),

or as a continuous around-the-clock mode of PD with continuous ambulatory peritoneal dialysis (CAPD). With CCPD the dialysis occurs over a specific time period, usually at night, making the patient independent of dialysis during the day. CCPD also has a lower risk of peritonitis because of less frequent accessing of the PD catheter throughout the day. However, clearance may not be as efficient. The benefit of CAPD is that it results in improved solute clearance, but the downside is that it often results in less ultrafiltration/ fluid removal. Therefore, in those patients who are anuric, CAPD is less preferable.

Complications of PD include hernias of the scrotum, the labia, or ventral/abdominal wall, which are associated with excessive abdominal distension. Such complications may result in loss of the ability to perform adequate PD. Peritoneal dialysis can also rarely result in transmission of peritoneal fluid into the pulmonary space (hydrothorax), resulting in significant pulmonary compromise. The most common complication of PD is peritonitis. Usual pathogens include gram-positive bacteria, followed by gram-negative bacteria, and even less commonly fungal infection. The more frequent the number of infections, particularly peritonitis caused by gram-negative organisms and/or fungus, the more likely the peritoneal membrane will sclerose, with resultant poor ultrafiltration and a decline in small solute clearance.

Risk factors for peritonitis include poor technique at placement and routine daily access, breaks in the PD system, and malnutrition. The younger the patient, the greater the loss of amino acids and immunoglobulins across the peritoneal membrane over time, resulting in a greater risk of malnutrition with the added increased risk of peritonitis. Therefore, in those patients with recurrent peritonitis, attention should focus on the individual's PD technique, with PD care and technique retraining/education, as well as additional attention to nutritional risk factors for peritonitis.

COMPLICATIONS OF END-STAGE RENAL DISEASE

Whether patients are treated chronically with HD or PD, attention to their vitamin D stores, anemia, nutrition, and growth is in order.

Renal Osteodystrophy

The past 25 years have witnessed great advances in vitamin D and calcium/phosphorous balance. Historically, calcium was used for phosphate binding and was associated with a higher incidence of developing coronary artery calcinosis. The newer generation of non–calcium-containing phosphate binders are equally effective yet have a lower risk of calcinosis.

The use of activated vitamin D is also important to maintain a balance of bone metabolism. The measurement of the patient's intact parathyroid hormone (iPTH) level is used by the vast majority of programs to look at the adequacy of vitamin D exposure. An iPTH level that is too low may result in adynamic renal bone disease; a PTH that is too high may result in bone loss secondary to renal osteodystrophy. An optimal iPTH level thus is roughly two to three times the upper limits of normal for the particular assay to maintain a balance between adynamic renal bone disease and renal osteodystrophy.

Anemia

Anemia in the ESRD population is caused by the inadequate production of erythropoietin, as well as insufficient absorption of oral iron. The use of recombinant erythropoietin (EPO) markedly improves hemoglobin/hematocrit levels in patients with ESRD. Newer, longer-acting formulations of erythropoietin (e.g., darbepoetin) are currently being considered for patients on dialysis. Darbepoetin is presently approved by the FDA for use in adult patients with chronic kidney disease and on dialysis. It is not yet formally approved for use in children, but some pharmacokinetic data exist. Treatment with darbepoetin improves hematocrit levels in patients with chronic kidney disease as effectively as recombinant EPO, and it has the added benefit of less frequent injections, which may improve compliance. This appears to be the case in children. With regard to decreased iron absorption in patients with ESRD, many programs currently treat HD and PD patients with scheduled intravenous iron infusions. The newer intravenous iron formulations (e.g., ferric gluconate) are much better tolerated than those used in the past with fewer side effects, making them easier to administer. Intravenous iron administration not only ensures compliance, it achieves adequate serum iron levels to maintain sufficient red cell production.

Growth

Poor growth in the patients with ESRD is multifactorial, often related to a malnourished state, inadequate vitamin D levels, renal osteodystrophy, anemia, as well as overall metabolic derangements (e.g., metabolic acidosis). Many programs use recombinant growth hormone as a way to improve overall growth in patients. Although the use of growth hormone is effective, it should *not* be considered a primary therapy. Without adequate nutritional intake, attention to vitamin D supplementation, as well as other risk factors associated with growth impairment, growth hormone may actually be detrimental or of no direct benefit. Therefore, administration of growth hormone should only be considered after all factors associated with growth impairment are addressed and treated properly.

Nutrition

Patients with ESRD are often anorexic because of diminished taste sensation, effects of elevated serum urea nitrogen levels, as well as significant dietary restrictions. Consideration of adequate nutritional intake should be determined by the urea reduction ratio.

These patients need to have roughly 20% to 30% more nutritional intake than their non-ESRD peers to achieve appropriate growth. Without adequate nutrition, patients with ESRD have a higher incidence of infections, significant growth impairment, and death compared to their non-ESRD peers.

Common Pitfalls

- Failure to refer a child when dialysis is needed
- Failure to weigh the pros and cons of different forms of dialytic therapy
- Failure to consider the issues that accompany both acute and chronic renal failure
- Failure to initiate and institute support systems for the child on dialysis

Communication and Counseling

Either acute or chronic dialysis is a major event with many concomitant ongoing issues. The patient and family must have ongoing support and communication with the team. Much formal learning needs to be imparted, and having didactic sessions and continual checks on understanding assures the best possible outcome for a child. For the child receiving acute dialysis, age-appropriate explanations are helpful; the family often is overwhelmed, and ongoing teaching and counseling are important. The child on chronic dialysis and his or her family need much input for the many decisions needed and for planning long-term care. A dialysis unit with pediatric expertise is optimal. The primary care physician, as well as the school and associates of the child and family, should all be involved in the care of children requiring chronic dialysis.

SUGGESTED READINGS

1. Barenbrock M, Hausberg M, Matzkies F, et al: Effects of bicarbonate- and lactate-buffered replacement fluids on cardiovascular outcomes in CVVH patients. Kidney Int 58:1751–1757, 2000. **The relation of replacement fluid in CVVH to outcome.**
2. Barletta GM, Kershaw DB, Mottes TA, et al: Intra-operative continuous renal replacement therapy in pediatric intensive care unit patients. J Am Soc Nephrol 14:731A, 2003. **Continuous renal replacement therapy in children.**
3. Brophy PD, Mottes TA, Kudelka TL, et al: AN–69 membrane reactions are pH-dependent and preventable. Am J Kidney Dis 38:173–178, 2001. **Article about membrane reactions.**
4. Bunchman TE, Maxvold NJ, Brophy PD: Pediatric convective hemofiltration: Normocarb replacement fluid and citrate anticoagulation. Am J Kidney Dis 42:1248–1252, 2003. **Article about the type of replacement fluid and management.**
5. Goldstein SL, Jabs K: Hemodialysis. In Avner ED, Harmon WE, Niaudet P (eds): Pediatric Nephrology, 5th ed. Philadelphia: Lippincott Williams & Wilkins, 2004, pp 1395–1410. **Useful chapter on hemodialysis in major text.**
6. Maxvold NJ, Bunchman TE: Renal failure and renal replacement therapy. Crit Care Clin 19:563–575, 2003. **Useful review.**
7. McBryde KD, Kudelka TL, Kershaw DB, et al: Clearance of amino acids by hemodialysis in argininosuccinate synthetase deficiency. J Pediatr 144:536–540, 2004. **Example of hemodialysis in inborn errors of metabolism.**
8. Papez K, Allred L, Mottes TA, et al: Hemodialysis (IHD) hemofiltration (HF) in pediatrics: A new approach to intoxication.

Presented at the June 2004 Pediatric Continuous Renal Replacement Therapy annual conference, Orlando, Florida. Abstract available at http://www.ltpro.com:80/pcrrt.com/confcab2004.htm. **Hemodialysis followed by hemofiltration blunts the rebound effect.**

9. Ronco C, Bellomo R, Homel P, et al: Effects of different doses in continuous veno-venous haemofiltration on outcomes of acute renal failure: A prospective randomized trial. Lancet 356:26–30, 2000. **Consideration of the amount of CVVH and outcome.**
10. Warady BA, Morgenstern BZ, Alexander SR: Peritoneal dialysis. In Avner ED, Harmon WE, Niaudet P (eds): Pediatric Nephrology, 5th ed. Philadelphia: Lippincott Williams & Wilkins, 2004, pp 1375–1394. **Helpful chapter in a major text.**

12 Infectious Diseases

FOCI OF INFECTION

Bacterial Meningitis

Alice Prince

KEY CONCEPTS

- Bacterial meningitis is a complex process involving systemic infection (bacteremia/sepsis) as well as central nervous system (CNS) infection.
- The primary pathophysiologic event is the disruption of the blood–brain barrier.
- Maintenance of adequate CNS and systemic perfusion is critical.
- Bactericidal antibiotics given in concentrations adequate to penetrate into the cerebrospinal fluid and to cover potentially antibiotic-resistant bacteria are essential.
- Strategies to control CNS inflammation, such as the administration of corticosteroids, are likely to be useful, especially if given very early in therapy.
- Fluid and electrolyte status must be carefully monitored.
- Effective vaccines are available to *prevent* common causes of bacterial meningitis.

Bacterial meningitis was a common disease of young infants and schoolchildren that dramatically decreased in prevalence with the widespread use of effective vaccines. However, it remains an important cause of morbidity and mortality. The major causes of bacterial meningitis are bacteria that produce polysaccharide capsules that require preformed, capsule-specific antibody for efficient phagocytosis. In hosts lacking either naturally acquired or vaccine-induced antibody, inhaled bacteria colonize and then invade mucosal surfaces, cause bacteremia or sepsis, and bind to receptors on the endothelial cells lining the capillaries that form the blood–brain barrier. The ensuing inflammatory response causes widespread disruption of the blood–brain barrier, the central event in the pathophysiology of bacterial meningitis. Administration of appropriate antibiotics, although usually lifesaving, may not be sufficient to prevent the significant neurologic morbidity that ensues in 5% to 40% of survivors.

The pathogenesis of bacterial meningitis is well studied. Potential pathogens colonize the upper respiratory tract of susceptible infants and young children. Neonates are colonized by the bacteria that compose the vaginal flora, such as *Escherichia coli* and group B streptococci. Older children and adolescents may become colonized by *Streptococcus pneumoniae* or *Neisseria meningitidis*. Endothelial cells in the meninges that are targeted by the bacteria initiate local proinflammatory signaling, recruiting the influx of polymorphonuclear leukocytes (PMNs). This inflammatory response in the meningeal space causes the clinical signs and symptoms of meningitis, namely headache, stiff neck, and increased intracranial pressure. In addition, persistent bacteremia results in the signs of systemic infection, fever, vasodilation, and hypoperfusion.

Expert Opinion on Management Issues

The successful management of bacterial meningitis requires an appreciation for the complex pathophysiology of this infection and the very real risk of permanent and potentially devastating neurologic sequelae. In addition to prescribing antimicrobial agents with high activity against the likely pathogens and pharmacokinetics that include the ability to cross the blood–brain barrier, meticulous attention to systemic and central nervous system (CNS) perfusion, fluid and electrolyte balance, and the control of inflammation are critically important. Children with bacterial meningitis are ill and usually require fluid resuscitation. They are often dehydrated or hypotensive because of decreased oral intake and vomiting, as well as the increased fluid requirements associated with fever and tachypnea. Sepsis may accompany meningeal infection, and activation of the clotting cascade is a common complication. The loss of blood–brain barrier function causes loss of local arteriolar autoregulatory function and the systemic blood pressure that maintains CNS perfusion. With ongoing sepsis and vasodilation it is often difficult to appreciate if the systemic blood pressure, particularly in an infant, is sufficient to maintain adequate perfusion. Fluid and electrolyte status must be carefully monitored, recognizing that a small fraction of patients may develop the syndrome of inappropriate antidiuretic hormone secretion, a complication far less frequent than hypotension or even septic shock. An intensive care setting with the capability of invasive monitoring techniques and frequent assessment and adjustment of fluid and electrolyte status is preferred for the management of these complications. The optimal treatment of bacterial meningitis requires much more than the selection of the correct antibiotic (Box 1, Box 2, Box 3).

ANTI-INFLAMMATORY AGENTS

Endothelial cells as well as professional immune cells are highly proficient in responding to bacterial components, cell wall fragments, peptidoglycan, and lipopolysaccharide (LPS). Through the expression of chemokines and cytokines and the upregulation of cell surface receptors, PMNs are recruited from the vasculature to attack the invading bacteria. However, the inflammatory process itself, opening of tight junctions, release of PMN products, and reactive oxygen intermediates and elastase is damaging to the CNS, and phagocytosis is inefficient in the cerebrospinal fluid (CSF) because of lack of antibody and complement.

Beyond the neonatal period (for which there are no controlled data), the administration of an anti-inflammatory agent (dexamethasone) immediately prior to antibiotics suppresses the inflammatory response evoked by intact bacteria as well as bacteria lysed by antibiotics. Although the use of steroids is still debated, controlled clinical trials performed in both children and adults indicate benefits ascribed to diminishing inflammation and few, if any, side effects if steroids are given

for the very limited period of time recommended (usually four doses).

ANTIBIOTICS

The choice of antibiotics depends on the age of the patient, social and epidemiologic characteristics, and immediate prior exposure to antibiotics. Consideration of local patterns of antimicrobial susceptibility is important. Agents to cover the most likely pathogens are used until a specific organism is isolated and susceptibility to antibiotics is known.

In neonates, ampicillin plus cefotaxime/ceftriaxone (non-premature infant, no indwelling catheters) is recommended. In infants, older children, and adolescents, cefotaxime/ceftriaxone and vancomycin (60 mg/kg in four divided doses) and/or rifampin (20 mg/kg daily) is necessary because penicillin-resistant *S. pneumoniae* are increasingly prevalent, and, although these organisms may be susceptible to levels of cefotaxime/ceftriaxone that are achievable in the blood, they may not be killed in the CSF, particularly if meningeal inflammation is decreased by the concomitant use of corticosteroids. Rifampin, which penetrates well in the absence of inflammation, can also be used in combination with the β-lactams.

PROPHYLAXIS

For high-risk individuals (household contacts likely to be exposed to secretions or mucous membranes, daycare or nursery school, mouth-to-mouth resuscitation) exposed to a confirmed case of *N. meningitidis*,

---

BOX 1 Organisms that Cause Meningitis

- Neonate—Group B streptococci, *Escherichia coli*, *Listeria monocytogenes* (intracellular pathogen: different pathophysiology than the other organisms)
- Infant—*Streptococcus pneumoniae*, *Neisseria meningitidis*, *Haemophilus influenzae* (type b; unvaccinated infants: other types as well)
- Older children/adolescents—*Neisseria meningitidis* *S. pneumoniae*: communal settings (dorms, military)
- Epidemic meningitis—*Neisseria meningitidis*: type A (sub-Saharan Africa)

BOX 2 Diagnosis of Meningitis

Neonate/Infant

- Fever or hypothermia
- Lethargy or irritability
- Vomiting
- Bulging fontanelle, stiff neck, positive Kernig sign

Older Child/Adolescent

- Fever
- Headache, photophobia
- Stiff neck (positive Kernig sign, positive Brudzinski sign)
- Mental status changes
- Vomiting

BOX 3 Cerebrospinal Fluid Findings

- Polymorphonuclear leukocytes (>10)
- Elevated protein
- Lowered glucose (less than half the blood glucose because of loss of blood–brain barrier function)
- Bacteria on Gram stain

BOX 4 Vaccines for Meningitis

- **_Haemophilus influenzae_ type b (Hib):** Conjugate vaccines given at 2, 4, and 6 months of age are highly effective against *H. influenzae* type b and have dramatically reduced the incidence of this once common disease.
- **Prevnar (_Streptococcus pneumoniae_):** A conjugate vaccine that includes coverages against seven common pneumococcal capsular types is routinely given to infants. However, because there are many other capsular types, this vaccine does not provide protection against all pneumococci.
- **_Neisseria meningitidis_:** A serogroup-specific vaccine consisting of purified bacteria capsular polysaccharide from group A, C, Y, and W–135 is available for children older than 2 years. A conjugate vaccine also was recently made available for children ages 11 to 18 years. Immunization is recommended for children at high risk (complement deficiency, asplenic hosts), travelers to endemic areas, and college students. No vaccine is currently available against type B capsular types associated with sporadic infections.

chemoprophylaxis within 24 hours of diagnosis of the primary case is recommended. Chemoprophylaxis may include rifampin, ceftriaxone, or ciprofloxacin (Box 4).

COMPLICATIONS

The resolution of the acute infection and sterilization of the CSF does not signify the end of treatment for meningitis. Depending on the age of the patient, *S. pneumoniae* is associated with the most severe neurologic sequelae, ranging from blindness, quadriplegias or hemiplegias, and psychomotor retardation to seizure disorders. Frequent complications include deafness or hearing impairment in approximately 10% to 20% of patients. Even children seemingly left unscathed by this infection are often found to have significant psychomotor delay and behavioral abnormalities, and they perform less well in school than matched controls.

Common Pitfalls

- Failure to hydrate these patients adequately may result in focal areas of hypoperfusion of the brain with resultant neurologic sequelae.
- Bleeding and clotting abnormalities are a common component of the pathophysiology of meningitis and may require therapy.
- Prolonged fever during the recovery phase of illness is not necessarily caused by ongoing bacterial infection, but it is more likely a result of persistent immune stimulation despite appropriate antimicrobial therapy.

Communication and Counseling

- Close neurologic follow-up including audiometry and monitoring language development is important.
- Awareness of an increased incidence of soft neurologic findings, such as attention-deficit disorders, may lead to early diagnosis and therapy.

SUGGESTED READINGS

1. De Gans J, van de Beek D: Dexamethasone in adults with bacterial meningitis. N Engl J Med 347:1549–1556, 2002. **A large clinical study demonstrating that early treatment with dexamethasone improves outcome in adults with bacterial meningitis.**
2. Odio CM, Faingezicht I, Paris M, et al: The beneficial effects of early dexamethasone administration in infants and children with bacterial meningitis. N Engl J Med 324:1525–1531, 1991. **One of the several studies demonstrating the benefits associated with dexamethasone in infants and children younger than 2 months with bacterial meningitis.**
3. Scheld WM, Koedel U, Nathan B, Pfister HW: Pathophysiology of bacterial meningitis: Mechanisms of neuronal injury. J Infect Dis 186:S225–S233, 2002. **A review of the pathophysiology of bacterial meningitis.**
4. van der Flier M, Geelen SPM, Kimpen JL, et al: Reprogramming the host response in bacterial meningitis: How best to improve outcome? Clin Microbiol Rev 16:415–429, 2003. **A comprehensive review of the current understanding of how bacteria activate inflammation and apoptosis in endothelial and neuronal cells.**

Cellulitis

Juan N. Walterspiel and Robert S. Baltimore

KEY CONCEPTS

- Cellulitis represents the spreading inflammatory reaction to an infection of the skin and the underlying soft tissues, usually caused by a breach in the integrity of the dermis.
- Diagnosis is based on physical examination and sometimes culture of the lesion and culture of the blood.
- In an otherwise well child, the most likely pathogens are *Staphylococcus aureus* and/or group A streptococci.
- Treatment is based on empirical treatment for the most likely cause of cellulitis followed by modification based on culture documentation of the etiology.
- The rate of methicillin-resistant *S. aureus* as a cause of superficial skin infections is rising and is a major cause of treatment failure.

12

Cellulitis is the acute, visible manifestation of the spreading inflammatory reaction to an infection of the skin and the underlying soft tissues. The point of entry for invading organisms can be an ulcer with poor perfusion, a dermatosis, or a forced breach of the dermis. The mechanics of injury include insect bites, teeth, thorns, splinters, weapons, surgical instruments, needles, catheters, tattooing, and body piercing. In young children and immunocompromised hosts, bacteremia provides a hematogenous route for cutaneous infection. Knowledge of the circumstances gives clues to the type of microorganism involved and makes the clinician aware of additional risk factors for tetanus, hepatitis, or human immunodeficiency virus (HIV) infection. Equally important in the evaluation are the circumstances of the host. Skin flora, human environment (e.g., hospital, long-term care, daycare), skin conditions (e.g., eczema, steroid application, exposure to water or corrosive agents), tissue perfusion and lymphatic drainage (e.g., pressure sores, diabetes, trauma, lymphedema), previous antibiotics that may select for resistant organisms, age (e.g., neonates, expected immunization status), and preceding immunosuppression can enter into the equation. The most common locations for cellulitis are the face and the extremities.

Diagnosis is made by observation and palpation. Localization, spread, pain, warmth, color, induration, and lymphatic drainage are assessed. Imaging is indicated if necrotizing fasciitis or osteomyelitis is suspected. Easily discernible irregular borders are seen in *Erysipelas*, a superficial infection caused by group A streptococci associated with significant induration (skin resembling *peau d'orange*, "orange peel"), lymphadenitis, and rapid progression. In most cases, however, the evolving borders of cellulitis are not as easy to assign. Whenever possible, the borders should be marked with a felt-tip pen to follow progression and facilitate the evaluation for subsequent observers. Table 1 lists the differential diagnoses.

TABLE 1 Differential Diagnoses of Cellulitis

Differential Diagnosis	Clinical Clues
Infectious	
Necrotizing fasciitis	
• Type I: Mixed infection of anaerobes plus facultative species such as streptococci or Enterobacteriaceae	Acute, rapidly developing infection of the deep fascia; marked pain, tenderness, swelling, often crepitus, bullae, and necrosis of underlying skin.
• Type II: Infection with group A streptococci	Acute infection, often accompanied by toxic shock syndrome; rapid progression of marked edema to violaceous bullae and necrosis of subcutaneous tissue, absence of crepitus.
Anaerobic myonecrosis (gas gangrene caused by *Clostridium perfringens*)	Rapidly progressive toxemic infection of previously injured muscle, producing marked edema, crepitus, and brown bullae showing large, gram-positive bacilli with scant polymorphonuclear cells: on radiography, extensive gaseous dissection of muscle and fascial planes; bacteremic spread of *Clostridium septicum* from occult colonic source can produce myonecrosis without penetrating trauma.
Cutaneous anthrax	Gelatinous edema surrounding eschar of anthrax lesion may be mistaken for cellulitis; anthrax lesions are painless or pruritic; epidemiologic factors are of importance.
Vaccinia vaccination	Erythema and induration around vaccination sites reaches peak at 10–12 days (slower than cellulitis); little to no toxicity; represents the cellular response to vaccinia.
Inflammatory, Neoplastic	
Insect bite (hypersensitivity response)	History of insect bite, local pruritus; absence of fever, toxicity, or leukocytosis.
Familial Mediterranean fever–associated cellulitis-like edema	Occurs in Sephardic Jews and persons from the Middle East who have had previous episodes of recurrent fevers with or without episodes of acute abdominal pain.
Fixed drug reaction	Skin erythema does not spread rapidly as in cellulitis, fever is low, if present; history of medication use.
Pyoderma gangrenosa (lesions starting in subcutaneous fat as acute panniculitis)	Lesions become nodular or bullous and ulcerate; occurs particularly in patients with inflammatory bowel disease or collagen vascular syndromes.
Sweet syndrome (acute febrile neutrophilic dermatosis)	Acute, tender erythematous pseudo-vesiculated plaques, fever, and neutrophilic leukocytosis; associated with cancer (hematologic); when on face may resemble erysipelas or periorbital cellulitis; corticosteroid responsive.
Kawasaki disease	Fever, conjunctivitis, acute cervical lymphadenopathy, oropharyngeal erythema, dermatitis on palms and soles, facial appearance and diffuse swelling may suggest periorbital cellulitis.
Well syndrome (eosinophilic cellulitis)	Urticaria-like lesion with central clearing; lesions progress slowly and persist for weeks or months; histologically, infiltration with eosinophils, peripheral eosinophilia in 50% of cases, recurrent.

Adapted from Swartz MN: Cellulitis. N Engl J Med 350:904–912, 2004. Copyright 2004 Massachusetts Medical Society. All rights reserved.

Expert Opinion on Management Issues

In selected cases it may be necessary to make an etiologic diagnosis. In such cases special cultures may be needed.

DIAGNOSIS

Cultures of Aspirates and Lesions

Culture of needle aspirates is not as rewarding as commonly assumed. The procedure leads to the identification of a likely pathogen in only approximately 29% of cases. In children, the yield may be slightly higher when the needle aspirate is obtained from the point of greatest inflammation instead of the leading edge.

Common organisms are *Staphylococcus aureus* and group A streptococci. Less common and dependent on the mode of entry, the circumstances of the host, and its age, are gram-negative bacilli, *Haemophilus influenzae* type b (Hib) in nonimmunized children, *Pasteurella multocida* in bite wounds (cats, dogs), and *Pseudomonas aeruginosa*, *Aeromonas* species, and *Acinetobacter* species where water and footwear exposure are involved. Table 2 lists the common specific circumstances, most likely organisms, and treatment.

Blood Cultures

Blood cultures have a low yield in otherwise normal children with cellulitis, but they should be obtained in those with buccal or periorbital cellulitis, in cases of salt- or freshwater contact, in patients who have a toxic appearance, and in those who are immunocompromised.

TABLE 2 Initial Treatment for Cellulitis at Specific Sites/Exposures

Specific Sites/Exposures	Bacterial Species to Consider in Addition to Streptococci and Staphylococci	Antimicrobial Therapy	Alternative Agents
Orbital cellulitis Buccal cellulitis	*Streptococcus pneumoniae;* *Haemophilus influenzae*	Ceftriaxone or cefotaxime plus vancomycin	Meropenem
Site of pressure sores	Aerobic gram-negative bacilli (Enterobacteriaceae, *Pseudomonas aeruginosa,* *Acinetobacter*); anaerobes (bacteroides, *Peptococcus*)	Ampicillin/sulbactam; amoxicillin/clavulanate	Meropenem or piperacillin/ tazobactam or ticarcillin/clavulanate
Human bites	Oral anaerobes (bacteroides species, Peptostreptococci); *Eikenella corrodens;* viridans streptococci; *Staphylococcus aureus*	Amoxicillin/clavulanate	Penicillin plus cephalosporin
Dog and cat bites	*Pasteurella multocida* and other *Pasteurella* species; *S. aureus,* *S. intermedius,* *Neisseria canis, Haemophilus felis,* *Capnocytophaga* *canimorsus*; anaerobes	Amoxicillin/clavulanate	Penicillin plus cephalosporin
Exposure to footwear, sneakers	*Pseudomonas aeruginosa*	Aminoglycoside, ciprofloxacin	Cefepime or ceftazidime or piperacillin/tazobactam or ticarcillin/clavulanate
Exposure to salt water of saltwater fish at site of injury	*Vibrio vulnificus*	Doxycycline	Cefotaxime; ciprofloxacin
Exposure to fresh water at site of lesion or after attachment of leeches	*Aeromonas* species	Ceftazidime plus gentamicin	Meropenem; ciprofloxacin
Exposure to meat animal carcass, fish, clams, veterinarian environment	*Erysipelothrix rhusiopathiae*	Amoxicillin; penicillin for bacteremia or endocarditis	Cefotaxime; ciprofloxacin

12

Imaging

Imaging is not routinely recommended, but radiography and CT are of value where location and probing suggest subjacent osteomyelitis. MRI may guide surgical intervention when necrotizing fasciitis is suspected. Sonography and CT are useful in detecting abscess formation and guiding draining procedures.

ANTIBIOTIC THERAPY

Uncomplicated Cellulitis

In an otherwise well child, the most likely pathogens are *S. aureus* and group A streptococci. Table 3 lists the suggested antimicrobial choices for oral treatment. The occurrence of community-acquired methicillin-resistant strains of *S. aureus* (MRSA) raises new issues about empirical treatment. Clindamycin is suggested as an alternative, but a physician has to be certain that resistance to clindamycin in the local area is significantly lower than the occurrence of MRSA. Such information is often not available and may not be current even if available. A consensus on what a reasonable threshold for resistance would be, or the actual risks and costs for failure, including a possible increase in pseudomembranous colitis, makes this decision difficult. Some strains of *S. aureus* also exhibit inducible resistance to clindamycin, increasing the complexity of testing and reporting. In addition, currently there is a lack of information concerning its clinical significance.

We suggest the standard oral empiric therapy should still be a first-generation cephalosporin in most communities. Table 3 lists first-line treatment, second-line agents for allergic patients, and choices for situations when the incidence of MRSA increases or an outbreak occurs.

Cellulitis in Immunocompromised Hosts

An immunocompromised state can result from concurrent varicella infection, uncontrolled HIV infection, chronic granulomatous diseases, and any of the genetically determined immunodeficiencies. Chemotherapy, steroids, bone marrow ablation, and post-transplant medications predispose to infection by a broad spectrum of organisms. These circumstances can result in altered and even delayed clinical manifestations of cellulitis with insidious spread. Every effort should be made to secure an etiology. Broad-spectrum empirical treatment, preferably with expert input, is recommended.

In neonates, specific sites of entry include scalp electrodes and the umbilical stump. Cultures from affected areas, blood, and cerebrospinal fluid (CSF) should be obtained. The routine antimicrobials for suspected sepsis, usually an aminoglycoside and ampicillin or cefotaxime, should be expanded to cover *S. aureus*. The latest local infection control information and policy should be consulted about whether vancomycin should be substituted for a penicillinase-resistant penicillin.

TABLE 3 Oral Antibiotics for Treatment of Uncomplicated Cellulitis (7–10 days)

Antibiotic Generic Name (Trade Name)	Route	Dose (mg/kg/day)	Interval	Maximum Daily Dose	Dosage Formulation	Comments
First-Line Agent						
Cephalexin (Keflex, Keftab)	PO	50–75	q6h	4 g	Suspension, 125, 250, 500 mg/5 mL; drops, 100 mg/mL; capsules, 250, 500 mg; tablets, 250, 500 mg	Other first- or second-generation oral cephalosporins are also effective.
Second-Line Agents for Patients Allergic to Cephalosporins						
Amoxicillin/ clavulanate (Augmentin)	PO	50–80	q8–12h	1.5 g	Suspension, 125, 200, 250, 400 mg/5 mL; ES 600 mg/5 mL Tablet, 250, 500, 875 mg XR 1 g	Loose stools.
Clindamycin (Cleocin)	PO	10–30	q6–8h	1.8 g	Capsules, 75, 150, 300 mg; suspension, 75 mg/5 mL	Inducible resistance requires additional testing; Risk for pseudomembranous colitis.
Clarithromycin (Biaxin)	PO	15	q12h	1 g	Tablets, 250, 500 mg; granules, 125, 250 mg/5 mL	Unpleasant taste.
Azithromycin (Zithromax)	PO	10 on day 1, then 5 for 4 more days	qd	1 g	Tablets, 250, 500 mg; suspension, 100, 200 mg/5 mL; capsules 250 mg	Inadequate blood levels; long persistence in cells favors development of resistance.
Linezolid (Zyvox)	PO	20	q12h	1.2 g	Tablets, 400 mg, 600 mg; suspension 100 mg/5 mL	Can cause transient bone marrow depression.
Cloxacillin (Cloxapen, Tegopen)	PO	100	q6h	4 g	Suspension, 125 mg/5 mL; capsules, 250, 500 mg/mL	Tablet hard to swallow.
Dicloxacillin (Dynapen, Pathocil)	PO	50	q6h	2 g	Suspension, 6.25 mg/5 mL; capsules, 125, 250, 500 mg	Tablet hard to swallow.
Methicillin-Resistant *S. aureus* Prevalence Significant/Outbreak Situation (choice must be based on resistance pattern)						
Clindamycin (Cleocin)	PO	10–30	q6–8h	1.8 g	Capsules, 75, 150, 300 mg; suspension, 75 mg/5 mL	Inducible resistance requires additional testing; risk for pseudomembranous colitis.
Trimethoprim-sulfamethoxazole (Bactrim, Septra)	PO	8–12 TMP 40–60 SMX	q12h	4 tablets or 2 double-strength tablets	Suspension, 40 mg/mL;* tablets, 80,* 160 mg*	Rare Stevens-Johnson syndrome.
Linezolid (Zyvox)	PO	20	q12h	1.2 g	Tablets, 400 mg, 600 mg; suspension, 100 mg/5 mL	Can cause transient bone marrow depression.

*TMP (trimethoprim) component.
MRSA, methicillin-resistant *Staphylococcus aureus*; PO, by mouth; q, every; qd, every day.

Periorbital/Orbital Cellulitis

The periorbital tissues expand easily and render cellulitis a dramatic event. The swelling may shut the eye, making an accurate distinction among an allergic reaction, periorbital cellulitis, and the dangerous vision-threatening orbital cellulitis challenging. Signs for orbital cellulitis are restriction in orbital mobility and, later, proptosis. When orbital mobility and absence of proptosis cannot be assessed, immediate imaging studies are indicated because a timely surgical decompression of the retro-orbital space can preserve vision. The organisms involved in periorbital and orbital cellulitis are derived from the respiratory flora, and in young children the spread occurs through the hematogenous route.

In the prevaccine era, periorbital cellulitis in infants and young children was commonly caused by Hib. This type of cellulitis is sometimes marked by a bluish tinge. Today, penicillin-resistant pneumococci must be considered. Because of the hematogenous route of infection, blood and CSF cultures should be obtained. The old adage "When in doubt, perform a lumbar puncture" applies particularly to this situation.

Periorbital cellulitis with a clearly defined entry lesion, such as a recent abrasion or an insect bite, makes group A streptococci or *S. aureus* more likely culprits, and a CSF culture would not be required in a normal host.

Animal/Human Bites

Bite injuries are characterized by crushed tissue (human, dog) or puncture wounds (cats, snakes). In both, skin flora is carried into the wound, mixed with the mouth flora of the biter. Puncture wounds are more prone to infection compared to crush wounds. Human bites pose a high risk for infection, presumably because the human mouth flora goes to the same host. A β-lactam/β-lactamase inhibitor combination (amoxicillin/clavulanic acid, ampicillin/sulbactam) is the recommended first choice to treat established cellulitis from bite wounds.

Puncture Wounds

The superficial appearance of puncture wounds often belies their pain. Soil contamination predisposes to polymicrobial infection that includes *Clostridium* species. Tetanus prophylaxis must be given where an inadequate immune status is noted. *Pseudomonas* species are notorious colonizers of footwear, and puncture wounds through footwear and on the feet raise the probability that this organism is involved. This location alone does not rule out *S. aureus* or group A streptococci, however. The osteochondritis that may follow cellulitis after puncture wounds on the feet requires surgical debridement because antimicrobial treatment alone is insufficient.

Children with Neurologic Impairment

Neurologic impairment can lead to pressure sores in contact areas. These and pressure points from orthopedic devices can give rise to cellulitis. Subjacent contiguous osteomyelitis, particularly in areas of diminished sensation, can ensue. Therapy in these situations requires debridement to remove necrotic tissue and procedures to restore an adequate blood supply. Surface cultures are not informative. Biopsies and deep cultures are required. A multitude of organisms, including coagulase-negative staphylococci, anaerobes, and gram-negative rods, are usually recovered. The choice of prolonged antimicrobial courses is often complicated by the resistance patterns associated with previous antimicrobial treatment and the flora encountered in long-term care facilities.

Common Pitfalls

- Complications from delayed treatment of cellulitis include bacteremia with seeding to other organs, heart valves, joints, and body cavities; systemic inflammatory response; and toxin-mediated manifestations, such as shock syndrome or scarlet fever.
- Lesions appearing similar to cellulitis can be misdiagnosed. The possibility of a deeper component

to the infection or a noninfectious condition (see Table 1) must be considered.

- Treatment failure may be caused by methicillin-resistant *S. aureus* as a cause of cellulitis and may require modification of antibiotic treatment.
- Local factors may predispose to recurrent cellulitis. When patients have interdigital dermatophyte infections, they should be treated with topical antifungal agents. Patients with peripheral edema should use support stockings and fastidious skin care.

Communication and Counseling

The inflammatory response in cellulitis may briefly increase as the organisms break down and is slow to resolve even under optimal antimicrobial therapy. It is therefore premature to consider changes from first-line therapy in an otherwise normal host until at least 3 days have passed without improvement.

Patients with risk factors for recurrent cellulitis caused by chronic skin conditions and disorders of lymphatic drainage should work out regimens for preventive care with their primary physicians, perhaps in consultation with a dermatologist.

SUGGESTED READINGS

1. Fleischer G, Ludwig S, Campos J: Cellulitis: Bacterial etiology, clinical features, and laboratory findings. J Pediatr 97:591–593, 1980. **Experience supporting the notion of hematogenous route of infection in children with facial cellulitis.**
2. Howe PM, Eduardo Fajardo J, Orcutt MA: Etiologic diagnosis of cellulitis: Comparison of aspirates obtained from the leading edge and the point of maximal inflammation. Pediatr Infect Dis J 6:685–686, 1987. **Describes experience that aspirates from the point of maximal inflammation have a higher yield.**
3. Swartz MN: Cellulitis. N Engl J Med 350:904–912, 2004. **An overview of cellulitis with calculation of an average yield of 29% from culture aspirates from several studies.**

Pneumonia

Marc D. Foca

KEY CONCEPTS

- The syndromic diagnosis of pneumonia may be necessary in the very young initially when physical examination is less revealing.
- The etiology of pneumonia varies with age and is frequently viral in the young infant.
- Standard laboratory diagnosis of bacterial infections using blood and sputum cultures is difficult in pediatric patients.
- Treatment is most often empirical and varies with age.
- Preventive measures reduce the incidence of certain viral and bacterial pathogens.
- The increasing prevalence of community-acquired methicillin resistant *Staphylococcus aureus* may change therapeutic management.

The diagnosis of pneumonia (inflammation of the lung parenchyma) in pediatric patients is common, especially in children younger than 5 years. Mortality in the developed world is generally low, but pneumonia accounts for more than 2 million pediatric deaths annually around the globe (20% of childhood mortality). Despite the importance of pneumonia as a clinical entity in pediatrics, there is little in the way of evidence-based guidelines for the diagnosis and management of this collection of disease entities.

Expert Opinion on Management Issues

DIAGNOSIS: SYNDROMIC

The World Health Organization (WHO) was the first to put clinical parameters for the diagnosis and management of lower respiratory tract infections (LRIs) into a usable format. The original criteria included cough, respiratory difficulty, tachypnea, and chest indrawing in combination to decide whether a patient needed admission to the hospital or could be treated as an outpatient. Tachypnea without any other signs or symptoms was considered an indicator of another condition, such as anemia, acidosis, or dehydration. Tachypnea with cough or respiratory difficulty was an indicator of less severe LRI, and chest indrawing was believed to be the best indicator of severe LRI with need for urgent hospitalization. Tachypnea was initially considered a respiratory rate greater than 50 in any child younger than 5 years, but this was later refined for greater sensitivity to be a respiratory rate greater than 60 in infants younger than 2 months, greater than 50 in children from 2 to 11 months of age, and greater than 40 in those from 1 to 5 years of age. Variations in respiratory rate due to fever are not included in these guidelines, but there is a modification for high-altitude diagnosis that includes pulse oximetry. These criteria are now used worldwide, and they are the basis for further discussions of this topic.

A Canadian task force in 1997 concluded that the absence of respiratory distress, tachypnea, rales, and decreased breath sounds excludes the diagnosis of pneumonia in a pediatric patient, but the British Thoracic Society (BTS) published the most comprehensive pediatric guidelines in 2002. Classic signs of pneumonia on physical examination, such as dullness to percussion, egophony, and whispered pectoriloquy, are of little value in the young pediatric patient; although they can be found in the older patient and should be elicited for localization of the affected pulmonary lobe, especially if chest radiography is not immediately available.

ETIOLOGY

The BTS estimates that up to a third of all cases of pneumonia in children are the result of viral infections, but dual infection with bacteria is common. As a child ages, bacterial infections become more prominent, with *Streptococcus pneumoniae* traditionally the most

---

> ### BOX 1   Frequently Isolated Pathogens by Age Group
>
> **All Age Groups**
> - Respiratory syncytial virus
> - Influenza
> - Cytomegalovirus
> - Parainfluenza
> - Adenovirus
> - Human metapneumovirus
> - Rhinovirus.
>
> **Neonates**
> - Group B *Streptococcus*
> - Gram-negative organisms
> - *Listeria monocytogenes*.
>
> **1 to 3 Months**
> - *Chlamydia trachomatis*
> - *Staphylococcus aureus*
> - *Streptococcus pneumoniae*.
>
> **4 Months to 5 Years**
> - *Streptococcus pneumoniae*
> - Nontypable *Haemophilus influenzae*
> - *Mycoplasma pneumoniae*.
>
> **5 Years and Older**
> - *Mycoplasma pneumoniae*
> - *Chlamydia pneumoniae*
> - *Streptococcus pneumoniae*.
>
> Adapted from Low DE, Pichichero ME, Schaad UB: Optimizing antibacterial therapy for community-acquired respiratory tract infections in children in an era of bacterial resistance. Clin Pediatr (Phila) 43(2):135–151, 2004.

important in the preschool-age group and *Mycoplasma pneumoniae* in the school-age group. Box 1 lists pathogens by age.

DIAGNOSIS: LABORATORY

Detection of viral pathogens today is aided by improved laboratory techniques, including direct fluorescence antibody (DFA) testing of nasopharyngeal washings and shell vial assays with more rapid detection times than standard viral cultures. These methods should be used for patients requiring admission to the hospital for purposes of isolation as well as to aid in the reduction of unnecessary antibiotic use. They are not generally required for the outpatient management of viral infections. Unfortunately, the detection of bacterial pathogens in pediatric patients remains problematic.

Blood cultures are very rarely positive, and it is difficult to perform adequate sputum sampling in the young patient. Urinary antigen tests to detect the pneumococcus are available, but their specificity in pediatric patients is low, and thus they are not used routinely. It is unnecessary to perform most laboratory tests in the management of an outpatient bacterial pneumonia. A complete blood count (CBC) with differential and, potentially, a chest radiograph should be adequate in most cases. Box 2 supplies the criteria for admission to the hospital. The workup for a patient requiring admission is more extensive and includes a

CBC with differential, a blood culture, a chest radiograph, an erythrocyte sedimentation rate or C-reactive protein to follow the course of therapy in a complicated pneumonia, and a urinary antigen test for the pneumococcus as well as the viral studies mentioned previously. If the patient is old enough to provide a good sputum sample, it should be obtained as well.

TREATMENT

In a healthy child, infections with viral pathogens generally require supportive care only and are not discussed here. Therapy for bacterial pathogens is largely empirical. Table 1 outlines by age the need for both outpatient and inpatient treatment.

PREVENTION

Children with underlying medical conditions that predispose to more severe viral infections (i.e., prematurity, chronic lung disease, reactive airway disease, congenital heart disease) and the immunocompromised should be given prophylaxis against the most common viral infection, respiratory syncytial virus (RSV), with monthly injections of the humanized monoclonal antibody product. In addition, all such affected children should receive influenza vaccination. Both strategies should follow American Academy of Pediatrics (AAP) and Red Book guidelines.

Prior to the advent of the seven-valent pneumococcal conjugate vaccine (PCV), the prevalence of *S. pneumoniae* isolates nonsusceptible (intermediately or highly resistant) to penicillin was rising dramatically. The organism acquires resistance to penicillin via conjugation of DNA fragments from cohabitating oral flora, which results in isolates with altered cell wall enzymes (penicillin-binding proteins [PBPs]) that have decreased affinity for β-lactam antibiotics. β-Lactamases are not involved in this process, and consequently, this mechanism of resistance can be overcome by increasing the oral dose of the β-lactam antibiotic used by the patient. Less often cited is the propensity of these penicillin nonsusceptible strains to also harbor resistance to the macrolides and the quinolones, making them potentially difficult to treat on an outpatient basis. Studies looking at the mortality from pneumonia caused by penicillin nonsusceptible strains of *S. pneumoniae* generally fail to show increased mortality with current therapies unless the isolate is highly resistant to both penicillin and cefotaxime. This is not true for infections such as meningitis where it is more difficult to obtain the antibiotic levels necessary to eradicate a resistant organism.

The previous 23-valent polysaccharide-based vaccine should not be used in children younger than 2 years because of the poor response to polysaccharides in this age group. PCV contains elements of the seven pneumococcal serotypes that cause 85% of invasive pneumococcal disease (IPD) conjugated to a protein carrier, and as a result, it can be used in routine childhood vaccination programs. The schedule of administration is 2, 4, 6, and 15 months. Initial studies performed after Food and Drug Administration (FDA) approval in 2000 indicated that the vaccine was effective in reducing the incidence of chest radiograph–documented pneumonia, especially in those children younger than 2 years with the highest incidence of IPD. Of note, studies now show a decrease in the racial/ethnic differences in IPD after

---

BOX 2 Hospital Admission Criteria

- Tachypnea (places the patient at risk for respiratory failure).
- Decreased oxygen saturation as measured by pulse oximetry or arterial blood gas.
- Grunting.
- Age: Neonates are always admitted; and young infants up to 4 months of age are often admitted.
- Failure to feed or evidence of dehydration.
- Evidence of pulmonary complication, such as empyema, abscess, or pneumatocele.

Adapted from British Thoracic Society guidelines.

TABLE 1 Initial Antimicrobial Regimens for Common Bacterial Pathogens by Age and Admission Status

Status	Neonate	1 mo–4 mo	4 mo–5 yr	5 yr and Older
Outpatient	No outpatient management	Often admitted unless Chlamydia is suspected: erythromycin, 20–50 mg/kg/day, divided q6 h	Amoxicillin, 80–100 mg/kg/day, divided bid-tid	Azithromycin, 12 mg/kg/day qd (max dose 500 mg) *or* amoxicillin, 80–100 mg/kg/day divided bid-tid
Inpatient	Ampicillin, 200 mg/kg/day divided q6 h, and cefotaxime, 150–200 mg/kg/day divided q6 h, *or* ceftriaxone, 100 mg/kg/day divided bid, *or* gentamicin, 6 mg/kg/day qd	Cefuroxime,* 200 mg/kg/day divided q8 h ± vancomycin,† 40 mg/kg/day divided q6h	Cefotaxime, 200 mg/kg/day, divided q8 h ± vancomycin, 40 mg/kg/day divided q6h	Cefotaxime, 200 mg/kg/day divided q8 h + azithromycin, 12 mg/kg/day qd (max dose 500 mg) ± vancomycin, 40 mg/kg/day divided q6 h

*Cefuroxime is a second-generation cephalosporin with improved activity against *Staphylococcus aureus*.
†The addition of vancomycin should be considered if a patient has rapid progression of disease while receiving appropriate empirical therapy, but every effort should be made to isolate a pathogen by performing pleurocentesis if a pleural effusion develops, a blood culture if there is a respiratory decompensation, and/or individualized imaging for a metastatic focus that might indicate a staphylococcal infection.
  bid, twice daily, q, every; qd, daily; qxh, every x hours; tid, three times per day.

introduction of PCV. African American children younger than 2 years had a rate of IPD of 340 per 100,000 prior to approval of PCV as compared to a rate of 170 per 100,000 in white children. After widespread institution of pneumococcal vaccination programs, this rate fell to a statistically nonsignificant level of 55.7 per 100,000 to 39.6 per 100,000, respectively. Vaccination also appears to lower the incidence of IPD in the older adult, probably through herd immunity, because colonization with pneumococcal isolates is more common in young children. Whether nonvaccine serotypes will replace vaccine serotypes in invasive infections and whether antibiotic resistance will decrease are still both open questions requiring further analysis in prospective cohorts.

Current evidence indicates that levels of drug resistance in nasopharyngeal isolates have not changed, despite a decrease in the isolation of vaccine serotypes. In addition, the Centers for Disease Control and Prevention database has not seen a change in resistance patterns, despite a decline in vaccine serotype isolation of 78% in children younger than 2 years.

Common Pitfalls

The greatest difficulty with the management of childhood bacterial pneumonia is that the causative organism is rarely isolated. Because of the problems with the laboratory diagnosis already described, therapy is most often empirical. However, with the increasing prevalence of community-acquired methicillin-resistant *S. aureus* (CA-MRSA), empirical therapy may need to be altered and/or more aggressive methods of pathogen isolation may be required. A reported 10% to 20% of CA-MRSA infections are pneumonia, and patients frequently develop an empyema and/or metastatic infection. Complications of bacterial pneumonia include pleural effusion, empyema, abscess formation, and pneumatocele, even in patients who are taking appropriate antibiotics. Although it remains reasonable to use antibiotics that cover the majority of suspected pathogens as outlined, it is prudent to perform pleurocentesis for culture and symptom relief when an effusion/empyema develops, and it may be necessary to perform a bronchoalveolar lavage (BAL) if the patient is not improving on empirical antimicrobials.

Communication and Counseling

Parents should be made aware that the complications just noted can occur at any time during therapy for pneumonia despite appropriate antibiotics. If a child has had symptomatic relief on oral therapy and then develops a new fever or symptoms of respiratory distress, reevaluation is needed for the development of complications that may prolong therapy, require more invasive diagnostic/therapeutic intervention, or demand the addition of alternate antibiotics. Parents also need to be told that certain viral infections (i.e., influenza and varicella) predispose to bacterial superinfection. If a patient is recovering from one of these infections and develops the new onset of fever or respiratory distress, an immediate evaluation for the development of a secondary pneumonia is necessary.

SUGGESTED READINGS

1. Black S, Shinefield H, Baxter R, et al: Postlicensure surveillance for pneumococcal invasive disease after use of heptavalent pneumococcal conjugate vaccine in Northern California Kaiser-Permanente. Pediatr Infect Dis J 23(6):485–489, 2004. **Analysis from the large database at Kaiser-Permanente.**
2. Black SB, Shinefield HR, Ling S, et al: Effectiveness of heptavalent pneumococcal conjugate vaccine in children younger than five years of age for prevention of pneumonia. Pediatr Infect Dis J 21(9):810–815, 2002. **One of the first post-licensure studies.**
3. Low DE, Pichichero ME, Schaad UB: Optimizing antibacterial therapy for community-acquired respiratory tract infections in children in an era of bacterial resistance. Clin Pediatr (Phila) 43(2):135–151, 2004. **Excellent review of pneumonia, the pathogens, and the management.**
4. Michelow IC, Olsen K, Lozano J, et al: Epidemiology and clinical characteristics of community-acquired pneumonia in hospitalized children. Pediatrics 113(4):701–707, 2004. **Large pre-PCV epidemiologic study of pneumonia isolates in children.**
5. Pelton SI, Loughlin AM, Marchant CD: Seven valent pneumococcal conjugate vaccine immunization in two Boston communities: Changes in serotypes and antimicrobial susceptibility among *Streptococcus pneumoniae* isolates. Pediatr Infect Dis J 23 (11):1015–1022, 2004. **Study showing that antimicrobial susceptibility of nasopharyngeal isolates has not changed.**
6. Pio A: Standard case management of pneumonia in children in developing countries: The cornerstone of the acute respiratory infection programme. Bull World Health Organ 81(4):298–300, 2003. **WHO criteria for the diagnosis of pneumonia.**
7. Schultz KD, Fan LL, Pinsky J, et al: The changing face of pleural empyemas in children: Epidemiology and management. Pediatrics 113(6):1735–1740, 2004. **Empyema incidence as a result of CA-MRSA.**
8. Song JH, Jung SI, Ki HK, et al: Clinical outcomes of pneumococcal pneumonia caused by antibiotic-resistant strains in Asian countries: A study by the Asian Network for Surveillance of Resistant Pathogens. Clin Infect Dis 38(11):1570–1578, 2004. **Large outcome study of resistant isolates.**
9. Talbot TR, Poehling KA, Hartert TV, et al: Reduction in high rates of antibiotic-nonsusceptible invasive pneumococcal disease in Tennessee after introduction of the pneumococcal conjugate vaccine. Clin Infect Dis 39(5):641–648, 2004. **Post-licensure study of antibiotic nonsusceptible isolates.**
10. Whitney CG, Farley MM, Hadler J, et al: Decline in invasive pneumococcal disease after the introduction of protein-polysaccharide conjugate vaccine. N Engl J Med 348(18):1737–1746, 2003. **Post-licensure study of invasive disease.**

Osteomyelitis

Paul Krogstad

KEY CONCEPTS

- Osteomyelitis is most common in childhood, especially in prepubertal children.
- Most cases result from hematogenous delivery of organisms.
- Gram-positive organisms are now the cause of most hematogenous infections in immunocompetent children.

- The diagnosis is usually confirmed by microbiologic tests (e.g., positive cultures from bone or soft tissue aspirates) and imaging (MRI or bone scanning).
- Therapy for most children is initially directed against gram-positive organisms.
- Serial monitoring of the erythrocyte sedimentation rate or serum levels of C-reactive protein is used to monitor the therapeutic response.
- With appropriate therapy, bony changes may not develop.

BOX 1 Differential Diagnosis

- Fracture
- Septic arthritis
- Rheumatic fever
- Sepsis
- Cellulitis
- Primary tumors of bone: Ewing sarcoma
- Leukemia
- Thrombophlebitis
- Bone infarction (sickle cell and Gaucher disease).

Infection of the tubular and flat bones of the skeleton occurs most commonly in early childhood and generally follows the hematogenous delivery of bacteria to bone marrow. In fully immunized, immunocompetent children, acute hematogenous osteomyelitis is most often caused by gram-positive pathogens such as *Staphylococcus aureus* and streptococci, although *Kingella kingae* is increasingly identified. In newborns, coliforms and coagulase-negative staphylococci are also common causes. Salmonella species predominate in children with sickle hemoglobinopathy. Less common causes of osteomyelitis include *Mycobacterium tuberculosis* and *Coccidioides immitis*. The long tubular bones are the usual sites of infection (femur, humerus, tibia, and fibula), although osteomyelitis may occur at any skeletal location. The presentation also varies by age, reflecting developmental changes in bone. In newborns, pus may rupture the thin loosely applied periosteum and spread into the overlying soft tissues. Older children and adolescents generally present with fever, localized pain, limp, and pain on passive or active movement.

Osteomyelitis also results from penetrating injuries of bone or spread of infection from adjacent tissues, and it has a more complex and unpredictable microbiology. Infection of bones of the foot may follow penetrating wounds of the foot, especially stepping on nails, toothpicks, or pins; prompt and complete debridement is essential and may permit a short course of antimicrobial therapy. Most cases of osteomyelitis require prolonged medical therapy. It is often possible to transition from intravenous to oral therapy, if compliance is assured.

Expert Opinion on Management Issues

DIAGNOSTIC EVALUATION

The diagnosis is generally made on clinical grounds, supplanted by a relatively small number of adjunctive tests. In neonates, infants, and young children, needle aspiration of the overlying soft tissue or incision and drainage of bone may yield the offending organism. Blood cultures should be obtained but are only positive in approximately half of all patients. In many patients, only an aspirate of bone yields a microbiologic diagnosis. A complete blood count, blood culture, erythrocyte sedimentation rate (ESR) and/or C-reactive protein (CRP), and conventional radiographs should always

be obtained at the time of evaluation and are an important tool in considering the broad differential diagnosis (Box 1). At the time of presentation, bony changes caused by osteomyelitis are seen in the majority of neonates, but soft tissue swelling is the only abnormality found in older children and adolescents. Radiographic evidence of bone destruction is not usually detected until 10 to 21 days after the onset of symptoms, and it may not be seen at all if antimicrobial therapy is initiated early in the disease.

If the diagnosis remains in doubt after initial evaluation, MRI is the imaging modality of choice, usually revealing evidence of metaphyseal inflammation. Without using ionizing radiation, it also delineates accurately subperiosteal or soft tissue collections of pus that might require surgical drainage, and it can identify sinus tracts for removal, thus providing more specific anatomic information than bone scanning, CT, or plain radiography. Radionuclide scanning historically was a valuable adjunct to the diagnosis of osteomyelitis, but it employs a radioactive tracer (usually ^{99m}Tc) and yields images of low resolution. Bone scans are often nondiagnostic in newborns. Gallium and tagged white blood cell scans do not offer any advantage over MRI and older radionuclide imaging approaches.

SURGICAL AND MEDICAL THERAPY

The need for surgical therapy must be promptly evaluated. Subperiosteal and soft tissue abscesses should be drained, and sequestra, if present, must be removed. These surgical procedures offer the opportunity to identify the pathogen(s) involved. Immobilization of the affected extremity or splinting may afford relief from pain and is sometimes used to prevent pathologic fractures from occurring when extensive bone involvement is detected by plain radiography.

Acute bacterial osteomyelitis should be initially treated with intravenous agents with potent activity against *S. aureus,* pneumococci, and group A streptococci. Nafcillin, oxacillin, or cefazolin are usually appropriate, but in areas where community-acquired methicillin-resistant *S. aureus* infections (CA-MRSA) are common, clindamycin or vancomycin should be used instead. If epidemiologic factors suggest the possibility of gram-negative pathogens (e.g., osteomyelitis in children with sickle cell disease or in newborns), a third-generation cephalosporin, such as cefotaxime or ceftriaxone, should be added to provide additional coverage.

Osteomyelitis caused by *Streptococcus pneumoniae* strains with decreased susceptibility to penicillin is successfully managed using a variety of agents, including ceftriaxone, vancomycin, and clindamycin. β-Lactam antibiotics, including oxacillin, nafcillin, and cephalosporins, are used in the successful treatment of *K. kingae*, but this organism is resistant to clindamycin. Because of the increasing frequency of drug-resistant pneumococci and CA-MRSA and the increasing reports of *K. kingae* in osteomyelitis, it is vital to attempt to identify the pathogen causing the infection.

Although once controversial, sequential use of intravenous and oral routes of administration of antibiotics has gained acceptance for the treatment of pediatric osteomyelitis. Completing treatment with oral therapy avoids the cost, pain, inconvenience, and hazards of long-term intravenous antibiotic administration. Oral therapy is most likely to succeed and is generally considered an acceptable option when the patient has the ability to swallow and retain medication, an etiologic agent has been identified, the laboratory is able to monitor degree of antibiotic absorption, and there is a clear clinical response to intravenously administered antibiotics. Although eschewed by some, therapeutic drug monitoring is generally recommended to demonstrate that adequate absorption of orally administered antibiotics is occurring. Rare patients have inadequate serum levels despite high oral dosage. If bacteria were isolated from the patient, a peak serum bactericidal titer of 1:8 or greater is sought. Alternatively, serum drug concentration assays for the drug may be used.

Both CRP and ESR rise during the first several days of antimicrobial therapy and then begin to decline. CRP generally normalizes within 7 to 10 days; the ESR falls more slowly. A slow decline of CRP values is associated with more extensive radiographic changes or persistent symptoms 1 to 2 months after discharge from the hospital. If bacteremia is documented, intravenous therapy is usually given for at least 7 days, but a change to oral therapy may be started when clinical examination, complete blood count (CBC), and CRP results all indicate a response to therapy; this pattern is often seen after 4 to 7 days. A typical transition is to switch from intravenous oxacillin to oral cephalexin or dicloxacillin. Treatment failures are common when treatment is given for less than 2 weeks. Consequently, most authorities recommend at least 4 to 6 weeks of treatment for hematogenous osteomyelitis, including the duration of both intravenous and oral therapy.

Common Pitfalls

Osteomyelitis may be confused for other infections or inflammatory disorders, particularly in cases of infections involving bones other than tubular bones. Osteomyelitis of the pelvis may be mistaken for septic arthritis of the hip, intra-abdominal infection, or other soft tissue disease. Infection of bones of the foot may be difficult to recognize, particularly if swelling is misinterpreted as a sign of superficial soft tissue disease. Chronic recurrent multifocal osteomyelitis, a chronic inflammatory disorder, is not linked to infection but initially may lead to prolonged courses of antimicrobial therapy. As noted earlier, oral medications can often be used for a portion of therapy for osteomyelitis, but treatment failures may occur in the event of poor adherence to therapy or poor drug absorption. However, weeks of intravenous therapy may be complicated by infection or other problems involved in the use of indwelling vascular catheters. Either oral or intravenous therapy for osteomyelitis may be complicated by antibiotic-associated diarrhea, *Clostridium difficile*–associated enterocolitis, bone marrow suppression, or other complications of prolonged exposure to antimicrobial therapy. The most serious complication of acute osteomyelitis is the development of chronic osteomyelitis, which usually requires meticulous debridement of devitalized bone and months of antimicrobial therapy.

Communication and Counseling

Osteomyelitis is a very serious illness with the potential to cause lifelong disability. Parents should be made aware of importance of adherence and good follow-up and counseled that treatment relapses, although infrequent, may occur years, even decades, after apparently successful therapy.

SUGGESTED READINGS

1. Jacobs RF, McCarthy RE, Elser JM: Pseudomonas osteochondritis complicating puncture wounds of the foot in children: A 10-year evaluation. J Infect Dis 160:657–661, 1989. **The authors describe their extensive experience with this disease, highlighting the complicated microbiology and the benefits of meticulous debridement.**
2. Krogstad PA: Osteomyelitis and septic arthritis. In Feigin R, Cherry JD, Demmler G, Kaplan SL (eds): Textbook of Pediatric Infectious Diseases, 5th ed. Philadelphia: WB Saunders, 2003. **Detailed description of the pathophysiology, evaluation, and treatment of acute and chronic osteomyelitis.**
3. Nelson JD: Acute osteomyelitis in children. Infect Dis Clin North Am 4(3):513–522, 1990. **A very large single-center experience showing the breadth of manifestations of the disease.**
4. Nelson JD: Toward simple but safe management of osteomyelitis. Pediatrics 99(6):883–884, 1997. **A well-referenced expert editorial that examines controversies in management.**
5. Roine I, Arguedas A, Faingezicht I, Rodriguez F: Early detection of sequela-prone osteomyelitis in children with use of simple clinical and laboratory criteria. Clin Infect Dis 24(5):849–853, 1997. **This study shows the utility of C-reactive protein measurements in managing osteomyelitis and identifying complications.**
6. Roine I, Faingezicht I, Arguedas A, et al: Serial serum C-reactive protein to monitor recovery from acute hematogenous osteomyelitis in children. Pediatr Infect Dis J 14(1):40–44, 1995. **This study demonstrates the utility of C-reactive protein measurements in the management of the disease, including the early identification of complications.**
7. Trobs R, Moritz R, Buhligen U, et al: Changing pattern of osteomyelitis in infants and children. Pediatr Surg Int 15(5–6):363–372, 1999. **A 30-year experience with osteomyelitis is described.**

Septic Arthritis

Paul Krogstad

KEY CONCEPTS

- Infectious arthritis in children is usually caused by bacteria.
- Most cases result from hematogenous delivery of organisms.
- Hip and shoulder joints must be promptly drained to avoid sequelae.
- Gram-positive organisms are now the cause of most cases in immunocompetent children and adolescents, although gonococcal infections must be considered in sexually active youths.
- The diagnosis is usually confirmed by microbiologic tests (e.g., positive cultures from joint fluid or blood, demonstration of organisms by Gram stain of joint fluid, elevated joint fluid, and white blood cell count).
- Intravenous therapy is used initially in most cases.
- Serial monitoring of the erythrocyte sedimentation rate (ESR) or serum level of C-reactive protein (CRP) is used to monitor the therapeutic response.
- Radiographs should be obtained at the start of therapy and repeated 2 to 3 weeks into therapy to look for signs of unsuspected osteomyelitis.

The terms *septic arthritis* and *acute suppurative pyarthrosis* are used interchangeably to refer to bacterial infections of the joints. Septic arthritis occurs at all ages, but it is particularly common in infants and young children. Septic arthritis usually results from hematogenous delivery of bacteria to the joint space, but it may also follow penetrating injuries or spread of infection from adjacent tissues. Prompt surgical drainage is a critical component of the therapy of septic arthritis of the shoulder and hip. Prolonged antimicrobial medical therapy is needed for most cases. Except in neonates, it is often possible to transition from intravenous to oral therapy if compliance is assured.

Expert Opinion on Management Issues

CLINICAL RECOGNITION

Almost all patients have fever and constitutional symptoms within the first few days of the infection. Lower extremity (knee, hip, and ankle) infections account for approximately 80% of all cases. In infants, in whom the hip is the most common joint involved, swelling, tenderness, and heat may be absent; the infant lies with the involved leg abducted and externally rotated, and joint effusion is present. In contrast, neonatal gonococcal infection in newborns may manifest with acute arthritis following nonspecific prodromal symptoms (poor feeding, irritability, and fever); the joints below the hip usually are involved (knee, ankles, and pedal metacarpophalangeal joints). Most children present with fever,

localized pain, limp, and pain on passive or active movement. During adolescence, the disseminated gonococcal infection (DGI) may manifest with fever, rash, and tenosynovitis or small-joint arthritis with minimal joint effusion. In adolescent girls, the illness often follows the onset of menses by a few days. Some patients with DGI develop frank septic arthritis indistinguishable from septic arthritis caused by other organisms.

Pyogenic sacroiliitis is often accompanied by tenderness detected by pressure applied over the sacrum during a digital rectal examination and by pain during simultaneous flexion, abduction, and external rotation at the hip.

DIAGNOSTIC EVALUATION

A complete blood count, erythrocyte sedimentation rate (ESR), and/or C-reactive protein (CRP) should be obtained at the time of evaluation. Blood cultures should always be obtained because they sometimes yield the pathogen when joint fluid cultures do not. Radiographs should also be obtained and are an important tool in considering the broad differential diagnosis (Box 1). The plain film is often normal in septic arthritis, although soft tissue swelling, dislocation or subluxation of the femoral head, muscle swelling, and loss of normal tissue planes may be identified. Ultrasound has high sensitivity for the detecting joint space effusions at the hip, and it may be helpful in deciding if hip joint aspiration is warranted. MRI is not usually used in the initial evaluation of septic arthritis, but it detects joint effusions with high sensitivity.

The joint fluid should be collected in a heparinized syringe so the large clot that usually forms in the fluid derived from patients with septic arthritis or juvenile rheumatoid arthritis does not preclude the enumeration of the leukocytes. Fluid aspirated from joint fluid is sent for cell count, Gram stain, and both aerobic and anaerobic cultures. Joint fluid normally contains 50 cells/mL or less. In septic arthritis, the joint fluid usually has a leukocyte count of more than 50,000 cells/mL, and the majority of the cells are polymorphonuclear granulocytes; it is unusual to find less than 20,000 cells/mL. A gram-stained smear of joint fluid aspirates must be examined carefully because joint fluid exerts a bacteriostatic effect on microorganisms and organisms that may be seen but may not grow in culture. However, one third of joint aspirates are sterile even when other clinical and laboratory findings indicate the presence of septic arthritis, including positive blood cultures. Inoculating cell lysis culture bottles may enhance the recovery of *Kingella kingae* and other organisms from joint fluid. Oropharyngeal, rectal, and urogenital cultures or nucleic acid detection assays for gonococcal DNA in urine may be needed to confirm the diagnosis of gonococcal arthritis.

SURGICAL AND MEDICAL THERAPY

Septic arthritis found in the hips or shoulders should be drained as soon as the diagnosis is apparent to prevent

BOX 1 Differential Diagnosis of Septic Arthritis

Related to Infections
Viral infections

- Adenovirus
- Erythrovirus (parvovirus) B19
- Hepatitis B
- Rubella
- Togaviruses
- Vaccinia
- Variola (smallpox)
- Varicella-zoster
- Enteroviruses

Fungal arthritis

- *Coccidiodes immitis*
- *Sporothrix schenckii*
- *Blastomyces dermatidis*
- *Candida* species

Other infections

- Lyme disease
- Tuberculous arthritis
- Obturator internus muscle abscess
- Epiphyseal osteomyelitis
- Deep cellulitis
- Bacterial endocarditis
- Septic bursitis

Reactive arthritis following bacterial infection

- *Shigella*
- *Salmonella*
- *Yersinia*
- *Chlamydia*

Noninfectious

- Post-traumatic
  - Thrombosis following femoral vein venipuncture
  - Fracture
  - Traumatic arthritis
  - Joint hemorrhage
- Legg-Calvé-Perthes disease
- Slipped femoral capital epiphysis
- Leukemia
- Lupus erythematosus
- Toxic synovitis
- Serum sickness
- Seronegative spondyloarthropathy
- Rheumatoid arthritis
- Rheumatic fever
- Henoch-Schönlein purpura
- Villonodular synovitis

plus gentamicin (or cefotaxime) are reasonable initial selections. Vancomycin should be substituted for the antistaphylococcal penicillin in infants who develop septic arthritis, particularly those with prolonged neonatal care, in view of the possibility of infection with coagulase-negative staphylococci.

For children older than 2 months, therapy must always include an antistaphylococcal agent such as β-lactamase–resistant penicillin (e.g., nafcillin or cloxacillin) or first-generation cephalosporin (e.g., cefazolin) or clindamycin. If methicillin-resistant *Staphylococcus aureus* or penicillin-resistant *Streptococcus pneumoniae* are suspected on the basis of local antimicrobial resistance, vancomycin or clindamycin should be used as the initial antistaphylococcal agent. In sexually active adolescents, the empirical coverage should include agents active against *Neisseria gonorrhoeae* (e.g., ceftriaxone or cefotaxime). Patients with sickle cell disease and other immunocompromised patients should be treated with a third-generation cephalosporin, such as ceftriaxone, in addition to the antistaphylococcal agent.

All researched antibiotics readily penetrate into the joint fluid. Injection of antibiotics into the joint space is usually unnecessary and may produce painful joint inflammation. If an effusion reaccumulates after initial drainage or aspiration, it should be removed by arthrocentesis, not only to make the patient more comfortable but also so serial assessment of therapy can be made. In newborns, therapy should be administered by the intravenous route for the entire course of therapy, but in older children, oral therapy may be used after a week or so of intravenous treatment has been administered. If oral medication is used to complete therapy, it is advisable to measure drug concentrations or determine the serum bacteriocidal titer to verify absorption. Although the exact duration of therapy needed to treat septic arthritis satisfactorily is not determined, 3 or more weeks of therapy are usually recommended. Some cases of presumed septic arthritis turn out to be cases of osteomyelitis of the epiphysis or metaphysis. Consequently, it is important to obtain follow-up radiographs 2 to 3 weeks into treatment of septic arthritis to look for evidence of periosteal new bone formation or lytic lesions in bone. As a rule of thumb, therapy can be stopped after 3 weeks if the erythrocyte sedimentation rate has returned to normal.

Common Pitfalls

Common pitfalls include delayed diagnosis of septic arthritis in infants, failure to recognize associated osteomyelitis, and failure to anticipate infection by unusual organisms. A high index of suspicion should be maintained in sick neonates in whom septic arthritis may occur without fever or other signs of current infection. The hip and the knee are the most commonly involved joints. Infants with septic arthritis of the hip may be irritable when the hip is manipulated during diaper changes, and they usually hold the thigh in a flexed, externally rotated, and abducted position. As noted earlier, septic arthritis may be associated with

sequelae. The need for surgical exploration should always be considered when septic arthritis follows penetrating injury, to ensure that radiolucent foreign bodies are not missed. In the treatment of septic arthritis of joints other than the hip and shoulder, open surgical drainage is not necessary and does not uniformly improve outcome. However, prompt aspiration of the joint to obtain synovial fluid for analysis and culture also decompresses the joint, usually making the patient more comfortable.

Septic arthritis in newborns is usually caused by the same pathogens involved in neonatal sepsis. Initial therapy should be directed against staphylococci, streptococci, and coliform bacteria. Oxacillin (or nafcillin)

osteomyelitis, particularly at the hip and shoulder. Unusual bacteria are more often found in immunocompromised hosts, including patients with sickle cell disease. *Brucella* infection may be encountered among foreign travelers or others with exposure to the organism, usually by consuming unpasteurized dairy products. Finally, pyogenic infections of a bursa (septic bursitis) may initially be misdiagnosed as septic arthritis.

Communication and Counseling

Septic arthritis has the potential to cause significant joint injury, particularly when the hip is involved. These sequelae include joint laxity, joint restriction, and leg-length discrepancy. Infants and those with longer durations of symptoms are more likely to develop sequelae, including hip dislocation. Prolonged follow-up may be needed to determine the extent of joint injury.

SUGGESTED READINGS

1. Del Beccaro MA, Champoux AN, Bockers T, et al: Septic arthritis versus transient synovitis of the hip: The value of screening laboratory tests. Ann Emerg Med 21:B1418–B1422, 1992. **Demonstrates that minimally elevated sedimentation rates are the norm for toxic synovitis.**
2. Holmes KK, Counts GW, Beaty HN: Disseminated gonococcal infection. Ann Intern Med 74(6):979–993, 1971. **An excellent description of DGI that clarifies the spectrum of arthritic involvement.**
3. Kallio MJ, Unkila-Kallio L, Aalto K, Peltola H: Serum C-reactive protein, erythrocyte sedimentation rate, and white blood cell count in septic arthritis of children. Pediatr Infect Dis J 16:411–413, 1997. **This study demonstrates the utility of C-reactive protein measurements in the diagnosis and management of the disease.**
4. Krogstad PA: Osteomyelitis and septic arthritis. In Feigin R, Cherry JD, Demmler G, Kaplan SL (eds): Textbook of Pediatric Infectious Diseases, 5th ed. Philadelphia: WB Saunders, 2003. **Detailed description of the pathophysiology, evaluation, and treatment of infectious arthritis.**
5. Tetzlaff TR, McCracken GJ, Nelson JD: Oral antibiotic therapy for skeletal infections of children: II. Therapy of osteomyelitis and suppurative arthritis. J Pediatr 92:485–490, 1978. **Now a classic study that demonstrates the safety of sequential intravenous and oral therapy for septic arthritis in children.**

Catheter-Associated Infections

Marc D. Foca

KEY CONCEPTS

- The pathogenesis of catheter-related infections and the organisms most frequently isolated depend on the catheter type.
- Prevention of infections requires attention to catheter care.
- Short-term catheters coated with antiseptics or antibiotics reduce colonization but do not definitively reduce blood stream infections (BSIs).
- The use of antibiotic or antiseptic flush/lock solutions to prevent infections in long-term catheters requires further study.
- Short-term catheters are generally removed once an infection is documented.
- The use of systemic antibiotics to prevent removal of a long-term catheter and to clear an infection is often attempted unless specific pathogens such as *Pseudomonas* and *Candida* species are isolated.
- Tunnel infections usually require catheter removal.

Short- and long-term intravascular catheters are used for a wide range of adjunctive therapies in pediatric patients, including administration of total parenteral nutrition and chemotherapy and facilitation of drawing blood. Short-term central venous catheters (CVCs) are nontunneled catheters placed under sterile conditions outside the operating room. They include, but are not limited to, double- and triple-lumen catheters and Swan-Ganz catheters for intracardiac pressure monitoring and are intended to remain in situ for 1 to 3 weeks, in hospitalized patients only. Long-term CVCs are devices placed in the operating suite by tunneling or implanting the catheter under the skin. They are intended to remain in situ for months to years and include the Broviac and Hickman catheters and implantable ports, and they may be used in outpatients.

Pathogenesis

The pathogenesis of blood stream infections (BSIs) related to both short- and long-term devices includes migration of potential pathogens from the skin at the exit site along the external surface of the catheter to the catheter tip, intraluminal migration of organisms from the catheter hub, contaminated infusates, or, rarely, infection of the catheter by hematogenous spread from a distant focus. In addition, bowel translocation of microorganisms with subsequent seeding of the catheter is proposed as a probable mechanism of catheter-related BSIs in patients, particularly those with short bowel syndrome. Short-term, noncuffed, nontunneled catheters are more prone to migration of organisms along the external surface of the catheter, and, as a result, they are infected by a greater proportion of skin flora, including coagulase-negative staphylococci and *Staphylococcus aureus*. Long-term, cuffed, and tunneled catheters are less likely to be infected by organisms along the external catheter surface because the cuff acts as a fibrotic dam to migration. Table 1 defines the different types of catheter-related infections.

Risk Factors

Multiple risk factors for catheter-related BSIs are identified. Catheters made from polyvinyl chloride or polyethylene are more prone to organism adherence than catheters made of Teflon or silicone elastomer. Short-term catheters inserted in the jugular vein have a greater risk of BSI than catheters placed in the subclavian vein. Multilumen catheters are at higher

12

TABLE 1 Definitions of Catheter-Related Infections

Infection Type	Definition
Catheter-related blood stream infection	Isolation of the same organism from semiquantitative or quantitative blood culture obtained through the catheter and from the peripheral blood of a patient with clinical symptoms of a blood stream infection (BSI) or defervescence after removal of the implicated catheter
Colonized catheter	Growth of >15 colony-forming units (CFU) (semiquantitative) or >10^3 CFU (quantitative) from a segment of the catheter removed under sterile conditions without accompanying signs or symptoms of infection
Exit-site infection	Erythema, tenderness, induration, or purulence within 2 cm of the exit site of the catheter along the catheter tract
Tunnel infection	Erythema, tenderness, induration, or purulence >2 cm from the exit site of the catheter
Pocket infection	Erythema and necrosis of the skin over the reservoir of a totally implanted device or purulent exudate in the pocket containing the device

risk of infection than single-lumen catheters. Catheters inserted by inexperienced personnel have a higher incidence of catheter-related infections. Short-term catheters have higher infection rates than long-term catheters. Neutropenia is an independent risk factor for catheter-related infections.

Expert Opinion on Management Issues

PREVENTION OF CATHETER-RELATED INFECTIONS

Short-Term Catheters

Maximal barrier precautions during insertion—including the use of sterile masks, gowns, gloves, and large sterile fields—significantly reduce the incidence of catheter-related BSIs. Appropriate care of catheters after insertion also reduces the incidence of infections. Prior to manipulation of the catheter, hand washing is mandatory. The exit site can be cleansed with 10% povidone-iodine before replacement of the dressing. A 2% chlorhexidine preparation is more effective in preventing catheter-related BSI than povidone-iodine. The use of a chlorhexidine patch to cover the exit site of short-term catheters is not yet fully evaluated. Sterile gauze or a transparent dressing can be used to cover the site. Preference is usually given to the transparent dressing because it makes it easier to evaluate the exit site. Dressings should only be changed when they are loose, soiled, or damp.

Infusion therapy teams that both insert and maintain catheters reduce the incidence of catheter-related BSIs and are cost effective. The responsibility of maintaining these devices (changing dressings), however, can be performed efficiently by trained ward staff. Although replacement by guide wire exchange reduces insertional complications, there appears to be a trend toward a higher rate of catheter-related BSI.

Catheters coated with either chlorhexidine/silver sulfadiazine or minocycline/rifampin may reduce infections. Both coatings are bactericidal. Use of these catheters for more than 10 days reduces their effectiveness because the antiseptic activity diminishes with time. Catheters coated only on the external surface are not expected to prevent intraluminal colonization.

Minocycline/rifampin-coated CVCs are also effective at reducing the incidence of colonization and BSIs when compared with an uncoated catheter. However, antibiotic-coated catheters are not used widely in pediatric patients.

No evidence indicates that scheduled periodic line changes over a guide wire decrease the incidence of catheter-related BSI when compared to removal and replacement of these devices as needed.

Long-Term Catheters

The long-term lines include the Broviac, Hickman, and the totally implanted devices. Because of their insertional technique and silicone rubber (Silastic) material, they can last far longer in situ. These lines are tunneled some distance subcutaneously and then a large vessel is cannulated. A cuff around the catheter is placed approximately 2 cm from the exit site, which eventually fibroses and acts as a physical barrier to the migration of organisms along the external surface of the catheter. The incidence of BSIs is reduced with the use of these catheters compared with short-term catheters. Care of the exit site is similar to that used for short-term catheters. Long-term catheters are not coated with chlorhexidine/silver sulfadiazine or antibiotics because the bactericidal activity of these agents diminishes over time and cannot last the lifetime of the catheter. For similar reasons, the use of a silver-impregnated cuff with long-term devices is not effective in reducing the number of BSIs.

Efforts at preventing infections in long-term catheters focus on reducing colonization of the intraluminal surface because catheters in place for more than 10 days are more likely to be contaminated by this route. Vancomycin instilled into the catheter lumen is effective in reducing gram-positive and gram-negative infections in these long-term lines. Concerns about resistance, however, limit widespread institution of this practice.

TREATMENT

Short-Term Catheters

If a catheter-related BSI is suspected, blood cultures should be obtained from all catheter lumens and a peripheral vein. Ideally, a short-term catheter should be removed when a catheter-associated infection is suspected. Replacement over a guide wire is permissible, however, if the catheter is required for patient care and the patient is stable. The catheter should be removed if an infection is documented by positive blood cultures. Many experts also recommend that if a catheter-related BSI is suspected, the initial line should be removed under sterile conditions, the tip placed into a sterile container, and semiquantitative tip cultures performed. If the tip culture is positive and a new line was placed over a guide wire, the newly placed catheter should be removed if signs and symptoms of infection persist. If a catheter is removed because of a documented infection, a new line should be placed in a different location. An alternative approach is removing all lines with a suspected infection or a documented mechanical dysfunction with reinsertion at a different location. Table 2 describes the indications for catheter removal.

Long-Term Catheters

Treatment of BSIs related to long-term catheters is more complex. When a catheter-related infection is suspected, blood cultures should be drawn from all lumens of the catheter and a peripheral vein. The duration of antibiotic therapy and the need for possible removal of the catheter are based on culture results. If the catheter culture is positive and the peripheral culture is negative, a short course (5 days for coagulase-negative staphylococci and 7 days for most other bacterial pathogens) is acceptable as long as the host is not immunocompromised and repeat cultures are negative. If the patient is also bacteremic, the duration of antimicrobials depends on the duration of bacteremia, and therapy may be prolonged by at least 1 week. Repeat cultures should be drawn before starting therapy if coagulase-negative staphylococci are isolated because of the possibility of contamination from a skin site. However, this might not always be practical in immunocompromised patients when empirical therapy is initiated prior to microbiology results.

It is now routine to attempt to treat an infection in a long-term catheter while the catheter is in place. However, in certain circumstances, immediate removal is indicated (see Table 2). Whether to remove a long-term catheter secondary to recrudescence of infection is more problematic. Most experts recommend line removal.

The choice of empirical antibiotics depends on the host, previous history of BSI, and nosocomial versus community-acquired pathogens. Although the choice of antibiotics for empirical coverage of short-term catheters is similar to that of long-term catheters in the hospital setting, short-term catheters are not used in outpatients, and therefore community-acquired pathogens are less often factored into the empirical coverage of short-term catheter infections. Many acceptable alternatives for empirical therapy and therapy for specific pathogens are available (Table 3 and Table 4). Febrile granulocytopenic patients with an indwelling catheter can be started on monotherapy with ceftazidime or cefepime. However, if local epidemiology demonstrates an increased prevalence of methicillin-resistant *S. aureus* or extended-spectrum β-lactamase (ESBL)–producing organisms (see Table 4), then vancomycin and/or a β-lactam agent with a β-lactamase inhibitor should be used as empirical therapy until culture results are known. Once a pathogen is identified, antibiotics should be directed against the susceptibility pattern of the pathogen, and vancomycin should be discontinued if not indicated. The utility of treating gram-negative infections with double coverage is only definitively proven in neutropenic patients and should not be instituted routinely. Further evaluation should be initiated for all patients who fail to clear their peripheral blood culture despite line removal or who remain persistently symptomatic despite negative blood cultures. This should include an echocardiogram, ophthalmology exam, and CT scan of the chest, abdomen, and head.

EXIT AND TUNNEL INFECTIONS

The treatment of exit and tunnel infections depends on the catheter in use. For short-term catheters, an exit-site infection associated with bacteremia should prompt catheter removal and the introduction of systemic as well as topical antimicrobials. If the exit-site infection is not associated with bacteremia, an attempt can be

TABLE 2 Indications for Removal of Short-Term versus Long-Term Catheters

Catheter	Indications for Prompt Removal	Removal Not Necessary If Clinical/ Microbiological Response to Treatment
Short term	Catheter-related blood stream infection Exit-site infection with bacteremia	Exit-site infection without bacteremia

Long term	Septic shock
	Tunnel infection
	Infections with *Candida* species, atypical mycobacteria, and possibly
	    Staphylococcus aureus or *Stenotrophomonas maltophilia*
	Failure to respond clinically/microbiologically after 48–72 h of
	    appropriate therapy
		Exit-site infection
		Uncomplicated bacteremia
		Organism amenable to treatment with
		    appropriate antimicrobials

TABLE 3 Empirical Therapy for Presumed Catheter-Related Infection

Type of Infection	Community Acquired	Nosocomial	Comments
Exit site	Triple antibiotic ointment or mupirocin; if systemic therapy required: oxacillin	Triple antibiotic ointment or mupirocin; if systemic therapy required: vancomycin	Systemic antibiotics should be adjusted once pathogen and sensitivities are known.
Tunnel	Oxacillin or vancomycin	Ticarcillin/clavulanate or piperacillin/tazobactam	Therapy for nosocomial tunnel infections should include *Pseudomonas aeruginosa* and *Staphylococcus aureus* coverage.
Blood stream	Oxacillin plus aminoglycoside or third-generation cephalosporin	Vancomycin plus aminoglycoside or third-generation cephalosporin	If local epidemiology or patient's previous antibiotic experience dictates broader gram-negative coverage, empirical therapy for nosocomial infections can be with ticarcillin/clavulanate or piperacillin/tazobactam.

TABLE 4 Therapy for Specific Pathogens

Pathogen	Antimicrobial Agent	Comments
Staphylococcus aureus	Oxacillin	
Methicillin-resistant *S. aureus*	Vancomycin	Many experts add an additional agent, such as rifampin or gentamicin, when this organism is identified.
Coagulase-negative staphylococci	Vancomycin	>85% are nosocomial and most are resistant to oxacillin.
Enterococcus species	Ampicillin or vancomycin	Linezolid or quinupristin/dalfopristin can be used in cases of vancomycin-resistant *Enterococcus faecium;* many experts add gentamicin when this organism is identified.
Viridans streptococci	Penicillin or vancomycin	Cause of septicemia and endocarditis in severely neutropenic patients.
Chromosomal β-lactamase-producing gram-negative bacilli*	Ticarcillin/clavulanate, piperacillin/tazobactam, aminoglycoside, or quinolone	
Extended-spectrum β-lactamase-producing gram-negative bacilli*	Imipenem or meropenem	
Stenotrophomonas maltophilia	Ticarcillin/clavulanate and trimethoprim/sulfamethoxazole	Many experts recommend line removal with this pathogen. A quinolone may also be an alternative.
Candida species	Amphotericin B or fluconazole, pending susceptibilities with an echinocandin as an alternative agent	Metastatic workup should be reserved for immunocompromised and those who fail to clear the organism quickly.

*Chromosomal β-lactamases usually encode a cephalosporinase that is either inducible or constitutively expressed and confers resistance to the third-generation cephalosporins. It is usually not inhibited by clavulanic acid, and it is possible to use several classes of antibiotics against these organisms. Extended-spectrum β-lactamases (ESBLs) are usually plasmid associated and often confer resistance to multiple classes of antibiotics. They are screened for by lack of susceptibility to cefpodoxime, ceftazidime, or aztreonam. The usual cutoff is a minimum inhibitory concentration (MIC) of 2 μg/mL or greater. Susceptibility to these antibiotics is improved in the presence of clavulanic acid. Although ESBL-producing organisms may appear susceptible to cefoxitin, this antibiotic should never be used to treat an ESBL-producing organism. Only imipenem is effective in this regard.

made to treat the infection with topical agents alone. The treatment of long-term catheter exit-site infections is essentially the same, except that unlike the short-term catheter, long-term catheters can be salvaged, even in the face of bacteremia, if the infection responds to appropriate antimicrobial therapy with sterilization of the blood culture and resolution of the local infection. Tunnel tract infections are seen with long-term catheters only. They require systemic antimicrobial therapy and usually necessitate catheter removal. Unless bacteremia is present, a trial of empirical therapy for *S. aureus* and *P. aeruginosa* is warranted if the patient is stable. If no improvement is noted, the catheter should be removed and the tract cultured. Antibiotics can then be tailored to the identified pathogen.

Common Pitfalls

Major complications of catheter infections include sepsis, septic emboli, endocarditis, endovascular infection including septic thrombophlebitis, abscess formation, and death. Prompt removal of the catheter and the initiation of prolonged antibiotic therapy are required. Catheter-related infections are associated with increased lengths of stay, higher medical costs, and mortality rates as high as 10% to 20%. Special attention should be given to the changing epidemiology of pathogens, outcomes of device-related infections for both short-term and long-term catheters, and the potential emergence of resistance under the pressure of new preventive strategies.

Communication and Counseling

Even with current technology, the morbidity and mortality associated with catheter infections remains significant. Short-term catheters should not be used in the outpatient setting. Caregivers must be appropriately educated about the proper techniques involved with antisepsis and with accessing long-term devices. In addition, caregivers must understand the urgency of a hospital-based evaluation when a child with an indwelling catheter develops a fever.

SUGGESTED READINGS

1. Darouiche RO, Raad II, Heard SO, et al: A comparison of two antimicrobial-impregnated central venous catheters. Catheter Study Group. N Engl J Med 340:1–8, 1999. **The first large-scale trial comparing the two major impregnated short-term catheters.**
2. Franklin JA, Gaur AH, Shenep JL, et al: In situ diagnosis of central venous catheter–related bloodstream infection without peripheral blood culture. Pediatr Infect Dis J 23:614–618, 2004. **This article adds to the debate concerning the usefulness of peripheral blood cultures for the diagnosis of blood stream infections.**
3. Gaur AH, Flynn PM, Giannini MA, et al: Difference in time to detection: A simple method to differentiate catheter-related from non-catheter-related bloodstream infection in immunocompromised pediatric patients. Clin Infect Dis 37:469–475, 2003. **The first prospective pediatric trial to look at this promising new technique for diagnosing catheter-related blood stream infections.**
4. Henrickson KJ, Axtell RA, Hoover SM, et al: Prevention of central venous catheter–related infections and thrombotic events in immunocompromised children by the use of vancomycin/ciprofloxacin/heparin flush solution: A randomized, multicenter, double-blind trial. J Clin Oncol 18:1269–1278, 2000. **The largest pediatric trial to date on the use of antibiotic flushes to prevent catheter-related infections.**
5. Mermel LA, Farr BM, Sherertz RJ, et al: Guidelines for the management of intravascular catheter-related infections. Clin Infect Dis 32:1249–1272, 2001. **Major treatment guidelines.**
6. O'Grady NP, Alexander M, Dellinger EP, et al: Guidelines for the prevention of intravascular catheter-related infections. Clin Infect Dis 35:1281–1307, 2002. **Major prevention guidelines.**
7. Veenstra DL, Saint S, Saha S, et al: Efficacy of antiseptic-impregnated central venous catheters in preventing catheter-related bloodstream infection: A meta-analysis. JAMA 281:261–267, 1999. **The first study to demonstrate the effectiveness of antiseptic catheters for the prevention of BSI.**

BACTERIAL INFECTIONS

12

Campylobacter

Theresa J. Ochoa and Thomas G. Cleary

KEY CONCEPTS

- *Campylobacter* species are fastidious organisms that are difficult to grow and identify.
- Although 14 species of *Campylobacter* can cause human disease, almost all illness (99%) is caused by a single species, *Campylobacter jejuni*.
- *Campylobacter* infection is common in the first years of life, especially in developing counties.
- *Campylobacter* can cause watery diarrhea or classic dysentery (high fever, bloody diarrhea, abdominal pain, and painful defecation).
- Most patients recover in less than 1 week, but 20% have a relapse or a prolonged or severe illness.
- *Campylobacter* infection can trigger a variety of neurologic syndromes, including Guillain-Barré syndrome, Miller-Fisher syndrome, and acute motor axonal neuropathy.

Campylobacter are gram-negative, spiral-curved flagellated rods that grow best under anaerobic or microaerophilic conditions (5% to 10% oxygen). They are typically cultured at 108°F (42°C). The high temperature of incubation is necessary because these organisms are particularly well adapted to live in the guts of birds. The organisms were not identified in fecal samples until it was recognized they are not tolerant of high oxygen and that they were being overgrown by other fecal flora. To isolate them it was necessary to add antibiotics to the media and culture in lower oxygen. Paradoxically, although they are fastidious, these organisms can survive for weeks in contaminated water.

Contaminated water, milk, and poultry are the major sources of infection in developed countries, although close contact with infected animals, including birds (especially chickens, geese, and ducks), cows, dogs, and cats can also lead to infection. Proper cooking kills the organisms, but foods normally eaten uncooked can be cross-contaminated during preparation. Person-to-person transmission is uncommon. In the United States, sporadic cases are typically caused by contact with contaminated poultry, whereas epidemics are usually caused by contaminated milk or water. The incubation period is 1 to 5 days.

In the United States, *Campylobacter* is the most common cause of bacterial gastroenteritis; an estimated 2.4 million cases occur each year. There is a bimodal age distribution, with a peak in the first year of life and a second peak in adults in the third decade.

These organisms cause watery diarrhea or inflammatory diarrhea with fever and positive fecal leukocytes. Illness can be virtually identical to that caused by *Shigella* species, with abdominal pain, nausea, vomiting, bloody stools, fever, and tenesmus. Abdominal pain can mimic that produced by appendicitis. Illness usually resolves in approximately 1 week, although it can last for up to 3 weeks and can sometimes recur. The differences in clinical presentation of various *Campylobacter* infections may reflect differing virulence genes in various strains. In the developing world, infection is very common; typically a child may be infected multiple times in the first few years of life. Initial infections are symptomatic but eventually, as immunity develops, colonization occurs. In developed countries, infected children are usually older and more symptomatic. Most patients clear the organism from stool within 2 weeks (mean 16 days), but some continue to excrete it for more than a year. The duration of fecal excretion is age related, with infants excreting longer than older children.

Although illness is usually self-limited, multiple adverse outcomes and complications are described. Death is uncommon in the developed world (124 deaths per year in the United States), but is a significant risk for children in the developing world. Sepsis is very infrequent. Febrile convulsions can occur during severe illness. *Campylobacter* is the most common cause of Guillain-Barré syndrome, although the risk is less than 1 per 1000 recognized *Campylobacter* infections. The episode of diarrhea may be as long as 12 weeks prior to onset of neurologic symptoms. Outcome appears to be worse than with the Guillain-Barré syndrome due to other causes. It can also trigger reactive arthritis and, rarely, other complications. Mucosa-associated lymphoma can be caused by *Campylobacter jejuni*; this malignancy can respond dramatically to antibiotics. Immunocompromised hosts can have severe illness that may recur despite appropriate treatment.

Expert Opinion on Management Issues

Therapy for gastroenteritis is directed first at fluid and electrolyte replacement and maintenance. Therapy should be intravenous if the child is in shock, is in a coma, or has an ileus, but otherwise it should be given orally. The World Health Organization oral rehydration solution (ORS) is accepted as the standard of care; commercially available oral rehydration solutions in the United States (e.g., Pedialyte) are acceptable alternatives. A key element of current management is early refeeding with breast milk or other age-appropriate food, beginning within 6 to 12 hours of initiation of oral rehydration therapy.

The role of antibiotics in general, and erythromycin therapy in particular, for gastrointestinal campylobacteriosis is debatable. The organisms are usually susceptible in vitro to macrolides such as erythromycin and azithromycin. It is clear that erythromycin shortens the duration of excretion in stool, but the effect on symptoms is less clear. Some studies suggest that children with *Campylobacter* dysentery benefit from erythromycin. However, other studies suggest that erythromycin has little effect on symptoms. The newer macrolides,

azithromycin and clarithromycin, have better tolerance and may be more effective. In adults, azithromycin seems to work as well as ciprofloxacin (the drug of choice for adults with susceptible strains). The ill-advised use of fluoroquinolones in animal feeds led to a rapid emergence of organisms resistant to this class of drugs. *Campylobacter* species grow slowly; identification may take 72 to 96 hours. Because late therapy of diarrheal disease is of doubtful benefit, empirical therapy may be more appropriate. Tetracycline for children 8 years or older is an alternative agent. Despite these controversies, antibiotics are often given; Table 1 lists the doses typically used. Illness that is prolonged, severe, or occurring in immunocompromised patients should be treated with antibiotics.

For the rare bacteremic infection, aminoglycosides, meropenem, or imipenem may be appropriate; doses similar to those used for other gram-negative rod bacteremia are presumed to be appropriate.

Common Pitfalls

- Overly optimistic expectations regarding antibiotic therapy may lead to disappointment. Therapy may result in little more than a shortening of duration of excretion.
- Although culture for *Campylobacter* should be part of a routine evaluation of fecal flora, stool cultures in small laboratories may not be set up on appropriate media (Butzler's, Skirrow's, or Campy-BAP) with appropriate incubation conditions (low O_2, 108°F [42°C]); the result can be failure to grow these fastidious organisms. Failure to diagnose the organism correctly can lead to inappropriate therapy that is costly, potentially toxic, and ineffective.

Communication and Counseling

There is a significant risk of acquiring *Campylobacter* enteritis during travel to less-developed countries. Families taking children to these countries should be instructed in methods of avoiding contaminated food and water. They should be encouraged to use bottled water or boiled water. Food should be consumed while steaming hot. Uncooked vegetables and fruits should be avoided unless the fruits can be peeled just prior to being eaten. Ice, like water in general, may be contaminated. Food purchased from street vendors is notoriously hazardous in terms of diarrheal risk. Hand washing should be discussed.

As with other forms of enteritis, careful attention to fluid and electrolyte state is important. Use of oral rehydration and early reinstitution of breast-feeding or other appropriate feeds is mandatory. Patients should not be starved for prolonged periods of time.

The pros and cons of antibiotic therapy should be discussed. Given the fact that benefit is often hard to show, parents should be informed of the data and involved in the treatment decisions. No vaccine is available for the prevention of campylobacteriosis.

TABLE 1 Therapy for *Campylobacter* Enteritis

Generic Name (Trade Name)	Dosage/Route/Regimen	Maximum Dose	Dosage Formulation	Common Adverse Reactions	Therapeutic Concentrations	Comments
Erythromycin ethylsuccinate (EES)	30–50 mg/kg/day divided q6–8h PO for 5 days	2 g/day (as base) or 3.2 g/day (as ethylsuccinate)	Suspension: 200, 400 mg/5 mL; oral drops: 100 mg/2.5 mL; chewable tabs: 200 mg; tabs: 400 mg	Nausea, vomiting abdominal pain, hepatitis, jaundice, rash	Absorption varies with the different salts.	May be effective in children with dysenteric disease if used early; many drug interactions; inhibit CYP 450 1A2 3A3/4 isoenzymes.
Ciprofloxacin (Cipro)	20 mg/kg/day divided q12h given IV; can be switched to oral after infection controlled; for 5 days	800 mg/day IV or 1.5 g/day orally	Suspension: 250/500 mg/5 mL; tablets: 100, 250, 500, 750 mg; injectable solution: 10 mg/mL	Theoretical risk of injury to growing cartilage; GI upset, renal failure, restlessness, rash, headache	Peak serum concentrations of 1–5 μg/mL after oral dose of 15 mg/kg.	Alternative when erythromycin cannot be used; drug of choice for adults.
Azithromycin (Zithromax)	12 mg/kg/day once daily PO on day 1, followed by 6 mg/kg/day once daily on days 2–5	500 mg/day	Suspension: 100 mg/5 mL, 200 mg/5 mL; tablets: 250, 500, and 600 mg	Rash, GI upset, nephritis		Efficacy shown in studies of adults.
Tetracycline (Sumycin, Tetram, Panmycin, etc.)	25–50 mg/kg/day divided q6h PO for 5 days	3 g/day	Suspension: 125 mg/5 mL; tablets: 250 and 500 mg	Nausea, vomiting, diarrhea, rash, pseudotumor cerebri; injury to growing bones and teeth		Contraindicated in children <8 years of age.

GI, gastrointestinal; IV, intravenous; PO, by mouth; q, every; qxh, every x hours.

12

SUGGESTED READINGS

1. Allos BM, Blaser MJ: *Campylobacter jejuni* and the expanding spectrum of related infections. Clin Infect Dis 20:1092–1099, 1995. **An excellent summary of both the common and uncommon manifestations of the various *Campylobacter* that are relevant to human disease.**

2. Kuschner RA, Trofa AF, Thomas RJ, et al: Use of azithromycin for the treatment of *Campylobacter* enteritis in travelers to Thailand, an area where ciprofloxacin resistance is prevalent. Clin Infect Dis 21(3):536–541, 1995. **This study shows that azithromycin is equivalent in efficacy to ciprofloxacin in adults with campylobacteriosis.**

3. Pai CH, Gillis F, Tuomanen E, Marks MI: Erythromycin in treatment of *Campylobacter* enteritis in children. Am J Dis Child 137 (3):286–288, 1983. **In contrast to the data of Salazar-Lindo, this randomized, prospective trial of treatment of *Campylobacter* enteritis in infants and children (like several other trials) showed an effect only on excretion but not symptoms in children treated with erythromycin ethyl succinate.**

4. Rees JH, Soudain SE, Gregson NA, Hughes RA: *Campylobacter jejuni* infection and Guillain-Barré syndrome. N Engl J Med 23; 333(3):1374–1379, 1995. **Summarizes data on patients with Guillain-Barré syndrome and Miller Fisher syndrome; it suggests that axonal degeneration, slow recovery, and severe residual disability are common with this form of neuropathy.**

5. Salazar-Lindo E, Sack RB, Chea-Woo E, et al: Early treatment with erythromycin of *Campylobacter jejuni*–associated dysentery in children. J Pediatr 109(2):355–360, 1986. **This randomized, double-blind placebo-controlled trial showed that the symptoms of children with Campylobacter dysentery improve with erythromycin ethyl succinate.**

Cholera

Jesica A. Neuhart and Russell W. Steele

KEY CONCEPTS

- Cholera continues to produce epidemic disease, primarily in developing countries.
- Recognition of this disease is important so correct therapy can be initiated and infection control measures rapidly implemented.
- Rehydration followed by adequate maintenance of hydration are keys to therapy.
- Antibiotics play only a minor role in treatment.
- Efforts to improve sanitation and hygiene must continue in order to prevent transmission.
- Two oral vaccines are currently available for use in endemic areas and for travelers but provide only 50% protection over 3 years.

Although rarely seen in the United States, cholera continues to be a cause of epidemic disease in many countries worldwide. In the United States, most cases are reported near the Gulf Coast, (e.g., Louisiana and Texas). *Vibrio cholerae* lives in coastal and brackish waters. Infection results from exposure to water or following ingestion of contaminated shellfish and crabs. In developing nations, cholera is usually acquired and spread by fecally contaminated water or food.

To date, cholera has caused seven pandemics involving millions of people and killing hundreds of thousands. The seventh pandemic began in Indonesia in 1961 and spread to Latin America in 1991. This pandemic remains today and has already affected 98 countries and a million people in the Americas alone.

V. cholerae is a gram-negative curved flagellated bacillus responsible for the disease cholera. Two biotypes exist: classical and El Tor. The El Tor biotype is responsible for the current pandemic and the classic type for those pandemics prior to 1961 and for disease in some areas of Bangladesh. Overall, more than 60 serogroups of *V. cholerae* exist, but only groups O1 and O139 cause disease of epidemic proportion.

After ingestion, *V. cholerae* organisms colonize the small intestinal epithelial cells but do not invade or alter the cells structurally. The secretory diarrhea characteristic of cholera is a result of the action of cholera toxin. The toxin increases sodium and bicarbonate secretion into the intestinal lumen and decreases intestinal absorption of sodium chloride and water.

The hallmark of cholera infection is diffuse, watery diarrhea. Patients pass large volumes of stool, sometimes more than 200 mL/kg/day, which leads rapidly to dehydration and electrolyte abnormalities. The descriptive term *rice water stools* was coined because of similarities in appearance to the water in which rice is cooked. Many patients also suffer from vomiting, which usually occurs early in the course of the illness. Some patients report intestinal cramping and abdominal pain. Usually fever is absent. Signs and symptoms of dehydration include tachycardia, hypotension, sunken eyes, skin tenting, "washerwoman's hands," scaphoid abdomen, decreased urine output, and mental status changes ranging from restlessness and irritability to lethargy and coma.

Definitive diagnosis is made by stool culture. Dark-field microscopy to visualize the organisms and stool antigen tests may also be used. A clinical diagnosis of cholera, however, requires immediate response because delayed treatment may result in increased morbidity and mortality.

Expert Opinion on Management Issues

The key to managing patients with cholera is fluid therapy. Fluid and electrolyte losses due to cholera toxin result in mild to severe dehydration. Because the amount and type of fluid therapy offered depends on the degree of dehydration demonstrated by the patient, classifying the degree of dehydration is the first step in management. Table 1 lists symptoms associated with mild, moderate, and severe dehydration.

Rehydration is the second step in cholera management. The rehydration phase should be completed in 3 to 6 hours. In patients with mild dehydration,

TABLE 1 Classification of Dehydration Based on Clinical Manifestations and Recommended Method of Treatment

Clinical Manifestation	Mild Dehydration	Moderate Dehydration	Severe Dehydration
Mental status	Alert and consolable	Restless or irritable	Lethargic, obtunded, stuporous, comatose
Pulse rate	Normal	Slightly increased	Increased/rapid
Pulse quality	Normal	Weak	Feeble, impalpable
Respiratory rate and character	Normal	Tachypneic	Tachypneic, deep, labored
Skin turgor	Normal (pinch retracts immediately)	Tenting (pinch retracts slowly)	None (pinch retracts very slowly)
Skin touch	Normal	Dry	Clammy
Mucous membranes (lips and buccal mucosa)	Moist	Dry	Parched, cracked
Eyes	Normal	Deep set	Sunken
Tears	Present	Reduced	Absent
Capillary refill	Normal	~ 2 sec	>3 sec
Fontanelle	Flat	Soft	Sunken
Urine output	Normal	Decreased, dark color	Scant, anuric
Fluid deficit (percentage of body weight and mL/kg of body weight)	Older child: 3% or 30 mL/kg; infant: 5% or 50 mL/kg	Older child: 6% or 60 mL/kg; infant: 10% or 100 mL/kg	Older child: 9% or 90 mL/kg; infant: 15% or 150 mL/kg
Treatment	ORS solution	ORS solution if tolerating oral intake; IV fluids if vomiting or stool losses exceed oral intake	IV fluids

IV, intravenous; ORS, oral rehydration salt.

Modified from Gunn VL, Nechyba C: The Harriet Lane Handbook, 16th ed. Philadelphia: Mosby, 2002: p 235; Bennish ML: Cholera: Pathophysiology, clinical features, and treatment. In Wachsmuth IK, Blake PA, Olsvik O (eds): *Vibrio Cholerae* and Cholera: Molecular to Global Perspectives. Washington, DC: American Society for Microbiology, 1994, p 238.

rehydration is completed orally using an oral rehydration salts (ORS) solution. Table 2 outlines the composition of the ORS solution. Moderately dehydrated patients who are able to tolerate oral administration of fluids should also receive replacement therapy by this route. Intravenous (IV) fluids are reserved for severely dehydrated patients and those who cannot tolerate the ORS solution. The volume of fluid given during rehydration phase is generally between 20 and 60 mL per kg in children. The World Health Organization (WHO) recommends a total of 100 mL per kg in the first 3 hours for children older than 1 year, with 30 mL per kg given as quickly as possible followed by 70 mL per kg over the next 2.5 hours. In children younger than 1 year, the same volume should be given over 6 hours. The rehydration phase continues until symptoms of dehydration resolve. Close monitoring of vital signs, peripheral perfusion, and mental status ensure effectiveness of therapy.

A maintenance hydration phase follows the replacement phase and can usually be provided with ORS solution, which is given at a rate that matches losses due to diarrhea plus insensible losses. Fluid requirements are highest in the first 24 hours of treatment, and often patients need up to 200 mL per kg or more. IV fluid administration is indicated in the maintenance phase in those patients who cannot tolerate ORS solution or in those experiencing diarrhea losses that exceed the amount a patient can take orally.

The World Health Organization (WHO) recommends lactated Ringer's (LR) solution as initial replacement therapy and in the maintenance phase when oral intake is not adequate. This solution most closely matches electrolyte concentrations lost in stool. Normal saline (NS) can be used but was found less effective in some studies. NS should be combined with ORS solution to replace bicarbonate losses.

Patients with moderate and severe dehydration require admission to a hospital/care facility so they can be closely monitored. Close attention should be paid to ongoing stool losses, vital signs, and urine output. Discharge criteria include a decrease or cessation of diarrhea and ability of the patient to mix and drink adequate amounts of ORS solution.

Oral therapy should be initiated as soon as possible in all patients. In patients with initial intolerance, ORS solution can be reintroduced every 2 hours after onset of treatment, and trials should continue frequently until it is tolerated. Both the glucose-based and rice-based formulas are effective and easily made. Solid foods should also be initiated as soon as the patient is tolerating the required fluids.

Antibiotics are not essential in the treatment of cholera but they do decrease the fluids needed during the maintenance phase secondary to decreased stool frequency. Antibiotics also shorten the illness. The drug of choice in adults and adolescents is doxycycline. Tetracycline can also be used but requires multiple doses. In young children and infants, erythromycin and trimethoprim-sulfamethoxazole are used. Fluoroquinolones have a role in treatment as well and provide an alternative to the prior-mentioned drugs. Table 3 describes the dosing. Antibiotics can be administered as soon as patients are tolerating oral intake and should be offered to those with severe cases of cholera.

TABLE 2 Composition of 10 Liters of Oral Rehydration Salt (ORS) Solution

Ingredient	Amount
Glucose-Based ORS Solution	
Sodium chloride (common salt	35 g
plus	
Glucose, anhydrous	200 g
or	
Sucrose (common sugar)	440 g
or	
Glucose, monohydrate	220 g
plus	
Trisodium citrate, dihydrated	29 g
or	
Sodium bicarbonate	25 g
plus	
Potassium chloride	15 g
In 10 L of water, completely dissolve the sugar and salts in the amounts shown here. Use the usual drinking water. Boiled water, cooled before use, or chlorinated water is best. If larger volumes are prepared, the amount of each ingredient should be increased proportionally. ORS solution should be used within 24 hours; after that time, unused solution should be discarded and fresh solution prepared.	
Rice-Based ORS Solution	
Sodium chloride (common salt	35 g
plus	
Trisodium citrate, dihydrated	29 g
or	
Sodium bicarbonate	25 g
plus	
Potassium chloride	15 g
To make 10 L of rice-based ORS solution, boil 500 g of rice powder in 11 L of water for 5 minutes. (The extra liter allows for water lost during the boiling.) Cool the liquid. Add ingredients shown here. Mix well. Rice-based ORS solution should be used within 8 to 12 hours, after which fresh solution should be prepared.	

Taken from World Health Organization: Guidelines for Cholera Control. Geneva: World Health Organization, 1993, p 22.

Several cholera vaccines, both parenteral and oral, exist today. The main indication for vaccination is to protect those at risk in endemic areas. WHO recommends vaccine for preemptive use in high-risk populations including, but not limited to, refugees in crowded camps and urban slum residents. Cholera vaccine is not required for entrance or exit from any country.

The parenteral vaccine made of inactivated *V. cholerae* O1 offers limited protective efficacy, a short duration of protection, and does not prevent transmission of cholera in stool. For these reasons, it is no longer recommended.

Two oral vaccines are currently in use: the killed WC/rBS vaccine and the live attenuated CVD 103-HgR vaccine. WC/rBS consists of killed whole-cell *V. cholerae* O1 with a recombinant B-subunit of cholera toxin. It has been available since the early 1990s, given in two doses separated by 10 to 14 days. WC/rBS confers a protection level of approximately 50% 3 years after immunization. The second oral vaccine is a live attenuated vaccine based on the *V. cholerae* strain CVD 103-HgR. It has been available for use since the mid–1990s and confers protection after a single dose.

Unfortunately, an ideal vaccine that conveys long-lasting immunity for both O1 and O139 strains does not exist. The protection offered by the oral vaccines is insufficient in children younger than 2 years. Neither oral vaccine is produced in the United States. For these reasons, only those at high risk for infection, such as emergency relief and health workers in refugee camps, should be immunized.

Common Pitfalls

- Failure to rehydrate patients properly may lead to complications such as renal failure and pulmonary edema.
- Failure to initiate prompt therapy can lead to complications and even death.
- Cholera patients require close and frequent monitoring to prevent repeated dehydration/shock states.

In moderate to severely dehydrated patients, IV access is often difficult to obtain; however, rehydration should begin immediately. If the patient is able to drink, ORS solution should be given while IV access is started. Other options for rehydration while waiting for IV access include hydration with ORS solution through an oral-gastric or nasogastric tube. In extreme cases an intraosseous needle should be used for rapid fluid administration. A severely dehydrated patient should never be allowed to decompensate further while attempting to place an IV line.

Patients with moderate to severe dehydration require frequent monitoring. If the patient continues to have poor pulses and tachycardia after rehydration, IV fluids should be continued at a high rate. Even after rehydration, patients need monitoring at least every 4 hours to ensure that fluid intake is enough to replace stool losses in addition to insensible losses. Repeated shock states due to dehydration can lead to acute renal failure and should be prevented. Young children and the elderly are at highest risk of this complication. If the patient continues to have very large stool output that cannot be maintained with ORS solution, an IV should be started. Monitoring urine output is also a good indication of hydration status.

In the rehydration phase, recommended IV fluids include LR and NS. Other polyelectrolyte solutions are not recommended for rapid administration in children. Overhydration without correction of metabolic acidosis can lead to pulmonary edema, which occurs most frequently when NS is used alone instead of in combination with ORS solution.

Antibiotics should be given to patients with severe diarrhea after rehydration. Antibiotics decrease stool volume and duration of illness, therefore shortening the length of hospitalization. There is no indication for using IV antibiotics, and oral medications are much more cost effective.

The clinician must also be aware of a condition called *cholera sicca*, which occurs in patients who have an ileus resulting from their illness. Watery stool accumulates in the paralyzed segment of intestine and causes

TABLE 3 Antibiotics Used in the Treatment of Cholera

Generic Name (Trade Name) Rx	Route/ Dosage/ Regimen	Maximum Dose	Dosage Formulas	Common Adverse Reactions	Comments
Tetracyclines (Inhibit bacterial protein synthesis by binding to the 30S ribosomal subunit)					
Doxycycline (Vibramycin, Periostat, and others) Rx	PO 300 mg × 1 in children >8 yr and adults	300 mg/24 hr	Caps/tabs: 20, 50, 100 mg; syrup: 50 mg/5 mL; suspension: 25 mg/5 mL	Risk of tooth enamel hypoplasia; GI symptoms; photosensitivity; rash; hypersensitivity	Outdated tetracyclines may cause Fanconi-like syndrome. Adjust dose in renal failure. Do not give with dairy products.
Tetracycline (Achromycin, Sumycin, Panmycin, and others) Rx	PO 12.5 mg/kg qid × 3 days; 500 mg qid × 3 days in children >8 yr and adults	3 g/24 hr	Caps/tabs: 250, 500 mg; suspension: 125 mg/ 5 mL	Tooth staining and decreased bone growth; GI symptoms; hepatotoxicity; rash; fever; photosensitivity	
Sulfonamides (Competitively inhibit bacterial enzymes responsible for synthesis of folic acid)					
Trimethoprim-sulfamethoxazole (Bactrim, Septra, Sulfatrim, and others) Rx	Doses based on TMP component; PO 4–5 mg/kg bid; 160 mg/dose bid in adults (>40 kg)	320 mg/24 hr	Tabs (regular strength): 80 mg TMP/400 mg SMX; tabs (DS): 160 mg TMP/800 mg SMX; suspension: 40 mg TMP/200 mg SMX per 5 mL	Rash; Hypersensitivity; blood dyscrasias; crystalluria; renal injury; hepatic injury; GI irritation	May cause hemolysis in patients with G6PD deficiency. Not recommended in infants < 2 mo. May cause Kernicterus in newborns.

TABLE 3—cont'd

Generic Name (Trade Name) Rx	Route/ Dosage/ Regimen	Maximum Dose	Dosage Formulas	Common Adverse Reactions	Comments
Quinolones (Inhibit DNA gyrase—an enzyme needed for DNA synthesis during bacterial replication)					
Ciprofloxacin (Cipro) Rx	PO 1 g × 1	1.5 g/24 hr	Tabs: 100, 250, 500, 750 mg; suspension: 250, 500 mg/5 mL	GI upset; renal failure; seizures; headache; rash; arthropathy*	Arthropathy demonstrated in animal studies and not in human subjects. Adjust dose in renal failure.
Macrolides (Inhibit bacterial protein synthesis by binding to the 50S ribosomal subunit)					
Erythromycin (Erythrocin, Pediamycin, E-mycin, EryPed, and others) Rx	PO 10 mg/kg tid × 3 days	Children: 2 g/24 hr Adults: 4 g/24 hr	Tabs: 250, 333, 500 mg; delayed-release tabs: 250, 333, 500 mg; EES suspension: 220, 400 mg/5 mL; oral drops: 100 mg/mL; chewable tabs: 125, 250 mg; tabs: 400 mg; Erythro Estolate suspension: 125, 250 mg/5 mL; oral drops: 100 mg/mL; chewable tabs: 125, 250 mg; tabs: 500 mg; caps: 125, 250 mg	GI side effects; hepatotoxicity	

bid, twice daily; DS, double strength; OTC, over the counter; PO, by mouth; qid, four times per day; Rx, prescription; SMX, sulfamethoxazole; TMP, trimethoprim.

distension of the bowel. Patients with this condition can manifest symptoms of severe dehydration before passing any stool, requiring immediate therapy.

Communication and Counseling

The key to preventing continuance of the cholera epidemic is proper sanitation and ensuring a safe water supply. Education of all individuals in epidemic areas is essential, emphasizing proper water safety, boiling and chlorination of drinking water, and construction of latrines to improve sanitation.

Travelers to epidemic areas should use simple precautions. Only boiled or bottled water should be used for drinking. Only fruits with removable peelings, such as oranges and bananas, should be consumed raw. All other foods, especially meats, should be cooked thoroughly and eaten while hot. Good hand washing is also a must.

If parents suspect cholera in their child, the precautions just described should continue and medical attention should be sought. As long as the disease is treated quickly, complications can be avoided and the prognosis remains excellent. Even children with severe dehydration recover completely after aggressive treatment.

SUGGESTED READINGS

1. Bennish ML: Cholera: Pathophysiology, clinical features, and treatment. In Wachsmuth IK, Blake PA, Olsvik O (eds): *Vibrio Cholerae* and Cholera: Molecular to Global Perspectives. Washington, DC: American Society for Microbiology, 1994, pp 229–255. **Pathophysiology, clinical manifestations, and a stepwise approach to the treatment of cholera.**
2. Carpenter CJ: The treatment of cholera: Clinical science at the bedside. J Infect Dis 1166:2–14, 1992. **Detailed history of cholera and its treatment.**
3. Centers for Disease Control and Prevention: Cholera. Available at http://www.cdc.gov/ncidod/dbmd/diseaseinfo/cholera_g.htm. **Basic information on cholera from the CDC. Site contains links to additional resources for cholera as well.**
4. Centers for Disease Control and Prevention: Update on cholera vaccines. 11 August 2003 Available at http://www.cdc.gov/travel/other/cholera-vaccine.htm. **Update on cholera vaccines.**
5. Fukuda JM, Yi A, Chaparro L, et al: Clinical characteristics and risk factors for *Vibrio cholerae* infection in children. J Pediatr 126:882–886, 1995. **Study of epidemic cholera and treatment of infected children in Lima, Peru.**
6. Guerrant RL, Benedito AC, Dillingham R: Cholera, diarrhea, and oral rehydration therapy: Triumph and indictment. Clin Infect Dis 37:398–405, 2003. **Description, history, and ongoing research on oral rehydration therapy.**
7. Raufman JP: Cholera. Am J Med 104:386–394, 1998. **Review article including brief epidemiology, treatment, prevention, and detailed information on the action of cholera toxin.**
8. Seas C, DuPont HL, Valdez LM, Gotuzzo E: Practical guidelines for the treatment of cholera. Drugs 51:966–973, 1996. **Detailed instruction on cholera management and treatment.**
9. World Health Organization: Cholera vaccines. Wkly Epidemiol Rec 16:117–124, 2001. **Detailed information on and recommendations for cholera vaccines.**
10. World Health Organization: Guidelines for Cholera Control. Geneva: World Health Organization, 1993. **Handbook on cholera, including brief history of disease, epidemiology, treatment, and prevention.**

Nontyphoidal *Salmonella*
Theresa J. Ochoa and Thomas G. Cleary

KEY CONCEPTS

- Gastroenteritis is the most common clinical manifestation of *Salmonella*. Diarrhea can be watery or bloody, with or without fever.
- Some *Salmonella* serotypes can invade the blood stream and seed distant organs. Bacteremia is more common in the newborn.
- The highest incidence rates of *Salmonella* occur in children younger than 5 years, especially those younger than 1 year.
- Antibiotic therapy of *Salmonella* gastroenteritis is generally not indicated. Multiple studies evaluating a variety of antibiotics show that antimicrobial therapy does not shorten the duration of symptoms. Antibiotics may prolong the period of fecal excretion, however. Some studies suggest these agents increase the duration of illness or cause serious adverse effects. Fecal excretion can lead to infection of close contacts, particularly when the individual handles food.
- Although the benefits are not clear, antibiotics are generally recommended for *Salmonella* gastroenteritis in the first 3 months of life, in immunocompromised hosts, and in patients who are toxic and potentially bacteremic.

There are more than 2000 serotypes of *Salmonella*. Current nomenclature considers them all as belonging to a single species (*Salmonella enterica*). There are important serotype-related differences in virulence. Obviously, *S. enterica* serotype Typhi and *S. enterica* serotypes Paratyphi A and B cause enteric fever (typhoid fever). But there are other more subtle virulence differences among serotypes. Some serotypes seem to be nonaggressive when they infect humans so they often are isolated from asymptomatic individuals, whereas others cause serious illnesses, including bloody diarrhea, blood stream invasion, and metastatic infection. For example, a strain of *S. enterica* serotype Senftenberg has been described that causes asymptomatic colonization of newborn infants. In contrast, both *S. enterica* serotype Dublin and *S. enterica* serotype Choleraesuis are commonly isolated from the blood stream. Gastroenteritis or bacteremia can occur with *S. enterica* serotype Dublin. Gastroenteritis is rare with *S. enterica* serotype Choleraesuis; bacteremia is the usual clinical manifestation of this serotype. In addition to organism-related virulence variation, there are differences in host susceptibility even to the same strain.

The most typical clinical manifestation of nontyphoidal *Salmonella* is gastroenteritis. Diarrhea caused by these organisms can be watery or bloody, with little fever or high fever. There may be headache, abdominal pain, malaise, vomiting, and chills. Illness may last for a few days or occasionally persist for weeks. Death is rare with *Salmonella* gastroenteritis in healthy children.

The organisms typically are high inoculum pathogens that require grossly contaminated food or water to cause symptomatic infection. Thus they generally do not spread easily to cause illness in close contacts of infected individuals. For example, daycare center outbreaks, although described, are uncommon. Animals are the usual reservoir (including poultry, livestock, and pets). Some serotypes are particularly associated with various reptiles, amphibians, cows, or birds. Eggs are important vehicles of infection. The incubation period usually is shorter than 72 hours.

The major complication of enteritis caused by these organisms is spread beyond the gut and mesenteric lymph nodes into the blood stream. The result can be sepsis, with or without seeding of distant organs. Any organ can be seeded during blood stream spread; however, the most common sites are the meninges and bones (particularly in sickle cell anemia). Major predisposing factors for severe or complicated disease include young age (particularly the first 3 months of life), reticuloendothelial system blockade (e.g., in hemoglobinopathies, malaria, schistosomiasis, bartonellosis, histoplasmosis), biliary and urinary tract abnormalities, colitis, congenital or acquired immunodeficiency diseases, and immunosuppressive drugs. Immunodeficiency diseases that predispose include phagocytic defects, such as chronic granulomatous disease; T cell defects, such as severe combined immune deficiency and human immunodeficiency virus (HIV); and defects in the interleukin (IL)-23/IL-12/interferon γ/STAT-1 pathway of Th1-mediated cellular immunity. Reactive arthritis, seen primarily in adults and less frequently in adolescents, can develop in HLA-B27–positive individuals; typically, it resolves without permanent residua.

Routine media are well suited for isolation of salmonella from stool as well as from normally sterile body fluids. Serologic studies generally are not helpful.

Expert Opinion on Management Issues

The mainstay of treatment, as with all forms of gastroenteritis, is management of nutritional and fluid/electrolyte status. Replacement of losses and early refeeding are central to management. The child who is in shock, coma, or has an ileus should be treated with intravenous fluids; other children with gastroenteritis should be treated with oral rehydration. The World Health Organization oral rehydration solution (ORS) or commercially available solutions, such as Pedialyte, can be used. The child should be restarted on feeding with breast milk or other age-appropriate foods within 6 to 12 hours of initiation of rehydration therapy.

For patients who require antibiotic therapy (for possible sepsis or extraintestinal focal infection), ceftriaxone is the usual choice; most nontyphoidal *Salmonella* infections in the United States are susceptible to ceftriaxone. Less than 5% of nontyphoidal *Salmonella* in the United States are currently resistant to multiple antibiotics. *S. enterica* serotype Typhimurium phage type 104 (DT104) is typically resistant to ampicillin, chloramphenicol, streptomycin, sulfonamides, and tetracyclines. This strain originated in Europe; it has spread to the United States, where it has become a common organism. Resistance to third-generation cephalosporins is rare; however, currently *S. enterica* serotype Newport is routinely resistant to ceftriaxone. The Newport strains typically have decreased susceptibility to ceftazidime, ampicillin, chloramphenicol, ceftriaxone, and cefotaxime; they are sensitive to ciprofloxacin, cefepime, and imipenem. Optimal choice of therapy for one of these infections is debatable but probably should be either cefepime or a fluoroquinolone.

Fluoroquinolone resistance is described in infected humans in the United States but is still rare. It is likely that with the 1993 licensing of this class of agents for use in veterinary medicine, resistance will eventually be a major issue. There are reports of resistant strains from Asia and Europe.

If antibiotics were previously started empirically based on a suspicion the child had an invasive pathogen such as *Shigella*, but the culture later demonstrates *Salmonella*, the antimicrobials should in general be stopped at that point.

Many extraintestinal *Salmonella* infections require prolonged antibiotic treatment to avoid relapse after therapy. Osteomyelitis should be treated a minimum of 4 to 6 weeks, and meningitis, a minimum of 4 weeks. Optimal duration for a bacteremia without documented organ involvement is not certain, although most authorities would recommend that antibiotics be given for 7 to 14 days. A poor response to therapy or evidence of relapse may require more prolonged treatment.

The diseases that predispose to *Salmonella* infection should be considered, particularly when extraintestinal infection is treated in an appropriate manner but repeatedly relapses. Such individuals typically require long-term suppressive therapy to prevent future relapses.

Because isolation of an unusual serotype may provide important epidemiologic clues to cause or suggest risk of additional cases, all *Salmonella* isolates should be serotyped by local public health authorities. Further decisions regarding the need for epidemiologic investigations should be made based on the results.

Common Pitfalls

- In the first few months of life, bloody diarrhea is often assumed to be caused by allergic proctitis: milk protein allergy/formula intolerance. However, *Salmonella* infections are very common in this age group. All episodes of bloody diarrhea should be evaluated for possible *Salmonella* even if the infant has no fever.
- Physicians often fail to caution families about exotic pets and the risk they pose to children.

Although most doctors are aware of the risk of turtles, there seems to be less awareness related to the risk of pet snakes, lizards, and amphibians. For example, more than half a million iguanas are imported into the United States annually; they are primarily used as family pets. Surveillance of iguanas indicates that they routinely excrete *Salmonella* species (especially *S. enterica* serotype Marina).

■ Isolation of an unusual serotype (*S. enterica* serotype Java, *S. enterica* serotype Stanley, *S. enterica* serotype Poona, *S. enterica* serotype Jangwani, *S. enterica* serotype Tilene, *S. enterica* serotype Litchfield, *S. enterica* serotype Manhattan, *S. enterica* serotype Pomona, *S. enterica* serotype Miami, *S. enterica* serotype Rubislaw, *S. enterica* serotype Marina, *S. enterica* serotype Wassenaar) suggests exposure to an exotic pet and should alert the physician to take appropriate action.

Communications and Counseling

Parents of infants and small children should be warned of the risk of exotic pets. They should be strongly encouraged to get rid of such animals to decrease the risk of the infant's becoming ill. Parents should be informed that even if the child does not have direct contact with the animal, risk remains. Serious infections have resulted, for example, when an iguana is in the house and the infant has never touched the animal or its cage.

Parents should be informed regarding the transmission of *Salmonella*. Good hand washing and care when handling foods should be encouraged. When a child in a daycare center develops nontyphoidal *Salmonella* infection, he or she should be excluded from the center until diarrhea has cleared; other children and adult staff need not be cultured if they are asymptomatic.

SUGGESTED READINGS

1. Gupta A, Fontana J, Crowe C, et al: Emergence of multidrug-resistant *Salmonella enterica* serotype Newport infections resistant to expanded-spectrum cephalosporins in the United States. J Infect Dis 1; 188(11):1707–1716, 2003. **Excellent summary of information regarding the U.S. data on the newly emerging multiply resistant pathogen *Salmonella enterica* serotype Newport.**
2. Mastroeni P: Immunity to systemic *Salmonella* infections. Curr Mol Med 2(4):393–406, 2002. **Overview of the integrated complex innate and acquired immune system activities that are required to protect the host from *Salmonella* infection.**
3. Ottenhoff TH, Verreck FA, Lichtenauer-Kaligis EG, et al: Genetics, cytokines and human infectious disease: Lessons from weakly pathogenic mycobacteria and salmonellae. Nat Genet 32(1):97–105, 2002. **Reviews the recent insights into genetic defects (in interleukin–12p40, interleukin–12R β 1, interferon-γ R1, interferon-γ R2, or STAT1) that cause increased susceptibility to mycobacteria and salmonellae.**
4. Reptile-associated salmonellosis—selected states, 1998–2002. MMWR Morb Mortal Wkly Rep 12; 52(49):1206–1209, 2003. **Increasing evidence suggests that amphibians (e.g., frogs, toads, newts, and salamanders), like reptiles, can pose risks for salmonellosis in humans.**
5. Threlfall EJ: Antimicrobial drug resistance in *Salmonella*: Problems and perspectives in food- and water-borne infections. FEMS Microbiol Rev 26(2):141–148, 2002. **Overview of the worldwide problem of antibiotic resistance, its relationship to inappropriate antimicrobial use in animals and people, and a description of the resistance patterns of the common currently circulating salmonellae.**

Shigellosis

Theresa J. Ochoa and Thomas G. Cleary

KEY CONCEPTS

■ Shigellosis occurs throughout the world because it is a low inoculum pathogen that is easily spread from person to person via contact. Because ingestion of as few as 10 organisms may cause severe disease, shigellosis commonly clusters in households, institutions, and daycare centers.

■ Although it can occur at any age, shigellosis is rare in neonates and in the first 6 months of life but common in the second through fourth years of life.

■ The classic case of dysentery is characterized by high fever, bloody diarrhea, abdominal pain, and painful defecation; however, prospective studies show that infection can be mild or even asymptomatic (half of infections lack bloody diarrhea).

■ Shigellosis in industrialized countries is more often caused by *Shigella sonnei* than *Shigella flexneri*; infection with *Shigella boydii* is very uncommon and *Shigella dysenteriae* (especially serotype 1) is rare. *S. sonnei* usually causes milder illness than *S. flexneri* or *S. dysenteriae*. In developing countries, *S. flexneri* is the most common species followed by *S. sonnei*

■ Empirical treatment should be given when shigellosis is strongly suspected; waiting for confirmation of the diagnosis results in late therapy that may have little effect on the clinical course.

■ Antibiotic resistance is common; knowledge of local resistance patterns can help in making empirical treatment decisions.

■ A negative stool culture does not exclude the diagnosis of shigellosis in a clinically compatible setting.

Shigellosis or bacillary dysentery is an infection by organisms of the genus *Shigella*. There are four serogroups or species (*Shigella dysenteriae, Shigella flexneri, Shigella boydii,* and *Shigella sonnei*). Although these organisms are conventionally grouped together, there are important variations in clinical features related to presence of specific virulence factors. For example, only *S. dysenteriae* serotype 1 always makes Shiga toxin; other shigellae either do not have the genes to make this toxin or make it only at low levels. Because this toxin damages vascular endothelium, it can cause unusually severe disease with complications such as hemolytic uremic syndrome. *S. flexneri* 2a makes an enterotoxin not made by other *Shigella* species. This may be an important determinant of the severity of dysentery caused by this serotype.

A broad spectrum of signs and symptoms are associated with infection by these organisms. Studies in which children in an endemic area (Mexico City) were cultured weekly during the first two years of life show that asymptomatic infection is as common as symptomatic illness. Many of the symptomatic infections are characterized by mild, nonspecific, watery diarrhea. However, the child who is recognized by physicians as having shigellosis typically has high fever, a toxic appearance, abdominal pain, and diarrhea. The extreme end of the clinical spectrum is characterized by painful defecation and passage of frequent low-volume stools containing blood and mucus.

Evaluation for shigellosis should be done in children who have some of the features of classic shigellosis. For example, a child who has high fever, a convulsion, and watery diarrhea should be cultured for *Shigella* even if no erythrocytes or leukocytes are found in the feces. Any child who has very high fever with watery diarrhea is a candidate to have shigellosis. Any child who has fecal leukocytes even with moderate fever is a candidate to have shigellosis. However, a child with grossly bloody diarrhea and no fever is less likely to have *Shigella* infection and far more likely to be infected with a Shiga toxin–producing *Escherichia coli* such as *E. coli* O157:H7.

The diagnosis of *Shigella* is conventionally made by stool culture. However, volunteer studies in adults show that stool cultures are often negative (20%) in patients known to be symptomatically infected with *Shigella*. Outbreaks of dysentery in closed populations also show that stool cultures are often falsely negative. Polymerase chain reaction (PCR) assay is positive for *Shigella* genes in feces of patients with dysentery significantly more often than is stool culture. Thus stool culture is useful when positive because it confirms the diagnosis and allows testing for susceptibility. A negative culture in a clinically compatible scenario is less helpful because it does not exclude the diagnosis. Nonspecific supportive data for the diagnosis of shigellosis include the presence of blood and leukocytes in feces. The peripheral blood leukocyte count is not consistently helpful because it can be high, low, or normal; there are more bands than segmented neutrophils in a minority of cases. Because of the inadequacy of stool cultures, a child with a scenario that strongly suggests shigellosis should be treated empirically while awaiting culture confirmation. Box 1 lists the complications of shigellosis.

Expert Opinion on Management Issues

As with all forms of infectious diarrhea, the mainstay of therapy is fluid and electrolyte replacement. Generally, the child who is not in shock or coma and does not have an ileus should be treated with oral rehydration. Classically, this has been done with the World Health Organization oral rehydrating solution (ORS), but

---

BOX 1 Complications of Shigellosis

- Dehydration (usually patients are more toxic than dry).
- Electrolyte abnormalities.
- Convulsions.
- Leukemoid reaction.
- Ileus, toxic megacolon, and intestinal perforation.
- Hemolytic uremic syndrome (seen only with *Shigella dysenteriae* serotype 1).
- Sepsis and bacteremia (rare except with *S. dysenteriae* serotype 1 in malnourished children)
- Ekiri syndrome or toxic encephalopathy (fulminant shigellosis with cerebral edema and death).
- Vaginitis (primarily with *Shigella flexneri*).
- Protein-losing enteropathy/malnutrition.
- Persistent diarrhea (uncommon).
- Reactive arthritis (primarily in adults who are HLA-B27 positive).

---

solutions commercially available in the United States (e.g., Pedialyte) are acceptable alternatives. It is key that refeeding with breast milk or other age-appropriate foods begins early (within 6 to 12 hours of onset of rehydration therapy). Important studies in the developing world emphasize not only the value of early refeeding but also, in the case of bacillary dysentery, the importance of high-protein feeds and supplementation with vitamin A and zinc.

Some experts recommend not treating shigellosis except when dysenteric disease occurs. However, this strategy can result in continuing spread to close contacts who may develop severe illness; such secondary cases might be prevented by treating index patients. We recommend empirical therapy whenever shigellosis is strongly suspected.

The usual empirical choice of therapy in children with suspected shigellosis is a third-generation cephalosporin, such as ceftriaxone. Oral third-generation cephalosporins, such as cefixime, are also effective. Cefixime is currently not available in the United States. A child who is ill with dysentery but allergic to third-generation cephalosporins or infected with an organism resistant to third-generation cephalosporins may be a candidate for treatment with a fluoroquinolone, such as ciprofloxacin, although these agents are generally not used in children. Nalidixic acid is used, particularly for S. *sonnei*, but data regarding its efficacy are contradictory; currently nalidixic acid is not available in the United States. Data suggest that azithromycin may be a useful alternate drug. Treatment with ampicillin, tetracycline, trimethoprim-sulfamethoxazole, or other sulfas is rarely appropriate given current susceptibility patterns. Table 1 gives examples of typical treatment regimens.

Common Pitfalls

- Many physicians are unaware of the spectrum of illness associated with *Shigella* infection. They fail to consider the diagnosis and culture for the pathogen because they consider it unlikely for the clinical scenario.

TABLE 1 Therapy for Shigellosis

Generic Name (Trade Name)	Dosage/Route/ Regimen	Maximum Dose	Dosage Formulation	Common Adverse Reactions	Therapeutic Concentrations	Comments
Ceftriaxone (Rocephin)	50 mg/kg/day IM or IV q24h for 5 days	2 g/day	Injection: 250 mg, 500 mg, 1 g, 2 g; contains 3.6 mEq Na/g of drug	Allergic reactions; cholelithiasis; sludging in gallbladder; jaundice	Peak serum concentration >300 μg/mL achieved after IV infusion of 75 mg/mL.	Current drug of choice for empirical therapy of severe dysentery in children.
Cefixime (Suprax)	8 mg/kg/day divided q12–24h PO for 5 days	400 mg/day	Tablets: 200 and 400 mg; suspension: 100 mg/5 mL	Diarrhea (up to 15%), nausea, abdominal pain, allergic reactions	Peak serum concentrations are 15% to 50% higher for the oral suspension versus the tablets.	Currently not available in the United States.
Ciprofloxacin (Cipro)	20–30 mg/kg/day divided q12h PO for 5 days	1.5 g/day	Suspension of 250 or 500 mg/5 mL; tablets: 100, 250, 500, 750 mg; injectable solution: 10 mg/mL	Theoretical risk of injury to growing cartilage; GI upset; renal failure, restlessness, rash, headache	Peak serum concentrations of 1–5 μg/mL after oral dose of 15 mg/kg.	Alternative when ceftriaxone, nalidixic acid, TMP/SMX, and ampicillin cannot be used.
Nalidixic acid (NegGram)	55 mg/kg/day divided q6h PO for 5 days	2 g/day	Suspension: 250 mg/5 mL; tablets: 250 mg, 500 mg and 1 g	Rash, GI upset, hepatoxicity, convulsions, increased intracranial pressure, arthralgia, myalgia		Not available in the United States; contraindicated in infants <3 months of age.
Trimethoprim-sulfamethoxazole (Bactrim, Septra, etc.)	10 mg/kg/day of the TMP component divided q12h PO for 5 days	320/1600 mg/day	Tablets: 80 mg TMP/ 400 mg SMX (regular strength), 160/800 (double strength); suspension: 40/200 per 5 mL; injectable: 16/80 per mL (may contain propylene glycol and benzyl alcohol)	Bone marrow suppression, rash, (rarely Stevens-Johnson syndrome): crystalluria, glossitis, nephrotoxic; hepatotoxic; GI upset; hemolysis in patients with G6PD deficiency; hyperkalemia in AIDS patients; not recommended for use in infants <2 mo of age (kernicterus risk)		Currently of limited value in the United States because of the high frequency of resistant *Shigella*; when the organism is known to be susceptible, it can be used.
Ampicillin (Omnipen, Principen, Totacillin, etc.)	100 mg/kg/day divided q6h PO, IV or IM for 5 days	4 g/day	Suspension: 125, 250 mg/5 mL; caps: 250, 500 mg; injectable: 3 mEq Na/g of IV prep	Diarrhea (20%), rash; allergic reactions; interstitial nephritis, pseudomembranous colitis		Currently of limited value in the United States because of the high frequency of resistant *Shigella*; when the organism is known to be susceptible, it can be used.
Azithromycin (Zithromax)	12 mg/kg/day once daily PO on day 1, followed by 6 mg/kg/day once daily on days 2–5	500 mg/day	Suspension: 100 mg/ 5 mL, 200 mg/5 mL; tablets: 250, 500, and 600 mg	Rash, GI upset, nephritis		Limited data in children.

AIDS acquired immune deficiency syndrome; G6PD, glucose–6-phosphate dehydrogenase; GI, gastrointestinal; IM, intramuscular; IV, intravenous; PO, by mouth; q, every; qxh, every x hours; SMX, sulfamethoxazole; TMP, trimethoprim.

12

- It is common for physicians to ignore epidemiologic data that could be very helpful. The age of the patient is relevant. A child in the first few months of life with bloody diarrhea and fever is very unlikely to have *Shigella* (*Salmonella* is more likely if intestinal infection is present); but a 13- to 48-month-old child with high fever and bloody diarrhea is at a very significant risk for being infected with *Shigella*. A clustering of cases of febrile bloody diarrhea in a family setting or daycare center is more likely to be *Shigella* than other pathogens; although clustering of cases could reflect ingestion of a contaminated meal, timing of cases may suggest person-to-person spread of the low inoculum pathogen.
- Physicians are often unaware of national and local changing resistance patterns. For example, trimethoprim-sulfamethoxazole has not been a reliable agent for shigellosis in the United States for nearly 10 years, but physicians continue to use it.

Communication and Counseling

Families (or daycare personnel) should be warned about the low inoculum size required to spread infection. The importance of hand washing in particular should be emphasized. If the infection occurs in a daycare center, special attention should be given to the specific duties of personnel; food and drink preparation should be done by different individuals than those involved in diapering of toddlers and toilet training. The potential for fomites (e.g., shared toys) serving as vehicles for transmission should be discussed.

Parents should be told that the child should be much improved within 24 hours of initiation of therapy. If the child is not better within 48 hours, a resistant organism may well be present or the presumptive diagnosis of shigellosis may be wrong. A change in treatment should be considered, even though culture confirmation and sensitivity data may not be available for several more days.

Individuals traveling to the developing world are at significant risk for acquiring shigellosis. Prospective travelers should be cautioned about the risk of contaminated food and water. Bottled water (carbonated) or boiled water as well as food served steaming hot is usually safe. No uncooked vegetables or fruits should be consumed except for fruits that can be peeled at the time of eating. Ice may be contaminated, so chilled drinks without ice are preferable. Food should not be purchased from street vendors. Hand washing should be encouraged. This strategy may prevent not only dysentery but also other food- and water-borne diseases common to the developing world.

There is no currently available vaccine, nor does it appear likely that one will be licensed in the foreseeable future. A variety of vaccine candidates are being studied, but thus far the constructs cause too many side effects and only result in narrow (serotype-specific), brief protection.

SUGGESTED READINGS

1. Ashkenazi S: Shigella infections in children: New insights. Semin Pediatr Infect Dis 15(4):246–252, 2004. **An excellent summary of current data on pathophysiology and treatment of shigellosis.**
2. Basualdo W, Arbo A: Randomized comparison of azithromycin versus cefixime for treatment of shigellosis in children. Pediatr Infect Dis J 22(4):374–377, 2003. **This trial demonstrates that azithromycin given for 5 days is as good as cefixime therapy.**
3. Guerrero L, Calva JJ, Morrow AL, et al: Asymptomatic *Shigella* infections in a cohort of Mexican children younger than two years of age. Pediatr Infect Dis J 13(7):597–602, 1994. **This study demonstrates the high frequency of asymptomatic and mild *Shigella* infection in prospectively studied Mexican children in the first 2 years of life.**
4. Hossain S, Biswas R, Kabir I, et al: Single dose vitamin A treatment in acute shigellosis in Bangladesh children: Randomised double blind controlled trial. BMJ 7; 316(7129):422–426, 1998. **This is one of a number of important randomized controlled trials that demonstrate the value of vitamin supplements or high-protein diets for shigellosis occurring either in areas where deficiencies are common or in children who are actually clinically malnourished.**
5. Sivapalasingam S, McClellan J, Joyce K, et al: Increasing antimicrobial resistance among shigella isolates in the United States, 1999–2000. PDF available for download at http://www.cdc.gov/narms/publications/2001/sivapalasingam_2001.pdf. **This CDC website (updated periodically) lists recent information regarding national trends in *Shigella* resistance patterns.**
6. Zimbabwe, Bangladesh, South Africa (Zimbasa) Dysentery Study Group: Multicenter, randomized, double blind clinical trial of short course versus standard course oral ciprofloxacin for *Shigella dysenteriae* type 1 dysentery in children. Pediatr Infect Dis J 21 (12):1136–1141, 2002. **This study suggests that *S. dysenteriae* type 1 can as safely be treated with short course (3 days) as with standard course (5 days) oral ciprofloxacin (15 mg/kg every 12 hours). Because of the morbidity and mortality associated with this serotype, a fluoroquinolone may be appropriate.**

Yersinia enterocolitica

Sarmistha B. Hauger

KEY CONCEPTS

- *Yersinia enterocolitica* is a zoonosis that can cause a variety of illnesses depending on host risk factors. Contaminated food, including refrigerated foods, may transmit infection.
- Enteritis is the most common presentation in young children; older children most often present with mesenteric adenitis or pseudoappendicitis. Adolescents and adults often present with postinfectious sequelae such as reactive arthritis.
- Bacteremia and extraintestinal complications are most common in infants younger than 3 months, immunocompromised hosts, persons with hemoglobinopathies or iron overload syndromes, and those on chelation therapy.
- Antibiotic therapy for self-limited enteritis and reactive arthritis is not usually warranted. Antibiotic therapy is indicated for high-risk hosts and extraintestinal complications.

Yersinia enterocolitica is a gram-negative bacillus that can cause a variety of human illnesses, including enteritis, sepsis, and reactive arthritis. It is a member of the genus *Yersinia*, which includes two other human pathogens: *Yersinia pestis* and *Yersinia pseudotuberculosis*. All of these infections are zoonoses; humans are accidental hosts. Many animals are important reservoirs of *Y. enterocolitica*. Pigs, in particular, are an important source of infection. People who handle or eat pork (especially pork intestines or chitterlings) have a risk of infection. Outbreaks are also traced to unpasteurized dairy products. Low levels of bacteria can grow at 39°F (4°C); therefore, even refrigerated foods and contaminated water can be a source of infection. *Y. enterocolitica* human infections are more common in cooler months and geographic zones, but they are reported from all parts of the world.

Pathophysiology

Y. enterocolitica has numerous virulence factors that directly affect the immune system. Pathogenic strains show resistance to complement-mediated phagocytosis, demonstrate cytotoxicity, and produce enterotoxin and lipopolysaccharide endotoxin. Most bacteria extract iron, an essential growth element, from transferrin by releasing siderophores. *Y. enterocolitica* does not produce siderophores but can use those made by other intestinal bacteria. In an extraintestinal environment, the bacteria can readily thrive in an environment of excess iron or exogenous siderophores, such as a chelating agent. Therefore, patients with iron overload syndromes and those under chelation therapy are two groups at special risk for *Y. enterocolitica* infection.

Clinical Manifestations

Y. enterocolitica causes various clinical presentations at different ages, depending on host risk factors (Table 1). Inapparent infection is infrequent, occurring in approximately 10% of cases. Enterocolitis with fever is the most common presentation in children younger than 5 years. The presentation is indistinguishable from other causes of colitis. Stools contain white blood cells and gross blood in up to 25% of patients. *Y. enterocolitica* is a cause of chronic diarrhea lasting longer than 2 weeks in infants and children. Complications such as bacteremia and extraintestinal infections are most often seen in infants younger than 3 months, immunocompromised patients, and in those with iron overload syndromes. Older children present with mesenteric adenitis and pseudoappendicitis. Intra-abdominal complications can occur, including intestinal perforation and toxic megacolon. *Y. enterocolitica* is reported as a cause of fever of unknown origin, granulomatous hepatitis, pancreatitis, pharyngitis, liver abscess, meningitis, osteomyelitis, cellulitis, erythema multiforme, and leukocytoclastic vasculitis. In adolescents and adults, postinfectious sequelae are common, including a polyarticular nonsuppurative reactive arthritis, the Reiter syndrome, ankylosing spondylitis, and erythema nodosum. Many of these patients are positive for the HLA-B27 antigen.

Diagnosis

Y. enterocolitica grows from a variety of body fluids. The frequency of isolation after illness decreases with time, with the best yield in the first 2 weeks of illness. Isolation is increased by use of selective cefsulodin-Irgasan-novobiocin (CIN) agar and cold enrichment. The microbiology laboratory should be alerted to the possibility of *Yersinia* infection so the proper steps can be taken to facilitate growth. Serologic methods are not useful for acute diagnosis and have poor sensitivity and specificity.

Expert Opinion on Management Issues

The value of antimicrobial therapy for self-limited *Y. enterocolitica* enteritis in children is not established; there does not appear to be a difference in clinical improvement in children treated with antibiotics versus those who were not treated. Indeed, bacterial relapse may be more common in children who are treated with antibiotics.

TABLE 1 Clinical Manifestations of *Yersinia enterocolitica* Human Infection

Clinical Manifestations	Host	Host Risk Factors
Enterocolitis	All ages	Most common in children <5 yr.
Enteritis with bacteremia or septicemia	Infant <3 mo; immunocompromised; iron overload syndromes; patients on chelation therapy	Poor immune response. Excess iron allows for bacterial growth.
Mesenteric adenitis or pseudoappendicitis	Older children Adults	None.
Postinfectious sequelae:	Adolescents/adults	
Reactive arthritis		HLA-B27 antigen positive.
Erythema nodosum		Female sex.

Adapted from Gomez HF, Cleary TG: *Yersinia* species. In Long SS, Pickering LK, Prober CG (eds): Principles and Practice of Pediatric Infectious Diseases, 2nd ed. New York: Churchill-Livingstone, 2003, p 840.

TABLE 2   Clinical Management of *Yersinia enterocolitica* Human Infection

Clinical Manifestations	Antibiotic Therapy
Enterocolitis (self-limited), healthy host	Not warranted
Enterocolitis with bacteremia or septicemia, immunocompromised host	Trimethoprim-sulfamethoxazole; third-generation cephalosporin; quinolone
Postinfectious syndromes	Not warranted

Antibiotic therapy should be reserved for patients with established sepsis, secondary foci of infection, and for those at risk for complications, such as infants younger than 3 months and patients with immunocompromise, hemoglobinopathies, iron overload syndromes, and those on chelation therapy.

The role of antibiotic therapy of reactive arthritis associated with *Y. enterocolitica* infections is unclear. *Yersinia* antigens may persist in peripheral blood cells for months after infection and are found in synovial tissue. However, the organism has not been cultured from such patients. One study showed a beneficial effect of quinolone therapy in resolution of symptoms. Further clinical studies need to be done before this can be a general recommendation. If antibiotic treatment is undertaken, it should be initiated earlier rather than later in the clinical course (Table 2).

Y. enterocolitica is sensitive in vitro to a variety of antibiotics, including trimethoprim-sulfamethoxazole, aminoglycosides, quinolones, tetracyclines, and third-generation cephalosporins. The organism is frequently β-lactamase positive and therefore resistant to the penicillins and first-generation cephalosporins. In most situations in children, oral trimethoprim-sulfamethoxazole or third-generation cephalosporin can be used; quinolones may be useful in adolescents and adults. Therapy with intravenous third-generation cephalosporins is indicated for the more severely ill patient.

Common Pitfalls

- Failure to obtain a complete food ingestion history.
- Failure to consider *Y. enterocolitica* as a possible pathogen in patients at high risk: infants younger than 3 months, those with immunocompromise or iron overload syndromes, and those on chelation therapy.
- Failure to alert the microbiology laboratory so laboratory methods can be undertaken to increase the yield of bacterial isolation.

Communication and Counseling

- All families with young infants and children with immunocompromise, hemoglobinopathies, iron overload syndromes, or on chelation therapy should be counseled about the possibility of infections related to food contamination, especially foods that are most often consumed during holidays, such as pork chitterlings.
- Adolescents and adults should be advised about the possibility of postinfectious syndromes, such as reactive arthritis or erythema nodosum, appearing approximately 1 month after enteric illness.

SUGGESTED READINGS

1. Abdel-haq NM, Asmar BI, Abuhammour WM, et al: *Yersinia enterocolitica* infection in children. Pediatr Infect Dis J 19:954–958, 2000. **Retrospective study defining role of *Yersinia* as a food-borne illness, as well as detailed clinical manifestations of illness in infants and children. Treatment section with details about therapy options.**
2. Cover TL, Aber RA: *Yersinia enterocolitica.* N Engl J Med 321:16–23, 1989. **Comprehensive and detailed review of the subject.**
3. Hoogkamp-Korstanje JA, Moesker H, Bruyn GA: Ciprofloxacin v. placebo for therapy of *Yersinia*-triggered reactive arthritis. Ann Rheum Dis 59(11):914–917, 2000. **Placebo-controlled trial of antibiotic therapy for *Yersinia*-triggered reactive arthritis, showing a benefit in clinical symptoms with therapy.**
4. Marks MI, Pai CH, Lefleur L: *Yersinia enterocolitica* gastroenteritis: Prospective study of clinical, bacterial and epidemiologic features. J Pediatr 96:26–31, 1980. **Clinical review of illness in children with good section on therapy issues.**
5. Pai CH, Gillis F, Toumanen E, et al: Placebo controlled double blind evaluation of trimethoprim-sulfamethoxazole treatment of *Yersinia enterocolitica* gastroenteritis. J Pediatr 104:308–311, 1984. **Double-blind trial showing no benefit of oral antibiotics on clinical symptoms and an increase in relapse rate in treated children.**

Anaerobic Infections

Itzhak Brook

KEY CONCEPTS

- Anaerobes are the predominant bacterial flora in the normal human skin and mucous membranes and therefore are a common cause of endogenous infections.
- Anaerobic infections are generally polymicrobial. Where anaerobes are mixed with aerobic organisms, therapy should provide for coverage of both types of pathogens.
- The isolation of anaerobes requires appropriate methods of collection, transportation, and cultivation of specimens. The lack of any of these methods can lead to inadequate recovery of anaerobes and inappropriate therapy.
- Treatment of anaerobic infections is complicated by the slow growth of anaerobic bacteria and the growing resistance of anaerobic bacteria to antimicrobials.
- The primary role of antimicrobials is to eliminate the pathogens and prevent local and systemic spread of the organism.
- Surgical drainage is of primary importance and includes debriding necrotic tissue, draining the pus,

improving circulation, alleviating the obstruction, and increasing the tissue oxygenation.
- The most effective antimicrobials against anaerobic organisms are metronidazole, the carbapenems, chloramphenicol, clindamycin, and the combination of an aminopenicillin and a β-lactamase inhibitor.

Infections in children caused by anaerobic bacteria may be serious and life-threatening. Anaerobes are the predominant components of the normal human skin and mucous membranes and therefore a common cause of endogenous bacterial infections. Exogenous infections can occur following introduction of these organisms into sterile body sites from the environment (through bites or trauma). Because of their fastidious nature, anaerobes are difficult to isolate and often overlooked. Failure to direct therapy against these organisms often leads to clinical failures. Their isolation requires appropriate methods of collection, transportation, and cultivation of specimens.

Anaerobic infections can occur in all body sites, including the central nervous system (i.e., meningitis, brain abscess); head and neck (i.e., chronic otitis, mastoiditis, and sinusitis, tonsillitis, and oropharyngeal abscesses); chest (i.e., aspiration pneumonia, lung abscess, empyema); abdomen (i.e., peritonitis, intra-abdominal abscesses); pelvis (i.e., pelvic inflammatory disease, and abscesses); skin (i.e., fasciitis, cellulites); and soft tissues (i.e., abscesses). They are also an important cause of neonatal infections, such as aspiration pneumonia, bacteremia, omphalitis, and cholangitis.

The recovery from an anaerobic infection depends on prompt and proper management. The principles of managing anaerobic infections include neutralizing toxins produced by anaerobes, preventing their local proliferation by changing the environment, and hampering their spread into healthy tissues.

Toxin neutralization by specific antitoxins may be employed, especially in infections caused by *Clostridium* species (tetanus and botulism). Controlling the environment is achieved by debriding necrotic tissue, draining the pus, improving circulation, alleviating the obstruction, and increasing the tissue oxygenation. Certain types of adjunct therapy, such as hyperbaric oxygen (HBO), may also be useful. The primary role of antimicrobials is to eradicate the pathogens and to limit the local and systemic spread of the organism(s). Antimicrobial therapy in many patients is the only form of therapy required; in others, it is an important adjunct to a surgical approach.

Expert Opinion on Management Issues

ACCEPTABLE INTERVENTIONS

Surgical Therapy

In many cases, surgical therapy is the most important and sometimes the only form of treatment required; in others, it is an adjunct to a pharmacologic approach. It includes draining abscesses, debriding necrotic tissues, decompressing closed space infections, and relieving obstructions. Without drainage, the infection may persist and serious complications can develop.

Antimicrobial Therapy

Appropriate management of mixed aerobic and anaerobic infections requires the administration of antimicrobials effective against both components. A number of factors should be considered when choosing appropriate antimicrobial agents. They should have efficacy against all target organisms, induce little or no resistance, achieve sufficient concentrations in the infected site, and have minimal toxicity and maximum stability.

When choosing antimicrobials for the therapy of mixed infections, their aerobic and anaerobic antibacterial spectrum (Tables 1, 2, and 3) and their availability in oral or parenteral form should be considered. Some antimicrobials have a limited range of activity. For example, metronidazole is active only against anaerobes (with the exception of non–spore-forming gram-positive rods) and therefore cannot be administered as a single agent for the therapy of mixed infections. Others (i.e., carbapenems) have wide spectra of activity against aerobes and anaerobes.

The selection of antimicrobials is simplified when reliable culture results are available. However, this may be difficult to achieve in anaerobic infections because of problems in obtaining appropriate specimens. Many patients are treated empirically on the basis of suspected, rather than established, pathogens. Fortunately, the types of organisms involved in many anaerobic infections and their antimicrobial susceptibility patterns tend to be predictable. But the pattern of resistance to antimicrobials may vary in a particular hospital, and resistance to antimicrobial agents may emerge while a patient is receiving therapy.

The susceptibility of the *Bacteroides fragilis* group to the frequently used antimicrobial drugs was studied systematically over the past two decades. These surveys fail to reveal strains resistant to chloramphenicol or metronidazole and minimal resistance (<1%) to carbapenems or the combinations of an aminopenicillin and a β-lactamase inhibitor, but resistance to other agents varies. The rate differs among various medical centers and generally increases with extensive use of some antimicrobial agents (penicillins, cephalosporins, and clindamycin).

Aside from susceptibility patterns, other factors influencing the choice of antimicrobial therapy include the pharmacologic characteristics of the various drugs, their toxicity, their effect on the normal flora, and bactericidal activity. Although identification of the infecting organisms and their antimicrobial susceptibility may be needed for selection of optimal therapy, the clinical setting and Gram-stain preparation of the specimen may indicate the types of anaerobes present in the infection as well as the nature of the infectious process.

TABLE 1 Antimicrobial Drugs of Choice for Anaerobic Bacteria

Bacteria Name	First Choice	Alternate Choices
Peptostreptococcus species	Penicillin	Clindamycin, chloramphenicol, cephalosporins
Clostridium species	Penicillin	Metronidazole, chloramphenicol, cefoxitin, clindamycin
Clostridium difficile	Vancomycin	Metronidazole, bacitracin
Gram-negative rods* (BL–)	Penicillin	Metronidazole, clindamycin, chloramphenicol
Gram-negative rods* (BL+)	Metronidazole, imipenem, a penicillin and β-lactamase inhibitor, clindamycin	Cefoxitin, chloramphenicol, piperacillin

BL, β-lactamase.
B. fragilis group; *Prevotella* species; *Porphyromonas* species; *Fusobacterium* species.

ANTIMICROBIAL AGENTS

Some classes of agents have poor activity against anaerobes. These include the aminoglycosides, the monobactams, and the older quinolones. The newer quinolones have improved efficacy against anaerobic bacteria. The most active ones are trovafloxacin, moxifloxacin, and gatifloxacin. However, these agents are not approved for use in children. Tables 1 through 4 show the antimicrobials suitable for use in anaerobic infections.

The available parenteral antimicrobials (Tables 3, 4, and 5) are clindamycin, metronidazole, chloramphenicol, cefoxitin, aminopenicillins (ticarcillin, ampicillin, piperacillin), a β-lactamase inhibitor (clavulanic acid, sulbactam, tazobactam), and carbapenems (imipenem, meropenem, ertapenem). An agent effective against gram-negative enteric bacilli (aminoglycoside) or an antipseudomonal cephalosporin (cefepime) is generally added to clindamycin, metronidazole, and, occasionally, cefoxitin when treating intra-abdominal infections (see Table 2). Penicillin is added to metronidazole in treating intracranial, pulmonary, and dental infections to cover for microaerophilic streptococci and *Actinomyces*. A macrolide is added to metronidazole in upper

TABLE 2 Antimicrobial Drugs Recommended for Therapy of Site-Specific Anaerobic Infections

Site	Surgical Prophylaxis	Parenteral	Oral
Intracranial	1. Penicillin[1] 2. Vancomycin[2]	1. Metronidazole[3] 2. Chloramphenicol	1. Metronidazole[3] 2. Chloramphenicol
Dental	1. Penicillin 2. Erythromycin	1. Clindamycin 2. Metronidazole,[3] chloramphenicol	1. Clindamycin, amoxicillin + CA 2. Metronidazole,[3] chloramphenicol
Upper respiratory tract	1. Cefoxitin 2. Clindamycin	1. Clindamycin 2. Chloramphenicol, metronidazole[3]	1. Clindamycin, amoxicillin + CA 2. Chloramphenicol, metronidazole[4]
Pulmonary	NA	1. Clindamycin[4] 2. Chloramphenicol, ticarcillin + CA, ampicillin + SU,[7] imipenem meropenem	1. Clindamycin[5] 2. Chloramphenicol, metronidazole,[4] amoxicillin + CA
Abdominal	1. Cefoxitin 2. Clindamycin[3]	1. Clindamycin,[6] cefoxitin,[3] metronidazole[3] 2. Imipenem meropenem, ticarcillin + CA	1. Clindamycin,[5] metronidazole[5] 2. Chloramphenicol, amoxicillin + CA
Pelvic	1. Cefoxitin 2. Doxycycline	1. Cefoxitin,[7] clindamycin[6] 2. Ticarcillin + CA,[7] ampicillin + SU,[7] metronidazole[7]	1. Clindamycin[7] 2. Amoxicillin + CA,[7] metronidazole[7]
Skin	1. Cefazolin 2. Vancomycin	1. Clindamycin, cefoxitin 2. Metronidazole[3] + methicillin	1. Clindamycin, amoxicillin + CA 2. Metronidazole[4]
Bone and joint	1. Cefazolin[8] 2. Vancomycin	1. Clindamycin, imipenem, meropenem 2. Chloramphenicol, metronidazole,[3] ticarcillin + CA	1. Clindamycin 2. Chloramphenicol, metronidazole[3]
Bacteremia with BLPB	NA	1. Imipenem, meropenem, metronidazole 2. Cefoxitin, ticarcillin + CA	1. Clindamycin, metronidazole 2. Chloramphenicol, amoxicillin + CA
Bacteremia with non-BLPB	NA	1. Penicillin 2. Clindamycin, metronidazole, cefoxitin	1. Penicillin 2. Metronidazole, chloramphenicol, clindamycin

[1]Drug(s) of choice.
[2]Alternative drugs.
[3]Plus penicillin.
[4]Plus a macrolide (erythromycin, azithromycin, or clarithromycin).
[5]Plus a quinolone (only in adults).
[6]Plus aminoglycoside.
[7]Plus doxycycline.
[8]In location proximal to the rectal and oral areas, use cefoxitin.
BLPB, β-Lactamase–producing bacteria; CA, clavulanic acid; NA, not applicable; SU, sulbactam.

respiratory infections to treat *Staphylococcus aureus* and aerobic streptococci. Penicillin is added to clindamycin to supplement its coverage against *Peptostreptococcus* species and other gram-positive anaerobes.

Doxycycline or a macrolide are added to most regimens in treating pelvic infections for chlamydia and mycoplasma. Penicillin is still the drug of choice for bacteremia caused by non–β-lactamase-producing bacteria (BLPB). However, other agents should be used for the therapy of bacteremia caused by BLPB.

Because the duration of therapy for anaerobic infections, which are often chronic, is generally longer than for infections caused by aerobic and facultative anaerobes, oral therapy is often substituted for parenteral therapy. The agents available for oral therapy are clindamycin, amoxicillin plus clavulanic acid, chloramphenicol, and metronidazole.

Clinical judgment, personal experience, safety, and patient compliance should direct the physician in the choice of the appropriate antimicrobials. The length of therapy ranges between 2 and 4 weeks but should be individualized depending on the response. In some cases, such as undrainable abscesses of the lungs, abdomen, or central nervous system, and osteomyelitis, treatment may be required for as long as 6 to 12 weeks but can often be shortened with proper surgical drainage.

URGENT INTERVENTIONS

Recovery from anaerobic infection depends on proper and prompt medical and surgical interventions. Surgery is urgently important in debriding necrotic tissues and decompressing closed space infections and relieving obstructions. This includes drainage of collected fluids (i.e., empyema, peritonsillar abscess). Management of deep-seated soft tissue infection includes surgical debridement, drainage, and vigorous surgical management. Improvement of oxygenation of the involved tissues through enhancement of blood supply and administration of HBO, especially in clostridial infection, may be helpful, although no formal evidence

demonstrates its benefit. Toxin neutralization by specific antitoxins may be employed, especially in infections caused by *Clostridium* species (tetanus and botulism).

Urgent interventions including life-support measures are needed in clostridial infections such as tetanus and botulism and necrotizing cellulitis and fasciitis. Other urgent interventions include fluid and electrolyte management in serious intra-abdominal and pelvic infections and respiratory care in patients with respiratory distress (i.e., aspiration pneumonia).

CONTROVERSIAL INTERVENTIONS

Using HBO in an infection of spore-forming gram-positive anaerobic rods is controversial. Several uncontrolled reports demonstrated efficacy in individual cases, but the efficacy of HBO is unproved in well-controlled studies. Using HBO in conjunction with other therapies is not contraindicated, except when it delays other essential procedures. Topical application of oxygen-releasing compounds may be useful.

Routine performance of antimicrobial susceptibility testing of anaerobes is controversial because it is very time consuming and in many cases unnecessary. Resistance to several antimicrobials, especially by anaerobic gram-negative bacilli and *Fusobacterium*, has increased over the past decade.

Screening of gram-negative bacilli isolates (particularly *Prevotella, Porphyromonas, Bacteroides,* and *Fusobacterium* species) for β-lactamase activity may be helpful. This can provide information regarding their penicillin susceptibility. However, occasional bacterial strains may resist β-lactam antibiotics through other mechanisms.

Susceptibility testing should be limited to anaerobes isolated from blood, bone, central nervous system, sterile body sites, and serious infections; those isolated in pure culture from properly collected specimens; those with particular epidemiologic or prognostic significance (e.g., *Clostridium difficile*); and those that

12

TABLE 3 Antimicrobial Agents Effective against Mixed Infection*

Antimicrobial Agent	Anaerobic Bacteria		Aerobic Bacteria	
	β-Lactamase-Producing Gram-negative Bacilli	Other Anaerobes	Gram-Positive Cocci	Enterobacteriaceae
Penicillin[†]	0	+ + +	+	0
Chloramphenicol[†]	+ + +	+ + +	+	+
Cephalothin	0	+	+ +	+ / −
Cefoxitin	+ +	+ + +	+ +	+ +
Imipenem/meropenem	+ + +	+ + +	+ + +	+ + +
Clindamycin[†]	+ + +	+ + +	+ + +	0
Ticarcillin	+	+ + +	+	+ +
Amoxicillin + Clavulanic acid[†]	+ + +	+ + +	+ +	+ +
Ticarcillin + Clavulanic acid	+ + +	+ + +	+ +	+ +
Metronidazole[†]	+ + +	+ +	0	0
Trovafloxacin[†]	+ +	+ +	+ +	+ + +

*Degrees of activity: 0 to + + +.
[†]Available also in oral form.

TABLE 4 Antibiotic Used for Treatment of Anaerobic Infections

Generic Name	Trade Name	Adult Regimen (Dose, Route, Dose Interval)	Pediatric (>3 mo) Regimen (Dose, Route, Dose Interval)	Common Side Effects
Clindamycin HCl	Cleocin HCl; Dalacin	150–300 mg PO q6–8h	10–30 mg/kg/day PO q6–8h	Diarrhea, *C. difficile* colitis, rash, neutropenia, blood dyscrasias, phlebitis
Clindamycin phosphate	Cleocin PO₄; Dalacin	600 mg IV q8h up to 2.7 g/day	20–40 mg/kg/day IM; IV q6–8h	Same
Chloramphenicol	Chloromycetin	250–500 mg PO q6h	50–75 mg/kg/day PO q4–6h	GI intolerance (oral), dose-related bone marrow suppression, aplastic anemia, fever, optic neuritis, *C. difficile* colitis, gray baby syndrome in infants
Chloramphenicol sodium succinate	Chloromycetin sodium succinate	0.5–2 g IV q6h, generally 1 g q6h	50–75 mg/kg/day IV q6h	Same
Doxycycline	Vibramycin, Doryx, Doxy-Caps, Doryx, Vibra-Tabs	100–200 mg PO or IV q12–24h	2–4 mg/kg/day PO IV q12h for day 1, then half the dose q24h	Dose-related GI intolerance, rash, liver and renal toxicity, elevation of CSF pressure in infants, photosensitivity, dental discoloration (<8 yr), diarrhea, candidiasis (thrush and vaginitis), *C. difficile* colitis, hemolytic anemia, phlebitis when given IV
Cefotetan disodium	Cefotan	1–2 g IM or IV q12h	40–80 mg/kg/day IV, IM q12h*	Phlebitis or pain at site, diarrhea, allergic reaction, *C. difficile* colitis, eosinophilia, serum sickness, hemolytic anemia, hepatic dysfunction, neutropenia, thrombocytopenia, CNS effects, anaphylaxis
Cefoxitin sodium	Mefoxin	0.5–2 g IM or IV q4–6h	80–160 mg/kg/day IV, IM q4–6h	Same
Metronidazole	Flagyl, Protostat Metric, Metro IV, Flagyl IV, MetroGel	250–500 mg PO q8h or 0.5–1.0 g PO q12h; 0.5–1 g IV q12h; topical: q12h	15–35 mg/kg/day PO q8h; 30–40 mg/kg/day IV q8h	GI intolerance, metallic taste, CNS toxicities, peripheral neuropathy, anticoagulant potentiation, disulfiram-like reaction with alcohol, phlebitis (IV use), insomnia
Vancomycin	Vancocin; Lyphocin, Vancoled, Vancor, Lyphocin, Vancocin HCl IV	125 mg PO q6–8h (for *C. difficile* colitis); 0.5–1 g IV q12h usually 2 g/day	40 mg/kg/day PO q6–8h (for *C. difficile* colitis); 40 mg/kg/day IV q6–8h	Phlebitis, with rapid infusion, red man syndrome, fever, allergic reaction, anaphylaxis, peripheral neuropathy, marrow suppression, oto- and nephrotoxicity

C. difficile, Clostridium difficile; CNS, central nervous system; CSF, cerebrospinal fluid; GI, gastrointestinal; IM, intramuscular; IV, intravenous; PO, by mouth; q*x*h, every *x* hours.

are clinically important and have variable susceptibilities. Antibiotics tested should include penicillin, a broad-spectrum penicillin, an aminopenicillin plus a β-lactamase inhibitor, clindamycin, chloramphenicol, a second-generation cephalosporin (e.g., cefoxitin), metronidazole, and a carbapenem.

Common Pitfalls

- Not obtaining or sending inappropriate specimens for anaerobic bacteria.
- Using an antimicrobial that is not effective against the pathogen(s) because of previous or newly developed antimicrobial resistance.
- Failure to debride and drain accumulated pus.

The proper management of anaerobic infection depends on appropriate documentation of the bacteria causing the infection. Without such an approach, the patient may be exposed to inappropriate, costly, and undesirable antimicrobials with adverse side effects. Failure to recover anaerobes may cause the clinician to direct therapy toward only the isolated aerobes. Some laboratories may fail to recover certain or all of the anaerobes present in a specimen. This can occur particularly when the specimen is not promptly placed under anaerobic conditions for transportation to the laboratory.

If care is not taken to avoid specimen contamination with normal flora, the results may be misleading. Because indigenous anaerobes are present in large number on the surfaces of skin and mucous

TABLE 5 Penicillins

Generic Name	Trade Name	Adult Regimen (Dose, Route, Dose Interval)	Pediatric (>3 mo) Regimen (Dose, Route, Dose Interval)	Common Side Effects
Natural Penicillins[†]				
Crystalline G potassium	Pfizerpen	0.5–5 million U, IV q4–6h	100,000–250,000 U/kg/day IV q4–6h	Anaphylaxis, rash, leukopenia, thrombocytopenia, hemolytic anemia; local reactions such as swelling; *C. difficile* colitis
Crystalline G sodium	Penicillin G sodium for injection	0.5–5 million U, IV q4–6h	100,000–250,000 U/kg/day IV q4–6h	Same
Penicillin G, Benzathine	Bicillin (in U.K.), Bicillin L-A	1.2–2.4 million U, IM, 1 dose	50,000 U/kg IM, 1 dose	Same
Penicillin G, Benzathine + procaine	Permapen, Bicillin C-R	1.2–2.4 million U, IM, 1 dose	50,000 U/kg IM, 1 dose	Same
Penicillin G, Procaine	Crysticillin, Pfizerpen, Wycillin	0.3–2.4 million U, IM q6–12h	25,000–50,000 U/kg/day IM q12–24h	Same
Phenoxymethyl penicillin (V)	Beepen VK, Betapen VK, Caropen VK, Pen-Vee K, Pen V, V-Cillin K, Wincillin, Veetids, Lanacillin VK, Ledercillin VK, Robicillin VK, Suspen	250–500 mg PO q6h	25–50 mg/kg/day PO q6–8h	Same, minor gastrointestinal (diarrhea) side effects
Aminopenicillins				
Ampicillin	Omnipen Principen Totacillin	250–500 mg PO q6h	50 mg/kg/day PO q8h	Hypersensitivity reaction, rash, anaphylaxis, incidence of rash higher in patients with mononucleosis) diarrhea, local reactions, seizures associated with renal insufficiency. *C. difficile* colitis
Ampicillin sodium	Omnipen-N Polycillin-N Totacillin-N	1–2 g IM, IV q4–6h (up to 8 g/day)	100–200 mg/kg/day IM, IV q6h	Same
β-Lactam and β-Lactamase Inhibitors				
Amoxicillin + clavulanate	Augmentin	250/62.5–500/125 mg PO q8h (Amoxicillin/ clavulanate) 875/125 mg PO q12h 2000/125 mg PO q12h	4:1 formulation 30 mg (Amox)/ kg/day PO q12h 7:1 formulation 45 mg q12h (Amox)/kg/day PO 14:1 formulation 90 mg (Amox)/ kg/day PO div q12h	Same as amoxicillin
Ampicillin + sulbactam	Unasyn	1–2 g IV q6h (Ampicillin)	100–200 mg/kg/day IV*	Same as ampicillin
Piperacillin + tazobactam	Zosyn	3 g (Piperacillin) IV q6h	240 mg (Piperacillin)/kg/day IV*	Same as piperacillin
Ticarcillin + clavulanic acid	Timentin	3–6 g (Ticarcillin) IV q4–6h, up to 24 g/day	200–300 mg/kg/day q4–6h	Same as ticarcillin
Carbapenems				
Imipenem/cilastatin	Primaxin	0.25–1 g IV q6h	60–100 mg/kg/day IM, IV q6h	Phlebitis, allergy, vomiting, diarrhea, eosinophilia, seizures (with CNS disorders and renal failure), transitory hypotension, *C. difficile* colitis
Meropenem	Merrem	1 g IV q8h	60 mg/kg/day IV q8h	Diarrhea, headache, rash, nausea, anaphylaxis, seizures, colitis, thrombocytopenia
Ertapenem	Invanz	1 g IM, IV q24h	30 mg/kg/day divided q12h, max 1 g/day	Diarrhea, nausea, headache

*Not recommended for children in the United States.
[†]1 unit (U) = 0.6 µg.
C. difficile, Clostridium difficile; CNS, central nervous system; IM, intramuscular; IV, intravenous; qxh, every x hours.

membranes, contamination of a specimen with normal flora can give misleading results. Materials appropriate for anaerobic cultures should be obtained using a technique that bypasses the normal flora. Acceptable specimens are needle aspirates and surgical specimens.

Antimicrobials often fail to cure the infection. Among the reasons for this are the development of bacterial resistance, achievement of insufficient tissue levels, incompatible drug interactions, and the development of an abscess. The abscess environment is detrimental to many antibiotics. The abscess capsule interferes with the penetration of drugs, and the low pH and the presence of binding proteins or inactivating enzymes (i.e., β-lactamase) may impair their activity. The low pH and the anaerobic environment within the abscess are especially unfavorable for the aminoglycosides and quinolones. However, an acidic pH, high osmolarity, and an anaerobic environment can also develop in the absence of an abscess.

Communication and Counseling

Communication can assist in the prevention and lead to institution of early therapy of conditions that may lead to anaerobic infection. Preventing oral flora aspiration by improving the neurologic status of the patient, repeated suctioning of oral secretion, improving oral hygiene, and maintaining lower stomach pH can reduce the risk of aspiration pneumonia and its complications. Skin and soft tissue infections can be prevented by irrigation and debridement of wounds and necrotic tissue, drainage of pus, and improvement of blood supply.

SUGGESTED READINGS

1. Brook I: The role of beta-lactamase-producing bacteria in the persistence of streptococcal tonsillar infection. Rev Infect Dis 6:601–607, 1984. **Describes the in vitro, in vivo, and clinical evidence supporting the role of β-lactamase–producing bacteria in persistence of the infection.**
2. Brook I: Pediatric Anaerobic Infections. 3rd ed. New York: Marcel Dekker, 2002. **Systematic textbook of anaerobic infections in newborns and older children, providing guidelines for diagnosis and treatment.**
3. Brook I: Microbiology and management of intra-abdominal infections in children. Pediatr Int 45:123–129, 2003. **Overview of the pathophysiology, microbiology, and principles of management of intra-abdominal infections.**
4. Finegold SM: Anaerobic bacteria in human disease. Orlando, Fla: Academic Press, 1977. **Thorough review of all publications on all types of anaerobic infections up to the year of publication.**
5. Goldstein EJ: Possible role for the new fluoroquinolones (levofloxacin, grepafloxacin, trovafloxacin, clinafloxacin, sparfloxacin, and DU–6859a) in the treatment of anaerobic infections: Review of current information on efficacy and safety. Clin Infect Dis 23: S25-S30, 1996. **Evaluation of the current susceptibility of anaerobic bacteria to new fluoroquinolones.**
6. Hoellman DB, Kelly LM, Credito K, et al: In vitro antianaerobic activity of ertapenem (MK–0826) compared to seven other compounds. Antimicrob Agents Chemother 46:220–224, 2002. **Updated study that evaluates the current susceptibility of anaerobic bacteria to newer antimicrobials.**
7. Sutter VL, Finegold SM: Susceptibility of anaerobic bacteria to 23 antimicrobial agents. Antimicrob Agents Chemother 10:736–752, 1976. **In-depth analysis of the susceptibility of all types of anaerobic bacteria to the most useful antimicrobials.**

Health Care–Associated Infections

Philip L. Graham III

KEY CONCEPTS

- *Health care–associated infection* (HAI) has replaced the term *nosocomial infection* reflecting the changing patterns of health care delivery.
- Surveillance for HAIs is one of the primary tasks of the health care epidemiology team.
- The transmission of viral illnesses, such as respiratory syncytial virus (RSV) and rotavirus, is particularly important in pediatric populations.
- Control measures include isolation of infected, colonized, or incubating patients; surveillance cultures to identify other cases; and cohorting.
- The most important procedure to prevent HAIs is hand hygiene.
- Expanded precautions designed for specific pathogens are an important second-tier defense against transmission of HAI.

Expert Opinion on Management Issues

HEALTH CARE EPIDEMIOLOGY ROLE

Health care–associated infection (HAI) has replaced the term *nosocomial infection*, reflecting the changing patterns of health care, which include a greater emphasis on outpatient care, short-stay units, and semiacute health care settings such as long-term care facilities. The morbidity and mortality (at least 88,000 deaths per year in the United States) as well as the costs (more than $6 billion per year) of the 2 million HAIs per year in the United States are well described. The health care epidemiology team is charged with a broad variety of patient safety tasks, many relating to HAIs. These tasks may be broadly categorized into identification of infections, surveillance, epidemiologic investigations, prevention, reporting, communication, and education. There is significant overlap among these, and the role is often changing as new challenges emerge, such as the threat of bioterrorism and highly resistant organisms such as glycopeptide-resistant *Staphylococcus aureus* (GRSA).

Children's hospitals and pediatric wards in general hospitals face special challenges in the control of HAIs. Standardized surveillance systems for HAIs (e.g., the National Nosocomial Infections Surveillance [NNIS] system) exist, but these are primarily designed for adult populations. Pediatric populations are affected by different pathogens and have different sites of infection than adults. Visiting family members play more of a role in transmission of HAIs than they do in adult hospitals.

SURVEILLANCE AND BENCHMARKING

Surveillance for HAIs is one of the primary tasks of the health care epidemiology team. Specific examples include surveillance for catheter-related blood stream infections (BSIs) in specific hospital locations (e.g., intensive care units) or in specific risk groups (e.g., infants of very low birth weight), other device-associated infections, and infections or colonization with multidrug resistant (MDR) pathogens of interest, such as methicillin-resistant *S. aureus* (MRSA) and vancomycin-resistant *Enterococcus* (VRE) species. The transmission of viral illnesses, such as respiratory syncytial virus (RSV) and rotavirus, is particularly important in pediatric populations because these and other viruses account for approximately 20% of all pediatric HAIs. In addition, practitioners' use of broad-spectrum antimicrobials, such as vancomycin and the carbapenems, can be an important contributor to the burden of resistance in bacterial infections and should be tracked and controlled. Surveillance efforts require thoughtful planning as to risk-stratified denominator data (e.g.,

catheter-days, patient-days, or birth weights) and a comparative benchmark (e.g., institution-specific historical data or national norms from a system like NNIS). Every hospital requires an individualized targeted surveillance plan suited to its needs and to local and national regulatory requirements. To be effective, this plan must include feedback to bedside clinicians.

OUTBREAK INVESTIGATIONS

One of the more visible roles of the hospital epidemiology team is in outbreak or cluster investigations. An *outbreak* is often difficult to delineate; in general, the presence of a pathogen in a host population at a significantly greater rate than usually expected is a reasonable working definition. *Significantly greater* depends greatly on the specific health care setting. For example, a single case of health care–associated varicella zoster or tuberculosis on an oncology ward warrants an investigation, whereas catheter-related BSIs with a specific organism in a neonatal intensive care unit (NICU) need to be above a previously defined norm to demand the same type of reaction. Evolving technologies, such as computerized surveillance, will dramatically increase the number of clusters of HAIs identified.

The first stages of an outbreak investigation include establishing a case definition (Table 1) and creating an epidemic curve. Figures 1 and 2 show examples of such a graph and of the relationship between the rates of infection and colonization during an outbreak period of *S. aureus* in a NICU. After this information is collected, control measures are activated, such as isolation of infected, colonized, or incubating patients; surveillance cultures to identify other cases; and cohorting known and newly detected cases together by room or ward assignment and by dedicated health care teams if

TABLE 1 Case Definition
Who? Which patients are involved?   **What?** What is the pathogen or type of infection?   **When?** What period of time?   **Where?** Which unit or type of patient is involved?   **How?** How is transmission occurring?

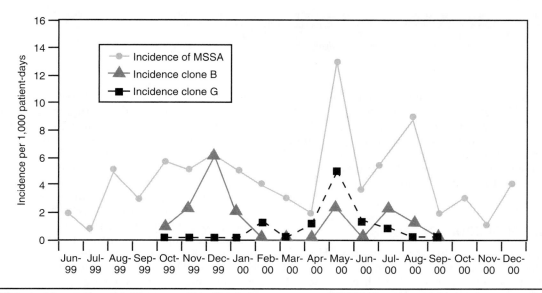

FIGURE 1. Incidence of methicillin-susceptible *Staphylococcus aureus* (MSSA) in a neonatal intensive care unit. Three periods of increased incidence of MSSA were observed, ranging from 6.4 to 13.5 cases of MSSA colonization/infection per 1000 patient-days. Two predominant clones were noted, clone "B" and clone "G," corresponding to the first two increased incidence periods.

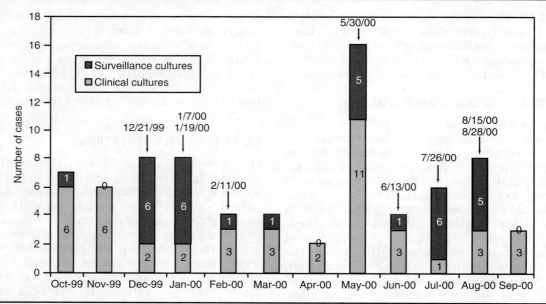

FIGURE 2. Clinical versus surveillance cultures. The distribution of clinical cultures versus surveillance cultures of the anterior nares for methicillin-susceptible *Staphylococcus aureus* (MSSA) during the study period is shown. The arrows show the dates of the surveillance efforts. The majority of cultures represent clinical cultures: 45 of 77 (58%).

TABLE 2 Extended Precautions*

Name of Expanded Precaution	Examples of Diseases	Personal Protective Equipment and/or Procedures Needed (All in Addition to Standard Precautions)
Contact	Draining skin infections; infection or colonization with MDR organisms such as MRSA and VRE, enteric pathogens in incontinent or diapered patients	Single room if available; gown, gloves, dedicated patient care equipment (e.g., thermometers and stethoscopes)
Droplet	Known or suspected *Neisseria meningitidis* disease; pertussis	Single room, mask (eye protection with face shield)
Airborne infection isolation	Tuberculosis	Single room with negative pressure, high-level respiratory protection (e.g., N95 mask)

*Patients should be placed on these precautions when they have suspected as well as proven disease. Some diagnoses such as severe acute respiratory syndrome (SARS) may require a combination of all three types of precautions. The primary method of decreasing/preventing HAIs remains Standard Precautions, including hand hygiene.

MDR, multidrug resistant; MRSA, methicillin-resistant *Staphylococcus aureus*; VRE, vancomycin-resistant *Enterococcus*.

feasible. Active surveillance must follow these control measures, and if they are not successful in stopping transmission, further interventions such as cultures of the environment and the staff must be performed. Molecular techniques, such as pulsed-field gel electrophoresis (PFGE), have significantly improved epidemiologists' ability to identify and control outbreaks and clusters.

POLICIES AND PROCEDURES

The most important procedure in preventing HAIs is enforcing specific precautions designed to prevent transmission of pathogens in the health care setting. The Healthcare Infection Control Practices Advisory Committee of the Centers for Disease Control and Prevention (HICPAC/CDC) has created evolving standards for prevention of HAIs. The 2004 version has finished the public comment stage at the time of this writing. Its draft form affirms a two-tiered approach, with Standard Precautions as the first tier or foundation for the prevention of transmission of infectious pathogens. Standard Precautions include hand hygiene, which is the single most effective tool for minimizing HAIs. Standard Precautions include use of personal protective equipment (PPE) for all contacts with blood, body fluids, nonintact skin, and mucous membranes. A proposed addition to Standard Precautions in this 2004 revision is "Respiratory Hygiene/Cough Etiquette." This includes education, signage, and source control measures (covering patients' mouths when coughing, surgical masks where appropriate, hand hygiene after contact with respiratory secretions, and spatial separation (>3 feet) of persons with respiratory infections in common waiting areas. The second tier of precautions is termed "Extended Precautions." The use of these is recommended when specific pathogens are known or suspected and includes "Contact Precautions," "Droplet Precautions," "Airborne Infection Isolation Precautions," and a "Protective Environment" for certain immunocompromised populations. Table 2 further describes contact, droplet, and airborne precautions. The most current recommendations may be found by accessing a link at the CDC website: http://www.cdc.gov/ncidod/hip

Common Pitfalls

The most common pitfalls in the identification and management of HAIs include failure to design and manage surveillance plans adequately, failure to identify and react quickly to outbreaks and emerging pathogens, and failure to implement and supervise a program of tiered infection control precautions.

Although the NNIS system is an excellent standard for many HAIs, it does not address health care–associated viral infections, nor has it tackled the difficult issue of quantifying the use of antimicrobials in pediatric populations. Pediatric hospitals or wards within hospitals must individualize such systems to their needs. At a minimum, the most prevalent HAIs in infants and children (i.e., catheter-related BSIs), must be tracked using specific denominators for catheter-days and birth weight. In addition, consideration should be given to examining rates of health care–associated viral infections (especially in high-risk areas such as oncology and transplant units) and MDR organisms.

Outbreaks are the most visible portion of the health care epidemiologist's job. Close attention to a well-run surveillance system and good communication with bedside clinicians and the microbiology laboratory is critical to identifying and controlling these potentially devastating events.

The tiered infection control system advocated by HICPAC/CDC serves as a general model from which individual units can create appropriate policies. The most common pitfall in the implementation of infection-control precautions is waiting for laboratory confirmation of a potentially transmissible pathogen prior to instituting precautions. Discontinuing infection-control precautions when a patient "rules-out" is significantly safer and less expensive than doing a postexposure investigation.

Communication and Counseling

Education and continuing education about hand hygiene and both Standard and Expanded Precautions are critical to ensure compliance of all health care and ancillary staff. Appropriate educational materials and clear signage in the health care setting are critical to these efforts. Communication among the key stakeholders in the patient-care process is necessary and desirable during outbreak situations and especially in the periods before, where prevention efforts can be best implemented. Key personnel from hospital epidemiology and infection control, infectious diseases, clinical microbiology laboratory, occupational health services, hospital administration, environmental services, safety departments, and bedside practitioners must have regular direct communication. One of the most effective tools in the prevention of HAIs is the practice where any member of the health care team is empowered to contact hospital epidemiology and infection control staff with concerns about practices or patterns that seem to need attention. No surveillance system, however enhanced, can replace real-time input from bedside caregivers.

SUGGESTED READINGS

1. Division of Healthcare Quality Promotion, CDC: National Nosocomial Infections Surveillance (NNIS) System Report, data summary from January 1992 through June 2003, issued August 2003. Am J Infect Control 31:481–498, 2003. **Update of surveillance from NNIS hospitals with explanations of how to apply NNIS procedures to individual institutions.**
2. Graham PL, Morel AS, Zhou J, et al: Epidemiology of methicillin-susceptible *Staphylococcus aureus* in the neonatal intensive care unit. Infect Control Hosp Epidemiol 23:677–682, 2002. **Examination of an outbreak of colonization and infection with a single clone of *Staphylococcus aureus* in a NICU with emphasis on methodology, including creating a case definition, infection control interventions, and molecular epidemiology using PFGE.**
3. Seigel J, Strausbaugh L, Jackson M, et al, for the Healthcare Infection Control Practices Advisory Committee CDC: DRAFT Guideline for Isolation Precautions; Preventing Transmission of Infectious Agents in Healthcare Settings. Accessed July 15, 2004, at http://www.cdc.gov/ncidod/hip/isoguide.htm. **Draft of update of HICPAC/CDC guidelines. This comprehensive discussion of the prevention of HAIs with emphasis on protective isolation is the gold standard for clinicians and health care epidemiologists.**

12

Infant Botulism

Sarah S. Long

KEY CONCEPTS

- Infant botulism occurs in infants when their gut may be transiently permissive to outgrowth of naturally acquired *Clostridium botulinum* spores.
- Infant botulism manifests as a neuroparalytic disease rather than as an infection.
- Infant botulism is the likely diagnosis in a child younger than 1 year who has constipation and then progressive symmetrical paralysis descending from muscles innervated by cranial nerves to those of the trunk and extremities.
- Bulbar paresis or palsy is essential to the clinical diagnosis of infant botulism.
- To manage cases of infant botulism optimally, BabyBIG should be acquired and administered urgently.

Infant botulism is a neuroparalytic disease that occurs in children younger than 1 year when seemingly natural events lead to acquisition of *Clostridium botulinum* spores, outgrowth of vegetative forms and production of neurotoxin in the intestine, and systemic absorption. The neurotoxin binds to peripheral cholinergic neurons, where it prevents release of acetylcholine. Progressive, descending symmetric flaccid paralysis ensues, initially involving muscles innervated by cranial nerves and then muscles of the trunk and limbs. It is not possible to have botulism without bulbar palsies. Preganglionic cholinergic synapses of the autonomic nervous system can also be affected, leading to dryness of eyes and mouth, fluctuating tachycardia and hypertension, flushing of the skin, and atony of the bowel and bladder. Clinical setting and manifestations of infant botulism are characteristic (Table 1), with variability only in rapidity of progression and degree of paralysis. Unless complications have occurred, the infant is afebrile. No signs of infection are apparent and laboratory tests are normal. Although a differential diagnosis should be considered, other possibilities fade when considering the rapid progression, absence of other neurologic signs, and presence of normal laboratory test results.

C. botulinum–produced neurotoxins type A and B are responsible for the vast majority of cases. Paralysis from types E and F, as well as disease caused by botulinal neurotoxins produced by other *Clostridium* species, are reported. Type A botulism is associated with consumption of spore-containing honey. Disease caused by neurotoxin type A and disease in formula-fed infants appears to be most severe. Sudden infant death is an occasional presentation.

TABLE 1 Typical Clinical Setting, Manifestations, and Diagnosis of Infant Botulism

Setting	Suburban/rural residence more than urban Soil disruption by construction Parents' work leading to daily contact with soil Infant usually is breast-fed Mean age onset in formula-fed infants: 7.6 wk Mean age onset in breast-fed infants: 13.8 wk
Symptoms (in order of progression)	Constipation Poor suck and feeble cry Loss of facial expression Ptosis Loss of head control Generalized weakness Gurgling (impaired swallowing) Choking (impaired gagging) Loss of extraocular movement Pupils midposition Decreased movement extremities against gravity
Differential diagnoses	Myasthenia gravis, Werdnig-Hoffmann disease, tick paralysis, brain stem encephalitis, drug ingestion or heavy metal poisoning, hypothyroidism
Laboratory diagnosis	Mouse lethality/neutralization test using sterile filtrate of stool (available at some state laboratories and at the Centers for Disease Control and Prevention)

Expert Opinion on Management Issues

ANTITOXIN AND ANTIBIOTIC THERAPY

BabyBIG, botulism immune globulin intravenous (human) (BIG-IV), should be administered urgently when infant botulism is diagnosed clinically. This purified immunoglobulin (Ig)G is derived from pooled plasma from persons immunized with pentavalent botulinum toxoid who were selected for their high titers of neutralizing antibody against botulinum neurotoxins A and B. Donors are screened for infectious diseases as is typical for blood donors. Additionally, the pooled plasma undergoes Cohn-Oncley fractionation, nanofiltration, and solvent/detergent treatment. In a double-blind, placebo-controlled study of BabyBIG conducted in California from 1992 to 1997, infants treated with BabyBIG within the first 3 days of hospital admission had significant reductions in mean length of hospitalization (2.6 weeks vs. 5.7 weeks), stay in intensive care (1.3 weeks vs. 3.6 weeks), mechanical ventilation (0.7 weeks vs. 2.4 weeks), and tube feeding (3.6 weeks vs. 10.0 weeks). Need for intubation was reduced two thirds. Adjusted to 2002 dollars, rounded mean hospital costs for placebo-treated patients was $151,000 versus $51,000 for those who received BabyBIG under protocol. In 2003, the U.S. Food and Drug Administration issued a license to the California Department of Health Services (CDHS) for BabyBIG. Release of BabyBIG still requires CDHS approval because supply is limited and it is a product of importance to national defense against bioterrorism. The CDHS Infant Botulism Program's telephone contact number is 510–231–7600 (24 hours a day). Additional information may be found online at www.infantbotulism.org. BabyBIG is distributed from a South California site; the January 2005 price was $45,300. The product is administered as a single dose intravenously.

Antibiotic therapy is indicated only to treat secondary bacterial infection. Clostridiacidal antibiotics show no apparent benefit or adverse effect on the course of paralysis, but in theory they could be detrimental if toxin is released during bacterial cell lysis prior to administration of BabyBIG. Aminoglycosidic agents are avoided because they contribute notably to neuromuscular blockade.

GENERAL SUPPORTIVE CARE

Almost all patients require observation under intensive care until nadir of neuromuscular function has passed. As paralysis progresses, upper airway occlusion, aspiration, or diaphragmatic paresis can occur suddenly. Many infants progress to require intubation (frequently with minimal ventilating support) prior to and for several days after administration of BabyBIG. Cardiac, respiratory, and oxygenation monitoring is essential. Appropriate positioning maximizes respiratory effort and ability to swallow secretions. The infant is placed supine on a flat surface with rostral elevation of the planar mattress at 30 degrees and with a thin roll to support normal curvature of the neck. The infant is repositioned from side to side periodically while supine. A cloth bumper placed below the buttocks prevents sliding and elevates the legs slightly to minimize venous pooling. Intubation should be performed preemptively when the ability to cough, gag, swallow, or move against gravity is impaired substantially. Careful attention to endotracheal tube size, technique of placement, air leak, and respiratory toilet prevents acquired subglottic stenosis and the need for tracheostomy. Extubation is appropriate when the infant has an adequate gag and swallow, normal respiratory function, and sustained movement of the extremities against gravity.

Enteral feedings are well absorbed and well tolerated because the paralytic effect apparently does not include the small bowel. Continuous small-volume nasoenteric feeding (with attention to residual volume) is begun within 48 hours of hospitalization, even in paralyzed infants, and is advanced over time to bolus feedings. Expressed human breast milk or formula is appropriate; the caloric need of the immobile ventilated infant is approximately two thirds that of healthy infants. Oral feedings are not resumed until swallowing function, protection of the airway, and sustained strength against gravity return and until bolus nasoenteral feedings are tolerated.

Weight, fluids, and electrolytes are monitored carefully through the nadir of motor function or to correct initial dehydration; the physician should observe for hyponatremia resulting from excessive secretion of antidiuretic hormone and other causes. Intravenous and urinary bladder catheterization is unnecessary and should be avoided because it carries risks of complications.

Constipation is a usual first symptom of infant botulism and can persist for months after hospital discharge. Cathartics, enemas, and enteral-activated charcoal intended to reduce the quantity of *C. botulinum* or toxin are ineffective. A softening agent, such as docusate (Colace), and glycerin suppositories can be helpful. Transient paralysis of the bladder is common. The Credé method for frequent emptying is effective and may reduce the risk of urinary tract infection.

Common Pitfalls

Apnea and aspiration are the major pitfalls in management, both of which should be avoidable by preemptive care as described earlier. Secondary infections are the most common complications. Increase in weakness after a period of stability or improvement can be the first indication of such an infection. Otitis media, sinusitis, pneumonia, and urinary tract infections are most common; targeted antibiotic therapy should be given only for specific indications. Unusually severe *C. difficile*–induced colitis and toxic megacolon complicating infant botulism are reported.

Profound hyponatremia with seizures can result from dehydration, from an antidiuretic hormone response to pneumonia or venous pooling, or from feeding of hyponatremic human milk (an occasional maternal response to stress). Monitoring of fluid intake and output and of serum electrolytes is required during the progression and at the height of disease.

Communication and Counseling

The prognosis for complete recovery from infant botulism is excellent. The severity and prolonged duration of the infant's impairment, however, pose challenges to the medical team, the family, and their interaction. Optimizing parents' participation in care of the infant affects this relationship positively.

Upon recovery, infants may be at heightened risk for strabismus. Observation and, when appropriate, intervention are required.

SUGGESTED READINGS

1. Arnon SS: Infant botulism. In Feigin RD, Cherry JD (eds): Textbook of Pediatric Infectious Diseases, 5th ed. Philadelphia: WB Saunders, 2004, pp 1758–1766. **Provides a detailed description of epidemiology, differential diagnosis, and management of infant botulism.**
2. Dworkin MS, Shoemaker PC, Anderson DE: Tick paralysis: 33 human cases in Washington state, 1946–1996. Clin Infect Dis 29:1435–1439, 1999. **Describes a case series of tick paralysis, a disorder mimicking botulism.**
3. Long SS: Epidemiologic study of infant botulism in Pennsylvania: Report of the infant botulism study group. Pediatrics 75:928–934, 1985. **Describes a case-control study by the striking geographic distribution of cases around but not in Philadelphia.**
4. Long SS: *Clostridium botulinum* (botulism). In Long SS, Pickering LK, Prober CP (eds): Principles and Practice of Pediatric Infectious Diseases, 2nd ed. New York: Churchill Livingstone, 2003, pp 984–991. **Provides a detailed description of epidemiology, differential diagnosis, and management of infant botulism.**
5. Long SS, Gajewski JL, Brown LW, et al: Clinical, laboratory, and environmental features of infant botulism in southeastern Pennsylvania. Pediatrics 75:935–941, 1985. **Delineates clinical manifestations, especially of cranial nerves and autonomic nervous system.**
6. Shapiro RL, Hatheway C, Swerdlow DL: Botulism in the United States: A clinical and epidemiologic review. Ann Int Med 129:221–228, 1998. **Summarizes types of botulism and sources of toxin, clinical manifestations, and management.**
7. Schechter R, Peterson B, McGee J, et al: *Clostridium difficile* colitis associated with infant botulism: Near-fatal case analogous to Hirschsprung's enterocolitis. Clin Infect Dis 29:367–374, 1999. **Describes a potentially life-threatening complication of hospitalization.**

12

Cat-Scratch Disease

Michael Giladi and Moshe Ephros

KEY CONCEPTS

- *Bartonella henselae* is the etiologic agent of cat-scratch disease (CSD).
- Ninety percent of patients present with regional lymphadenopathy (typical CSD); 10% have disease involving other organs, such as neuroretinitis and encephalitis (atypical CSD).

KEY CONCEPTS—cont'd

- In most CSD cases, whether typical or atypical, spontaneous resolution occurs in 2 to 4 months.
- Culture of lymph nodes or other tissues are rarely positive. Serology is the mainstay of diagnosis. Polymerase chain reaction (PCR) performed on lymph node tissue or pus is highly sensitive and specific.
- Data on the efficacy of antibiotic therapy in CSD are limited, and in mild to moderate cases antibiotics are not indicated. Azithromycin had a favorable effect in a small comparative study and may be considered in more severe cases of typical CSD.
- Doxycycline combined with rifampin may shorten the disease course of neuroretinitis. A similar regimen can be used for other serious manifestations (e.g., encephalitis and hepatosplenic CSD), although data to support this approach are lacking.
- Lymph node aspiration is indicated therapeutically when suppuration occurs.

Bartonella henselae is the major etiologic agent of cat-scratch disease (CSD). Apparently healthy domestic and stray cats bacteremic with *B. henselae* constitute the major reservoir of this pathogen. Other animals, particularly dogs, are implicated as possible reservoirs of *B. henselae,* but reports are anecdotal and evidence essentially circumstantial. History of close cat or, more commonly, kitten contact is reported in approximately 90% of CSD patients, but only half of these patients experience a scratch or bite. The exact mechanism of cat-to-human transmission of *B. henselae* is not clear. Cat-to-cat transmission by infected cat fleas does occur; however, evidence of cat-to-human transmission by fleas is lacking.

Typical CSD, which occurs in approximately 90% of cases, is characterized by subacute regional lymphadenopathy, mostly involving the head, neck, or upper extremities. Lymph nodes are usually tender, and in approximately 15%, suppuration occurs. Approximately one third to half of patients has fever. A cutaneous papule or pustule, often referred to as a primary or inoculation lesion, usually develops within 1 or 2 weeks at the site of a cat scratch or bite. Adenopathy develops 1 to 8 weeks later. The prolonged course of CSD lymphadenopathy, particularly when accompanied by fever, night sweats, weight loss, and liver or spleen involvement, may resemble lymphoma or other malignant processes, and consequently it can lead to unnecessary, extensive, costly, and sometimes invasive diagnostic procedures.

Atypical CSD occurs in approximately 10% of CSD patients and includes the Parinaud oculoglandular syndrome, neuroretinitis, encephalitis, isolated cranial and peripheral neuropathies (e.g., facial palsy), transverse myelitis, erythema nodosum, hepatic and splenic abscesses or granulomatous inflammation, fever of unknown origin, pneumonitis, pulmonary nodules, and musculoskeletal manifestations including osteomyelitis and arthropathy. In most cases, whether typical or atypical, spontaneous resolution occurs in 2 to 4 months, although a prolonged course lasting more than a year sometimes occurs. Although *B. henselae* endocarditis shares similar epidemiologic characteristics with CSD and may be regarded as another manifestation of atypical CSD, this interesting topic is not within our scope here.

Laboratory corroboration of the clinical diagnosis of CSD is sometimes difficult, and more than one technique is often needed to establish the diagnosis. Serology is the mainstay, and acute and convalescent sera are often required. Table 1 presents the methods used to confirm CSD diagnosis. These tests replace the skin test that was poorly standardized and carried a potential risk for transmission of infectious agents.

TABLE 1 Diagnosis of Cat-Scratch Disease

Test	Advantages	Disadvantages
Serology: immunofluorescence antibody test (IFAT)	Sensitivity of 84%–95% and specificity of 94%–98% when performed at CDC; does not require an invasive procedure.	Results are inconsistent and less satisfactory in studies performed in Europe, perhaps because of higher background seroprevalence; seroconversion may occur >3 wk after disease onset; most experience is with IgG and not IgM.
Serology: ELISA/enzyme immunoassay	Sensitivity of 85% with an outer membrane antigen-based EIA when IgG and/or IgM positive; specificity 98%; does not require an invasive procedure.	Seroconversion may occur >3 wk after disease onset; limited experience compared with IFAT; several different assays with variable sensitivity and specificity.
Histopathology of lymph nodes	Necrotizing granulomatous lymphadenitis is characteristic, although not specific.	Low sensitivity and specificity; requires an invasive procedure.
Warthin-Starry silver stain of affected lymph node	Can identify purported *Bartonella* spp. in tissue.	Low sensitivity, not specific; requires an invasive procedure.
Culture of pus or tissue aspirated from lymph nodes	High specificity.	Low sensitivity, isolation of *B. henselae* is very rare; requires an invasive procedure.
PCR of pus or tissue aspirated from lymph nodes	High sensitivity and specificity.	Available in referral laboratories; requires an invasive procedure.

CDC, Centers for Disease Control and Prevention; EIA, enzyme immunoassay; ELISA, enzyme-linked immunoabsorbent assay; Ig, immunoglobulin; PCR, polymerase chain reaction.

Expert Opinion on Management Issues

DRUG THERAPY

Antimicrobial susceptibility studies, using various methods, demonstrate that *B. henselae* is susceptible in vitro to most antibacterial agents, including penicillins, cephalosporins, tetracyclines, macrolides, aminoglycosides, fluoroquinolones, rifampin, chloramphenicol, and trimethoprim-sulfamethoxazole. Unfortunately, in vitro results do not necessarily predict the in vivo response to therapy. Treatment of immunocompetent patients with CSD with a variety of β-lactams (both penicillins and cephalosporins) appears largely ineffective. Several reasons may explain such a discrepancy between in vitro testing and clinical outcome:

- Regional lymphadenitis, the hallmark of typical CSD, may be caused by the host's immune response rather than because of a direct toxic effect by *B. henselae*. The failure to isolate *B. henselae* from lymph nodes in the presence of positive PCR for *B. henselae* DNA, except in very rare occurrences, suggests that in most cases there are no viable organisms at the time biopsy or aspirate is performed.
- Most antimicrobials studied show a lack of bactericidal effect, except gentamicin and perhaps rifampin.
- Human and cat studies show that *Bartonella* species may occupy particular niches in the host (e.g., sequestration in erythrocytes) that are protected from antimicrobials.

Antibiotic regimens for *Bartonella* infections are therefore determined empirically, based on published case reports, expert experience, and clinical studies that are mostly retrospective and with limited follow-up. There have been anecdotal reports of the utility of various antimicrobial agents in the treatment of CSD, and a large retrospective study found that patients treated with rifampin, ciprofloxacin, gentamicin, or trimethoprim-sulfamethoxazole had a shorter disease course compared with patients treated with other antibiotics or not treated at all. Most experts agree, however, that typical CSD does not respond to antibiotic therapy. Only azithromycin was evaluated in a small prospective, double-blind, placebo-controlled study of immunocompetent patients with typical CSD. An 80% decrease of initial lymph node volume, as determined using three-dimensional ultrasonography at entry and at weekly intervals, was documented in 7 of 14 azithromycin-treated patients compared with 1 of 15 placebo-treated controls during the first 30 days of observation ($P = .026$). After 30 days there was no significant difference in rate or degree of resolution between the two groups. There was no difference in any other clinical parameter between the two groups, and data regarding the role of azithromycin in preventing any of the atypical manifestations complicating CSD are lacking.

Because of the limited data on the role of azithromycin in treatment of CSD and the self-limited nature of this disease, supporting a universal recommendation to treat immunocompetent patients with typical CSD with azithromycin is difficult. Most experts would therefore agree not to give antimicrobials for mild and moderate cases of typical CSD, particularly if spontaneous improvement has begun. CSD is diagnosed in any patients 2 to 3 weeks or longer after disease onset when fever has resolved and the pain associated with lymphadenopathy is improving. There is no indication for antibiotic treatment in these patients. In more severe cases, such as when lymphadenopathy is large and painful, sometimes to the degree of severe limitation of the shoulder motion (in axillary lymphadenopathy) or difficulty walking (in inguinal lymphadenopathy), or when fever, malaise, and other systemic symptoms are significant and prolonged, azithromycin seems to be a reasonable choice (Table 2). Alternative regimens include doxycycline, with or without rifampin, or gentamicin.

In rare cases of *B. henselae* bacteremia associated with CSD in normal hosts, at least 4 weeks of therapy with either a macrolide or doxycycline is probably indicated. Treatment may be extended to 2 to 3 months if fever or bacteremia is persistent or recurrent. Aminoglycosides may also play a role in the treatment of *B. henselae* bacteremia.

Although corticosteroids are reported anecdotally to be administered to patients with CSD, apparently with some success, corticosteroids cannot be recommended for CSD because of lack of adequate data. Data are even less satisfactory regarding treatment of atypical CSD.

12

TABLE 2 **Treatment of Cat-Scratch Disease**

Disease	Suggested Antibiotic Treatment
Typical CSD	
Mild to moderate disease	Treatment not necessary.
Severe local disease (large, painful, prolonged, lymphadenitis) or significant systemic symptoms (fever, malaise)	Children: Oral azithromycin, 10 mg/kg on day 1, 5 mg/kg/day on days 2–5. Adults: Oral azithromycin, 500 mg on day 1, 250 mg/day on days 2–5.
Neuroretinitis*	Children: Oral doxycycline,† 1 mg/kg (max 100 mg) bid, and rifampin, 10–15 mg/kg/day in 1–2 doses (max 300 mg bid), for 4–6 wk. Adults: Oral doxycycline, 100 mg bid, and rifampin, 300 mg bid (or 600 qd), for 4–6 wk.
Encephalitis and other severe atypical manifestations	See text.

*One study supports treatment of neuroretinitis in adults. Treatment of encephalitis seems reasonable assuming similar pathogenesis.

†CSD-associated neuroretinitis is rare in children; data on treatment in children ≤8 years of age are lacking. See text.

bid, twice daily; qd, daily.

The Parinaud oculoglandular syndrome is, in fact, preauricular regional lymphadenopathy with granulomatous conjunctivitis and may be treated with antimicrobials using the same severity-related approach as with typical CSD. The role of antimicrobial therapy for CSD-associated neuroretinitis is controversial. In one study, comparing seven adult patients with CSD with neuroretinitis to historic controls, treatment with doxycycline and rifampin shortened the disease course and hastened visual recovery. In another study, final visual acuity was similar in 10 patients who were treated with various oral and parenteral antibiotics, sometimes in conjunction with steroids, and in 13 untreated patients. Despite the limited data, it is difficult to withhold treatment in the presence of retinal involvement, which is often associated with a significant visual disturbance. The demonstration of *B. henselae* bacteremia in a small number of patients with neuroretinitis adds weight to the argument for antimicrobial intervention. We usually begin treatment with doxycycline and rifampin, based on history of cat contact and clinical manifestations suggestive of CSD neuroretinitis, even before laboratory confirmation of CSD. In untreated patients we see for the first time at a later stage of neuroretinitis, when spontaneous improvement is noticed, as often occurs when the ophthalmologist waits for serologic confirmation, we usually withhold treatment. Data regarding treatment of children younger than 8 years are lacking; however, azithromycin or clarithromycin with or without rifampin seems to be a reasonable substitution when a prolonged course of a tetracycline is contraindicated. Steroids have been used as an adjunct to antibiotics in treating the ocular manifestations of CSD. However, comparative studies are needed before recommendations regarding steroid use in CSD neuroretinitis can be made.

No evidence supports the use of antibiotic therapy in CSD encephalopathy. However, both the severity of this complication and the assumption that encephalopathy may share a similar pathogenesis with neuroretinitis for which antibiotics may be beneficial support treating CSD encephalitis with antibiotics. Intravenous doxycycline with or without rifampin seems to be a reasonable choice. Corticosteroids are shown anecdotally to improve clinical manifestations of encephalitis, but in the absence of controlled studies the role of steroids in CSD encephalopathy is difficult to evaluate. There are no studies to support recommendations for other, often severe, atypical CSD manifestations, such as osteomyelitis, hepatic or splenic abscess, or granulomatous hepatitis; using the same antibiotic regimens as for other severe CSD manifestations is a reasonable option, however.

OTHER MEASURES

Analgesics or nonsteroidal anti-inflammatory drugs can be used to control pain associated with lymphadenopathy, and local warm compresses are reported by patients to diminish discomfort. Aspiration is indicated in patients with suppuration of the affected lymph node or nodes, diagnosed either clinically or with the aid of ultrasonography. A 16- to 18-gauge needle is used to puncture the skin overlying the suppuration. Local anesthetic is usually not necessary in adolescents and adults; however, children may benefit from the use of local anesthetic creams (e.g., EMLA 5% [lidocaine/prilocaine]) and even midazolam. Relief of pain usually occurs following the aspiration of pus. Pus is odorless and thick, with a beige-yellowish color and sometimes blood tinged, and it should be sent for bacterial and mycobacterial stains and cultures, cytology, and, if available, for *B. henselae* polymerase chain reaction (PCR). Culture of *B. henselae* may be attempted in reference laboratories. Surgical excision or removal of involved lymph nodes for treatment purposes should be discouraged to avoid sinus formation and chronic drainage.

WHEN TO PERFORM LYMPH NODE BIOPSY

Lymph node biopsy is justified when the diagnosis is in doubt and malignancy has to be ruled out. Such clinical circumstances may occur when acute and convalescent sera are tested negative for anti–*B. henselae* antibodies more than 4 weeks after onset of lymphadenopathy (as occur in 10% to 20% of CSD patients) without spontaneous regression in lymph node size and particularly when fever, night sweats, or weight loss accompany lymphadenopathy. In cases in which CSD is likely (history of a recent cat scratch, presence of a primary lesion, regional tender lymphadenitis following an acute flu-like illness), a fine-needle aspiration may be adequate. The presence of inflammatory cells or granulomas is reassuring, and PCR performed on the aspirated material can identify *B. henselae* DNA and confirm the diagnosis of CSD. When clinical and epidemiologic data are less supportive of the diagnosis of CSD, lymph node biopsy rather than fine-needle aspiration is preferred. In *B. henselae*–seronegative patients with severe complications, such as neuroretinitis, early lymph node biopsy with PCR testing is often recommended because rapid diagnosis facilitates the initiation of early antibiotic therapy.

Common Pitfalls

- Inquiring about a cat scratch or a cat bite rather than cat contact may lead to the erroneous dismissal of CSD diagnosis. A significant proportion of CSD patients report cat contact without injury. This may be particularly true with head and neck lymphadenopathy, which is often associated with hugging and kissing a cat.
- One must keep an open mind to the possibility of transmission of *B. henselae* from other animals such as dogs.
- In young children (<2 years of age), chronic or subacute head and neck lymphadenitis is most often caused by nontuberculous mycobacteria. When epidemiology is appropriate, *Myobacterium tuberculosis* must also be considered.
- To rule out malignancy, patients with regional lymphadenopathy often undergo unnecessary

extensive, costly, and sometimes invasive diagnostic procedures, even when malignancy is unlikely, when nodes are painful, sometimes floridly inflamed, and even suppurative.

■ Serology, the most commonly used diagnostic method, may be negative during the first 2 to 3 weeks of disease and sometimes even longer. Approximately 10% to 20% of patients with CSD remain seronegative even when tested later.

■ Avoid referring patients with CSD with suppurative lymph nodes to surgeons who tend to incise and drain nodes instead of aspirate them with a needle. Incision may lead to chronic draining sinuses.

Communication and Counseling

CSD is usually a self-limited disease with a good prognosis. When the diagnosis is confirmed, patients and their parents should be reassured there is no need for further diagnostic evaluation.

What to Do with the Cat

Removal of the cat from the home or the immediate environment is usually not necessary when one acquires CSD. The infected individual is considered to be protected from reinfection, and infection of another family member by the same cat is unusual because transmission of *B. henselae* from cats to humans is inefficient. Thus outbreaks are rare in households. Exceptions include two groups of patients: those with a predisposition to endocarditis (e.g., those with valvular disease), who are at risk of acquiring *Bartonella* endocarditis, and immunocompromised patients, particularly human immunodeficiency virus (HIV)-infected persons, who may acquire *B. henselae*–related and potentially life-threatening infections, such as bacillary angiomatosis, peliosis, or bacteremia. These patients should be advised to avoid cat contact, particularly when another family member has had CSD, because the cat suspected of being the source of *B. henselae* is presumably bacteremic with *B. henselae* and therefore infectious. Control of flea infestation in cats may interrupt cat-to-cat and theoretically cat-to-human transmission of *B. henselae*.

SUGGESTED READINGS

1. Anderson BE, Neuman MA: *Bartonella* spp. as emerging human pathogens. Clin Microbiol Rev 10:203–219, 1997. **A comprehensive review of the microbiologic and clinical aspects of Bartonella species, including B. henselae.**
2. Bass JW, Freitas BC, Freitas AD, et al: Prospective randomized double blind placebo-controlled evaluation of azithromycin for treatment of cat-scratch disease. Pediatr Infect Dis J 17:447–452, 1998. **Although limited by small number of patients enrolled, this is the only prospective, comparative, placebo-controlled study of antibiotic treatment for CSD.**
3. Bass JW, Vincent JM, Person DA: The expanding spectrum of *Bartonella* infections: II. Cat-scratch disease. Pediatr Infect Dis J 16:163–179, 1997. **A comprehensive review of cat-scratch disease.**
4. Reed JB, Scales DK, Wong MT, et al: *Bartonella henselae* neuroretinitis in cat scratch disease. Diagnosis, management, and sequelae. Ophthalmology 105:459–466, 1998. **This retrospective analysis demonstrates a possible benefit of antibiotics in the treatment of CSD-associated neuroretinitis.**
5. Rolain JM, Brouqui P, Koehler JE, et al: Recommendations for treatment of human infections caused by *Bartonella* species. Antimicrob Agents Chemother 48:1921–1933, 2004. **Comprehensive and up-to-date review of treatment options and recommendations according to the ranking system of the Infectious Disease Society of America practice guidelines.**

Diphtheria

Barbara W. Stechenberg

KEY CONCEPTS

■ Diphtheria should be considered in patients with appropriate epidemiologic contact, especially with evidence of adherent membrane formation (that bleeds on scraping) in the respiratory tract.

■ Disease is most severe in unimmunized persons. It may be mild or asymptomatic in partially or fully immunized persons.

■ Diagnosis of diphtheria should be based initially on clinical findings because delay in therapy may be associated with serious complications.

■ Accurate diagnosis requires isolation of the organism. The laboratory must be alerted so appropriate culture media are inoculated. Material from beneath the membrane and/or a portion of the membrane should be obtained for culture. Presumptive diagnosis can be made by identifying gram-positive rods in a Chinese character distribution on Gram stain.

■ Suspected cases should be reported immediately to local and state public health authorities. Recovered diphtheria bacilli should be tested for toxigenicity by a recommended laboratory.

Diphtheria is an acute infectious disease caused by toxigenic strains of *Corynebacterium diphtheriae* and, less commonly, *Corynebacterium ulcerans*. Symptomatic diphtherial infection is caused by local noninvasive inflammation of the respiratory tract or skin and by local and systemic effects from the potent exotoxin. Any part of the respiratory tract may be affected, with tonsillar or pharyngeal involvement accounting for two thirds of cases. Onset is usually insidious, associated with low-grade fever, malaise, and sore throat. Table 1 presents specific clinical presentations. Box 1 shows complications.

Humans are the only reservoir for the organism, which is spread by close contact with infectious material, either directly or via droplets. Asymptomatic carriers may transmit the organism. Diphtheria, distributed worldwide, is endemic in many developing countries, including Turkey, Bangladesh, India, and areas of Africa, Asia, South America, and the Caribbean, particularly Haiti and the Dominican Republic.

TABLE 1　Clinical Manifestations of Diphtheria

Tonsillopharyngeal	Mild erythema progresses to white patches, then to adherent pseudomembrane.
Nasal	Usually mild with development of serosanguineous or seropurulent nasal discharge.
Laryngeal	Hoarseness and cough may occur alone or with other respiratory tract involvement.
Tracheobronchial	Usually results from downward spread and may cause additional respiratory compromise.
Cutaneous	Primary chronic, nonhealing ulcers with a dirty gray membrane or colonization of preexisting dermatoses.

TABLE 2　Antitoxin Treatment

- Obtain antitoxin from the National Immunization Program of the Centers for Disease Control and Prevention (CDC).
- Test for sensitivity to horse serum.
- Desensitize if necessary.
- Determine dose by site and size of membrane, duration of illness, and degree of toxic effects.

Laryngeal or pharyngeal involvement of ≤48 h	20,000–40,000 U
Nasopharyngeal lesions	40,000–60,000 U
Extensive disease of ≥3 days or diffuse swelling of neck	80,000–120,000 U
Cutaneous diphtheria	120,000–140,000 U

BOX 1　Complications of Diphtheria

- Respiratory compromise
- Systemic toxicity: risk usually proportional to severity of local lesions
  - Cardiac
    - Electrocardiographic changes
    - Myocarditis
  - Neurologic
    - Local neuropathies
    - Cranial nerve neuropathies
  - Peripheral neuritis

A large outbreak of more than 150,000 cases occurred in the 1990s in the newly independent states of the former Soviet Union.

In the prevaccine era, children were at highest risk, but today diphtheria primarily affects adolescents and adults. Diphtheria is prevented on a community-wide basis by universal active immunization. Primary immunization for children younger than 7 years consists of a combination of diphtheria toxoid with tetanus toxoid and pertussis antigen. Continuing immunity requires regular booster injections of diphtheria toxoid (with tetanus toxoid) every 10 years.

Expert Opinion on Management Issues

The outcome in patients with diphtheria depends on prompt initiation of therapy. Treatment combines administration of antitoxin with antibiotic therapy. Diphtheria antitoxin is a hyperimmune equine antiserum. It only binds and inactivates free toxin before it enters the cells, so it must be given early as a single rapid intravenous dose. Because the condition of a patient with diphtheria may deteriorate quickly, the antitoxin should be given based on the clinical diagnosis even before culture or toxigenicity results are available. Consultation with experts at the Centers for Disease Control and Prevention (CDC) is imperative to discuss diagnosis and treatment and to obtain antitoxin. The dose of antitoxin is determined empirically by considering the size and site of the diphtheria membrane, the duration of illness, and the degree of toxic effects. Soft diffuse cervical lymphadenitis (so-called bull neck) suggests moderate to severe involvement. Table 2 lists the dose ranges for antitoxin. There is an approximately 10% risk of hypersensitivity and/or serum sickness. Before administration antitoxin, tests for sensitivity to horse serum should be performed with a scratch test of a 1:1000 dilution of antitoxin in saline solution. If the patient is found to be sensitive to the equine serum, desensitization with slowly advancing doses, preferably by the intravenous route, are necessary before proceeding with the full intravenous dose.

Antibiotics are not a substitute for treatment with antitoxin, although antibiotic therapy kills the organism, which slows the spread of local infection and prevents transmission. Penicillin and erythromycin are effective therapy against most strains of *C. diphtheriae*. They also are effective in eradicating group A streptococci, which may be present in up to 30% of cases. Penicillin may be given as aqueous penicillin G, at 100,000 to 150,000 U/kg/day in four divided doses intravenously, or as procaine penicillin, 25,000 to 50,000 U/kg/day (maximum 1.2 million U) in two divided doses intramuscularly. Treatment is continued for 14 days. When the patient can tolerate oral medications, penicillin V, 125 to 250 mg four times a day, may be used to complete the course. Erythromycin, 40 mg/kg/day (maximum 2 g per day) in four divided doses for 14 days, is an acceptable alternative. Some erythromycin resistance is documented, but it is uncommon and its epidemiologic significance unknown. End point of therapy is documentation of two negative cultures at least 24 hours apart after completion of therapy.

Supportive measures include serial electrocardiographic monitoring and careful airway management. Isolation should consist of standard and droplet precautions until two cultures are negative for *C. diphtheriae*. Patients with diphtheria should be immunized during convalescence because infection may not confer immunity.

Management of contacts is very important and requires coordination with local public health authorities. Close contacts should be identified promptly. All close contacts, regardless of immunization status, should be observed closely for 7 days for evidence of disease; cultured for *C. diphtheriae,* and started on antimicrobial prophylaxis with oral erythromycin, 40 to 50 mg/kg/day for 7 days, or a single intramuscular injection of benzathine penicillin G (600,000 U for those <30 kg and 1.2 million U for those weighing >30 kg). Follow-up cultures should be obtained from contacts found to be carriers at a minimum of 2 weeks after therapy completion. Immunization status should be assessed, and those with incomplete immunizations should receive appropriate vaccine. For those previously immunized who have not received a booster within the last 5 years, a booster dose should be given.

Common Pitfalls

- It is important to recognize the signs and symptoms of diphtheria in a patient with potential exposure, particularly those in contact with communities where diphtheria is endemic.
- Early involvement of public health authorities for contact evaluation and acquisition of antitoxin is critical to prevent morbidity in the patient and to prevent spread among contacts.
- Failure to maintain immunization rates at more than 80% is a potential pitfall. Preparations with both diphtheria and tetanus toxoids for wound management should be used as appropriate for age to help ensure diphtheria immunity. Regular 10-year boosters for adolescents and adults should be encouraged.
- Travelers to countries with endemic or epidemic diphtheria should have their diphtheria immunization status reviewed and updated as necessary.

Communication and Counseling

Parents need to be educated about the importance of diphtheria immunization to prevent the disease. The safety and efficacy of the vaccine must be emphasized. If a case of diphtheria is suspected, parents need to understand the importance of swift action to decrease morbidity and mortality and to identify contacts to limit spread.

SUGGESTED READINGS

1. American Academy of Pediatrics: Antibiotics of Animal Origin (Animal Antiserum). Pickering L (ed): Red Book: 2003 Report of the Committee on Infectious Disease, 26th ed. Elk Grove Village, Ill: American Academy of Pediatrics, 2003, pp 60–63. **Includes protocol for sensitivity and desensitization testing.**
2. American Academy of Pediatrics: Diphtheria. Pickering L (ed): Red Book: 2003 Report of the Committee on Infectious Disease, 26th ed. Elk Grove Village, Ill: American Academy of Pediatrics, 2003, pp 263–266. **AAP guidelines for diphtheria diagnosis and treatment.**
3. Bisgard KM, Hardy IR, Popovic T, et al: Respiratory diphtheria in the United States, 1980 through 1995. Am J Public Health 88:787–791, 1998. **Describes epidemiologic, laboratory, and clinical features of diphtheria cases over a 15-year period in the United States.**
4. Farizo KM, Strebel PM, Chen RT, et al: Fatal respiratory disease due to *C. diphtheriae*: Case report and review of guidelines for management, investigation, and control. Clin Infect Dis 16:59–68, 1993. **Guidelines for contact evaluation and management.**
5. Galaska A: The changing epidemiology of diphtheria in the vaccine era. J Infect Dis 1815:52–59, 2000. **Describes the resurgence of diphtheria, socioeconomic factors, and the shift in age.**
6. Kadirova R, Kartoglu HU, Strebel PM: Clinical characteristics and management of 676 hospitalized diphtheria cases, Kyrgyz Republic, 1995. J Infect Dis 181(Suppl.):S110–S115, 2000. **Describes large group of hospitalized patients with diphtheria, their presentation and complications.**
7. Kheen R, Phan NG, Solomon T, et al: Penicillin vs. erythromycin in the treatment of diphtheria. Clin Infect Dis 27:845–850, 1998. **Open-label randomized trial in Vietnamese children with diphtheria showed a shorter duration of fever with penicillin.**
8. Mattos-Giaraldi AL, Moreira LO, Damasco PV, et al: Diphtheria remains a threat to health in the developing world—an overview. Mem Inst Oswaldo Cruz 98:987–993, 2003. **Discusses the waning of immunity to diphtheria and endemicity in large areas of the world.**

Gonococcal Infections

Kenneth Bromberg

KEY CONCEPTS

- Gonorrhea can be a perinatally acquired infection that manifests as ophthalmia neonatorum, scalp abscess, or disseminated infection.
- Gonorrhea manifests differently in prepubescent children. Boys may have a swollen penis, and girls may have vaginitis rather than cervicitis.
- Gonococcal infections in postpubertal patients are similar in presentation to adults.
- Gonococcal infections are associated with sexual abuse in individuals who are not sexually active.

Gonorrhea (the term used for infections caused by *Neisseria gonorrhoeae)* can be a perinatally acquired infection manifested as conjunctivitis (ophthalmia neonatorum). Maternal infection during pregnancy can result in prematurity and fetal demise. In the United States, perinatally acquired gonorrhea is an uncommon infection because of the identification and treatment of infected mothers before delivery and the use of ocular prophylaxis (silver nitrate, tetracycline, or erythromycin). However, when prenatal care does not occur, prenatally acquired gonorrhea is more common. Ophthalmia neonatorum associated with gonorrhea is less frequent than ophthalmia caused by *Chlamydia,* but it is a much more serious infection and associated with systemic spread and perforation of the globe.

Infection can also be secondary to fetal monitoring (scalp abscess). Mucosal surfaces, such as the nasopharynx, the rectum, the vagina, and the urethra, can also be infected. Dissemination from any of these sites can occur with spread, via the blood, to joints or the central nervous system (in newborns). Outside of the neonatal period, spread can manifest as a perihepatitis

TABLE 1 Uncomplicated Gonorrhea Infection beyond the Neonatal Period in Prepubertal Children Who Weigh Less than 45 kg

Name	Dosage/Route/Regimen	Maximum Dose	Dose Route	Common Adverse Reactions	Comments
Ceftriaxone	125 mg once	125 mg	IM	Pain at injection site	
Spectinomycin	40 mg/kg	2 g	IM	Pain at injection site	May not eliminate nasopharyngeal infection

IM, intramuscular.

TABLE 2 Uncomplicated Gonorrhea Infection (Cervix, Urethra, and Rectum) in Children and Adolescents Who Weigh More than 45 kg

Name	Dosage/Route/Regimen	Maximum Dose	Dose Route	Common Adverse Reactions	Therapeutic Considerations	Comments
Ceftriaxone	125 mg IM once	125 mg	IM	Pain at injection site		
Cefixime	400 mg PO once	400 mg	Oral suspension 100 mg/5 mL or 400-mg tablets (not currently available)	None with single dose		
Quinolones						
Ciprofloxacin	500 mg PO once			None with single dose	Resistance from certain geographic areas currently rules against this class of antibiotics.	Quinolones are not currently indicated in children <18 years of age but can be used when other options are not available.
Ofloxacin	400 mg once					
Levofloxacin	250 mg once					

IM, intramuscular; PO, by mouth.

(Fitz-Hugh–Curtis syndrome), presumably from the cervix via the peritoneal space.

Gonorrhea in prepubescent children manifests differently than in those who are sexually mature. Gonococcal infection in children outside the neonatal period implies sexual abuse. In prepubescent girls, vaginitis is the most common sign, as opposed to cervicitis, which occurs after puberty in girls and women. Boys can have a swollen penis. In boys after puberty, dysuria associated with a urethral discharge is the typical symptom. Infection in females may be asymptomatic.

The gonorrhea attack rate is highest in women between 15 and 19 years of age and in men between 20 and 24 years of age. Rates in African Americans are 30 times higher than those in whites and 11 times higher than rates in Hispanics. Incarcerated youth tend to have higher rates of sexually transmitted infection (STI), including gonorrhea, than the general population.

Expert Opinion on Management Issues

Diagnosis is critical in the management of gonococcal infections. Outside of the neonatal period, diagnosis has medicolegal implications. In prepubertal patients, specimens should be obtained from the site of suspected infection (eye in ophthalmia, vaginal discharge in vaginitis). Outside the newborn period, abuse should be suspected and additional samples obtained from the pharynx, genitals (vagina in girls and urethral discharge in boys who have evidence of urethritis or from a urethral swab if no discharge exists), and rectum (rectal specimen without obvious fecal contamination).

Gram stain of an infected site with a visible discharge or a normally sterile site may be of value in the initial diagnosis. For example, gram-negative diplococci of the appropriate morphology are an adequate basis for beginning therapy for gonococcal ophthalmia neonatorum. Therapy for gonococcal ophthalmia is ceftriaxone, 25 to 50 mg/kg intravenously (IV) or intramuscularly (IM) in a single dose, not to exceed 125 mg. The adult dose is 1 g IM in a single dose. Treatments are listed in Tables 1, 2, and 3.

Common Pitfalls

It is crucial to inoculate the specimen directly onto selective media to prevent drying and to provide carbon

TABLE 3 Therapy for Complicated Gonococcal Infections: Disseminated Gonococcal Infection (DGI)

Name	Dosage/Route/ Regimen	Maximum Dose	Dose Route	Common Adverse Reactions	Therapeutic Considerations	Comments
Ceftriaxone	50 mg/kg/day	1 g <45 kg 2 g >45 kg	IM	Biliary sludge with long-term use	7 days for arthritis or bacteremia; 10–14 days for meningitis or endocarditis	Consultation with an infectious diseases expert is usually indicated in cases of meningitis or endocarditis.

IM, intramuscular.

dioxide (CO_2) in the form of a candle jar or other CO_2-generating system. These systems may require incubation for the generation of CO_2. Direct inoculation is preferred over any system involving transport. Isolation from nonsterile sites should be on selective media such as modified Thayer-Martin agar to inhibit other flora. Some gonococci currently are resistant to antibiotics in the selective media (vancomycin), so the maximal isolation of organisms requires both a selective and nonselective plate. However, such an approach is not practical. Sterile sites such as cerebrospinal fluid and joints do not require selective media; chocolate media is the ideal choice.

Although newer methods involving amplified DNA detection (nucleic acid amplification test) are used for the diagnosis of gonococcal infections, standard culture done correctly is as sensitive as these newer tests. In addition, because of the medicolegal aspects of a diagnosis of gonococcal infection (child abuse), culture represents the gold standard regarding specificity. A test other than culture is not approved for diagnosis in children, so only culture should be used in children. These tests may be used in sexually active adolescents. A discussion of the fine line between sexual abuse and sexual activity in minors is beyond the scope of this article.

In addition, gonococcal isolates (from the child and any other associated isolates from suspected abusers) should be preserved by freezing at −94°F (−70°C) for possible further evaluation. Before preservation, all isolates should be confirmed by tests involving two different principles (biochemical, enzyme substrate, DNA detection, or serologic). Gonococci tend to self-destruct (autolyse) beyond 48 hours of growth, so they must be harvested for confirmation and storage while they are still viable.

One STI is often associated with others. If chlamydial infection cannot be ruled out, therapy is indicated in most instances of infection with the gonococcus.

Gonococci are occasionally confused with meningococci, both of which can cause septic arthritis or tenosynovitis with skin manifestations (without arthritis). These are both referred to as DGI (disseminated gonococcal infection) when caused by the gonococcus. Skin lesions might not yield the organism by bacterial culture.

Gonococcal endocarditis is now rare and may manifest with aspects of DGI (as described). Chronic infection with terminal complement deficiency may be associated with endocarditis, perhaps because of the persistence of bacteremia.

Conjunctivitis related to sexual activity can be caused by the gonococcus, although a less severe form is associated with the meningococcus, both of which look similar on Gram stain and can be confused in a microbiology laboratory. Both should be treated immediately with ceftriaxone to prevent destruction of the globe.

Communication and Counseling

The identification of an STI in a sexually active adolescent should trigger appropriate education about human immunodeficiency virus (HIV) infection and testing. The identification of gonococcal infection in the newborn period also identifies a mother at risk.

Treatment of DGI is usually successful, but repeated infections strongly suggest underlying immunodeficiency (terminal complement deficiency). Pelvic inflammatory disease is associated with a decreased rate of fertility.

SUGGESTED READINGS

1. Centers for Disease Control and Prevention: Sexually transmitted diseases treatment guidelines 2002. MMWR Recomm Rep 51 (RR–6):36–42, 2002. **Latest sexually transmitted diseases (STDs) guidelines. Check online at http://www.cdc.gov/ mmwr/preview/mmwrhtml/rr5106a1.htm for updates.**
2. Committee on Infectious Diseases, American Academy of Pediatrics (AAP): Gonococcal infections. In Pickering LK (ed): 2003 Red Book: Report of the Committee on Infectious Diseases, 26th ed. Elk Grove Village, Ill: American Academy of Pediatrics, 2003. **Latest AAP recommendations.**
3. Iverson CJ, Wang SA, Lee MV, et al: Fluoroquinolone resistance among *Neisseria gonorrhoeae* isolates in Hawaii, 1990–2000: Role of foreign importation and increasing endemic spread. Sex Transm Dis 31:702–708, 2004. **Typical report of growing bacterial resistance.**
4. Rawstron SA, Bromberg K, Hammerschlag MR: STD in children: Syphilis and gonorrhea. Genitourin Med 69:66–75, 1993. **A good overview about STDs as they relate to children.**
5. Robertson AA, Thomas CB, St. Lawrence JS, Pack R: Predictors of infection with *Chlamydia* or gonorrhea in incarcerated adolescents. Sex Transm Dis 32:115–122, 2005. **Discusses STD issues in high-risk pediatric populations: incarcerated adolescents.**

12

Leprosy (Hansen Disease)

Roland V. Cellona, Robert H. Gelber, and Ma. Victoria F. Balagon

KEY CONCEPTS

- The worldwide annual incidence of new leprosy cases remains relatively stable at 700,000, which almost entirely originate from the developing world.
- Morbidity and social stigma are largely a consequence of the unique tropism of the disease. Among all bacteria, *Mycobacterium leprae* invades and causes pathology in peripheral nerves, resulting in disabilities and/or deformities.
- Leprosy presents a clinical spectrum of varied clinical signs and symptoms, pathology, infectivity, and reactional states, and it dictates optimal therapeutic regimens.
- Immunologically mediated reactional states frequently complicate the course of the disease and require specific therapeutic intervention.
- Early diagnosis and the institution of effective therapy prevent deformity, and most patients can proceed with their lives uninterrupted.
- Psychosocial counseling, a culturally sensitive issue in many countries, and the care of any resulting deformities or disabilities are crucially important.

Leprosy (Hansen disease) is a chronic, immunologically mediated infectious disease caused by *Mycobacterium leprae*. The causative organism is an obligate intracellular bacillus, morphologically indistinguishable from other acid-fast bacilli, and it does not grow on artificial media. Clinical manifestations mainly affect the skin and peripheral nerves, but the route of transmission remains unclear. Although transmission is generally believed to be by nasal droplets spread from person to person, other sources, such as from infected soil or from insect vectors, are possible. Leprosy is not highly contagious and generally requires close, prolonged, often household contact with a patient with high bacterial load. Most individuals are naturally immune, and infection does not generally progress to actual disease. Medical personnel working with patients are not at risk, and nosocomial transmission does not occur.

The mean age of onset of clinical leprosy is in the second decade. It affects all age groups but is uncommon in infancy. However, children infected in infancy have a greater risk of progression to disease. Clinical leprosy is more common in males than in females in a ratio of 2:1. The incubation period, although usually 2 to 5 years, can be more than 30 years from infection.

The disease presents a spectrum of clinical, pathologic, immunologic, and bacteriologic types ranging from mild to severe. The particular type of disease encountered in individual patients determines prognosis, reactional states, and the intensity of antimicrobial therapy required. At the milder tuberculoid pole of the spectrum of leprosy, patients have one or few hypopigmented, anesthetic, well-marginated macules and, if present, asymmetrical neuropathy involving one or a few nerve trunks. In this type of the disease, cell-mediated immunity is intact, few bacilli are present, and reversal reactions (RRs) but not erythema nodosum leprosum (ENL) can occur. On the other pole of the leprosy spectrum is the more severe lepromatous type, in which symmetrical indurated skin lesions, nodules, or plaques are present. However, symmetrical acral-distal neuropathy appears late. These patients may have both RRs and ENL *M. lepra* reactions, absence of *M. lepra*–specific cellular immunity but not generalized anergy, and a high bacterial load. For ease of classification and management of the disease in the field, the World Health Organization (WHO) classified leprosy into two types of a somewhat analogous system: the milder paucibacillary (PB) leprosy for patients with five or fewer skin lesions and the more severe multibacillary (MB) leprosy for patients with more than five skin lesions. Fortunately, the vast majority of children develop the milder PB leprosy.

For diagnostic purposes, the clinician should look for the cardinal signs of the disease, any one of which is sufficient to establish a diagnosis. These include a localized area of sensory deficit (e.g., anesthetic lesion), nerve enlargement, demonstration of *M. leprae* in the skin or peripheral nerves, and granuloma within dermal nerves or nerve trunks.

Expert Opinion on Management Issues

Successful treatment requires not only proper antimicrobial therapy but also proper management of reactional states and reconstructive and cosmetic surgery for disabilities and deformities. Because of the stigma associated with the disease, mindfulness of the psychosocial and cultural problems the patients usually encounter is necessary for continued integration in society and a salutary outcome.

In 1943, the sulfones, of which dapsone became the prime candidate, although only bacteriostatic for *M. leprae,* were used as monotherapy worldwide for all forms of leprosy with generally good results. The emergence of clinically relevant levels of drug resistance surprisingly was found to be quite low. However, the recommended therapy was very long and even for life in lepromatous patients. In 1970, rifampin was found to be profoundly bactericidal for *M. leprae,* and multidrug regimens, evolved largely by the WHO and combining rifampin, dapsone, and another bacteriostatic agent, clofazimine, came into being. This made possible a shorter duration of treatment, currently no more than 1 year of therapy. Unfortunately, high relapses occur on these regimens, which are largely confined to MB patients with high bacterial load. Although ethionamide/prothionamide and certain aminoglycosides are bacteriostatic, and minocycline, clarithromycin, and several fluoroquinolones are bactericidal for *M. leprae* (although not nearly as potent as rifampin), none of these are used significantly in the treatment of leprosy.

TABLE 1 Recommended Pediatric Doses of Common Antileprotics and Regimens*

	Age of Patient		
Drug	**2–5 yr**	**6–12 yr**	**13–18 yr**
Dapsone	25 mg 3×/wk	25 mg/day	50 mg/day
Rifampin	150 mg/daily or monthly	300 mg/daily or monthly	600 mg/daily or monthly
Clofazimine			
Low dose	50 mg 2×/wk	50 mg 3×/wk	50 mg/day
High dose	50 mg 2×/wk	100 mg once/mo then 50 mg 3×/wk	150 mg once a month then 50 mg/day

	Paucibacillary (Tuberculoid)		Multibacillary (Lepromatous)	
	WHO	**More Intensive**	**WHO**	**More Intensive**
Regimen	Rifampin (monthly supervised), then dapsone (unsupervised)	Dapsone	Rifampin, clofazimine high dose, dapsone (monthly supervised) then dapsone, clofazimine low dose, (unsupervised)	Rifampin daily, dapsone (3 yr), then dapsone (lifelong)
Duration of treatment	6 mo	5 yr	1 yr	Lifelong

*Recommended dose of drugs varies with patient's age and/or body weight.
WHO, World Health Organization.

TABLE 2 Summary of Major Side Effects of Common Antileprosy Drugs

Drug	Major Side Effects
Dapsone	Hemolytic anemia; agranulocytosis; skin rashes; gastrointestinal complaints; sulphone syndrome (erythematous morbilliform rash with later exfoliative dermatitis, fever, lymphocytosis with atypical lymphocytes, hemolytic anemia, lymphadenopathy, and hepatitis), which requires immediate discontinuation of dapsone and systemic corticosteroids.
Rifampin	Hepatotoxicity; flu-like syndrome; thrombocytopenia; renal failure; gastrointestinal complaints; significant drug interactions; red-orange urine discoloration.
Clofazimine	Skin pigmentation; gastrointestinal complaints; small bowel obstruction; diminished sweating and tearing.
Ethionamide	Gastrointestinal complaints; hepatotoxicity.
Aminoglycosides	VIII cranial nerve toxicity; renal toxicity; administration for no longer than 1 year.
Clarithromycin	Gastrointestinal intolerance.

Of these bactericidal agents, only clarithromycin is acceptable in children.

The optimal antimicrobial therapy of leprosy depends largely on the type of disease encountered and available resources of the local health services, which globally remains unresolved. Consequential issues related to decision making center on the frequency and importance of drug resistance and the late relapse, which occurs, in our experience, almost entirely in patients with a high bacterial load and on average more than 10 years after the completion of therapy. Certainly, multidrug therapy for lepromatous leprosy (MB type) and a longer duration of treatment is required than for tuberculoid leprosy (PB type). The WHO regimens are generally reliable both for PB and MB patients having low bacterial loads but not in those with a higher bacterial load. Table 1 details the recommended doses of the commonly used antimicrobials used to treat pediatric patients and the regimens of both the WHO and what we find reliably effective in the United States. The WHO regimen's unique call for rifampin once monthly is primarily because daily rifampin is prohibitively expensive for countries where

leprosy is endemic. Rifampin is profoundly bactericidal for *M. leprae*, far more than other agents, and the doubling time of *M. leprae* is uniquely long, 14 days, as opposed to 1 day for *Myobacterium tuberculosis*. Alternatively, an initial more intensive phase by using the newer, more bactericidal agents and maintaining the WHO-recommended regimens for longer periods is worthy of consideration. Table 2 summarizes the toxicities and side effects of each of the antimicrobials used to treat pediatric patients.

REACTIONS

Lepra reactions are varied signs and symptoms of inflammation brought about by patient's immunologic response to *M. leprae* antigens. They may occur before, during, or even after effective chemotherapy. There are two distinct types of lepra reactions: Type 1, or RR, is cell-mediated immunity (CMI) mediated and occurs in approximately half of midspectrum borderline patients in treatment. Type 1 reactions often begin during the first few months of treatment. Clinically, RRs manifest as inflamed existing lesions, appearance of new lesions,

TABLE 3 Treatment for Type 1 and Type 2 Reactions in Children

Type of Reaction	Corticosteroids	Clofazimine	Thalidomide
Type 1	0.5–1 mg/kg/day. Initially attempt to taper off over 2–3 mo.	Ineffective.	Ineffective.
Type 2	0.3–1 mg/kg/day. Initially attempt to discontinue in 2 wk; reinstitute if recurrent.	50–100 mg/daily until controlled off corticosteroids, then taper to 50 mg 2–3×/wk. Increase as needed if reaction recurs.	50–300 mg nightly (no more than 100 mg nightly in children <20 kg); reinstitute if recurrent.

neuritis, and, on occasion, low-grade fever. Type 2 reactions, or erythema nodosum leprosum (ENL), is associated with immune complexes. It occurs in approximately half of patients with lepromatous leprosy and most commonly first occurs in the later part of year 1 of therapy. Its most common clinical manifestations are crops of painful erythematous papulonodules usually affecting the extensor surfaces of the extremities. Also, it may result in fever and neuritis and, less commonly, arthritis, uveitis, lymphadenitis, orchitis, and even frank glomerulonephritis. ENL may last for a few months to as long as 2 to 3 years and generally is more debilitating than the type 1 reaction.

A patient in reaction should continue taking antileprosy drugs. In addition, a patient with type 1 reaction should be given corticosteroids (prednisone) at an initial dose of 0.5 to 1 mg/kg/day depending on the severity of reaction, tapering slowly to a dose of 0.3 mg/kg/day for several months to avoid a recurrence. Thalidomide is the drug of choice for ENL. However, if thalidomide is not available, using the same initial dose recommended for type 1 reaction, corticosteroids (prednisone) are also effective. Also, for severe cases of ENL, clofazimine is of some value in decreasing steroid requirements. When new ENL lesions cease appearing, therapy can be discontinued in a few weeks, but if the process appears recurrent, patients should be maintained on the lowest dose of prednisone or thalidomide required to prevent recurrence.

Fortunately, because the majority of childhood leprosy is of the tuberculoid type and reactional states generally occur in borderline leprosy, reactions are not as much of a problem in children as in adults. Table 3 summarizes the recommended treatment for type 1 and type 2 reactions in children.

PROPHYLAXIS

Children in prolonged, intimate contact with a lepromatous leprosy patient are at risk of developing leprosy. Inasmuch as the use of dapsone as chemoprophylaxis is, at most, marginally effective, these children should be examined annually by an experienced leprologist for a period of 5 to 7 years.

VACCINES

No specific vaccines are available for leprosy. Bacille Calmette-Guérin (BCG) vaccine, similar to its use for tuberculosis, is variably effective in different locales but never reliably so. Because *M. leprae* contains large amounts of immunosuppressive lipids and polysaccharides, protein vaccines that show promise in mice may in the future prove useful in humans.

Common Pitfalls

Unfortunately, in many parts of the world where leprosy is endemic, health services and a reliable supply of medication are wanting. Also, there is a recent trend to integrate leprosy care from specialized vertically organized programs to the general health services. This shift certainly has some virtues, but as a result, the care of leprosy patients is losing priority. Resources and the medical expertise to diagnose the infection and perform and interpret skin smears and biopsies, as well as the skill to treat patients and their complications, are compromised. The priority and care of leprosy patients in the general health services often is inadequate to a salutary outcome.

Communication and Counseling

Because of its unnecessary social stigma, patients, their families, and the community at large must be intensively educated and counseled. From the outset and on an ongoing basis, patients and their families must internalize the fact that the affected individual can and should lead a normal life in the community, need not be isolated, and will not likely become deformed and disabled. Furthermore, the importance of compliance with a therapeutic regimen and the knowledge of the signs and symptoms of both reactional states and drug toxicities must be explained carefully and thoroughly to avoid their potentially deleterious complications.

SUGGESTED READINGS

1. World Health Organization: Chemotherapy of Leprosy for Control Programmes [Report of a WHO study group 1982], Technical report series no. 675, 1982. **A rationale for the WHO regimens.**
2. Gelber RH, Balagon VF, Cellona RV: The relapse rate in MB leprosy patients treated with 2-years of WHO-MDT in not low. Int J Lepr Other Mycobact Dis 72:493–500, 2004. **Underscores the late and high relapse rates in MB patients treated with 2-year WHO multidrug therapy (MDT), particularly with patients with a high bacterial burden.**
3. Gelber RH, Rea TH: Leprosy (Hansen's disease). In Mandell GL, Bennett JE, Dolin R (eds): Principles and Practice of Infectious Diseases, vol. 2: Philadelphia: Churchill Livingstone, 2000, pp 2608–2614. **A textbook chapter on leprosy.**

4. Hastings RC: Leprosy, 2nd ed. Edinburgh: Churchill Livingstone, 1994. **A book devoted to several aspects of leprosy.**
5. McDougal AC, Yuasa Y: A New Atlas of Leprosy. Tokyo: Sasakawa Memorial Health Foundation, 2000. **Photographs with descriptions of lesions and histopathology.**
6. Ridley DS, Jopling WH: Classification of leprosy according to immunity. Int J Leprosy 34:155–173, 1966. **Describes the clinical, histologic, and immunologic leprosy spectrum.**
7. Srinivasan H: Prevention of Disabilities in Patients with Leprosy (A Practical Guide). Geneva: World Health Organization, 1993. **Describes the different disabilities encountered in leprosy patients and their appropriate preventive measures.**

Listeriosis

Kavita S. Seth and Sharon A. Nachman

KEY CONCEPTS

- **Intrapartum disease**
  - T cell–mediated immunity is slightly impaired, therefore prone to listerial bacteremia (usually in third trimester at 26 to 30 weeks' gestation).
  - Central nervous system (CNS) infection is rare during pregnancy.
  - Maternal bacteremia: acute febrile illness with myalgias, arthralgias, headache, and backache.
  - Can result in premature labor, stillbirth, neonatal death, spontaneous abortion (granulomatosis infantiseptica).
  - Early diagnosis and antimicrobial treatment during pregnancy can result in birth of healthy infant.
- **Neonatal disease**
  - One of three major causes of neonatal sepsis.
  - High fatality rate (3% to 50%).
  - Similar to presentations of group B streptococcal disease (early-onset and late-onset sepsis).
- **CNS infection**
  - An estimated 30% to 55% of patients with *Listeria bacteremia* have associated meningitis.
  - High mortality (22%) in patients with serious underlying disease.
  - Postinfectious movement disorders and seizures are common (meningoencephalitis).
  - Healthy adults may present with rhombencephalitis (brain stem).
  - Macroscopic brain abscesses: 10% of listerial CNS infections.
- **Endocarditis: usually in adults (approximately 7.5% of listerial infections)**
  - Native valve and prosthetic valve disease associated with high rate of septic complications.
  - Mortality rate of approximately 50%.
- **Localized disease (rare)**
  - Conjunctivitis, skin infection, lymphadenitis.
  - Bacteremia can lead to peritonitis, cholecystitis, hepatitis, splenic abscess, pleuritis, pericarditis, osteomyelitis, and endophthalmitis.
- **Acute gastroenteritis**
  - Antecedent gastrointestinal symptoms prior to development of listerial bacteremia or CNS infection.

Listeria monocytogenes was first isolated by Murray and associates in 1926 in infected laboratory rabbits and guinea pigs. In 1936, the first case of human disease causing perinatal infection was reported. Since the 1960s, the organism has been implicated as the causative agent in many outbreaks of food-borne disease in both North America and Europe. *L. monocytogenes* remains an uncommon cause of illness in the general population but is isolated with increasing frequency in neonates, pregnant women, persons 65 years of age and older, and immunosuppressed patients.

L. monocytogenes is a small, facultatively anaerobic, non–spore-forming, gram-positive rod with a characteristic tumbling motility. The genus *Listeria* has six species, of which *L. monocytogenes* is the main human pathogen.

L. monocytogenes is distributed widely in the environment. The organism tolerates low temperatures, high salt concentrations, and high pH, which allows for replication in soil, water, sewage, manure, animal feed, and contaminated refrigerated foods. Outbreaks and sporadic infections occur as a result of food-borne transmission. Foods contaminated with *Listeria* include unwashed raw vegetables; unpasteurized milk; soft cheeses; prepared meats, such as hot dogs, deli meat, and pâté; undercooked poultry; and fish. The mean incubation period for food-borne listeriosis is approximately 3 weeks.

Neonatal disease results from transplacental or ascending infection or exposure during delivery because of asymptomatic fecal and vaginal carriage in pregnant women (Table 1). Maternal exposure results in abortion, preterm delivery, and fetal death. Nosocomial nursery outbreaks also occur. The incubation period for neonatal disease varies from 1 day to more than 3 weeks.

L. monocytogenes activates T cell–mediated immunity. The memory T cells provide an acquired resistance to listerial infection. This association with the T cell–mediated immunity explains the clinical association between listerial infections and conditions associated with impaired cellular immunity, including malignancies, immunosuppressive therapy, acquired immunodeficiency syndrome (AIDS), and pregnancy.

Diagnosis of *Listeria* infection is based on isolation of the pathogen from blood, cerebrospinal fluid, meconium, gastric washings, placenta, amniotic fluid, and other infected tissue specimens, including joint, pleural, or pericardial fluid. Cultures of feces are not helpful in diagnosis because carriage of the organism may occur without clinical disease. *Listeria* species can be mistaken for a contaminant or saprophyte because of morphologic similarity to diphtheroids and streptococci.

Expert Opinion on Management Issues

DRUG THERAPY

No controlled trials have established a drug of choice or duration of therapy for listerosis. Recommendations regarding therapy are based on data from in vitro

TABLE 1 Features of Early-Onset versus Late-Onset Neonatal Listeriosis

Characteristic	Early Onset (0–5 days)	Late Onset (>5 Days)
Onset of disease	Infected in utero	Infant colonized at birth, with delayed onset of infection or due to cross-infection
Major symptoms observed	Septicemia	Meningitis
Mortality rate	15%–50%	10%–20%
Infant status	Usually occurs in premature child with low birth weight	Usually occurs in infants apparently healthy at birth
Conditions	Respiratory distress, cyanosis, apnea, pneumonia, widespread microabscesses	Fever, poor feeding, irritability, leukocytosis, diarrhea
Possible contaminated sites	External ear, nose, throat, meconium, amniotic fluid, placenta or blood, lung, gut	Cerebrospinal fluid; blood and superficial cultures may be negative
Maternal fever and isolation of *Listeria monocytogenes* from maternal sites	About 50% of cases	0%–5% of cases

From Farber JM, Peterkin PI: *Listeria monocytogenes*, a food-borne pathogen. Microbio Rev 55:476–511, 1991.

TABLE 2 Intravenous Therapy for Listerial Infection

Clinical Syndrome	Antibiotics	Dosage	Minimum Duration of Therapy
Meningitis	Ampicillin *plus* gentamicin	200 mg/kg q4h 5 mg/kg q8h	3 weeks
Brain abscess or rhombencephalitis	Ampicillin *plus* gentamicin	200 mg/kg q4h 5 mg/kg q8h	6 weeks
Endocarditis	Ampicillin *plus* gentamicin	200 mg/kg q6h 5 mg/kg q6h	4–6 weeks
Bacteremia	Ampicillin	200 mg/kg q6h	2 weeks

Note: Patients allergic to penicillin and who do not have endocarditis can be treated with trimethoprim-sulfamethoxazole alone (15 mg/kg of trimethoprim q6–8h). Patients with endocarditis should be desensitized to ampicillin and treated as shown in table.
From Posfey-Barbe KM, Wald ER: Listeriosis. Pediatr Rev 25:151–159, 2004.

susceptibility testing, animal models, and clinical experience. Prompt administration of antibiotic therapy is required for prevention of death or severe sequelae, although sequelae may occur despite prompt antimicrobial therapy.

Antibiotic resistance is low for *L. monocytogenes* strains. Isolates of *L. monocytogenes* generally are susceptible to a wide range of antibiotics except for cephalosporins. Therapeutic success is impeded by particular biologic behavior of the facultative intracellular nature of the organism. Other factors that need to be considered include location of infection, penetration across the blood-brain barrier, and host factors.

L. monocytogenes demonstrates tolerance to some antibiotics in vitro, with the minimal bactericidal concentration (MBC) more than fourfold the minimal inhibitory concentration (MIC). Antibiotics commonly recommended for treatment include ampicillin, penicillin, erythromycin, and tetracycline. These antibiotics are bacteriostatic for *Listeria* in the blood. Other antibiotics effective for eradication of listerial infections, trimethoprim-sulfamethoxazole (TMP/SMX), aminoglycosides, and rifampin, are bactericidal.

Ampicillin is generally considered the preferred agent for treatment of listeriosis. Because the β-lactams are bacteriostatic, the combination with aminoglycosides, in particular gentamicin, is recommended. The combination has a synergistic effect on most *Listeria* strains and therefore exerts better and more rapid killing. This combination is recommended for treatment of all cases of listerial meningitis and endocarditis as well as treatment of listerial infections in patients with impaired T-cell function (Table 2).

Resistance to penicillin derivatives is not yet detected under natural conditions. Penicillin and ampicillin have good affinity for penicillin-binding protein 3 (PBP3) of *Listeria*, which causes cell death. However, *Listeria* is resistant to cephalosporins because of weak affinity for PBP3 targets.

For patients intolerant of penicillins, TMP/SMX is thought to be the best alternative single agent. This combination is bactericidal for *Listeria* species, and outcomes associated with its use appear at least comparable to the combination therapy of ampicillin and gentamicin. However, TMP/SMX cannot be used in the treatment of perinatal listeriosis because of the concern of bilirubin toxicity with sulfonamides.

Only in rare cases is resistance to macrolides, gentamicin, trimethoprim, or rifampin detected. These are plasmid mediated. Streptomycin and kanamycin, which do not play a role in therapy, have similar resistance profiles. Most quinolone and macrolide antibiotics are bacteriostatic only. In vivo studies with these agents are not promising and therefore should be avoided for treatment of listerial infections.

Vancomycin has been used in a few penicillin- and sulfa-allergic patients with some success, but experience is limited. In some cases, patients on therapy with vancomycin develop listerial meningitis. Vancomycin should only be used to treat bacteremia or endocarditis in penicillin-allergic patients.

Rifampin is active in vitro and penetrates into phagocytic cells; therefore it is speculated to be effective against intracellular *Listeria* species. Rifampin does penetrate into cerebrospinal fluid and could help eradicate the intracellular bacteria and cure infection.

In vitro studies of some antibiotic combinations for treatment of listeriosis have been variable. When erythromycin is combined with penicillin, ampicillin, or gentamicin in in vitro testing, all combinations are antagonistic. Combinations with amoxicillin or ampicillin or TMP/SMX with rifampin are also antagonistic in in vitro studies. Ampicillin plus gentamicin is the most reliable synergistic combination and remains the recommended initial therapy for listeriosis.

Duration of therapy depends on the clinical syndrome, presence of underlying disease, and response to therapy (see Table 2). The currently recommended duration of therapy is 2 weeks for bacteremia without CSF abnormalities and 3 weeks for meningitis, even in the absence of CNS or CSF abnormalities.

PREVENTIVE MEASURES

No vaccine is available for listerial infections. Standard infection control precautions are recommended when caring for patients with listerial infection.

The incidence of listeriosis has decreased substantially since 1989 when U.S. regulatory agencies began surveillance for *L. monocytogenes* in ready-to-eat processed meats and enforced regulations prohibiting the sale of contaminated meats ("zero-tolerance policy"). Since then, the number of cases of listerial infections has dropped dramatically.

The Centers for Disease Control and Prevention established dietary recommendations for preventing food-borne listeriosis in 1992. They are similar to those for other food-borne illnesses (Box 1).

In 2001, the Department of Agriculture developed a joint plan to reduce the number of listerial infections by 50% by 2005. Listeriosis has been a nationally notifiable disease since 2001. Cases of listeriosis should be reported to the regional health department to facilitate early recognition and control of common-source outbreaks.

Common Pitfalls

Complications of nonperinatal listerial disease, including disseminated intravascular coagulation, acute respiratory distress syndrome, and rhabdomyolysis with acute renal failure, are reported infrequently. Episodes of reinfection rarely occur.

Most of the antimicrobials used for treatment of listeriosis are able to interact with the extracellular bacteria and reduce the bacterial load. In the immunocompetent host, the body's defense system rids itself of the residual bacteria. However, in immunosuppressed hosts, these bacteria may trigger an exacerbation by

---

BOX 1 Dietary Recommendations for Food-Borne Listeriosis

For All Persons

- Thoroughly cook raw food from animal sources (beef, pork, poultry).
- Thoroughly wash raw vegetables before eating.
- Keep uncooked meats separate from vegetables, cooked foods, and ready-to-eat foods.
- Avoid consumption of raw (unpasteurized) milk or foods made from raw milk.
- Wash hands, knives, and cutting boards after handling uncooked foods.

Additional Recommendations for Persons at High Risk* for Listeriosis

- Avoid soft cheeses (Mexican-style, feta, Brie, Camembert, and blue-veined cheese); no need to avoid hard cheeses, processed cheeses, cream cheese, including slices and spreads, cottage cheese, or yogurt.
- Reheat leftover foods or ready-to-eat foods (hot dogs) until steaming hot before eating.
- Avoid refrigerated pâtés and other meat spreads, or heat/reheat these foods until steaming; no need to avoid canned or shelf-stable pâté and meat spreads.
- Avoid foods from delicatessen counters (prepared salads, meats, cheeses) or heat/reheat these foods until steaming before eating.

---

*Immunocompromised, by illness or medications, pregnant women, persons ≥65 years old.

From Lorber B: Listeriosis. Clin Infect Dis 24:1–11, 1997. Reprinted with permission of the University of Chicago Press.

12

---

multiplying and residing intracellularly, and consequently, the body's own defense mechanisms may not be able to eradicate the residual bacteria. Therefore, in spite of adequate recommended antibiotic therapy for listeriosis, a high mortality rate or recurrence after initial improvement may occur. Rifampin may be able to counteract the intracellular bacteria but at the same time may interfere with the action of ampicillin on extracellular *Listeria*. Therapeutic failure is usually not due to the antimicrobial resistance but rather is caused by the stage of the infection or complication as a result of the patient's underlying disease.

Communication and Counseling

Listeriosis has a high case fatality rate. Precise morbidity and mortality data for *L. monocytogenes* infection are not available. Perinatal listerial infection may result in abortion or stillbirth. Fetal mortality rates probably are high with gestational listeriosis, although the relative risk of intrauterine death is not known.

Among reported cases of early-onset sepsis in North America, the mortality rate is approximately 40%. Most survivors appear to be normal; however, sequelae are related to complications of prematurity, pneumonia, and sepsis. Late-onset sepsis has a mortality rate of less than 10%. Listerial meningitis may have a more favorable outcome than other types of bacterial meningitis, although hydrocephalus and mental retardation are reported. Beyond the newborn period, outcome of listerial infection depends on the underlying disease and management.

SUGGESTED READINGS

1. American Academy of Pediatrics: *Listeria monocytogenes* infections. In Pickering LK (ed): Red Book: 2003 Report of the Committee on Infectious Diseases, 26th ed. Elk Grove Village, Ill: American Academy of Pediatrics, 2003, pp 405–407. **Brief overview of listeriosis in pediatrics.**
2. Bortolussi R, Mailman T: Listeriosis. In Feigin RD, Cherry JD Demmler GJ, Kaplan SL (eds): Textbook of Pediatric Infectious Diseases, 5th ed. Philadelphia: Elsevier, 2004, pp 330–336. **Review of Listeria infections in children.**
3. Farber JM, Peterkin PI: Listeria monocytogenes, a food-borne pathogen. Microbiol Rev 55:476–511, 1991. **Detailed review of epidemiology and clinical manifestations of *L. monocytogenes* as a food-borne pathogen.**
4. Hof H: Therapeutic options. FEMS Immunol Med Microbiol 35:203–205, 2003. **Therapy and mechanism of antimicrobial therapy for listeriosis.**
5. Hof H, Nichterlein T, Kretschmar M: Management of listeriosis. Clin Microbiol Rev 10:345–357, 1997. **Detailed description of the properties and mechanism of the bacteria and antimicrobials used for therapy of listeriosis.**
6. Lorber B: Listeriosis. Clin Infect Dis 24:1–11, 1997. **Describes clinical syndrome and therapy of listeriosis.**
7. Posfey-Barbe KM, Wald ER: Listeriosis. Pediatr Rev 25:151–159, 2004. **Concise review of listerosis in pediatrics.**
8. Taege AJ: Listeriosis: Recognizing it, treating it, preventing it. Cleve Clin J Med 66:375–380, 1999. **Describes the epidemiology, clinical manifestations, treatment, and prevention of listerial infections.**
9. Temple ME, Nahata MC: Treatment of listeriosis. Ann Pharmacother 34:656–661, 2000. **Review of currently accepted treatment options for listeriosis.**

Lyme Disease

Eugene D. Shapiro

KEY CONCEPTS

- In each of the different stages of Lyme disease, affected patients have characteristic objective signs of infection (e.g., an erythema migrans rash, facial nerve palsy, or frank synovitis).
- Patients with *only* nonspecific symptoms and no abnormalities on examination are very unlikely to have Lyme disease regardless of the results of tests for antibodies to *Borrelia burgdorferi*.
- Misdiagnosis is the most common reason for failure of treatment.
- Tests for antibodies to *B. burgdorferi* should not be done if the prior probability of Lyme disease is low (such as in patients with only nonspecific complaints and no objective signs of infection).
- Antimicrobial prophylaxis for tick bites is not recommended routinely.
- Persistence of nonspecific symptoms after treatment is not an indication for additional treatment with antimicrobials.
- Benefit of prolonged (>1 month) treatment with an antimicrobial is not demonstrated for patients with any stage of Lyme disease.

Lyme disease, caused by the spirochete *Borrelia burgdorferi,* is the most common vector-borne illness in the United States. In the Northeast and the Upper Midwest, it is transmitted by *Ixodes scapularis* (the black-legged tick commonly known as the deer tick). It is much less common in the Pacific states, where it is transmitted by *Ixodes pacificus* (the western black-legged tick). In recent years, increases in the reported incidence of Lyme disease have been accompanied by increases in publicity about the illness in the press (and on the Internet), at times accompanied by near hysteria about both its risks and complications. This publicity, combined with a high frequency of misdiagnoses, contributes to anxiety about Lyme disease that is out of proportion to the morbidity it actually causes.

The clinical manifestations of Lyme disease are divided into three stages: early localized disease, early disseminated disease, and late disease. Patients may present with signs of either early disseminated or of late disease without having had manifestations of earlier stages of the illness. Early localized disease is marked by the characteristic erythema migrans rash (which may or may not be accompanied by fever and/or viral-like symptoms). Early disseminated disease is characterized most often by multiple erythema migrans; it also may manifest as palsy of a cranial nerve (especially palsy of the facial nerve). Meningitis (sometimes accompanied by papilledema) or, even more rarely, carditis (clinically manifest as heart block) may also occur in this stage of the illness. Late Lyme disease is characterized by oligoarthritis that usually affects the knee.

Expert Opinion on Management Issues

TREATMENT

Box 1 and Table 1 show the recommended regimens for treatment of Lyme disease.

Early Localized Disease

A limited number of clinical trials of treatment for Lyme disease have been conducted, so in many instances the appropriate minimal duration of therapy is unknown. The preferred drugs are doxycycline or amoxicillin. Cefuroxime is the preferred alternative drug. Although macrolides are used to treat early Lyme disease, they are not as effective as the three preferred drugs and should be used only if all of those agents are contraindicated.

The potential benefits of doxycycline include better penetration into the central nervous system (CNS) than alternative oral agents and the fact that it is effective treatment for ehrlichiosis, another illness that may occur as a coinfection with Lyme disease because it is also transmitted by *I. scapularis*.

Early Disseminated Disease

A study in which doxycycline (100 mg twice daily orally for 21 days) was compared with ceftriaxone (2 g per day

---

BOX 1 Recommended Duration and Mode of Antimicrobial Treatment of Lyme Disease

Early Localized Disease (Localized Erythema Migrans)

- Treat orally for 14 to 21 days (in some patients, 10 days may be sufficient).

Early Disseminated Disease

- Multiple erythema migrans
  - Treat orally for 21 days.
- Neurologic disease
  - Isolated VII nerve or other cranial nerve palsy (no evidence of meningitis). Treat orally for 21 days (doxycycline preferred if no contraindications). Some would treat as for meningitis.
  - Meningitis (with or without encephalitis or radiculoneuritis). Treat intravenously with ceftriaxone, cefotaxime, or penicillin for 14 to 21 days.
- Carditis
  - First- or second-degree heart block. Treat orally for 21 days.
  - Third-degree heart block or other evidence of severe carditis: Treat as for meningitis.

Late Disease (Arthritis)

- First episode: Treat orally (doxycycline or amoxicillin preferred) for 28 days. Nonsteroidal anti-inflammatory drugs may be a useful adjunct to treatment.
- Second episode: If swelling persists or recurs after 2 months, most would repeat a course of oral treatment. Some would use ceftriaxone or other intravenous treatment for 14 to 21 days.

---

intravenously for 14 days) to treat patients with early disseminated Lyme disease found no significant difference in the outcomes of the two groups. Because it is less expensive, more convenient, and associated with fewer adverse effects, orally administered treatment is recommended except for patients with meningitis or severe carditis (e.g., third-degree heart block). No evidence indicates that antimicrobial treatment affects the outcome of the facial nerve palsy caused by Lyme disease, which usually resolves either completely or with only minor residua in 2 to 6 weeks. Treatment of patients with facial nerve palsy is designed to prevent other manifestations of Lyme disease. Corticosteroids are not indicated to treat patients with facial nerve palsy caused by Lyme disease. If the eye does not close completely, drops to lubricate the eye should be administered several times a day.

Late Disease

Most experts treat Lyme arthritis with orally administered doxycycline (amoxicillin for those younger than 8 years) unless these drugs are contraindicated.

PREVENTION

Antimicrobial Prophylaxis for Tick Bites

Because the risk of Lyme disease from a recognized tick bite is low (2% to 3%), even in the most highly endemic areas, routine administration of antimicrobial prophylaxis to persons bitten by a deer tick is not recommended. In the rare instances in areas where the risk of Lyme disease is high and a person older than 8 years is bitten by a nymphal-stage deer tick that is engorged (i.e., that has fed for more than 48 to 72 hours), it might be reasonable to administer a single dose of 200 mg of doxycycline to try to prevent infection with *B. burgdorferi*. It should be given with food to minimize nausea.

Other Measures

No vaccine is currently available. Limited data suggest that personal protective measures, such as the use of insecticide before entering tick-infested areas and searching for and removing ticks from the body after leaving such areas, are somewhat effective.

Common Pitfalls

MISDIAGNOSIS

Misdiagnosis of Lyme disease is a major problem and the most common reason for failure of treatment. Because the sensitivity of culture for *B. burgdorferi* is poor and it is necessary for patients to undergo an invasive procedure such as a biopsy or a lumbar puncture to obtain appropriate samples for culture, it rarely is indicated in normal clinical practice. Consequently, if an erythema migrans rash is not present, the diagnosis of Lyme disease usually rests on the demonstration of antibodies to *B. burgdorferi* in the patient's serum.

The sensitivity and the specificity of antibody tests for Lyme disease vary substantially. The accuracy of widely used commercial test kits is much poorer than that of tests performed by reference laboratories. Likewise, the reproducibility of most commercially available antibody tests for Lyme disease is poor. Although the use of a Western immunoblot to confirm a positive quantitative test result for antibodies improves the specificity of serologic testing for Lyme disease, false-positive results of the immunoblot, especially for IgM antibodies, are not uncommon. Most important, as with any diagnostic test, the predictive value of antibody tests for Lyme disease depends highly on the prevalence of the infection among patients who are tested. Unfortunately, because many people, including physicians, have the erroneous belief that nonspecific symptoms *alone* (e.g., headache, fatigue, or arthralgia) may be a manifestation of Lyme disease, patients with only nonspecific symptoms frequently demand to be tested for Lyme disease, and some physicians routinely order tests for Lyme disease on such patients. However, because the specificities of even excellent antibody tests for Lyme disease are far from perfect, the vast majority (>95%) of positive test results in patients without specific signs of Lyme disease are false-positive results. Nevertheless, an erroneous diagnosis of Lyme disease, based on the results of these tests, is made frequently, and such patients often are treated unnecessarily with antimicrobials. Physicians should not routinely order antibody tests for Lyme disease as screening tests for patients with only nonspecific symptoms; nor should

TABLE 1 Antimicrobials to Treat Lyme Disease

Generic Name (Trade Name)	Dosage/Route/ Regimen	Maximum Dose	Formulations	Common Adverse Reactions	Comments
β-Lactams (Destroy cell wall of bacteria)					
Amoxicillin (Amoxil, Polymox, Trimox, others)	50 mg/kg/day PO divided into 3 doses/day	500 mg/dose	PO	Diarrhea, rash	
Cefuroxime axetil (Ceftin)	30 mg/kg/day PO divided into 2 doses/day	500 mg/dose	PO	Nausea, rash	
Ceftriaxone (Rocephin)	50–100 mg/kg/day IV in 1 dose/day	2 g/day	IV or IM	Diarrhea, rash, biliary sludging	
Cefotaxime (Claforan)	150–200 mg/kg/day IV divided q8h	8–9 g/day	IV	Rash, diarrhea	
Penicillin G (Pfizerpen; others)	200,000–400,000 U/kg/day IV divided q4h	18–24 million U/day	IV	Rash	
Tetracyclines (Inhibit protein synthesis by binding to 30s subunit of bacterial ribosome)					
Doxycycline (Doryx, Vibramycin)	2–4 mg/kg/day PO divided into 2 doses/day	100 mg/dose (200 mg single dose for prophylaxis of tick bite in older children)	PO	Nausea	Some patients develop sun-induced dermatitis so should protect skin from sun; do not use in children <8 yr or in pregnant or lactating women.
Tetracycline	20–50 mg/kg/day PO divided into 4 doses/day	500 mg/dose	PO	Nausea	Do not use in children <8 yr or in pregnant or lactating women.
Macrolides (Inhibit protein synthesis by binding to 50s subunit of bacterial ribosome)					
Erythromycin (numerous)	30 mg/kg/day PO divided into 4 doses/day	500 mg/dose	PO	Nausea	Interactions with a number of drugs metabolized by P450 system.
Clarithromycin (Biaxin)	15 mg/kg/day PO divided into 2 doses/day	500 mg/dose	PO	Nausea, diarrhea	Interactions with a number of drugs metabolized by P450 system.
Azithromycin (Zithromax)	10 mg/kg/day PO in 1 dose/day	600 mg	PO	Nausea, jaundice	Interactions with a number of drugs metabolized by P450 system.

IM, intramuscular; IV, intravenous; PO, by mouth; q*x*h, every *x* hours.

they order such tests for patients who have not been in endemic areas.

PERSISTENT NONSPECIFIC SYMPTOMS

Symptoms such as fatigue, arthralgia, and myalgia sometimes persist for some time after completion of a course of treatment for Lyme disease. These nonspecific symptoms, which may accompany or may follow more specific symptoms and signs of Lyme disease but virtually never are the sole manifestations, usually resolve over a period of weeks. In many of the clinical trials of treatment of Lyme disease, most of the so-called failures of treatment were patients who continued to complain of nonspecific symptoms that are highly prevalent in the population. Persons who are labeled as having Lyme disease may be more likely to report minor nonspecific symptoms than persons who never had Lyme disease. It is important to distinguish true treatment failures (patients with objective signs of persistent infection on examination) from persons with fibromyalgia or chronic fatigue, neither of which is likely to benefit from additional antimicrobial treatment. Indeed, no evidence indicates that prolonged treatment with antimicrobials offers any benefit over conventional treatment, but considerable evidence shows that prolonged treatment can be associated with significant adverse side effects. Because antibodies against

B. burgdorferi usually persist after successful treatment, there is no reason to routinely obtain follow-up tests of antibody concentrations in a patient in whom Lyme disease has been confirmed.

JARISCH-HERXHEIMER REACTION

In a small proportion of patients, a Jarisch-Herxheimer reaction, marked by increased fever and worsening myalgia, may occur 24 to 48 hours after treatment begins, presumably because of the release of toxins associated with lysis of the organisms. The reaction usually resolves within 24 to 48 hours. Antimicrobial treatment should be continued. Nonsteroidal anti-inflammatory drugs may help relieve the symptoms.

PATIENTS WITH FACIAL NERVE PALSY

There is controversy about whether patients with facial nerve palsy due to Lyme disease should undergo a lumbar puncture routinely and whether they should be treated with antimicrobials administered parenterally. Some patients without apparent involvement of the CNS may have pleocytosis or other abnormalities of the cerebrospinal fluid (CSF), including persons with solitary erythema migrans and no apparent involvement of the CNS. Nevertheless, treatment with an antimicrobial administered orally is virtually always highly successful. Likewise, patients with isolated facial nerve palsy and no apparent involvement of the CNS do very well if treated orally. Treatment with doxycycline is preferred, if possible, because of its relatively good penetration into the CNS, although treatment with amoxicillin is also effective. I do not routinely recommend performing a lumbar puncture in patients with facial nerve palsy due to Lyme disease unless they have signs or symptoms of involvement of the CNS (e.g., severe headache, papilledema, nuchal rigidity), although some experts do routinely recommend a lumbar puncture. If a lumbar puncture is performed and inflammation is evident, the patient should be treated as for meningitis. If the diagnosis of facial nerve palsy due to Lyme disease is based solely on serology, there must be good evidence that Lyme disease is the cause of the palsy, especially if the palsy does not resolve in the usual manner (both because of the possibility of a false-positive antibody test result for Lyme disease and because there are other treatable causes of facial nerve palsy, such as acoustic neuroma or lymphoma).

ARTHRITIS

Treatment with a single course of an orally administered antimicrobial is usually successful. However, particularly if there was a delay before treatment was initiated and chronic synovitis has developed, it may take several months before the inflammation resolves completely. If inflammation persists for 2 to 3 months after the initial treatment, most experts prescribe a second 4-week course of an orally administered antimicrobial (some recommend 2 to 4 weeks of parenteral treatment with ceftriaxone). Nonsteroidal anti-inflammatory agents also may be useful. If inflammation persists despite two courses of antimicrobial treatment, other causes of arthritis have to be ruled out.

COINFECTIONS

Because both human granulocytic ehrlichiosis and babesiosis are also transmitted by Ixodes ticks, coinfection with these agents, although uncommon, can occur in patients with Lyme disease. Babesiosis rarely is a problem except in patients who are asplenic or immunocompromised. Ehrlichiosis should be considered in patients who are severely ill and who are leukopenic and/or thrombocytopenic.

Communication and Counseling

Because there is so much misinformation about Lyme disease in the media and on the Internet (including statements that Lyme disease cannot be cured), patients and parents need reassurance that the prognosis for children treated for Lyme disease is excellent. I ask parents their biggest fears about this infection so misconceptions can be addressed directly. The other situation that arises frequently is the need to explain to a parent that a child with only chronic, nonspecific symptoms, such as fatigue or arthralgia, does not have active Lyme disease, regardless of whether antibody test results are positive or negative. Some can accept and understand this reality and others cannot. But stating that Lyme disease is not the cause of a child's problems does not mean the child does not have problems; nor does it mean the child is consciously malingering. Rather, it simply means that Lyme disease is not the cause of the symptoms and treating such a child with antimicrobials is not likely to be of any benefit.

SUGGESTED READINGS

1. Klempner MS, Hu LT, Evans J, et al: Two controlled trials of antibiotic treatment in patients with persistent symptoms and a history of Lyme disease. N Engl J Med 345:85–92, 2001. **Randomized, double-blind clinical trial of long-term antibiotic treatment of persons who thought they had chronic Lyme disease. Study demonstrated no benefit of long-term antibiotic treatment of these patients.**
2. Nadelman RB, Nowakowski J, Fish D, et al: Prophylaxis with single-dose doxycycline for the prevention of Lyme disease after an *Ixodes scapularis* tick bite. N Engl J Med 345:79–84, 2001. **Study showing the effectiveness of a single dose of doxycycline in preventing Lyme disease in persons bitten by a deer tick.**
3. Seltzer EG, Shapiro ED: Misdiagnosis of Lyme disease: When not to order serologic tests. Pediatr Infect Dis J 15:762–763, 1996. **Brief article that demonstrates the poor positive predictive value of tests for Lyme disease when the prior probability of Lyme disease is low.**
4. Shapiro ED: Doxycycline for tick bites—not for everyone. N Engl J Med 345:133–134, 2001. **Editorial that discusses the limitations of the study cited (reference 2) by Nadelman and colleagues and explains why routine use of prophylactic antimicrobials for tick bites is not recommended.**
5. Shapiro ED: Long-term outcomes of persons with Lyme disease. Vector Borne Zoonotic Dis 2:279–281, 2002. **Brief review of the**

studies of the long-term outcomes of persons with Lyme disease.

6. Shapiro ED, Gerber MA: Lyme disease. Clin Infect Dis 31:533–542, 2000. **Comprehensive clinical review of Lyme disease.**

7. Wormser GP, Nadelman RB, Dattwyler RJ, et al: Infectious Diseases Society of America Practice Guidelines for the Treatment of Lyme Disease. Clin Infect Dis 31(Suppl. 1):S1–S14, 2000. **Official practice guidelines for the treatment of Lyme disease from an expert panel that represents the Infectious Disease Society of America.**

Meningococcal Disease

Steven Black and Henry R. Shinefield

KEY CONCEPTS

- Invasive meningococcal disease is most likely to occur in infants, young children, and adolescents, particularly first-year college students.

- Antibiotics should be started immediately in patients with a clinical presentation consistent with meningococcal disease, such as fever and purpura, without waiting for laboratory confirmation of the diagnosis. Because the symptoms of meningococcal disease can overlap with meningitis or sepsis caused by other organisms, an antibiotic with broad coverage, such as cefotaxime or vancomycin, should be considered.

- Chemoprophylaxis is indicated for all high-risk contacts of the index patient within 24 hours of case identification. The index patient should also be treated to eradicate nasopharyngeal carriage.

- A quadrivalent polysaccharide vaccine is available in the United States, although the vaccine is not effective in children younger than 2 years and does not protect against serotype B disease. Three conjugate vaccines against serotype C are available in Europe and Canada; quadrivalent (A, C, Y, W135) conjugate vaccines are in development. Vaccines against serotype B are available in Latin America and New Zealand but are of limited effectiveness.

Neisseria meningitidis is a gram-negative diplococcal bacterium capable of causing both sporadic and epidemic disease. The human nasopharynx is the only known reservoir for *N. meningitidis*, which is spread though contact with nasopharyngeal secretions, such as by kissing or sharing eating utensils. Exposure to *N. meningitidis* is widespread, and 5% to 15% of the population carries meningococci at any given time, although only a small percentage develops invasive disease. Most individuals have developed bactericidal antibodies against *N. meningitidis* by the time they are 20 years of age; as a result, the highest incidence of meningococcal disease occurs in infants and young children, with another peak in adolescence when social contact increases. Individuals with deficiencies in complement function or who are functionally or anatomically asplenic are at higher risk of meningococcal disease; however, other forms of immunodeficiency do not appear to increase the risk. Viral respiratory infections and exposure to tobacco smoke are also associated with increased risk of meningococcal disease.

Although at least 13 serotypes of meningococci are identified, five serogroups (A, B, C, Y, and W135) cause the majority of disease worldwide. In the United States, serotypes B and C are the most prevalent, each accounting for approximately one third of meningococcal disease, with serotype Y accounting for an additional one quarter. In Europe, serotype C is most common; in sub-Saharan Africa, serogroup A predominates.

Meningococcal Disease

Infection with *N. meningitidis* can result in a wide range of effects, from asymptomatic carriage to shock, organ failure, and death. The most common forms of meningococcal disease are meningitis and meningococcemia, although other presentations, such as arthritis, myocarditis, and conjunctivitis, also occur. In meningitis, the predominant symptoms are headache, fever, photophobia, and generalized achiness. Stiff neck is also common except in young infants, and seizures occur in approximately 20% of patients. Although meningococcal meningitis is uniformly fatal if left untreated, the case fatality rate is reduced to approximately 5% with appropriate antibiotic treatment. By contrast, the case fatality rate for meningococcemia remains at 10% to 40% despite aggressive treatment. The meningococcal endotoxin is produced very quickly, resulting in rapid disease progression, with the development of hypotension, organ failure, and even death occurring as early as a few hours after infection.

The early symptoms of meningococcemia are commonly fever and rash, which may take the form of petechiae, purpura, or maculopapules. The presence of spreading purpura indicates severe disease. As *N. meningitidis* spreads, the released endotoxin binds to macrophages, stimulating the release of various cytokines and subsequently activating a procoagulation state. This in turn leads to disseminated intravascular coagulation (DIC), thrombosis, ischemia, and infarction of the skin, digits, and organs. The endotoxin also activates complement, resulting in vasodilation, capillary leakage, and eventual hypotension or pulmonary edema. Thus severe bleeding may coexist with thrombosis, complicating the choice of therapies. Severe metabolic abnormalities, including hypokalemia, hypocalcemia, hypomagnesemia, and hypophosphatemia, may also be present, as can impaired myocardial function. Sequelae, including limb loss, hearing loss, or neurologic disability, are present in 11% to 19% of survivors of meningococcal disease.

DIAGNOSIS

For both therapeutic and public health reasons, the presence and strain of the meningococci responsible for invasive disease must be confirmed. A positive antigen test in the context of an illness consistent with meningococcal disease suggests a probable case, which is further supported by the isolation of gram-negative diplococci from blood or cerebrospinal fluid

(CSF). However, confirmation of a diagnosis of meningococcal disease requires the isolation of *N. meningitidis* from sites that are usually sterile, such as blood, CSF, synovial fluid, pleural fluid, pericardial fluid, or petechial or purpuric lesions. If antibiotics are given before blood or CSF are cultured, it may be difficult to obtain live bacteria to confirm the presence or type of meningococci by culturing. Newer techniques, such as polymerase chain reaction (PCR) (nested or real time) and enzyme-linked immunoabsorbent assay (ELISA), allow the identification of meningococci for several days after the initiation of antibiotic therapy. Isolation of *N. meningitidis* from a throat, nasopharyngeal, or conjunctival swab does not confirm meningococcal disease because *N. meningitidis* can be part of the normal commensal flora of these regions.

Expert Opinion on Management Issues

URGENT INTERVENTIONS

Because of the fulminant nature of meningococcemia, immediate intravenous (or intramuscular, if intravenous access is not available) treatment with antibiotics (Table 1) is necessary if there is any indication of meningococcal disease.

ACCEPTED INTERVENTIONS

Treatment of Complications

The first treatment priority should be basic life support and administration of antibiotics, after which secondary disorders can be addressed. Common complications of meningococcal disease include shock, increased intracranial pressure (ICP), and gangrene. Volume replacement with human albumin solution or isotonic sodium chloride solution at 20 mL/kg should be initiated if shock is present. If this is insufficient, both inotropic support with dopamine, dobutamine, or adrenaline (see Table 1) and endotracheal intubation and ventilation may be necessary. Ventilation, sedation, and correction of biochemical imbalances are used to manage ICP; note that administration of mannitol can be dangerous in patients with shock. Amputations or skin grafts may be necessary if gangrene develops in the extremities.

Prevention of Secondary Cases

To prevent the spread of meningococcal disease from the index patient, the close contacts of the patient (Box 1) must be identified quickly, ideally within 24 hours after identification of the index patient, and offered chemoprophylaxis with an antibiotic that will clear nasopharyngeal carriage of meningococcal strains. Because penicillin is not effective for this purpose, rifampin, ceftriaxone, ciprofloxacin, or sulfadiazine should be used instead (see Table 1). If the index patient was treated with penicillin, an additional course of antimicrobials should be administered to eliminate carriage before the patient leaves the hospital.

CONTROVERSIAL INTERVENTIONS

A number of studies show that dexamethasone reduces hearing loss following bacterial meningitis caused by *Haemophilus influenzae* and *Streptococcus pneumoniae*. Although no data are available regarding the efficacy of dexamethasone in meningococcal meningitis, there is no reason to think it would not also be effective in meningococcal meningitis.

Protein C is an anticoagulant that is depleted in patients with meningococcal disease. A recombinant form of activated protein C (drotrecogin alfa [activated]; Xigris, Eli Lilly) was approved by the U.S. Food and Drug Administration in 2002 for the reduction of mortality in adults with severe sepsis; however, few patients in the clinical trials had sepsis caused by *N. meningitidis*, and the safety and efficacy of the drug is not established in children. Furthermore, the use of protein C is associated with increased bleeding. Similar findings are reported for the use of heparin.

Antiendotoxin therapies were also investigated. Two monoclonal antibodies against endotoxin (HA-1A and E5) were not efficacious in improving the disease course. A randomized clinical trial of recombinant bactericidal permeability-increasing protein (rBPI), a molecule that binds endotoxin and is cytotoxic to gram-negative bacteria, showed trends toward improved outcomes, but the trial did not have sufficient power to detect significant differences in morbidity or mortality.

VACCINATION

Although several polysaccharide vaccines are available in Europe, the only vaccine currently available in the United States is a quadrivalent vaccine against the capsular polysaccharides of types A, C, Y, and W135 (Menomune, Aventis Pasteur) (Table 2). The vaccine is well tolerated and recommended for individuals at high risk, such as those with complement deficiencies, functional or anatomic asplenia, or those traveling to areas with epidemic meningococcal disease. It is also given routinely to military recruits and offered to many college students. However, this vaccine has two major limitations: It does not protect against serotype B, the most common cause of invasive meningococcal disease in the United States, and, like other polysaccharide vaccines, it is poorly immunogenic in the highest risk group, children younger than 2 years. In addition, the protection afforded by the polysaccharide vaccine is short lived.

The B polysaccharide is very similar to endogenous sialic acid antigens and is not immunogenic. To circumvent this difficulty, vaccines against serotype B are based on bacterial components other than the polysaccharide, such as outer membrane vesicles. One such vaccine is available in Latin America, and another was approved for use in New Zealand to combat an ongoing group B epidemic, although no prospective efficacy trials have been performed using this vaccine. Other group B vaccines, including one delivered as a nasal spray, are in development.

Polysaccharides conjugated to proteins are immunogenic in very young children and were developed for a

TABLE 1 Medications for Meningococcal Disease

Generic Name (Trade Name) Rx	Route/Dosage/Regimen	Maximum Dose	Dosage Formulations	Common Aftereffects	Comments
Meningococcal Infection Antibiotics (Therapeutic)					
Penicillin G (Pfizerpen)* Rx	IV or IM First dose: <1 yr: 300 mg (1.2 million U)* 1–9 yr: 600 mg (2.4 million U)* >10 yr (including adults): 1.2 g (4.8 million U)*	1.2 g	Powder	Hypersensitivity reactions; anaphylaxis	
Cefotaxime (Claforan) Rx	IV or IM 1 mo to 12 yr: 50 to 180 mg/kg/d divided into 4 or 6 doses (higher doses for severe infections, including meningitis)	12 g/day	Powder	Local reactions, colitis, diarrhea, nausea, vomiting, hypersensitivity	
Ceftriaxone (Rocephin) Rx	IV or IM Initial dose 100 mg/kg, followed by 100 mg/kg/day (in 1 or 2 doses) for 7 to 14 days	4 g	Powder	Local reactions, eosinophilia, thrombocytosis, leukopenia, diarrhea	
Chloramphenicol* (Chloromycetin) Rx	IV First dose: <12 yr: 25 mg/kg >12 yr and adult: 1.2 g				For use in patients with allergies to penicillin and cephalosporins.
Rifampin (Rifadin) Rx	PO, 2 days <1 mo: 5 mg/kg q12h ≥1 mo: 10 mg/kg q12h Adults: 600 mg q12h		Capsule		Not indicated for the treatment of meningococcal infection; for prophylaxis only; not recommended for pregnant women.
Ciprofloxacin* (Cipro) Rx	Adults: single oral dose of 500 mg <18 yr: not recommended				Causes cartilage damage in animals; not recommended for use in children or pregnant women.
Ceftriaxone* (Rocephin) Rx	Single IM dose <12 yr: 125 mg >12 yr and adults: 250 mg			Local reactions, eosinophilia, thrombocytosis, leukopenia, diarrhea	
Sulfadiazine (Microsulfon)	PO, 2 days Adults: 500 mg qid <1 yr: 125 mg qid 1–12 yr: 250 mg qid				Use only if strain is known to be susceptible.
Shock Vasopressors					
Dopamine (Intropin)	IV 5–20 µg/kg/min; 5 µg/kg/min every few minutes titrated until response	50 µg/kg/min	Solution		
Dobutamine (Dobutrex) Rx	IV 5–20 µg/kg/min, 5 µg/kg/min every few min titrated until response		Solution		
Epinephrine* (adrenaline)	IV 0.1–5 µg/kg/min				
Increased Intracranial Pressure Glucocorticoids (Anti-inflammatory and immunosuppression)					
Dexamethasone* (Decadron) Rx	IV 0.4 mg/kg qd for 4 days				Also sometimes used for adrenal insufficiency. Administer with first dose of antibiotics for meningitis to prevent hearing loss.

*From Faust S, Levin M: Meningococcal infections. eMedicine. Last updated January 26, 2005. Available at http://www.emedicine.com/ped/topic1412.htm. Accessed November 4, 2005.

IM, intramuscular; IV, intravenous; PO, by mouth; qd, every day; qid, four times per day; qch, every x hours; Rx, prescription.

From Faust S, Levin M: Meningococcal infections. eMedicine. Last updated November 2, 2003. Available online http://www.emedicine.com/ped/topic1412.htm. Accessed August 20, 2004.

TABLE 2 Meningococcal Vaccines

Name	Manufacturer	Type	Serotypes	Availability
Mengivac	Aventis Pasteur	Polysaccharide	A, C	Europe
Menomune	Aventis Pasteur	Polysaccharide	A, C, Y, W135	Europe, United States, Canada
AC Vax	GSK Biologicals	Polysaccharide	A, C	Europe
ACWY Vax	GSK Biologicals	Polysaccharide	A, C	Europe
Meningitec	Wyeth Vaccines	Conjugate (CRM$_{197}$)*	C	Europe, Canada
Menjugate	Chiron Vaccines	Conjugate (CRM$_{197}$)*	C	Europe, Canada
NeisVac-C	Baxter Immuno	Conjugate (tetanus toxoid)	C	Europe, Canada
	Finlay Institute/GSK	Outer membrane vesicles	B	Latin America
	Various	Outer membrane vesicles	B	In development
	Various	Conjugate	A, C, Y, W135	In development

*CRM$_{197}$ is a nontoxic derivative of diphtheria toxin.

BOX 1 Recommendations for Chemoprophylaxis

If Any of the Following Criteria Are Met during the 7 Days before Illness Onset

- Household contacts
- Daycare contacts
- Close social contact (e.g., kissing, sharing eating utensils)
- Mouth-to-mouth resuscitation
- Endotracheal tube placement

Not Necessary

- Schoolmates or work colleagues without exposure to patient's nasal or oral secretions
- Health care personnel not in contact with patient's nasal or oral secretions

Drugs Effective for Chemoprophylaxis

- Rifampin
- Ciprofloxacin
- Ceftriaxone
- Sulfadiazine (if susceptible)

- Early symptoms of meningococcemia may include only fever and rash, which can resemble other severe bacterial, rickettsial, or viral infections; other patients present only with pneumonia or with uncommon manifestations such as arthritis or conjunctivitis.
- Meningococcemia can progress very quickly. Therefore, if meningococcal disease is suspected, aggressive antibiotic therapy must be started immediately, without waiting for diagnostic confirmation.

Communication and Counseling

Public education campaigns could raise awareness that a meningococcal vaccine is available. Improving the public's recognition of the symptoms of meningococcal disease might also result in the initiation of antibiotics earlier in the disease course. Close contacts of a case patient should be identified quickly and cautioned to seek care immediately if any suspicious signs or symptoms emerge, even if they are receiving chemoprophylaxis.

number of diseases, such as *H. influenzae* and *S. pneumoniae*. Three conjugate vaccines against *N. meningitidis* serotype C are licensed in Europe and Canada (see Table 2). In 1999, the United Kingdom was the first to introduce one of these meningococcal conjugate vaccines into a routine vaccination schedule; the vaccine was also offered to all children younger than 18 years, with those younger than 1 year or those 15 to 17 years of age given priority. After 4 years, they found the vaccine was 83% to 100% effective against serotype C disease across the various age groups and time since vaccination. A notable exception was that infants given routine vaccination at 2, 3, and 4 months were no longer protected after 1 year. This suggests that a booster dose before 2 years of age should be considered for children vaccinated as infants. Various quadrivalent conjugate vaccines are also in development.

Common Pitfalls

- Misdiagnosis is a potential pitfall that can lead to a critical delay in appropriate treatment. In particular, young children may not present with typical symptoms of meningitis.

SUGGESTED READINGS

1. Bryant PA, Li HY, Zaia A, et al: Prospective study of a real-time PCR that is highly sensitive, specific, and clinically useful for diagnosis of meningococcal disease in children. J Clin Microbiol 42:2919–2925, 2004. **Comparison of the usefulness of nested PCR, real-time PCR, and culturing of blood or CSF for the identification of meningococcal disease.**
2. Centers for Disease Control and Prevention: Prevention and control of meningococcal disease and meningococcal disease and college students: Recommendations of the Advisory Committee on Immunization Practices (ACIP). MMWR Morb Mortal Wkly Rep 49(RR-7):1–20, 2000. **Governmental recommendations on preventing and treating meningococcal disease in the general population and in college students.**
3. Committee on Infectious Diseases, American Academy of Pediatrics, Infectious Diseases and Immunization Committee, Canadian Paediatric Society: Meningococcal disease prevention and control strategies for practice-based physicians. Pediatrics 97:404–412, 1996. **Definitions of relevant terms and practical advice for recognizing, treating, and preventing meningococcal disease.**
4. Faust S, Levin M: Meningococcal infections. eMedicine. Last updated January 26, 2005. Available online at http://www.

12

emedicine.com/ped/topic1412.htm (accessed November 4, 2005). **Step-by-step clinical guide to diagnosing and treating pediatric meningococcal infections.**

5. Granoff DM, Feavers IM, Borrow R: Meningococcal vaccines. In Plotkin SA, Orenstein WA (eds): Vaccines, 4th ed. Philadelphia: WB Saunders, 2004, pp 959–987. **Detailed descriptions of meningococcal disease, available treatments, and vaccines that are available or under development.**

6. Katial RK, Brandt BL, Moran EE, et al: Immunogenicity and safety testing of a group B intranasal meningococcal native outer membrane vesicle vaccine. Infect Immunol 70:702–707, 2002. **Report of an early trial of a serotype B vaccine that is delivered nasally rather than parenterally.**

7. Levin M, Quint PA, Goldstein B, et al: Recombinant bactericidal/permeability-increasing protein (rBPI$_{21}$) as adjunctive treatment for children with severe meningococcal sepsis: A randomised trial. Lancet 356:961–967, 2000. **Clinical trial of an antiendotoxin treatment for meningococcemia.**

8. Offit PA, Peter G: The meningococcal vaccine—public policy and individual choices. N Engl J Med 349:2353–2356, 2003. **Discussion of why the public in the United States is not aware of the meningococcal vaccine and what can be done about it.**

9. Rennels M, King J Jr, Ryall R, et al: Dosage escalation, safety and immunogenicity study of four dosages of a tetravalent meningococcal polysaccharide diphtheria toxoid conjugate vaccine in infants. Pediatr Infect Dis J 23:429–435, 2004. **Report of a phase 1 trial of a meningococcal conjugate vaccine against serotypes A, C, Y, and W135.**

10. Trotter CL, Andrews NJ, Kaczmarski EB, et al: Effectiveness of meningococcal serogroup C conjugate vaccine 4 years after introduction. Lancet 364:365–367, 2004. **Evaluation of the effectiveness of a meningococcal conjugate vaccine across various age groups in Britain in the first 4 years after introduction.**

Nontuberculosis *Mycobacterium* Infections

Elaine J. Abrams and Lisa-Gaye Robinson

KEY CONCEPTS

- Nontuberculous mycobacteria (NTM) are ubiquitous in the environment.
- Person-to-person transmission of NTM has not been documented.
- The most common clinical syndrome in children is lymphadenitis.
- NTM infections in children may have clinical features similar to those caused by *Mycobacterium tuberculosis*.
- Surgical intervention is often warranted and curative for some manifestations.
- Multidrug prolonged therapy is used for essentially all NTM infections.
- Disseminated infections with NTM almost exclusively occur in children with impaired cell-mediated immunity.

Nontuberculous mycobacteria (NTM) infections are caused by a heterogeneous group of more than 50 species within the *Mycobacterium* genus excluding *Mycobacterium tuberculosis, Mycobacterium bovis, Mycobacterium microti,* and *Mycobacterium africanum.* NTMs are ubiquitous in the environment and can be easily recovered from soil, plants, house dust, water, food, and domestic and wild animals. Person-to-person transmission of NTMs is not documented; however, nosocomial spread is described. It is increasingly reported that cystic fibrosis patients may be colonized with NTM. The major clinical syndromes include lymphadenitis; skin, soft tissue, and skeletal infections; pulmonary infections; catheter infections; and disseminated disease (Table 1). Cervical lymphadenitis is the most common of these syndromes in children. Disseminated disease is almost always associated with impaired cell-mediated immunity, most commonly HIV/AIDS (human immunodeficiency virus/acquired immune deficiency syndrome).

The ubiquity of these organisms makes distinguishing colonization from infection/disease challenging. Clinical suspicion and careful interpretation of diagnostic tests are important when determining pathogenicity of a recovered NTM. Recovery of NTM from a sterile site is the most reliable diagnostic test. Unlike bacteria, recovery from a draining sinus tract is usually clinically significant. Specific therapy depends on the clinical syndrome, the species causing the infection, drug-susceptibility testing, and the host's immune function. Surgical intervention is often warranted and curative for some manifestations. Most NTM strains are resistant to first-line antituberculous drugs. Multidrug prolonged therapy (Table 2) is used for essentially all NTM infections other than some cases of *Mycobacterium marinum* skin infections.

NTM infections in children may have clinical features similar to those caused by *M. tuberculosis* (MTB). Therefore, an important consideration in the management of children with suspected NTM is exclusion of MTB disease.

Expert Opinion on Management Issues

LYMPH NODE INFECTION

Lymphadenitis is the most common clinical manifestation of NTM infection in children. The cervical lymph nodes are most commonly involved. *Mycobacterium avium* complex (MAC) accounts for the majority of infected nodes. Local infections can lead to chronic draining sinus tracts and disfiguring scars. Incision and drainage of a node suspected to be NTM for diagnostic and treatment purposes can lead to unacceptably high rates of draining fistulas/recurrences and therefore is not recommended. Total excisional biopsy of the involved nodes without antibiotics is the treatment of choice and prevents recurrence. Antimicrobial therapy with clarithromycin or azithromycin with either ethambutol or rifabutin and close observation may be considered for cases in which the family refuses surgery, disease has recurred, or surgical excision was incomplete.

TABLE 1 Nontuberculosis Mycobacterial Disease Spectrum and Treatment

Clinical Syndrome	Predominant Species	Treatment	Duration
Lymphadenitis	MAC	Complete surgical excision. If not possible or disease recurs, consider clarithromycin or azithromycin combined with either ethambutol or rifabutin.	Undefined. Depends on clinical response (usually several months).
Skin, soft tissue infections	*Myobacterium marinum, Myobacterium fortuitum, Myobacterium chelonae,* * *Myobacterium abscessus*	None, if minor. Rifampin, doxycycline, clarithromycin, or trimethoprim-sulfamethoxazole. More extensive lesions may require surgical debridement. Excision of tissue. Initial therapy with amikacin plus cefoxitin, IV for 2–4 wk, followed by erythromycin, clarithromycin, doxycycline, or ciprofloxacin orally.	≥3 mo.
Skeletal infections	MAC, *Myobacterium kansasii, M. fortuitum*	Surgical debridement is paramount for treatment and diagnosis. Use species-specific treatment regimens as outlined for other syndromes.	18–24 mo.
Catheter infections	*M. fortuitum, M. chelonae, M. abscessus*	Catheter removal. Initial therapy with amikacin plus cefoxitin, IV for 2–4 wk, followed by erythromycin, clarithromycin, doxycycline, or ciprofloxacin orally.	6–12 wk.
Pulmonary infections	MAC, *M. kansasii, M. abscessus*	Clarithromycin or azithromycin plus ethambutol with rifampin or rifabutin. Extensive disease may require addition of amikacin or streptomycin. Surgical resection may be required. Isoniazid, rifampin, and ethambutol (if HIV infected and on HAART, replace rifampin with rifabutin or clarithromycin).	18–24 mo with at least 12 mo of culture-negative therapy (if rifampin resistant or HIV infected, treat for at least 15 culture-negative mo).
		Clarithromycin, amikacin, and cefoxitin, or a multidrug regimen based on susceptibility testing. May require surgical resection.	6 mo.
Disseminated infections	*Mycobacterium avium–intracellulare* complex	Clarithromycin or azithromycin plus ethambutol. A third and/or fourth agent may be added in severe cases (rifabutin, amikacin, streptomycin, or a fluoroquinolone).	Indefinite.

*Initial therapy with clarithromycin alone or in combination with another agent is successful for infections with *M. chelonae.*
HAART, highly active antiretroviral therapy; HIV, human immunodeficiency virus; IV, intravenous; MAC, *Mycobacterium avium* complex.

12

SKIN, SOFT TISSUE, AND SKELETAL INFECTIONS

Cutaneous infections with NTM occur following local trauma. *Mycobacterium marinum* is the most common cause of localized cutaneous infection. Minor lesions caused by *M. marinum* often require no treatment and can be managed with simple observation. Many of these lesions resolve spontaneously over several months. Persistent or more extensive lesions may require antimicrobial treatment regimens. Rifampin, doxycycline, clarithromycin, or trimethoprim-sulfamethoxazole for a minimum of 3 months is successful. More extensive lesions may require surgical debridement.

Less common causes of cutaneous infections include *Mycobacterium fortuitum, Mycobacterium abscessus,* and *Mycobacterium chelonae.* The most predictable effective therapy for these infections is surgical removal of all involved tissue and any foreign body. Adjuvant antimicrobial therapy is usually recommended for infections with these species. Susceptibility testing may be helpful to guide adjunctive antimicrobial therapy. However, drug susceptibility is not standardized and may not necessarily correlate with clinical outcomes.

The initial antimicrobial therapy should consist of intravenous amikacin and cefoxitin for at least 2 to 4 weeks. When clinical improvement is noted, an oral agent, preferably one to which the organism is susceptible, can be used. Initial therapy with clarithromycin alone or in combination with another agent is successful for infections with *M. chelonae.* The minimum duration of therapy for cutaneous infections is not well defined but should be individualized according to the patient, clinical response, and extent of infection. An extended duration of at least 6 months is usually recommended.

NTM infection of bone, bursa, and tendon sheaths usually results from direct inoculation after penetrating trauma or surgical procedures. The most common agents are *Mycobacterium kansasii, M. fortuitum,* and MAC. Management requires surgical debridement for both diagnosis and therapy. Drug therapy is aimed at the etiologic agents and usually required for a prolonged period (see Table 2).

PULMONARY INFECTIONS

Pulmonary infection with NTM is rare in children. It is described in children with cystic fibrosis and those

TABLE 2 Commonly Used Antimycobacterial Agents

Drug	Dose (mg/kg/day)	Maximum Daily Dose	Route	Adverse Reactions/Comments
Amikacin	7.5–10 qd or 15–20 q8h	1.5 g	IM/IV	Ototoxicity/nephrotoxicity.
Azithromycin	10–20 bid	500 mg	PO/IV	GI disturbance, hepatitis.
Cefoxitin	80–160 q4–6h	12 g	IM/IV	Rash and nephrotoxicity. Some experts recommend administration with probenecid to increase concentration.
Ciprofloxacin	20–30 q12h PO; 10–20 q12h IV	1500 mg PO/800 mg IV	PO/IV	Not FDA approved in children <18 yr for potential risk of arthropathy. Consider risks and benefits. GI upset. CNS toxicity.
Clarithromycin	15–30 q12h	1 g	PO	GI disturbance, hepatitis. Levels can be decreased by rifabutin and some protease inhibitors.
Doxycycline	2–4 q12h	200 mg	PO/IV	GI upset, rash, photosensitivity. May cause tooth enamel hypoplasia and discoloration in children <8 yr, therefore not recommended in this age group unless life-threatening infection without other treatment options.
Erythromycin	40 q6h	4 g	PO	GI disturbance.
Ethambutol	15–25 qd	2.5 g	PO	Optic neuritis, peripheral neuropathy, rash.
Ethionamide	10–20 qd	1	PO	GI disturbances; hepatotoxicity or hypersensitivity reaction.
Isoniazid	10–15 qd	300	PO	Hepatitis, peripheral neuropathy. Supplement with vitamin B_6 if malnourished, chronically ill, pregnant, breast-feeding, or has a meat- or milk-deficient diet.
Rifabutin	5–10 qd	300	PO	
Rifampin	10–20 qd	600	PO/IV	Orange coloration of body fluids; vomiting, hepatitis, thrombocytopenia, or influenza-like illness.
Streptomycin	15 qd or 20–40 q8h for the initial 2–3 mo, then 15 2–3 times per wk	1 g	IM	Ototoxicity/ nephrotoxicity.
Trimethoprim-sulfamethoxazole	8–20 mg of TMP q12h	2 g	PO/IV	Hematologic effects, fever, rash, Stevens-Johnson syndrome.

bid, twice daily; CNS, central nervous system; FDA, Food and Drug Administration; GI, gastrointestinal; IV, intravenous; PO, by mouth; q, every; qd, daily; qxh, every x hours; TMP, trimethoprim.

infected with HIV, but it is also reported in immunocompetent children without underlying pulmonary disease. The most common organism is MAC, with *M. kansasii* and *M. abscessus* causing some disease. Signs and symptoms are not unlike pulmonary tuberculosis (TB) disease. The diagnosis should be suspected in a child who is not responding to treatment for TB disease. The recommended treatment of MAC pulmonary infection consists of clarithromycin or azithromycin with rifampin or rifabutin plus ethambutol. Amikacin or streptomycin can be used in complicated or extensive disease. The duration of therapy is 18 to 24 months and at least 12 months after conversion of sputum cultures to negative. Pulmonary resection may be necessary in some cases and is most successful when disease is localized to one lobe of the lung. Treatment of HIV-negative hosts is usually successfully (60% to 90%), with drug intolerance the major reason for failure.

The recommended treatment for *M. kansasii* is isoniazid, rifampin, and ethambutol. A minimum duration of 18 months, with at least 12 months of culture-negative therapy, is advised. HIV-infected individuals and rifampin-resistant cases should be treated for at least 15 culture-negative months.

M. abscessus pulmonary infections are usually resistant to cure. Six-month regimens consisting of clarithromycin, cefoxitin, and amikacin or a multidrug regimen based on susceptibility testing can produce significant clinical improvements but often do not result in microbiologic eradication. Surgical resection may be indicated.

CATHETER INFECTIONS

Children with long-term central intravenous, peritoneal, or shunt catheters are at risk for NTM infections. The most common species are *M. fortuitum, M. chelonae,* and *M. abscessus.* Successful treatment requires both catheter removal and prolonged antimicrobial therapy (6 to 12 weeks). Catheter tunnel infections often require surgical excision of the tissue surrounding the infected tunnel to prevent recurrence. Initial intravenous therapy with amikacin and cefoxitin for at least the first 2 to 4 weeks is recommended. Imipenem can usually be substituted for isolates resistant to cefoxitin. Tobramycin is more active in vitro than amikacin against *M. chelonae.* When clinical improvement is noted and susceptibilities are available, the regimen can be switched to a susceptible oral agent.

DISSEMINATED INFECTIONS

Disseminated infections with NTM almost exclusively occur in children with impaired cell-mediated immunity. The most common cause of disseminated disease, particularly those infected with HIV, is MAC, which occurs at a higher CD4 cell count among younger HIV-infected children than older children or adults. The common symptoms include recurrent fever, weight loss or failure to thrive, neutropenia, night sweats, fatigue, chronic diarrhea, malabsorption, and abdominal pain. Treatment of disseminated MAC should be done in consultation with an expert in pediatric HIV. Combination therapy with a minimum of two drugs is recommended. Clarithromycin or azithromycin plus ethambutol is the preferred initial regimen. In patients with severe symptoms, some experts add a third and, in some situations, a fourth agent to the regimen (rifabutin, amikacin, streptomycin, or a fluoroquinolone). Coadministration of rifabutin with highly active anti-retroviral therapy (HAART) drugs metabolized by the cytochrome P enzyme may require dose adjustments. Clofazimine is not effective and should not be used for MAC disease. The empirical regimen can be adjusted according to the results of in vitro susceptibility testing.

Clinical improvement may take 4 to 6 weeks, but it may take up to 12 weeks to eliminate the organism from the blood. Antiretroviral therapy should be optimized. Options for patients who fail multidrug macrolide-containing regimens are very limited. Despite the presence of macrolide resistance, most experts suggest continuation of a macrolide because macrolide-sensitive organisms are likely to be present. The addition of at least two new agents in the salvage setting is desirable. Current guidelines recommend lifetime chronic suppressive dual-maintenance therapy for MAC among HIV-infected children after recovery from MAC disease. However, discontinuation of such secondary prophylaxis is safe in adults receiving HAART after immunologic recovery.

PROPHYLAXIS

Prophylaxis against MAC should be offered to HIV-infected children at risk for developing primary MAC disease. This risk is determined by CD4+ cell count and varies with age. Monotherapy with either azithromycin or clarithromycin is the recommended regimen. Rifabutin is an acceptable alternative but should not be used unless tuberculosis is excluded. A blood culture for MAC should be obtained prior to beginning the prophylaxis to exclude disseminated MAC. MAC prophylaxis is recommended for children with the following CD4+ cell thresholds: children older than 6 years, less than 50 CD4+ cells per mm^3; those 2 to 6 years old, 75 CD4+ cells per mm^3; those 1 to 2 years old, less than 500 CD4+ cells per mm^3; and children younger than 12 months, 750 CD4+ cells per mm^3. The discontinuation of primary prophylaxis in HIV-infected adults with immune recovery is safe; however, the safety of discontinuing primary MAC prophylaxis in similar children has not been studied.

Common Pitfalls

Most strains of NTM are resistant to the most common first-line antituberculosis agents. NTMs demonstrate in vitro susceptibility to many individual drugs within various classes; however, they have a propensity to develop drug resistance during monotherapy. Choosing an active multidrug regimen is particularly challenging because drug susceptibility testing is not standardized and may not necessarily correlate with clinical outcomes. Moreover, the multidrug treatment courses are prolonged, with often undefined duration, and they are fraught with adverse reactions, drug-drug interactions, and poor adherence to treatment that compromise a successful outcome. For the HIV-infected child, failure to initiate prophylaxis when recommended can lead to development of disseminated infection.

Communication and Counseling

Children with NTM infections often require surgical intervention as part of their diagnostic and therapeutic management. Parents should to be educated about the need for surgery and the associated complications. The importance of prolonged multidrug adjunctive antimicrobial treatment must be explained to the caregivers. In addition, they should be aware that susceptibility testing and/or clinical outcome may warrant changing the antimicrobials over time.

SUGGESTED READINGS

1. Albright JT, Pransky SM: Nontuberculous mycobacterial infections of the head and neck. Pediatri Clin North Am 50:503–514, 2003. **Detailed review of NTM lymphadenitis in children.**
2. American Academy of Pediatrics: Nontuberculous *Mycobacteria*. In Pickering LK (ed): 2003 Red Book: Report of the Committee on Infectious Diseases, 26th ed. Elk Grove Village, Ill: American Academy of Pediatrics, 2003, pp 642–660. **Governmental recommendations for treatment of NTMs in children.**
3. American Thoracic Society: Diagnosis and treatment of disease caused by nontuberculous *Mycobacteria*. Am Rev Respir Dis 156 (Suppl.):1–25, 1997. **Official statement guidelines for NTM infections by the American Thoracic Society.**
4. Saiman L: The mycobacteriology of non-tuberculous mycobacteria. Paediatr Respir Rev 5(Suppl. A):S221–S223, 2004. **Brief review of the mycobacteriology of NTM.**

Bordetella pertussis (Whooping Cough)

James D. Cherry and Rick E. Harrison

KEY CONCEPTS

- Pertussis occurs in association with both primary infection and reinfections with *Bordetella pertussis*.
- The clinical manifestations of pertussis in young infants are often not recognized as caused by *B. pertussis* infection, and therefore specific treatment is delayed.
- The usual source of infection in infants is an adult family member who has a cough illness not recognized as caused by *B. pertussis* infection.

12

KEY CONCEPTS—cont'd

- The prophylactic use of macrolide antibiotics is highly effective in preventing pertussis in unimmunized infants.
- Treatment of *B. pertussis* infections with macrolide antibiotics early in their course (catarrhal stage and the beginning of the paroxysmal stage) shortens the illness.
- Treatment of full-blown pertussis has little effect on its severity or duration but decreases the risk of spread of *B. pertussis* to contacts.
- The reservoir of *B. pertussis* is its endemic presence as cough illnesses in adolescents and adults.
- Present multicomponent Tdap (tetanus toxoids, diphtheria, and acellular pertussis) vaccines, which contain pertactin, are effective in controlling pertussis in children.
- Multicomponent Tdap vaccines for adolescents and adults, if universally used, will decrease adolescent and adult pertussis and the spread of *B. pertussis* to infants.

Whooping cough (pertussis) is a highly contagious, acute infectious illness of the respiratory tract caused by *Bordetella pertussis*. Similar illness can also occasionally be caused by these other related species: *Bordetella parapertussis*, *Bordetella holmesii*, and *Bordetella bronchiseptica*. Effective pertussis vaccines have been available for more than 60 years, and the rate of pertussis is dramatically reduced in populations in which the vaccines are used universally to immunize children.

Immunity against *B. pertussis* infection and illness, whether the result of vaccination or natural infection, is not long lasting, so both primary infections and reinfections occur regularly. Clinical manifestations of infection vary by age and by previous experience with the organism (i.e., vaccination or infection).

Classic pertussis occurs in children between 1 and 10 years of age as a primary infection. It is a three-stage illness (catarrhal, paroxysmal, and convalescent) that lasts 4 to 12 weeks. The specific manifestations are paroxysmal cough, lack of significant fever, no systemic illness, coryza but no significant pharyngitis, post-tussive vomiting, post-tussive whoop, and leukocytosis with an absolute lymphocytosis. Approximately 18% to 25% of primary infections result in milder cough illnesses, which last approximately 21 days or less. Common complications of classic pertussis include pneumonia (primary *B. pertussis* infection or secondary infection with other bacteria), otitis media, seizures, and encephalopathy.

Pertussis in infancy, particularly in neonates, is frequently severe. Apnea is common and seizures caused by hypoxia are common; pneumonia is frequent and severe, and often pulmonary hypertension occurs. Pulmonary hypertension in association with extreme leukocytosis with a marked lymphocytosis is a common finding in neonates and young infants who die from *B. pertussis* infection. The etiology of pulmonary hypertension in pertussis is unclear. Leukocyte thrombi were found in the pulmonary vascular system in a fatal case, which leads to the suggestion that leukocyte plugging may be responsible for the hypertension. Several *B. pertussis* toxins (adenylate cyclase toxin, pertussis toxin, and tracheal cytotoxin) may have a role in pathogenesis.

Prolonged cough illnesses caused by *B. pertussis* infection are common in adults, and these illnesses are most often not recognized as pertussis. These coughing adults are a frequent source of infection in infants.

In spite of a continued high level of immunization of children in the United States, the rate of reported pertussis has increased over the last two decades. This is because of a greater awareness of pertussis and perhaps also the use of some less-efficacious vaccines between 1985 and the present.

Primary infection with *B. parapertussis* in children produces an illness similar to that caused by *B. pertussis*. However, the severity of illness caused by *B. parapertussis* is less than that caused by *B. pertussis* infection, and the duration is somewhat shorter.

Expert Opinion on Management Issues

DIAGNOSIS

Table 1 reviews the diagnosis of pertussis. The hallmark for the diagnosis is a positive culture from a nasopharyngeal specimen. This specimen is collected by either nasopharyngeal aspiration or a specific nasopharyngeal swab with a flexible wire shaft and a calcium alginate fiber tip. Nasal wash specimens are also often used, but dilution reduces their sensitivity. Throat cultures and nasal cultures are not satisfactory for the recovery of *B. pertussis*. The specimen for culture should be plated on Regan-Lowe agar (or other specific media) immediately or placed in Regan-Lowe transport medium and then shipped to the laboratory. The main reason for the failure to isolate *B. pertussis* from a case seen within 2 weeks of illness onset is improper collection of the specimen (failure to touch the ciliated epithelium of the pharyngeal wall with the swab or catheter).

TABLE 1 Criteria for Diagnosis of Pertussis

Clinical characteristics (paroxysmal cough illness of ≥2 weeks' duration with no or minimal fever)

Leukocytosis ($>11,100/mm^3$) with absolute lymphocytosis ($>6300/mm^3$)

Positive DFA on nasopharyngeal specimen

Positive culture or PCR on nasopharyngeal specimen

Demonstration of a significant titer rise of IgG antibody to PT between an acute-phase and convalescent-phase serum specimen by ELISA

Demonstration by ELISA of a significantly high single–IgG antibody titer to PT in adolescents, adults, and children who have not received a pertussis immunization within the previous one year

DFA, direct fluorescent antibody; ELISA, enzyme-linked immunosorbent assay; Ig, immunoglobulin; PCR, polymerase chain reaction; PT, pertussis toxin.

Direct fluorescent antibody (DFA) testing of nasopharyngeal specimens is used for rapid diagnosis of *B. pertussis* infection, but this method lacks both sensitivity and specificity. Today many laboratories use polymerase chain reaction (PCR), which is rapid, more sensitive than culture, and when rigidly controlled has good specificity. Many laboratories now only use PCR without backup culture. Although this is generally satisfactory, clinically it is less than optimal because it does not allow the study of organisms for antibiotic resistance or for epidemiologic purposes.

As noted in Table 1, *B. pertussis* infection can be diagnosed by enzyme-linked immunosorbent assay (ELISA) by the detection of immunoglobulin G (IgG) antibody to pertussis toxin (PT). The most practical test is the use of a high single-serum titer, which is offered in some commercial laboratories.

ANTIMICROBIAL THERAPY

The mainstay of antimicrobial treatment over the last 30 years is oral erythromycin (Table 2). Treatment during the catarrhal stage and early paroxysmal stage of illness shortens the duration of symptoms, whereas initiation of therapy later in the paroxysmal stage usually does not benefit the patient. However, all patients should be treated to shorten the period of individual contagiousness.

One large study suggests a 7-day course of erythromycin is as effective as a 14-day course. In neonates, the use of erythromycin occasionally is associated with the occurrence of hypertrophic pyloric stenosis. *B. pertussis* strains resistant to erythromycin have been noted on very rare occasions. These strains were also resistant to other macrolides but sensitive to trimethoprim-sulfamethoxazole.

Trimethoprim-sulfamethoxazole is recommended for use in children who cannot tolerate erythromycin or in situations of demonstrated resistance. Trimethoprim-sulfamethoxazole is not recommended for first-line treatment because it has not been studied adequately.

Azithromycin and clarithromycin are also effective for the treatment of pertussis. Because most adolescents and adults do not tolerate erythromycin well, we suggest using either azithromycin or clarithromycin to treat these older patients.

The treatment of patients infected with *B. parapertussis* or *B. holmesii* is the same as already described for *B. pertussis* infections. *B. bronchiseptica* infections can be treated with trimethoprim-sulfamethoxazole because this species is likely to be resistant to erythromycin.

OTHER THERAPY

The mainstay of supportive care is the avoidance of factors that provoke attacks of coughing. These factors include a noisy environment, unnecessary examination, strangers, excessive brightness of room lighting, noxious odors, and the supine position. Because vomiting is a problem and food intake stimulates coughing episodes, careful attention to adequate hydration and nutrition is necessary. Patients are sometimes treated with corticosteroids or salbutamol, but no evidence indicates efficacy for either modality, and the former increases the risk of secondary infections.

In the hospital, tenacious secretions should be removed by gentle suction. Well-humidified oxygen should be administered to patients with pneumonia and significant respiratory distress. Therapy for the respiratory and cardiovascular failure seen with severe pertussis in infants has limited success with high mortality rates, despite the use of pulmonary artery vasodilators and even extracorporeal membrane oxygenation (ECMO). A review of all pediatric patients placed on ECMO revealed a mortality rate of more than 70%. A single case report used a double volume exchange transfusion to reduce the leukocyte load with subsequent improvement in oxygenation and survival. Current therapy should include meticulous ventilatory management to avoid ventilator-induced lung injury and consideration of leukocyte-reducing measures such as exchange transfusion. Nitric oxide may be used, although response is variable. High doses of vasopressors may be required for the vascular failure seen in severe pertussis. ECMO may be considered if contraindications do not exist, although overall survival remains poor.

ISOLATION AND PROPHYLACTIC MEASURES

Close contacts of patients (household members, those in daycare centers, playmates) should be protected from infection by the administration of erythromycin for 14 days. This regimen should be started as soon after exposure as possible and is highly effective. The index case must be treated promptly to shorten communicability and therefore limit the spread of

---

TABLE 2 Antimicrobial Agents for the Treatment and Prevention* of Pertussis

Children

Erythromycin[†]: 40–50 mg/kg/day for 14 days q6h (max dose 2 g/day)
Azithromycin: 10 mg/kg day 1, 5 mg/kg days 2–5 as single dose/day (max 500 mg day 1, 250 mg days 2–5)
Clarithromycin: 15–20 mg/kg in 2 divided doses for 7 days (max dose 1g/day)
Trimethoprim-sulfamethoxazole: 8–12 mg/kg trimethoprim, 40–60 mg/kg sulfamethoxazole /day in 2 doses for 14 days (max dose 320 mg of trimethoprim)

Adults

Azithromycin: 500 mg day 1, 250 mg days 2–5 as single dose/day
Clarithromycin: 1 g/day in 2 divided doses for 7 days
Trimethoprim-sulfamethoxazole: 320 mg trimethoprim, 1.6 g sulfamethoxazole/day in 2 doses for 14 days

---

max, maximum; q*x*h, every *x* hours.
*Prophylactic dose is the same as the treatment dose.
[†]Recent data suggest that a 7-day treatment course is effective.

TABLE 3 Composition of Three Dtap Vaccines for Children Currently Available in the United States

Vaccine (Trade name)	*B. pertussis* Antigens (μg/dose)				Aluminum (mg/dose)	Preservative	Diphtheria Toxoid*	Tetanus Toxoid*
	PT	FHA	PRN	FIM				
Tripedia	23.4	23.4			0.17	Thimerosal	6.7	5
Infanrix†	25	25	8		0.50	Phenoxyethanol	25	10
Daptacel	10	5	3	5	0.33	Phenoxyethanol	15	5

*Limit of flocculation per dose.
†Also available as Pediarix, a Dtap, inactivated poliovirus, and hepatitus B combination vaccine.
Dtap, diphtheria, tetanus toxoid, and acellular pertussis; FHA, filamentous hemagglutinin; FIM, fimbriae 2,3; PRN, pertactin; PT, (toxoid) pertussis toxin.

infection. Immunization of children younger than 7 years who have not completed their vaccination series for pertussis should also be carried out.

For adults it is better to use azithromycin or clarithromycin for prophylaxis because these antibiotics are better tolerated than erythromycin. An alternative approach for adult contacts is to follow them closely and only treat with macrolides at the first sign of respiratory illness.

IMMUNIZATION

Pertussis can be well controlled by the universal use of pertussis vaccines in infants and children. Up-to-date recommendations for pertussis immunization are available form the Committee on Infectious Diseases of the American Academy of Pediatrics and the Advisory Committee on Immunization Practices (ACIP) of the Centers for Disease Control and Prevention. These recommending groups present a complete discussion of indications, schedules, vaccine reactions, and contraindications and therefore the information is not included here.

At present, three Tdap (diphtheria, tetanus toxoids, and acellular pertussis [adsorbed]) vaccines for children are available in the United States (Table 3). These three vaccines vary in the number of *B. pertussis* htheria toxoid they contain, as well as other minor differences.

Of the three vaccines, only Infanrix and Daptacel contain pertactin. Data indicate that multicomponent Tdap vaccines that contain pertactin are more efficacious than Tdap vaccines with only PT or PT and FHA (filamentous hemagglutinin).

The recommendation for Tdap vaccines for children in the United States currently consists of a five-dose schedule, with doses at 2, 4, 6, and 12 to 20 months and 4 to 6 years of age. The efficacy of Infanrix and Daptacel following the first three doses against mild as well as typical pertussis is approximately 75%. The reactogenicity of these two vaccines after each of the first three doses is mild and similar. Local redness and induration after booster doses tend to be greater in Infanrix recipients compared with Daptacel recipients. Contraindications for further doses of Tdap vaccines are the occurrence of an immediate anaphylactic reaction or encephalopathy within 7 days of vaccine administration.

Two adolescent and adult Tdap vaccines are available in the United States. Boostrix contains 2.5 Lf (flocculation units) diphtheria toxoid, 5.0 Lf tetanus toxoid, 8.0 μg PT toxoid, 8.0 μg FHA, and 2.5 μg PRN (pertactin) per dose; it is approved for preadolescents and adolescents 10 through 18 years of age. Adacel contains 2 Lf diphtheria toxoid, 5 Lf tetanus toxoid, 2.5 μg PT toxoid, 5 μg FHA, 3 μg PRN, and 5 μg FIM (fimbriae 2,3) per dose; it is approved for adolescents and adults 11 through 64 years of age. The widespread use of these vaccines will decrease the spread of pertussis from adolescents and adults to unprotected infants.

Common Pitfalls

- Failure to recognize the common occurrence of atypical pertussis in adolescents and adults as the source of infection in unimmunized infants.
- Failure to diagnose pertussis in neonates because the presenting findings of apnea and seizures lead to other etiologic considerations.
- Failure to obtain proper specimens for culture.
- Hospitalized infants seem to improve and are often discharged home too soon, which often leads to severe episodes of coughing with hypoxia and readmission to the hospital.

SUGGESTED READINGS

1. Cherry JD, Heininger U: Pertussis other *Bordetella* infections. In Feigin RD, Cherry JD Demmler GJ, Kaplan S (eds): Textbook of Pediatric Infectious Diseases, 5th ed. Philadelphia: WB Saunders, 2004, pp 1588–1608. **Detailed review of all aspects of pertussis.**
2. Cherry JD, Olin P: Commentaries: The science and fiction of pertussis vaccines. Pediatrics 104:1381–1384, 1999. **Indicates misconceptions relating to vaccine efficacy and serologic correlates of immunity.**
3. Halasa NB, Barr FE, Johnson J, et al: Fatal pulmonary hypertension associated with pertussis in infants: Does extracorporeal membrane oxygenation have a role? Pediatrics 112:1274–1278, 2003. **Describes aspects of pulmonary hypertension in pertussis in infants.**
4. Mattoo S, Cherry JD: Molecular pathogenesis, epidemiology, and clinical manifestations of respiratory infections due to *Bordetella pertussis* and other *Bordetella* subspecies. Clin Microbiol Rev (in press). **Up-to-date complete review of all aspects of *Bordetella* species.**

5. Romano MJ, Weber MD, Weisse ME, et al: Pertussis pneumonia, hypoxemia, hyperleukocytosis, pulmonary hypertension: Improvement in oxygenation after a double volume exchange transfusion. Pediatrics 114:264–266, 2004. **Speculates on the role of hyperleukocytosis in pulmonary hypertension.**

Staphylococcal Infections

Susan E. Crawford and Robert S. Daum

KEY CONCEPTS

- Approximately 30% of people are colonized by *Staphylococcus aureus.*
- Community-acquired methicillin-resistant *S. aureus* (CA-MRSA) is now responsible for the majority of community *S. aureus* infections in many geographic locales.
- β-Lactams can no longer be considered empirical therapy for suspected *S. aureus* infections in many centers.
- Culture and susceptibility testing is necessary to assess methicillin susceptibility and guide therapy for *S. aureus* infections.

Staphylococcus aureus is a major pathogen that causes a wide spectrum of community and nosocomial infections and toxinoses. Asymptomatic nasal or skin colonization of *S. aureus* occurs in about 30% to 40% of healthy children. Several other staphylococcal species, such as *Staphylococcus epidermidis,* are human commensals and cause occasional clinical concern by persistently adhering to devices such as indwelling venous catheters and prosthetic cardiac valves.

A wide spectrum of clinical disease can be attributed to *S. aureus.* Mucosal or skin injury allows *S. aureus* to cause localized skin and soft tissue infection or invasive disease. The species causes skin and soft tissue, ocular, respiratory, intravascular, bone and joint infections, as well as necrotizing fasciitis, central nervous system infections, shock, and disseminated intravascular coagulation. Additionally, toxic shock syndrome, staphylococcal scalded skin syndrome, and food poisoning syndromes may be mediated by *S. aureus* toxins.

Nearly all *S. aureus* isolates have a plasmid encoding β-lactamase that mediates resistance to penicillin and other compounds like amoxicillin that are hydrolyzed by that enzyme. Semisynthetic penicillins, such as methicillin, oxacillin, and cephalosporins, are relatively resistant to β-lactamase–mediated hydrolysis and until recently could be relied on for empirical treatment of most community-acquired *S. aureus* infections. These β-lactams work by binding to a penicillin-binding protein, thus inhibiting bacterial peptidoglycan (cell wall) synthesis. Methicillin-resistant *Staphylococcus aureus* (MRSA) isolates appeared in the 1960s and 1970s and increased in frequency largely in hospital environments, where they now account for the majority of nosocomial *S. aureus* infections, including ventilator-associated pneumonia, bacteremia associated with intravascular devices, and postoperative wound infections.

The term *MRSA* implies resistance to all β-lactam antibiotics, including penicillins and cephalosporins. MRSA isolates produce a penicillin-binding protein called PBP2a that has a low affinity for β-lactams. In the presence of PBP2a, bacterial cell wall synthesis can proceed even when β-lactams are present. Vancomycin has become the drug most often used to treat hospital-acquired MRSA (HA-MRSA) infections and is termed the "antibiotic of last resort." The recent emergence of vancomycin-intermediate *S. aureus* (VISA) and vancomycin-resistant *S. aureus* (VRSA) isolates has led to new challenges in the treatment of MRSA infections.

At many centers the epidemiology of MRSA has changed. Once confined to people with known risk factors, including recent hospitalization, surgery, or chronic disease, MRSA now appears in the community in healthy people with no known MRSA risk factors. Although some community-acquired MRSA (CA-MRSA) infections represent so-called hospital MRSA strains migrating into the community, new CA-MRSA strains are now recognized that have distinct molecular features and antibiotic-resistance profiles. These CA-MRSA isolates are frequently susceptible to non–β-lactam antimicrobials, including clindamycin, trimethoprim-sulfamethoxazole, and tetracycline; they cause a disease spectrum similar to community-acquired methicillin-susceptible *S. aureus* (CA-MSSA) disease. Previously healthy children frequently present with CA-MRSA skin infections, such as boils or abscesses, or more serious infections, such as osteomyelitis, pyomyositis, necrotizing pneumonia, and sepsis. Surveillance at Texas Children's Hospital in Houston revealed that both the absolute number of *S. aureus* infections and the proportion of MRSA infections increased in the years 2001 to 2004. At this hospital and others, MRSA now accounts for more than 70% of all community-acquired *S. aureus* infections. The recent emergence and rapid increase in CA-MRSA prevalence has led to greater complexity in the treatment of suspected *S. aureus* community-acquired infections in children.

Expert Opinion on Management Issues

Table 1 summarizes the syndrome-specific antimicrobial treatment of *S. aureus* infections. Because CA-MRSA is an increasingly frequent cause of infections in previously healthy children, providers can no longer assume that suspected *S. aureus* infections are caused by β-lactam–susceptible organisms. Because the CA-MRSA epidemic has not affected all areas equally, practitioners must now monitor their community *S. aureus* ecology. Local resistance rates can be tracked by monitoring hospital clinical microbiology laboratory reports and outbreaks investigated by local public health departments. Culture of the infection site to identify the causative isolate and its antibiotic susceptibility is strongly recommended. Empirical antibiotic treatment should reflect the local rate of methicillin resistance and the clinical consequences of choosing suboptimal therapy transiently before culture results are known.

METHICILLIN-SUSCEPTIBLE *STAPHYLOCOCCUS AUREUS*

Infections caused by MSSA isolates are best treated with a β-lactamase–resistant β-lactam, such as oxacillin, nafcillin, cloxacillin, or dicloxacillin, or a first-generation cephalosporin, such as cefazolin or cephalexin. Appropriate β-lactams are available for intravenous and oral administration; β-lactams are generally well tolerated, although the oral formulations have a poor taste. Dose- and duration-related neutropenia can occur with β-lactam use but are reversible when the drug is discontinued. β-Lactams are more bactericidal than vancomycin in the treatment of MSSA infections and are preferred agents once it is known that the isolate is susceptible.

TABLE 1 Treatment of *Staphylococcus aureus* Syndromes

Syndrome	Empirical Antibiotic Treatment Recommendations in Areas with High CA-MRSA Prevalence	Empirical Antibiotic Treatment Recommendations in Areas with Low CA-MRSA Prevalence	Other Treatments
Skin and Soft Tissue Infection			
Impetigo	Topical mupirocin if uncomplicated, tid × 7 days; if complicated or widespread, PO or IV clindamycin × 7 days.	Topical bacitracin if uncomplicated, tid × 7 days; if complicated or widespread, PO or IV β-lactam × 7 days.	Washing and good hygiene to prevent spread.
Abscess	In uncomplicated cases, particularly when the abscess is small, antibiotics may not be necessary after incision and drainage; if antibiotic treatment is required, Clindamycin PO/IV tid × 10 days. TMP-SMX and doxycycline are used with success.	If antibiotic treatment is required, oxacillin or cefazolin IV or dicloxacillin or cephalexin PO × 10 days.	Incision and drainage is an important component of therapy.
Cellulitis	Clindamycin IV/PO for uncomplicated cases.	Oxacillin or cefazolin IV with transition to dicloxacillin or cephalexin PO.	
Conjunctivitis	Topical sulfacetamide drops; avoid quinolones because resistance develops readily. Many isolates resistant to erythromycin, especially MRSA.	Topical sulfacetamide drops because many MSSA isolates are resistant to erythromycin.	
Invasive Syndromes			
Catheter-associated intravascular infection	Vancomycin.	Oxacillin/nafcillin.	Removal of catheter.
Endocarditis	Vancomycin (some experts add gentamicin for 5–14 days after diagnosis).	Oxacillin (some experts add gentamicin for 5–14 days after diagnosis).	Surgical intervention may be needed if clinical response inadequate.
Osteomyelitis	Clindamycin/vancomycin.	Oxacillin.	May need surgical debridement in complicated cases.
Septic arthritis	Clindamycin/vancomycin.	Oxacillin.	Drainage of joint effusion, emergently for hip involvement.
Pneumonia	Vancomycin.	Oxacillin.	May need thoracentesis, decortication for empyema.
Sepsis	Vancomycin + (?) clindamycin	Oxacillin.	Supportive treatment, pressors, (?) IVIG.
Toxinoses			
Toxic shock syndrome	Vancomycin ± clindamycin to inhibit protein synthesis.	Oxacillin ± clindamycin.	Supportive treatment, pressors if needed. IVIG often used, although benefit unproven.

CA-MRSA, community-acquired methicillin-resistant *Staphylococcus aureus*; IV, intravenous; IVIG, intravenous immunoglobulin; MSSA, methicillin-resistant *Staphylococcus aureus*; PO, by mouth; tid, three times per day; TMP-SMX, trimethoprim-sulfamethoxazole; (?), unproven therapy.

HOSPITAL-ACQUIRED METHICILLIN-RESISTANT *STAPHYLOCOCCUS AUREUS*

Infections caused by HA-MRSA often require treatment with intravenous vancomycin, a compound that binds to precursor peptidoglycan and thereby prevents bacterial cell wall synthesis. Vancomycin is generally well tolerated but requires serum level monitoring, especially when used with other nephrotoxic agents. An infusion-related syndrome called *red man syndrome* is characterized by flushing, pruritus, chest pain, muscle spasms, and occasionally hypotension. It can almost always be managed by slowing the rate of infusion or pretreating with antihistamines (diphenhydramine or hydroxyzine). Ototoxicity is attributed to vancomycin but is rarely well documented and is probably associated with older preparations. Nephrotoxicity is almost always reversible; preexisting renal failure may worsen. There is no vancomycin preparation for intramuscular administration, and oral vancomycin is not absorbed. Vancomycin–intermediate resistant strains and vancomycin-resistant strains have emerged and probably occur more frequently than is recognized because clinical laboratories seldom perform optimal testing to detect them.

BEYOND VANCOMYCIN

Linezolid is a new oxazolidinone antibiotic that inhibits bacterial protein synthesis. It is approved for treatment of MRSA infections such as skin and soft tissue infections or pneumonia in children. Linezolid is probably not effective in the prevention or treatment of endocarditis. Available for intravenous or oral administration, it is well tolerated, with nausea, vomiting, and diarrhea occasionally observed. Leukopenia, anemia, and thrombocytopenia can occur, and leukocyte, hemoglobin, and platelet counts should be monitored weekly. Its good absorption makes it useful once a patient is clinically stable and able to take oral medication. Linezolid is very expensive and not routinely stocked at many pharmacies. Table 2 lists additional newer options for the treatment of *S. aureus* infections.

Daptomycin has received no evaluation in children and cannot be used to treat pneumonia; only a parenteral form is available.

COAGULASE-NEGATIVE STAPHYLOCOCCI

Coagulase-negative staphylococci (CoNS), such as *S. epidermidis,* are generally more resistant than *S. aureus,* and in clinical situations such as central catheter–associated bacteremia or endocarditis, treatment with vancomycin is often required. Rifampin and gentamicin may be added as initial therapy if endocarditis seems likely.

COMMUNITY-ACQUIRED METHICILLIN-RESISTANT *STAPHYLOCOCCUS AUREUS*

The emergence of CA-MRSA isolates presents new dilemmas in choosing antibiotic therapy for suspected staphylococcal infections. Because CA-MRSA isolates are often susceptible to non–β-lactam antibiotics, older antibiotics, such as clindamycin, trimethoprim-sulfamethoxazole, and tetracyclines, are used to treat CA-MRSA infections, the last in children older than approximately 9 years. The use of the bacteriostatic agent clindamycin requires consideration of possible resistance even when an isolate tests susceptible. To address this possibility, clinical microbiology laboratories now perform a D test when an MRSA isolate is susceptible to clindamycin but resistant to erythromycin. A positive D test suggests that clindamycin may select resistant strains in vivo, and treatment failure may therefore occur. Clindamycin should probably not be used to treat *S. aureus* endocarditis. Studies evaluating and comparing the efficacy of clindamycin, trimethoprim-sulfamethoxazole, and other antibiotics in treatment of CA-MRSA in children have not been performed.

TOXIN-MEDIATED DISEASE

Many experts advocate clindamycin as primary or adjunctive therapy in the treatment of presumed

TABLE 2 Antimicrobials Used in Treatment of *Staphylococcus aureus* Infections

Antimicrobial	Mechanism of Action	Target
β-Lactams	Bind to penicillin binding protein, arrest cell wall synthesis	MSSA
Trimethoprim-sulfamethoxazole	Inhibits synthesis of dihydrofolic acid	MSSA, CA-MRSA
Clindamycin	Arrests protein synthesis	MSSA, CA-MRSA; possible benefit in toxin-mediated disease
Vancomycin	Inhibits bacterial cell wall synthesis	MSSA, HA-MRSA, CA-MRSA
Linezolid	Prevents formation of 70S initiation complex for translation; arrests protein synthesis	MSSA, HA-MRSA, CA-MRSA; possible benefit in toxin-mediated disease
Daptomycin	Binds to bacterial cell membrane and causes depolarization of membrane potential; indirectly inhibits protein, DNA, and RNA synthesis	MSSA, HA-MRSA, VISA, VRSA
Quinupristin/dalfopristin	Arrests protein synthesis	MSSA; possible benefit in toxin-mediated disease

CA-MRSA, community-acquired methicillin-resistant *Staphylococcus aureus*; HA-MRSA, hospital-acquired methicillin-resistant *Staphylococcus aureus*; MSSA, methicillin-resistant *Staphylococcus aureus*; VISA, vancomycin-intermediate *Staphylococcus aureus*; VRSA, vancomycin-resistant *Staphylococcus aureus*.

toxin-mediated *S. aureus* diseases such as toxic shock syndrome and sepsis. This approach has theoretical benefit because clindamycin inhibits protein synthesis and may therefore decrease toxin production. Additionally, some experts believe that pooled intravenous immunoglobulin (IVIG) may contain antibodies directed against *S. aureus* toxins, and these antibodies can bind and neutralize toxins. In vivo data are not available.

Common Pitfalls

Clinicians are strongly encouraged to monitor the local prevalence of CA-MRSA to guide empirical therapy; empirical antibiotic therapy should target MRSA in a child with skin and soft tissue infection, severe pneumonia, or sepsis in areas where CA-MRSA has become prevalent.

When isolated from blood, *S. aureus* should not be considered a procedural contaminant. Bacteremia may be transient, and *S. aureus* can seed multiple organs if not treated aggressively.

Communication and Counseling

Many healthy children carry *S. aureus* in the nose, and most infections occur with the endogenous strain. At this time, eradication of nasal carriage cannot be routinely recommended. Hand washing and wound site hygiene are the best current measures to prevent wound infections and transmission of *S. aureus*. Decolonization with intranasal mupirocin is occasionally attempted in patients with recurrent MRSA infections, but long-term success rates are not encouraging. Body washes used to eradicate MSSA from the skin, such as chlorhexidine, are probably even less successful in decolonizing MRSA. Some experts use both modalities to attempt decolonization, but the low success rate limits such attempts to selected cases. The antibody response to *S. aureus* infections is not well characterized, and infection by the same organism can recur.

SUGGESTED READINGS

1. Herold BC, Immergluck LC, Maranan MC, et al: Community-acquired methicillin-resistant *Staphylococcus aureus* in children with no identified predisposing risk. JAMA 279:593–598, 1998. **One of the first papers to describe clinical features of community-acquired MRSA and its appearance in children without risk.**
2. Jain A, Daum RS: Staphylococcal infections in children: Part 1. Pediatr Rev 20:183–191, 1999. **Introduces the epidemiology, pathogenesis, host defenses, and infectious syndromes of *S. aureus*.**
3. Jain A, Daum RS: Staphylococcal infections in children: Part 2. Pediatr Rev 20:219–227, 1999. **The second part of this series of review details clinical infections of *S. aureus* and coagulase-negative staphylococci.**
4. Jain A, Daum RS: Staphylococcal infections in children: Part 3. Pediatr Rev 20:261–265, 1999. **The third part of this series of reviews *S. aureus* toxinoses and treatment of *S. aureus* infections.**
5. Kaplan SL, Hulten KG, Gonzalez BE, et al: Three-year surveillance of community-acquired *Staphylococcus aureus* infections in children. Clin Infect Dis 40:1785–1791, 2005. **Documents the increase in both the absolute number of *S. aureus* infections and the proportion of those caused by CA-MRSA in a children's hospital.**
6. Lowy FD: Staphylococcus aureus infections. N Engl J Med 339:520–532, 1998. **Comprehensive review on the pathophysiology and clinical features of *S. aureus* infections.**
7. Naimi TS, LeDell KH, Borchardt SM, et al: Comparison of community- and health care-associated methicillin-resistant *Staphylococcus aureus* infection. JAMA 290:2976–2984, 2003. **Compares the clinical syndromes, antibiotic susceptibility, genotypes, and toxin gene presence of community-acquired MRSA with hospital-acquired MRSA.**

Group A Streptococcal Infections

Michael A. Gerber

KEY CONCEPTS

- The diagnosis of group A β-hemolytic streptococcal (GABHS) pharyngitis should be suspected on clinical and epidemiologic grounds and then supported by performance of a throat culture or rapid antigen detection test (RADT).
- A negative RADT result should be confirmed with a throat culture result unless the physician has determined in his or her own practice that the RADT used is comparable to a throat culture.
- Antimicrobial therapy for patients with GABHS pharyngitis can prevent acute rheumatic fever, suppurative sequelae, and transmission to close contacts, and it can shorten the clinical course.
- On the basis of its narrow spectrum of antimicrobial activity, the infrequency with which it produces adverse reactions, and its modest cost, penicillin is the drug of choice for the treatment of patients with GABHS pharyngitis who are not allergic to it.
- The majority of asymptomatic patients who have GABHS remaining in their upper respiratory tract after completing a course of appropriate antimicrobial therapy are streptococcal carriers.

Group A β-hemolytic streptococci (GABHS), also known as *Streptococcus pyogenes*, are among the most common pathogenic bacteria isolated from children. They are associated with a wide variety of infections and disease states and are the most common cause of bacterial pharyngitis. GABHS are also the cause of two potentially serious nonsuppurative complications, rheumatic fever and acute glomerulonephritis, that may occur after uncomplicated infections.

Human beings are the natural reservoir for GABHS. These bacteria are highly communicable and can cause disease in normal individuals of all ages who do not have type-specific immunity against the particular serotype involved. Disease in neonates is uncommon, probably because of maternally acquired antibodies. The incidence of GABHS pharyngitis is highest in children older than 3 years, especially in young school-age children. GABHS pharyngitis occurs most often in the northern regions of the United States, especially during the winter and early spring. Children with untreated acute pharyngitis spread GABHS by airborne salivary droplets and nasal discharge. Transmission is favored by close proximity, and therefore the school and the home are important environments for spread. The incubation period for pharyngitis is usually 2 to 5 days. Children are usually not infectious 24 hours after appropriate antimicrobial therapy is initiated.

Expert Opinion on Management Issues

When attempting to decide whether to perform a microbiologic test on a patient presenting with acute pharyngitis, clinical and epidemiologic findings should be considered before the test is performed (Box 1). Testing usually is not necessary for patients with acute pharyngitis whose clinical and epidemiologic features suggest a viral etiology, but the signs and symptoms of GABHS and viral pharyngitis overlap broadly. Thus the clinical diagnosis of GABHS pharyngitis cannot be made with certainty even by the most experienced physicians, and an accurate diagnosis depends on the performance of a throat culture or a rapid antigen detection test (RADT).

Culture of a throat swab on a sheep blood–agar plate remains the standard for the documentation of the presence of GABHS in the upper respiratory tract and for the confirmation of the clinical diagnosis of acute GABHS pharyngitis. If performed correctly, a single throat swab cultured on a blood-agar plate has a sensitivity of 90% to 95% in detecting the presence of GABHS in the pharynx.

A disadvantage of culturing a throat swab on a blood-agar plate is the delay (overnight or longer) in obtaining the culture result. RADTs can identify GABHS directly from throat swabs. Although these RADTs are more expensive than the blood-agar culture, they offer the advantage of speed over the traditional procedure. Rapid identification and treatment of patients with GABHS pharyngitis can both reduce the risk of the spread of GABHS, allowing the patient to return to school or work sooner, and reduce the acute morbidity of this illness.

The great majority of the RADTs currently available have an excellent specificity of 95% or greater when compared with blood-agar plate cultures. This means that false-positive test results are unusual, and therapeutic decisions can be made on the basis of a positive test with confidence. Unfortunately, the sensitivity of most of these tests is between 80% and 90% (or even lower) when compared with the blood-agar plate culture. Therefore, negative RADTs should be confirmed by a blood-agar plate culture. Newer tests may be more sensitive than other RADTs and perhaps even as sensitive as blood-agar plate cultures. However, in view of conflicting data, physicians who elect to use any RADT in children and adolescents without culture backup of negative results should do so only after confirming in their own practice that the RADT is comparable in sensitivity to the throat culture.

A throat culture or RADT cannot distinguish between patients with bona fide streptococcal infections and those who are streptococcal carriers. Patients who are streptococcal carriers pose no danger to themselves or to others. They do not develop acute rheumatic fever and they rarely transmit this organism. Consequently, they do not need to be identified or treated. To minimize the number of streptococcal carriers who are cultured and subsequently treated unnecessarily with antimicrobials, the physician should perform throat cultures or RADTs selectively, taking into consideration the specific clinical and epidemiologic findings (see Box 1). In addition, only sick household contacts of a patient with GABHS pharyngitis should be cultured and, if positive, treated, unless the immediate family has a history of rheumatic fever.

Antimicrobial therapy for patients with GABHS pharyngitis can prevent acute rheumatic fever, suppurative sequelae (e.g., peritonsillar abscess, retropharyngeal abscess), and transmission to close contacts, and it can shorten the clinical course. GABHS are exquisitely sensitive to penicillin, and resistant strains have never been encountered. Thus penicillin is the drug of choice (except in penicillin-allergic individuals) for pharyngeal infections as well as for their suppurative complications. Treatment with oral penicillin V in doses of 500 to 1000 mg daily in two or three divided doses is appropriate, but it must be taken for a full 10 days even though these children usually appear to have recovered in 3 or 4 days. Amoxicillin suspension is often used in place of penicillin V suspension as oral therapy for young children because it is more palatable; the efficacy appears to be equal. The major problem with oral therapy is the risk that the drug will be

---

> ### BOX 1 Clinical and Epidemiologic Findings
>
> **Features Suggestive of Group A β-Hemolytic Streptococcal Pharyngitis**
> - Sudden onset
> - Sore throat
> - Fever
> - Inflammation of pharynx and tonsils
> - Patchy, discrete exudate
> - Tender, enlarged anterior cervical lymph nodes
> - Headache
> - Nausea, vomiting, abdominal pain
> - Patient between 5 and 15 years of age
> - Presentation in winter or early spring
> - Exposure to well-documented case of group A β-hemolytic streptococcal (GABHS) pharyngitis
> - High prevalence of GABHS infections in community
>
> **Features Suggestive of Viral Pharyngitis**
> - Cough
> - Coryza
> - Diarrhea
> - Conjunctivitis
> - Characteristic exanthems
> - Characteristic enanthems

discontinued before the 10-day course is completed. When oral treatment is prescribed, the necessity of completing a full course of therapy must be emphasized. If the parents seem unlikely to comply because of family disorganization, difficulties in comprehension, or other reasons, parenteral therapy is indicated. A single intramuscular injection of benzathine penicillin G, 600,000 IU for patients weighing less than 60 pounds (27 kg) and 1.2 million IU for those 60 pounds (27 kg) or more, is the most efficacious and often the most practical method of treatment. Its only disadvantage is soreness around the site of injection that may last for several days. The local reaction is diminished when benzathine penicillin G is combined with procaine penicillin G. However, when this combination is used in a single injection, an adequate amount of benzathine penicillin G must be administered.

Erythromycin is the drug of choice for patients allergic to penicillin. The dosage is erythromycin estolate, 20 to 40 mg/kg/day, or erythromycin ethylsuccinate, 40 mg/kg/day, both for 10 days. Although there have been recent isolated reports of high rates of macrolide resistance among isolates of GABHS in the United States, no evidence indicates this is widespread at present. Although routine susceptibility testing of GABHS is not currently recommended, physicians should be aware of local patterns of antimicrobial resistance.

A 10-day course of a narrow-spectrum oral cephalosporin is an acceptable alternative for patients allergic to penicillin. However, because a substantial proportion of penicillin-allergic patients are also allergic to cephalosporins, the latter should not be given to patients with an immediate-type hypersensitivity to penicillin. The additional cost of cephalosporins and their broader spectrum of antibacterial activity compared with penicillin preclude their routine use in patients with GABHS pharyngitis who are not allergic to penicillin. Sulfonamides and the tetracyclines are contraindicated in patients with GABHS pharyngitis.

Most oral antimicrobials must be administered for the conventional 10 days to achieve maximal pharyngeal eradication rates of GABHS, but certain newer agents have been reported to achieve comparable bacteriologic and clinical cure rates when given for 5 days or less. Definitive results from comprehensive studies are not available to allow final evaluation of these proposed shorter courses of oral antimicrobial therapy, however, so they cannot be recommended at this time. In addition, these antimicrobials have a much broader spectrum than penicillin, and most, even when administered for short courses, are more expensive.

Preliminary investigations demonstrate that once-daily amoxicillin therapy is effective in the treatment of GABHS pharyngitis. Once-daily amoxicillin therapy, because of its low cost and relatively narrow spectrum, could become an alternative regimen for the treatment of GABHS pharyngitis if its effectiveness is confirmed by additional investigations.

Suppurative complications of GABHS pharyngitis from the spread of GABHS to adjacent structures were very common before antimicrobial therapy became available. Cervical adenitis, peritonsillar abscess, retropharyngeal abscess, otitis media, mastoiditis, and sinusitis still occur in children in whom the primary illness has gone unnoticed or in whom treatment of the pharyngitis was inadequate. GABHS pneumonia can rarely occur. Acute rheumatic fever and acute poststreptococcal glomerulonephritis are both nonsuppurative sequelae of infections with GABHS that occur after an asymptomatic latent period. They are both characterized by lesions remote from the site of the GABHS infection. However, acute rheumatic fever and acute glomerulonephritis differ in their clinical manifestations, epidemiology, and potential morbidity. In addition, acute glomerulonephritis can occur after a GABHS infection of either the upper respiratory tract or the skin, but acute rheumatic fever can only occur after an infection of the upper respiratory tract.

Some reports note a higher incidence of failures to eradicate GABHS from the upper respiratory tract following recommended courses of appropriate antimicrobial therapy, despite demonstrated sensitivity of GABHS to these antimicrobials. The reasons for these bacteriologic failures are unclear. For patients who have received oral penicillin, poor compliance always should be considered a possible explanation. Evidence suggests that most of the patients in whom treatment fails are streptococcal carriers and not truly infected. Routine reculturing of asymptomatic individuals who have completed a full course of appropriate antimicrobial therapy thus is not indicated. Reculturing of asymptomatic individuals, and retreating if they are positive, should be considered if any if any of the following are present: questionable compliance, a history of rheumatic fever in the immediate family, many cases of poststreptococcal glomerulonephritis in the community, an outbreak of GABHS pharyngitis in a closed or semiclosed community, or intrafamily back-and-forth transmission of GABHS pharyngitis.

Common Pitfalls

- The throat culture or an RADT cannot distinguish between patients with bona fide streptococcal infections and those who are streptococcal carriers.
- In general, oral antimicrobial therapy for GABHS pharyngitis taken for less than 10 days is associated with a significantly increased failure rate.
- Poor compliance always has to be considered as a possible explanation for failure to eradicate GABHS from the upper respiratory tract after a course of appropriate oral antimicrobial therapy.
- Routine reculturing of asymptomatic individuals who have completed a full course of appropriate antimicrobial therapy is not indicated.

Communication and Counseling

Most children with acute pharyngitis have a viral infection and do not benefit from antimicrobial therapy. Therefore, a throat culture or RADT should be performed only on those children with clinical and epidemiologic findings suggestive of GABHS pharyngitis; only those children with a positive throat culture or RADT should receive antimicrobial therapy. Although the patient may be entirely well after a few days of oral antimicrobial therapy, the antimicrobial therapy must be continued for a full 10 days to be effective. In general, repeat throat cultures or RADT should be performed only on those children who have a recurrence of the clinical findings suggestive of GABHS pharyngitis.

SUGGESTED READINGS

1. Bisno AL: Group A streptococcal infections and acute rheumatic fever. N Engl J Med 325:783–793, 1991. **Review of group A streptococcal infections including acute pharyngitis.**
2. Bisno AL: Acute pharyngitis. N Engl J Med 344:205–211, 2001. **Review of all forms of acute pharyngitis including GABHS pharyngitis.**
3. Bisno AL, Gerber MA, Gwaltney JM, et al: Practice guideline for the diagnosis management of group A streptococcal pharyngitis. Clin Infect Dis 35:113–125, 2002. **Update of Infectious Diseases Society of America practice guideline first published in 1997.**
4. Gerber MA, Shulman ST: Rapid diagnosis of pharyngitis caused by group A streptococci. Clin Microbiol Rev 17:571–580, 2004. **Comprehensive review of the current status of rapid diagnostic testing for GABHS pharyngitis.**
5. Gerber MA, Tanz RR: New approaches to the treatment of group A streptococcal pharyngitis. Curr Opin Pediatr 13:51–55, 2001. **Critical review of the antimicrobial options available for the treatment of GABHS pharyngitis.**
6. Kaplan EL, Gerber MA: Group A, group C, group G beta-hemolytic streptococcal infections. In Feigin RD, Cherry JD Demmler GJ, Kaplan SL (eds): Textbook of Pediatric Infectious Diseases, 5th ed. Philadelphia: WB Saunders, 2004, pp 1142–1156. **Comprehensive review of β-hemolytic streptococcal infections.**

Group B Streptococcal Infections

Carol J. Baker and Morven S. Edwards

KEY CONCEPTS

- Group B streptococcal (GBS) disease should be considered as a possible etiologic agent in all infants with suspected sepsis or focal infection until 3 months of age and in premature infants until postconceptional age of 3 months.
- After obtaining a culture of blood, cerebrospinal fluid (CSF), and, if present, any focal site of infection (e.g., bone, joint, abscess), empirical antimicrobial therapy should be initiated while awaiting the culture results. The interval between onset of signs of sepsis and death from fulminant GBS disease can be as short as 12 hours.
- Attention to details of supportive therapy, including tissue perfusion, fluid balance, mechanical ventilation, seizure control, and surgical drainage, as needed, are crucial to optimizing the outcome in young infants with GBS infections.
- High inocula of GBS in the CSF require a high dosage of β-lactam antimicrobials to achieve rapid killing of the organism in the CSF.
- GBS are uniformly susceptible to penicillin G, which is the drug of choice for treatment of GBS infections.
- Infants remain colonized at mucous membrane sites after successful treatment for invasive infection. Thus recurrent disease is a possibility (estimated frequency, 1%).

Group B streptococcal (GBS) infections are caused by *Streptococcus agalactiae*, a gram-positive bacterium that colonizes the gastrointestinal and genitourinary tracts of healthy adults and the upper respiratory tract of neonates and infants. Infants at risk for GBS infection are those exposed to the organism shortly before or during the delivery process or postnatally. Colonization at mucous membrane sites in infancy may precede the development of invasive infection by days, weeks, or occasionally months. Neonates with early-onset GBS infection typically present during the first few hours (approximately 93% of cases within 24 hours) or week of life with signs of sepsis. A subset of neonates presents with respiratory distress and has chest radiographic findings characteristic of congenital pneumonia, respiratory distress syndrome, or transient tachypnea of the newborn. Infants with late-onset GBS infection present from 7 days to 3 months of age with signs that can include fever, poor feeding, and lethargy. In some of these infants findings are consistent with extension of bacteremic infection to the meninges (seizures), bones or joints (swelling, pain, and decreased movement), or the lymph nodes (enlargement of lymph nodes with overlying cellulitis). In premature infants with an extended stay in the neonatal intensive care unit, the age at which late-onset infection occurs extends to 6 months of age (or 3 months' postconceptional age). These infections usually manifest as bacteremia without a focus and are designated as late, late-onset disease. Table 1 summarizes the features of GBS infection in neonates and young infants.

A comprehensive program of intrapartum antibiotic prophylaxis (IAP) to prevent early-onset GBS infection was endorsed by the American Academy of Pediatrics (AAP) and the American College of Obstetrics and Gynecology (ACOG) in 1996 in collaboration with the Centers for Disease Control and Prevention (CDC). By 2002, the implementation of IAP resulted in a dramatic (approximately 75%) reduction in the incidence of early-onset neonatal GBS disease, and it was clear from accumulated evidence that culture-based antenatal screening to select women for IAP prevented more cases of early-onset GBS neonatal disease than identification based on risk factors. Revised CDC recommendations include vaginal and rectal cultures for GBS in all pregnant women at 35 to 37 weeks' gestation and administration of IAP to all GBS-colonized women unless a cesarean delivery occurs in the absence of labor or amniotic membrane rupture. Figure 1 shows the indications for IAP to prevent perinatal GBS disease under this universal culture screening strategy.

TABLE 1 Features of Group B Streptococcal Infections in Infancy

Feature	Early Onset (<7 days)	Late Onset (7–89 days)	Late, Late Onset (>3 mo)
Median age at onset	1 h	27 days	Unknown
Maternal obstetric complications	Common	Uncommon	Varies
Frequency of gestation <37 wk	Frequent (30%)	Uncommon	Common
Clinical presentations	Septicemia (25%–30%)	Meningitis (25%–35%)	Bacteremia without a focus (common)
	Meningitis (5%–10%)	Bacteremia without a focus (60%–65%)	Bacteremia without a focus (common)
	Respiratory distress (35%–55%)	Osteoarthritis (5%)	
Serotypes	Ia, Ib, II, III, V	III (~75%)	Unknown
Mortality rate	(5%–10%)	2%–6%	Low

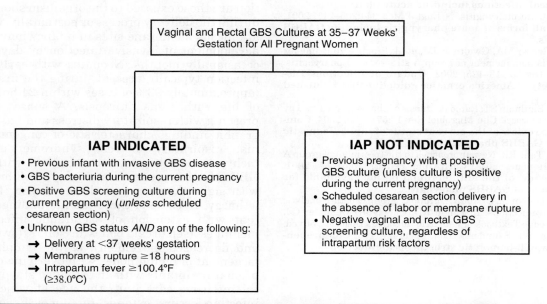

FIGURE 1. Algorithm adapted from the Centers for Disease Control and Prevention 2002 recommendations for the prevention of early-onset group B streptococcal (GBS) infection in neonates. IAP, intrapartum antibiotic prophylaxis.

Expert Opinion on Management Issues

NEWBORNS WITH MOTHERS RECEIVING INTRAPARTUM ANTIBIOTIC PROPHYLAXIS

Figure 2 presents an approach to the management of newborns born to women who received IAP to prevent early-onset GBS disease. If a woman has received intrapartum treatment for suspected chorioamnionitis, her newborn infant should have a full evaluation for systemic infection and receive treatment for suspected neonatal sepsis, pending culture results. Infants with clinical signs of sepsis should receive a full diagnostic evaluation and empirical therapy. Infants for whom a limited evaluation is performed (complete blood count, blood culture, and chest radiograph, if respiratory signs are present) and those for whom no diagnostic evaluation is required should be observed in the hospital for at least 48 hours. An exception to this duration of observation is for healthy-appearing infants who were delivered at 38 weeks' gestation or later and whose mothers received appropriate IAP (e.g., penicillin, ampicillin, or cefazolin 4 or more hours before delivery). These infants can be discharged home after 24 hours under the care of a person able to comply with instructions for home care, to communicate by telephone with a health care facility, and to return promptly to the hospital if signs of sepsis appear.

EMPIRICAL THERAPY FOR SUSPECTED INFECTIONS

Table 2 shows the treatment for GBS infection. Initial therapy for suspected early-onset infection is ampicillin and gentamicin for the treatment of GBS as well as other potential pathogens. If vancomycin and

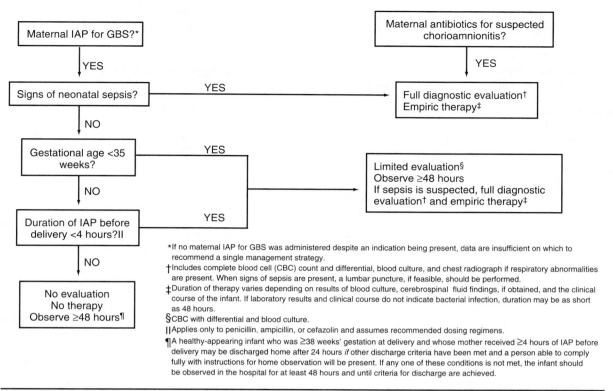

FIGURE 2. Algorithm adapted from Centers for Disease Control and Prevention 2002 recommendations for the management of newborn infants born to women given intrapartum antibiotic prophylaxis to prevent early-onset group B streptococcal (GBS) disease. IAP, intrapartum antibiotic prophylaxis.

TABLE 2 Antimicrobial Therapy for Neonatal Group B Streptococcal Infections

Type of Infection	Antibiotic (Dose)	Duration
Suspected meningitis (initial empirical therapy)	Ampicillin (300 mg/kg/day) *plus* Gentamicin (5–7.5 mg/kg/day)	Until cerebrospinal fluid sterility and penicillin susceptibility documented
Suspected sepsis* (initial empirical therapy)	Ampicillin (150 mg/kg/day) *plus* Gentamicin (5–7.5 mg/kg/day)*	Until blood stream sterility documented
Bacteremia	Penicillin G (200,000 U/kg/day)	10 days
Meningitis	Penicillin G (450,000–500,000 U/kg/day)	14–21 days
Arthritis	Penicillin G (200,000 U/kg/day)	2–3 wk
Osteomyelitis	Penicillin G (200,000 U/kg/day)	3–4 wk
Endocarditis	Penicillin G (300,000 U/kg/day)	4 wk

*Assumes lumbar puncture to exclude meningitis has been performed and that cerebrospinal fluid has no detectable abnormalities.

gentamicin are employed for empirical therapy of suspected late-onset infection, this regimen is adequate for infants with late- or late, late-onset GBS bacteremia, but vancomycin does not penetrate the blood-brain barrier well, and spread of GBS to the meninges may occur. If late-onset meningitis is a consideration or if infants are critically ill, ampicillin, at the dosages shown in Table 2, should be included in the regimen. The combination of ampicillin and gentamicin is more effective than ampicillin alone in the in vitro and in vivo killing of most GBS strains. Gentamicin should be continued until sterility of the blood and cerebrospinal fluid (CSF) is documented. This usually results in combination therapy for the first 4 or 5 days of treatment.

SPECIFIC THERAPY FOR GROUP B STREPTOCOCCAL DISEASE

Penicillin is the antibiotic of choice for the treatment of infections caused by GBS, including meningitis, because GBS remain uniformly susceptible to penicillin. The optimum dose and duration (see Table 2) are dictated by the focus of infection. Treatment should be administered exclusively by the parenteral route. Controlled clinical data are insufficient to support a recommendation to shorten the duration of parenteral antimicrobial therapy. The high dose of penicillin recommended for the treatment of GBS meningitis (450,000 to 500,000 U/kg/day) is based on the high bacterial inoculum (10^7 to 10^8 colony-forming units per milliliter) that may be found in the CSF. This dose is safe to employ even in infants of very low birth weight. Potential toxicity of penicillin should be monitored by performing a CBC (complete blood count), blood urea nitrogen, creatinine, and urinalysis one to two times per week.

Meningitis is best managed with repeated CSF evaluations to monitor the progress of resolution of active infection and the inflammatory process. It is our practice to perform a repeat lumbar puncture (LP) 24 to 48 hours after the initiation of therapy to document sterility of the CSF. A persistently positive CSF culture indicates either a very high bacterial inoculum, obstructive hydrocephalus, or (rarely) another focus of infection in the central nervous system (CNS). We advocate repeating an LP on the 14th day of therapy before discontinuing penicillin therapy. The finding of a high CSF protein (>150 mg/dL) or ongoing predominance of neutrophils (>35%) is an indication to continue penicillin for an additional week of treatment. A CT scan of the head with contrast enhancement performed near the anticipated end of therapy should be obtained to determine whether cerebritis persists or an abscess is present. These findings require additional therapy.

PREVENTIVE MEASURES

Further reduction in the incidence of early-onset GBS disease can be expected with wide implementation of the guidelines for universal antenatal screening of all pregnant women by vaginal and rectal cultures for GBS at 35 to 37 weeks' gestation and the administration of penicillin to all GBS culture–positive women. Candidate protein-polysaccharide conjugate GBS vaccines have proved safe and immunogenic in clinical trials. Hope for prevention of late-onset GBS disease through maternal immunization awaits the licensure of GBS vaccines. Currently, no known measures are available to prevent either late-onset GBS infection or recurrent disease.

Common Pitfalls

- The initial sign of GBS sepsis in otherwise healthy term infants may be an episode of poor feeding, fussiness, or an apparently self-limited episode of apnea. Caregivers should have a high index of suspicion for sepsis and a low threshold for evaluation and provision of empirical antibiotic treatment within the first month of life.
- Failure to perform LP when clinical signs suggest sepsis is a potential pitfall. The blood culture can be sterile in as many as 15% of newborn infants with meningitis.
- Caregivers should understand that seizures in infancy may not manifest as tonic-clonic movements. Compromise of oxygen supply to the brain may occur when seizure activity is not appreciated and controlled with anticonvulsant therapy. Tonic activity and abnormal eye movements should

raise a high index of suspicion in infants suspected of having GBS infection.

Communication and Counseling

Most children with GBS sepsis or bone and joint infection and a majority of those with GBS meningitis recover uneventfully. Most of those who experience sequelae either as a consequence of septic shock in the acute phase of illness or from damage to the CNS from meningitis have an abnormal neurologic examination when antimicrobial therapy is completed. It is important to discuss with the parents or guardians of all children recovering from GBS infection the possibility of invasive infection recurring. The prognosis for those with an abnormal neurologic examination after therapy is guarded. All infants recovering from GBS meningitis should have testing of hearing and vision as well as close assessment of developmental milestones so early childhood intervention can optimize function when developmental delay is evident. Mothers who have had an infant with either early- or late-onset GBS disease should be counseled to receive IAP with all subsequent pregnancies, so there is no need for ongoing assessment of their GBS colonization status.

SUGGESTED READINGS

1. Baker CJ, Edwards MS: Group B streptococcal conjugate vaccines. Arch Dis Child 88:375–378, 2003. **Comprehensive review of the safety and immunogenicity of the GBS polysaccharide-protein conjugate vaccines in adults, including pregnant women.**
2. Centers for Disease Control and Prevention: Prevention of perinatal group B streptococcal disease. MMWR Morb Mortal Wkly Rep 51(RR-11):1–22, 2002. **This comprehensive review of the prevention of early-onset GBS disease in neonates and GBS morbidity in their mothers provides the gold standard prevention method for physicians, microbiology laboratories, and health care epidemiologists.**
3. Escobar GJ, Li D-K, Armstrong MA, et al: Neonatal sepsis workups in infants ≥2000 grams at birth: A population-based study. Pediatrics 106:256–263, 2000. **Assessment of neonatal sepsis evaluations in the era of intrapartum antibiotic prophylaxis for GBS underscores the need for hospital observation given the poor sensitivity and specificity of the CBC and blood culture.**
4. Kanto WP, Baker CJ: New recommendations for prevention of early-onset group B streptococcal disease in newborns. Pediatr Rev 24:219–221, 2003. **This review of the 2002 CDC GBS guidelines provides further detail about the evaluation and management of neonates born to women given IAP.**
5. Schrag SJ, Zell ER, Lynfield R, et al: A population-based comparison of strategies to prevent early-onset group B streptococcal disease in neonates. N Engl J Med 347:233–239, 2002. **Results from this seminal study comparing risk factor- to culture-based methods shows the antenatal culture screening method is superior and the basis on which the recommendation for universal GBS culture screening in all pregnant women stands.**
6. Schrag SJ, Zywicki S, Farley MM, et al: Group B streptococcal disease in the era of intrapartum antibiotic prophylaxis. N Engl J Med 342:15–20, 2000. **Prospective multicenter surveillance study of the incidence of early- late-onset GBS disease in the United States from 1993 through 1999 that demonstrates a significant reduction of early-onset but not late-onset disease with maternal IAP.**

Helicobacter pylori Infection

L. Arturo Batres and Benjamin D. Gold

KEY CONCEPTS

- *Helicobacter pylori* infection, one of the most prevalent infections worldwide, is particularly common in developing countries and immigrant populations in industrialized nations.
- The infection is associated with gastritis, duodenal ulcers, and, to a lesser extent, gastric ulcers. Infection with *H. pylori* significantly increases the risk of gastric adenocarcinoma and mucosa-associated lymphoid tissue (MALT) lymphoma.
- *H. pylori* infection occurs in childhood, and although most children remain asymptomatic, gastroduodenal disease can occur in the pediatric patient.
- Histology of the gastric mucosa obtained at upper endoscopy with biopsy is currently the standard for the diagnosis in the United States.
- The preferred regimen includes a proton pump inhibitor and a combination of two antibiotics for 14 days.

Helicobacter pylori is a gram-negative, flagellated bacillus, curved or spiral in shape, with microaerophilic properties. Infection with *H. pylori* was first described in 1982 in association with antral gastritis and duodenal mucosal ulceration in adults. Subsequently, the infection was shown to have a causal role in gastritis, duodenal ulcers, and, to a lesser extent, gastric ulcers. *H pylori* infection has been determined to be strongly linked to development of gastric adenocarcinoma and mucosa-associated lymphoid tissue (MALT) lymphoma. A number of factors confer virulence to infected *H. pylori* strains. These bacterial virulence factors include a cytotoxin-associated gene (*cag*A), part of a series of genes within the *H. pylori* genome called the *cag* pathogenicity island that promotes, among other processes, interleukin-induced inflammation; a vacuolating cytotoxin-associated gene (*vac*A) that causes degeneration of the epithelium, increasing its permeability; and the enzyme urease (encoded by the *ure* gene) that protects the bacteria from stomach acid and releases a toxic ammonium ion. Several host factors predispose to the infection, including Lewis blood group antigens, poor hygienic conditions (i.e., poor sanitation), low socioeconomic status, and crowded conditions. In particular, the prevalence of *H. pylori* infection is higher in developing compared to developed countries and in immigrant populations in industrialized nations, including the United States. At present, the impact of breast-feeding compared to formula feeding on infection acquisition remains unclear.

H. pylori infection is considered the most prevalent infection worldwide. An estimated 50% or more of the world's population is infected, and it is more common in developing countries. The mode of transmission is not definitively characterized, but is believed to occur via gastro–oral, oral–oral, and fecal–oral routes. The inoculum size and incubation period requisite for infection persistence are not known. In addition, the natural reservoir is human; however, the infection may be propagated by fecally contaminated water. Zoonotic or vector-borne infection, although previously investigated, are not definitive routes of transmission.

H. pylori is primarily acquired during childhood, and in the majority of individuals, unless treated, it lasts for a person's lifetime. Most of the infected children are asymptomatic. However, vomiting and abdominal pain may be associated with *H. pylori* infection and ulcer disease. It remains unknown if recurrent abdominal pain and nonulcer dyspepsia are related to *H. pylori* infection in children. Manifestations outside the upper intestinal tract, such as anemia, growth retardation, and chronic urticaria, are reported with *H. pylori* infection.

Expert Opinion on Management Issues

TESTING

Table 1 presents the diagnostic tests for *H. pylori*. Histology with staining of the gastric mucosa when obtained by upper endoscopy with biopsies is considered the standard for the diagnosis of *H. pylori* infection. The best location for biopsies is the midantrum at the level of the lesser curvature. If a child undergoes endoscopy while concurrently taking antisecretory agents (e.g., a proton pump inhibitor or histamine–2 receptor antagonist), biopsies should be obtained from both the antrum and the gastric corpus for optimal yield of detecting *H. pylori* infection. A variety of stains are used on the gastric biopsies to reveal detection of *H. pylori* organisms, including Giemsa, silver stains, and other modified stains like the Genta stain.

Urea breath testing has good sensitivity and specificity, and at present it is considered the gold standard for diagnosis in children suspected of having *H. pylori* in Europe. This test relies on the cooperation of the patient and may be difficult to perform in children, particularly those younger than 5 years. The breath test measures active infection and can be used as a test to document success or failure of eradication therapy.

Several serologic and whole blood tests have been evaluated, including Western blot, immunoassays, and enzyme-linked immunoabsorbent assay (ELISA). The Western blot test appears the most reliable; however, not all of the serologic and whole blood tests are validated for use in children in the United States. Blood tests are currently not recommended for clinical use and are particularly poor for post-treatment monitoring (i.e., as a test for cure).

The stool antigen is an immunoassay with good specificity and sensitivity, and in some studies it demonstrates utility for evaluating eradication after treatment. The original stool antigen test was a polyclonal assay, which was found to be variable in the United States and Europe. However, data evaluating a number of second-generation monoclonal stool assays demonstrate great promise for this test in the clinical arena once validation studies are performed.

TABLE 1 Tests for *Helicobacter pylori* Infection

Test	Description
Invasive Tests	
Histology	Gold standard. Multiple biopsies from different locations of the stomach mucosa. Organisms can be identified on hematoxylin-eosin stain; better identification occurs with special staining, such as Warthin-Starry silver, Giemsa, Steiner, or Genta stains.
Rapid urease test	The urease enzyme of *H. pylori* produces a pH color change in the indicator. Complements histology.
Bacterial culture	The bacteria grow at 98.6°F (37°C) for 2 to 5 days with media using microaerobic conditions. Useful for antibiotic sensitivity. Recovery rates are variable. Expensive, labor intensive, not available commercially.
PCR of bacterial DNA	Can detect *H. pylori* in water, body fluids, and tissue. Expensive; not available commercially.
Noninvasive Tests	
Urea breath test	Uses radiolabeled ^{14}C urea or urea tagged with ^{13}C. False positive if urease producing organisms are from the mouth. Technically difficult in some patients. Can remain positive up to 4 weeks after treatment.
Serum antibody	Detects serum immunoglobulin G indicative of past or current exposure to *H. pylori*. Remains positive after treatment; not recommended for post-treatment monitoring. Not clinically recommended for use in children.
Stool antigen	Enzyme immunoassay. Can detect eradication 7 days after completing treatment.

PCR, polymerase chain reaction.

TABLE 2 Recommended Treatment of *Helicobacter pylori* infection

Drug Name	Dosage/Route/Regimen	Maximum Dose	Formulation	Common Adverse Reaction
Proton Pump Inhibitors (irreversibly inhibit H⁺,K⁺-ATPase pump in the parietal cell, interfering with the hydrochloric acid secretion)				
Omeprazole (Prilosec, Prilosec OTC)	PO: 0.7–3.3 mg/kg/day div bid or 20 mg bid	Max: 3.3 mg/kg/day or 20 mg bid	Capsule: 10, 20, 40 mg. Tablet: 20 mg. Bicarbonate solution can be prepared.	Diarrhea, headaches, constipation, nausea, vomiting
or				
Lansoprazole (Prevacid)	PO: 0.7–1.5 mg/kg/day div bid or 15 mg bid	Max: 1.5 mg/kg/day or 15 mg bid	Capsule: 15, 30 mg. Oral solution: 15, 30 mg. Disintegrating tablet: 15, 30 mg.	Diarrhea, headaches, constipation, nausea, vomiting
Plus Two of the Following Antibiotics:				
Antibiotics (bacteriostatic or bactericidal properties against *H. pylori*)				
Amoxicillin (Amoxil, Trimox, Polymox, and others)	PO: 50 mg/kg/day div bid or 1g bid	Max: 1 g bid	Suspension: 125, 200, 250, 400 mg/5 mL. Tablet: 500, 875 mg. Chew tab: 125, 200, 250, 400 mg. Capsule: 250, 500 mg.	Rash, diarrhea
Clarithromycin (Biaxin)	PO: 15 mg/kg/day div bid or 500 mg bid	Max: 500 mg bid	Suspension: 250–500 mg/5 mL. Tablet: 250, 500 mg.	Diarrhea, nausea, arrhythmias, headaches
Metronidazole (Flagyl, Metro, and others)	PO: 20 mg/kg/day div bid or 500 mg bid	Max: 500 mg bid	Tablet: 250, 500 mg. Suspension can be prepared.	Nausea, diarrhea, peripheral neuropathy
Tetracycline* (Achromycin and others)	PO: 50 mg/kg/day div bid or 500 mg bid	Max: 500 mg bid	Tablet: 500 mg.	Nausea, rash, photosensitivity

*Contraindicated in children younger than 12 years of age.
bid, twice daily; div, divided; max, maximum; PO, by mouth.

TREATMENT

Eradication of the organism is recommended when active infection is confirmed by histology. Table 2 shows the treatment for *H. pylori* infection. The preferred regimen includes a proton pump inhibitor and a combination of two antibiotics for 10 to 14 days. The only two proton pump inhibitors approved for children and labeled for *H. pylori* eradication are omeprazole and lansoprazole. Rabeprazole is labeled for eradication of *H. pylori* in adult patients but not in children. Even though pantoprazole and esomeprazole are not labeled for *H. pylori* eradication, studies demonstrate similar efficacy of these drugs when compared to omeprazole and lansoprazole.

The recommended length of therapy for children infected with *H. pylori* is 14 days, although some courses of 7 days are described. The shorter durations do not yield greater than 85% eradication rates, however, and thus are not recommended at present. Studies show better eradication rates with twice-daily dosing of both the proton pump inhibitor and the two antibiotics. This is because of increased patient compliance, since noncompliance is one of the two most common reasons for treatment failures.

Antibiotic resistance of *H. pylori* to the different antibiotics, the second most common reason for treatment failure, is reported worldwide. In the United States, resistance to metronidazole can be as high as 25%; in other parts of the world, resistance is as high as 95% (e.g., Bangladesh). The resistance of clarithromycin and amoxicillin appears to be lower overall. Resistance to clarithromycin worldwide is higher in children infected by *H. pylori* compared to adults; once a strain is resistant to clarithromycin, there is cross-resistance to all other macrolide antibiotics, which can dramatically affect treatment success. Resistance to two antibiotics is reported in 5% of the cases. The antibiotic resistance appears related to the frequent use of antimicrobial agents for other childhood conditions.

Common Pitfalls

■ Inadequate or inappropriate use of diagnostic tests (e.g., nonvalidated diagnostic tests, inaccurate diagnostic tests) can lead to improper diagnosis and treatment and increases the prevalence of antibiotic resistance.
■ Failure to take the proton pump inhibitor with the antibiotics, as well as poor compliance with the antibiotic regimen, are other potential pitfalls leading to increased treatment failure.
■ Reinfection rates can be high if family members, particularly children younger than 6 years, caregivers, and other close contacts, are infected.
■ Resistance to antibiotics, especially clarithromycin and metronidazole, is important to consider if failure to eradicate the infection occurs.

Communication and Counseling

Most patients recover from the gastroduodenal disease associated with *H. pylori* infection after treatment. Reinfection needs to be considered if symptoms persist. Some patients may require maintenance on a proton pump inhibitor after antibiotic therapy is completed. Infection is more common in crowded conditions and during travel in endemic areas. Standard precautions are recommended for hospitalized patients and for those traveling to endemic areas or exposed to persons from those parts of the world. Patients need to be educated about the importance of compliance with the antibiotic regimen in eradicating the organism and preventing gastric cancer in the future. Public health measures, such as improved housing, sanitation, and proper nutrition, are important in contributing to the reduction of the overall infection burden, especially in developing countries.

SUGGESTED READINGS

1. Crone J, Gold BD: *Helicobacter pylori* infection in pediatrics. Helicobacter 9:49–56, 2004. **Review of epidemiology, diagnosis, and treatment of *H. pylori* in children.**
2. Duck WM, Sobel J, Pruckler JM, et al: Antimicrobial resistance incidence and risk factors among *Helicobacter pylori*–infected persons, United States. Emerg Infect Dis 10:1088–1094, 2004. **Presents a comprehensive report of the antibiotic resistance of *H. pylori* in the United States in children and adults.**
3. Gold BD, Colletti RB, Abbott M, et al: *Helicobacter pylori* infection in children: Recommendations for diagnosis and treatment. J Pediatr Gastroenterol Nutr 31:490–497, 2000. ***H. pylori* guidelines of the North American Society for Pediatric Gastroenterology and Nutrition.**
4. Makristathis A, Hirschl AM, Lehours P, Megraud F: Diagnosis of *Helicobacter pylori* infection. Helicobacter 9:7–14, 2004. **Reviews the usefulness and limitations of each diagnostic test for *H. pylori* infection in adults.**

Syphilis

Sarah Anne Rawstron

12

KEY CONCEPTS

■ Syphilis is a systemic sexually transmitted disease (STD) that may also be transmitted transplacentally to infants.
■ Adults and adolescents present with symptoms of primary, secondary, or tertiary syphilis, or neurosyphilis, or they may have no symptoms and present with latent syphilis (reactive serologic tests only).
■ Infants with congenital syphilis may present with symptoms at delivery, but most often they are asymptomatic. Because no definitive laboratory tests are available to make the diagnosis in asymptomatic infants, the maternal history of syphilis and treatment is pivotal in making evaluation and treatment decisions in the infant.
■ Children with syphilis diagnosed outside the neonatal period either have congenital or acquired syphilis. Any child with acquired syphilis should be considered a case of sexual abuse and reported to child welfare authorities.
■ Treatment for syphilis at all stages remains parenteral preparations of penicillin G.
■ No alternatives to penicillin therapy are available for congenital syphilis and pregnant women with syphilis.
■ Nontreponemal serologic tests are used to follow the response of therapy.
■ All patients with syphilis should be tested for human immunodeficiency virus (HIV).

Syphilis, a systemic disease caused by the spirochete bacterium *Treponema pallidum,* can be either congenital or acquired. Congenital syphilis is acquired from a mother with syphilis who has had either no treatment or inadequate treatment for syphilis during pregnancy. Acquired syphilis is a sexually transmitted disease (STD), and patients may present with symptoms of primary syphilis (painless chancres and ulcers at the inoculation site); secondary syphilis (rash, mucocutaneous lesions, and adenopathy); or tertiary syphilis (cardiac, neurosyphilis, or gummatous lesions). Many patients with syphilis are asymptomatic and the diagnosis is made by serologic testing (latent syphilis). Those infections acquired within the preceding year are defined as early latent syphilis, with all other cases either late latent syphilis or latent syphilis of unknown duration. Congenital syphilis is also a systemic disease, similar to secondary syphilis in presentation (hepatosplenomegaly, skin rash, mucocutaneous lesions, neurosyphilis, bone lesions), or infants may be asymptomatic with the diagnosis made based on serologic findings and history of maternal syphilis and lack of adequate maternal therapy.

The diagnosis of syphilis can be made definitively if spirochetes are identified in lesions, exudates, or tissues using Darkfield examination or direct fluorescent antibody tests (useful in primary and secondary syphilis and occasionally congenital syphilis if lesions are present). However, most patients have the diagnosis of syphilis made presumptively based on results of serologic tests. Two types of serologic tests for syphilis are used: nontreponemal tests (e.g., rapid plasma reagent [RPR] and Venereal Disease Research Laboratory [VDRL] tests) and specific treponemal tests (e.g., fluorescent treponemal antibody absorption [FTA-ABS] and *T. pallidum* particle agglutination [TP-PA]). Both types of tests are required to make the diagnosis (both tests need to be reactive), because false-positive nontreponemal tests may occur secondary to many medical conditions (e.g., lupus) and false-positive treponemal tests can occur in other diseases caused by spirochetes (e.g., Lyme disease).

Nontreponemal test results are reported quantitatively as titers, and the titers usually correlate with disease activity and are very useful in monitoring the results of therapy. A clinically significant change in titer is at least a fourfold change (two tube dilutions), for example 1:8 to 1:32 or 1:16 to 1:64. Monitoring of individual patients should use the same test (e.g., RPR) preferably by the same laboratory, because VDRL and RPR tests are not directly comparable, with RPR titers often higher than VDRL. Nontreponemal titers usually become nonreactive after treatment, particularly if treatment is given early in the course of the disease. However, some patients retain reactive serology at low titer for long periods of time, even for life, which is called the *serofast reaction*.

Treponemal tests, in contrast, usually remain reactive for life, even after appropriate therapy, although some patients treated during primary syphilis may revert to nonreactive treponemal tests after 2 to 3 years. Treponemal tests are not quantitated and should not be used to assess treatment response.

Some patients with HIV may have atypical serologic results, either unusually low or high or fluctuating titers, although most patients with HIV have typical serologic results that are reliable for diagnosis and monitoring treatment response.

A reactive VDRL-CSF test is the standard test to diagnose neurosyphilis, as long as the cerebrospinal fluid (CSF) does not have substantial contamination with red blood cells. However, it is a highly specific but insensitive test to diagnose neurosyphilis. The diagnosis of neurosyphilis can also be made based on a combination of reactive serologic tests and CSF abnormalities (e.g., elevated white cell count or protein), or a reactive VDRL-CSF test with or without clinical manifestations.

Expert Opinion on Management Issues

DRUG THERAPY

Penicillin remains the antibiotic of choice for treatment of all stages of syphilis. Infants and children with congenital syphilis and pregnant women with syphilis should be treated only with penicillin regimens, even if this requires desensitization when there is a history of penicillin allergy. No other alternatives are recommended by the Centers for Disease Control and Prevention (CDC).

Adults and adolescents with acquired syphilis should receive penicillin treatments according to their stage of syphilis, but alternative antibiotic regimens can be considered for patients who are allergic to penicillin, including doxycycline, tetracycline, and ceftriaxone for patients with primary or secondary syphilis. Close follow-up is recommended for patients given these nonpenicillin regimens because the efficacy of alternative regimens is not well documented.

The Jarisch-Herxheimer reaction should be anticipated and discussed with patients being treated for syphilis. This adverse reaction is an acute febrile reaction often associated with headache and myalgia that occurs in the first 24 hours of therapy. It occurs most often in patients with early syphilis. Antipyretics may be used, but no evidence indicates they prevent this reaction. Pregnant women in particular should be advised that they may develop premature labor and/or fetal distress if they develop a Jarisch-Herxheimer reaction, and they should seek medical attention if this occurs, although treatment should not be delayed because stillbirth can also be an outcome of untreated maternal syphilis.

PRIMARY AND SECONDARY SYPHILIS

Box 1 describes the treatment for adults and adolescents. Any younger children with clinical manifestations of primary and secondary syphilis must have acquired their infection recently, and they should be assessed for other STDs, including HIV. After the newborn period, children with syphilis should have a CSF examination to detect asymptomatic neurosyphilis, and birth and maternal records should be reviewed

---

BOX 1 Primary and Secondary Syphilis

Adults and Adolescents

- Benzathine penicillin G, 2.4 million U IM in a single dose

Children

- Benzathine penicillin G, 50,000 U/kg IM up to maximum adult dose in a single dose

Alternatives for Penicillin-Allergic Adults

- Doxycycline, 100 mg PO bid for 14 days
- Tetracycline, 500 mg PO qid for 14 days
- Ceftriaxone, 1 g daily IM or IV, 8–10 days (not a single dose)
- Azithromycin, 2-g single dose PO

bid, twice daily; IM, intramuscular; IV, intravenous; PO, by mouth; qid, four times per day.

BOX 2

Early Latent Syphilis

- Adults and adolescents—Benzathine penicillin G, 2.4 million U IM in a single dose
- Children—Benzathine penicillin G, 50,000 U/kg IM up to a maximum adult dose in a single dose

Late Latent Syphilis or Latent Syphilis of Unknown Duration

- Adults and adolescents—Benzathine penicillin G, 7.2 million U total, administered as three doses of 2.4 million U IM each at 1-week intervals
- Children—Benzathine penicillin G, 150,000 U/kg total, administered as three doses of 50,000 U/kg IM (up to maximum adult dose of 2.4 million U), each at 1-week intervals
- Alternatives for penicillin-allergic adults
  - Doxycycline, 100 mg PO bid for 28 days
  - Tetracycline, 500 mg PO qid for 28 days

bid, twice daily; IM, intramuscular; IV, intravenous; PO, by mouth; qid, four times per day.

---

to assess if they have congenital or acquired syphilis. If, after evaluation, they are assessed as having primary or secondary syphilis, they should be treated as described in Box 1.

Follow-up

After treatment, patients should be reexamined at 6 and 12 months, and serologic tests should be repeated (using the same type of nontreponemal test used initially). Expected findings are a fourfold decline in nontreponemal titers within 6 months.

LATENT SYPHILIS

Latent syphilis is defined as serologic evidence of syphilis without any signs or symptoms of disease. Early latent syphilis is diagnosed if during the preceding year the patient had a documented seroconversion, unequivocal symptoms of primary or secondary syphilis, or his or her sex partner had primary, secondary, or early latent syphilis. All other patients have late latent syphilis or syphilis of unknown duration and should be managed as if they have late latent syphilis. The height of the serologic titer cannot be used to distinguish early latent from late latent syphilis, although higher titers are usually seen in patients with early latent syphilis.

Adults and Adolescents

Before treatment, all patients with latent syphilis should be evaluated clinically for tertiary disease (iritis, gumma, aortitis). In addition, a lumbar puncture should be performed in patients with any neurologic or ophthalmologic signs or symptoms, evidence of tertiary disease, treatment failure, or HIV infection with late latent syphilis or syphilis of unknown duration. Box 2 shows the treatment of patients with normal CSF examination findings (if performed).

Follow-up

Quantitative nontreponemal tests should be repeated at 6, 12, and 24 months. Retreatment (after a lumbar

---

BOX 3

Tertiary Syphilis

- Benzathine penicillin G, 7.2 million U total, administered as three doses of 2.4 million U IM, each at 1-week intervals

Neurosyphilis

- Aqueous crystalline penicillin G, 18–24 million U per day, administered as 3–4 million U IV q4h or continuous infusion, for 10–14 days
- Alternative regimen (if compliance with therapy can be assured)
  - Procaine penicillin, 2.4 million U IM qd
    plus
  - Probenecid, 500 mg orally qid, both for 10–14 days
- Alternatives for penicillin-allergic adults
  - Ceftriaxone, 2 g daily either IM or IV for 10–14 days (possibility of cross-reactivity between ceftriaxone and penicillin; may need skin testing to confirm penicillin allergy and desensitization if necessary)

IM, intramuscular; IV, intravenous; PO, by mouth; q, every; qd, once daily.

---

puncture is performed) is recommended for patients whose titers rise fourfold after therapy, a high titer ($\geq$1:32) fails to fall fourfold within 12 to 24 months, or signs and symptoms attributable to syphilis develop.

TERTIARY SYPHILIS

Tertiary syphilis includes cardiovascular syphilis and gummatous lesions but not neurosyphilis. This condition is rare in children because lesions take years to develop. Before therapy, patients with tertiary syphilis should have a CSF examination. It is advised to manage these patients in consultation with an expert. Box 3 lists treatment recommendations.

NEUROSYPHILIS

Central nervous system involvement can occur at any stage of syphilis. Any patient with syphilis and clinical evidence of neurologic involvement (meningitis, motor or sensory signs, ophthalmic or auditory symptoms, cranial nerve palsies, cognitive dysfunction) should have a CSF examination. All patients with neurosyphilis should be tested for HIV. Patients with neurosyphilis or syphilitic eye disease (uveitis, neuroretinitis, optic neuritis) should be treated with the regimens described in Box 3.

Follow-up

A CSF examination should be repeated every 6 months until the cell count is normal in any patient with an initial CSF pleocytosis. CSF-VDRL and protein should also be followed, but these tend to fall more slowly.

SYPHILIS DURING PREGNANCY

Serologic tests for syphilis should be performed on all pregnant women at their first prenatal visit. In communities with a high prevalence of syphilis, a repeat serologic test should be performed at 28 weeks and at delivery, in addition to the early screening. No infant should leave the hospital without the results of a maternal serologic test performed at least once during pregnancy and preferably again at delivery. Any pregnant woman with a reactive serologic test for syphilis should be considered infected, unless there is adequate documentation of treatment and sufficient decline in serologic tests after therapy in her medical chart (not simply a verbal history of therapy).

Penicillin is the only treatment recommended for pregnant women, there are no recommended alternatives, and, if necessary, pregnant women with syphilis should be desensitized and treated with penicillin. Treatment during pregnancy should be with the penicillin regimen appropriate for her stage of syphilis. Some experts recommend a second dose of benzathine penicillin G, 2.4 million U intramuscularly (IM) 1 week after the initial dose, for women with primary, secondary, and early latent syphilis. Follow-up is particularly important in women treated for syphilis during pregnancy, and all treatment and follow-up serologic tests should be clearly documented in the chart. This information should be given to the pediatrician when the infant is born because diagnosis and treatment decisions are based on this information.

CONGENITAL SYPHILIS

Congenital syphilis is the result of untreated or inadequately treated maternal syphilis. The most effective way to prevent congenital syphilis is to identify syphilis in pregnant women through routine testing early in pregnancy. Routine testing of cord or neonatal blood is not recommended because there can be false-positive and false-negative results of these specimens in comparison with maternal blood, which is preferred for testing.

Evaluation of Infants

Making the diagnosis of congenital syphilis at birth is difficult because most infants do not have symptoms at delivery, and the diagnostic tests used are insensitive. Serologic testing of the infant merely reflects maternal antibody status in most infants, which makes interpretation of serologic tests difficult. Treatment decisions are usually based on the history of syphilis treatment and follow-up in the mother and on any evidence of congenital syphilis in the child.

All infants born to mothers with reactive nontreponemal and treponemal tests should have a serologic test performed on infant serum (not cord blood because of contamination from maternal blood). Nontreponemal tests are recommended, but a treponemal test is unnecessary because the mother's reactivity in both nontreponemal and treponemal tests already indicates she has syphilis. No IgM tests are currently available commercially to aid the diagnosis of congenital syphilis.

In addition to serologic testing, all infants born to mothers with syphilis should be examined carefully for any signs of infection (e.g., nonimmune hydrops, hepatosplenomegaly, rash, jaundice, rhinitis, pseudoparalysis of an extremity). If possible, pathologic specimens of placenta or umbilical cord should be examined for treponemes with specific fluorescent antibody staining. Any skin or mucous membrane lesions should also be evaluated with direct fluorescent antibody staining. Further evaluation of the infant depends on the adequacy of the maternal treatment and follow-up for syphilis.

Decisions on further evaluation of the infant and treatment can be difficult and may require the advice of a pediatric infectious disease specialist. The 2002 CDC guidelines are helpful in describing four common scenarios encountered in practice. Scenario 1 is an infant with highly probable congenital syphilis (abnormal physical findings, treponemes detected, or infant serologic titer fourfold maternal titer). These infants should have a lumbar puncture performed (CSF cell count, protein, and CSF-VDRL), complete blood count (CBC) with differential and platelet count, and other tests as clinically indicated (long bone radiograph, chest radiograph, liver function tests, cranial ultrasound, ophthalmologic examination, and auditory brainstem response). We usually recommend a radiograph of the knee routinely. Box 4 describes the recommended therapy for these infants. If more than 1 day of therapy is missed, the full 10-day course needs to be restarted. Few data are available on antibiotics other than penicillin, and although the CDC prefers a full 10-day course of penicillin, even in cases where ampicillin was used initially for possible sepsis, we have treated many infants with combined ampicillin and penicillin courses successfully. Close serologic follow-up is important if regimens other than the recommended ones are used to assess adequacy of therapy.

Scenario 2 describes an infant with normal physical findings, a serum nontreponemal serologic test the same as or less than fourfold maternal titer, and a maternal history of inadequate or no treatment for

BOX 4 Congenital Syphilis Treatment

Scenario 1

Infants with proven or highly probable disease

- Aqueous crystalline penicillin G, 100,000–150,000 U/kg/day administered as 50,000 U/kg/dose IV q12h during the first 7 days of life and q8h thereafter for a total of 10 days.
  or
- Procaine penicillin G, 50,000 U/kg/dose IM in a single daily dose for 10 days.

Scenario 2

Infants with normal physical examinations, serologic titer ≤ maternal titer, and inadequate maternal therapy

- Same as scenario 1 (10 days aqueous crystalline penicillin or procaine penicillin).
  or
- Benzathine penicillin G, 50,000 U/kg/dose IM in a single dose (*only* if normal CSF, CBC, radiographs, and good follow-up; some specialists prefer the 10 days of parenteral therapy if the mother has untreated early syphilis at delivery).

Scenario 3

Infants with normal physical examination, serologic titer the same as or fourfold less than maternal titer, and adequate maternal therapy

- Benzathine penicillin G, 50,000 U/kg/dose IM in a single dose. (Some specialists do not treat the infant but provide close serologic follow-up.)

Scenario 4

Infants with normal physical examination, serologic test the same as or fourfold less than maternal titer, adequate maternal therapy before pregnancy, and stable low titer

- No treatment is required, but some specialists treat with benzathine penicillin G, 50,000 U/kg as a single IM injection, particularly if follow-up is uncertain.

CBC, complete blood count; CSF, cerebrospinal fluid; IM, intramuscular; IV, intravenous; q, every.

---

follow-up. Lack of follow-up plays a large part in treatment decisions.

Scenario 3 describes infants with normal physical examinations and serum nontreponemal serologic titers the same or fourfold less than the maternal titer, whose maternal history includes treatment during pregnancy that was appropriate for her stage of pregnancy, administered more than 4 weeks before delivery, with an appropriate fourfold fall in titer after therapy and no evidence of reinfection or relapse. In these cases, no further evaluation of the infant is recommended (see Box 4).

Scenario 4 describes infants with normal physical examinations and serum nontreponemal serologic titers the same as or fourfold less than the maternal titer, whose mother has documented adequate therapy before pregnancy, and the mother's nontreponemal titer has remained low and stable before and during pregnancy and at delivery (VDRL ≤1:2 or RPR ≤1:4). No further evaluation is recommended for these infants (see Box 4).

Because of lack of specific diagnostic tests at birth to determine infection, and often difficult and uncertain social circumstances, we advise overtreatment in cases where follow-up is uncertain. We prefer treating with 10 days of parenteral therapy rather than risk not treating an infant with congenital syphilis.

Follow-up

All infants with reactive nontreponemal serologic tests should be followed carefully with repeat examinations and serologic follow-up every 2 to 3 months until the test is nonreactive or decreased fourfold (we recommend until nonreactive). The expected findings are a fall in nontreponemal titer by 3 months of age and nonreactive nontreponemal tests by 6 months of age. If the infant was treated after the neonatal period, the titers are expected to fall more slowly, but if the titers remain stable or increase after 6 to 12 months of age, the child should be evaluated with an examination of the CSF and treated with 10 days of parenteral penicillin G.

Treponemal tests are not used to evaluate treatment response because (as in adults) infants infected with syphilis may retain a reactive treponemal test for a long time (there are few published data available). Passively transferred maternal treponemal tests may be present in infants for up to 15 months of age (according to the CDC), and the CDC considers a reactive treponemal test after 18 months of age as diagnostic of congenital syphilis. If the nontreponemal test is nonreactive at 18 months of age, no further evaluation or treatment is recommended. However, if both nontreponemal and treponemal tests are reactive at 18 months of age, the CDC recommends reevaluation (including CSF evaluation) and treatment for congenital syphilis.

Any infant with an initial abnormal CSF evaluation should have a repeat CSF evaluation every 6 months until the results are normal. Retreatment should be given to children with abnormal CSF results not explained by another illness or a reactive CSF-VDRL.

syphilis, inadequate documentation of treatment, treatment less than 4 weeks before delivery, or the mother's titer did not fall fourfold after therapy. These infants should be further evaluated with a lumbar puncture (CSF-VDRL, cell count, and protein), CBC with differential and platelets, and long bone radiographs. The performance of the lumbar puncture is important in treatment decisions in these infants. If a lumbar puncture is not performed, or the CSF is not interpretable because the tap was bloody, the infant should be treated in the same way as those with highly probable congenital syphilis, either crystalline penicillin G or procaine penicillin for 10 days. For infants who have received a full evaluation, including lumbar puncture and long bone radiographs and CBC, with normal results, the CDC also recommends an alternative therapy (one dose of benzathine penicillin G, 50,000 U/kg/dose IM in a single dose). However, our preference in these infants at higher risk of having congenital syphilis is to give them 10 days of therapy, and we only rarely recommend a single dose of benzathine penicillin to infants whose mothers have a history that strongly suggests they will bring the child for

Penicillin Allergy

Penicillin allergy is not an issue in neonates, but it may be a problem in older infants and children, although it is still less common than in adults. No recommended alternatives to penicillin in children are available, and if there is a strong history of penicillin allergy, the child should be desensitized and treated with penicillin. There are insufficient data on using other antibiotics such as ceftriaxone for treating children with syphilis. If a nonpenicillin regimen is used, the patient should have close serologic and CSF follow-up.

Human Immunodeficiency Virus

Infants born to mothers with syphilis and HIV are treated the same as those with only syphilis. There are insufficient data on infants in this situation, but no published data suggest the evaluation or management of these infants should be any different. Close follow-up is of course most important in evaluating these infants.

EVALUATION AND TREATMENT OF OLDER INFANTS AND CHILDREN

Children sometimes have reactive serologic tests for syphilis after the neonatal period (more than 1 month of age). In these cases, maternal serology and records and birth records should be reviewed to assess if this condition is congenital or acquired syphilis. Any child at risk for congenital syphilis should be fully evaluated, including a CSF evaluation, CBC with differential and platelets, and other tests as clinically indicated (see highly probable congenital syphilis scenario 1) and should be tested for HIV. Box 5 describes the recommended therapy for treatment of older infants and children with congenital syphilis.

Serologic tests for syphilis are sometimes performed on children who are suspected victims of sexual abuse and may lack physical findings of primary or secondary syphilis. Reactive tests for syphilis (a reactive nontreponemal and a reactive treponemal test) in children may indicate either evidence of congenital syphilis or acquired syphilis. Congenital syphilis is likely only in children who have a documented history of syphilis in the neonatal period; otherwise, the assumption must be that the child has acquired syphilis after this period and has been sexually abused, which should be reported to the local child welfare agency.

In these cases, children with syphilis diagnosed after the newborn period should have a CSF examination to detect asymptomatic neurosyphilis. In addition, a CBC with differential and platelet count plus other tests as clinically indicated (e.g., long bone radiographs, etc.) should be performed. Treatment of children with acquired syphilis depends, as it does for adults, on the stage of syphilis (see primary and secondary syphilis). If distinguishing between congenital and acquired syphilis is difficult because of lack of information, the child should be fully evaluated for congenital syphilis and treated for 10 days with a regimen of parenteral penicillin (see Box 5), which is essentially the same as the adult regimen for treating neurosyphilis.

Preventive Measures

Syphilis is an STD, and transmission occurs only when mucocutaneous lesions are present, usually in the first year of infection. Prevention involves safe sex practices, including condom use, although condom use alone cannot prevent the transmission of syphilis if the primary chancre is not in the genital area or if significant sexual contact takes place before placing the condom. The main preventive health-care measure used is contact tracing and treatment of sexual partners.

Congenital syphilis is almost entirely prevented by early prenatal care and diagnosis and treatment of syphilis in pregnancy. In communities with high syphilis prevalence, repeating maternal syphilis screening at 28 weeks and at delivery is also helpful to identify new maternal infections so therapy can be started as soon as possible.

Common Pitfalls

- Patients with primary syphilis may have nonreactive serologic tests. The best diagnostic test in these patients is a darkfield examination or direct fluorescent antibody testing of the lesion. Darkfield examination is usually only available now in STD clinics, so primary physicians may have difficulty making this diagnosis.
- Patients with high titers, such as in secondary syphilis, may have a false-negative nontreponemal serologic test (the prozone phenomenon), if only an undiluted serum specimen is sent. Practitioners should ask for the test to be performed on diluted specimens.
- Pregnant women should always be screened for syphilis during pregnancy. Any reactive serologic test should be taken seriously, not ignored, and treatment should be given promptly.
- When evaluating the mother's history of treatment and follow-up titers, only well-documented information should be used to make evaluation and treatment decisions in the infant. A verbal history of therapy is not adequate and often inaccurate.
- Knowledge of the mother's serologic status should be confirmed before any infant leaves the hospital. Cord or infant serum samples are not a substitute

---

BOX 5 Treatment of Older Infants and Children

- Aqueous crystalline penicillin G, 200,000–300,000 U/kg/day IV, administered as 50,000 U/kg q4-6h for 10 days.
- Some experts also suggest giving a single dose of benzathine penicillin G, 50,000 U/kg IM, following the 10-day course of IV penicillin.

IM, intramuscular; IV, intravenous; q, every.

for maternal samples because they are falsely negative in approximately a third of cases and thus infants with potential congenital syphilis are not identified.

- In making treatment decisions in the infant, often the most important information is the likelihood of follow-up. In infants in scenario 2, where congenital syphilis remains quite possible, 10 days of procaine penicillin should be given (visiting nurses can give the remaining daily doses at home after discharge to finish the 10-day course).

Communication and Counseling

Because syphilis is an STD, it is crucial to communicate to the patient the importance of safe sex practices as well as the importance of follow-up to ensure treatment was adequate. Pregnant women with syphilis found on routine screening may be shocked at the news. They may require significant counseling to cope with all the implications of having an STD and an unfaithful sexual partner and concerns about their infant. The outcome for infants with congenital syphilis is good (although the data on outcomes in infants with neurosyphilis are unclear; older literature suggests a poor outcome in some, and there are few modern data), which should be communicated to the parents, as well as emphasizing the importance of follow-up to ensure adequacy of therapy. Children with acquired syphilis (not congenital syphilis) have been sexually abused and should receive extensive counseling to help them cope. Usually counseling is initiated as part of the child abuse evaluation and therapy when the child welfare agency is informed of the case.

SUGGESTED READINGS

1. American Board of Pediatrics: Syphilis. In Pickering LK (ed): Red Book: 2003 Report of the Committee on Infectious Diseases, 26th ed. Elk Grove Village, Ill: American Academy of Pediatrics, 2003, pp 595–607. **Readily available resource with practical guidelines.**
2. Augenbraun MH: Treatment of syphilis 2001: Nonpregnant adults. Clin Infect Dis 35(Suppl 2):S187–S190, 2002. **Review of the data used to compile the 2002 STD treatment guidelines for adults.**
3. Bromberg K, Rawstron S, Tannis G: Diagnosis of congenital syphilis by combining *Treponema pallidum*–specific IgM detection with immunofluorescent antigen detection for *T. pallidum*. J Infect Dis 168:238–242, 1993. **A study evaluating diagnostic tests for congenital syphilis.**
4. Centers for Disease Control and Prevention: Brief report: Azithromycin treatment failures in syphilis infections—San Francisco, California, 2002–2003. MMWR Morb Mortal Wkly Rep 53 (0):197–198, 2004. **Important first case reports of clinical failures with azithromycin.**
5. Centers for Disease Control and Prevention: Sexually Transmitted Diseases Treatment Guidelines—2002. MMWR Recomm Rep 51 (RR-6):1–80, 2002. **Definitive resource for up-to-date guidelines on evaluation and treatment.**
6. Lukehart SA, Godornes C, Molini BJ, et al: Macrolide resistance in *Treponema pallidum* in the United States and Ireland. N Engl J Med 351:154–158, 2004. **Identification of a mutant gene conferring functional azithromycin resistance in T. pallidum in a single patient and prevalence of this resistance gene in four different geographical sites. This has important implications for azithromycin therapy.**
7. Wendel GD, Sheffield JS, Hollier LM, et al: Treatment of syphilis in pregnancy prevention of congenital syphilis. Clin Infect Dis 35 (Suppl. 2):S200–S209, 2002. **Review of the data used to compile the 2002 STD treatment guidelines for pregnant mothers.**

Tetanus Neonatorum

Jeanette R. Pleasure and Elias Abrutyn

KEY CONCEPTS

- The epidemiology of neonatal tetanus (NT) reveals it is still a major cause of morbidity and mortality in developing areas of the world. There is high mortality and marked underreporting throughout the developing world. Immunization with tetanus toxoid during pregnancy, usually given with diphtheria toxoid, is inexpensive (approximately $0.15 per dose) and protective for both mother and infant.
- Neonatal tetanus has virtually disappeared in developed countries, where adults are affected most commonly. The incidence has decreased markedly as a result of widespread immunization. Only two cases have occurred in the United States in the last decade.
- The pathogen, *Clostridium tetani*, is abundant in soil and in the feces of domestic animals, horses, and humans, and is even found in homes. Toxin production depends on the carriage of a specific plasmid not found in all strains.
- The mechanism of disease is the production of spastic paralysis from blockade of inhibitory synapses by the neurotoxin tetanospasmin, secreted by the organisms.
- The clinical picture of neonatal tetanus is that of an infant who was initially well and became unable to suck, with development of stiffness or convulsions between days 3 and 28 of life. As in adult disease, the clinical picture is the means of diagnosis.
- Management of neonatal tetanus should take place in an intensive care unit where artificial ventilation is available. Metronidazole and benzodiazepines are the mainstays of drug therapy. There are so few cases of neonatal tetanus in developed countries that cues for care may be based on the latest management used in adult cases. Evidence-based studies are not likely to develop.

Tetanus neonatorum remains a health challenge in areas of the world that are riddled with poverty, lack of education, social upheaval, armed conflict, or deficient health systems. This noncommunicable disease is endemic in the developing world, particularly in Southeast Asia, which accounts for approximately half the cases, and Africa, which accounts for almost one third of the cases of neonatal tetanus (NT) worldwide.

In 2003, the director-general of the World Health Organization (WHO) noted that 20% of the 57 million deaths worldwide in 2002 occurred in children younger than 5 years, and 98% of these deaths occurred in developing countries. NT is found in 90 countries and

TABLE 1 Neonatal Tetanus in the United States During the Last Decade

Date and State	Maternal and Birth Factors	Clinical Course	Treatment	Outcome
1995 Tennessee*	• Mother: 30 yr of age, Mexican-born, had one tetanus immunization at 12 yr of age. • Prenatal care in Mexico early in gestation and five visits to Tennessee obstetrician in final 6 wk. • Birth: male, labor induced, sterile care of umbilical cord, discharged after 24 h of age post removal of cord clamp and application of isopropyl alcohol, cloth binder around abdomen on day 7. • Home: near pasture; father's job: feeding cattle and pigs on a farm.	• Isopropyl alcohol to cord a few times/day • Day 3–4: foul-smelling discharge from umbilicus • Day 6: irritable, poor feeding, stiff muscles • Day 7: admitted to hospital with tight masseter muscles, difficulty swallowing, opisthotonus • Cord anaerobic culture: Gram+ bacilli; not further identified	• Penicillin G, IV 100,000 U/kg/day, divided q6h • Human tetanus immunoglobulin IM, 500 U • Human tetanus immunoglobulin SC around umbilicus, 250 U • Intubation, paralysis, ventilated for 1 mo; another mo in hospital because of poor feeding, hypertonia	• Developmentally normal for age later in first year of life
• 1998 Montana†	• Mother: 32 yr of age, U.S. born, never vaccinated because of philosophical beliefs. • Prenatal care: licensed direct-entry midwife (distinct from certified nurse midwife). • Birth: female, cesarean delivery in local hospital; standard umbilical cord care with isopropyl alcohol, discharged at 3 days of age. Midwife supplied "Health and Beauty Clay" for umbilical care at home: unsterile, dispensed from local store to midwives from large container, to accelerate drying of the cord • Home: rural, adjacent to horse pasture, dog went back and forth between house and pasture.	• Clay applied to umbilicus 3×/day with clean cotton-tipped swab. • Day 7–8: foul-smelling discharge from umbilicus. • Day 9: unable to nurse, difficulty opening jaw for 10 h, admitted to hospital. Trismus, in-creased tone, hyperresponsive to stimuli. • Cord culture: Clostridia (perfringens and sporogenes), Staphylococcus, Streptococcus, and Bacillus species.	• Penicillin G, IV 300,000 U/kg/day for 10 days • Tetanus immune globulin IM, 500 U • Intubated on hospital day 3, ventilated for 12 days • Discharged 17 days later	• Developmentally normal at 7 mo of age

*From Craig AS, Reed GW, Mohon RT, et al: Neonatal tetanus in the United States: A sentinel event in the foreign-born. Pediatr Infect Dis J 16:955–959, 1997.

†From Centers for Disease Control and Prevention: Neonatal tetanus—Montana, 1998. MMWR Morb Mortal Wkly Rep 47:928–930, 1998.

IM, intramuscular; IV, intravenous; q, every; SC, subcutaneous.

accounts for half of neonatal deaths and one quarter of infant deaths worldwide.

As a result of immunization, tetanus is a rarity in developed countries. Vaccine became available in 1923, but routine tetanus toxoid immunization was first widely used during World War II. Tetanus became reportable in the United States in 1947 when the incidence was 3.9 cases per million population and mortality 91%. Data from the Centers for Disease Control and Prevention (CDC) for 1998 to 2000 confirmed an average annual incidence of 43 (0.16 cases per million) and mortality down to 18%. In 2003, the CDC compiled only 11 cases of tetanus in the United States up until October.

Approximately 80 cases of NT were reported annually in the 1950s in the United States, followed by a dramatic drop in the 1960s, and just 31 have been reported since 1972. No infant deaths from tetanus have occurred for many years, and just two cases of NT were reported in the last decade (Table 1). Both of these children were delivered in hospitals and had sterile care of their umbilical cords until reaching home. Each lived in rural homes where the bacteria were most likely acquired. It is noteworthy that both involved underimmunized mothers. One lived in Mexico until 8 years before the birth of her affected infant in Tennessee. She had previously delivered two infants in California, representing missed opportunities to be immunized. Obstetrical practices in Tennessee were subsequently surveyed to find out if prenatal patients were asked about their vaccination status. Only 14% of 103 practices reported asking their patients routinely for a specific history of tetanus immunizations. This is important information when caring for immigrants, especially in rural areas. Mexican Americans born outside the United States have two thirds the rate of tetanus immunity compared to those born within the United States.

The Missoula, Montana, health department investigated the second NT case (see Table 1) and released an advisory to health care workers in the area to highlight the importance of tetanus toxoid vaccination in pregnant women and to caution against the use of nonsterile substances for umbilical cord care.

The Pathogen

Clostridium tetani, a nonencapsulated organism, is an obligate anaerobic motile gram-positive rod. It readily forms endospores at one end, giving a characteristic appearance variously described as a squash racket, club, or drumstick. Spores need anaerobic conditions to germinate, so wounds that are necrotic or contain a foreign body are particularly supportive environments. The spores are stable and resist disinfectants and drying, but they are destroyed by autoclaving, iodine, or hydrogen peroxide. Complete eradication of tetanus is unlikely to ever occur. In contrast to communicable viruses such as smallpox and polio that require human hosts, *C. tetani* is abundant in soil and in the feces of domestic animals, horses, and humans, and is even found in homes.

Diagnosis is based solely on the clinical features of the patient. The organisms are relatively noninvasive and rarely found in the blood or in the wound. The wound may be minor, even inapparent (e.g., injury from a rose thorn or middle ear infection), with little local reaction and no purulence. *C. tetani* is difficult to culture, and finding the organism in culture is not definitive evidence it is producing toxin. A plasmid contains the necessary DNA for toxin production, but it is not carried by all strains.

Mechanism of Disease

Tetanus and botulinum neurotoxins are the most potent toxins known. Whereas botulism is a flaccid paralysis caused by inhibition of acetylcholine release at skeletal neuromuscular junctions, tetanus produces predominantly a spastic paralysis from preferential blockade of inhibitory synapses.

C. tetani synthesizes two exotoxins: a hemolysin with unclear function and a water-soluble neurotoxin termed *tetanospasmin,* or tetanus neurotoxin (TeNT). TeNT is translated and synthesized as an inactive polypeptide chain of 151 kDa and then cleaved by a bacterial protease to form a light chain (LC, 43 kDa) and heavy chain (HC, 107 kDa). TeNT diffuses to axon terminals of peripheral motor nerves and cranial nerves, and the HC binds to gangliosides at neuromuscular junctions. The LC enters neurons, is internalized within vesicles, and reaches the ventral horn or cranial motor nuclei by fast retrograde axonal transport. Transport occurs first in motor, then sensory, and, later, autonomic nerves. Via transsynaptic spread, the LC passes further to other neurons in the spinal cord or brain.

Presynaptic inhibitory interneurons and presynaptic neurons of the sympathetic system are thus affected. A single catalytic atom of zinc is bound to the LC and is essential for intracellular inhibition of neurotransmitter release. Zinc chelation can detoxify TeNT in vitro. The LC is an endopeptidase that specifically cleaves synaptic proteins known as *synaptobrevins* or *vesicle-associated membrane proteins* (VAMP-1 and -2). Docking of synaptic vesicles to the plasma membrane at nerve endings is inhibited, and exocytosis of presynaptic vesicles containing transmitter is hampered.

Release of the inhibitory neurotransmitters γ-aminobutyric acid (GABA) and glycine is prevented, resulting in intermittent muscle spasms. Agonist and antagonist muscles contract simultaneously and produce especially severe pain. Weakness between intense spasms and cranial nerve paralyses or myopathies are thought to result from some inhibition of acetylcholine release at the neuromuscular junction.

The Clinical Picture

With no characteristic laboratory findings, tetanus is diagnosed clinically. There are four forms of tetanus: neonatal, cephalic (rare, severe), local (rare, mild), and generalized (at least 80% of all cases). Shorter incubation periods occur if infected sites are close to the central nervous system (CNS); these cases are more severe with higher fatality rates. Manifestations also depend somewhat on the concentration of toxin, which in turn depends on inoculum size and growth conditions in the tissues. Low concentration may lead to localized tetanus. The length of the neuronal pathway determines progression. Shorter nerves are affected first (face, jaw, and paraspinal muscles) and longest nerves later. NT quickly becomes severe generalized disease that usually requires respiratory support.

The prototypic infant with NT feeds and cries normally in the first 2 days of life and becomes ill between days 3 and 28 of life, manifested by inability to suck and development of stiffness or convulsions. Generalized tetanus typically starts with rigidity and spasm of masseter muscles, producing trismus or so-called lockjaw; as facial muscles are affected, risus sardonicus may be seen as a grimace through clenched teeth, with a closed mouth and raised eyebrows. Other muscles gradually go into spasm, including those of the neck, thorax, back, and extremities. Finally there is opisthotonus, abdominal rigidity, and the possibility of apnea related to pharyngeal spasm. The first week is characterized by spasms and increasingly severe rigidity. Painful, convulsion-like spasms may be triggered by relatively minor sensory stimuli or emotional changes.

In the second week, severe disease is associated with autonomic dysregulation (hypo- or hypertension, flushing, arrhythmias) that may last 1 to 2 weeks. Spasms decrease after 3 weeks, but stiffness may persist much longer. A classic triad is proposed: rigidity, muscle spasms, and autonomic dysfunction. Beyond the neonatal period, the differential diagnosis includes strychnine poisoning and dystonic reactions to medications.

The umbilicus is the usual portal of entry in the neonate. A variety of traditions increase contamination, such as delivery on earth or straw, application of animal dung or ghee (clarified butter) to the umbilical stump, and continuous bundling of the infant in sheepskin for a week after application of cow dung to the abdomen and legs. Elective procedures such as circumcision and ear piercing are other routes of contamination, prevented to great extent by topical antibiotics.

Low levels of education and poor prenatal care are markers for inadequate maternal immunization. Adequate tetanus immunization before conception or during prenatal care is important because it is protective against maternal tetanus as well as NT.

Pathologic evaluation shows no specific gross or histologic abnormalities. Changes caused by terminal hypoxia and autonomic dysfunction are found in fatal cases. Survival without sequelae is typical in patients given modern intensive care.

Expert Opinion on Management Issues

Prophylaxis (Box 1) occurs most notably when transplacental antibody reaches the fetus. Care of the affected infant (Boxes 2 and 3) includes removal of the source of TeNT (necrotic tissue debrided, umbilicus cleansed), neutralization of circulating toxin with antitoxin, and provision of supportive care until tetanospasmin already fixed in tissue is metabolized. Penicillin, used for many years, is now considered suboptimal therapy because it inhibits GABA(A) receptors (as do other β-lactams). Many of the drugs used in care of adults may be of use on an individual basis in affected infants. Small non–evidence-based studies suggest that magnesium sulfate infusions in adults effectively decrease the duration of spasms and ventilator requirement. Certainly, calcium and magnesium levels should be tested in these infants and any low values corrected; aiming for supranormal levels is controversial.

BOX 1 Strategies for Prevention of Neonatal Tetanus

- Check immunization status of all pregnant women:
  - Give primary series of Td (tetanus and diphtheria toxoid) if uncertain or negative history, consisting of three doses: the first two doses at least 4 weeks apart and the third dose 6 to 12 months after the second dose. Two doses are remarkably protective for the infant.
  - Give one dose of Td if mother has received primary series and last vaccination was 10 years ago or longer.
- Be aware of the interventions especially lacking and needed in developing countries:
  - Skilled delivery attendant
  - Promotion of clean delivery and umbilical care
  - Prenatal education about the signs and severity of neonatal tetanus and its total preventability
- Explore each case for root causes and potential changes in risky behaviors.

Common Pitfalls

Failure to recognize the diagnosis causes delay in specific therapy. Other diagnoses to be treated and ruled out in the neonate include sepsis, seizures, meningitis, and hypocalcemic tetany. Intensive care will be needed and transport arranged. Ventilator support and intravenous lines are used and may lead to respiratory complications, such as pneumothorax, chronic lung disease in the neonate, and increased nosocomial infections. Prolonged hospitalization raises the risk for complications and becomes a major financial burden. In contrast, immunization costs mere cents!

BOX 2 Initial Management of Neonatal Tetanus

- Transport to a level III neonatal intensive care unit (NICU) with ventilator capacity.
- Assess for severe dysphagia with danger of aspiration, apnea, or unremitting spasms. If dysphagia is present:
  - Benzodiazepine sedation (diazepam, 0.1–0.2 mg/kg IV q4–6h, or lorazepam, 0.05–0.1 mg/kg/dose IV over 2–5 min, or midazolam, 0.05–0.1 mg/kg/dose IV over 2–3 min). Action: GABA(A) agonists.
  - Follow by paralysis with vecuronium bromide, initial 0.1 mg/kg/dose IV, maintenance 0.03–0.15 mg/kg/dose IV q1–2h PRN, or pancuronium bromide, initial 0.2 mg/kg/dose IV, maintenance 0.05–0.1 mg/kg/dose IV q0.5–4h PRN as needed, endotracheal intubation, and ventilation. May follow with drugs via IV drip for continued spasms. Consider tracheostomy after several weeks if prolonged intubation and irritation of airway are extreme.
- Human tetanus immune globulin (HTIG), 500 U IM; possible SC infiltration around the wound (not evidence based). Give after sedation; neutralizes circulating TeNT; may shorten course of disease by preventing diffusion into CNS.
- Metronidazole, 15 mg/kg/day, in two doses/day (double if 7 days of age) IV (PO) for 7–10 days.
- Quiet, darkened room, minimal stimuli to decrease spasms.
- Clean umbilicus thoroughly to remove source of more toxin.
- Fluids and parenteral nutrition. May progress later to enteral feeds. Adequate fluids to prevent acute renal failure associated with rhabdomyolysis. Extra calories needed for excessive activity and autonomic output. Follow with electrolytes; give calcium and magnesium if decreased.

CNS, central nervous system; IM, intramuscular; IV, intravenous; PO, by mouth; q, every; SC, subcutaneous; TeNT, tetanus neurotoxin.

BOX 3 Subacute Care for the Infant with Neonatal Tetanus

- Care for autonomic instability as needed:
  - Hypotension: dopamine, 2–20 µg/kg/min intravenously.
  - Hypertension: Apresoline, clonidine, morphine.
- Taper sedation and blockade over 14–21 days. Gradually increased doses may become habituating; must avoid withdrawal.
- Request consultations as needed.
- Immunize after recovery as appropriate for age. Tetanus toxin is a poor immunogen, and even previous infection does not guarantee immunity.

Be aware of complications: bone fractures, ruptured tendons, asphyxia, muscle hematomas, rhabdomyolysis, renal compromise.

Communication and Counseling

Enhanced awareness of NT would lead to more complete reporting and fuller national and statewide surveillance data. All cases of NT should be investigated to uncover correctable factors that could improve maternal vaccine delivery or reduce contamination.

SUGGESTED READINGS

1. Bleck TP: Tetanus: Pathophysiology, management and prophylaxis. Dis Mon 37:556–603, 1991. **A classic treatment of tetanus including its interesting history.**
2. Centers for Disease Control and Prevention: Neonatal tetanus—Montana, 1998. MMWR Morb Mortal Wkly Rep 47:928–930, 1998. **Report of a case born to an unvaccinated U.S. native.**
3. Cook TM, Protheroe RT, Handel JM: Tetanus: A review of the literature. Br J Anaesth 87:477–487, 2001. **A review of clinical findings, complications, and management.**
4. Craig AS, Reed GW, Mohon RT, et al: Neonatal tetanus in the United States: A sentinel event in the foreign-born. Pediatr Infect Dis J 16:955–959, 1997. **Report of case that occurred in Tennessee to an infant of a Mexican-born undervaccinated mother.**
5. Gunn VL, Nechyba C (eds) The Harriet Lane Handbook: A Manual for Pediatric House Officers, 16th ed. Philadelphia: Mosby, 2002. **Excellent source for pediatric and neonatal drug dosages.**
6. Jong-wook L: Global health improvement and WHO: Shaping the future. Lancet 362:2083–2088, 2003. **The director-general of WHO views the world's health challenges of the last few decades and his concerns for the future.**
7. McQuillan GM, Kruszon-Moran D, Deforest A, et al: Serologic immunity to diphtheria and tetanus in the United States. Ann Intern Med 136:660–666, 2002. **Data from the Third National Health and Nutrition Examination Survey (NHANES III).**
8. Sheffield JS, Ramin SM: Tetanus in pregnancy. Am J Perinatol 21:173–182, 2004. **Tetanus in pregnancy should be treated like tetanus in other settings.**
9. Thwaites CL, Farrar JJ: Preventing and treating tetanus. BMJ 326:117–118, 2003. **Subtitled "The challenge continues in the face of neglect and lack of research." An editorial written by two physicians from Vietnam whose hospital admits 300 patients with tetanus per year.**
10. Turton K, Chaddock JA, Acharya KR: Botulinum and tetanus neurotoxins: Structure, function and therapeutic utility. Trends Biochem Sci 27:552–558, 2002. **A remarkably complete review of the mechanisms of action of the clostridial neurotoxins.**

Tuberculosis

Lisa-Gaye Robinson and Wafaa M. El-Sadr

KEY CONCEPTS

- Children with latent tuberculosis (TB) infections serve as a pool for future TB cases.
- When a young child has a new diagnosis of TB disease or has a newly positive tuberculin skin test, it is a sentinel event and most likely indicates transmission from an adult or adolescent with the disease. Investigation of such cases by a local health department is warranted.
- Treatment for latent tuberculosis infection (LTBI) should not be started until TB disease has been excluded.

- Treatment for TB disease requires a multidrug regimen to avoid the development of resistance.
- In addition to the multidrug regimen, treatment requires a prolonged course to ensure the elimination of persistent bacilli to prevent treatment failures and relapse.
- Successful treatment for LTBI and TB disease requires strict adherence to the prescribed regimen. Directly observed therapy (DOT) is recommended.

Tuberculosis (TB) is a multifaceted disease caused primarily by infection with the organism *Mycobacterium tuberculosis* (MTB). MTB is usually transmitted through inhalation of droplets from an individual with TB disease. TB is also rarely caused by *Mycobacterium bovis,* transmitted via ingestion of unpasteurized milk. Infection with either organism does not progress to disease in the majority of patients. The likelihood that a child will develop disease if infected is inversely related to the age at which infection occurs. Children younger than 1 year are at greatest risk for progression to disease (43%), and those between 1 and 5 years of age have a risk of 24%, both alarmingly high rates of progression.

Treatment of children with latent tuberculosis infection (LTBI) or TB disease is warranted not only for the individual child but also from a public health perspective. Children with LTBI serve as a pool for future TB cases. Moreover, a child with TB disease or tuberculin skin test (TST) conversion is a sentinel event and most likely indicates transmission from an adult or adolescent with disease. Involvement of the local health department is critical to identification of the source case as well as identification of contacts for the child. Prevention of new cases of TB in children is a critical component in the attempt to eliminate the disease in the United States.

TB in children often manifests in an occult manner without the typical symptomatology reported in the adolescent and adult populations. Approximately 50% of children with pulmonary TB disease are asymptomatic at the time of diagnosis. Fever, cough, weight loss, and night sweats are not commonly reported, although the youngest children are more likely to be symptomatic. Thus diagnosis of TB in children requires a high level of suspicion and appropriate clinical, immunologic, radiographic, and microbiologic evaluations. A significant proportion of TB cases in children are diagnosed clinically and are not laboratory-confirmed cases. An understanding of the local epidemiology (where the patient was diagnosed and/or where the patient most likely acquired the infection) is useful in choosing the most effective antituberculosis regimen.

Expert Opinion on Management Issues

TREATMENT OF LATENT TUBERCULOSIS INFECTION

Treatment for LTBI should not be started before TB disease is excluded. Thus a chest radiograph must be

TABLE 1 Recommended Treatment Regimens for Tuberculosis

TB Manifestation	Regimen	Minimum Duration	Comments
LTBI			
• INH susceptible	INH daily or intermittently (DOT only)	9 mo	
• INH resistant/RIF susceptible	RIF daily	6 mo	
• INH/RIF resistant	Usually two susceptible second-line agents	Prolonged	Consult a TB expert.
Pulmonary TB	INH, RIF, PZA, and either ethambutol or an aminoglycoside daily for 2 mo, followed by 4 mo INH and RIF (can be given two times per wk by DOT)	6 mo	DOT is strongly recommended. The fourth drug can be discontinued as soon as the susceptibilities are determined. Resistant strains may require unfamiliar second-line drugs and require up to 2 years of treatment and should be done in conjunction with a TB expert.
Extrapulmonary TB	INH, RIF, PZA, and either ethambutol or an aminoglycoside daily for 2 mo, followed by 7–10 mo INH and RIF (can be given two times per wk by DOT)	9–12 mo	DOT and resistance comments remain the same as above. Cervical lymph node TB disease can be treated for 6 mo. Steroids are recommended for meningitis and may be considered for other forms of extrapulmonary TB (see text).

DOT, directly observed therapy; INH, isoniazid; LTBI, latent tuberculosis infection; PZA, pyrazinamide; RIF, rifampin; TB, tuberculosis.

obtained *and* interpreted prior to starting treatment. If possible, identification of the source case and the drug susceptibility pattern of the source case's isolate of MTB should be obtained. Administration of isoniazid (INH) daily for 9 months (270 doses) is the preferred regimen if the source case has an INH-susceptible organism or the susceptibility is unknown (Table 1). Adherence to required doses of treatment is critical. If treatment needs to be prolonged because of missed doses, the INH daily regimen should be completed within a 12-month period. Experts recommend retreatment if the patient received less than 6 months of INH within a 9-month period. Intermittent (twice- or thrice-weekly) INH for 9 months can be used if directly observed therapy is used to ensure adherence. To avoid hepatotoxicity missed doses should not be added to the subsequent day's dose if the patient is receiving daily therapy. Although liquid INH may be easier logistically to deliver in young children, this formulation is associated with abdominal pain and/or diarrhea in more than 50% of children. INH is available as scored 100-mg and 300-mg tablets, which are easily crushed and dispensed in soft foods (e.g., pudding, gelatin, or infant food) and much better tolerated. Rifampin (RIF) is the preferred alternate regimen if the source case has an INH-resistant and RIF-susceptible organism or INH is not tolerable despite efforts to alleviate mild side effects. Vitamin B$_6$ is recommended for breast-fed infants, children or adolescents on milk- and meat-deficient diets, those with human immunodeficiency virus (HIV) infection, pregnant adolescents, or those who experience paresthesias while taking INH.

Treatment of LTBI in a child exposed to an infectious source case with MDR (multidrug resistant) TB should be done in consultation with an expert in pediatric TB. Directly observed therapy (DOT) is strongly recommended for treatment of all children and adolescents

with MDR LTBI. Consultation with an expert in pediatric TB and pediatric HIV for treatment of LTBI in a child with HIV infection who is receiving antiretroviral therapy is advised.

Parents/caregivers and patients should be educated at each visit about signs and symptoms of hepatotoxicity and other potential adverse reactions. They should be instructed to stop medications immediately if symptoms consistent with hepatotoxicity develop and to return immediately to the provider for assessment. Monthly face-to-face evaluation to assess adherence, missed doses, evidence of adverse reactions, or progression to TB disease should be performed.

Liver function tests during treatment of LTBI in children and adolescents are not necessary unless signs or symptoms of hepatotoxicity develop. However, in patients at risk for development of hepatotoxicity (e.g., patients with underlying liver disease or those receiving other hepatotoxic drugs), liver function tests should be obtained 1 and 3 months after initiation of treatment for LTBI. It is not necessary to obtain a chest radiograph at the completion of treatment of LTBI unless signs and symptoms of TB disease develop.

TREATMENT OF CHILD WITH A NEGATIVE TUBERCULIN SKIN TEST WITH KNOWN EXPOSURE (WINDOW PROPHYLAXIS)

Window prophylaxis is recommended in children 5 years of age or younger who were exposed to an adult or adolescent with TB disease and have an initial negative screening TST. This is not an unusual scenario because TST conversion after exposure and infection with *M. tuberculosis* may take 6 to 12 weeks. Thus early initiation of treatment for latent TB infection is recommended in these younger children who are at particularly high risk for progression to TB disease after infection. A second TST should be repeated at the end of the window (12 weeks after end of known exposure to the TB case) to determine if TST conversion occurred. If TST conversion did not occur, it suggests the child was not infected, and treatment for LTBI can be discontinued. Some experts recommend completing the 9-month prophylaxis in children younger than 1 year. In addition, even in the absence of TST conversion among exposed immunosuppressed children younger than 5 years, treatment for LTBI should be continued for 9 months.

TREATMENT OF TUBERCULOSIS DISEASE

The treatment of TB disease requires a multidrug regimen with a prolonged course to ensure the elimination of persistent bacilli to prevent treatment failures and relapse. The antimycobacterial agents should ideally be bactericidal and kill both intracellular and extracellular *M. tuberculosis*. RIF is considered the most active agent for treatment of TB and kills dormant extracellular bacteria. INH similarly kills extracellular organisms. Pyrazinamide (PZA) kills intracellularly. Six months is the minimum duration of treatment for pulmonary and extrapulmonary lymph node disease, whereas disseminated, meningeal, and musculoskeletal disease requires at least 9 to 12 months of treatment.

The standard of care in the United States for adults with TB disease has evolved in most jurisdictions to beginning an initial four-drug regimen because of concern about possible isoniazid resistance (Table 2). The initial 2-month regimen for TB disease in children is the same for all disease presentations (see Table 1). The initial treatment is empirical and usually presumptive in the absence of confirmatory laboratory results. A four-drug regimen, consisting of INH, RIF, PZA, and either ethambutol or an aminoglycoside as the fourth drug, is recommended (Table 3). If susceptibility results are received within the first 2 months of therapy and demonstrate a pansusceptible isolate, the fourth drug (usually ethambutol) can be discontinued. If the source case is identified, susceptibility of the source case's isolate should be sought and the therapy modified accordingly. The goal of the initial 2 months

of daily therapy is to offer the most effective bactericidal activity, with the goal of rapidly decreasing the number of viable organisms (sterilization) and thereby decreasing morbidity and transmission. The initial multidrug therapy also diminishes the likelihood of the emergence of drug resistance.

At the end of the initial 2 months of therapy, sterilization should be achieved and drug susceptibilities should be available from the patient or source case isolate. If this information is not available and risk factors for possible drug resistance are not present, the remaining 4 to 10 months of treatment (which can be can be administered twice weekly if DOT is available) can be completed with INH and RIF. *M. bovis* strains are typically resistant to PZA and can be treated with 9 to 12 months of INH and RIF alone if the organism is susceptible to these two agents (with 2 months of ethambutol during the initial phase).

Therapy for drug-resistant TB disease requires varied regimens based on susceptibility of the isolate and typically requires longer treatment. Tuberculosis caused by an INH monoresistant isolate may be treated using RIF, PZA, and ethambutol for the disease-appropriate duration of treatment. Disease caused by a PZA monoresistant isolate should be treated using INH, RIF, and ethambutol for at least 9 months. Children with an RIF-monoresistant or a multidrug-resistant strain (resistant to both INH and RIF) require treatment with at least three active second-line drugs for a period of 18 to 24 months (see Table 3). Children with resistant TB disease should be managed in conjunction with an expert in pediatric tuberculosis.

Corticosteroids are recommended for children with tuberculous meningitis. Steroids should be considered in children with pleural and pericardial effusions, severe miliary disease, and endobronchial disease. Steroids must always be administered in conjunction with antituberculous drugs. An initial dose of 1 to 2 mg/kg of prednisone daily for 1 to 2 weeks and tapered over 4 to 6 weeks is suggested.

Vitamin B_6 is recommended for breast-fed infants, children, or adolescents on milk- and meat-deficient diets, those with HIV infection, pregnant adolescents, or those who experience paresthesias while receiving antituberculous treatment. The recommended dose is 25 to 50 mg/day given as a single daily dose. Vitamin B_6 is also recommended for patients receiving ethionamide or cycloserine. Higher dosages (50 to 100 mg) should be prescribed for patients receiving cycloserine to prevent peripheral neuropathy caused by this agent.

Patients should be followed monthly during treatment for disease progression and drug toxicity. Routine laboratory evaluation is not warranted unless the patient develops symptoms of toxicity, has underlying liver disease, or is taking medications that may potentiate liver damage. A chest radiograph should be obtained at the end of TB therapy. This film may not be normal, but significant improvement should be evident. Clinical and radiographic follow-up 1 year after completion of treatment for TB disease is recommended to ensure continued resolution.

TABLE 2 Persons at Increased Risk for Drug-Resistant Tuberculosis Infection or Disease

Contacts of a patient with drug-resistant contagious tuberculosis disease

Foreign-born persons from countries with high rates of resistant tuberculosis

Residents of areas where the prevalence of drug-resistant *Mycobacterium tuberculosis* is documented as high (defined by most experts as isoniazid-resistance rates >4%)

Persons with a history of treatment for tuberculosis disease (or whose source case for the contact received such treatment)

Persons whose source case has positive smears for acid-fast bacilli or cultures after 2 mo appropriate antituberculosis therapy

TABLE 3 Recommended Drugs for Tuberculosis in Children

Drugs	Formulations	Daily Dosage (Maximum)	Twice Weekly Dose (Maximum)	Adverse Reactions
First-Line Drugs				
Isoniazid*	Tablets: 100, 300 mg Syrup: 10 mg/mL Injection: 100 mg/mL	10–20 mg/kg PO (300 mg)	20–40 mg/kg (900 mg)	Elevated transaminases, hepatitis, or peripheral neuropathy
Rifampin*	Capsules: 150, 300 mg Syrup: 10, 15 mg/mL Injection: 600 mg	10–20 mg/kg PO (600 mg)	10–20 mg/kg (600 mg)	Orange coloration of body fluids, vomiting, hepatitis, thrombocytopenia, or influenza-like illness
Pyrazinamide*	Tablets: 500 mg	20–30 mg/kg PO (2 g)	40–50 mg/kg (4 g)	Hyperuricemia, skin rash, joint manifestation, or hepatotoxicity
Ethambutol†	Tablets: 100 mg Tablets: 400 mg	15–25 mg/kg PO (1.6 g)	25–50 mg/kg (4.0 g)	Rash, vision loss, or color blindness
Streptomycin	Vial: 1 g Vial: 4 g	20–40 mg/kg IM (1 g)	20–40 mg/kg (1.5 g)	Ototoxicity, nephrotoxicity
Second-Line Drugs				
Capreomycin	Vial: 1 g	15–30 mg/kg IM (1 g)		Ototoxicity, nephrotoxicity
Ciprofloxacin‡	Tablets: 100, 250, 500, 750 mg Syrup: 250, 500 mg/5 mL	20–30 mg/kg PO in 2 divided doses (1.5 g) PO		Gastrointestinal disturbance, headache, psychosis, rash, or photosensitivity
Cycloserine	Capsules: 250 mg	15–20 mg/kg PO in 2 divided doses (1 g)		Psychosis, personality changes, seizures, or rash
Ethionamide	Tablets: 25 mg	15–20 mg/kg PO in 2 divided doses (1 g)		Gastrointestinal disturbances, hepatotoxicity, or hypersensitivity reaction
Kanamycin	Vial: 75, 500 mg, 1 g	15–30 mg/kg IM (1 g)		Ototoxicity, nephrotoxicity
Para-aminosalicylic acid	Packets: 4 g	150–200 mg/kg PO (12 g)		Gastrointestinal disturbances, hepatotoxicity, or hypersensitivity reaction

*Rifamate (Aventis Pharmaceuticals, Bridgewater, NJ) is a capsule containing 150 mg of isoniazid and 300 mg of rifampin. Two capsules provide the usual adult (>50 kg) daily doses of each drug. Rifater is a capsule containing 50 mg of isoniazid, 120 mg of rifampin, and 300 mg of pyrazinamide.

†Twice-weekly dosing, 50 mg/kg; thrice-weekly dosing, 25–30 mg/kg. Dose-related optic toxicity less of a concern at 15 mg/kg daily dose used in younger nonverbal children whose vision cannot be easily monitored.

‡Fluoroquinolones are currently not licensed for use in persons younger than 18 years; their use in this age group necessitates assessments of the potential risks and benefits.

IM, intramuscular; PO, by mouth.

Common Pitfalls

It is imperative to exclude TB disease prior to treatment for LTBI. Failure to do so may lead to monotherapy in a child with TB disease, which could potentially result in development of INH-resistant or INH/RIF-resistant isolates and complicate eventual treatment of the patient. Because approximately 50% of children with pulmonary tuberculosis are asymptomatic at the time of TB diagnosis, careful assessment is needed to distinguish latent TB infection from TB disease. The diagnosis of TB disease in a child is often a clinical diagnosis without the benefit of confirmatory culture or information on susceptibility of the source case isolate. This complicates the treatment of TB in children and underscores the need to pay careful attention to the local epidemiology and drug susceptibility of TB cases in the community to assist in the choice of antituberculous agents as part of empirical therapy.

The most daunting pitfall of the treatment of LTBI or TB disease is the challenge of adherence to prolonged therapy. Failure to adhere to treatment hampers the effectiveness of the treatment in the individual patient and is a public health risk for the community, resulting in TB cases in the future and/or development of resistant organisms. For this reason, standard of care for those with TB disease demands the use of DOT, if available. It is equally imperative that efforts be focused on promotion and monitoring of adherence to treatment of LTBI. Education about the importance of adherence should be provided to the child and caregiver. Adherence-enhancing strategies, including enablers and incentives, should be used. Most importantly, child-friendly programs should be developed. Available resources for DOT for LTBI should prioritize DOT for children younger than 3 years, those with HIV infection, close contacts of cases of TB disease, those who are immunocompromised, or those with a history of poor adherence. If resources allow, all children should be considered for DOT. School-based DOT through school nurses should be used, if available.

Communication and Counseling

Parents/caregivers and patients who completed treatment for LTBI should be informed that future tuberculin skin testing is unnecessary, but if such a test is inadvertently performed in the future, it is safe. Children who successfully complete treatment for LTBI rarely develop TB disease, and those who complete treatment for pansusceptible or INH-resistant TB disease have very low relapse rates and excellent prognoses. However, children who do not complete treatment, who have MDR-TB, or whose antituberculous regimen did not include RIF are at risk of progression or reactivation and therefore require closer follow-up. In all cases, parents/caregivers and patients should be educated about the signs and symptoms of TB disease and instructed to return promptly to their provider if such signs or symptoms develop. Written documentation of TST results and evidence of completion of LTBI or TB treatment should be provided.

SUGGESTED READINGS

1. American Academy of Pediatrics: Tuberculosis. Pickering LK (ed): 2003 Red Book: Report of the Committee on Infectious Diseases, 26th ed. Elk Grove Village, Ill: American Academy of Pediatrics, 2003, pp 642–660. **Governmental recommendations for treatment of tuberculosis in children.**
2. Ampofo K, Saiman L: Pediatric tuberculosis. Pediatr Ann 31 (2):98–108, 2002. **Comprehensive review of tuberculosis in children.**
3. Loeffler AM: Pediatric tuberculosis. Semin Respir Infect 18 (4):272–291, 2003. **Comprehensive review of tuberculosis in children.**
4. Pediatric Tuberculosis Collaborative Group: Targeted tuberculin skin testing and treatment of latent tuberculosis infection in children and adolescents. Pediatrics 114:1175–1201, 2004. **American Academy of Pediatrics guidelines for screening, targeted testing, and treating latent tuberculosis in children and adolescents.**

Tularemia

Richard F. Jacobs

KEY CONCEPTS

- Tularemia is a tick-borne infection that has important regional disease distribution.
- A thorough physical examination identifies a papular-based ulcer with associated regional lymphadenitis that is a hallmark of disease.
- Ulceroglandular and glandular forms (no skin lesion) of the disease are frequent; tularemia affects children in the cervical lymph node chain most commonly.
- The diagnosis relies on serologic testing, but exclusion of other causes of acute regional lymphadenitis can be important.
- Presumptive therapy in clinically compatible cases may be required.

Tularemia is an acute, febrile, zoonotic illness that is distributed widely in the Northern Hemisphere, with numerous infections occurring in humans over relatively large areas of the United States, Europe, and Asia. It is a disease of small animals, but humans are highly susceptible hosts. *Francisella tularensis* is a small, nonmotile, gram-negative coccobacillary organism divided into two types: *F. tularensis* biovar *tularensis* (type A) and *F. tularensis* biovar *palaearctica* (type B).

F. tularensis biovar *tularensis* is found predominantly in North America, is highly virulent, and causes severe disease in mammals and mild to severe disease in humans. *F. tularensis* biovar *palaearctica* is found in Asia, Europe, and North America, frequently linked to environmental sources and waterborne diseases of rodents, and commonly acquired by airborne spread, with less virulence in mammals. Tularemia is a ubiquitous organism found in the Northern Hemisphere between 30 and 71 degrees north latitude. It has been reported throughout the United States, but it occurs most commonly in the western and south central states. The major vector of *F. tularensis* is the tick, and the disease is seen primarily in children and young adults during the major tick seasons of spring, summer, and early fall. The disease is transmitted to humans by vector (e.g., ticks, lice, fleas, deer flies, mosquitoes), animal bites, or ingestion of infected, inadequately cooked animal tissues or contaminated water. *Amblyomma americanum* (Lone Star tick), *Dermacentor andersoni* (wood tick), and *Dermacentor variabilis* (dog tick) are the main reservoirs for *F. tularensis*.

F. tularensis gains access to the human body through the skin, conjunctiva, oropharynx, respiratory tract, or gastrointestinal tract. It spreads by lymphatics or hematogenously, and bacteremia usually develops during the first week of infection. Skin, regional lymph nodes, liver, spleen, and lungs can be involved, and the lesions can occur in the gastrointestinal tract and the central nervous system. After a tick bite, a hallmark presentation for *F. tularensis* infection is the resultant eschar, ulcer, or papule with regional lymphadenitis. Seroconversion may take 1 or 2 weeks after infection. Despite reports of recurrent disease, the initial infection with *F. tularensis* usually confers long-term immunity. The average incubation period for tularemia is 3 to 4 days (range, 1 to 21 days).

The onset of symptoms typically is abrupt, with a temperature usually greater than 103°F (39.4°C), chills, pharyngitis, myalgias, arthralgias, nausea and vomiting, and, occasionally, headaches, cough, and photophobia. The predominant signs of tularemia include regional lymphadenopathy or lymphadenitis; an ulcer, eschar, or papule at the site of tick embedment; and hepatosplenomegaly. In untreated cases of tularemia, fever may persist for 2 to 3 weeks or longer. No characteristic peripheral blood profile is established for tularemia. A variety of skin rashes (macular, morbilliform, pustular, and erythema nodosum) are described, but the predominant feature is regional lymphadenopathy or lymphadenitis.

TABLE 1 Clinical Types and Presentation of Tularemia

Type of Disease	(%)	Clinical Sign or Symptom	(%)
Ulceroglandular	45	Lymphadenopathy	96
Glandular	25	Fever (≥101°F [38.3°C])	87
Oculoglandular	2	Pharyngitis	43
Pneumonic	14	Ulcer, eschar, papule	45
Oropharyngeal	4	Myalgias, arthralgias	39
Typhoidal	2	Nausea, vomiting	35
Unclassified	6	Hepatosplenomegaly	35

Adapted from Jacobs RF, Condrey YM, Yamauchi T: Tularemia in adults and children: A changing presentation. Pediatrics 76:818, 1985.

The classification of six forms of tularemia depends on the portal of entry. The distribution of the clinical manifestations of tularemia in children in one large series was 45% ulceroglandular, 25% glandular, 14% pneumonic, 4% oropharyngeal, and 2% oculoglandular and typhoidal, with 6% of the cases remaining unclassified (Table 1). The most common forms of tularemia are ulceroglandular and glandular, in which organisms gain access through the skin, usually after a tick bite. Approximately 2 days after the onset of symptoms, the regional lymph nodes become tender and swollen. Within 24 hours, a painful, swollen papule develops distal to the regional nodes. This papule ruptures and progresses to ulceration and eschar. In children, regional lymphadenopathy typically is seen in the cervical area, and in adults it occurs in the inguinal area, probably reflecting the most frequent sites of tick bites. Glandular tularemia is identical to the ulceroglandular form, except the portal of entry cannot be identified. The other four forms of tularemia are relatively uncommon compared with the ulceroglandular and glandular types.

The diagnosis of tularemia is suggested by the history and aided by the physician's awareness in endemic areas. In nonendemic areas, the diagnosis of tularemia may be difficult. History of contact, although often unavailable, should take into account the season of the year, the clinical manifestations of the disease, the unresponsiveness to antibiotics not effective against tularemia, and the endemic rate of disease in that area. The diagnosis is confirmed by serologic tests. The commercially available standard agglutination test is reliable. Microagglutination and an enzyme immunoassay using outer membrane proteins are now the standard tests because of their enhanced sensitivity compared with the standard agglutination test. Unfortunately, they do not provide a diagnosis early in the course of disease. Agglutinating antibody titers often are not detectable until the second week of illness (days 10 to 14). In some cases, seroconversion is not described until 4 to 6 weeks of illness. A fourfold increase in the specific agglutination titer confirms the diagnosis, but a presumptive diagnosis should be considered with acute titers of 1:160 or greater.

Expert Opinion on Management Issues

ACCEPTED INTERVENTIONS

Table 2 describes the antibiotic treatment of tularemia. Streptomycin is considered the drug of choice. The recommended regimen of 30 to 40 mg/kg/day divided into two daily intramuscular injections for a 7-day course is effective. An alternative regimen is streptomycin at a dosage of 30 to 40 mg/kg/day administered intramuscularly for the first 3 days, with subsequent reduction to 15 to 20 mg/kg/day given intramuscularly for the final 4 days. A Jarisch-Herxheimer reaction is sometimes observed in the beginning of therapy with aminoglycosides. In severe cases or if a child does not establish an afebrile, asymptomatic course within a few days, extension of treatment beyond 7 days is indicated and should be based on clinical assessment. Streptomycin-resistant strains are reported, but they are rare. Defervescence and symptomatic response is prompt, usually within several days. The response may be somewhat delayed if the lymph nodes have progressed to suppuration.

Gentamicin has become a more popular choice for treatment. In hospitalized children, intravenous gentamicin at standard dosages of 2.5 mg/kg/dose given every 8 hours (or 5.0 mg/kg/dose every 12 hours) for 7 days is used. If clinical defervescence does occur, outpatient management with intravenous or intramuscular gentamicin can be pursued. Consideration for once- to twice-daily dosing of gentamicin (5.0 mg/kg/dose) is currently recommended by some experts based on their clinical experience. The streptomycin guidelines for length of therapy with time to defervescence and symptom relief should be used in gentamicin therapy. Although no randomized trial data exist to compare aminoglycoside versus quinolone treatment of tularemia, ciprofloxacin is used successfully. Fluoroquinolones, specifically ciprofloxacin, are now recommended by some experts for the treatment of tularemia in older adolescents and adults. The use in children is anecdotal with successful results in small numbers, but most of the experience was in Scandinavia with the less virulent serotype.

TABLE 2 Antibiotic Treatment of *Francisella tularensis*

Drug Name	Dosage
Streptomycin	30–40 mg/kg/day divided q12h IM for 7 days
Streptomycin*	Alternate dosing: 30–40 mg/kg/day for 3 days followed by 15–20 mg/kg/day
Gentamicin	7.5 mg/kg/day divided q8h IM or IV
Gentamicin*	10 mg/kg/day divided q12h
Tetracycline†	2–4 mg/kg/day (maximum 100 mg/dose) PO or IV
Ciprofloxacin‡	20–30 mg/kg/day divided q12h PO or IV

*Alternate dosing based on personal experience.
†Usually doxycycline preparation; reported higher relapse rate.
‡Recommended by some experts; used successfully in Scandinavia; possible differences in serotypes may account for this response.
IM, intramuscular; IV, intravenous; PO, by mouth; q*x*h, every *x* hours.

Common Pitfalls

- Tularemia has a short incubation period, so serologic testing is commonly negative until at least the second week of illness.
- Clinicians should notify laboratory personnel if cultures are ordered because of the potential laboratory hazard for aerosolization.
- Tularemia can manifest like many other causes of acute cervical lymphadenitis in children, but it does not respond to β-lactam antibiotic therapy.
- Ceftriaxone failures are well described despite in vitro testing that would indicate a susceptible organism.
- The many clinical manifestations of tularemia can make the diagnosis challenging, especially in regions of the United States that do not see this infection often.
- Treatment with a tetracycline antibiotic has a relatively high relapse rate.
- Late suppuration of lymph nodes occurs in up to 25% of cases but they do not usually contain live organisms, and it is not a reason to retreat the patient.

Communication and Counseling

Prevention of human tularemia depends on the prevention of contact with vectors and protection during the handling of contaminated animal tissues. Children should be cautioned against handling sick or dead rabbits or rodents. Rabbit or rodent carcasses should be disposed of by burial or incineration. Rubber gloves should be worn when preparing game animals. Children who live in tick-infested areas should have their skin and hair checked frequently for the presence of ticks, which should be removed carefully and appropriately. Children in an area of tick endemism should wear clothing with tightly fitting cuffs at the ankles and wrists. In endemic areas, tick repellents to prevent the attachment and feeding of ticks on children should be used appropriately.

SUGGESTED READINGS

1. Baker CN, Hollis DG, Thomsberry C: Antimicrobial susceptibility testing of *Francisella tularensis* using a modified Mueller-Hinton broth. J Clin Microbiol 22:212–215, 1985. **Provides antibiotic minimum inhibitory concentration (MIC) sensitivity testing of tularemia isolates.**
2. Centers for Disease Control and Prevention: Tularemia—Oklahoma 2000. MMWR Morb Mortal Wkly Rep 50:704–706, 2001. **Describes the prevalence and regional distribution of cases of tularemia.**
3. Ikaheimo I, Syrjala H, Karhukorpi J, et al: In vitro antibiotic susceptibility of *Francisella tularensis* isolated from humans and animals. J Antimicrob Chemother 46:287–290, 2000. **Provides additional MIC sensitivity testing on tularemia isolates.**
4. Jacobs RF, Condrey YM, Yamauchi T: Tularemia in adults and children: A changing presentation. Pediatrics 76:818–822, 1985. **Describes the disease presentation in children compared to adults.**
5. Jacobs RF, Narain JP: Tularemia in children. Pediatr Infect Dis 1:487–491, 1983. **Describes tularemia in children and addresses management issues.**
6. Johansson A, Berglund L, Gothefors L, et al: Ciprofloxacin for treatment of tularemia in children. Pediatr Infect Dis J 19:449–453, 2000. **One of the first descriptions of ciprofloxacin treatment of tularemia in Scandinavia.**
7. Mason WL, Eigelsbach HT, Little SF, et al: Treatment of tularemia, including pulmonary tularemia with gentamicin. Am Rev Respir Dis 121:39–45, 1980. **Addresses the issue of gentamicin usage for the treatment of tularemia.**
8. Pullen RL, Stuart BM: Tularemia analysis of 225 cases. JAMA 129:495–500, 1945. **A large series describing tularemia in adults and some children with outcomes.**

Typhoid Fever

Theresa J. Ochoa and Thomas G. Cleary

KEY CONCEPTS

- Infection is acquired through the fecal–oral route. Illness begins after a 3- to 60-day incubation period (typically 7 to 14 days).
- Typhoid fever is variable in its clinical course. The classic case is characterized by gradual onset of high fever, headache, anorexia, malaise, abdominal pain, and hepatosplenomegaly. Constipation occurs in approximately 50% of cases; diarrhea occurs in approximately 30% of patients.
- Most infections in the United States are acquired during travel; more than 80% of cases have a history of travel in the previous 6 weeks, with ingestion of contaminated food or water the presumed method of acquisition.
- Domestically acquired infections may be traced to a chronic carrier. The person who is the source of infection may have been infected years before.

Typhoid fever (enteric fever) usually is caused by *Salmonella typhi* and less often by other invasive *Salmonella*, including *Salmonella paratyphi* A and *Salmonella paratyphi* B. Occasionally other serotypes of *Salmonella* can cause a very similar illness. Typhoid fever is a protracted bacteremic illness characterized by insidious onset of fever, constitutional symptoms (headache, malaise, anorexia, lethargy), abdominal pain and tenderness, and hepatosplenomegaly. The older child or adult with typhoid has a gradually increasing fever up to 104°F to 104.5°F (40°C to 40.5°C) that becomes hectic during the first week. Spiking fevers may continue for a month or more, if left untreated. Even after resolution of fever, patients may feel weak and tired for months. During the febrile illness, the child feels very ill and has severe headache, anorexia, weakness, and myalgia. Delirium, psychosis, confusion, or coma may occur. On occasion, children may have cough. Older children and adults are often constipated; younger children commonly have diarrhea. Relative bradycardia may be found on exam. Occasionally, rose spots (millimeter-sized maculopapular lesions) are seen on the trunk.

Most complications develop during the second or third week of illness. Major complications include gastrointestinal bleeding, intestinal perforation, shock, meningitis, seizures, and death (currently a rare outcome; in the era before antibiotics, mortality was approximately 20%). Other complications include acalculous cholecystitis, hepatitis, osteomyelitis, arthritis, pneumonia, pyelonephritis, myocarditis, parotitis, and orchitis. The relapse rate is 5% to 20%, even when appropriate therapy is given. Relapses typically are milder than the initial illness. Chronic carriers excrete *Salmonella* in stools for more than 1 year. Approximately 1% to 6% of infected individuals become chronic biliary tract carriers and an important source of infection to their contacts. Women are much more likely than men to be chronic carriers, reflecting their higher incidence of gallbladder disease.

Expert Opinion on Management Issues

Choice of therapeutic agent has become debatable as multiply resistant organisms have emerged. In the past, chloramphenicol given for 2 weeks was the norm. In much of the world, the low cost of this approach still makes it the appropriate first-line therapy. The major risks of this therapy are bone marrow suppression and a high frequency of relapse after completion of treatment. If chloramphenicol is used, blood counts should be followed.

The development of multiply resistant *S. typhi* in many areas has led to study and use of other regimens. Trimethoprim-sulfamethoxazole, ampicillin, third-generation cephalosporins, fluoroquinolones, and azithromycin are all effective if the organism is not resistant in vitro. However, although typhoid bacilli are sensitive in vitro to aminoglycosides, first-generation cephalosporins (e.g., cephalothin), and second-generation cephalosporins (e.g., cefazolin, cefamandole), these drugs should not be used for treating typhoid because clinically they often fail.

Travel history and knowledge of local resistance patterns are now key to decisions regarding treatment. The vast majority of travel-related cases are acquired during visits to Mexico, India, the Philippines, Pakistan, Bangladesh, or Haiti. The Indian subcontinent is a particularly high-risk destination for travelers, because of both the risk of infection and the risk that infection may be caused by a multiply resistant organism. Such organisms may be resistant to ampicillin, chloramphenicol, trimethoprim-sulfamethoxazole, and, in some cases, ciprofloxacin. The high frequency of travel-related multiply resistant organisms dictates that current empirical therapy for typhoid fever be either ceftriaxone or ciprofloxacin. If the patient is known to have a susceptible strain, treatment with ampicillin, chloramphenicol, or trimethoprim-sulfamethoxazole is reasonable. A variety of regimens have been studied in randomized clinical trials. Table 1 provides examples of typical treatment schedules used in the United States (chloramphenicol is not shown because the oral preparation is no longer available in this country).

Optimal dose and duration of therapy with ceftriaxone are open to debate. Conventionally, treatment is given as one or two doses per day for 10 to 14 days. However, shorter courses may be adequate; one regimen consists of ceftriaxone, 75 mg/kg/day (maximally 2 g per day) intravenously in two doses, until defervescence, after which an additional 5 days of treatment is given. Courses as short as 3 to 5 days have been studied but appear to have a higher risk of relapse. Multiresistant organisms require a longer course of treatment.

Fluoroquinolones, such as ciprofloxacin, may have special advantages. Therapy is typically given for approximately 7 days. However, very short courses of therapy, as little as 2 to 5 days, are effective and appear to be associated with lower rates of recurrent disease than traditional chloramphenicol therapy (relapse rate approaching zero vs. 10% to 20% relapse with chloramphenicol). However, these short courses of therapy are much less effective when the organisms are resistant to nalidixic acid. In fact, even more traditional, longer courses of therapy with a fluoroquinolone may fail when the organism is resistant to nalidixic acid; in vitro susceptibility to fluoroquinolones therefore must be interpreted with great caution if the organism is resistant to nalidixic acid. The fluoroquinolones are not recommended for use in children younger than 18 years because of concerns about cartilage damage; however, large clinical pediatric studies in patients with typhoid fever suggest that toxicity is rare and treatment highly effective.

A single daily dose of azithromycin (10 mg/kg/day; maximum, 500 mg/day) for 7 days is effective in typhoid fever, but there is less experience with this regimen than with either ceftriaxone or ciprofloxacin. Depending on the setting (e.g., cephalosporin-allergic child, organism resistant to nalidixic acid), azithromycin may be a reasonable alternative.

TABLE 1 Therapy for Typhoid Fever

Generic Name (Trade Name)	Dosage/Route/Regimen	Maximum Dose	Dosage Formulation	Common Adverse Reactions	Therapeutic Concentrations	Comments
Ceftriaxone (Rocephin)	75 mg/kg/day IM or IV in one or two daily doses for 10–14 days.	Up to 4 g/day can be used in serious infections in adults.	Injection: 250 mg, 500 mg, 1 g, 2 g; contains 3.6 mEq Na/g of drug.	Allergic reactions; cholelithiasis; sludging in gallbladder; jaundice	Peak serum concentration greater than 300 μg/mL are achieved after IV infusion of 75 mg/mL.	Current drug of choice for empirical therapy of typhoid in children.
Ciprofloxacin (Cipro)	20–30 mg/kg/day divided q12h IV; can be switched to oral after infection is controlled; therapy typically 7–14 days.	800 mg/day may be used IV or 2.5 g/day PO.	Suspension: 250 or 500 mg/5 mL; tablets: 100, 250, 500, 750 mg; injectable solution: 10 mg/mL.	Theoretical risk of injury to growing cartilage; GI upset, renal failure, restlessness, rash, headache	Peak serum concentrations of 1–5 μm/mL after oral dose of 15 mg/kg.	Alternative when ceftriaxone cannot be used.
Azithromycin (Zithromax)	10 mg/kg/day once daily PO for 7 days.	500 mg/day.	Suspension: 100 mg/5 mL, 200 mg/5 mL; tablets: 250, 500, and 600 mg.	Rash, GI upset, nephritis		Reasonable alternative after ceftriaxone and ciprofloxacin.
Trimethoprim-sulfamethoxazole (Bactrim, Septra, etc.)	10 mg/kg/day of the TMP component in two divided doses; treatment usually 10–14 days.	320/1600 mg/day.	TMP/400 mg SMX (regular strength, 160/800 mg (double strength); Suspension: 40/200 mg per 5 mL; Injectable: 16/80 mg per mL (may contain propylene glycol and benzyl alcohol).	Bone marrow suppression, rash, (rarely Stevens-Johnson syndrome); crystalluria, glossitis, nephrotoxic; hepatotoxic; GI upset; hemolysis in patients with G6PD deficiency; hyperkalemia in AIDS patients; not recommended for use for <2 mo (kernicterus risk)		Acceptable choice when the organism is susceptible.
Ampicillin (Omnipen, Principen, Totacillin, etc.)	100–200 mg/kg/day IV or IM divided q6h; treatment usually continued for 10–14 days; amoxicillin may be given orally to complete therapy.	12 g/day IV/IM.	Suspension 125, 250 mg/5 mL; caps: 250, 500 mg; injectable: contains 3 mEq Na/g of IV prep.	Diarrhea (20%), rash; allergic reactions; interstitial nephritis, pseudomembranous colitis		Acceptable choice when the organism is susceptible.

AIDS, acquired immune deficiency syndrome; GI, gastrointestinal; G6PD, glucose-6-phosphate dehydrogenase; IM, intramuscular; IV, intravenous; PO, by mouth; q, every; qxh, every x hours.

Severe typhoid (with delirium, obtundation, stupor, coma, or shock) should be treated with corticosteroids as well as antibiotics. Dexamethasone (3 mg/kg intravenously followed by eight doses of 1 mg/kg given every 6 hours) decreases fatality from 56% to 10% in these serious infections.

Carriers should be decolonized to remove the risk of infection to their contacts and to decrease the possible long-term risk of biliary tract cancers. Management consists of either a prolonged course (up to 6 to 8 weeks) of an oral antibiotic to which the organism is susceptible or cholecystectomy. High-dose intravenous ampicillin or oral amoxicillin combined with probenecid may be used for eradication of the carrier state, assuming the organism is susceptible.

Two vaccines are currently available to the U.S. public. The Ty21a oral vaccine is highly effective and has minimal risk. The Vi capsular polysaccharide vaccine is injected and has more side effects but similar efficacy. Boosters are required every 2 to 5 years (depending on which vaccine is used) if the child is returning to a risk area. Vaccination must be completed well before travel to be effective. Vaccine is recommended for travel to the Indian subcontinent and high-risk areas of Asia, Africa, and Latin America. Recent information suggests that vaccine should be considered even for quite short visits to very high-risk areas. Unfortunately, no vaccine is currently licensed for children younger than 2 years, even though in endemic areas they represent a significant portion of cases. Updated information regarding vaccine use is found online at a Center for Disease Control and Prevention (CDC) website: (http://www2.ncid.cdc.gov/travel/yb/utils/ybGet.asp?section=dis&obj=typhoid. htm).

Common Pitfalls

- Although disease may be very severe in infants, children younger than 5 years may have a milder, less distinctive illness, often misdiagnosed as a viral syndrome.
- Culture from multiple sites should be submitted for suspected typhoid fever. During the first week of illness, the yield of blood and bone marrow cultures is high and the yield of stool and urine cultures is low. During subsequent weeks, the yield of blood culture decreases and the yield of stool and urine cultures increases.
- Among the various diagnostic modalities, bone marrow culture has the highest yield (approximately 80%). Usually other cultures are obtained before bone marrow (blood, urine, stool, rose spot), but the lower yield often forces the physician to obtain the marrow.
- Stool cultures are more important in children than in adults with typhoidal syndromes because there is a higher yield in children (60% vs. 27%).
- Diagnosis confirmed by culture is preferred over diagnosis suggested by serologies. *Salmonella* agglutinins ("febrile agglutinins," Widal test) may suggest the diagnosis, but because of false-positive

and false-negative results, these tests are not recommended.

- Failure to take into account the local resistance pattern of the country where infection was acquired can lead to delay in initiating appropriate therapy.
- Clinical failures or relapses can occur following treatment with fluoroquinolones if the isolate is resistant in vitro to nalidixic acid. In vitro susceptibilities must be interpreted with caution.
- Failure to vaccinate a child and other family members prior to their visiting an endemic area remains a shortcoming of care. Tourists and business travelers rarely acquire typhoid; families visiting relatives and friends abroad are at highest risk.

Communication and Counseling

The vaccines are approximately 50% to 80% effective, so families anticipating travel should be instructed in other commonsense measures in addition to being vaccinated. Travel instructions regarding typhoid are relevant, particularly if the family is going into rural areas rather than the usual tourist routes. Information should be given about the risk of contaminated food and water. Bottled water (especially carbonated water) or boiled water is usually safe, as is food served steaming hot. Tourists should be discouraged from eating uncooked vegetables or fruits that cannot be peeled at the time of eating. Ice is frequently unsafe, so drinks chilled in a refrigerator are preferable to drinks served with ice. Food purchased from street vendors is often contaminated. Hand washing before meals and after using the toilet should be encouraged. Adherence to such measures has the advantage not only of decreasing the risk of typhoid but also that of more common travel-related infections, such as diarrheas related to *Escherichia coli*, cholera, dysentery, and hepatitis A.

Once an infection is diagnosed in a family, the parents should be informed that the organism may be excreted in stool for a prolonged time, and this excretion is associated with a risk of additional cases in close contacts. If there are food handlers in the family, care should be taken to ensure they are not carriers before they return to work. If an individual with typhoid is identified in a daycare center, other children and staff should be cultured. If infection is diagnosed in a child younger than 5 years, the child should be excluded from daycare until three negative stool cultures are obtained. For older children and adult daycare staff, return to the center is appropriate 1 day after diarrhea resolves. A child who is hospitalized with typhoid should be isolated until therapy is completed and three stool cultures, separated by at least 48 hours, are negative. The risk of symptomatic relapse should also be discussed; a recurrence of fever should immediately lead to reconsultation with the physician. Cases should be reported to public health authorities so outbreaks can be recognized and dealt with.

SUGGESTED READINGS

1. Ackers ML, Puhr ND, Tauxe RV, Mintz ED: Laboratory-based surveillance of *Salmonella* serotype *typhi* infections in the United States: Antimicrobial resistance on the rise. JAMA 283 (20):2668–2673, 2000. **Approximately 25% of isolates (primarily related to travel) were resistant to one or more antimicrobials, with 17% resistant to five or more agents, including ampicillin, chloramphenicol, and tri-methoprim-sulfamethoxazole. No resistance to ciprofloxacin or ceftriaxone was observed, but 7% of isolates were resistant to nalidixic acid, a pattern associated with clinical failures or relapses following treatment with a fluoroquinolone.**
2. Hosoglu S, Aldemir M, Akalin S, et al: Risk factors for enteric perforation in patients with typhoid fever. Am J Epidemiol 160 (1):46–50, 2004. **In multivariate analysis, male sex, leukopenia, inadequate treatment prior to admission, and short duration of symptoms were highly associated with perforation.**
3. Katz DJ, Cruz MA, Trepka MJ, et al: An outbreak of typhoid fever in Florida associated with an imported frozen fruit. J Infect Dis 186(2):234–239, 2002. **This outbreak of typhoid related to imported fruit points out the risk of a globalized food supply. Travel or exposure to carriers are not the only way to get infected in the United States.**
4. Renuka K, Kapil A, Kabra SK, et al: Reduced susceptibility to ciprofloxacin and *gyr*A gene mutation in North Indian strains of *Salmonella enterica* serotype *typhi* and serotype *paratyphi* A. Microb Drug Resist 10(2):146–153, 2004. **The gyrA gene mutation confers resistance to nalidixic acid and reduces susceptibility to ciprofloxacin. Testing using traditional disk diffusion methods may not detect resistance and result in delay in initiation of appropriate treatment.**
5. Steinberg EB, Bishop R, Haber P, et al: Typhoid fever in travelers: Who should be targeted for prevention? Clin Infect Dis 39(2):186–191, 2004. **This review of cases of typhoid fever reported to the CDC between 1994 and 1999 defined the current epidemiology of travel-related typhoid and the need to reevaluate current vaccine policy.**

VIRAL INFECTIONS

Cytomegalovirus Infections

Gail J. Demmler

KEY CONCEPTS

- Infection with cytomegalovirus (CMV) is common and may be classified as primary or recurrent; as symptomatic or asymptomatic; and as a congenital, perinatal, postnatal, or health care–associated infection.
- Sources of CMV infection include transplacental transmission from mother to fetus; cervical secretions and body fluids, especially urine, saliva, human milk, and semen; blood products; and organ or marrow transplants.
- Congenital CMV infection affects approximately 1% of newborns and is diagnosed by detection of the virus within the first 3 weeks of life; 90% are asymptomatic or silently infected at birth, and 10% have symptoms including growth retardation, hepatosplenomegaly, petechiae, thrombocytopenia, and direct hyperbilirubinemia.
- Congenital CMV infection is a leading cause of childhood deafness. Developmental and motor disabilities and visual impairment also may occur in severely affected newborns.
- CMV infection in healthy individuals is usually asymptomatic, but it may cause fever, malaise, hepatitis, pneumonitis, or a mononucleosis syndrome.
- CMV infection in immunocompromised individuals can be asymptomatic but may be associated with fever with leukopenia syndrome, esophagitis, colitis, hepatitis, encephalitis, retinitis, rejection in transplant recipients, and graft-versus-host disease in marrow transplant recipients.

- Viral culture, DNA and antigen detection, serology, and histology all may be used to detect CMV infection. Definitive diagnosis of CMV disease requires presence of virus and cytomegalic inclusion cells in tissue.
- Treatment of active CMV infection with antiviral medication suppresses viral replication and resolves symptoms of CMV-associated disease, but it does not "cure" infection. Early, preemptive, or prophylactic antiviral treatment, as well as passive immunoprophylaxis with CMV hyperimmune globulin, may reduce risk of disease in high-risk patients.
- Prevention strategies include reducing host exposure to CMV by use of CMV-seronegative donors for human milk, transfusions, and transplants; hygienic precautions to avoid direct contact with saliva and urine; and immediate and careful hand washing if exposure occurs.
- No vaccine is licensed for prevention of CMV infection or disease.

Cytomegalovirus (CMV) is a ubiquitous virus that commonly infects individuals of all ages, backgrounds, races, and ethnicities. Most infections with CMV are asymptomatic, but in special patients, such as the unborn fetus and the immunocompromised, this virus can cause serious life-threatening or permanently disabling disease. Infections with CMV that are acquired for the first time, called primary infections, are more likely to produce symptoms. Individuals who have experienced primary CMV infections may also experience recurrent infections, through reactivation of the individual's CMV strain they originally acquired or, less commonly, when they are reinfected with another strain of CMV. Recurrent infections with CMV also may produce signs, symptoms, and sequelae in the patient, but they are usually less frequent and less severe than primary infections.

Cytomegalovirus is common worldwide, with no seasonal occurrences. It infects individuals of all ages, but important periods of acquisition are the fetus stage; newborn, infancy and toddler years; adolescence; and childbearing years (Box 1). Approximately 1% of all newborns in the United States are congenitally infected with CMV, and most individuals become infected by the time they reach middle adulthood years. Risk factors for acquiring CMV infection include inges-

---

BOX 1 Sources of Cytomegalovirus Infections

Mother to Infant
- Congenital
- Cervicovaginal secretions
- Human milk

Person to Person
- Saliva and urine (transmission within daycare and families)
- Cervicovaginal and seminal secretions (sexual transmission)

Associated with Health Care
- Transfusions
- Transplantation
- Person to person (rare)

TABLE 1 Signs, Symptoms, and Sequelae of Congenital CMV Infections in Symptomatic (S) and Asymptomatic (A) Newborns

Signs and Symptoms at Birth	S	A
Non-CNS		
• Intrauterine growth retardation	+	±
• Hepatosplenomegaly	+	—
• Petechiae or purpura	+	—
• Pneumonitis	+	—
• Hepatitis	+	—
• Thrombocytopenia	+	±
• Hyperbilirubinemia	+	—
• Hemolytic anemia	+	—
CNS		
• Microcephaly	+	—
• Intracranial calcifications	+	+
• Ventriculomegaly	+	—
• Periventricular leukomalacia	+	—
• Vasculitis	+	—
• Seizures	+	—
Sensory		
• Hearing loss	+	+
• Chorioretinitis	+	—
• Optic atrophy	+	—
Sequelae after Birth		
• Progressive hearing loss	+	+
• Vision loss	+	—
• Mental retardation	+	—
• Learning disorders	+	±
• Motor disabilities	+	—

CMV, cytomegalovirus; CNS, central nervous system.

---

tion of human milk from a CMV-seropositive mother or milk bank donor; blood product transfusions or marrow, stem cell, or solid organ transplantation from CMV-seropositive donors; and close or intimate contact in the daycare or family setting with another individual who is actively infected and shedding CMV. Newborns congenitally infected with CMV are usually asymptomatic at birth but may experience progressive deafness during childhood. Newborns with symptomatic congenital CMV infection may have a variety of clinical manifestations at birth, and they commonly experience permanent neurologic or sensory sequelae (Table 1). Most CMV infections in healthy infants, toddlers, adolescents, and adults are asymptomatic, but immunocompromised individuals, especially those with abnormalities in their T-cell–mediated cellular immunity, may experience CMV-associated syndromes, such as fever with leukopenia syndrome, esophagitis, hepatitis, pneumonitis, encephalitis, and sight-threatening retinitis.

Infection with CMV is most commonly diagnosed by viral culture or detection of viral DNA or antigen. Detection of CMV immunoglobulin (Ig) M antibody production, when accompanied by a CMV IgG seroconversion, demonstrates primary CMV infection. Active recurrent CMV infections in previously CMV IgG seropositive individuals and recent primary infections in individuals whose previous CMV serostatus is unknown are suggested by detection of CMV by culture, or DNA or antigen detection methods, as well as CMV IgM antibody production. However, because infection with CMV is very common, diagnosis of CMV-associated disease is best demonstrated by detection of the virus accompanied by histopathologic changes, such as cytomegalic inclusions cells, in the tissue of those affected with end-organ damage.

Disease associated with CMV can be treated with antiviral medications, such as ganciclovir, valganciclovir, foscarnet, and cidofovir. Because these medications have significant toxicity, treatment is usually reserved for immunocompromised patients and some newborns. Also, despite treatment, infection with CMV is lifelong and may recur for indefinite periods of time.

Preemptive therapy with antiviral medications administered at the time of laboratory-diagnosed CMV infection, but before symptoms and signs of disease occur, prevents or modifies CMV-associated disease in transplant recipients. Prophylaxis with antiviral medications or CMV-specific Ig preparations also reduces risk of serious CMV disease in CMV-seronegative transplant recipients who receive marrow, stem cells, or solid organs from CMV-seropositive donors. Prevention of CMV infection by vaccination is not yet possible. Thus current prevention strategies are based on risk reduction and include use of CMV-seronegative donors, whenever possible, for blood products, human milk, and transplants. In addition, hygienic practices that reduce direct exposure to saliva and urine of young children and include hand washing after exposure to these secretions should be practiced by women of childbearing age, especially if they are pregnant.

TABLE 2 Antiviral Therapy Options for Treating CMV Infection and Disease

Treatment	Dose	Interval	Route	Duration
Ganciclovir				
Induction*	5 mg/kg	q12h	IV	2–3 wk
Maintenance	5 mg/kg	q24h (3–5 times/wk)	IV/PO	Indefinite
Congenital	6 mg/kg	q12h	IV	6 wk
Valganciclovir				
Induction*	900 mg	q12h	PO	2 wk
Maintenance	900 mg	q24h	PO	Indefinite
Congenital	Investigational			
Foscarnet				
Induction*	60 mg/kg	q8h	IV	2–3 wk
Maintenance	90 to 120 mg/kg	q24h	IV	Indefinite
Congenital	Not recommended			
Cidofovir				
Induction*	5 mg/kg	q7days	IV	2 wk (2 doses)
	1 mg/kg	q3days	IV	2 wk (6–8 doses)
Maintenance*	5 mg/kg	q14days	IV	10 wk (5 doses)
Congenital	Not recommended			

*Adjust for renal function.
CMV, cytomegalovirus; IV, intravenous; PO, by mouth; q*x*h, every *x* hours.

Expert Opinion on Management Issues

CONGENITAL INFECTIONS

Treatment of newborns congenitally infected with CMV is a controversial issue, and the decision to administer antiviral medication to these infants remains at the discretion of the clinician. Treatment with antiviral medication should be considered if the newborn has signs at birth of active viral sepsis syndrome, severe pneumonitis requiring oxygen supplementation or mechanical ventilation, severe or persistent thrombocytopenia, or active sight-threatening chorioretinitis. Antiviral therapy temporarily reduces or eliminates active viral replication and helps these newborns resolve and heal end-organ disease. However, the role of short-term treatment in the newborn period in improving long-term audiologic and developmental outcome is less clear, and experts differ on this issue.

A 6-week course of ganciclovir administered in doses of 6 mg/kg every 12 hours appears to improve hearing, maintain normal hearing, and prevent hearing deterioration for the first 6 to 12 months of life (Table 2). It also may improve growth and head circumference and hasten resolution of hepatitis during this time period. It is not clear whether the effects of early treatment are long lasting or prevent late progression of hearing loss. In addition, treatment is also significantly associated with absolute neutropenia, severe enough in many cases to require dosage adjustment or cessation of therapy to reverse. Care also should be taken to avoid infiltration of the medication into tissues surrounding veins because it can cause severe ulceration. Some

experts recommend use of oral ganciclovir or valganciclovir for extended periods of time, up to months or years, in children with hearing loss associated with congenital infection. This form of treatment is usually administered with the hope of halting progressive hearing loss. Unfortunately, no controlled trials are available to assess the true benefit of this approach, and experience remains limited and anecdotal. In addition to antiviral therapy, management of infants with congenital CMV disease also includes supportive care of severely ill infants, with ventilatory and pressor support, seizure control, and platelet transfusions.

Long-term management of symptomatic infants includes periodic assessments of hearing, vision, motor skills, growth, and development, with early interventions by therapists and tutors as appropriate (Box 2). Hearing loss may be treated with preferential seating and school accommodations, hearing aids, and cochlear implants if deafness is severe, bilateral, and nonresponsive to hearing aids. Some severely affected infants also may have feeding difficulties, either in the immediate newborn period or during the first 3 years of life, so growth and nutrition should be carefully monitored and adjustments in caloric intake and diet made to meet the child's needs. Feeding by gastrostomy tube (G-tube) also may be necessary if the child is severely delayed and does not have sufficient oropharyngeal coordination to take sufficient calories by the traditional oral route. Infants born with asymptomatic congenital CMV infection appear to have normal growth and development and are at minimal risk for eye disease; however, because up to 15% of these children develop progressive hearing loss, they should receive annual hearing assessments through 18 years of age and appropriate interventions, if hearing loss is documented.

BOX 2 **Evaluation and Management of a Newborn with Congenital Cytomegalovirus Infection**

At Birth

- Clinical evaluations
- Physical and neurologic examination
- Ophthalmologic examination
- Hearing evaluation (diagnostic auditory brainstem-evoked responses)
- Laboratory evaluations
  - Complete blood count, differential, platelet count
  - Alanine transaminase
  - Total and direct bilirubin
  - Urine or saliva cytomegalovirus culture

Follow-Up Treatment Indicated in Selected Patients

- Annual physical, growth, and neurodevelopmental assessments
- Periodic hearing evaluations
- Ophthalmologic examinations (only if retinitis or optic atrophy seen at birth)
- Early interventions as indicated
- Routine immunizations as indicated (provided no other contraindications)

Prevention of congenital CMV infection depends, in part, on prevention of primary CMV infection in pregnant women. Congenital infection that occurs as a result of a maternal recurrent infection, especially a reactivation infection, is not preventable at this time.

INFECTIONS IN THE PREGNANT WOMAN AND FETUS

Women with serologic evidence of a primary infection during pregnancy should be referred to a perinatologist for counseling and prenatal diagnosis. Serial fetal ultrasound examinations should be performed to assess fetal growth and development. Amniotic fluid may be sampled for detection of CMV by viral culture and DNA polymerase chain reaction (PCR) tests. Collection of amniotic fluid as early as 20 weeks' gestation may be used to diagnose fetal infection, and, when coupled with serial ultrasounds, it may provide useful information about whether or not the fetus has an asymptomatic infection or symptomatic disease. A negative amniocentesis does not exclude CMV infection in the fetus, however. Treatment of the pregnant woman or the infected fetus with antiviral medication is currently not recommended. However, some women may choose termination of the pregnancy if severe neurologic involvement is documented early in the pregnancy. If the pregnancy is continued, the newborn's urine should be cultured for CMV to confirm congenital infection.

Prevention of CMV infection in the pregnant woman remains controversial, and a CMV vaccine is not yet available. However, many experts suggest screening women of childbearing age for serologic evidence of past CMV infection (CMV IgG antibody), and they recommend education regarding behavioral and hygienic precautions that may reduce their risk of acquiring the virus during pregnancy.

INFECTIONS IN THE IMMUNOCOMPROMISED HOST

therapy. Treatment of CMV-associated disease in the immunocompromised patient involves a 2- to 3-week period of induction therapy with an intravenous medication such as ganciclovir to halt viral replication and allow recovery from disease. In special circumstances, foscarnet and/or cidofovir may be used (see Table 2). Induction therapy is almost always followed by a reduced-dosage schedule of intravenous or oral maintenance Duration depends on the patient's clinical and immunologic condition. Maintenance therapy may be necessary for only a brief period if the patient's clinical condition and immune status, especially T cell function, are good, or it may be required for months or years if a chronic condition such as graft-versus-host disease, chronic rejection, or acquired immunodeficiency syndrome (AIDS) is present. If the patient does not show clinical and virologic improvement during induction treatment or if CMV-associated disease recurs during maintenance therapy, a resistant strain of CMV may be present, and foscarnet may be added to the antiviral regimen. Because most ganciclovir-resistant CMV strains exhibit cross-resistance to cidofovir, its use should be reserved for special circumstances. In addition, the patient's immune suppression should be assessed, and other coinfections and comorbid conditions should be treated.

Prevention of CMV disease in immunocompromised hosts is important and may be accomplished through a CMV-negative organ or marrow donor selection process, use of CMV seronegative or leukocyte-depleted blood products, pre- and post-transplant prophylaxis with CMV Ig or antiviral medications, and post-transplant viral surveillance accompanied by preemptive antiviral therapy when evidence of an active infection is detected. A CMV vaccine is not currently available; however, research continues in this area.

Common Pitfalls

- Treatment of congenital CMV infection has a small but measurable benefit for some newborns, yet it requires a commitment to central venous access, frequent clinical follow-up visits, and periodic laboratory assessments. Approximately half of treated newborns develop significant neutropenia and require dosage adjustment or cessation of ganciclovir.
- Diagnosis of primary or past CMV infection in a pregnant woman does not necessarily mean the fetus will be infected or have disease. CMV infection in the fetus does not always mean disease or poor outcome after birth. Therefore, prenatal diagnosis of CMV infection should be considered only if patient and doctor understand how the knowledge will be used for the benefit of the infant.
- CMV infection is common in the immunocompromised patient, and establishing the role CMV is playing, if any, in disease requires clinical correlation with careful virologic documentation in the organ involved.

- CMV infection is lifelong, and disease has serious consequences in the immunocompromised patient. However, treatment is associated with significant side effects, including hematologic and renal toxicities. Because CMV infection cannot be cured, the goal is to achieve a balance between CMV and the host.
- Prevention of CMV infection or disease through immunization is not available, and prevention by behavioral and hygienic practices may not prevent all exposures and/or be effective in all individuals. Thus CMV infections remain common and are an important public health problem.

Communication and Counseling

Resources are available for families and health care workers who care for infants with congenital CMV infection and disease, for pregnant women with CMV infection who desire to know the risks to their fetus, for women of childbearing years who wish to reduce their risk of acquiring CMV during pregnancy, and for immunocompromised individuals who require prolonged or investigational treatments (available online at http://www.cdc.gov, http://www.aap.org, and http://www.bcm.tmc.edu/pedi/infect/cmv).

SUGGESTED READINGS

1. Adler SP, Finney JW, Manganello AM, et al: Prevention of child-to-mother transmission of cytomegalovirus by changing behaviors: A randomized controlled trial. Pediatr Infect Dis J 15:240–246, 1996. **Describes a randomized, clinical trial evaluating the effects of a behavioral hygienic strategy to reduce risk of CMV infection in women of childbearing age.**
2. Cannon MJ, Davis KF: Washing our hands of the congenital cytomegalovirus disease epidemic. BMC Public Health 5(1):70 2005, (E-pub ahead of print.). **A plea for public health officials to promote education and hygienic strategies for prevention of congenital CMV infection.**
3. Demmler GJ: Summary of a workshop on surveillance for congenital cytomegalovirus disease. Rev Infect Dis 13:315–329, 1991. **Summarizes current knowledge regarding the public health problem of congenital CMV infection and disease in the United States and provides the basis for the National Congenital CMV Registry.**
4. Demmler GJ: Congenital cytomegalovirus infection treatment. Pediatr Infect Dis J 22(11):1005–1006, 2003. **Reviews management recommendations for newborns with congenital CMV infection and disease.**
5. Demmler GJ: Screening for congenital cytomegalovirus infection: A tapestry of controversies. J Pediatr 146(2):162–164, 2005. **Discusses current controversies surrounding the benefits and challenges associated with routine screening of newborns for congenital CMV infection.**
6. Kimberlin DW, Lin CY, Sanchez PJ, et al: Effect of ganciclovir therapy on hearing in symptomatic congenital cytomegalovirus disease involving the central nervous system: A randomized, controlled trial. J Pediatr 143(1):16–25, 2003. **This landmark article describes the only large, randomized, multicenter clinical trial evaluating treatment of neonates with congenital CMV disease. It demonstrates that early treatment protects against progressive and late-onset hearing loss but is associated with hematologic side effects.**
7. Michaels MG, Greenberg DP, Sabo DL, Wald ER: Treatment of children with congenital cytomegalovirus infection with ganciclovir. Pediatr Infect Dis J 22:504–509, 2003. **This controversial article describes anecdotal nonrandomized experience of one center in treating infants with ganciclovir for extended periods of time to prevent hearing loss progression associated with congenital CMV disease.**
8. Noyola DE, Demmler GJ, Nelson CT, et al: Early predictors of neurodevelopmental outcome in symptomatic congenital cytomegalovirus infection. J Pediatr 138(3):325–331, 2001. **Provides a numerical scoring system for clinicians to use that predicts neurodevelopmental outcome in childhood from characteristics of the newborn, such as head size, CT findings, and eye disease at birth.**
9. Ross SA, Boppana SB: Congenital cytomegalovirus infection: Outcome and diagnosis. Semin Pediatr Infect Dis 16(1):44–49, 2005. **Reviews current understanding of diagnosis and predictors of outcome in infants born with congenital CMV infection.**
10. Schleiss MR: Antiviral therapy of congenital cytomegalovirus infection. Semin Pediatr Infect Dis 16(1):50–59, 2005. **Reviews antiviral options to treat CMV infections.**

Enteroviruses
Carrie L. Byington

KEY CONCEPTS

- Enteroviruses (EVs) are ubiquitous viruses that frequently infect humans and result in seasonal outbreaks and sporadic cases of disease.
- The majority of EV infections are asymptomatic.
- The clinical presentations of symptomatic EV disease are diverse and include nonspecific febrile illness; self-limited infections, such as herpangina and conjunctivitis; more serious infections, including aseptic meningitis; and life-threatening infections, including encephalitis, myocarditis, and sepsis-like syndromes.
- Neonates are at greatest risk for severe EV infections.
- Rapid diagnosis of EV infections is best achieved through polymerase chain reaction (PCR) testing. Blood and cerebrospinal fluid (CSF) are the most commonly tested specimens.
- For confirmation of enterovirus type, culture-based methods are most commonly used. The best specimens for culture include throat swabs, stool, blood, and CSF.
- No approved treatments for EV infections are available, although intravenous immunoglobulin preparations and the antiviral agent pleconaril are used experimentally.

The nonpolio enteroviruses, including coxsackieviruses A and B, echoviruses, and the numbered enteroviruses, are common causes of fever and illness in infants and children. Nonpolio enteroviruses are one of the most common causes of fever in infants 1 to 90 days of age, accounting for approximately 25% of admissions for suspected sepsis overall and 40% to 50% during the summer and fall months.

The clinical manifestations of enteroviral infections are broad and range from asymptomatic infections to nonspecific febrile illnesses that resolve quickly, to more serious diseases such as aseptic meningitis, to life-threatening infections such as encephalitis, acute flaccid paralysis, myocarditis, and neonatal hepatitis. Enteroviral (EV) infections are also proposed triggers of chronic diseases such as diabetes mellitus and multiple sclerosis, but these associations remain unproven.

More than 60 antigenically distinct nonpolio enteroviruses exist. These are single-stranded RNA viruses and members of the family Picornaviridae. Transmission most often occurs by the fecal–oral route. Children are the most commonly infected because they often lack type-specific antibody protection, and their habits facilitate spread of virus in family groups, child-care settings, and schools.

EV infections are common worldwide. In temperate climates, such as the United States, there is a seasonal distribution, with the majority of EV infections occurring during the summer and fall months. Fecal contamination of swimming pools or water parks may facilitate transmission during the summer months. In tropical climates, EV infections occur year round.

Specific Enteroviral Illnesses

Diagnosis of enteroviral illnesses is given in Table 1.

NEONATAL DISEASE

In the neonatal period, EV infections may be severe. These infections are usually acquired during the perinatal period from an infected mother. The most common EV types causing neonatal infection are echoviruses and coxsackieviruses.

Infants with congenital EV infection most often present in the first week of life and may be ill at birth. These infants have evidence of hepatitis and coagulopathy and may also have manifestations of central nervous system disease or myocarditis. The untreated mortality for neonatal EV infections is reported to be between 0% and 83% depending on the population studied. Neonates with both coagulopathy and myocarditis have higher mortality rates. Neonates who have onset of infection in the first 2 weeks of life are more likely to die than those with infection in the second week of life. Similarly, infants who acquire EV infection congenitally have higher mortality rates than neonates who acquire the same infection via nosocomial transmission during nursery outbreaks. These findings may reflect both viral loads associated with different modes of transmission and the influence of type-specific antibody on infection severity.

MYOCARDITIS

Many enterovirus types are associated with myocarditis, but coxsackieviruses B1 through B5 are the most frequently diagnosed. Signs and symptoms of acute myocarditis may be subtle and include fatigue, chest pain, and exercise intolerance. Arrhythmia may be the presenting sign of myocarditis and may result in sudden death. The long-term outcomes of survivors of myocarditis caused by EV infection are thought to be good; however, they are not well documented because in most cases of myocarditis, the etiology is never determined.

ASEPTIC MENINGITIS

EV infections are one of the most common causes of aseptic meningitis. Outbreaks of aseptic meningitis may occur in temperate climates in the summer and fall months. Symptoms include fever, headache, nuchal rigidity, and vomiting. Outbreaks of meningitis attributed to echovirus types 9, 13, 18, and 30 have been reported in the United States and Europe. Several outbreaks were traced to a contaminated water source. The majority of cases of aseptic meningitis caused by EV infection have a good outcome.

ENCEPHALITIS

EV infections, especially those caused by echoviruses, may result in encephalitis. In cases of encephalitis in which an etiologic agent is identified, enteroviruses account for approximately 2% of infections. The encephalitis associated with enteroviruses may be less severe than that seen with the herpesviruses. The neurologic outcome of EV encephalitis in survivors is generally favorable. Encephalitis may be chronic in patients with immune compromise, especially agammaglobulinemia.

PLEURODYNIA (BORNHOLM DISEASE)

Pleurodynia is classically reported to occur in epidemics, but sporadic cases do occur. The coxsackie B viruses are often responsible for outbreaks of pleurodynia, but many EV types can cause disease. The majority of those affected are younger than 30 years. Symptoms include sudden onset of spasmodic chest pain associated with fever. The pain may be severe and confused with angina. Physical examination may reveal a pleural friction rub. The chest radiograph is invariably normal. The illness may be biphasic with asymptomatic periods between episodes of chest pain. Patients occasionally develop aseptic meningitis or myocarditis in association with pleurodynia.

ENTEROVIRUS 71 INFECTIONS

Enterovirus 71 was discovered in 1969 and is recognized as a cause of severe EV infection in children, especially those younger than 5 years. Outbreaks are described in countries in the Asia-Pacific region, including Taiwan, Malaysia, Singapore, and Australia. Sporadic cases are documented in Europe as well as in North and South America. EV 71 infection usually results in hand, foot, and mouth disease, a self-limited illness, but other outbreaks are associated with brain stem encephalitis and resultant neurogenic pulmonary edema. These infections are rapidly progressive and have a high mortality rate. Acute flaccid paralysis is also associated with EV 71 infection and must be

TABLE 1 Diagnosis of Enterovirus Infections

Historical Information	Neonatal Infection	Aseptic Meningitis	Myocarditis	Enterovirus 71	Chronic Enterovirus Infections in the Immune Compromised
	Season? Maternal febrile illness, especially with rash, near time of delivery? Severe abdominal pain in mother prior to delivery?	Season? Exposure to contaminated water source (swimming, camping)?	Season?	Season? Travel to Asia or other areas experiencing outbreak? Contact with herpangina or hand, foot, mouth cases?	Agammaglobulinemia?
Signs and symptoms seen in patient	Fever, hypothermia, lethargy, poor feeding, respiratory distress, heart failure, arrhythmia, jaundice, hepatitis, coagulopathy, rash.	Fever, headache, nausea, vomiting, photophobia.	Fever, fatigue, chest pain, exercise intolerance, tachycardia unexplained by fever, tachypnea.	Oral lesions, brain stem encephalitis, pulmonary edema, acute flaccid paralysis.	Meningoencephalitis, polymyositis, or dermatomyositis-like illness, arthritis
Duration of illness	Symptoms appear within first 14 days of life and resolve within 7 days in mild cases but may require weeks in severe cases.	Days, illness may be biphasic with nonspecific febrile illness or pleurodynia followed by improvement and after several days meningitis.	Days to weeks required for recovery of cardiac function.	Days required for recovery from acute illness, although weeks to months may be needed for full recovery. Neurologic damage may be permanent.	Months to years
Differential diagnosis	Sepsis secondary to bacterial infection, herpes simplex infection, adenovirus infection.	Bacterial meningitis; Herpes simplex infection.	Noninfectious congestive heart failure or arrhythmia.	Poliomyelitis, West Nile virus infection.	
Laboratory diagnosis	PCR for enterovirus of blood and/or CSF, viral culture of throat, respiratory, stool, CSF, or blood specimen for typing.	PCR for enterovirus of blood and/or CSF, viral culture of throat, respiratory, stool, CSF, or blood specimen for typing.	PCR or viral culture of cardiac tissue; viral testing of nasopharynx or stool may suggest but does not prove diagnosis.	PCR of CSF; culture of CSF, nasopharynx, stool, demonstration of type specific IgM or fourfold rise in IgG antibody in serum.	PCR of CSF

CSF, cerebrospinal fluid; Ig, immunoglobulin; PCR, polymerase chain reaction.

12

distinguished from poliomyelitis and infection with West Nile virus. MRI may reveal lesions in the anterior horn cells of the spinal cord. Children who recover from EV 71 may have permanent neurologic sequelae.

Diagnosis

EV infections are most readily diagnosed by the polymerase chain reaction (PCR). PCR testing of both blood and cerebrospinal fluid (CSF) may be diagnostic of acute infection. In one study of 666 infants 1 to 90 days of age who had PCR testing of both blood and CSF specimens, test results were concordant in 93%. Real-time PCR assays are available in some clinical and many reference laboratories in the Unites States. Results of PCR testing are usually available within hours and can favorably impact the management of the patient.

In clinical laboratories without PCR technology, culture for enteroviruses can be performed but requires multiple cell lines and is time-consuming, usually yielding results in 5 to 10 days. More rapid culture results can be obtained by using centrifugation-enhanced antigen detection in commercially manufactured shell vials.

Expert Opinion on Management Issues

ACCEPTED INTERVENTIONS

Isolation

Patients with EV infections can shed virus in stool for several weeks; therefore, contact precautions are needed to reduce transmission of virus in hospital settings. Isolation is especially critical for neonates managed in an intensive care setting. Multiple nursery outbreaks with resultant neonatal fatalities are reported that can be traced to infected newborns or their caregivers. Special consideration must be given to the fact that the ill neonate's mother may also be infected with enterovirus and should not be allowed to have contact with other infants in the nursery. In all cases of EV infection, family members and health care providers should observe good hand-washing practices.

Supportive Care

The majority of patients with EV infections have self-limited illnesses and require no specific care. However, for more serious infections, especially those resulting in hospitalization, supportive care is beneficial. Intravenous fluids can be given to maintain hydration. For those with aseptic meningitis, pain control may be an important issue and narcotic pain relievers may be needed for a short time to relieve headache. Antipyretics can be given to manage fever; however, in patients with hepatitis, care must be taken to avoid further injury to the liver.

URGENT INTERVENTIONS

In neonates and children with life-threatening EV disease, treatment includes measures designed to maintain hemodynamic stability and to correct the manifestations of illness caused by the infection. Neonates with disseminated EV disease often have hepatitis and coagulopathy associated with bleeding. These infants frequently require transfusions of blood products, including platelets and fresh-frozen plasma. The administration of vitamin K may also be necessary. Infants and children with encephalitis should be monitored for seizures and treated with anticonvulsants if needed. Children with myocarditis may require inotropic support.

Intravenous immune globulin (IVIG) is used to treat immunocompromised children, especially those with agammaglobulinemia who may have chronic EV meningitis. IVIG is also used to treat severe neonatal infections, although conclusive data regarding efficacy are lacking. The suggested doses of IVIG given to neonates with disseminated infection range from 500 mg per kg to 2 g/kg in an effort to provide neutralizing antibody directed toward the most common EV serotypes (Table 2).

OTHER INTERVENTIONS

In cases of severe neonatal EV infection, anecdotal evidence supports the use of maternal plasma for the treatment of the neonate. In cases of congenital EV infection caused by rare serotypes of enterovirus, maternal serum may contain type-specific neutralizing antibody in greater quantity than that found in commercial IVIG preparations.

Antiviral therapy for EV disease approved by the Food and Drug Administration (FDA) is not available in the United States. The investigational drug pleconaril was used in the past on a compassionate basis for the treatment of severe EV disease in both immunocompetent and immunodeficient hosts. Pleconaril, at the time of this writing, is no longer available for compassionate use in the United States, but it may be released in the future. Individual clinicians can contact Schering-Plough through their drug information service at 1–800–526–4099 (See Table 2).

TABLE 2 Potential Treatments for Serious Enterovirus Infections

Treatment	Dosage
Intravenous immune globulin (IVIG)	500 mg to 2 g/kg usually as a single dose, but lower doses may be repeated.
Pleconaril oral suspension	Pediatric dosage: 5.0 mg/kg per dose q8h for 7–10 days. Adult dosage: 200 mg or 400 mg per dose q8h for 7–10 days.

q*x*h, every *x* hours.

In a study of the treatment of enterovirus 71, children with severe disease, including neurogenic pulmonary edema and acute flaccid paralysis, benefited from advanced supportive care delivered in an intensive care setting. Milrinone treatment improved the outcomes of children younger than 5 years with pulmonary edema (mortality 36% vs. 92%, $P = 0.005$). Pleconaril treatment did not change the outcome of severe enterovirus 71 diseases.

Common Pitfalls

- Severe EV infection in the neonate may mimic bacterial disease or other serious, but potentially treatable viral infections such as herpes simplex and adenovirus. It is critical that clinicians test for these and offer treatment with antibiotics and acyclovir while awaiting the results of bacterial and viral assays.
- In cases of acute flaccid paralysis, EV infection, primarily caused by enterovirus 71, must be distinguished from West Nile virus infection. Survivors of severe enterovirus 71 infection may have significant neurologic morbidity and potentially could benefit from early rehabilitation services.
- Infants and children with EV infections may shed these viruses in their stool for several weeks and can potentially infect others. Hand hygiene is especially important in families with immunocompromised individuals, especially those with agammaglobulinemia, because these individuals may experience severe and chronic EV infections.

Communication and Counseling

Most EV infections are self-limited and require no treatment. Good hygiene should be stressed in family and hospital settings to prevent further transmission of the virus. For those with severe EV infections, especially neonates, the prognosis is guarded. However, for neonates who survive acute illness, the majority do recover fully. Unfortunately, this is not the case for children who survive serious enterovirus 71 infections and may have significant neurologic morbidity.

SUGGESTED READINGS

1. Abzug MJ: Prognosis for neonates with enterovirus hepatitis and coagulopathy. Pediatr Infect Dis J 20:758–763, 2001. **Prognosis of EV disease.**
2. Abzug MJ: Presentation, diagnosis, and management of enterovirus infections in neonates. Paediatr Drugs 6:1–10, 2004. **Excellent review of neonatal EV disease.**
3. Amvrosieva TV, Titov LP, Mulders M, et al: Viral water contamination as the cause of aseptic meningitis outbreak in Belarus. Cent Eur J Public Health 9:154–157, 2001. **Description of water as source of EV outbreak.**
4. Aseptic meningitis outbreak associated with echovirus 9 among recreational vehicle campers—Connecticut, 2003. MMWR Morb Mortal Wkly Rep 53:710–713, 2004. **Description of EV outbreak associated with camping.**
5. Byington CL, Taggart EW, Carroll KC, Hillyard DR: A polymerase chain reaction–based epidemiologic investigation of the incidence of nonpolio enteroviral infections in febrile and afebrile infants 90 days and younger. Pediatrics 103:E27, 1999. **Epidemiology of EV disease in febrile infants.**
6. Enterovirus surveillance—United States, 2000–2001.MMWR Morb Mortal Wkly Rep 51:1047–1049, 2002. **Surveillance data for United States.**
7. Glaser CA, Gilliam S, Schnurr D, et al: In search of encephalitis etiologies: Diagnostic challenges in the California Encephalitis Project, 1998–2000. Clin Infect Dis 36:731–742, 2003. **Description of viral causes of encephalitis, including EV disease.**
8. Ho M, Chen ER, Hsu KH, et al: An epidemic of enterovirus 71 infection in Taiwan. Taiwan Enterovirus Epidemic Working Group. N Engl J Med 341:929–935, 1999. **Description of EV 71 disease.**
9. Huang CC, Liu CC, Chang YC, et al: Neurologic complications in children with enterovirus 71 infection. N Engl J Med 341:936–942, 1999. **Description of neurologic complications of EV 71 infection.**
10. Klespies SL, Cebula DE, Kelley CL, et al: Detection of enteroviruses from clinical specimens by spin amplification shell vial culture and monoclonal antibody assay. J Clin Microbiol 34:1465–1467, 1996. **Description of shell vial technology for identification of EV disease.**
11. Lipson SM, David K, Shaikh F, Qian L: Detection of precytopathic effect of enteroviruses in clinical specimens by centrifugation-enhanced antigen detection. J Clin Microbiol 39:2755–2759, 2001. **Description of shell vial technology for identification of EV disease.**
12. Modlin JF: Perinatal echovirus infection: Insights from a literature review of 61 cases of serious infection and 16 outbreaks in nurseries. Rev Infect Dis 8:918–926, 1986. **Description of nursery outbreaks due to EV infection.**
13. Nolan MA, Craig ME, Lahra MM, et al: Survival after pulmonary edema due to enterovirus 71 encephalitis. Neurology 60:1651–1656, 2003. **Sequelae of EV infection.**
14. Outbreaks of aseptic meningitis associated with echoviruses 9 and 30 and preliminary surveillance reports on enterovirus activity—United States, 2003. MMWR Morb Mortal Wkly Rep 52:761–764, 2003. **Epidemiology of EV infection in the United States.**
15. Pichichero ME, McLinn S, Rotbart HA, et al: Clinical and economic impact of enterovirus illness in private pediatric practice. Pediatrics 102:1126–1134, 1998. **Documents common nature of EV infection.**
16. Rittichier K, Bryan P, Bassett K, et al: Diagnosis and outcomes of enterovirus infections in young infants. Pediatr Infect Dis J 24:546–550, 2005. **Diagnosis and prognosis of EV.**
17. Rotbart HA, Webster AD: Treatment of potentially life-threatening enterovirus infections with pleconaril. Clin Infect Dis 32:228–235, 2001. **Use of pleconaril in EV infection.**
18. Verboon-Maciolek MA, Nijhuis M, van Loon AM, et al: Diagnosis of enterovirus infection in the first 2 months of life by real-time polymerase chain reaction. Clin Infect Dis 37:1–6, 2003. **Documents importance of EV infection as cause of fever in infants.**
19. Wang SM, Lei HY, Huang MC, et al: Therapeutic efficacy of milrinone in the management of enterovirus 71–induced pulmonary edema. Pediatr Pulmonol 39:219–223, 2005. **Use of milrinone to treat EV 71 disease.**

Infectious Mononucleosis

Ben Z. Katz

KEY CONCEPTS

- Epstein-Barr virus (EBV) is responsible for all heterophil-positive and most heterophil-negative cases of infectious mononucleosis (IM).
- The classic symptom triad of IM is fever, lymphadenopathy, and pharyngitis.

Infectious mononucleosis (IM) is usually an acute, benign lymphoproliferative disease. Epstein-Barr virus (EBV) is responsible for all heterophil-positive and most heterophil-negative cases of IM. Other causes of heterophil-negative IM include cytomegalovirus, toxoplasmosis, hepatitis A and B, adenovirus, human immunodeficiency virus (HIV), rubella, and human herpesvirus 6.

The classic symptom triad of IM is fever, lymphadenopathy, and pharyngitis. Typical laboratory findings include lymphocytosis with atypical lymphocytes and the presence of heterophil antibodies. After a 4- to 6-week incubation period, the illness begins with a 3- to 5-day prodrome of malaise, headache, and fatigue, typically followed by the onset of the triad. Additional symptoms can include anorexia, nausea, vomiting, periorbital or facial edema, and generalized lymphadenopathy, which is usually symmetrical. Splenomegaly occurs by the second or third week of illness in approximately half of all cases; rarely, splenic rupture can occur, which can be fatal. Hepatomegaly occurs in 10% to 15% of cases, with hepatitis occurring in approximately 5%. Up to 15% of individuals with IM have a rash that may be erythematous, maculopapular, morbilliform, scarlatiniform, or urticarial, especially if ampicillin or one of its derivatives is given. Other symptoms may include arthritis or jaundice. Complications are uncommon but can be neurologic (seizures, cranial nerve palsies, aseptic meningitis, encephalitis, optic neuritis, transverse myelitis, infectious polyneuritis [Guillain-Barré syndrome], psychosis, or acute cerebellar ataxia); hematologic (hemolytic or aplastic anemia, thrombocytopenic purpura, agranulocytosis, or agammaglobulinemia); cardiac (pericarditis or myocarditis); pulmonary (cough or atypical pneumonia); or renal (glomerulonephritis, acute renal failure, or acute interstitial nephritis).

IM is a self-limited disease in nearly all individuals. The acute symptoms usually resolve in 2 to 6 weeks, with the fatigue persisting for up to 12 months in approximately 10% of individuals. It is extremely rare for IM to recur in an otherwise healthy individual.

Saliva is the main vehicle for transmission of EBV, the major etiologic agent of IM. Transmission usually requires direct and prolonged contact with infected oropharyngeal secretions, with salivary exchange the presumed main mode of transmission. The infection begins with viral replication in the oropharyngeal epithelial cells and then spreads to local B lymphocytes, which then disseminate throughout the reticuloendothelial system, resulting in a vigorous T-cell response. The atypical lymphocytes produced in IM are T cells directed against EBV-infected B cells. It is believed most of the clinical manifestations of IM are due to this T-cell immune response, which may explain why young children, whose immune responses are not completely developed, usually are asymptomatic with primary EBV infection.

The diagnosis of IM is usually based on the clinical picture, 10% atypical lymphocytosis, and positive heterophil serology. Most adolescents and adults have most or all of these features as well as an abnormal white count. Many infected individuals also have mild thrombocytopenia and elevated hepatocellular enzymes. The positive heterophil is usually measured as a positive monospot test. False-positive heterophil tests are reportable. False-negative tests do occur, especially in younger children. If IM is suspected and heterophil antibodies are negative, specific titers for EBV, including viral capsid antigen (VCA), early antigen (EA), and Epstein-Barr nuclear antigen (EBNA), as well as serologies for cytomegalovirus and toxoplasmosis, should be sent. Acute EBV infection is characterized by the presence of both IgM and IgG VCA antibodies, EA antibodies, and the absence of EBNA antibodies. If liver function tests are elevated, serology for hepatitis A and B should be considered. If risk factors are present, HIV antibodies should be checked. A throat culture is indicated in patients with pharyngitis or tonsillitis.

Expert Opinion on Management Issues

General, supportive management of IM consists of bed rest and acetaminophen (10 to 15 mg/kg every 4 to 6 hours), aspirin (10 to 15 mg/kg every 4 to 6 hours), or nonsteroidal anti-inflammatory agents, such as ibuprofen (5 to 10 mg/kg every 6 to 8 hours), as needed. Saline gargles can be useful to treat the sore throat; in severe cases, codeine (0.5 to 1 mg/kg every 4 to 6 hours) or meperidine (Demerol) (1 to 1.5 mg/kg every 3 to 4 hours) may be required. Quarantine is not indicated. A short, tapering course of corticosteroid therapy (e.g., 2 mg/kg of prednisone for 5 days, 1 mg/kg for 5 days, and then 0.5 mg/kg for 5 days) should be considered for treatment of severe cases of IM characterized by hemolysis, respiratory embarrassment, or thrombocytopenic purpura.

Antiviral therapy is not recommended for acute IM in the normal host. Parenteral acyclovir can reduce the level of oropharyngeal EBV replication; however, EBV replication returns to previously high levels after cessation of treatment, there is little or no reduction in the number of EBV-infected B cells in the peripheral circulation, and little effect is observed clinically. High-dose oral acyclovir combined with steroids also decreases oropharyngeal shedding while it is given but not thereafter, and it has absolutely no discernible effect clinically. Ganciclovir and other agents are too toxic to have a role in the treatment of IM in the normal host.

Common Pitfalls

Symptomatology varies with the infected individual's age at the time of primary infection. Younger children usually have atypical, inapparent, or mild infections.

Although corticosteroids may have a beneficial effect by improving symptoms of pharyngitis or lymphadenopathy within 24 hours in many instances, caution is warranted. Infection is self-limited in nearly all cases without any therapy, and the long-term effects of steroids on the normal immune response to EBV are unknown. In addition, rare reports of neurologic or septicemic complications following steroid use have appeared. Use of steroids in atypical or antibody-negative cases is inappropriate because the diagnosis of a lymphoma can then be confounded.

Ampicillin and related drugs should be avoided when treating secondary bacterial complications because of its association with rash in individuals with IM. Contact sports should be eschewed until patients are fully recovered and as long as splenomegaly is evident because of the rare possibility of splenic rupture.

Communication and Counseling

Older adolescents and young adults are often quite ill with IM. Approximately 25% of patients with IM still have some symptoms (e.g., fatigue) at 6 months, and 10% may linger for up to 1 year. Nevertheless, the prognosis is nearly uniformly excellent.

SUGGESTED READINGS

1. Anderson J, Britton S, Ernberg I, et al: Effect of acyclovir on infectious mononucleosis: A double-blind, placebo-controlled study. J Infect Dis 153:283–290, 1986. **Given parenterally, acyclovir had only a modest effect when several clinical variables were combined.**
2. Evans AS: Infectious mononucleosis and related syndromes. Am J Med Sci 276:325–339, 1978. **A classic of epidemiology in clinical medicine.**
3. Jenson HB: Acute complications of Epstein-Barr virus infectious mononucleosis. Curr Opin Pediatr 12:263–268, 2000. **A thorough review.**
4. Katz BZ: Update on chronic fatigue syndrome and Epstein-Bar virus. Pediatr Ann 31:741–744, 2004. **Discusses the most recent literature related to persistent fatigue following IM.**
5. Katz BZ, Miller G: Epstein-Barr virus infections. In Katz SL, Gershon AA, Hotez PJ (eds): Krugman's Infectious Diseases of Children, 11th ed. Philadelphia: Mosby, 2004, pp 143–159. **A detailed discussion of IM and other more serious manifestations of EBV infection in normal and immunocompromised hosts.**
6. Tynell E, Aurelius E, Brandell A, et al: Acyclovir and prednisolone treatment of acute infectious mononucleosis: A multicenter, double-blind, placebo-controlled study. J Infect Dis 174:321–331, 1996. **The same group studied high-dose oral acyclovir and could discern no clinical benefit.**
7. van der Horst C, Joncas J, Ahronheim G, et al: Lack of effect of peroral acyclovir for the treatment of acute infectious mononucleosis. J Infect Dis 164:788–792, 1991. **Oral acyclovir also does not have any clinical effect when used without steroids.**
8. Waldo RT: Neurologic complications of infectious mononucleosis after steroid therapy. Southern Med J 74:1159–1160, 1981. **Two case reports of neurologic complications of IM beginning shortly after a brief course of tapered steroids was completed.**

Severe Acute Respiratory Syndrome (SARS)

Anne Moscona

KEY CONCEPTS

- Severe acute respiratory syndrome (SARS) is caused by a novel coronavirus.
- SARS spreads primarily by close person-to-person contact and by airborne dissemination.
- The incubation period of SARS is 2 to 10 days; 95% of patients develop symptoms within 10 days.
- The World Health Organization and the Centers for Disease Control and Prevention (CDC) have established case definitions for SARS that should be used in evaluating patients.
- There are no specific treatment recommendations for SARS yet available except for supportive care.
- Various antiviral and other therapeutic agents are under investigation.
- Vaccines are in development but not currently available.
- Experimental passive immunization strategies hold promise for prophylaxis against SARS in exposed people and are being studied.
- Infection control measures are key in preventing the spread of SARS. These include measures carried out globally, in the community, in hospitals, and in the home.
- The CDC website provided in this chapter maintains updated information on evolving recommendations and should be consulted regularly.

12

In late 2002, cases of a severe atypical pneumonia of unknown etiology were reported in the People's Republic of China, and similar cases were subsequently detected in individuals in Hong Kong, Vietnam, and Canada during February and March 2003. The World Health Organization (WHO) issued a global alert for this illness, which was designated "severe acute respiratory syndrome," or SARS. The disease rapidly spread to more than 25 countries and sickened thousands of people by April 2003. The global medical and scientific communities engaged in a cooperative effort that led to rapid progress in understanding and diagnosing the disease.

A novel coronavirus was identified and proved to be the causative agent of SARS. SARS appears to spread primarily by close person-to-person contact; however, airborne SARS coronavirus spread, in which droplets of smaller size remain suspended in the air, likely also occurs. The incubation period is 2 to 10 days. Because 95% of patients develop symptoms within 10 days, after possible exposure an individual should be monitored for the development of symptoms for at least this length of time. Most cases of SARS thus far are identified in individuals who cared for or lived with a patient or had direct contact with infectious material from an infected person.

The infection results in an acute interstitial pneumonia, in many cases progressing to fatal lung disease. In general, SARS begins with a fever higher than 100.4°F (>38.0°C). Other symptoms may include headache, malaise, body aches, and mild respiratory symptoms. After 2 to 7 days, a lower respiratory phase begins with the onset of a dry, nonproductive cough or dyspnea, which may be accompanied by or progress to hypoxemia. The case fatality rate may be as high as 50%. Chest radiographs may be normal during the febrile prodrome; however, in a substantial proportion of patients the respiratory phase is characterized by focal interstitial infiltrates progressing to generalized, patchy, interstitial infiltrates.

Both the WHO and the Centers for Disease Control and Prevention (CDC) established case definitions for SARS (Box 1; http://www.who.int/csr/sars/casedefinition/en/; and http://www.cdc.gov/ncidod/sars/casedefinition.htm). A suspected case is defined by the WHO as an individual presenting with fever higher than 100.5°F (>38°C) plus cough or difficulty breathing, plus either close contact with a person who has a diagnosis of SARS and/or history of travel or residence in an area with recent local transmission of SARS within 10 days of symptom onset. Patients with a fatal unexplained acute respiratory illness fitting these epidemiologic criteria who did not have an autopsy performed also are classified as suspected cases. A probable case is defined as a suspected case with chest radiograph findings of pneumonia or acute respiratory distress syndrome (ARDS), a suspected case positive for the SARS virus in one or more laboratory assays, or a suspected case with an unexplained respiratory illness resulting in death with an autopsy demonstrating the pathology

of ARDS without an identifiable cause. The CDC case definition differs only slightly, in that radiographic findings are included along with respiratory symptoms for severe cases, and the definition begins with a respiratory illness without known etiology. The surveillance CDC case definition also includes detailed laboratory criteria. Enzyme-linked immunosorbent assay (ELISA) testing for immunoglobulin (Ig) G antibody to the SARS virus is positive in most cases, but a limitation to serologic testing is that the appearance of antibodies is delayed, making it less useful for acute diagnosis. The sensitivity of virus culture is lower than that for real-time polymerase chain reaction (RT-PCR) for organism detection in clinical specimens; however, the currently available rapid diagnostic tests are not sufficiently sensitive for early diagnosis. The sensitivity may be improved with RT-PCR, and work is ongoing to standardize both PCR and ELISA testing for SARS.

Continuously updated data on this illness are available on the WHO and CDC websites (http://www.who.int/csr/sars/en/ and http://www.cdc.gov/ncidod/sars/index.htm, respectively), which are excellent sources for current information.

Expert Opinion on Management Issues

SUPPORTIVE AND EMPIRICAL THERAPY

No specific treatment recommendations for SARS are yet available except for meticulous supportive care, and currently no approved antiviral drugs are effective against coronaviruses. Empirical therapy may include presumptive coverage for causative agents of community-acquired pneumonia of unclear etiology; however, antibiotics have proven ineffective in treating SARS.

ANTIVIRALS AND OTHER THERAPEUTIC AGENTS UNDER INVESTIGATION

Antiviral agents, including ribavirin, oseltamivir, and lopinavir-ritonavir, were used in ill patients, but the efficacy of these drugs is not clearly demonstrated. Ribavirin was administered most extensively; however, it was subsequently shown to have no activity against the SARS virus in vitro and is also associated with significant toxicity. Most attempted treatment regimens include corticosteroids, also without documentation of their efficacy.

Several other treatments are under evaluation and may provide treatment options in the future. Interferon-alfa inhibits the SARS virus in vitro. One small study suggested that therapy with interferon alfacon–1 plus corticosteroids produces more rapid improvement than treatment with corticosteroids alone. In another small study, the use of inhaled nitric oxide appeared promising. Other agents, including glycyrrhizin, an active ingredient found in licorice roots, and small molecule inhibitors of the SARS coronavirus protease, are under active investigation.

PREVENTION: ACTIVE IMMUNIZATION STRATEGIES UNDER DEVELOPMENT

At present, several approaches to SARS vaccination are under evaluation. These include animal immunization experiments using adenoviral vectors carrying SARS structural proteins, using DNA vaccines, using recombinant modified vaccinia virus Ankara (rMVA) expressing the SARS-CoV spike protein, and using attenuated parainfluenza virus that expresses the spike protein. No vaccine is as yet being tested in humans; however, this is likely to be under way in the near future.

PREVENTION: IMMUNOPROPHYLAXIS

Passive administration of antibodies is another possible approach to preventing SARS, based on the rationale that neutralizing antibodies, reactive in vitro against the SARS virus, develop in most patients with SARS. Experiments in an animal model showed that human neutralizing monoclonal antibody against SARS virus decreased lung SARS virus replication more than 1000-fold in ferrets. The animals did not develop macroscopic lung lesions, and three of four did not shed virus in pharyngeal secretions. In vitro, a human monoclonal antibody to the spike protein effectively neutralized the virus. If further studies confirm these promising results, such antibodies may be useful for prophylaxis against SARS in exposed people, reduction of spread of infection from person to person, or even for therapy.

PREVENTION: INFECTION CONTROL

Rapid institution of rigorous infection control measures was critical in controlling the global and local spread of SARS. Patients with SARS pose a significant risk of transmission to close household contacts and healthcare personnel in close contact. Infection control is made more difficult because not all patients are sick enough to require hospitalization, and this means that rigorous adherence to voluntary measures to avoid exposing others in the community is needed. Clinicians evaluating suspected cases should use standard precautions (hand hygiene), together with airborne (N95 respirator) and contact (gowns and gloves) precautions, and refer to the updated infection control guidelines on the CDC website listed later. For family members caring for a person with SARS, the CDC has developed infection control recommendations for patients with suspected SARS in the household. These basic precautions should be followed for 10 days after respiratory symptoms and fever are gone. During that time, SARS patients should limit interactions outside the home (not go to work, school, or other public areas). The duration of time before or after onset of symptoms during which a patient with SARS can transmit the disease to others is unknown.

The guidelines given here (Box 2) are in accord with the current recommendations from the CDC; the CDC website maintains updated information and should be consulted (http://www.cdc.gov/ncidod/sars/ic.htm).

BOX 2 Infection Control Strategies

In the Hospital

- Isolate patients in negative pressure rooms.
- Ensure that health care workers and visitors wear masks (N–95 respirator), gowns, gloves, and protective eyewear.
- Exclude health care workers who develop fever and/or respiratory symptoms within 10 days of exposure to a SARS patient from work.
- Ensure that the health care workers who have these symptoms remain out of work for a full 10 days after fever and respiratory symptoms have resolved.

In the Community

- Persons with suspected SARS should stay at home and not go out for any reason.
- The CDC advises that people remain at home for 10 days after resolution of fever and other symptoms.
- Household contacts should:
  - Carefully wash their hands.
  - Wear gloves for contact with bodily fluids.
  - Not share utensils.
  - Not use the same bedding as the patient unless it has been properly washed.
  - Consider using surgical masks for close contact.

CDC, Centers for Disease Control and Prevention; SARS, severe acute respiratory syndrome.

Hospitalized SARS patients should be isolated in negative pressure rooms, and health care workers and visitors should wear masks (N95 respirators if possible) as well as gowns, gloves, and protective eyewear to protect against contact transmission. Health care workers who develop fever and/or respiratory symptoms within 10 days of exposure to a patient with SARS need to stay home from work and remain out of work for a full 10 days after the fever and respiratory symptoms resolve. In the community, the key to control is that patients with suspected SARS stay at home and not go outside for any reason. The patient should remain at home for a full 10 days after resolution of the fever and other symptoms. Careful hand washing should be practiced by all household contacts in the home, and gloves should be used for contact with bodily fluids. Utensils and bedding should not be shared. Surgical masks may be considered either for the at-home patients or their household contacts.

PREVENTION: TRAVEL

Because of the rapid worldwide spread of SARS and the local geographic outbreaks, travel recommendations were developed. For individuals who must travel to an area with SARS, the CDC advises that travelers in an area with SARS wash their hands frequently and avoid close contact with large numbers of people as much as possible to minimize the possibility of infection. The CDC does not currently recommend the routine use of masks or other personal protective equipment while in public areas. During the initial outbreak, WHO issued a travel advisory against nonessential travel to Guangdong Province, China, and Hong Kong, and the CDC added all of China, Hong Kong, Hanoi, and Singapore to the advisory. Both agencies recommended postponing all but essential travel to these areas during the epidemic.

Common Pitfalls

The most common foreseeable pitfall is failure to observe proper infection control practices, including voluntary isolation, because these measures are at present the only effective method for controlling spread of the SARS virus.

Communication and Counseling

To avoid the pitfall just described, alertness of the community to news of outbreak activity and education of health-care workers and caregivers in infection control measures are of foremost importance. Instructions on voluntary measures such as isolation and rigorous hand washing require frequent reinforcement to be effective. Clinicians should keep the relevant websites close at hand to obtain the most current information on recommendations.

SUGGESTED READINGS

1. Centers for Disease Control Prevention: Revised U.S. surveillance case definition for severe acute respiratory syndrome (SARS) and update on SARS cases—United States and worldwide, December 2003. MMWR Morb Mortal Wkly Rep 52 (49):1202–1206, 2003. **This reference provides the detailed laboratory criteria useful for the diagnosis of SARS.**
2. Chen L, Liu P, Gao H, et al: Inhalation of nitric oxide in the treatment of severe acute respiratory syndrome: A rescue trial in Beijing. Clin Infect Dis 39(10):1531–1535, 2004. Epublication, October 22, 2004. **This study in six patients showed the possible utility of inhaled nitrous oxide (NO).**
3. Drosten C, Gunther S, Preiser W, et al: Identification of a novel coronavirus in patients with severe acute respiratory syndrome. N Engl J Med 348(20):1967–1976, 2003. Epublication, April 10, 2003.
4. Fouchier RAM, Kuiken T, Schutten M, et al: Aetiology: Koch's postulates fulfilled for SARS virus. Nature 423(6937):240, 2003. **This study clearly established the etiologic association between the SARS coronavirus and SARS.**
5. Ksiazek TG, Erdman D, Goldsmith CS, et al: SARS Working Group. A novel coronavirus associated with severe acute respiratory syndrome. N Engl J Med 348(20):1953–1966, 2003. **Together with the next reference, this study identified SARS CoV as associated with the disease and thus the most likely causative agent.**
6. Rota PA, Oberste MS, Monroe SS, et al: Characterization of a novel coronavirus associated with severe acute respiratory syndrome. Science 300(5624):1394–1399, 2003. **This work provided initial characterization of the SARS CoV.**
7. Stroher U, DiCaro A, Li Y, et al: Severe acute respiratory syndrome–related coronavirus is inhibited by interferon-alfa. J Infect Dis 189(7):1164–1167, 2004. Epublication, March 12, 2004. **This small study offers hope that interferon-alfa treatment will be a therapeutic option.**
8. Sui J, Li W, Murakami A, et al: Potent neutralization of severe acute respiratory syndrome (SARS) coronavirus by a human mAb to S1 protein that blocks receptor association. Proc Natl Acad Sci USA 101(8):2536–2541, 2004. **This paper provides the key theoretical justification for pursuing studies of passive immunization using human monoclonal antibodies.**
9. ter Meulen J, Bakker AB, van den Brink EN, et al: Human monoclonal antibody as prophylaxis for SARS coronavirus infection in ferrets. Lancet 363(9427):2139–2141, 2004. **This work provides initial evidence, in an animal model, that passive immunization may be effective for preventing SARS.**
10. World Health Organization: Severe acute respiratory syndrome (SARS): Multi-country outbreak. Available online at http://www.who.int/csr/don/2003_04_25/en/. **The initial report of the outbreak.**

Herpes Simplex Virus

David W. Kimberlin

KEY CONCEPTS

- Herpes simplex virus type 1 (HSV-1) and herpes simplex virus type 2 (HSV-2) establish latency following primary infection and thus remain in the host's body forever.
- Under certain circumstances, viral reactivation from latency leads to symptomatic recurrent disease or asymptomatic viral shedding.
- Asymptomatic viral shedding accounts for a significant proportion of cases of viral transmission, both for genital herpes and for orolabial HSV infections.
- Disease manifestations from HSV-1 and HSV-2 infections relate to the site of infection and the age and immunologic status of the host.

Virology and Epidemiology

VIROLOGY

The two distinct types of herpes simplex virus (HSV) are HSV type 1 (HSV-1) and HSV type 2 (HSV-2). Two biologic properties of HSV that directly influence human disease are neurovirulence and latency. *Neurovirulence* refers to the affinity with which HSV is drawn to and propagated in neuronal tissue. This can result in profound disease with severe neurologic sequelae. *Latency* refers to the persistence of the viral genome in neural ganglia throughout the life of the host. Events such as physical or emotional stress, fever, ultraviolet light, and tissue damage can result in reactivation of latent virus, with resultant asymptomatic infection or clinically apparent disease. Disease manifestations from HSV–1 and HSV–2 infections relate to the site of infection and the age and immunologic status of the host (Tables 1 and 2).

EPIDEMIOLOGY

HSV-1 is found most commonly in the oropharynx, although any organ system can be involved. Seroprevalence rates increase throughout childhood and adolescence, with 20% to 40% of children seropositive for HSV-1 by 5 years of age. By 60 years of age, however, up to 90% of persons are seropositive for HSV-1

TABLE 1 Therapeutic Management of Nongenital HSV Infections

Drug	Primary Oro- pharyngeal HSV Infections (Gingivostoma- titis; HSV-1)	Recurrent Oro- pharyngeal HSV Infections (Herpes labialis; HSV-1)	Other Primary HSV Skin Infec- tions (HSV-1)	HSV Keratitis or Keratocon- junctivitis (HSV-1)	CNS Infection (beyond neo- natal period; HSV-1)	Neonatal HSV (HSV–2 or HSV-1)	Mucocutaneous HSV Infections in Immuno- compromised Patients (HSV-2 or HSV-1)
Acyclovir	600 mg/m²/dose PO qid × 10 days (adult max: 200 mg/dose PO 5×/ day).	15 mg/kg/day div q8h until able to switch to PO; 200 mg/dose PO 5×/ day × 7–10 days.	*Eczema herpeticum:* 10 mg/kg/dose PO 3–5×/day × 5–7 days (adult max: 200 mg/dose PO 5×/day) *Whitlow:* 200 mg/ dose PO 5×/day× 10 days		30 mg/kg/day div q8h IV × 14–21 days (some experts recommend 45–60 mg/kg/ day).	60 mg/kg/day div q8h IV × 14–21 days	*Mild:* 15 mg/kg/ day div q8h until able to switch to PO; then 10–20 mg/kg/dose PO 5×/day × 10–21 days (adult max 200 mg/dose PO 5×/day) *Moderate to severe:* 15 mg/ kg/day (or 750 mg/m²/day) div q8h × 10–21 days
Valacyclovir		2 g PO bid for 1 day.					
Famciclovir			*Whitlow:* 125 mg/ dose PO bid				
Penciclovir (Denavir)	Apply topically q2h during waking hours × 4 days.						
Trifluridine				1 drop q2h (max 9 drops/day) until cornea is re- epithelialized; then q4h for an additional 7 days (max 21 days)			
Vidarabine				Thick strip of ointment (1.25 cm) q3h until cornea is completely re- epithelialized; then bid for an additional 7 days			

bid, twice daily; CNS, central nervous system; div, divided; IV, intravenous; max, maximum; PO, by mouth; qid, four times per day; q*x*h, every *x* hours.

TABLE 2 Therapeutic Management of Genital Herpes Simplex Virus Infections (HSV–2 or HSV–1)*

Drug	First Clinical Episode (treat orally for 7–10 days[†])	Episodic Recurrent Infection[‡] (treat orally for 5 days)	Oral Suppressive Therapy	Episodic Recurrent Infection in HIV-Infected Persons (treat orally for 5–10 days)	Oral Suppressive Therapy in HIV-Infected Persons	Advantages	Disadvantages
Acyclovir	200 mg 5×/day *or* 400 mg tid	200 mg 5×/day *or* 800 mg bid	400 mg bid	200 mg 5×/day *or* 400 mg tid	400–800 mg bid or tid	Less expensive; smaller tablets; liquid formulation available	Less convenient dosing regimens
Valacyclovir	1000 mg/ bid	500 mg bid[§] *or* 1000 mg 1×/day	500 mg 1×/day[¶] *or* 1000 mg 1×/day	1000 mg bid	500 mg bid	More convenient dosing regimens	More expensive; larger caplet
Famciclovir	250 mg tid	125 mg bid	250 mg bid	500 mg bid	500 mg bid	More convenient dosing regimens; smaller tablet	More expensive

*Modified from Sexually Transmitted Diseases Treatment Guidelines 2002. MMWR-Morbidity & Mortality Weekly Report 51(RR6):12–17, 2002.
[†]The range of duration of therapy relates to differences in treatment durations in the original clinical studies. If the shorter course of therapy is initially prescribed, the patient should be reevaluated toward the end of treatment. Therapy should be continued if new lesions continue to form, if complications develop, or if systemic signs and symptoms have not abated.
[‡]When started within 24 hours of the recurrence.
[§]Three-day course of therapy is also acceptable.
[¶]For patients with nine or fewer recurrences per year.
bid, twice daily; tid, three times per day.

antibodies. At any given time, 1% of normal children and 1% to 5% of normal adults excrete HSV-1 asymptomatically and therefore are capable of transmitting HSV to susceptible contacts.

HSV-2 causes 75% to 80% of the cases of genital HSV infections in the United States. Since the late 1970s, seroprevalence rates for HSV-2 in the United States have increased by 30%. Among Americans 30 years of age or older, one in four has HSV-2, although most do not realize they are infected. In a potentially positive development, data suggest that HSV-2 seroprevalence rates have leveled off and may even be declining in certain age groups.

Expert Opinion on Management Issues

OROPHARYNGEAL HSV INFECTION

Primary oropharyngeal HSV-1 infection (gingivostomatitis) occurs most commonly in young children between 1 and 3 years of age. It is usually asymptomatic. The incubation period ranges from 2 to 12 days, with an average of 4 days. Symptomatic disease is characterized by fever to 104°F (40°C), oral lesions, sore throat, fetor oris, anorexia, cervical adenopathy, and mucosal edema. Oral lesions initially are vesicular but

rapidly rupture, leaving 1- to 3-mm shallow gray-white ulcers on erythematous bases. These lesions are distributed on the hard palate, the anterior portion of the tongue, along the gingiva, and around the lips (Fig. 1). In addition, the lesions may extend down the chin and neck because of drooling. Primary gingivostomatitis results in viral shedding in oral secretions for an average of 7 to 10 days. Virus can be isolated from the saliva of asymptomatic children and adults as well.

Recurrent oropharyngeal HSV-1 infection (herpes labialis) is frequently preceded by a prodrome of pain, burning, tingling, or itching. Painful vesicles typically occur at the vermillion border of the lip (Fig. 2). Recurrences occur only rarely in the mouth or on the skin of the face of immunocompetent patients. As with primary HSV-1 infection, recurrent infection may occur in the absence of clinical symptoms.

Treatment of primary gingivostomatitis in pediatric patients using oral acyclovir (see Table 1) decreases time to cessation of symptoms by 30% to 50% and time to lesion healing by 20% to 25%. Oral acyclovir has a more modest effect in the treatment of recurrent herpes labialis, and treatment of these patients should be individualized. In general, therapeutic benefit is enhanced if treatment is initiated as soon as possible after onset of symptoms, preferably within 24 to 48 hours of onset of the recurrence. Topical penciclovir

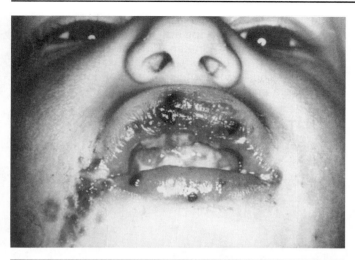

FIGURE 1. Herpes simplex gingivostomatitis. (From Whitley RJ: Herpes simplex virus. In Fields BN, Knipe DM, et al: Virology, 2nd ed. New York, Raven Press, pp 1843–1847, 1990.)

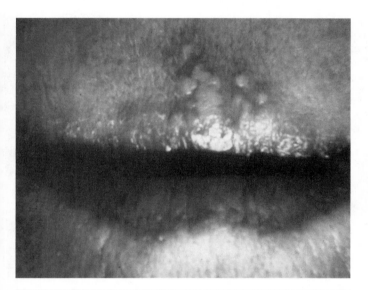

FIGURE 2. Recurrent herpes simplex labialis. (From Whitley RJ: Herpes simplex virus. In Fields BN, Knipe DM, et al: Virology, 2nd ed. New York, Raven Press, pp 1843–1847, 1990.)

(Denavir) for the treatment of recurrent herpes labialis (see Table 1) reduces time to healing and duration of pain by approximately half a day.

GENITAL HSV INFECTION

Local and systemic symptoms associated with primary HSV-2 and HSV-1 are generally of equal intensity. A classical clinical presentation of primary infection is that of macules and papules, progressing to vesicles, pustules, and ulcers. Skin ulcers crust; mucous membrane lesions heal without crusting. The majority of patients with primary genital herpes, however, do not experience these classic symptoms.

The overwhelming majority of both men and women with *clinically apparent* first-episode genital HSV-2 disease have localized symptoms such as pain at the site of the lesions and tender regional adenopathy. Constitutional symptoms, such as fever, headache, malaise, and myalgias, are present in two thirds of women and approximately 40% of men with clinically apparent first-episode genital HSV-2 disease. First-episode non-primary infections (acquisition of HSV-2 in persons with preexisting HSV-1 antibody, or, more rarely, vice versa) generally result in fewer systemic symptoms than first-episode primary infections (acquisition of HSV-1 or -2 in persons with no preexisting HSV antibody).

Recurrences of genital HSV-2 infection may be symptomatic or, more commonly, asymptomatic, with asymptomatic viral shedding accounting for much of the transmission of HSV. The duration of viral shedding is shorter with recurrences than with primary infection, and fewer lesions are present. Within 12 months of diagnosis, 90% of patients with documented first-episode genital HSV-2 infection have at least one recurrence. Regardless of viral type and whether or not suppressive therapy is employed, recurrence rates decrease over time.

Table 2 presents treatment options for the management of genital HSV infections. Acyclovir, famciclovir, and valacyclovir therapies are all equally efficacious in the treatment of genital HSV infections and in antiviral suppression of viral reactivation from latency.

OTHER PRIMARY HSV SKIN INFECTIONS

Alteration in the barrier properties of skin, as occurs in atopic dermatitis, can result in localized HSV skin infection (eczema herpeticum). Localized cutaneous HSV infection following trauma is known as herpes gladiatorum (wrestler's herpes or traumatic herpes); HSV infection of the digits results in herpetic whitlow.

OCULAR HSV INFECTION

Herpetic infection of the eye usually manifests as either a blepharitis or a follicular conjunctivitis. As disease progresses, branching dendritic lesions develop. Symptoms include severe photophobia, tearing, chemosis, blurred vision, and preauricular lymphadenopathy. Topical antiviral therapy is effective in the treatment of ocular HSV infection (see Table 1). An ophthalmologist should always be involved in the care of such patients.

CENTRAL NERVOUS SYSTEM HSV INFECTION BEYOND THE NEONATAL PERIOD

Herpes simplex encephalitis (HSE) is the most common cause of sporadic fatal encephalitis, with approximately 1250 cases of HSE in the United States each year, virtually all of which are caused by HSV-1. HSE is a necrotizing encephalitis with widespread hemorrhagic necrosis throughout infected brain parenchyma, particularly the temporal lobe. The manifestations of HSE in the older child and adult are indicative of the areas of the brain affected. Although no signs are pathognomonic, a progressively deteriorating level of consciousness, fever, abnormal cerebrospinal fluid (CSF) indexes, and focal neurologic findings in the absence of other causes should make this disease highly suspect. A burst suppression pattern on electroencephalogram is characteristic of HSV encephalitis (periodic lateralizing epileptiform discharges [PLEDS]).

In untreated patients, mortality exceeds 70%, and only 2.5% of survivors return to normal neurologic function. Even with the use of antiviral therapy (see Table 1), substantial mortality and morbidity remain, with 19% of patients dying and 62% of survivors having residual neurologic sequelae. Patients with a Glasgow Coma Scale score of less than 6, those older than 30 years, and those with encephalitis for longer than 4 days have a poorer outcome.

NEONATAL HSV INFECTION

Herpes simplex virus disease of the newborn is acquired in one of three distinct time intervals: intrauterine (in utero), peripartum (perinatal), and

TABLE 3 Diagnostic Tests for Herpes Simplex Virus (HSV) Infection and Disease

Diagnostic Modality	Description	Sensitivity and/or Specificity	Utility in Clinical Practice	Source(s) of Specimen
Cytology	Cytologic examination of cells from skin or mucous membrane.	Sensitivity, 60%–70%.	May be useful for presumptive diagnosis.	Maternal cervix; genital lesion(s); infant skin, mouth, conjunctivae, or corneal lesion
Serology	Detection of antibody. Two type-specific antibody assays manufactured by Focus Technologies, Inc., have received FDA approval: the HerpeSelect HSV-1 and HSV-2 ELISA and the HSV-1 and HSV-2 Immunoblot tests. Several additional tests that claim to distinguish between HSV-1 and HSV-2 antibody are commercially available, but high cross-reactivity rates, because of their use of crude antigen preparations, significantly limit their utility.	HerpeSelect HSV-2 ELISA: sensitivity, 96%–100%; specificity, 97%–98%. HerpeSelect HSV-2 Immunoblot: sensitivity, 97%–100%; specificity, 98%. Type-specific tests for HSV-1 tend to be 5%–10% less sensitive than their HSV-2 counterparts.	Beyond the infantile period, establishes prior infection with HSV-1 and/or HSV-2. Does not distinguish site of infection. Could be considered in patients with symptomatic genital disease with lesions in an advanced stage of healing and patients with risk factors for HSV but no history of genital herpetic lesions. Not useful for diagnosis of neonatal HSV disease.	Blood
Viral culture	Specimen collected, transferred in appropriate viral transport media on ice to a diagnostic virology laboratory, and inoculated into cell culture systems, which are then monitored for cytopathic effects characteristic of HSV replication.	≈ 95% of vesicular genital lesions grow HSV, compared with 70% of ulcerative lesions and 30% of crusted lesions.	The definitive diagnostic method of establishing HSV disease outside of the CNS.	Skin vesicles, oropharynx, CSF, urine, blood, stool or rectum, oropharynx, and conjunctivae
Polymerase chain reaction	Detection of viral DNA by molecular amplification.	Neonatal HSV CNS disease: sensitivity, 75%–100%; specificity, 71%–100% HSE beyond the neonatal period: Sensitivity, 95–100%; specificity, 94%.	The gold standard for documenting CNS HSV disease.	CSF; cutaneous or mucous membrane lesions

CNS, central nervous system; CSF, cerebrospinal fluid; FDA, Food and Drug Administration; HSV, herpes simplex virus.

postpartum (postnatal). Among infected infants, the time of transmission for the overwhelming majority (approximately 85%) of neonates is in the peripartum period. An additional 10% of infected neonates acquire the virus postnatally, and the final 5% are infected with HSV in utero. HSV infections acquired either peripartum or postpartum can be further classified as encephalitis, with or without skin involvement (CNS disease); disseminated infection involving multiple organs, including the CNS, lung, liver, adrenal glands, skin, eye, and/or mouth (disseminated disease); and disease localized to skin, eyes, and/or mouth (SEM disease). Current mortality following neonatal HSV disease ranges from 0% (SEM) to 5% (CNS) to 20% (disseminated). Seventy percent of survivors of CNS disease experience neurologic morbidity, compared with 20% of disseminated survivors and 0% to 5% of SEM survivors.

Intravenous acyclovir is the treatment of choice for neonatal HSV disease (see Table 1). The primary apparent toxicity associated with the use of this dose of intravenous acyclovir is neutropenia.

HSV IN THE IMMUNOCOMPROMISED HOST

Patients compromised by immunosuppressive therapy, underlying disease, or malnutrition are at increased risk for severe HSV infection. Disseminated disease may occur with widespread dermal, mucosal, and visceral involvement. Alternatively, disease may remain localized but persist for much longer periods of time than would be seen in immunocompetent hosts. Such patients should be treated with intravenous or oral acyclovir, depending on severity of disease (see Table 1).

Common Pitfalls

SUPPRESSIVE THERAPY FOLLOWING DISEASE BEYOND THE NEONATAL PERIOD

Neonatal HSV disease and HSV CNS infections beyond the neonatal period are managed acutely with intravenous acyclovir (see Table 1). The potential value of subsequent oral suppressive therapy with acyclovir or valacyclovir is under investigation currently by the NIAID (National Institute of Allergy and Infectious Diseases) Collaborative Antiviral Study Group. Currently, however, no evidence exists to suggest that suppressive oral acyclovir or valacyclovir therapy is beneficial in preventing neurologic complications in either of these disease populations.

ANTIVIRAL RESISTANCE

Compared with the prevalence of genital herpes, resistant HSV infections are distinctly rare. Currently, most isolates resistant to acyclovir, valacyclovir, or famciclovir are recovered from immunocompromised persons. Acyclovir-resistant isolates are usually resistant to famciclovir also but typically remain susceptible to foscarnet and cidofovir. Nevertheless, monitoring in research laboratories for resistant isolates from immunocompetent persons is warranted as antiviral agents against HSV are increasingly used.

VACCINE DEVELOPMENT

An HSV-2 glycoprotein D subunit vaccine was recently demonstrated to be safe and, in women who were HSV-1 and -2 seronegative prior to vaccination, mod-

12

TABLE 4 Telephone and Online Resources for Herpes Information

Organization	Telephone Information	Website
American Social Health Association (ASHA)	800–230–6039 (Resource Center) 919–361–8488 (Patient Herpes Hotline)	www.ashastd.org (ASHA website) www.ashastd.org/hrc (Herpes Resource Center website) www.ashasdt.org/hrc/helpgrp1.html (HELP support groups for people in the United States, Canada, and Australia with genital herpes)
The Centers for Disease Control and Prevention (CDC)	800–227–8922 National STD Hotline	www.cdc.gov (CDC website) www.cdc.gov/nchstp/dstd/dstdp.html (CDC fact sheet on STDs)
Planned Parenthood	800–230–7526	www.plannedparenthood.org
GlaxoSmithKline		www.herpeshelp.com www.herpesweb.net www.harduherpes.nu (in Swedish)
Novartis		www.cafeherpe.com www.genitalherpes.com www.herpes.com.au (Australia)
National Institutes of Health		www.nih.gov (NIH website) www.niaid.nih.gov/dmid/stds (NIAID fact sheet on STDs)
American Herpes Foundation		www.herpes-foundation.org
International Herpes Management Forum		www.ihmf.org
DAC Consultants		www.herpesdiagnosis.com
International Herpes Alliance		www.herpesalliance.org
Association Herpes		www.herpes.asso.fr (in French)

STD, sexually transmitted disease.

estly effective in preventing clinically apparent HSV-1 or -2 genital herpes disease. Efficacy was not seen in men, or in women with preexisting HSV-1 antibodies. Additional investigation of this vaccine in HSV-1 and -2 seronegative women is under way.

Communication and Counseling

Despite the advances in our understanding of the natural history of genital herpes, its diagnosis (Table 3), and its management, considerable shame, embarrassment, and stigma remain among infected persons. A number of resources are available to patients with genital herpes (Table 4), and their use should be encouraged. Similarly, having an infant with neonatal HSV infection can place stress on the parents' relationship that cannot be overstated. Professional counseling for the parents should be encouraged from the outset when an infant is being treated for neonatal HSV disease.

SUGGESTED READINGS

1. Kimberlin DW: Neonatal herpes simplex infection. Clin Microbiol Rev 17(1):1–13, 2004. **Detailed overview of the current diagnosis and management of neonatal HSV infections.**
2. Kimberlin DW, Rouse DJ: Genital herpes. N Engl J Med 350 (19):1970–1977, 2004. **Detailed overview of the current diagnosis and management of genital HSV infections.**
3. Wald A, Corey L, Cone R, et al: Frequent genital herpes simplex virus 2 shedding in immunocompetent women. Effect of acyclovir treatment. J Clin Invest 99:1092–1097, 1997. **Investigation of asymptomatic shedding of HSV in women.**
4. Whitley RJ, Cobbs CG, Alford CA Jr, et al: Diseases that mimic herpes simplex encephalitis. Diagnosis, presentation, and outcome. JAMA 262:234–239, 1989. **Extremely useful differential diagnosis for HSV CNS infections beyond the neonatal period.**
5. Whitley RJ, Kimberlin DW, Roizman B: Herpes simplex viruses. Clin Infect Dis 26:541–555, 1998. **Overview of the biology and disease pathogenesis of HSV infections.**

Human Immunodeficiency Virus Infection

Elaine J. Abrams

KEY CONCEPTS

- Human immunodeficiency virus (HIV) infection in children is most often acquired perinatally during pregnancy, delivery, and postpartum through breast-feeding.
- Without treatment, HIV disease manifestations can be rapid and fatal, particularly during infancy and early childhood.
- The use of antiretroviral and supportive therapies, including prophylaxis against opportunistic infections, significantly reduces HIV-related morbidity and mortality.
- Three or more antiretroviral medications, targeting different steps in the life cycle of the HIV virus, must be used in combination to minimize the likelihood of the

development of genetic mutations conferring resistance to specific agents.
- Clinical status, immune function, and the level of virologic replication guide the decisions about when to initiate and when to change treatment regimens.
- Adherence to antiretroviral regimens presents significant challenges to children and their families and warrants close monitoring and support.

A broad spectrum of disease ranging from asymptomatic infection to acquired immunodeficiency syndrome (AIDS) is caused by the retrovirus HIV, human immunodeficiency virus. Infection with HIV results in a gradual deterioration of immune function and increased susceptibility to infectious complications and malignancies. Of the estimated 2.5 million children living with HIV worldwide, the vast majority were infected through mother-to-child transmission (MTCT). The virus can be transmitted from an HIV-infected mother to her child during pregnancy, labor and delivery, and postpartum through breast-feeding. Adolescents are at risk for acquiring HIV infection through high-risk behaviors such as unprotected sex, particularly men having sex with men, and intravenous drug use.

Without treatment, disease manifestations can be rapid and fatal during infancy and early childhood. High levels of HIV replication and rapid loss of CD4+ cells leave the infant at risk for a variety of severe clinical manifestations, including *Pneumocystis carinii* pneumonia (PCP), HIV encephalopathy, failure to thrive, chronic diarrhea, severe thrush, and recurrent bacterial infections. Some children follow a less fulminant course of disease, including a small subset who may remain asymptomatic until late childhood. Most children, however, manifest some findings, including diffuse lymphadenopathy, hepatosplenomegaly, rashes, and impaired growth and cognitive development.

HIV infection has no cure, so the most effective approach to pediatric HIV disease focuses on prevention of MTCT. More than 21 antiretroviral medications are licensed for treatment of HIV infection, although not all of them are approved for or are suitable for children. The availability of antiretroviral treatment, however, has transformed pediatric HIV disease from a rapidly fatal infection to a chronic disease. The use of prophylactic regimens against several common infections like PCP and *Mycobacterium avium* complex (MAC) has also contributed to the decreased incidence of opportunistic infections. Additionally, the management of noninfectious complications of HIV, such as impaired growth and nutrition as well as neurologic and behavioral abnormalities, has further enhanced the care and treatment of children infected with HIV.

Expert Opinion on Management Issues

The core of HIV management entails the use of antiretroviral medications to interrupt specific steps in the life cycle of the virus. Use of multiple agents targeting different steps in the cycle minimizes the likelihood of

TABLE 1 Indications for Initiation of Antiretroviral Treatment in Children <12 Months of Age

Clinical Category	CD4+ Cell Percentage	Plasma HIV RNA Copy Number*	Recommendation
Symptomatic (clinical category A, B, or C)	<25% (immune category 2 or 3)	Any value	Treat
Asymptomatic (clinical category N)	<25% (immune category 1)	Any value	Consider treatment[†]

HIV, human immunodeficiency virus.

*Plasma HIV RNA levels are higher in HIV-infected infants than in older infected children and adults and may be difficult to interpret in infants younger than 12 months of age because overall HIV RNA levels are high and there is overlap in HIV RNA levels between infants who have and infants who do not have rapid disease progression.

[†]Because HIV infection progresses more rapidly in infants than in older children or adults, some experts would treat all HIV-infected infants younger than 6 months or younger than 12 months of age, regardless of clinical, immunologic, or virologic parameters.

TABLE 2 Indications for Initiation of Antiretroviral Treatment in Children 1 Year and Older with HIV Infection

Clinical Category	CD4+ Cell Percentage	Plasma HIV RNA Copy Number	Recommendation
AIDS (clinical category C)	<15% (immune category 3)	Any value	Treat
Mild to moderate symptoms (clinical category A or B)	15–25%* (immune category 2 or 3)	≥100,000 copies/mL[†]	Consider treatment
Asymptomatic (clinical category N)	>25% (immune category 1)	<100,000 copies/mL[†]	Many experts would defer therapy and closely monitor clinical, immune, and viral parameters.

*Many experts would initiate therapy if the CD4+ cell percentage is between 15% and 20% and would defer therapy but increase monitoring frequency in children with a CD4+ cell percentage of 21% to 25%.

[†]There is controversy among pediatric HIV experts regarding the plasma HIV RNA threshold warranting consideration of therapy in children in the absence of clinical or immune abnormalities. Some experts would consider initiating therapy in asymptomatic children if plasma HIV RNA llevels were between 50,000 and 100,000 copies/mL.

AIDS, acquired immunodeficiency syndrome; HIV, human immunodeficiency virus.

12

the development of genetic mutations conferring resistance to specific agents. The goals of antiretroviral treatment are to maximize suppression of viral replication, minimize the development of resistance, and restore or maintain immune integrity and function.

The decision about when to initiate treatment requires consideration of several critical variables, including the child's age, risk of disease progression, drug toxicities, and the ability of the child and family to adhere to treatment. The amount of measurable virus, HIV RNA viral load, and the degree of immune suppression are *not* reliable predictors of disease progression in infants younger than 12 months. It is currently recommended that all infants with symptomatic disease and any degree of immune suppression begin antiretroviral treatment; treatment can be postponed for those who are asymptomatic with normal immune function (Table 1). Some experts, however, believe that all infants with HIV infection should be started on therapy as soon after diagnosis as possible. The Working Group on Antiretroviral Therapy and Medical Management of Children with HIV Infection meets regularly to develop guidelines for antiretroviral treatment for children in the United States. Guidelines are revised as new treatment data become available.

CD4+ lymphocyte subset count and percentage as well as HIV RNA viral load are reasonably predictive of the risk of HIV disease progression in older children. It

is recommended that children older than 1 year with AIDS or advanced immune suppression begin treatment independent of HIV RNA viral load (Table 2). Children with symptomatic disease and/or moderate immune suppression and/or HIV RNA viral load equal to 100,000 copies should be considered for treatment, whereas those without symptoms, who have intact immune function and an HIV RNA viral load less than 100,000 copies per mL, can postpone initiation. For those not on treatment, frequent monitoring of clinical status, CD4+ number and percentage, and HIV RNA viral load is recommended.

The choice of treatment regimen is guided by the imperative to provide a fully suppressive regimen and to maximize the likelihood that the child will maintain strict adherence. Currently it is recommended that a child starting treatment begin therapy with two nucleoside reverse transcriptase inhibitors in combination with either a protease inhibitor or a non-nucleoside reverse transcriptase inhibitor (Table 3). The specific drugs to prescribe vary by age, weight, and medication formulation. Recommendations for specific drugs are also frequently reviewed and updated by the Working Group.

Monitoring of drug toxicity and medication efficacy should be done at regular intervals. Monitoring is generally more frequent, every 2 to 4 weeks, immediately after initiation and can safely be decreased to every 3 to

TABLE 3   Recommended Antiretroviral Regimens for Initial Therapy for HIV Infection*

Protease Inhibitor–Based Regimens

Strongly recommended	Two NRTIs[†]
Alternative recommendation	Two NRTIs[†] *plus* amprenavir (children ≥4 years old) or indinavir

Non-nucleoside Reverse Transcriptase Inhibitor–Based Regimens

Strongly recommended	Children >3 years: Two NRTIs[†] *plus* efavirenz (± nelfinavir)
	Children ≤3 years or who cannot swallow capsules: Two NRTIs[†] *plus* nevirapine)
Alternative recommendation	Two NRTIs[†]

Nucleoside Analogue–Based Regimens

Strongly recommended	None
Alternative recommendation	Zidovudine *plus* lamivudine *plus* abacavir
Use in special circumstances	Two NRTIs

Other Regimens

Not recommended	Monotherapy
	Certain two-NRTI combinations
	Two NRTIs *plus* saquinavir soft or hard gel capsule as a sole protease inhibitor
Insufficient data to recommend	Two NRTIs[†] *plus* delavirdine
	Dual protease inhibitors, including saquinavir soft or hard gel capsule with low-dose ritonavir, with the exception of lopinavir/ritonavir
	NRTI *plus* NNRTI *plus* protease inhibitor
	Tenofovir-containing regimens
	Enfuviritide (T–20)-containing regimens
	Atazanivir-containing regimens
	Fosamprenavir-containing regimens

*These regimens are as of 2005.

†Dual NRTI combination recommendations:

Strongly recommended choices: Zidovudine plus didanosine or lamivudine; or stavudine plus lamivudine

Alternative choices: Abacavir plus zidovudine or lamivudine; or didanosine plus lamivudine

Use in special circumstances: Stavudine plus didanosine; or zalcitabine plus zidovudine

Insufficient data: Tenofovir- or emtricitabine-containing regimens

Not recommended: Zalcitabine plus didanosine, stavudine, or lamivudine; or zidovudine plus stavudine

±, with or without; HIV, human immunodeficiency virus; NRTI, nucleoside analogue reverse transcriptase inhibitor; NNRTI, non-nucleoside analogue reverse transcriptase inhibitor.

4 months when the child is stable. Side effects vary with treatment regimen, but gastrointestinal dysfunction, bone marrow suppression, and hepatic toxicity are the most common. Elevations of serum lipids, cholesterol, and triglycerides are reported with increasing frequency in children receiving antiretroviral regimens, raising concerns about the long-term risk of cardiovascular disease.

The determination of treatment failure can be difficult and varies with the special circumstances of each child. Many children continue to maintain clinical benefit despite inadequate viral suppression and immune restoration. However, ongoing viral replication in the presence of antiretroviral drugs leads to the development of resistance mutations. Because resistance mutations to one drug within a specific class or category of treatment may confer resistance to other drugs within the same class, the development of these mutations can affect the efficacy of future treatments. General considerations for treatment failure include immunologic, virologic, and clinical response. For children receiving their first regimen, most experts define treatment failure based on viral load parameters. The decision to change a second or third regimen often requires evidence of clinical and/or significant immunologic deterioration. The goals of treatment for children who have failed multiple regimens are different from those initiating treatment for the first time:

focusing on maximizing clinical health and immune function rather than viral suppression. Inadequate adherence is often the major reason for treatment failure. Adherence should be thoroughly assessed prior to any decision to change treatment regimen.

The choice of treatment regimen for children who have failed prior therapy should be guided by resistance testing. Genotypic testing detects specific HIV genetic variants; phenotypic testing measures the viral isolate's ability to grow in the presence of the drug. Resistance testing is most informative if it is obtained while the child is receiving the failing regimen. Choosing a new regimen should be done in consultation with an HIV expert who is familiar with the interpretation of these tests as well as the nuances of the different interactions of medications. For example, the pharmacokinetic interactions of two drugs may increase blood levels beyond the inhibitory levels and counterbalance the impact of the resistance mutations. Treatment regimens for children with multiple-drug resistance mutations may require innovative strategies, such as cycling different regimens or inclusion of new experimental therapies.

Providing prophylaxis against opportunistic infections is a critical component of HIV care (Table 4). Current recommendations suggest that all HIV-infected infants begin trimethoprim-sulfamethoxazole (TMP-SMX) prophylaxis for the prevention of PCP at 4

TABLE 4 Prophylaxis Regimens for Children with HIV Infection

Indication	Medication	Alternatives
Pneumocystis carinii	**Trimethoprim-sulfamethoxazole (TMP-SMX)** 150/750 mg/m^2/day in 2 divided doses PO tiw on consecutive days Single dose PO tiw on consecutive days 2 divided doses PO qd 2 divided doses PO tiw on alternate days	**Dapsone** 2 mg/kg (max: 100 mg) PO qd 4 mg/kg (max: 200 mg) PO qw **Atovaquone** (1–3 mo, >24 mo of age) 30 mg/kg PO qd (4–24 mo) 45 mg/kg PO qd
	Aerosolized Pentamidine (≥5 yr) 300 mg via Respirgard II nebulizer, monthly **Clarithromycin** 7.5 mg/kg (max: 500 mg) PO bid	
Mycobacterium avium complex	**Azithromycin** 20 mg/kg (max: 1200 mg) PO qw 5 mg/kg PO qd (max 250 mg)	

bid, twice daily; HIV, human immunodeficiency virus; max, maximum; PO, by mouth; qd, every day; qw, every week; tiw, three times per week.

to 6 weeks of life and continue throughout the first year. Initiation of cotrimoxazole (TMP-SMX) at older ages should be guided by CD4 number and percentage: CD4+ less than 500 cells per μL or less than 15% for children 1 to 5 years of age; CD4+ less than 200 μL or less than 15% for children older than 6 years. Dapsone, atovaquone, and pentamidine are alternative medications for PCP prophylaxis. Children with advanced immune suppression should also be given prophylaxis to prevent MAC disease: CD4+ less than 750 cells per μL for children younger than 1 year; CD4+ less than 500 cells per μL for children 1 to 2 years of age; CD4+ less than 75 cells per μL for children 2 to 6 years of age; CD4+ less than 50 cells per μL for children older than 6 years. Clarithromycin and azithromycin are both used for this purpose. Children with recurrent bacterial infections may benefit from bacterial prophylaxis with daily antibiotics. Clinicians may opt to use amoxicillin or TMP-SMX, although the efficacy of these treatments has not been tested in children receiving highly active antiretroviral therapy. Prophylaxis or suppressive treatment for recurrent or chronic herpes simplex virus and varicella zoster virus infections may be indicated for individual children.

Care and treatment of children with HIV infection must be comprehensive, recognizing that the infection can affect multiple organ systems. Many children manifest nutritional and growth abnormalities. Central nervous system disease can result in physical, developmental, and behavioral disabilities. Multidisciplinary care and access to appropriate specialty services is critical to optimize the health of the HIV-infected child.

Common Pitfalls

Failure to recognize the obstacles to adherence to antiretroviral therapy can have significant negative consequences. A high degree of adherence is critical for success of treatment, but there are many reasons why

children and families may have periods of inadequate adherence. Most regimens require daily or twice-daily administration of multiple liquids and pills, many of which are difficult to administer and tolerate. High pill burden and side effects, particularly gastrointestinal complaints, are often cited as reasons for missed doses. Also, as children with HIV become adolescents, their ability to continue uninterrupted treatment is often challenged by developmental pressures such as the need to be like peers. The commitment of an adult family member to supervise and ensure daily treatment of a child or teen is a critical component of HIV care.

Treating HIV as a chronic viral infection without recognizing the complex developmental and psychological consequences of the disease can also result in unforeseen consequences. Pediatric HIV infection in the United States affects primarily children of ethnic minorities living in impoverished communities. HIV may be only one of multiple complex issues affecting the lives of these children, including poverty, violence, and under-resourced educational systems. Furthermore, HIV continues to be associated with significant stigma that can affect the child's acceptance and support within the family and community.

Communication and Counseling

HIV infection of childhood can now be managed effectively using a variety of antiretroviral, prophylactic, and supportive treatments. The landscape of drug availability is quickly changing and requires vigilance on the part of the practitioner to remain abreast of the latest developments. Effective treatment requires the establishment of a vital partnership with the child and the family to ensure honest communication and shared decision making. As children grow from infancy through adolescence, each developmental stage presents new challenges to adherence and the maintenance of optimal health and well-being.

SUGGESTED READINGS

1. Centers for Disease Control and Prevention: 1994 revised classification system for human immunodeficiency virus infection in children less than 13 years of age. MMWR Recomm Rep 43(RR–2): 1–10, 1994. **Provides the pediatric clinical and immunologic classification system currently used in the United States.**

2. Dunn D, and HIV Paediatric Prognostic Markers Collaborative Study Group: Short-term risk of disease progression in HIV-1-infected children receiving no antiretroviral therapy or zidovudine monotherapy: A meta-analysis. Lancet 362(9396):1605–1611, 2003. **The largest study in untreated children to examine the predictive value of CD4+ percentage and HIV RNA viral load for risk of progression to AIDS or death.**

3. McComsey GA, Leonard E: Metabolic complications of HIV therapy in children. AIDS 18:1738–1768, 2004. **Provides a comprehensive overview of metabolic complications associated with HIV treatment in children.**

4. 2001 USPHS/IDSA Guidelines for the Prevention of Opportunistic Infections in Persons Infected with Human Immunodeficiency Virus. November 2001. Accessed October 26, 2005. Available online at http://aidsinfo.nih.gov/guidelines/op_infections/OI_112801.html. **Provides guidelines for prophylaxis and treatment of opportunistic infections in adults and children.**

5. Working Group on Antiretroviral Therapy and Medical Management of HIV Infected Children: Guidelines for the Use of Antiretroviral Agents in Pediatric HIV Infection. Accessed January 17, 2004. PDF available for download at http://aidsinfo.nih.gov/guidelines/pediatric/PED_032405.pdf. **A living document frequently updated by HIV experts providing guidelines for antiretroviral treatment in children.**

Influenza Virus

Kenneth M. Zangwill

KEY CONCEPTS

- Influenza infection is a common infection in all age groups, and children younger than 2 years are at the greatest risk of hospitalization among all children.
- Antiviral medications are available, but their usefulness is limited.
- Inactivated and live, attenuated influenza vaccines are generally safe and effective for use in children.
- Vaccination coverage rates for influenza vaccine are quite low; every effort should be made to vaccinate at-risk children.

Influenza virus is an important cause of annual morbidity and mortality in the United States and worldwide. Each year, approximately 10% of adults and up to 15% to 40% of children experience symptomatic influenza caused by type A or B; type C is not a common pathogen in humans. Children younger than 2 years of age, especially those younger than 6 months, are at the greatest risk for hospitalization for influenza of any age group younger than 65 years. This is especially true among children with coexisting chronic cardiopulmonary diseases. From a public health perspective, school-age children are the most important transmitters of influenza virus within communities. Each year, influenza epidemics result in significant school absenteeism and substantial adult lost work time, with accompanying important economic losses. Since 1997, when avian-to-human influenza virus transmission was first identified, global pandemic planning has accelerated vaccine development for pandemic strains, stockpiling of antivirals, and increased viral surveillance for influenza infection among humans and nonhuman reservoirs.

Typical clinical influenza illness in children begins with the acute onset of fever, rhinorrhea, and headache followed very soon thereafter by cough and lassitude, a syndrome that may last for several days. Abdominal symptoms such as vomiting and pain are more commonly seen than in adults. Most patients recover without complication, although bacterial superinfection may occur in children following influenza infection (e.g., otitis media, pneumonia). Other known manifestations and potential complications include laryngotracheobronchitis, bronchiolitis, myositis, toxic shock syndrome (usually associated with *Staphylococcus aureus* coinfection), myocarditis or pericarditis, and central nervous system (CNS) syndromes, the most serious of which is encephalitis. Despite the availability of several antivirals, disease prevention by vaccination remains the best strategy for control of this infection. Two types of influenza vaccines are available, but vaccine coverage among pediatric and many adult high-risk groups is quite low (e.g., 9% to 25% among children with asthma).

Expert Opinion on Management Issues

A general approach to influenza prevention and treatment in clinical practice requires planning prior to its expected winter season onset and an assessment of the availability of vaccine. A plan for identification of high-risk children should be developed so they (or their contacts) may be vaccinated and/or receive antiviral prophylaxis.

ANTIVIRAL MEDICATION

Anti-influenza medications are used to prevent or treat influenza. Currently four medications are available: amantadine, rimantadine, zanamivir, and oseltamivir. Amantadine and rimantadine are M2 channel inhibitors active against type A strains; zanamivir and oseltamivir are neuraminidase inhibitors active against both types A and B strains (Table 1). As prophylactic agents, these drugs are 70% to 90% effective, and typically they are used seasonally in a specific individual for primary protection or for contacts of an infectious case to prevent secondary disease transmission. For the former purpose, prophylactic medication can be considered in the following scenarios:

- Patients who cannot receive influenza vaccine, in which case the drug should be administered at least during the peak influenza season, if not longer (this may be a period of several weeks if coverage through the season is desired by the physician or patient).

TABLE 1 Antivirals for Influenza Virus Infection

Name (Trade Name)	Treatment Dosage	Prophylactic Dosage	Maximum Dose	Dosage Formulations	Common Adverse Reactions	Comments
Amantadine* (Symmetrel)	1–9 yr: 5 mg/kg/day div bid for 3–5 days ≥10 yr: 100 mg bid‡ for 3–5 days	1–9 yr: 5 mg/kg/day div bid ≥10 yr: 100 mg bid‡	150 mg/day	Tablet and syrup	No common adverse events in children. Rarely, CNS excitation§ and exacerbation of underlying seizure disorder, worse with renal insufficiency.	Type A only
Rimantadine* (Flumadine)	≥18 yr, but often used by clinicians in children using the same dose and duration as amantadine	1–9 yr: 5 mg/kg/day div bid ≥10 yr: 100 mg bid‡	150 mg/day	Tablet and syrup	No common adverse events in children. CNS excitation§ and exacerbation of underlying seizure disorder; some nausea and vomiting. Less than with amantadine; worse with renal insufficiency.	Type A only
Oseltamivir† (Tamiflu)	≥1 yr: if ≤15 kg, 30 mg bid; >15–23 kg, 45 mg bid; >23–40 kg, 60 mg bid; >40 kg, 75 mg bid for 5 days If ≥13 yr: 75 mg bid	≥13 yr: 75 mg bid		Capsule and suspension	10%–15% of children may develop nausea and/or vomiting, usually only after early dose(s). This side effect can be tempered by taking the drug with food.	Types A and B
Zanamivir† (Relenza)	≥7 yr, 2 inhalations bid for 5 days	Not recommended		Blister pack for inhalation	Some bronchospasm reported in adults with preexisting airways disease.	Types A and B

*Amantadine and rimantadine antivirals: inhibition of viral M2 channel function, thus limiting viral intracellular uncoating and replication.
†Oseltamivir and zanamivir antivirals: inhibition of viral neuraminidase, thus limiting spread of virus from cell to cell.
‡For children <40 kg, 5 mg/kg/day, regardless of age, is advised.
§This may include nervousness, insomnia, difficulty with concentration.
bid, twice daily; div, divided.

- Patients who receive vaccine after the season has started and need to be covered for 2 weeks to allow for an adequate immune response to develop post-vaccination. Antivirals do not affect the immune response to vaccine in this scenario.
- Patients who are immunosuppressed and may not respond to the vaccine adequately (e.g., patients infected with human immunodeficiency virus [HIV] or those receiving cancer chemotherapy).

When using antivirals for contacts of an index case, individuals targeted should include those at high risk of morbidity, including unvaccinated persons older than 65 years or younger than 2 years; those living in assisted living situations; those with chronic cardiopulmonary, metabolic, and/or renal diseases; and those with hemoglobinopathy or who are otherwise immunosuppressed. Also, an antiviral should be considered for unvaccinated health care providers who may interact with high-risk patients.

As a group, antivirals are of modest usefulness for therapeutic purposes in that none is effective when used beyond 2 days from the onset of clinical symptoms, and each is approximately 70% to 90% effective in lessening the duration of symptoms by only 0.5 to 1.5 days in uncomplicated disease. Amantadine and rimantadine are only effective against type A influenza; the neuraminidase inhibitors (zanamivir and oseltamivir) are active against both types A and B. The clinical decision to use these drugs requires several points of information. The most important is the likelihood of influenzal disease in the individual patient. This can be definitively determined at the point of care by viral culture, but more practical and timely is use of rapid diagnostic testing which is approximately 70% to 80% sensitive and 80% to 90% specific for influenza. In the absence of such testing, the diagnostic sensitivity and specificity of the presence of cough, headache, and pharyngitis in a child in the winter has a sensitivity and specificity of approximately 80% for a diagnosis of influenza. Further, treatment decisions need to consider the local epidemiologic information on the frequency and type of virus circulating in the community, particularly because type B is not treated by all antivirals.

Oseltamivir and zanamivir are significantly more expensive than amantadine and rimantadine. Side effects of these medications are generally uncommon. Nausea and vomiting may occur with oseltamivir, but it usually resolves after the first doses and can be ameliorated when taken with food. Zanamivir is not recommended for those with underlying airway disease because of some reports of bronchospasm in adults, but it can be used cautiously in this setting if deemed necessary. Amantadine and rimantadine can cause CNS excitation (nervousness, insomnia, and increased seizures in children with epilepsy), the most serious of which are usually only seen at high doses or among those with renal disease (which impacts on drug elimination). All of the drugs except zanamivir need to be adjusted for severe renal insufficiency. Each is available in a liquid form except for zanamivir, which is a disk inhaler and therefore not appropriate for young children (see Table 1). Resistance may quickly develop during amantadine or rimantadine use, but this is not yet established as an important problem with zanamivir or oseltamivir. In general, for children with risk factors for more severe disease (such as children taking corticosteroids or chemotherapy), antiviral therapy may be more liberally used.

Nonspecific therapies for influenza should focus on rest, maintenance of adequate hydration, and pain relief as needed. Physical rest is probably helpful, given the systemic nature of the symptoms and anecdotal reports of extreme activity resulting in death among infected military recruits. Maintenance of adequate hydration may facilitate mucociliary viral clearance. Pain relief should not include aspirin products given the known association between influenza virus infection and Reye syndrome. There are reports suggesting the topical zinc preparations may ameliorate symptoms in viral upper respiratory infections, but data are lacking for influenza virus. Other alternative therapies (e.g., herbs) are not adequately studied in children to recommend specifically. Symptomatic treatments for upper respiratory complaints in younger children (i.e., decongestants, antihistamines, cough suppressants) are generally ineffective and may be counterproductive.

VACCINATION

Two types of influenza vaccines currently are available for use in the United Sates for adults and children. The older type, developed before World War II, consists of inactivated influenza viruses and is administered intramuscularly. The second, licensed in 2003, contains live, attenuated viral strains and is administered as a large-droplet intranasal spray. Each year these vaccines are formulated with three viral strains (A/H1N1, A/H3N2, and B) based on viral surveillance data from around the world.

Both vaccines are effective in preventing influenza-like illnesses, hospitalization for cardiopulmonary conditions, visits to health care providers, use of health

---

BOX 1   General Indications and Contraindications for Inactivated Influenza Vaccine

- Groups for whom influenza vaccine is recommended:
  - Persons 50 years and older or children between 6 months and 2 years of age.
  - Contacts of infants younger than 6 months.
  - Pregnant women.
- Persons with and contacts of persons with:
  - Chronic cardiopulmonary, renal, or metabolic (e.g., diabetes) disease.
  - Immunosuppressive conditions including human immunodeficiency (HIV) infection.
  - Hemoglobinopathies.
  - Chronic aspirin use in children 6 months to 18 years of age.
  - Those living in assisted living facilities.
  - Anyone interested in vaccine should receive influenza vaccine.
- Contraindications
  - Previous severe anaphylactic reaction to egg protein or other components of the vaccine.

TABLE 2 Specific Use Differences between Inactivated and Live, Attenuated Influenza Vaccines

	Inactivated Vaccine	Live, Attenuated Vaccine
Route.	Intramuscular.	Intranasal spray.
Age indication.	≥6 mo.[†]	5–49 yr; healthy only.[†]
Give to immunosuppressed persons?	Yes.[*]	No.
Give to immunocompetent contacts of an index case?	Yes.	Yes.
Give to contacts of immunosuppressed persons?	Yes.	Inactivated vaccine preferred.
Give with another live viral vaccine?	Yes.	Separate by 1 mo.
Give to pregnant women?	Yes.	No.
History of previous Guillain-Barré syndrome.	Avoid if GBS occurred within 6 wks of previous influenza vaccination *and* low risk for severe influenza.	No.
Give with antivirals?	Yes.	Wait at least 2 days after stopping antiviral to give vaccine. Wait 2 wk after vaccine to give antivirals.
Give to breast-feeding woman?	Yes.	No.
Schedule.	6–35 mo: One 0.25-mL dose. 3–8 yr: One 0.5-mL dose. 9–12 yr: One 0.5-mL dose. >12 yr: One 0.5-mL dose.	5–49 yr: One dose.

*Wait until 3 weeks after last dose of chemotherapy and the peripheral white count is recovering to maximize immunogenicity.
†Two doses separated by at least 1 month (inactivated) and 6 to 10 weeks (live, attenuated) are recommended for children receiving primary immunization.

care resources, antibiotic use, incidence of concomitant otitis media, work loss, and school and work absenteeism. The potential economic benefits of influenza vaccination (among all age groups) are often underappreciated among clinicians and policymakers and include direct costs of health care and indirect costs (including lost wages and extra caregiving due to illness). Influenza vaccination should be widely promoted and implemented by clinicians.

Influenza vaccine is recommended for those at increased risk for morbidity and mortality following infection as noted in Box 1. Because one vaccine is inactivated and the other merely attenuated, their specific uses need to be individualized to certain situations (Table 2). One dose is given for any child who has ever previously received influenza vaccine and two doses are required—1 month apart for inactivated vaccine and 6 to 10 weeks apart for attenuated vaccine—if the child has not previously received influenza vaccine (primary immunization). If such a child receives only one dose of vaccine in a given flu season, the following year that child should still receive only one dose.

Despite the general awareness of influenza infection, vaccine coverage rates for high-risk children are disappointing. For example, among children with asthma (perhaps the largest pediatric group at risk), vaccine coverage in the United States is no more than 25%. This phenomenon is primarily due to misconceptions about the burden of influenza illness and the safety, efficacy, and effectiveness of the vaccines.

Common Pitfalls

Although influenza is a condition well known to clinicians, several pitfalls in its management and prevention occur with frequency. These include the following:

- Failure to consider influenza as the etiologic agent in children with so-called colds and other more unusual presentations.
- Antiviral medication may be used too late in the illness to impact reliably on symptomatology.
- Some rapid diagnostic tests do not detect both influenza types A and B, so the laboratory should be consulted when specimens are obtained.
- Because national recommendations focus on vaccination of all children younger than 2 years, those at high risk who are older than 6 months may be missed.
- Forgetting that children older than 5 years may receive the live, attenuated vaccine in lieu of the shot if preferred by the patient or family.
- Not identifying contacts of high-risk children (especially asthmatics and those younger than 6 months) who otherwise should be vaccinated.
- Failure of a clinical practice to plan for influenza prevention before the season starts.
- Antiviral medication and vaccination may not work if a new pandemic emerges.

Communication and Counseling

Influenza infections occur every year, young children are at particular risk for hospitalization, and school-age children are efficient transmitters of the virus within communities. Most children recover uneventfully and antivirals have limited usefulness. Practitioners should plan vaccination strategies aggressively to target high-risk groups and their contacts. Parents should understand that vaccination and identification of high-risk contacts of a child with influenza are important to themselves and their family.

12

SUGGESTED READINGS

1. Centers for Disease Control and Prevention (CDC): Prevention and control of influenza: Recommendations of the Advisory Committee on Immunization Practices (ACIP). MMWR Mor Mortal Wkly Rep 54(RR08):1–40, July 29, 2005. **Governmental general recommendations on the use of influenza vaccines and antivirals.**
2. Matheson NJ, Symmonds-Abrahams M, Sheikh A, et al: Neuraminidase inhibitors for preventing and treating influenza in children. Cochrane Database Syst Rev 3:CD002744 2003. **Rigorous evaluation of the safety and efficacy of neuraminidase inhibitors for prophylaxis and treatment of influenza in children.**
3. Englund JA: Antiviral therapy of influenza. Semin Pediatr Infect Dis 13:120–128, 2002. **Good summary of antivirals for prophylactic and therapeutic use against influenza virus.**
4. Rennels MB, Meissner HC; Committee on Infectious Diseases: Technical Report: Reduction of the influenza burden in children. Pediatrics, 110(6), 2002. PDF available for download at http://pediatrics.aappublications.org/cgi/reprint/110/6/e80. **Comprehensive summary from the American Academy of Pediatrics about the burden of influenza disease in children, complications of clinical disease, and the available vaccines.**
5. Uyeki TM: Influenza diagnosis and treatment in children: A review of studies on clinically useful tests and antiviral treatment for influenza. Pediatr Infect Dis J 22:164–177, 2003. **Comprehensive summary of the use of diagnostic testing and antiviral treatment for influenza.**
6. Zangwill KM, Belshe RB: Safety and efficacy of trivalent inactivated influenza vaccine in young children: A summary for the new era of routine vaccination. Pediatr Infect Dis J 23:189–200, 2004. **Comprehensive summary of the safety of inactivated and live, attenuated influenza vaccines in pediatric populations.**

Measles

Robert T. Perry and Walter A. Orenstein

KEY CONCEPTS

- Measles remains common in many countries in Europe, Africa, and Asia, although it is virtually eliminated from the Americas.
- Diagnosis should be confirmed by immunoglobulin (Ig) M serology, and specimens should be taken for virus isolation.
- Measles may be prevented if measles vaccine or Ig is given in the first days after exposure.
- Vitamin A is the only treatment shown to reduce the risk of complications or death after measles.
- All children should receive two doses of measles vaccine in the form of measles-mumps-rubella (MMR) vaccine, the first at 12 months of age and the second at 4 to 6 years of age.

Measles is a viral illness marked by a prodrome of fever and respiratory symptoms, including cough, coryza, and nonpurulent conjunctivitis, followed by a typical maculopapular erythematous rash. Koplik spots, an enanthema on the buccal mucosa, are whitish papules on a bluish base that appear 1 to 2 days before the onset of rash and are considered pathognomonic for measles. In normal hosts, the prodromal period lasts 2 to 4 days; the rash is present for roughly 1 week and ends with a fine desquamation of the skin. The rash usually begins centrally and spreads to the limbs. Confirming the clinical diagnosis with serologic testing is essential in countries such as the United States, where the incidence of measles is low and the possibility of other clinically similar conditions is consequently high.

Although most people recover from measles without complications or sequelae, measles virus can have a profound effect on the respiratory and gastrointestinal (GI) epithelium, the immune system, the nervous system, and vitamin A levels. In the United States, measles infections result in complications such as otitis media (in 7% of cases), diarrhea (6%), pneumonia (6%), encephalitis (0.15%), and subacute sclerosing panencephalitis (SSPE) (1 in 100,000). Death occurs in 1 to 3 of every 1000 cases, with infants and adults at higher risk than children.

In the developing world, case fatality rates can be 5% to 15% and are related to overcrowded living conditions, malnutrition, and inadequate health care. In these situations, the disease is associated with a more intense, occasionally hemorrhagic rash ("black measles"); significant inflammation of the oral and GI mucosa leading to decreased oral intake and diarrhea; an increased risk of secondary bacterial infections, notably pneumonia and otitis media; and sometimes blindness from keratitis and coexisting vitamin A deficiency.

In the prevaccine era, up to 90% of all children in the United States had measles sometime before 15 years of age. In the late 1950s, an average of 450 deaths from measles was reported each year. With widespread vaccination, the number of cases and deaths in the United States has fallen dramatically. Since 1998, the number of reported cases has been 100 or fewer per year, and only 2 acute deaths from measles have been reported since 1992. Worldwide, measles is still a killer and caused an estimated 30 to 40 million cases and 611,000 deaths in 2002. Although measles is currently not endemic in the United States, numerous imported cases are detected and reported each year, many of them leading to limited domestic spread.

Primary Prevention

Measles can be effectively prevented through vaccination, as shown by the dramatic decline in cases and deaths in the United States. An attenuated live virus vaccine was introduced in the United States in 1963, and further attenuated strains were introduced in 1965 (Schwarz) and in 1968 (Moraten). Currently, vaccination in the United States uses the Moraten strain, together with live attenuated rubella and mumps vaccines, a combination forming the MMR vaccine (MMR II). It is also available as single-antigen measles (Attenuvax) and in combination with rubella vaccine (MR-Vax II). MMR is the vaccine of choice and induces immunity to measles in 95% or more of children when given at 12 to 15 months of age. The current recommendation by the Advisory Committee on Immunization Practices (ACIP) and the Centers for Disease Control and Prevention (CDC) is for two vaccinations, the first at 12 to 15 months and the second at 4 to 6 years of age. For unvaccinated older children or young adults, administration of two doses of vaccine at least 1 month apart is recommended (see the ACIP recommendations for detailed information).

After vaccination with MMR, common adverse events are fever (5% to 10%), transient rash (5%), joint pains or arthritis (in 1% of children and 10% to 25% of postpubertal women), and parotitis (1% to 2%). More severe reactions, such as anaphylaxis, encephalopathy, idiopathic thrombocytopenic purpura, and febrile seizures, are extremely rare. An Institute of Medicine review reviewed the suspected link between MMR vaccination and autism and concluded that "the body of epidemiologic evidence favors rejection of a causal relationship between the MMR vaccine and autism." Persons who should not receive MMR vaccine include women who are pregnant or plan to become pregnant within 3 months of vaccination, people with a history of anaphylaxis to neomycin or gelatin, those with thrombocytopenia or thrombocytopenic purpura, and those with evidence of immunodeficiency. MMR vaccine should be given to people with asymptomatic human immunodeficiency virus (HIV) infection without severe immunosuppression because vaccination against measles has not led to severe adverse reactions, and clinical measles can be life-threatening. Vaccination with MMR should be deferred if the potential vaccinee has received blood or blood products during the past few months before the anticipated vaccination (see the ACIP recommendations for detailed information).

Expert Opinion on Management Issues

GENERAL PRINCIPLES

In the vast majority of cases, measles resolves without specific treatment and leaves few sequelae. Therapy should be aimed at alleviating symptoms and preventing complications. People with measles should receive antipyretics and extra fluids during the febrile period and cough suppressants as necessary. In most cases, return to work, school, or daycare is permitted by the fifth day after onset of the rash. In hospitalized cases, airborne isolation precautions should be in place for 4 days after onset of the rash in otherwise healthy children or for the duration of the illness in immunocompromised children.

In a systematized review of the published literature, prophylactic antibiotics were found ineffective in preventing secondary bacterial infections. However, if fever persists more than 2 to 3 days after appearance of the rash or recurs after an initial defervescence, or if other symptoms of infection develop, the patient should be thoroughly reevaluated, including collection of appropriate samples for bacterial and viral culture. If any signs of secondary bacterial infection are noted, prompt treatment with antibiotics should begin.

URGENT INTERVENTIONS: SECONDARY PREVENTION

When exposure to measles occurs in someone not already immune who is at risk for serious disease, administration of immune globulin (IG) or measles-containing vaccine can prevent or attenuate the disease. Vaccination with monovalent measles vaccine or, if not available, MMR within 72 hours of exposure may provide protection from measles and is the preferred method of secondary prevention in children 12 months of age or older. Children 6 to 12 months of age who are household contacts of a measles case should also be vaccinated if it can be done within 72 hours of initial exposure. Because the original measles case is frequently not confirmed within this period, IG is recommended for susceptible household contacts who were not vaccinated within 72 hours of initial exposure (see later). Infants vaccinated when younger than 12 months should receive two additional doses of measles-containing vaccine beginning on or after their first birthday, with at least 28 days between doses. Pregnant women, immunocompromised people, or others with contraindications to vaccination should not receive measles vaccine but should instead receive IG if prophylaxis is needed.

For nonimmune people at high risk of measles or its complications, Ig administered within 6 days of exposure can prevent or attenuate measles. The dose is 0.25 mL/kg body weight (0.5 mL/kg body weight for immunocompromised persons) given intramuscularly. In all situations, the maximal dose of Ig is 15 mL. This method should not be used to control epidemics in schools and communities; vaccination should be used instead. A person receiving intravenous immune globulin (IVIG) should need no further administration of IG if the last dose was at least 100 mg/kg and given within 3 weeks before exposure. Persons with HIV are found to lose vaccine-induced immunity and suffer from severe measles if disease develops. Regardless of current antiretroviral therapy regimens, HIV-infected people exposed to measles who are not receiving regular IVIG infusions or whose last dose of IVIG does not meet the criteria just described should still be considered for IG prophylaxis. Barring contraindications to vaccination, those who receive IG should receive MMR vaccine 5 to 6 months after the IG dose.

The most important step in secondary prevention of measles is to report suspected cases to state or local public health authorities as required by law or regulation in every state of the United States and in many other countries. State and local public health departments can assist in the laboratory confirmation of measles, identification of contacts, provision of vaccine or IG to exposed susceptible persons, and collection and shipment of samples for viral isolation. Measles is no longer endemic in the United States, and aggressive public health intervention, together with high levels of vaccine coverage, can prevent outbreaks from internationally imported cases. The first step is to notify the local health department of suspected measles cases so secondary spread can be interrupted quickly.

VITAMIN A

Measles virus infection is associated with a sharp drop in serum vitamin A levels in children worldwide, including in the United States. This acute lowering of vitamin A levels may lead to xerophthalmia and blindness; in fact, measles is one of the major infectious causes of blindness worldwide. Lower levels of vitamin A in children with measles also increase the risk of other complications and death from measles. A meta-analysis of clinical trials of vitamin A supplementation for children with measles showed significant reductions in morbidity and mortality when children were given vitamin A supplementation when they arrived at the hospital, with the effects most pronounced in children younger than 2 years. Even though these children did not have overt signs of vitamin A deficiency, more than 50% had levels of vitamin A in the deficient range when evaluated for acute measles. Studies in the United States showed that between 50% and 60% of children with acute measles also have levels of vitamin A in the deficient range. The American Academy of Pediatrics therefore recommends vitamin A supplementation for children with measles in the circumstances and in the doses listed in Box 1.

TREATMENT OF COMPLICATIONS

Otitis Media

Otitis media is a frequent complication of measles that should be treated with antibiotics (as it is in patients without measles).

Diarrhea

Diarrhea is another common complication of measles and should be managed symptomatically to prevent dehydration (as it is for children without measles). Bacterial cultures of the stool may be helpful, although antibiotic therapy should be used only when warranted by culture results and the clinical condition of the patient.

Laryngotracheobronchitis (Croup)

Steroids are a safe and effective therapy for croup in children without measles. However, rare cases of measles inclusion body encephalitis are reported in children in whom measles developed while taking prolonged courses of steroid therapy. Although it is unlikely that the short courses of steroids used for croup would also lead to measles complications, it is prudent to monitor closely those children who receive this therapy for croup in the context of measles. In more severe or complicated cases, children with measles-associated croup may have additional complications, such as lower respiratory tract infections and bacterial tracheitis. These conditions are treated successfully in the same manner as cases not associated with measles, although viral pneumonitis should be considered in children with lower respiratory infections not responding to antibiotics.

Pneumonia

Pneumonia is a common and sometimes severe complication of measles that causes up to half of measles-associated deaths. It may be direct infection of the lungs by measles virus; secondary viral infection, typically adenovirus; secondary bacterial infection; or all three. Because this mix of viral and bacterial etiologies is difficult to differentiate, it is best to give antibiotics to all children with measles and clinical or radiologic evidence of pneumonia. The bacteria implicated in pneumonia secondary to measles are generally similar to those often found in the same community. Pneumonia in malnourished children and nosocomial pneumonia are more likely to be caused by gram-negative bacilli such as *Klebsiella* or *Pseudomonas*. All children with measles-associated pneumonia should receive vitamin A in addition to appropriate antibiotics.

In vitro, ribavirin is active against measles virus. In a few patients with severe primary measles-associated pneumonia, ribavirin has been tried as a small-particle aerosol, intravenously, and via both routes. The results are inconclusive, and ribavirin has not been evaluated for measles pneumonitis in controlled clinical trials. Randomized, double-blind, placebo-controlled studies using oral ribavirin in children with measles were conducted in Mexico, Brazil, and the Philippines. The groups receiving ribavirin had a reduction in the duration and degree of symptoms with no adverse reactions, but the magnitude of the reduction was small, and the studies did not include children with pneumonia or other severe complications. The U.S. Food and Drug Administration has not approved ribavirin for use in the treatment of measles or its complications. The adverse reaction most frequently reported with intravenous administration in humans is anemia, although seizures are also described. In the small number of cases of aerosol administration of ribavirin for measles pneumonitis, few adverse events were reported. However, in critically ill infants with respiratory syncytial virus pneumonitis, this route of administration is associated with worsening of pulmonary and cardiovascular function, although it is not clear whether the adverse events were a result of the severity of the underlying disease or of the aerosol administration of ribavirin.

Encephalitis

Measles causes three neurologic syndromes:

- Acute, immune-mediated encephalitis (postinfectious encephalitis) that develops during or within weeks to months of the measles rash in otherwise healthy older children.
- Acute encephalitis from direct infection of the brain by measles virus in immunocompromised hosts (measles inclusion body encephalitis) that develops several months after measles and progresses to death in most cases.
- SSPE from direct infection of the brain by measles virus in a normal host, with measles inclusion bodies in the brain and high levels of antimeasles antibodies in the cerebrospinal fluid. SSPE develops an average of 7 years after the initial measles infection and typically progresses to death in months to years.

For all types of postmeasles encephalitis, patients should receive symptomatic and supportive care. For postinfectious encephalitis, no specific treatment exists. Measles inclusion body encephalitis is treated with various agents, including interferons, ribavirin, and IVIG. Case reports document successes and failures with each of these therapies, but none of them show clear scientific evidence of effectiveness. A multicenter open-label randomized trial found no differences in SSPE progression or 6-month survival between patients treated with inosiplex (Isoprinosine) versus inosiplex plus intraventricular interferon alfa–2b. Although one third of each treatment group had a stable or improving disease course, compared to the authors' expected rate of 5% to 10% in untreated cases, the true effects of the treatments are not clear because 33% of patients treated with inosiplex and 53% of patients treated with inosiplex and interferon did not comply with the study protocol or were lost to follow-up, and 12% received so-called escape medications. Although SSPE has been treated with many other agents, the variable course of this disease, together with the lack of concurrent controls, make it difficult to assess the results of different therapies. In view of the rarity of SSPE, it would be helpful to enter all new patients in the registry maintained by Dr. Paul Dyken in Alabama.*

---

*Paul Dyken, MD, World SSPE Registry, P.O. Box 70191, 283 Wingfield Drive, Mobile, Alabama, USA, 36670-0191; pdyken@aol.com; telephone (U.S.) 334-478-6424; fax (U.S.) 334-476-8277.

Common Pitfalls

Young infants, adults, pregnant women, and people with impaired cellular immunity have a higher risk of complicated measles infection, especially primary measles viral pneumonia and measles inclusion body encephalitis. In addition, those with impaired immunity may not have a rash, or the rash may not have the typical appearance, thus delaying recognition and treatment of the disease. It would be prudent to monitor these patients closely because early recognition and treatment of measles and its complications appear, at least in case reports, to increase the chance of successful recovery. In immunocompromised individuals, negative measles serologic results may not reliably indicate the absence of measles virus infection, and during the initial evaluation, samples of urine, nasopharyngeal aspirate, or blood lymphocytes should be sent for viral culture and direct fluorescent antigen staining. In complicated cases, more invasive procedures, such as bronchoalveolar lavage, open lung biopsy, or brain biopsy, may be necessary to make the diagnosis.

Important Note

Given the paucity of clinical trials and the varying treatment regimens used in patients with measles, all cases of encephalitis and pneumonia that are severe or involve patients with compromised immunity should be managed in consultation with infectious disease and other appropriate specialists. Issues in measles case management are reviewed in articles by Hussey and Duke (see Suggested Readings).

Communication and Counseling

Most children with measles recover uneventfully, and those with complications should recover with proper antibiotic and supportive treatment. However, the prognosis for children with encephalitis or SSPE is very guarded. Parents should be counseled that the MMR vaccine is safe, and the weight of scientific evidence is against any association between receipt of MMR vaccine and autism. They should also know that the vaccine is effective in preventing complications and deaths from measles, and their children should receive two doses of vaccine, the first at 12 months of age and the second at 4 to 6 years of age.

SUGGESTED READINGS

1. American Academy of Pediatrics: Committee on Infectious Diseases and Committee on Pediatric AIDS: Measles immunization in HIV-infected children. Pediatrics 103:1057–1060, 1999. **Practice guideline from the AAP on measles immunization of HIV-infected children.**
2. American Academy of Pediatrics: Measles. In Pickering LK (ed): Red Book: 2003 Report of the Committee on Infectious Diseases, 26th ed. Elk Grove Village, Ill: American Academy of Pediatrics, 2003, pp 419–429. **AAP recommendations for control and management of measles.**
3. Banks G, Fernandez H: Clinical use of ribavirin in measles: A summarized review. In Smith RA, Knight V, Smith JAD (eds): Clinical Applications of Ribavirin. Orlando, Fla: Academic Press,

1984, pp 203–209. **Reviews three studies of ribavirin in children with uncomplicated measles.**

4. D'Souza RM, D'Souza R: Vitamin A for treating measles in children (Cochrane Review). In The Cochrane Library, Issue 2. Chichester, UK: John Wiley, 2004, pp 1–21. **Meta-analysis showing reduced morbidity and mortality after measles when children are given vitamin A at the time of rash onset.**

5. Duke T, Mgone CS: Measles: Not just another viral exanthem. Lancet 361:763–773, 2003. **Review of virology, pathophysiology, and clinical issues with measles; discusses problem of measles in infants too young for vaccination; reviews success of various control strategies; proposes areas for future research.**

6. Frieden TR, Sowell AL, Henning KJ, et al: Vitamin A levels and severity of measles—New York City. Am J Dis Child 146:182–186, 1992. **Observational study of vitamin A levels and risk of measles complications.**

7. Gascon GG: Randomized treatment study of inosiplex versus combined inosiplex and intraventricular interferon-alpha in subacute sclerosing panencephalitis (SSPE): International multicenter study. J Child Neurol 18(12):819–827, 2003. **Results of multicenter, randomized trial of treatment for SSPE.**

8. Hussey GA, Clements CJ: Clinical problems in measles case management. Ann Trop Paediatr 16:307–317, 1996. **Reviews rates, typical time course, causative organisms, and treatments used for measles complications.**

9. Immunization Safety Review Committee, Board on Health Promotion and Disease Prevention, Institute of Medicine: Immunization Safety Review: Measles-Mumps-Rubella Vaccine and Autism. Washington, DC: National Academy Press, 2004. **Reviews laboratory and epidemiologic data bearing on the linkage between the receipt of MMR vaccine and the development of autism.**

10. Moss WJ, Clements CJ, Halsey NA: Immunization of children at risk of infection with human immunodeficiency virus. Bull World Health Organ 81:61–70, 2003. **Reviews data on safety, immunogenicity, and efficacy of childhood vaccines in HIV-infected children.**

11. Papania MJ, Orenstein WA: Defining and assessing measles elimination goals. J Infect Dis 189(Suppl. 1):S23–S26, 2003. **Defines criteria for measles elimination in the United States and outlines the application of those criteria to current surveillance data.**

12. Perry RT, Halsey NA: The clinical significance of measles: A review. J Infect Dis 189(Suppl. 1):S4–S16, 2004. **Describes clinical features and complications and reviews factors influencing complication rates and death rates.**

13. Shann F: Meta-analysis of trials of prophylactic antibiotics for children with measles: Inadequate evidence. BMJ 314:334–336, 1997. **Meta-analysis showing no benefit of prophylactic antibiotic administration to children with uncomplicated measles.**

14. Watson JC, Hadler SC, Dykewicz CA, et al: Measles, mumps, and rubella—vaccine use and strategies for elimination of measles, rubella, and congenital rubella syndrome and control of mumps: Recommendations of the Advisory Committee on Immunization Practices (ACIP). MMWR Morb Mortal Wkly Rep 47(RR–8):1–57, 1998. **Critical reference on measles prevention with guidelines for both immunoglobulin and measles vaccine use.**

Parvovirus Infection

William C. Koch

KEY CONCEPTS

- Infection with the human parvovirus B19 (B19) is usually mild and self-limited and does not require treatment.
- No antiviral agent is available.
- Infections in immunocompromised patients may lead to chronic infections with more serious symptoms.
- Patients with anemia secondary to chronic B19 infection may benefit from administration of intravenous immunoglobulin (IVIG).
- Children with erythema infectiosum (EI) and adults with arthropathy are not infectious.
- Patients presenting with a transient aplastic crisis (TAC) or chronic anemia are usually viremic and therefore potentially infectious and should be isolated in the hospital setting.

The human parvovirus B19 (B19) is one of the smallest DNA viruses known to cause disease in humans and the only member of the Parvovirus family proven to cause symptomatic infection in humans. There are many other animal parvoviruses, some of which are important pathogens in mammals (e.g., canine parvovirus, feline panleukopenia virus). However, as a group, these viruses are very species specific: Other mammalian parvoviruses do not infect humans, and B19 does not infect other animals. The primary cellular target for B19 infection is an erythroid precursor near the pronormoblast stage. Viral replication within these cells results in cell lysis with progressive loss of these erythroid precursors. B19 infection leads to a temporary arrest of erythropoiesis with a loss of reticulocytes on the peripheral blood smear and red cell aplasia of the bone marrow. In an immunocompetent patient this is a transient effect and, assuming a normal red cell life span, it usually results in only a mild drop in serum hemoglobin that recovers without noticeable clinical effects. Because of this tropism for red cell precursors, this virus was placed in a genus separate from the other mammalian parvoviruses and is referred to as *Erythrovirus* B19 for purposes of taxonomic classification.

Infection with B19 is common and worldwide. The incidence of infection is highest among children from 5 to 15 years of age. Infections can continue to occur throughout life in seronegative individuals and are especially prevalent in adults who have contact with children either at home, in daycare, or at work (e.g., schoolteachers). B19 infections occur sporadically throughout the year with a seasonal peak in the late winter and early spring. Infection is transmitted primarily by contact with respiratory secretions and possibly through large droplet spread. The virus can be found in respiratory secretions during periods of viremia in experimental infection in humans.

Humoral immune responses appear to be of primary importance in controlling infection with B19. Experimental infection in normal volunteers is followed by a brisk viremia after a 6- to 8-day incubation period accompanied by mild, nonspecific symptoms. Disappearance of the virus from the blood corresponds with the appearance of B19-specific antibodies: Anti-B19 immunoglobulin (Ig) M appears first, followed by antiviral IgG, which is neutralizing and leads to clearance of the viremia. These IgG antibodies persist for life and are protective against reinfection. Individuals with

TABLE 1 Major Clinical Manifestations Associated with Parvovirus B19 Infection

Diseases	Primary Patient Groups
Diseases Associated with Acute Infection	
Erythema infectiosum (fifth disease)	Normal children
Polyarthropathy	Normal adolescents and adults
Transient aplastic crisis	Patients with hemolytic anemia or other condition of accelerated erythropoiesis
Papular-purpuric "gloves and socks" syndrome	Normal children and adults
Diseases Associated with Chronic Infection	
Persistent anemia (red cell aplasia)	Immunodeficient or immunocompromised children and adults
Nonimmune hydrops fetalis	Fetal infection (especially at <20 weeks' estimated gestational age)
Congenital anemia	Fetal infection

Adapted from Young NS, Brown KE: Parvovirus B19. N Engl J Med 350:588, 2004. Copyright 2004 Massachusetts Medical Society. All rights reserved. Adapted 2006 with permission.

defects in immunoglobulin production are at risk for persistent infection with B19.

Most infections with B19 are mild or asymptomatic and self-limited. The most common clinical manifestation of infection is erythema infectiosum (EI), or fifth disease, a benign rash illness of children. B19 causes a number of other clinically diverse syndromes in other patient groups (Table 1). Clinical manifestations of infection vary depending on the status of the host, and B19 can cause chronic infections in some. Infection in individuals with accelerated erythropoiesis or rapid red cell turnover leads to a transient red cell aplasia or transient aplastic crisis (TAC). First associated with the TAC of sickle cell disease, this is now described in most types of hemolytic anemia and a variety of other conditions that have an increased rate of red cell turnover. Infection in immunocompromised patients who are unable to generate adequate neutralizing antibody responses can lead to chronic infection, usually manifested as chronic anemia. Primary infection in a pregnant woman can result in fetal infection, leading to fetal hydrops, especially with infection during the first half of gestation. Other disease syndromes, such as EI or polyarthropathy of adults, become clinically evident after the period of viremia has passed and presumably are related to the immune response to infection.

The diagnosis of the most common manifestations of B19 infection usually does not require laboratory confirmation. EI is usually diagnosed based on recognition of the characteristic rash and a compatible history. The diagnosis of a typical transient aplastic crisis in a patient known to have sickle cell disease is based primarily on the hematologic profile and does not require virologic tests.

Serologic tests are available for the diagnosis of B19 infection when needed. Detection of B19 IgM is the best serologic marker of acute/recent infection on a single serum sample. B19-specific IgM is detectable within 1 to 2 days after symptoms develop and remains detectable for approximately 2 to 3 months. Anti-B19 IgG is detectable within a few days after the appearance of IgM and persists for life. In this regard, B19 IgG serves as a marker of past infection or immunity. Demonstration of B19 IgG in the absence of IgM, even in high titer,

is not diagnostic of recent infection. Seroconversion of B19 IgG from negative to positive on paired sera can also be used to confirm recent infection.

In immunodeficient or immunosuppressed patients whose ability to make specific antibody responses is impaired, serologic diagnosis is unreliable. These patients are unable to generate a neutralizing antibody response and so can develop a chronic infection with a persistent viremia. Diagnosis of B19 infection in these patients requires methods to detect viral particles or viral DNA, such as nucleic acid hybridization or polymerase chain reaction (PCR). Viral culture is not useful because B19 does not grow in standard cell cultures. Virus can be also be detected by PCR in the blood of patients with TAC prior to the development of specific antibodies, in umbilical cord blood and amniotic fluid of infected fetuses, and at low levels in the blood of some normal individuals for months after infection.

Expert Opinion on Management Issues

No specific antiviral agent is available for B19 infections and rarely would one be needed. Children with a rash typical of EI do not require specific therapy because all should recover uneventfully. Likewise, polyarthropathy in normal adults is self-limited and does not lead to joint destruction. Symptomatic therapy with nonsteroidal anti-inflammatory drugs (NSAIDs) may be helpful. Symptoms should resolve within 2 to 4 weeks for most patients, although in rare cases they may persist for months and be confused with the onset of other forms of chronic arthritis.

Patients with a transient aplastic crisis or red cell aplasia are generally ill when they present with fever, pallor, tachycardia, and signs of high-output heart failure. Rash is rare. Most require hospitalization and supportive care with red blood cell (RBC) transfusion and intravenous fluids until stable.

Infections in immunocompromised patients may respond to treatment with intravenous immunoglobulin (IVIG). In such patients, the virus can be demonstrated in the serum by PCR or other methods, and measurable

12

B19-specific IgG is lacking. Most commercial lots of IVIG contain levels of anti-B19 IgG sufficient to neutralize the circulating virus and allow for viral clearance. Treatment usually leads to improvement of symptoms (usually increased reticulocyte counts and serum hemoglobin) and improvement or resolution of viremia. Doses reported with good outcomes include 400 mg/kg/day for 5 to 10 days or 1 g/kg/day for 3 days. In patients in whom the immune system is not likely to recover (e.g., those with AIDS, congenital immunodeficiency syndromes, etc.), periodic reinfusions may be necessary. However, IVIG may not always be necessary. In patients undergoing cytotoxic chemotherapy for malignancies, cessation of the immunosuppressive therapy alone may result in the development of neutralizing antibodies and subsequent clearance of viremia leading to resolution of the anemia. In patients with HIV/AIDS, clearance of B19 infection is reported with immune reconstitution after initiation of highly active antiretroviral therapy (HAART).

Pregnant women with B19-induced fetal hydrops diagnosed intrauterinely are treated with intrauterine blood transfusions with reported success. However, there are attendant risks to this sort of procedure. Also, fetal hydrops, although associated with a high mortality, is not uniformly fatal and may resolve prior to delivery. Treatment of such women with intrauterine transfusion or IVIG cannot be routinely recommended until prospective studies are done. Recommendations for the management of pregnant women diagnosed with a primary B19 infection are published in the obstetric literature.

IVIG should not be given as treatment for B19-associated polyarthropathy because no studies support its use. In fact, immunocompromised patients treated with IVIG for chronic anemia secondary to chronic B19 infection are reported to develop other immune-mediated symptoms of B19 infection like arthritis and rash. Treatment with IVIG is reported for a variety of other conditions associated with B19 infections. Such treatment is controversial because the relationship between the virus and these conditions is not definitively established.

No vaccine is currently licensed. A recombinant viral capsid vaccine is being studied in phase I trials. No published studies support postexposure prophylaxis with IVIG in immunocompromised children or pregnant women.

Common Pitfalls

The most common pitfall of care is in making an accurate diagnosis of acute B19 infection. B19-specific IgM develops within a few days of viremia and lasts for up to 2 to 3 months; demonstration of B19 IgM in serum is the best serologic marker of acute/recent infection. Development of B19 IgG occurs within a week but remains positive for life. Many kits are available commercially to test for B19 antibodies, but they use various antigens and their sensitivity and specificity varies, especially IgM tests.

For immunocompromised patients at risk for chronic infection, demonstration of the viral genome is necessary because these patients are not able to make appropriate antibody responses. B19 DNA can be detected with PCR or DNA hybridization, methods that are not routinely available and may require sending specimens to a reference laboratory. Because low levels of B19 DNA can be detected in the blood of normal patients for a period of time after a resolved infection, this may cause some diagnostic confusion. It may be necessary to find a laboratory that employs a quantitative method of PCR. Giving IVIG to patients with aplastic anemia or other hematologic conditions suspected to be caused by B19 based on equivocal IgM results or low-level PCR positivity is costly and risks masking other findings and ultimately delaying diagnosis of other conditions.

Communication and Counseling

The majority of B19 infections are mild or asymptomatic, and most patients recover without difficulty and without need for treatment. For children with EI, exclusion from school is not beneficial because they are beyond the period of infectivity. Immunity gained following infection appears to be durable and lifelong, so immunologically normal patients are not expected to have another infection with B19. This is true for patients with TAC because it is usually a unique event. The polyarthropathy associated with B19 does not lead to permanent erosive damage in the affected joints.

The risks of infection during the first half of pregnancy have been described. Pregnant women (or those attempting pregnancy) who are exposed to children with EI at home or at work should be referred to their health care provider for counseling regarding their risk and further studies and monitoring of the pregnancy. B19 infection is not teratogenic.

SUGGESTED READINGS

1. Adler SP, Harger JH, Koch WC: Parvovirus. In Faro F, Soper DE (eds): Infectious Diseases in Women. Philadelphia: WB Saunders, 2001, pp 100–115. **A thorough review of infection in pregnancy and management options.**
2. American Academy of Pediatrics: Parvovirus B19. In Pickering LK (ed): Red Book: Report of the Committee on Infectious Diseases, 26th ed. Elk Grove Village, Ill: American Academy of Pediatrics, 2003, pp 459–461. **AAP recommendations for control of B19 infection in various settings.**
3. Anderson LJ: Treatment prevention of human parvovirus B19 disease. In Anderson LJ, Young NS (eds): Human Parvovirus B19. Basel: Karger, 1997, pp 137–144. **Discussion of potential treatment and preventive measures.**
4. Ballou WR, Reed JL, Noble W, et al: Safety and immunogenicity of a recombinant parvovirus B19 vaccine formulated with MF59C.1. J Infect Dis 187(4):675–678, 2003. **Report of a phase I B19 vaccine trial in humans.**
5. Frickhofen N, Abkowitz JL, Safford M, et al: Persistent B19 parvovirus infection in patients infected with human immunodeficiency virus type 1 (HIV–1): A treatable cause of anemia in AIDS. Ann Intern Med 113:926–933, 1990. **Case reports that describe treatment and response.**
6. Heegaard ED, Brown KE: Human parvovirus B19. Clin Microbiol Rev 15:485–505, 2002. **Detailed review of the microbiology of the virus.**
7. Koch WC: Fifth (human parvovirus) and sixth (herpesvirus 6) diseases. Curr Opin Infect Dis 14:343–356, 2001. **Review**

including discussion of reported unusual manifestations of infection.

8. Koch WC, Massey G, Russell EC, et al: Manifestations and treatment of human parvovirus B19 infection in immunocompromised patients. J Pediatr 116:355–359, 1990. **Clinical cases emphasizing varied presentations in immunocompromised patients and response to therapy.**

9. Smith PT, Landry ML, Carey H, et al: Papular-purpuric gloves and socks syndrome associated with acute parvovirus B19 infection: Case report and review. Clin Infect Dis 27:164–168, 1998. **Illustrative case report with a review of the syndrome.**

10. Young NS, Brown KE: Parvovirus B19. N Engl J Med 350:586–597, 2004. **Recent review of the virus with an emphasis on mechanisms of disease, including section on treatment.**

Respiratory Syncytial Virus

Maria-Arantxa Horga and Anne Moscona

KEY CONCEPTS

- Respiratory syncytial virus (RSV) is the leading cause of lower respiratory tract infection (LRTI) in young children.
- One hundred percent are infected at least once by 3 years of age.
- Clinical presentation ranges from upper respiratory tract infection (URTI) to LRTI.
- Predisposing factors for enhanced disease include prematurity, young age, cardiopulmonary disease, immunodeficiency, metabolic disease, and some neuromuscular disorders.
- Diagnosis is done with viral culture and rapid antigen detection methods (DFA [direct fluorescent antibody], ELISA [enzyme-linked immunoabsorbent assay]); PCR (polymerase chain reaction) in the future.
- Management of RSV infection is supportive and symptomatic for most children, to ensure adequate oxygenation and hydration; severe illness requires hospitalization.
- A trial of bronchodilator therapy early in the course of disease may be beneficial.
- Corticosteroids should be considered in infants who have underlying chronic lung disease or prior wheezing episodes.
- Ribavirin, currently the only antiviral agent available for the treatment of RSV, is of very limited use and should only be considered in certain settings.
- RSV vaccines are under development but not currently available.
- Passive immunoprophylaxis with an RSV antibody preparation (palivizumab [Synagis]) protects children at high risk for severe RSV disease.
- Immunoprophylaxis should be considered for children at risk for severe RSV infection: infants and young children with bronchopulmonary dysplasia, prematurity, and hemodynamically significant congenital heart disease.
- Infection-control practices are critical for preventing nosocomial spread of RSV.

Respiratory syncytial virus (RSV) is the leading cause of acute lower respiratory tract infection (LRTI) in young children and was recently recognized as an important pathogen in adults and immunocompromised patients as well. Management of RSV infections poses an important economic burden in the United States, accounting for more than 120,000 inpatient admissions each year. RSV is responsible for as much as 25% of excess wintertime mortality, previously attributed to influenza.

RSV outbreaks occur in a distinctive seasonal pattern. In temperate climates, the RSV season begins in late fall and continues until midspring, with a winter peak between January and March. Each community is affected every year, and the attack rate in young children is high: 50% of children in their first year of life are infected with RSV in their first winter season, and by 3 years of age, almost 100% of children are infected at least once. Primary infection is generally symptomatic, ranging from mild upper respiratory tract infection (URTI) to severe LRTI. RSV causes repeated infections throughout an individual's lifetime, with an annual risk rate close to 20%. Primary infection fails to establish permanent immunologic memory but leads to cumulative partial immunity with decreased severity of the clinical manifestations in older children and adults.

The clinical presentation of RSV infection generally begins with upper respiratory symptoms, such as nasal discharge, pharyngitis, and cough. Fever is common during the first 4 days of illness. Progression to the lower respiratory tract causes bronchiolitis and pneumonia in 30% to 70% of young children after primary exposure, with wheezing and rales on physical examination. Younger and premature infants can present with apnea. As the illness progresses, dyspnea and hypoxemia may develop, and some children progress to severe respiratory failure. In severe disease, radiograph findings are consistent with hyperinflation and diffuse interstitial pneumonitis. Risk factors predisposing to serious disease include underlying medical conditions, such as prematurity, cardiopulmonary disease, immunodeficiency, metabolic disease, and some neuromuscular disorders. However, most patients presenting with RSV bronchiolitis are normal full-term infants in the first 3 months of life, and pediatricians are posed with the challenge of evaluating and predicting the need for hospitalization and further therapy in this population (Box 1).

The diagnosis of RSV infection is made by isolating the virus in tissue culture or identifying the virus in

---

BOX 1 **Indications to Hospitalize Respiratory Syncytial Virus Infection Patient**

- Toxic appearance, poor feeding, lethargy, and dehydration
- Moderate to severe respiratory distress, as indicated by one or more of the following signs: nasal flaring, intercostal retraction, tachypnea and/or dyspnea, cyanosis
- Hypoxemia (oxygen saturation <95% on room air) with or without hypercapnia (arterial carbon dioxide tension >45 mm Hg)
- Atelectasis or consolidation on chest radiograph
- Parents unable to care for the child at home

respiratory tract secretions. Nasopharyngeal (NP) secretions are a good source of diagnostic material, even if the disease appears to be limited to the lower respiratory tract. Rapid identification of RSV antigen can be achieved using commercially available kits for rapid screening that have on average a sensitivity and specificity of 80% to 90%. These tests are performed directly in NP secretions by either using fluorescent-conjugated antibody (RSV DFA [direct fluorescent antibody]) or by enzyme-linked immunosorbent assay (ELISA) with a monoclonal antibody. Multiplex quantitative reverse transcription-PCR (polymerase chain reaction)-enzyme hybridization assay can identify a panel of respiratory viruses and differentiate between RSV viral subtypes A and B. PCR-based technology may provide a useful contribution to diagnosis and subtyping of RSV in the future.

Expert Opinion on Management Issues

SUPPORTIVE THERAPY

For most infants, management of RSV infection is supportive and symptomatic, with the goal of ensuring adequate oxygenation and hydration. Assessment of the risk for progression to severe disease must include the presence of underlying conditions, the overall clinical status of the child, and importantly the measurement of oxygen saturation, which, if found to be less than 95% by pulse oximetry, is a reliable objective predictor of progression to severe disease. Children with severe disease may require hospitalization, and although there are no established criteria, a number of useful published guidelines are available (see Box 1).

BRONCHODILATORS

The use of α- and β-adrenergic agonists to prevent hypoxemia and to maintain airway patency remains controversial. Taken together, the evidence from large randomized trials and meta-analyses does not suggest a benefit from bronchodilator therapy in infants with bronchiolitis. However, the individual response to these therapies is variable, with approximately half of infants responding to inhaled β-agonists, and their use may be assessed in each individual case. It is now recognized that a subset of patients may benefit more and improve when bronchodilator therapy is given early in the course of their disease. Because there is little toxicity from therapy, most experts recommend a trial of inhaled (nebulized) bronchodilators if bronchospasm is clinically apparent, with discontinuation of therapy if clinical improvement is not rapid.

ANTI-INFLAMMATORY DRUGS

RSV disease is the result of a balance between cellular damage mediated by the viral pathogen and injury caused by the immune response of the host. Because of this element of inflammation, corticosteroids were considered and studied for the treatment of RSV acute respiratory infection, but to date whether they provide benefit in different subgroups of children with bronchiolitis is uncertain. Most studies that evaluated the effect of systemic corticosteroids in hospitalized healthy infants showed no significant benefit in terms of length of stay, although there was some trend toward benefit; however, some studies showed more of a benefit if corticosteroids were administered early in the course of illness. Although routine corticosteroid use is not recommended in healthy infants hospitalized with a first episode of mild to moderate bronchiolitis, corticosteroids should be considered in infants who have underlying chronic lung disease and in those with prior wheezing episodes. In those cases, a short course of prednisolone or prednisone (1 to 2 mg/kg/day in one dose or divided into two doses per day for 3 to 7 days) may be given. In addition to corticosteroids, the use of other anti-inflammatory compounds such as NSAIDs (nonsteroidal anti-inflammatory drugs) is currently under investigation.

ANTIVIRALS

The role of antivirals in the treatment of RSV infection remains uncertain because some studies fail to show a correlation between viral load and disease severity, whereas others suggest that reduced viral levels correlate with improved clinical outcomes. These findings are not surprising in view of the significant role that proinflammatory responses play in the pathogenesis of this virus. Data obtained from animal models and human subjects indicate that antivirals should be used very early in the course of the disease to be effective.

Ribavirin is currently the only antiviral agent available for the treatment of children with RSV lower respiratory tract disease. Although ribavirin is a nucleoside analogue that has good activity against RSV in vitro, clinical studies examining its effect in children are conflicting. In addition, ribavirin is expensive, hard to administer, and must be given at very early time points during the course of the disease to have any significant benefit. As a result, its use in children remains highly controversial, and it should only be considered for certain target populations. The Committee on Infectious Diseases of the American Academy of Pediatrics (AAP) reassessed indications for ribavirin therapy and recommended that decisions regarding the use of ribavirin administration should be made on the basis of particular clinical circumstances (e.g., underlying congenital heart disease, lung disease, immunosuppression, need for mechanical ventilation) and physicians' experience (Box 2).

Studies in RSV-infected lung transplant recipients suggest that combined ribavirin with intravenous immunoglobulin (IVIG) and steroids can reduce mortality, length of mechanical ventilation, and incidence of bronchiolitis obliterans. Although combined ribavirin and intravenous immunoglobulin is not supported by a prospective, randomized study, this treatment is now used regularly.

BOX 2 High-Risk Groups for Severe Respiratory Syncytial Virus Disease

Ribavirin therapy should be considered in the following groups of patients:

- Complicated congenital heart disease (including pulmonary hypertension)
- Chronic lung disease (cystic fibrosis, bronchopulmonary dysplasia)
- Premature infants (<37 weeks' gestational age) and infants younger than 6 weeks
- Underlying immunosuppressive disease or therapy (AIDS, severe combined immunodeficiency syndrome, transplant recipients)
- Severely ill infants with or without mechanical ventilation
- Hospitalized patients at high risk for progression to severe disease because of age (<6 weeks), or underlying condition such as multiple congenital anomalies and some neurologic or metabolic diseases (cerebral palsy, myasthenia gravis)

Ribavirin is administered as an aerosol. The recommended treatment regimen is to administer the drug at 20 mg/mL for 12 to 18 hours a day. An alternative intermittent regimen of 60 mg/mL for 2 hours a day three times daily was well tolerated, showing similar efficacy. The suggested length of treatment is 3 to 7 days, which may vary according to the clinical response. The aerosol can be delivered to mechanically ventilated infants through an endotracheal tube or to nonmechanically ventilated infants using an infant oxygen hood, face mask, or oxygen tent. Bronchospasm and sudden worsening of the pulmonary and cardiovascular function are documented during ribavirin administration.

Ribavirin is a category X drug and contraindicated during pregnancy and lactation. Health care personnel should be informed, and unnecessary occupational exposure should be avoided.

Several new antivirals against RSV are currently being investigated, including Chinese herbal extracts, F protein fusion inhibitors, and benzimidazoles. In addition, novel experimental approaches to inhibit RSV replication include the use of antisense oligonucleotides and RNA interference (iRNA) technology. These approaches, although promising, are still in relatively early stages of development.

ANTIBODY PREPARATIONS AS THERAPY

The use of IVIG with a high neutralizing activity against RSV (RSVIG) and monoclonal antibody are not beneficial in the treatment of RSV in hospitalized infants and young children. RSVIG has been discontinued. Studies using an RSV-specific humanized monoclonal antibody (palivizumab, effective in prophylaxis and discussed in detail later) also failed to improve outcome when used as therapy.

PREVENTION: ACTIVE IMMUNIZATION

RSV vaccine development was hampered in the past by several factors:

- Severe disease occurs in young infants, whose responses to vaccines are diminished by passively acquired maternal antibody and relative immunologic immaturity.
- Natural infection does not protect against reinfection with RSV.
- Early experiences with a formalin-inactivated RSV vaccine resulted in enhanced disease.

However, given the observation that the severity of LRTI decreases with repeated infections, the impetus for developing an RSV vaccine is strong.

At present, several approaches to RSV vaccination are under evaluation. Of the various approaches evaluated in animal models, two demonstrated promise in clinical trials: purified F protein (PFP) subunit vaccines and live attenuated vaccines. Live attenuated vaccines pose the challenge of finding a balance between underattenuation (and subsequent induction of inefficient immunologic responses) or overattenuation, which may result in disease, especially in the younger infants. Live cold-passaged (cp), temperature-sensitive (ts) RSV vaccines (called cpts vaccines) containing many attenuating mutations are currently attractive candidates for live attenuated RSV vaccines. One such cpts, the 248/404 vaccine candidate, was safe and immunogenic in RSV-seronegative infants as young as 6 months. However, this candidate was not sufficiently attenuated in 4- to 12-week-old infants, and newer cpts vaccine candidates are currently under development.

Subunit vaccines, although not viable for infants and therefore of limited use in the normal population, may provide a suitable approach to vaccination in immunosuppressed populations at high risk of severe RSV infection, although at present these vaccines are only being evaluated in seropositive children. One of the viral surface glycoproteins, the fusion protein (F), was used as the antigen for development of subunit vaccines (PFP–1, PFP–2, and PFP–3). These vaccines are moderately immunogenic and well tolerated in healthy seropositive children older than 12 months, children older than 12 months with cystic fibrosis, and children older than 12 months with chronic lung disease of prematurity. A meta-analysis of studies on PFP–1 and PFP–2 studies suggested these vaccines reduce the incidence of RSV infections but not of LRTI. Further studies are required to evaluate these vaccines in specific target populations. Other potential vaccine candidates currently under development include subunit vaccines containing other viral proteins including G and M.

PREVENTION: IMMUNOPROPHYLAXIS

Until effective vaccines for RSV are widely available, passive immunoprophylaxis with RSV antibody preparations can protect children at high risk for severe RSV disease. A humanized monoclonal antibody (palivizumab (Synagis, MedImmune, Gaithersburg, Md) directed against the RSV fusion protein affords moderate protection to premature infants who are at high risk for severe RSV disease. This preparation cuts the risk of hospitalization by 41%, the length of hospital

---

BOX 3 AAP Recommendations for Severe Respiratory Syncytial Virus Immunoprophylaxis Using Palivizumab

Patients with congenital heart disease most likely to benefit from RSV immunoprophylaxis:
- Infants receiving medication to control heart failure
- Infants with moderate to severe pulmonary hypertension
- Infants with cyanotic heart disease

Not indicated for:
- Infants with hemodynamically insignificant heart disease
- Infants with lesions adequately corrected by surgery who do not require ongoing medications
- Infants with mild cardiomyopathy not receiving medical therapy

AAP, American Academy of Pediatrics.

BOX 4 Respiratory Syncytial Virus Prevention Strategies

- Frequent hand washing
- Isolation from contacts with respiratory infection
- Avoidance of secondary smoke, daycare, crowds, and siblings during RSV season
- Cohorting of hospitalized patients with RSV
- Prophylaxis with palivizumab for high-risk patients

---

admission by 53%, and the length of intensive care stay by 44%. Palivizumab is given monthly as a single intramuscular injection of 15 mg/kg once a month during the RSV season; duration of therapy and indications for prophylaxis depend on gestational age and presence or absence of chronic lung disease (Box 3).

The AAP recommends that immunoprophylaxis be considered for the groups of children who are at risk for severe RSV infection. These include infants and young children with bronchopulmonary dysplasia, prematurity, and hemodynamically significant congenital heart disease. In addition to these conditions, other factors that may influence the decision to administer immunoprophylaxis include the presence of other conditions that predispose to respiratory illness (e.g., neurologic disease), distance to and availability of hospital care for severe respiratory illness, logistical difficulties of monthly administration, and cost. Administration in the home setting may increase adherence to the schedule and should be encouraged.

If immunoprophylaxis is given, it should continue throughout the RSV season, even after the infant becomes old enough that prophylaxis is no longer indicated. Immunoprophylaxis also should continue even if the infant experiences an RSV infection. High-risk infants may be hospitalized more than once during an RSV season and different RSV strains may co-circulate in a community. Palivizumab does not interfere with immunizations.

In October 2003, MedImmune submitted an investigational new drug application to the FDA to evaluate MEDI–524 (Numax), another monoclonal antibody that may be 20 times more active than palivizumab. This antibody is currently in two phase III clinical studies that began in November 2004. Similar approaches using other monoclonal antibodies are in different stages of clinical development.

PREVENTION: INFECTION CONTROL

Nosocomial spread of RSV in the hospital setting is a serious problem because the virus can spread rapidly in the hospital environment, despite routine infection control procedures. Infection can also occur through contact with large droplet aerosols or fomites. The virus can survive on fomites, such as countertops or diaper-changing stations, for 4 to 7 hours, and the survival time in humid environments can exceed 24 hours. As many as 40% of hospitalized children may become infected during an RSV outbreak. In the hospital setting, these features of RSV mandate that strict isolation (gown, glove, mask) and rigorous hand-washing precautions be enforced until the child has stopped shedding RSV from the respiratory tract as documented by culture or by rapid antigen study. Additional important measures include education of caregivers and cohorting of infected patients when practical to prevent nosocomial transmission (Box 4).

Common Pitfalls

The most common pitfall is failure to observe proper infection control practices and resultant nosocomial infection with disease in children who cannot afford this complication. Because observation of the recommended procedures is highly effective at preventing nosocomial infection, this pitfall should be avoidable in many settings. Another pitfall is failure to administer appropriate prophylaxis to susceptible infants. Because the benefit of passive immunoprophylaxis (currently with pavlizumab) in the vulnerable population is now well established, every effort needs to be made to increase awareness of and adherence to the recommendations.

Communication and Counseling

Most infants and children with RSV infection recover uneventfully; however, the contribution of these infections to subsequent development of reactive airway disease in susceptible children remains unknown. This interaction between viral infection and subsequent airway disease is an area of active investigation. To avoid the pitfalls just described, education of health care workers and caregivers in infection control measures is of foremost importance. Instructions on isolation and rigorous hand washing require frequent reinforcement to be effective.

SUGGESTED READINGS

1. American Academy of Pediatrics Committee on Infectious Diseases and Committee of Fetus and Newborn: Prevention of respiratory syncytial virus infections: Indications for the use of

palivizumab and update on the use of RSV-IGIV. Pediatrics 102:1211–1216, 1998. **Provides the rationale, discussion, and recommendations for the use of passive immunoprophylaxis.**

2. American Academy of Pediatrics: In Respiratory syncytial virus. Pickering LK (ed): Red Book 2003: The Report of the Committee on Infectious Diseases, 26th ed. Elk Grove Village, Ill: American Academy of Pediatrics, 2003, pp 523. **Details the suggested uses of ribavirin in RSV infection.**

3. Maggon K, Barik S: New drugs and treatment for respiratory syncytial virus. Rev Med Virol 14:149–168, 2004. **Excellent summary of the state of the art for antivirals and other developments in therapy for RSV.**

4. Polack FP, Karron RA: The future of respiratory syncytial virus vaccine development. Pediatr Infect Dis J 23:S65–S73, 2004. **Review and discussion of the state of the art in RSV vaccine development.**

5. Puppe W, Weigl JA, Aron G, et al: Evaluation of a multiplex reverse transcriptase PCR ELISA for the detection of nine respiratory tract pathogens. J Clin Virol 30(2):165–174, 2004. **Discusses a diagnostic modality that will likely be very useful for rapid diagnosis of RSV and other respiratory infections.**

6. Revised indications for the use of palivizumab and respiratory syncytial virus immune globulin intravenous for the prevention of respiratory syncytial virus infections. Pediatrics 112(6 Pt 1):1442–1446, 2003. **Presents the modifications to the original recommendations for the use of passive immunoprophylaxis.**

7. Saez-Llorens X, Moreno MT, Ramilo O, et al: Safety and pharmacokinetics of palivizumab therapy in children hospitalized with respiratory syncytial virus infection. Pediatr Infect Dis J 23 (8):707–712, 2004. **Details the outcome of efforts to use monoclonal antibody preparations to treat ill inpatients.**

8. Schmidt AC, Johnson TR, Openshaw PJM, et al: Respiratory syncytial virus other pneumoviruses: A review of the international symposium—RSV 2003. Virus Research 106:1–13, 2004. **Key paper on recent developments in treatment, including efforts to combine antivirals with antibody treatment.**

9. Thompson WW, Shay DK, Weintraub E, et al: Mortality associated with influenza and respiratory syncytial virus in the United States. JAMA 289(2):179–186, 2003. **Report that raises awareness of the impact of RSV and influenza on morality in children in the United States.**

Rotavirus Infections

David I. Bernstein

KEY CONCEPTS

- Oral rehydration therapy (ORT) with oral rehydration solutions is the mainstay of treatment of mild to moderate and many cases of severe dehydration (those who can take oral fluids).
- Intravenous therapy may be indicated for the more severe cases, especially if the child is obtunded.
- Therapy with so-called clear fluids, such as fruit juices, tea, carbonated beverages, or homemade solutions, is not appropriate.
- Continuation of breast-feeding and rapid return to a regular diet improves recovery.
- Antibiotics and antimotility and antisecretory agents are not indicated for children.

Rotaviruses are the most common cause of severe infantile gastroenteritis around the world. In the United States, rotavirus infections account for approximately 50,000 hospitalizations and 500,000 office visits; worldwide more than 500,000 deaths annually are attributed to rotavirus. Direct medical costs in the United States are an estimated $100 to $400 million annually; indirect costs may be as high as $1 billion. Transmission of rotavirus is by the fecal–oral route and occurs in almost all children worldwide by 3 to 5 years of age. Infection is most common in children 6 to 24 months of age but can occur earlier, especially in poorer countries, and it is also responsible for a small percentage of adult gastroenteritis. In temperate climates, the disease is most common in the winter and fall. An unexplained pattern of disease in North America occurs annually, with infections beginning in Mexico and the southwest United States in mid to late fall and traveling across the continent to end in the Northeast in the spring.

Typical symptoms, which can be mild or severe, include diarrhea, vomiting, and fever that progress rapidly to dehydration. Compared to other viral causes of gastroenteritis, rotavirus infections are more severe and more often lead to dehydration and hospitalization.

No specific antiviral therapies are available for treatment, and thus therapy relies on correction of the fluid deficit with oral rehydration or, more rarely, intravenous (IV) therapy. Because of the associated morbidity and mortality and the lack of specific therapies for these infections, rotavirus is a leading target for vaccine development. Unfortunately, the first licensed rotavirus vaccine, RotaShield, was withdrawn from the market because of an association with intussusception. Two other vaccines, however, may be licensed within the next 2 to 3 years.

Potential Complications

Rotavirus infection is associated with several other clinical manifestations, including viremia and systemic spread, encephalitis and meningitis, various upper and lower respiratory tract infections, hepatitis, neonatal necrotizing enterocolitis, and perhaps intussusception.

Expert Opinion on Management Issues

Treatment of rotavirus gastroenteritis, and dehydration caused by gastroenteritis in general, is aimed first at restoration of the fluid deficit and then maintenance, which includes replacement of ongoing losses and resumption of adequate dietary intake. The mainstay of therapy is oral rehydration therapy (ORT) with glucose electrolyte solutions. The glucose in the solution enhances the absorption of sodium and water through the intestine. A variety of oral solutions are available in the United States and around the world and generally are similar to those proposed by the World Health Organization (WHO), but they differ substantially from other commonly used liquids (Table 1). A reduced osmolarity ORT was recommended and distributed by the WHO in 2002 (see Table 1).

Following an assessment of the level of dehydration, ORT is initiated to correct the deficit over a period of

12

TABLE 1 Composition of Commercial Oral Rehydration Solutions (ORS) and Commonly Consumed Beverages

Oral Rehydration	Carbohydrate (g/L)	Sodium (mmol/L)	Potassium (mmol/L)	Base* (mmol/L)	Osmolarity (mOsm/L)
Electrolyte Solution					
WHO (2002)	13.5	75	20	30	245
WHO (1975)	20	90	20	30	311
Enfalyte	30	50	25	34	200
Pedialyte	25	45	20	30	250
Rehydrate	25	75	20	30	305
CeraLyte	40	50–90	20	30	220
Commonly Used Beverages†					
Apple juice	120	0.4	44	N/A	730
Coca-Cola Classic	112	1.6	N/A	13.4	650

*Actual or potential bicarbonate (e.g., lactate, citrate, or acetate).
†Not appropriate for diarrhea treatment.
N/A, not available; WHO, World Health Organization.
Adapted from King CK, Glass R, Bresee JS, Duggan C: Centers for Disease Control and Prevention: Managing acute gastroenteritis among children: Oral rehydration, maintenance, and nutritional therapy. MMWR Recomm Rep 52:1–16, 2003.

approximately 4 hours. Current recommendations are to administer 50 to 100 mL of ORT per kg body weight. Following rehydration, regular diets can be resumed and supplemented with ORT to replace ongoing losses. Regular diets are the child's preferred, usual, and age-appropriate diet. They are generally more effective than restricted or progressive diets, and gut rest is not indicated. If the child is vomiting, feedings should be restricted to small amounts given more frequently.

If dehydration is more severe and especially if the child is obtunded, IV fluids are indicated. If IV access is not available, nasogastric administration of ORT should be considered. Lactated Ringer's solution, normal saline, or a similar solution should be administered (20 mL/kg body weight) until perfusion and mental status return to normal. Close observation is mandatory during this period. For patients with severe dehydration or suspected hypo- or hypernatremic dehydration, serum electrolytes, bicarbonate, blood urea nitrogen, creatinine, and glucose levels should be obtained. When the patient's level of consciousness returns to normal, ORT therapy can usually be initiated to correct the remaining deficits and replace the ongoing losses.

POTENTIAL THERAPIES (NOT CURRENTLY RECOMMENDED)

Other experimental approaches to treatment are also being evaluated. Trials suggesting beneficial effects using passive administration of oral immunoglobulins, probiotics, and bismuth subsalicylate have all been published. Racecadotril (acetorphan), an enkephalinase inhibitor with antisecretory and antidiarrheal properties, decreases stool output by approximately 50% in children with rotavirus infection.

PREVENTION

Trials of rotavirus vaccines began just 10 years after rotavirus was identified as the leading cause of gastroenteritis in children. Most vaccines have been live attenuated viruses administered orally to induce both local and systemic antibodies and protection. The vaccine licensed in 1998 contained four live attenuated rotaviruses; three viruses were reassortant, with 10 genes from a rhesus (monkey) rotavirus (RRV) and 1 gene (VP7) from three human strains, and one was RRV itself. This vaccine was effective but associated with intussusception and withdrawn from the market in 1999. This void may soon be filled by two other vaccines. A live attenuated oral vaccine based on reassortants between a bovine strain and human strains is finishing extensive evaluations in the United States and may be available from Merck & Co. within 1 to 2 years. It is expected this vaccine will not induce intussusception because bovine strains replicate less well than human or monkey strains in children and this vaccine is less likely to cause fever than the RRV-based vaccine.

The second oral vaccine, based on a single attenuated human strain, has undergone extensive evaluation in Latin America and indeed was approved for marketing in Mexico in June 2004. It is hoped that licensure in several other Latin American countries will follow within the year, followed by other countries in Europe, Asia, and Africa. Whether this vaccine will be available in the United States is unclear. It is expected this vaccine will not cause intussusception because most studies suggest that human rotaviruses do not do so, and this vaccine also induces less fever than the RRV-based vaccine. Whether the association of RRV-based vaccines and intussusception is unique to RRV is unclear, but this question should be resolved with the use of both new vaccines and postmarketing surveillance.

Common Pitfalls

- Use of clear liquids, juices, or other common beverages for treatment of diarrhea instead of oral rehydration solutions.

- Failure to return to regular diet as soon as possible
- Failure to use small-volume feedings if patient is vomiting
- Failure to instruct families to return if symptoms persist over several days or worsen significantly
- Use of antibiotics or antimotility drugs

Communication and Counseling

As discussed in the management section, careful explanation of the benefits of ORS compared to other commonly used beverages and the need to maintain breast-feeding and return to normal diet should be emphasized. The need for limited frequent volumes of ORS for those patients who are vomiting is also important. Parents should be encouraged to return if signs of more severe dehydration are seen or if symptoms continue or worsen over several days.

SUGGESTED READINGS

1. American Academy of Pediatrics, Provisional Committee on Quality Improvement, Subcommittee on Acute Gastroenteritis: Practice parameter: The management of acute gastroenteritis in young children. Pediatrics 97:424–435, 1996. **Excellent source for information on gastroenteritis and rehydration therapies.**
2. Bernstein DI, Sack DA, Rothstein E, et al: Efficacy of live, attenuated, human rotavirus vaccine 89–12 in infants: A randomised placebo-controlled trial. Lancet 354:287–290, 1999. **Evaluates the predecessor of one of the new potential rotavirus vaccines.**
3. Choice Study Group: Multicenter, randomized, double-blind clinical trial to evacuate the efficacy and safety of a reduced osmolarity oral rehydration salts solution in children with acute watery diarrhea. Pediatrics 107:613–618, 2001. **Compares reduced osmolarity oral rehydration to standard WHO solution.**
4. Clark HF, Bernstein DI, Dennehy PH, et al: Safety, efficacy, and immunogenicity of a live, quadrivalent human-bovine reassortant rotavirus vaccine in healthy infants. J Pediatr 144:184–190, 2004. **Evaluates predecessor of one of the new potential rotavirus vaccines.**
5. Cohen MB, Mezoff AG, Laney DW, et al: Use of a single solution for oral rehydration and maintenance therapy of infants with diarrhea and mild to moderate dehydration. Pediatrics 95:639–645, 1995. **Discusses the use of oral rehydration and return to regular diet.**
6. Fayad IM, Hashem M, Duggan C, et al: Comparative efficacy of rice-based and glucose-based oral rehydration salts plus early reintroduction of food. Lancet 342:772–775, 1991. **Discusses benefits of early return to regular diet.**
7. Figueroa-Quintanilla D, Salazar-Lindo E, Sack RB, et al: A controlled trial of bismuth subsalicylate in infants with acute watery diarrheal disease. N Engl J Med 328:653–658, 1993. **Provides evidence for potential therapy using bismuth subsalicylate.**
8. Guarino A, Canani RB, Russo, et al: Oral immunoglobulins for treatment of acute rotaviral gastroenteritis. Pediatrics 93:12–16, 1994. **Provides evidence for potential use of oral immunoglobulin for treatment.**
9. King CK, Glass R, Bresee JS, Duggan C; Centers for Disease Control Prevention: Managing acute gastroenteritis among children: Oral rehydration, maintenance, and nutritional therapy. MMWR Recomm Rep 52:1–16, 2003. **Excellent source for information on gastroenteritis and rehydration therapies.**
10. Nager AL, Wang VJ: Comparison of nasogastric and intravenous methods of rehydration in pediatric patients with acute dehydration. Pediatrics 109:566–572, 2002. **Supports use of nasogastric rehydration if IV not available.**
11. Peter G, Myers MG: National Vaccine Advisory Committee; National Vaccine Program Office. Intussusception rotavirus and oral vaccines: Summary of a workshop. Pediatrics 110:e67, 2002. **Summarizes our understanding of rotavirus vaccines and intussusception.**
12. Salazar-Lindo E, Santisteban-Ponce J, Chea-Woo E, Guiterrez M: Racecadotril in the treatment of acute watery diarrhea in children. N Engl J Med 343:463–467, 2000. **Provides evidence for potential therapy using racecadotril.**
13. Staat MA, Azimi PH, Berke T, et al: Clinical presentation of rotavirus infection among hospitalized children. Pediatr Infect Dis J 21:221–227, 2002. **Describes clinical signs and symptoms of hospitalized patients.**
14. Van Niel CW, Feudtner C, Garrison M, et al: *Lactobacillus* therapy for acute infectious diarrhea in children: A meta-analysis. Pediatrics 109:678–684, 2002. **Provides evidence for potential therapy using Lactobacillus.**

West Nile Virus

William Borkowsky

KEY CONCEPTS

- Symptomatic West Nile virus (WNV) disease occurs more commonly in the geriatric population and is rare in the pediatric population.
- Symptomatic disease is most often seen as aseptic meningitis with fever and headache, but it can also manifest as meningoencephalitis and, rarely, as facial palsy, other cranial neuropathies, or axonal neuropathy, such as Guillain-Barré syndrome. Non-CNS (central nervous system) syndromes involving heart, pancreas, and liver inflammation are seen rarely.
- Symptoms of WNV disease are indistinguishable from other causes of CNS disease, such as enteroviruses and other flavivirus (Japanese encephalitis virus, St. Louis encephalitis virus) causes.
- Most individuals with symptomatic disease improve with time, although residual deficits may persist for more than a year. Immunocompromised individuals are both more likely to demonstrate symptomatic disease and for that disease to result in death.

West Nile Virus (WNV) infection is a single-stranded, positive-sense, arthropod-borne (i.e., by *Culex* species) flavivirus disease that was first identified in a febrile adult from Uganda in 1937. It is endemic in Africa, with sporadic outbreaks in the Mideast (Israel in the 1950s and 1990s), Europe (France in the 1960s and Romania in the 1990s), South Africa (in the 1970s), and India (in the 1980s). WNV is closely related serologically to St. Louis encephalitis virus and by nucleic acid to Kunjin virus (previously known to cause encephalitis in Australia). Seroprevalence levels approach 40% in many regions of the world. There appear to be two lineages of WNV worldwide, one endemic to Africa that produces mild illness and another that is associated with worldwide distribution and can cause meningoencephalitis and other CNS syndromes. The latter lineage also causes significant death of bird species such as crows.

The virus infects birds, resulting in viral amplification to levels sufficiently high to allow its transmission to humans and other mammals such as horses. No human-to-human transmission is documented other than a single case of documented in utero transmission, a probable transmission via breast milk, and several instances of transfusion and solid organ transplantation infection in the recipients.

During 1999, WNV was introduced to North America, resulting in a cluster of patients with encephalitis. Subsequent seroepidemiologic studies revealed that approximately 80% of those infected were asymptomatic. Moreover, fewer than 1% of those infected developed CNS disease at all.

Expert Opinion on Management Issues

Supportive care should allow for spontaneous recovery in the majority of symptomatic individuals, particularly the pediatric population. Nonrandomized trials of ribavirin and interferon alfa have produced largely descriptive information without evidence of proven efficacy. Because CNS symptoms may mimic those of treatable neurotropic viruses, such as herpes simplex virus (HSV), it would be prudent to include such therapy (e.g., acyclovir) until a diagnosis of WNV is established. Hyperimmune plasma and γ-globulin are efficacious in the prevention and treatment of WNV-challenged mice in a dose- and time-dependent manner. In contrast, pooled plasma or intravenous immunoglobulin (IVIG) from individuals without high titers of antibody to WNV are ineffective.

In order to address whether antibody alone could treat WNV, congenic mice that were pure B-cell deficient or both B- and T-cell deficient were treated with polyclonal antibodies that reacted with WNV. Increased survival time and decreased mortality rate were seen in wild-type and B-cell deficient mice when given immune but not nonimmune immunoglobulin. Using immune mouse serum for prophylaxis, the investigators noted some protection of the B-cell deficient mice that waned with time. The protective effect in the B- and T-cell deficient mice was even shorter. Using the same serum for treatment of the B-cell deficient mice also increased survival time and decreased mortality even when given after infection was present. Moreover, it also prevented the seeding of virus to the brain. Anecdotal treatment of encephalitic immunocompromised humans suggests virologic suppression in one and clinical improvement in the other.

Common Pitfalls

- Do not omit treatment for "treatable" causes of encephalitis (e.g., HSV).
- Do not assume WNV infection is unlikely in dry climates because collections of water (e.g., swimming pools) are breeding grounds for mosquitoes.

Communication and Counseling

Parents need to be told that the best way to avoid dealing with WNV is to minimize contact with mosquitoes, using clothing cover and/or insect repellent. Areas of standing water need to be drained. It should be reinforced that children and adolescents are rarely affected with clinical CNS symptoms, despite serologic evidence of infection with WNV.

SUGGESTED READINGS

1. Ben-Nathan D, Lustig S, Tam G, et al: Prophylactic and therapeutic efficacy of human intravenous immunoglobulin in treating West Nile virus infection in mice. J Infect Dis 188(1):5–12, 2003. **Full protection was achieved when the infected mice were treated with pooled plasma or IVIG obtained from healthy Israeli blood donors that contained WNV-specific antibodies. These results indicate that antibodies play a major role in protection and recovery from WNV infection.**
2. Engle MJ, Diamond MS: Antibody prophylaxis and therapy against West Nile virus infection in wild-type and immunodeficient mice. J Virol 77(24):12941–12949, 2003. **This murine study suggests that although antibody suppresses viremia when given before and after viral challenge, T cells are important in clearing viremia after the antibody wanes.**
3. Haley M, Retter AS, et al: The role for intravenous immunoglobulin in the treatment of West Nile virus encephalitis. Clin Infect Dis 37(6):e88–e 90, 2003. **High-titer IVIG sterilized the cerebrospinal fluid of WNV in a patient with chronic lymphocytic leukemia.**
4. Hamdan A, Green P, et al: Possible benefit of intravenous immunoglobulin therapy in a lung transplant recipient with West Nile virus encephalitis. Transpl Infect Dis 4(3):160–162, 2002. **High-titered IVIG therapy of a lung-transplant recipient with serologically confirmed WNV encephalitis resulted in rapid improvement within 24 hours and complete disappearance of signs and symptoms within 48 hours.**

Human Papillomavirus

William Borkowsky

KEY CONCEPTS

- Fifty percent of women upon becoming sexually active contract a genital human papillomavirus (HPV) infection within 2 years.
- Genital warts fall into one of four phenotypes: classic condyloma acuminata, flat warts, papular warts, and keratotic warts.
- Anogenital warts are frequently diagnosed in children, and their incidence in prepubertal children is increasing. Modes of transmission of HPV to the anogenital area include perinatal, autoinoculation and heteroinoculation, sexual abuse, and possibly indirect transmission via fomites.
- The prevalence of HPV infection in pregnancy varies between 5.4% and 68.8%. The populations with the highest risk, also among pregnant women, are those younger than 26 years.

- Infrequently, children born to mothers with HPV infection associated with condyloma later develop laryngeal infection that may compromise their airway.
- Benign skin lesions associated with HPV (typically HPV 1–4) include common warts (verruca vulgaris), plantar warts, and flat warts.

Human papillomavirus (HPV) belongs to the family Papovaviridae, affecting a variety of species, although infections are species specific. The more than 100 types are distinguished by the differences in their DNA. All HPV target epithelial cells, both squamous and mucosal. Infection is most often painless and asymptomatic but also prone to malignant transformation. The DNA encodes nine genes with *early genes* and *late genes*. Two of the early genes, E6 and E7, produce proteins that bind and help degrade p53 and retinoblastoma (Rb) family proteins, respectively, resulting in a proliferative state. Another early gene, E5, enhances epidermal growth factor. Late genes L1 and L2 encode capsid proteins. Different HPV types are classified as low risk for malignancy (e.g., 6,11, 42, 43, 44) or high risk (e.g., 16, 18, 31, 33, 35, 45, 51, 52, 56, 58, 59). The early genes of the high-risk HPVs are more efficient in p53 and Rb binding than those from low-risk HPVs. Certain types of HPV cause selective infection of nongenital or anogenital infections, the latter further differentiated into those with proliferative or oncogenic potential. Other types are associated with genetic diseases (i.e., epidermodysplasia verruciformis [EV]) and immunocompromised hosts. Benign skin lesions associated with HPV (typically HPV 1–4) include common warts (verruca vulgaris), plantar warts, and flat warts.

HPV infection is the most common sexually transmitted disease in the world, resulting in an estimated 5.5 million cases of infection annually, and it accounts for an estimated 11% of the global cancer incidence in women. Fifty percent of women upon becoming sexually active contract a genital HPV infection within 2 years. The lifetime risk of contracting a genital HPV infection is estimated to be 80%, but very few of these women develop cervical cancer, which is linked with HPV infection in more than 90% of cases. As a result, HPV detection at a single moment is of limited clinical value in the triage of patients with abnormal cervical scrapes or during follow-up after treatment for carcinoma in situ. Sexual contacts of patients with genital warts should be evaluated for warts.

HPV-16 is the most prevalent type detected in cervical cancer. Along with types 18, 31, 33, and 45, it is labeled a class I carcinogen. In addition to cervical cancer, HPVs are also associated with the malignant transformation of other mucosal and skin cancers. HPV is implicated in the pathogenesis of 15% to 23% of head and neck squamous cell carcinomas as well as most oropharyngeal carcinomas. Thus the combination of the malignant potential of HPV and its high prevalence of infection confers to it an importance of generalized clinical and virologic significance.

Genital warts fall into one of four phenotypes: classic condyloma acuminata, pointed or coliform in shape; flat warts, seen on the cervix; papular warts, which are smooth; and keratotic warts, which have a thick, horny appearance. Anogenital condylomata acuminata are the most frequent clinical manifestation of genital HPV infection, affecting both women and men. Biopsy of warts involving the cervix are required to rule out invasive cervical cancer.

Anogenital warts are frequently diagnosed in children, and their incidence in prepubertal children is increasing. Modes of transmission of HPV to the anogenital area include perinatal, autoinoculation and heteroinoculation, sexual abuse, and possibly indirect transmission via fomites. Childhood sexual abuse was thought previously to be the most common mode of transmission, and HPV types 6 and 11 were most often detected. Recent studies suggest that perinatal infection and autoinoculation or heteroinoculation may be much more prevalent than originally thought. Spontaneous resolution is seen in more than 50% of cases over a 5-year observation period.

The prevalence of HPV infection in pregnancy varies between 5.4% and 68.8%. The populations with the highest risk, also among pregnant women, are those younger than 26 years. Infrequently, children born to mothers with HPV infection associated with condyloma later develop laryngeal infection that may compromise their airway.

The natural history of HPV infection with or without treatment varies from spontaneous regression to persistence. The most important mechanism for wart regression appears to be cell-mediated immunity. Cytokines released by keratinocytes or cells of the immune system may play a part in the induction of an effective immune response against HPV infection and the subsequent regression of lesions. Currently, cervical HPV DNA is detected by means of polymerase chain reaction (PCR) and sandwich capture molecular hybridization methods.

Epidermodysplasia verruciformis (EV), a rare genetic disease, is associated with HPV types not usually seen in those without defects in cell-mediated immunity. EV undergoes oncogenesis in a quarter to half of affected children, particularly in areas exposed to sunlight.

Expert Opinion on Management Issues

GENITAL WARTS

In 2002, the Centers for Disease Control and Prevention (CDC) issued guidelines for the treatment of sexually transmitted diseases. Box 1 shows therapies specific for HPV.

Treatment Methods

Podofilox (Condylox Gel; Oclassen Dermatologics, Carona, Calif) is an antimitotic compound, more purified than podophyllin. It results in local reactions such as erythema, swelling, and erosions in half of those

---

BOX 1   Treatment Recommendations for Genital Warts

Patient-Applied Therapies

- Podofilox 0.5% solution applied twice daily for 3 days, to cover a surface area not to exceed 10 cm² followed by a 4-day rest period; *or*
- Imiquimod cream, applied to lesions overnight, three times a week for up to 16 weeks.

Therapy Administered by Health Care Provider

- Surgical excision, cryotherapy with liquid nitrogen, podophyllin resin (10%–25%) in tincture of benzoin, bichloracetic acid (BCA) or trichloroacetic acid (TCA) (80%–90%).
- Alternative treatments include laser vaporization and intralesional interferon.

---

treated. Clearance rates range from 50% to 90%, with some relapsing to give a long-term clearance in 30% to 60% of those treated. Treatment with this compound is not recommended for pregnant women or for use in the vagina or anus.

Imiquimod is an immune modulator, resulting in increased local release of cytokines that include interferon, tumor necrosis factor, interleukin (IL)-2, IL-6, IL-8, and IL-12. It also increases anti-HPV cytolytic activity of the immune system. Complete responses range from 24% to 79%, with responses in women occurring twice as often as in men. Lesions shrink even in those not classified as a complete responder.

Podophyllin resin is neurotoxic and should not be used on mucosal surfaces because it may be absorbed. It should be dried after application and washed off after 6 hours. It results in erythema and pain within 48 hours. Clearance rates vary from 30% to 80%, with frequent relapses.

Bichloracetic/trichloroacetic acid (BCA/TCA) can be used on both keratinized and mucosal epithelial sites. It can be used in pregnancy. It results in a frosted lesion and may result in painful areas with significant erythema and swelling. Petrolatum or zinc can be used to protect the surrounding area from the caustic effects. Clearance rates as high as 80% can be seen after several applications.

Nitrous oxide and liquid nitrogen are used successfully for cryotherapy. The colder nitrous oxide is required for cervical lesions, whereas liquid nitrogen is adequate for vaginal or anal growths. Clearance rates up to 90% may be seen when treatment is administered weekly, with relapse rates approaching 40%. Cryotherapy is acceptable therapy in the pregnant woman.

Surgical excision with scalpel or cautery is probably the first-line treatment for very large lesions, particularly those causing obstruction of the vagina or anus. Clearance rates approach 70%, with relapses particularly at the surgical margins.

Laser vaporization with a carbon dioxide (CO₂) laser is more effective than electrocautery, with clearance rates that approach 90%, relapses again occurring at the margins of therapy. Laser therapy may be the treatment of choice for pregnant women.

Alternative Methods

Trials of topical interferon for mucosal lesions resulted in clearance rates of 40% to 90%, with minimal side effects. Systemic interferon (given intramuscularly or subcutaneously) results in no better outcome than other modalities, with significant influenza-like symptoms in the recipients. Intralesional interferon (interferon alfa-n3 is administered 0.05 mL per wart, twice weekly for up to 8 weeks; interferon alfa-2b is given in 0.1 mL injections per lesion three times a week for 3 weeks) resulted in clearance rates of 35% to 80%, with relapse rates approaching 20%. None of the interferons appear to be superior to the others, but all are quite expensive.

The antimetabolite 5-fluorouracil (5-FU) is used topically and intralesionally. Response rates are variable, with rates from 29% to 83%. Relapses occur in up to a third of the responders. Treatment with this modality can cause pain, erythema, ulcerations, and skin discoloration.

Cidofovir, a nucleotide analogue with activity against a host of DNA viruses, given as a 1% gel, is used for the therapy of warts that occur in the immunocompromised and are rather resistant to typical treatment modalities. Complete responses are seen in approximately 20%, with an additional 50% demonstrating reductions in lesion size.

Therapeutic vaccination to increase cell-mediated immune responses to HPV early and late antigens were performed on a small scale with some limited success. Additional trials with modified vaccines are in progress.

LARYNGEAL PAPILLOMA

HPV laryngeal infection typically involves types 6 and 11. A national registry, involving 600 patients from 22 tertiary-care pediatric centers has been established. The mean age of diagnosis was 4 years of age. Treatment of laryngeal papillomatosis was based on surgery, especially on CO₂ laser and shaver. Interferon alfa was the drug of choice in patients whose response to surgery was poor. However, neither interferon nor other antiviral drugs were able to eradicate the virus from laryngeal mucosa. Approximately 75% of treated children maintained stable disease over time, and only 18% had no evidence of disease for at least a year. Susceptibility to recurrent disease may be increased in those with HLA DRB1*0301 (present in half of patients). Most recently, cidofovir intralesional injections were studied in both children and adults. When given in multiple intervals, remissions were achieved in the majority of patients. However, complete remission was achieved in only 20% and 36% of juvenile-onset and adult-onset disease, respectively.

COMMON AND UNCOMMON SKIN WARTS

Spontaneous regression in immunocompetent individuals may occur in up to 70% of children over the course of 2 years. Consequently, treatment should be an option only in those with painful or disfiguring lesions. Treatment with keratolytic agents, such as salicylic acid, in a variety of solvents are usually effective. When nonprescription preparations fail, the periodic use of 25% TCA often succeeds. Liquid nitrogen cryotherapy or electrodesiccation with curettage is often painful but very effective when used on distal extremity lesions.

Newer Therapies

Oral cimetidine (30 to 40 mg/kg/day) is somewhat effective in treating multiple viral warts. It activates Th1 cells to produce IL-2 and IFN-γ, and their expression correlates with wart remission. EV treated with oral cimetidine (40 mg/kg/day) also shows a marked improvement after 3 months of therapy, with no relapse at a 6-month follow-up.

Imiquimod 5% cream applied twice a day by the patients or by their parents to therapy-resistant, long-lasting (2 to 7 years) common warts in children resulted in total clearance in 16 of 18 patients; 2 showed partial improvement. The mean duration of treatment was 5.8 months. Two of the 14 patients in whom a follow-up was performed showed a small number of new warts after a period of at least 1 year without recurrence.

Common Pitfalls

- Podophyllin resin is contraindicated in pregnancy and for use on mucosal surfaces, the vagina, and anus.
- Because 5-FU is a mutagen and teratogen, treatment should not be applied to those who are pregnant.
- Because of unacceptable side effects and superior alternatives, many therapies are now avoided. These include topical bacillus Calmette-Guérin (BCG), dinitrochlorobenzene, bleomycin, cantharidin, glutaraldehyde and formaldehyde, salicylic acid, monochloroacetic acid, diphencyprone, and squaric acid dibutylester.
- HPV DNA can be released in the smoke plumes of CO_2 lasers, possibly endangering the respiratory tract of the surgeon.

Communication and Counseling

External genital HPV disease is not necessarily caused by sexual activity. Such warts may resolve spontaneously or with self-applied treatments. Cervical HPV infection is caused by sexual activity. Most of these infections clear without intervention in the adolescent and young adult, but they need monitoring. Certain HPV strains have a predilection for causing premalignant and malignant conditions. These strains are different from the ones that cause genital warts. Repeated histologic evidence of atypical cells on Papanicolaou smear requires gynecologic intervention. Individuals with immunosuppression are particularly susceptible to advanced HPV disease.

Skin warts invariably go away, either spontaneously or with medical help. Warts that grow on the larynx are difficult to treat and typically require multiple treatments over months to years.

SUGGESTED READINGS

1. Berry JM, Palefsky JM: A review of human papillomavirus vaccines: From basic science to clinical trials. Front Biosci 8:s333–s345, 2003. **Reviews the various types of vaccines in development.**
2. Centers for Disease Control and Prevention: Sexually transmitteddiseases guidelines. MMWR Morb Mort Wkly Rep 51(RR-6): 53–57, 2002. **A good review of HPV and non-HPV treatment.**
3. Corona Gutierrez CM, Tinoco A, et al: Therapeutic vaccination with MVA E2 can eliminate precancerous lesions (CIN 1, CIN 2, and CIN 3) associated with infection by oncogenic human papillomavirus. Hum Gene Ther 15(5):421–431, 2004. **A recent example of the potential for therapeutic vaccination.**
4. Gelder CM, Williams OM, Hart KW, et al: HLA class II polymorphisms and susceptibility to recurrent respiratory papillomatosis. J Virol 77(3):1927–1939, 2003. **As in the case of most chronic infectious disease, genetic predispositions are identifiable.**
5. Koutsky LA, Ault KA, et al: A controlled trial of a human papillomavirus type 16 vaccine. N Engl J Med 347(21):1645–1651, 2002. **Excellent large-scale trial that gives a hint of the potential prophylactic efficacy of vaccination in patients 16 to 23 years of age.**
6. Naiman AN, Ceruse P, Coulombeau B, Froehlich P: Intralesional cidofovir and surgical excision for laryngeal papillomatosis. Laryngoscope 113:2174–2181, 2003. **Reports on the use of cidofovir in lesions that have resisted other forms of therapy.**
7. Woodman CB, Collins S, et al: Natural history of cervical human papillomavirus infection in young women: A longitudinal cohort study. Lancet 357(9271):1831–1836, 2001. **Excellent review of the natural history of cervical HPV infection.**
8. Wright TC Jr, Cox JT, Massad LS, et al: ASCCP-Sponsored Consensus Conference: 2001 consensus guidelines for the management of women with cervical cytologic abnormalities. JAMA 287 (16):2120–2129, 2002. **Offers potential management options as well as consensus opinion regarding the best options.**

12

Rubella

Gustavo H. Dayan, Susan E. Reef, and Walter A. Orenstein

KEY CONCEPTS

- Rubella is an exanthematous disease with an incubation period ranging from 14 to 21 days.
- The disease is spread by respiratory secretions, and a person is usually contagious from 7 days before to 5 to 7 days after rash onset.
- Rubella is usually a mild rash illness; however, when acquired during pregnancy, it may result in spontaneous abortions, fetal death, stillbirths, or congenital rubella syndrome (CRS), especially when infection occurs during the first trimester of pregnancy.
- The most common congenital defects associated with CRS are hearing impairment, cataracts, and heart defects.
- Vaccination is the most effective way to prevent rubella and CRS. Rubella vaccine is usually available combined in the mumps, measles, rubella vaccine (MMR). In the United States, two doses of MMR are recommended for

Continued

KEY CONCEPTS—cont'd

children, one at 12 to 15 months of age and the second at 4 to 6 years of age.
- Vaccination is also recommended for susceptible adults. Rubella immunity should be assured in women of childbearing age and adults more likely to be in contact with rubella cases, such as health care and child-care personnel.
- Rubella vaccine should not be given to pregnant women. However, if a pregnant woman is vaccinated inadvertently, termination of pregnancy is not recommended because the risk to the fetus appears to be extremely low, if it exists at all.

Rubella, also known as German measles, is an exanthematous disease caused by the rubella virus, a member of the togavirus family and the genus *Rubivirus*. Rubella is transmitted through direct contact or droplets shed from the respiratory secretions of infected persons. The disease is moderately contagious; an infected person may shed virus from 7 days before to 5 to 7 days after rash onset. The incubation period ranges from 14 to 21 days and is usually 16 to 18 days. Symptoms of rubella are often mild, and up to 50% of infections may be subclinical or inapparent. Infected persons may have a prodromal illness, which consists of low-grade fever, malaise, mild conjunctivitis, and lymphadenopathy, particularly occipital and postauricular. The maculopapular erythematous rash of rubella usually appears first on the face and the neck and then progresses from head to foot. The rash, which may be pruritic, usually lasts 1 to 3 days. Transient arthralgia or arthritis may occur in up to 70% of women with rubella; however, it is uncommon in children and men. Other rare complications are thrombocytopenic purpura, which occurs in approximately 1 per 3000 cases, and encephalitis, occurring in 1 per 5000 cases. In addition, orchitis, neuritis, and Guillain-Barré syndrome are rarely reported.

Although rubella is usually a mild rash illness, it may result in serious consequences when a pregnant woman becomes infected, particularly during the first trimester of pregnancy. Rubella infection during pregnancy can result in spontaneous abortion, fetal death, stillbirth, and a constellation of birth defects known as congenital rubella syndrome (CRS). Up to 85% of infants born to mothers infected with rubella virus during the first 10 weeks of gestation develop CRS. The most common congenital defects are hearing impairment; eye defects, such as cataracts, glaucoma, retinopathy, and microphthalmia; and heart defects, such as patent ductus arteriosus, peripheral pulmonic stenosis, and ventricular septal defect. Other manifestations include low birth weight, microcephaly, mental retardation, hepatosplenomegaly, purpura, and radiolucent bone disease. Delayed manifestations of CRS, such as diabetes mellitus or progressive encephalopathy, may appear later in childhood. Infants with CRS may shed virus from body secretions for up to 1 year.

Rubella is now rare in the United States (only 7 cases were reported in 2003), but it is common throughout the world. Failure to keep up high levels of population immunity through vaccination runs the risk of a return of endemic disease.

Live attenuated rubella vaccine was licensed for use in the United States in 1969. Since 1979, the RA 27/3 (grown in human diploid fibroblasts) is the only strain in use in the United States. An immune response to rubella is induced in 95% or more of vaccinees after a single dose administered at or after 12 months of age. More than 90% of vaccinated persons with one dose have long-term, probably lifelong, protection against rubella infection. Rubella vaccine is available as a single-antigen vaccine, combined with measles vaccine, or combined with mumps, measles, rubella vaccine (MMR). Two doses of MMR vaccine are recommended routinely in the United States, the first one at 12 to 15 months of age and the second dose at 4 to 6 years of age in accordance with the routine two-dose measles immunization schedule. The second dose may be administered before the recommended age if at least 4 weeks have elapsed since the first dose. Table 1 presents the indications and contraindications for rubella vaccine. Approximately 5% to 15% of susceptible children may develop fever 5 to 12 days after MMR vaccination. Rash can occur in 5% of MMR recipients, and lymphadenopathy can also occur. Arthralgia and transient arthritis are infrequent in vaccinated children; however, joint symptoms may occur in approximately 25% of postpubertal females. The onset is 1 to 3 weeks after

---

TABLE 1 Indications and Contraindications for Use of Rubella Vaccine

Indications

- Healthy children ≥12 mo of age, even if immunocompromised or pregnant susceptibles are in the household.
- Healthy susceptible adults. Vaccination should be emphasized in the following groups:
  - Postpubertal nonpregnant females. Postpartum vaccination is recommended if women are found susceptible during serologic prenatal screening.
  - Child-care personnel.
  - Health care personnel.
  - Military personnel.

Contraindications

- Severe allergic reaction following a prior dose of rubella vaccine or to a vaccine component (e.g., gelatin, neomycin).
- Pregnancy should be avoided for 4 wk after rubella vaccination.
- Immunodeficiency or immunosuppression.
- Cancer chemotherapy: Vaccination should be deferred until 3 mo after chemotherapy discontinuation.
- Corticosteroids: >2 mg/kg/day (or its equivalent) for ≥14 days. Vaccination should be deferred until 1 mo after therapy discontinuation.
- Human immunodeficiency virus (HIV) severely immunocompromised patients (i.e., low CD4+ T-lymphocyte counts or low percentage of total circulating lymphocytes).
- Receipt of antibody or blood products: Vaccine should be given 2 wk before or deferred for at least 3 mo following administration of an antibody-containing blood product. Vaccine may be given at the same time as anti-Rho; however, serologic test is recommended 6–8 wk after vaccination to ensure immune response.

vaccination, and symptoms may persist for 1 day to 3 weeks. Even though studies from one institution reported chronic arthropathy following rubella vaccination, other studies do not support a role for rubella vaccine in chronic joint disease. Other adverse events, such as polyneuropathy and carpal tunnel syndrome, are also reported rarely. Thrombocytopenia may infrequently occur, especially after administration of MMR.

Expert Opinion on Management Issues

The clinical diagnosis of rubella is not reliable because rash illnesses from other causes may mimic rubella infection. Diagnosis based on clinical symptomatology misses the high proportion of subclinical infections. Therefore, rubella diagnosis relies on laboratory evidence of rubella infection. Serology is the most common laboratory diagnostic method; however, other laboratory techniques, such as viral isolation and reverse transcription–polymerase chain reaction (RT-PCR) techniques, are also available.

POSTNATALLY ACQUIRED INFECTION

Rubella serologic diagnosis depends on the demonstration of rubella-specific IgM antibody in acute specimens or a fourfold or greater increase in rubella IgG antibodies between acute and convalescent sera.

Rubella-specific immune globulin (Ig) M antibodies usually rise shortly after the onset of rash, but they may not be detectable until 5 days after rash onset. IgM antibodies usually peak 1 week after rash onset and persist for 8 to 12 weeks. Low concentrations can be detected for much longer if sensitive tests are used. Because IgM may be negative if collected within the first 4 days following rash onset, a second test may be necessary. False-positive rubella-specific IgM results may occur in persons with parvovirus infection, with a positive heterophile test for mononucleosis, or with a positive rheumatoid factor.

Confirming the diagnosis through a significant rise in IgG rubella-specific antibodies is most likely to be helpful if the acute specimen is obtained within 7 days of rash onset followed by a convalescent specimen approximately 10 days later. The first (acute phase) and second (convalescent phase) specimens should be tested simultaneously in the same laboratory.

Different serologic tests are available for laboratory confirmation of rubella infection. Enzyme immunoassays (EIAs) for rubella IgM and IgG antibodies are the most commonly used, but other serologic methods, such as hemagglutination inhibition, immunofluorescent antibody assays, and latex agglutination, are also available. In addition, the avidity of IgG antibodies can also be tested. Avidity gradually increases within 1 to 2 months after the illness. Therefore, low-avidity IgG antibody in serum is a marker of recent infection, and high avidity is a marker of past infection. A positive IgM detected in an asymptomatic person without a

known exposure to rubella and a history of a prior positive IgG test or documentation of rubella vaccine may be a false positive. Avidity testing may be most useful in these circumstances to confirm acute rubella infection. This may be particularly important for pregnant women. The algorithm in Figure 1 shows how to use IgG and avidity testing to determine whether a positive IgM is a true or false positive.

Rubella virus can be isolated from throat, nasal, urine, and cerebrospinal fluid specimens from persons with rubella infection. Virus can be isolated from the nasopharynx during the prodromal period until 2 weeks after rash onset, although the possibility of virus recovery is low by 4 days after the rash onset.

Oral-fluid tests can detect rubella-specific IgM or rubella RNA by RT-PCR, but its widespread use depends on the availability of suitable commercial assays.

There is no specific treatment for rubella. Although Ig following exposure may abort or mitigate clinical symptoms and signs, it does not prevent viremia and fetal infection. Administration of Ig should only be considered for confirmed seronegative women who continue with their pregnancy. If Ig is used, it should be administered as soon as possible following exposure, ideally within 72 hours. Suspected or confirmed cases of rubella should be reported to state or local public health authorities according to their regulations.

CONGENITALLY ACQUIRED INFECTION

Congenital rubella infection can be diagnosed by demonstration of rubella-specific IgM antibody in the newborn. IgM can also be obtained by cordocentesis in fetal blood if prenatal diagnosis is required. Approximately 20% of infected infants tested for rubella IgM may not have detectable titers before 1 month of age. Thus infants with symptoms consistent with CRS who test negative soon after birth should be retested after 1 month of age.

Although rubella-specific IgG is detectable at birth in newborns with CRS, maternally derived rubella-specific IgG is also present in children without CRS. Diagnosis of CRS can be confirmed if IgG titers do not decline at the rate expected based on decay of passively derived IgG. Alternatively, persistence of IgG antibodies beyond 6 months of age, which can be detected in 95% of infants with CRS, is also supportive of the diagnosis. In addition, low-avidity IgG antibody matures slowly in children with CRS and might persist in some cases beyond the second birthday.

In infants with CRS, rubella virus can be isolated from nasopharyngeal, urine, or cerebrospinal fluid specimens. Isolation of virus is generally positive during the first month of life, but virus excretion declines gradually during infancy, making CRS diagnosis difficult after 1 year of age.

The detection of viral RNA by RT-PCR is particularly useful for detecting fetal rubella infection. The method is both sensitive and specific. A negative RT-PCR in amniotic fluid, chorionic villus samples, or other fetal material suggests the fetus is not infected.

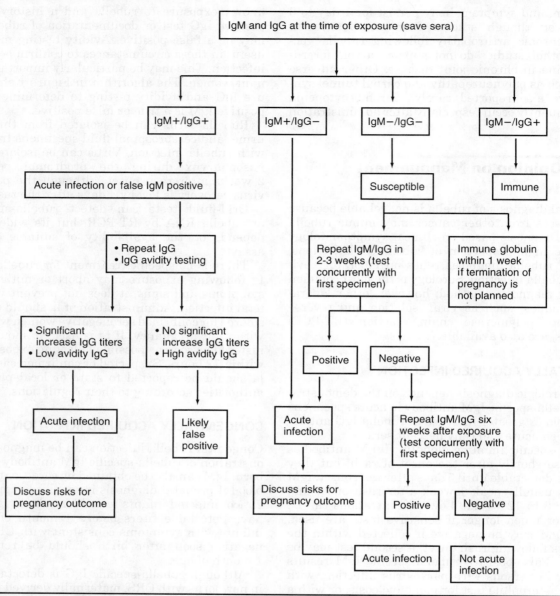

FIGURE 1. Algorithm for evaluation of pregnant women exposed to rubella. Ig, immune globulin.

There is no specific therapy for CRS; however, children with CRS should be evaluated to detect specific abnormalities and referred to specialists to provide early intervention.

Common Pitfalls

■ Failure to assess rubella immunity status, particularly in women of childbearing age (WCBA). Susceptible women should be vaccinated. Evidence of immunity generally consists of a positive rubella IgG test or documentation of receipt of rubella vaccine on or after the first birthday. Because the consequences of rubella infection in pregnancy are so great and rubella vaccine is not 100% effective, it may be reasonable to consider only a positive IgG test as acceptable evidence of immunity for pregnant women.

■ Failure to follow up on identified susceptible women to ensure they are vaccinated as soon as eligible (e.g., for pregnant women in the postpartum period).

■ Failure to suspect and confirm rubella in persons presenting with acute rash illness. This is particularly important in travelers, women who may be pregnant, and persons who come in contact with pregnant women.

Communication and Counseling

Rubella vaccine is the most effective way to prevent rubella before exposure. Exposed nonpregnant persons without documentation of at least one dose of rubella vaccine or proof of rubella immunity by serology should be vaccinated. Vaccine does not prevent illness postexposure. However, for theoretical reasons, there may be some benefit if vaccine is administered shortly after exposure. Moreover, it can be protective for future exposures if exposure did not result in infection. The algorithm presented in Figure 1 can be used to evaluate pregnant women exposed to rubella. If infection is documented, the risks of rubella infection during pregnancy and possible options for their care should be discussed. The diagnosis of fetal infection can be confirmed by detection of the virus in fetal specimens.

Children with postnatally acquired infection should be excluded from school or child care for 7 days after rash onset. For hospitalized patients, droplet precautions are recommended 7 days after rash onset in addition to standard precautions. Infants with CRS should be considered infectious during the first year of life unless two nasopharyngeal or urine cultures taken at least 1 month apart are negative for rubella virus. CRS cases should be managed with contact isolation and cared for by persons immune to rubella. Caregivers should be counseled to avoid contact of infants with CRS with susceptible pregnant contacts.

SUGGESTED READINGS

1. Banatvala JE, Brown DWG: Rubella. Lancet 363:1127–1137, 2004. **Describes pathogenesis, clinical features, laboratory diagnosis, and epidemiology of rubella.**
2. Bottiger B, Jensen IP: Maturation of rubella IgG avidity over time after acute rubella infection. Clin Diagn Virol 8(2):105–111, 1997. **Study showing changes over time of the avidity of rubella IgG antibodies after acute rubella infection.**
3. Centers for Disease Control and Prevention: Control and prevention of rubella: Evaluation and management of suspected outbreaks, rubella in pregnant women, and surveillance for congenital rubella syndrome. MMWR Recomm Rep 50(RR–12): 30, 2001. **Recommendations for management of rubella outbreaks and pregnant women with rubella.**
4. Centers for Disease Control and Prevention: Measles, mumps, and rubella—vaccine use and strategies for elimination of measles, rubella, and congenital rubella syndrome and control of mumps. Recommendations of the Advisory Committee on Immunization Practices (ACIP). MMWR Recomm Rep 47(RR–8):1–57, 1998. **Recommendations for control of rubella by immunization.**
5. Freij BJ, South MA, Sever JL: Maternal rubella and the congenital rubella syndrome. Clin Perinatol 15(2):247–257, 1988. **Describes association of rubella infection and congenital rubella syndrome and provides a good description of congenital rubella syndrome.**
6. Herrman KL: Available rubella serologic tests. Rev Infect Dis 7: S108–S112, 1985. **Review of sensitivity and specificity of different laboratory techniques.**
7. Miller E, Cradock-Watson JE, Pollock TM: Consequences of confirmed maternal rubella at successive stages of pregnancy. Lancet 2:781–784, 1982. **Indicates consequences of rubella infection at different stages in pregnancy.**
8. Plotkin SA, Reef S: Rubella vaccine. In Plotkin SA, Orenstein WA (eds): Vaccines. Philadelphia: WB Saunders, 2004, pp 389–440. **Detailed description of rubella disease and vaccine.**
9. Reef SE, Frey TK, Theall K, et al: The changing epidemiology of rubella in the 1990s: On the verge of elimination and new challenges for control and prevention. JAMA 287(4):464–472, 2002. **Describes the changes in epidemiology of rubella in the United States.**

Varicella-Zoster Infections

Anne A. Gershon

KEY CONCEPTS

- Both varicella (chickenpox) and zoster (shingles) are caused by varicella-zoster virus (VZV).
- Live attenuated varicella vaccine was licensed for routine use for healthy children in 1995 in the United States, and since that time the incidence of varicella and its complications have decreased. Varicella vaccine is not recommended for use in immunocompromised patients.
- Varicella vaccine is extremely safe. The most common adverse effects are mild rash in an estimated 5% of children approximately 1 month after vaccination. Unless the rash is extensive and/or severe, contagion to others is unlikely to occur.
- Outbreaks of mild varicella are reported among vaccinated children years after vaccination.
- Otherwise healthy adolescents and adults who have not been vaccinated and who develop varicella should receive acyclovir (ACV) therapy, usually by the oral route. Immunocompromised patients usually require treatment with intravenous ACV.
- Passive immunization with varicella-zoster immune globulin (VZIG) is usually reserved for varicella-susceptible immunocompromised children who were closely exposed to persons with either varicella or zoster.

12

Both varicella (chickenpox) and zoster (shingles) are caused by varicella-zoster virus (VZV). Patients with varicella present with fever and a vesicular pruritic rash that is most concentrated on the face, body, and chest. The illness is frequently mild, although complications may occur, especially in adults and immunocompromised patients. Months to years after vaccination, approximately 10% of persons nevertheless may develop mild varicella. Following varicella, the virus may become latent but does not manifest further symptoms. In approximately 15% of people, however, the latent virus reactivates to cause zoster; often this occurs decades after varicella. Zoster after vaccination is rare. Zoster manifests as a unilateral, often painful, vesicular rash in a dermatomal distribution. It is as contagious to others as varicella. Zoster is most common in persons older than 60 years and the immunocompromised. Table 1 presents diagnostic points concerning VZV infection. Box 1 shows complications of varicella.

Live attenuated varicella vaccine was licensed for routine use in healthy children in the United States in 1995. Most states now require this vaccine for entry into school or daycare. Box 2 presents indications and contraindications for use of varicella vaccine. Approximately 5% of vaccines develop a mild varicella-like rash approximately 1 month after vaccination. This rash is very rarely contagious. Should spread to others occur, the contact illness is mild or subclinical. No antiviral

TABLE 1 Diagnosis of Varicella-Zoster Virus Infections

	Varicella	Zoster
Important historical information	Was patient immunized? When?	Was patient immunized? When?
	Has patient had varicella previously?	Has patient previously had varicella? When?
	Was patient exposed to someone with varicella or zoster? When?	
	Is patient otherwise healthy?	Is patient otherwise healthy?
	Are there other varicella-susceptibles in the household?	Are there varicella-susceptibles in the household?
Characteristic rash	Generalized, but preponderantly on head and trunk; fewer on extremities	Unilateral, initially localized to one to three dermatomes; may develop a few generalized lesions
	Pruritic, with vesicles	
	Lesions in all stages of development in any one area of skin: maculopapules, vesicles, pustules, scabs	Painful or pruritic
Duration of illness	5–7 days	Up to several weeks
Differential diagnosis (in order of frequency)	Insect bites, contact dermatitis, HSV infection, rickettsialpox, smallpox	HSV infection, contact dermatitis
Laboratory diagnosis	Direct immunofluorescence of smear of vesicle to demonstrate VZV antigen, culture for VZV, PCR, acute and convalescent titers to demonstrate rise in antibody titer to VZV	Same as for varicella

HSV, herpes simplex virus; PCR, polymerase chain reaction, VZV, varicella-zoster virus.

BOX 1 Complications of Varicella

- Bacterial superinfection (1 in 3000–5000 cases), requires antibiotic therapy
  - Group A β-hemolytic streptococci
  - Staphylococci
- Central nervous system complications
  - Ataxia (1 in 4000 cases), usually transient
  - Encephalitis (1 in 100,000 cases), associated with long-term sequelae

BOX 2 Indications and Contraindications for Varicella Vaccine

Healthy, older than 1 year

- Vaccinate child even if there are immunocompromised or pregnant susceptibles in the household.
- Vaccinate healthy susceptibles who were not immunized previously and were recently exposed to VZV.
- Vaccine may be administered concomitantly with MMR vaccine using separate sites and syringes or as MMRV. Vaccine may also be administered with DPT and polio vaccines.

Contraindications

- Pregnancy, immunocompromised, allergic to vaccine components such as gelatin.
  - Acceptable to immunize if patient with HIV infection has <25% CD4 cells.
  - Defer vaccination in individuals receiving 20 mg/kg of prednisone (or its equivalent) daily, until steroids stopped for at least 3 mo.
- After VZIG, defer vaccination for 5 mo; after IVIG for Kawasaki disease, withhold varicella vaccination for 11 mo.
- After vaccination: unnecessary to determine VZV antibodies; routine ELISA tests lack sensitivity for this purpose.

DPT, diphtheria, pertussis, and tetanus (vaccine); ELISA, enzyme-linked immunoabsorbent assay; HIV, human immunodeficiency virus; IVIG, intravenous immune globulin; MMR, mumps, measles, rubella (vaccine); VZIG, varicella-zoster immune globulin; VZV, varicella-zoster virus.

Expert Opinion on Management Issues

ACCEPTED INTERVENTIONS

Box 3 shows the treatment of VZV infections. The preferred drug is acyclovir (ACV), which is available for oral use as a suspension (200 mg/5 mL) and also as tablets of 200 and 800 mg. An intravenous (IV) formulation is also available for treatment of immunocompromised patients. ACV is remarkably well tolerated. Side effects include nausea and other gastrointestinal complaints in 20% and central nervous system symptoms (headache, agitation) in 5%. Rapid infusion by the IV route is associated with renal toxicity, which can be avoided by slow administration to the well-hydrated patient.

Otherwise healthy children with varicella are not routinely treated with ACV because the illness is usually mild. Because second cases are often more

therapy is necessary to treat this rash, except if it occurs in an immunocompromised patient who was immunized inadvertently. Rare CNS manifestations (ataxia, encephalitis) after vaccination have not been found to be caused by the vaccine virus (strain Oka). One injection is given for patients 1 to 12 years of age; two doses, 4 to 8 weeks apart, are given to those who have reached their 13th birthday.

Recently a formulation of measles-mumps-rubella-varicella (MMRV) was licensed by the FDA in the United States. About 15 % of vaccinated children develop a breakthrough case of varicella in the years after vaccination. This is usually a very mild infection but is contagious to others.

BOX 3 **Treatment of Varicella and Zoster**

Acyclovir (ACV):
- Pediatric dose: 80 mg/kg qid PO for 5 days; IV: 500 mg/m^2 tid for 7–10 days
- Adult dose: 800 mg PO five times a day for 5–7 days; IV: 10 mg/kg tid

Adolescents with zoster:
- Valacyclovir: 1 g PO tid for 7 days
- Famciclovir: 500 mg PO tid for 7 days

IV, intravenously; PO, orally; qid; four times daily; tid, three times daily.

---

severe than first cases in a family, treatment may be given to these children, although studies do not show a significant modification in the illness. Otherwise healthy adolescents and adults who develop varicella should receive ACV therapy by the oral route. For the rare person who does not respond adequately to oral medication, the IV route may be used. Immunocompromised patients should be treated with ACV. Highly immunocompromised patients should be treated intravenously; for less immunocompromised patients, the oral route may be tried first. Newer antivirals, such as valacyclovir and famciclovir, are not approved for use in children or for varicella; however, adolescents with zoster may be given these medications.

Fever is best treated with acetaminophen. Aspirin should not be given because of the risk of Reye syndrome. Nonsteroidal anti-inflammatory drugs may be linked to an increase in serious bacterial infections and should therefore be avoided.

URGENT INTERVENTIONS

Healthy varicella susceptibles may be vaccinated even if they were recently exposed to the illness. The sooner this is accomplished, the more effective the vaccine. Because not every exposure results in disease, however, the vaccine could be given even longer than 5 days after the exposure.

If oral antiviral therapy is contemplated, it should be instituted within 24 hours after rash onset for varicella and within 72 hours after rash onset for zoster. For immunocompromised patients with VZV infection, IV therapy should be started as soon as possible after rash onset for best results.

For exposed immunocompromised patients who have intimate exposures to VZV infection, passive immunization with varicella-zoster immune globulin (VZIG) should be given as soon as possible, ideally within 3 days of the exposure. VZIG may be administered as long as 5 days after exposure but may not modify the disease in these patients.

The dose is 125 U per 10 kg body weight, with a maximum dose of 625 U, given intramuscularly. It is necessary to wait at least 3 months after giving VZIG to

immunize with the mumps, measles, rubella (MMR) vaccine.

CONTROVERSIAL INTERVENTIONS

Routine treatment of otherwise healthy children with varicella or zoster with ACV is not recommended because ACV alters the course of illness only marginally. Nevertheless, some physicians continue to use it. Routine vaccination to avoid varicella is preferred.

Common Pitfalls

- Failure to administer routine vaccination is a potential pitfall. Now that the vaccine has been approved for this indication for 10 years, it is potentially dangerous not to vaccinate a child. Unvaccinated children have a high probability of growing up to be susceptible adults because the opportunity for exposure to wild-type VZV continues to decrease in the United States.
- Serologic testing after vaccination is not useful because the available ELISA tests are not usually sensitive enough to identify immunity following vaccination.
- Immunocompromised patients should not receive live attenuated varicella vaccine. They are best protected from varicella by immunizing the varicella susceptibles in their families and use of VZIG.
- It is possible that vaccination of persons who have had varicella will protect against zoster. This is currently the subject of a large double-blind research study, in which very high titer vaccine is being used. Until the results of this study become available, immunization to prevent zoster should not be performed.
- Failure to administer ACV promptly to adolescents, adults, or immunocompromised patients with varicella could potentially lead to development of severe infection in these high-risk individuals.
- The dose of ACV used to treat VZV infections is higher than that used to treat infections with herpes simplex virus (HSV). Strict attention must be paid to the correct dose of ACV when treating VZV infections.
- For patients with possible bacterial superinfections, it is important to try to identify the causative organism and to institute antibiotic therapy rapidly, in case the superinfecting organism is invasive group A streptococci.

Communication and Counseling

Most children with varicella or zoster recover uneventfully. Most with serious bacterial complications who are treated aggressively recover. Those who develop the alarming symptom of ataxia recover, but the prognosis for those with encephalitis is guarded. Parents need to be educated about the safety and efficacy of varicella vaccine to avoid these complications. Present information also suggests that vaccinees are less likely to develop zoster than those who have had natural infection.

SUGGESTED READINGS

1. Balfour HH, Kelly JM, Suarez CS, et al: Acyclovir treatment of varicella in otherwise healthy children. J Pediatr 116:633–639, 1990. **Study showing the efficacy of orally administered antiviral treatment of varicella.**
2. Balfour HH, Rotbart H, Feldman S, et al: Acyclovir treatment of varicella in otherwise healthy adolescents. J Pediatr 120: 627–633, 1992. **Study showing the efficacy of orally administered antiviral treatment of varicella in adolescents.**
3. Centers for Disease Control and Prevention: Prevention of varicella: Recommendations of the Advisory Committee on Immunization Practices (ACIP). MMWR Morb Mortal Wkly Rep 45:1–36, 1996. **Governmental recommendations for control of varicella by immunization.**
4. Centers for Disease Control and Prevention: Prevention of varicella. MMWR Morb Mortal Wkly Rep 48:1–6, 1999. **Additional governmental recommendations for control of varicella by immunization.**
5. Gershon A, Takahashi M, Seward J: Live attenuated varicella vaccine. In Plotkin S, Orenstein W (eds): Vaccines, 4th ed. Philadelphia: WB Saunders, 2003, pp 783–823. **History and extremely detailed description of varicella vaccine, VZIG, acyclovir.**
6. Gershon AA: Live-attenuated varicella vaccine. Infect Dis Clin North Am 15:65–81, 2001. **Detailed description of the use of varicella vaccine.**
7. Laupland KB, Davies HD, Low DE, et al: Invasive group A streptococcal disease in children and association with varicella-zoster virus infection. Ontario Group A Streptococcal Study Group. Pediatrics 105:E60, 2000. **Describes severe bacterial superinfections associated with varicella.**
8. Seward JF, Watson BM, Peterson CL, et al: Varicella disease after introduction of varicella vaccine in the United States, 1995–2000. JAMA 287:606–611, 2002. **Indicates how use of vaccine has decreased the incidence of varicella by both personal and herd immunity.**
9. Sharrar RG, LaRussa P, Galea S, et al: The postmarketing safety profile of varicella vaccine. Vaccine 19:916–923, 2000. **Postlicensure study indicating the safety of varicella vaccine and the rarity of zoster following it.**
10. Zerr DM, Rubens CE: NSAIDs and necrotizing fasciitis. Pediatr Infect Dis J 18:724–725, 1999. **Describes the association of nonsteroidal anti-inflammatory drugs (NSAIDs) and serious bacterial superinfection after varicella.**

Viral Meningitis and Encephalitis

Mark J. Abzug

KEY CONCEPTS

- Many viral causes of meningitis and encephalitis have characteristic epidemiologies that are clues to their diagnosis.
- In general, viral meningitis manifests similarly, regardless of etiology. Infants and young children have nonspecific symptoms, such as fever, irritability, lethargy, anorexia, and emesis.
- Viral encephalitis is manifested in younger children by irritability and/or lethargy, often following a nonspecific febrile illness. Older children may develop headache, altered consciousness, disorientation, unusual behavior, abnormal speech, bizarre movements, and emotional outbursts, along with fever, nausea, vomiting, myalgias, and photophobia.
- The differential diagnosis of meningitis and encephalitis is broad and includes infections, medication-induced meningitis, connective tissue disease, metabolic derangements, malignancy, toxins, and hemorrhage.
- CSF exam, imaging, electroencephalography, and viral testing may assist in diagnosis.

Meningitis refers to an inflammatory process of the meninges, reflected by an alteration of cerebrospinal fluid (CSF) parameters. Viral meningitis is the most common cause of so-called aseptic meningitis, meningitis in which common bacterial pathogens are not isolated.

Encephalitis, an inflammatory condition that affects brain parenchyma, is typically a more severe illness. Encephalitis may be acute, caused by viral invasion of the central nervous system (CNS) and/or by an inflammatory response to a virus, or it may be postinfectious (acute disseminated encephalomyelitis), in which an autoimmune process characterized by demyelination follows a viral illness or vaccination.

Many viral infections of the CNS are best referred to as meningoencephalitis, characterized by inflammation in meninges and brain tissue. The estimated 8000 to 13,000 cases of aseptic meningitis and 20,000 cases of encephalitis reported annually in the United States, most of which are caused by viral infections, likely reflect under-reporting. In newer series, the etiology of viral meningitis and encephalitis was identified in up to 55% to 70% and 25% to 65% of cases, respectively. Of viral meningitis and encephalitis cases with proven etiology, the majority are caused by enteroviruses. Other important causes include arboviruses (transmitted by arthropod vectors, e.g., mosquitoes or ticks), herpes simplex virus (HSV), influenza virus, rabies virus, varicella-zoster virus, Epstein-Barr virus, human immunodeficiency virus (HIV), and adenovirus (Tables 1 and 2). The differential diagnosis for meningitis and encephalitis is listed in Box 1.

In general, viral meningitis manifests similarly, regardless of etiology. Infants and young children have nonspecific symptoms, such as fever, irritability, lethargy, anorexia, and emesis. Findings of meningeal inflammation (e.g., nuchal rigidity, bulging fontanelle, or photophobia) are frequently absent. In older children, signs of meningeal inflammation are more common, often accompanying fever, headache, and emesis. Focal neurologic findings and seizures are uncommon presenting findings. However, approximately 10% of children hospitalized with enterovirus meningitis have acute complications (e.g., seizures, obtundation, increased intracranial pressure, and inappropriate

TABLE 1 Etiologies and Epidemiology of Viral Meningitis and Encephalitis

Etiology	Epidemiology
Enteroviruses	85%–95% of viral meningitis and up to 80% of encephalitis of proven etiology. Majority in children, especially <1 yr of age. Epidemic during warm seasons in temperate climates. Enterovirus 71 infections frequently in regional outbreaks (e.g., Asia since late 1990s). Poliovirus infection decreased with widespread immunization.
Arboviruses	≈5% of viral meningitis; important cause of encephalitis. Prevalent during warm and/or wet seasons when mosquitoes and ticks active. Agents: La Crosse virus (M ≈ E); St. Louis encephalitis virus (≈15%, up to 35%–60% in children, of symptomatic cases manifest as meningitis; lower incidence and severity of encephalitis in children); Eastern equine encephalomyelitis virus (E > M); Western equine encephalomyelitis virus (E > M); Venezuelan equine encephalitis virus (E > M); West Nile virus (<1% of infections with neurologic illness; neurologic syndromes include meningitis in ~ 29% and encephalitis in ~ 63%; lower incidence and severity of neurologic disease in children; regional outbreaks, e.g., United States since late 1990s); Colorado tick fever virus (meningitis in up to 18%; encephalitis uncommon); Japanese encephalitis virus (most important epidemic encephalomyelitis; prevalent in Asia; E > M); Powassan, Rocio, Murray Valley, Kyasuma Forest, Jamestown Canyon, California encephalitis, tick-borne encephalitis, Ilheus, Snowshoe Hare, and Rift Valley viruses.
Herpes simplex virus	≈1%–3% of viral meningitis, primarily with type 2 primary genital infection; less frequently with primary type 1 genital infection, nonprimary genital infection (either type), or without recent genital disease. Mollaret meningitis (recurrent, benign aseptic meningitis) associated with type 2 infection without signs of genital infection and occasionally with type 1 or with Epstein-Barr virus. ~10% of encephalitis in United States (primarily type 2 in neonates and type 1 outside the neonatal period); one third of cases <20 yr of age. Most common focal viral encephalitis in nonepidemic settings.
Influenza virus	Rare cause of meningitis; important cause of encephalitis, including acute necrotizing encephalopathy reported predominantly in children in Asia (also linked to human herpesvirus 6, measles, parainfluenza, and mycoplasma).
Rabies virus	Relatively uncommon in United States (raccoon, fox, bat, skunk bites); important encephalitis in developing countries (dogs, cats).
Varicella-zoster virus	Meningitis, encephalitis, cerebellar ataxia with chickenpox, cutaneous zoster, or zoster without skin lesions.
Human immunodeficiency virus	Transient meningitis during primary infection (acute retroviral syndrome); transient or chronic meningitis or encephalitis during chronic infection; opportunistic infections.
Mumps virus	Leading cause of meningitis in prevaccine era; meningitis and encephalitis now uncommon in developed countries.
Measles virus	Meningitis in ≈ 30% of cases; meningitis and encephalitis decreased with immunization.
Rubella virus	Encephalitis decreased with immunization.
Lymphocytic choriomeningitis virus	Meningitis and encephalitis more common in developing countries; transmitted by rodent secretions.
Acute disseminated encephalomyelitis	Days to weeks after influenza, measles, varicella-zoster, other respiratory virus infections, or vaccinations.
Other	Human herpesvirus 6 (M, E), Epstein-Barr virus (M, E), cytomegalovirus (M, E), adenovirus (M, E), parainfluenza virus (M), rotavirus (M, E), encephalomyocarditis virus (M, E), parvovirus B19 (M, E), rhinovirus (M), coronavirus (M), simian herpes B virus (E), human T-lymphotropic virus (E), JC virus (E), yellow fever virus (E), Lassa fever virus (E), Nipah virus (E), Australia bat *Lyssavirus* (E).

E, encephalitis; M, meningitis.

antidiuretic hormone secretion). Illness can last for 1 to 2 weeks.

Viral encephalitis is manifested in younger children by irritability and/or lethargy, often following a nonspecific febrile illness. Older children may develop headache, altered consciousness, disorientation, unusual behavior, abnormal speech, bizarre movements, and emotional outbursts, along with fever, nausea, vomiting, myalgias, and photophobia. Focal or, more commonly, generalized neurologic abnormalities (e.g., seizures and motor deficits) may be present. Disease may progress to extreme lethargy, stupor, or coma.

Expert Opinion on Management Issues

Supportive care is the mainstay of therapy for viral meningitis and encephalitis. In young children, especially those younger than 1 year, difficulty in distinguishing bacterial and viral meningitis usually prompts hospitalization and parenteral antibiotics until bacterial cultures are negative and/or an alternative diagnosis is made (e.g., by a positive CSF polymerase chain reaction [PCR] test for enterovirus) (Table 3). Neonates or other immunocompromised patients with enterovirus meningitis may require supportive treatment for disseminated disease, including myocarditis, pericarditis, hepatitis, and coagulopathy. In older, otherwise healthy children who are not very ill, the presumptive diagnosis of viral meningitis can frequently be made based on clinical appearance and CSF profile (e.g., mononuclear predominance on an initial specimen or a repeat lumbar puncture obtained 8 to 24 hours later). The lumbar puncture itself may relieve symptoms such as headache, emesis, and irritability.

Hospitalization and empirical antibacterial therapy are generally indicated for children who appear ill (including those requiring intravenous [IV] hydration or

TABLE 2 Clinical Features of Selected Viral Meningitides and Encephalitides

Virus	Clinical Features
Enterovirus	Rash (macular, maculopapular, petechial, vesicular), enanthem, conjunctivitis, respiratory symptoms, pleurodynia, pericarditis, myocarditis, diarrhea, myalgias may accompany. Fever may be biphasic; meningeal or neurologic symptoms during second phase. Encephalitis usually generalized, although focal seizures and abnormalities may occur (especially neonates). Systemic illness, severe encephalitis in neonates; severe disease less common beyond neonatal period. Chronic meningitis or meningoencephalitis with waxing and waning neurologic symptoms, and, frequently, fatal outcome, with agammaglobulinemia or hypogammaglobulinemia. Enterovirus 71 associated with hand-foot-mouth disease, herpangina, neurologic disease (meningitis, brain stem encephalitis, myelitis/acute flaccid paralysis, Guillain-Barré syndrome); severe brain stem encephalitis in children <5 yr. Findings include myoclonic jerks, tremors, ataxia, limb weakness, cranial nerve palsy, seizures, altered consciousness, increased intracranial pressure, CSF pleocytosis, pulmonary edema/hemorrhage, cardiac failure, myocarditis, neurogenic shock.
Herpes simplex virus	Encephalitis in ≈50% of neonatal infections. CNS-only disease frequently begins in temporal lobe, then becomes bitemporal. Encephalitis with disseminated disease more commonly diffuse. Findings include seizures (focal and generalized), lethargy, irritability, tremors, anorexia, temperature instability, bulging fontanelle. Encephalitis beyond neonatal period typically febrile, focal encephalitis with necrosis and hemorrhage. Tropism for temporal lobe (aphasia, anosmia, temporal lobe seizures, other focal findings); disease can be widespread and bilateral. Other findings include headache, emesis, altered consciousness, bizarre behavior, personality changes, disorientation, ataxia. Focal features not always present.
West Nile virus	Meningitis frequently mild, particularly in children. Severe findings include altered consciousness; asymmetrical muscle weakness, flaccid paralysis, areflexia (poliomyelitis syndrome); ataxia, cranial nerve palsies (brain stem involvement); sensory deficits; hyperreflexia; optic neuritis; polyradiculitis; seizures (uncommon); abnormal movements; transverse myelitis; Guillain-Barré syndrome. Focal temporal lobe disease mimics herpes encephalitis. Fever, emesis, maculopapular rash (especially children) frequent.
Influenza virus	Acute necrotizing encephalopathy characterized by fever, altered consciousness, seizures, rapid progression to coma, elevated CSF protein (usually without pleocytosis). Predilection for thalamus and brain stem. Mortality ≈30%; severe sequelae in survivors.
Lymphocytic choriomeningitis virus	Occasionally severe; spectrum includes transverse myelitis, hydrocephalus, encephalitis.
Human herpesvirus 6	Meningoencephalitis with confusion, headache, seizures. May be focal and mimic herpes encephalitis.
Acute disseminated encephalomyelitis (postinfectious encephalitis)	Findings reflect areas of brain involved; often multifocal. Spectrum includes transverse myelitis, optic neuritis, cerebellar ataxia, peripheral neuritis.

CNS, central nervous system; CSF, cerebrospinal fluid.

BOX 1 Differential Diagnosis of Meningitis and Encephalitis

The differential diagnosis of meningitis and encephalitis is broad:

- Bacterial etiologies (*Streptococcus pneumoniae, Neisseria meningitidis, Haemophilus influenzae, Mycobacterium tuberculosis,* syphilis, Lyme disease, leptospirosis, borreliosis, brucellosis, *Bartonella henselae, Mycoplasma pneumoniae, Mycoplasma hominis,* rickettsioses)
- Parameningeal foci (brain abscess, subdural or epidural empyema)
- Parasitic infection
- Fungal infection
- Kawasaki disease
- Medication-induced meningitis (nonsteroidal anti-inflammatory agents, immune globulin, sulfa antibiotics, carbamazepine, cytosine arabinoside, OKT3)
- Connective tissue disease (systemic lupus erythematosus)
- Metabolic derangements (hepatic encephalopathy, uremia, inborn errors, leukodystrophy)
- Malignancy
- Toxin
- Hemorrhage

CSF exam, imaging, electroencephalography, and viral testing may assist in diagnosis.

---

aggressive pain control), children in whom it cannot readily be distinguished whether meningitis is viral or bacterial, and patients with signs of encephalitis. Presumptive treatment for *Mycobacterium tuberculosis* infection may also be appropriate if the exposure history, clinical presentation, and CSF and imaging results are suggestive. General measures include providing a quiet environment, analgesics for headache, antiemetics, anticonvulsants if indicated, and IV fluids and medications for patients with significantly depressed consciousness. For severely affected patients, intensive care is indicated, including intubation to protect the airway, respiratory support as necessary, and monitoring. Cerebral edema or inappropriate antidiuretic hormone secretion can be managed with mild fluid restriction. Head of bed elevation; fluid restriction; hyperventilation; osmotic (mannitol) and loop diuretics; and control of temperature, pain, and seizures are used for management of increased intracranial pressure.

Few specific antiviral therapies are available for viral meningitis and encephalitis. Acyclovir can be used to hasten recovery from HSV meningitis, although

TABLE 3 Diagnostic Tests for Viral Meningitis and Encephalitis

Test	Utility and Interpretation
CSF examination	Indicated in suspected meningitis or encephalitis unless contraindicated by concern for space-occupying lesion or increased intracranial pressure. Meningitis: low-grade pleocytosis (100–1000 WBC/mm^3, occasionally <100 WBC/mm^3 or ≥ 2000 cells/mm^3); polymorphonuclear leukocytes may predominate early, becoming mononuclear in 8–48 h; protein normal or slightly increased (occasionally quite elevated); glucose normal or slightly low (occasionally very depressed). Encephalitis: predominantly mononuclear pleocytosis; elevated protein; normal glucose; ≈3%–5% normal CSF profile; increased RBCs may be seen with HSV.
Imaging	Excludes alternative diagnoses (e.g., brain abscess and tumor); demonstrates distribution of viral-induced disease. Focal disease, especially temporal lobe, suggests HSV, although may be seen with other viruses (e.g., arboviruses, Epstein-Barr virus, enteroviruses, influenza, mumps). Imaging may be normal early with HSV; sensitivity of MRI >CT. High-signal intensity lesions in brain stem suggest enterovirus 71. Bilateral thalamic lesions and multifocal symmetric lesions in brain stem tegmentum, putamina, medulla, cerebral periventricular white matter, cerebellum on MRI suggest influenza-associated acute necrotizing encephalopathy. Thalamic, basal ganglia, midbrain, and brain stem lesions characteristic of Japanese and eastern equine encephalitides. Demyelination often prominent in acute disseminated encephalomyelitis.
EEG	Useful for distinguishing encephalitis versus metabolic encephalopathy. Abnormal temporal lobe activity (spike and slow wave activity, periodic lateralizing epileptiform discharges) characteristic of HSV.
Viral cultures	CSF viral culture yield in encephalitis <meningitis; 65%–75% overall sensitivity of culture for enteroviruses; enteroviruses can be isolated from CSF of young infants lacking pleocytosis. CSF, serum viral cultures usually negative in enterovirus 71 encephalitis; throat and stool culture, serology higher yield. CSF viral culture positive in 25%–40% of neonates (throat, blood, urine, stool may also be positive) and <2% of older children and adults with HSV.
PCR	Sensitive and specific for enterovirus meningitis, encephalitis; rapid diagnosis reduces unnecessary therapies, hospital stay, costs. Detects persistent enterovirus infection in agammaglobulinemic patients with chronic meningoencephalitis despite negative cultures. CSF PCR may be negative in EV71 encephalitis; throat and stool may have higher yields. Sensitivity and specificity of CSF PCR = 95%–99% and ≥94%, respectively, in older children/adults with HSV (remaining positive in >80% up to 1 wk into therapy, falling to <20% after 2 wk of treatment); PCR may be negative in the first few days of illness. Sensitivity and specificity of CSF PCR = 75%–100% and 71%–100%, respectively, in neonates with HSV; positive PCR at end of treatment associated with increased rate of death or neurologic impairment. CSF PCR may be useful for diagnosis of other agents (e.g., cytomegalovirus, varicella-zoster virus, human herpesvirus 6, JC virus), some arboviruses [low sensitivity for West Nile virus]). PCR of saliva for rabies virus is highly sensitive.
Serology	Detection of serum and CSF antibodies against many viruses (e.g., most arboviruses) possible; frequently requires acute and convalescent specimens (helpful epidemiologically but not for acute patient management). Useful to define the extent of enterovirus 71 outbreaks. For some agents (e.g., West Nile virus and Japanese encephalitis virus), serum and CSF IgM assays useful for rapid diagnosis.
Other	Brain biopsy infrequently performed with advent of PCR testing but may be useful if diagnosis uncertain. Immunostain (skin at nape of neck, corneal impression, buccal mucosa, brain) useful for rabies.

CSF, cerebrospinal fluid; EEG, electroencephalography; HSV, herpes simplex virus; IgM, immunoglobulin M; PCR, polymerase chain reaction.

12

the outcome of herpes meningitis without encephalitis is excellent even without antiviral therapy. Empirical therapy with acyclovir (30, up to 45 to 60 mg/kg/day IV divided every 8 hours) for possible HSV encephalitis should be considered in children with encephalitis, especially in the presence of fever and focal findings on clinical exam, imaging, or electroencephalography (see Table 3). A 14- to 21-day course is indicated if HSV infection is confirmed or clinical and neurodiagnostic studies are strongly suggestive (see Table 3). Acyclovir (60 mg/kg/day IV divided every 8 hours) should be presumptively administered to neonates presenting with encephalitis (with or without focal findings) and continued for 21 days (and until an end-of therapy CSF PCR is negative) if HSV disease is proven or considered likely. Acyclovir (varicella-zoster virus), ganciclovir (cytomegalovirus, human herpesvirus 6), and foscarnet (human herpesvirus 6, cytomegalovirus) are available for other herpesvirus infections.

The experimental agent pleconaril was investigated for enterovirus meningitis, acute encephalitis, and chronic meningoencephalitis in agammaglobulinemic patients, with some evidence of benefit; however, it is not currently available. For the latter entity, intraventricular, intrathecal, and IV immune globulin are used to suppress or stabilize disease. Patients with severe enterovirus 71 disease are managed with close monitoring, fluid restriction, osmotic diuretics, and cardiorespiratory support. IV immune globulin, corticosteroids, interferon-alfa, and pleconaril have been tried, but none has been proven effective. Influenza encephalitis is treated with antivirals (e.g., amantadine, rimantadine, oseltamivir), corticosteroids, and immune globulin, without definitive proof of efficacy. Unproven therapies for West Nile virus encephalitis include ribavirin, interferon, immune globulin, and corticosteroids; therapeutic trials are in progress. No specific proven therapies are available for encephalitis caused by rabies virus, Japanese encephalitis virus, or arboviruses. Corticosteroids and IV immune globulin are frequently used to treat acute disseminated encephalomyelitis, without proof of efficacy. Regardless of etiology, rehabilitative therapy and neurodevelopmental follow-up are frequently necessary after the acute phase of encephalitis.

Common Pitfalls

- Children receiving antibiotics prior to diagnosis of meningitis represent a management challenge because it can be difficult to distinguish "partially treated bacterial meningitis" from viral meningitis based on clinical appearance, CSF profile, and bacterial cultures. These children usually require hospitalization and antibacterial treatment pending viral diagnostic and bacterial antigen studies. If bacterial meningitis cannot be discounted based on clinical and laboratory results, a complete course of antimicrobial therapy is frequently necessary.
- Although newer laboratory techniques facilitate making an etiologic diagnosis, many cases, especially of encephalitis, defy specific diagnosis.
- Satisfactory clinical outcome of HSV encephalitis requires a high index of suspicion and early empirical treatment with acyclovir.
- The prognosis for encephalitis patients can be difficult to predict early in the course of illness.

Communication and Counseling

The prognosis for viral meningitis is generally favorable; permanent sequelae are uncommon, although fatigue, irritability, and decreased concentration may take weeks to resolve. Older reports suggest that enterovirus meningitis in very young infants may have sequelae (e.g., speech and language delay, intellectual deficits, and motor abnormalities), but newer larger series do not suggest long-lasting deficits.

The prognosis for patients with encephalitis is variable, depending on severity of illness and extent of brain involvement, patient age, and etiology; and often difficult to predict. Sequelae may include intellectual, motor, visual, or auditory deficits and seizures. In one series of non-neonatal herpes encephalitis treated with acyclovir, 19% died and 62% of survivors had sequelae. Age older than 30 years, Glasgow Coma Scale less than 6, and neurologic symptoms lasting longer than 4 days prior to treatment were associated with worse outcome. Relapses occasionally occur. In neonates with herpes encephalitis, mortality is generally less than 15%, but up to two thirds of survivors are impaired. Severe enterovirus encephalitis may be associated with poor outcome in neonates. Poor outcome beyond the neonatal period is uncommon, except for enterovirus 71 neurologic and cardiopulmonary disease, which is associated with significant mortality and sequelae, including hypoventilation, facial palsy, dysphagia, and paresis. Severe West Nile virus encephalitis is associated with a 10% fatality rate, higher in persons older than 65 years. Rare deaths are reported in children, and long-lasting sequelae (e.g., weakness, paralysis, and learning difficulties) can occur. Mortality rates of up to 30% and sequelae in an estimated 50% of survivors with Japanese encephalitis are reported. Rabies encephalitis is nearly uniformly fatal. For other viruses, outcomes are generally favorable, although fatalities or significant sequelae occur. Acute disseminated encephalomyelitis may be associated with significant mortality or sequelae.

Methods to reduce acquisition and/or circulation of viral agents that cause meningoencephalitis include routine immunization (mumps, measles, rubella; poliovirus; varicella-zoster; influenza), immunization targeted to residents and travelers in endemic regions (Japanese encephalitis, yellow fever), immunization for persons at risk of animal exposures (rabies), animal immunization (eastern, western, and Venezuelan equine encephalitis; West Nile virus; rabies), and public health (insecticides, larvicides) and personal protective measures (reduced outdoors exposure at dawn and dusk, long pants and long-sleeved shirts, diethyltoluamide (DEET)-containing repellents) to prevent arbovirus infections.

SUGGESTED READINGS

1. Bonthius DJ, Karacay B: Meningitis and encephalitis in children: An update. Neurol Clin 20:1013–1038, 2002. **Discussion of selected etiologies of meningitis and encephalitis, including lymphocytic choriomeningitis virus, West Nile virus, and human herpesvirus 6.**
2. Chang L, Hsia S, Wu C, et al: Outcome of enterovirus 71 infections with or without stage-based management: 1998–2002. Pediatr Infect Dis J 23:327–331, 2004. **Discussion of EV 71–associated neurologic disease and decreased fatality using a standardized treatment protocol based on disease stage.**
3. Kennedy PGE: Viral encephalitis: causes, differential diagnosis, and management. J Neurol Neurosurg Psychiatry 75 (Suppl 1): i10–i15, 2004. **Description of the causes, differential diagnosis, and management of viral encephalitis.**
4. Kimberlin DW: Herpes simplex virus infections of the central nervous system. Semin Pediatr Infect Dis 14:83–89, 2003. **Review of neonatal herpes simplex disease and herpes simplex encephalitis, with an emphasis on diagnostic techniques.**
5. Lipton JD, Schafermeyer RW: Central nervous system infections. The usual and the unusual. Emerg Med Clin North Am 13:417–443, 1995. **Discussion of several important categories of CNS infections, including viral meningitis and herpes simplex encephalitis.**
6. Rotbart HA: Viral meningitis. Semin Neurol 20:277–292, 2000. **Comprehensive review of important etiologies of viral meningitis, with an emphasis on enteroviruses.**
7. Vidwan G, Bryant K, Puri V, et al: West Nile virus encephalitis in a child with left-side weakness. Clin Infect Dis 37:e91–e94, 2003. **Description of West Nile virus encephalitis in a child, with a review of other reported pediatric cases.**
8. Watson JT, Gerber SI: West Nile virus: A brief review. Pediatr Infect Dis J 23:355–358, 2004. **Brief overview of West Nile virus epidemiology, clinical manifestations, laboratory diagnosis, therapy, and prevention.**
9. Weitkamp J, Spring MD, Brogan T, et al: Influenza A virus–associated acute necrotizing encephalopathy in the United States. Pediatr Infect Dis J 23:259–263, 2004. **Description of a case of influenza-associated acute necrotizing encephalopathy in the United States, with a review of the disease entity.**
10. Whitley RJ, Gnann JW: Viral encephalitis: Familiar infections and emerging pathogens. Lancet 359:507–514, 2002. **Discussion of pathogenesis and diagnosis of viral encephalitis, with focus on herpes simplex virus, rabies virus, arboviruses, and enteroviruses.**
11. Whitley RJ, Kimberlin DW: Viral encephalitis. Pediatr Rev 20:192–198, 1999. **Overview of viral encephalitis, with a discussion of important etiologies and an emphasis on herpes simplex virus.**

FUNGAL INFECTIONS

Aspergillosis

Kavita S. Seth and Sharon A. Nachman

KEY CONCEPTS

- Clinical manifestations of immunocompetent patients include allergic bronchopulmnoary aspergillosis, aspergillomas (fungal balls), otomycosis (nonallergic colonization), and fungal sinusitis.
- Clinical manifestations of immunocompromised patients include invastive aspergillosis.
- Route of transmission is inhalation of conidia (spores).
- Person-to-person spread does not occur.
- Diagnosis of aspergillosis encompasses clinical features, radiologic findings, and histologic identification in tissue.

Aspergillosis was first described as a human disease by Sluyter in 1847. However, the diverse clinical manifestations of aspergillosis were not described until 1952, and only recently was the importance of aspergillosis infection in immunosuppressed patients recognized. The widespread use of antimicrobials and immunosuppressive agents has resulted in systemic disseminated aspergillosis and an overall increase in incidence of aspergillosis infection.

Aspergillus species are ubiquitous molds that form on decaying vegetation and in soil. More than 180 species within the genus *Aspergillus* are described to date. *Aspergillus fumigatus* and *Aspergillus flavus* are the most common pathogens, and *Aspergillus nidulans*, *Aspergillus niger*, and *Aspergillus terreus* account for most of the remainder. *Aspergillus* is frequently isolated from the air because spores are lightweight, resistant to desiccation, and easily dispersed. Inhaled airborne conidia (spores) can be recovered from sputum for several days after exposure.

Aspergillosis infection comprises a variety of manifestations, including noninvasive and invasive disease (Box 1). The principal entities range from allergic bronchopulmonary aspergillosis (ABPA) or sinusitis, to pulmonary aspergilloma, to invasive aspergillosis that disseminates from the lungs to distal organs in severely immunocompromised patients.

Diagnosis of aspergillosis should be based on clinical and radiographic evidence of infection at a given site, isolation and identification of *Aspergillus* from the site, and histologic identification in the tissue. Suggestive of diagnosis is microscopic examination, which identifies dichotomously branched and septate hyphae. Definitive diagnosis is made by isolation of *Aspergillus* species in culture. The organism usually is not recovered from blood but is isolated readily from lung, sinus, and skin biopsy specimens.

BOX 1 Clinical Manifestations of Aspergillosis

Clinical manifestations in immunocompetent patients

- Allergic bronchopulmonary aspergillosis (ABPA)
  - Hypersensitivity to the fungus *Aspergillus fumigatus* in patients with underlying chronic asthma and cystic fibrosis
  - Manifestations include episodic wheezing, expectoration of brown mucus plugs, low-grade fever, eosinophilia, and transient pulmonary infiltrates
- Aspergillomas (fungal balls)
  - Usually benign saprophytic colonization of the lung with *Aspergillus* in patients with underlying lung disease (cystic fibrosis)
  - Semi-invasive aspergillosis is tissue invasion of *Aspergillus* in patients with mild to moderate degrees of immune suppression
- Otomycosis (nonallergic colonization)
  - Colonization of the external auditory canal by a fungal mat that produces a dark discharge (swimmer's ear)
- Fungal sinusitis
  - Allergic, saprophytic (fungal ball within the sinus), or invasive
  - Allergic sinusitis manifestations include allergic rhinitis, nasal polyposis, recurrent sinusitis, and occasionally asthma
  - Indolent form of invasive sinusitis occurs with chronic infection where there is high or persistent exposure to environmental molds

Clinical manifestations in immunocompromised patients

- Invasive aspergillosis
  - Risks for development of invasive disease includes underlying disease or medical intervention that impairs neutrophil function: Chronic granulomatous disease, human immunodeficiency virus (HIV) infection, congenital or acquired immunodeficiency, cytotoxic chemotherapy, and immunosuppressive therapy including prolonged corticosteroid use.
  - Most common site of invasive disease is pulmonary involvement manifested as necrotizing bronchopneumonia or hemorrhagic infarction because of the propensity to invade blood vessels.
  - Single or multiple abscesses, granulomata, or lobar infiltrates are occasionally present.
  - Dissemination to other organs can occur rarely.

Expert Opinion on Management Issues

DRUG THERAPY

The antifungal agents currently available for treatment of aspergillosis include deoxycholate amphotericin B, three lipid-based preparations of amphotericin B, itraconazole, oral and intravenous triazoles (voriconazole and posaconazole), and echinocandins (caspofungin acetate) (Table 1).

Therapy of invasive aspergillosis can be prophylactic; empirical based on clinical suspicion, particularly in the immunocompromised; or specific because of certainty of diagnosis. Intravenous therapy is usually preferred initially in the acutely ill.

Amphotericin B is the standard of treatment for life-threatening and severe infections. In general, studies show an overall response rate of 37% (range, 14% to 83%). Lipid-based formulations are often used in patients who develop nephrotoxicity on amphotericin B and in patients with marginal renal function or on other nephrotoxic drugs. The only clear advantage of lipid formulation amphotericin over conventional amphotericin is the slight decrease in nephrotoxicity and fewer infusion-related reactions, but no data indicate improved efficacy.

Itraconazole is a good alternative in those patients intolerant of amphotericin B. Two recent studies show a complete response rate of 39% and improved clinical symptoms of 63%. A logical sequence of therapy is to start with intravenous therapy until disease progression is arrested and then switch to the oral formulation. The oral form of itraconazole is an alternative to intravenous amphotericin in patients who are likely to adhere to prescribed therapy, unlikely to have problems with absorption, and who are not receiving drugs that interact with itraconazole or cannot be easily managed. Itraconazole is an inhibitor of the cytochrome P–450 enzyme and has important drug interactions, such as rifampin, phenytoin, carbamazepine, and phenobarbital. Any drug handled by the cytochrome P–450 pathway

should be closely monitored. Children and infants usually require a higher dosing (Table 2).

Voriconazole, a second-generation triazole and synthetic derivative of fluconazole, with both oral and parenteral bioavailability, has both fungicidal and fungistatic activity against *Aspergillus*. This drug is recommended for use in patients refractory to or intolerant of conventional antifungal therapy. Voriconazole is the only antifungal that inhibits *Aspergillus* conidiation and also has good cerebrospinal fluid (CSF) penetration. A review of 42 children with invasive aspergillus treated with voriconazole showed that the drug was well tolerated and had an overall response rate of 43%. A recent large prospective study demonstrates the superiority of voriconazole over amphotericin B as initial therapy for invasive aspergillosis, in terms of response rate, survival rate, and safety. Patients who initially received voriconazole had a better response rate (53%) compared with those initially receiving amphotericin B (32% response rate). Survival rates also improved with voriconazole (71%) versus amphotericin B (58%). Voriconazole was better tolerated than amphotericin B, with fewer adverse effects, fewer severe adverse events, and less discontinuation of therapy because of adverse events.

Caspofungin acetate (echinocandin), a glucan synthesis inhibitor, was approved by the Food and Drug Administration (FDA) for the treatment of invasive aspergillosis in patients who are refractory or intolerant of other therapies. A recent open-labeled, noncomparative, multicenter trial demonstrates the safety and efficacy of caspofungin for invasive aspergillosis. Of the 90 patients enrolled, 85.5% of the cases were refractory to standard therapy and yielded an overall favorable response rate of 45%. These patients were not necessarily refractory to voriconazole therapy. Caspofungin

---

TABLE 1 Selected Antifungal Agents with Activity against *Aspergillus*

Drug Class, Drug Name (Brand Name)	Formulation
Polyene	
Amphotericin B deoxycholate (Fungizone)	IV
Amphotericin B lipid complex (Abelcet)	IV
Amphotericin B colloidal dispersion (Amphocil; Amphotec)	IV
Liposomal Amphotericin B (AmBisome)	IV
Triazole	
Itraconazole (Sporanox)	PO, IV
Voriconazole (Vfend)	PO, IV
Echinocandin	
Caspofungin (Cancidas)	IV

IV, intravenous; PO, orally.

TABLE 2 Recommended Therapeutic Dosages for Invasive Aspergillosis

Drug	Dosage
Amphotericin B deoxycholate	1.0–1.5 mg/kg/day
Amphotericin B lipid complex	5 mg/kg/day
Amphotericin B colloidal dispersion	3–5 mg/kg/day
Liposomal amphotericin B	1–5 mg/kg/day
Itraconazole	PO: Loading dose: 800 mg for 3 days or 600 mg for 4 days Maintenance dose: 400 mg/day IV: 8–12 mg/kg/day
Voriconazole	Loading dose: 6 mg/kg IV q12h (2 doses) Maintenance dose: IV: 4 mg/kg q12h PO: (<40 kg) 100 mg q12h; (>40 kg) 200 mg q12h
Caspofungin	Initial 70 mg/m² IV, then 50 mg/m² IV

IV, intravenous; PO, orally; q*x*h, every *x* hours.

therapy was well tolerated by most patients, and drug-related toxicity was minimal.

Combination therapy that uses amphotericin with azoles may be successful in the future; however, this approach has had limited success in case reports. The role and efficacy of this combination is not established in invasive aspergillosis. The combination of echinocandins with triazoles remains hopeful; however, further studies are required.

The optimal duration of therapy for invasive aspergillosis is unknown and depends on the extent of disease, response to therapy, and underlying disease or immune status. Practice guidelines suggest that initial therapy be continued until the infection is stabilized radiographically and microbiologically, and that maintenance therapy with an alternative, perhaps less toxic, oral formulation be considered until complete resolution of radiographic findings and immune reconstitution.

The mainstay of management of ABPA is systemic corticosteroids and not antifungals. Although corticosteroids induce remission acutely, recurrent exacerbations continue to occur despite maintenance treatment with steroids, and the effect of corticosteroids on preservation of lung function is unknown. Although the role of antifungal therapy is unclear, only two antifungal agents are known to be efficacious for ABPA when used in conjunction with steroids: amphotericin B and the azoles (itraconazole and ketoconazole). Itraconazole use demonstrated a significant fall in markers of systemic immune activation and a reduction in markers of airway inflammation, requiring decreased use of steroids. Itraconazole, dosed at 200 to 400 mg/day for 16 to 32 weeks, resulted in reduction in corticosteroid dependence, circulating IgE, and improvement in pulmonary function. Longer term trials are needed before a firm recommendation can be made for treatment of ABPA with adjunctive itraconazole therapy. Ketoconazole reduces immune activation and symptoms but has no effect on lung function.

BEHAVIORAL/PSYCHOLOGICAL/SURGICAL THERAPY

Surgical excision is successful in the treatment of children with *Aspergillus* sinusitis, cerebral mycetoma, infected prosthetic valves, and localized pulmonic infections. Surgical resection combined with antifungal therapy is also used in endocarditis, bone infections, cutaneous aspergillosis, and endophthalmitis. For most other sites of *Aspergillus* infection, surgical debridement is not advantageous over medical therapy alone.

There is no consensus concerning treatment of aspergilloma; however, definitive therapy of aspergilloma is considered to be surgical resection in patients with life-threatening hemoptysis and normal pulmonary function. Pulmonary resection is associated with high mortality and morbidity because of the vascular pulmonary adhesions and possibility of aspergillus infection of the postsurgical space. Alternative treatment options for aspergillomas include radiation therapy, intracavitary or endobronchial instillation of

antifungal agents, inhaled nebulized antifungals, and systemic antifungals. Several retrospective, unblinded studies demonstrate that itraconazole is an efficacious modality of treatment for aspergilloma. The semi-invasive form of aspergilloma may necessitate systemic antifungal therapy because of the extrapulmonary extension of disease.

Therapy of fungal sinusitis can vary depending on the disease manifestation and the degree of immunocompetence of the host. Allergic sinusitis treatment requires surgical drainage with adjunctive therapy with nasal corticosteroids and saline douches for alleviation of allergic symptoms. A definitive role for systemic therapy is not established; however, antifungal therapy or systemic corticosteroids may decrease recurrence after drainage. Surgical debridement is the mainstay of therapy for fungal balls or mycetoma in the sinuses. Systemic antifungal therapy has no clear role except in the event of development of invasive disease. Chronic indolent invasive sinusitis in immunocompetent hosts requires surgical debridement and drainage and possible prolonged antifungal therapy. Invasive sinusitis, usually in the immunocompromised host, requires adequate surgical drainage and resection of tissues and bone when necrosis or extensive infection occurs, combined with antifungal therapy and withdrawal of immunosuppression.

In addition to antifungal therapy, other adjunctive modalities for therapy or prophylaxis in the neutropenic or immunocompromised host are under study. These include granulocyte transfusions, colony-stimulating factors, macrophage colony-stimulating factor, granulocyte-macrophage colony stimulating factor, or interferon-γ. These are not recommended for routine therapeutic use. Proof of increased survival is not demonstrated with any of these adjunctive modalities.

PREVENTIVE MEASURES

Preventive measures for invasive aspergillosis in immunosuppressed or neutropenic patients focus on attempts to reduce exposure to *Aspergillus* spores. Environmental measures reported to be effective include placement of suitable barriers between patient-care areas and construction sites, cleaning of air-handling systems, repair of faulty airflow, and replacement of contaminated air filters. High-efficiency particulate air filters and laminar flow rooms markedly decrease the risk of conidia in patient-care areas. Antifungal prophylaxis with amphotericin B nasal spray is effective in controlling respiratory or sinus colonization in neutropenic patients and is used in bone marrow transplant patients to reduce invasive aspergillosis. Prophylactic itraconazole with or without nasal amphotericin B in preliminary studies was effective for patients with prolonged granulocytopenia or chronic granulomatous disease from fatal aspergillosis.

Common Pitfalls

A few diagnostic pitfalls with regard to noninvasive aspergillosis include lack of specificity of fungal morphologic features in histologic samples and confusion of pathologic diagnosis with an etiologic diagnosis.

The therapeutic pitfall for invasive aspergillosis is that the optimal duration of therapy remains unknown. The treatment for noninvasive ABPA, combination therapy with itraconazole and inhaled corticosteroids, may induce adrenal suppression. Itraconazole may then potentiate other known side effects of corticosteroids, such as osteoporosis or cataract formation.

Communication and Counseling

Aspergillus species are now considered important fungal pathogens in both immunocompetent and immunosuppressed patients. There has been an increase of invasive aspergillosis because of an overall increase of the immunosuppressed population. Prevention of invasive aspergillosis in immunosuppressed patients requires reduction of exposure to *Aspergillus* spores in the environment. The introduction of new antifungals with variable activity against molds emphasizes new therapeutic alternatives other than amphotericin B. The role of the new antifungals in pediatric patients needs to be defined by large well-designed, prospective clinical trials.

SUGGESTED READINGS

1. American Academy of Pediatrics: Aspergillosis. Pickering LK (ed): Red Book: 2003 Report of the Committee on Infectious Diseases, 26th ed. Elk Grove Village, Ill: American Academy of Pediatrics, 2003, pp 208–210. **Brief overview of aspergillosis in children.**
2. Blum MD, Wiedermann BL: Aspergillus infections. In Feigin RD, Cherry JD, Demmler GJ, Kaplan SL (eds): Textbook of Pediatric Infectious Diseases, 5th ed. Philadelphia: Elsevier, 2004, pp 2550–2560. **Review of aspergillus infections in children.**
3. Herbrecht R, Denning DW, Patterson TF, et al: Voriconazole versus amphotericin B for primary therapy of invasive aspergillosis. N Engl J Med 357:408–415, 2002. **Study comparing the efficacy, safety, and tolerability of voriconazole with those of amphotericin B for primary therapy of invasive aspergillosis.**
4. Maertens J, Raad I, Petrikkos G, et al: Efficacy and safety of caspofungin for treatment of invasive aspergillosis in patients refractory to or intolerant of conventional antifungal therapy. Clin Infect Dis 39:1563–1571, 2004. **Study indicating the efficacy and safety of caspofungin in the treatment of invasive aspergillosis.**
5. Marr KA, Patterson T, Denning D: Aspergillosis: Pathogenesis, clinical manifestations, and therapy. Infect Dis Clin North Am 16:875–894, 2002. **Epidemiology and pathogenesis of diseases caused by Aspergillus** and diagnosis and therapy of invasive disease.
6. Steinbach WJ, Stevens DA: Review of newer antifungal and immunomodulatory strategies for invasive aspergillosis. Clin Infect Dis 37(Suppl 3):S157–S187, 2003. **Detailing the newer antifungals and immunomodulatory therapies for treatment of invasive aspergillosis.**
7. Stevens DA, Kan VL, Judson MA, et al: Practice guidelines for diseases caused by *Aspergillus*. Clin Infect Dis 30:696–709, 2000. **Extensive discussion of therapeutic recommendations for invasive aspergillosis, pulmonary aspergilloma, and ABPA.**
8. Walsh TJ, Lutsar I, Driscoll T, et al: Voriconazole in the treatment of aspergillosis, sebopsoriasis and other invasive fungal infections in children. Pediatr Infect Dis J 21:240–248, 2002. **Comprehensive report of the efficacy and safety of voriconazole in pediatric patients with invasive fungal infections.**
9. Wark PA, Gibson PG, Wilson AJ: Azoles for allergic bronchopulmonary aspergillosis associated with asthma. Cochrane Database Syst Rev 3:CD001108, 2004. **Discusses the efficacy of azoles in the treatment of ABPA.**

Blastomycosis: Recognition, Diagnosis, and Management

L. Joseph Wheat and John F. Marcinak

KEY CONCEPTS

- Blastomycosis is an endemic mycosis often overlooked until the patient is severely ill.
- The clinical spectrum of illness is variable, including asymptomatic infection, acute or chronic pneumonia, and disseminated disease. The skin, bones, and genitourinary system are the most frequent sites of extrapulmonary disease.
- Once suspected, knowledge of the strengths and limitations of the diagnostic tools is needed to make a prompt diagnosis. Rapid diagnosis can be achieved by cytologic evaluation of body fluids or tissues and by detection of a glycoprotein antigen in body fluids using a new immunoassay.
- Preferred treatment regimens include amphotericin B or itraconazole and should be tailored to the severity of the illness and immune status of the patient.
- Children treated with itraconazole or other azoles should be followed closely in the outpatient setting and monitored closely for adherence to therapy.

Blastomycosis, caused by the dimorphic fungus *Blastomyces dermatitidis*, is an important endemic mycosis in certain areas of the Americas that often afflicts children. In the United States, the highest attack rates are in Minnesota, Wisconsin, Alabama, Arkansas, Tennessee, Mississippi, and Missouri, often within so-called hyperendemic areas. Most patients do not recall exposure to the organism, but exposure is usually associated with outdoor activities bringing the individual into contact with water or soil. Because the clinical findings are not specific, blastomycosis is often overlooked. Difficulty in establishing the diagnosis poses a significant problem in children with the infection, and the average time to diagnosis is more than 2 months. Misdiagnosis as community-acquired pneumonia is common. Patients also may present with diffuse pulmonary infiltrates associated with respiratory failure, the acute respiratory distress syndrome (ARDS). In pediatric cases with pulmonary involvement, the chest radiographic findings may be indistinguishable from a bacterial process. The radiographic findings in children include nodules, focal or diffuse infiltrates or consolidation, cavities, pleural effusion associated with rib involvement, and hilar adenopathy.

Extrapulmonary dissemination is common in blastomycosis, usually in association with pulmonary involvement. Dissemination is usually recognized late in the course in patients who present with chronic illness. Skin lesions are the most common manifestations, followed by bone and genitourinary tract involvement. Central nervous system (CNS) involvement is uncommon, manifesting as meningitis or mass lesions. Blastomycosis during pregnancy presents a unique challenge because of the risk of transplacental infection and the teratogenic potential of triazole therapies.

Cultures provide the definitive diagnosis of blastomycosis, but growth may be slow, limiting the value for early diagnosis. In adults, cytology is useful for diagnosis in most cases with higher sensitivity for cytology (93.2%) compared to KOH (potassium hydroxide [stain]) preparation (48%) or histopathology (85%). Fungal serology in blastomycosis is limited by lack of accurate methods and not recommended by most experts because tests lack both sensitivity and specificity. A newly described antigen detection assay also is useful for rapid diagnosis. Using an enzyme immunoassay directed against *B. dermatitidis* antigen, antigenuria was detected in 93% of cases of disseminated or pulmonary blastomycosis. Cross-reactivity occurs in specimens from patients with histoplasmosis.

The recommended approach includes collection of specimens from the respiratory tract and extrapulmonary sites for cytology and fungal culture and collection of urine for antigen detection in cases of suspected pulmonary and/or disseminated blastomycosis. Table 1 presents guidelines for diagnosis. Cross-reactivity with *Histoplasma* antigens must be recognized, but the two mycoses usually can be distinguished by isolation of the fungus in culture, morphologic differences in cytology or histopathology, or clinical and epidemiologic characteristics. In patients with suspected pulmonary blastomycosis when antigen tests and cytology of respiratory specimens are negative, open-lung biopsy may be required.

Expert Opinion on Management Issues

Treatment is indicated in most patients with blastomycosis. In patients without underlying immunosuppression with isolated pulmonary infection, the course may be self-limited and observation is appropriate, with careful monitoring for progression. Treatment also is recommended in pregnant women to reduce the risk of transplacental infection. Table 2 summarizes the guidelines for treatment.

Antifungal therapy is highly effective if initiated before the infection becomes advanced. Amphotericin B and itraconazole are both effective, with response rates above 90% when initiated before patients become severely ill. Response to fluconazole appears to be lower than to itraconazole, although not directly compared. Concern was raised about the effectiveness of the azoles (most commonly ketoconazole) in pediatric patients, based on poor results when used alone or after a short course of amphotericin B. Single cases of pediatric patients with extrapulmonary disease successfully treated with amphotericin B followed by itraconazole are reported, however.

In the Infectious Diseases Society of America (IDSA) guideline document, amphotericin B is recommended for severe cases and itraconazole for others. A prolonged course of amphotericin B is preferred, acknowledging that a shorter course followed by itraconazole is an alternative regimen. Given the effectiveness of itraconazole and the cost, toxicity, and inconvenience of

---

TABLE 1 **Guidelines for Diagnosis of Blastomycosis**

Test	Cytology, Histopathology, and Fungal Culture	*Blastomyces* Antigen Enzyme Immunoassay (EIA)
Sputum	+	−
Bronchoscopy specimens	+	+
Biopsy specimens*	+	−
Urine	−[†]	+
Cerebrospinal fluid (CSF)	+[‡]	+[‡]
Other body fluids	+[§]	+[§]

*Skin lesions or other involved tissues if biopsy performed. Of note is that higher risk, invasive procedures may be delayed pending analysis of other specimens if the patient is not severely ill.
[†]Routine cytologic evaluation or fungal culture of urine is not recommended, but the genitourinary tract is often involved in disseminated cases, and analysis should be considered if the urine sediment is abnormal or there is evidence of involvement of the genitourinary tract.
[‡]CSF should be examined if there are neurologic or mental status abnormalities in the absence of evidence for increased intracranial pressure.
[§]Abnormal fluid collections should be tested by cytology, fungal culture, and antigen detection.

TABLE 2 **Guidelines for Treatment of Blastomycosis**

Clinical Parameter	Regimen
Pregnancy Immunosuppression Meningitis Moderate to severe disease in the nonimmunocompromised patient	Lipid amphotericin B 3-5 mg/kg/day or deoxycholate amphotericin B 0.7-1.0 mg/kg/day until clinically improved and ready for outpatient therapy.
	Full course of amphotericin B (≥35 mg/kg) or lipid formulation (≥105 mg/kg) if life-threatening infection, meningitis, or pregnancy.
Mild non-CNS disease in nonimmunocompromised and nonpregnant patient	Itraconazole, 5 mg/kg qd or bid for at least 6 mo and until resolution of clinical findings and antigenuria.
Continuation following response to amphotericin B	Lifelong suppressive therapy if persistent immunosuppression or repeated relapse.
Failure or intolerance of itraconazole	Fluconazole, 10 mg/kg qd, or posaconazole, 5 mg/kg bid, or voriconazole, 2.5 mg/kg bid.

bid, twice daily; CNS, central nervous system; qd, every day.

intravenous amphotericin B, perhaps itraconazole should be the treatment of choice, reserving amphotericin B for patients sufficiently ill to require hospitalization or who are pregnant. Following improvement in response to amphotericin B, early transition to itraconazole may be more appropriate than prolonged treatment with amphotericin B, except in pregnancy and CNS infection.

Itraconazole is recommended for mild cases in nonimmunocompromised patients and after improvement with amphotericin B in other cases. Itraconazole and other triazoles are teratogenic and should not be used in pregnancy, leaving amphotericin B the drug of choice. Therapy should last at least 6 months and until all clinical findings resolve. Based on experience in histoplasmosis, it may be prudent to continue therapy until resolution of antigenuria. Patients with osteomyelitis should receive at least 1 year of treatment with an azole. Measurement of itraconazole blood levels is recommended during the first few weeks of therapy to establish adequate drug exposure, with care also to exclude co-administration of medications that reduce itraconazole levels. Levels are expected to be in the range of 1 to 5 µg per mL. Although the itraconazole oral solution has several advantages, including ease of administration in young children and superior absorption to the capsule formulation, its taste is unpleasant to some patients. This characteristic of the oral solution may impair adherence.

Choice between the standard deoxycholate and more expensive but better tolerated lipid formulations of amphotericin B requires consideration in immunosuppressed patients and those with more severe manifestations. Mortality is high in the immunocompromised host and in those with respiratory failure, despite treatment with amphotericin B. By analogy to histoplasmosis, response rate and survival were higher in acquired immunodeficiency syndrome (AIDS) patients treated with liposomal than with deoxycholate amphotericin B.

Relapse occurs in 10% or more of patients with blastomycosis, most often because of inadequate drug exposure or duration of therapy. If relapse follows an inadequate course of therapy, treatment should be repeated with careful attention to adherence, optimization of dosage based on measuring itraconazole drug levels, and avoidance of drug interactions. Itraconazole has an excellent safety profile in children. The most common adverse effect, gastrointestinal upset, is usually mild and transient. Drug interactions that may reduce itraconazole exposure include those that reduce gastric acidity or stimulate hepatic cytochrome 3A4 enzyme metabolisms. The reduction in absorption caused by medications that reduce gastric acidity can be overcome by using the oral solution. Another reason for poor adherence is the high cost of itraconazole, so some families fail to purchase the medication or do not administer it as directed.

Alternative agents may be needed in patients who fail itraconazole because of inability to achieve therapeutic drug concentrations or who do not tolerate it. Other oral agents to consider include fluconazole, voriconazole, and posaconazole. Fluconazole at high dosage is effective as initial therapy in nearly 90% of cases in adults. Of note is that *Histoplasma capsulatum* has developed resistance to fluconazole during therapy in patients with AIDS, with resultant treatment failure. Whether fluconazole resistance will develop during treatment in blastomycosis is unknown. Voriconazole and posaconazole also are active against *B. dermatitidis*, with MIC90s (minimum inhibitory concentration for 90% of isolates) of 0.25 versus 0.06 µg/mL, respectively. Posaconazole is effective in murine models of blastomycosis, but neither it nor voriconazole have been studied in humans for this indication. The echinocandins (e.g., caspofungin) have not been studied in animal models or humans and should not be used for treatment of blastomycosis. Chronic suppressive therapy with itraconazole may be indicated in those with AIDS or severe immunosuppression because frequent relapses occur.

Common Pitfalls

Failure to consider the diagnosis of blastomycosis in children with persistent pulmonary symptoms and pneumonia leads to delay in treatment and risk for progression of disease. Relying on serology to make the diagnosis of blastomycosis can result in failure to establish the correct diagnosis as well as overdiagnosis.

Failure to treat children with life-threatening or CNS disease with the full course of amphotericin B therapy can result in failure. Other pitfalls include treating children with itraconazole without measuring drug levels, not determining if other medications are being taken that can reduce absorption of itraconazole, not scheduling close outpatient follow-up, and not paying attention to the issue of adherence, which increases risk for relapse.

Communication and Counseling

Most children with acute or chronic pneumonia as well as extrapulmonary disease with blastomycosis recover if they receive appropriate antifungal therapy. Parents of children who receive itraconazole should be informed of the importance of measuring blood levels of itraconazole, the common adverse effects of the medication, and the possible unpleasant taste of the oral suspension. Parents must be involved in medication administration and attention to adherence because the treatment is prolonged. All patients should be observed for relapse for at least 1 year following therapy.

SUGGESTED READINGS

1. Alkrinawi S, Reed MH, Pasterkamp H: Pulmonary blastomycosis in children: Findings on chest radiographs. Am J Roentgenol 165:651–654, 1995. **Detailed description of the radiographic findings in 16 children with culture-proven blastomycosis.**
2. Chapman SW, Bradsher RW Jr, Campbell GD Jr, et al: Practice guidelines for the management of patients with blastomycosis. Clin Infect Dis 30:679–683, 2000. **Evidence-based guidelines for the treatment of blastomycosis from the National Institute of Allergy and Infectious Diseases Mycoses Study Group and the Infectious Diseases Society of America.**

3. Chapman SW, Lin AC, Hendricks KA, et al: Endemic blastomycosis in Mississippi: Epidemiological and clinical studies. Semin Respir Infect 12:219–228, 1997. **Review of epidemiology, clinical findings, and outcome of therapy in well-characterized cases of blastomycosis.**

4. Davies SF, Sarosi GA: Epidemiological and clinical features of pulmonary blastomycosis. Semin Respir Infect 112:206–218, 1997. **Excellent chest radiographs of pulmonary blastomycosis.**

5. Dismukes WE, Bradsher RW Jr, Cloud GC, et al: Itraconazole therapy for blastomycosis and histoplasmosis. Am J Med 93:489–497, 1993. **Clinical trial establishing role of itraconazole for treatment of blastomycosis.**

6. Durkin M, Witt J, LeMonte A, et al: Antigen assay with the potential to aid in diagnosis of blastomycosis. J Clin Microbiol 42:4873–4875, 2004. **Description of antigen testing for diagnosis of blastomycosis.**

7. Gupta AK, Cooper EA, Ginter G: Efficacy and safety of itraconazole use in children. Dermatol Clin 21:521–535, 2003. **Good review of drug interactions and safety profile of itraconazole in children.**

8. Johnson PC, Wheat LJ, Cloud GA, et al: Safety and efficacy of liposomal amphotericin B compared with conventional amphotericin B for induction therapy of histoplasmosis in patients with AIDS. Ann Intern Med 137:105–109, 2002. **Clinical trial showing advantage of liposomal amphotericin B for treatment of disseminated histoplasmosis, as background for its potential use for treatment of blastomycosis in patients with more severe clinical manifestations.**

9. Lemos LB, Guo M, Baliga M: Blastomycosis: Organ involvement and etiologic diagnosis. A review of 123 patients from Mississippi. Ann Diagn Pathol 4:391–406, 2000. **Good review of laboratory diagnosis of blastomycosis.**

10. Schutze GE, Hickerson SL, Fortin EM, et al: Blastomycosis in children. Clin Infect Dis 22:496–502, 1996. **Reviews ten children with blastomycosis, five with isolated pulmonary disease, four requiring open-lung biopsy for diagnosis.**

Candidiasis

Natalie Neu and Christine J. Kubin

KEY CONCEPTS

- Candidiasis may occur in both immunocompetent and immunocompromised hosts. Systemic invasive disease usually only occurs in immunocompromised individuals or individuals with specific risk factors.
- Speciation and susceptibility testing of the *Candida* species is an important tool for antifungal management. Most species are susceptible to amphotericin B and fluconazole. Exceptions to this are *Candida lusitaniae,* which is intrinsically resistant to amphotericin and requires treatment with an azole agent, and *Candida krusei,* which is intrinsically resistant to fluconazole.
- Prophylactic therapy with an azole agent (e.g., fluconazole) is common in certain at-risk populations. This has implications for the development of more resistant *Candida* species.

Candida is a yeast, which on culture media appears as a white, creamy smooth colony. Infections with *Candida* species may occur in both immunocompetent and immunocompromised hosts. Although *Candida albicans* is the most common species in the past 20 years, other species have increased in prevalence because of antibiotic and antifungal pressures. Other significant species include *Candida parapsilosis, Candida glabrata, Candida tropicalis, Candida krusei, Candida guilliermondii,* and *Candida lusitaniae. Candida* species may colonize the gastrointestinal tract and can cause disease when a host has an increased susceptibility to infection and a high organism burden. Conditions that can increase susceptibility to candidal infection include chemotherapy and corticosteroids (abnormal cellular immunity), human immunodeficiency virus (HIV) infection (decreased CD4 counts), diabetes mellitus, endocrine disorders, congenital immune deficiencies, foreign bodies (including intravascular catheters and urinary catheters), and broad-spectrum antibiotics in which normal flora is decreased, leading to an overgrowth of *Candida* in the intestines.

Candida infections can be cutaneous, mucocutaneous, or systemic. *Candida* infections usually occur from an endogenous source but may be transmitted from person to person (e.g., during childbirth and sexual contact). Diagnosis is made by direct examination with potassium hydroxide (KOH) and by culture on Sabouraud agar. Fermentation and agglutination reactions are useful for determining the *Candida* species. Successful therapy for candidiasis requires treatment of the host immune system and the infection itself, which often includes removal of foreign bodies (e.g., catheters). Prophylactic therapy for children at risk for fungal disease (e.g., preterm infants, HIV-infected children), especially those on broad-spectrum antimicrobials, is becoming the mainstay of therapy. Although fungal susceptibility testing in not yet standardized, testing should be done to help guide management.

Expert Opinion on Management Issues

Table 1 lists the currently available antifungal agents, their primary clinical indication, Food and Drug Administration (FDA) approval, and other specific comments. The Infectious Disease Society of America has published guidelines for the treatment of candidiasis. Table 2 is adapted from the treatment guidelines presented in *Clinical Infectious Diseases* in 2004.

MUCOCUTANEOUS CANDIDAL DISEASES

Mucocutaneous candidiasis includes oral, esophageal, cutaneous diaper dermatitis, and vaginal types. If initial therapy with topical medications fails, treatment should be changed to an oral azole antifungal. Oral azoles include fluconazole, ketoconazole, voriconazole, or itraconazole. If itraconazole is used, the solution is preferred because it is better absorbed than itraconazole capsules. Oral polyenes (nystatin and amphotericin B) are also effective. Esophageal disease does not respond to topical therapy, and thus oral or intravenous therapy is needed. Alternative therapy or therapy for refractory cases includes the use of intravenous antifungal agents. Some patients with mucocutaneous

12

TABLE 1 Systemic Antifungal Agents, Mechanism of Action, and Indications for Use

Class	Drug	Mechanism of Action	Formulation	FDA-Approved Indications for *Candida* species	FDA-Approved Dosing for Pediatric Use	Comments
Triazole	Fluconazole	Inhibits C–14a methylation of lanosterol in fungi by binding to CYP–450 enzymes leading to reduced concentrations of ergosterol, a sterol comprising the fungal membrane.	PO and IV	Vaginal, oropharyngeal, and esophageal candidiasis; prophylaxis in patients receiving bone marrow transplants or cytotoxic chemotherapy.	Yes	Extensive clinical experience with this drug; well tolerated. Activity against most *Candida* species, but fluconazole-resistant strains have emerged (susceptibility testing recommended).
Triazole	Itraconazole		PO and IV	None	No	Few studies evaluating its use in invasive candidiasis; no pediatric studies using IV formulation. Significant phlebitis with IV preparation. Caution with IV formulation in patients with creatinine clearance <30 mL/min as cyclodextrin component accumulates. Significant drug interactions via cytochrome P–450 enzyme system. Oral solution better absorbed than oral capsules.
Triazole	Voriconazole		PO and IV	Candidemia and invasive candidiasis; esophageal candidiasis.	No	Activity against fluconazole-resistant *Candida* species but cross-resistance reported. Limited data in pediatric patients. Significant drug interactions via cytochrome P–450 enzyme system. Caution with IV formulation in patients with creatinine clearance <50 mL/min as cyclodextrin component accumulates. Visual disturbances common early in therapy but usually no need to discontinue therapy.
Echinocandin	Caspofungin	Blocks synthesis of β–1,3-D-glucan, an essential component of the cell wall that leads to disruption of the cell wall integrity and cell death.	IV only	Candidemia and invasive candidiasis; esophageal candidiasis; empirical antifungal therapy for patients with fever and neutropenia.	No	Activity against *Candida* species including fluconazole-resistant strains. Some *Candida parapsilosis* do not clinically respond well to caspofungin. Some studies with small numbers of patients appear to show safety and efficacy in pediatrics.

Class	Agent	Mechanism of action	Route	Use		Comments
Polyene	Amphotericin B deoxycholate (conventional)	Binds to sterols in fungal cytoplasmic membranes and creates pores and channels which increase cell membrane permeability and lead to cell death.	IV only	Invasive fungal infections (systemic candidiasis).	No	Considered the standard for antifungals and used successfully in pediatric patients. Activity against most *Candida* species (including azole-resistant strains). *Candida lusitaniae* usually resistant.
Lipid-associated formulations of amphotericin B	Lipid complex (ABLC; Abelcet)		IV only	Invasive fungal infections.	Yes	Approval as second-line therapy for those intolerant (renal dysfunction) or those with refractory disease. Less nephrotoxicity, but higher cost compared to conventional amphotericin B.
	Colloidal dispersion (ABCD; Amphotec)		IV only		Yes	Similar toxicity to conventional amphotericin B and rarely used.
	Liposomal (L-AmB; AmBisome)		IV only	Empirical antifungal therapy for patients with fever and neutropenia; *Candida* species infection in patients refractory to amphotericin B deoxycholate or with renal impairment or toxicity that precludes the use of amphotericin B deoxycholate.	Yes	Less infusion-related side effects compared to lipid complex amphotericin B (Abelcet) without premedications, but higher cost.

FDA, Food and Drug Administration; IV, intravenous; PO, by mouth.

TABLE 2 Treatment Guidelines for Candidiasis

Condition	Therapy			Comments
	Primary	**Alternative**	**Duration**	
Candidemia				
Non-neutropenic Adults	AmB, 0.6–1.0 mg/kg/day IV; or Flu, 400–800 mg/day IV or PO; or Casp[1]	AmB, 0.7 mg/kg/day, plus Flu, 800 mg/day for 4–7 days, then Flu, 800 mg/day	14 days after last positive blood culture and resolution of signs and symptoms.	Remove all intravascular catheters, if possible.
Children	AmB, 0.6–1.0 mg/kg/day IV; or Flu, 6 mg/kg q12h IV or PO; LFAmB, 3–5 mg/kg/day[2]	Casp	14–21 days after resolution of signs and symptoms and negative repeat blood cultures.	PK data in children for Casp are not available.[3]
Neonates	AmB, 0.6–1.0 mg/kg/day IV; or Flu, 5–12 mg/kg/day IV; LFAmB, 3–5 mg/kg/day	Casp	14–21 days after resolution of signs and symptoms and negative repeat blood cultures.	PK data in neonates for Casp are not available.
Neutropenia	AmB, 0.7–1.0 mg/kg/day IV; or LFAmB, 3.0–6.0 mg/kg/day; or Casp	Flu, 6–12 mg/kg/day IV or PO	14 days after last positive blood cultures and resolution of signs and symptoms and resolved neutropenia.	Removal of all intravascular catheters is controversial in neutropenic patients; gastrointestinal source is common.
Chronic disseminated candidiasis (hepatosplenic)	AmB, 0.6–0.7 mg/kg/day or LFAmB, 3–5 mg/kg/day	Flu, 6 mg/kg/day or Casp	3–6 mo and resolution or calcification of radiologic lesions.	Flu may be given after 1–2 wk of AmB therapy if clinically stable or improved.
Disseminated cutaneous neonatal candidiasis	AmB, 0.5–1.0 mg/kg/day	Flu, 6–12 mg/kg/day	14–21 days after clinical improvement.	Treat as for neonatal candidemia.
Endocarditis	AmB, 0.6–1.0 mg/kg/day IV; or LFAmB, 3.0–6.0 mg/kg/day plus 5-FC, 25–37.5 mg/kg PO q6h (adjusted for serum level of 40–60 μg/mL)	Flu, 6–12 mg/kg/day PO or IV; Casp	At least 6 wk after valve replacement; if no surgery is performed, long-term suppression may be necessary.	In adults, valve replacement is almost always necessary; surgery in premature neonates is usually not necessary; right-sided lesion; long-term suppression may be necessary.

Osteomyelitis and arthritis	AmB, 0.6–1.0 mg/kg/day IV; Flu, 6–12 mg/kg/day (if susceptible isolate)	—	Initial treatment with AmB, 2–3 wk, followed by 6–12 mo.
Meningitis	AmB, 0.6–1.0 mg/kg/day IV; or LFAmB, 3.0–6.0 mg/kg/day plus 5-FC, 25–37.5 mg/kg PO q6h (adjusted for serum level of 40–60 µg/mL)	LFAmB, Flu for follow-up or long-term suppression	Minimum 4 wk. Surgical debridement is critical for successful therapy. Removal of all neurosurgical prosthetic devices.
Endophthalmitis	AmB, 0.7–1.0 mg/kg/day IV; or Flu, 6–12 mg/kg/day PO or IV (limited data)	—	6–12 wk after surgery. Vitrectomy is usually performed when vitreitis is present.
Oropharyngeal	Clo, 10 mg 5 times/day, or Nys, 200,000–400,000 U 5 times/day (4 times/day for younger children), or Flu, 100–200 mg/day PO	Itr, 200 mg/day PO, or AmB, 1 mL q6h PO,[4] or AmB, >0.3 mg/kg/day IV,[4] or Casp, 50 mg/day IV[4]	7–14 days after clinical improvement. Long-term suppression with Flu (200 mg/day) in patients with AIDS and a history of OPC is acceptable and does not appear to lead to Flu resistance.
Esophageal	Flu, 100–200 mg/day PO or IV/ Flu for children: 3–6 mg/kg/day PO or IV, or Itr, 200 mg/day; Itr for children: 2.5 mg/kg/day oral solution	Vor, 4 mg/kg q12h IV or PO; AmB, 0.3–0.7 mg/kg/day IV,[5] or Casp[5]	14–21 days after clinical improvement. IV therapy is necessary for patients with severe and/or refractory esophagitis.
Genital candidiasis	Topical azoles (e.g., clotrimazole, nystatin, Terazol, etc.)	Oral Flu, 150 mg; boric acid (600-mg gelatin capsule daily)	1–7 days for topical therapy; oral: 1 day; boric acid: 14 days. May need longer course of oral therapy.

[1]Casp dosing in adults consists of 70-mg loading dose followed by 50 mg IV daily.

[2]The use of LFAmB has been studied and used in pediatric patients in treatment of candidemia. This information appears in the text of the guidelines.

[3]Casp dosing of 50 mg/m²/day provides comparable concentration time curves in pediatric patients (2–12 yr). Two articles support this dosing: Walsh T, Adamson P, Siebel N, et al: Pharmacokinetics of caspofungin in pediatric patients. In 42nd Interscience Conference on Antimicrobial Agents and Chemotherapy, M–896, 2002. Washington, DC: American Society of Microbiology, 2002. (Abstract 395); and Cesaro S, Toffolutti T, Messina C, et al: Safety and efficacy of caspofungin and liposomal amphotericin B, followed by voriconazole in young patients affected by refractory invasive mycosis. Eur J Haematol 73:50–55, 2004.

[4]AmB IV and PO/IV Casp for refractory or pharyngeal candidiasis are FDA-approved indications in adults. No FDA indication for pediatrics.

[5]Vor, AmB, and Casp are FDA approved in adults for severe and/or refractory esophageal candidiasis. Clinical experience and dosing available for use of voriconazole in children 12 years and older for esophageal candidiasis.

AIDS, acquired immune deficiency syndrome; AmB, conventional deoxycholate amphotericin B; Casp, caspofungin; Clo, clotrimazole; 5-FC, 5-flucytosine; Flu, fluconazole; Itr, itraconazole; IV, intravenous; LF, lipid formulation; LFAmB, amphotericin B; Nys, nystatin; OPC, oral pharyngeal candidiasis; PK, pharmacokinetic; PO, by mouth; qxh, every x hours; Vor, voriconazole.

Adapted from Pappas P, Rex J, Sobel J, et al: Guidelines for treatment of candidiasis. Clin Infect Dis 38:161–189, 2004.

candidiasis relapse, and some require chronic prophylaxis to prevent recurrences. In a healthy host without risk factors, the presence of mucocutaneous (specifically esophageal candidiasis) should be evaluated for immune deficiency (e.g., HIV testing). Disseminated cutaneous neonatal candidiasis in a preterm infant requires intravenous therapy with amphotericin or alternatively fluconazole. Although vaginal candidiasis is common in adolescents on birth control, the possibility of pregnancy and immune deficiency in this age group should be explored.

HEMATOGENOUS DISSEMINATED CANDIDAL INFECTIONS

Candida may disseminate hematogenously to other organs, including the eyes, liver, spleen, heart, lungs, kidneys, meninges, and bones. Infections often begin as catheter-related infections, and thus early removal of the catheter is critical to contain the dissemination of the infection. All patients with candidemia should have an ophthalmologic examination to rule out retinal disease. This examination should preferably occur when the infection is under control and unlikely to have further hematogenous spread. Likewise, in a neonate with candidemia, the spinal fluid should be examined to rule out meningitis because this will also change the length of therapy. In neutropenic patients, the ophthalmologic examination must be repeated when the patient recovers white blood cells.

Patients with persistent fevers and those with neutropenia should have CT scans of the lungs, liver, spleen, and kidneys to rule out disseminated disease. Ultrasound may also be useful for diagnosis and therapeutic monitoring of renal candidiasis. Candiduria may be an initial sign of disseminated candidal disease. However, it is most often associated with an indwelling catheter. Removal of the catheter and treatment for 7 to 14 days with fluconazole for high-risk patients (symptomatic, neutropenic, infant of low birth weight, patients with renal allografts, and patients who will undergo urologic manipulations) are recommended. Table 2 reviews the key management issues for disseminated infections.

Common Pitfalls

Treatment for candidiasis is often started empirically. Therapy needs to be monitored and altered for efficacy, safety, and drug interactions. Evaluating isolates for susceptibility is crucial for successful therapy and should be performed by a laboratory with clinical experience in fungal susceptibility testing. New antifungal agents are being developed, but often safety and efficacy studies are not performed in pediatric populations. Caution must be used in applying adult pharmacokinetic data to the use of these new antifungal agents in the pediatric population.

Communication and Counseling

Candidiasis is a serious condition that usually occurs in children with preexisting medical conditions that place them at risk for this infection. Parents need to be aware of the possibility of candidal infections complicating the care of critically ill hospitalized children. Over the last 5 years, the number of antifungal agents that are effective in treating serious candidal infections has increased; however, some of these therapies are not yet studied in the pediatric population. Physicians need to be aware of the pediatric populations most at risk for candidal disease. Physicians might consider surveillance for candidemia in high-risk patients and the use of prophylactic antifungal agents in those at high risk for disease. Management of patients with candidemia should occur in consultation with an infectious disease specialist.

SUGGESTED READINGS

1. Ellis M, Al-Abdely H, Sandridge A, et al: Fungal endocarditis: Evidence in the world literature, 1965–1995. Clin Infect Dis 32:50–62, 2001. **Overview of the changes presented in the literature of fungal endocarditis with an emphasis on clinical presentations, risk factors, fungal organisms, and therapeutic management.**
2. Hughes W, Armstrong D, Bodey G, et al: 2002 guidelines for the use of antimicrobial agents in neutropenic patients with cancer. Clin Infect Dis 34:730–751, 2002. **The Infectious Disease Society of America guidelines on the use of antimicrobials and antifungal agents in neutropenic patients.**
3. Kaufman D, Boyle R, Hazen K, et al: Fluconazole prophylaxis against fungal colonization and infection in preterm infants. N Engl J Med 345:1660–1666, 2001. **Prospective randomized clinical trial showing the efficacy of prophylactic fluconazole in the prevention of fungal colonization and invasive disease in infants weighing less than 1000 g.**
4. Pappas P, Rex J, Sobel J, et al: Guidelines for treatment of candidiasis. Clin Infect Dis 38:161–189, 2004. **Evidence-based guidelines for the treatment of candidal infections organized by disease state with a thorough description of each antifungal agent now available.**
5. Saiman L, Ludington E, Pfaller M, et al: Risk factors for candidemia in neonatal intensive care unit patients. Pediatr Infect Dis J 19:319–332, 2000. **National multicenter prospective cohort study evaluating the incidence and risk factors for neonatal candidemia.**
6. Walsh T, Witcomb P, Piscitelli S, et al: Safety, tolerance, and pharmacokinetics of amphotericin B lipid complex in children with hepatosplenic candidiasis. Antimicrob Agents Chemother 41:1944–1948, 1997. **The first study to investigate the safety, tolerance, and pharmacokinetics of lipid complex amphotericin in children.**

Coccidioidomycosis

Ziad M. Shehab

KEY CONCEPTS

- The diagnosis of coccidioidomycosis requires a high index of suspicion. A good history should be obtained regarding living or passing through endemic areas of the Southwest.
- Pulmonary coccidioidomycosis is usually an asymptomatic infection.

- Symptoms of fever, cough, fatigue, and/or pleuritic chest pain occur in 40% of infected individuals. The illness is usually self-limited.
- Extrapulmonary dissemination occurs in 0.5% of infected individuals. The rate of dissemination is higher among those of Filipino or African American ancestry.
- Extrapulmonary dissemination usually involves the central nervous system, bones, or cutaneous structures.
- Diagnostic tests include serology, microscopic inspection of tissue specimens, and fungal cultures of lower respiratory secretions or tissue specimens.
- All immunocompromised individuals and all those with disseminated disease require therapy, typically with an azole.

Coccidioidomycosis is an endemic mycosis of the southwestern United States caused by the dimorphic fungus *Coccidioides immitis*. In the United States, it is distributed in the Lower Sonoran Life Zone, which includes the deserts of California, Arizona, New Mexico, and western Texas. The organism lives in the superficial layers of the soil and becomes aerosolized during windstorms or when the soil is disrupted. The initial infection is acquired via the respiratory route. In most patients, the infection remains localized to the lungs and hilar nodes. In 0.5% of infected individuals, dissemination to extrapulmonary sites occurs, typically the central nervous system, musculoskeletal system, or the skin. The majority of cases are diagnosed in the endemic areas of the Southwest; however, 10% to 15% of cases are identified elsewhere.

Sixty percent of primary infections are subclinical or resemble a mild upper respiratory tract infection. Approximately 1 to 3 weeks after exposure, 40% of infected individuals develop symptoms of a mild febrile respiratory illness, of an influenza-like syndrome, or of a severe lower respiratory tract infection manifested by pneumonic infiltrates, sometimes pleural effusions, and rarely pericarditis. The illness is usually subacute and self-limited but may be severe in some patients. The clinical presentation is most commonly that of cough and fever often associated with chest pain, chills, dyspnea, and fatigue. Fever occurs in approximately half the patients. Findings of eosinophilia, severe pleuritic chest pain, and cutaneous manifestations, such as erythema nodosum or erythema multiforme, are helpful clues. Radiologically, single or multiple bronchopneumonic infiltrates are the most common findings. They are accompanied by hilar adenopathy in 20% of the cases. Small pleural effusions are common. These findings are self-limited in 90% to 95% of individuals and do not require any specific therapy. Cavities and nodule formation develop later in approximately 5% of patients. The cavities can lead to abscesses or to pyopneumothoraces. A miliary pattern on chest radiograph is sometimes seen and represents hematogenous dissemination. Calcifications are seen in 10% of nodules and are usually single. Primary cutaneous infection is rare and usually self-limited.

Disseminated infection is unusual and occurs in 0.5% of infected individuals. It is more common in young infants, immunosuppressed individuals, and children of certain ethnic groups, especially those of Filipino, Chinese, African American, and Hispanic origin. Meningitis is often the only site of extrapulmonary disease and may manifest early on with a picture of aseptic meningitis. More commonly, it appears later with manifestations of headache, ataxia, and sometimes signs of hydrocephalus. Osteomyelitis is usually chronic, and it is multifocal in 40% of cases. It typically involves the long bones, vertebrae, metacarpals and metatarsals, and skull. Cutaneous dissemination manifests with cold abscesses, ulcers, and chronic sinus tract formation or with verrucous lesions, typically around the nasolabial fold. Coccidioidomycosis can also occur during pregnancy and is usually associated with significant complications. People with T cell deficiencies and organ transplant recipients are at risk for more severe disease including dissemination. They may also experience reactivation of a latent infection leading to significant pulmonary or extrapulmonary disease.

The diagnosis is established by direct demonstration of the organism on culture or stains; alternatively, the infection can be diagnosed by demonstration of immunoglobulin (Ig) M or IgG antibodies in the serum or in the spinal fluid.

Expert Opinion on Management Issues

Antifungal therapy is given to a minority of patients with coccidioidomycosis. The decision to treat takes into consideration a variety of factors, such as the severity of the illness, ethnicity, immunologic status, and risk of dissemination (Box 1).

UNCOMPLICATED PRIMARY PULMONARY INFECTION

Coccidioidal disease is self-limited in more than 90% of children with primary infection. These children do not need antifungal therapy. Healthy individuals who present with a pulmonary infiltrate or an asymptomatic thin-walled nodule or a cavity do not need any

---

BOX 1   Indications for Antifungal Therapy in Coccidioidomycosis

- Significant weight loss
- Night sweats >3 wk
- Extensive pulmonary infiltrates
- Hilar adenopathy: prominent or persistent
- Paratracheal adenopathy
- Symptoms >2 mo
- Coccidioidal complement fixation titer >1:16
- Evidence of extrapulmonary dissemination
- Immunodeficiency (especially T cell)
- Neoplasm
- Neonates and young infants
- Pregnancy, especially third trimester
- Severe primary infection in certain ethnic groups, especially Filipinos and African Americans

antifungal therapy, even though they may have positive cultures from sputum or from resected surgical specimens. These patients can be safely observed and require clinical, serologic, and radiologic follow-up for at least 1 year to document resolution of disease and to look for evidence of any dissemination.

Therapy is reserved for those with significant weight loss, night sweats lasting longer than 3 weeks, extensive infiltrates (more than half of one lung or bilateral disease), prominent or persistent hilar adenopathy, symptoms lasting longer than 2 months, or coccidioidal complement fixation titers of more than 1:16. Therapy is also indicated for pregnant women, especially those with disease in the third trimester of pregnancy or in the perinatal period; neonates; and very young children. Treatment should be considered for persons at high risk of dissemination, such as children of Filipino or African ancestry. The therapy consists of a 3- to 6-month course of an oral azole, usually fluconazole or itraconazole. Fluconazole is given as a single daily dose of 10 to 12 mg/kg, and itraconazole is given at 5 mg/kg twice a day. Itraconazole levels should be monitored because the bioavailability of the drug is variable.

COMPLICATED PNEUMONIA

Patients with symptomatic pulmonary cavities manifested by local discomfort, secondary fungal or bacterial infections, or hemoptysis may benefit from a course of azole therapy. Alternatively, surgical resection of the cavity is a good alternative to chronic antifungal therapy. Individuals with a ruptured cavity leading to a pyopneumothorax should receive antifungal therapy in addition to a lobectomy.

The finding of reticulonodular or miliary infiltrates on chest radiograph suggests hematogenous dissemination and is frequently associated with the presence of an immunodeficiency. These patients should be started on amphotericin B. The treatment can be changed to an azole once improvement is apparent. These children should be evaluated for the presence of immunodeficiency. Therapy should be continued for at least 1 year; in the case of immunodeficient patients, suppressive therapy should be lifelong (Table 1).

Patients with chronic pneumonia are treated with azoles. Surgical resection may be indicated if the disease is localized and significant hemoptysis occurs.

EXTRAPULMONARY DISSEMINATION

All patients with extrapulmonary disease should receive antifungal therapy, which is usually initiated with amphotericin B for rapidly progressive infections. The azoles have largely replaced amphotericin B in more chronic forms of the disease.

Amphotericin B is generally started at a dose of 0.5 mg/kg/day, which is rapidly escalated in 1 to 2 days to 1 mg/kg/dose. The dose is given intravenously over 2 to 4 hours. Its administration is usually preceded by 20 mL/kg of normal saline. A premedication regimen of acetaminophen and chlorphenhydramine is used to decrease the drug's side effects. Meperidine (1 mg/kg) is the drug of choice for amphotericin-induced chills. Nephrotoxicity is common and manifested by decreased glomerular filtration, renal potassium and magnesium wasting, and renal tubular acidosis. Initially, monitoring of renal function is necessary daily. After a period of time, the frequency of administration

TABLE 1 Antifungal Agents Used in the Treatment of Coccidioidomycosis

Generic Name (Trade Name)	Dosage/Route/ Regimens	Maximum Dose	Dosage Formulations	Common Adverse Reactions	Comments
Amphotericin deoxycholate (Amphotec)	1 mg/kg/day IV for a total dose of 35 mg or more	Undefined	IV.	Fever, chills, decreased glomerular filtration rate, hypokalemia, hypomagnesemia	Liposomal preparations may be good substitutes in children who cannot tolerate amphotericin B.
Ketoconazole (Nizoral)	10 mg/kg/day for ≥6 mo	800 mg	200-mg tablet; liquid formulation can be prepared with limited shelf half-life.	GI upset, suppression of pituitary adrenal axis	
Fluconazole (Diflucan)	10–12 mg/kg PO or IV; single daily dose	800 mg	Tablet (50, 100, 150, or 200 mg). Oral suspension: (10 mg/mL or 40 mg/mL). IV: 20 mg/mL.	GI symptoms in <10% of children	Bioequivalence between oral and intravenous drug; may be teratogenic.
Itraconazole (Sporanox)	10 mg/kg divided bid	400 mg	Tablet: 100 mg. Oral suspension: 10 mg/mL. IV: 10 mg/mL.	GI upset in 10% of patients	Numerous drug interactions. Tablet: Improved bioavailability with meals. Oral liquid: Better bioavailability in fasted state.

bid, twice daily; GI, gastrointestinal; IV, intravenous; PO, by mouth.

can be changed to three times per week. In cases of prolonged use of amphotericin, the insertion of a central venous catheter obviates the common side effects of phlebitis. Once the patient improves, typically after a period of a few weeks, therapy can be changed to an oral azole. Doses of up to 25 mg/kg or more are used. Amphotericin's cerebrospinal fluid penetration is limited and its intrathecal administration can be complicated by arachnoiditis.

MENINGITIS

Fluconazole is the drug of choice in the treatment of meningeal coccidioidal infections, with itraconazole as an alternative. These azoles supersede the use of ketoconazole, which penetrates poorly into the cerebrospinal fluid. The usual starting dose of fluconazole is 400 mg/day in adults or 10 to 12 mg/kg/day in children. Adults can be treated with daily doses as high as 800 to 1000 mg of fluconazole or 400 to 600 mg of itraconazole. Treatment with azoles is lifelong because relapse rates are very high after discontinuation of therapy. Hydrocephalus is a common complication of meningitis in children and often the presenting symptom. It requires shunting for decompression of the ventricles. Intrathecal or intraventricular administration of amphotericin has no role, except possibly in patients who do not respond to the azoles. The role of voriconazole remains to be defined; case reports suggest it might have a role in patients failing fluconazole therapy.

NONMENINGEAL DISSEMINATION

Cutaneous dissemination is readily treated with azoles. Large soft tissue abscesses require drainage. Osteomyelitis requires long-term chemotherapy and is best treated with drainage and curetting of the involved bone, when feasible. Studies in adults indicate that itraconazole is more effective than fluconazole for this form of dissemination and equivalent to amphotericin therapy. Fluconazole has excellent bioavailability and can be given once a day with meals, a major advantage over itraconazole, which is given twice a day, erratically absorbed, and ideally given on an empty stomach. As a result, I continue to use fluconazole in younger children as the primary azole with all forms of disseminated disease. Treatment is usually given for at least 1 year. In all forms of dissemination, therapy is guided by the clinical response and the monitoring of coccidioidal complement fixation titers.

Common Pitfalls

- Failure to consider the diagnosis of coccidioidomycosis, especially in areas where coccidioidomycosis is not endemic, is a major pitfall.
- Rarely, serologic diagnosis may lag behind the development of symptoms, making the diagnosis difficult to establish.
- Failure to maintain immunosuppressed individuals on suppressive antifungal therapy may lead to reactivation of infection.

- Failure to diagnose and treat immunosuppressed individuals promptly may lead to rapid progression of disease.

Communication and Counseling

Most children with coccidioidomycosis make an uneventful recovery without the administration of any antifungal therapy. Those with complicated infections and immunosuppressed individuals need antifungal therapy, which is typically long term and, in the case of meningitis, lifelong.

SUGGESTED READINGS

1. Dewsnup DH, Galgiani JN, Graybill JR, et al: Is it ever safe to stop azole therapy for *Coccidioides immitis* meningitis? Ann Intern Med 124:305–310, 1996. **A paper documenting very high relapse rate of meningitis if therapy is stopped.**
2. Drutz DJ: Amphotericin in the treatment of coccidioidomycosis. Drugs 26:337–346, 1983. **Reviews the use of amphotericin for the treatment of coccidioidal infections.**
3. Galgiani JN, Ampel NM, Catanzaro A, et al: Practice guidelines for the treatment of coccidioidomycosis. Clin Infect Dis 30:658–661, 2000. **Current practice guidelines.**
4. Galgiani JN, Catanzaro A, Cloud GA, et al: Comparison of oral fluconazole and itraconazole for progressive nonmeningeal coccidioidomycosis. A randomized double blind trial. Ann Intern Med 133:676–686, 2000. **The only randomized trial of coccidioidal therapy.**
5. Graybill JR, Stevens DA, Galgiani JN, et al: Itraconazole treatment of coccidioidomycosis. NIAID Mycoses Study Group. Am J Med 89:282–290, 1990. **Results of itraconazole trials in the treatment of coccidioidomycosis.**
6. Shehab ZM, Britton H, Dunn JH: Imidazole therapy of coccidioidal meningitis in children. Pediatr Infect Dis J 7:40–44, 1988. **Early studies of imidazole therapy of coccidioidal meningitis without the use of amphotericin B in children.**

12

Cryptococcus neoformans
William V. La Via

KEY CONCEPTS

- The major risk factor for invasive cryptococcosis is altered cell-mediated immunity; however, it can affect individuals with no demonstrable immune defect.
- Infection is linked with exposure to pigeon (and other avian) feces as well as eucalyptus trees.
- Patients with meningoencephalitis are often afebrile without nuchal rigidity, and the chronic presentation can wax and wane for months with completely asymptomatic periods.
- Early symptoms of meningoencephalitis include headache, nausea, dizziness, irritability, and personality changes.
- In patients with these symptoms, a positive environmental exposure history should prompt an evaluation for cryptococcal meningoencephalitis.
- Cryptococcal antigen in the cerebrospinal fluid (CSF) is the most sensitive way to make the diagnosis of central

Continued

nervous system (CNS) infection; India Ink examination is the least sensitive.
- Opening pressure (OP) should be measured at the time of lumbar puncture (LP) and, if elevated, followed daily until normal. If it is persistently more than 400 mm H_2O, a lumbar drain may be required.

Cryptococcus neoformans is a budding yeast that most commonly affects immunocompromised persons but may also affect immunocompetent individuals. Regardless of immune status, it rarely affects individuals before the onset of puberty. It is not clear why the pediatric population is less commonly affected by this pathogen.

C. neoformans is divided into two subspecies, composed of four serotypes (A, B, C, and D) that vary in their ability to cause disease. Two of these make up the subspecies *gatti* (B and C), which appears to be more likely to cause invasive disease and more often affects immunocompetent persons. This subspecies is found most commonly in tropical and subtropical regions and associated with eucalyptus trees. In the United States, it is most common in California, and worldwide it is seen in Southeast Asia, Australia, Africa, and South America. The other subspecies, *C. neoformans* variant *neoformans,* is composed of the remaining serotypes (A and D). Serotype A causes more than 95% of the cases in immunocompromised individuals. It is found in high concentration in pigeon feces, soil, decaying wood, and is also isolated from some fruits. Numerous virulence factors contribute to the ability of this fungus to cause invasive disease. Capsular polysaccharide antigen, the most important of these factors, is known to inhibit the host inflammatory response. Other pathogen-specific virulence factors include melanin and mannitol.

Acquisition most likely occurs via the respiratory route. In conditions found in nature, the organism is weakly encapsulated and of appropriate size (<2 μm) for alveolar deposition. Once in the lungs, the organisms are rehydrated and acquire thick polysaccharide capsules that help evade the host immune response. In immunocompetent individuals, pulmonary symptoms associated with exposure are usually mild and self-resolving. Progressive pulmonary disease can develop, and if identified in a patient, it requires further evaluation for invasive disease. This should include serum cryptococcal antigen, fungal blood culture, and, if available, sputum culture. If any of these are positive, cerebrospinal fluid (CSF) examination for cryptococcus is mandatory. Immunocompromised patients (Box 1) are at highest risk for invasive disease and need careful evaluation to exclude central nervous system (CNS) disease regardless of the results of the laboratory evaluations just mentioned.

The most worrisome site of invasion is the CNS. Cryptococcal meningoencephalitis can be acute or chronic in presentation and is characterized by headache, nausea, dizziness, irritability, and personality changes, which, if not recognized, can progress to confusion, clumsiness, and somnolence or obtundation.

BOX 1 Predisposing Risk Factors for Invasive Infection Caused by *Cryptococcosis neoformans*

- Acquired immune deficiency syndrome (AIDS) (80%–90%)
- Transplantation
- Lymphoreticular malignancy
- Sarcoidosis
- Diabetes mellitus
- Collagen vascular disease

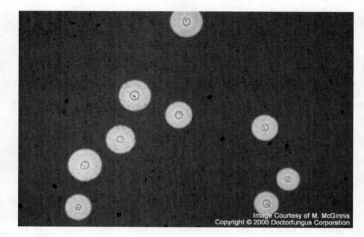

FIGURE 1. India ink staining of *Cryptococcal neoformans* in cerebrospinal fluid. (Image courtesy of www.doctorfungus.org©2005.)

TABLE 1 Sensitivity of Laboratory Studies for Detection of *Cryptococcus neoformans* in the Cerebrospinal Fluid (CSF)

Laboratory Study	Sensitivity
India ink	≈50%
Culture*	≈75%
Antigen†	
Latex agglutination	≈95%
EIA	≈95%

*Culture of 5 to 10 mL of cerebrospinal fluid on three occasions.
†False positives are usually 1:8 or less and can be caused by *Trichosporon beigelii* or *Capnocytophaga canimorsus.*
EIA, enzymatic immunoassay.

In the chronic presentation, symptoms can wax and wane for weeks to months with relatively symptom-free intervals. Acute presentation correlates with more profound immunosuppression. The diagnosis is secured by CSF examination. Usually, the opening pressure is elevated, glucose is low, protein is elevated, and white blood cell (WBC) count is more than 20/mm^3. Eosinophilia is occasionally present in the CSF. Antigen testing for the polysaccharide antigen, culture, and India ink staining (Fig. 1) are used to identify cryptococcal meningoencephalitis (Table 1). Other sites of dissemination are skin, bone, genitourinary, and, rarely, conjunctival granuloma. Skin lesions closely resemble molluscum contagiosum.

BOX 2 Treatment for Cryptococcosis in Non–HIV-Infected Patients

Cryptococcal Disease, Treatment Regimen

- Pulmonary.
- Mild to moderate symptoms or culture-positive specimen.
- Fluconazole, 10–12 mg/kg/day, 6–12 mo.
- Itraconazole, 10 mg/kg/day, 6–12 mo.
- Amphotericin B, 0.5–1 mg/kg/day, 3–4 wk.
- Severe symptoms and immunocompromised hosts.
- Treat like CNS (central nervous system) disease.

Central Nervous System

- Induction/consolidation: amphotericin B, 0.7–1 mg/kg/day, plus flucytosine, 100 mg/kg/day for 2 wk, then fluconazole, 10–12 mg/kg/day for minimum 10 wk.
- Amphotericin B, 0.7–1 mg/kg/day, plus flucytosine, 100 mg/kg/day for 6–10 wk.
- Amphotericin B, 0.7–1 mg/kg/day for 6–10 wk.
- Lipid formulation of amphotericin B, 3–6 mg/kg/day for 6–10 wk.

BOX 3 Treatment for Cryptococcosis in HIV-Infected Patients

Cryptococcal Disease, Treatment Regimen

- Pulmonary
- Mild to moderate symptoms or culture-positive specimen
- Fluconazole, 10–12 mg/kg/day, lifelong
- Itraconazole, 10 mg/kg/day, lifelong
- Fluconazole, 10–12 mg/kg/day, plus flucytosine, 100–150 mg/kg/day for 10 wk

Central Nervous System

- Induction/consolidation: amphotericin B, 0.7–1 mg/kg/day, plus flucytosine, 100 mg/kg/day for 2 wk, then fluconazole, 10–12 mg/kg/day for a minimum of 10 wk
- Amphotericin B, 0.7–1 mg/kg/day, plus flucytosine, 100 mg/kg/day for 6–10 wk
- Amphotericin B, 0.7–1 mg/kg/day for 6–10 wk
- Fluconazole, 10–12 mg/kg/day for 10–12 wk
- Itraconazole, 10 mg/kg/day for 10–12 wk
- Fluconazole, 10–12 mg/kg/day, plus flucytosine, 100–150 mg/kg/day for 6 wk
- Lipid formulation of amphotericin B, 3–6 mg/kg/day for 6–10 wk
- Maintenance:
  - Fluconazole, 6–10 mg/kg/day PO qd, lifelong
  - Itraconazole, 6 mg/kg/day PO bid, lifelong
  - Amphotericin B, 1 mg/kg IV 1–3 times/wk, lifelong

bid, twice daily; IV, intravenously; PO, orally; qd, every day.

Expert Opinion on Management Issues

IMMUNOCOMPETENT PATIENTS

Asymptomatic persons with a positive sputum culture can be managed by careful observation or, alternatively, by 3 to 6 months of fluconazole therapy. For pulmonary disease with mild to moderate symptoms, treatment for 6 to 12 months is indicated. If the patient has cryptococcemia (serum antigen titer >1:8), urinary tract, or cutaneous disease, fluconazole should be administered for 6 to 12 months after excluding CNS disease with a lumbar puncture (LP). For CNS disease, see Box 2.

IMMUNOCOMPROMISED PATIENTS

Patients with pulmonary disease need to have CNS involvement carefully excluded. Evaluation should include an LP and careful evaluation for other sites of dissemination, including a serum cryptococcal antigen measurement. If disease is limited to the lungs, less aggressive regimens are acceptable (Box 3). Patients with CNS disease need lifelong therapy after an aggressive induction/consolidation regimen (see Box 3). The CNS maintenance regimen should consist of daily fluconazole (10 to 12 mg/kg) or amphotericin B 1 mg/kg intravenously one to three times per week, lifelong. In the regimens just described, itraconazole can be substituted for fluconazole; however, erratic absorption, more common drug interactions, and poor palatability make it a less attractive choice than fluconazole.

Common Pitfalls

In addition to failure to consider the diagnosis, the most common pitfall is failure to manage elevated intracranial pressure appropriately once cryptococcal meningoencephalitis is identified. An opening pressure (OP) of more than 200 mm H_2O is associated with a poorer outcome. When identified, daily LP to decrease OP by 50% is needed until OP is below 200 mm H_2O. If the OP is more than 400 mm H_2O, a lumbar drain may be required. Steroids, acetazolamide, and mannitol are not beneficial in this setting.

Culture negativity is the only reliable indicator of success. Neither serum nor CSF antigen titers correlate with successful eradication. Also, low-grade pleocytosis may persist for up to 6 months. A normal LP after 1 year of therapy is a good indication of relative cure. Patients should be followed closely for 1 year after therapy to monitor for relapse.

Communication and Counseling

Once the diagnosis of cryptococcosis is established, the chronic nature of this infection and importance of adherence to prescribed regimens should be emphasized, as well as the need for long-term follow-up even after completion of therapy. For patients whose underlying condition dictates lifelong therapy, adherence to prescribed regimens and regular follow-up are equally important. Therefore, a solid physician/patient partnership is necessary for successful disease suppression and will lead to the best quality of life for the patient.

SUGGESTED READINGS

1. Larsen RA, Leal MA, Chan LS: Fluconazole compared with amphotericin B plus flucytosine for cryptococcal meningitis in AIDS. A randomized trial. Ann Intern Med 113:183–187, 1990. **Demonstrates the superiority of using an amphotericin-containing regimen at the onset of treatment for meningitis versus an all-fluconazole regimen.**

12

2. Leenders AC, Reiss P, Portegies P, et al: Liposomal amphotericin B (AmBisome) compared with amphotericin B, both followed by oral fluconazole in the treatment of AIDS-associated cryptococcal meningitis. AIDS 11:1463–1471, 1997. **Demonstrates the use of liposomal amphotericin for treatment of cryptococcal meningitis.**
3. Mitchell DH, Sorrell TC, Allworth AM, et al: Cryptococcal disease of the CNS in immunocompetent hosts: Influence of cryptococcal variety on clinical manifestations and outcome. Clin Infect Dis 20:611–616, 1995. **Examines the clinical differences between infections with the two subspecies of Cryptococcus.**
4. Powderly WG, Cloud GA, Dismukes WE, Saag MS: Measurement of cryptococcal antigen in serum and cerebrospinal fluid: Value in the management of AIDS-associated cryptococcal meningitis. Clin Infect Dis 18:789–792, 1994. **Demonstrates the minimal utility of cryptococcal antigen for predicting long-term outcome.**
5. Saag MS, Graybill RJ, Larsen RA, et al: Practice guidelines for the management of cryptococcal disease. Infectious Diseases Society of America (IDSA). Clin Infect Dis 30:710–718, 2000. **IDSA guidelines for management of Cryptococcal disease, the basis of all the treatment recommendations in this chapter.**

Histoplasmosis*

Duane R. Hospenthal

KEY CONCEPTS

- Histoplasmosis is a common fungal infection endemic to the Mississippi and Ohio River valleys.
- Most infections are asymptomatic or produce very mild respiratory symptoms.
- Most symptomatic infections resemble influenza and do not require antifungal therapy.
- Children 2 years or younger are at risk for disseminated (life-threatening) infection.
- Disseminated infection manifests with fever, splenomegaly and/or hepatomegaly, and anemia.
- Amphotericin B is the drug of choice for severe disease.

Histoplasmosis is a fungal infection commonly affecting persons residing in the central or eastern United States. An estimated 500,000 new cases occur annually. Most frequently the cause of asymptomatic or self-limited pulmonary infection, *Histoplasma capsulatum* can also cause life-threatening disseminated infection in immunocompetent children younger than 2 years and in immunocompromised persons of any age.

Epidemiology

Histoplasmosis exists in most temperate areas of the world, with large endemic areas in the United States and in Central and South America. The area of highest prevalence is the Ohio and Mississippi River valleys of the United States. The primary etiologic agent is the dimorphic fungus *Histoplasma capsulatum* (variant *capsulatum*), a fungus found in the soil and other organic debris enriched by bird or bat guano. Disease is initiated by the inhalation of aerosolized conidia (asexual spores) often following disruption of contaminated soils or debris. Exposure to soil or debris in areas where birds (e.g., starlings, chickens) roost or in caves harboring bats are common sources of infection. Because the conidia can be carried long distances by the wind, sometimes the source of low-level exposures is not readily apparent.

Clinical Manifestations

Infection is generally mild or asymptomatic but may be life-threatening (Box 1). Disease occurs 3 to 21 (average 14) days after exposure. Intensity of exposure (number of conidia) and host immune status are the two most important factors that determine the severity of disease. Following initial exposure, the fungus is transported to the lymphatic system via alveolar macrophages. This is followed by hematogenous dissemination that only rarely results in disseminated infection.

Symptomatic infection is primarily limited to the lungs, and the only residual from initial dissemination in most exposed persons is splenic and hepatic granulomata seen as small calcifications on radiograph. With low-level exposures, 90% to 99% of persons develop mild disease that is ignored or they do not develop symptoms at all. An estimated 1% to 10% develop self-limited symptomatic infection, virtually always limited to the lungs. Acute pulmonary infection is the most common syndrome of symptomatic histoplasmosis.

BOX 1 Common Histoplasmosis Syndromes

Asymptomatic Pulmonary Infection
- Risk factors: immunocompetent, low inoculum
- Presentation: no symptoms or mild respiratory symptoms
- Differential diagnosis: viral respiratory infection
- Diagnosis (past infection): chest radiograph findings of scattered lung, spleen and/or liver calcifications, skin test positivity

Acute Pulmonary Infection
- Risk factors: high inoculum
- Presentation: fever, cough, pleuritic chest pain, headache, chills, myalgias, fatigue, chest radiograph with diffuse patchy infiltrates and/or hilar or mediastinal adenopathy
- Differential diagnosis: influenza
- Diagnosis: culture of sputum; urine antigen in severe cases

Disseminated Histoplasmosis
- Risk factors: immunocompetent and ≤2 yr of age or immunosuppressed (any age)
- Presentation: fever, splenomegaly and/or hepatomegaly, anemia, other hematologic abnormalities, cough, pulmonary infiltrates, diffuse lymphadenopathy, elevated lactate dehydrogenase (LDH) and transaminases
- Differential diagnosis: leukemia, aplastic anemia, failure to thrive, hypercalcemia
- Diagnosis: culture of blood, bone marrow, liver, or splenic biopsy, urine or serum antigen testing

---

*Disclaimer: The views expressed herein are those of the author and do not reflect the official policy or position of the Department of the Army, Department of Defense, or the U.S. government. The author is an employee of the U.S. government. This work was prepared as part of his official duties and, as such, there is no copyright to be transferred.

Manifesting similar to influenza, acute pulmonary histoplasmosis generally is self-limited and requires no specific therapy or hospitalization. With high-level exposures, most people develop symptomatic infection including disseminated disease. Disseminated infection is estimated to occur in 1 of every 2000 infections, and in adults most commonly in association with acquired immunodeficiency syndrome (AIDS). In children, disseminated infection occurs in the setting of immunocompromise (commonly leukemia) as well, but it may also occur in the youngest of this population, even without detectable immune deficiency. Life-threatening infection in immunocompetent children of 2 years or younger is coined *disseminated histoplasmosis of infancy*. Untreated, this infection, as with all disseminated disease in the immunocompromised, carries a nearly 100% mortality.

Chronic pulmonary histoplasmosis is unlikely in children; it appears restricted to older adults with underlying chronic lung disease. Ten percent of symptomatic adults present with self-limited rheumatologic syndromes (polyarthritis and/or erythema nodosum) or pericarditis. Other more rare manifestations include granulomatous mediastinitis, fibrosing mediastinitis, and central nervous system (CNS) infections.

Diagnosis

Diagnosis of histoplasmosis begins with a high degree of suspicion in persons who live in or have recently traveled to endemic areas (Box 2). A history of any exposure that may be associated with high level of inoculum should be sought.

Visualization of the small (2 to 4 µm), usually intracellular, yeasts of *H. capsulatum* in sputum and other aspirates, tissue biopsies, or blood buffy coat can support the diagnosis of a fungal infection, but confirmation with culture or serologic methods is needed. At room temperature and in nature, *H. capsulatum* exists as a whitish mold consisting of hyphae and micro- and macroconidia. The microconidia are the infectious particles. In the infected host and at 98.6°F (37°C) in the laboratory, *H. capsulatum* exists as small budding yeasts. Conversion of the mold form to yeast in the laboratory is not always easy to accomplish, requiring specific media, time, and sometimes a bit of luck. This procedure has been mostly replaced by the use of commercial DNA probes to confirm identification of the organism in its mold form. Unfortunately, it may still take up to 6 weeks for *H. capsulatum* to grow in culture, especially from sputum. This recovery is more rapid in disseminated infection from sources such as bone marrow, spleen, or liver. The use of lysis centrifugation blood cultures also improves the sensitivity of and shortens the time to recovery.

Skin testing can be used as a diagnostic test, but it should be limited to use in children younger than 5 years and in persons from outside of the endemic areas with recent exposure. Skin test reactivity takes several weeks to develop and persists for many years, and the majority of adults in an endemic area test

> **BOX 2 Diagnosis of Histoplasmosis**
>
> **Direct Observation**
> - Sputum smear, bone marrow, spleen, or liver aspirate, tissue biopsy, blood buffy coat.
> - Small (2–4 µm), usually intracellular yeasts, best seen with Gomori methenamine silver (GMS) or periodic acid Schiff (PAS) stain.
>
> **Culture**
> - Sputum, bone marrow, spleen or liver aspirate, tissue biopsy, or blood.
> - Whitish mold producing hyphae, microconidia, and macroconidia.
> - Temperature-dependent dimorphism.
> - DNA probe available commercially to identify mold in laboratory culture.
>
> **Antigen Testing**
> - Urine, serum.
> - Urine testing more sensitive.
> - Higher detection rate in disseminated or severe acute pulmonary disease.
> - May be used to monitor therapeutic success and detect relapse.
>
> **Serology**
> - Serum.
> - Complement fixation (CF), immunodiffusion (ID), and others.
> - Fourfold increase or titer ≥1:32 consistent with acute infection.
> - Takes weeks to become positive; may cross-react with other fungal infections; may remain positive for several years.
>
> **Skin Testing**
> - Easy to use.
> - Very high positivity rate in adults in endemic areas.
> - Remains reactive for many years.
> - May be useful in those potentially exposed in endemic area who have not resided in these areas.
> - May be useful in children younger than 5 yr because they are less likely to be positive.

positive for past infection. This test may cross-react with other fungal infections and may cause other *Histoplasma* serologies to falsely become positive.

Serologies, including complement fixation (CF) and immunodiffusion (ID), may be useful in documenting infections, although they are often negative at the time of presentation. These tests also may persist for several years. A fourfold rise in CF titer or a titer of 1:32 or greater is compatible with acute infection. The *Histoplasma* antigen test can be quite helpful in the diagnosis and follow-up of histoplasmosis, especially disseminated disease. This test is usually positive early in severe or disseminated infection, allowing earlier diagnosis. Serial measurements of the antigen in urine and/or blood are quite predictive of disease response and relapse.

Expert Opinion on Management Issues

ACCEPTED INTERVENTIONS

Histoplasmosis treatment guidelines are published by the Infectious Diseases Society of America (IDSA).

TABLE 1 Treatment of Histoplasmosis

Infection	Therapy
Asymptomatic pulmonary infection	No therapy
Acute pulmonary infection	
Mild to moderate, symptoms <4 wk	No therapy
Mild to moderate, symptoms >4 wk	Itraconazole, 6–12 wk
Severe	Amphotericin B ± corticosteroids, then itraconazole, 12 wk
Disseminated infection	
Mild to moderate, non-AIDS	Itraconazole, 6–18 mo
Mild to moderate, AIDS	Itraconazole, lifelong*
Severe, non-AIDS	Amphotericin B, then itraconazole, 6–18 mo
Severe, AIDS	Amphotericin B, then itraconazole, lifelong*
Chronic pulmonary infection, meningitis, granulomatous mediastinitis	Antifungal therapy
Rheumatologic manifestations, pericarditis, fibrosing mediastinitis	No therapy

*Accumulating data in adult patients support discontinuation of lifelong therapy after immune reconstitution with antiretroviral therapy.

These provide the practitioner with suggestions as to which patients require antifungal therapy and what agents appear most appropriate. No guidelines are currently available for the treatment of children. The IDSA guidelines provide suggestions based on disease severity. Amphotericin B is suggested for all severe disease, at least until clinical response is achieved (Tables 1 and 2). Follow-up therapy with itraconazole is then suggested, with the exception of meningitis, for which fluconazole is suggested because of its cerebrospinal fluid (CSF) penetration. In mild to moderate disease requiring therapy, itraconazole is suggested as initial therapy. Ketoconazole is also used, but drug cost is the only advantage of this agent, and no liquid formulation is available in the United States.

Nonsteroidal anti-inflammatory agents can be used in mild to moderate pericarditis and severe rheumatologic manifestations. Corticosteroids are suggested in severe pericarditis.

URGENT INTERVENTIONS

Diagnosis and assessment of severity of disease should be the most urgent intervention. Those individuals with acute pulmonary disease who present with hypoxemia

TABLE 2 Antifungal Drugs Used in Histoplasmosis Therapy

Generic Name (Trade Name) Rx	Dosage/ Route/ Regimen	Maximum Dose	Dosage Formulations	Common Adverse Reactions	Comments
Polyene Antifungals (Disrupt fungal cell membranes by binding to ergosterol and creating pores)					
Amphotericin B (Fungizone) Rx	IV: 0.5–1.0 mg/kg/ day	Max: 1 mg/kg/ day	Injection	Renal dysfunction, hypokalemia, hypomagnesemia, fever, chills, rigors, headache, anemia	May replace with azole therapy when patient has clinically improved.
Liposomal amphotericin B (AmBisome) Rx, amphotericin B lipid complex (Abelcet) Rx, amphotericin B colloidal dispersion (Amphotec) Rx	IV: 3 mg/kg/day	Max: unknown	Injection	As above; reduced renal toxicity	
Azole Antifungals (Inhibit fungal cell membrane synthesis by interfering with ergosterol synthesis)					
Itraconazole (Sporanox) Rx	PO: 5 mg/kg/day in one or two doses	Max: 12 mg/kg	Oral solution: 10 mg/ mL Capsules: 100 mg Injection: 3.33 mg/ mL	Hepatotoxicity, gastrointestinal upset, multiple drug–drug interactions	Loading dose: 4 mg/kg tid × 3 days; levels should be monitored during prolonged therapy.
Ketoconazole (Nizoral) Rx	PO: 3.3–6.6 mg/ kg/day	Max: unknown	Tablets: 200 mg	Hepatotoxicity, gastrointestinal upset, multiple drug–drug interactions	
Fluconazole (Diflucan) Rx	PO: 6–12 mg/kg/ day IV: 6–12 mg/kg/ day	Max: unknown	Oral solution: 10 or 40 mg/mL Tablets: 50, 100, 150, and 200 mg Injection: 2 mg/mL	Hepatotoxicity, gastrointestinal upset	Appears less effective than other azoles in histoplasmosis; use limited to meningitis.

IV, intravenous; PO, by mouth, Rx, prescription; tid, three times per day.

and those believed to have disseminated disease should be started promptly on antifungal therapy (Table 2). Amphotericin B is recognized as the drug of choice in all with severe disease. Lipid-based formulations may be substituted for conventional amphotericin B. One study showed improved survival in persons with disseminated infection and AIDS treated with liposomal amphotericin B as compared to the conventional drug.

CONTROVERSIAL INTERVENTIONS

Experts suggest the addition of corticosteroids in severe acute pulmonary infection, although the effectiveness of this intervention is not supported by controlled clinical trials. As with *Pneumocystis* pneumonia, the inflammatory host response is believed to play a role in the hypoxemia seen in severe diffuse pulmonary infection. Treatment of fibrosing mediastinitis with antifungal agents is also controversial. Neither antifungal therapy nor surgery has proved effective in this rare complication of histoplasmosis. Chiefly because of the poor outcome of this manifestation and the safety of the newer azole antifungals, it is suggested that therapy be tried in persons who have elevated erythrocyte sedimentation rates or CF titers of 1:32 or more.

Common Pitfalls

Adrenal insufficiency may be seen as a complication of disseminated histoplasmosis. Close monitoring of hospitalized patients should include testing of adrenal corticosteroid production if insufficiency is suspected. In children, gastrointestinal bleeding is reported commonly in disseminated infection. As reported earlier, skin testing may cause false-positive serologic testing, and both skin and serologic testing may not accurately differentiate acute from past infection.

Communication and Counseling

Untreated patients and their parents should be instructed to follow up with their health care provider for antifungal therapy if their symptoms worsen or persist longer than 4 weeks. Immunocompromised individuals should avoid caves, chicken coops, and areas where bird roosts are being disrupted, such as building, excavation, and demolition sites. Persons treated for disseminated infection need close follow-up for several years. Those with AIDS and disseminated infection may need lifelong suppressive antifungal therapy.

SUGGESTED READINGS

1. Adderson EE: Histoplasmosis in a pediatric oncology center. J Pediatr 144:100–106, 2004. **Review of 78 children with and without cancers and with a diagnosis of histoplasmosis at a cancer center.**
2. de Repentigny L, Ratelle J, Leclerc J, et al: Repeated-dose pharmacokinetics of an oral solution of itraconazole in infants and children. Antimicrob Agents Chemother 42:404–408, 1998. **Report of the use and safety of oral itraconazole solution given to 26 children, 6 months to 12 years of age.**
3. Fojtasek MF, Kleiman MB, Connolly-Stringfield P, et al: The *Histoplasma capsulatum* antigen assay in disseminated histoplasmosis in children. Pediatr Infect Dis J 13:801–805, 1994. **Review of the use of the Histoplasma antigen test in children.**
4. Johnson PC, Wheat LJ, Cloud GA, et al: Safety and efficacy of liposomal amphotericin B compared with conventional amphotericin B for induction therapy of histoplasmosis in patients with AIDS. Ann Intern Med 137:105–109, 2002. **Direct comparison of liposomal and conventional amphotericin B in adult patients with disseminated histoplasmosis and AIDS.**
5. Maxson S, Jacobs RF: Community-acquired fungal pneumonia in children. Semin Respir Infect 11:196–203, 1996. **Excellent review of fungal pneumonias in children.**
6. Müller FMC, Groll AH, Walsh TJ: Current approaches to diagnosis and treatment of fungal infections in children infected with human immunodeficiency virus. Eur J Pediatr 158:187–199, 1999. **Excellent review of fungal infections of children with HIV/AIDS.**
7. Odio CM, Navarrete M, Carrillo JM, et al: Disseminated histoplasmosis in infants. Pediatr Infect Dis J 18:1065–1068, 1999. **Description of the presentation and treatment of 40 cases of disseminated histoplasmosis of infancy.**
8. Tobón AM, Franco L, Espinal D, et al: Disseminated histoplasmosis in children: The role of itraconazole therapy. Pediatr Infect Dis J 15:1002–1008, 1996. **Description of the use of itraconazole in seven children with disseminated histoplasmosis of infancy.**
9. Wheat J: Histoplasmosis: Recognition and treatment. Clin Infect Dis 19(Suppl. 1):S19–S27, 1994. **Excellent general review of histoplasmosis.**
10. Wheat J, Sarosi G, McKinsey, et al: Practice guidelines for the management of patients with histoplasmosis. Clin Infect Dis 30:688–695, 2000. **IDSA guidelines for the treatment of histoplasmosis.**

12

Mucormycosis

Shirley Jankelevich

KEY CONCEPTS

- Mucormycosis occurs primarily in patients with predisposing conditions; premature infants are at risk for cutaneous and gastrointestinal (GI) mucormycosis.
- The clinical presentation is influenced by site of infection(s) and underlying medical conditions; presentation is usually nonspecific, making clinical diagnosis difficult.
- Angioinvasiveness of the fungi results in vessel thrombosis, tissue necrosis, extension to adjacent organs, and hematogenous dissemination.
- Blood cultures are rarely, if ever, positive and radiologic and histologic tissue diagnoses are needed.
- Radical surgical excision and long-term treatment with an amphotericin-based therapy are required.
- Mortality is very high.

Mucormycosis is a group of uncommon, opportunistic, and most often fatal infections caused by the filamentous fungi in the order of Mucorales. The most common species causing disease are *Rhizopus, Rhizomucor, Cunninghamella,* and, less commonly, *Apophysomyces, Saksenaea, Mucor,* and *Absidia.* These fungal pathogens are ubiquitous in the environment. Infection of the sinuses, nasopharynx, and lungs is usually

TABLE 1 Most Common Clinical Forms of Mucormycosis, Initial Infection Sites, Complications, Clinical Manifestations, and Differential Diagnoses

Most Common Clinical Form	Initial Site Infected	Complications	Common Clinical Manifestations*	Differential Diagnosis
Rhino-orbito-cerebral	Paranasal sinus, palate.	Necrosis of nasal mucosa, turbinates, hard palate; invasion of orbit; cerebral abscesses; thrombosis of cavernous sinus or retinal, cerebral or carotid arteries.	Bloody rhinorrhea, epistaxis, sinus tenderness, facial pain, headache, cranial nerve (CN) dysfunction (predominantly CN V and VII), loss of consciousness.	*Aspergillus* infection, orbital tumor.
Pulmonary	Often unilateral in upper lobe of lung.	Endobronchial obstruction, cavitation, pneumonia, lobar collapse, pulmonary artery thrombosis and erosion, direct invasion to mediastinum; may lead to disseminated infection.	Dyspnea, cough, hemoptysis, pleuritic chest pain.	*Aspergillus* infection, bland pulmonary embolism.
Cutaneous/soft tissue†	Primary cutaneous infection or may be secondary to hematogenous spread from distant infection.	Extension to subcutaneous tissue, muscle, fat, fascial planes, bone; may lead to disseminated infection.	Primary cutaneous. Superficial presentation: vesicles or pustules, hemorrhagic ulcer, eschar, necrosis. Gangrenous presentation: gangrenous cellulitis and ulceration. Hematogenous spread: erythematous nodular lesions with necrotic centers.	Bacterial skin infections, progressive necrotizing lesions of the skin, ecthyma gangrenosum.
Disseminated	Paranasal, pulmonary, GI tract, skin.	May lead to infection of any tissue or organ system.		
Gastrointestinal (GI)‡	Can affect any portion of the GI tract.	Perforation; NEC; dissemination.		Can mimic a variety of diseases of GI tract depending on the site of infection, including intra-abdominal abscess.
Other	Heart, kidney, bone, joint, mediastinum, bladder, other.			

*Common clinical manifestations depend on the extent of infection.
†Risk factors include compromised integrity of skin (trauma, burns) with introduction of spores, prematurity.
‡Risk factors include severe protein malnutrition, prematurity, underlying GI infection (amebiasis, typhoid fever).
GI, gastrointestinal; NEC, necrotizing enterocolitis.

acquired following inhalation of fungal spores. Fungal spores may also contaminate skin wounds and the gastrointestinal (GI) tract. There is no evidence of direct person-to-person spread. If conditions are favorable for fungal growth, which occurs in persons with metabolic acidosis of deficient or defective macrophages and neutrophils, for example, hyphae invade the blood vessels, resulting in thrombosis, ischemia, or hemorrhagic necrosis of tissue. Mucormycosis may be widely disseminated and occur in one or more organ systems simultaneously. Infection can also spread through tissue planes to adjacent tissue and organs.

The most common syndromes in adults and children are rhino-orbito-cerebral, pulmonary, cutaneous/soft tissue, disseminated, and GI mucormycosis (Table 1). Certain syndromes are more commonly found in patients with specific underlying conditions, such as diabetes mellitus (DM), metabolic acidosis, hematologic malignancies, prolonged neutropenia, organ or bone marrow transplantation; prematurity, renal insufficiency, deferoxamine therapy, iron overload, compromised integrity of skin, trauma, systemic lupus erythematosus (SLE) with high-dose steroids, severe protein malnutrition, and intravenous drug abuse (IVDA). Specific risk factors for GI mucormycosis include altered gastric pH because of H_2-receptor antagonists, corticosteroid therapy, preexisting gastric ulcers, and local trauma to the gastric mucosa because of nasogastric catheters. Mucormycosis rarely occurs in persons with human immunodeficiency virus (HIV) unless accompanied by IVDA or severe neutropenia. Rarely, no predisposing conditions are found. Infection may be chronic and slowly progressive, but most often fulminant, resulting in death unless there is early, aggressive institution of treatment.

Premature neonates are at risk for mucormycosis of the skin and GI tract. Primary cutaneous mucormycosis of premature infants of very low birth weight is associated with the use of broad-spectrum antibiotics, corticosteroid therapy, and respiratory distress

TABLE 2 Medications for the Treatment of Mucormycosis*

Medication	Dosage/ Route/ Regimen	Dosage Formulation	Common Adverse Reactions	Comments
Amphotericin B deoxycholate (Fungizone B)[†‡]	1.0–1.5 IV mg/kg/day	Injectable	Acute infusion-related reactions (chills, fever, hypoxia, hypotension, nausea, tachypnea); nephrotoxicity; hypokalemia; anaphylaxis	Acute infusion-related reactions can be managed by pretreatment with antihistamines, corticosteroids, and/or decreasing the rate of infusion. A test dose with careful clinical monitoring is advisable when starting first course of treatment with amphotericin B deoxycholate.
Liposomal Amphotericin B (AmBisome)[†‡]	5.0 mg/kg/day		Nephrotoxicity; acute infusion-related reactions; hypokalemia; anaphylaxis	Decreased but not diminished incidence of acute infusion-related reactions, nephrotoxicity, and hypokalemia relative to amphotericin B deoxycholate. Per FDA, AmBisome is approved only for the following: empirical therapy for presumed fungal infection in febrile neutropenic patients; treatment of cryptococcal meningitis in HIV-infected patients; treatment of patients with *Aspergillus* species, *Candida* species, and/or *Cryptococcus* species; and pediatric patients >1 mo of age.
Amphotericin B lipid complex (ABLC, Abelcet)[†‡]	5.0 mg/kg/day		Acute infusion-related reactions; nephrotoxicity; hypokalemia; anaphylaxis	Decreased but not diminished incidence of acute infusion-related reactions and nephrotoxicity relative to amphotericin B deoxycholate. Per FDA, Abelcet is approved for the treatment of invasive fungal infections in patients who are refractory to or intolerant of conventional amphotericin B therapy.
Amphotericin B colloidal dispersion (ABCD, Amphotec)[†‡]	5.0 mg/kg/day		Acute infusion-related reactions; nephrotoxicity; hypokalemia: anaphylaxis	Decreased but not diminished incidence of nephrotoxicity and hypokalemia. relative to amphotericin B deoxycholate. Incidence of acute infusion-related reactions similar to that of amphotericin B deoxycholate. Acute infusion-related reactions can be managed by pretreatment with antihistamines, corticosteroids, and/or decreasing the rate of infusion. A test dose with careful clinical monitoring is advisable when starting first course of treatment with amphotericin B colloidal dispersion. Per FDA, Amphotec is approved only for the treatment of invasive aspergillosis in patients in whom renal impairment or unacceptable toxicity precludes the use of amphotericin B deoxycholate in effective doses, and in patients with invasive aspergillosis in whom prior amphotericin B deoxycholate therapy has failed.

*Amphotericin-based formulations are polyene macrolides that bind to sterols in the fungal cell membrane and generate spores, resulting in altered membrane permeability.
[†]Careful monitoring of laboratory renal, hepatic, electrolyte, and hematologic tests should be done throughout therapy.
[‡]Interactions with the following drugs may cause serious toxicity or decrease effectiveness: antineoplastic agents, corticosteroids/corticotrophin, cyclosporine/tacrolimus, digitalis, flucytosine, imidazoles, other nephrotoxic drugs, skeletal muscle relaxants.
FDA, Federal Drug Administration; HIV, human immunodeficiency virus; IV, intravenous.

syndrome. The infection has often occurred at sites where adhesive dressing, invasive catheters, monitor leads, wooden tongue depressors used as limb splints, or other devices contaminated with fungal spores caused local trauma to skin, allowing spores to germinate. Rapid widespread dissemination usually followed initial infection. Despite debridement and systemic amphotericin B, mortality remained very high.

GI mucormycosis in neonates most often occurs in the stomach and colon and less frequently in the small bowel and esophagus. GI mucormycosis is associated with preparation of oral medications with a wooden tongue depressor contaminated with Mucorales species. GI mucormycosis may disseminate and extend to the abdominal wall and adjacent organs. It can easily be confused with necrotizing enterocolitis (NEC).

Mortality is 60% to 80%, approximately five to seven times higher than that from NEC.

Diagnosis

Presentation of mucormycosis is usually nonspecific. The only clinical syndrome that may have a specific presentation is rhino-orbito-cerebral *Mucor*, in which necrotic lesions may be seen in the nares and hard palate. Mucormycosis should be considered in any patient with associated predisposing conditions who does not respond to therapy for usual infections and diseases. Radiologic studies such as CT and MRI help determine the location and extent of infection. Fungal cultures of sputum, urine, blood, cerebrospinal fluid (CSF), and swabs of tissue are rarely positive. Tissue specimens sent for fungal culture often do not grow fungal organisms because homogenization of tissue prior to plating destroys the fungal cell wall. If mucormycosis is considered, the microbiologic laboratory must be informed so the tissue specimen can be prepared appropriately. Histologic examination of infected tissue showing invasion by broad, ribbon-like pauciseptate hyphae with right-angle branching is necessary for diagnosis. Unfortunately, the diagnosis is most often made postmortem.

Expert Opinion on Management Issues

Correction of predisposing conditions, such as metabolic acidosis, neutropenia, malnutrition, and immunosuppression, to the extent possible is necessary. A combination of prolonged medical and extensive, often disfiguring, surgery is essential to effect a cure for all clinical syndromes of mucormycosis except for superficially infected skin lesions in a normal host. Often repeated radical debridement of all infected and necrotic tissue needs to be performed.

Intravenous amphotericin B deoxycholate remains the standard medical therapy for mucormycosis, although no controlled trials have been conducted because of the low incidence of mucormycosis (Table 2). Doses of 1 to 1.5 mg/kg/day of amphotericin B deoxycholate, often with a total of 2 to 4 g, are recommended until resolution of infection is seen. If nephrotoxicity occurs, lipid formations of amphotericin B should be considered, although there is less experience with these formulations for the treatment of mucormycosis. Adjunctive therapy with hyperbaric oxygen may provide some benefit, but no comparative clinical studies have assessed its effectiveness. Failure to provide early, prolonged, and adequate therapy results in dissemination or relapse and death. Treatment failure may also occur because of the decreased susceptibility of certain species of Mucorales to amphotericin B or the inability of amphotericin B to achieve adequate levels in infected tissue because of thrombosis and necrosis. Because of the possibility of recurrence, each patient must have careful clinical and radiologic follow-up.

Common Pitfalls

- Failure to consider mucormycosis in a patient with a predisposing medical condition who has not responded to standard therapy.
- Lack of specificity of clinical presentation for mucormycosis and difficulty in isolating *Mucor* from usual laboratory specimens.
- Inability to correct underlying predisposing conditions.
- Failure to provide early, aggressive medical and surgical treatment or proper follow-up after completion of treatment.

Communication and Counseling

Recurrence of mucormycosis and mortality remains very high in patients whose underlying medical conditions cannot be corrected. Proper management requires early recognition of infection, aggressive diagnostic studies, and treatment as well as correction of underlying predisposing medical conditions. Despite adequate treatment, mortality remains high. No effective preventive therapy is available other than the use of high-efficiency particulate air (HEPA) filters in patients with severe neutropenia.

SUGGESTED READINGS

1. Deray G: Amphotericin B nephrotoxicity. J Antimicrob Chemother 49(Suppl 1):37–41, 2002. **Review of toxicity of amphotericin B–based formulations.**
2. Goldman RD, Koren G: Amphotericin B nephrotoxicity in children. J Pediatr Hematol Oncol 26(7):421–426, 2004. **Review of toxicity of amphotericin B–based formulations with emphasis on pediatric pharmacokinetics.**
3. Hamilton JF, Bartkowski HB, Rock JP: Management of CNS mucormycosis in the pediatric patient. Pediatr Neurosurg 38(4):212–215, 2003. **Case report of rhinocerebral mucormycosis in a child with information on the surgical treatment.**
4. Lee FYW, Mossad SB, Adal KA: Pulmonary mucormycosis: The last 30 years. Arch Intern Med 159:1301–1309, 1999. **Extensive review of published cases of isolated pulmonary mucormycosis: diagnosis, treatment, and outcome.**
5. Nissen MD, Jana AK, Cole MJ, et al: Neonatal gastrointestinal mucormycosis mimicking necrotizing enterocolitis. Acta Paediatr 88(11):1290–1293, 1999. **Case report and brief review of published cases of neonatal gastrointestinal mucormycosis manifesting in a manner similar to NEC.**
6. Oh D, Notrica D: Primary cutaneous mucormycosis in infants and neonates: Case report and review of the literature. J Pediatr Surg 37(11):1607–1611, 2002. **Case report and detailed review of reported cases of primary cutaneous mucormycosis in infants and neonates.**
7. Prabhu RM, Patel R: Mucormycosis and entomophthoramycosis: A review of the clinical manifestations, diagnosis, and treatment. Clin Microbiol Infect 10(Suppl. 1):31–47, 2004. **Excellent review of mucormycosis and its diagnosis and treatment.**
8. Shah D, Peters KR, Reuman PD: Recovery from rhinocerebral mucormycosis with carotid artery occlusion: A pediatric case and review of the literature. Pediatr Infect Dis J 16(1):68–71, 1997. **Case report of rhinocerebral mucormycosis complicated by carotid artery thrombosis and detailed review of reported cases.**

CHLAMYDIAL INFECTIONS

Chlamydial Infections

Margaret R. Hammerschlag

KEY CONCEPTS

- Chlamydial species are ubiquitous and occur in practically every mammalian, avian, and probably reptilian and amphibian species.
- *Chlamydia trachomatis* is the most common sexually transmitted pathogen in the United States. Adolescent girls, 15 to 19 years of age, have the highest rates of infection, often higher than 20%.
- The major clinical syndromes associated with *C. trachomatis* infection include mucopurulent cervicitis and pelvic inflammatory disease in women, urethritis and epididymitis in men, but the majority of genital infections caused by *C. trachomatis* are asymptomatic, more than 70% in women.
- *C. trachomatis* can be transmitted during delivery from an infected mother to her infant, who may develop conjunctivitis or pneumonia.
- The introduction of highly sensitive and specific nucleic acid amplification tests (NAATs) for detection of *C. trachomatis,* combined with systematic screening and treatment of pregnant women, has resulted in a marked decrease of perinatally acquired *C. trachomatis* infection in infants.
- NAATs allow for use of noninvasive specimens, such as urine, and self-collected vaginal swabs, which facilitate the screening of adolescents in nontraditional settings such as schools.
- *Chlamydia pneumoniae* is a frequent cause of community-acquired respiratory infection, including pneumonia, in children and adult, but clinically, *C. pneumoniae* pneumonia cannot be differentiated from pneumonia caused by other organisms, including *Mycoplasma pneumoniae.*
- *Chlamydia psittaci* infection (psittacosis) should be suspected in individuals who develop pneumonia following exposure to sick birds.

Chlamydiae are obligate intracellular pathogens that have established a unique niche within the host cell. The order contains one genus, *Chlamydia,* with four recognized species: *Chlamydia trachomatis, Chlamydia psittaci, Chlamydia pneumoniae,* and *Chlamydia pecorum,* of which *C. trachomatis* and *C. pneumoniae* are significant human pathogens. *C. psittaci* is a major avian pathogen and an important zoonosis in humans. The results of new taxonomic analysis using the 16S and 23S rRNA genes suggest splitting the genus *Chlamydia* into two genera: *Chlamydia* and *Chlamydophila.* Two new species, *Chlamydia muridarum* and *Chlamydia suis,* would join *C. trachomatis. Chlamydophila* would contain *Chlamydophila pecorum, Chlamydophila pneumoniae,* and *Chlamydophila psittaci,* and three new species split off from *C. psittaci: Chlamydia abortus, Chlamydia caviae,* and *Chlamydia felis.*

Chlamydiae are characterized by a unique developmental cycle with morphologically distinct infectious and reproductive forms: elementary body (EB) and reticulate body (RB). Chlamydiae also share a group-specific lipopolysaccharide antigen and use host adenosine triphosphate (ATP) for the synthesis of chlamydial protein. Although chlamydiae use the host cell's pool for three of four nucleoside triphosphates, they do encode functional glucose-catabolizing enzymes, which can be used for generation of ATP, but for some reason these genes are turned off. All chlamydiae also encode an abundant protein called the major outer membrane protein (MOMP, or OmpA) that is surface exposed in *C. trachomatis* and *C. psittaci,* but apparently not in *C. pneumoniae.* The MOMP is the major determinant of the serologic classification of *C. trachomatis* and *C. psittaci* isolates.

Understanding the life cycle of chlamydia is important because it explains the potential problems with diagnosis and treatment. Following infection, the infectious EBs, which are 200 to 400 μm in diameter, attach to the host cell by a process of electrostatic binding and are taken into the cell by endocytosis that does not depend on the microtubule system. Within the host cell, the EB remains within a membrane-lined phagosome. The phagosome does not fuse with the host cell lysosome. The EBs then differentiate into RBs that undergo binary fission, and after approximately 36 hours, the reticulate bodies differentiate back into EBs, and infectivity increases. At approximately 48 hours, release may occur by cytolysis or by a process of exocytosis or extrusion of the whole inclusion, leaving the host cell intact. Unlike other bacteria, the life cycle is prolonged, 48 to 72 hours versus 20 minutes. Thus treatment requires multiple-dose regimens, for 5 to 14 days, depending on the species and site of infection. Single-dose azithromycin is effective for treatment of genital *C. trachomatis* infection because it has a half-life in tissue of 5 to 7 days. However, single-dose azithromycin is not effective in eradicating *C. pneumoniae* from the respiratory tract. The ability to cause prolonged, often subclinical, infection is one of the major characteristics of chlamydiae.

Expert Opinion on Management Issues

TREATMENT OF *CHLAMYDIA TRACHOMATIS* INFECTIONS

Box 1 shows the recommended treatment regimens for *C. trachomatis* infection. Single-dose azithromycin or 7-day courses of doxycycline are the first-line drugs of choice for the treatment of uncomplicated genital infections in male and female adolescents and adults. The results of clinical trials demonstrate that azithromycin and doxycycline are equally effective. Alternatives include erythromycin or levofloxacin, also for 7 days. Azithromycin has the advantage of a single-dose regimen, which improves compliance; however, doxycycline has an advantage in cost. There is less experience with use of levofloxacin. Sexual partners should also be treated. Patients do not need to be retested for *C. trachomatis* after completing treatment with azithromycin or doxycycline unless symptoms persist or reinfection is thought likely.

The most effective method for control of perinatal chlamydial infection is screening and treatment of pregnant women. The Centers for Disease Control and Prevention (CDC) currently recommends either amoxicillin or erythromycin base as first-line regimens for treatment of *C. trachomatis* infection in pregnant women. Single-dose azithromycin is listed as an alternative regimen with the caveat that data on its use are insufficient to recommend its use routinely in pregnant women. However, clinical experience and preliminary data suggest that azithromycin is safe and effective. Reasons for failure of maternal treatment to prevent infantile chlamydial infection include poor compliance and reinfection from an untreated sexual partner.

Oral erythromycin suspension (ethylsuccinate) is the therapy of choice for the treatment of chlamydial conjunctivitis and pneumonia in infants. It provides better and faster resolution of the conjunctivitis and also treats any concurrent nasopharyngeal infection, which prevents the development of pneumonia. Additional topical therapy is not needed. The efficacy of this regimen ranges from 80% to 90%; as many as 20% of infants may require another course of therapy. Erythromycin at the same dose for 2 to 3 weeks is the treatment of choice for pneumonia and does result in clinical improvement as well as elimination of the organism from the respiratory tract. An association between treatment with oral erythromycin and infantile hypertrophic pyloric stenosis is reported in infants younger than 6 weeks who were given the drug for prophylaxis after nursery exposure to pertussis. Data on use of other macrolides (azithromycin or clarithromycin) for the treatment of neonatal chlamydia infection are limited. One small study suggested that a short course of azithromycin, 20 mg/kg/day orally, one dose daily for 3 days, was as effective as 2 weeks of erythromycin.

Lymphogranuloma venereum (LGV) is a sexually transmitted disease caused by the L_1, L_2, and L_3 serotypes of *C. trachomatis*. The infection is characterized

---

BOX 1 Treatment of *Chlamydia trachomatis* Infections

Infections in Adolescents and Adults
- Recommended regimens
  - Azithromycin, 1 g PO in a single dose

  or

  - Doxycycline, 100 mg PO bid for 7 days
- Alternative regimens
  - Erythromycin base, 500 mg PO qid for 7 days

  or

  - Erythromycin ethylsuccinate, 800 mg PO qid for 7 days

  or

  - Levofloxacin, 500 mg PO qd for 7 days

Infections in Pregnancy
- Recommended regimens
  - Erythromycin base, 500 mg PO qid for 7 days

  or

  - Amoxicillin, 500 mg PO tid for 7 days
- Alternative regimens
  - Erythromycin base, 250 mg PO qid for 14 days

  or

  - Erythromycin ethylsuccinate, 800 mg PO qid for 7 days

  or

  - Erythromycin ethylsuccinate, 400 mg PO qid for 14 days

  or

  - Azithromycin, 1 g PO, single dose

Infections in Infants: Conjunctivitis and Pneumonia
- Recommended regimen
  - Erythromycin base or ethylsuccinate, 50 mg/kg/day PO divided into four doses daily for 14 days
- Alternative regimen
  - Azithromycin suspension, 20 mg/kg/dose PO once a day for 3 days

Infections in Older Children
- Erythromycin suspension, 50 mg/kg/day qid PO to a maximum of 2 g a day for 7 days
- Children >8 yr of age: tetracycline, 25 to 50 mg/kg/day qid PO for 7 days

  or

- Azithromycin, 1 g PO as a single dose, may also be used in children who weigh >45 kg and/or >8 yr of age

---

bid, twice daily; PO, by mouth; qid, four times per day; tid, three times per day.

---

by an initial genital papule or ulcer that is transient, followed by the development of inguinal adenopathy, which may break down and form fistulas. These findings are most common in men. Because the lymphatic drainage of the vulva is to the retroperitoneal nodes, women are more likely to be seen in the tertiary stage of the disease with rectovaginal fistulas and strictures. Tetracycline, 500 mg four times daily, or doxycycline, 100 mg twice daily, should be given for 3 to 6 weeks.

TREATMENT OF *CHLAMYDIA PNEUMONIAE* INFECTIONS

Data on the response of *C. pneumoniae* to antimicrobial therapy are limited. Most of the treatment studies of pneumonia caused by *C. pneumoniae* published

---

BOX 2 Treatment of *Chlamydia pneumoniae* Infections

Adolescents and Adults

- Doxycycline, 100 mg bid PO for 14 to 21 days

or

- Tetracycline, 250 mg qid PO for 14 to 21 days

or

- Azithromycin, 1.5 g PO over 5 days

or

- Levofloxacin, 500 mg/day, PO or IV for 7 to 14 days

or

- Moxifloxacin, 400 mg/day, PO or IV for 10 days

Children

- Erythromycin ethylsuccinate suspension, 50 mg/kg/day for 10 to 14 days

or

- Clarithromycin suspension, 15 mg/kg/day for 10 days

or

- Azithromycin suspension, 10 mg/kg on day 1 followed by 5 mg/kg/day once daily on days 2–5

---

bid, twice daily; IV, intravenous; PO, by mouth; qid, four times per day.

BOX 3 Diagnosis and Treatment of *Chlamydia psittaci* Infections

CDC Case Definitions (2000)

Confirmed Case of Psittacosis

- Requires a compatible clinical illness, usually with a good history of avian exposure.
- Laboratory confirmation can be made by one of the three following methods:
  - Culture of *C. psittaci* from respiratory secretions
  - Fourfold increase in complement fixation (CF) or microimmunofluorescence (MIF) titer in sera collected at least 2 wk apart
  - MIF immunoglobulin (Ig) M titer of >16.

Probable Case of Psittacosis

- Should be epidemiologically linked to a confirmed case.

or

- A single CF or MIF antibody titer of >32 in at least one serum should be obtained after onset of symptoms.

Treatment for Adults and Children Older than 8 yr

- Tetracycline, 500 mg q6h PO for 7 to 10 days

or

- Erythromycin, 50 mg/kg/day up to 2 g/day for 7 to 10 days

CDC, Centers for Disease Control and Prevention; PO, by mouth; qxh, every x hours.

---

so far relied entirely on diagnosis by serology; thus microbiologic efficacy could not be assessed. Results of two pediatric multicenter pneumonia treatment studies found that 10-day courses of erythromycin and clarithromycin and 5 days of azithromycin suspension were equally efficacious, eradicating the organism in 79% to 86% of the children. Quinolones, including levofloxacin and moxifloxacin, also demonstrated 70% to 80% efficacy in eradicating *C. pneumoniae* from adults with community-acquired pneumonia. Box 2 shows the suggested regimens for the treatment of *C. pneumoniae* pneumonia.

TREATMENT OF *CHLAMYDIA PSITTACI* INFECTIONS

Box 3 shows the current CDC recommendations for the diagnosis and treatment of psittacosis. Tetracycline remains the drug of choice; anecdotal evidence suggests that erythromycin may be less effective.

Common Pitfalls

- Failure to treat sexual partners is the major reason for treatment failures of genital *C. trachomatis* infection, especially in adolescents.
- Although NAATs are the diagnostic method of choice for genital *C. trachomatis* infection in adolescents and adults, they are not approved for use in genital or rectal sites from children, especially for evaluation of children who are suspected victims of sexual assault or abuse.
- Definitive diagnosis of *C. pneumoniae* infections requires isolation of the organism in tissue culture, which is predominantly limited to a small number of research laboratories.
- There are no FDA-approved NAATs for detection of *C. pneumoniae* or FDA-approved serologic tests.

12

Serologic testing is not appropriate for diagnosis of *C. trachomatis* infections because chlamydial infections are frequently subclinical and of long duration. Various antibody tests are offered by several commercial laboratories for the diagnosis of *C. trachomatis* infections, but the CDC strongly recommends against their use. There are currently three FDA-approved NAATs for detection of *C. trachomatis* (Table 1) but no FDA-approved serologic tests for *C. trachomatis*. Although NAATs are now the standard for diagnosis of *C. trachomatis* infections in adolescents and adults, they are not approved for rectogenital sites in children. As of this writing, only culture is recommended for detection of *C. trachomatis* in children being evaluated for suspected sexual abuse. Inappropriate use of non-culture tests, especially first-generation enzyme immunoassays (EIAs) and direct fluorescent antibody tests (DFAs), are associated with many false-positive results. The DNA probe assay (Pace 2, Gen-Probe) is not an amplification test. The EIAs, DFAs, and DNA probe assays are less sensitive than culture; in contrast, the currently available NAATs may be 10% to 30% more sensitive than culture when used for urethral and cervical specimens from adults. The 2003 CDC Sexually Transmitted Disease Guidelines suggests a NAAT could be used if culture is not available, providing that any positive result be confirmed by a different NAAT targeting a different gene sequence. However, because most laboratories only perform one test, confirmation with a second test is probably not an option for most practitioners.

There are also no FDA-approved serologic tests for *C. pneumoniae*. Studies in children demonstrate a very

TABLE 1 NAATs for Diagnosis of *Chlamydia trachomatis* Infection

Assay	DNA/ RNA	Approved Indications
Polymerase chain reaction (Amplicor, Roche)	DNA	Female: cervix, urine Male: urethra, urine
Strand displacement amplification (Probe TEC, Becton Dickson)	DNA	Female: cervix, urine Male: urethral, urine
Transcription-mediated amplification (*Chlamydia* Amplifier Test, Gen-Probe)	RNA	Female: cervix, urine, vagina Male: urethra, urine

NAAT, nucleic acid amplification test.

poor correlation between serology and culture in children with community-acquired pneumonia caused by *C. pneumoniae*; as many as 70% of these children will be seronegative. A number of commercial laboratories are also offering in-house polymerase chain reaction (PCR) assays for diagnosis of *C. pneumoniae* infection. However, these assays are not standardized, and none are validated or approved by the FDA. Several multicenter studies demonstrated major problems with both inter- and intralaboratory reproducibility with in-house PCRs for detection of *C. pneumoniae* in clinical specimens. Unfortunately, diagnosis remains syndromic.

Communication and Counseling

Because *C. trachomatis* is a sexually transmitted infection, every effort must be made to treat the sexual partner, and the patient should be counseled to avoid unprotected sexual activity. Similarly, the diagnosis of *C. trachomatis* conjunctivitis or pneumoniae in an infant implies that both parents are probably infected and should be referred for treatment.

SUGGESTED READINGS

1. Black CM: Current methods of laboratory diagnosis of *Chlamydia trachomatis* infection. Clin Microbiol Rev 10:160–184, 1997. **Detailed review of diagnostic methods.**
2. Block S, Hedrick J, Hammerschlag MR, Cassell GH: *Mycoplasma pneumoniae* and *Chlamydia pneumoniae* in pediatric community-acquired pneumonia. Comparative efficacy and safety of clarithromycin vs. erythromycin ethylsuccinate. Pediatr Infect Dis J 14:471–477, 1995. **Controlled treatment study of C. pneumoniae pneumonia in children that used culture and assessed microbiologic efficacy.**
3. Boman J, Gaydos CA, Quinn TC: Molecular diagnosis of *Chlamydia pneumoniae* infection. J Clin Microbiol 37:3791–3799, 1999. **Detailed review of molecular methods for diagnosis of C. pneumoniae.**
4. Centers for Disease Control and Prevention: Compendium of measures to control *Chlamydia psittaci* infection among humans (psittacosis) and pet birds (avian chlamydiosis). MMWR Recomm Rep 49(RR-8):3–17, 2000. **Government recommendations for control and diagnosis of C. psittaci infections.**
5. Centers for Disease Control and Prevention: Sexually transmitted diseases treatment guidelines 2006. MMWR Recomm Rep (in preparation). **Government recommendations for diagnosis and treatment of sexually transmitted infections.**
6. Centers for Disease Control and Prevention: Screening tests to detect *Chlamydia trachomatis* and *Neisseria gonorrhoeae* infections—2002. MMWR Recomm Rep 51(RR-15):1–40, 2002. **Governmental recommendations for use of screening tests for C. trachomatis and N. gonorrhoeae.**
7. Dowell SF, Peeling RW, Boman J, et al: Standardizing *Chlamydia pneumoniae* assays: Recommendations from the Centers for Disease Control and Prevention (USA) and the Laboratory Centre for Disease Control (Canada). Clin Infect Dis 33:492–503, 2001. **Report and recommendations of CDC conference on diagnostic methods for C. pneumoniae.**
8. Hammerschlag MR, Ajl S, Laraque D: Inappropriate use of nonculture tests for the detection of *Chlamydia trachomatis* in suspected victims of child sexual abuse: A continuing problem. Pediatrics 104:1137–1139, 1999. **Describes several cases of false-positive results with nonculture tests for C. trachomatis in children being evaluated for suspected sexual abuse.**

RICKETTSIAL INFECTIONS

Ehrlichiosis (Anaplasmosis)

Eugene D. Shapiro

KEY CONCEPTS

- A high level of suspicion is necessary to make the diagnosis of ehrlichiosis because most symptoms are nonspecific.
- Doxycycline should be used for children who are seriously ill, even if they are younger than 8 years, because the drug is very effective and ehrlichiosis is potentially life-threatening.
- Chronic ehrlichiosis is not recognized as a clinical entity. Persons with infection that need treatment are generally acutely ill.

In the United States, two major causes of ehrlichiosis affect humans:

1. Human monocytic ehrlichiosis (HME), caused by *Ehrlichia chaffeensis*

2. Human granulocytic ehrlichiosis (HGE), caused by *Anaplasma phagocytophilum* (formerly called *Ehrlichia equi*)

Ehrlichia ewingii is a less common cause of HGE. All three organisms are obligate intracellular bacteria and belong to the family Anaplasmataceae. Ticks are the vector for ehrlichiosis. The primary vector for *E. chaffeensis* and *E. ewingii* is *Amblyomma americanum*, the lone star tick. Most cases of HME (and of HGE caused by *E. ewingii*) occur in the southern, central, and mid-Atlantic states, although cases do occur in other areas. The vector for *A. phagocytophilum,* the most common cause of HGE, is *Ixodes scapularis* (the deer tick) or *Ixodes pacificus* (on the Pacific Coast), the ticks that are the vectors for Lyme disease and babesiosis. Most cases of HGE occur in southern New England, the mid-Atlantic states, and the upper Midwest (Wisconsin, Michigan, and Minnesota). As with most tick-borne infections in temperate climates, the highest incidence of infection occurs during the peak months of human exposure to ticks—from April to September.

Despite differences in the cells they infect, the clinical manifestations of HME and HGE are similar. Serosurveys indicate that a diagnosis of ehrlichiosis is not made in most children who are infected, presumably because they have symptoms thought to be caused by a viral infection that resolves spontaneously. In children in whom the diagnosis is made, fever and headache are the most common manifestations of the illness, followed by myalgia, nausea, vomiting, and arthralgia. Rash occurs in approximately a third of children with HME but in only approximately 10% of those with HGE. Leukopenia, thrombocytopenia, and elevated liver enzymes occur in most patients.

Diagnosis requires a high level of suspicion because most of the signs and symptoms of ehrlichiosis are nonspecific. The diagnosis is established in the proper clinical and epidemiologic setting if the organism can be seen in the blood of a patient (morulae inside the cytoplasm of leukocytes in Giemsa-stained smears of blood), by a positive result of a polymerase chain reaction (PCR) assay, or by a fourfold or greater rise in concentrations of antibody in acute and convalescent samples of serum (obtained at least 1 month apart).

Expert Opinion on Management Issues

Table 1 shows the drugs to treat ehrlichiosis. Tetracyclines are the drugs of choice to treat severe ehrlichiosis. Doxycycline usually is preferred because it can be administered twice a day. Tetracyclines usually are not recommended for children younger than 8 years because of the potential for discoloring permanent teeth; however, because ehrlichiosis is potentially fatal if untreated and tetracyclines are uniformly effective, prompt treatment of even young children with a tetracycline is encouraged if the child is severely ill. Moreover, evidence indicates that a short course of doxycycline does not discolor permanent teeth. For children younger than 8 years with less severe infection or for those who cannot tolerate a tetracycline, rifampin is an effective alternative agent.

Common Pitfalls

COINFECTIONS

Because both Lyme disease and babesiosis are transmitted by the same tick that transmits *A. phagocytophilum* (the cause of HGE), coinfection with either or both of these agents may occur. These diagnoses should be considered in patients who have atypical features of ehrlichiosis.

TABLE 1 Antimicrobials to Treat Ehrlichiosis

Generic Name (Trade Name)	Dosage/Route/Regimen	Maximum Dose	Formulations	Adverse Reactions	Comments
Tetracyclines (Inhibit protein synthesis by binding to 30s subunit of bacterial ribosome)					
Doxycycline (Doryx, Vibramycin)	3–4 mg/kg/day PO div two doses/day. Treat for 3–5 days after fever resolves.	100 mg/dose	PO	Nausea	Some patients develop sun-induced dermatitis so should protect skin from sun.
Tetracycline	20–50 mg/kg/day PO, div four doses/day Treat for 3–5 days after fever resolves.	500 mg/dose	PO	Nausea	Doxycycline preferred, especially in children <8 yr of age.
Rifampin (Inhibits protein synthesis by binding to DNA-dependent RNA polymerase)					
Rifampin (Rifadin)	20–40 mg/kg/day PO, div two doses/day Treat for 3–5 days after fever has resolved.	600 mg/dose	PO	Nausea	Interactions with a number of drugs metabolized by P-450 system; turns secretions red and may stain soft contact lenses permanently.

div, divided; PO, by mouth.

MISDIAGNOSIS

No chronic form of ehrlichiosis exists. However, infection that either is asymptomatic or indistinguishable from a self-limited viral infection apparently is relatively common because serosurveys indicate that many children in endemic areas are infected although the illness is never diagnosed. A single positive immunoglobulin (Ig) G antibody test result in a child who is not acutely ill likely means either a false-positive test result or past infection. No evidence indicates that antimicrobial treatment is indicated for such children.

Communication and Counseling

Patients and parents should be reassured that antimicrobial treatment of ehrlichiosis is highly successful and there is no chronic or recurrent form of infection.

They should also be counseled on personal protective measures (including avoiding tick-infested areas when possible, short-term use of insect repellent, and use of protective clothing such as long pants) to avoid tick bites in the future.

SUGGESTED READINGS

1. Bakken JS: Human granulocytic ehrlichiosis. Clin Infect Dis 34:554–560, 2000. **Comprehensive review of HME.**
2. Jacobs RF, Schutze GE: Ehrlichiosis in children. J Pediatr 131:184–192, 1997. **Reviews HME in children in the south-central United States.**
3. Krause PJ, Corrow CL, Bakken JS: Successful treatment of human granulocytic ehrlichiosis in children using rifampin. Pediatics 112:e252–e253, 2003. **Reports success with the use of rifampin to treat HGE.**
4. Lantos P, Krause PJ: Ehrlichiosis in children. Sem Pediatr Infect Dis 13:249–256, 2002. **Reviews ehrlichiosis in children.**
5. Olano JP, Walker DH: Human ehrlichioses. Med Clin North Am 86:375–392, 2002. **Excellent review of ehrlichiosis in humans.**

HELMINTH INFECTIONS

Cysticercosis

Linda S. Yancey, Susan H. Wootton, and A. Clinton White

KEY CONCEPTS

- Cysticercosis is primarily caused by exposure to feces from human carriers of the pork tapeworm. It is *not* caused by contact with pigs or undercooked pork.
- Antiepileptics are the first line of therapy in any case of symptomatic seizures.
- Seizures in the parenchymal form of neurocysticercosis are caused by the host immune reaction to the dying parasite.
- Calcified cysts have already died, and thus treating this form of the disease with antiparasitic agents is not beneficial.

The pork tapeworm, *Taenia solium*, is a widespread human and animal pathogen affecting mainly the developing world. The life cycle of the organism requires passage though both humans and pigs, resulting in one porcine and two distinct forms of human disease depending on the portion of the parasitic life cycle in which infection occurs. One of the two forms of human disease, neurocysticercosis, is the most common cause of acquired epilepsy worldwide. The optimal treatment for neurocysticercosis depends on the number and location of lesions within the central nervous system (CNS).

Intestinal taeniasis, carriage of the mature tapeworm in the human intestine, is commonly asymptomatic, and carriers may not be aware of the infection. The adult worm sheds proglottids and eggs that are passed intermittently with stool. When these eggs are ingested by a human or pig, the larvae leave the eggs and migrate through the gut wall into the tissues of the host. These cysticerci survive for months to years evading the host immune system. Parasitism of the CNS causes most morbidity in human disease and is referred to as neurocysticercosis (Fig. 1).

Although cysticercosis is associated classically with areas where pigs are allowed to forage freely, growth in global immigration has led to an increase in the presentation of neurocysticercosis in areas where it is not endemic. In the United States, areas with large immigrant populations, especially those from Mexico, South America, and Central America, have an increased incidence of the disease.

Identification and treatment of tapeworm carriers is vital to controlling the transmission of neurocysticercosis because cysticercosis is acquired via fecal–oral spread from a human carrier of the adult tapeworm. Thus contact with pigs or pork is not necessary for infection to occur.

The mainstay for diagnosis remains neuroimaging. Both CT and MRI scans are useful in the diagnosis. Both are able to detect degenerating parenchymal lesions, but MRI is more sensitive for detection of cysticerci in the

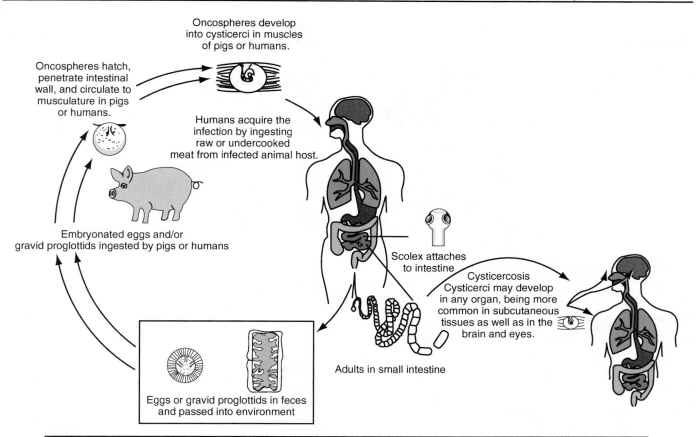

FIGURE 1. Taenia solium life cycle.

ventricles or cisterns and for visualization of the scolex. CT is better at detecting calcified lesions and more readily available in most areas (Tables 1 and 2). Serologic tests are plagued by poor sensitivity.

Expert Opinion on Management Issues

Neurocysticercosis was traditionally treated as a single disease entity. However, the parasite has the ability to migrate to virtually any area of the CNS from freely floating in the ventricles to the parenchyma of the brain. Additionally, the parasite burden an individual patient can carry varies from a single to hundreds of cysts of differing ages. This results in a wide spectrum of presentations, varying in severity from asymptomatic, incidentally noted infection to life-threatening disease. The clinical presentation, pathogenesis, and optimal treatment for neurocysticercosis vary depending on the number and location of lesions within the brain and the nature of the host inflammatory response (Table 3).

PARENCHYMAL DISEASE

Solitary Enhancing Lesions

Intraparenchymal cysts are the most common form of neurocysticercosis in children, accounting for approximately 75% of cases. On imaging studies, viable cysticerci appear as fluid collections 1 to 2 cm in diameter, isodense with cerebrospinal fluid (CSF). In some cases, the scolex may be seen as a 1- to 2-mm mural nodule. Although viable, the intraparenchymal cysts seldom produce symptoms because the parasite uses a variety of mechanisms to blunt or evade the host immune response. Thus viable cysticerci lack the local inflammation that is the hallmark of the symptomatic disease, and the parasitic infection per se does not cause symptoms.

The cysticerci are eventually attacked by the host's immune system, and the intense local inflammation results in seizure activity. It is during this stage of the disease that most pediatric patients present. The classic setting is that of new-onset seizures in a previously healthy child associated with a single enhancing lesion seen on brain scan.

The prognosis for patients with single enhancing lesions is excellent. Seizure recurrence is infrequent when patients are on adequate levels of antiepileptic drugs, which can usually be tapered after the patients are asymptomatic and the lesions resolve. The role of antiparasitic drugs (e.g., albendazole, 15 mg/kg/day for 7 days) in patients with single enhancing lesions is controversial. Because the host immune attack on an already dying parasite causes the symptoms, antiparasitic treatment has only limited benefit. Controlled trials suggest a possible role for a short course of

TABLE 1 Revised Diagnostic Criteria for Neurocysticercosis

Category	Criteria
Absolute	Histologic demonstration of the parasite from biopsy of a brain or spinal cord lesion
	Cystic lesions showing the scolex on CT or MRI
	Direct visualization of subretinal parasites by funduscopic examination
Major	Lesions highly suggestive of neurocysticercosis on neuroimaging studies*
	Positive serum EITB† for the detection of anticysticercal antibodies
	Resolution of intracranial cystic lesions after therapy with albendazole or praziquantel
	Spontaneous resolution of small single enhancing lesions‡
Minor	Lesions compatible with neurocysticercosis on neuroimaging studies§
	Clinical manifestations suggestive of neurocysticercosis‖
	Positive CSF ELISA for detecting of anticysticercal antibodies or cysticercal antigens
	Cysticercosis outside the CNS¶
Epidemiologic	Evidence of a household contact with *Taenia solium* infection
	Individuals coming from or living in an area where cysticercosis is endemic
	History of frequent travel to disease-endemic areas

*CT or MRI showing cystic lesions without scolex, enhancing lesions, or typical parenchymal brain calcifications.

†Enzyme-linked immunoelectrotransfer blot assay using purified extracts of *Taenia solium* antigens, as developed by the Centers for Disease Control and Prevention.

‡Solitary ring-enhancing lesions measuring >20 mm in diameter in patients presenting with seizures, a normal neurologic examination, and no evidence of an active systemic disease.

§CT or MRI showing hydrocephalus or abnormal enhancement of the leptomeninges, and myelograms showing multiple filling defects in the column of contrast medium.

‖Seizures, focal neurologic signs, intracranial hypertension, and dementia.

¶Histologically confirmed subcutaneous or muscular cysticercosis, plain X-ray films showing cigar-shaped soft-tissue calcifications, or direct visualization of cysticerci in the anterior chamber of the eye.

CNS, central nervous system; CSF, cerebrospinal fluid; CT, computed tomography; EITB, enzyme-linked immunoelectrotransfer blot; ELISA, enzyme-linked immunosorbent assay.

From Garcia HH, Evans CA, Nash TE, et al: Current consensus guidelines for treatment of neurocysticercosis. Clin Microbiol Rev 15(4):747–756, 2002.

TABLE 2 Revised Degrees of Certainty for the Diagnosis of Neurocysticercosis

Diagnostic Certainty	Criteria
Definitive	Presence of one absolute criterion
	Presence of two major plus one minor and one epidemiologic criterion
Probable	Presence of one major plus two minor criteria
	Presence of one major plus one minor and one epidemiologic criterion
	Presence of three minor plus one epidemiologic criterion

From Garcia HH, Evans CA, Nash TE, et al: Current consensus guidelines for treatment of neurocysticercosis. Clin Microbiol Rev 15(4):747–756, 2002.

In some cases, patients present with multiple parenchymal cysts, at least one of which shows some radiologic signs of inflammation. In such cases, antiparasitic medications (e.g., albendazole, 15 mg/kg/day for 7 to 14 days, along with steroids) appear beneficial in reducing the long-term incidence of seizures.

Calcifications

A significant risk factor for persistent seizures is the presence of a residual calcification at the site of an old cysticercus. In such cases, it is not the presence of viable parasite but rather the presence of residual parasitic antigen that triggers the local inflammation and results in seizures. Patients with persistent calcifications are at a much higher risk for continued seizure activity. Patients with seizures caused exclusively by persistent calcifications do not benefit from antiparasitic drugs because they no longer have living parasites. Antiepileptic medications are beneficial; however, the optimal duration of therapy is unclear and may need to be lifelong.

EXTRAPARENCHYMAL DISEASE

Ventricular Neurocysticercosis

Cysticerci may also be found floating in the ventricles or basilar cisterns. Viable cysticerci can cause mechanical obstruction of the foramina, leading to the blockage of CSF flow and intracranial hypertension. Once the cysts begin to succumb to the host immune system, they may adhere to surrounding tissues and cause local inflammation, which can cause damage to the adjacent tissue.

In cases of obstructive hydrocephalus, shunting or other forms of surgery to relieve intracranial pressures are critically important. Open craniotomy, used in the past, is associated with both short-term and long-term morbidity. Neuroendoscopy provides a preferred and less invasive approach. In general, endoscopic cysticercus removal should be performed without prior antiparasitic drug treatment because the inflamed cysticerci can adhere to the ventricular wall or become more friable, preventing complete removal.

corticosteroid treatment for patients with a single enhancing cysticercus. If antiparasitic drugs are used, a funduscopic examination should be performed beforehand to exclude intraocular parasites.

Cysticercal Encephalitis and Multiple Parenchymal Cysticerci

A small group of patients infected with multiple cysticerci develop diffuse cerebral edema from the inflammatory response to the parasites. These patients should be treated with anti-inflammatory drugs, such as corticosteroids. In this context, antiparasitic drugs are contraindicated because of the potential to increase the already brisk host inflammatory response.

TABLE 3 Guidelines for Use of Antiparasitic Treatment in Neurocysticercosis

Type	Infection Burden	Recommendations	Evidence
Parenchymal Neurocysticercosis			
Viable (live cysts)	Mild (1–5 cysts)	1. Antiparasitic treatment, with steroids.	II–3
		2. Antiparasitic treatment; steroids used only if side effects related to therapy appear.	II–3
		3. No antiparasitic treatment; neuroimaging follow-up.	II–3
	Moderate (>5 cysts)	Consensus: antiparasitic treatment with steroids.	II–3
	Heavy (>100 cysts)	1. Antiparasitic treatment with high-dose steroids.	III
		2. Chronic steroid management; no antiparasitic treatment; neuroimaging follow-up.	III
Enhancing lesions (degenerating cysts)	Mild or moderate	1. No antiparasitic treatment; neuroimaging follow-up.	I
		2. Antiparasitic treatment with steroids.	II–3
		3. Antiparasitic treatment; steroids only if side effects develop.	II–3
	Heavy (cysticercotic encephalitis)	Consensus: no antiparasitic treatment; high-dose steroids and osmotic diuretics.	III
Calcified cysticerci	Any number	Consensus: no antiparasitic treatment.	
Extraparenchymal Neurocysticercosis			
Ventricular cysticercosis		Consensus: neuroendoscopic removal, when available. If not available:	III
		1. Cerebrospinal fluid diversion followed by antiparasitic treatment, with steroids.	III
		2. Open surgery (mainly for ventricle cysts).	III
Subarachnoid cysts, including giant cysts or racemose cysticercosis, and chronic meningitis		Consensus: antiparasitic treatment with steroids, ventricular shunt if there is hydrocephalus.	II–3
Hydrocephalus with no visible cysts on neuroimaging		Consensus: ventricular shunt; no antiparasitic treatment.	III
Spinal cysticercosis, intra- or extramedullary*		Consensus: primarily surgical; anecdotal reports of successful use of albendazole with steroids.	III
Ophthalmic cysticercosis*		Consensus: surgical resection of cysts.†	II–3

*Given the rarity of these presentations, treatment was discussed based on the published literature.

†Experience in the use of albendazole with methylprednisolone for treatment of retinal cysticercosis and as a presurgical treatment for intravitreal cysticercosis has been published but not yet replicated.

Copyright © 2002, American Society for Microbiology.

Available online at http://www.pubmedcentral.nih.gov/articlerender.fcgi?tool=pubmed&pubmedid=12364377#figures-tables-sec, Table 4.

Garcia HH, et al: Current consensus guidelines for treatment of neurocysticercosis. Clin Microbiol Rev 15(4):747–756, 2002.

12

Patients treated only with ventriculoperitoneal shunting have a higher rate of shunt failure than those also treated with corticosteroids and antiparasitic drugs. Thus the combination of shunting plus chemotherapy is also a viable option. Case series have identified some patients treated with only chemotherapy and steroids. However, this approach should generally be discouraged because it carries the risk of development of acute hydrocephalus from cysticerci and/or accompanying inflammation causing obstruction.

Subarachnoid Neurocysticercosis

The growth of cysts that form in the basilar cisterns and gyri is not limited by surrounding tissue, and they can achieve diameters of several centimeters. The cysticerci often lose the scolex and may grow as a cluster of cystic lesions (termed *racemose cysticercosis*). Disease may result from mass effect from large cysticerci, particularly if there is surrounding cerebral edema. Cysticerci in the basilar cistern can also be accompanied by arachnoiditis, leading to CSF outflow obstruction, communicating hydrocephalus vasculitis,

and stroke. The basilar area is difficult to reach via surgical techniques. Consensus recommendations are to treat with a combination of antiparasitic drugs (e.g., albendazole, 15 mg/kg/day usually for more than 28 days) and steroids. Patients often also require CSF diversion procedures for intracranial hypertension.

Common Pitfalls

- Failure to obtain cranial imaging in patients in whom neurocysticercosis should be suspected. The detection of neurocysticercosis requires a high degree of clinical suspicion, especially in the case of the more serious extraparenchymal form of the disease. Patients with unexplained new-onset seizures or hydrocephalus should be considered for cranial imaging, especially if they, their family, or their friends are from an endemic area.
- Failure to treat symptoms of increased intracranial pressure aggressively. Regardless of the cause, any patient with increased intracranial pressure should be treated aggressively to relieve pressure.

For patients with obstructive hydrocephalus, this usually requires surgery (e.g., endoscopic removal or placement of a shunt).

■ Treatment of calcific disease with antiparasitic drugs. Because calcified cysts have already died, antiparasitic treatment is of no further benefit. If, however, viable cysts are detected on imaging studies, there is some argument for the use of antiparasitic agents. This decision should be made on a case-by-case basis.

■ Failure to obtain adequate follow-up. The common form of neurocysticercosis seen in the United States is that of a single degenerating lesion. Such lesions generally remain symptomatic as long as there is inflammation around the site; generally a year after the onset of seizures. Thus antiepileptic therapy could be stopped once the inflammation, seen on cranial imaging, subsides. This treatment decision should be made in conjunction with a neurologist and depends on the neuroradiologic findings, the patient's history of seizures, and the presence of residual calcification.

Communication and Counseling

The diagnosis of a parasitic infection, especially one involving the brain and having such a severe manifestation as seizures, can be very upsetting to both patients and their parents. It should be stressed that the most common form of neurocysticercosis, a solitary degenerating intraparenchymal lesion, has an excellent long-term prognosis. In one case series, the lowest overall mortality rate of any age group was in those patients younger than 14 years. Most patients respond well to antiepileptic medications and are able to taper these over time with a low risk of residual seizure activity. Patients with cysticercosis (in the absence of taeniasis) cannot spread the disease to others and do not need to be isolated from friends, family, or other patients.

SUGGESTED READINGS

1. Bergsneider M, Nieto JH: Endoscopic management of intraventricular cysticercosis. In Singh G, Prabhakar S (eds): *Taenia solium* Cysticercosis: From Basic to Clinical Science. Oxford: CABI, 2002, pp 399–410. **An overview of the pathogenesis and management of intraventricular disease.**
2. Del Brutto OH, Rajshekhar V, White AC Jr, et al: Proposed diagnostic criteria for neurocysticercosis. Neurology 57(2):177–183, 2001. **Consensus criteria for the diagnosis of neurocysticercosis from the Neurocysticercosis Working Group.**
3. Garcia HH, Pretell EJ, Gilman RH, et al: A trial of antiparasitic treatment to reduce the rate of seizures due to cerebral cysticercosis. N Engl J Med 350(3):249–258, 2001. **Large randomized clinical trial in adults examining the role of antiparasitic medications in seizure reduction in patients with neurocysticercosis.**
4. Garcia HH, Evans CA, Nash TE, et al: Current consensus guidelines for treatment of neurocysticercosis. Clin Microbiol Rev 15(4):747–756, 2002. **Guidelines for the treatment of neurocysticercosis from the Neurocysticercosis Working Group.**
5. Garcia HH, Del Brutto OH: *Taenia solium* cysticercosis. Lancet 362(9383):547–556, 2003. **Broad overview of cysticercosis.**
6. Nash TE, et al: Calcific neurocysticercosis and epileptogenesis. Neurology 62:1934–1938, 2004. **Review of the pathogenesis and treatment of the calcific form of the disease.**
7. Psarros TG, Krumerman J, Coimbra C: Endoscopic management of supratentorial ventricular neurocysticercosis: Case series and review of the literature. Minim Invasive Neurosurg 46(6):331–334, 2003. **Case series examining the role of minimally invasive endoscopic management of ventricular neurocysticercosis.**
8. Singhi P, Jain V, Khandelwal N: Corticosteroids versus albendazole for treatment of single small enhancing computed tomographic lesions in children with neurocysticercosis. J Child Neurol 19(5):323–327, 2004. **Pediatric study showing benefit to combination steroids and albendazole.**
9. Stringer JL, Marks LM, White AC Jr, Robinson P: Epileptogenic activity of granulomas associated with murine cysticercosis. Exp Neurol 183(2):532–536, 2003. **An animal model noting that seizures caused by neurocysticercosis are caused by the host immune response in epileptogenesis.**

Soil-Transmitted Helminth Infections

Peter J. Hotez, Jeff M. Bethony, and Simon Brooker

KEY CONCEPTS

■ Soil-transmitted helminth (STH) infections, caused by the nematodes (roundworms) *Ascaris lumbricoides* and *Trichuris trichiura* and the hookworms *Necator americanus* and *Ancylostoma duodenale,* are among the most common infections in developing countries.

■ Schoolchildren typically have the highest intensity of STH infection (highest worm burden) of any single group.

■ Chronic and intense STH infections in childhood lead to deficits in physical growth, cognition, intellect, school performance, and school attendance.

■ Treatment of STH infections in childhood with a single dose of a benzimidazole anthelminthic (BZA), either mebendazole or albendazole, results in temporary worm burden reductions with resulting improvements in health and education. This observation provides the basis of international school-based control programs.

■ In North America and Europe, the most common STH infections are caused by the nematodes *Enterobius vermicularis,* which causes pinworm infection, and *Toxocara canis,* which causes visceral and ocular larva migrans. The treatment and management goals and approaches for the treatment of these infections are different from STH infections in developing countries.

Soil-transmitted helminth (STH) infections are among the most common infections in the developing world. In these areas, the most prevalent of these parasitic nematodes (roundworms) are *Ascaris lumbricoides,* *Trichuris trichiura* and the hookworms *Necator americanus* and *Ancylostoma duodenale.* In North America and Europe, extensive surveillance data for parasitic diseases are not available. However, the existing

TABLE 1 Classes of Intensity for STH Infections

STH Infection	Light-Intensity Infections	Moderate-Intensity Infections	Heavy-Intensity Infections
Ascariasis	1–4999 epg	5000–49,999 epg	≥50,000 epg
Trichuriasis	1–999 epg	1000–9999 epg	≥10,000 epg
Hookworm infection	1–1999 epg	2000–3999 epg	≥4000 epg

epg, eggs per g feces; STH, soil-transmitted helminth.
From World Health Organization: Report of a WHO Expert Committee: Prevention and control of schistosomiasis and soil-transmitted helminthiasis. WHO Technical Report Series 912. Geneva: World Health Organization, 2002.

BOX 1 Major Anthelminthic Drugs Used for Mass Chemotherapy in Developing Countries

- Albendazole: Single dose, 400 mg (reduced to 200 mg for children between 12 and 24 mo of age)
- Mebendazole: Single dose, 500 mg
- Levamisole: Single dose, 2.5 mg/kg
- Pyrantel pamoate: Single dose, 10 mg/kg (not effective for trichuriasis)

BOX 2 Health and Educational Consequences of School-age Deworming with BZA Drugs in Developing Countries

- Improved iron and hemoglobin status
- Improved physical growth
- Improved cognition
- Higher educational achievement
- Reduced school absenteeism
- Reduced community transmission (ascaris and trichuris infections only)

BZA, benzimidazole anthelminthic.

evidence indicates that pinworm infection caused by *Enterobius vermicularis* and zoonotic infection caused by the canine roundworm *Toxocara canis* are probably the most common STH infections in these regions.

Morbidity is closely related to the number of worms a person harbors; those with light infections generally have no symptoms or signs of infection, whereas those with heavy infections suffer the greatest morbidity. In the case of ascaris, trichuris, and hookworm, the World Health Organization (WHO) distinguishes light, moderate, and heavy STH infections by estimating the number of eggs released by adult female worms living in the gastrointestinal tract (Table 1). In contrast, because pinworm eggs do not typically appear in the feces and *T. canis* migrating tissue larvae do not develop to egg-producing adults in humans, it is more difficult to define heavy worm burdens for these two STH infections. A major epidemiologic feature of STHs is an aggregated distribution in human communities where most individuals harbor a few worms and a minority of people harbor a majority. As a general rule, approximately 80% of the worm burden is harbored by 20% of the host population. For *Ascaris*, *Trichuris*, *Enterobius*, and probably *Toxocara* infections, infection intensities are highly age dependent, with schoolchildren typically harboring the heaviest infections of any single group. A large body of evidence indicates that schoolchildren with moderate and heavy STH infections exhibit deficits in physical growth, as well as cognition and intellectual development. In addition, some studies indicate that STH infections result in reduced school attendance. Therefore, STH infections have an educational as well as an economic impact.

Fortunately, much of this morbidity can be prevented and reversed through repeated chemotherapy with anthelminthic drugs. The most commonly used drugs are of the benzimidazole anthelminthic (BZA) class, mebendazole and albendazole, although both are less effective against hookworm and trichuriasis than against ascariasis. In addition, older drugs such as pyrantel pamoate (not effective for trichuriasis) and levamisole are also still in use in some developing countries (Box 1). Several studies conducted throughout the developing world show that treatment with a BZA reduces worm burdens and subsequently improves iron and hemoglobin status, physical growth,

cognition, educational achievement, school absenteeism, as well as a major consequence for the entire community, namely reduced ascaris and trichuris transmission (Box 2). Although debate continues about the precise health impact of infection, the demonstrable impact of BZAs, along with the relative low cost, high efficacy, and ease of delivery, prompted passage of a resolution at the 2001 World Health Assembly, which urges member states to administer anthelminthic chemotherapy regularly to at least 75% of all schoolchildren at risk for morbidity by 2010. In time, this could become an enormous global health program.

Expert Opinion on Management Issues

GENERAL COMMENTS

Box 3 lists the major drugs used for the treatment of STH infections. The BZAs have largely replaced pyrantel pamoate and other agents as first-line treatment for STH infections. The two major BZAs used for human STHs, mebendazole and albendazole, cause death of susceptible STHs through a slow process that does not result in their clearance from the intestine until a few days after treatment. The primary activity of these drugs is to inhibit microtubule polymerization by binding to the unique β-tubulin of these invertebrates. The BZAs have only limited solubility in water; in the case of albendazole, absorption is enhanced by coingestion of fatty foods.

Although albendazole and mebendazole are widely considered equivalent, some important differences can be noted between the two agents. In addition to differential susceptibilities of different STHs to these agents

---

BOX 3 Clinical Sequelae and Complications of Moderate and Heavy STH Infections

- STH infections (general)
  - Physical growth retardation
  - Intellectual retardation
  - Cognitive deficits
- Ascariasis
  - Intestinal obstruction
  - Hepatobiliary ascariasis
- Trichuriasis
  - Trichuris colitis
  - Trichuris dysentery syndrome
  - Rectal prolapse
- Hookworm infection
  - Iron-deficiency anemia
  - Protein-losing enteropathy
- Enterobiasis
  - Pruritus
- Toxocariasis
  - Visceral larva migrans
- Hepatomegaly
- Pneumonitis
- Cerebritis
  - Ocular larva migrans
- Retinitis
  - Covert toxocariasis
- Wheezing (asthma)
- Seizures

STH, soil-transmitted helminth.

(specified later), the therapeutic activities of mebendazole are largely confined to the gastrointestinal tract. In contrast, albendazole is metabolized in the liver to a sulfoxide derivative, which has potent anthelminthic activity and is widely distributed in the tissues. This explains why albendazole is preferred for the treatment of tissue-dwelling helminths, including toxocara. In the doses used to treat STHs, neither BZA causes significant systemic toxicity in routine clinical use, although transient abdominal pain, diarrhea, nausea, dizziness, and headache occur on occasion. Rarely, long-term use results in bone marrow suppression, alopecia, and hepatotoxicity. Both BZAs are embryotoxins and teratogens in laboratory animals. This finding previously curtailed their use in pregnancy and for infants (see later).

In the United States, albendazole is approved only for the treatment of neurocysticercosis and echinococcosis and should be considered investigational for the purpose of treating STH infections. Outside the United States, albendazole and mebendazole are widely available as generic drugs. In many developing countries, both BZAs can be purchased in bulk, so the delivery costs exceed the actual drug costs. Although it is convenient to consider all STH infections as a single entity, important differences warrant a separate discussion for each STH (Table 2).

ASCARIASIS

Rare in temperate climates, *Ascaris lumbricoides* is the most common STH with 1221 million cases worldwide.

The highest worm burdens occur in schoolchildren. Heavy ascaris infections can lead to serious complications, including acute intestinal obstruction and hepatobiliary ascariasis. However, because of their large size, even a single adult worm can cause significant mechanical damage and warrants treatment. Microscopic examination of unconcentrated feces is usually adequate to diagnose ascariasis. Both mebendazole and albendazole are highly efficacious for ascaris infection. When heavy infections occur, transient symptoms of abdominal pain, distention, and diarrhea can occur in association with the expulsion of adult ascaris worms.

ENTEROBIASIS

Human pinworm infection remains a common pediatric problem in temperate climates. Although pinworms do not produce serious symptoms, pruritus ani, the most common clinical feature of enterobiasis, results in irritation and excoriation of the perianal skin. In rare cases, adult pinworms may migrate into the female genitourinary system, where they may cause vaginitis. The diagnosis of enterobiasis is established by visualization of adult worms or eggs in the perianal region. The cellophane tape or "Scotch tape" test is a reliable method for detecting parasite eggs. The drug of choice for pinworm infection is a single dose of mebendazole, albendazole, or pyrantel pamoate. The dose should be repeated in 2 weeks. In the United States, pyrantel pamoate is available as an over-the-counter (OTC) treatment for pinworm (Pin-X [Effcon]) in most chain pharmacies. It can also be ordered by calling Effcon Laboratories, Inc. (800-722-2428). Because all family members are usually affected, treatment of the entire household may be recommended. Occasionally, parents report a recurrence of symptoms following two treatments with a BZA. In such cases, the health care provider should document true recurrence of infection by repeat diagnosis.

HOOKWORM INFECTION

The two major human hookworms, *Necator americanus* and *Ancylostoma duodenale*, occur in an estimated 740 million people worldwide. Adult hookworms cause intestinal blood loss, so moderate and heavy infections can produce sufficient blood loss to cause iron-deficiency anemia. In many parts of Africa (and presumably, elsewhere) where iron stores are depleted, hookworm can significantly contribute to anemia. Unlike ascaris and trichuris infections, heavy infections with hookworm occur commonly in both adults (including pregnant women) and children. Microscopic examination of unconcentrated feces is usually adequate to diagnose hookworm infection.

On an individual basis, the two major goals of therapy are nutritional support for children with iron deficiency and removal of the adult hookworms with a BZA. The former may require replacement therapy with an iron salt preparation. In rare cases, anemia is severe enough to warrant transfusion. Either mebendazole or albendazole is considered a first-line

TABLE 2 Treatment of Soil-Transmitted Helminth Infections

Generic Name (Trade Name)	Dose	Maximum Dose	Formulation	Adverse Effects
Ascariasis				
Albendazole (Albenza)*	Pediatric and adult dose: 400 mg once (reduced dose in children 12–14 months of age)		Tablets	Abdominal pain, nausea, vomiting, headache, elevated transaminases
Mebendazole (Vermox)†	Pediatric and adult dose: 100 mg bid × 3 days or 500 mg once		Chewable tablets	Abdominal pain, diarrhea, rash, elevated transaminases
Pyrantel pamoate (Pin-X)‡	Pediatric and adult dose: 11 mg/kg once	1 g	Suspension	Nausea, diarrhea, vomiting
Enterobiasis				
Albendazole (Albenza)*	Pediatric and adult dose: 400 mg once; repeat in 2 wk (reduced dose in children 12–14 months of age)		Tablets	Abdominal pain, nausea, vomiting, headache, elevated transaminases
Mebendazole (Vermox)†	Pediatric and adult dose: 100 mg once; repeat in 2 wk		Chewable tablets	Abdominal pain, diarrhea, rash, elevated transaminases
Pyrantel pamoate (Pin-X)‡	Pediatric and adult dose: 11 mg/kg once; repeat in 2 wk	1 g	Suspension	Nausea, diarrhea, vomiting
Hookworm Infection				
Albendazole (Albenza)*	Pediatric and adult dose: 400 mg once (reduced dose in children 12–14 months of age)		Tablets	Abdominal pain, nausea, vomiting, headache, elevated transaminases
Mebendazole (Vermox)†	Pediatric and adult dose: 100 mg bid × 3 days		Chewable tablets	Abdominal pain, diarrhea, rash, elevated transaminases
Pyrantel pamoate (Pin-X)‡	Pediatric and adult dose: 11 mg/kg × 3 days	1 g	Suspension	Nausea, diarrhea, vomiting
Toxocariasis				
Albendazole (Albenza)*	Pediatric and adult dose: 400 mg bid × 5 days		Tablets	Abdominal pain, nausea, vomiting, headache, elevated transaminases
Trichuriasis				
Albendazole (Albenza)*	Pediatric and adult dose: 400 mg qd × 3 days (reduced dose in children 12–14 months of age)		Tablets	Abdominal pain, nausea, vomiting, headache, elevated transaminases
Mebendazole (Vermox)†	Pediatric and adult dose: 100 mg bid × 3 days		Chewable tablets	Abdominal pain, diarrhea, rash, elevated transaminases

*GlaxoSmithKline.
†McNeil Consumer.
‡Effcon.
bid, twice daily.

12

treatment for hookworm infection. However, a single dose of mebendazole achieves a cure rate of only 21%, in contrast to higher though variable rates for albendazole. Therefore, albendazole is probably superior to mebendazole in reducing hookworm burdens in children. Some authorities believe *N. americanus* is less susceptible to BZAs than *A. duodenale*, so repeated dosing with albendazole may also be required. Because hookworm larvae of *A. duodenale* may be arrested in the muscles and enter the gastrointestinal tract at a later time, the health care provider should be alert to the possibility of recurrence of hookworm infection. Such recurrence can take place several months after the patient receives specific anthelmintic chemotherapy, even after leaving an endemic area. The frequency of this phenomenon is unknown. In clinical practice, it is not routinely feasible to distinguish between the two species of hookworm.

TOXOCARIASIS

Toxocariasis is a common infection of dogs worldwide. It is also a relatively common zoonosis in North America and Europe, as well as in some developing countries, including Brazil. In the United States, up to 50% of inner-city children are seropositive as measured by enzyme-linked immunosorbent assay. Toxocariasis is particularly common among migrants from Puerto Rico. Human toxocara infection occurs via the accidental ingestion of embryonated eggs, which are common in the external environment. After egg ingestion, the larvae migrate through the tissues until they are ultimately overcome by the host inflammatory response. Most children are asymptomatic following exposure to toxocara eggs. However, others develop larva migrans syndromes, including visceral larva migrans (VLM), ocular larva migrans (OLM), or covert toxocariasis. It has been conjectured that the severity of symptoms is related to the size of the inoculum, the frequency of egg ingestion, the intensity of the host inflammatory response, and the migratory pattern of the parasite in the infected host.

VLM, which most commonly occurs in toddlers and young children, is associated with an eosinophilic pneumonitis accompanied by cough, fever, wheezing, and infiltrates on chest radiographs. Hepatomegaly and other extrapulmonary manifestations are infrequent. Occasionally, seizures occur in association with larval migrations in the brain and resultant cerebritis. Children with VLM often have leukocytosis, eosinophilia, and hypergammaglobulinemia. The diagnosis of VLM is established by clinical findings and a confirmatory enzyme immunoassay. The treatment of VLM with anthelminthic drugs is reserved for patients with severe, persistent, or progressive symptoms. Albendazole is the drug of choice. A 5-day course of treatment with this drug is recommended.

OLM usually occurs in older children and presents with unilateral vision loss sometimes accompanied with a strabismus. OLM is an inflammatory monocular disease associated with retinochoroiditis, optic papillitis, and endophthalmitis. In some cases retinal detachment can occur. In contrast to VLM, the enzyme immunoassay is frequently negative in OLM. Diagnosis therefore requires the assistance of an experienced ophthalmologist who can recognize the characteristic granulomas, larval tracks, and accompanying inflammation on funduscopic examination. Medical management is frequently not helpful in the treatment of OLM, except for the use of topical or systemic steroids when appropriate. Specific surgical management is sometimes required.

The term *covert* or *occult toxocariasis* is used to describe patients with some but not all of the findings of VLM. The identification of pulmonary infiltrates, wheezing, and eosinophilia in some children with covert toxocariasis led some investigators to postulate that *T. canis* is an underappreciated environmental cause of asthma in inner cities. The role of albendazole in the treatment of covert toxocariasis is unknown.

TRICHURIASIS

The common whipworm *Trichuris trichiura* is responsible for 795 million cases worldwide. Heavy trichuris infection results in colitis and dysentery. Rectal prolapse can occur as a result of severe and frequent straining during defecation. Microscopic examination of unconcentrated feces is usually adequate to diagnose trichuriasis. Either mebendazole or albendazole is the drug of choice for the treatment of trichuriasis. However, when used in a single dose during mass chemotherapy efforts, albendazole is considered more efficacious for the treatment of trichuriasis. Generally, multiple dosing of BZA drugs is required to reduce trichuris worm burdens. Although pyrantel pamoate is effective for ascaris and hookworm infections, it is not effective in the treatment of trichuriasis.

Common Pitfalls

Cimetidine inhibits BZA metabolism and may result in an increase in plasma concentrations of BZAs. Steroids also affect the metabolism of BZAs.

Both albendazole and mebendazole showed embryotoxic and teratogenic activity in pregnant rats at a single oral dose approximately equal to the human dose. In view of these findings, the use of BZAs is not recommended in pregnant women. However, in postmarketing surveys on women who inadvertently consumed mebendazole during the first trimester of pregnancy, the incidence of spontaneous abortion and malformation did not exceed that in the general population. There are no corresponding controlled studies of albendazole in pregnancy, so it should only be used in pregnancy if the potential benefit justifies the risk to the fetus. An estimated 44 million pregnant women are infected with hookworms. Iron deficiency anemia in pregnancy is linked to a number of adverse outcomes that affect maternal and child health. Therefore, the WHO recommends treatment of hookworm with BZAs during the second and third trimesters of pregnancy.

The BZAs have not been extensively studied in children younger than 2 years; therefore, the relative benefits and risks should be considered in this age group. The use of BZAs in children younger than 24 months for the treatment of STHs was reviewed. The review was based on an informal consultation convened by the WHO in Geneva in April 2002 to review the treatment of children younger than 24 months for STH infections. It was concluded that "while systems for the absorption, distribution, metabolism and elimination of drugs do not fully develop until children are in their second year of life . . . current knowledge reveals that the incidence of side effects linked to BZAs in young children are likely to be the same as older children. Accordingly . . . albendazole and mebendazole may be used to treat children as young as 12 months if local circumstances show that relief from ascariasis and trichuriasis is justified" (Montresor et al., 2003, p 223).

In endemic areas, STH reinfection rapidly occurs following treatment, and therefore frequent and periodic treatments are often necessary to maintain low worm burdens in susceptible populations. A report that the efficacy of BZAs may diminish with frequent and periodic use caused concerns about the possible emergence of BZA drug resistance, a phenomenon well documented among STHs of livestock. To date, however, BZA drug resistance is not yet shown to occur among human STHs.

Communication and Counseling

Parents should be educated about how specific STH infections may be transmitted, particularly for enterobiasis because it can be transmitted by fecal–oral contact. Following diagnosis of enterobiasis in a child, it is common to recommend scrupulous hygienic measures, including the washing of clothes with hot water. However, no direct evidence indicates that such practices are effective.

SUGGESTED READINGS

1. Albonico M, Bickle Q, Ramsan M, et al: Efficacy of mebendazole and levamisole alone or in combination against intestinal nematode infections after repeated targeted mebendazole treatment in Zanzibar. Bull World Health Organ 81:343–352, 2003. **Provides evidence that the efficacy of a benzimidazole anthelminthic drug could diminish following frequent and periodic use.**
2. Bennett A, Guyatt H: Reducing intestinal nematode infections: Efficacy of albendazole and mebendazole. Parasitol Today 16:71–74, 2000. **Reviews published data on cure rates and egg reduction rates in the treatment of Ascaris lumbricoides, Trichuris trichiura, and hookworm.**
3. De Silva NR: Impact of mass chemotherapy on the morbidity due to soil-transmitted nematodes. Acta Trop 86:197–214, 2003. **Summarizes the impact of worm burden reductions on child development.**
4. De Silva NR, Brooker S, Hotez PJ, et al: Soil-transmitted helminth infections: Updating the global picture. Trends Parasitol 19:547–551, 2003. **Outlines the global burden of disease caused by STH infections.**
5. DeSilva N, Guyatt H, Bundy D: Anthelmintics. A comparative review of their clinical pharmacology. Drugs 53:769–788, 1997. **Review of clinical pharmacology.**
6. Despommier D: Toxocariasis: Clinical aspects, epidemiology, medical ecology, and molecular aspects. Clin Microbiol Rev 16:265–272, 2003. **Updates the current literature on human toxocariasis.**
7. Dickson R, Awasthi S, Williamson P, et al: Effects of treatment for intestinal helminth infection on growth and cognitive performance in children: Systematic review of randomized trials. BMJ 320:1697–1701, 2000. **Summarizes the effects of anthelminthic drug treatment on growth and cognitive performance of in children.**
8. Horton J: Global anthelminthic chemotherapy programs: Learning from history. Trends Parasitol 19:405–409, 2003. **Summarizes previous attempts to control helminth morbidity through mass chemotherapy programs.**
9. Hotez PJ: Reducing the global burden of human parasitic diseases. Comp Parasitol 69:140–145, 2002. **Outlines the need for a U.S. nationwide survey for parasitic infections.**
10. Hotez PJ, Brooker S, Bethony JM, et al: Current concepts: Hookworm infection. N Engl J Med 351:799–807, 2004. **Summarizes the major morbidities caused by human hookworm infection and approaches to its control.**
11. Montresor A, Awasthi S, Crompton DWT: Use of benzimidazoles in children younger than 24 months for the treatment of soil-transmitted helminthiasis. Acta Trop 86:223–232, 2003. **Discusses the safety of albendazole and mebendazole in children younger than 2 years.**
12. Pawlowski Z: Toxocariasis in humans: Clinical expression and treatment dilemma. J Helminthol 75:299–305, 2001. **Summarizes the controversial issues in the management and treatment of human toxocariasis.**
13. Sabrosa NA, de Souza EC: Nematode infections of the eye: Toxocariasis and diffuse unilateral subacute neuroretinitis. Curr Opin Ophthalmol 12:450–454, 2001. **Summarizes the management and treatment of ocular toxocariasis.**
14. Sharghi N, Schantz P, Hotez PJ: Toxocariasis: An occult cause of childhood asthma, seizures, and neuropsychological deficit? Semin Pediatr Infect Dis 11:257–260, 2000. **Summarizes current knowledge of covert toxocariasis.**
15. The Medical Letter on Drugs and Therapeutics. Drugs for Parasitic Infections August 2004. The Medical Letter, Inc. Available at http://www.themedicalletter.com/restricted/articles/w1189c.pdf (accessed September 26, 2005). **Up-to-date recommendations on drug selections and doses.**
16. World Health Organization: Report of a WHO Expert Committee: Prevention and control of schistosomiasis and soil-transmitted helminthiasis, WHO Technical Report Series 912. Geneva: World Health Organization, 2002. **Summarizes WHO's recommendations for controlling the morbidity of STH infections with anthelminthic drugs, as well as a resolution calling for STH control at the World Health Assembly in 2001.**

Schistosomiasis

Ronald E. Blanton

KEY CONCEPTS

- Major morbidities with *Schistosoma mansoni* and *Schistosoma japonicum* include portal hypertension in the presence of good liver function.
- Major morbidities with *Schistosoma haematobium* are hydronephrosis, nonfunctioning kidneys, and bladder cancer.
- Schistosomiasis is also associated with pulmonary hypertension, transverse myelitis, seizures, hepatomegaly, genitourinary granulomatous swellings, bloody diarrhea, malnutrition, and anemia.
- There is no natural sterile immunity, so reinfection is common.
- Praziquantel, the only drug readily available, is effective against all species.
- Higher doses are recommended for treatment of *S. japonicum* and *Schistosoma mekongi*.
- Resistance is uncommon, and most cases respond to retreatment.
- Oxamniquine is a suitable alternative when praziquantel resistance is suspected for *S. mansoni*.

Schistosomiasis is the collection of morbidities caused most commonly by three species of flatworms: *Schistosoma mansoni*, *Schistosoma haematobium*, and *Schistosoma japonicum*. Less common are *Schistosoma intercalatum* and *Schistosoma mekongi* infections. *S. mansoni* has the widest distribution, with endemic areas throughout much of Africa and the Middle East. It is also the only human schistosome in the Americas. *S. haematobium* is also common in Africa and the Middle East, sometimes overlapping with *S. mansoni*. *S. japonicum* is endemic to East Asia, primarily China, Indonesia, and the Philippines. Infection with each species produces distinct clinical characteristics related to parasite biology and location within the host. Transmission requires that contaminated feces or urine come in contact with fresh water and specific snail species. Infected snails eventually shed developmental stages of the parasite infective for humans and/or domestic animals in the case of *S. japonicum*. Schistosomes do not multiply in humans; therefore, repeated exposure to contaminated water is necessary to develop heavy infections.

In humans, the adult parasites live within the mesenteric venous bed (*S. mansoni* and *S. japonicum*) or the vesicular veins (*S. haematobium*). The eggs produced by mated worm pairs provoke strong immune reactions that resolve by local fibrosis, which may occlude portal flow of the ureters. Hepatosplenomegaly in childhood is associated with *S. mansoni* and *S. japonicum*, as are hepatic fibrosis, portal hypertension, and bleeding esophageal varices. Because of massive egg production, *S. japonicum* infections may produce portosystemic shunts early in infections with the resultant ectopic location of eggs in the lung (pulmonary

12

hypertension) or brain (epilepsy). With *S. haematobium* infection, granulomatous inflammation around eggs deposited in the urinary tract produces microscopic or frank hematuria. Ectopic location of *S. haematobium* eggs results in genital granulomas, although all species may produce eggs that lodge near the spinal cord to produce transverse myelitis. All human schistosome infections may be associated with bloody diarrhea, may aggravate malnutrition, and may be a source of anemia. Severe morbidity is found in only 5% to 10% of those infected. Hundreds of millions are infected worldwide, however, so schistosomiasis ranks among the most important public health problems in developing countries. Nonhuman schistosomes found in North America produce skin irritation (swimmer's itch) when juvenile parasites penetrate and die in the skin. These do not develop into adults, however.

Sterile immunity does not naturally exist, and reinfection often follows treatment. Infection can be diagnosed by examination of stool or urine, by rectal biopsy, and by serum or urine antigen assays. The extent of disease in the liver or urinary tract is best evaluated by ultrasound.

Expert Opinion on Management Issues

DRUG THERAPY

General Principles

Currently, only three drugs can be considered for treatment of schistosomiasis: praziquantel, oxamniquine, and artemether (Table 1). Of these, only praziquantel is approved for use in the United States and in active production. Fortunately, praziquantel is effective as a single dose, inexpensive (<$0.10 per dose), broad spectrum, and well tolerated. All of these drugs are administered orally.

Every infected individual should be treated regardless of intensity of infection, but treatment is rarely an emergency. The objective of therapy is foremost for prevention of chronic morbidity. Even where rapid reinfection is the rule, a single round of chemotherapy has long-term beneficial effects. Hepatic fibrosis as a result of *S. mansoni* infection or bladder pathology from *S. haematobium* both show benefit from a brief period of treatment, even many years after regular

therapy is discontinued. Praziquantel is a category B agent and presumed safe in pregnancy. The World Health Organization (WHO) recommends its use in women of childbearing age as well as in pregnant and lactating women who are infected.

Public Health Strategies

Strategies for large-scale treatment vary, but most strategies focus on schoolchildren whether or not the control program is school based, because this age group has the highest intensity of infection. The most expensive approaches require parasitologic diagnosis for everyone in the community or, in the case of *S. haematobium*, a dipstick assay for hematuria, followed by treatment of those infected. This is selective therapy in the strict sense. Even more selectively, diagnosis and treatment may be restricted to children between 7 and 15 years of age, the group with the highest intensity of infection and with the best chance for reversal of morbidity. Mass chemotherapy, by contrast, usually begins with a parasitologic survey of a sample of children, and if the infection rate is above 50%, all members of a community or all schoolchildren are treated. The mass chemotherapy approach saves on the cost in time and money of parasitologic examination taking into account the insensitivity of parasitologic diagnosis. Light infections can be difficult to diagnose by a single stool examination. A single dose of either praziquantel or oxamniquine has an apparent cure rate of 70% to 90%, with a 90% to 95% egg reduction in those not cured. Treatment failure is positively correlated with the initial infection intensity.

The side effects of praziquantel and oxamniquine are very similar and appear to be primarily related to host response to dying parasites (i.e., the higher the intensity of infection, the more likely side effects will occur). Mild nausea, vomiting, and diarrhea are common.

Dosing and Schedules

Praziquantel is effective against all species of schistosomes as well as many other flukes and tapeworms. Immature parasites are relatively resistant, and adult females are the most susceptible. The drug is generally provided as a 600-mg pill. Egypt produces a praziquantel syrup for pediatric use, and one is under development in Brazil. Standard dosing for *S. mansoni* and

TABLE 1 Treatment of Schistosomiasis				
Drug	**Schistosome Species**	**Stage and Sex**	**Other Parasites**	**Dose**
Praziquantel	*Schistosoma mansoni* *Schistosoma haematobium* *Schistosoma japonicum*	Adult female	Most adult cestodes	40 mg/kg 40 mg/kg 60 mg/kg divided into 2 doses × 1 d
Oxamniquine	*S. mansoni*	Immature and adult males	None	15 mg/kg (adult) 20 mg/kg (child)
Artemether	*S. japonicum* *S. mansoni* *S. haematobium*	Immature females	Malaria	6 mg/kg 6 mg/kg 6 mg/kg

S. haematobium is 40 mg/kg as a single dose; however, 60 mg/kg in two doses that can be administered within hours of each other is recommended for *S. japonicum* and *S. mekongi*. Depending on the objectives of therapy, repeated dosing over a short period of time increases cure rates.

Oxamniquine is active only against *S. mansoni*. It is more active against immature and male parasites than praziquantel. The drug reaches peak levels after a few hours, with a mean half-life of 90 minutes, and it is primarily eliminated in the urine. It is supplied as a 250-mg capsule or a 50 mg/mL syrup. A relative tolerance to the drug in some parts of Africa cannot be well explained by either host or parasite differences. It is primarily used in South America at a single dose of 15 mg/kg. For children weighing less than 30 kg, 20 mg/kg is given in two divided doses. In much of Africa, 30 to 60 mg/kg is recommended, but 15 mg/kg is again effective in West Africa. Although oxamniquine was still available in Brazil as of 2004, production has stopped and stocks will likely be exhausted within 5 years. Oxamniquine is rarely associated with seizures, largely in those with preexisting epilepsy.

Artemether is not currently in use for schistosomes. It is effective primarily against immature stages of *S. japonicum* and *S. mansoni*, less so for *S. haematobium*. Its suggested use is for prophylaxis every 2 to 3 weeks at a dose of 6 mg/kg ($\approx$\$1.2 per adult) to produce a 50% to 25% reduction in infection. Artemether is not as effective as praziquantel. It should not be used for schistosomiasis where there is the possibility of inducing malarial resistance to this drug (i.e., most of sub-Saharan Africa, where schistosomiasis is most prevalent).

Drug Resistance

Resistance to any of these drugs is uncommon and in most cases should not be a consideration in treatment. Drug tolerance can be produced, however, in the laboratory, and rare field isolates also show relative tolerance. In practice, cure rates are always less than 100%, but most initial failures respond to repeat treatment. There have been two well-studied instances of apparent resistance to praziquantel. In an area of new transmission in Senegal, cure rates were only 30% to 40%, although a 95% reduction was still found in the number of eggs in stool. This apparent failure was thought to be primarily the result of intense transmission and the presence of immature parasites in many individuals, because the efficacy of praziquantel is low for between 2 days and 4 weeks after infection. Retreatment with praziquantel or use of oxamniquine was successful. Some parasite isolates from this focus and a focus in Egypt, however, did show increased tolerance to praziquantel. General experience and mathematical models indicate that resistance to this drug will continue to be slow to develop.

SURGERY

Portal hypertension due to *S. mansoni* or *S. japonicum* can be life-threatening. Unlike this condition caused by toxins or viral infections, hepatic function usually remains intact in schistosomal fibrosis; thus the ability to clot, control bleeding, and other synthetic hepatic functions are intact. Surgery is a last resort. Even with some advanced disease, praziquantel treatment reduces the inflammatory response, much fibrosis regresses in children, and portal hypertension resolves or is reduced, making surgery unnecessary. Indications for surgery are large or repeated hemorrhage or hypersplenism with splenic sequestration. Conservative treatment consists of endoscopic sclerosis or clipping of varices. The TIPS (transjugular intrahepatic portosystemic shunt) procedure is not recommended in most cases because the risk of intrahepatic complications is significant, and occlusion of the prosthesis usually occurs within the first year. Splenorenal shunt or ligation of the posterior gastric vessels, together with subtotal or total splenectomy and autologous implantation, are the most used invasive approaches. Long-term recurrence of esophageal bleeding or, rarely, hemorrhage from visceral varices are among the complications of this surgery.

PREVENTIVE MEASURES

The developmental history of schistosomes is a cycle of transmission between humans and an appropriate snail host and back to humans. A break anywhere in the cycle interrupts transmission. Thus, sanitation, economic development, treatment of human infections, and snail control are the keys to prevention. There are hopes for a vaccine, but none appears to be on the horizon in the short term. Education is beneficial when aimed at sanitation measures and awareness of available treatment. Instructions about abstinence from contact with water may not be productive because many essential activities involve water contact. In tropical countries, essential activities appear to include swimming for children younger than 15 years. Studies conducted two decades ago on St. Lucia established the usefulness of major sanitation measures, such as piped water, for control of many diseases including schistosomiasis, but drug therapy was the most cost effective in the short term.

Common Pitfalls

False positives are rarely a problem in the direct microscopic diagnosis of schistosome infections. As discussed, however, stool eggs can be difficult to observe in light infections, and the effect of community-wide treatment is often to convert heavy infections to light infections, thus underestimating the prevalence. Apparent resistance to praziquantel where there is high transmission is likely to represent the presence of immature parasites. Retreatment or switching to oxamniquine, if still available, is usually effective.

Communication and Counseling

Ninety percent of those infected have no overt symptoms. There is a good prognosis following treatment, especially in those with light infections (<100 eggs per g feces or 10 mL urine). The reversibility of many lesions in childhood is complete following treatment.

SUGGESTED READINGS

1. Cioli D, Pica-Mattoccia L: Praziquantel. Parasitol Res 90(Suppl 1): S3–S9, 2003. **Excellent short review of praziquantel's history, pharmacology, available brands, and its future.**
2. Gryseels B, Mbaye A, De Vlas SJ, et al: Are poor responses to praziquantel for the treatment of *Schistosoma mansoni* infections in Senegal due to resistance? An overview of the evidence. Trop Med Int Health 6:864–873, 2001. **Presents an analysis of an outbreak demonstrating apparent praziquantel resistance and concludes from the data that true genetically transmitted resistance did not play a role.**
3. King CH, Muchiri EM, Ouma JH: Evidence against rapid emergence of praziquantel resistance in *Schistosoma haematobium*, Kenya. Emerg Infect Dis 6:585–594, 2000. **Analysis of a long-term treatment program and review of the literature that estimates the time to development of resistance to praziquantel at 10 years based on modeling current usage rates.**
4. Magnussen P: Treatment and re-treatment strategies for schistosomiasis control in different epidemiological settings: A review of 10 years' experiences. Acta Trop 86:243–254, 2003. **Evidence-based discussion of treatment approaches in a developing country setting. A range of options is discussed depending on transmission pattern and resources.**
5. Stelma FF, Sall S, Daff B, et al: Oxamniquine cures *Schistosoma mansoni* infection in a focus in which cure rates with praziquantel are unusually low. J Infect Dis 176:304–307, 1997. **Demonstrates the usefulness of oxamniquine in a setting where there is relative praziquantel resistance.**
6. Subramanian AK, Mungai P, Ouma JH, et al: Long-term suppression of adult bladder morbidity and severe hydronephrosis following selective population chemotherapy for *Schistosoma haematobium*. Am J Trop Med Hyg 61:476–481, 1999. **Long-term follow-up (7 to 13 years after treatment) shows substantially reduced bladder and kidney pathology in treated versus untreated individuals.**
7. World Health Organization: The Control of Schistosomiasis. Second Report of the WHO Expert Committee. Geneva: World Health Organization, 1993. **Covers a wide range of topics, including control strategies, cost analysis, parasite genetics, sanitation, and chemotherapy. Recommendations and analyses are still applicable today for most countries.**
8. World Health Organization: Report of the WHO Informal Consultation on the Use of Praziquantel during Pregnancy/Lactation and Albendazole/Mebendazole in Children under 24 Months. Geneva: World Health Organization, 2002. **Emphasizes the relative risk of leaving women of childbearing age and pregnant and lactating women out of treatment programs versus the very low risk of drug-related complications and concludes that these groups should be treated.**

Trichinellosis (Trichinosis)

Melissa R. Held and Michael Cappello

KEY CONCEPTS

- Trichinellosis is a food-borne zoonosis affecting at least 10 million people worldwide.
- Early diagnosis requires a high index of suspiciozn, and the differential diagnosis includes visceral larva migrans (toxocariasis), schistosomiasis, rheumatologic disorders, viral encephalitis, typhoid fever, and leptospirosis.
- Complications are rare, usually occurring in the first 2 to 3 weeks following infection.
- Diagnosis is confirmed by serologic testing or histologic analysis of a muscle biopsy specimen.
- Treatment of symptomatic cases should include both anthelminthic therapy and systemic glucocorticoids.

Epidemiology and Life Cycle

Trichinellosis (also known as trichinosis) is a zoonotic infection caused by nematode parasites of the genus *Trichinella*. The majority of human cases are caused by *Trichinella spiralis*, although infections with *Trichinella pseudospiralis*, *Trichinella papuae*, *Trichinella nativa*, and *Trichinella murrelli* are reported. An estimated 10 million people or more worldwide are at risk, and sporadic outbreaks are reported in the United States. Most human infections result from ingestion of contaminated meat, including pork, bear, horse meat, or other wild game containing encysted larvae. Host digestive enzymes degrade the cyst wall, releasing larvae that quickly invade the columnar epithelium of the small intestine. After molting to the adult stage (4 to 5 days), the worms mate, and females release newborn larvae into the lumen of the gut. These larvae penetrate the intestinal mucosa, invade small vessels and/or lymphatics, and arrest within various tissues. The most common location of the disseminated larvae is somatic muscle, although other organs, including the heart, brain, lung, and kidneys, may also be involved. Upon reaching their final destination, larvae may persist for months to years within a specialized host-derived structure called the *nurse cell*.

Stages of Infection

Each stage of *Trichinella* infection is associated with specific symptoms attributable to tissue invasion by the parasite and/or the host immune response. Initial symptoms usually appear between 7 and 14 days following ingestion of contaminated meat, although incubation periods of up to 30 days are reported. The acute stage of infection, characterized by the invasion of intestinal epithelium by excysted larvae, is often asymptomatic. Heavily infected individuals, however, may experience a variety of gastrointestinal symptoms, including diarrhea, nausea, and abdominal pain. These symptoms are often associated with a systemic illness that is most likely attributable to the effects of newborn larvae as they disseminate throughout the body. Fever is a nearly universal feature of acute trichinellosis, present in up to 90% of infected individuals during the first week of illness. The dissemination phase of infection is also associated with a number of nonspecific symptoms, including myalgia, dysphagia, swelling of the upper extremities and torso, as well as central nervous system (CNS) disturbances (dizziness, headache, visual disturbances, neurasthenia, and paralysis of the ocular muscles). These symptoms usually resolve at 4 to 6 weeks postinfection, at which time the adult females within the intestine stop excreting larvae. Acute infection is followed by a convalescent stage, which is usually asymptomatic.

Expert Opinion on Management Issues

DIAGNOSIS

The diagnosis of trichinellosis is based on clinical grounds in the setting of a positive serology or tissue diagnosis. Trichinellosis should be considered in any patient who presents with fever, periorbital edema, and muscle tenderness. Individuals presenting with this particular constellation of signs and symptoms should be asked about recent ingestion of wild game or undercooked meat. Laboratory findings include a leukocytosis with a predominance of eosinophils. Although eosinophilia generally correlates with the intensity of infection, its absence in heavily infected individuals signifies a poor prognosis. Elevation of circulating muscle enzymes, including lactate dehydrogenase (LDH) and creatine phosphokinase (CPK), can also be seen. The diagnosis is most frequently confirmed using serologic tests directed at a variety of *Trichinella* antigens, although seroconversion may not occur for up to 3 weeks after infection. It is recommended that serum samples be sent to the U.S. Centers for Disease Control and Prevention for accurate measurement of anti-*Trichinella* antibodies using enzyme immunoassay (EIA). Information about this service is available online (www.dpd.cdc.gov/dpdx/Default.htm) or by telephone (770–488–4431). The diagnosis of trichinellosis can also be confirmed by histologic examination of a muscle biopsy specimen, although this is usually not necessary.

TREATMENT

Most symptoms of mild to moderate infection resolve without specific intervention. Thus, the role of anthelminthic therapy in the management of trichinellosis remains controversial. However, most experts concur that heavily infected or symptomatic individuals warrant therapy directed at the parasite, as well as the host inflammatory response. Benzimidazole anthelmintic, including thiabendazole, mebendazole, and albendazole, demonstrate variable efficacy in the treatment of human trichinellosis. Thiabendazole is no longer recommended because of its unfavorable side-effect profile. Mebendazole (Vermox; McNeil Pharmaceuticals) is the current drug of choice for treatment of trichinellosis in children and adults. The pediatric dose is 200 to 400 mg orally twice daily for 10 to 15 days. Side effects include abdominal pain, diarrhea, and urticaria. Albendazole (Albenza; GlaxoSmithKline) is an acceptable alternative and administered at a dose of 400 mg orally twice daily for 10 to 15 days. Side effects of albendazole include abdominal pain, alopecia, and elevated serum transaminase levels. Both

mebendazole and albendazole are approved by the U.S. Food and Drug Administration, but they are considered experimental for this indication. In addition, the use of benzimidazoles is not recommended for children 0 to 2 years of age, although data are emerging to suggest that both mebendazole and albendazole are safe in this age group. Glucocorticoids are often used in treatment of the acute stage of trichinellosis because they suppress signs and symptoms of immediate-type hypersensitivity. It is generally recommended that prednisone be administered with anthelminthics, at a total daily dose of up to 60 mg per day.

Common Pitfalls

Complications from trichinellosis are rare and usually occur during the acute phase of illness as larvae disseminate to somatic tissues. Myocarditis, which may develop in up to 20% of infections, can lead to congestive heart failure and serious arrhythmias. CNS invasion by migrating larvae may result in encephalitis or focal neurologic deficits, which may be evident on brain-imaging studies. Pneumonitis may develop in heavily infected individuals as large numbers of larvae migrate through the pulmonary vasculature. Early diagnosis is essential in preventing long-term complications of trichinellosis because serious sequelae are generally more likely to occur in those patients in whom treatment is delayed.

Communication and Counseling

Although complications may be severe, the vast majority of patients with trichinellosis recover fully, even without specific therapy. Nonetheless, the noted increase in travel-associated trichinellosis underlines the need for physicians to counsel patients traveling to endemic areas regarding cautious consumption of locally prepared or stored meat products. Thorough cooking of meat, proper animal husbandry techniques, and regulation of meat production are associated with a decrease in the incidence of trichinellosis in the United States. Cooking meat to an internal temperature of 170°F (76.7°C) or freezing at 5°F (−15°C) for 3 weeks kills encysted larvae. But freezing meat from some game animals may not effectively kill larvae, and these should be thoroughly cooked. Trichinellosis is a reportable disease in the United States, and physicians should notify state health officials of confirmed or suspected cases.

SUGGESTED READINGS

1. Ancelle T, Dupouy-Camet J, Desenclos JC, et al: A multifocal outbreak of trichinellosis linked to horse meat imported from North America to France in 1993. Am J Trop Med Hyg 59:615–619, 1998. **Describes 538 cases of trichinellosis linked to contaminated horse meat.**
2. Bruschi F, Murrell KD: New aspects of human trichinellosis: The impact of new *Trichinella* species. Postgrad Med J 78:15–22, 2002. **Describes newly recognized species of *Trichinella* that are pathogenic for humans.**

12

3. Centers for Disease Control and Prevention (CDC): Trichinellosis associated with bear meat—New York and Tennessee. MMWR Morb Mortal Wkly Rep 53(27):606–610, 2003. **Report of an outbreak of trichinellosis traced to consumption of bear meat.**
4. Centers for Disease Control and Prevention: DPDx: Laboratory identification of parasites of public health concern. Available online at http://www.dpd.cdc.gov/dpdx/Default.htm (accessed November 11, 2005). **This website provides instructions for submitting samples to the CDC for serologic diagnosis of Trichinella infection.**
5. Drugs for parasitic infections. Med Lett Drugs Ther 46:1–12, 2004. **Most recent recommendations for treatment of trichinellosis.**
6. Dupouy-Camet J, Kociecka W, Bruschi F, et al: Opinion on the diagnosis and treatment of human trichinellosis. Expert Opin Pharmacother 3:1117–1130, 2002. **Detailed review of the clinical spectrum of trichinellosis.**
7. Gamble HR, Pozio E, Bruschi F, et al: International Commission on Trichinellosis: Recommendations on the use of serological tests for the detection of Trichinella infection in animals and man. Parasite 11:3–13, 2004. **Summary of currently available serologic assays for detecting Trichinella infection.**
8. Watt G, Saisorn S, Jongsakul K, et al: Blinded, placebo-controlled trial of antiparasitic drugs for trichinosis myositis. J Infect Dis 182:371–374, 2000. **Report of a randomized study of 46 adults treated for trichinellosis.**

PROTOZOA

Babesiosis

Peter J. Krause

KEY CONCEPTS

- Babesiosis is caused by intraerythrocytic protozoa that are transmitted by *Ixodes* ticks.
- Clinical manifestations of babesiosis generally are mild, especially in children, but they range from subclinical illness to fulminating disease resulting in death.
- Treatment consists of clindamycin and quinine or atovaquone and azithromycin for 7 to 10 days.
- Exchange transfusion or partial exchange transfusion should be considered in children experiencing severe babesiosis.

Babesiosis is an emerging tick-borne disease caused by intraerythrocytic protozoa with clinical features similar to those of malaria. Worldwide, more than 90 species in the genus *Babesia* infect a wide variety of wild and domestic animals. Several species are known to cause disease in humans. *Babesia microti* is endemic in the northeastern and northern midwestern United States. WA-1, originally isolated from a resident of Washington state and closely related to *Babesia gibsoni*, was reported in Washington and California. MO-1 was isolated from a resident of Missouri and is closely related to *Babesia divergens,* a species known to cause human disease in Europe. The clustering of cases of human *B. microti* infection in the United States contrasts with the sporadic occurrence of the disease in Europe, Africa, and Asia. Because *Ixodes scapularis* (also known as *Ixodes dammini*) is the vector for *B. microti*, as well as the causative agents of Lyme disease and of human granulocytic anaplasmosis, co-infection may occur. Rarely, babesiosis may be transmitted perinatally or through blood transfusion.

The clinical manifestations of babesiosis range from subclinical illness to fulminating disease resulting in death. Children generally experience mild disease. Patients at increased risk of severe babesiosis include those who lack a spleen, patients infected with human immunodeficiency virus (HIV), and those older than 50 years. Overt signs and symptoms begin after an incubation period of 1 to 6 weeks from the beginning of tick feeding. The unengorged *I. scapularis* nymph is approximately 2 mm in length, and there often is no recollection of a tick bite. In most cases, a gradual onset of malaise, anorexia, and fatigue is followed by intermittent temperature to as high as 104°F (40°C) and one or more of the following: chills, sweats, myalgia, arthralgia, nausea, and vomiting. Babesiosis should be suspected in any patient with unexplained febrile illness who has recently lived or traveled in an endemic region during the months of May to September with or without a history of tick bite. Box 1 summarizes the diagnosis of babesiosis.

Expert Opinion on Management Issues

ACCEPTED INTERVENTIONS

Box 2 summarizes the current recommended treatment for babesiosis. The combination of clindamycin and quinine for 7 to 10 days is the treatment of choice. This combination frequently produces untoward reactions, such as tinnitus, vertigo, and gastrointestinal upset. Treatment failures are reported in patients with splenectomy, HIV infection, and those receiving concurrent corticosteroid therapy. In the first prospective study of antimicrobial therapy for babesiosis, the combination of atovaquone and azithromycin was compared with that of clindamycin and quinine for treatment of adults with *B. microti* infection. Atovaquone and azithromycin were found to be as effective in clearing parasitemia and resolving symptoms as

---

BOX 1 Diagnosis of Babesiosis

Epidemiology
- Residence in or travel to an endemic area.
- *Ixodes scapularis* tick bite.

Symptoms
- Chills, sweats, myalgia, arthralgia, nausea, and vomiting.
- Less common: emotional lability and depression, hyperesthesia, headache, sore throat, abdominal pain, conjunctival injection, photophobia, weight loss, and nonproductive cough.

Signs on Physical Examination
- Fever, splenomegaly, hepatomegaly, pallor.

Laboratory Diagnosis
- Identification of the causative agent in Giemsa-stained peripheral blood smears.
- Fourfold rise in babesial antibody in acute or convalescent sera or identification of serum babesial IgM antibody.
- Amplification of babesial DNA in blood using polymerase chain reaction.

BOX 2 Treatment of Babesiosis

Antibiotics
- Regimen for children, adolescents, or adults:
  - Clindamycin, 20 mg/kg/day IV or PO q8h (maximum: 600 mg q6h)

  and
  - Quinine, 25 mg/kg/day PO q6–8h (maximum: 650 mg q6–8h)
  - Treat for 7 to 10 days
- Alternative regimen for adolescents and adults:
  - Atovaquone, 750 mg q12h

  and
  - Azithromycin, 500–600 mg on day 1 and 250 mg/day thereafter
  - Alternative dose: 1000 mg on day 1 and 500–600 mg/day thereafter
  - Treat for 7 to 10 days

Exchange Transfusion
- Exchange transfusion or partial exchange transfusion for severe cases

---

IV, intravenous; PO, by mouth; q*x*h, every *x* hours.

---

clindamycin and quinine when given by mouth for 7 days. Significantly fewer adverse effects were associated with the atovaquone and azithromycin combination. Three fourths of patients receiving clindamycin and quinine experienced adverse drug reactions, and a third were forced to decrease the dose or to discontinue the medication. By contrast, only 15% in the azithromycin and atovaquone group experienced symptoms consistent with adverse drug reaction, and none required a decrease in dosage or discontinuation of medication. Anecdotal evidence suggests the atovaquone and azithromycin combination is effective for treatment of adolescents.

URGENT INTERVENTIONS

For severe cases with high parasitemia (>5%), significant hemolysis, or renal or pulmonary compromise, clindamycin should be administered intravenously, and exchange or partial exchange transfusion should be considered.

CONTROVERSIAL INTERVENTIONS

For those few patients who do not respond to clindamycin and quinine or atovaquone and azithromycin, pentamidine (240 mg/day given intravenously in addition to orally administered quinine) and cotrimoxazole (3 g/day given by mouth) might be considered because they were found to be moderately effective in clearing parasitemia and symptoms in an adult patient infected with *B. divergens*.

Common Pitfalls

- The diagnosis of babesiosis should be firmly established before instituting specific therapy. Expectant therapy is not justified in children unless there is at least some supportive laboratory evidence of infection.

- Treatment with a single antibiotic is not effective.
- Failure to institute exchange or partial exchange transfusion in a patient experiencing a severe babesial infection may end in a fatal outcome. Children rarely experience such severe infections.
- Coinfection with Lyme disease and/or human granulocytic anaplasmosis should be considered in children experiencing babesiosis. Appropriate diagnostic and therapeutic measures should be initiated. Coinfected patients may benefit from the addition of doxycycline therapy because neither clindamycin and quinine nor atovaquone and azithromycin are effective for the treatment of Lyme disease or human granulocytic anaplasmosis.

Communication and Counseling

Children experiencing babesiosis should be monitored closely during therapy. In most cases, improvement occurs within 1 or 2 days after antiprotozoal therapy is begun. Symptoms generally completely resolve within 1 or 2 months after clindamycin and quinine or atovaquone and azithromycin therapy is completed. In severely ill patients, the hematocrit and percentage of erythrocytes parasitized should be monitored daily or every other day until the patient improves and the parasitemia decreases to less than 5%. Some patients may have persistence of low-grade parasitemia for months following antibiotic therapy. Because low-grade parasitemia may be difficult to detect on thin blood smear, the more sensitive polymerase chain reaction (PCR) for amplifying parasite DNA should also be considered. We suggest retreatment of patients with antibabesial therapy if patients show evidence of parasitemia in their blood for more than 3 months after initial therapy.

Prevention of babesiosis can be accomplished by avoiding areas in May through September where ticks, deer, and mice are known to thrive. Those at increased risk in endemic areas, such as asplenic individuals, should avoid tall grass and brush where ticks may abound. Use of clothing that covers the lower part of the body and is sprayed or impregnated with diethyltoluamide (DEET), dimethyl phthalate, or permethrin (Permanone) is recommended for those who are exposed to the foliage of endemic areas, but care must be taken with repeated use of high-concentration products. A search for ticks on people and pets should be carried out and the ticks removed as soon as possible. The latter is accomplished best with tweezers by grasping the mouth parts without squeezing the body of the tick.

SUGGESTED READINGS

1. Jacoby GA, Hunt JV, Kosinski KS, et al: Treatment of transfusion-transmitted babesiosis by exchange transfusion. N Engl J Med 303:1098–1100, 1980. **Early study describing the use of exchange transfusion in a patient experiencing severe babesiosis.**
2. Krause PJ: Babesiosis. Med Clin North Am 86:361–373, 2002. **Detailed description of babesiosis.**
3. Krause PJ, Lepore T, Sikand VK, et al: Atovaquone and azithromycin for the treatment of babesiosis. N Engl J Med 343:1454–1458, 2000. **The first prospective study of antimicrobial therapy for babesiosis.**
4. Krause PJ, Telford S, Spielman A, et al: Concurrent Lyme disease and babesiosis: Evidence for increased severity and duration of illness. JAMA 275:1657–1660, 1996. **The first prospective study of the epidemiologic and clinical features of babesiosis and Lyme disease co-infection.**
5. Krause PJ, Spielman A, Telford S, et al: Persistent parasitemia following acute babesiosis. N Engl J Med 339:160–165, 1998. **Compares persistent parasitemia in treated and untreated patients experiencing babesiosis.**
6. Krause PJ, Telford SR III, Pollack RJ, et al: Babesiosis: An under-diagnosed disease of children. Pediatrics 89:1045–1048, 1992. **The first prospective study of babesiosis in children.**
7. Raoult D, Soulayrol L, Toga B, et al: Babesiosis, pentamidine, and cotrimoxazole [letter to the editor]. Ann Intern Med 107:944, 1987. **The only report of pentamidine and cotrimoxazole therapy for babesiosis.**
8. Wittner M, Rowin KS, Tanowitz HB, et al: Successful chemotherapy of transfusion babesiosis. Ann Intern Med 96:601–604, 1982. **The first report of successful antimicrobial treatment for babesiosis.**

Intestinal Protozoa

David I. Rappaport, Jane Atkins, and David P. Ascher

KEY CONCEPTS

- *Giardia lamblia*
  - *Giardia lamblia* is the most common cause of chronic diarrhea in travelers.
  - Symptoms may mimic those of irritable bowel syndrome.
  - Infection in immunocompromised patients should be promptly identified and treated.
  - Prevention strategies consist of water treatment and basic hygienic measures.
  - Emerging resistance to metronidazole may necessitate alternative therapies.
- *Cryptosporidium*
  - *Cryptosporidium parvum*, of particular importance in immunosuppressed and malnourished children, is transmitted via contaminated water, occasionally causes outbreaks, and resists most water treatment methods.
  - Nitazoxanide represents the only FDA-approved therapy for *C. parvum*.
- *Dientamoeba* and *Blastocystis*
  - *Dientamoeba fragilis* represents an important, often unrecognized, and easily treatable cause of gastrointestinal symptoms; its hosts are often co-infected with *Enterobius vermicularis*.
  - *Blastocystis hominis* is of questionable pathogenicity and, as an isolated finding, generally requires no treatment.

GIARDIA LAMBLIA

The flagellate protozoan *Giardia lamblia*, also known as *Giardia duodenalis* or *Giardia intestinalis*, represents the most common intestinal protozoan. Travel to endemic areas constitutes an important risk factor for contracting *G. lamblia*. Although classified as zoonotic, most infections appear to be acquired via fecal–oral transmission or via contaminated water, especially from mountain streams (Table 1). Outbreaks of *G. lamblia* caused by contaminated water supplies have been described. Ingestion of cysts, which are relatively resistant to changes in temperature and chlorination, leads to a release of two trophozoites per cyst upon reaching the small intestine. Patients typically shed cysts and trophozoites intermittently in the stool. Diagnosis may be established via a number of modalities, including stool microscopy, stool enzyme immunoassay (EIA), and duodenal biopsy or aspiration (see Table 1). Sensitivity and specificity of EIA approximate 90% to 100%.

Patients with immunosuppressive conditions or cystic fibrosis demonstrate increased susceptibility to *G. lamblia*, and those in facilities such as daycare centers or homes for the disabled may also be at higher risk. Children younger than 5 years and adults 30 to 40 years of age seem to be at highest risk of contracting clinically apparent disease. Clinical manifestations range from asymptomatic carriage to acute or chronic gastrointestinal complaints, such as diarrhea, flatulence, weight loss, and malabsorption (see Table 1). Other symptoms may include epigastric pain, abdominal distention, nausea, anorexia, and, rarely, arthritis. Symptoms may resemble those of irritable bowel syndrome. Hospitalization, although relatively unusual, may be required for hypovolemia associated with significant diarrhea. Invasive disease is rare. Carriage of *G. lamblia* in children rarely causes overt gastrointestinal manifestations but may lead to growth impairment.

TABLE 1 Clinical and Diagnostic Characteristics of Giardiasis and Cryptosporidiosis

Characteristic	Giardiasis	Cryptosporidiosis
Important historical information and exposures	Recent travel Campers, hikers, or backpackers Daycare attendance Institutionalized patients	Recent travel Recreational water parks Swimming pools Daycare attendance Farm animal exposure (especially young calves)
Underlying illnesses predisposing to infection	Immunodeficiency AIDS Humoral immunodeficiencies (IgA deficiency and hypogammaglobulinemia) Cystic fibrosis Crohn disease	Immunodeficiency AIDS Primary T-cell immunodeficiencies Malnutrition Immunosuppression Transplant patients Childhood leukemia and lymphoma
Incubation period	1–4 wk	2–14 days (median 7 days)
Clinical syndromes	Asymptomatic infection Acute watery, nonbloody diarrhea associated with abdominal pain; usually afebrile Chronic intermittent diarrhea characterized by flatulence, foul-smelling stools, abdominal distention with anorexia, and weight loss	Asymptomatic infection Acute self-limited, watery, nonbloody diarrhea associated with abdominal cramping, fatigue, vomiting, anorexia, weight loss, and fever Chronic severe diarrhea resulting in malnutrition and severe dehydration Extraintestinal disease (pancreas, biliary, and pulmonary) seen in immunocompromised hosts
Laboratory diagnosis	Direct microscopic exam of stool EIA Aspiration of duodenal fluid String test or Entero-Test* Duodenal biopsy	Modified Kinyoun acid-fast stain EIA Immunofluorescent assay Polymerase chain reaction (research only) Biopsy of intestinal or extraintestinal tissue

*HDC Corporation, San Jose, Cal.
AIDS, acquired immune deficiency syndrome; EIA, enzyme immunoassay.

Expert Opinion on Management Issues

TREATMENT

Box 1 lists the treatment options for giardiasis. Historically, metronidazole or furazolidone represented treatments of choice for uncomplicated *G. lamblia* infection. Furazolidone is commercially unavailable in the United States, as is quinacrine. Metronidazole demonstrates efficacy of approximately 60% to 100% in adults. Tinidazole is chemically similar to metronidazole and now approved by the U.S. Food and Drug Administration (FDA). It may be better tolerated than metronidazole, and the tablet may be crushed. Albendazole is an alternative therapy, although resistance to metronidazole and albendazole may coexist. Neither metronidazole nor albendazole is available in suspension, so administration to younger children may be inconvenient. Treatment of children in settings such as daycare centers is generally unwarranted because reinfection frequently occurs. Paromomycin, an aminoglycoside, represents the treatment of choice in pregnant women. Nitazoxanide, a newer nitroimidazole, displays effectiveness against both metronidazole-sensitive and metronidazole-resistant organisms and is available in a 100 mg per 5 mL suspension. This drug appears to be well tolerated and demonstrates activity against a variety of parasitic organisms. Treatment of asymptomatic carriers is generally not indicated unless the child is in close contact with an immunocompromised individual. Significant dehydration may require hospitalization and intravenous fluid therapy.

PREVENTIVE MEASURES

Travelers to endemic areas must recognize the risk of acquiring *G. lamblia*. Proper water treatment on both an individual and large scale is important. Travelers should consider consuming only bottled water in certain areas. Campers, hikers, and backpackers should avoid drinking from surface water sources (streams, lakes, or rivers). Boiling of water kills the infective cyst form, as well as other enteric pathogens. Large-scale water filtration typically prevents transmission. On an individual basis, water treatment options include heating water to 158°F (70°C) for 10 minutes or the use of iodine purification tablets for 8 hours, although neither measure kills all cysts definitively. Proper sewage disposal and diaper disposal are critical steps to prevent outbreaks in communities and daycare centers, respectively. The importance of rigorous hand washing cannot be overemphasized. Breastfeeding may be protective against *G. lamblia* in infants.

Common Pitfalls

- Intermittent shedding in stool may cause falsely negative stool microscopy. Examination of three or more stools every other day is recommended.
- The *Giardia* EIA on a single stool is more sensitive than direct stool microscopy but misses infection or coinfection with other protozoan pathogens if used alone.
- Travelers must be warned that iodination or chlorination of water may be insufficient to eradicate *G. lamblia* cysts.

BOX 1 Therapeutic Alternatives for Intestinal Parasites

Giardia lamblia

Treatments of choice

- Metronidazole: 15 mg/kg/day div tid × 5 days (max: 250 mg tid)
- Nitazoxanide: 1–3 yr: 100 mg bid × 3 days; 4–11 yr: 200 mg bid × 3 days; ≥12 yr: 500 mg bid
- Tinidazole†: 50 mg/kg once (max: 2 g/dose)

Alternatives

- Albendazole: 10 mg/kg/day qd × 5 days (max: 800 mg/day)
- Paromomycin: 25–35 mg/kg/day div tid × 7 days
- Furazolidone*: 6 mg/kg/day div qid × 7 days (max: 100 mg qid)
- Quinacrine*: 6 mg/kg/day div tid × 5 days (max: 100 mg tid)

Cryptosporidium parvum

- Nitazoxanide: 1–3 yr: 100 mg bid for 3 days; 4–11 yr: 200 mg bid × 3 days; ≥12 yr: 500 mg bid

Dientamoeba fragilis

- Iodoquinol: 30–40 mg/kg/day div tid × 20 days (max: 2 g/day)
- Paromomycin: 25–35 mg/kg/day div tid × 7 days
- Tetracycline‡: 40 mg/kg/day div qid × 10 days (max: 2g/day)
- Metronidazole: 20–40 mg/kg/day div tid × 10 days (max: 2g/day)

Blastocystis hominis

- Metronidazole: 750 mg tid × 10 days§
- Iodoquinol: 650 mg tid × 20 days§
- Trimethoprim-sulfamethoxazole: 1 double-strength tab bid × 7 days§
- Nitazoxanide: 1–3 yr: 100 mg bid × 3 days; 4–11 yr: 200 mg bid × 3 days; ≥12 yr: 500 mg bid

---

*Currently unavailable in United States, although quinacrine may be compounded by Panorama Compounding Pharmacy, Van Nuys, Cal. (800–247–9767), or Medical Center Pharmacy, New Haven, Conn. (203–688–6816). Furazolidone is manufactured by Riviera in Austria and Norwich-Eaton in Israel.

†Ornidazole, a similar drug unavailable in the United States, may also be used.

‡Not used in pregnancy or in children younger than 8 yr.

§Dose for adult patients because pediatric data are lacking.

bid, twice daily; div, divided; max, maximum; tid, three times per day; qd, every day; qid, four times per day.

Communication and Counseling

Travelers, campers, and hikers should be educated about the risk of acquiring *G. lamblia* and must be vigilant about the water they ingest. Most infected children are asymptomatic or have mild disease and recover uneventfully. Particular attention should be paid to the hydration status of younger children with significant diarrhea. In cases of chronic diarrhea, a history of travel prior to symptom onset should be sought. Preventive steps, such as hand washing, waste disposal, and water treatment, represent important individual and public health measures to decrease the risk of infection.

Cryptosporidium

Cryptosporidium parvum, an intracellular protozoan, represents a particular problem in children in developing countries and in those with immunosuppressive conditions such as human immunodeficiency virus (HIV). The organism is transmitted primarily via contaminated water and less commonly via food and person to person. Outbreaks, particularly associated with contaminated municipal water supplies, are not rare; one such outbreak affected 400,000 persons in Milwaukee in 1993.

Patients may present with profuse diarrhea and associated malnutrition as well as systemic symptoms such as fever, abdominal pain, and anorexia. Individuals may also be asymptomatic. The organism displays an affinity for the jejunum and terminal ileum. Malnutrition represents an important risk factor for significant disease, and long-term consequences in children in developing countries may include diminished intellectual function and physical fitness. Patients with T cell dysfunction (primary T cell immunodeficiency, acquired immune deficiency virus [AIDS], bone marrow and solid organ transplantation, leukemia, and lymphoma) are at risk for severe intestinal and extraintestinal infection. Extraintestinal sites of infection include the pancreas as well as the biliary and respiratory tracts. Cholangitis associated with *C. parvum* is the most common extraintestinal manifestation (see Table 1).

The modified Kinyoun acid-fast stain historically represented the gold standard for diagnosing cryptosporidiosis. This method is relatively insensitive and not included in routine stool examination for ova and parasites. Enzyme immunoassay and immunofluorescent assay demonstrate considerably higher sensitivity. Polymerase chain reaction (PCR) is the most sensitive methodology and can be used on both clinical and environmental samples but is available for research use only (see Table 1).

Expert Opinion on Management Issues

TREATMENT

Recent data in children with *C. parvum* suggest that a 3-day course of nitazoxanide, 100 mg twice a day, may be effective in reducing clinical symptoms and eradicating the organism. This treatment demonstrates increased efficacy in HIV-negative children and in those with good nutrition. Improvement of the nutritional status of children infected with *C. parvum* represents a key aspect of therapy but may prove difficult because of socioeconomic conditions and because the infection itself decreases nutrient absorption. If a 3-day course of nitazoxanide is ineffective, a 6-day course may increase rates of cure, although data are few. Azithromycin combined with paromomycin may demonstrate some effectiveness, although nitazoxanide is preferred. Optimal duration of therapy for immunocompromised patients is not known. Immunocompromised patients may require extended antimicrobial therapy and repeat examination of the stool to document clearance. In HIV-infected patients, anti-HIV therapy improves outcomes associated with *C. parvum* by reconstitution of immune function. Reduction of immunosuppression may be required in transplant patients.

PREVENTIVE MEASURES

Prevention of *C. parvum* remains challenging because the organism is resistant to most forms of water treatment. The Centers for Disease Control and Prevention recommends boiling water for 1 minute or filtering with pore size less than 1 μm if concerns about water safety arise. Ensuring safe drinking water, especially for those with immunosuppressive conditions, is critical. Other steps include avoidance of farm animals and of ingestion of water from swimming pools.

Common Pitfalls

- *Cryptosporidium* may be missed on routine stool microscopy for ova and parasites unless specifically requested.
- If clinically unimproved after a 3-day course of nitazoxanide, patients with documented *C. parvum* infection should probably be treated for another 3 days.
- *Cryptosporidium* oocysts are resistant to the low level of chlorine used in municipal water systems. Proper water filtration requires removal of particles less than 1 μm.
- Sand filtration systems used by many pools are not adequate for removal of *Cryptosporidium* oocysts.

Communication and Counseling

Patients with decreased immune function may be especially affected by *C. parvum*. Travelers, especially those who are immunosuppressed, must be meticulous about the water and food they ingest and must exercise rigorous hygienic measures. HIV-positive patients must understand the importance of daily anti-HIV medication. Prevention of *C. parvum* outbreaks in municipal water supplies remains a public health concern. Teaching children about the importance of steadfast hand washing remains the most critical step to prevent the acquisition of gastrointestinal protozoa.

Dientamoeba and *Blastocystis*

Dientamoeba fragilis is a flagellate and, despite its name, is not related to *Entamoeba histolytica*. The life cycle of this organism involves a trophozoite stage but apparently no cyst stage. Infection with this organism may be more common than generally appreciated, even in developed countries. One study investigating children and caregivers in Toronto daycare centers suggested *D. fragilis* may be more common than *G. lamblia* in this population, especially in children 7 to 10 years of age. This study identified cat ownership as a potential risk factor. Persons who reside in institutions are also at higher risk for *D. fragilis*. This organism, probably transmitted via the fecal–oral route, is often associated with *Enterobius vermicularis* infection. Patients may complain of diarrhea, abdominal pain, flatulence, or anorexia. Identification of *D. fragilis* on stool specimen may prove difficult because detection of the trophozoite requires preservation with polyvinyl alcohol soon after collection before staining with trichrome or similar stain. Several stool samples may be required.

Blastocystis hominis, a relatively common intestinal protozoan, was long considered a commensal. Newer studies question this assertion. Difficulties in assessing its pathogenicity include a high proportion of patients co-infected with a variety of other organisms as well as the often self-limited nature of the illness. Symptoms ascribed to *B. hominis* include diarrhea and abdominal pain, although many asymptomatic patients demonstrate *B. hominis* in their stool. Travel to a developing country represents an important risk factor for acquisition of the organism. Initial reports correlating a high concentration of *B. hominis* in the stool with more significant clinical findings have been largely discredited.

Expert Opinion on Management Issues

TREATMENT

Treatment of *D. fragilis* may involve one of a number of drugs as shown in Box 1. Iodoquinol is not available in a liquid formulation or in all locations. Doxycycline and erythromycin are also reported to be effective. If trophozoites remain present after a standard course of therapy, a longer course may be required. Secnidazole, although not widely available and not FDA approved, may represent a viable therapeutic alternative at a dose of 30 mg/kg once (maximum 2 g). Secnidazole is manufactured by Ache in Brazil and other corporations outside the United States.

B. hominis acquisition is often associated with travel to developing nations. Data suggesting the effectiveness of nitazoxanide in eradicating the organism and improving intestinal symptoms in Mexican children are difficult to interpret because of the efficacy of the medication against a variety of pathogens. Box 1 lists the potential treatments.

PREVENTIVE MEASURES

Incidence of *D. fragilis* infection may be lowered by general sanitary measures, especially in travelers and in daycare centers and other similar institutions. Maintaining cleanliness of the perineal region may lower the risk of *E. vermicularis* and thus *D. fragilis*.

Limited understanding of the life cycle of *B. hominis* precludes specific prevention strategies apart from general hygienic measures, especially among travelers to developing nations.

Common Pitfalls

- *D. fragilis* infection is not rare, and detection of trophozoites may require special staining.
- Significant symptoms in patients with *B. hominis* should prompt a search for alternative etiologies of intestinal pathology.

Communication and Counseling

Patients and parents should be counseled that *B. hominis* in the stool may not be causative in cases of significant gastrointestinal symptoms. *D. fragilis* infection is common and easily treatable with a number of medications. Rigorous hygienic measures constitute the most important means of preventing the acquisition of gastrointestinal protozoa.

SUGGESTED READINGS

Giardia lamblia

1. Adagu IS, Nolder D, Warhust DC, Rossignol JF: In vitro activity of nitazoxanide and related compounds against isolates of *Giardia intestinalis, Entamoeba histolytica,* and *Trichomonas vaginalis.* J Antimicrob Chemother 49:103–111, 2002. **Laboratory evaluation of efficacy of nitazoxanide against these organisms, especially as compared to metronidazole.**
2. D'Anchino M, Orlando D, De Feudis L: *Giardia lamblia* infections become clinically evident by eliciting symptoms of irritable bowel syndrome. J Infect 45:169–172, 2002. **Controlled study of giardiasis in patients with and without irritable bowel syndrome (IBS), suggesting that many patients with symptomatic giardiasis may have IBS and may respond to IBS therapy.**
3. Fraser D, Bilenko N, Deckelbaum RJ, et al: *Giardia lamblia* carriage in Israeli Bedouin infants: Risk factors and consequences. Clin Infect Dis 30:419–424, 2000. **Cohort study of a population in which *G. lamblia* carriage is nearly universal; suggests that carriage is not associated with overt disease but may result in slowed growth.**
4. Lebwohl B, Deckelbaum RJ, Green PHR: Giardiasis. Gastrointest Endosc 57(7):906–913, 2003. **A review of epidemiology, clinical findings, diagnosis, and treatment, with particular emphasis on diagnosis via endoscopic modalities.**
5. Upcroft P, Upcroft JA: Drug targets and mechanisms of resistance in the anaerobic protozoa. Clin Microbiol Rev 14(1):150–164, 2001. **Extensive review of drug therapies and resistance to *Giardia duodenalis, Entamoeba histolytica,* and *Trichomonas vaginalis.***
6. Yereli K, Balcioglu IC, Ertan P, et al: Albendazole as an alternative therapeutic agent for childhood giardiasis in Turkey. Clin Microbiol Infect 10(6):527–529, 2004. **Randomized, prospective study comparing albendazole versus metronidazole, demonstrating 90% parasite eradication in each group.**

Cryptosporidium parvum

1. Amadi B, Mwiya M, Musuku J, et al: Effect of nitazoxanide on morbidity and mortality in Zambian children with cryptosporidiosis: A randomised controlled trial. Lancet 360:1375–1380, 2002. **Randomized study suggests that 3-day course of nitazoxanide may be effective in a developing country, especially in HIV-negative patients, and a 6-day course may be even more so.**
2. Guerrant DI, Moore SR, Lima AA, et al: Association of early childhood diarrhea and cryptosporidiosis with impaired physical fitness and cognitive function 4–7 years later in a poor urban community in northeast Brazil. Am J Trop Med Hyg 61:707–713, 1999. **Highlights potential long-term consequences of *C. parvum* infection among nutritionally deficient Brazilian children.**
3. Huang DB, Chapell C, Okhuysen PC: Cryptosporidiosis in children. Semin Pediatr Infect Dis 15:253–259, 2004. **Comprehensive review of cryptosporidiosis in children.**
4. Hunter PR, Nichol G: Epidemiology and clinical features of cryptosporidium infection in immunocompromised patients. Clin Microbiol Rev 15:145–154, 2002. **Review of the epidemiology and clinical features of cryptosporidiosis in immunocompromised patients.**
5. Leav BA, Mackay M, Ward HD: *Cryptosporidium* species: New insights and old challenges. Clin Infect Dis 36(7):903–908, 2003.

Review of epidemiologic, clinical, diagnostic, and therapeutic approaches to *Cryptosporidium* infection.

6. MacKenzie WR, Schell WL, Blair K, et al: Massive outbreak of waterborne *Cryptosporidium* infection in Milwaukee, Wisconsin: Recurrence of illness and risk of secondary transmission. Clin Infect Dis 21:57–62, 1995. **Describes large-scale *Cryptosporidium* outbreak because of contaminated water supply.**
7. Rossignol JF, Ayoub A, Ayers MS: Treatment of diarrhea caused by *Cryptosporidium parvum*: A prospective randomized, double-blind, placebo-controlled study of nitazoxanide. J Infect Dis 184:103–106, 2001. **Double-blind, placebo-controlled study in immunocompetent children, adolescents, and adults in Egypt, concluding that nitazoxanide is effective for *C. parvum* alone and in co-infections with other parasites.**

Dientamoeba fragilis

1. Butler WP: *Dientamoeba fragilis*: An unusual intestinal pathogen. Dig Dis Sci 41(9):1811–1813, 1996. **Case report of a 32-year-old and discussion of epidemiology, diagnosis, and therapy of *D. fragilis*.**
2. Dickinson E, Cohen MA, Schlenker MK: *Dientamoeba fragilis*: A significant pathogen. Am J Emerg Med 20(1):62–63, 2002. **Case report of 5-year-old girl with *D. fragilis* and review of its characteristics.**
3. Girginkardesler N, Coskun S, Balcioglu IC, et al: *Dientamoeba fragilis*, a neglected cause of diarrhea, successfully treated with secnidazole. Clin Microbiol Infect 9(2):110–113, 2003. **Prospective study of Turkish adults and children with single-dose secnidazole; children received one-time dose of 30 mg per kg; eradication noted in 97%.**
4. Keystone JS, Yang J, Grisdale D, et al: Intestinal parasites in metropolitan Toronto day-care centres. Can Med Assoc J 131:733–735, 1984. **Sample of Toronto daycare attendees and staff, revealing that both *D. fragilis* and *G. lamblia* are endemic in these groups.**

Blastocystis hominis

1. Ok UZ, Girginkardesler N, Balcioglu C, et al: Effect of trimetho-prim-sulfamethoxazole [TMP-SMX] in *Blastocystis hominis* infection. Am J Gastroenterol 94(11):3245–3247, 1999. **A prospective cohort study in which symptomatic children and adults were treated with TMP-SMX and demonstrated clinical improvement (92%) and microbiologic eradication (95%).**
2. Shlim DR, Hoge CW, Rajah R, et al: Is *Blastocystis hominis* a cause of diarrhea in travelers? A prospective controlled study in Nepal. Clin Infect Dis 21:97–101, 1995. **Investigates travelers and expatriates in Nepal, concluding that higher concentration of organisms is not associated with higher likelihood of symptoms.**

Miscellaneous

1. Drugs for parasitic infections: Med Lett Drugs Ther 46:1–12, 2004. **Detailed therapeutic alternatives for a variety of parasitic infections, including adult and pediatric dosages.**

Leishmaniasis, American Trypanosomiasis, African Trypanosomiasis

Jonathan Berman

KEY CONCEPTS

- Leishmaniasis, American trypanosomiasis, and African trypanosomiasis, parasitic diseases spread by biting insects, are generally acquired when the traveler visits the endemic region in which transmission is occurring.

- Almost all cases are acquired by travel abroad. Transmission is rare but possible for cutaneous leishmaniasis in Texas and American trypanosomiasis in a few southern states.
- Because these parasites persist in the blood, infection can be acquired by a contaminated blood transfusion, and infected persons should not donate blood for specified periods of time.
- Diagnosis requires thinking of the disease and then identifying the parasite in infected tissues or fluids.
- Treatment requires unusual agents, which are often toxic and may be ineffective. Effective patient management requires consultation with an expert on the disease.

The clinical diseases caused by infection with kinetoplast-containing parasites are the leishmaniases, African trypanosomiasis, and American trypanosomiasis. Although these phylogenetically related parasites are each spread by the bite of insects, the interaction of the three parasites with the human host are as dissimilar as that of *Neisseria meningitidis* and *Neisseria gonorrhoeae*. Leishmania infect the skin and visceral reticuloendothelial system (liver/spleen/bone marrow); African trypanosomes most importantly affect the central nervous system (CNS); American trypanosomes affect the heart and gastrointestinal (GI) system. The incidence of these infections in developed nations is determined by the frequency with which travelers from such nations intrude into the respective endemic environments in which parasite transmission is occurring. By far the preponderance of such infections in the U.S. population is caused by the *Leishmania*.

Leishmaniasis

Leishmaniasis is spread by sandflies and presents as either a dermatologic or a visceral disease. There are typically 50 to 100 cases of leishmaniasis per year, of which 90% are cutaneous, in the U.S. population. Infection by dermatologic species in Asia and southern Europe (the Old World) or Central and South America (the New World) begins as a small papule but then evolves over 2 to 4 months into a skin ulcer often covered with a scab, at which point the patient typically first seeks medical attention. If untreated, the ulcer heals with scarring in approximately 2.5 months (Old World) or 6 to 18 months (New World). Inoculation into the skin of visceral species does not lead to dermatologic symptoms because these species spread to and infect the liver, spleen, and bone marrow. Continued multiplication in those organs leads to a presentation of fever, hepatosplenomegaly, and pancytopenia. Typical presenting values in moderate cases of visceral leishmaniasis are spleens that are 7 cm below the left costal margin, total white counts of 3500/mm^3, and platelets of 120,000/mm^3. Once symptomatic, visceral leishmaniasis does not self-cure, and severe cases can be rapidly fatal. Death is usually caused by intercurrent pneumonia or gastroenteritis in the setting of immunocompromise because of pancytopenia. Diagnosis of the leishmaniases is classically made by visualizing the parasites in Giemsa stains of lesion biopsies or aspirates, although a dipstick test (recombinant K39) to see if plasma contains anti-leishmanial antigen is both sensitive and specific for visceral leishmaniasis.

American Trypanosomiasis

Infection with *Trypanosoma cruzi* via bite of the reduviid bug gives rise to American trypanosomiasis (Chagas disease). Acute local symptoms at the bite site and acute systemic symptoms subside in a few months, and infected patients enter the indeterminate phase in which there is lifelong low-grade parasitemia but no symptoms. Years or decades after the initial infection, the chronic phase with conduction abnormalities and enlargement of the heart and GI system occurs in 10% to 30% of patients. In an endemic region, children are involved in the sense that initial infection and then indeterminate disease occurs in a sizable percentage, perhaps 5%, of the pediatric population. Chagas disease is very rare in the United States. There may be 100,000 Latin American immigrants in the United States with indeterminate disease due to *T. cruzi*. Very few of these individuals become symptomatic. Prior to 1993, nine cases of imported acute *T. cruzi* infections were reported to the Centers for Disease Control and Prevention (CDC). In addition, *T. cruzi* is maintained by mammalian hosts and reduviid bugs in some southern U.S. states, and there were five reported cases, four of which were in infants, of autochthonous infections. An important threat is the spread of *T. cruzi* to previously uninfected persons via contaminated blood transfusions from persons in the asymptomatic indeterminate phase of infection. Diagnosis during the acute initial infection is made by visualizing the parasite in Giemsa-stained blood. Diagnosis during the indeterminate or chronic phase is made by detecting antibodies to *T. cruzi* in serum.

African Trypanosomiasis

African trypanosomiasis (sleeping sickness) is caused by infection with *Trypanosoma brucei gambiense* or *Trypanosoma brucei rhodesiense*. These parasites are transmitted by the tsetse fly from the human reservoir living in African rain forests (West African disease caused by *T. brucei gambiense*) or the animal reservoir, including those in game parks (East African disease caused by *T. brucei rhodesiense*). It is rare for U.S. populations to intrude on these habitats, and since 1994, the CDC is aware of 16 cases of *T. brucei rhodesiense* and 5 cases of *T. brucei gambiense*, all in adults, treated in the United States. Stage 1 disease for both West and East African disease consists of a painful chancre at the site of parasite inoculation, hematogenous and lymphatic spread of the parasite, and intermittent fever. CNS involvement (stage 2 disease) is often initially manifested by indifference and sleepiness (so-called sleeping sickness), although auditory and visual hallucinations, decreased arm coordination, parkinsonian gait, and a wide variety of other neurologic signs are seen eventually. *T. brucei rhodesiense* disseminates to the CNS in weeks to months, whereas *T. brucei gambiense* disseminates more slowly in months to years. Diagnosis is made by visualizing the parasite in lymph nodes, buffy coat, and cerebrospinal fluid (CSF).

Expert Opinion on Management Issues

The classic treatment agent for the leishmaniases is pentavalent antimony, available under the trade name Pentostam from the CDC (Table 1). Efficacy is typically more than 90%. Side effects are typically myalgias and arthralgias (without arthritis) in approximately 75% of patients, abdominal pain in an estimated 33% of cases, laboratory evidence of hepatitis (~40% of cases) and pancreatitis (85% of cases), and mild T-wave flattening on electrocardiogram (ECG).

Alternative agents for antimony-treatment failures in visceral disease are amphotericin B and AmBisome (Liposomal amphotericin B). AmBisome is registered with the U.S. Food and Drug Administration (FDA)

for visceral leishmaniasis and is the preferred agent because of its lower toxicity. Miltefosine is the first oral agent for visceral leishmaniasis and has demonstrable efficacy in children. Miltefosine is not yet registered in the United States but might be obtainable from the manufacturer (Zentaris, Frankfurt, Germany).

Cutaneous leishmaniasis is an ultimately self-healing disease, so for cutaneous disease, the side effects of the standard 20 days of antimonial therapy approximate the morbidity of the disease itself. Because *Leishmania major* in the Old World and *Leishmania mexicana* in the New World typically heal more quickly than the other forms of cutaneous disease, for ulcers that can be clearly ascribed to these species of *Leishmania*, a short course of antimony (10 days), treatment with fluconazole, or simple observation is the best choice. For ulcers ascribed to other species or for which the species is unknown, the full course of antimony should be used.

For visceral disease, fever should remit in 1 week, parasites should be absent by the end of therapy, and the spleen should diminish by 75% by that time. The physical manifestations of cutaneous infection may take time to improve, even after the parasites are eliminated. By 6 weeks after the end of therapy, the lesion should diminish by 75%. For both visceral and cutaneous leishmaniasis, the patient needs to be followed for 6 months (ideally, 12 months) to demonstrate complete lesion healing and lack of clinical relapse.

AMERICAN TRYPANOSOMIASIS TREATMENT ISSUES

Benznidazole may decrease the parasite load but not eliminate the infection as determined by polymerase chain reaction (PCR) of the blood. Nifurtimox is the only anti–*T. cruzi* agent available in the United States from the CDC. Treatment of the trypanosomiases is given in Table 2.

TABLE 1 Treatment of the Leishmaniases

Type	Recommended	Alternative
Cutaneous Leishmaniasis		
Old World		
Rural or known *L. major*	Fluconazole PO, 200 mg/day × 6 wk Pentostam IV, 20 mg/kg/day × 10 days	Observe
Urban or unknown	Pentostam IV, 20 mg/kg/day × 20 days	Observe
New World		
Mexico or known *L. mexicana*	Pentostam IV, 20 mg/kg/day × 10 days	Observe
Other regions or known *L. braziliensis* complex	Pentostam IV, 20 mg/kg/day × 20 days × 7 injections	Pentamidine, 2 mg/kg qod
Visceral Leishmaniasis		
	Pentostam IV, 20 mg/kg/day × 28 days AmBisome IV, 3 mg/kg on days 1, 2, 3, 4, 5, 14, 21 Amphotericin B IV, total dose of 20 mg/kg (1 mg/kg qod for 20 injections) Miltefosine PO, 2.5 mg/kg/day × 28 days	

IV, intravenous; *L.*, *Leishmania*; PO, by mouth; qod, every other day.

TABLE 2 Treatment of the Trypanosomiases

Disease	Recommended Treatment
Chagas disease	Nifurtimox from CDC, ≈15 mg/kg/day × 90–120 days Benznidazole in Latin America, 7.5 mg/kg/day × 60 days
African trypanosomiasis stage 1 (normal CSF)	Suramin, 20 mg/kg IV on days 1, 3, 7, 14, 21 Pentamidine, 4 mg/kg/day IM or IV × 10 days
West African stage 2 (abnormal CSF)	Melarsoprol, 2.2 mg/kg/day × 10 days Eflornithine, 400 mg/kg/day IV × 14 days
East African stage 2 (abnormal CSF)	Melarsoprol, 18–25 mg/kg IV × 1 mo

CDC, Centers for Disease Control and Prevention; CSF, cerebrospinal fluid; IM, intramuscular; IV, intravenous.

AFRICAN TRYPANOSOMIASIS TREATMENT ISSUES

Stage 1 infection is treated with pentamidine or suramin, drugs that poorly treat disease of the CNS. Stage 2 (CNS disease) was classically treated with melarsoprol, an organic arsenical. Newer treatment schedules may make it possible to diminish the toxicity of this agent, at least for West African disease because of *T. brucei gambiense*. Eflornithine, obtained from the WHO, is the preferred agent for West African (*T. brucei gambiense*) stage 2 disease.

Common Pitfalls

Leishmaniasis, American trypanosomiasis, and African trypanosomiasis together have an incidence of less than 100 cases per year in the United States and probably less than 20 cases per year in the pediatric population. A high index of suspicion is needed for these diseases. Consideration of travel history in patients with chronic skin ulcer or fever with hepatosplenomegaly (leishmaniasis) or meningoencephalitis (African trypanosomiasis) is needed to initiate correct diagnostic tests.

Leishmaniasis, American trypanosomiasis, and African trypanosomiasis are exotic diseases treated with drugs that are, with few exceptions, equally exotic. A good rule is to treat only after consultation with a specialist with previous experience with these unusual diseases and drugs. In many cases, the only method to access preferred therapy is via the CDC or the WHO.

Communication and Counseling

Leishmania, African trypanosomes, and American trypanosomes are present in the circulation, and patients should not donate blood for specified periods of time (specifics can be obtained from the CDC) after diagnosis and treatment.

SUGGESTED READINGS

1. Alrajhi AA, Ibrahim EA, De Vol EB, et al: Fluconazole for the treatment of cutaneous leishmaniasis caused by *Leishmania major*. N Engl J Med 346:891–895, 2002. **Reports the first success in a placebo-controlled trial of an oral therapy for Old World cutaneous leishmaniasis.**
2. Bhattacharya SK, Jha TK, Sundar S, et al: Efficacy and tolerability of miltefosine for childhood visceral leishmaniasis in India. Clin Infect Dis 38:217–221, 2004. **Extends the use of miltefosine to the pediatric population.**
3. Burri C, Nkunku S, Merolle A, et al: Efficacy of new, concise schedule for melarsoprol in treatment of sleeping sickness caused by *Trypanosoma brucei gambiense*: A randomized trial. Lancet 355:1419–1425, 2000. **Describes a short, yet effective course of melarsoprol for West African CNS disease.**
4. Carvalho SFG, Lemos EM, Corey R, Dietze R: Performance of recombinant K39 in the diagnosis of Brazilian visceral leishmaniasis. Am J Trop Med Hyg 68:321–324, 2003. **Describes a serologic test that obviates the need for a parasitologic test for visceral leishmaniasis.**
5. Herwaldt BL, Grijalva MJ, Newsome AL, et al: Use of PCR to diagnose the fifth reported US case of autochthonous transmission of *Trypanosoma cruzi*, in Tennessee 1998. J Infect Dis 181:395–399, 2000. **Reviews the particulars of pediatric infection in the United States with *T. cruzi*.**
6. Kirchhoff LV: American trypanosomiasis (Chagas' disease)—a tropical disease now in the United States. N Engl J Med 329:639–644, 1993. **Overview of Chagas disease as it pertains to the U.S. population.**
7. Sahlas DJ, MacLean JD, Janevski J, Detsky AS: Out of Africa. N Engl J Med 347:749–753, 2002. **Dramatic presentation of African trypanosomiasis at a U.S. medical center.**
8. Sundar S, Jha TK, Thakur CP, et al: Oral miltefosine for Indian visceral leishmaniasis. N Engl J Med 347:1739–1746, 2002. **Presents the first effective oral treatment for visceral leishmaniasis.**

Malaria
Chandy C. John

KEY CONCEPTS

- Take time to teach parents of the child traveling to malaria-endemic areas about effective protection measures and chemoprophylaxis against malaria. If possible, refer them to a travel clinic.
- Evaluate any child traveler with fever and malaria exposure within the past year for malaria.
- Treat malaria early to avoid complications. When in doubt, treat.
- Admit the child with severe or complicated malaria to an intensive care unit for treatment with intravenous quinidine.
- Assess for and treat hypoglycemia, lactic acidosis, and severe anemia in the patient with severe malaria.
- Evaluate and treat children with a sepsis-like syndrome for coexistent bacteremia.
- Refer to the website of the Centers for Disease Control and Prevention (www.cdc.gov/malaria/diagnosis_treatment/tx_clinicians.htm) or call the malaria hotline (770–488–7788) for the latest updates on treatment of patients with malaria.

Malaria is a leading infectious cause of morbidity and mortality. An estimated 300 to 500 million clinical cases occur each year, causing between 1.5 and 2.7 million deaths. Four *Plasmodium* species cause malaria: *Plasmodium falciparum*, *Plasmodium vivax*, *Plasmodium ovale*, and *Plasmodium malariae*. *P. falciparum* causes the most severe disease. In the United States, almost all of the approximately 1000 cases of malaria reported annually to the Centers for Disease Control and Prevention (CDC) occur in travelers to or immigrants from malaria-endemic countries, although rare cases of local transmission have been reported.

Children, especially infants, often do not exhibit the classic malaria paroxysm, with its cold, hot, and sweating phases. Nonspecific symptoms, such as fever, lethargy, decreased appetite, and listlessness, are common in children. Vomiting, loose stools, and abdominal pain are also very common. Fevers may be intermittent or continuous, rather than the 48-hour (*P. vivax*, *P. ovale*) or 72-hour (*P. malariae*) fever patterns classically

---

BOX 1 Manifestations of Severe Malaria

Primary Manifestations

- Prostration (unable to sit or stand; in infants, unable to breast-feed)
- Impaired consciousness
- Respiratory distress
- Severe anemia (hemoglobin <5 mg/dL)
- Multiple seizures
- Jaundice
- Hemoglobinuria
- Circulatory collapse
- Abnormal bleeding
- Pulmonary edema

Supporting Manifestations

- Hypoglycemia
- Hyperparasitemia (>250,000 parasites/μL)
- Hyperpyrexia (temperature >102°F [39.5°C])
- Renal failure

---

described. Children with *P. falciparum* often have daily fevers. Hepatomegaly and splenomegaly are seen in approximately half of all children with acute malarial disease.

Nonimmune children with *P. falciparum* malaria often develop complications from the disease. The World Health Organization (WHO) lists 10 defining criteria and additional supporting criteria for severe malaria (Box 1). The most common of these complications in children are those involving the central nervous system (CNS) (coma and repeated convulsions), metabolic dysfunction (hypoglycemia and acidosis), severe malarial anemia, and respiratory distress. Mortality increases as the number of malarial complications increases. Children with malaria caused by *P. vivax* and *P. ovale* may appear ill, but complications other than anemia are uncommon in these children.

Examination of Giemsa-stained thick and thin blood smears remains the primary method of diagnosis for malaria. Thick smears are more sensitive in detecting parasites, but thin smears are necessary for *Plasmodium* species identification and allow estimation of the degree of peripheral blood parasitemia. Lab findings that support the diagnosis include a normocytic, normochromic anemia, and thrombocytopenia. New immunochromatographic tests looking for *P. falciparum* histidine-rich protein–2 (HRP2) and parasite enzyme lactate dehydrogenase are fairly sensitive and specific (>90%), but they are still inferior to microscopy. Parasite messenger RNA (mRNA) or DNA polymerase chain reaction (PCR) testing is more sensitive than microscopy and allows parasite species and strain identification, but at present it remains a research tool.

Expert Opinion on Management Issues

APPROACH

Treatment of malaria differs depending on whether it involves semi-immune individuals living in a malaria-endemic area or nonimmune individuals who have not had persistent exposure to *P. falciparum* throughout their lives. The primary difference is that semi-immune individuals may have relatively mild disease even with very high levels of parasitemia, and they can often be treated as outpatients. Treatment of the nonimmune individual is the focus here. In assessment of the nonimmune child with suspected malaria, appropriate evaluation and treatment depend on the answers to these three questions:

1. Does the child have malaria caused by *P. falciparum*?
2. Was the child exposed to malaria in an area with chloroquine-resistant malaria parasites?
3. Does the child have evidence of complications of malarial disease?

DRUG TREATMENT

Severe Malaria Caused by Chloroquine-Resistant *P. falciparum*

Chloroquine-resistant *P. falciparum* is present in most malaria-endemic areas, including Africa, Asia, and South America. In the United States, intravenous (IV) quinidine is the drug of choice for all children with severe *P. falciparum* malaria. In malaria-endemic countries, quinine (IV/IM [intravenous/intramuscular]), artesunate (IV/IM), and artemether (IM) are the drugs of choice for severe chloroquine-resistant *P. falciparum* malaria. These medications are currently unavailable in the United States. Treatment can be completed with the oral forms of quinine or artemisinin. Treatment of *P. falciparum* infection with any of these drugs alone is associated with recrudescence of infection, which is decreased if doxycycline, sulfadoxine/pyrimethamine, or clindamycin is used at the end of treatment (Table 1). However, increasing sulfadoxine/pyrimethamine resistance may soon make this drug ineffective as adjunctive therapy, and in children who acquire malaria in sub-Saharan Africa, clindamycin or doxycycline should be used instead.

Uncomplicated Malaria Caused by Chloroquine-Resistant *P. falciparum*

Atovaquone/proguanil (Malarone), quinine, and mefloquine are the three drugs available in the United States for treatment of uncomplicated chloroquine-resistant *P. falciparum* malaria. The high efficacy and modest side-effect profile of atovaquone/proguanil make it the drug of choice for treatment of uncomplicated malaria in children in the United States. Oral quinine is an acceptable alternative to atovaquone/proguanil, but its side effects of cinchonism and its bitter taste make compliance with treatment an issue. As noted previously, treatment with doxycycline or sulfadoxine-pyrimethamine is recommended at the end of quinine treatment, and this adjunctive treatment allows 3-day quinine treatment for many children with uncomplicated malaria (Table 2). Children who acquire *P. falciparum* infection in sub-Saharan Africa

TABLE 1 Drug Treatment of Severe *Plasmodium falciparum* Malaria in Children

Drug	Dosage/Route/Regimen*	Maximum Dose	Dosage Formulations	Common Adverse Reactions	Comments
Quinidine gluconate *or*	10 mg/kg salt loading dose in normal saline over 1–2 h IV followed by continuous infusion at 0.02 mg/kg/min, IV, with ECG monitoring, until able to take oral medication or for 7 days.	600 mg	Injection	Monitor patient for hypoglycemia.	Monitor QT interval; slow infusion rate if QT prolonged by >25% of baseline value. Use with caution in patients on other cardiac medications. Do not use loading dose if patient on mefloquine or quinine therapy in the last 24 h.
Quinine dihydrochloride *or*	20 mg/kg salt over 4 h, then 10 mg/kg over 2–4 h, q8h, IV, until able to take oral medication or for 7 days.	600 mg	Injection	Cinchonism (nausea, dysphoria, tinnitus, and high-tone deafness) resolves with cessation of therapy. Monitor patient for hypoglycemia.	Do not use loading dose if patient on mefloquine or quinine therapy in the last 24 h. Side effects.
Artesunate *or*	2.4 mg/kg first dose, then 1.2 mg/kg at 12 h and 24 h, then 1.2 mg/kg qd, IV or IM, until able to take oral medication or for 7 days.	—	Injection	Minimal side effects (occasional nausea, vomiting, dizziness).	Not available in the United States.
Artemether *plus*	3.2 mg/kg day 1, then 1.6 mg/kg IM qd until able to take oral medication or for 7 days. Do not give IV.	—	Injection	Minimal side effects (occasional nausea, vomiting, dizziness).	Not available in the United States.
Doxycycline *or*	3 mg/kg/day PO qd × 7 days. (1 tablet = 200 mg)	200 mg	Tablet	Photosensitivity, vaginitis, nausea, vomiting.	Do not use in children <8 yr of age or pregnant women.
Sulfadoxine/ pyrimethamine *or*	Single PO dose on the last day of quinine therapy: 5–10 kg: 1/2 tablet; 11–20 kg: 1 tablet; 21–30 kg: 1½ tablets; 31–40 kg: 2 tablets; >40 kg: adult dose (3 tablets).	3 tablets	Tablet	Rare risk of Stevens-Johnson syndrome.	
Clindamycin	10 mg/kg/dose PO in 3 doses × 7 days. (1 tablet = 900 mg)	900 mg	Tablet	Rare risk of pseudomembranous colitis. Liquid form is unpleasant tasting.	Frequent drug resistance in sub-Saharan Africa (see text).

*All pediatric doses are given up to a maximum of the adult dose.
ECG, electrocardiogram; IM, intramuscular; IV, intravenous; max, maximum; PO, by mouth; qxh, every x hours; qd; every day.

should be treated with either 3 days of quinine plus 7 days of doxycycline or 7 days of quinine plus 7 days of clindamycin. Sulfadoxine-pyrimethamine should not be used in these children because of increasing resistance to sulfadoxine-pyrimethamine in Africa. Children who acquire *P. falciparum* infection in border areas of Thailand (where low-level quinine resistance is endemic), who have persistent parasitemia more than 1%, or who receive clindamycin as their adjunctive therapy should receive the full 7-day course of quinine treatment. Children frequently vomit after receiving quinine, especially if they are febrile when receiving the drug. Acetaminophen and sponge bathing prior to administration of oral quinine may decrease the likelihood of vomiting. If a child vomits within 1 hour of receiving quinine, the dose should be repeated. Increasing mefloquine resistance and significant CNS side effects with treatment dosages make mefloquine an inferior alternative to quinine and atovaquone/-proguanil.

Combination therapies containing artemisinin derivatives are likely to become first-line therapy for uncomplicated chloroquine-resistant *P. falciparum* infection in malaria-endemic areas. A number of dosage

TABLE 2 Drug Treatment of Uncomplicated Malaria in Children

Drug	Dosage/Route/Regimen*	Maximum Dose	Dosage Formulations	Common Adverse Reactions	Comments
Chloroquine-Resistant *Plasmodium falciparum*					
Quinine sulfate *or*	8.3 mg/kg base or 10 mg/kg salt q8h × 3–7 days (see text) 1 tab = 500 mg base.	500 mg (base)	Tablet	See Table 1. Also bitter taste.	See Table 1
Artesunate *or*	4 mg/kg/day on day 1, 2 mg/kg on days 2 and 3, 1 mg/kg on days 4–7 (1 tab = 50 mg)	200 mg	Tablet	See Table 1	See Table 1
Artemether *plus*	Regimen same as artesunate (1 cap = 40 mg).	200 mg	Capsule	See Table 1	See Table 1
Doxycycline or sulfadoxine/pyrimethamine (SP) or clindamycin	See Table 3 for doxycycline, SP, and clindamycin dosages.	See Table 3	See Table 1	See Table 1	See Table 1
Artemether, or artesunate *plus* mefloquine	4 mg/kg/day × 3 days as for mefloquine alone (dosage below).	200 mg			
Atovaquone/proguanil	11–20 kg: 1 adult tab qd × 3 days. 21–30 kg: 2 adult tabs qd × 3 days. 31–40 kg: 3 adult tabs qd × 3 days. >40 kg (adult dose): 4 adult tabs qd × 3 days. (Adult tabs: 250 mg atovaquone/100 mg proguanil.)	4 adult tabs	Tablet	Nausea, vomiting, headache (generally mild), rare transaminase elevations.	Contraindicated in patients with renal failure (creatinine clearance <30 mL/min). Take with food or a milky drink.
Artemether/lumefantrine	10–14 kg: 1 tab q8h × 2 doses, then q12h × 4 doses. 15–24 kg: 2 tabs q8h × 2 doses, then q12h × 4 doses. 25–34 kg: 3 tabs q8h × 2 doses, then q12h × 4 doses. >35 kg: 4 tabs q8h × 2 doses, then q12h × 4 doses. (1 tab = 120 mg lumefantrine/20 mg artemether.)	4 tabs	Tablet	Side effects similar to those of artemether alone.	Not available in the United States.

Mefloquine	15 mg/kg base × 1; 10 mg/kg base 8–24 h later. (1 tab = 250 mg base.)	1250 mg	Tablet	Do not use mefloquine to treat patients who have taken mefloquine as prophylaxis. Do not use in individuals with depression or other psychiatric disorders or seizure disorders. Do not use in conjunction with quinine or quinidine.	High-level mefloquine resistance exists in border areas of Thailand; other medications should be used in patients acquiring malaria in these areas.

All *Plasmodium* Species Except Chloroquine-Resistant *Plasmodium falciparum*

| Chloroquine phosphate | 10 mg base/kg (16 mg salt/kg) × 1; 5 mg base/kg (8 mg salt/kg) 6 h later, then 5 mg base/kg (8 mg salt/kg) q24h × 2 days. Adult dose: 600 mg base (1000 mg salt), then 300 mg base (500 mg salt) 6 h later, then 300 mg base (500 mg salt) q24h × 2 days. (Tablets available in 2 doses: 1 tab = 150 mg base/250 mg salt (generic) *or* 1 tab = 300 mg base/500 mg salt.) | 600 mg (base) | Tablet | Nausea, dysphoria, may exacerbate psoriasis, pruritus in dark-skinned individuals. Rarely, cerebellar or neuropsychiatric syndromes. | If not available, hydroxychloroquine sulfate can be used, at the same *base* dosage (200 mg hydroxychloroquine salt = 155 mg base). If parenteral therapy required, treat as for severe *P. falciparum* malaria. High-level *P. vivax* chloroquine resistance reported in Oceania and India; consider alternative treatment (see text). |

P. vivax and *P. ovale* (prevention of relapse)

| Primaquine phosphate | 0.5 mg/kg/day base × 14 days. Adult dose: 30 mg base qd × 14 days. (1 tab = 15 mg base or 26.3 mg salt.) | 30 mg (base). | Tablet. | Screen for G6PD deficiency and do not give primaquine if present (see text). | Primaquine is given for eradication of liver stage parasites and should be given at the end of chloroquine treatment. |

*All pediatric doses are given up to a maximum of the adult dose.
G6PD, glucose-6-phosphate dehydrogenase; q*x*h, every *x* hours; qd, every day.

regimens of these therapies are used (see Table 2). It is likely that fixed-combination therapy will eventually standardize dosage regimens. A fixed combination of artesunate and lumefantrine was formulated by Novartis and is now available in developing countries but not in the United States.

Severe or Uncomplicated Malaria Caused by Chloroquine-Susceptible *P. falciparum*

At the time of publication, chloroquine-susceptible *P. falciparum* was still present in the Middle East, Central America north of the Panama Canal, Haiti, and the Dominican Republic, but this may change. The CDC website (www.cdc.gov) and malaria hotline (770–488–7788) have up-to-date information on malaria drug resistance in every country. Chloroquine-susceptible malaria requiring parenteral treatment should be treated identically to severe chloroquine-resistant malaria (see Table 2). Chloroquine-susceptible *P. falciparum* malaria amenable to oral treatment should be treated with chloroquine. If there is any doubt whether chloroquine resistance is present in the area malaria was acquired, therapy should be given as for chloroquine-resistant malaria.

Malaria Caused by *P. vivax*, *P. ovale*, and *P. malariae*

Chloroquine is the initial drug of choice for *P. vivax*, *P. ovale,* or *P. malariae* malaria. In some areas of Oceania, high-level chloroquine resistance is reported in *P. vivax*. Quinine, artemisinin derivatives, and atovaquone/proguanil show efficacy in small clinical studies, but treatment of a patient with *P. vivax* with medications other than chloroquine should be done in consultation with the CDC or a malaria treatment expert. Patients with *P. vivax* and *P. ovale* malaria should also receive a 2-week course of primaquine to eradicate dormant liver stages of these parasites. Individuals with glucose-6-phosphate dehydrogenase (G6PD) deficiency may experience massive hemolysis with primaquine administration and should not receive primaquine. No effective alternatives to primaquine for liver-stage parasite eradication are currently available.

Adjunctive Therapy for Severe *P. falciparum* Malaria

Antipyretics (acetaminophen) should be given to all children unless there are signs of liver failure. Hypovolemia should be corrected with IV fluids or colloid. Patients with symptomatic anemia (e.g., in congestive heart failure) or a hemoglobin level of 5 mg/dL or below should be transfused. Hypoglycemia should be corrected with a 50% dextrose bolus, and IV solutions for children with severe malaria should contain at least 5% dextrose.

Lactic acidosis should be addressed by aggressive treatment of malarial infection, volume repletion if the patient is dehydrated, and transfusion of blood as appropriate. Some experts suggest administration of sodium bicarbonate if the patient's blood pH is less than 7.1. However, others would not advocate sodium bicarbonate administration even at this pH because it can cause a paradoxical tissue acidification. Preliminary studies suggest that dichloroacetate (DCA) may ameliorate malaria-induced lactic acidosis, but larger studies are required before this can be recommended as standard therapy.

A randomized clinical trial of prophylactic phenobarbital in children with cerebral malaria demonstrated increased deaths in the phenobarbital group, despite better control of seizures. Future trials may yield alternative drugs or dosages for effective prophylaxis against seizures in children, but at present prophylactic anticonvulsants are not recommended in children. If convulsions do occur, they should be treated with IV diazepam. Recurrent seizures should be treated with phenobarbital or phenytoin, following the standard treatment for status epilepticus.

Bacterial superinfection, including pneumonia, bacteremia, and meningitis, may occur in children with severe malaria, although it appears to be less common in children than in adults. In children with acute clinical deterioration or a sepsis-like picture, a blood glucose level should be checked, blood cultures drawn, and broad-spectrum antibiotics initiated.

At present, the usefulness of other interventions, such as mannitol, deferoxamine, pentoxifylline, dextran, and antibodies against tumor necrosis factor, is not clear. Corticosteroids, heparin, and cyclosporine appear to be harmful and should not be used.

CONTROVERSIES IN MANAGEMENT

The role of exchange blood transfusion in malaria therapy is controversial. Large prospective randomized, controlled studies have not been done, and probably will not be done, in nonimmune individuals, and the results of other studies are largely anecdotal. A meta-analysis of exchange transfusion trials failed to demonstrate a benefit to exchange transfusion. Many clinicians believe nonetheless that exchange transfusion is likely to be beneficial to individuals with severe malaria and a high percentage of parasitized erythrocytes. One review recommends that exchange transfusion be performed in the seriously ill patient with a parasitemia level higher than 15%, and it should be considered in the patient with parasitemia in the 5% to 15% range if the patient has other signs of poor prognosis.

Certain guidelines state that even children with *severe* malaria can be given a 3-day course of quinidine/quinine if they receive doxycycline or sulfadoxine/pyrimethamine at the end of quinidine/quinine treatment. The full 7-day course of quinidine/quinine plus terminal doxycycline or sulfadoxine/pyrimethamine or clindamycin is reserved in these guidelines for children with severe malaria who have traveled to an area with quinine resistance (currently Southeast Asia). Because no prospective studies on the efficacy of the 3-day regimen in nonimmune children with *severe* malaria are available, many experts treat all children with severe malaria with a 7-day course of quinidine/quinine plus terminal doxycycline, sulfadoxine/pyrimethamine, or clindamycin, regardless of the area in which the child became infected.

Use of oral atovaquone/proguanil rather than oral quinine to follow up IV quinidine treatment in children with severe malaria is an attractive option because atovaquone/proguanil has far fewer side effects than quinine and is more palatable. Anecdotally, such treatment is effective, but no studies have been performed to date using this combination of drug treatments, so it cannot be routinely recommended.

PREVENTION

Protection from mosquitoes is an important part of malaria prevention for individuals who travel to or live in malaria-endemic areas. The *Anopheles* mosquito feeds from dusk to dawn. Travelers should remain in well-screened areas, wear clothing that covers most of the body, sleep under a bed net (ideally one impregnated with permethrin), and use insect repellants with diethyltoluamide (DEET) during these hours.

Repellants with 20% to 30% DEET (not >30%) should be used for children up to every 6 hours as needed. Systemic toxicity with DEET is rare in children and appears related to excessive use.

Chemoprophylaxis is the cornerstone of malaria prevention for nonimmune children who travel to malaria-endemic areas (Table 3). Weekly mefloquine is the drug of choice for malaria chemoprophylaxis in children traveling to areas with chloroquine-resistant *P. falciparum*. The lack of a liquid or suspension formulation sometimes makes mefloquine administration difficult. Mefloquine is better tolerated by children if it is disguised in other foods, such as chocolate syrup or applesauce. Adults have a 10% to 25% incidence of sleep disturbances and dysphoria with mefloquine, but these side effects appear to be less common in children. Daily atovaquone/proguanil (Malarone) is preferred for children traveling to malaria-endemic areas for less than 2 weeks because it needs to be taken only 1 day prior to departure, during the travel period, and 7 days after travel. Daily doxycycline is another alternative for prophylaxis, but it cannot be used in children younger than 8 years. Daily primaquine is used successfully as malaria prophylaxis, but it should be taken only with CDC guidance and if other options are unsuitable. In areas

12

TABLE 3 Malaria Chemoprophylaxis for Children

Drug	Dosage/Route/Regimen	Maximum Dose	Dosage Formulations	Common Adverse Reactions	Comments
Chloroquine-Resistant *P. falciparum*					
Mefloquine	<15 kg: 1/8 tab/wk. 15–19 kg: 1/4 tab/wk. 20–30 kg: 1/2 tab/wk. 31–45 kg: 3/4 tab wk. >45 kg: 1 tab/wk. (1 tab = 228 mg base/250 mg salt.)	1 tab	Tablet	See Table 1.	Take 2 wk prior to travel, during travel, and for 4 wk after travel.
Atovaquone/Proguanil	11–20 kg: 1 *pediatric* tab once daily. 21–30 kg: 2 *pediatric* tabs once daily. 31–40 kg: 3 *pediatric* tabs once daily. >40 kg: 1 *adult* tab once daily (Pediatric tabs: 62.5 mg atovaquone/25 mg proguanil; Adult tabs: 250 mg atovaquone/100 mg proguanil.)	1 adult tab	Tablet	See Table 1.	Take 1 day prior to travel, during travel, and for 7 days after travel.
Doxycycline	2 mg/kg daily. (1 tab = 100 mg.)	100 mg	Tablet	See Table 1.	Take 1–2 days prior to travel, during travel, and for 4 wk after travel.
Chloroquine-Susceptible *P. falciparum*					
Chloroquine	5 mg base/kg/wk. Tablets available in 2 doses: 1. 1 tab = 150 mg base/250 mg salt *or*, 2. 1 tab = 300 mg base/500 mg salt.	300 mg base	Tablet	See Table 1.	Take 2 wk prior to travel, during travel, and for 4 wk after travel.

where malaria remains chloroquine susceptible, chloroquine is the drug of choice for prophylaxis. The CDC website and hotline number listed earlier are useful resources for determining the current malaria prophylaxis guidelines for specific countries. Travelers should be reminded that no prophylaxis is completely effective.

Numerous malaria vaccine trials are in progress, using components of pre-erythrocytic and erythrocytic malarial antigens, but currently no malaria vaccine is available for travelers' prophylaxis.

Common Pitfalls

- Accurate diagnosis of malaria requires a microscopist with experience in reading malaria slides. If there is no one at your institution, consult the CDC.
- Repeat blood smears at least three times before ruling out the diagnosis of malaria.
- Coinfection with multiple *Plasmodium* species may occur. Any child who has traveled to an area with *P. vivax* or *P. ovale* should receive primaquine treatment as terminal prophylaxis, even if the smear shows only *P. falciparum*. Conversely, any child with severe or complicated malaria who has been to a *P. falciparum*–endemic area should be presumed to have *P. falciparum* infection, even if the smear shows only another malaria species.
- If a child vomits less than an hour after administration of a dose of quinine, mefloquine, or atovaquone/proguanil, the dose should be repeated once. If the child vomits more than an hour after administration, no repeat dose is necessary.
- When writing prescriptions for chloroquine, quinine, mefloquine, and primaquine, be very careful to note on the prescription whether you are prescribing a dose of the *base* or *salt* form of the drug.
- Make sure that parents understand how to give medications, particularly unpleasant-tasting medicines like quinine or mefloquine, which are often more palatable in a vehicle like chocolate syrup or applesauce.

Communication and Counseling

Parents of children traveling to malaria-endemic areas must be thoroughly informed about the importance of preventative measures and chemoprophylaxis for malaria. They must also be made aware that if their child develops fever during the trip or up to a year afterward, the child should be evaluated immediately for malaria. Early treatment is the key to prevention of malaria complications.

SUGGESTED READINGS

1. John CC: Drug treatment of malaria in children. Pediatr Infect Dis J 22:649–651, 2003. **Concise summary of drug treatment options for children with malaria.**
2. Newton CR, Krishna S: Severe falciparum malaria in children: Current understanding of pathophysiology and supportive treatment. Pharmacol Ther 79:1–53, 1998. **Comprehensive overview relating adjunctive treatment to severe malaria pathogenesis.**
3. Stauffer W, Fischer PR: Diagnosis and treatment of malaria in children. Clin Infect Dis 37:1340–1348, 2003. **Includes a helpful algorithm for initial assessment and management of the child with suspected malaria.**
4. Warrell DA: Management of severe malaria. Parassitologia 41:287–294, 1999. **Nicely summarizes various trials of ancillary treatments for severe malaria.**
5. White NJ: The treatment of malaria. N Engl J Med 335:800–806, 1996. **A well-organized review of treatment options for uncomplicated and severe malaria in adults and children.**
6. World Health Organization, Communicable Diseases Cluster: Severe falciparum malaria. Trans R Soc Trop Med Hyg 94(Suppl 1):S1–S90, 2000. **Most recent WHO monograph on the classification, pathogenesis, diagnosis, and treatment of severe malaria.**

Pneumocystis jiroveci Pneumonia (PCP)

Heather J. Zar

KEY CONCEPTS

- *Pneumocystis jiroveci* pneumonia (PCP) is a common severe opportunistic infection in patients infected with HIV (human immunodeficiency virus). Children with T-cell dysfunction or those on immunosuppressive therapy are also at risk for PCP.
- The clinical presentation, chest radiology abnormalities, and laboratory findings are nonspecific.
- Diagnosis requires special stains and microscopy for identification of *Pneumocystis* in a respiratory specimen.
- Treatment with trimethoprim-sulfamethoxazole (TMP-SMX) should be initiated when PCP is suspected. Corticosteroids should be added for moderate or severe illness.
- Prophylaxis can effectively prevent PCP in susceptible children. TMP-SMX is the prophylactic agent of choice.

Pneumocystis jiroveci pneumonia (PCP) is an opportunistic infection, occurring predominantly in immunosuppressed children. PCP was described initially in malnourished or premature European infants during World War II. Subsequently, cases have been reported in children with primary immunologic disorders, in those receiving immunosuppressive therapy, and in children with primary immune deficiencies, with underlying malignancy. More recently, PCP has emerged as one of the most common serious opportunistic infections in children infected with HIV (human immunodeficiency virus); however, in developed countries, the incidence of PCP has declined following the introduction of chemoprophylaxis and antiretroviral therapy.

P. jiroveci is host specific for humans; infection is usually limited to the lungs. Rarely, disseminated disease in the context of severe immunosuppression or overwhelming infection occurs. Among HIV-infected children, PCP occurs most commonly in infants 3 to 6 months of age. The number or percentage of CD4 T lymphocytes is a useful predictor of PCP but is less reliable in those younger than 1 year.

The clinical course of PCP is variable, depending on the child's host defense mechanisms. Infection may produce a spectrum of respiratory disease; the onset may be insidious with slow progression or acute with a fulminant course. Symptoms include tachypnea, fever, dyspnea, and cough. The cough is characteristically nonproductive; auscultation of the lungs is usually normal, although crepitations, rhonchi, or wheezing may

occur. HIV-infected infants usually present with an acute, severe illness characterized by prominent and progressive hypoxia and increasing respiratory difficulty. No specific clinical features can distinguish children with PCP from those with other lower respiratory tract infections. Coinfection with bacterial, viral, or fungal pathogens may also occur.

No radiologic or laboratory abnormalities are specific for PCP. The chest radiograph usually shows a diffuse interstitial pattern that progresses to alveolar opacification (Fig. 1); however, hyperinflation, focal infiltrates, cavities, a miliary pattern, pneumothoraces, or a normal appearance may also occur. Serum lactate dehydrogenase (LDH) may be markedly elevated (>1000 IU/L), but this is nonspecific and may reflect the extent of lung involvement.

Definitive diagnosis requires identification of *P. jiroveci* cysts or trophozoites in lower respiratory tract secretions. Open lung or transbronchial biopsy are the most reliable diagnostic procedures, but they may be hazardous, particularly in severely ill patients. Less invasive procedures, including bronchoalveolar lavage or sputum induction, are useful for diagnosis. Nasopharyngeal aspirates may yield *P. jiroveci* in cases of severe infection. Because *P. jiroveci* cannot be cultured, special stains are used to identify the organism. Silver methenamine, toluidine blue, or calcofluor white are useful for staining cyst forms; Giemsa, modified Wright-Giemsa, or modified Papanicolaou stains identify trophozoites. Fluorescein-conjugated monoclonal antibodies provide a more sensitive stain for detecting both the cyst and trophozoite forms. Polymerase chain reaction (PCR) techniques have a high sensitivity and specificity and may improve diagnostic accuracy, but they are currently a research tool.

Expert Opinion on Management Issues

TREATMENT

Timely and effective therapy should be given to any child with suspected infection because untreated PCP is usually fatal. The recommended treatment is intravenous (IV) trimethoprim-sulfamethoxazole (TMP-SMX) for 2 to 3 weeks (Table 1). IV therapy is preferable for severely ill children, but oral treatment can be substituted if there is mild disease or once clinical improvement occurs, provided that patients do not have malabsorption. The response to therapy may take 5 to 7 days. Adverse reactions to TMP-SMX occur in approximately 15% of cases, but treatment should only be discontinued if reactions are severe.

IV pentamidine may be used as an alternative drug for children who cannot tolerate TMP-SMX or who have not responded to therapy (see Table 1). Pentamidine is associated with a high incidence of adverse reactions, including pancreatitis, alterations in blood glucose, renal dysfunction, fever, neutropenia, and hypotension. Other alternative agents include atovaquone, dapsone with trimethoprim, trimetrexate

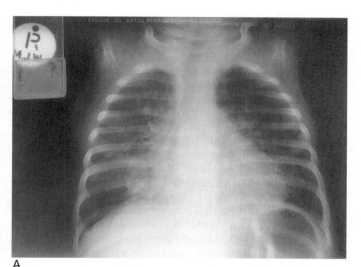

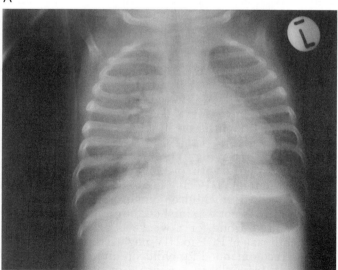

FIGURE 1. Chest radiographs of an HIV-infected infant with PCP showing progression of interstitial infiltrates to alveolar opacification. *A,* presenting chest radiograph; *B,* progression of interstitial infiltrates and alveolar organization within 24 hours.

TABLE 1 Treatment of *Pneumocystis* Pneumonia in Children

Drug	Dose	Route	Comments
Trimethoprim-sulfamethoxazole (TMP-SMX)	15–20 mg/kg TMP with 75–100 mg/kg SMX per day given q6h	IV *or* oral	IV is first choice. Oral therapy only if mild disease or once clinical improvement occurs.
Pentamidine	4 mg/kg/day, once daily	Intravenous	In those who cannot tolerate TMP-SMX or who do not respond after 5–7 days. High incidence of side effects. Should not be administered with didanosine because of risk of pancreatitis.
Atovaquone	30–45 mg/kg/day	Oral	Limited experience in children.
Dapsone and trimethoprim	No studies in children of established doses	Oral	Limited experience in children.
Primaquine and clindamycin	No studies in children of established doses	Oral	Limited experience in children.

IV, intravenous; q*x*h, every *x* hours.

TABLE 2 Indications for *Pneumocystis* Pneumonia Prophylaxis for HIV-infected Children

Age	CD4 T Lymphocyte Count*
4–6 wk to 12 mo[†]	All patients irrespective of CD4 count
1–5 yr	<500 cells/mL *or* if percentage is less than 15%
>5 yr	<200 cells/mL *or* if percentage is less than 15%

HIV, human immunodeficiency virus.

*If CD4 measurements are unavailable, prophylaxis should be given to all symptomatic children.

†HIV-exposed children should receive prophylaxis for 4 to 6 weeks to 4 months; thereafter prophylaxis may be discontinued if HIV infection has been excluded.

glucuronate with leucovorin, and clindamycin with primaquine, but little information is available on the efficacy or tolerability of these regimes in children. Mutations in *P. jiroveci* dihydropteroate synthase genes (a key enzyme target of TMP-SMX) may occur, especially in HIV-infected patients with PCP taking TMP-SMX prophylaxis. However, the clinical importance of mutant strains is unclear, and the response to TMP-SMX treatment is variable.

Corticosteroids are beneficial, improving oxygenation and reducing the incidence of respiratory failure, when used early in the course of PCP in hypoxic HIV-infected adults. Although no controlled trials on the use of corticosteroids in children have been performed, use is reported to improve survival compared with historical controls. Corticosteroids are therefore recommended in children with moderate to severe PCP. The optimal dose and duration have not been determined, but a recommended regime is prednisone, 2 mg/kg for 7 to 10 days, with tapering doses over the next 10 to 14 days.

Appropriate supportive therapy and treatment of copathogens are important in the management of PCP. Oxygen should be administered to all hypoxic children; many children may also require intensive care support and positive pressure ventilation.

PREVENTION

PCP is a preventable illness, and prophylaxis should be provided to children at risk. Prophylaxis is recommended for all HIV-exposed infants from 4 to 6 weeks of age; prophylaxis should be discontinued once infants are reliably confirmed to be HIV negative. Infants who are HIV infected or those whose HIV status remains unknown should continue prophylaxis for the first year of life. Thereafter, prophylaxis should be given to HIV-infected children with severe immunosuppression as reflected by CD4 T lymphocyte measurements (Table 2). Prophylaxis is also indicated for children with rapidly declining CD4 counts or those with severe clinical disease (Centers for Disease Control and Prevention [CDC] category C or World Health Organization [WHO] category III or IV disease). When CD4 counts are unavailable, prophylaxis is recommended for children with symptomatic HIV infection. Lifelong prophylaxis should be initiated following an episode of PCP. Recent data suggest that prophylaxis may be safely withdrawn in HIV-infected children older than 2 years who have sustained immune reconstitution for at least 6 months on highly active antiretroviral therapy (HAART).

Children receiving chronic immunosuppressive therapy or those with primary immune deficiencies that are related to HIV should also receive prophylaxis. The risk of PCP in children on chronic oral corticosteroid therapy is not established, but a dose of 16 mg or more of prednisone for 8 weeks is associated with a significant risk of PCP in HIV-negative adults. Prophylaxis is recommended for children after hematopoietic stem cell transplants for at least 6 months after engraftment.

The recommended prophylactic regimen is oral TMP-SMX three times a week; alternative dosage schedules or drugs may be used if TMP-SMX is poorly tolerated (Table 3).

TABLE 3 Drugs for *Pneumocystis* Pneumonia Prophylaxis in Children

Drug	Dose	Route	Comments
Trimethoprim-sulfamethoxazole (TMP-SMX)	150 mg/m² TMP with 750 mg/m² SMX per day given bid thrice weekly *or* single dose daily, thrice weekly, *or* bid, 7 days per week	PO	First choice.
Dapsone	2 mg/kg daily *or* 4 mg/kg weekly	PO	Higher incidence of PCP with weekly therapy.
Pentamidine	300 mg monthly *or* Aerosol administered via Respirgard II nebulizer. Only recommended in children ≥5 yr.		AerosoL
	4 mg/kg q2–4wk	IV	IV form associated with adverse effects.
Atovaquone	30 mg/kg daily	PO	If <3 mo or >24 mo of age.
	45 mg/kg daily		If 3–24 mo of age.

Common Pitfalls

Children with PCP may be coinfected with bacterial or viral pathogens; additional antimicrobial therapy for these should be used when appropriate. The use of corticosteroids in children who are infected with other pathogens such as cytomegalovirus (CMV) may be detrimental; thus, a careful search for other respiratory pathogens should be undertaken even when *P. jiroveci* is identified.

Failure to administer prophylaxis to susceptible children could result in PCP with severe consequences. Knowledge of the mother's HIV status and early postnatal identification of HIV-infected infants is necessary for effective prevention of PCP because prophylaxis should be initiated at 4 to 6 weeks of age. HIV-infected children should have periodic monitoring of immune function, particularly CD4 measurements, to determine whether prophylaxis is indicated after 1 year of age. Failure to identify children who have altered immunity that is not HIV related or who are receiving chronic immunosuppressive therapy such as oral corticosteroids as being at risk for PCP may lead to omission of prophylaxis.

Long-term use of TMP-SMX prophylaxis may affect the antimicrobial resistance patterns of bacteria, limiting the use of this antibiotic for childhood bacterial infections. Long-term TMP-SMX prophylaxis may promote the development of mutant *P. jiroveci* isolates. However, the effect of mutant strains on clinical illness and outcome from PCP is controversial.

Communication and Counseling

Long-term prophylaxis for PCP is necessary for many HIV-infected and immunosuppressed children. Children who have had an episode of PCP require lifelong prophylaxis. Children and their caregivers should be informed about the efficacy of chronic prophylaxis; ongoing communication and support of children and their families is necessary to promote adherence to prophylaxis. The incidence of side effects to TMP-SMX is high in HIV-infected children, and alternative prophylactic

regimes may be needed, as outlined earlier. Prophylaxis should be integrated into a comprehensive package of care for children with HIV or other chronic underlying immunosuppressive diseases.

SUGGESTED READINGS

1. American Academy of Pediatrics: *Pneumocystis jiroveci* infections. In Pickering LK (ed): *Red Book* 2003: Report of the Committee on Infectious Diseases, 26th ed. Elk Grove Village, Ill: American Academy of Pediatrics, 2003, pp 500–505. **Summary of the clinical features, diagnosis, treatment, and prevention of PCP in children.**
2. Hughes WT: *Pneumocystis carinii* pneumonia: New approaches to diagnosis, treatment, and prevention. Pediatr Infect Dis J 10:391–399, 1991. **A review of available diagnostic, therapeutic, and preventative options for PCP.**
3. Masur H, Kaplan JE, Holmes KK: Guidelines for preventing opportunistic infections among HIV-infected persons—2002. Recommendations of the U.S. Public Health Service and the Infectious Diseases Society of America. Ann Intern Med 137(5 Pt 2):435–478, 2002. **Recommendations for PCP prophylaxis in HIV-exposed and -infected children living in developed countries.**
4. Thomas CF, Limper AH: *Pneumocystis* pneumonia. N Engl J Med 350(24):2487–2498, 2004. **Review of the clinical and epidemiologic features of PCP with emphasis on new understanding of the biology of *Pneumocystis* and the host response to infection.**
5. Wakefield AE: *Pneumocystis carinii*. Br Med Bull 61:175–188, 2002. **Review of the biology of the parasite and use of molecular techniques to study the epidemiology of infection and facilitate diagnosis and detection of mutant strains.**
6. World Health Organization; UNAIDS: Provisional WHO/UNAIDS recommendations on the use of cotrimoxazole prophylaxis in adults and children living with HIV/AIDS in Africa. Afr Health Sci 1(1):30–31, 2001. **WHO/UNAIDS recommendations for PCP prophylaxis for HIV-exposed and -infected children living in Africa.**
7. World Health Organization: Statement on use of cotrimoxazole as prophylaxis in HIV exposed and HIV infected children. November 2004. Available at http://www.who.int/3by5/mediacentre/news32/en/. **Joint WHO/UNAIDS/Unicef statement on use of cotrimoxazole as prophylaxis in HIV-exposed and HIV-infected children.**
8. Zar HJ: Prevention of HIV-associated respiratory disease in developing countries: Potential benefits. Int J Tuberc Lung Dis 7(9):820–827, 2003. **Review of the epidemiology of PCP in HIV-infected children and prophylactic strategies for developing countries.**

12

Toxoplasmosis

Jeffrey L. Jones

KEY CONCEPTS

- Humans become infected with *Toxoplasma gondii* by ingestion of undercooked contaminated meat, ingestion of soil or water contaminated with cat feces, infection transplacentally leading to congenital toxoplasmosis, and transplantation or transfusion.
- Symptoms are usually mild or unapparent in children (infected after birth) and adults with normal immune systems.
- Congenitally infected infants are usually asymptomatic at birth, but up to 80% develop neurologic or ocular disease by the third decade of life.
- Classic symptoms are chorioretinitis, intracranial calcifications, hydrocephalus, and convulsions. They occur in only a minority of infants with congenital toxoplasmosis.
- In immunocompromised persons, toxoplasmosis can lead to severe encephalitis, pneumonitis, myocarditis, retinitis, or other types of disseminated disease. Prophylactic therapy is needed for those with severe immunosuppression.
- Diagnosis is usually made or greatly assisted by antibody detection tests, or, in the case of fetal toxoplasmosis, detection of *Toxoplasma* DNA in amniotic fluid.
- Treatment is most frequently provided for pregnant women with acute infection to prevent or treat fetal infection, congenitally infected infants, immunosuppressed persons, and acute and recurrent ocular disease.
- Food-, water-, soil-, and cat feces–related hygiene are the principal means of toxoplasmosis prevention.

Toxoplasma gondii is a ubiquitous protozoan that infects most species of warm-blooded animals, including humans. In the United States, 22.5% of adolescents and adults have antibodies to *T. gondii* that indicate chronic infection. Seroprevalence increases with age and varies markedly in different populations. There are three stages of this obligate intracellular parasite:

1. Tachyzoite, which rapidly proliferates and destroys cells during acute infection
2. Bradyzoite, which multiplies slowly and forms tissue cysts
3. Oocyst, which can survive months to years in the environment and is resistant to disinfectants and freezing.

Members of the cat family (Felidae) are the definitive host for *T. gondii*. After tissue cysts or oocysts are ingested by a cat, the sexual cycle takes place in the intestinal mucosa and millions of oocysts are shed in the feces for several weeks. The oocysts take 1 to 5 days to sporulate and become infectious.

Humans usually become infected when they:

- Ingest tissue cysts in raw or undercooked meat (especially pork, mutton, or wild game)
- Inadvertently ingest oocysts from contaminated soil (for example, soil on uncooked fruits or vegetables), cat litter, or contaminated water
- Become infected through transplacental transmission leading to congenital toxoplasmosis.

Although less common, humans can also become infected by transplantation or transfusion or by accidental inoculation in the laboratory. After infection, the tachyzoite stage rapidly multiplies intracellularly, destroys host cells, enters the blood and lymphatic vessels, and is carried to distant sites where it invades other cells that develop into the chronic cyst form. The tachyzoite can invade all mammalian cells; however, the chronic cyst form has a propensity for brain, muscle, and heart tissue.

Clinical Manifestations

Symptoms of acute infection are generally mild or inapparent in children and adults with normal immune systems. Ten percent to 20% of those infected may develop symptoms such as lymphadenopathy, fever, sore throat, fatigue, and malaise that resolve in weeks to months. Chorioretinitis occurs in up to 2% of those infected in the United States; however, in some areas of the world it has been documented in more than 15% of persons with acute *T. gondii* infection, which may represent infection with more virulent strains. Of the three major genetic types of *T. gondii*, based on restriction fragment length polymorphism (RFLP) analysis of the surface antigen coding region, type I is more commonly associated with severe ocular disease. Although immunocompetent persons usually have a self-limited illness, rare instances of severe manifestations such as encephalitis and hepatitis have been documented.

Women infected with *T. gondii* before conception, with rare exception do not transmit the infection to their fetuses. However, women newly infected during pregnancy can transmit the infection across the placenta, leading to congenital infection of the fetus. The risk of congenital infection is lowest (10% to 25%) when maternal infection occurs during the first trimester and highest (60% to 90%) when maternal infection occurs during the third trimester. However, the disease is generally more severe the earlier in pregnancy that fetal infection occurs. Congenitally infected infants may have one or more of the classic symptoms, including chorioretinitis, intracranial calcifications, and hydrocephalus; or they may have other signs and symptoms such as microcephaly, convulsions, hepatomegaly, jaundice, splenomegaly, lymphadenopathy, thrombocytopenia, fever, anemia, maculopapular rash, spasticity and palsies, deafness, and growth retardation. However, most (80%–90%) congenitally infected infants do not have signs or symptoms detected on physical examination at birth. Nevertheless, approximately 80% of untreated congenitally infected infants develop chorioretinitis or neurologic symptoms in later childhood or by the third decade of life.

In immunocompromised persons, *T. gondii* infection can reactivate, leading to severe encephalitis, pneumonitis, myocarditis, retinitis, and other types of disseminated disease. Reactivated toxoplasmosis leading to toxoplasmic encephalitis is one of the most common severe neurologic infections in patients with the acquired immunodeficiency syndrome (AIDS). Symptoms can include those of meningoencephalitis or a mass lesion. Transplacental infection with toxoplasmosis has been documented after reactivation of chronic infection in pregnant women with AIDS. Transplant (particularly cardiac) recipients are also at risk of toxoplasmosis. Screening of donor and recipient blood for *Toxoplasma* antibodies is important; a seronegative recipient who receives a heart from a seropositive donor requires prophylactic treatment and close observation.

Diagnosis

GENERAL AND PREGNANT WOMEN

Because toxoplasmosis can only rarely be documented by the observation of parasites in patient specimens, antibody detection tests are the main source of diagnostic information. More commonly available tests include enzyme immunoassays (EIAs), agglutination tests, and indirect fluorescent antibody (IFA) tests. Positive immunoglobulin (Ig) G antibody tests are indicative of an infection occurring in the past, whereas positive IgM antibody tests indicate an infection occurring more recently. However, some IgM antibody tests can stay positive for 18 months or more, or give false-positive reactions. When clinicians are attempting to determine whether or not *T. gondii* infection occurred in a woman during her pregnancy, a serologic profile done in a reference laboratory—including the avidity test, differential agglutination, Sabin-Feldman dye test, IgM EIA, IgA EIA, and IgE EIA, and, if indicated, repeat titers—is helpful in attempting to determine the timing of infection. Serologic diagnosis must be confirmed at a reference laboratory before potentially toxic drugs or amniocentesis for *T. gondii* infection diagnosis are considered for a pregnant woman. When serologic test results indicate a potential *T. gondii* infection during pregnancy, diagnosis of congenital toxoplasmosis in the fetus is usually accomplished by amniocentesis and DNA polymerase chain reaction (PCR) testing of amniotic fluid at a reference laboratory from 18 weeks of gestation onward.

INFANTS

In the newborn, diagnosis of *Toxoplasma* infection is made with a combination of serologic testing (IgG, IgM, and IgA antibodies), parasite isolation, and evaluation of cerebrospinal fluid (CSF) (glucose, protein, cells, total IgG antibody, *Toxoplasma*-specific IgG and IgM antibodies, and direct examination for tachyzoites). In addition, an infant suspected of having congenital toxoplasmosis should have a thorough general, neurologic, and ophthalmologic examination and a CT scan of the head. Positive *Toxoplasma*-specific IgM or IgA is diagnostic of congenital infection. Although occasionally placental leak can lead to a false-positive IgM test in the infant, repeat testing in approximately 10 days can help resolve the diagnosis because the half-life of IgM is only 3 to 5 days. Maternal IgG antibodies in the newborn's peripheral blood reflect infection in the mother; however, persistent or increasing IgG antibody levels in the infant compared with the mother measured by the dye test or IFA test provide strong evidence of congenital infection. Persistence of a positive IgG test result in the infant beyond 1 year of life confirms congenital infection, whereas a negative IgG test at 1 or more years of age essentially rules out congenital infection.

Demonstration of serum antibodies in the newborn that are directed against unique *Toxoplasma* epitopes on immunoblot that are not found in the mother provides diagnostic evidence for congenital infection. In addition, direct demonstration of the parasite by isolation (mouse inoculation or tissue culture) and amplification of *T. gondii*–specific DNA (e.g., PCR of CSF, peripheral blood, or urine) are used to diagnose infection in infants. Infants born to women who have serologic evidence of infections with human immunodeficiency virus (HIV) and *Toxoplasma* should be evaluated for congenital toxoplasmosis.

IMMUNOSUPPRESSED PERSONS

Diagnosis of toxoplasmosis in immunosuppressed persons is confirmed by identifying the organism replicating in tissue histologically or cytologically, by isolation, or by identification of nucleic acids in sites such as amniotic fluid, CSF, bronchoalveolar fluid, or placenta in which the organism would not be expected to reside in the chronic cyst form. Most persons with AIDS who are chronically infected with *T. gondii* have demonstrable antibodies. Presumptive diagnosis of toxoplasmic encephalitis can be made in HIV-infected persons with severe immunosuppression using the following criteria:

- Recent onset of neurologic abnormality consistent with intracranial disease or a reduced level of consciousness
- Evidence of a mass lesion by brain imaging that enhances by contrast media (usually multiple lesions)
- Positive serum antibody antibodies to *T. gondii*
- Response to anti-*Toxoplasma* therapy

OCULAR DISEASE

Ocular toxoplasmosis is usually diagnosed by characteristic eye lesions and positive serum antibodies. Detection of DNA in the ocular fluids using PCR, demonstration of the parasite by isolation or histopathology, or local production of antibody are also used to demonstrate active ocular toxoplasmosis.

Expert Opinion on Management Issues

Physicians most frequently treat *T. gondii* infection in the following patients:

- Pregnant women with acute infection to prevent or treat fetal infection
- Congenitally infected infants
- Immunosuppressed persons, usually with reactivated disease
- Patients with acute or recurrent ocular disease

Drugs are also prescribed for preventive or suppressive treatment in HIV-infected persons. The currently recommended drugs work primarily against the actively dividing tachyzoite form of *T. gondii* and do not eradicate organisms in tissue cysts (bradyzoites).

The most common drug combination used to treat congenital toxoplasmosis consists of pyrimethamine and a sulfonamide (sulfadiazine is recommended in the United States), plus folinic acid in the form of leucovorin calcium to protect the bone marrow from the toxic effects of pyrimethamine. Pyrimethamine inhibits dihydrofolate reductase, which is important in the synthesis of folic acid and produces a reversible depression of the bone marrow. Sulfonamides inhibit synthesis of dihydrofolic acid, also important in the synthesis of folic acid. The two drugs work synergistically against *T. gondii*. Because of toxicity, therapy with pyrimethamine and sulfadiazine is not generally recommended for use in pregnant women before the 18th week of gestation. After the 18th week, pyrimethamine and sulfadiazine may be given if fetal infection is confirmed by amniocentesis. Spiramycin (available through the U.S. Food and Drug Administration [FDA], 301–443–2127 or 301–796–1600) is recommended for pregnant women with acute toxoplasmosis when fetal infection has not been confirmed in an attempt to prevent transmission of *T. gondii* from the mother to the fetus. Table 1 gives specific doses.

Randomized prospective studies of treatment during acute infection in pregnant women have not been performed. Some researchers question the effectiveness of treatment during pregnancy in preventing congenital infection or sequelae in infants. One hypothesis for the lack of effectiveness is that *T. gondii* tachyzoites transform into bradyzoites within days of infection, probably coinciding with the serologic and cell-mediated responses. Therefore, by the time an infection is detected in a pregnant woman, tachyzoites may have already been transmitted to the fetus, inflicted damage, and been converted to encysted bradyzoites that do not respond to therapy. Nevertheless, a recent multicenter observational study found that the treatment of acute *T. gondii* infection in pregnancy was associated with a reduction of sequelae in infants, but not a reduction in maternal-fetal transmission. Pyrimethamine and sulfadiazine (plus folinic acid) are also the drugs generally used to treat infants with congenital toxoplasmosis and have led to improved outcomes compared with historic controls. In the United States, therapy for congenitally infected infants is usually given for the first year of life (see Table 1).

In immune-suppressed persons with toxoplasmosis, a regimen of pyrimethamine and sulfadiazine plus folinic acid is also the preferred treatment. Clindamycin is a second alternative for use in combination with pyrimethamine in those who cannot tolerate sulfonamides. Because relapse often occurs after toxoplasmosis in HIV-infected patients, maintenance therapy (secondary prophylaxis) with pyrimethamine plus sulfadiazine (first choice) or pyrimethamine plus clindamycin (alternative) is recommended for the life of the patient. The role of alternative drugs in the treatment of systemic toxoplasmosis has not been fully defined by controlled trials. In general, alternative drugs should be used in combination with pyrimethamine. These alternative drugs include atovaquone, dapsone, azithromycin, and clarithromycin.

HIV-infected persons should be tested for IgG antibodies to *Toxoplasma* soon after the diagnosis of HIV infection to detect latent infection with *T. gondii*. *Toxoplasma*-seronegative persons who are not taking a *Pneumocystis* pneumonia (PCP) prophylactic regimen known to be active against toxoplasmic encephalitis should be retested for IgG antibody to *Toxoplasma* when their CD4+ T-lymphocyte count (per μL) declines to the level of severe immunosuppression (<12 months, <750 [or percent of total lymphocytes <15]; 1–5 years, <500 [or percent of total lymphocytes <15]; 6–12 years, <200 [or percent of total lymphocytes <15]; adolescents/adults <100) to determine whether they have seroconverted. For prophylaxis to prevent an initial episode of *T. gondii* in IgG antibody–positive adolescents/adults with CD4+ T-lymphocyte counts less than 100 cells/μL (or severe immunosuppression as defined previously in infants and children), trimethoprim-sulfamethoxazole is recommended as the first choice. Alternatives are dapsone plus pyrimethamine or atovaquone with or without pyrimethamine. Folinic acid is given with all regimens including pyrimethamine.

HIV-infected children older than 12 months of age who qualify for PCP prophylaxis and who are receiving an agent other than trimethoprim-sulfamethoxazole or atovaquone should have serologic testing for *Toxoplasma* antibody (BIII), because alternative drugs for PCP prophylaxis might not be effective against *Toxoplasma*. Severely immunosuppressed children who are not receiving trimethoprim-sulfamethoxazole or atovaquone who are found to be seropositive for *Toxoplasma* should be administered prophylaxis for both PCP and toxoplasmosis (i.e., dapsone plus pyrimethamine). HIV-infected children with a history of toxoplasmosis should be administered lifelong prophylaxis to prevent recurrence. The safety of discontinuing primary or secondary prophylaxis in HIV-infected children receiving highly active antiretroviral therapy (HAART) has not been studied extensively. However, prophylaxis against toxoplasmic encephalitis should be discontinued in adult and adolescent patients who have

TABLE 1 Guidelines for Treatment of *Toxoplasma gondii* Infection

Manifestation of Infection	Medication	Dosage	Duration of Therapy
In pregnant women with acute toxoplasmosis			
First 21 wk of gestation or until term if fetus is not infected	Spiromycin[1]	1 g q8h without food	Until fetal infection is documented or excluded at 21 wk; if documented, in alternate months with pyrimethamine, leucovorin, and sulfadiazine
If fetal infection is confirmed after 18th wk of gestation	Pyrimethamine *plus*	Loading dose: 100 mg/day in 2 div doses for 2 days Maintenance:50 mg/day	As for no fetal infection[2]
	Sulfadiazine *plus*	Loading dose: 75 mg/kg/day in 2 div doses (max 4 g/day) for 2 days Maintenance:100 mg/kg/day in 2 div doses (max 4 g/day)	As for no fetal infection[2]
	Leucovorin (folinic acid)	10–20 mg qd[3]	During and for 1 wk after pyrimethamine therapy
In infants			
Congenital *T. gondii* infection[4]	Pyrimethamine[4] *plus*	Loading dose: 2 mg/kg/day for 2 days Maintenance:1 mg/kg/day for 2 or 6 mo,[5] then this dose every MWF[4]	1 yr[6]
	Sulfadiazine[4] *plus*	100 mg/kg/day in 2 div doses	1 yr[6]
	Leucovorin[4]	10 mg tiw[3]	During and for 1 wk after pyrimethamine therapy
	Corticosteroids[7] (prednisone) have been used when cerebrospinal fluid protein is ≥1 g/dL and when active chorioretinitis threatens vision	1 mg/kg/day in 2 div doses	Until resolution of elevated (≥1 g/dL) CSF protein level or active chorioretinitis that threatens vision
In older children			
Active chorioretinitis	Pyrimethamine *plus*	Loading dose: 2 mg/kg/day (max 50 mg) for 2 days Maintenance: 1 mg/kg/day (max 25 mg)	Usually 1–2 wk beyond the time that signs and symptoms have resolved
	Sulfadiazine *plus*	Loading dose: 75 mg/kg Maintenance: 50 mg/kg q12h	As for pyrimethamine
	Leucovorin	10–20 mg tiw[3]	During and for 1 wk after pyrimethamine therapy
	Corticosteroids[7]	As for corticosteroids in congenital *T. gondii* infection	As for corticosteroids in congenital *T. gondii* infection

12

Adapted from Remington JS, McLeod R, Thulliez P, et al: Toxoplasmosis. In Remington JS, Klein JO (eds): Infectious Diseases of the Fetus and Newborn Infant, 5th ed. Philadelphia: WB Saunders, 2001, p 293.

CSF, cerebrospinal fluid; div, divided; max, maximum; MWF, Monday, Wednesday, Friday; qd, daily; q*x*h, every *x* hours; tiw, three times a week

[1]Available only on request from the U.S. Food and Drug Administration; phone number 301–443–5680 (see text for alternative phone numbers).

[2]The only studies are Daffos F, Mirlesse V, Hohlfeld P, et al: Toxoplasmosis during pregnancy. Lancet 344:541, 1994, and Daffos F, Forestier F, Capella-Pavlovsky M, et al: Prenatal management of 746 pregnancies at risk for congenital toxoplasmosis. N Engl J Med 318:271–275, 1988. However, because Daffos and colleagues found pyrimethamine-sulfadiazine therapy to be superior to spiramycin for treatment of the fetus, continued therapy with pyrimethamine, sulfadiazine, and leucovorin should be considered in the third trimester. This regimen has been used extensively in France and appears to be safe and feasible. Alternatively, in the United States, daily administration of pyrimethamine (50 mg/day) and sulfadiazine (1 g q6h) plus leucovorin (10 mg) administered every other day to the mother has been used in the treatment of a limited number of fetuses in utero. this treatment was begun after the 18th week of gestation and continued until birth of the infant. Subsequent treatment of the infant is the same as that described under treatment of congenital infection. This appears to have been feasible and safe treatment for a small number of patients. When the diagnosis of infection in the fetus is established earlier, we suggest that sulfadiazine be used alone until approximately 20 weeks of gestation, at which time pyrimethamine should be added to the regimen

[3]Adjusted for megaloblastic anemia, granulocytopenia, or thrombocytopenia; blood cell counts, including platelets, should be monitored as described in the text.

[4]Optimal dosage, feasibility, and toxicity are being evaluated or planned in the ongoing Chicago-based National Collaborative Treatment Trial; telephone number 773–834–4152.

[5]These two regimens are currently being compared in a randomized manner in the National Collaborative Treatment Trial. Data are not yet available to determine which, if either, is superior. Both regimens appear to be feasible and relatively safe.

[6]The duration of therapy is unknown for infants and children, especially those with AIDS.

[7]Corticosteroids should be used only in conjunction with pyrimethamine, sulfadiazine, and leucovorin treatment and should be continued until signs of inflammation (high CSF protein [>1 g/dL]) or active chorioretinitis that threatens vision have subsided. Dosage can then be tapered and discontinued Use only with pyrimethamine, sulfadiazine, and leucovorin.

responded to HAART with an increase in CD4+ T-lymphocyte counts to greater than 200 cells per μL for at least 3 months. Some experts would obtain an MRI of the brain as part of their evaluation to determine whether discontinuation of therapy is appropriate. Because specifics of prevention and prophylactic treatment of opportunistic infections such as toxoplasmosis can change from year to year, before therapy is given the latest USPHS/IDSA Guidelines for the Prevention of Opportunistic Infections in Persons Infected with HIV (see Suggested Readings) should be consulted.

Pyrimethamine and sulfadiazine are often used to treat ocular toxoplasmosis. Clindamycin, in combination with other antiparasitic medications is also frequently used for treatment of ocular disease. A variety of newer agents have been tried in the treatment of ocular toxoplasmosis including atovaquone, rifabutin, trovafloxacin, azithromycin, and clarithromycin. In addition to antiparasitic drugs, physicians may add corticosteroids to reduce ocular inflammation. However, the optimal treatment for ocular toxoplasmosis remains to be defined by controlled trials. To reduce the recurrences of toxoplasmic retinochoroiditis, intermittent trimethoprim-sulfamethoxazole therapy is used in some settings.

Common Pitfalls

- Failure to inform pregnant women and immunosuppressed persons about how to prevent toxoplasmosis
- Failure to confirm a positive *T. gondii* IgM test at a reference laboratory before starting therapy for acute infection in a pregnant woman
- Failure to prescribe folinic acid and monitor the peripheral blood cell counts for bone marrow depression in regimens that contain pyrimethamine

Communication and Counseling

Pregnant women and immunosuppressed persons should be counseled about how to prevent toxoplasmosis. Recommendations for prevention of *T. gondii* and other food-borne illnesses include:

- Food should be cooked to safe temperatures (beef, lamb, and veal roasts and steaks to at least 145°F [62.7°C]; pork, ground meat, and wild game to 160°F [71°C]; poultry to 180°F [82°C]).
- Raw fruits and vegetables should be peeled or washed thoroughly before eating.
- Cutting boards, dishes, counters, utensils, and hands should always be washed with hot soapy water after they have contacted raw meat, poultry, seafood, or unwashed vegetables.
- Pregnant women and immunosuppressed persons should wear gloves when gardening and during any contact with soil or sand—because cat waste might be in soil or sand—and wash their hands afterward.
- Pregnant women and immunosuppressed persons should avoid changing cat litter if possible; if no one else is available to change the cat litter, pregnant women and immunosuppressed persons should wear gloves and then wash hands thoroughly.
- The litter box should be changed daily because *T. gondii* oocysts require a day or more to become infectious.
- Pregnant women and immunosuppressed persons should be encouraged to keep their cats inside and should not adopt or handle stray cats.
- Cats should be fed only canned or dried commercial food or well-cooked table food, not raw or undercooked meats.
- People should avoid drinking potentially contaminated water, especially when traveling to developing countries.

SUGGESTED READINGS

1. Centers for Disease Control and Prevention: Preventing congenital toxoplasmosis. MMWR Morb Mortal Wkly Rep 49(RR–2): 57–75, 2000. **Overview of congenital toxoplasmosis with Centers for Disease Control and Prevention congenital toxoplasmosis prevention guidelines.**
2. Guidelines for preventing opportunistic infections among HIV-infected persons—2002: Recommendations of the U.S. Public Health Service and the Infectious Diseases Society of America. MMWR Recomm Rep 14(51):(RR–8):1–52, 2002. **Authoritative source of information about primary and secondary prophylaxis for toxoplasmosis in HIV-infected persons.**
3. Holland GN: Ocular toxoplasmosis: A global reassessment. Part I: Epidemiology course of disease. Am J Ophthalmol 136(6):973–988, 2003.
4. Holland GN: Ocular toxoplasmosis: A global reassessment. Part II: Disease manifestations and management. Am J Ophthalmol 137(1):1–17, 2004. **This two-part series presents a thorough review of ocular toxoplasmosis.**
5. Jones J, Lopez A, Wilson M: Congenital toxoplasmosis. Am Fam Physician 67:2131–2138, 2003. **Overview of congenital toxoplasmosis including biology, epidemiology, screening, serologic diagnosis, treatment, and prevention.**
6. Luft BJ, Chua A: Central nervous system toxoplasmosis in HIV pathogenesis, diagnosis, and therapy. Cur Infect Dis Rep 2: 358–362, 2000. **Review of central nervous system toxoplasmosis in HIV-infected persons.**
7. McAuley J, Boyer KM, Dushyant P, et al: Early and longitudinal evaluations of treated infants and children and untreated historical patients with congenital toxoplasmosis; the Chicago collaborative treatment trial. Clin Infect Dis 18:38–72, 1994. **Clinically related article covering therapy and evaluation of infants and children with congenital toxoplasmosis.**
8. Montoya JG: Laboratory diagnosis of *Toxoplasma gondii* infection and toxoplasmosis. J Infect Dis 185(Suppl 1):S73–S82, 2002. **Practical overview of laboratory diagnosis for a variety of clinical situations.**
9. Montoya JG, Liesenfeld O: Toxoplasmosis. Lancet 363:1965–1976, 2004. **Current review of toxoplasmosis with treatment guidelines for pregnant women, infants, ocular toxoplasmosis, and toxoplasmic encephalitis in persons with AIDS.**
10. Remington JS, McLeod R, Thulliez P, et al: Toxoplasmosis. In Remington JS, Klein JO (eds): Infectious Diseases of the Fetus and Newborn Infant, 5th ed. Philadelphia: WB Saunders, 2001, pp 205–346. **Thorough authoritative presentation on all clinical aspects of toxoplasmosis with emphasis on the fetus and newborn.**

MISCELLANEOUS INFECTIONS

Idiopathic Pain Syndromes and Chronic Fatigue Syndrome

Lisa Imundo

KEY CONCEPTS

- Symptoms of fatigue and nonspecific pain occur frequently in teenagers.
- Children can develop chronic fatigue syndrome (CFS) or pain syndromes. These syndromes are characterized by disability and pain out of proportion to physical findings.
- Important differences exist between children and adults in the nature and impact of these syndromes and their management.
- CFS can threaten adolescents' physical, emotional, and intellectual development and disrupt education and social and family life.
- A prompt and authoritative diagnosis is needed, and appropriate evaluation must rule out infectious, rheumatologic, endocrinologic, and psychological diagnoses.
- No effective pharmacologic treatment for CFS is available; described multidisciplinary regimens improve functional outcome and school attendance.

As many as 30% of children experience significant fatigue and chronic or recurrent musculoskeletal pain. The symptom may have many causes, and the differential diagnoses are quite broad in children. They include infectious and metabolic conditions; growing pains; overuse injuries; hyperextensibility; and orthopedic, arthritic, and genetic syndromes. A subset of chronic or recurrent pain or more debilitating fatigue called the idiopathic pain syndromes and chronic fatigue syndrome (CFS) is discussed here.

Idiopathic pain syndromes and CFS are characterized by a lack of physical or laboratory findings, despite severe disabilities. Indeed, the degree of pain and disability in these groups is strikingly high compared to children with juvenile arthritis or other classical rheumatic conditions. Chronic pain, disability out of proportion to physical findings, the sensation of pain to nonpainful stimuli, psychological distress, inappropriate affect, significant family history of disability or chronic pain, the presence of multiple other somatic complaints, similar demographic profile of patients/families, and enmeshment with the mother are typical associations of the idiopathic pain syndromes.

An important, clearly defined etiologic component of the idiopathic pain syndromes and CFS is depression. Although it is often clear to the physician that unexplained physical symptoms in an adolescent suffering mood changes, loss of interest in normal activities, and withdrawal to home or bed are not typical symptoms of a physical illness, parents of these patients may ascribe these behavioral changes to a mysterious physical disease rather than to classical forms of depression with somatization. Indeed, an important problem in reaching the diagnosis of idiopathic pain syndrome is the presumed but often unproven association of the painful symptom with known physically isolatable causes of diseases. For example, the terms *fibromyalgia syndrome (FMS), reflex sympathetic dystrophy (RSD),* and *chronic fatigue syndrome (CFS)* are all subsets of the idiopathic pain syndromes, and they suggest associations with rheumatic, neurologic, and infectious etiologies, respectively. However, these associations are not fully established or else poorly describe the presentation of the patient. The overlap of the idiopathic pain syndromes and CFS with depression is, in contrast, a well-documented etiology.

Given the lack of certain etiology and a large number of associated illnesses, idiopathic pain syndromes have been called by many names, despite the possibility that they all represent variations of a common process. In addition, each has a long list of synonyms. *Fibromyalgia* is a descriptive term for a syndrome of widespread musculoskeletal pain, fatigue, and multiple discrete painful points (also called generalized pain syndrome, fibrositis, myofascial pain syndrome, pain amplification syndrome, and diffuse widespread myofascial pain). RSD is also called localized pain syndrome, reflex neurovascular dystrophy, causalgia, and Sudeck atrophy.

A further problem in understanding the idiopathic pain syndrome and establishing reliable categories is that current definitions derive from adult patients and do not necessarily fit similar-appearing diseases of children. Some authors suggest that precise classification in children with pain and fatigue is not necessary because overlap in clinical presentation is frequent, and all children with pain syndromes respond to a similar treatment program.

Despite the confusion of description, classification, and etiology, it is reassuring that the experienced clinician can recognize and diagnose the idiopathic pain syndrome, based on the history and physical examination and a minimum amount of testing. The following text focuses on CFS, but the unifying themes stressed in this introduction should not be overlooked.

Expert Opinion on Management Issues

CFS is defined as debilitating fatigue lasting longer than 6 months. The criteria for CFS overlap with those for FMS and depression (Box 1). Similar to FMS, *fibromyalgia* is a descriptive term for a syndrome of widespread musculoskeletal pain, fatigue, and multiple discrete painful points. Demographics indicate a predominance of female, white, middle-class patients. The age of onset of CFS is 20 to 50 years, but children from 7 to 20 years of age are reported. As with other idiopathic pain syndromes, it is not clear that the existing definition should be extended to children. Many adolescent patients do have a history of premorbid problems in school attendance or poor school performance, but after the onset of the illness, the average length of school missed is 1 year, a massive amount of disability compared to other diseases. This is the most severe consequence of the illness.

Most patients describe onset after a preceding illness with pharyngitis and fever. Up to one third continue to complain of low-grade fevers, pharyngitis, adenopathy, and weakness, but the fevers are usually not documented on examination. No infectious etiology is identified to date despite rigorous epidemiologic studies. Likewise, a postinfectious process is postulated but has never been proved. Eight percent of patients with CFS have psychological and neuropsychological complaints, such as fatigue, difficulty sleeping, abdominal pain, cognitive difficulty, and inability to tolerate activity. Many patients with CFS were found previously to suffer from depression and anxiety and somatoform disorders, but the current criteria of CFS require the exclusion of diagnosable psychiatric illnesses. Other possible occult causes of fatigue must also be excluded, such as drug or alcohol abuse, as well as other medical conditions, such as hepatitis, mononucleosis, thyroid disease, and rheumatologic or inflammatory conditions including inflammatory bowel disease.

A detailed history and physical examination is usually diagnostic; routine screening laboratory tests should include complete blood count (CBC), chemistry panel, erythrocyte sedimentation rate (ESR), and uric acid (U/A). Some children may require additional testing of thyroid function, muscle enzymes, Epstein-Barr virus (EBV), and/or Lyme titers depending on the clinical situation. These patients routinely have normal or negative laboratory or radiologic tests, and no underlying physiologic pathology can be demonstrated.

Some patients occasionally may have mildly abnormal laboratory tests that do not correlate with the patient's level of disability and pain. Parents may focus undue attention on mild laboratory abnormalities, such as a positive antinuclear antibody (ANA) or a low immunoglobulin (Ig) A level, as the explanation of the child's problems. Some physicians may inadvertently promote this notion by continuing to test these children and referring them to multiple specialists. In sum, there is some support for placing CFS into the idiopathic pain syndrome category because the approach to the diagnosis and treatment is similar.

TREATMENT AND PROGNOSIS

Management of CFS (like other pain syndromes) requires a comprehensive treatment plan that takes into account factors that influence the perception of and adaptation to fatigue and pain, such as cultural and behavioral/psychiatric components (Box 2).

Alternative therapies are not proven to improve symptoms. To date, pharmacologic interventions remain largely ineffective. There have been several prospective studies of treatment for CFS. Antibiotic treatment, acyclovir, and intravenous immunoglobulin

---

BOX 1 Chronic Fatigue Syndrome Case Criteria

Fatigue
- New onset of unexplained fatigue >6 mo
- Not the result of ongoing exertion
- Not substantially alleviated by rest
- Results in a substantial reduction in activities

Sympton Criteria (at least four of eight):
- Cognitive dysfunction
- Sore throat
- Tender cervical or axillary lymph nodes
- Myalgia
- Multijoint arthralgia without swelling or redness
- Headaches of a new pattern
- Unrefreshing sleep
- Postexertional malaise

Adapted from Fukuda K, Straus SE, Hickel I, et al: The chronic fatigue syndrome: A comprehensive approach to its definition and study. International Chronic Fatigue Syndrome Study Group. Ann Intern Med 121:953–959, 1994.

BOX 2 Management Approach to Chronic Fatigue Syndrome

- Assure the patient and family that:
  - Symptoms are typical for diffuse pain or fatigue syndromes.
  - These syndromes are difficult to treat, but the long-term outcome is good and better than in adults.
  - The goal is to optimize function and minimize disability despite continuing symptoms.
- The treatment protocol includes:
  - An educational protocol with written material for patients
  - Mandatory school attendance
  - Physical therapy with aerobic exercises to steadily increase endurance
- Psychological support with:
  - Evaluation for coexisting conditions (depression, anxiety, and school phobia)
  - Behavioral treatment of sleep disturbances (biofeedback, self-hypnosis, relaxation techniques)
  - Improving coping and communication skills
- Medications include:
  - Nonsteroidal anti-inflammatory drugs (NSAIDs)
  - Tramadol hydrochloride
  - Tricyclic antidepressants at low doses at night as a soporific
  - Antidepressants if indicated

have each proved ineffective. Fludrocortisone has not proved beneficial in patients with coexisting neurally mediated hypotension. However, medication may have a role in normalizing sleep, and low-dose antidepressants are helpful in adults and children with FMS. Antidepressants have not been studied in children with CFS.

Graded exercise and cognitive behavioral therapy are both effective in lessening symptoms in adults. Although there is no effective pharmacologic treatment, simply labeling patients with the diagnosis of CFS allows them to stop their search for other illnesses and have less fear of the unknown. Patients should be told that their condition is not mysterious or made up; they should be frequently examined, especially at times of increased fatigue or pain, and they should be reassured that their bodies are actually fine. They must be supported in their successful reentry to school by providing whatever accommodations are needed, such as an extra set of schoolbooks, a modified physical education program, or permission to begin classes later in the morning.

On long-term follow-up, these children do not develop any other diseases. No treatment protocols are completely successful, but incorporating psychological support and exercise reduces disability. A higher percentage of children than adults improve. Limited studies in children indicate improvement in symptoms and resumption of function in the majority of patients after 2 years. Neither the rate of relapse nor long-term functional outcome is known.

Common Pitfalls

- Failure to reasonably investigate and exclude occult diagnoses, including psychological diagnosis
- Failure to consider CFS and pain syndromes as a diagnosis in a child or adolescent
- Removal from activities and school by the medical practitioner without any diagnosis or rehabilitation plan
- Failure to recognize that mild laboratory abnormalities do not lead to debilitating fatigue

Communication and Counseling

When disability exceeds visible evidence of organic disease, the child must be directed back to full activities. Repeated studies demonstrate that long school absence for any reason indicates a poor prognosis for later achievement in life. Occasionally, the child, the family, and their physicians limit the child's activities (or accede to suggestion or demand for limitations), and the practitioner is then confronted with a totally disabled child without any evidence of organic disease. The current treatment regimen should employ a coordinated team of experienced professionals and include aggressive physical therapy and rehabilitation with endurance training, psychological intervention to improve communication and adjustment to symptoms, pain

management with a pharmacologic component as needed, and school accommodation. Overall, the prognosis for idiopathic pain syndromes and chronic fatigue in children is good, especially if appropriate treatment is initiated in a timely manner.

SUGGESTED READINGS

1. Benjamin S, Morris S, McBeth J, et al: The association between chronic widespread pain and mental disorder: A population-based study. Arthritis Rheum 43(3):561–567, 2000. **Important reminder to fully assess a patient with fatigue for occult psychiatric disease.**
2. Croft P, Burt J, Schollum J, et al: More pain, more tender points: Is fibromyalgia just one end of a continuous spectrum? Ann Rheum Dis 55(7):482–485, 1996. **Excellent population survey of musculoskeletal complaints and fatigue in a Canadian province.**
3. Isenberg D, Miller J: Adolescent Rheumatology. London; Malden, Mass: Dunitz, 1999. **Unified multidisciplinary treatment with very aggressive physical therapy is recommended here with outcome results reported.**
4. Jacobs JC: Pediatric Rheumatology for the Practitioner, 2nd ed. New York: Springer-Verlag, 1992. **Excellent diagnostic guide with vivid clinical descriptions.**
5. Malleson PN, Fung MY, Rosenberg AM: The incidence of pediatric rheumatic diseases: Results from the Canadian Pediatric Rheumatology Association Disease Registry. J Rheumatol 23(11):1981–1987, 1996. **Excellent population survey of musculoskeletal complaints and fatigue in a Canadian province.**
6. Martinez-Lavin M: Is fibromyalgia a generalized reflex sympathetic dystrophy? Clin Exp Rheumatol 19(1):1–3, 2001. **This paper makes the case of reclassifying pain and fatigue syndromes into one continuous spectrum of disease.**
7. Patel MX, Smith DG, Chalder T, Wessely S: Chronic fatigue syndrome in children: A cross-sectional survey. Arch Dis Child 88(10):894–898, 2003. **Most adolescent patients showed significant improvement over 2 years; school absence was the most consistent problem.**
8. Viner R, Christie D: Fatigue and somatic symptoms. BMJ 330:1012–1015, 2005. **Practical approach to the treatment of CFS in adolescent patients.**

12

Bioterrorism

David Markenson and Irwin Redlener

KEY CONCEPTS

- Possible biologic agents are classified according to availability, potential for morbidity and mortality, and ease of dissemination.
- The natural history and management of injuries and exposures depend on the agent and the route of exposure.
- Vaccines are available for anthrax and smallpox; antitoxins are available for botulism.

Terrorism preparedness is a highly specific component of general emergency preparedness. In addition to the unique pediatric issues involved in general emergency preparedness, terrorism preparedness must consider several additional issues, including the unique vulnerabilities of children to various agents as well as the limited availability of age- and weight-appropriate antidotes and treatments. Although children may respond more rapidly to therapeutic intervention, they are at the same time more susceptible to various agents and conditions and more likely to deteriorate if not carefully monitored.

The release of chemical or biologic toxins would disproportionately affect children through several mechanisms. For example, because children become dehydrated easily and possess minimal reserve, they are at greater risk than adults when exposed to agents that may cause diarrhea or vomiting. Agents that might cause only mild symptoms in an adult could lead to hypovolemic shock in an infant. Another example involves the unique respiratory physiology of children. Many of the agents used for both chemical and biologic attacks are aerosolized (e.g., sarin, chlorine, or anthrax). Because children have faster respiratory rates than adults, they are exposed to relatively greater dosages and would suffer the effects of these agents much more rapidly than adults. Many biologic and chemical agents are absorbed through the skin. Because children have more permeable skin and more surface area relative to body mass than adults, they receive proportionally higher doses of agents that either affect the skin or are absorbed through the skin. In addition, because the skin of children is poorly keratinized, vesicants and corrosives result in greater injury to children than to adults.

It is well known that children may exhibit different effects of biologic agents. Here are some examples:

- Smallpox: Lack of immunity in children, whereas some adults who were vaccinated as children may still possess some degree of immunity.
- Trichothecenes: The data show that children may be more susceptible.
- Melioidosis: Children manifest unique parotitis.
- Anthrax: Recent and older data support the concept that children are less susceptible to the effects of anthrax.

In addition to the differences in clinical presentation of biologic agents, children also may present different incubation periods following exposure. For many agents, the incubation period is shorter for children. Consequently, surveillance systems based on symptoms in children may yield earlier detection, which can lead to earlier containment and mitigate the effects of a bioterrorism agent.

Lastly, there may be issues with the antibiotics of choice for bioterrorist agents. Many medications, although used in children, are not indicated for children by the U.S. Food and Drug Administration (FDA). Although this does not pose a problem for health care providers, several government programs, such as the Strategic National Stockpile, may only stock items for the FDA-approved indications. In addition, certain medications may have an absolute contraindication to use in children and others may have relative contraindications.

Biologic weapons are referred to as the "poor person's nuclear bomb" because they are easy to manufacture, can be deployed without sophisticated delivery systems, and have the ability to kill or injure hundreds of thousands of people. A range of biologic agents could be used as weapons of terror, and the actual clinical syndrome will vary depending on the type of agent, its virulence, route of the exposure, and susceptibility of the victim to infection. In contrast to chemical, conventional, and nuclear weapons that generate immediate effects, biologic agents are generally associated with a delay in the onset of illness, and therefore they may not be recognized in their initial stages. A covert release of a contagious biologic agent has the potential for large-scale spread before detection. For some infectious agents, secondary and tertiary transmission may continue for weeks or months after the initial attack. Both infected persons and the "worried well" would seek medical attention, with a corresponding need for medical supplies, diagnostic tests, and hospital beds. Simple devices such as crop-dusting airplanes or small perfume atomizers are effective delivery systems for biologic agents. The biologic agents that are considered likely candidates for weaponization include bacteria, viruses, rickettsia, fungi, and preformed toxins.

Expert Opinion on Management Issues

The Centers for Disease Control and Prevention (CDC) separates bioterrorist agents into three categories (A, B, and C) in order of priority based on the combined factors of availability, potential for morbidity and mortality, and ease of dissemination (Table 1).

Although virtually any microorganism has the potential to be used as a biologic weapon, most would be difficult to weaponize and disseminate effectively. So, although those listed in Table 1 are possible candidates for weaponization, the biologic agents most likely to be used as possible terrorist agents are *Bacillus anthracis* (anthrax), *Brucella* species (brucellosis), *Clostridium botulinum* (botulism), *Francisella tularensis* (tularemia), *Yersinia pestis* (plague), Ebola virus, variola (smallpox), the hemorrhagic fever viruses, and *Coxiella burnetii* (Q fever).

ANTHRAX

Anthrax has been extensively developed as a biologic weapon and is considered the most likely candidate for a biologic release. Recent history in New York City, Connecticut, and Florida shows that the use of anthrax as a terrorism agent is not a theoretical possibility but a reality. The causative organism, *Bacillus anthracis,* is a gram-positive sporulating rod. Anthrax cannot be transmitted person to person. Because the initial symptoms of anthrax are nonspecific and experience with the disease among physicians is uncommon, anthrax may be misdiagnosed. The first indication of an aerosol exposure may be groups of patients presenting with severe influenza-like disease with a high case-fatality

TABLE 1 CDC Categories, Definitions, and Pathogens

Category	CDC Definition	Pathogens
Category A	High-priority agents include organisms that pose a risk to national security because they have the following characteristics: Can be easily disseminated or transmitted from person to person Result in high mortality rates and have the potential for major public health impact Might cause public panic and social disruption Require special action for public health preparedness.	Anthrax (*Bacillus anthracis*) Botulism (*Clostridium botulinum* toxin) Plague (*Yersinia pestis*) Smallpox (variola major) Tularemia (*Francisella tularensis*) Viral hemorrhagic fevers (Filoviruses [e.g., Ebola, Marburg] and Arenaviruses [e.g., Lassa, Machupo])
Category B	Second highest priority agents include those with the following characteristics: Are moderately easy to disseminate Result in moderate morbidity rates and low mortality rates Require specific enhancements of the CDC's diagnostic capacity and enhanced disease surveillance.	Brucellosis (*Brucella* species) Epsilon toxin of *Clostridium perfringens* Food safety threats (e.g., *Salmonella* species, *Escherichia coli* O157:H7, *Shigella*) Glanders (*Burkholderia mallei*) Melioidosis (*Burkholderia pseudomallei*) Psittacosis (*Chlamydia psittaci*) Q fever (*Coxiella burnetii*) Ricin toxin from *Ricinus communis* (castor beans) Staphylococcal enterotoxin B Typhus fever (*Rickettsia prowazekii*) Viral encephalitis (Alphaviruses [e.g., Venezuelan equine encephalitis, eastern equine encephalitis, western equine encephalitis]) Water safety threats (e.g., *Vibrio cholerae, Cryptosporidium parvum*)
Category C	Third highest priority agents include emerging pathogens that could be engineered for mass dissemination in the future because of these characteristics: Availability Ease of production and dissemination Potential for high morbidity and mortality rates and major health impact.	Emerging infectious diseases such as Nipah virus and Hantavirus

CDC, Centers for Disease Control and Prevention.
Adapted from the table available from Centers for Disease Control and Prevention online. Available at www.bt.cdc.gov

12

rate. After a few hours or days, and possibly some improvement, the condition then progresses to fever, dyspnea, and eventually shock. A widened mediastinum consistent with lymphadenopathy or hemorrhagic mediastinitis is common. Usually, no evidence of bronchopneumonia exists. The symptoms (warning signs) of anthrax are different depending on the type of the disease:

- Cutaneous: The first symptom is a small sore that develops into a blister. The blister then develops into a skin ulcer with a black area in the center. The sore, blister, and ulcer do not hurt.
- Gastrointestinal: The first symptoms are nausea, loss of appetite, bloody diarrhea, and fever, followed by severe stomach pain.
- Inhalation: The first symptoms of inhalation anthrax resemble cold or flu symptoms and can include a sore throat, mild fever, and muscle aches. Later symptoms include cough, chest discomfort, shortness of breath, tiredness, and muscle aches.

PLAGUE

Plague, caused by *Yersinia pestis,* is also considered a potential bacterial weapon. Unlike anthrax, pneumonic plague can be highly contagious, and if untreated, mortality can be as high as 100%. The pneumonic form of plague would be the primary form seen after purposeful aerosol dissemination of the organism. The bubonic form would be seen after purposeful dissemination through the release of infected fleas. The typical sign of the most common form of human plague is a swollen and very tender lymph gland, accompanied by pain. The swollen gland is called a *bubo.*

Bubonic plague should be suspected when a person develops a swollen gland, fever, chills, headache, and extreme exhaustion and has a history of possible exposure to infected rodents, rabbits, or fleas. A person usually becomes ill with bubonic plague 2 to 6 days after being infected. When bubonic plague is left untreated, plague bacteria invade the blood stream. As the plague bacteria multiply in the blood stream, they spread rapidly throughout the body and cause a severe and often fatal condition. Infection of the lungs with the plague bacterium causes the pneumonic form of plague, a severe respiratory illness. The infected person may experience high fever, chills, cough, and breathing difficulty and may expel bloody sputum. If plague patients are not given specific antibiotic therapy, the disease can progress rapidly to death. Recovery from the disease may be followed by temporary immunity.

TABLE 2 Recommended Therapy and Prophylaxis of Anthrax in Children

Form of Anthrax	Category of Treatment (Therapy or Prophylaxis)	Agent and Dosage
Inhalational	Therapy[a] Patients who are clinically stable after 14 days can be switched to a single oral agent (ciprofloxacin or doxycycline) to complete a 60-day course[b] of therapy.	Ciprofloxacin[c] 10–15 mg/kg IV q12h (max 400 mg/dose) *or* Doxycycline 2.2 mg/kg IV (max 100 mg) q12h *and* Clindamycin[d] 10–15 mg/kg IV q8h *and* Penicillin C[e] 400–600 U/kg/day IV div q4h
Inhalational	Post-exposure prophylaxis (60-day course[b])	Ciprofloxacin[f] 10–25 mg/kg PO (max 500 mg/dose) q12h *or* Doxycycline 2.2 mg/kg (max 100 mg) PO q12h
Cutaneous, endemic	Therapy[g]	Penicillin V 40–80 mg/kg/day PO div q6h *or* Amoxicillin 40–80 mg/kg/day PO div q8h *or* Ciprofloxacin 10–15 mg/kg PO (max 1 g/day) q12h *or* Doxycycline 2.2 mg/kg PO (max 100 mg) q12h
Cutaneous (in setting of terrorism)	Therapy[g]	Ciprofloxicin 10–15 mg/kg PO (max 1 g/day) q12h *or* Doxycycline 2.2 mg/kg PO (max 100 mg) q12h
Gastrointestinal	Therapy[g]	Ciprofloxacin[f] 10–25 mg/kg PO (max 500 mg/dose) q12h *or* Doxycycline 2.2 mg/kg (max 100 mg) PO q12h

[a]In a mass casualty setting, in which resources are severely limited, oral therapy may need to be substituted for the preferred parenteral option. This may be most acceptable for ciprofloxacin because it is rapidly and well absorbed from the gastrointestinal tract with no substantial loss from first-pass effect.

[b]Children may be switched to oral amoxicillin (40–80 mg/kg/day divided q8h) to complete a 60-day course (assuming the organism is sensitive). We recommend that the first 14 days of therapy or postexposure prophylaxis, however, include ciprofloxacin and/or doxycycline regardless of age. A three-dose series of vaccine may permit shortening of the antibiotic course to 30 days.

[c]Levofloxacin or ofloxacin may be acceptable alternatives to ciprofloxacin.

[d]Rifampin or clarithromycin may be acceptable alternatives to clindamycin as drugs that target bacterial protein synthesis. If ciprofloxacin or another quinolone is used, doxycycline may be used as a second agent because it also targets protein synthesis.

[e]Ampicillin, imipenem, meropenem, or chloramphenicol may be acceptable alternatives to penicillin as drugs with good CNS penetration.

[f]According to most experts, ciprofloxacin is the preferred agent for PO prophylaxis.

[g]Ten days of therapy may be adequate for endemic cutaneous disease. However, a full 60-day course is recommended in the setting of terrorism because of the possibility of concomitant inhalational exposure.

CNS, central nervous system; div, divided; PO, by mouth; qxh, every x hours.

This table was created from recommendations developed by the Columbia University Mailman School of Public Health National Center for Disaster Preparedness at the Pediatric Disaster and Terrorism National Consensus Conference, and in part it is based on reviewed reference materials from the American Academy of Pediatrics, Centers for Disease Control and Prevention, Food and Drug Administration, and the Infectious Disease Society of America and published as Markenson D, Redlener I: Pediatric Disaster and Terrorism National Consensus Conference: Executive Summary. National Center for Disaster Preparedness, 2003.

The organism probably remains viable in water and in moist meals and grains for several weeks.

SMALLPOX

There are two clinical forms of smallpox. Variola major is the severe and most common form, with a more extensive rash and higher fever. The four types of variola major smallpox are ordinary (the most frequent type, accounting for 90% or more of cases), modified (mild and occurring in previously vaccinated persons), flat, and hemorrhagic (the last two are rare and very severe). Historically, variola major has an overall fatality rate of approximately 30%; however, flat and hemorrhagic smallpox usually are fatal. Variola minor is a less common presentation of smallpox and a much less severe disease, with death rates historically of 1% or less. A person with smallpox is sometimes contagious with onset of fever (prodrome phase), but the person becomes most contagious with the onset of rash. The infected person is contagious until the last smallpox scab falls off. Generally, direct and fairly prolonged face-to-face contact is required to spread smallpox from one person to another. Smallpox also can be spread through direct contact with infected bodily fluids or contaminated objects such as bedding or clothing. Rarely, smallpox is spread by virus carried in the air in enclosed settings such as buildings, buses, and trains. Humans are the only natural hosts of variola. Smallpox is not known to be transmitted by insects or animals.

Exposure to the virus is followed by an incubation period during which people do not have any symptoms and may feel fine. This incubation period averages approximately 12 to 14 days, but can range from 7 to 17 days. During this time, people are not contagious. A rash emerges first as small red spots on the tongue and in the mouth. These spots develop into sores that break open and spread large amounts of the virus into the mouth and throat. At this time, the person becomes most contagious. Around the time the sores in the mouth break down, a rash appears on the skin, starting on the face and spreading to the arms and legs and then to the hands and feet. The rash usually spreads to all parts of the body within 24 hours. As the rash appears, the fever usually falls and the person may start to feel better. By the third day of the rash, the rash becomes raised bumps. By the fourth day, the bumps fill with a thick, opaque fluid and often have a depression in the center that looks like the umbilicus (a major distinguishing characteristic of smallpox). Fever often rises again at this time and remains high until scabs form

TABLE 3 Recommended Therapy and Prophylaxis in Children for Additional Select Diseases Associated with Bioterrorism

Disease	Therapy or Prophylaxis	Treatment, Agent, and Dosage[a]
Smallpox	Therapy	Supportive care
	Prophylaxis	Vaccination may be effective if given within the first several days after exposure
Plague	Therapy	Gentamicin 2.5 mg/kg IV q8h *or*
		Streptomycin 15 mg/kg IM q12h (max 2 g/day; only available for compassionate use and in limited supply, but preferred agent) *or*
		Doxycycline 2.2 mg/kg IV q12h (max 200 mg/day) *or*
		Ciprofloxacin 15 mg/kg IV q12h *or*
		Chloramphenicol[b] 25 mg/kg q6h (max 4 g/day)
	Prophylaxis	Doxycycline 2.2 mg/kg IV q12h *or*
		Ciprofloxacin[c] 20 mg/kg PO q12h
Tularemia	Therapy	Same as for plague
Botulism	Therapy	Supportive care; antitoxin may halt progression of symptoms but is unlikely to reverse them
Viral hemorrhagic fevers	Therapy	Supportive care; ribavirin may be beneficial in select cases[d]
Brucellosis	Therapy[e]	TMP/SMX 30 mg/kg PO q12h *and*
		Rifampin 15 mg/kg q24h *or*
		Gentamicin 7.5 mg/kg IM qd ×5

[a]In a mass casualty setting, parenteral therapy might not be possible. In such cases, oral therapy (with analogous agents) may need to be used.

[b]Concentration should be maintained between 5 and 20 mcg/mL; some experts recommend that chloramphenicol be used to treat patients with plague meningitis because chloramphenicol penetrates the blood–brain barrier. Use in children younger than 2 years may be associated with adverse reactions but might be warranted for serious infections.

[c]Other fluoroquinolones (levofloxacin, ofloxacin) may be acceptable substitutes for ciprofloxacin; however, they are not approved for use in children.

[d]Ribavirin is recommended for Arenavirus, Bunyavirus, and may be indicated for a viral hemorrhagic fever of an unknown etiology, although not FDA approved for these indications. For IV therapy, use a loading dose: 30 kg IV once (maximum dose, 2 g), then 16 mg/kg IV q6h for 4 days (maximum dose, 1 g) and then 8 mg/kg IV q8h for 6 days (maximum dose, 500 mg). In a mass casualty setting it may be necessary to use oral therapy. For oral therapy, use a loading dose of 30 mg/kg PO once, then 15 mg/kg/day PO in two divided doses for 10 days.

[e]For children younger than 8 years. *For children older than* 8 years, adult regimens are recommended. Oral drugs should be given for 6 weeks. Gentamicin, if used, should be given for the first 5 days of a 6-week course of TMP/SMX (trimethoprim/sulfamethoxazole).

CDC, Centers for Disease Control and Prevention; FDA, Food and Drug Administration; IV, intravenous; PO, by mouth; q*x*h, every *x* hours.

This table was created from recommendations developed by the Columbia University Mailman School of Public Health National Center for Disaster Preparedness at the Pediatric Disaster and Terrorism National Consensus Conference and in part is based on reviewed reference materials from the American Academy of Pediatrics, Centers for Disease Control and Prevention, Food and Drug Administration, and Infectious Disease Society of America and published as Markenson D, Redlener I: Pediatric Disaster and Terrorism National Consensus Conference: Executive Summary. National Center for Disaster Preparedness, 2003.

12

over the bumps. The bumps become pustules—sharply raised, usually round and firm to the touch as if there is a small round object under the skin. The pustules begin to form a crust and then scab. By the end of the second week after the rash appears most of the sores have scabbed over. Most scabs will have fallen off 3 weeks after the rash appears. The person is contagious to others until all of the scabs have fallen off.

Because smallpox was eradicated globally in 1980 and children are no longer being immunized, more than 80% of the adult population and 100% of children are susceptible to variola virus. The currently licensed smallpox vaccine (Dryvax; Wyeth, Philadelphia, Pa) makes no mention in its package insert of an approved age range. In practice, until the early 1970s, this vaccine was administered to children of 1 year of age. The CDC currently recommends against vaccination of children younger than 1 year. In reality, all contraindications to smallpox vaccination are relative. After bona fide exposure, even the youngest infants should be vaccinated.

Despite the lack of FDA indications for some medications and relative contraindications for some, recommended agents can be used in response to category A agents. These recommendations represent FDA-indicated medications—they do not have an FDA indication for children but literature and medical judgment support their use, acceptable alternatives, or valid reasons to use an agent despite its relative contraindications (Tables 2 and 3). As part of effective pediatric preparedness for bioterrorism events, one must not only have these agents for pediatric use but must maintain them in forms that allow pediatric administration. This includes the availability of liquid preparations but also staff and facilities for dosing to accommodate different-weight children and to reconstitute the liquid medications.

In addition to the medications described in the event of bioterrorism, immunotherapy and immunoprophylaxis may have to be considered. These agents also have unique pediatric considerations because many of them are not used or may not be FDA indicated for children (Box 1).

Common Pitfalls

One of the key elements in terrorism preparedness is early detection of any possible terrorism event. The most likely scenario involves exposure in a community,

---

BOX 1 Immunotherapy and Immunoprophylaxis

- Anthrax: The currently licensed anthrax vaccine (anthrax vaccine adsorbed [AVA]; Bioport, Lansing, Mich) is approved for persons 18 to 65 years of age. This vaccine may have a limited role as an adjunct to postexposure chemoprophylaxis, although data are limited. In such an event, potential benefit will have to be weighed against unproven risk to children. This vaccine has limited potential for use in a civilian preexposure setting, but future studies of new-generation vaccines should include children.
- Smallpox: The currently licensed smallpox vaccine (Dryvax; Wyeth, Philadelphia, Pa) makes no mention in its package insert of an approved age range. In practice, until the early 1970s, this vaccine was administered to children of 1 year of age. The Centers for Disease Control and Prevention (CDC) currently recommends against vaccination of children younger than 1 year. All contraindications to smallpox vaccination are relative. After bona fide exposure or known usage of weaponized smallpox, even the youngest exposed at-risk infants should be vaccinated. Moreover, future studies of new-generation vaccines must include children.
- Botulism: A licensed trivalent (types A, B, E) antitoxin is available through the CDC. This antitoxin is to be used in children of any age known to have been exposed to botulinum toxin of the appropriate serotypes. An IND pentavalent (types A-E) botulinum immune globulin (human) is available through the California Department of Health specifically for the treatment of infantile botulism. The study of this product must be continued and that licensure pursued.
- Plague: No licensed plague vaccine is currently in production. A previously licensed vaccine was approved only for persons 18 to 61 years of age. There is little, if any, role for this or similar vaccines in a bioterrorist context.

BOX 2 Important Clues that May Signal a Biologic Emergency

- A single suspected case of an uncommon disease
- Single or multiple cases of a suspected common disease or syndrome that does not respond to treatment as expected
- Clusters of a similar illness occurring in the same time frame in different locales
- Unusual clinical, geographical, seasonal, or temporal presentation of a disease and/or unusual transmission route
- Unexplained increase in incidence of an endemic disease
- Unusual illness that affects a large disparate population or is unusual for a population or age group
- Unusual pattern of illness or death among animals or humans
- Sudden increase in the following nonspecific illnesses: pneumonia, flulike illness, or fever with these atypical features:
  - Bleeding disorders
  - Unexplained rashes and mucosal or skin irritation, particularly in adults
  - Neuromuscular illness, such as muscle weakness and paralysis
  - Diarrhea

Adapted from materials developed by the Centers for Disease Control and Prevention and the American Medical Association.

---

which may manifest with subtle symptoms and signs and unusual patient presentations in terms of numbers of diseases. Physicians must function continually as part of a surveillance system to provide for early detection of any bioterrorism agent.

To enhance detection and treatment capabilities, pediatricians should be familiar with the clinical manifestations, diagnostic techniques, isolation precautions, treatment, and prophylaxis for likely causative agents. For some of these agents, delay in medical response could result in a potentially devastating number of casualties. Physicians must have an increased level of suspicion regarding the possible intentional use of biologic agents as well as an increased sensitivity to reporting those suspicions to public health authorities. Clinicians should report noticeable increases in unusual illnesses, symptom complexes, or disease patterns (even without definitive diagnosis) to public health authorities (Box 2).

SUGGESTED READINGS

1. Committee on Environmental Health and Committee on Infectious Diseases: Chemical-biological terrorism and its impact on children. Pediatrics 105:662–670, 2002. **Review article from the American Academy of Pediatrics that covers key concepts related to children and chemical and biologic terrorism.**
2. Lillibridge SR, Bell AJ, Roman RS: Centers for Disease Control and Prevention bioterrorism preparedness and response. Am J Infect Control 27:463–464, 1999. **Review article of the public health system's preparedness efforts.**
3. Markenson D, Redlener I: Pediatric Disaster and Terrorism National Consensus Conference: Executive Summary. National Center for Disaster Preparedness, 2003. **This document presents a comprehensive set of emergency preparedness guidelines and treatment recommendations for children. These guidelines represent the only national guidelines for emergency preparedness that address the unique needs of children.**
4. Redlener I, Markenson D: Disaster and terrorism preparedness: What pediatricians need to know. Adv Pediatr 50:1–37, 2003. **This article presents a general overview of emergency preparedness for pediatricians.**
5. American Academy of Pediatrics: Children, terrorism and disasters. Available at www.AAP.org/Terrorism (accessed November 10, 2005). **Page on the American Academy of Pediatrics website that contains all the AAP resources and information on pediatric aspects of preparedness.**
6. Centers for Disease Control and Prevention: Emergency preparedness and response. Available at www.bt.cdc.gov (accessed November 10, 2005). **CDC website that contains compendium of all CDC publications related to emergency preparedness and has a page dedicated to pediatric resources and issues.**
7. National Center for Disaster Preparedness: Home page. Available at www.ncdp.mailman.columbia.edu (accessed November 10, 2005). **This website offers a comprehensive compendium of emergency preparedness resources and has a specific program dedicated to addressing the unique needs of children.**

Antibacterial Therapies

Lisa Saiman

KEY CONCEPTS

- Prior to choosing an antimicrobial agent, review host characteristics, the site of infection, and comorbid conditions to determine the potential pathogens associated with the infection.

KEY CONCEPTS—cont'd

- Consider if an infection is community or hospital acquired, and be familiar with local epidemiologic factors including clinical presentations of specific pathogens and resistance patterns.
- Obtain cultures, whenever feasible, and review all results to guide treatment.
- When treating empirically prior to culture results, use an adequate dose to avoid exposing bacteria to subinhibitory concentrations of antibiotics that will promote the emergence of resistance.
- If possible, change to an antibiotic with a narrower spectrum of activity as soon as culture results are available to avoid placing selective pressure on the host's flora.
- Use the shortest treatment course that will result in a clinical cure to minimize the emergence of resistance.
- Remove a foreign body that has become infected to achieve clinical cure.
- Educate patients and their families about the judicious use of antibiotics.
- Do not treat viral illnesses with antibiotics.
- Review patterns of antimicrobial use by individual practitioners to improve antibiotic stewardship.

TABLE 1 Choosing an Antimicrobial Agent

Factor	Examples
Host	Age
	Immunization status
	Drug allergies
Site of infection	Central nervous system
	Abscess
	Foreign body
Comorbid conditions	Immune status
	Underlying diseases
	Renal function
	Hepatic function
Epidemiologic factors	Community-acquired versus health-care–acquired infection
	Prevalence of resistance
	Foreign birth
	Travel history
	Pets
	Ill contacts

The development of antibiotics was truly a remarkable feat in the evolution of the control of infectious diseases. The appropriate choice of antibiotics considers the host characteristics, the clinical presentation, comorbid conditions, and local epidemiologic factors. Despite enormous advances in antibiotic development over the past 40 years, resistance to antibiotics has developed with remarkable speed, which threatens our ability to control and cure some infectious agents. Perhaps most alarming, resistance has emerged in both hospital- and community-acquired pathogens. Thus, antibiotic management involves not only the appropriate choice of antimicrobial agents to treat infections, but control strategies that promote the judicious use of antibiotics in efforts to slow the development of resistance and preserve this precious resource.

Expert Opinion on Management Issues

Choosing the correct antimicrobial agent requires consideration of numerous factors that should be reviewed prior to selection of an agent and includes host characteristics, the site of infection, and comorbid conditions (Table 1). For instance, young infants are more vulnerable to certain pathogens such as *Streptococcus pneumoniae* or *Neisseria meningitidis* and more likely to develop meningitis. The immune status of a patient should be considered. For example, patients with sickle cell anemia are at increased risk of bacteremia caused by encapsulated organisms such as *S. pneumoniae* or osteomyelitis caused by *Staphylococcus aureus* or *Salmonella* species. Neutropenic hosts are vulnerable to invasive disease caused by endogenous flora.

The clinical presentation must be distinguished as viral or bacterial. If an infection is thought most likely to be caused by a bacterial pathogen, a differential diagnosis of the types of bacteria that could be responsible should be considered to determine if gramnegative or gram-positive bacteria are more likely. Viral infections rarely require antiviral agents, particularly in otherwise healthy hosts.

It is critical to be very familiar with local epidemiologic factors, which include patterns of resistance among specific pathogens. For decades it was appreciated that hospital-acquired pathogens may be highly resistant to antibiotics because of both acquired and intrinsic resistance. Hospital-acquired multidrug-resistant pathogens may be endemic or associated with outbreaks, and they frequently require newer, more costly agents for effective treatment, such as linezolid for vancomycin-resistant enterococci or meropenem for extended-spectrum β-lactamase–producing *Klebsiella pneumoniae*. Although community-acquired pathogens are generally more susceptible to antimicrobial agents than hospital-acquired pathogens, most recently pathogens in the community have developed increasing rates of resistance, such as penicillin-resistant *S. pneumoniae,* community-acquired methicillin-resistant *S. aureus* (MRSA), or cephalosporin-resistant *Salmonella* species. In addition, patterns of health-care delivery have blurred the margins between the hospital and community because long-term health-care facilities, home care, and outpatient management of many chronic illnesses are commonplace. Patients cared for in these settings can introduce multidrug-resistant pathogens into the hospital.

EMPIRICAL VERSUS TARGETED THERAPY

Most infections are initially treated empirically, and the factors just cited must be considered when choosing an antimicrobial agent. Although infections in the community are often treated without obtaining cultures (e.g., pneumonia, otitis media, skin and soft tissue infections), depending on local epidemiology, cultures should be obtained in some infections. For example, in

12

locales with high rates of community-acquired MRSA, skin and soft tissue infections should be cultured to identify the pathogen, particularly in the setting of recalcitrant infections.

The numerous classes of antibiotics each have advantages and limitations. Table 2 shows examples of some of the antibiotics commonly used in pediatric patients and provides examples of their spectrum of activity. A detailed discussion of specific management of infections is beyond the scope of this chapter. Other chapters in this text detail treatment guidelines for specific infections.

Once a pathogen is identified, the antimicrobial susceptibilities should be reviewed, and, if possible, an agent with narrower coverage should be selected. For example, many *Escherichia coli* or enterococcal strains may be susceptible to ampicillin. Patients on broader antibiotics, such as third-generation cephalosporins or vancomycin, should be changed to a narrower agent to minimize selective pressure on host flora. Broader spectrum agents are not more effective antibiotics for a pathogen that is susceptible to a narrower spectrum agent, and they have the disadvantages of inducing resistance, costing more, and often only being available intravenously.

MECHANISMS OF RESISTANCE

The three major mechanisms of resistance include modification of the drug by an enzyme, mutations in the target of action, or changes in permeability of the antibiotic into the bacterial cell (Table 3). Often, a pathogen may harbor more than one mechanism working in concert.

Common Pitfalls

When a patient fails to improve clinically despite antibiotics, the following possibilities should be considered:

- Is the patient receiving the agent and is the proper dose prescribed? Thus, it is critical to review antibiotic orders and adherence to the prescribed treatment including missed doses.
- Is the pathogen susceptible to the agent? Patients may be infected with more than one pathogen or the antimicrobial susceptibility pattern may be unusual, have changed, or in vitro activity may not predict in vivo efficacy. Extended-spectrum β-lactamase–producing strains may appear susceptible to piperacillin tazobactam in vitro, but this agent can fail in vivo.
- Is the agent getting to the site of infection? The presence of a foreign body or abscess may preclude effective treatment.
- Is the host unable to control the infection despite appropriate antibiotics? Additional agents may be warranted to treat bacteremia in a neutropenic host, or endocarditis or immune adjuvants may prove useful such as granulocyte-stimulating factor.

TABLE 2 Classes of Antibiotics

Class	Examples of Agents	Spectrum of Activity
β-Lactam agents		
Penicillins	Penicillin	Community-acquired GPC
		Group A streptococci, *Streptococcus pneumoniae,** Enterococcal species
	Ampicillin	Community-acquired GNB
		Escherichia coli, Haemophilus. influenzae
	Oxacillin	*Staphylococcus aureus*[†]
β-lactam + β-lactamase inhibitors	Amoxicillin plus clavulanate, ampicillin plus sulbactam, piperacillin plus tazobactam	*S. aureus,* β-lactamase–producing *E. coli, H. influenzae* Hospital-acquired GNB
Cephalosporins		
First generation	Cephalexin	*S. aureus*[†]
Second generation	Cefoxitin	GPC, GNB, anaerobes
Third generation	Cefotaxime	GNB, PCN-R *S. pneumoniae*
Fourth generation	Ceftazidime Cefepime	GNB, *Pseudomonas aeruginosa*
Other Classes		
Carbapenems	Imipenem Meropenem	Multidrug-resistant, hospital-acquired GNB, including ESBL-producing GNB
Aminoglycosides	Gentamicin Tobramycin Amikacin	Community- and hospital-acquired GNB
Macrolides	Erythromycin Azithromycin Clarithromycin	*Chlamydia, Mycoplasma,* group A streptococci, *S. pneumoniae*
Quinolones	Ciprofloxacin	GNB; best for *P. aeruginosa*
	Levofloxacin	GPC and GNB
Oxalidioxones	Linezolid	Vancomycin-resistant GPC
Glycopeptides	Vancomycin Daptomycin	PCN and oxacillin-resistant GPC

*Increasing resistance to penicillin.
[†]Increasing resistance to methicillin in community-acquired strains.
ESBL, extended spectrum β-lactamase; GNB, gram-negative bacilli; GPC, gram-positive cocci; PCN, penicillin.

- Is there another explanation for the clinical presentation, such as a viral infection, drug fever, rejection of a transplant, or graft-versus-host disease?

Communication and Counseling

The appropriate use of antibiotics and reducing antimicrobial resistance are areas of great public health

TABLE 3 Mechanisms of Antimicrobial Resistance

Mechanism	Examples	Presence in Pathogens
Modification of drug	β-lactamases	*Staphylococcus aureus* resistance to oxacillin *Klebsiella pneumoniae* resistance to ampicillin
	Aminoglycoside-modifying enzymes	*Pseudomonas aeruginosa* resistance to gentamicin
Mutation in target	Ribosomal mutations	Resistance to aminoglycosides
	DNA gyrase mutations	Resistance to quinolones
Permeability changes	Efflux pumps	Multidrug resistance in *P. aeruginosa*
	Loss of porins	Resistance to imipenem

implications. Numerous methods are used to control the emergence of antibiotic resistance in both community and health care settings. Community efforts include limiting the use of antibiotics for empirical treatment of otitis media in Europe and the United States in certain lower risk populations or limiting use of erythromycin to decrease macrolide resistance in group A streptococci in Finland. Educational efforts for health care providers and patients focus on promoting an increased understanding that viral illnesses, such as upper respiratory tract infections, bronchitis, and gastroenteritis, rarely require antibiotics. There has also been an increasing appreciation that some animal husbandry practices, such as routinely including prophylactic antibiotics in feed, can promote antibiotic resistance in human pathogens. Finally, many hospitals have antibiotic control programs that limit treatment selection to a narrow panel of agents and require approval for broader spectrum agents. Such programs may also limit the duration of empirical treatment in the setting of negative cultures and make recommendations for the duration of treatment for proven infections.

SUGGESTED READINGS

1. Berild D, Ringertz SH, Aabyholm G, et al: Impact of an antibiotic policy on antibiotic use in a pediatric department. Individual based follow-up shows that antibiotics were chosen according to diagnoses and bacterial findings. Int J Antimicrob Agents 20 (5):333–338, 2002. **Review of the issue by one of world's experts in the perils of antibiotic resistance.**
2. Levy SB: Antibiotic resistance: Consequences of inaction. Clin Infect Dis 33(Suppl. 3):S124–S129, 2001. **Review of principles to guide responsible antibiotic usage, particularly among gram-positive cocci, and discussion of new antimicrobial agents.**
3. Lieberman JM: Appropriate antibiotic use and why it is important: The challenges of bacterial resistance. Pediatr Infect Dis J 22 (12):1143–1151, 2003. **Review of current strategies and treatment options for common community infections (e.g., pneumonia, otitis media) to maximize judicious use and cure, minimize resistance, and avoid treatment of viral illnesses.**
4. Low DE, Pichichero ME, Schaad UB: Optimizing antibacterial therapy for community-acquired respiratory tract infections in children in an era of bacterial resistance. Clin Pediatr 43(2):135–151, 2004. **Large survey demonstrating enormous variability in local epidemiology.**
5. Raymond J, Aujard Y: Nosocomial infections in pediatric patients: A European, multicenter prospective study. European Study Group. Infect Control Hosp Epidemiol 21(4):260–263, 2000. **Thoughtful descriptions of the relationship between animal husbandry practices/agriculture and resistant human pathogens.**
6. Shea KM: Antibiotic resistance: What is the impact of agricultural uses of antibiotics on children's health? Pediatrics 112(1 Pt 2):253–258, 2003. **Excellent review of the subject that provides good examples of pharmacokinetic profiles for specific antimicrobial agents.**
7. Singh J, Burr B, Stringham D, Arrieta A: Commonly used antibacterial and antifungal agents for hospitalised paediatric patients: Implications for therapy with an emphasis on clinical pharmacokinetics. Paediatr Drugs 3(10):733–761, 2001. **Overview of the scope of antimicrobial resistance in general pediatrics as opposed to hospital-based practices.**
8. Zaoutis T, Dawid S, Kim JO: Multidrug-resistant organisms in general pediatrics. Pediatr Ann 31(5):313–320, 2002. **Excellent example of the successes, challenges, and pitfalls in antibiotic control in pediatric hospitals.**

Antifungal Therapies

Valerie J. Waters and Alice Prince

12

KEY CONCEPTS

- Fungal infections range in severity from trivial superficial infections, such as athlete's foot, to severe life-threatening systemic mycoses.
- Definitive diagnosis depends on obtaining specimens for staining, culture, and sensitivity testing.
- Antifungal therapy is often used empirically in high-risk patients.
- Amphotericin B is the gold standard for treatment of severe fungal infections.
- Lipid formulations of amphotericin B are associated with less nephrotoxicity and fewer electrolyte abnormalities and infusion-related reactions than conventional amphotericin B.
- Azoles and echinocandins are less toxic and highly effective for specific indications.

Fungal infections in hospitalized children are increasingly common and associated with mortality rates as high as 29% in one pediatric study population with candidemia. Recognition of fungal species as potential pathogens is important to ensure prompt institution of therapy. Although some fungal infections (e.g., aspergillosis and mucormycosis) primarily affect immunocompromised hosts, such as those with neutropenia or impaired cell-mediated immunity, other systemic mycoses, such as histoplasmosis or coccidioidomycosis, can occur in patients with no underlying disease or predisposing factors (Table 1). Systemic mycoses

TABLE 1 Predisposing Factors for Fungal Infections

Fungal Infection	Predisposing Host Factors
Primary systemic mycoses	
Histoplasmosis	No predisposing factors
Coccidioidomycosis	Travel to endemic areas
Blastomycosis	
Paracoccidioidomycosis	
Opportunistic mycoses	
Invasive candidiasis	Traumatized skin
Invasive aspergillosis	Chronic granulomatous disease
Cryptococcosis	Impaired cell-mediated immunity
Mucormycosis (*Mucor* species, *Rhizopus* species, *Rhizomucor* species)	Neutropenia
	Malnutrition

TABLE 2 Diagnosis of Fungal Infections

Diagnostic Test	Limitations
Stains	
KOH (potassium hydroxide)	Can be difficult to see fungal elements.
Calcofluor	Clearly stains cell walls but requires fluorescent microscope.
Gomori methenamine silver (GMS)	Stains cell wall striking brown/black.
Periodic acid–Schiff	Fungi must be viable to stain.
Gram stain	Stains yeast cells but not hyphae.
Culture	
Sabouraud dextrose agar	Growth may take 4–6 wk.
Brain heart infusion (BHI) agar	Blood culture requires large inoculum.
Rapid Methods	
Galactomannan enzyme immunoassay	Only for *Aspergillus*. Variable sensitivity and specificity.

occur through inhalation of spores, whereas cutaneous mycoses are usually caused by direct inoculation of the organism. The resulting clinical illness can vary widely in type and severity of infection.

Definitive diagnosis of fungal infection requires tissue for staining and culture. The appearance of the specimen on staining can be suggestive of the etiology because most fungi can be divided into either yeasts (e.g., *Candida*), which reproduce by budding, or molds (e.g., *Aspergillus*), which are composed of tubular structures called *hyphae*. The traditional stain for fungi is the KOH (potassium hydroxide) wet mount stain, but the Gomori methenamine silver (GMS) and periodic acid–Schiff stains, both of which stain the cell wall, are also useful (Table 2). Cultures should be

maintained for 4 to 6 weeks, and sensitivity testing should be done to aid in treatment decisions.

With the recent introduction of new antifungal agents, there are several options in choosing antifungal therapy. This review focuses on three major classes of antifungal drugs with their indications, dosage and administration, and common adverse events (Table 3).

Expert Opinion on Management Issues

AMPHOTERICIN B

Amphotericin B has been available for more than 40 years. Because of its efficacy in the treatment of a wide range of mycoses, including invasive candidiasis, aspergillosis, cryptococcal meningitis, and mucormycosis, it remains the gold standard for treatment of severe fungal infections. Conventional amphotericin B, however, causes significant nephrotoxicity, infusion-related reactions, and electrolyte abnormalities that limit the dose and therapeutic concentrations that can be achieved. Lipid-based formulations of amphotericin, such as ABLC (amphotericin B lipid complex) and liposomal amphotericin, are much better tolerated. To maintain equivalent efficacy, higher doses of the lipid formulations must be given than conventional amphotericin. The lipid formulations concentrate in the liver, spleen, and lungs, making them particularly useful in invasive infections in these tissues. ABLC and liposomal amphotericin provide either equivalent or improved efficacy in the treatment of a wide range of fungal infections. ABLC and liposomal amphotericin are comparable in terms of efficacy and toxicity, but the latter may have greater central nervous system (CNS) penetration.

AZOLES

Fluconazole is a first-generation azole developed in the 1990s. It is widely used for susceptible species of *Candida*-causing invasive and mucosal infections. It is well absorbed from the gastrointestinal tract, and the oral formulation is very well tolerated. Other indications include cryptococcal meningitis and fungal prophylaxis in immunosuppressed patients. Fluconazole-resistant fungal species, such as *Candida glabrata* and *Candida krusei,* are not infrequent, especially in patients receiving long-term therapy. As an inhibitor of a cytochrome P450–dependent enzyme, fluconazole also affects the metabolism of drugs such as phenytoin and cyclosporine.

The drug voriconazole is fungicidal for *Aspergillus*, *Scedosporium,* and *Fusarium* species and is fungistatic against *Candida* species, including fluconazole-resistant strains. Like fluconazole, voriconazole is available in both intravenous and oral formulations that have excellent bioavailability. In invasive aspergillosis, treatment with voriconazole is associated with a better clinical response, improved survival, and fewer severe side effects than treatment with conventional amphotericin. Voriconazole is also an effective, well-tolerated

TABLE 3 Antifungal Therapies

Drug	Dose	Maximum	Formulations	Adverse Effects
Amphotericin B (Binds to ergosterol, altering cell membrane permeability causing cell death)				
Amphotericin B deoxycholate (Fungizone) Rx	IV: 0.3–1 mg/kg/day qd	1.5 mg/kg/day	Injection: 50-mg vial	Chills, fever, nausea, nephrotoxicity, electrolyte disturbances
ABLC (Abelcet) Rx	IV: 5 mg/kg/day qd	12–15 mg/kg/day	Injection: 100-mg vial	Fever, chills, nausea, less nephrotoxicity than amphotericin B
Liposomal amphotericin B (AmBisome) Rx	IV: 3–5 mg/kg/day qd	12–15 mg/kg/day	Injection: 50-mg vial	Less fever, chills, and nephrotoxicity than amphotericin B
Azoles (Inhibit ergosterol synthesis by inhibiting cytochrome P450 enzyme)				
Fluconazole (Diflucan) Rx	PO: 3–6 mg/kg/day qd IV: 3–6 mg/kg/day qd Cl_{Cr} <30 mL/min: 1.5–3 mg/kg/day	1600 mg/day	Tablet: 50, 100, 150, 200 mg Oral suspension: 50, 200 mg/5 mL Injection: 200-, 400-mg vial	Nausea, headache, skin rash, increased SGOT
Itraconazole (Sporanox) Rx	IV: 200 mg/dose q12h ×4 doses, then PO: 400 mg/day bid	400 mg/day	Capsule: 100 mg Oral suspension: 10 mg/mL	Nausea, vomiting, diarrhea, hepatotoxicity, hypokalemia
Voriconazole (Vfend) Rx	PO: <40 kg: 400 mg/day ×1 day, then 200 mg/day bid; >40 kg: 800 mg/day ×1 day, then 400 mg/day bid IV: 6 mg/kg/dose q12h ×2 doses, then 4 mg/kg/dose q12h	12 mg/kg/dose		Blurred vision, hepatotoxicity, skin rash
Echinocandins (Inhibit glucan synthesis, disrupting cell wall)				
Caspofungin (Cancidas) Rx	IV: 70 mg/m^2 ×1 dose, then 24 h later, 50 mg/m^2/day in qd dosing	70 mg/day	Injection: 50-,70-mg vial	Fever, nausea, vomiting

ABLC, amphotericin B lipid complex; Cl_{Cr}, creatinine clearance; IV, intravenous; max, maximum; PO, by mouth; qxh, every x hours; qd, every day; Rx, prescription; SGOT, serum glutamic-oxaloacetic transaminase.

treatment choice for refractory or less common invasive fungal infections such as sebopsoriasis and fusariosis.

ECHINOCANDINS

Caspofungin inhibits glucan synthesis, necessary to maintain the fungal cell wall structure, thereby distinguishing it from amphotericin B and the azoles that target ergosterol and the fungal cell membrane. Caspofungin is fungicidal against *Candida* species, making it an excellent choice for empirical therapy of suspected candidal infections that may be fluconazole resistant. Because of its mechanisms of action, caspofungin, when combined with either amphotericin B or azoles in vitro or in animal studies, rarely displays antagonism, suggesting that such combinations may be effective clinically. Unlike azoles, caspofungin does not inhibit the P450 enzyme, and its interaction with other drugs is minimal. In invasive candidiasis, caspofungin is reported to be at least as effective and better tolerated than conventional amphotericin B. Caspofungin may also be used as salvage therapy of invasive aspergillosis in patients who are refractory to other therapies. Caspofungin should not be used for the treatment of meningitis or brain abscess because it has limited CNS penetration.

Common Pitfalls

- With the availability of less toxic drugs, presumptive antifungal therapy should not be delayed in patients at high risk of systemic fungal infection.
- Amphotericin B, preferably the lipid formulation, should be used for the treatment of invasive mycoses until the fungal species is identified and sensitivity testing is available.
- Possible drug interactions must be considered when instituting azole therapy.
- Caspofungin should not be used for CNS infections because of poor penetration.

Definitive diagnosis of fungal infections and choosing an appropriate treatment depend on obtaining specimens for staining and culture because not all antifungal agents have the same spectrum of activity. Lipid formulations of amphotericin B should be used in patients with renal impairment and to avoid toxicity. Some species of *Candida* are intrinsically resistant to fluconazole and potential drug interactions, and hepatotoxicity should be considered before instituting azole therapy.

Communication and Counseling

With the development of an increasing number of antifungal agents, numerous choices are available for treatment of invasive mycoses, but knowledge of their side effects is crucial to prevent toxicity. Parents need to be informed about both the desired effects and possible adverse reactions of each specific antifungal drug.

SUGGESTED READINGS

1. Anaissie EJ, Darouiche RO, Abi-Said D, et al: Management of invasive candidal infections: Results of a prospective, randomized, multicenter study of fluconazole versus amphotericin B and review of the literature. Clin Infect Dis 23:964–972, 1996. **Study showing equivalent efficacy and improved tolerance of fluconazole compared to amphotericin B in the treatment of invasive candidiasis.**
2. Deresinski SC, Stevens DA: Caspofungin. Clin Infect Dis 36:1445–1457, 2003. **Review of pharmacology and clinical uses of caspofungin.**
3. Herbrecht R, Denning DW, Patterson TF, et al: Voriconazole versus amphotericin B for primary therapy of invasive aspergillosis. N Engl J Med 347:408–415, 2002. **Study showing improved response, survival, and tolerance of voriconazole compared to amphotericin B in the treatment of invasive aspergillosis.**
4. Johnson LB, Kauffman CA: Voriconazole: A new triazole antifungal agent. Clin Infect Dis 36:630–637, 2003. **Review of pharmacology and clinical uses of voriconazole.**
5. Martino R: Efficacy, safety and cost-effectiveness of amphotericin B lipid complex (ABLC): A review of the literature. Curr Med Res Opin 20:485–504, 2004. **Detailed review of clinical trials on efficacy and safety of different amphotericin formulations.**
6. Mora-Duarte J, Betts R, Rotstein C, et al: Comparison of caspofungin and amphotericin B for invasive candidiasis. N Engl J Med 347:2020–2029, 2002. **Study showing equivalent efficacy and improved tolerance of caspofungin compared to amphotericin B in the treatment of invasive candidiasis.**
7. Perfect JR, Marr KA, Walsh TJ, et al: Voriconazole treatment for less-common, emerging, or refractory fungal infections. Clin Infect Dis 36:1122–1131, 2003. **Study showing clinical response to voriconazole in the treatment of refractory or less common fungal infections.**

Antiviral Therapies

Soren Gantt and Lisa M. Frenkel

KEY CONCEPTS

- Antiviral agents offer treatment for herpesvirus, hepatitis B and C, influenza, and a few other viral infections.
- Antiviral compounds act against specific steps in viral replication metabolism, augment the host immune response against infection, or destroy virally infected tissues.
- Antiviral therapy typically does not eliminate infection in the absence of an effective host immune response.
- Familiarity with the indications, dosage, and adverse effects of a given antiviral agent is central to its safe and effective use.

Specific antiviral agents first became available in the 1950s. Multiple classes of antivirals have since been developed, some with broad efficacy. Therapies limit viral infections by various means: They may interfere with specific metabolic functions of the targeted virus, augment the host's immune response, or destroy the infected tissues. The antivirals used clinically for treatment of viral infections, as of late 2004, are described here, including data regarding their clinical usefulness and toxicity. Table 1 indicates whether data supporting clinical use of agents were derived from randomized, controlled trials or observational studies, and Table 2 provides information regarding drug formulations and dosing. A large number of agents, 20 within four pharmaceutical classes as of late 2004, are now available for the treatment of human immunodeficiency virus type 1 (HIV–1). These drugs and the vaccines and immunoglobulins used to prevent viral infections are discussed in the chapters addressing each infection.

Expert Opinion on Management Issues

NUCLEOSIDE ANALOGUES

Modified nucleosides and nucleotides that masquerade as DNA or RNA building blocks were developed as antiviral drugs. These inhibit viral replication and, in doing so, the spread of infection within a host. These agents are not virucidal, and some degree of host immunity is required to contain or eliminate the infection once the drug limits viral replication.

As a group, many nucleoside/nucleotide analogues are highly toxic because of effects on cellular DNA replication and transcription. The first nucleoside, idoxuridine, is toxic if used systemically; however, it, and the more potent trifluorothymidine (also called trifluridine), are useful as topical agents to inhibit replication of herpes simplex virus (HSV) in the eye. Both idoxuridine and trifluridine are used for treatment of keratitis caused by vaccinia virus.

Nucleoside analogues that are preferentially activated by viral enzymes have significantly less toxicity. The HSV and varicella zoster virus (VZV) thymidine kinases activate acyclovir and its prodrug, valacyclovir; penciclovir and its prodrug, famciclovir; and ganciclovir and its prodrug, valganciclovir. A cytomegalovirus (CMV) kinase activates ganciclovir and valganciclovir. The prodrugs markedly increase oral bioavailability, with drug levels reaching those achieved by intravenous (IV) dosing of the parent compound. Currently, none of the prodrugs are available in suspension, although pharmacokinetic studies of a suspension of valganciclovir are ongoing. The pill formulations of valacyclovir and valganciclovir are made into extemporaneous suspensions for administration to young

TABLE 1 Type of Evidence Supporting Antiviral Treatments

Antiviral Treatment	Strength of Evidence
Nucleoside and Nucleotide Analogues	
Idoxuridine	2 = HSV keratitis; 2, 3 = vaccinia keratitis.
Trifluorothymidine	1 = HSV keratitis; 2, 3 = vaccinia keratitis.
Penciclovir	1 = HSV mucocutaneous.
Acyclovir	1 = HSV mucocutaneous, encephalitis, and neonatal infections; varicella zoster virus; 2 = HSV meningitis and esophagitis, oral hairy leukoplakia, simian B herpesvirus.
Valacyclovir	1 = HSV mucocutaneous, varicella zoster virus.
Famciclovir	1 = HSV mucocutaneous, varicella zoster virus.
Ganciclovir	1 = CMV retinitis, pneumonitis, colitis, and congenital infection; prophylaxis and preemptive therapy of CMV disease.
Valganciclovir	1 = CMV retinitis; 1 = prophylaxis of CMV disease.
Ribavirin	1 = RSV, HCV; 2 = parainfluenza viruses, measles.
Lamivudine	1 = chronic HBV infection; 2 = HTLV–1.
Emtricitabine	2 = HBV.
Cidofovir	1 = CMV retinitis; 2 = papillomas, BK virus hemorrhagic cystitis, acyclovir-resistant CMV and VZV, adenovirus; 3 = smallpox treatment and prophylaxis.
Adefovir	1 = chronic HBV.
Tenofovir	2 = chronic HBV.
Other Antiviral Agents	
Foscarnet	1 = CMV retinitis; acyclovir-resistant mucocutaneous HSV; 2 = CMV disease (nonretinitis).
Fomivirsen	1 = CMV retinitis.
Amantadine	1 = influenza A.
Rimantadine	1 = influenza A.
Oseltamivir	1 = influenza A and B.
Zanamivir	1 = influenza A and B.
Pleconaril	1 = picornaviral upper respiratory infection; 1 = enteroviral meningitis; 2 = severe picornaviral infection.
Immune Modulators	
Interferon-α	1 = chronic HCV and HBV infection, genital warts (HPV); 2 = laryngeal papillomatosis.
Imiquimod	1 = external genital warts; 1 = molluscum contagiosum.
Immunoglobulins	Ig: 1 = HAV exposure, measles exposure.
	IVIG and CMVIG: 1 = treatment of CMV pneumonitis (with ganciclovir).
	RIG: 1 = rabies exposure.
	IVIG: 1 = treatment of neonatal enteroviral infection; 2 = treatment of enteroviral infection in patients with hypo/agammaglobulinemia.
	HBIG: 1 = HBV and HCV exposures.
	VZIG: 1 = VZV.
Physical Treatments	
Salicylic acid/ keratolytics	1 = cutaneous warts, external genital warts; 2 = molluscum contagiosum.
Liquid nitrogen	2 = cutaneous and genital papillomatosis (HPV), molluscum contagiosum.
Duct tape	1 = cutaneous warts (HPV).
Laser therapy	2 = cutaneous, genital and laryngeal papillomatosis (HPV).
Electrocautery	2 = cutaneous, genital and laryngeal papillomatosis (HPV).
Antimetabolites	2 = cutaneous and genital papillomatosis (HPV), molluscum contagiosum.
Podophyllin, podophyllotoxin	1 = cutaneous and genital papillomatosis (HPV), molluscum contagiosum.

1, effective in randomized controlled trial(s); 2, case series and anecdotal reports; 3, in vitro data suggest antiviral effect at drug levels achieved in humans.
CMV, cytomegalovirus; CMVIG, cytomegalovirus immunoglobulin; HAV, hepatitis A virus; HBIG, hepatitis B immunoglobulin; HBV, hepatitis B virus; HCV, hepatitis C virus; HPV, human papillomavirus; HSV, herpes simplex virus; HTLV, human T-cell leukemia virus; Ig, immunoglobulin; IVIG, intravenous immunoglobulin; RIG, rabies immunoglobulin; RSV, respiratory syncytial virus; VZIG, varicella-zoster immunoglobulin; VZV, varicella zoster virus.

children; however, the pharmacokinetics and dosing of these agents are not yet determined.

Acyclovir, valacyclovir, and famciclovir are primarily used for treatment and prevention of serious herpes simplex virus (HSV) and varicella zoster virus (VZV) disease. These agents also have in vitro activity against Epstein-Barr virus (EBV) and variable effects on disease associated with EBV infection. Resistance to these agents occurs through mutations in the viral thymidine kinase and, less commonly, the viral DNA polymerase. Cross-resistance to foscarnet and cidofovir is rare with mutations in thymidine kinase, but it may occur with mutations of the polymerase gene. Clinically relevant resistance is unusual in immunocompetent individuals but not uncommon in severely immunocompromised hosts (e.g., patients with AIDS [acquired immune deficiency syndrome]).

The bioavailability of acyclovir is approximately 25%; therefore the IV route is recommended for severe infections, such as neonatal HSV infections and VZV infections in immunocompromised individuals. Acyclovir distributes widely into body fluids and obtains cerebrospinal fluid (CSF) levels that are approximately 50% of plasma levels.

TABLE 2 Dosing and Adverse Reactions of Commonly Used Antiviral Agents

Drug	Indication	Dose	Adverse Reactions/Comments
Idoxuridine	HSV and vaccinia keratitis in adults and adolescents	0.1% solution: 1 drop q1h during the day and q2h during the night, or 1 drop per min for 5 min q4h day and night. 0.1% ointment: a thin strip (≈1 cm) of ointment q4h, for max 21 days.	Local irritation, corneal clouding, lacrimal punctal occlusion, punctate keratopathy. Teratogenic in animals; use with caution in pregnancy.
Trifluorothymidine (trifluridine)	HSV keratoconjunctivitis and recurrent epithelial keratitis >6 yr of age	1% solution: 1 drop q2h (max 9 drops/day), for max 21 days.	Transient local irritation, palpebral or stromal edema, punctate keratopathy, keratitis sicca, increased intraocular pressure. Teratogenic in animals; use with caution in pregnancy.
Penciclovir	Herpes labialis	1% cream to affected area q2h while awake for 3 to 5 days.	Local skin reactions. Apply at earliest indication of disease.
Famciclovir	Mucocutaneous HSV in adolescents and adults	Primary: 250–500 mg PO tid for 7–10 days. Recurrent: 125–500 mg PO bid for 7 days. Chronic suppression: 250 mg PO bid for up to 1 yr. 500 mg PO bid-tid for 10 days.	Well tolerated. Nausea, diarrhea, rash, confusion, hallucinations, neutropenia, elevated hepatic transaminases occur uncommonly.
Acyclovir	Zoster Neonatal HSV HSV encephalitis (non-neonate) HSV infection in immunocompromised or critically ill patients Mucocutaneous HSV	20 mg/kg IV q8h for ≥21 days. 10 mg/kg IV q8h for 14–21 days. 5–10 mg/kg IV q8h. Primary: 10 mg/kg PO 5 times/day (max 1.2 g/day) for 7–10 days. Recurrent: 5–10 mg/kg PO 5 times/day (max 1.2 g/day) for 5 days. Suppression: 15 mg/kg PO 2–5 times/day (max 1.2 g/day) for up to 1 yr; then reassess.	Nephrotoxicity, neutropenia, lethargy, headache, encephalopathy, nausea, vomiting. Ensure adequate hydration to reduce risk of nephrotoxicity. Adjust dosage in renal failure.
Valacyclovir	Varicella (with risk for severe infection) and zoster Mucocutaneous HSV in adolescents and adults	10 mg/kg q8h IV; 20 mg/kg q6h PO. Primary: 1000 mg PO bid for 5 days. Secondary: 500 mg PO bid for 3 days. Chronic suppression: 500–1000 mg PO qd for up to 1 yr; then reassess.	See acyclovir.
Ganciclovir	Zoster in adolescents and adults Treatment or prevention of CMV in immunocompromised host	1000 mg PO tid for 7 days. Induction: 5–6 mg/kg IV q12h for 14–21 days. Maintenance: 5–6 mg/kg IV qd (or 1000 mg PO tid with food for adolescents and adults).	Neutropenia common, thrombocytopenia, behavioral changes, nephrotoxicity, elevated transaminases, rash. Teratogenic and embryotoxic. Ganciclovir-induced neutropenia often reversible with G-CSF. Adjust dosage in renal insufficiency.
Valganciclovir	Symptomatic congenital CMV CMV retinitis in adults	6 mg/kg IV q12h for 6 wk. Induction: 900 mg PO bid for 21 days. Maintenance: 900 mg PO qd.	Adverse effects similar to ganciclovir, and diarrhea. Take with food. Adjust dosage in renal insufficiency.
Ribavirin	Treatment of hepatitis C Severe RSV infections	25–36 kg: 200 mg PO q AM and q PM; >36–49 kg: 200/400; >49–61 kg: 400/400; >61–75 kg: 400/600; >75 kg: 600/600; Continuous aerosolization of 20 mg/mL (6 g reconstituted with 300 mL of sterile water) via small-particle aerosol generator (SPAG-2) for 12–18 h/day for 3 to 7 days.	Anemia, irritability, depression. Given in combination with Interferon-alfa-2b. Teratogenic, mutagenic, and embryotoxic—contraindicated in pregnancy. Not recommended in severe renal impairment. Rash, conjunctivitis, worsening respiratory function, bronchospasm, headache. Teratogenic, mutagenic, and embryotoxic—contraindicated in pregnancy; concern for environmental exposure. Ribavirin should be administered in well-ventilated rooms (at least 6 air changes/h).
Lamivudine	Treatment of chronic hepatitis B in children ≥2 yr of age	3 mg/kg PO qd (max 100 mg/dose)	Well tolerated. Headache, fatigue, diarrhea, rash are uncommon. Adjust dose in renal insufficiency.
Cidofovir	CMV and adenovirus infections in immunocompromised hosts	Induction: 5 mg/kg IV once per week for 2 wk with probenecid. Maintenance: 5 mg/kg IV every other week or 3 mg/kg once per week with probenecid.	Nephrotoxicity in ≈50% of patients, neutropenia, ocular toxicity. Risk of nephrotoxicity reduced with hydration and probenecid, given PO 3 h before, and 2 and 8 h after each dose of cidofovir. Check urinalysis and renal function before each dose. Adjust dosage if renal insufficiency or proteinuria occurs. Ophthalmologic monitoring recommended.

Drug	Indication	Dosage	Comments
Adefovir	Chronic hepatitis B in adults	10 mg PO qd.	Well tolerated. Renal toxicity may occur; follow renal function. Exacerbation of hepatitis may occur after discontinuation. Adjust dosage in renal insufficiency. Use with caution in pregnancy.
Foscarnet	CMV disease	Induction: 60 mg/kg IV q8h for 21 days. Maintenance: 90–120 mg/kg IV qd.	Renal toxicity in ≈one third of patients. Risk of renal toxicity reduced with prehydration and slow infusion over 2 h.
	Acyclovir-resistant HSV infections	40 mg/kg IV q8h.	
Fomivirsen	CMV retinitis in adults	Induction: 330 µg intravitreal injection q wk for two doses. Maintenance: 330 µg intraocular injection q mo.	Uveitis, iritis, vitritis, conjunctival hyperemia, conjunctivitis, increased intraocular pressure, cataracts, corneal edema, abnormal vision, optic neuritis, vitreous hemorrhage. Ocular inflammation occurs in ≈25% of patients. Avoid use in patients who have recently (2–4 wk) been treated with either IV or intravitreal cidofovir because of the risk of exaggerated ocular inflammation.
Amantadine	Influenza A prophylaxis and treatment	5 mg/kg PO qd; max dose: 200 mg/day.	CNS symptoms (behavioral changes, dizziness, hallucinations, seizures) rare in children; nausea, vomiting. Prophylaxis may be administered for up to 6 wk after first vaccine dose, 2 wk after the second dose; administer a 10-day course of therapy following exposure; for symptomatic treatment, administer within 48 h of symptom onset for 3–7 days or until ≥48 h after asymptomatic. Adjust dosage in renal insufficiency.
Rimantadine	Influenza A prophylaxis and treatment	2.5 mg/kg PO bid; max dose: 150 mg/day.	See amantadine (CNS symptoms may be less frequent than for amantadine).
Oseltamivir	Treatment of influenza A and B, ≥1 yr of age	2 mg/kg PO bid; max: 75 mg/dose.	Nausea, vomiting. Treatment should be started within 48 h of symptom onset. Adjust dosage in renal impairment.
	Prophylaxis of influenza A and B, ≥13 yr of age	2 mg/kg PO qd.	Nausea, vomiting. Adjust dosage in renal impairment.
Zanamivir	Treatment and prophylaxis of influenza A and B, >7 yr of age	2 Diskhaler inhalations (10 mg total) bid for 5 days.	Not recommended for use in patients with underlying respiratory disease, such as reactive airway disease, because of risk of bronchospasm.
Pleconaril	Picornaviral infection	5 mg/kg PO q8h.	Well tolerated, but experience is limited. Crystalluria was noted after high single doses; urinalysis is recommended during prolonged therapy.
Interferon	Papilloma, anogenital warts	Interferon alfa-2b or alfa-n3; inject 1 million U (0.1 mL) into lesion 3 times/wk for 3 wk.	Painful, local irritation. Dilute to 10 MU/mL to avoid hypertonicity. Used in refractory cases (e.g., in AIDS patients).
	Chronic hepatitis B	Adults: Interferon alfa-2b 5 MU SC qd or 10 MU qd 3 times/week. Children: Interferon alfa-2b 5–6 MU/m² SC 3 times/wk.	Influenza-like syndrome, fever, headache, myalgia, nausea, and anorexia occurs in almost all patients initially, but often resolves within a few wk of treatment. Depression, mental status changes, bone marrow suppression, and elevated liver enzymes can also result.
	Chronic hepatitis C	Adults: PEG-interferon alfa-2a1, 80 µg SC q wk, or PEG-interferon alfa-2b, 1.5 µg/kg SC q wk. Children: Interferon alfa-2b, 5–6 MU/m² SC 3 times/wk.	As above. Given in combination with ribavirin.
Imiquimod	Anogenital warts, condyloma acuminata in adolescents and adults	Apply 3 times/wk on alternative days prior to bedtime and wash off after 8 h. Continue treatment until total clearance for 16 wk.	Local irritation common. Avoid use of excessive amounts of cream. Instruct patients to apply imiquimod to external or perianal warts; not for vaginal use. Apply a thin layer to the wart area and rub in until the cream is no longer visible. Do not occlude the application site. May increase sunburn susceptibility; patients should protect themselves from the sun. Contraindicated in pregnancy.
	Common warts in adolescents and adults	Apply once daily prior to bedtime, 5 days/wk for 6 wk. Treatment area should include a 1-cm margin of skin around the lesion. Leave on skin for 8 h, then wash.	
Podophyllin, Podofilox	Anogenital warts, condyloma acuminata	25% podophyllin in tincture of benzoin (Podocon 25); apply once weekly and wash off after 1–4 h, for up to 6 wk. Podofilox: apply bid for 3 days followed by no treatment for 4 days; repeat cycle 4–6 times as necessary.	Local skin irritation common. Contraindicated in pregnancy. Warts recur in ≈ one third of cases within 1 mo of treatment.
Cantharidin	Warts, molluscum contagiosum	Apply directly to lesion, cover with nonporous tape, remove tape in 24 h, reapply if necessary.	Dermal irritation, dermal burns, acantholysis.

AIDS, acquired immune deficiency syndrome; bid, twice daily; CMV, cytomegalovirus; CNS, central nervous system; G-CSF, granulocyte colony-stimulating factor; HSV, herpes simplex virus; IV, intravenous; max, maximum; MU, million units; PO, by mouth; q, every; qxh, every x hours; qd, every day; RSV, respiratory syncytial virus; SC, subcutaneous; tid, three times per day.

Acyclovir, valacyclovir, and famciclovir have excellent safety profiles; however, neutropenia occasionally occurs, with increased frequency in infants. Acyclovir is not teratogenic to the human fetus, but it is unknown whether it is carcinogenic. These agents are renally excreted and require dose modification for renal insufficiency. Importantly, in dehydrated individuals, acyclovir, valacyclovir, and famciclovir may precipitate in the renal tubules, leading to acute tubular necrosis. Therefore, hydration is recommended to minimize the risk of drugs crystallizing. In addition, when high doses are administered, serum creatinine levels and absolute neutrophil counts should be assessed at least weekly to monitor for toxicity.

Vidarabine is an older nucleoside analogue that effectively inhibits HSV and VZV replication. However, it is rarely used because acyclovir had superior or equivalent efficacy and less toxicity in comparative trials.

Ganciclovir and its prodrug, valganciclovir, are used to prevent and treat serious infections caused by cytomegalovirus, and less commonly infections caused by EBV, human herpesvirus type 6 (HHV–6), HHV–7, HHV–8, hepatitis B virus (HBV), and adenoviruses. CMV resistant to ganciclovir can be selected, most commonly with mutations in the *UL97* gene encoding a viral kinase that phosphorylates ganciclovir, but also with mutations in the *UL54* gene that encode the viral DNA polymerase. Strains with *UL97* mutations remain susceptible to foscarnet, whereas *UL54* mutants may be resistant to foscarnet and/or cidofovir. Ganciclovir penetrates the blood–brain barrier with concentrations reaching approximately 40% of plasma. Ganciclovir is renally excreted, and doses should be reduced in patients with renal insufficiency. Neutropenia is the most common ganciclovir-associated toxicity, which can be successfully managed by administration of granulocyte colony-stimulating factor (G-CSF). In preclinical trials in animals, ganciclovir was teratogenic, carcinogenic, and associated with testicular atrophy; however, the extent to which these toxicities are manifest in humans is not yet determined.

Ribavirin is a nucleoside analogue that inhibits messenger RNA (mRNA) formation in a broad spectrum of RNA and DNA viruses. Ribavirin is used most commonly in the treatment of HCV and in some centers for treatment of respiratory viruses. In infants, ribavirin can favorably modify severe respiratory syncytial virus (RSV) infections, when aerosolized drug is initiated early. Aerosolized ribavirin is also used to treat influenza, parainfluenza, and measles infections, and to limit the progression of upper respiratory tract infections in immunocompromised individuals. Resistance to ribavirin is uncommon. Ribavirin can be administered by aerosol, orally or intravenously, with approximately 70% of plasma levels passing into the CSF. Ribavirin accumulates in red blood cells and is associated with anemia, primarily in association with oral and IV administration. Otherwise, ribavirin has a few minor adverse effects, including irritation of the mucous membranes with aerosol administration using a mask or tent, and bronchospasm. During mechanical ventilation, inadvertent high pressures are generated

if ribavirin precipitates and causes malfunction of mechanical valves. Ribavirin is metabolized by the liver and excreted by the kidney. Systemic use is not recommended in severe renal impairment. Ribavirin was found to be teratogenic and mutagenic in preclinical trials in animals. Thus, its use is contraindicated in pregnancy, and health care workers should avoid exposure to aerosols of ribavirin.

Lamivudine (3TC or LMV) and emtricitabine (FTC), a congener with a longer half-life, are nucleoside analogues with principal action through DNA chain termination. Both are used most commonly for their antiretroviral activity. However, both also inhibit replication of hepatitis B virus (HBV), and lamivudine decreases human T-cell leukemia virus 1 (HTLV–1) load. Resistance to lamivudine and emtricitabine is selected rapidly, although not as rapidly with HBV as with HIV–1. Trials of dual- or triple-drug therapy are in progress. Lamivudine and emtricitabine are well tolerated, with few, if any, adverse effects. Both are primarily excreted by the kidney; thus, dosing should be adjusted for renal insufficiency.

Cidofovir is a nucleotide analogue with preferential inhibition of viral over cellular DNA polymerases. The polymerases of essentially all DNA viruses are inhibited by cidofovir, although its most specific activity is toward CMV and other herpesviruses. Viral resistance to cidofovir is uncommon. The half-life of cidofovir is prolonged, and infrequent dosing is a clinical advantage of this agent. Penetration into the CSF and brain is likely, although largely unstudied. Cidofovir is excreted through the kidney. It is associated with an extremely high rate of nephrotoxicity. Serum creatinine and development of proteinuria should be monitored closely to detect renal impairment. Cidofovir should be administered with saline loading and probenecid to minimize renal toxicity. Cidofovir is contraindicated in individuals with marginal renal function because of the high risk of renal failure. Neutropenia and ocular toxicity are also common and require close monitoring. Cidofovir was carcinogenic and embryotoxic in preclinical animal studies.

Adefovir and tenofovir are nucleotide analogues that inhibit HBV and other DNA polymerases. Adefovir is effective in the treatment of compensated and uncompensated chronic hepatitis B infection in adults, including cases in which lamivudine failed because of resistance. Preliminary studies suggest greater suppression of HBV with tenofovir compared to adefovir. Renal toxicity occurs with high-dose adefovir; however, it is uncommon at dosing recommended for treatment of HBV. Tenofovir exhibits less nephrotoxicity; however, monitoring of renal function is recommended with both agents. Tenofovir is associated with diminished bone density. Both agents are excreted by the kidney, and therefore dosing adjustments are required with renal insufficiency.

PYROPHOSPHATE ANALOGUES

Foscarnet is a pyrophosphate analogue that inhibits DNA polymerase, with greater binding to the viral compared to cellular polymerases. Foscarnet inhibits the replication of herpesviruses and HBV. It crosses into the CSF, and levels attain approximately 60% that of plasma. Renal toxicity is commonly induced by foscarnet. Also, the divalent ions, specifically magnesium and calcium, are bound by the drug, which may result in a myriad of symptoms because of metabolic disorders, including seizures and cardiac dysrhythmias. Hydration, saline, and prolongation of infusions may diminish toxicities. In preclinical trials, foscarnet was mutagenic and associated with bone abnormalities.

ANTISENSE RNA AND DNA

An antisense DNA, fomivirsen, is effective for treatment of CMV retinitis. It acts by inhibiting the translation of the viral immediate-early proteins essential for virulence. Fomivirsen is administered via direct intravitreal injection and associated with a relatively high rate of local adverse effects. Generally, fomivirsen is used when CMV retinitis does not respond to standard therapies or when these therapies are not tolerated or they are contraindicated. Fomivirsen can be used in combination with valganciclovir.

TRICYCLIC AMINES

Amantadine and rimantadine inhibit the uncoating and assembly of the influenza A viral membrane. Both drugs effectively reduce illness when administered early (<48 hours of symptoms) in the course of disease, and provide prophylaxis to individuals who are immunocompromised or for other reasons do not benefit from vaccine-induced immunity. These agents do not inhibit influenza B viruses effectively, and they reportedly have poor activity against avian influenza viruses but inhibit hepatitis C virus (HCV). Drug-resistant influenza A virus is selected after only a few days of exposure to the drugs. The resistant viruses are transmissible and cause illness. CSF levels reach approximately half those in serum. Amantadine is excreted in the urine, whereas rimantadine is metabolized in the liver prior to renal excretion. Amantadine doses should be reduced for renal insufficiency, and rimantadine reduced for both renal and hepatic insufficiency. Adverse central nervous system (CNS) effects can occur with both drugs but are more common with amantadine.

NEURAMINIDASE INHIBITORS

Oseltamivir and zanamivir are analogues of *N*-acetyl-neuraminic acid, the cellular receptor of influenza viruses, and inhibit the neuraminidase of both influenza A and B viruses. Inhibition of the viral neuraminidase diminishes viral access to human respiratory cells and budding of new viral particles from infected cells. Both agents offer effective prophylaxis from influenza, and they shorten the duration of symptoms of influenza if administered within 48 hours of the onset of illness. Mutations altering either the viral neuraminidase or the hemagglutinin can confer resistance to these drugs.

Viral resistance was detected in 5% to 8% of children treated with oseltamivir. Zanamivir-resistant virus is extremely rare, although it was documented after prolonged administration to an immunocompromised child. Oseltamivir is absorbed well following oral dosing. It is available as a suspension with dosing recommendations for children 1 year or older. The drug is generally well tolerated but associated with nausea and vomiting.

Oseltamivir passes into the CNS. Oseltamivir is eliminated via the kidney, and thus dosing should be adjusted for renal insufficiency. Zanamivir is poorly absorbed by the oral route and therefore only available as an inhaled powder, which limits its use to children older than 7 years. Adverse effects of zanamivir include cough and, less commonly, bronchospasm, so it should be avoided in patients with reactive airway disease. Serum levels of zanamivir are extremely low or undetectable after inhaled administration.

MISCELLANEOUS ANTIVIRAL AGENTS

Pleconaril, an investigational agent, interferes with the attachment and uncoating of picornaviruses (enteroviruses and rhinoviruses). It is currently available in clinical trials or by requests for "compassionate use." A modicum of clinical efficacy was demonstrated in treatment of adults with the common cold (1 day) and enteroviral meningitis. In case series, pleconaril was associated with improvement in a series of serious enteroviral infections, such as chronic meningitis, myocarditis, poliomyelitis, and disseminated neonatal disease. Controlled trials of pleconaril are ongoing in infants with enteroviral sepsis syndrome. Pleconaril is orally bioavailable and concentrates in brain, liver, and nasal epithelium. Adverse effects are limited to rare and mild gastrointestinal symptoms and headache.

IMMUNE MODULATORS

Immune modulators are substances that directly or indirectly affect the immune response. The role of immune modulators in the prevention and treatment of viral infections typically involves the replacement or augmentation of factors that increase antiviral immune activity. The antiviral actions of interferon-α (IFN-α), immunoglobulin preparations, and imiquimod are discussed briefly here and in the chapters addressing each specific disease.

IFN-α is a protein cytokine produced in response to a variety of stimuli, including viral infections. Primarily, IFN-α is used to treat chronic HCV and, on occasion, HBV infections. HCV treatment combines ribavirin with IFN-α. Pegylated (PEG) IFN-α has a longer half-life and is more effective compared to the standard preparation for treatment of HCV. Injection of IFN-α into external genital warts and refractory or severe tracheal condyloma caused by human papillomavirus (HPV) has variable success. Systemically administered IFN-α is associated with a high rate of adverse effects, most of which are dose dependent. An influenza-like syndrome occurs in virtually all patients, and it often subsides with continued treatment. Bone marrow suppression, neuropsychiatric symptoms (depression, anxiety, emotional lability, agitation), and elevated hepatic transaminases are also common. Intralesional IFN-α is associated with local discomfort and inflammation and mild systemic effects.

Imiquimod is a synthetic compound that has no direct antiviral activity. Rather its activity likely results from stimulating the release of interferons, interleukins, and tumor necrosis factor (TNF) from dendritic cells and macrophages that enhance a local cellular immune response. Imiquimod is effective in treatment of genital and perianal papillomavirus, and preliminary studies suggest efficacy for treatment of molluscum contagiosum. It is applied topically three times per week. Local inflammation at the site of application is common. Systemic reactions with malaise and myalgia are rarely reported.

IMMUNOGLOBULINS

Passive immunization with polyclonal and monoclonal immunoglobulin preparations is used to prevent and, less commonly, to treat viral infections. Examples of postexposure use include polyclonal γ-globulin for hepatitis A and measles, and specific immune globulin against hepatitis B, varicella, vaccinia, and rabies. Intravenous immunoglobulin (IVIG) and CMV-immunoglobulin are used to treat CMV pneumonitis. In addition, limited data demonstrate efficacy for treatment of enteroviral infections with IVIG in neonates and hypo- and agammaglobulinemic patients. Anaphylactic shock is the most serious adverse reaction associated with the use of immunoglobulins, and it occurs more frequently with IV administration.

PHYSICAL TREATMENTS

A variety of physical interventions are used to treat cutaneous warts (verrucae) caused by human papillomaviruses (HPV). These are divided into keratolytics, such as salicylic acid preparations, and destructive therapies, such as liquid nitrogen or cantharidin. Many of these treatments are also effective for treatment of molluscum contagiosum, caused by a poxvirus, which also is treated by curettage. Typically, both warts and molluscum regress spontaneously in immunocompetent individuals; however, the process may take years. Treatment can hasten resolution, although recurrences are common.

Destructive therapies work by causing necrosis of virus-infected epithelial cells, through physical or toxic insult. Of these, liquid nitrogen cryotherapy is the most commonly employed. Small lesions are frozen for 10 seconds; thicker lesions may be frozen for up to 60 seconds during two or more freeze-thaw cycles. Cryotherapy may be too painful for young children to tolerate.

Mild irritation of the treated area occurs during the subsequent days, and inflammation of the adjacent tissues occurs with more treatment. Liquid nitrogen should be used cautiously on the digits, especially near superficial nerves, because freezing could result in permanent neuropathy and in the periungual region could result in permanent nail dystrophy. Hypopigmentation may occur in the area treated, warranting a cautious approach to dark-skinned individuals.

Covering warts with duct tape may be more effective than cryotherapy. Treatment consists of occluding lesions with duct tape for 6 days, removing the tape, soaking and debriding the wart with an emery board or pumice stone, and then leaving the wart uncovered on the sixth night. The duct tape is then reapplied the next morning, and the cycle is repeated until resolution or for a maximum of 2 months.

Cantharidin is the extract of a blister beetle toxin that is used as a topical vesicant and results in intradermal blisters. The initial application is painless, so multiple lesions can be easily treated. Because of the risk of damaging unaffected skin, cantharidin should be applied by a clinician and then covered with an occlusive dressing. The treatment should be washed off after 4 hours. Blistering occurs, which can be painful. Care should be taken to avoid secondary infection of lesions. After ulcers heal, treatment with a salicylic acid preparation for an additional 5 to 7 days may reduce the risk of recurrence.

Simple curettage may be effective for isolated warts or molluscum. Electrocautery and laser treatments are also effective for large or refractory warts, but they require anesthesia and incur greater risks of scarring.

ANTIMITOTICS AND ANTIMETABOLITES

Podophyllin resin and its purified derivative podophyllotoxin are used for the topical treatment of anogenital HPV. These agents have antimitotic activity, causing tissue necrosis. Both agents produce irritation to proximal normal tissues. Recurrences are common following treatment. Antimetabolites, including bleomycin and 5-fluorouracil (5-FU), are also used to treat HPV. They are applied directly to lesions, usually twice a week, and inhibit the cellular proliferation induced by HPV. Evidence for efficacy of bleomycin and 5-FU is limited. None of these agents are virus specific, and, except for podophyllotoxin, they are applied by health care providers because of the risk of damage to unaffected skin. Use of effective contraception is recommended for women of childbearing age using these antimitotics and antimetabolites, and all are contraindicated during pregnancy.

Common Pitfalls

- Certain viral infections may have serious morbidity or result in death. These serious infections should be managed with guidance of the relevant specialist(s) (e.g., gastroenterology for chronic viral hepatitis, ophthalmology for ocular HSV, and infectious diseases for CNS or neonatal HSV infections and management of infections in neonates and immunocompromised children).

- To prevent the spread of viral infections, the appropriate infection control practices should be observed.
- Treatment for influenza should be initiated within 48 hours of the onset of symptoms.
- Certain antiretroviral agents can cause serious adverse reactions. Toxicity may be minimized by administration practices and limiting exposure to the agent when monitoring of laboratory tests reveals intolerance.
- Destructive treatments for warts and molluscum are painful. They can scar and are associated with high recurrence rates.

Communication and Counseling

As with any medical treatment, the rationale and risks and benefits of antiviral therapy should be communicated to patients and their families. Similarly, clear and effective communication regarding the correct use of these agents is crucial for optimal treatment. The specific indication for treatment should determine the details of these discussions.

SUGGESTED READINGS

1. Amir J, Harel L, Smetana Z, Varsano I: Treatment of herpes simplex gingivostomatitis with acyclovir in children: A randomised double-blind placebo controlled study. Br Med J 314:1800–1803, 1997. **Study showing efficacy of acyclovir for HSV gingivostomatitis in children.**
2. Couch RB: Prevention and treatment of influenza. N Engl J Med 343(24):1778–1787, 2000. **Review of the use of anti-influenza drugs for prophylaxis and therapy.**
3. Demmler GJ: Antiviral agents. In Feigin RD, Cherry J, Demmler GJ, Kaplan S (eds): Textbook of Pediatric Infectious Diseases, 5th ed. Philadelphia: WB Saunders, 2004, pp 3048–3074. **Detailed overview of antiviral agents with extensive references.**
4. Hochman JA, Balistreri WF: Chronic viral hepatitis: Always be current. Pediatr Rev 24(12):399–410, 2003. **Review of HBV and HCV infections in children with information on treatment.**
5. Kimberlin DW, Lin CY, Jacobs RF, et al: Safety and efficacy of high-dose intravenous acyclovir in the management of neonatal herpes simplex infections. Pediatrics 108(2):230–238, 2001. **Study showing increased efficacy of high-dose (60 mg/kg/day) acyclovir for neonatal HSV.**
6. Kimberlin DW, Lin CY, Sanchez PJ, et al: Effect of ganciclovir therapy on hearing in symptomatic congenital cytomegalovirus disease involving the central nervous system: A randomized, controlled trial. J Pediatr 143(1):16–25, 2003. **Study showing efficacy of ganciclovir therapy for selected cases of congenital CMV infection.**
7. Naesens L, De Clercq E: Recent developments in herpesvirus therapy. Herpes 8(1):12–16, 2001. **Additional details on drugs with activity against herpesviruses including those in development.**
8. Randolph AG, Wang E: Ribavirin therapy for respiratory syncytial virus lower respiratory tract infection: A systematic overview. Arch Pediatr Adolesc Med 150:942–947, 1996. **Review of studies of ribavirin for RSV pneumonia.**
9. Rotbart HA: Pleconaril treatment of enterovirus and rhinovirus infections. Infect Med 17:488–494, 2000. **Review of the use of pleconaril in picornaviral infections.**
10. Wiley DJ, Douglas J, Beutner K, et al: External genital warts: Diagnosis, treatment, and prevention. Clin Infect Dis 35(Suppl. 2):S210–S224, 2002. **Review that includes clinical evidence for therapies for external genital HPV.**

Infections in Daycare Environments

Dennis A. Clements

KEY CONCEPTS

- Daycare facilities are described as either small family, large family, or a child-care center (see Table 1). With or without licensing requirements, there are still principles of infection contagiousness that eclipse our ability to legislate.
- The fundamental concepts to keep in mind are that children are separated by age (see Table 2). Of necessity, this arrangement clusters susceptible children. The youngest children are cohorted and because they are immunologically and experientially naïve, any new infection has the ability to spread to every child.
- Small children are kept in relatively close environments, and hence the potential to spread infection by air, contact, or shared objects is enhanced. Studies introducing objects with genetically marked viruses on inanimate objects in daycare show that by the end of 8 hours, a majority of the children in the room are carrying the virus, and by the next day, half of their parents are also.
- Because children younger than 3 years are frequently in diapers, the opportunity for fecal–oral spread of organisms is high. Even with the best staff hygiene, children tend to have their hands in their mouths, then their mouths, then objects in the room. Without a 1:1 ratio of staff to child, it is impossible to prevent this potential transmission route.
- These children also need help with their toileting issues from the staff, and even with the best intentions, other children may be in various degrees of distress during a routine diapering episode. Thus, well-intentioned hygiene technique may be broken because of circumstances that are difficult for the staff to control.
- This potential for infection transmission can be partially overcome by separation of diaper changers and food handlers, and, in fact, many daycare centers actually have their food prepared elsewhere and delivered to the daycare by a unit separate from their own.
- Because of the potential for infections to spread among the children, consideration must be given to whether antibiotics are really required for an infection. In these close environments, with the increased frequency of infection, if antibiotics are used routinely there is considerable pressure for resistant organisms to survive and spread.

Infections in daycare children have become a subject of great importance. More and more children spend time in daycare, whether in a small family setting or a large daycare center (Table 1). Both parents are working, either for personal growth or for financial survival. There are also an increasing number of single parents who need daycare for their children. Thus, their children need to be cared for by someone else. Regardless of the type of daycare setting, these children are at increased risk of infection. Their immature and

12

undeveloped immune systems are placed in an environment where they are exposed to multiple and frequent infectious agents. This leads to a number of issues we need to understand so we can minimize the impact on the child, the other children in the daycare, and the parents.

Several principles are extremely important to understand the circumstances children encounter in daycare. Most crucial is that daycare centers by their nature cluster susceptible individuals (Table 2), children who are mostly immunologically naïve, so that when an infection is introduced into the daycare setting, it can eventually make the rounds of the entire room and possibly the facility. Then eventually (usually 2 years), enough new immunologically naïve children enter daycare, so when the same infection reappears, it can pass once again from child to child.

Another significant principle of infection in daycare is the close proximity of all of the participants, both children and adults (Table 3). Infections spread by the oral route can easily pass from individual to individual. And, although good hand-washing and diaper-changing hygiene are encouraged and indeed transpire most of the time, emergency falls and crying do occur that

can interrupt this preferred technique because of the demands to take care of the child.

Studies show that with the introduction of a marked virus on a toy to a daycare room of toddlers in the morning, it can be cultured from 80% of the children by the end of the day and 50% of the parents by the next morning. Obviously, transmission can be very rapid.

Generally, infants and toddlers in daycare have a new viral infection approximately every 3 to 4 weeks and manifest symptoms of illness approximately every 2 months. This repeated acquisition of infections may not allow the child's physiology to return to a steady state, so some children appear to be prone to otitis media.

And lastly, the frequency of illness and possible secondary bacterial complications make these children much more prone to antibiotic treatment, which makes the appearance of antibiotic-resistant organisms much more likely.

Expert Opinion on Management Issues

ACCEPTED INTERVENTIONS

If antibiotics are needed, using ones with the narrowest spectrum possible is preferred. The judicious use of

TABLE 1 Classification of Daycare

Type of Daycare	Number of Children	Licensing Required
Small family child-care homes	<7	Uncommon
Large family child-care homes	7–12	Occasional
Child-care center	>12 in nonresidential setting	Always

Adapted from American Academy of Pediatrics: Children in out-of-home child care. In Pickering LK (ed): 2003 Red Book. Elk Grove Village, Ill: American Academy of Pediatrics, 2003, p 124.

TABLE 2 Grouping of Children

Description	Age	No. Children per Room	Child-to-Staff Ratio
Infants	Up to 1 yr	10	3:1
Toddlers	12–35 mo	15	4:1
Preschoolers	36–59 mo	20	6:1
Schoolchildren	5–12 yr	25	8:1

Adapted from American Academy of Pediatrics: Children in out-of-home child care. In Pickering LK (ed): 2003 Red Book. Elk Grove Village, Ill: American Academy of Pediatrics, 2003, p 124.

TABLE 3 Modes of Transmission of Organisms in Child-Care Settings

Usual Route of Transmission	Bacteria	Viruses	Other
Fecal–oral	*Campylobacter, Clostridium difficile, Escherichia coli* O157:H7, *Salmonella, Shigella, Aeromonas, Plesiomonas*	Astroviruses, caliciviruses, enteric adenoviruses, enteroviruses, hepatitis A, rotavirus, Norwalk	*Cryptosporidium parvum, Enterobius vermicularis, Giardia lamblia*
Respiratory	*Bordetella pertussis, Haemophilus influenzae* type b, *Mycobacterium tuberculosis, Neisseria meningitides, Streptococcus pneumonia,* group A streptococcus	Adenovirus, influenza, measles, mumps, metapneumovirus, parainfluenza, parvovirus B19, respiratory syncytial virus, rhinovirus, rubella, varicella-zoster	—
Person-to-person	Group A streptococcus, *Staphylococcus aureus*	Herpes simplex, varicella-zoster	Agents causing pediculosis, scabies, and ringworm
Contact with body fluids	—	Cytomegalovirus, herpes simplex	—
Blood-borne	—	Hepatitis B, hepatitis C, HIV	—

HIV, human immunodeficiency virus.
Adapted from American Academy of Pediatrics: Children in out-of-home child care. In Pickering LK (ed): 2003 Red Book. Elk Grove Village, Ill: American Academy of Pediatrics, 2003, p 125.

BOX 1 Inclusion: No Reason to Exclude from Daycare

- URTI without fever or other significant constitutional symptoms
- Viral conjunctivitis
- Rash without fever
- HIV infection
- CMV infection
- HBV infection

CMV, cytomegalovirus; HBV, hepatitis B virus; HIV, human immunodeficiency virus; URTI, upper respiratory tract infection.
From American Academy of Pediatrics: Children in out-of-home child care. In Pickering LK (ed): 2003 Red Book. Elk Grove Village, Ill: American Academy of Pediatrics, 2003, pp 127, 128.

BOX 2 Exclusion: Reason to Exclude from Daycare

- Illness that requires care greater than available from staff present
- Fever, lethargy, irritability, shortness of breath, or crying that suggests significant illness
- Rash with constitutional symptoms unless determined to be noncontagious and does not require excess care
- Impetigo until 24 h of treatment (assumes sensitive to antibiotic)
- Group A streptococcal pharyngitis until 24 h on antibiotics
- Mouth sores with drooling (assumed to be viral and contagious)
- Purulent conjunctivitis: red with purulent discharge until adequately treated
- Head lice until after first treatment and no mobile lice are seen
- Scabies until after treatment
- Varicella while febrile or with vesicular lesions
- Pertussis until after 5 days of antibiotic treatment (14 days total required)
- Hepatitis A infections, until 1 wk after onset of symptoms of illness
- Tuberculosis until physician confirms child is noncontagious
- Diarrhea with blood or mucus
- *Shigella* or Shiga toxin–producing infections (*Escherichia coli* O157:H7) until two stool cultures are negative and diarrhea subsides
- Vomiting twice in last 24 h unless noninfectious

From American Academy of Pediatrics: Children in out-of-home child care. In Pickering LK (ed): 2003 Red Book. Elk Grove Village, Ill: American Academy of Pediatrics, 2003, pp 127, 128.

BOX 3 Controlling Infection in Daycare

- Hand washing between every child encounter
- Separate personnel for food handling and other child-care contact (e.g., diaper changing)
- Food preparation in a room separate from where children frequent (or have it catered)
- Continually maintaining adequate immunization (not just at admission to daycare)
- Considering hepatitis A vaccine (presently approved for 2 years of age and older)
- Exclusion of children with specific diseases (see Box 2)
- Cohorting of sick children at the site
- Antibiotic treatment when indicated (including prophylaxis)
- Facility closed/accepting no new children until disease subsides if necessary

From American Academy of Pediatrics: Children in out-of-home child care. In Pickering LK (ed): 2003 Red Book. Elk Grove Village, Ill: American Academy of Pediatrics, 2003, pp 135–137.

BOX 4 Immunizations* for Children in Daycare

- Diphtheria, tetanus toxoids, and acellular pertussis (DTaP)
- Diphtheria
- Pertussis
- Tetanus
- Polio
- Hepatitis B
- Mumps, measles, rubella (MMR)
- Varicella
- Influenza (yearly)
- Possibly hepatitis A

*These immunizations need to be current at the time of admission and kept current after admission.
From American Academy of Pediatrics: Children in out-of-home child care. In Pickering LK (ed): 2003 Red Book. Elk Grove Village, Ill: American Academy of Pediatrics, 2003, pp 135–137.

---

antibiotics is vital in daycare centers. With the potential for multiple contacts, the liberal use of antibiotics increases the likelihood of selection of resistant organisms.

Symptomatic treatment of most gastrointestinal illnesses is preferred. Children with organisms that shed Shiga toxin (*Shigella* and *Escherichia coli* O157:H7) should be excluded from daycare until they have two confirmed negative stool cultures to prevent spread of these organisms.

Most viral illnesses are contagious for several days before symptoms manifest, so exclusion during the symptomatic period is not warranted unless symptoms are such that the child requires more care than the staff ratios permit.

Separation of age groups may prevent spread of some infections. Older children with antibody to certain diseases may not get sick themselves but may be carrying an organism that can be devastating to younger children. This was the case with *Haemophilus influenzae* type b (Hib) before the use of the conjugate Hib vaccine.

Children should not be in contact with reptiles in the daycare setting. The carriage of *Salmonella* species by reptiles is extremely high. The diarrheal illness caused by reptiles can produce blood and mucus. Antibiotic treatment is not usually warranted unless fever or young age suggests it is required. Treatment may prolong the carrier state after the initial infection, so the child's stool may be contagious for a longer period of time.

Viral infections, although frequent in and of themselves, do not require that a child be restricted from daycare (parvovirus, respiratory syncytial virus [RSV], rhinovirus, parainfluenza, metapneumovirus, coronavirus, adenovirus, rotavirus, astrovirus, cytomegalovirus [CMV], Epstein-Barr virus [EBV], human immunodeficiency virus [HIV]). However, some infections, such as hepatitis A and varicella, require that

BOX 5 Immunizations/Screening for Daycare Employees

- Tetanus-diphtheria (toxoid; adult type) (Td)
- Diphtheria booster
- Tetanus booster
- Mumps, measles, rubella (MMR)
- Polio
- Influenza (yearly)
- Hepatitis B
- Varicella if no previous infection
- Tuberculosis (PPD [purified protein derivative] screening for tuberculosis yearly)
- Possibly hepatitis A

From American Academy of Pediatrics: Children in out-of-home child care. In Pickering LK (ed): 2003 Red Book. Elk Grove Village, Ill: American Academy of Pediatrics, 2003, pp 134, 135.

those around them receive prophylaxis (vaccination with or without immunoglobulin) if they themselves are seronegative.

Pharyngitis caused by group A β-hemolytic streptococcus should be treated, and the child should not be readmitted until after 24 hours of antibiotics. Young children with streptococcal pharyngitis may manifest abdominal and head pain rather than sore throat.

Being up to date on immunizations is the most useful preventative strategy. Hib vaccine virtually eliminates *H. influenzae* type b infection. Conjugate pneumococcal vaccine has greatly reduced bacterial sepsis in children and somewhat reduced the incidence of bacterial otitis media. Varicella vaccine has greatly reduced chickenpox disease and almost eliminated significant disease from this virus. This vaccine can be used in the susceptible child even after the first few days of exposure to reduce the disease caused by the wild virus. Rotavirus vaccine, when available, significantly reduces the morbidity caused by rotavirus disease.

Head lice (pediculosis) and scabies (*Sarcoptes scabiei* mite) in children require keeping them out of daycare until they have completed treatment. Scabies requires a 5% permethrin cream (1% lindane and 10% crotamiton are also options) left on overnight. A second course occasionally is required. Consideration should also be given as to whether the child also needs treatment for impetigo if excoriation from the itching is extensive.

Impetigo in daycare children is an increasing problem. Impetigo caused by *Staphylococcus aureus* is increasingly resistant to antibiotics. In some areas, up to 50% of the *Staphylococcus* isolated is methicillin-resistant *S. aureus* (MRSA). If initial treatment with amoxicillin-clavulanate or cephalexin does not work, culture, along with a change to treatment with clindamycin or trimethoprim-sulfamethoxazole, is sometimes warranted.

URGENT INTERVENTIONS

Few emergencies in daycare require immediate intervention. Of utmost importance is the presence of a child in daycare who has a meningococcal disease. Once the diagnosis is certain, all children and adults in close contact with the patient should receive chemoprophylaxis (rifampin, ciprofloxacin, and ceftriaxone are all appropriate). Close contact is considered household members/contacts, daycare classmates, those who have shared water glasses/drinks, or other intimate contact. Casual contact or no direct exposure to oral secretions excludes one from needing chemoprophylaxis. *H. influenzae* type b is rarely seen today, but if a case is present in the daycare center, the same rules would apply. The youngest children may be in various stages of completing their Hib vaccinations, so chemoprophylaxis is warranted unless the Hib series is complete.

Hepatitis A exposure in daycare, either from a child or adult, warrants immunoglobulin therapy, and if the child is at least 2 years of age, consideration for hepatitis A vaccination (two injections required 6 months apart). Children are frequently asymptomatic when infected, so they are a danger to their parents if the infection goes undetected.

Varicella is increasingly less frequent, and the immunization can be given to children 1 year and older, but if a child is older than 1 year and exposed to wild-type varicella and has not had the immunization, it can be given within the first 1 to 4 days and modification of the natural disease would be expected.

Tuberculosis (TB) in children is uncommon, and most infants do not have a productive cough, but their caregivers can easily infect these young children and need to be screened yearly. If an adult or child is found to have TB, all children need to be screened with a purified protein derivative (PPD) and monitored closely. Anyone positive for TB with a productive cough needs to be sent home until he or she is no longer contagious after appropriate antibiotic treatment. Children with TB are more likely to manifest systemic illness because they do not compartmentalize the infection just to their lungs.

If pertussis is diagnosed in the daycare, everyone needs to receive antibiotic prophylaxis, and the index case should not return to daycare until after 5 days of appropriate antibiotic therapy.

CONTROVERSIAL INTERVENTIONS

Although purulent conjunctivitis is a reason for antibiotic treatment and exclusion from daycare until improvement, viral conjunctivitis is not a reason for exclusion. Many other children in the daycare have the same viral illness, whether or not they manifest conjunctivitis, and antibiotic eye drops do nothing to change the course of disease in the daycare or the disease in the child. Nevertheless, this exclusion seems to be a common daycare requirement.

Otitis media is a common complication of an upper respiratory infection, and a certain percentage do go on to be bacterial infections, but immediate antibiotic treatment is not always necessary. Pus, erythema, and a bulging eardrum are more likely to be bacterial, and most would initiate antibiotic treatment. Fluid behind and mild erythema of the eardrum may profit from watchful waiting.

Common Pitfalls

- Not separating food handlers from diaper changers in the daycare setting
- Not having children adequately immunized and continuously monitoring the immunizations received
- Not washing hands after every child encounter
- Not washing with 10% bleach after diaper changing or other body fluid contamination
- Not having adequate staff to handle age and activities of children
- Not having adequately trained personnel to carry out all the precautions just described
- Not keeping children of different ages separated as much as possible

Communication and Counseling

The important information for parents and daycare centers to understand is that young children are repeatedly colonized with viruses and bacteria. Bacteria in general follow a virus introduction, generally in the pharynx. Some children manifest more symptoms than others when they are ill. The amount of fever in particular can vary considerably among children with the same illness. Thus, sending children home to avoid infecting others is rarely beneficial because it was during the prodrome that the children were the most contagious. So the first principle is to send children home when the care they warrant is more than can be provided.

The second principle is that children pass infections from child to child, but daycare providers can be accomplices if they do not wash adequately after every child encounter. Separating the food handlers from the diaper changers is the ultimate separation. Because each child cannot have one provider (as may occur at home), hand washing is absolutely essential.

For the few infections that do need isolation (see earlier), the children should be sent home until there is relatively little chance of their being contagious with that organism.

Lastly, keeping staff and children appropriately immunized will keep vaccine-preventable infections to a minimum.

SUGGESTED READINGS

1. American Academy of Pediatrics: Children in out-of-home child care. In Pickering LK (ed): 2003 Red Book. Elk Grove Village, Ill: American Academy of Pediatrics, 2003, pp 123–137. **This summary of infections by the American Academy of Pediatrics is the pediatrician's guide to how to handle daycare infections. Updated frequently.**
2. Jiang X, Dai X, Goldblatt S, et al: Pathogen transmission in child care settings studied by using a cauliflower virus DNA as a surrogate marker. J Infect Dis 177(4):881–888, 1998. **Description of the rapid transmission of a surrogate marker virus in daycare setting.**
3. Pickering LK, Bartlett AV, Reves RR, et al: Asymptomatic rotavirus before and after rotavirus diarrhea in children in daycare centers. J Pediatr 112:361–365, 1988. **Description of the asymptomatic carriage common in daycare. Although this article describes rotavirus, it is true of multiple other pathogens.**
4. Reves RR, Morrow AL, Bartlett AV, et al: Child daycare as a risk factor for acute diarrheal disease. Am J Epidemiol 137:97–107, 1993. **Review of the risk for diarrheal diseases in daycare.**
5. Reves RR, Pickering LK: Impact of child daycare on infectious diseases in adults. Infect Dis Clin North Am 6(1):239–250, 1992. **Review of the infections that adults may acquire from children in daycare.**
6. Wald ER, Guerra N, Byers C: Frequency and severity of infections in daycare. Three-year follow-up. J Pediatr 118:509–514, 1991. **Description of how common respiratory infections are in the daycare environment.**

12

13

Hematology

Iron-Deficiency Anemia

Marianne McPherson and Jennifer Tender

KEY CONCEPTS

- Iron-deficiency anemia is a late manifestation of a prolonged iron deficit.
- Children ages 1 to 2 years and adolescent girls are at highest risk for iron-deficiency anemia.
- Iron deficiency is associated with developmental delays, behavioral disturbances, and learning impairments that may be irreversible.
- Dietary counseling and screening are the keys to prevention and identification of iron deficiency in infants and children.
- Children with mild to moderate anemia may be presumed to have iron deficiency without other testing and started on iron supplementation if they are at high risk due to their age or dietary history.
- If a patient fails to respond to iron therapy or the history does not suggest iron deficiency, an alternate explanation for anemia should be considered.

Iron deficiency is the most common pediatric hematologic disorder and nutritional deficiency worldwide and can result in significant and possibly irreversible developmental and behavioral consequences. Iron deficiency is often detected only after the development of iron-deficiency anemia, a late finding that occurs after a prolonged period of total body iron depletion. In the United States, the prevalence of iron-deficiency anemia has declined over the past two decades because of the introduction of iron-fortified infant formulas and cereals. Toddlers and adolescent girls, however, continue to be at high risk because of their rapid growth and inadequate iron intake as well as blood loss from menses among adolescent girls.

Iron deficiency affects 7% of children ages 1 to 2 years, 9% of nonpregnant girls 12 to 15 years old, and 16% of nonpregnant girls 16 to 19 years old (Fig. 1). In contrast, iron-deficiency anemia occurs in only 2% of toddlers and adolescent girls, making anemia a relatively insensitive indicator of iron deficiency.

In addition to being an essential element for oxygen transport and storage, iron is also a cofactor for enzymes controlling cellular respiration, central nervous system (CNS) myelination, and dopamine synthesis. As the body becomes iron depleted, iron is prioritized to assist with hemoglobin synthesis at the expense of its other cellular functions, allowing neurologic damage to occur before anemia is noted.

In the initial stages, iron stores in the reticuloendothelial cells of the bone marrow and liver are depleted. Ferritin, the major iron-storage protein of the body, declines in direct relation to the amount of stored iron. Serum ferritin accurately reflects total body stores of iron in the absence of liver disease, infection, and inflammatory disease. As stores continue to be depleted, the serum level of iron decreases. The incorporation of iron is a rate-limiting step in the synthesis of heme from its precursor protoporphyrin. As serum iron decreases, zinc becomes incorporated into protoporphyrin in place of iron. Laboratories measure this compound as either zinc protoporphyrin (ZPP) or free erythrocyte protoporphyrin (FEP), a molecule created in vitro when zinc is removed from ZPP. In an attempt to compensate for low serum iron, the liver synthesizes more transferrin, the body's major iron-transport protein. The serum's total iron-binding capacity (TIBC), which reflects the availability of iron-binding sites on transferrin, increases, and the percent saturation of transferrin decreases. When iron binding is decreased, hemoglobin synthesis is impaired, leading to the development of a microcytic hypochromic anemia. This ineffective process of hematopoiesis results in poikilocytosis, a wide variation in size and shape of the red blood cells (RBCs), reflected by a high RBC distribution width (RW).

Children with iron-deficiency anemia may have irritability, decreased exercise tolerance, weakness, and pica. Many with iron deficiency and iron-deficiency anemia show few or no signs or symptoms (Table 1).

Iron deficiency is rare in full-term infants younger than 6 months of age even if there is inadequate iron intake because of significant iron stores accumulated in the liver and bone marrow during gestation. Approximately 80% of these stores are acquired during the third trimester, leaving preterm infants more susceptible to iron deficiency.

Expert Opinion on Management Issues

PRIMARY PREVENTION

Because of the potential for developmental, cognitive, and behavioral harm, the goal of pediatricians should be

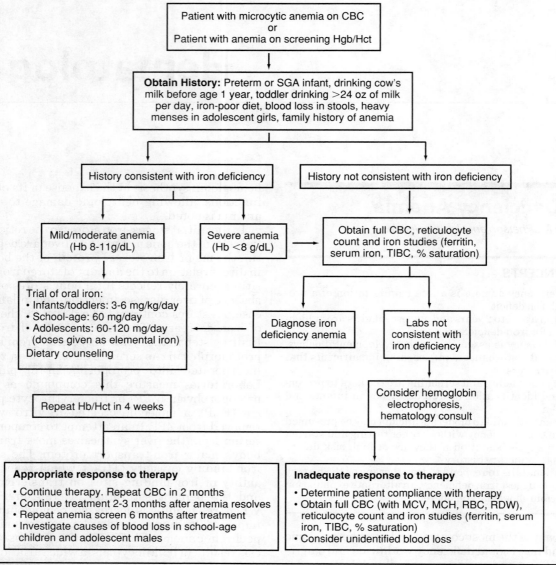

FIGURE 1. Diagnosis and management of iron-deficiency anemia. CBC, complete blood count; Hct, hematocrit; Hgb, hemoglobin; labs, laboratory findings; MCH, mean cell hemoglobin; MCV, mean corpuscular volume; RBC, red blood cell; RDW, red (blood cell) distribution width; SGA, small for gestational age; TIBC, total iron-binding capacity. (Adapted from Lane P, Nuss R: Microcytic anemia. In Berman S, (ed): Pediatric Decision Making. Philadelphia: BC Decker, 1996.)

to prevent iron deficiency. To reduce the risk of iron deficiency in infancy, exclusive breast-feeding for the first 6 months of life should be encouraged. Although breast milk has less iron than formula has (0.5 mg/L in breast milk versus 10–12.8 mg/L in iron-fortified formula), approximately half of the iron in breast milk is absorbed, while only 7% to 12% of iron in cow's milk formula and 1% to 7% of the iron in soy-based formula is absorbed. Infants who are partially breast-fed or receive no breast milk should always receive iron-fortified formula, as the intake of nonfortified formulas or whole cow's milk places infants at high risk of iron deficiency.

By the age of 6 months, when full-term infants' maternally derived iron stores have been depleted, breast-fed infants need supplementation with iron-rich foods such as fortified cereals and/or meats or iron drops to provide an additional 1 mg/kg/day of elemental iron. To enhance absorption of dietary iron, infants should also receive at least one serving per day of food rich in vitamin C. Preterm infants or infants of low birth weight, in whom iron stores are depleted earlier, require a greater *total* amount of iron (approximately 4 mg/kg/day of elemental iron). Therefore, in addition to breast milk or formula, preterm infants' diets should be supplemented with approximately 2 mg/kg per day of elemental iron until 12 months of age.

In preschool children ages 1 to 5 years, pediatricians should assess dietary iron intake and emphasize limiting intake of cow's milk to 16 to 24 ounces per day. Cow's milk inhibits absorption of iron because of its low iron and high calcium content. In addition, milk protein can irritate the GI tract, causing occult blood loss.

TABLE 1 Laboratory Findings and Signs/Symptoms Associated with Iron Deficiency and Iron-Deficiency Anemia

	Iron Depletion	Iron Deficiency	Iron Deficiency Anemia	Severe Iron Deficiency Anemia
Ferritin	Decreased	Decreased	Very low	Very low
Serum iron	Normal	Decreased	Decreased	Very low
TIBC	Normal	Increased	Increased	Increased
% saturation	Normal	Decreased	Decreased	Decreased
FEP or ZPP	Normal	Increased	Increased	Increased
Hemoglobin	Normal	Normal	Decreased	Very low
Symptoms	None	Early cognitive deficit	Mild cognitive deficits	Cognitive deficits
			Decreased exercise tolerance	Decreased exercise tolerance
			Weakness	Weakness
			Pica	Pica
Signs	None	None	Mild pallor	Pallor
				Systolic murmurs
				Tachycardia
				Cardiac dilatation
				Blue sclerae
				Koilonychia
				Angular stomatitis

FEP, free erythrocyte protoporphyrin; TIBC, total iron-binding capacity; ZPP, zinc protoporphyrin.

SECONDARY PREVENTION

Although anemia is a late indicator of iron deficiency, use of earlier indicators for screening is often prohibited by cost and feasibility. In communities with significant rates of iron deficiency anemia or a patient population with risk factors such as low income or recent immigration, universal screening for anemia is recommended for infants between the ages of 9 and 12 months and again 6 months later. Preterm or low birth weight infants should be screened by the age of 6 months. In communities or pediatric practices that have less than a 5% rate of anemia among children 1 to 2 years old, physicians may selectively screen only infants with risk factors for anemia. Children with risk factors include:

- Infants who were preterm or low birth weight
- Infants who received nonfortified formula or cow's milk before the age of 12 months
- Breast-fed infants who did not receive adequate supplemental iron after 6 months
- Children with medical problems such as chronic disease or inflammation, blood loss, or restricted diet
- Children taking medications that interfere with iron absorption, such as tetracycline, antacids, or calcium supplements

Selective screening should occur at the same ages as universal screening.

Past the age of 2 years, the prevalence of iron deficiency declines; therefore, most children do not require screening until adolescence. Screening should be considered in 2 to 12-year-olds, however, who have low dietary intake of iron, excessive milk ingestion, or a history of iron deficiency.

The Centers for Disease Control and Prevention (CDC) recommends screening all females older than 12 years for anemia every 5 to 10 years or annually if at high risk for anemia because of menorrhagia, low dietary iron, or history of anemia. The American Academy of Pediatrics recommends annual screening of all menstruating girls and one screen of adolescent boys during their peak growth spurt.

TREATMENT

When mild to moderate anemia (defined by hemoglobin approximately 8 to 11 g/dL) is discovered, a pediatrician may make a presumptive diagnosis of iron-deficiency and initiate supplementation with 3 to 6 mg/kg per day of elemental iron (Table 2). This course is appropriate as long as the patient's age and diet are consistent with an increased risk of iron deficiency and the patient does not have a known hematologic disease. Hemoglobin and hematocrit or a complete blood count (CBC) should be retested after 4 weeks of therapy. An increase in hemoglobin (Hb) of 1 g/dL or an increase in hematocrit of 3% is considered diagnostic of iron-deficiency anemia without further workup. Iron therapy should then be continued and a hemoglobin or hematocrit rechecked two months later. After the anemia resolves, the patient should continue iron therapy for another 2 to 3 months to replete the body's iron stores. A final hemoglobin or hematocrit should be rechecked 6 months after successful treatment. If the patient does not show an adequate response to initial treatment, other causes of microcytic anemia such as a thalassemia syndrome, lead toxicity, or other hemoglobinopathy must be considered (Table 3). Practitioners should also consider poor compliance or unidentified blood loss as reasons for treatment failure.

In patients with severe anemia (defined as hemoglobin less than 8 g/dL) or patients with adequate iron intake, it is appropriate to obtain iron studies (serum ferritin, serum iron, TIBC, and % iron saturation), a CBC (with red blood cell count [RBC], mean corpuscular volume [MCV], and RDW), and reticulocyte count to rule out other diagnoses. Quantitative hemoglobin

TABLE 2 Medication Table for Iron Preparations

Generic Name (Trade Name)	Dosage	Maximum Dose of Elemental Iron	Dosage Formulations	Relative Cost	Common Adverse Reactions	Comments
Ferrous sulfate (20% elemental iron) (Fer-in-Sol) Rx, (Feosol) Rx	Preterm infants: PO: 2–4 mg elem Fe/kg/day div qd-bid Children: PO: 3–6 mg elem Fe/kg/day div qd-tid Adults: PO: 60 mg elem Fe bid-qid	Neonates: 15 mg/day Adult: 240 mg/day	Drops: 125 mg (15 mg Fe)/0.6 mL, Syrup: 90 mg (18 mg Fe)/5 mL, Elixir: 220 mg (44 mg Fe)/5 mL Tablet: 195 mg (39 mg Fe), 300 mg (60 mg Fe), 324 mg (65 mg Fe), Capsule: 250 mg (50 mg Fe)	$	Constipation, dark stools, nausea, epigastric pain. Liquid preparations may stain teeth.	All liquid preparations contain alcohol except Fer-in-Sol drops.
Ferrous gluconate (12% elemental iron) (Fergon) Rx	Children: PO: 3–6 mg elem Fe/kg/day div qd-tid Adults: PO: 60 mg elem Fe bid-qid	Neonates: 15 mg/day Adults: 240 mg/day	Elixir: 300 mg (34 mg Fe)/5 mL Tablet: 240 mg (27 mg Fe), 300 mg (34 mg Fe), 320 mg (37 mg Fe), 325 mg (38 mg Fe), Capsule: 86 mg (10 mg Fe) Sustained-release capsule: 320 mg (37 mg Fe)	$	Constipation, dark stools, nausea, epigastric pain. Liquid preparations may stain teeth.	
Ferrous bis-glycinate chelate/polysaccharide-iron complex (Niferex) Rx	Children: PO: 3–6 mg elem Fe/kg/day div qd-tid Adults: PO: 60 mg elem Fe bid-qid	Neonates: 15 mg/day Adults: 240 mg/day	Tablet: 50 mg Fe Capsule: 150 mg Fe Elixir: 100 mg Fe/5 mL	$$	Constipation, dark stools, nausea, epigastric pain. Liquid preparations may stain teeth.	Less constipation and better absorption.

bid, twice daily; div, divided; elem, elemental; Fe, iron; PO, orally; qd, every day; qid, four times a day; Rx, prescription.

TABLE 3 Microcytic Anemias

Diagnosis	MCV	RBC Number	RDW	Ferritin	TIBC
Iron-deficiency anemia	Low or normal	Low	High (>14%)	Low	High
Thalassemia trait	Low	Normal to high	Normal (<14%)	Normal	Normal
Viral suppression or Chronic disease	Normal or low	Low	Normal	High	Low
Lead poisoning	Low or normal	Low	Normal to high	Normal or high	Normal

MCV, mean corpuscular volume; RBC, red blood cell; RDW, red (blood cell) distribution width; TIBC, total iron-binding capacity.

electrophoresis may also be indicated based on history and lab values. Consider referring these patients to a hematologist for further evaluation.

Common Pitfalls

- Failure to screen at-risk infants and children for iron deficiency prevents identification of an avoidable cause of developmental delay.
- Iron deficiency is not the only cause of microcytic anemia. If a patient's anemia fails to respond to iron therapy, other causes such as thalassemia minor, lead poisoning, or chronic disease should be considered (see Table 3).
- In patients with anemia as a result of thalassemia syndrome, sickle cell disease, or other hemoglobinopathy, iron deficiency should not be diagnosed and the child should not be given iron therapy.
- Iron-deficiency anemia in school-age children, adolescent males, and other children with adequate dietary iron may be due to unidentified sources of GI blood loss such as a bleeding Meckel diverticulum, inflammatory bowel disease, peptic ulcer, or hookworm or other parasites. Rarely, pulmonary hemosiderosis may be an unidentified source of blood loss.

Communication and Counseling

Patients and parents or caretakers need nutritional counseling on dietary sources of iron. There are two forms of dietary iron—heme iron, found in meat, fish, and poultry, and nonheme iron found in foods such as beans, spinach, and dark green vegetables, tofu, dried fruit, and iron-fortified cereals. Heme iron is absorbed two to three times more readily than nonheme iron. Iron absorption is enhanced by vitamin C and is inhibited by calcium, tea, and bran.

Iron deficiency in infancy and early childhood is associated with delays in motor and mental development and an increased risk of behavioral problems that may persist into later childhood despite correction of anemia. In later childhood and adolescence, iron deficiency has been associated with lower performance on tests of memory, verbal learning, and mathematics. Parents need to be aware of the importance of both treating and preventing iron deficiency to avoid negative impacts on development, learning, and behavior.

ACKNOWLEDGEMENTS

The authors wish to thank Dr. Naomi Luban for reviewing this manuscript.

SUGGESTED READINGS

1. Centers for Disease Control and Prevention: Iron deficiency—United States, 1999–2000. MMWR Morb Mortal Wkly Rep 51:897–899, 2002. **This is the most recent report from the National Health and Nutrition Examination Survey (NHANES 1999–2000) on the prevalence of iron deficiency by age and sex in the United States.**
2. Centers for Disease Control and Prevention: Recommendations to prevent and control iron deficiency in the United States. MMWR Recomm Rep 47(RR–3):1–29, 1998. **These are the most recent guidelines from the CDC on prevention, screening, and treatment of iron deficiency.**
3. Idjradinata P, Pollitt E: Reversal of developmental delays in iron-deficient anaemic infants treated with iron. Lancet 341:1–4, 1993. **This paper shows improvement in mental and motor test scores in infants with iron-deficiency anemia after treatment with ferrous sulfate.**
4. Iron deficiency. In Kleinman RE (ed): Pediatric Nutrition Handbook, 5th ed. Elk Grove Village, Ill: American Academy of Pediatrics, 2004, pp 299–312. **This chapter provides information on causes and consequences of iron deficiency, diagnosis, and AAP recommendations on dietary prevention, screening, and treatment.**
5. Zlotkin S: Clinical Nutrition: The role of nutrition in the prevention of iron deficiency anemia in infants, children and adolescents. CMAJ 168:59–63, 2003. **This paper describes the adverse effects of anemia and provides dietary guidelines for the prevention and treatment of iron deficiency.**

13

Megaloblastic Anemia

Yih-Ming Yang

KEY CONCEPTS

- Megaloblastic anemia is characterized by megaloblastic changes in the bone marrow due to unbalanced biosynthesis in the nucleus and cytoplasm secondary to defects in deoxyribonucleic acid (DNA) synthesis.
- The hematologic features of megaloblastic anemia (macrocytic anemia accompanied by various degrees of neutropenia and thrombocytopenia) are merely a manifestation of a systemic disease caused by an underlying defect in DNA synthesis.
- Not all erythrocyte macrocytosis is caused by vitamin B_{12} or folate deficiency.

KEY CONCEPTS—cont'd

- The type of vitamin deficiency responsible for megaloblastic anemia should be precisely identified in order to provide proper replacement therapy and prevent disastrous consequences.

Megaloblastic anemia is a group of disorders characterized by macrocytic anemia secondary to megaloblastic changes in the bone marrow. Megaloblastic changes are hematologic features of asynchrony between nuclear and cytoplasmic maturation due to the arrest of nuclear maturation while normal cytoplasmic ribonucleic acid (RNA) production and protein synthesis continue. The unbalanced biosynthesis in the nucleus and cytoplasm affects not only hematopoiesis but also all proliferating cells. It is prudent to understand that hematologic features of megaloblastic anemia are merely manifestations of a systemic disease caused by an underlying DNA defect.

It is also important to recognize the difference between erythrocyte macrocytosis and megaloblastic anemia. Erythrocyte macrocytosis is a hematologic finding that simply indicates that the size of red blood cells is larger than normal. Megaloblastic anemia is a state of megaloblastic changes that gives specific hematologic features. Common causes of macrocytic anemia are shown in Box 1.

Clinicians should be aware that clinical manifestations of megaloblastic anemia in infants and children caused by deficiencies of either vitamin B_{12} or folate are often subtle and nonspecific. Decreased activity, loss of appetite with minimal weight loss, nausea, and constipation may be observed. Infants may present with failure to thrive or delay in mental development. A neurologic syndrome of vitamin B_{12} deficiency, known as *subacute combined degeneration of the spinal cord*, may be present without evidence of anemia and with serum vitamin B_{12} level above the range of deficiency.

Expert Opinion on Management Issues

ACCEPTED INTERVENTIONS

Patients presenting with severe anemia may not require transfusion unless the degree of anemia is profound or there are associated signs of circulatory collapse or cardiopulmonary decompensation. It is important to identify the cause of megaloblastic anemia and to define the underlying nature of the deficiency. This makes it possible to eliminate some underlying causes of the disease, such as discontinuation of drugs that interfere with vitamin metabolism, or treatment of parasite infestation or bacteria overgrowth in the terminal ileum that result in defective vitamin absorption. It is also critical to precisely identify the type of vitamin deficiency that is responsible for megaloblastic anemia. An approach to diagnosis of megaloblastic anemia is shown in Box 2. This allows for proper vitamin replacement therapy and prevents disastrous consequences. Folic acid therapy should not be administered to patients with megaloblastic anemia until a diagnosis of folic acid deficiency is established.

BOX 1   Common Causes of Macrocytic Anemia

Non-megaloblastic Macrocytic Anemia

- Hemolytic anemia, post-hemorrhagic anemia
- Liver disease, obstructive jaundice
- Post splenectomy
- Hypothyroidism
- Down syndrome
- Aplastic anemia, Diamond-Blackfan anemia

Megaloblastic Anemia

- Vitamin B_{12} (cobalamin) deficiency
- Dietary insufficiency
- Pernicious anemia (with presence of anti-IF antibody)
- Absence of or abnormal intrinsic factor
- Abnormal absorption of B_{12}/intrinsic factor complex caused by surgical resection of ileum, regional enteritis, celiac disease, tropical sprue, Imerslund syndrome, or competitive parasites or bacteria
- Transcobalamin II deficiency
- Metabolic disorders caused by nitrous oxide inhalation or inborn enzyme errors
- Folic acid deficiency
- Dietary insufficiency
- Increased requirement in chronic hemolytic anemia during infancy and pregnancy and in patients on anticonvulsants
- Abnormal absorption caused by sprues or inherited defects
- Antifolates such as methotrexate and pyrimethamine
- Inherited defects of folate metabolism such as dihydrofolate reductase deficiency

Other Causes

- Drug interference with DNA metabolism such as 6-mercaptopurine and hydroxyurea
- Metabolic disorders such as orotic aciduria
- Secondary to HIV infection

IF, intrinsic factor.

BOX 2   Approach to Diagnosis of Megaloblastic Anemia

Initial Approach

- High index of suspicion for unexplained clinical manifestations that may be associated with megaloblastic anemia
- Recognition of hematologic patterns of megaloblastic anemia based on CBC, included MCV, and peripheral blood smear findings
- Bone marrow examination
- Serum vitamin B_{12} and folic acid levels
- Diet history, maternal history, medication and surgical history

Specific Tests

- Serum methylmalonic acid; elevated in vitamin B_{12} deficiency
- Serum homocysteine; elevated in vitamin B_{12} or folic acid deficiency
- Reticulocyte count, serum lactate dehydrogenase, and iron, for follow-up of initial therapeutic response
- For undetermined causes: Further testing for less-common causes of megaloblastic anemia, such as inborn error of metabolism and HIV infection

CBC, complete blood count; HIV, human immunodeficiency virus; MCV, mean corpuscular volume.

The use of therapeutic doses of folic acid for patients with vitamin B_{12} deficiency may produce transient and partial response. However, the neurologic complications of vitamin B_{12} deficiency will not be corrected and may be aggravated by folic acid treatment.

URGENT INTERVENTIONS

Infants presenting with severe megaloblastic anemia may be critically ill. These patients often require emergency treatment before a definitive diagnosis is established. A 24-hour urine sample for the measurement of methylmalonic acid and homocysteine, as well as a blood sample for serum folate and vitamin B_{12} concentration and red cell folate concentration should be performed immediately. A portion of the urine sample should be stored for further testing. Patients then can be treated with daily parenteral vitamin B_{12} (250 μg) and folic acid (3–5 mg). If there is no clinical response in 2 to 3 days, other rare DNA synthesis defects, such as orotic aciduria, should be considered. Administration of large doses of vitamin B_{12} to a patient with profound anemia may result in severe hypokalemia. Providing sufficient potassium and beginning treatment with an initial low dose of vitamin B_{12} (0.2 μg/kg up to 10 μg/kg per day for 2 days) are recommended to prevent this life-threatening complication. Cerebral vascular accident following treatment for profound anemia has been reported. No specific measures to prevent this complication have been established. A judicious use of a small volume of red cell transfusions to achieve partial correction of the profound anemia as part of initial treatment should be considered.

Treatment

VITAMIN B_{12} DEFICIENCY

Because vitamin B_{12} is widely present in foods, deficiency of vitamin B_{12} caused by dietary insufficiency is rare and is easily treated with dietary supplementation. Most cases of vitamin B_{12} deficiency are caused by inadequate absorption due either to absent or abnormal intrinsic factor or to a defect at the terminal ileal absorption site. A treatment outline for vitamin B_{12} deficiency is presented in Box 3. Parenteral administration of B_{12} is generally required for these patients throughout life. Vitamin B_{12} (cyanocobalamin/hydroxocobalamin) is administered in a dose of 0.2 μg/kg up to 10 μg subcutaneously daily for 2 to 7 days. A larger dose of vitamin B_{12}, 1000 μg subcutaneously, is then given daily for 7 days starting 1 week after initiation of treatment, followed by 100 μg subcutaneously once a week for 1 month. Because the optimal treatment doses of vitamin B_{12} in children are not well established, patients should be followed closely to ensure good response to treatment in the first week, particularly in the first 2 to 3 days. Follow-up with serum concentration of vitamin B_{12} is necessary.

Vitamin B_{12}, 100 μg subcutaneously, should be given monthly for life to patients with pernicious anemia or congenital absence of nonfunctional intrinsic factor.

A defect at the terminal ileal absorption site is generally the result of resection of the ileum or diseases

---

BOX 3 **Treatment of Megaloblastic Anemia Caused by Vitamin B_{12} or Folic Acid Deficiency**

Vitamin B_{12} Deficiency
- Vitamin B_{12} (cyanocobalamin) 0.2 μg/kg up to 10 μg SC qd for 7 days
- Verify laboratory and clinical response in 2 to 7 days.
- Follow with 100 μg SC qd for 1 week, then 100 μg SC qw for 1 month.
- For patients who cannot absorb vitamin B_{12} from the diet, vitamin B_{12} should be continued at 100 μg SC monthly.

Transcobalamin Deficiency
- Vitamin B_{12} (cyanocobalamin) 100 μg weekly

Folic Acid Deficiency
- Folic acid 200 μg PO qd
- Verify initial laboratory and clinical response during the first week of therapy.
- Follow with 1 mg PO qd.

Combined Vitamin B_{12} and Folic Acid Deficiency
- Vitamin B_{12} 0.2 μg/kg up to 10 μg SC qd for 2–7 days
- Folic acid 1 mg PO qd for 7 days
- Continue with both agents, following the regimen described for individual deficiencies.
- For patients with profound anemia, see the section on urgent intervention.

PO, orally; qd, daily; qw, weekly; SC, subcutaneously.

---

involving the terminal ileum such as regional enteritis. Because vitamin B_{12} malabsorption may occur after resection of a small section of ileum, prophylactic use of vitamin B_{12} may be indicated after an ileal resection or bypass procedure. In patients with small bowel bacterial overgrowth, vitamin B_{12} deficiency may be temporarily corrected by administration of tetracyclines or other appropriate antibiotics. Surgical resection of proximal small bowel lesions is frequently required to eliminate the bacterial competition for dietary B_{12}. In fish tapeworm–induced megaloblastic anemia, both expulsion of fish tapeworm and administration of vitamin B_{12} are needed to effectively correct the anemia. Treatment with parenteral vitamin B_{12} for patients with Imerslund syndrome can correct anemia but not proteinuria. The institution of a gluten-free diet can manage malabsorption of vitamin B_{12} caused by celiac disease.

Patients with transcobalamin II deficiency develop more severe anemia in early infancy compared to those with other causes of vitamin B_{12} deficiency. Large parenteral doses of vitamin B_{12} ranging from 500 to 1000 μg 2 to 3 times weekly are generally required to produce adequate response and maintain optimal control of deficiency. Some patients with methylmalonic aciduria secondary to cobalamin coenzyme defects may respond to massive doses of parenteral vitamin B_{12} (1000 to 2000 μg daily). Intrauterine treatment can be given for congenital methylmalonic aciduria when the condition is diagnosed prenatally and is known to be vitamin B_{12} responsive by family history. For patients with mutase deficiency induced methylmalonic aciduria, protein restriction to limit the amino acids that use the propionate pathway is essential. Special formula containing no valine, isoleucine, methionine, and threonine is recommended. Administration of vitamin B_{12} is ineffective for this condition. Megaloblastic anemia may be caused by repeated or prolonged exposure (more than 6 hours) to nitrous oxide. This condition can be corrected by vitamin B_{12} treatment.

FOLIC ACID DEFICIENCY

Like vitamin B_{12}, folic acid is widely distributed in plants and animal products, and pure dietary insufficiency is rare. However, because of limited body store, folate deficiency may develop in conditions with increased folic acid requirements such as in chronic hemolytic anemia and during infancy and pregnancy. Infants are at high risk for developing severe folic acid deficiency when they are fed exclusively with goat's milk, because it contains very little folic acid. Administration of oral folic acid is effective in correcting folic acid deficiency of all causes. Some folic acid is absorbed even in malabsorption syndromes. A treatment outline for folate deficiency is presented in Box 3. Folic acid, 200 µg orally daily, is sufficient to give optimal response in patients with megaloblastic anemia caused by folic acid deficiency. Initial laboratory and clinical response must be verified during the first week of therapy. Folic acid is then administered orally at 1 mg daily for a duration based on the cause of the deficiency, though a 2-week treatment will give optimal clinical response and replenish body storage for most patients. The parenteral preparation is usually reserved for patients who are unable to take the oral form. Folinic acid (leucovorin), a form of tetrahydrofolate, is indicated for the treatment of toxicity induced by antifolate agents such as methotrexate.

Duration of therapy depends on the underlying cause of the deficiency. Dietary insufficiency needs to be treated for 3 to 4 months until a new generation of red blood cells has been produced and body stores of folic acid are replenished. Longer duration of treatment is required if dietary habits that produce the folic acid deficiency are not corrected. Treatment should be continued throughout the duration of increased requirement states. Folic acid is commonly recommended for patients with severe chronic hemolytic anemia because of increased demand associated with limited body stores and because borderline serum folate concentration has been observed in a significant portion of this population. Megaloblastic anemia caused by orotic aciduria can be corrected by the administration of pharmacologic doses of uridine.

RESPONSE TO TREATMENT

The clinical and hematologic response to vitamin B_{12} and folic acid is prompt and may be dramatic. The patient's activity is increased, appetite improved, a sense of well-being restored, and interest in surroundings may reappear within a couple days of the start of treatment. Metabolic abnormalities such as elevated serum lactate dehydrogenase and iron levels are corrected in 2 days. Elevated serum methylmalonic acid and homocysteine return to normal in 1 week. Reticulocytes start to increase in 3 days and reach maximal levels in 7 days. Hemoglobin level begins to rise in 1 week and often returns to normal in 3 to 6 weeks if no complications develop. The neutrophils and platelets increase within 3 days and return to normal in 7 days. The hypersegmentation of neutrophils disappears within 7 to 14 days. Mean corpuscular volume (MCV) may further increase initially because of reticulocytosis and then decrease by 5 fL over 2 weeks. Megaloblastic changes in the marrow improve within 24 to 48 hours. Neurologic abnormalities caused by vitamin B_{12} deficiency improve slowly over a period of 1 to 6 months.

ROUTINE SUPPLEMENTATION OF FOLIC ACID AND VITAMIN B_{12}

The association between folic acid deficiency and neural tube defects is well established. An oral folic acid supplement provided in the periconceptional period (from the time of conception to 1 month of gestation) significantly reduces the incidence of neural tube defects. The problem, however, is that half of pregnancies are unplanned, so there is no opportunity to plan for and provide folic acid supplementation. The indication for prophylaxis with folate or vitamin B_{12} is shown in Box 4.

Common Pitfalls

- Some clinical manifestations and hematologic features of megaloblastic anemia may not be readily recognized because of the uncommon occurrence of this hematologic disorder.
- Unawareness of nonmegaloblastic macrocytosis may prevent proper evaluation of this condition.
- All effort should be made to precisely diagnose the type of megaloblastic anemia before the treatment is started unless urgent intervention is truly indicated.
- Although most neural tube defects can be prevented by providing folic acid supplementation, half of pregnancies are unplanned.

Communication and Counseling

Most megaloblastic anemia in children is caused by vitamin B_{12} or folic acid deficiency. Children generally

---

BOX 4 Indications for Prophylaxis with Folic Acid or Vitamin B_{12}

Folic Acid Prophylaxis
- All women planning a pregnancy
- Pregnant and lactating women
- Premature infants
- Patients with chronic hemolytic anemia
- Patients taking antifolate therapy, such as methotrexate, for nonmalignant disorders

Vitamin B_{12} Prophylaxis
- Infants of mothers with pernicious anemia
- Vegetarians
- Infants on special diets

respond well to specific treatment with rapid clinical improvement. Caution should be taken for identifying persistent subtle initial clinical manifestations in infants and in pursuing precise diagnosis before treatment is initiated.

SUGGESTED READINGS

1. Czeizel AE, Dudas I: Prevention of the first occurrence of neural-tube defects by periconceptual vitamin supplementation. N Engl J Med 327:1832–1835, 1992. **An observation of neural tube defect prevention by folic acid supplementation.**
2. Davenport J: Macrocytic anemia. Am Fam Physician 53:155, 1996. **A concise general review for clinicians; covers information primarily for adults.**
3. Kamen BA, Meyers PA: Megaloblastic anemia. In Miller DR, Baehner RL (eds): Blood Diseases in Infancy and Childhood, 7th ed. St. Louis: Mosby, 1995, pp 220–240. **A thorough review addressing the biochemical, pathophysiological, and clinical aspects of Vitamin B_{12} and folic acid deficiencies and other causes of megaloblastic anemia.**
4. Schorah CJ, Smithells RW, Scott J: Vitamin B_{12} and anencephaly. Lancet 1:880, 1980. **A classic documentation of the association between neural tube defects and folic acid.**
5. Whitehead UM, Resenblatt DS, Cooper BA: Megaloblastic anemia. In Nathan D, Orkin S, Ginsburg D, Look A (eds): Nathan Oski's Hematology of Infancy and Childhood, 6th ed. Philadelphia: WB Saunders, 2003, pp 419–455. **A comprehensive review of the basic and clinical aspects of megaloblastic anemia.**

Hemolytic Anemias

Roger L. Berkow and Jeffrey H. Schwartz

KEY CONCEPTS

- Hemolytic anemias are caused by increased destruction of red blood cells.
- Diagnosis of hemolytic anemia requires evidence of increased destruction of red blood cells (such as spherocytes and schistocytes or other abnormal red blood cell forms on the peripheral blood smear, jaundice, and/or splenomegaly) and increased production of red blood cells in response to the increased destruction (such as increased reticulocytes and polychromasia on the peripheral blood smear).
- Extrinsic hemolytic anemias are generally acute processes that are responsive to treatment.
- Intrinsic hemolytic anemias are lifelong processes with variable severity. Treatment is preventative and supportive. Patients should receive folic acid.
- Referral and/or consultation with a pediatric hematologist is often helpful.

Anemia caused by increased destruction of red blood cells is termed hemolytic anemia. There are many different mechanisms of red blood cell destruction, but the final common pathway is hemolysis. In general, hemolytic anemias can be classified into processes intrinsic or extrinsic to the red blood cell. Intrinsic processes are inherent to the red blood cell and are caused by abnormalities of the red blood cell membrane, cytoplasmic enzymes,

or hemoglobin. These processes are variable in their severity and are lifelong (disorders of hemoglobin are presented in other chapters in this book and are not discussed here.) Extrinsic processes, on the other hand, are acquired and caused by factors external to the red blood cell. These disorders can be acute (self-limited) or chronic and can have variable severity. They are most frequently a result of damage to the red blood cell membrane by antibodies or mechanical stress.

Expert Opinion on Management Issues

There are relatively few management options (Table 1) for hemolytic anemias, but a thorough understanding of the underlying mechanism causing the hemolytic anemia is critical to choosing the most appropriate management. Once hemolytic anemia is established by the presence of anemia and an elevated reticulocyte count, a Coombs test is essential. The direct Coombs test (direct antiglobulin test [DAT]) will determine if the anemia is caused by an immune-mediated process in almost all cases. There are rare cases in which an autoimmune or isoimmune hemolytic anemia will have a negative DAT because the level of antibody is below the detection limits of the test. In the presence of a positive DAT, further testing will elucidate whether the process is warm reactive (immunoglobulin [Ig] G), which is the most common form of autoimmune hemolytic anemia (AIHA), or cold reactive. Cold reactive processes can be associated with IgM and rarely IgG (the so-called Donath-Landsteiner antibody). In the absence of a known underlying cause of the hemolysis, the AIHA is referred to as primary. Secondary AIHA can be caused by autoimmune diseases (evaluation of antinuclear antibody [ANA], for example, should be considered), infection (including mycoplasma and viral agents), drugs, and other causes.

MANAGEMENT

The management of primary AIHA depends on the severity of the anemia and the specific antibody, if any, identified, as well as treatment of any identified underlying cause such as infection or exacerbation of an autoimmune disorder. A mild and stable anemia may require observation only. AIHA however, may manifest with a rapidly developing and life-threatening anemia requiring emergent treatment. The first line of treatment, when necessary, is steroids. It is thought that steroids inhibit the FCR-mediated clearance of sensitized red blood cells in the acute period and over time inhibit antibody production. Once the anemia has stabilized, the steroid dose can be tapered over several weeks.

Second-line therapy is often intravenous γ-globulin (IVIG) or plasma exchange transfusion; IgM-positive AIHA responds better to plasma exchange than IgG-mediated AIHA. Transfusion is warranted only if the patient is unstable and/or the degree of anemia is rapidly worsening. Transfusions in patients with AIHA can be challenging because it may be difficult to find compatible blood because of the presence of circulating antibodies.

TABLE 1 Management Options for Hemolytic Anemia

Generic Name	Dosage/Route/Regimen	Maximum Dose	Dosage Formulations	Common Adverse Reactions	Therapeutic Concentrations	Comments
Deferoxamine	IV: 24 h continuous infusion: 50–150 mg/kg/day; SC: 8–12 h Infusion: 40–60 mg/kg/day	6 g/day 2 g/day	Injection: 500 mg, 2 g	Flushing, localized pain and erythema, visual and hearing changes	NA	
Folic acid	PO: infants: 0.1 mg/day <4 yr: 0.3 mg/day >4 yr: 0.4 mg/day	1 mg	Tablet: 0.4 mg, 0.8 mg, 1 mg	None	NA	
IVIG	IV: 500–1000 mg/kg/day × 1–2 days	None	Injection (varies with manufacturer): 0.5 g, 1 g, 2.5 g, 5 g, 10 g	Malaise, blood pressure changes, fever, aseptic meningitis	NA	May repeat as necessary.
Penicillin	PO: <5 yr: 125 mg bid ≥5 yr: 250 mg bid	NA	Solution: 125 mg/5 mL, 250 mg/5 mL; Tablet: 250 mg, 500 mg	Rash, allergic reaction	NA	
Prednisone (or equivalent)	PO or IV: 1–2 mg/kg/day	None	Injection (varies with manufacturer): 40 mg, 125 mg, 500 mg; Solution: 1 mg/mL, 5 mg/mL; Tablet: 1 mg, 2.5 mg, 5 mg, 10 mg, 20 mg, 50 mg	Hyperglycemia, increased appetite, insomnia	NA	Maintain starting dose for 2 wk then wean off slowly.
Transfusion	5–15 mL/kg	None	NA	None	NA	Volume and rapidity of infusion vary with underlying problem.

IV, intravenous; IVIG, intravenous immunoglobulin; NA, not applicable; PO, orally; SC, subcutaneous.

BOX 1 Risks of Splenectomy

- Postsplenectomy sepsis
- Penicillin-resistant pneumococci
- Ischemic heart disease and stroke (in HS)
- Pulmonary hypertension

In this case, choosing the least incompatible blood may be necessary. Patients may also hemolyze the transfused blood. In chronic AIHA, splenectomy has been used with some success but the benefits and risks should be carefully considered (Box 1 gives a review of the risks of splenectomy). Consultation with a pediatric hematologist is recommended when AIHA is suspected.

The neonate with an immune-mediated hemolytic anemia deserves special consideration. Commonly referred to as *alloimmune* or *isoimmune hemolytic disease* of the newborn, this condition is caused by transplacental passage of maternal antibodies against fetal red blood cells. Most cases of severe hemolytic anemia are caused by Rh 13 incompatibility, whereas ABO incompatibility only rarely causes severe hemolysis. Knowledge of maternal blood type and Rh status, as well as past pregnancy history and anti-Rh antibody titer, is essential for proper management. The first line of treatment for Rh incompatibility is anti-Rh immunoglobulin administration to the mother at approximately week 28 of gestation. Fetal red blood cell transfusions may be used in severe cases of intrauterine hemolysis, especially if there is a history of a previous pregnancy complicated by alloimmunization. Blood should be group O, Rh-negative, cross-matched against the mother's blood, cytomegalovirus (CMV)-negative, and irradiated. Early delivery of the fetus may be necessary, if possible waiting until at least 36 weeks' gestation. In the neonate, exchange transfusion may be necessary to prevent kernicterus, especially if the cord blood hemoglobin is less than 11 g/dL or the cord blood bilirubin is greater than 4 mg/dL. Blood should be ABO-compatible with the neonate, Rh-negative, irradiated, and cross-matched against the mother. In neonates with ABO incompatibility with the mother, careful monitoring of the hemoglobin, hematocrit, and bilirubin level is important in determining appropriate therapy.

Nonimmune-mediated extrinsic causes of hemolysis include microangiopathic hemolytic anemia (MAHA), in addition to idiopathic and secondary causes. MAHA is the final common pathway for intravascular hemolysis caused by fragmentation of normal red blood cells, most commonly, because red blood cells adhere to fibrin deposited in the microvasculature and are injured by the shear force of the blood flow. The many underlying causes of MAHA include disseminated intravascular coagulation (DIC), thrombotic thrombocytopenic purpura (TTP), hemolytic-uremic syndrome (HUS), drugs, solid organ and bone marrow transplantation, vasculitis, and localized vascular abnormalities. Red blood cell transfusion may be necessary in the case of severe anemia, but it will likely result in hemolysis of the transfused cells, similarly to the endogenous cells. Platelet transfusions, on the other hand, may worsen the situation by increasing the propagation of fibrin-platelet aggregates, leading to further aggregation and consumption. Bleeding is, ironically, not a significant problem, so platelet transfusions should only be used as a life-saving effort. Fresh-frozen plasma may be helpful in TTP because of the congenital deficiency of the von Willebrand factor cleaving protease (vWFCP), and plasma exchange may be helpful in TTP because of the acquired inhibitor of the vWFCP.

Intrinsic hemolytic anemias can be classified as disorders of the red blood cell membrane, enzymes, or hemoglobin. Hemoglobinopathies and thalassemias are discussed in the chapters "Sickle Cell Disorders" and "Thalassemia," respectively. Treatment modalities for the intrinsic hemolytic anemias are preventive and supportive. The most common membrane disorders are hereditary spherocytosis (HS) and hereditary elliptocytosis (HE), both of which involve abnormalities of the cytoskeletal support of the cell membrane. While the severity of anemia in HS can vary from mild to severe, HE is rarely severe enough to require intervention. HS is inherited as an autosomal dominant trait, although 15% to 20% of patients present without a family history. Patients with HS typically tolerate a hemoglobin as low as 8.0 without needing transfusion support, but symptomatic anemia could dictate the necessity of transfusion. Splenectomy should be considered in patients with severe HS requiring multiple transfusions and will resolve the anemia in almost all patients. This should be avoided until at least age 5 (see Box 1). Patients with HS can present in the neonatal period with prolonged jaundice, but they may present with an asymptomatic anemia at 1 to 2 years of age. With viral illness, some patients develop either an accelerated hemolysis or an arrest of red blood cell production (aplastic crisis) and may require transfusion support. Because of chronic hemolysis, these patients can also develop gallbladder disease and should have an ultrasound performed at least every 5 years and prior to splenectomy.

There are several red blood cell enzyme defects that lead to hemolysis. Glucose–6-phosphate dehydrogenase (G6PD) deficiency is the most common disorder, occurs in individuals of Mediterranean, Middle Eastern, and African descent, and is inherited as an X-linked trait. Numerous mutations of this enzyme have been described. Patients with G6PD deficiency are normally asymptomatic, but with an oxidative challenge, hemoglobin is damaged, leading to varying degrees of hemolysis associated with irritability, dark or red urine, jaundice, and splenomegaly. Primary prevention by avoiding stimuli is the most important component of managing these patients (Box 2 provides a listing of common stimuli). Patients with G6PD deficiency may require transfusions for a hemoglobin of less than 7.0 g/dL or less than 9.0 g/dL with associated hemoglobinuria. These patients should be well hydrated and monitored closely for renal failure during a hemolytic crisis. Infants with G6PD can develop severe neonatal jaundice requiring aggressive management including exchange transfusion to prevent kernicterus.

Pyruvate kinase deficiency is the second most common disorder of red blood cell enzymes. The severity ranges

---

BOX 2 Common Stimuli Exacerbating G6PD Deficiency

- Fava beans
- Antimalarial agents (primaquine, pamaquine, chloroquine)
- Sulfonamides and sulfones
- Other antibacterial agents (nitrofurans, chloramphenicol, p-aminosalicylic acid)
- Antihelmintics (β-naphthol, stibophen, niridazole)
- Analgesics (aspirin, phenacetin)
- Other (vitamin K, naphthalene, probenecid, dimercaprol, methylene blue)

G6PD, glucose–6-phosphate dehydrogenase (deficiency).

---

from mild to severe, and these patients require transfusion less frequently. Splenectomy may be helpful in patients with severe disease but will not completely correct their anemia. These patients should also avoid the chronic use of salicylates (because they can deplete ATP, exacerbating the severity of the disease).

Common Pitfalls

- Review of the peripheral blood smear is essential when evaluating a hemolytic anemia because many clues to the correct diagnosis can be found. Unnecessary evaluations and delay in appropriate treatment can result from not reviewing the peripheral blood smear.
- A careful assessment of the risks and benefits of splenectomy should be reviewed prior to recommending the procedure.
- Postsplenectomy patients should be treated with prophylactic penicillin.
- Patients should be placed on folic acid to prevent relative folic acid deficiency.
- Patients requiring frequent transfusions may develop iron overload (usually seen after 100–150 mL/kg total blood exposure). Serum ferritin should be followed and liver biopsy considered. Iron chelation with deferoxamine may be necessary.

Communication and Counseling

There is great variability in the severity of hemolytic anemias ranging from mild and clinically insignificant to life threatening. Patients with acute immune-mediated processes most frequently recover but can be chronic and can present with a rapid life-threatening anemia. Microangiopathic hemolytic anemias may be severe and life threatening, but an understanding of the underlying mechanism and appropriate treatment will usually lead to a full recovery. The intrinsic membrane and enzyme defects are lifelong and vary significantly in severity. Exacerbations are generally responsive to transfusion. Patients with HS will usually respond to splenectomy with improvement in the anemia, although the underlying defect in the red blood cell persists.

SUGGESTED READINGS

1. Gallagher PG, Lux SE: Disorders of the erythrocyte membrane. In Nathan DG, Orkin SH, Ginsburg D, Look AT (eds): Hematology of Infancy and Childhood, 6th ed. Philadelphia: WB Saunders, 2003, pp 560–604. **Reviews hemolytic anemias associated with erythrocyte membrane defects.**
2. Liley HG: Immune hemolytic disease. In Nathan DG, Orkin SH, Ginsburg D, Look AT (eds): Hematology of Infancy and Childhood, 6th ed. Philadelphia: WB Saunders, 2003, pp 56–85. **Reviews immune-mediated hemolytic anemias during the neonatal period.**
3. Luzzatto L: Glucose–6-phosphate dehydrogenase deficiency hemolytic anemia. In Nathan DG, Orkin SH, Ginsburg D, Look AT (eds): Hematology of Infancy and Childhood, 6th ed. Philadelphia: WB Saunders, 2003, pp 721–742. **Reviews G6PD deficiency in detail.**
4. Mentzer WC: Pyruvate kinase deficiency disorders of glycolysis. In Nathan DG, Orkin SH, Ginsburg D, Look AT (eds): Hematology of Infancy and Childhood, 6th ed. Philadelphia: WB Saunders, 2003, pp 685–720. **Reviews congenital and acquired disorders of glycolysis associated with hemolytic anemia.**
5. Ware RE: Autoimmune hemolytic anemias. In Nathan DG, Orkin SH, Ginsburg D, Look AT (eds): Hematology of Infancy and Childhood, 6th ed. Philadelphia: WB Saunders, 2003, pp 521–559. **Reviews autoimmune hemolytic anemias in detail.**

Thalassemia

Naveen Qureshi and Elliott Vichinsky

KEY CONCEPTS

- The diagnosis of thalassemia should be confirmed with appropriate tests.
- Transfusion therapy suppresses ineffective erythropoiesis and prevents complications of severe anemia.
- Iron should be removed with iron-chelating agents.
- Complications must be appropriately treated.
- Bone marrow transplantation is used to correct hematopoiesis.
- The disease may be prevented by antenatal diagnosis and genetic counseling.

The thalassemias are a heterogeneous group of single gene disorders in which the production of normal hemoglobin is suppressed partially or completely because of defective synthesis of β- or α-globin chains. The clinical severity depends on the number of defective globin chains, the amount of globin expression from an individual gene and other genetic characteristics. The disease varies from uniformly fatal (α thalassemia major) to very mild. Beyond hydrops fetalis, thalassemia major is the most severe form of thalassemia. It manifests with growth failure, progressive pallor, hepatosplenomegaly, and bony changes during infancy. It is often fatal in the first few years of life if transfusion therapy is not initiated. Patients with the heterozygous form β- or α-thalassemia trait are at the other end of the severity spectrum. These mildly anemic, asymptomatic patients are at risk for having affected offspring and require genetic counseling. Between these two extremes are thalassemia intermedia patients, who do not initially require chronic transfusion therapy but suffer varying clinical manifestations of thalassemia. Their clinical course is deceptively severe and often deteriorates with age. These patients should be followed closely for complications of ineffective erythropoiesis and organ failure.

Because of wide clinical variability, a definitive diagnosis is essential to properly manage the thalassemia patient. The initial evaluation starts with hemoglobin red cell indices, reticulocyte count, and iron studies. A microcytic anemia without iron deficiency usually indicates thalassemia. The screening tests are then followed by a hemoglobin electrophoresis and quantitative hemoglobin A2 and F. An elevated fetal hemoglobin or A2 level with decreased (or absent) hemoglobin A1 are noted in β-thalassemia disorders. Outside the neonatal period, α-thalassemia disorders may have normal hemoglobin electrophoresis and is often a diagnosis of exclusion. Both α- and β-globin disorders require confirmatory studies including DNA testing. Determination of both α- and β-mutations in patients is helpful because of the coinheritance of genetic modifiers (e.g., a triplication), which alter the clinical severity and, therefore, the recommended treatment.

Expert Opinion on Management Issues

Over the last 3 decades, thalassemia major has been treated with regular red blood cell (RBC) transfusion support in an effort to prevent severe anemia and suppress endogenous ineffective erythropoiesis. Blood transfusions are also indicated for thalassemia intermedia patients who, despite maintaining hemoglobin more than 6 g/dL, develop dysmorphic skeletal features, growth failure, organ failure, and significantly impaired quality of life. Transient events such as Parvovirus infection may occur, suppressing erythroid production. Therefore, a single incident of severe anemia requiring transfusion should not be the sole justification for chronic transfusions. Safe transfusion therapy involving expanded red blood cell antigen matched, leukodepleted, packed RBC transfusions at 2- to 5-week intervals are intended to maintain pretransfusion hemoglobin levels more than 9 g/dL. To obtain extended RBC antigen–matched blood, an RBC phenotype should be planned prior to the initiation of transfusion therapy. Following transfusion, close observation for febrile, allergic, and hemolytic reactions is required. Early detection of alloimmunization by serial monitoring Coombs testing is recommended.

The treatment of thalassemia major has improved dramatically over the last 2 decades, leading to a sharp increase in survival rates and significant improvements in quality of life. Nonetheless, patients with thalassemia major may suffer medical problems from the disease itself or its therapy.

Hypersplenism can develop and results in increased anemia or transfusion requirements. If the number of RBC units transfused to maintain a desired level of hemoglobin increases, hypersplenism should be suspected. The detection of hypersplenism requires the hemoglobin and the number of units transfused to be monitored closely in all patients. Splenectomy is considered in both the nontransfused patient who develops worsening anemia and the transfused patient with increasing transfusion requirements. Splenectomy should be considered when the amount of blood required to maintain hemoglobin levels increases by 1.5 times or more than 225 mL/kg/year. Splenectomy carries the risk of developing serious infections postoperatively, especially in the infant. Thromboembolic events and pulmonary hypertension are also increased in splenectomized patients. These complications may be minimized by the routine use of aspirin or low-dose anticoagulants.

Iron overload is a major cause of morbidity for both transfused and nontransfused thalassemia patients. Early detection of iron overload, whether from red cell transfusions or increased gastrointestinal iron absorption, is essential to prevent organ damage. Determination of serial serum ferritin levels alone is not adequate for monitoring iron overload because it is often inaccurate in predicting total iron body stores. Direct measurement of hepatic iron by liver biopsy is recommended throughout therapy to detect iron overload. New noninvasive techniques to quantify liver iron are becoming available. The superconducting quantum interference device (SQUID) is the most accurate noninvasive method to determine the degree of iron overload. MRI for iron overload is currently being developed but is not yet proven reliable. Chronic transfusion therapy, elevated ferritin, and high hepatic iron are indications for chelation (Box 1). All patients with hepatic iron concentration more than 7 mg/g dry weight require chronic chelation. Ferritin levels higher than 2500 mg/L and hepatic iron more than 15 mg/g dry weight are associated with early cardiac mortality and therefore require immediate intervention. Moreover, iron-overloaded thalassemia patients suffer from complications in multiple organ systems, requiring frequent surveillance for complications (Table 1).

Cardiac disease is the major cause of death in thalassemia patients and can be fatal in the second decade of life. In the absence of effective iron chelation, patients often develop arrhythmia and congestive heart failure. Annual cardiac function assessments including echocardiogram, 12-lead electrocardiogram (ECG), and Holter ECG are recommended after the age of 10 years. Reversal of iron overload is the most important factor in prevention and treatment. Pulmonary hypertension is common in patients without iron-induced cardiomyopathy and may be secondary to anemia, hemolysis, and thrombosis. Improved transfusion therapy and nitric oxide–modulating drugs may be very useful.

Endocrine dysfunction caused by iron deposition results in hypothyroidism, hypoparathyroidism, diabetes,

---

BOX 1 Indications for Chelation

- 1–2 years of transfusion history
- Serum ferritin >1000 ng/dL
- Hepatic iron ≥7 mg/g dry weight

TABLE 1 Complications and Surveillance of Iron-Overloaded Thalassemia Patients

Complication and Organ System	Screening Modalities
Cardiac disease	12-lead ECG, CXR, echocardiogram; baseline at age 10 yr, then q2yr; 24-hour Holter, transtelephonic event recorder
Endocrine disorder	Tanner staging, height and weight measurements, bone age;
Thyroid, hypoparathyroid	TSH, T4, Cortrosyn stimulation, PTH, calcium, magnesium, phosphorus,
Diabetes mellitus	Vitamin D, fasting blood glucose, oral glucose tolerance,
Hypogonadism, osteoporosis	IGF–1, IGF BP–3, bone density DEXA
Liver disease	Hepatitis serologies (HBV, HCV, EBV, CMV)
Infectious disease	HIV, CMV, EBV, HBV, HCV, *Yersinia enterocolitica*; liver function tests

BP, binding protein; CMV, cytomegalovirus; CXR, chest radiograph; DEXA, dual energy x-ray absorptiometry; EBV, Epstein-Barr virus; ECG, electrocardiogram; HBV, hepatitis B virus; HCV, hepatitis C virus; HIV, human immunodeficiency virus; IGF, insulin-like growth factor; PTH, parathyroid hormone; TSH, thyroid-stimulating hormone.

BOX 2 Complications of Desferal Therapy*

- High frequency hearing loss
- Severe local reaction
- Vision/retinal damage
- Allergy
- Delayed linear growth, especially <3 yr
- Gastrointestinal symptoms
- *Yersinia enterocolitica* infection
- Tinnitus
- Metaphyseal dysplasia
- Renal failure
- Renal calculus

*Listed in descending order in recent Thalassemia Clinical Research Network–based study among 309 thalassemia patients.

Data from Cunningham M, Macklin EA: Complications of ß thalassemia major in North America. Blood 104:34–39, 2004.

---

gonadal failure, growth failure, and osteoporosis. Prevention, with annual endocrine screening, effective chelation, nutritional supplements, and exercise are required. Treatment with specific hormone replacement therapy for endocrine deficiencies and bisphosphonates for osteoporosis are recommended.

Liver toxicity can occur as a direct consequence of iron toxicity and/or from transfusion-acquired hepatitis. Once hepatic dysfunction has been documented, rapid iron chelation and treatment of hepatitis is critical for preservation of liver function. Hepatitis C can often be adequately treated with pegylated interferon and ribavirin. Patients who have chronic hepatitis B or C should be monitored for development of hepatocellular carcinoma with alpha-fetoprotein and hepatic ultrasounds annually.

Infections are the second most common cause of death in thalassemia major. Transmission of viral infections via blood transfusions is possible. Bacterial infections including *Streptococcus pneumoniae* and *Yersinia enterocolitica* may be fatal. The latter is an iron-dependent bacterium, and infection often manifests with abdominal pain and fever. Immunization for pneumococcus, *Haemophilus influenzae*, hepatitis (A, B), and influenza are indicated. Following splenectomy, penicillin prophylaxis is required.

CURRENT ACCEPTED THERAPY FOR THALASSEMIA-RELATED HEMOSIDEROSIS

Iron chelation therapy with desferrioxamine therapy has increased patient survival and is the most effective therapy for the treatment of iron overload. Nonetheless, desferal chelation in high doses can lead to toxicity and complications (Box 2). Noncompliance is the major factor for ineffectiveness of therapy. Desferrioxamine toxicity is affected by age, total body iron stores, dose, and duration of therapy. The standard dose is 25 to 40 mg/kg for children as an 8 to 12 hour slowly delivered subcutaneous infusion for 5 to 7 days per week, with a goal to keep serum ferritin less than 1000 µg/mL. Lower doses are given to young children less than 3 years of age. Ascorbic acid on the days of desferrioxamine infusion enhances iron excretion. High-dose short-term infusions increase toxicity without improved efficacy. Severe iron overload (ferritin >2500 µg/L or liver iron >15 mg/g dry weight) may be treated with continuous infusions of desferrioxamine at 50 mg/kg/day (maximum 6 g/day). Desferal toxicity monitoring requires annual hearing and ophthalmology examinations. Orally effective iron chelators are currently undergoing clinical trials. Deferiprone is available outside the United States for patients with contraindications to desferrioxamine. ICL 670 is completing efficacy and safety trials and appears promising.

Limiting iron intake helps to minimize hemosiderosis. Nutritional counseling to avoid iron rich diets and supplementation with tea is useful. Tea reduces iron absorption from food. Experimental red cell pheresis treatment may significantly decrease transfusion induced iron overload and is in clinical trial.

EMERGING THERAPIES

In healthy thalassemia patients, bone marrow transplantation (BMT) and cord blood transplantation from human leukocyte antibody (HLA)-matched sibling donors offers a 91% event-free survival. BMT should be considered at an early age before complications of hemosiderosis have developed. Before transfusion therapy is initiated, patients should be counseled and HLA typed in anticipation of possible BMT. Recently, preimplantation genetic diagnosis (PGD) has been used to obtain HLA-matched donors for BMT of an affected sibling.

Although this method raises new hope for cure, it is costly and unreliable, and it raises ethical and psychosocial issues. Chemotherapy (hydroxyurea, decitabine, and butyrate) may correct the anemia by increasing fetal hemoglobin synthesis. However, inconsistent responses and toxicity have prevented clinical use. Correction of β-thalassemia by gene therapy has not entered clinical trials.

Common Pitfalls

Thalassemia is a complex chronic disease that requires early detection and continued surveillance for improved outcomes. Failure of timely transfusion and maintaining pretransfusion hemoglobin may promote ineffective erythropoiesis. Similarly, failure of effective iron chelation owing to lack of compliance or improper dosing may lead to complications of iron overload. Failure to treat infections, provide penicillin prophylaxis, and administer appropriate vaccinations to thalassemia patients who have undergone splenectomy places the patient at grave risk for serious and life-threatening infections. Heart and liver disease as well as endocrinopathies are morbid complications that may ensue caused by failure of early diagnosis, detection, and therapy. Overall, inappropriate blood transfusion therapy, lack of blood safety, and suboptimal chelation may promote development of medical problems such as osteoporosis, diabetes, and chronic infections that may potentially worsen the quality of life.

Communication and Counseling

As with other chronic illnesses, thalassemia patients face considerable challenges, from financial hardship and absence from school and work to significant issues with self-esteem and assurance. All significantly affect the quality of life of the patients. Because of the genetic inheritance of thalassemia, prevention of disease involves identification of thalassemia carriers at risk and subsequent genetic counseling of affected couples. Starting lifelong transfusions and chelation has a major impact on the patient and family. Compliance with the therapy is probably the most important factor in reducing the morbidity of chronic transfusion therapy. Support from a child-life or social work program is helpful to achieve compliance with chelation therapy. An individualized protocol for initiating chelation therapy is also helpful in maintaining compliance. Effective nursing, child-life services, and psychological support services are needed in order to encourage compliance and a smooth transition to this lifelong therapy.

SUGGESTED READINGS

1. Cunningham M, Macklin EA: Complications of ß thalassemia major in North America. Blood 104:34–39, 2004. **Current clinical complications of β-thalassemia patients in North America.**
2. Lo L, Singer ST: Thalassemia: Current approach to an old disease. Pediatr Clin North Am 49:1165–1191, 2002. **Discusses the approach for recognition, diagnosis, and management of the thalassemias, and reviews new prospects of therapy.**
3. Olivieri N, Brittenham G: Iron-chelating therapy and the treatment of thalassemia. Blood 89:739–761, 1997. **Overview of therapeutic options for treatment of thalassemia.**
4. Singer ST, Wu V, Mignacca R: Alloimmunization and erythrocyte autoimmunization in transfusion-dependent thalassemia patients of predominantly Asian descent. Blood 96:3369–3373, 2000. **RBC antigen screening and use in prevention of alloimmunization.**

Sickle Cell Disorders
Lee M. Hilliard and Thomas H. Howard

KEY CONCEPTS

- Sickle cell disorders are heterogeneous hemoglobinopathies with variable phenotypic expression.
- Sickle hemoglobin (HbS) polymerizes in the deoxygenated state causing hemolysis and vasoocclusion.
- In the pediatric age group, acute, episodic complications occur secondary to hemolysis and vasoocclusion. The resulting organ damage that begins in the first year of life ultimately leads to organ failure, typically in adulthood.
- Newborn screening and comprehensive care improve outcomes in sickle cell disease.
- Although decreased in incidence by newborn screening and prophylactic penicillin, infection remains the leading cause of death in young children with sickle cell disease.
- Sickle cell disease is the leading cause of stroke in childhood.
- Recently introduced interventions such as hydroxyurea, transcranial Doppler (TCD) evaluation for stroke risk, and stem cell transplant (SCT) offer the potential to decrease morbidity and mortality and improve quality of life.

Sickle cell disorders are a heterogeneous group of inherited hemoglobinopathies characterized by:

- Inheritance of two abnormal β-globin genes, at least one of which is the sickle cell hemoglobin (HbS) gene
- Expression of HbS as the majority hemoglobin (Hb)

The HbS gene mutation (β^S) causes a single amino acid substitution (valine for glutamine) in the sixth residue of the β-globin protein. The existence of unique β^S haplotypes (different nucleotide sequences in the noncoding regions of the gene) demonstrate that the β^S mutation occurred independently in at least four different regions in Africa and Asia. The specific β^S haplotypes inherited contribute to the clinical heterogeneity of sickle cell disorders. Other factors affecting phenotypic expression of the sickle syndromes are coinheritance of varied α-globin gene numbers, genetic factors affecting fetal hemoglobin (HbF) production, and the coinheritance of the hemoglobin C (HbC) and β-thalassemia genes. The most common disorders are hemoglobin SS disease (HbSS), hemoglobin S-β thalassemia disease (HbS/β^0thal, HbS/β^+thal), and hemoglobin SC disease (HbSC).

The characteristic sickle-shaped red blood cells were first described by Herrick in 1910. This distinct shape occurs because HbS ($\alpha_2\beta_2^S$) is insoluble in the deoxygenated state. Thus, crystal polymers called *tactoids* are formed in red blood cells (RBCs) in a deoxygenated environment. This polymer formation distorts the biconcave disc RBCs into sickled cells. Because sickle RBCs are less deformable, premature lysis occurs (hemolytic anemia), which drastically shortens the sickle RBC life span from the normal 120 days to 10 to 15 days. Sickle RBCs also episodically occlude microvascular circulation. These two processes, hemolysis and vasoocclusion in various organs, are responsible for the clinical manifestations of sickle cell disorders. Clinical severity and laboratory parameters of the sickle cell disorders vary between and within each genotype and can range from largely asymptomatic to life-threatening even in infancy.

In general, the order of severity of clinical manifestations of the sickle cell disorders is as follows from severe to mild:

- HbSS and HbS/β^0thal
- HbSC
- HbS/β^+thal

In most cases, disease severity parallels the HbS percentage in the disorder. However, identification of all HbS disorders at birth through newborn screening teaches that the heterogeneity of severity within any one genotype is astounding. For example, although HbSC is a milder disorder, the frequency of painful vasoocclusive crisis (VOC) in a small percentage of individuals with HbSC disease equals that of severe HbSS individuals. In contrast, nearly 40% of HbSS patients experience no painful VOCs in any given year.

Expert Opinion on Management Issues

PREVENTIVE AND COMPREHENSIVE CARE

Comprehensive care is known to improve outcomes for patients with sickle cell disease. Standard comprehensive care should include:

- Extensive parental education regarding appropriate genetic counseling and recognition of and response to fever, symptoms of severe anemia, acute development of splenomegaly, stroke symptoms, painful VOC, dactylitis, and respiratory symptoms
- Access to psychosocial services
- Annual stroke prevention screens for 2- to 16-year-olds by transcranial Doppler (TCD) to determine the time-averaged mean maximal velocity (TAMM) in major intracranial vessels (TAMM >200 cm/sec indicates high risk of stroke)
- Evaluation for coexisting medical problems that lower O_2 saturations and intensify the sickling phenomenon, such as reactive airway disease and obstructive sleep apnea
- Assessment of abdominal pain, which includes ultrasonography for gallstones

- Identification of patients more likely to experience a severe clinical course by careful tracking of white count, Hb, hematocrit, reticulocyte count, history of dactylitis, and the annual frequency of painful VOC and acute chest syndrome (ACS).

Measures aimed at prevention of infection also have a significant impact on lessening morbidity and mortality from sickle cell disease. Predisposition to sepsis with encapsulated organisms (*Streptococcus pneumoniae, Haemophilus influenzae*) caused by functional and anatomic asplenia, impaired antibody production, and opsonin availability is common in patients younger than 5 years old. Historically, infection is a leading cause of mortality in patients younger than 20 years old with sickle cell disorders. The natural history of pneumococcal infection in younger children with sickle cell disease may be altered by institution of conjugate pneumococcal vaccine (Prevnar), but the effect of this intervention on a large scale is not yet reported. (Prior to the development of conjugate pneumococcal vaccine, children with sickle cell disease who are younger than 2 years of age were not immunized against pneumococcus because younger children do not mount an effective immune response to polysaccharide antigens.)

Measures that decrease the risk of sepsis-related mortality are:

- Rigorous adherence to immunization schedules (Prevnar, *Haemophilus influenzae* type b conjugate [Hib] vaccine, and if older than 24 months, the 23 valent polysaccharide vaccine [Pneumovax 23])
- Daily oral penicillin prophylaxis (125 mg twice daily if younger than 3 years of age; 250 mg twice daily if older than 3 years of age)
- Parental education to immediately seek medical attention for a temperature ≥101°F (38.3°C)
- Commitment by medical personnel to carefully evaluate febrile patients with physical exam, chest radiograph, and blood cultures.
- Use of parenteral antibiotics for young, febrile patients (as an inpatient or outpatient depending upon evaluation)
- Awareness of the possibility of sepsis with penicillin-resistant pneumococci

PAINFUL VASOOCCLUSIVE CRISES

The hallmark of sickle cell disease is painful VOC of bone or bone marrow that manifests as intense episodes of pain especially localized to the lower back and the extremities. VOC may follow infections or marked changes in ambient temperature. Pathophysiologically, VOC is thought to occur when sickle cells occlude the microvasculature of bone or bone marrow. Repeated vasoocclusion can cause avascular necrosis of bone—most commonly in the femoral head, the humeral head, or the clavicular head at the sternoclavicular joint. VOC, particularly in the femur, may increase the risk of ACS because of fat embolism.

Because pain is subjective in nature, accurate assessment is difficult and depends on patient self-report supplemented by physical findings, laboratory data, and diagnostic procedures as indicated. There are several pain-assessment instruments, such as the Wong-Baker Faces Pain Rating scale, which is particularly useful for evaluating the pain level of younger children. Although VOC is by far the most common reason for pain in sickle cell disease, physicians must be vigilant in reviewing an appropriate differential with each episode so as not to miss other problems such as gallstones, appendicitis, ACS, or osteomyelitis.

Treatment of pain in sickle cell disease falls into two major categories: (1) Acute pain episodes and (2) chronic or recurring pain episodes. For patients with acute pain who have exhausted their home care options, treatment consists of aggressive hydration (2200–2500 mL/m^2 of dextrose 5% in water solution [D5W] with half normal saline $\pm$ potassium chloride [KCl]), limited administration of nonsteroidal anti-inflammatory drugs (NSAIDs) such as ketorolac or ibuprofen, and use of parenteral narcotics, usually morphine sulfate. Narcotics may be given as pulse, continuous intravenous (IV) infusion, or by patient-controlled anesthesia (PCA) device. Historically, meperidine (Demerol) was the drug of choice; however, recent evidence suggests that parenteral meperidine should be avoided as first-line treatment of acute pain because of central nervous system (CNS) toxicity from its metabolite, normeperidine. Normeperidine has a long half-life, is cleared more slowly in sickle cell disease, and is a CNS irritant. Therefore, its accumulation can cause a spectrum of problems ranging from irritable mood to seizures.

Physicians must also be aware that patients receiving narcotic treatment for VOC are at increased risk for ACS. This risk can be reduced by the use of incentive spirometry. Oxygen saturation should be monitored in all patients on parenteral narcotics. While a more extensive review of pain management is beyond the scope of this chapter, excellent guidelines and algorithms for pain management are available in the National Institutes of Health (NIH)-sponsored monograph, *The Management of Sickle Cell Disease* (see Suggested Readings). These guidelines focus on the importance of rapidly titrated pain medications, cautious monitoring of O$_2$ saturations, and thoughtful transitions from IV to oral outpatient management of pain.

For individuals with chronic or recurring pain (usually defined as more than three emergency department visits or hospital admissions for VOC and/or frequent school absences for home pain), medical professionals should consider the use of hydroxyurea. Hydroxyurea (HU) is a DNA clastic agent first reported by Charache and colleagues in 1995 to decrease by 50% the occurrence of VOC and ACS in adult patients with sickle cell disease. Subsequently, in 1998, the Food and Drug Administration approved the first drug for the prevention of painful episodes in adult sickle cell patients. A Phase II trial (Ped HUG) showed that HU could be safely administered to children with sickle cell disease between the ages of 5 and 15 years. A phase III trial is under development to evaluate the effect of HU on organ function in very young children. However, if HU is used, it is the authors' opinion that management of this medication should be done in consultation with a hematologist. Care must be taken to monitor HU dosage and blood counts as well as to inform patients of all known and potential side effects including the theoretical possibility of leukemogenesis. The most severely affected individuals who fail HU should be considered for SCT if a related allogeneic donor is available.

ACUTE CHEST SYNDROME

ACS is the combined findings of a new pulmonary infiltrate on chest radiograph and fever. The patient may experience tachypnea, dyspnea, chest pain, or other chest symptoms and usually has decreased oxygen saturations. ACS can be caused by lung infection with microorganisms such as pneumococcus, mycoplasma, chlamydia, or parvovirus B19. ACS may also occur secondary to lung infarction caused by sickle cells occluding pulmonary microvasculature or the combination of infection and infarction. As mentioned previously, fat embolism in patients with VOC, particularly of the femur, is a recently recognized cause of ACS.

Patients with any pulmonary symptom, hypoxemia, bone pain, or fever should have a chest radiograph and are at risk for developing ACS. Because deoxygenation induces HbS polymerization and both lung infection and infarction lower O$_2$ saturation, either etiologic event can initiate a rapidly progressive cycle of lung injury, worsening hypoxia, sickling, infarction, and more lung injury, which leads to complete lung opacity, severe hypoxemia, and mechanical ventilation. This progression may occur over a period of hours. Therefore, the guiding principles in ACS management are:

- Recognize ACS early by anticipating circumstances in which ACS may occur (fever, VOC, any chest complaint or hypoxemia).
- Treat with IV antibiotics that cover pneumococci, chlamydia, and mycoplasma.
- Hydrate adequately with maintenance fluids, but avoid overhydration.
- Carefully monitor for progression of ACS with frequent physical exams, continuous pulse oximetry measurements, and repeated daily chest radiographs.
- Use transfusions appropriately.

Recommendations regarding indications for transfusion in ACS vary, but most hematologists would agree that transfusion for patients with an oxygen requirement, respiratory symptoms, or rapid progression of ACS is indicated. For severe or rapidly progressive cases, RBC exchange, best performed by erythrocytapheresis, is indicated. Repeated ACS in sickle cell disease is a hallmark of disease severity and is associated with deterioration of lung function over time. ACS is a major cause of death in adolescence and early adulthood. Therefore, if repeated ACS occurs, patients should be evaluated for coexisting medical problems like asthma or obstructive sleep apnea, and, if found, these problems should be aggressively managed. Persons who experience more than two ACS episodes per year are candidates for HU. If a patient with recurrent ACS does not improve with HU, allogeneic SCT should be considered. As with VOC and stroke, these alternative therapies should be pursued only with careful monitoring and with advice of a hematologist who specializes in sickle cell care.

SEVERE ANEMIA AND ACUTE TRANSFUSION

Sickle cell anemia is a chronic hemolytic anemia that produces rigid cells that are trapped and destroyed in the spleen, thus requiring continuous, rapid production of reticulocytes. Dramatic worsening of anemia occurs in sickle cell disease when reticulocytosis ceases—a condition known as aplastic crisis. Aplastic crisis is commonly caused by parvovirus B19 infection, which destroys erythroid precursors, decreases reticulocyte count, and heightens anemia. Other viruses and some drugs can cause aplastic crisis. Anemia can also be exacerbated if the spleen (and occasionally the liver) acutely entraps sickled cells and increases in size, a condition known as a sequestration crisis. Both aplastic crisis and sequestration crisis cause profound, life-threatening anemia.

Acute splenic sequestration crisis describes massive, acute splenomegaly often with fever, severe anemia, shock, and thrombocytopenia. The treatment for both aplastic crisis and a sequestration crisis is acute simple transfusion of packed RBCs. In splenic sequestration, rapid recirculation of entrapped cells may result in a greater-than-expected increase in hematocrit; thus frequent monitoring and careful calculation of amount of blood transfused is indicated. However, if the patient is in shock, rapid restoration of blood volume is indicated. Splenic sequestration usually occurs in children younger than 2 years who have HbSS disease, and it is often recurrent and life-threatening. Therefore, most hematologists now recommend chronic transfusion until splenectomy can be performed (depending on the patient's age). This approach reduces the patient's risk of sepsis. In addition, an important preventive measure to limit mortality from splenic sequestration is to educate parents in spleen palpation. Splenic sequestration may also occur in older children with milder sickle syndromes such as HbSC and HbSβ⁺thal. While splenic sequestration events in patients with milder sickle syndromes are usually not life threatening, they may be chronic and eventually necessitate splenectomy.

Transfusion in sickle cell disease is not without risks and complications. Transfusion increases blood viscosity; therefore, caution must be taken to not raise the hematocrit more than 35%, as higher hematocrits increase the risk of hyperviscosity and stroke. Chronic transfusion is associated with the certainty of iron overload, and infectious disease risk still exists with any transfusion of blood products. Another consideration in transfusion of SCD patients is the possibility of alloimmunization. Alloimmunization occurs when patients receive transfusions of packed red blood cells (PRBCs) that have red cell antigens the patient lacks. For example, many African American patients are negative for RBC antigens such as E, and this antigen is common in the pool of volunteer RBC donors. Therefore, if a patient

negative for E receives E-positive blood, the patient is likely to form an anti-E antibody. Up to 60% of adult patients receiving chronic transfusions have RBC antibodies, many of which are against multiple antigens. Thus, transfusion becomes very difficult, if not eventually impossible. Transfusion of RBCs phenotypically matched for the more common and immunogenic RBC antigens is known to decrease this risk. Therefore, when possible, RBCs phenotypically matched for the antigens C, D, E, Kell, and Duffy should be used in the transfusion of patients with sickle cell disease. Because determination of RBC phenotype is time-consuming, phenotyped packed red blood cells (PRBCs) may not be available in the acute setting unless the patient's RBC phenotype is previously determined.

Another transfusion issue unique to the sickle cell population is adequate preparation of the patient for anesthesia and surgical procedures. Patients should be adequately prepared for anesthesia to decrease their risk of ACS. A study on aggressive versus conservative transfusion regimens in the preoperative management of sickle cell patients showed that conservative transfusion (Hgb >10 g/dL) was adequate for all but high-risk surgical procedures. (It is also important to note that during nothing-by-mouth [NPO] status, sickle cell patients dehydrate more easily secondary to poor urine concentrating ability. Therefore, the above-mentioned study used a minimum of 6 hours of preoperative hydration for all NPO patients.)

STROKE AND SECONDARY STROKE PREVENTION

Sickle cell disease is the leading cause of stroke in childhood. Stroke is most common in HbSS disease. Peak incidence in childhood occurs between 2 and 5 years of age. Infarctive stroke is more common than hemorrhagic stroke in the pediatric age group.

In children with sickle cell disease, the most common symptom of stroke is hemiparesis. However, patients may also have visual and language disturbance, seizures, or altered levels of consciousness. Transient ischemic attacks (TIAs), although sometimes difficult to recognize in children, may also occur.

In most cases, clinical evaluation is adequate to diagnose stroke in children with sickle cell disease. In early ischemia, CT scans may be negative. MRI with diffusion-weighted imaging (DWI) provides much better detail than CT and can detect ischemia at the time of presentation. However, because MRI is time consuming and often requires sedation, its use in the acute setting is not recommended unless the diagnosis is in doubt.

Although there are no controlled studies, the accepted acute treatment for pediatric sickle cell patients with stroke is transfusion to lower the HbS level. Exchange transfusion (manual or automated) is recommended to obtain an HbS level less than 30% while avoiding hyperviscosity from higher hematocrits. After acute treatment, patients are maintained on chronic transfusion to reduce the risk of secondary stroke. Complications of chronic transfusion (as discussed earlier) are iron overload, alloimmunization, and transmission of infectious diseases. Because of these complications, stroke patients are candidates for SCT.

PRIMARY STROKE PREVENTION

Transcranial Doppler (TCD) examination is a noninvasive screening method known to predict stroke risk in children with sickle cell disease by evaluating intracranial blood flow velocity. The Stroke Prevention Trial in Sickle Cell Anemia (STOP) study demonstrated that for patients at high risk of stroke (TCD velocity >200 cm/sec), stroke occurrence is significantly reduced by chronic transfusion. A subsequent trial, STOP II, was undertaken to determine whether chronic transfusion for primary stroke prevention can be stopped at 30 months and still reduce stroke risk. This study was terminated early in November 2004 because a significant number of children randomized to cease transfusion had reversion of TCD to abnormal levels. Two of the children randomized off transfusion had a stroke. Thus, further research is needed to test alternative therapies for stroke prevention given the known long-term complications of chronic transfusion.

"SILENT" INFARCTS

Children with sickle cell disease and no evidence of clinical stroke may have infarcts noted on MRI. These "silent" infarcts are associated with poor performance on neuropsychological testing. A current study is under way to evaluate the impact of chronic transfusion on outcome for these patients.

Common Pitfalls

Pitfalls in management of sickle cell disease fall into three categories:

1. Failure to institute appropriate preventative measures and preventative education for patients and families
2. Failure to recognize and aggressively treat known complications of the sickle syndromes
3. Failure to judiciously evaluate patients for newer therapies or failure to institute newer evaluations such as TCD

However, newer therapies with potential risk such as HU and SCT must be used with caution and with detailed knowledge of sickle cell disease. Decisions regarding these therapies should be made in conjunction with a pediatric hematologist.

Communication and Counseling

Education is an integral part of care for families and patients with sickle cell disease. Parents should be educated about the inheritance of sickle cell disease and preventive measures to reduce morbidity and mortality. Parents and patients should learn to recognize complications of the disease and to respond promptly to their symptoms.

SUGGESTED READINGS

1. Adams RJ, McKie VC, Hsu L, et al: Prevention of a first stroke by transfusions in children with sickle cell anemia and abnormal results on transcranial Doppler ultrasonography. N Engl J Med 339:5–11, 1998. **This study showed that stroke risk in childhood sickle cell disease could be accurately predicted with TCD and significantly decreased by chronic transfusion.**
2. Charache S, Terrin ML, Moore RD, et al: Effect of hydroxyurea on the frequency of painful crisis in sickle cell anemia. N Engl J Med 332:1317–1322, 1995. **First randomized trial demonstrating the efficacy of hydroxyurea in decreasing the occurrence of vasoocclusive crisis.**
3. Gaston MH, Verter JI, Woods G, et al: Prophylaxis with oral penicillin in children with sickle cell anemia. A randomized trial. N Engl J Med 314:1593–1599, 1986. **This paper demonstrates the efficacy of penicillin prophylaxis to decrease morbidity and mortality from pneumococcal sepsis. Its publication gave the impetus for institution of universal newborn screening of neonates.**
4. Gill FM, Sleeper LA, Weiner SJ, et al: Clinical events in the first decade in a cohort of infants with sickle cell disease. The Cooperative Study of Sickle Cell Disease. Blood 86:776–783, 1995. **This paper represents an excellent comprehensive natural history study of pediatric sickle cell complications.**
5. National Institutes of Health. National Heart, Lung and Blood Institute. The Management of Sickle Cell Disease. NIH Publication No. 02–2117, 4th ed, June 2002. **This publication provides a concise, yet comprehensive guide to management of medical complications of sickle cell disease as well as references that encompass important papers on clinical aspects of sickle cell disease.**
6. Ohene-Frempong F, Weiner SJ, Sleeper LA, et al: Cerebrovascular accidents in sickle cell disease: Rates and risk factors. Blood 91:288–294, 1998. **This paper gives a comprehensive report of the natural history of stroke in sickle cell disease.**
7. Platt O, Thorington BD, Brambilla DJ, et al: Pain in sickle cell disease: Rates and risk factors. N Engl J Med 325:11–16, 1991. **This paper gives a comprehensive review of the natural history of painful crisis in sickle cell disease.**
8. Rosse WF, Gallagher D, Kinney TR, et al: Transfusion and alloimmunization in sickle cell disease. The Cooperative Study of Sickle Cell Disease. Blood 76:1431–1437, 1990. **This study represents a comprehensive evaluation of the development of alloimmunization in sickle cell disease.**

Disorders of Coagulation, Platelet Number, and Function

Michael Briones and Thomas C. Abshire

KEY CONCEPTS

- Hemophilia is characterized by spontaneous bleeding manifested by hemarthrosis, surgical/trauma bleeds, intracranial hemorrhage, and intramuscular bleeds.
- The clinical severity of hemophilia depends on factor VIII or IX level.
- Treatment of hemophilia requires prompt recombinant factor replacement.
- von Willebrand disease (vWD) is the most common inherited bleeding disorder.
- vWD is caused by either a quantitative or qualitative defect of the von Willebrand factor (vWF) protein.
- Idiopathic thrombocytopenia purpura (ITP) is a diagnosis of exclusion from a long list of causes of thrombocytopenia.

KEY CONCEPTS—cont'd

- Disseminated intravascular coagulation (DIC) is always secondary to an underlying disorder.
- The key therapeutic approach to DIC is treatment of the underlying disease.

Hemostasis is defined as the control of bleeding from an injury and involves the interaction of the blood vessel, circulating platelets, formation of fibrin by the coagulation factors, and regulation of the extension of the newly formed clot. The process is usually set in motion by tissue injury and exposure of cell membrane tissue factor (TF) in vivo. TF interacts with factor VII (FVII), resulting in conversion of FVII to the active protease VIIa. TF functions as a cofactor for FVIIa, enhancing its enzymatic activity several orders of magnitude. This FVIIa/TF complex (TFC) also directly activates precursor zymogens factor X (FX) and additional FVII and factor IX (FIX). Activated X (Xa) in concert with factor Va now initiates the conversion of prothrombin (factor II) to thrombin (Fig. 1). The initial TF-VIIa complex produces a small thrombin burst that is quickly inhibited by tissue factor pathway inhibitor (TFPI). However, the small amount of thrombin produced is enough to activate FXI as well as FV, factor VIII (FVIII), and platelets and dramatically augment the formation of Xa with resultant production of more thrombin. Importantly, the initiation of coagulation via TF-FVIIa and subsequent propagation by intrinsic Xa are both necessary to achieve optimal activation of the coagulation system. Thrombin (IIa) also functions to cleave fibrinogen to fibrin and activate factor XIII (FXIII) resulting in a more stable cross-linked clot. The differential diagnosis of abnormal coagulation is given in Box 1.

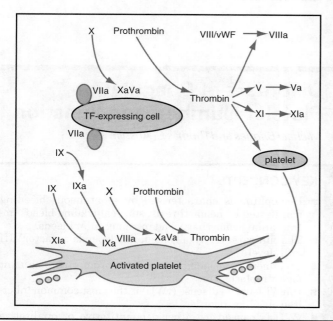

FIGURE 1. Model of normal hemostasis depicting essential role of tissue factor-factor VIIa in initiating thrombin generation and subsequent interaction of factors VIII, IX, and XI on the surface of the platelet with resultant larger thrombin burst. F, factor; TF, tissue factor.

Expert Opinion on Management Issues

HEMOPHILIA A (FACTOR VIII DEFICIENCY)

FVIII is a 320-kD glycoprotein that circulates in plasma as a stable complex with von Willebrand factor (vWF). Its function, when proteolytically activated by Xa or thrombin, is as a cofactor to accelerate the activation of X by factor IXa (FIXa). The genetic deficiency of FVIII is known as hemophilia A, and the incidence is 1:5000 live male births. The gene is located on the long arm of X chromosome at Xq28. Approximately 50% of persons with severe FVIII deficiency (<1% level) have an inversion mutation as the causative defect. Clotting factor is dosed in units of activity. One unit of FVIII per kg of body weight raises the plasma level of FVIII by approximately 2%. The half-life of FVIII is approximately 12 hours.

HEMOPHILIA B (FACTOR IX DEFICIENCY)

FIX is a vitamin K–dependent factor with a molecular weight of 57,000 that circulates as a single-chain glycoprotein proenzyme. FIX is activated by factor XIa or VIIa-TF in the presence of cofactors (FVIII, Ca^+, phospholipids) and converts X to Xa. Like hemophilia A, FIX deficiency is an X-linked recessive bleeding disorder. The gene-encoding FIX is located near the terminus of the long arm of chromosome X. Approximately 1:30,000 males are affected, with many mutations. Clotting factor

---

BOX 1 Differential Diagnoses of Abnormal Coagulation Tests

Isolated Prolonged aPTT in Order of Prevalence
- Lupus anticoagulant (not associated with bleeding)
- Heparin contamination
- Factor VIII or IX deficiency
- Factor XII deficiency (not associated with bleeding)
- Factor XI deficiency
- Inhibitors to factors VIII, IX, and XI

Isolated Prolonged PT
- Factor VII deficiency
- Mild multiple factor deficiency (II, V, or X) or liver disease

Prolonged aPTT and PT
- Liver disease
- Vitamin K deficiency
- Factor X, II, V deficiency
- High-dose heparin

Prolonged aPTT, PT and Thrombocytopenia
- DIC
- Liver disease
- Dilutional coagulopathy (massive blood transfusion)

Normal aPTT, PT, and Platelet Count
- von Willebrand disease
- Platelet function disorders

---

aPTT, activated partial thromboplastin time; DIC, disseminated intravascular coagulation; PT, prothrombin time.

is likewise dosed in units of activity, where one unit of FIX per kg raises the plasma level by approximately 1%. The half-life of FIX is approximately 24 hours.

Severe hemophilia patients (FVII and FIX deficiency) have factor levels less than 1% and are at risk for spontaneous hemorrhage. Bleeding complications seen in severe hemophiliacs include recurrent hemarthrosis; large soft tissue and muscle bleeds; and intracranial, gastrointestinal, and genitourinary bleeds. Those with moderate hemophilia (factor levels between 1% and 5%) and mild hemophilia (factor levels 6%–30%) are at low risk of spontaneous hemorrhage but usually have bleeding after trauma or surgery. The mainstay of hemophilia treatment and/or prevention of acute hemorrhage is replacement therapy of FVIII or FIX to hemostatic levels.

The target factor level is determined by the type and severity of the bleed (Table 1). There are two types of factor concentrates, plasma-derived and recombinant factor. All factor concentrates have undergone viral attenuation. These procedures have eliminated transfusion-associated human immunodeficiency virus (HIV), hepatitis B and C infections, and contamination from nonlipid envelope viruses (e.g., hepatitis A, parvovirus). Recombinant factor replacement is the agent of choice in North America. The long-term complications in hemophilia patients are hemophilic arthropathy, inhibitor formation, and infections (often seen when central venous catheters are used to administer factor). Patients may have recurrent hemorrhage into one or more joints that can lead to chronic effusions, joint space narrowing, and resultant end-stage arthropathy. Treatments include aggressive on-demand (3 or 4 infusions of factor) target joint therapy and prophylactic therapy to prevent bleeding. Synovectomy (surgical or radioisotopic) is reserved for joints that are not amenable to factor replacement therapy.

Inhibitory alloantibodies occur in 25% of patients with hemophilia A and 3% of those with hemophilia B. These antibodies are usually immunoglobulin (Ig) G antibodies and predominantly the IgG4 subtype. Patients with new onset inhibitors become clinically evident when they no longer respond adequately to factor replacement or if their bleeding symptoms seem out of proportion to their typical pattern of bleeding. Patients with inhibitors of less than 5 BU are low-titer inhibitors and can often be treated with high doses of factor, whereas those with greater than 5 BU are high-titer inhibitors. Patients with high-titer inhibitors should be treated with "by-passing agents" such as activated prothrombin complex concentrates (aPCCs) (e.g., FEIBA [FVIII-inhibiting bypassing agent] and recombinant FVIIa [NovoSeven]). Long-term treatment of FVIII inhibitors requires high doses of daily FVIII to induce immune tolerance.

TABLE 1 Therapy for Hemophilia A and B

Site of Hemorrhage	Factor Dosing Hemophilia A	Factor Dosing Hemophilia B	Hemostatic Factor Level (%)	Comments
Joint	20–50 U/kg/dose q12–24h × 3–4 doses	40 U–100 U/kg/dose	40–100	Physical therapy is important adjunct.
Central nervous system	50 U/kg/dose, then 25 U/kg q12h or continuous factor infusion of 4–5 U/kg/h for 10–14 days	100 U/kg/dose q24h for 10–14 days	80–100	If suspected, give factor first and then imaging studies. Follow daily FVIII/14 levels.
Muscle	20 U–50 U/kg/dose or 25 U/kg q12h or q24h	40 U–100 U/kg/dose	40–100	Monitor closely for compartment syndrome.
Iliopsoas	50 U/kg/dose, then continuous factor infusion of 4–5 U/kg/h for 7–10 days	100 U/kg/dose q24h for 7–10 days	80–100	Can develop significant blood loss.
Oral Mucosal	25 U/kg/dose	50 U/kg/dose	50	Use of antifibrinolytic agent is important adjunct. Aminocaproic acid (100 mg/kg/dose qid for 5–7 days).
Trauma/Surgery	50 U/kg/dose, then 25 U/kg q12h or continuous factor infusion of 4–5 U/kg/h for 10–14 days	100 U/kg/dose q24h for 10–14 days	80–100	Follow daily FVIII/FIX levels.
Genitourinary		50–100 U/kg as needed	50–100	Hydration recommended first. Antifibrinolytic agents are contraindicated. Prednisone 1–2 mg/kg/day for 5–7 days. Renal ultrasound.

qid, four times a day; qxh, every x hours; FVIII, factor VIII; FIX, factor IX; u, units.

VON WILLEBRAND DISEASE

von Willebrand disease (vWD) is the most common inherited bleeding disorder with an incidence of 1 in 100 people. Unlike hemophilia, which is X-linked and usually affects males, vWD is autosomal dominant (although type 3 vWD is recessive). Females and males are equally affected. The disease is caused by either a quantitative or qualitative defect in von Willebrand factor. At sites of vascular injury, vWF provides a major adhesive link between platelets and the vascular wall by binding to specific receptors on the platelets (GPIb) as well as to the subendothelium, via collagen and heparin-like substances. vWF also serves as a carrier for FVIII in plasma, stabilizing and localizing FVIII to sites of platelet plug and fibrin clot formation, thus prolonging FVIII half-life and facilitating the delivery of FVIII to sites of vascular injury. Bleeding manifestations are usually mucocutaneous such as epistaxis, oral cavity bleeding, and menorrhagia.

The diagnosis of vWD is based upon the bleeding history of the patient and the family history, and is supported by corresponding laboratory findings. Appropriate laboratory testing includes von Willebrand factor antigen (vWFAg), ristocetin cofactor activity, vWF multimer studies, FVIII activity and blood type. The blood type influences interpretation of normal values of vWF. Type 1 vWD is the most common variety, affecting 70% of patients, and is a proportional quantitative reduction of vWF. It is usually treated with DDAVP (desmopressin). Type 2 subtypes are qualitative defects of the vWF and can manifest as either mild or severe bleeding. Type 2 patients need treatment with factor concentrates containing vWF but some also respond to DDAVP. Type 3 vWD is almost complete absence of the vWF protein. Accordingly, these patients are clinically similar to patients

with severe hemophilia and are treated with factor replacement that is high in vWF (Table 2).

FACTOR XI DEFICIENCY

Hereditary factor XI (FXI) deficiency is inherited in an autosomal manner, with heterozygous patients demonstrating levels ranging from 20% to 60% and homozygous deficiency showing levels less than 15%. Bleeding severity does not correlate well with the level of FXI. Bleeding manifestations usually consist of mucosal type bleeding and postsurgical bleeding. There is a high prevalence of this disorder in the Ashkenazi Jewish population. Treatment necessitates replacement with fresh-frozen plasma (FFP). There are FXI concentrates available in Europe that occasionally are associated with thrombotic complications.

RARE FACTOR DEFICIENCIES

Congenital deficiencies of factors II, V, VII, X are all extremely rare (1:1 million) but should be suspected in patients with a personal or family history of factor deficiency bleeding where common hemophilias (FVIII, FIX, FXI) have been ruled out. Some of these deficiencies are more common in certain ethnic groups. Treatment is usually with FFP. Recombinant FVIIa is considered the off-label treatment of choice for patients with FVII deficiency.

PLATELET DISORDERS

Thrombocytopenia

Thrombocytopenia is defined as a platelet count less than 150,000/µL. Thrombocytopenia may be classified as secondary to increased destruction of platelets,

---

TABLE 2 Therapy for von Willebrand Disease

Type	Treatment of Choice	Spontaneous Bleeding Episodes and Surgery	Adjunctive Therapy
Type I	DDAVP	0.3 µg/kg/dose in 30 mL normal saline IV over 30 min. *or* Stimate: 1 spray if < 50 kg 2 sprays if > 50 kg	Aminocaproic acid (Amicar) 100 mg/kg/dose q6h for 5 to 7 days. Maximum dose 30 g/day. Hormonal therapy such as estrogen for menorrhagia.
Type IIA	Factor VIII-VWF concentrates *or* DDAVP	20 to 50 Units/kg IV q12–24h depending on severity	Aminocaproic acid (Amicar). Hormonal therapy such as estrogen for menorrhagia. Some patients may respond to DDAVP.
Type IIB	Factor VIII-VWF concentrates	20 to 50 Units/kg IV q12–24h depending on severity	Aminocaproic acid (Amicar). DDVAP is a relative contraindication.
Type IIM	Factor VIII-VWF concentrates	20 to 50 Units/kg IV q12–24h depending on severity	Aminocaproic acid (Amicar). Hormonal therapy such as estrogen for menorrhagia.
Type IIN	DDAVP and factor VIII-VWF concentrates	See doses for desmopressin and factor replacement	Aminocaproic acid (Amicar). Hormonal therapy such as estrogen for menorrhagia.
Type III	Factor VIII-VWF concentrates	20 to 50 Units/kg IV q12–24h depending on severity	Aminocaproic acid (Amicar). Hormonal therapy such as estrogen for menorrhagia.

DDAVP, desmopressin; IV, intravenously; q*x*h, every *x* hours.

sequestration, or decreased production. The degree of symptoms is directly related to the degree of thrombocytopenia. It is important to understand whether the thrombocytopenia is part of a systemic disease or if it is an isolated event. A thorough history and physical examination as well as careful examination of the complete blood count and interpretation of the blood smear are necessary to the evaluation. Box 2 lists possible causes of thrombocytopenia. Bleeding manifestations of thrombocytopenia are usually petechiae and ecchymosis. More significant bleeding includes mucous membrane bleeding (epistaxis, gastrointestinal, and menorrhagia), intracranial hemorrhage, as well as the more immediate-type surgical bleeding.

Immune-Mediated Thrombocytopenia

Idiopathic thrombocytopenia purpura (ITP), also known as immune thrombocytopenic purpura, is a common cause of thrombocytopenia in children. Patients can present with petechiae, purpura, and mucosal bleeding or be totally asymptomatic and only discovered on routine blood count. The diagnosis of ITP is a diagnosis of exclusion. The peak age is 2 to 4 years. The disorder affects males and females equally. In children, there is usually a history of a preceding viral syndrome that manifests 2 to 3 weeks later with purpura and petechiae. The majority of children with ITP (80%) recover spontaneously, generally within 6 months. The diagnosis of ITP is made when the history, physical examination, complete blood count, and peripheral smear exclude other causes of thrombocytopenia. Management consists of either careful observation or medication to raise the platelet count. The goal in treatment is to prevent major bleeding. Various therapies include steroids (prednisone, dexamethasone), intravenous immunoglobulin (IVIG) and anti-D (WinRho) (Table 3). Splenectomy, immunosuppression (cyclosporin, vincristine, cyclophosphamide), and anti-CD20 antibody (rituximab) are reserved for refractory ITP and chronic ITP.

Neonatal alloimmune thrombocytopenia purpura (NATP) is analogous to Rh disease of the newborn. Alloantibodies are produced by the mother to a specific antigen on fetal platelets that the mother is lacking. The most common antigen is Pl^{A1} (HPA–1a). The incidence of NATP is approximately 1 in 1000 deliveries. The diagnosis should be suspected in a newborn that presents with petechiae and ecchymosis but otherwise looks well. Twenty percent of infants with NATP have an associated intracranial hemorrhage. The platelet count is usually less than 50,000 within 24 hours of birth, and response to random donor platelet transfusion is poor. Therapy consists of prompt diagnosis, platelet typing of the mother and father, and therapy with IVIG, Pl^{A1} negative platelets, or washed maternal platelets. Another form of neonatal immune thrombocytopenia is secondary to maternal ITP. The maternal antibodies cross the placenta and react with the infant's platelets. These antibodies are directed against the platelet-associated glycoproteins. There is less incidence of intracranial hemorrhage in this disorder. Therapy is supportive with IVIG. In both NATP and maternal ITP, the disorder resolves in 3 to 4 months with disappearance of maternal antibody.

Hereditary Platelet Function Defects

Platelets contribute to hemostasis and the formation of the primary hemostatic plug by providing:

- Adequate numbers for surface activation of the coagulation process
- Secretion of important components for recruitment of more platelets
- Release of promoters of endothelial repair

Platelet function abnormalities can be classified as defects in adhesion (Bernard-Soulier syndrome), defects in aggregation (Glanzmann thrombasthenia), defects in secretion (storage pool defect), and disorder of the procoagulant surface (Scott syndrome). As with other platelet-vessel disorders, patients present with easy bruising, mucocutaneous bleeding, menorrhagia, and immediate postsurgical bleeding. Diagnosis is based upon appropriate history and physical examination as well as abnormal screening tests of platelet function (prolonged closure time with PFA–100). If the history is suggestive of a bleeding disorder and von Willebrand testing is normal, platelet aggregation testing should be performed, even if the

---

BOX 2 Causes of Thrombocytopenia in Infants and Children

Increased Platelet Destruction/Sequestration

- Immune thrombocytopenia
  - Neonatal alloimmune thrombocytopenia
  - Maternal ITP
  - Idiopathic thrombocytopenia purpura
  - Autoimmune thrombocytopenia
  - Drug induced
  - Malignancy
- Nonimmune
  - DIC syndromes
  - Infections (bacterial, viral, fungal)
  - Kasabach-Merritt syndrome
  - HUS/TTP
  - Cardiac diseases especially valvular dysfunction (e.g. aortic stenosis)
  - Hypersplenism

Decreased Platelet Production

- Aplastic anemia
  - Fanconi anemia
  - TAR
  - Congenital amegakaryocytosis
- Marrow infiltrative process
  - Leukemias
  - Solid tumor metastasis
  - Myeloproliferative disorders
  - Osteopetrosis
  - Histiocytosis syndromes

Hereditary Thrombocytopenias

- Bernard-Soulier syndrome
- Montreal platelet syndrome
- Chediak-Higashi syndrome
- Wiskott-Aldrich syndrome
- Gray platelet syndrome
- May-Hegglin anomaly

DIC, disseminated intravascular coagulation; HUS, hemolytic uremic syndrome; ITP, idiopathic thrombocytopenic purpura; TAR, thrombocytopenia with absent radii.

TABLE 3 Diagnosis and Therapy for Selected Platelet Disorders

Type	Diagnosis	Therapy	Comments
Immune thrombocytopenia			
NAIT	Severe thrombocytopenia in a well-appearing neonate Maternal platelet antibody positive Maternal PI^{A1} antigen negative	Maternal platelets transfusion IVIG 1g/kg	Cranial ultrasound to rule out hemorrhage.
Maternal ITP	Severe thrombocytopenia Maternal history of ITP	IVIG 1g/kg	Cranial ultrasound.
ITP	Severe thrombocytopenia in a well-appearing child No other cause for thrombocytopenia	Observation IVIG 1 g/kg/dose once WinRho (Anti-D) 25–60 µg/kg dose IV (depends on Hgb level) Prednisone 2 mg/kg/day × 7–14 days, tapered	Treat if there is active mucosal bleeding. Patient must be Rh+. Consider bone marrow aspiration.
Platelet function defects			
Defect in platelet receptor: Glanzmann thrombasthenia Bernard-Soulier syndrome	Platelet aggregation study	Recombinant FVIIa (NovoSeven) 90–120 µg/kg/dose Aminocaproic acid	Platelet transfusion for severe, life-threatening bleeding (risk of alloimmunization).
Defect in granule content/storage pool deficiency Grey platelet syndrome Quebec platelet Hermansky-Pudlak release defects	Platelet aggregation study	DDAVP 0.3 µg/kg/doses IV in 30–50 mL of saline over 30 min or Stimate (intranasal DDAVP) 1 spray for patients <50kg; 2 sprays for patients >50 kg Aminocaproic acid	

DDAVP, desmopressin; ITP, idiopathic thrombocytopenic purpura; IV, intravenously; IVIG, intravenous immunoglobulin; NAIT, neonatal alloimmune thrombocytopenia.

BOX 3 Causes of Disseminated Intravascular Coagulation

- Sepsis or severe infection
  - Any microorganism
- Trauma
  - Severe tissue injury
  - Head injury
  - Fat embolism
- Malignancy
  - Solid tumors
  - Acute leukemias (for example, acute promyelocytic leukemia)
- Vascular abnormalities
  - Hemangiomas
  - Large vessel aneurysm
- Obstetrical
  - Placenta abruption
  - Amniotic fluid embolism
  - Pregnancy induced hypertension
  - Retained fetus
- Toxins
  - Snake bites
  - Recreation drug
  - Transfusion reactions
  - Transplant rejection
- Liver failure

PFA–100 is normal. Consultation with a pediatric hematologist would be instructive. Therapy may include DDAVP, antifibrinolytic agents, platelet transfusions, or,

as an off label use, recombinant FVIIa (NovoSeven) (see Table 3).

Disseminated Intravascular Coagulation

Disseminated intravascular coagulation (DIC) is a syndrome characterized by systemic intravascular activation of coagulation leading to widespread fibrin deposition in the circulation. The massive ongoing activation of coagulation results in the depletion of platelets and coagulation factors leading to bleeding and thrombosis. DIC is not a disease but a syndrome, which is always secondary to an underlying disorder. Several disease states may lead to the development of DIC (Box 3). The two general mechanisms by which DIC is initiated are:

- A systemic inflammatory response leading to activation of the cytokine network and subsequent activation of coagulation (e.g., sepsis or major trauma)
- Release or exposure of procoagulant material in the bloodstream (acute promyelocytic leukemia or obstetrical causes).

In clinical practice, the diagnosis of DIC can be made by a combination of laboratory tests consisting of platelet count and measurement of the prothrombin time (PT), partial prothrombin time (PTT), fibrinogen, and fibrin degradation product (D dimer and or fibrin split products [FSPs]). Serial testing is usually more helpful than single laboratory results. There is a downward trend of the platelet count and fibrinogen, consumption of coagulation factors, prolongation of PT and PTT, and elevation of the fibrin degradation products. The foundation of therapy in DIC is the treatment of the underlying disorder. The efficacy of replacement therapy with plasma products and platelets has not been proven in randomized controlled trials but replacement therapy clinically appears to be a rational therapy. Heparin therapy is controversial at best. Recent reports of recombinant activated protein C appear to be promising in patients with sepsis related DIC.

Common Pitfalls

- Normal screening tests such as PT, PTT, and platelet count do not rule out a significant bleeding disorder.
- Detailed questioning concerning the patient/family history is usually not performed and is likely the most important part of evaluating a patient with a possible bleeding disorder.
- Laboratory results can be spurious secondary to poor collection technique, poor handling, and errors from laboratories not experienced in coagulation disorders.

When Do You Need a Referral?

A hematologist should be consulted when:

- The patient or the family has a history of a possible bleeding disorder such as easy bruising, menorrhagia, postoperative bleeding, hematomas, or other mucosal bleeding symptoms such as nosebleeds or mouth (gum and teeth) bleeding.
- The patient has abnormal screening bleeding tests.
- A patient with a known bleeding disorder requires the services of a comprehensive bleeding disorder clinic.

Communication and Counseling

The patient and family history should determine the evaluation for a bleeding disorder. If the initial bleeding screen is normal, a significant coagulation defect may still be present.

SELECTED READINGS

1. Andrew M, Vegh P, Johnston M, et al: Maturation of the hemostatic system during childhood. Blood 80:1998–2005, 1992. **Review of pediatric normal hemostasis and disease condition pertinent to each age group.**
2. British Committee for Standards in Haematology: Guidelines for the investigation and management of idiopathic thrombocytopenic purpura in adults, children and in pregnancy. Br J Haematol 120:574–596, 2003. **A good guideline for the diagnosis and management of ITP.**
3. George JN, Shattil SJ: The clinical importance of acquired abnormalities of platelet function. N Engl J Med 324:27, 1991. **Extensive discussion of platelet function defects and its management.**
4. George JN, Woolf SH, Raskob GE, et al: Idiopathic thrombocytopenic purpura: A practice guideline developed by explicit methods for the American Society of Hematology. Blood 88:3–40, 1996. **Excellent and extensive evidence-based review of diagnosis, testing, and management of ITP in both children and adults.**
5. Goodnight S, Hathaway WE: Disorders of Hemostasis and Thrombosis: A Clinical Guide. New York: McGraw Hill, 2001. **Excellent, concise overview of coagulation, from normal hemostasis to clinical conditions in hemostasis and thrombosis covering both pediatric and adult patients.**
6. Mannucci PM: How I treat patients with von Willebrand disease. Blood 97:1915–1919, 2001. **Reviews von Willebrand disease and its management.**
7. Marcel L: Current understanding of disseminated intravascular coagulation. Br J Haematol 124, 567–576, 2004. **A good review article discussing the pathophysiology, diagnosis, and treatment of DIC.**

Deep Venous Thrombosis with and without Pulmonary Embolism

Eric F. Grabowski

KEY CONCEPTS

- Deep venous thromboses (DVTs) in children are frequently accompanied by silent pulmonary emboli that should always be considered in the evaluation of a DVT.
- Low-dose thrombolytic therapy is comparatively safe and efficacious, in contrast to high-dose therapy used for symptomatic pulmonary emboli, stroke, and acute myocardial infarction, which carries a significant bleeding risk.
- While Doppler ultrasound is extremely useful in the extremities, CT venography or magnetic resonance angiography (MRA) is often required for identification and characterization of DVTs in veins of the abdomen or chest.
- The evaluation for hypercoagulability should also include structural factors, including vascular anomalies associated with the May-Thurner syndrome, thoracic outlet syndrome, and the anomalous (atretic) inferior vena cava.
- Counseling for risk for recurrent DVT should take into consideration the good prognosis for children with at most a single risk factor in the setting of a reversible systemic illness. Conversely, children with chronic inflammatory conditions/diseases and multiple risk factors warrant long-term anticoagulation therapy.

13

Major deep venous thromboses (DVTs) are less frequent in children than in adults. Nonetheless, the incidence as either a secondary or primary diagnosis is at least 1 in 100,000 per year. The management of such thromboses is critical if the postphlebitic syndrome and recurrent thromboses are to be avoided in later life. In addition, 16% to 20% of such DVTs are associated with silent or clinically significant pulmonary emboli. This chapter reviews:

- Management of DVTs with respect to imaging studies

- Evaluation for congenital risk factors
- Upfront thrombolytic versus anticoagulation therapy
- Special considerations for pulmonary emboli

DVTs in children frequently arise from a combination of an underlying hypercoagulability risk factor and an acquired risk factor or trigger. Although pulmonary emboli are possible in the seemingly well child, they are seen much more often in an acute care setting.

Expert Opinion on Management Issues

DIAGNOSTIC CONSIDERATIONS

Imaging Modalities

Useful imaging modalities include duplex ultrasonography and color Doppler flow imaging, CT with contrast enhancement, magnetic resonance angiograms (MRAs), and venography. Real-time ultrasound is noninvasive and effective in demonstrating the presence or absence of residual blood flow in DVTs in the extremities. This modality is also able to identify thrombi adherent to the ends of indwelling catheters. However, venography remains the gold standard. It is superior to ultrasonography in the detection of thrombi at the ends of umbilical artery and vein catheters. Furthermore, venography may be the optimal means of assessing chronic venous insufficiency. With regard to pulmonary emboli, a baseline ventilation-perfusion scan is warranted in cases of a major DVT to exclude silent pulmonary emboli. Symptomatic pulmonary emboli may be assessed by pulmonary angiography with multidetector CT (spiral CT) or a ventilation-perfusion scan.

Evaluation for Hypercoagulability

Certain natural inhibitors of coagulant and fibrinolytic enzymes are known to play critical roles in the control of hemostasis. Heterozygous antithrombin III deficiency, for example, is an autosomal defect characterized by repeated episodes of venous thrombosis, with or without pulmonary emboli. Inhibition of serine esterase activity by antithrombin III accounts for its effects not only on thrombin but also on activated forms of factors XII, XI, IX, and X.

Activated protein C and its cofactor, protein S, are now recognized as significant modulators of fibrinolysis and thrombosis. Children and adults who are heterozygous for deficiencies (generally to the 50% range) of either protein are at increased risk for thrombosis. Synthesis is vitamin K–dependent and occurs in the liver (protein C) or in both the liver and the endothelium (protein S). Protein C, a glycoprotein, is activated by the thrombomodulin-thrombin complex on the endothelial cell surface, thereby becoming a serine protease with both anticoagulant and profibrinolytic activities. In the presence of protein S, activated protein C degrades the thrombin-activated forms of factors V and VII and neutralizes a circulating inhibitor of tissue-plasminogen activator. Tissue-plasminogen activator, in turn, converts plasminogen into the enzyme plasmin. Recently, a mutant factor V has been identified, known as factor V Leiden, which resists degradation by activated protein C. Hence, the presence of this mutant factor V is also known as activated protein C resistance and may be screened for by a clotting assay based upon resistance to clotting in the presence of added, activated protein C. The mutation involves the replacement of arginine by glutamine at position 506 of the factor V molecule. Present in one factor V gene in nearly 5% of the white population, this mutation confers a relative thrombosis risk of 6.6.

More recently, a mutant prothrombin (prothrombin G20210A polymorphism) has been reported that has prevalence in the white population of 2% to 3%. Although it confers a relative thrombosis risk of 2.8, a laboratory screening test for this mutation is not yet available. The definitive test at present for either factor V Leiden or prothrombin G20210A is a polymerase chain reaction (PCR)-based assay. Other congenital plasma phase conditions to consider include an elevated lipoprotein(a), hyperhomocysteinemia, a decreased or dysfunctional plasminogen, and dysfibrinogenemia.

Of current interest is the identification of individuals who are compound heterozygotes, that is, who are heterozygous for two of the conditions given in the previous paragraph at once. Examples include heterozygosity for both factor V Leiden and protein C deficiency, and heterozygosity for both factor V Leiden and hyperhomocysteinemia. Of special interest are individuals who are homozygous for either factor V Leiden or prothrombin G20210A and are heterozygous for one of the other conditions. I follow several teenagers who have such compound risk factors. Uncommon homozygous deficiencies of antithrombin III, protein C, and protein S all have been described, but these conditions lead rapidly in the perinatal period to purpura fulminans and death unless a major effort is undertaken to reverse the deficiency with, as appropriate, antithrombin III concentrate, protein C concentrate, and fresh-frozen plasma (FFP), followed by lifelong anticoagulation. Thus, these conditions are not likely to be seen for the first time in the older child.

Acquired conditions predisposing to thrombosis include a lupus-like anticoagulant, the presence of anticardiolipin antibodies, the presence of antibodies to protein C and/or S (reported following cases of varicella), certain systemic conditions (nephrotic syndrome, diabetes mellitus, dehydration, use of estrogens), trauma, malignancy (more in adults), and placement of a central venous catheter.

Pulmonary Emboli

While clinically significant in a minority of the cases in Table 1, pulmonary emboli should always be considered, as these may be silent and require special follow-up. Symptomatic pulmonary emboli (e.g., those with dyspnea and tachypnea, or even a simple oxygen requirement) may go unrecognized as such if not considered in the differential diagnosis of acute chest pain. This is especially true if there are no symptoms to suggest an origin from pelvic veins or from a lower or, less commonly, upper

TABLE 1 Intensive Care Cases Seen at Massachusetts General Hospital

Patient/Age/Sex	Risk Factor(s)	Therapy
MD/7/M	Catheter, nephrotic syndrome	IV heparin
AM/11/F	Catheter, factor V Leiden, seizure disorder	Urokinase with heparin
KM/8/f	Multiple catheters, seizure disorder, aspiration pneumonia	Urokinase with heparin
LL/15/F	Factor V Leiden, ATIII deficiency, appendicitis	Urokinase with (catheter directed) heparin
TH/12/M	AML, L-asparaginase therapy, catheter	Urokinase with heparin
MB/1/M	Catheter, dKA	Urokinase with heparin, then t-PA
AR/16/F	Factor V Leiden, catheter, Crohn disease	t-PA with heparin
GB/17/F	Sepsis and DIC (Lemierre syndrome)	LMW heparin, then coumadin
BH/12/M	Mastoiditis	LMW heparin, then coumadin
AE/18/F	Birth control pills, smoking	Heparin, then coumadin

AML, acute myeloid leukemia; ATIII, antithrombin III; DIC, disseminated intravascular coagulation; DKA, diabetic ketoacidosis; IV, intravenous; LMW, low molecular weight; t-PA, tissue plasminogen activator.

extremity. I am aware of at least one instance in which an ultimately fatal pulmonary embolism (PE) went unsuspected because the affected child had sickle cell disease, was identified as having chest pain, but was thought to be having a vasoocclusive crisis. Any massive PE warrants high-dose thrombolytic therapy when such therapy is not contraindicated (see "Thrombosis for Massive Pulmonary Embolism").

TREATMENT

Thrombolysis

In most cases of DVTs, thrombolytic therapy may be considered safe front-line therapy, unless a significant bleeding risk exists or there has been recent surgery. In the latter cases, the preferred approach is anticoagulation with either low molecular weight heparin (LMWH) or standard, unfractionated heparin. In the absence of a significant bleeding risk, thrombolytic therapy has promise of becoming the preferred approach, especially with PE or occlusion of a major vein, because of the better opportunity to preserve organ (lung) function and/or the function of the venous valves. In addition, clot resolution may be faster. Fresh thrombi respond better to thrombolytics than old ones do; however, clots as old as 2 weeks have lysed either partially or completely.

Thrombolytics

Available thrombolytic agents include streptokinase, recombinant prourokinase, and tissue-plasminogen activator (t-PA). All these agents activate plasminogen, converting it to the fibrinolytic enzyme plasmin. Under investigation is the agent Agkistrodon contortrix, which does not require plasminogen. Streptokinase may be associated with allergic reactions with rechallenge and, therefore, is not recommended for children, especially if there has been a recent streptococcal infection. Recombinant prourokinase is currently not widely available. t-PA is effective in acute coronary occlusions and massive pulmonary emboli, although with an increased risk of hemorrhagic stroke at the high dosages (1 mg/kg over 1–2 hours) employed. Recent experience with t-PA in the lysis of arterial and venous thromboses with lower

dosing over a more extended period (e.g., 0.03 mg/kg for 12 to 48 hours) indicates that such dosing is likely to be equally effective for DVTs and nonmassive PEs yet much safer. The risk of significant hemorrhage with such dosing is likely to be a fraction of 1%.

Indications for thrombolytics are extensive DVT, massive PE (see "Thrombolysis for Massive Pulmonary Embolism"), PE not responding to heparin therapy, and demonstrated "freely floating" thrombus on the outer surface of an indwelling central venous catheter that makes simple catheter removal a potential cause of PE.

Contraindications to thrombolytic therapy include active bleeding, surgery or organ biopsy (e.g., liver, kidney) within the previous 10 days, neurosurgery within the previous 3 weeks, and an underlying bleeding diathesis (e.g., hemophilia, disseminated intravascular coagulation [DIC]). However, if the underlying bleeding diathesis can be corrected, as with factor replacement for hemophilia, thrombolysis can become an option.

Thrombolysis for Deep Venous Thromboses

For children older than age 3 months, 0.03 mg/kg/hour should be given intravenously (IV) to a maximum total dose of 3 mg/hour, without a loading dose. Radiographic and laboratory evidence of fibrinolysis should be monitored to adjust the infusion rate upward by 20% increments for greater efficacy (if no bleeding) or downward (in the event of minor bleeding). t-PA should be accompanied by either low-dose standard unfractionated heparin, at 5 to 10 U/kg/hour without a loading dose, or low molecular weight heparin (LMWH) (e.g., dalteparin at 50 U/kg subcutaneously [SC] twice daily). (Table 2 provides a comparison of these agents.) This serves the purpose of inactivating any clot-bound thrombin released by thrombolysis itself. Use of LMWH is particularly indicated for patients without adequate venous access or for those with serum albumins much below 2 g/dL (see "Anticoagulant Therapy"), keeping in mind the greater difficulty in reversing LMWH in the event of hemorrhage.

Imaging should be performed at least every 12 hours, and t-PA (and any standard unfractionated heparin) should be stopped when the clot has resolved or 48 hours has elapsed, whichever comes first.

TABLE 2 Comparison of Standard and Low Molecular Weight Heparins

Heparin	Standard Unfractionated Heparin	Low Molecular Weight Heparin
Molecular weight	12,000–15,000	4,000–7,000
Half-life, min	60	120–180
Binds to plasma proteins and blood cells	Yes	Weakly
Inactivates thrombin	Yes	Weakly
Monitoring	aPTT, anti-factor Xa level	Anti-factor Xa level

aPTT, activated partial thromboplastin time.

For term infants younger than age 3 months, there appears to be a need for a somewhat higher dose of t-PA, in the range of 0.045 mg/kg/hour. Similarly, the doses of heparin and LMWH are higher (e.g., 7–14 U/kg/hour for heparin, and 75 U/kg SC twice daily for dalteparin). Again, however, one should evaluate the relative risk to life versus risk of hemorrhage.

Thrombolysis for Massive Pulmonary Embolism

Massive PE is characterized by cardiogenic shock, profound hypoxemia, impending respiratory failure, and/or an anatomically large PE on pulmonary angiography or chest CT. It seems reasonable to extend this definition to include normotensive patients with PE who have moderate or severe right ventricular dysfunction on echocardiography, although the matter remains controversial. Because pediatricians see so few massive pulmonary emboli, it is critical in this situation to enlist the guidance and support of a medical pulmonology service. For massive PE, the U.S. Food and Drug Administration (FDA) has approved for adults a dosing regimen of 100 mg t-PA as a continuous IV infusion over a 2-hour period. One might consider for older children a dose extrapolated from that for adults and based on surface area and weight of 2 mg/kg over 2 hours. The risk of intracranial hemorrhage with such doses in adult patients is approximately 3%.

Any such patients, of course, need to be managed in an intensive care setting, because they will require oxygen support, correction of abnormal arterial blood gases, monitoring of oxygen saturation, and pain control.

Thrombolysis for Cerebral Sinus Thrombosis

A special situation arises when a child suffers cerebral sinus thrombosis involving multiple sinuses (e.g., as suggested by involvement of the torcula) with risk to drainage from cortical veins. In the absence of intracerebral hemorrhage, the author has twice used low-dose t-PA (for 60- and 72-hour durations), along with low-dose unfractionated heparin, with complete reperfusion of the involved sinuses and without hemorrhage. Much of the benefit appeared to occur toward the end of the thrombolysis period.

Long-Term Management

When t-PA is discontinued, one should immediately start therapeutic LMWH, preferably with bid injections. The platelet count should be monitored because of a small risk of thrombocytopenia with this agent. Beginning with day 3 of LMWH, the child should be converted to oral warfarin, beginning with 0.15 mg/kg/day (Box 1), with a target International Normalized Ratio (INR) of 2 to 3 for DVT, and of 3 to 4 for PE or massive DVT. The LMWH may be discontinued when the INR is greater than 2.0 or greater than 3.0, respectively, on two successive determinations. The INR may be less frequently monitored at this point. Warfarin therapy should be continued for 3 to 6 months. A longer (e.g., 6 to 12 months, if not indefinite) duration of such therapy may be indicated in the presence of one or more of the risk factors listed in Box 2.

Thrombolytic Failure

If t-PA fails to eliminate the thrombus or a large part of it, one should revert to therapeutic standard heparin for 3 to 7 days to allow time for the thrombus to organize ("stabilize") to the point where embolization is much less likely. Catheter-directed thrombolysis, balloon angioplasty, or surgical thrombectomy are other options (see "Other Considerations").

BLEEDING WHILE ON THERAPY

For local or minor bleeding, use compresses, topical thrombin, and/or topical collagen. When the patient experiences severe or life-threatening bleeding while receiving thrombolytic therapy, the thrombolytic agent and heparin should be stopped. Administer cryoprecipitate (0.2 U/kg), which replaces fibrinogen. Consider reversing the thrombolytic process by using epsilon-aminocaproic acid (Amicar) at a dose of 50 to 100 mg/kg IV or orally (PO) (maximum of 4 g). When significant bleeding occurs while the patient is receiving heparin, stop the heparin. Administer protamine. When the patient experiences significant bleeding while receiving warfarin, the warfarin should be stopped and FFP administered.

Other Considerations

For patients who fail systemic thrombolysis, who have contraindications to thrombolysis, or who require more aggressive therapy than anticoagulation alone, consider catheter-directed thrombolysis, balloon angioplasty (a form of surgical thrombectomy), placement of a filter, and surgical thrombectomy. Catheter-directed thrombolysis and/or balloon angioplasty may have a particularly

BOX 1 Anticoagulants

Heparin, Standard Unfractionated

- 50–75 U/kg IV bolus, then
- 25–28 U/kg/h in newborns
- 15–20 U/kg/h in older children and adults

Heparin, Low Molecular Weight

- 1.5 mg (or 150 U)/kg q12h subcutaneously for newborns
- 1.0 mg (or 100 U)/kg q12h subcutaneously for older children and adults

Coumadin (Warfarin Sodium)

- 0.3 mg/kg/day PO for newborns
- 0.15 mg/kg/day PO for older children
- 0.1 mg/kg/day PO for adults

IV, intravenously; PO, orally; qxh, every x hours.

BOX 2 Risk Factors Warranting a Longer Duration of Anticoagulation

- Acquired or congenital plasma-phase risk factors, excluding the presence of factor V Leiden or prothrombin G20210A alone.
- The presence of an uncorrectable vascular structural anomaly.
- The absence of an obvious triggering event for the DVT, or the presence of a triggering event that cannot be removed, such as inflammatory bowel disease or recurrent pancreatitis. Examples of triggering events that can be removed include use of oral contraceptives, smoking, or a central venous access device.
- The occurrence of a second DVT.
- A DVT virtually completely occluding the deep vein in question at presentation, especially if markers of thrombosis and inflammation such as the d dimer or factor VIII level remain elevated for 6 weeks or more.

important role in the teenager with thoracic outlet syndrome, or with chronic recurrent deep venous thrombosis. Removable catheter-placed filters have a role in selected older children who cannot be immediately anticoagulated, such as trauma victims with life-threatening hemorrhage. Anticoagulation can be started as soon as it is judged safe. The filters can be removed up to 6 months or longer following placement, provided they are free of clot and no new thrombus is being generated (normal D-dimer level). Pneumatic compression of unaffected lower extremities with pneumatic "boots" should be employed with patients who are immobilized for any prolonged period.

Anticoagulant Therapy

When thrombolytic therapy is contraindicated or not desired by a given patient or child's family, anticoagulation with either standard unfractionated heparin or LMWH may be undertaken (for a comparison, see Table 2). Standard unfractionated heparin with (ATIII) is a potent antithrombin that also possesses anti-factor IXa and anti-factor Xa activity in addition to a tendency to bind to cellular surfaces and plasma proteins. Its potency depends in part on the level of plasma proteins (potency diminishes with an increase in acute phase reactants,

yet increases with serum albumin levels below 2 g/dL) and the state of endothelial cells in a given patient. In acute inflammatory states, for example, heparin resistance may be seen, a state that is not so much resistance as decreased bioavailability. In such a situation, dosing should not be based on the partial thromboplastin time (PTT), but rather on levels of circulating anti-factor Xa activity (heparin levels). LMWHs, however, are derived from standard heparin by various methods of depolymerization. These heparins bind antithrombin III (ATIII), but have a much weaker antithrombin activity compared with standard heparin while retaining anti-factor Xa and anti-factor IXa actions. In addition, LMWHs are minimally cell-membrane or plasma-protein bound. Consequently, dosing is more straightforward and predictable. Little monitoring is required for anticoagulant efficacy, aside from an anti-factor Xa level 2 to 3 days into therapy. Box 1 summarizes age-dependent dosing for these two classes of agents. Both standard heparin and LMWH are metabolized more rapidly in the newborn and have a greater distribution volume in the newborn. Heparin conceptually remains the more potent anticoagulant of the two. However, DVTs that are neither massive nor complicated by PE are now being managed safely with LMWH. Some patients may even be managed on an outpatient basis following initial evaluation.

Common Pitfalls

- Doppler flow ultrasound is less sensitive than CT venography, MRA, or venography especially in the abdomen and upper venous system. This is because of the presence in the abdominal and chest cavities of air-filled loops of bowel and the lungs themselves, respectively. In these locations, CT with contrast enhancement or MRA is preferred in older children and adults.
- Hypercoagulability evaluations are often compromised by the acute phase reactants accompanying acute DVTs. Protein S levels are notoriously falsely lowered in any clotting-based assay because of the sensitivity of these assays to the factor VIII level, which is often elevated. Lipoprotein(a) levels may similarly be somewhat elevated acutely. Protein C levels may be transiently lowered because of consumption in the thrombotic process. Anticardiolipin antibodies may be only transiently positive, especially in young children (e.g., <10 years of age).
- With thrombolysis, reduce the rate of standard heparin infusion in the presence of low serum albumin, and reduce the dose of LMWH in the presence of renal compromise. If the serum albumin is low (of the order of 2 g/dL, as in patients with nephrotic syndrome or with other causes of protein wasting), the infusion rate should be reduced to 2.5 to 5 U/kg/hour or even less because of the greater bioavailability of heparin with low total serum protein. The rate of heparin infusion should not lead to a significant prolongation of the PTT. Similarly, the dose of LMWH should be lowered because of delayed excretion with renal impairment (follow anti-factor Xa levels).

- Duration of therapy should not, with presently available data, be determined by the presence of factor V Leiden or prothrombin G20210A alone.
- Precautions should be followed to minimize bleeding risk. During thrombolytic or anticoagulation therapy, one should avoid intramuscular injections, minimize physical therapy or patient manipulation, avoid concurrent use of aspirin or other antiplatelet agents, avoid urinary catheterization, refrain from performing rectal temperatures, and avoid arterial punctures. Blood samples should be obtained from a peripheral vein or a previously inserted catheter. The platelet count should be maintained above 50,000/μL.

Communication and Counseling

Childhood DVT often results in the postthrombotic syndrome, caused by venous occlusion and loss of competence of the venous valves and characterized by chronic swelling, pain, and limb disability. Whereas the overall incidence is estimated at 20%, in very high-risk populations, such as children with nearly completely occluded veins at presentation and with persistence in elevations in markers of thrombosis and inflammation such as the d dimer, this percentage can approach 80%. Affected children and their parents need to be counseled regarding the use of support/compression stockings, the importance of physical therapy and physical activity, and appropriate modifications in lifestyle.

Children with specific plasma-phase disorders predisposing to thrombosis—or even vascular structural anomalies—require longer follow-up, given the risk of recurrence and the need to balance a sufficient duration of anticoagulation with bleeding risks. Those who have had a significant PE can be at especial risk of pulmonary compromise and long-term right heart dysfunction.

Finally, it is important to provide affected children and their families with information regarding support groups, such as the National Alliance for Thrombosis and Thrombophilia (NATT) and the Coalition to Prevent Deep-Vein Thrombosis.

SUGGESTED READINGS

1. Goldhaber SZ: Thrombolysis for PE. N Engl J Med 347:1131–1132, 2002. **This is an excellent review of indications for high-dose t-PA.**
2. Grabowski EF, Corrigan JJ: Hemostasis: General considerations. In Miller DR, Baehner RL (eds): Blood Diseases of Infancy and Childhood. St. Louis: Mosby, 1995, pp 849–865. **Blood rheology and basic hemostasis are integrated in this overview.**
3. Journeycake JM, Manco-Johnson MJ: Thrombosis during infancy and childhood: What we know and what we do not know. Hematol Oncol Clin North Am 18:1315–1338, 2004. **This is a good review for pediatric DVT.**
4. Prandoni P, Lensing A, Cogo A, et al: The long-term clinical course of acute deep venous thrombosis. Ann Int Med 125:1–7, 1996. **This interesting paper focuses on recurrent DVT and its risk factors.**
5. Wang M, Hays T, Balasa V, et al. Pediatric Coagulation Consortium. Low-dose tissue plasminogen activator thrombolysis in children. J Pediatr Hematol Oncol 25:379–386, 2003. **This article summarizes the safe use of low-dose t-PA in several pediatric centers.**

Inherited Forms of Aplastic Anemia: The Inherited Bone Marrow Failure Syndromes

Blanche P. Alter

KEY CONCEPTS

- Approximately 25% of children with aplastic anemia have an underlying genetic etiology.
- Acquired and inherited aplastic anemias have critical differences in medical management.
- Hematopoietic stem cell protocols differ between acquired and inherited aplastic anemia.
- Several of the inherited aplastic anemias are associated with a high risk of leukemia and/or specific solid tumors.

Patients who present with aplastic anemia may have an acquired or an inherited etiology for their bone marrow failure. The genetic disorders must be considered and ruled out before assuming that the disorder is acquired. Many of the genetic aplastic anemias are associated with specific physical abnormalities that often lead to the correct diagnoses, and thus careful physical examination should be performed. The combination of these findings with the blood counts and bone marrow aspirates, biopsies, and cytogenetics may reveal the most likely diagnosis and identify the degree of severity of the hematopoietic problem. Mutant genes have been identified for many of the disorders, and mutation testing is often useful for final confirmation of the diagnosis, genetic counseling, prenatal diagnosis, and choice of a related, syndrome-negative, stem cell transplant donor. Details about these syndromes can be found in textbook chapters listed in Suggested Readings.

The most common of the rare inherited bone marrow failure syndromes (IBMFSs) (Table 1) associated with pancytopenia is Fanconi anemia (FA). Approximately 75% of the reported patients have characteristic birth defects, such as short stature, café au lait spots, radial ray deformities, abnormal kidneys, hearing defects, and others. Even in the absence of these features, the diagnosis of FA should be considered in any child with aplastic anemia, as well as in adults if there is any possibility of this diagnosis. Patients with dyskeratosis congenita (DC) may present with cytopenias during childhood or adolescence, whereas the pathognomonic abnormal fingernails and toenails, reticular skin pigmentation, and leukoplakia often develop during adolescence or adulthood.

The other inherited bone marrow failure syndromes may manifest with single cytopenias. Patients with Diamond-Blackfan anemia (DBA) have pure red cell aplasia that is usually apparent in infancy, although milder cases have been identified later, including in adults. Approximately 25% have abnormal thumbs, and more than 50% have short stature. It is very unusual for DBA patients to develop full-blown aplastic anemia. Shwachman-Diamond syndrome (SDS) is characterized by malabsorption because of exocrine pancreatic insufficiency

TABLE 1 Inherited Bone Marrow Failure Syndromes*

Syndrome	Age, Years	Sex	Family History	Major Characteristic Features	Hematology/Oncology	Specific Diagnostic Test	Genetics (Genes)
Fanconi anemia	0->50	M=F	Siblings	Skin pigmentation, short stature, triangular face, abnormal thumbs/radii, microcephaly, abnormal kidneys, decreased fertility	Macrocytosis, thrombocytopenia, anemia, neutropenia, hypocellular marrow MDS, leukemia, solid tumors, liver tumors	Chromosome breaks in cells cultured with DNA cross-linkers	Autosomal/X-linked recessive (>12 FANC genes)
Dyskeratosis congenita	0->50	M>F	Male relatives, parents, siblings	Dyskeratotic nails, Lacey reticular rash, oral leukoplakia	Macrocytosis, thrombocytopenia, anemia, neutropenia, hypocellular marrow. MDS, leukemia, solid tumors	None (short telomeres may be useful)	X-linked (DKC1), autosomal dominant (TERC, TERT), ? autosomal recessive
Diamond-Blackfan anemia	0->50	M=F	Parents	Short stature, abnormal thumbs	Macrocytosis, anemia, reticulocytopenia, erythroid hypoplasia in marrow MDS, leukemia, solid tumors	Elevated red cell adenosine deaminase (ADA)	Autosomal dominant (RPS19 in 25%)
Shwachman-Diamond syndrome	0-5	M=F	Siblings	Short stature, malabsorption	Neutropenia; myeloid hypoplasia in marrow MDS, leukemia	Decreased serum trypsinogen and isoamylase	Autosomal recessive (SBDS)
Severe congenital neutropenia	0-1	M=F	Parents	Severe infections in infancy	Neutropenia; promyelocyte arrest in marrow MDS, leukemia	None	Autosomal dominant (ELA-2, GFI-1)
Thrombocytopenia and absent radii	0	M=F	Siblings	Absent radii with thumbs present	Thrombocytopenia; decreased megakaryocytes in marrow Leukemia	Arm x-ray	Autosomal recessive
Amegakaryocytic thrombocytopenia	0-5	M=F	Siblings	Petechiae	Thrombocytopenia; decreased megakaryocytes in marrow Aplastic anemia, MDS, leukemia	None	Autosomal recessive (MPL)

*Some patients with these syndromes have no family history, and none of the physical or hematologic features.
MDS, myelodysplastic syndrome; ?, no gene found.
From Alter BP: Bone marrow failure: A child is not just a small adult (but an adult may have a childhood disease). Hematology (Am Soc Hematol Educ Program) 2005:97–104.

and neutropenia. The pancreatic function sometimes improves with age, and the neutropenia may become milder. However, SDS patients may also develop pancytopenia. Patients with severe congenital neutropenia (SCN) do not have a unique physical phenotype. The diagnosis depends on severe neutropenia (<200 neutrophils per mm^3) in infancy, associated with a marrow myeloid differentiation arrest at the promyelocyte/myelocyte stage. These infants may have severe pyogenic infections. Newborns with thrombocytopenia and absent radii

(TAR) syndrome present with neonatal thrombocytopenia and the characteristic forearm deformities. These children usually show improved platelet counts after the first year, and there are no reports of development of aplastic anemia. In contrast, children with amegakaryocytic thrombocytopenia (amega) do not usually have birth defects, but have severely low platelet counts, and often evolve into aplastic anemia.

Figure 1 shows the algorithm for the diagnosis of FA. The gold standard is the detection of chromosome breaks in dividing cells that are cultured with a DNA cross-linker such as diepoxybutane (DEB) or mitomycin C (MMC). The test is usually positive in blood T lymphocytes stimulated to divide with phytohemagglutinin. However, approximately 10% of patients with FA have hematopoietic somatic mosaicism, in which genetic reversion has occurred in differentiated or pluripotent stem cells, and the progeny of these cells are resistant to cross-link damage, as are normal cells. If the suspicion of FA remains high, skin fibroblasts can be used for the diagnostic test.

There are no diagnostic tests for the other syndromes that are as sensitive and specific as the FA test, and clinical acumen is critical. Demonstration of short telomeres in blood cells of patients with DC may be helpful but is currently a research study. Patients with DBA often have elevated red cell adenosine deaminase (ADA), but this test is not useful if the patient has recently received transfusions, and there are some family members without clinical DBA who have increased ADA. Patients with SD usually have low serum trypsinogen and isoamylase levels or other evidence of exocrine pancreatic insufficiency. The diagnoses of SCN, amega, and TAR are based on clinical examinations, blood counts, and bone marrow examinations.

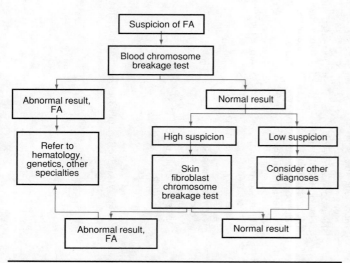

FIGURE 1. Fanconi anemia (FA) diagnostic algorithm. (From Alter BP: Bone marrow failure: A child is not just a small adult [but an adult may have a childhood disease]. Hematology [Am Soc Hematol Educ Program] 2005:97–104.)

TABLE 2 Management Guidelines

Syndrome	When to Treat	Pharmaceutical Treatment	Transfusions	Stem Cell Transplant	Spontaneous Improvement
Fanconi Anemia	Hb <8 g/dL, or ANC <1000/mm^3, or platelets <30,000/ mm^3	Androgens, usually oxymetholone 2–5 mg/kg/day G-CSF, ~5 mcg/kg/day	Packed red cells or platelets as needed	Bone marrow, or cord blood	Rare
Dyskeratosis congenita	Hb <8 g/dL, or ANC <1000/mm^3, or platelets <30,000/ mm^3	Androgens, usually oxymetholone 2–5 mg/kg/day G-CSF, ~5 mcg/kg/day	Packed red cells or platelets as needed	Bone marrow, or cord blood	Rare
Diamond-Blackfan Anemia	Hb <8g/dL	Prednisone, 2–5 mg/kg/day	Packed red cells	Bone marrow, or cord blood	~25%
Shwachman-Diamond syndrome	ANC <1000/mm^3	G-CSF, 5–10 mcg/kg/day		Bone marrow, or cord blood	No
Severe congenital neutropenia	ANC <1000/mm^3	G-CSF, 5–10 mcg/kg/day		Bone marrow, or cord blood	No
Thrombocytopenia absent radii	Platelets <15,000/mm^3	None	Platelets as needed	Bone marrow, or cord blood	Most patients
Amegakaryocytic thrombocytopenia	Hb <8 g/dL, or ANC <1000/mm^3, or platelets <30,000/ mm^3	Androgens, usually oxymetholone 2–5 mg/kg/day G-CSF, ~5 mcg/kg/day	Packed red cells or platelets as needed	Bone marrow, or cord blood	No

Hb, hemoglobin; ANC, absolute neutrophil count; G-CSF, granulocyte colony-stimulating factor.
From Alter BP: Bone marrow failure: A child is not just a small adult (but an adult may have a childhood disease). Hematology (Am Soc Hematol Educ Program) 2005:97–104.

TABLE 3 Risk of Neoplasia

Syndrome	Leukemia	Solid Tumors
Fanconi anemia	Acute myeloid leukemia	Head and neck squamous cell carcinomas; gynecologic, esophageal, brain tumors
Dyskeratosis congenita	Acute myeloid leukemia	Head and neck and anogenital carcinomas
Diamond-Blackfan anemia	Acute myeloid leukemia	Osteogenic sarcomas
Shwachman-Diamond syndrome	Acute myeloid leukemia	No
Severe congenital neutropenia	Acute myeloid Leukemia	No
Thrombocytopenia and absent radii	Acute myeloid Leukemia	No
Amegakaryocytic thrombocytopenia	Acute myeloid leukemia	No

From Alter BP: Bone marrow failure: A child is not just a small adult (but an adult may have a childhood disease). Hematology (Am Soc Hematol Educ Program) 2005:97–104.

Expert Opinion on Management Issues

Research and family support groups for some of the inherited marrow syndromes have convened expert panels to develop consensus guidelines for management of the disorders. Table 2 summarizes the major indications for treatment and the types of treatment that can be considered. There is no evidence beyond the expert level, because the advice is based on case reports and consensus panels, and not on retrospective or prospective cohort studies. The FA recommendations are available online and in a book published by the Fanconi Anemia Research Fund. Results from an international consensus conference on SDS were also published recently. To date there have not been similar consensus guidelines for the other disorders, and thus physicians must rely on textbooks and on consultation with more experienced colleagues. There are several centers to which patients might be referred for diagnostic and management expertise. In particular, if stem cell transplant is being considered, it is advisable to send patients to transplant centers with expertise in the specific syndrome.

Common Pitfalls

The appropriate diagnosis is critical for management of patients with any of the inherited syndromes. Although patients with acquired aplastic anemia might respond to treatment with immunosuppressive agents, such as antithymocyte globulin and cyclosporine A, patients with the inherited disorders will not respond, and precious time may be lost. If a hematopoietic stem cell transplant is chosen, the preparation that is used in acquired aplastic anemia is most likely to be toxic to patients with FA, DC, DBA, and SDS, although it may be tolerated by those with amega and perhaps TAR.

However, patients with aplasia as a consequence of FA, DC, amega, or SDS who do not have a good transplant donor may respond to treatment with androgens, granulocyte-colony stimulating factor (G-CSF), erythropoietin, or some combination. Corticosteroids are specifically effective only in DBA patients. Although in general we try to avoid transfusions of blood products unless necessary (to avoid sensitization that may jeopardize a future transplant), platelet transfusions may be critical for prevention of hemorrhage during the first year in TAR infants, who are likely to improve with time. In all cases that do require blood products, one must avoid using related donors to prevent sensitization.

Communication and Counseling

The diagnosis of the appropriate syndrome must be made as soon as possible to guide therapeutic options, and to begin to discuss prognosis and other complications that might ensue, such as leukemia or solid tumors (Table 3). Families must be offered genetic counseling, including:

- Opportunities for examination of all family members who are at risk of having the disorder in a milder form, or of being nonpenetrant carriers
- Estimates of recurrence risks in future pregnancies
- The possibilities of prenatal diagnosis and in vitro fertilization and preimplantation diagnosis

The counseling should be provided by experts who are familiar with all of the possible inheritance patterns, and who understand these rare disorders.

SUGGESTED READINGS

1. Alter BP: Inherited bone marrow failure syndromes. In Nathan DG, Orkin SH, Look AT, Ginsburg D (eds): Nathan and Oski's Hematology of Infancy and Childhood, 6th ed. Philadelphia: WB Saunders, 2003, pp 280–365. **Most recent comprehensive review of the inherited bone marrow failure syndromes.**
2. Owen J, Frohnmayer L, Eiler ME (eds): Fanconi Anemia: Standards for Clinical Care, 2nd ed. Eugene, Ore: Fanconi Anemia Research Fund, 2003. **Recommendations for diagnosis and care in FA.**
3. Fanconi Anemia Research Fund: Available online at http://www.fanconi.org. **Website of the Fanconi Anemia Research Fund, with links to their published books and newsletters.**
4. Rothbaum R, Perrault J, Vlachos A, et al: Shwachman-Diamond syndrome: Report from an international conference. J Pediatr 141:266–270, 2002. **Recommendations for diagnosis and care in SDS.**
5. Young NS, Alter BP: Aplastic Anemia: Acquired and Inherited. Philadelphia: WB Saunders, 1994. **Comprehensive review of acquired and inherited aplastic anemias.**

13

Acquired Aplastic Anemia

Neelam Giri and Blanche P. Alter

KEY CONCEPTS

- Acquired aplastic anemia (AA) is a rare disorder that may be rapidly fatal if left untreated.
- Diagnosis is confirmed by demonstration of peripheral blood pancytopenia and bone marrow aplasia.
- Inherited bone marrow failure should be excluded by specific tests because the management differs.
- Support with red blood and platelet transfusions may be required.
- Bone marrow transplant from an HLA-identical sibling is the treatment of choice for severe and very severe AA, and is curative in more than 75% of cases.
- For patients who lack a sibling donor and for those with moderate AA who are transfusion-dependent, immunosuppression with antithymocyte globulin and cyclosporine is the first line of therapy, resulting in greater than 50% long-term survival.

Aplastic anemia (AA) is a rare disorder, characterized by peripheral blood pancytopenia and a hypocellular bone marrow. Other causes of pancytopenia, such as hypersplenism, marrow infiltration by premalignant or malignant cells (myelodysplastic syndrome [MDS], leukemia, or metastatic cancer), infection (e.g., tuberculosis), or collagen vascular disease must be ruled out. Approximately 75% of patients with AA have the acquired form (Box 1, and see chapter entitled "Inherited Forms of Aplastic Anemia"). Factors implicated in the development of acquired AA include radiation, drugs and chemicals, viruses, toxins, and autoimmune disorders. However, in the majority of cases, no specific cause can be identified; these are termed *idiopathic*. A genetic predisposition may exist that increases the likelihood of bone marrow failure after an environmental insult. Approximately 5% to 10% of cases occur following an episode of hepatitis in which no known viral pathogen or drug has been identified. The reported incidence of acquired AA is two per million per year in Europe and North America, and the incidence is two to three times higher in East Asia.

Aplastic anemia is defined by the presence of bone marrow hypoplasia plus at least two of the following cytopenias:

1. Hemoglobin less than 10 g/dL
2. Platelet count less than 50×10^9/L
3. Neutrophil count less than 1.5×10^9/L

The disease varies from moderate AA (MAA) to severe AA (SAA) based on the severity of pancytopenia (Table 1). Patients with SAA who have a neutrophil count of less than 0.2×10^9/L are considered to have very severe AA (VSAA). The assessment of disease severity is important for treatment decisions and has prognostic significance. Patients with bi- or trilineage cytopenias that do not meet the criteria listed previously are not classified as AA. However, they should have their blood counts monitored because of the risk that they will develop AA.

Bone marrow failure in AA results from an immune-mediated destruction of hematopoietic progenitors. Clinical evidence for this includes circulating cytotoxic lymphocytes and an increased production of cytokines such as γ-interferon and tumor necrosis factor.

Clinical manifestations are related to the severity and duration of the underlying pancytopenia. Early symptoms often include easy bruising and/or mucosal hemorrhage caused by thrombocytopenia. Anemia may lead

---

BOX 1   Classification of Aplastic Anemia

Acquired Aplastic Anemia

Secondary Aplastic Anemia

- Radiation
- Drugs and chemicals
  - Regular effects: cytotoxic agents, benzene
  - Idiosyncratic reactions: Chloramphenicol
- Viruses
  - Epstein-Barr virus (infectious mononucleosis)
  - Hepatitis without an identified virus
  - Human immunodeficiency (HIV)
- Immune diseases
  - Eosinophilic fasciitis
  - Hypoimmunoglobulinemia
  - Thymoma and thymic carcinoma
  - Graft-versus-host disease (GvHD)
- Paroxysmal nocturnal hemoglobinuria
- Pregnancy

Idiopathic Aplastic Anemia

- Nonsteroidal antiinflammatory drugs
- Antiepileptics, gold, other drugs and chemicals

Inherited Aplastic Anemia

- Fanconi anemia
- Dyskeratosis congenita
- Shwachman-Diamond syndrome
- Amegakaryocytic thrombocytopenia
- Reticular dysgenesis
- Familial aplastic anemias
- Preleukemia (e.g., monosomy 7)
- Nonhematologic syndromes (Down, Dubowitz, Seckel)

Adapted from Young NS, Alter BP: Aplastic Anemia: Acquired and Inherited. Philadelphia: WB Saunders, 1994, p 9.

TABLE 1   Definition of Aplastic Anemia

Category	Definitions
Aplastic anemia (AA)	Hypocellular bone marrow and at least two of: 1. Hemoglobin <10 g/dL 2. Platelets $<50 \times 10^9$/L 3. Neutrophils $<1.5 \times 10^9$/L
Severe AA (SAA)	Hypocellular bone marrow with cellularity <25% or with <30% hematopoietic cells and at least two of: 1. Neutrophils $<0.5 \times 10^9$/L 2. Platelets $<20 \times 10^9$/L 3. Reticulocytes $<40 \times 10^9$/L
Very severe AA (VSAA)	SAA with neutrophils $<0.2 \times 10^9$/L
Moderate AA (MAA)	Moderate cytopenias and hypocellular bone marrow not meeting the criteria for SAA

to fatigue and reduced activity. Infection is a less frequent presentation. However, in the presence of severe neutropenia, fever, mouth sores, and even life-threatening infections can develop rapidly. Lymphadenopathy and hepatosplenomegaly are uncommon and suggest other underlying causes. A preceding history of jaundice may indicate hepatitis-associated AA. A careful history for exposure to drugs, chemicals, and pesticides in the preceding 6 months should be obtained in all cases.

Expert Opinion on Management Issues

Investigations required to confirm the diagnosis of acquired AA and to exclude other possible causes of pancytopenia are listed in Box 2. The complete blood count often reveals a low platelet, hemoglobin, and neutrophil count, although in early stages only thrombocytopenia may be seen. Anemia may be macrocytic or normocytic, and the absolute reticulocyte count is low. Fetal hemoglobin may be high, suggesting "stress hematopoiesis." Serum transaminase levels may be elevated in hepatitis-associated AA. Serology testing for hepatitis A, B, and C, cytomegalovirus (CMV), Epstein-Barr virus (EBV, parvovirus B19, and human immunodeficiency virus (HIV) is indicated to investigate known viral causes. Paroxysmal nocturnal hemoglobinuria (PNH) should be excluded by flow cytometry; phosphatidylinositol glycan (PIG) anchored proteins such as CD55 and CD59 are deficient in PNH. Iron, vitamin B_{12}, and folate levels should be measured to exclude nutrient deficiencies. Specific inherited bone marrow syndromes such as Fanconi anemia must be ruled out (see the chapter "Inherited Forms of Aplastic Anemia"). Bone marrow examination should include both aspiration (for morphology) and biopsy (for cellularity). In AA the bone marrow is hypocellular, with prominent fat spaces and reduced hematopoietic

cells with or without an apparent increase in lymphocytes and plasma cells. Dysplastic or immature cells may indicate MDS or leukemia. Cytogenetic analysis should be performed to look for abnormal clones consistent with those diagnoses.

The treatment of AA involves supportive care to prevent complications of pancytopenia and specific therapy aimed at curing the disease. The choice of therapy depends on the severity of the disease and the availability of a matched sibling bone marrow donor (Figure 1). Although spontaneous recovery may rarely occur, definitive treatment should be initiated as soon as possible to reduce the risk of infection, hemorrhage, and alloimmunization.

Supportive care with platelet transfusions is given to maintain the platelet count above $10 \times 10^9/L$ to prevent life-threatening intracranial or gastrointestinal hemorrhages. Packed red blood cell transfusions should be used if the hemoglobin is below 8 g/dL. Directed donor transfusions from family members should be avoided, and all blood products should be irradiated and leukodepleted to reduce the risk of sensitization to minor histocompatibility antigens. The risk of bacterial and fungal infections (particularly aspergillosis) is proportional to the degree and duration of neutropenia. Bacterial, fungal, and *Pneumocystis* prophylaxis may be used according to institutional guidelines. All infections should be promptly treated with the appropriate systemic antimicrobials.

Bone marrow transplantation (BMT) from a matched sibling donor is the treatment of choice for pediatric patients, and offers a greater than 75% probability of cure. HLA typing should be done on the patient, parents, and all siblings at the time of diagnosis to identify a possible donor. Current conditioning regimens use immunoablative and non–radiation-based therapy. The standard protocol includes cyclophosphamide, 50 mg/kg per day × 4 days, in combination with antithymocyte globulin (ATG), 30 mg/kg/day × 3 days. Graft-versus-host disease

---

BOX 2 Laboratory Tests Recommended for the Diagnosis of Aplastic Anemia

- Complete blood count, differential, and peripheral smear morphology
- Reticulocyte count
- Hemoglobin F %
- Bone marrow aspirate, biopsy, and cytogenetics
- Peripheral blood chromosome breakage study to exclude Fanconi anemia
- Flow cytometry for CD55 and CD59 to exclude PNH
- Vitamin B_{12} and folate levels
- Liver function tests
- Viral studies: hepatitis A, B, C; EBV; CMV; HIV
- Tests for collagen vascular diseases (e.g. antinuclear antibody and anti-ds DNA)
- Chest x-ray
- Abdominal ultrasound scan

CMV, cytomegalovirus; EBV, Epstein-Barr virus; HIV, human immunodeficiency virus; PNH, paroxysmal nocturnal hemoglobinuria.
Modified from Marsh JC, Ball SE, Darbyshire P, et al., on behalf of the British Committee for Standards in Haematology: Guidelines for the diagnosis and management of acquired aplastic anaemia. Br J Haematol 123:783, 2003.

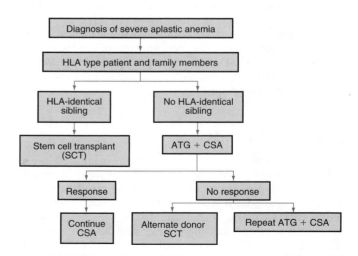

FIGURE 1. Treatment algorithm for severe acquired aplastic anemia. ATG, antithymocyte globulin; CSA, cyclosporine A; HLA, human leukocyte antigen; SCT, stem cell transplant.

(GvHD) prophylaxis includes cyclosporine A (CSA) and methotrexate. The main risks associated with BMT include graft failure in 5% to 10% of patients and GvHD in approximately 25% of patients. Older patient age and exposure to large numbers of blood transfusions may be risk factors for graft failure. The increased intensity of pretransplant conditioning regimens and a slower tapering of post-transplant immunosuppression have been associated with reduced graft rejection. Although a lower incidence and less severe GvHD are seen in children than in adults, mortality from GvHD continues to be a problem. Newer transplant regimens aimed at further intensifying the pretransplant and post-transplant immunosuppression are currently being explored.

Immunosuppressive therapy (IST) is indicated for the approximately 75% of patients with severe or very severe AA who do not have an HLA-matched sibling donor and for patients with moderate AA who are transfusion-dependent. IST with ATG (either horse or rabbit) and cyclosporine with or without granulocyte colony-stimulating factor (G-CSF) or granulocyte-macrophage colony-stimulating factor (GM-CSF) is associated with response rates of approximately 80%, with current 5-year survival rates of approximately 75%. Responses usually occur within the first 3 months. Although most patients show improved blood counts and become transfusion independent, complete normalization of peripheral blood and bone marrow is rarely achieved. Relapses occur in up to 30% of patients. With longer duration of use and slower tapering of cyclosporine, the relapse rate may be reduced. Side effects from ATG include anaphylaxis, urticaria, fever, chills, thrombocytopenia, and serum sickness. Corticosteroids are usually given along with ATG to reduce these side effects. Cyclosporine may cause renal dysfunction, hypomagnesemia, hypertension, and neurotoxicity. There is an up to 40% risk of late clonal bone marrow diseases including acute myeloid leukemia (AML), MDS (5%–10%), or PNH (10%–15%) after IST. For patients who fail to respond to IST or relapse after treatment, matched unrelated donor BMT, or further courses of immunosuppression remain treatment options.

Other treatment regimens, including the use of high-dose steroids and androgens, have been tried in the past without much success. Treatment with ATG or cyclosporine alone is inferior to the combination of the two drugs. Immunosuppression with cyclophosphamide alone is associated with high mortality caused by prolonged and persistent neutropenia.

Common Pitfalls

Every effort should be made to exclude inherited causes of bone marrow failure before the institution of specific treatment, as failure to diagnose these syndromes may result in death as a result of an ineffective treatment. Delay in treatment of AA increases the risk of death from hemorrhage or infection, and treatment with BMT or IST in the presence of serious infection or uncontrolled bleeding is associated with high mortality. Only irradiated and leukocyte-reduced blood products should be used to avoid sensitization. Cytomegalovirus

(CMV)-negative patients should not receive CMV-positive blood products because of the risk of transmission of the virus.

Androgens, lithium, or isolated use of high-dose steroids should be avoided as primary treatment modalities because these have no beneficial hematological responses in acquired AA. Likewise, the use of growth factors such as G-CSF, GM-CSF, and erythropoietin as single modality treatment should be discouraged.

Communication and Counseling

Aplastic anemia is a rare disease. Treatment is very intensive and is generally instituted in a specialized center that may be far away from the patient's primary residence. The patient and the family should be made aware of the chronic nature of the disease, prolonged treatment, slow recovery, and risks of relapse and late clonal disorders such as MDS, leukemia, and PNH.

Education and emotional and psychological support for the patient and the family are of great importance. The Aplastic Anemia & MDS International Foundation, Inc. (http://www.aamds.org/aplastic/) serves as a resource for patient assistance and emotional support and provides educational materials, family support conferences, and updated medical information.

SUGGESTED READINGS

1. Marsh JC, Ball SE, Darbyshire P, et al., on behalf of the British Committee for Standards in Haematology: Guidelines for the diagnosis and management of acquired aplastic anaemia. Br J Haematol 123:782–801, 2003. **Recommendations of a committee of experts.**
2. Shimamura A, Guinan E: Acquired aplastic anemia. In Nathan DG, Orkin SH, Look AT, Ginsburg D (eds): Nathan Oski's Hematology of Infancy and Childhood, 6th ed. Philadelphia: WB Saunders, 2003, pp 256–279. **Most recent comprehensive review of acquired aplastic anemia.**
3. Young NS, Alter BP: Aplastic Anemia Acquired and Inherited. Philadelphia: WB Saunders, 1994. **Comprehensive review of acquired and inherited aplastic anemias.**
4. Young NS: Acquired aplastic anemia. Ann Intern Med 136:534–546, 2002. **Describes mechanisms of immune-mediated marrow failure and current treatments.**

Neonatal and Childhood Neutropenia

Maria Luisa Sulis, Erin Morris, and Mitchell S. Cairo

KEY CONCEPTS

- Neutropenia in neonates and children is usually secondary to production defects or accelerated destruction and may be congenital or acquired.
- Myelopoietic growth factors have been used successfully for congenital and/or chronic neutropenias secondary to production defects.
- Granulocyte transfusions may be an important modality of therapy in selected acute forms of neonatal and childhood neutropenias.

- Blood and marrow transplantation may be curative in selected forms of chronic neutropenia that fail standard medical management.
- Acute and long-term complications of chronic neutropenia include severe infectious morbidity, myelodysplasia, and acute leukemia transformation.

Neutropenia is defined as a decrease in the number of neutrophils and bands in the peripheral blood below 1500 cells/μL in children older than 1 year of age and below 1000 cells/μL in infants between 2 months and 1 year. The degree of neutropenia and its duration are the most important factors in assessing the risk of developing severe bacterial and fungal infections. The degree is classified as mild, moderate, or severe based on neutrophil and band counts of 1500 to 1000, 1000 to 500, or <500/μL, respectively. Any associated impairment of the host defense such as defects in cell-mediated and humoral immunity or alteration of the skin and mucosal barrier needs to be considered when estimating the risk of contracting severe infections. The increased incidence and severity of bacterial sepsis in the neonate is indeed related to both quantitative and qualitative abnormalities of the phagocytic cellular immunity, such as impaired oxidative metabolism, chemotaxis, phagocytosis, and bacterial killing, in addition to the limited pool of neutrophil progenitors.

The most common infections that develop in the setting of neutropenia are cutaneous infections (cellulitis, furunculosis), pneumonia, otitis media, stomatitis, perirectal infections, and septicemia. Fever may frequently be the only sign of infection, because the usual signs and symptoms of inflammation are diminished in the settings of neutropenia. The most common infectious agents are *Staphylococcus aureus*, *Escherichia coli*, and *Pseudomonas* species.

The etiologies of neutropenia can be classified in two groups: (1) Neutropenia secondary to an intrinsic defect of the myeloid cells and (2) neutropenia caused by extrinsic factors. The mechanisms responsible for the extrinsic defects leading to chronic neutropenias are largely unknown. Generally, the symptomatology of intrinsic causes of neutropenia manifests in early age with recurrent infections that may be more or less severe according to the disease. Patients with severe congenital neutropenia (Kostmann syndrome) or reticular dysgenesis tend to acquire severe infections that frequently evolve into sepsis, whereas in patients with cyclic neutropenia or Shwachman syndrome, the infections, although frequent, are rarely severe or fatal. Supportive care and, in many of these syndromes, granulocyte colony-stimulating factor (G-CSF) is the standard treatment for severe neutropenia secondary to intrinsic defects. Neutropenia secondary to extrinsic defects includes a broad spectrum of etiologies and a variety of clinical presentations. Hepatitis A and B, respiratory syncytial virus, influenza A and B, Epstein-Barr virus, cytomegalovirus, and others are the most common causes of neutropenia in children. These forms of neutropenia tend to resolve spontaneously and usually do not represent a significant risk of developing severe bacterial infections. On the contrary, neutropenia secondary to drugs (penicillin, phenytoin, and quinidine) can be very worrisome, and immediate discontinuation of the medication is usually necessary. Autoimmune neutropenia can be either idiopathic or secondary to infections, medications, or part of a systemic autoimmune disease. Bacterial infections are common but usually mild.

The largest population of neutropenic patients occurs in children receiving chemotherapy or myeloablative therapy. As mentioned previously, the risk of developing severe, life-threatening bacterial infections is mostly, but not solely, related to the degree as well as to the duration of neutropenia. Despite marked improvement in supportive care and the use of granulocyte colony-stimulating factor (G-CSF) and granulocyte-monocyte colony-stimulating factor (GM-CSF), bacterial and fungal infections remain a major cause of morbidity and mortality in neutropenic patients.

In general, management of all neutropenic patients includes careful attention to the identification and prompt treatment of suspected or proven infections. Good skin and oral hygiene is also an important component of the care of these patients. Appropriate use of myelopoietic growth factors, antibiotics, granulocyte transfusions, and/or bone marrow transplantation has played a fundamental role in the successful management of patients with severe neutropenia and is discussed in further detail later in this chapter.

Expert Opinion on Management Issues

MYELOPOIETIC GROWTH FACTORS

GM-CSF and G-CSF are growth factors that regulate the production and differentiation of myelopoietic progenitor cells into mature phagocytes. In particular, G-CSF acts on relatively late progenitors that have already committed to the neutrophil lineage, whereas GM-CSF acts on earlier progenitors that will yield both neutrophils and monocytes. The American Society of Clinical Oncology has updated the guidelines for the judicious use of human recombinant GM-CSF (250–500 μg/m^2/day) and G-CSF (5–10 μg/kg/day) in patients with cancer; however, these guidelines are mostly for adults and clear recommendations for pediatric patients are lacking. Many studies have evaluated the efficacy of myelopoietic growth factors as primary prophylaxis in children with hematologic malignancies. All studies have shown that the use of G-CSF or GM-CSF shortens the duration of neutropenia and frequently the degree of neutropenia. The analysis of other clinical parameters that may be considered as surrogate for infectious complications, such as fever, incidence of documented infections, duration of antibiotic therapy, and days of hospitalization has for the most part demonstrated an advantage following the use of prophylactic growth factors. However, no study has shown a survival benefit in CSF-treated children. Less data are available on the advantage of CSF following chemotherapy for the treatment of solid tumors; although a reduction in the duration of neutropenia is clearly shown,

TABLE 1 Doses and Route of Administration of G-CSF and GM-CSF

Type of Neutropenia	G-CSF Dose (μg/kg) and Administration	GM-CSF Dose (μg/kg) and Administration	Time of Initiation of Myelopoietic Growth Factors
Severe chronic neutropenia	Start at 5 μg/kg/day and escalate q2wk SC	Insufficient data	At discretion of the physician
Chemotherapy induced neutropenia	5 μg/kg/day SC or IV	250 μg/m²/day SC or IV	1–5 days after the end of chemotherapy administration

*Subcutaneous route is preferred.
G-CSF, granulocyte colony-stimulating factor; GM-CSF, granulocyte-monocyte colony-stimulating factor; IV, intravenous; q, every; SC, subcutaneous.

no definite benefit in clinical endpoints has been reported. Outside of clinical trials, the use of myelopoietic growth factors should be reserved for children receiving dose-intensive chemotherapy with an expected incidence of febrile neutropenia above 40%. In addition, the routine use of growth factors in patients with fever and neutropenia or neutropenia and documented infection is not recommended. However, in certain circumstances in which clinical deterioration can be expected, the use of growth factors seems reasonable, even in the absence of definite proven benefit.

The use of myelopoietic growth factors has had a major impact in both the prognosis and quality of life of patients with malignant disease and with severe chronic neutropenia. The vast majority of patients with chronic neutropenia respond to G-CSF, however, its routine prophylactic use is recommended only for those diseases associated with frequent, severe, and/or life-threatening infections. Data from the Severe Chronic Neutropenia International Registry show that more than 90% of patients with severe congenital neutropenia treated in clinical trials and all the patients with cyclic and idiopathic neutropenia responded to G-CSF administration. There was an increase in absolute neutrophil count greater than 1×10^9 and a decrease in the incidence and severity of infectious complications as well as the use of antibiotics. The effective median dose of daily G-CSF varied from 3.5 to 11.5 μg/kg/day, but higher doses may be required especially for patients with Kostmann disease. The goal should be to keep the neutrophil and band count between 1.5 and 10×10^9 per liter. Adverse effects associated with the use of G-CSF in patients with severe chronic neutropenia include bone pain, mild thrombocytopenia, osteoporosis and osteopenia, splenomegaly, vasculitis, and glomerulonephritis. Whether the development of leukemia reported solely in patients with congenital neutropenia is related to the use of G-CSF is still controversial, because conversion to myelodysplastic syndrome (MDS)/acute myeloblastic leukemia (AML) was reported prior to the use of G-CSF. Whether G-CSF induces or favors the leukemic transformation or prolongs survival, therefore, allowing more time for a predisposition to transform into AML, is still unknown. For patients with neutropenia associated with lower risk of severe infections, such as immune neutropenia and Shwachman syndrome, the use of G-CSF is recommended in the settings of severe, life-threatening infections or routinely, as prophylaxis, for subgroups of patients who

seem to have more frequent and serious infections. G-CSF, in this latter situation, may be used at lower dosage and daily dosage may not be required.

Neonates, and in particular preterm infants, are extremely susceptible to severe infections that represent a major cause of morbidity and mortality. The role of CSFs (in particular GM-CSF) both as prophylactic and therapeutic treatment has been studied in this group of patients. Two randomized, controlled studies showed that GM-CSF administered prophylactically caused an increase of the circulating neutrophils and a trend toward decreased culture-proven infections; however, the difference in confirmed infections between the treated and untreated groups was not significant. Similar results were obtained when G-CSF was administered to septic neonates. The routine use of CSF in neonates, prophylactically or therapeutically, is not recommended at this time. Table 1 gives information on doses and administration of G-CSF and GM-CSF.

MANAGEMENT OF FEVER AND NEUTROPENIA

Fever is defined as a single oral temperature of 100.4°F (38.0°C) or that same temperature for 1 hour. Neutropenia is defined as a neutrophil count of less than 500 cells/mm³ or a count of less than 1000 cells/mm³ that is decreasing over time. For all patients who meet these criteria, prompt evaluation and administration of antibiotics within an hour is mandatory; afebrile, neutropenic patients who have signs or symptoms suggestive of an infection should be handled in the same way. The Infectious Disease Society of America has published guidelines to assist physicians in the treatment of neutropenic patients with cancer who develop unexplained fever. Symptoms and signs of infection may be minimal or absent; however, a careful search for subtle symptoms and signs especially at sites most commonly involved is of paramount importance. These sites are the oropharynx, periodontium, lungs, perineum and anus, skin, and vascular catheter access sites. Blood cultures for bacteria and fungi should be obtained immediately, whereas other specimens should be cultured only if clinically indicated (stool samples, urinary culture, and CSF culture); similarly, a chest radiograph should be obtained in the presence of signs and symptoms of respiratory tract infection. Complete blood count, serum creatinine, blood urea, and transaminases should be checked at

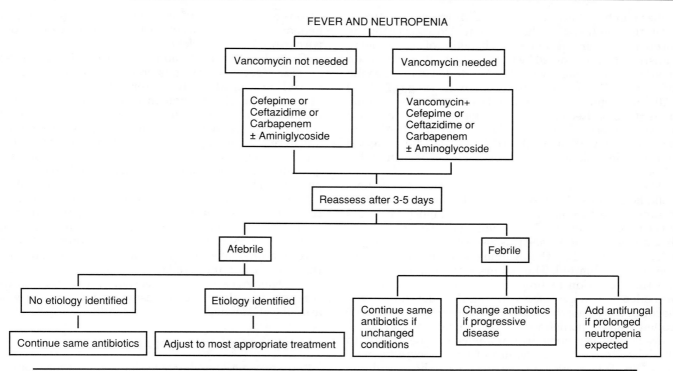

FIGURE 1. Empiric antibiotic therapy in children with fever and neutropenia.

presentation and at least every 3 days once antibiotic therapy has been initiated.

Gram-positive bacteria today account for 60% to 70% of documented infections; usually they cause more indolent infections except for *S. aureus, S. viridans,* and resistant pneumococcus, which may cause fulminant and, at times, fatal infections if not treated promptly. Severe life-threatening infections are more commonly caused by gram-negative bacteria (*Pseudomonas aeruginosa, E. coli, Klebsiella* species). All pediatric patients with fever and neutropenia should be treated with broad-spectrum intravenous antibiotics in inpatient settings; no definitive recommendations are currently available for outpatient, oral antibiotic treatment in low-risk patients.

In the selection of initial antibiotic treatment the type, frequency, and antibiotic susceptibility of bacterial isolates from other patients in that same hospital need to be considered. At presentation, the physician should decide whether the additional use of vancomycin in the initial empiric therapy is needed. Generally, it is reasonable to include vancomycin in the initial therapy if a catheter infection is suspected, and if there is known colonization with penicillin-resistant pneumococcus or methicillin-resistant *S. aureus.* It is also reasonable to include vancomycin in the initial therapy if a gram-positive bacterium is identified in the blood culture, even if the final identification is not available, in the presence of hypotension and probably also in the presence of severe mucositis. If a gram-positive bacterium is not identified and the patient has been clinically stable since presentation, vancomycin can be discontinued after 24 to 48 hours. If the patient does not qualify for the use of vancomycin, then monotherapy with a cephalosporin (cefepime or

ceftazidime) or a carbapenem (meropenem or imipenem-cilastatin) should be initiated; the addition of an aminoglycoside (gentamicin, tobramycin, amikacin) should be considered in complicated cases.

The subsequent management depends on whether a causative bacterium is identified, the clinical condition of the child changes, and the neutropenia is resolved or is expected to be prolonged (Fig. 1). The addition of antifungal therapy (amphotericin B) is recommended in the case of a child with persistent fever and neutropenia after 5 days of broad-spectrum antibiotics and in whom prolonged neutropenia (7 days) is expected. It is critical to closely monitor these patients for possible changes in their clinical condition or emergence of new signs or symptoms that can further guide the therapy. If the fever persists for more than 3 days, the patients need to be reassessed to attempt to identify factors that may explain the nonresponse to the initial empiric therapy. Review of all the cultures, chest radiograph, culture of additional blood samples or other specimens, diagnostic imaging, antibiotic serum levels, and, most importantly, a careful physical examination need to be done.

GRANULOCYTE TRANSFUSION

The use of allogeneic granulocyte transfusions to treat patients with severe neutropenia and/or granulocyte dysfunction with presumed or documented severe bacterial or fungal infection has been limited by the small amount of granulocytes collected by leukapheresis from unstimulated donors. The patients in whom the transfusion of granulocytes reduced mortality are the neonates with severe neutropenia and sepsis. This is likely because of the higher number of granulocytes per kilogram transfused, given the small size of the recipient. More recently, the enthusiasm over the potential benefits of granulocyte transfusion is supported by the finding that mobilization of allogeneic donors with G-CSF and dexamethasone induces a collection of neutrophils in the range of 3 to 10 $\times 10^{10}$ neutrophils, compared to 4 to 6×10^9 from unstimulated donors. Recent studies suggest that successful collections are obtained following administration of dexamethasone (8 mg orally [PO]) and G-CSF (5 μg/kg) to allogeneic donors 12 hours before the scheduled collection.

The advantage of granulocyte transfusion to treat neutropenic children with severe infection not responding to supportive care is still controversial, mostly because of the lack of recent well-designed trials. The majority of the studies that addressed this issue were conducted 2 to 3 decades ago, when the available supportive care was clearly more limited. The donors were not stimulated, and the collection techniques impaired the activity of the collected cells. A few recent small studies have led to discordant results; therefore, in the absence of large controlled studies, no definite recommendations can be delivered. However, some useful advice can be offered to physicians considering the use of granulocyte transfusions (Box 1). Granulocyte transfusion can be considered for the selected group of patients with severe neutropenia and bacterial sepsis or fungal or yeast infection in whom antibacterial and antifungal treatment has failed and in whom neutropenia is expected to last for at least 3 weeks. At least 2 to 3 $\times 10^{10}$ granulocytes should be transfused daily for a minimum of 5 days; granulocytes should be transfused as soon as possible after collection and should be obtained, when possible, from a compatible donor. Convincing data from several randomized, controlled studies support the use of granulocyte transfusion in septic neonates. The survival from sepsis was markedly improved in the group of neonates who received 0.5 to 1 $\times 10^9$ granulocytes compared to the neonates who received supportive care alone or supportive care and immunoglobulins.

Granulocyte transfusion is associated with several adverse reactions to be considered when assessing its potential benefits. Mild adverse reactions mostly consisting of fever occur with an incidence of 5% to 13% and can be limited by premedication with antipyretics and corticosteroids. Of greater concern is the respiratory distress and development of pulmonary infiltrates that have been reported in up to 57% of patients receiving prophylactic granulocyte transfusion compared to 27% in untreated patients. The etiology is not clear, but it is probably related to fluid overload, leukoagglutination, sequestration of granulocytes at sites of infection, or microembolization. The concomitant use of granulocyte transfusion and amphotericin B is also known to potentially cause severe pulmonary reactions, and it is recommended that they be administered at least 8 hours apart. Finally, cytomegalovirus (CMV) infection can be transmitted through granulocyte transfusion and, therefore, when available, CMV-negative donors should be preferred.

BONE MARROW TRANSPLANTATION

Only a very small number of patients with severe congenital or acquired neutropenia have been treated with bone marrow transplantation. The advent of myelopoietic growth factors has significantly improved the life of patients affected by severe neutropenia, so that the risk related to bone marrow transplantation is not justified. Bone marrow transplantation should be considered for patients with severe neutropenia who do not respond to even high doses of G-CSF.

Common Pitfalls

- Failure to evaluate and treat febrile neutropenic patients promptly.
- Failure to recognize subtle signs and symptoms of infections caused by decreased inflammatory response in neutropenic patients.
- Routine use of vancomycin as initial empiric treatment of febrile neutropenic patients is not recommended, as it predisposes to emergence of resistant organisms. Its use is warranted only in selected patients.
- Inadequate collection of granulocytes or failure to administer them as soon as obtained decreases the benefit of granulocyte transfusion.
- Inadequate screening of donors for infectious diseases exposes the recipient to possible CMV infection.
- Concomitant administration of granulocytes and amphotericin B can cause severe respiratory distress in the recipient.
- Administration of G-CSF to patients with severe congenital neutropenia may increase the risk of leukemic transformation. Routine screening for emergence of translocations or monosomy 7 is recommended.

BOX 1 Recommendations for Granulocyte Transfusion in Children and Neonates

Indication

Neonates and children with severe neutropenia and presumed or proven sepsis not responding to standard therapy and with expected prolonged neutropenia

Dose of PMN to be transfused

$\geq 0.75-1.0 \times 10^{10}$/dose

Schedule

Daily until recovery of ANC ≥ 500/mm^3

Adverse reactions

Fever, chills
Respiratory distress
CMV infection

ANC, absolute neutrophil count; CMV, cytomegalovirus; PMN, polymorphonuclear neutrophil.

Communication and Counseling

Severe infections are the most frequent and feared complications occurring in neutropenic patients. Families need to be educated to seek immediate medical care when fever or clinical changes occur. Combined efforts of hematologists, oncologists, and the infectious disease teams are fundamental to guaranteeing the most comprehensive and complete care to children with severe neutropenia.

SUGGESTED READINGS

1. Cairo MS, Agosti J, Ellis R, et al: A randomized, double-blind, placebo-controlled trial of prophylactic recombinant human granulocyte-macrophage colony-stimulating factor to reduce nosocomial infections in very low birth weight neonates. J Pediatr 134:64–70, 1999. **Largest trial on the prophylactic use of GM-CSF in 264 neonates of very low birth weight.**
2. Dale DC, Cottle TE, Fier CJ, et al: Severe chronic neutropenia: Treatment and follow-up of patients in the Severe Chronic Neutropenia International Registry. Am J Hematol 72:82–93, 2003. **Update on treatment and follow-up of 853 patients with severe chronic neutropenia; data were collected from the Severe Chronic Neutropenia International Registry.**
3. Hughes WT, Armstrong D, Bodey GP, et al: 2002 guidelines for the use of antimicrobial agents in neutropenic patients with cancer. Clin Infect Dis 34:730–751, 2002. **The latest recommendations on the use of antimicrobials in neutropenic patients with cancer from the Infectious Disease Society of America.**
4. Lehrnbecher T, Welte K: Hematopoietic growth factors in children with neutropenia. Br J Haematol 116:28–56, 2002. **Comprehensive review on the use of growth factors in children with neutropenia of different etiologies.**
5. Ozer H, Armitage JO, Bennett CL, et al: 2000 update of recommendations for the use of hematopoietic colony-stimulating factors: Evidence-based clinical practice guidelines. American Society of Clinical Oncology Growth Factors Expert Panel. J Clin Oncol 18:3558–3585, 2000. **The latest version of the guidelines and recommendations for the use of colony-stimulating factors from the ASCO.**
6. Satwani P, Bessmertny O, Morris E, et al: Prophylactic use of myelopoietic growth factors in children after myelosuppressive and myeloablative therapy. Curr Hematol Reports 2:480–490, 2003. **Updated review of most significant pediatric studies on the use of growth factors following myelosuppressive and myeloablative therapy.**
7. Sulis ML, Harrison L, Cairo MS: Granulocyte Transfusion in the neonate child. In Hillyer CD, Luban N, Strauss RG (eds): Handbook of Pediatric Transfusion Medicine. San Diego: Elsevier, 2004, pp 167–180. **Overview of granulocyte mobilization and collection methods, indications for the therapeutic and prophylactic use of granulocyte transfusion in pediatric patients, and side effects.**

Complications of Blood Transfusion

Naomi L. C. Luban

KEY CONCEPTS

- Transfusions of blood and blood products result in both infectious and noninfectious complications.
- Infectious complications include transmission of bacteria, viruses, protozoa, prions, and parasites.

- Processes have been implemented to decrease many infectious risks, but some remain.
- Noninfectious complications of transmissions are also important; metabolic complications are of particular concern for neonates but immunologic complications, both humoral and cellular, may affect a child of any age.
- Blood salvage, use of growth factors, limiting unnecessary laboratory testing, and evidence-based justification of the need to transfuse may decrease donor exposures and reduce transfusion-associated disease.

In the 1980s and 1990s, the recognition of and devastating consequences of transmission of viruses by transfusion changed blood donor collection and transfusion practices. Blood donor screening prior to donation, technological innovations in laboratory testing of donor blood with sensitive immunoassays and nucleic acid–based amplification assays, improved viral inactivation methods for pooled plasma components, and the use of evidence-based criteria to determine transfusion need have been implemented. Although the blood supply in the United States has an unprecedented level of safety, it remains vulnerable to emerging infections, like West Nile virus, severe acute respiratory syndrome (SARS), and other infections resulting from global epidemics and noninfectious hazards of transfusion (NISHOTs). Mosquito-borne infections like malaria, dengue, and West Nile virus may be acquired during travel or through domestic transmission. Immigrant donors from Central and South America can transmit *Trypanosoma cruzi*; those from the Middle East can carry leishmania, and those from the United Kingdom may carry variant Creutzfeldt-Jacob disease. Standardized testing does not exist for these pathogens. New technology including mass-produced nucleic acid chips and nanoassays may provide a cost-effective alternative to current donor testing algorithms in the future.

Among infants and children, the most important NISHOTs include hyperkalemia as a metabolic complication, transfusion-acquired graft-versus-host disease (TA-GvHD), and other immunologic consequences of transfusion, iron overload in children on hypertransfusion protocols, and plasticizers' toxicity as an example of blood-derived chemical exposures. Such adverse complications require proactive selection of blood, specialized processing, and surveillance for long-term consequences; no pretransfusion testing is possible to obviate these complications. Pathogen reduction and artificial blood and platelets would be ideal ways to obviate transfusion complications but are years away from pediatric use.

Expert Opinion on Management Issues

INTERVENTIONS

Neonates have a long post-transfusion expected survival. Therefore, long intervals may pass before a specific infectious disease develops. Post-transfusion hepatitis C, for example, may take 10 to 20 or more years to progress to cirrhosis and liver failure in an adult, but have a very different clinical course in the neonate or young child. Because of their long expected survival, neonates as a group, derive a proportionally greater benefit from reducing the risks of long-term adverse effects of transfusion.

Neonates have primarily passive, maternally transmitted immunity to transfusion-transmissible agents such as the hepatitis viruses, Epstein-Barr, and cytomegalovirus (CMV) because of a lack of intrauterine exposure and a limited capacity for innate fetal antibody production. As passively acquired antibody titers decrease, neonates may become susceptible to these more unusual transfusion-acquired infections. Cell-mediated immunity—notably, T-lymphocyte response and cytokine production—is also not fully established in newborns. Thus, the transfused neonate's ability to control and eliminate viable, functioning donor lymphocytes contained in blood components may be compromised. If allowed to engraft, transfused lymphocytes can proliferate and result in TA-GvHD. γ Irradiation of cellular blood components will abrogate TA-GvHD. Some institutions irradiate components for all neonatal transfusions to ensure that any neonate who might require irradiated products, but who may not yet be diagnosed with a specific disease (i.e., those with suspected or confirmed T-cell–mediated immunodeficiencies), receives them. Based on immunologic immaturity, infants weighing less than 1200 g may also receive irradiated products. There are no definitive data establishing the need for irradiation for all neonatal transfusions or for large-volume transfusions (e.g., extracorporeal membrane oxygenation, exchange transfusion, major surgery). Granulocytes given to neonates for sepsis should be irradiated as well as any donation from a family member, intrauterine transfusion, and transfusions to neonates who have received intrauterine transfusions. It is not necessary to irradiate blood for neonates with human immunodeficiency virus infection.

Defects in cell-mediated immunity also contribute to the adverse consequences of viral infections in the neonatal period. In hospitalized newborns of CMV-seronegative mothers, transfusion is the primary route by which CMV is acquired, whereas newborns of seropositive mothers often acquire CMV perinatally. Most adult transfusion recipients are immune secondary to naturally acquired infection and suffer little or no morbidity from post-transfusion CMV. Only immunologically challenged patients, such as those receiving hematopoietic stem cell transplants or ablative chemo/radiotherapy, can develop significant disease from CMV; reactivation of preexisting infection rather than new infection from transfusion is often the source. Like the severely immune-compromised adult, transfusion-acquired CMV, particularly in a sick or premature neonate without passive immunity, may progress to hepatitis, viral sepsis, or lethal CMV pneumonia.

Transfusion-associated CMV is preventable with CMV reduced-risk blood and blood components by using either CMV-seronegative or third-generation leukocyte-reduced products. The Association Bulletin 97–2 of the American Association of Blood Banks (AABB) suggests that all neonates weighing less than 1200 g, regardless of CMV serostatus, should receive CMV-reduced-risk components because of loss of passively acquired immunity over time even in seropositive neonates. Although the available evidence suggests that seropositive infants of low birth weight are not at increased risk of transfusion-transmitted CMV disease, any infant receiving an intrauterine transfusion or transfusion following intrauterine transfusion and CMV-seronegative pregnant women requiring transfusion should receive reduced-risk products because primary CMV infection during pregnancy may pose significant risk to the fetus.

The indications for and benefits of blood administration to neonates are not founded in strong scientific observations and clinical trials, but rather reflect experience and example. As a result, although there are several thoughtfully prepared sets of guidelines for neonatal transfusion, most are based on common practice and best guesses. There is a continuing need for critical assessment and reevaluation of the indications for transfusion in newborns and older children.

THE STORAGE LESION AND NEONATAL TRANSFUSION

Acute transfusion complications are often the result of metabolic consequences of product storage and infusion of the anticoagulant-preservative solution. A storage lesion occurs for both red blood cells and platelets, and increases over the course of storage. Selection of blood and blood products for both small-volume and massive transfusions is often predicated on concerns over the storage lesion.

POTASSIUM

The potassium (K^+) level in plasma in 35-day-old, refrigerator-stored red blood cell (RBC) units may reach 78.5 mmol/L in blood collected in citrate-phosphate-dextrose (CPD) solutions. In the newer anticoagulant preservative adenine-saline (AS) solutions, the K^+ ranges from 45.6 to 50 mmol/L at 42 days. RBCs irradiated and stored at refrigerator temperature for 28 days have higher K^+ levels. When administered as small-volume transfusions of 10 to 15 mL/kg, this quantity of K^+ is relatively insignificant, but fatal cardiac arrhythmias have been associated with hyperkalemia during neonatal exchange transfusion and following rapid infusion during surgery. Renal failure, low cardiac output, and intra-arterial transfusion may predispose to transfusion-associated hyperkalemia. Irradiation as close to the time of transfusion as possible decreases the risk of hyperkalemia. In adults receiving more than one blood volume during a 24-hour period, hypokalemia has been noted. This occurs because Na-K–dependent adenosine triphosphate shifts are activated in vivo, red blood cells exchange intracellular sodium for extracellular K^+, and a sink for K^+ results. Alkalosis from metabolized citrate can result in further potassium shifts into cells in exchange for hydrogen ions. Similar phenomena have not been reported in infants to date (Table 1).

TABLE 1 Some Complications of Transfusion Unique to Infants and Children

Observation	Implications	Recommendations
A high proportion of patients are transfused.*	High total donor exposures per patient.	Assigned limited donor programs and unit practices are effective.
Routine transfusion volumes are relatively large.*	Increased risk of transfusion-acquired infection.	Routine screening for transfusion-related infections and complications may be fruitful.
Recipient's blood volume is small relative to standard blood products and equipment.	Potassium, citrate, volume, cold temperature, and preservative toxicity might be increased.	Give routine transfusions over 2 to 4 hours; specially select and prepare components for rapid or massive transfusion.
	Dividing products may be required.	Carefully coordinate preparation with transfusion volumes and timing.
	Plasma-incompatible platelet transfusion is more likely to cause hemolysis.	ABO-identical or plasma-compatible platelets are preferred.
	Blood loss through phlebotomy for laboratory tests is a major cause of anemia.	Small-volume replacement transfusions used most often in smallest and sickest infants.
Red-cell-reactive antibodies are passively acquired from mother or by transfusion.*†	Anti-A and anti-B titers may not correspond to the patient's ABO group.	Test for anti-A and anti-B if non–group-O red cells are to be given, or if non–group-AB plasma or platelets have been transfused and potentially incompatible red cells are to be given.
Recipient has a long post-transfusion life expectancy.	There is the risk of hemolytic anemia in the infant of selected infant-mother pairs.	Cross-match with maternal sample whenever possible; select and prepare transfusion as if for mother and patient simultaneously.
Recipient has a defective humoral immune response.*†‡	Increases the likelihood of surviving long enough to develop disease from transfusion-transmitted infection.	Seek lowest infectious risk donors, components, and preparations.
Recipient has a defective cellular immune response.*†‡	Infant recipients are unlikely to form red cell antibodies.	Vigilance by health care providers for post-transfusion disease is needed.
	Recipient's ability to contain donor lymphocytes may be limited.	Assume negative antibody detection test results through neonatal period if initially negative and no major transfusion episodes in interval.
	Viral infections acquired as a neonate are more likely to progress to systemic illness.	Gamma irradiation is recommended to avoid GvHD.
		Cytomegalovirus-reduced risk is recommended.

*More of an issue for hospitalized neonates.
†More of an issue for affected fetuses.
‡More of an issue for older children with congenital or acquired immunodeficiencies.
ABO, blood group system of groups A, AB, B, and O. GvHD, graft-versus-host disease.

13

2,3-DIPHOSPHOGLYCERATE

Levels of intraerythrocytic 2,3-diphosphoglycerate (2,3-DPG) affect the ability of red cells to release oxygen at any given pH. With progressive storage, 2,3-DPG levels decrease by more than 50%, resulting in a decreased ability to off-load oxygen to the tissues. In adults, 2,3-DPG is gradually restored over several hours following routine transfusion. In one study of premature infants receiving small-volume transfusions, quantitative 2,3-DPG was measured weekly. Results were similar in infants transfused with fresh citrate-phosphate-dextrose-adenine (CPDA–1) and stored AS–1 RBCs, suggesting that, at least in this setting, infants can effectively maintain 2,3-DPG post-transfusion. Of note, untransfused infants in this study had higher 2,3-DPG levels, as would be expected in infants with higher fetal hemoglobin concentrations.

COLD STORAGE

RBCs are stored at 33.8°F to 42.8°F (1°C to 6°C). Rapid infusion of cold RBCs can result in hypothermia and cardiac arrhythmia/asystole. In infants, transfusion of cold blood is associated with apnea, hypotension, and hypoglycemia. Small-volume transfusions are rarely associated with physiologic instability induced by cold blood but massive transfusions, exchange transfusions, and some intraoperative transfusions call for blood-warming devices. Microwave ovens and other devices that do not have strict quality checks on the heating device should never be used because heating may be inconsistent and hemolysis may result.

DILUTIONAL HEMOSTATIC DYSFUNCTION

Dilutional hemostatic dysfunction results from the massive transfusion of many units of RBCs from which platelets and plasma have been removed. Dilutional hemostatic dysfunction is characterized by thrombocytopenia, hypofibrinogenemia, and prolongation of both the prothrombin time and partial thromboplastin time; fibrin degradation products are often present, and coagulation factor proteins are reduced except for factor VIII (unless there is severe, concomitant disseminated intravascular coagulation). Clinically, the patient may present with microvascular bleeding or oozing from sites of injury, venipuncture sites, and mucosal surfaces.

ADVERSE EFFECTS OF ANTICOAGULANT/ PRESERVATIVE SOLUTIONS

The RBC anticoagulant and preservative solutions adenine-saline (AS-1, AS-3, and AS-5) permit storage of RBCs to 42 days and allow for maximum plasma extraction. The concentration of the AS solution is highest in the freshest blood and decreases over time as the constituents diffuse into the RBCs and are used to maintain red cell integrity. The average hematocrit of RBCs collected in AS solutions is approximately 60%, and the flow rate is more rapid because the component is less viscous. The metabolic and physiologic safety of these solutions as small-volume transfusions has been demonstrated in infants of very low birth weight in several studies. However, the lower hematocrit of the product means that the transfusion volume needed to achieve a hemoglobin increment comparable to that achieved by transfusing a red cell product with a hematocrit of $75 \pm 5\%$ (i.e., RBCs stored in CPD-A1 or CPD) must be increased. In massive transfusion, theoretical concerns of osmotic load and diuresis, hyperglycemia, hypernatremia, and hypoalbuminemia remain; no clinical trials confirming the safety of the different AS-added solutions have been performed to date. Consequently, for large-volume transfusions (i.e., >25 mL/kg), it is customary to either avoid their use or centrifuge the blood unit to remove the solution prior to transfusion.

DECREASING DONOR EXPOSURE IN THE NEONATE

Although most infants weighing more than 1500 g will not require transfusion during their neonatal stay, almost all infants weighing less than 1000 g have a transfusion requirement that results in one or several donor exposures. As each donor exposure provides further infectious and immunologic risk, efforts to decrease the donor exposures have resulted in changes in practices. For several years, fresh (e.g., <7-day-old) group O, Rh-negative blood was the preferred component. Now, by using a sterile connecting device and multiple aliquot bags, dedicating one unit to one or more infants, and using RBCs until outdate, practitioners can reduce donor exposure without adverse clinical outcome. The use of washed RBC units should be limited to infants with immunoglobulin (Ig) A deficiency or T activation of red cells, or to those in renal failure for whom the anticoagulant-preservative solution and K^+ load would be detrimental.

TRANSFUSION IRON OVERLOAD

Transfusion iron overload occurs in patients on chronic transfusion therapy for hemoglobinopathies and hypoproliferative or dyserythropoietic anemias. Free iron radicals have direct and indirect damaging effects on lipid membranes, organelles, and DNA. Many organs are adversely affected including the heart, liver, pituitary, pancreas, thyroid, ovary, testis, and adrenal glands, causing end-organ failure. Iron chelation with parenterally administered deferoxamine, usually administered by slow subcutaneous infusion over 8 to 12 hours, 6 nights per week with oral vitamin C can reduce body iron load. Additional intravenous infusions may be needed for patients with severe iron overload, cardiac dysrhythmias, and poor left ventricular function and those with active hepatitis C and those who are awaiting bone marrow transplantation. Some patients who cannot tolerate subcutaneous infusions may receive regular intravenous deferoxamine. Periodic quantitative liver iron measurements—obtained on liver biopsy specimens, superconducting quantum interference device susceptometer (SQUIDS), and magnetic biosusceptometry, when available—are used to establish efficacy and modify therapy. New pharmacologic therapies, some oral, are in active clinical trials.

BACTERIAL CONTAMINATION

Bacterial contamination of blood accounts for as many as 500 to 750 fatalities annually. Although all blood components are susceptible to contamination and transfusion-associated septic complications, platelets that are stored at room temperature are especially prone to bacterial contamination. Predominant organisms are skin flora (staphylococci, aerobic and anaerobic, diphtheroid, bacilli, streptococci, and gram-negative bacilli) and, less often, occult bacteremia in the donor. Based on surveillance methods, it has been estimated that 1000 to 3000 platelet units per year may be contaminated with bacteria. The number of septic episodes resulting from transfusion of these units is unknown as prospective surveillance is not routine. As of March 2004, all blood-collection establishments instituted methods to limit and detect bacterial contamination of platelet products.

FEBRILE NONHEMOLYTIC TRANSFUSION REACTION (FNHTR)

Acute reactions to blood and blood products are defined as adverse events occurring during a transfusion or a few hours after. These transfusion reactions are classically defined as acute hemolytic, febrile nonhemolytic (FNHTR), allergic, hypotensive, or bacterial. FNHTR is the most commonly reported adverse event with a frequency of 0.5% to 0.38%, depending on the product and recipient patient population. FNHTRs have been reported with both red blood cell and platelet transfusions but are more commonly reported with platelets. Cytokine accumulation secondary to breakdown of white blood cells in the product is thought to be the primary cause. Chills, a sense of cold, and rigors with a 0.5°F (1°C) increase in temperature, with or without fever, are the signs and symptoms most often reported. Recent studies using a third-generation prestorage leukoreduced filter demonstrate effective reduction in the incidence of these reactions with both RBC and platelet products. Because of studies that support reduction in FNHTR incidence, platelet alloimmunization rates, and possibly prion transmission, leukoreduction has gained favor; however, the clinical risk to benefit ratio remains to be determined.

Common Pitfalls

- There is no hemovigilence program in the United States, so identification of both acute and long-term transfusion transmitted complications is limited in scope.
- There are no large or multi-institutional trials of either blood and blood component indications or outcome, especially morbidity in infants and children. Until such studies are established, guidelines have been developed from small studies with questionable statistical power.
- The use of recombinant erythropoietin has limited usefulness, especially for premature infants in preventing transfusion or decreasing donor exposure.
- The emergence of pathogen inactivation methods to treat cellular blood components may expose infants and children to chemical compounds whose long-term toxicity is yet unknown.

Communication and Counseling

Most families sign specific informed consent for blood and blood component transfusions, but they are unaware of the true risks, benefits, and alternatives to transfusion. The American Academy of Pediatrics has prepared a brochure for parents that outlines risks; some hospitals have educational handouts for families. However, new pathogens are emerging, making continuous surveillance for possible transfusion-associated cases a necessity, and emphasizing practitioner vigilance in reporting suspected transfusion complications.

SUGGESTED READINGS

1. Dzik WL: Emily Cooley Lecture 2002: Transfusion safety in the hospital. Transfusion 43:1190–1197, 2003. **Reviews noninfectious hazards of transfusion.**
2. Fridey JL (ed): Standards for Blood Banks and Transfusion Services, 22nd ed. Bethesda, Md: American Association of Blood Banks, 2003. **Provides standards in use of licensed transfusion services and blood collection facilities.**
3. Gibson BE, Todd A, Roberts I, et al: Transfusion guidelines for neonates and older children. Br J Haematol 124:433–453, 2004. **British guidelines for transfusion indications.**
4. King KE, Shirey RS, Thoman SK, et al: Universal leukoreduction decreases the incidence of febrile nonhemolytic transfusion reactions to RBCs. Transfusion 44:25–29, 2004. **An effectiveness study of rates of FNHTRs over time while blood transfusion practices changed in a single institution.**
5. Leukocyte reduction for the prevention of transfusion-transmitted cytomegalovirus (TT-CMV). Bethesda, Md: American Association of Blood Banks, 1997. Association Bulletin 97–2. **Reviews articles to date and makes recommendations on patient populations that would benefit.**
6. Luban NLC, Strauss RG, Hume HA: Commentary on the safety of red cells preserved in extended-storage media for neonatal transfusions. Transfusion 31:229–235, 1991. **Mathematical analysis of small- versus large-volume transfusions for toxicity from anticoagulant preservative solutions.**
7. Luban NLC: Neonatal red blood cell transfusions. Curr Opin Hematol 9:533–536, 2002. **Reviews evidence-based studies of neonatal transfusion.**
8. Nichols WG, Price TH, Gooley T, et al: Transfusion-transmitted cytomegalovirus infection after receipt of leukoreduced blood products. Blood 101:4195–4200, 2003. **Questions whether leukoreduced RBCs are equivalent to CMV negative in at-risk population of adult hematopoietic stem cell transplantation (HSCT) patients.**
9. Roseff SD, Luban NLC, Manno CS: Guidelines for assessing appropriateness of pediatric transfusion. Transfusion 42:1398–1413, 2002. **Prepared by a subcommittee of pediatric transfusion medicine physicians; details published studies and advises how to establish hospital-specific guidelines.**
10. Strauss RG, Burmeister LF, Johnson K, et al: AS–1 red cells for neonatal transfusions: A randomized trial assessing donor exposure and safety. Transfusion 36:873–878, 1996. **Demonstrates safety of small volume transfusion using prestorage solution.**

14   Endocrine System

Hypopituitarism and Growth Hormone Therapy

Jennifer L. Robbins and Sally Radovick

KEY CONCEPTS

- Short stature is defined as height at least 2.5 standard deviations below the mean (−2.5 SD), or height less than the third percentile.
- Growth hormone therapy is accepted for growth hormone deficiency or insufficiency, chronic renal insufficiency (pretransplantation), Turner syndrome, adults with growth hormone deficiency, adults with acquired immunodeficiency syndrome wasting, Prader-Willi syndrome, and children born small for gestational age without adequate catch-up growth by 2 years.
- Growth hormone therapy is most controversial for children with idiopathic short stature.
- The dose of growth hormone, most often administered via daily subcutaneous injection, is 0.17 to 0.33 mg/kg/week.
- Side effects of growth hormone therapy include local irritation, local or generalized edema, pseudotumor cerebri, slipped capital femoral epiphysis, and impaired glucose tolerance.
- For the duration of growth hormone therapy, patients are monitored every 3 to 4 months. Insulin-like growth factor-1 and insulin-like growth factor–binding protein-3 are monitored every 6 to 12 months, and bone age determinations are made annually.
- Growth hormone therapy should be continued until final adult height is reached; then growth hormone sufficiency should be re-evaluated.
- Ethical considerations may surround the decision to treat patients with growth hormone.

The hormones produced by the anterior pituitary gland play central roles in the endocrine control of growth. These include growth hormone (GH), or somatotropin, prolactin (PRL), thyroid-stimulating hormone (TSH), or thyrotropin, follicle-stimulating hormone (FSH), luteinizing hormone (LH), and adrenocorticotropin (ACTH). GH secretion is pulsatile after the newborn period, and the pulsatility is regulated from the hypothalamus by both growth hormone–releasing hormone (GHRH), which stimulates GH release, and somatostatin (or somatotropin release-inhibiting factor

[SRIF]), which inhibits GH release. GH acts by stimulating the synthesis of insulin-like growth factor-1 (IGF-1), mainly in the liver, which increases throughout childhood. Insulin-like growth factor-binding protein-3 (IGFBP-3) is a member of the family of binding proteins that carry insulin-like growth factors to target cells and interact with IGF receptors. After puberty, GH release continues but generally decreases with age.

Deficiencies in the GH axis can occur at many levels. Congenital GH deficiency (GHD) can occur with or without other pituitary hormone deficiencies. Congenital GHD occurs in 1/4000 to 1/10,000 live births and can manifest with normal birth weight and length; in the newborn period with micropenis in boys, hypoglycemia, conjugated hyperbilirubinemia, or hepatitis; and later with growth failure, delayed dentition, delayed bone age, increased abdominal fat and decreased muscle mass, thin hair, poor nail growth, and a high-pitched voice. Congenital GHD, especially with other pituitary hormone deficiencies, can be associated with holoprosencephaly, septo-optic dysplasia, or other midline defects. Other causes of GHD can be acquired, such as pituitary tumors or prior radiation therapy.

Nonendocrine causes of short stature include constitutional delay of growth and development, in which patients ultimately attain normal stature, but are *late bloomers*, and familial short stature, in which growth velocity is normal, but short stature is genetic. Other abnormalities, such as malnutrition, systemic chronic disease, intrauterine growth retardation, small for gestational age (SGA), and chromosomal abnormalities can contribute to short stature. Finally, when the height is 2.5 standard deviations below the mean (−2.5 SD), with no known cause for the short stature, the patient has idiopathic short stature (ISS).

Expert Opinion on Management Issues

DIAGNOSTIC DILEMMAS LEAD TO THERAPEUTIC DILEMMAS

GH is difficult to measure because it is secreted in a pulsatile manner with peak amplitudes occurring during sleep and has a very brief half-life. Evaluating for GHD is a burdensome process and results are difficult to interpret and are inconclusive. As a general guideline, any patient whose height is −2 SD below the mean or lower and/or who has a growth velocity less than 10th percentile over 6 months to 1 year (after the age of 2 years) warrants further workup to determine the basis of the short stature. This evaluation should include a complete history and physical examination, with special attention to family history of GHD, combined pituitary hormone deficiency (CPHD), or midline defects. Additionally, personal or family history of inflammatory bowel disease, celiac disease, thyroid disease, or other chronic illness that could contribute to short stature should be obtained.

Initial workup should include chemistries, liver function tests, erythrocyte sedimentation rate, and complete blood count (workup for a chronic illness); measurements of height, weight, and growth velocity; bone age, thyroid function tests, IGF-1, and IGFBP-3. IGF-1 and IGFBP-3 are both GH-dependent, easily measurable, and, unlike GH, not diurnally variable. IGF-1 levels (and to a lesser degree IGFBP-3 levels) depend on sexual maturity, age, and nutritional status; they are not interpretable in the setting of malnutrition or chronic illness. In terms of determining GH sufficiency, IGF-1 and IGFBP-3 levels are very helpful: If both levels are above the 50th percentile, GH deficiency is not likely, and further testing is not warranted.

In contrast, levels that are not clearly sufficient may warrant growth hormone stimulation testing (GHST). Multiple growth hormone stimulation tests exist. Unfortunately, each test is somewhat difficult to carry out, and the results may be difficult to interpret and unreliable. Because of the lack of precision in growth hormone testing, provocative GH testing is recommended only in those patients for whom there is a high clinical suspicion of GH deficiency. At this time, although GHST is cumbersome, two abnormal tests remains the standard criterion for making a diagnosis of GH deficiency.

TREATMENT LOGISTICS

GH dosing is calculated per kilogram body weight per week and generally falls between 0.17 and 0.33 mg/kg/week. In the United States, children are usually treated with approximately 0.3 mg/kg/week, divided per day, and provided as a daily subcutaneous injection. Final height outcome is generally good, but serum IGF-1 levels are generally higher than average during therapy.

Side effects of GH therapy include edema secondary to salt and water retention and pseudotumor cerebri. Edema and headache usually resolve when therapy is discontinued, and if therapy is reintroduced slowly, often these symptoms do not recur. Slipped capital femoral epiphysis occurs with increased incidence in patients with acquired GHD, as opposed to idiopathic GH deficiency. GH therapy is also associated with impaired glucose tolerance, but an increased incidence of diabetes mellitus has only been seen with patients who have Turner syndrome or brain tumors.

Children treated with GH are usually monitored with clinical visits 3 to 4 times per year. Interval history (checking for trouble with or adjustment to GH administration, psychosocial status, screening for symptoms of side effects) and physical examination should be performed, including height, weight, calculated height velocity, and pubertal stage. IGF-1 and IGFBP-3 levels are followed for adequacy of treatment and as an indication of adherence to the medication, because they should normalize. Bone age determinations are done annually, to continue to assess the patient's growth potential.

Duration of treatment is generally continued at least until final adult height is reached, at which time reassessment of GH sufficiency should be performed to determine if continuation of therapy may be indicated. GH therapy in adults with GHD has been associated with reduction in body fat and overall improvement in body composition, exercise tolerance, and bone mineral density. In patients with acquired GHD, such as that secondary to irradiation or brain tumor, or panhypopituitarism, GHD in adulthood can be assumed, and therapy may be continued for life.

DETERMINING WHO SHOULD BE TREATED

The difficulty in diagnosing GHD also produces a therapeutic challenge. If the tests are not accurate, how can the decision to treat be made? Consideration of patient benefit, clinical decision making, evaluation of GH function, and predicted adult height currently contribute to decisions to treat children with recombinant GH therapy. The U.S. Food and Drug Administration (FDA) has approved GH treatment for the following conditions:

- GHD or insufficiency (presumably proven with two inadequate responses to provocative GHST)
- Chronic renal insufficiency prior to transplantation
- Turner syndrome
- Adults with GHD
- Adults with AIDS wasting
- Prader-Willi syndrome
- Children who were SGA at birth and who have not achieved adequate catch-up growth by the age of 2 years
- As of 2003 (the most recent condition), children with ISS who have height at least 2.25 SD below the mean (−2.5 SD or less) and are unlikely to achieve normal stature.

The use of GH treatment for many of these conditions, such as Turner syndrome, even if the patients cannot be proven to be GH-deficient, is widely accepted among clinicians; whereas its use for ISS has been disputed. The FDA approval of GH treatment for children with ISS is based on two studies, a randomized placebo-controlled study done by Leschek and associates and a yet-unpublished dose-response study done by Wit and colleagues. Additionally, Finkelstein and associates published a meta-analysis of the studies so far which have looked specifically at children with ISS.

In Leshcek's study, GH-sufficient children with ISS were randomized to receive GH or placebo at 0.22 mg/kg/week, divided into three doses per week. Thirty-three subjects were available for adult height measurements; the mean duration of treatment was 4.4 years, and the mean final height in the treatment group was 3.7 cm greater than that in the placebo group. This study was limited by the small sample size and the inclusion of patients who were SGA in the ISS group, who are generally considered in a different category clinically, both by clinicians and the FDA. Also, the dosing interval standard had changed to daily dosing during the course of the study because of reported improved efficacy and better physiologic approximation. In Wit's study, patients with ISS received one of three increasing doses of GH, six times per week, for an average duration of 6.5 years. The mean final height was up to 3 to 4 inches higher than predicted. In Finkelstein and colleagues' meta-analysis, the average height gained was 4 to 6 cm for children with ISS. In looking at the cost-benefit ratio, this response approximates a cost of $35,000 per inch of height gained from GH therapy in children with ISS. These studies all have limitations and only re-emphasize the need to make treatment decisions for patients with idiopathic short stature on a case by case, clinical basis, at least until better standards are developed with a large, multicenter analysis with current dosage and interval standards.

Common Pitfalls

Ethical considerations surround the decision to treat any patient with GH. In some patients, such as those with severe GHD, the benefits may clearly outweigh the risks, but in patients with ISS, in whom the benefits may be less clear, the decision often falls into a gray area. The presumption, by some, of treating patients with ISS is that achievement of a greater adult height will prevent poor psychosocial outcomes. Many studies have tried to examine the effects of short stature on psychosocial functioning. To date, no definitive evidence has been found that short stature itself has a negative impact on psychosocial well-being or overall daily function. It is difficult to study this group. Referral to a pediatric endocrinologist itself may affect patients' views about being short, even if they are normal short patients. It is difficult to assess a child's well-being without relying on parental opinion, which introduces another level of bias. Ultimately, longitudinal studies, beginning in childhood and continuing into adulthood, need to be done with short children, referred and nonreferred, examining objective and subjective measures of psychosocial function and daily societal function.

Communication and Counseling

The dispute about treating children with ISS with recombinant GH has many aspects. First, it is difficult to prove that patients who have GH insufficiency, or mild GHD, based on their provocative tests, are different from those with ISS. It is accepted that some patients who are GH-sufficient fail provocative testing, and some who are later found to be deficient have adequate

provocative testing results. How then, can we universally accept GH therapy for those with GHD or GH insufficiency, but deny it for those with idiopathic short stature? The FDA approval of GH treatment for patients with ISS may be considered by some to be a clinical formality, but possibly a financial necessity. Clinical decisions to treat or not have always been made—with GH provocative testing playing a role in the decision but not necessarily driving it—on an individual basis. Clinicians have chosen, with families and patients, to treat patients with ISS, or possibly not to treat patients with some degree of GH insufficiency, based on the predicted final height, age, and pubertal stage at initial evaluation as well as other clinical parameters. One of the barriers to treating patients who are in need of GH therapy has always been financial. Insurance companies and Medicaid are not always willing to pay for this very expensive and invasive therapy. With FDA approval for treatment of patients with ISS, clinicians may be given an opportunity to argue successfully for insurance coverage for patients for whom GH therapy is clinically indicated but for whom necessity could not previously be defended under an FDA-approved category. The consequences of the FDA approval of GH therapy for children with ISS could also lean in another direction. This approval could open floodgates from families or patients who are frustrated with short stature and who may be willing to pay for treatment, but for whom treatment may or may not be indicated. It is critically important that this approval not be seen as a *tabula rasa* for anyone wanting or "needing" GH therapy, but be considered based on each clinical scenario, with the recognition that some patients with ISS may actually have biochemical GH deficiency that has not been clinically or biochemically documented.

SUGGESTED READINGS

1. Botero D, Evliyaoglu O, Cohen LE: Hypopituitarism. In Radovick S, MacGillivray MH (eds): Contemporary Endocrinology: Pediatric Endocrinology: A Practical Clinical Guide. Totowa, NJ: Humana Press, 2003, pp 3–36. **This chapter reviews hypopituitarism and its causes, GHD, GHST, and management.**
2. Leschek EW, Rose SR, Yanovski JA, et al: Effect of growth hormone treatment on adult height in peripubertal children with idiopathic short stature: A randomized, double-blind, placebo-controlled trial. J Clin Endocrinol Metab 89:3140–3148, 2004. **This paper is a randomized, placebo-controlled study of patients with ISS and the effects of GH treatment.**
3. Rosenfeld RG, Cohen P: Disorders of growth hormone/insulin-like growth factor secretion action. In Sperling MA (ed): Pediatric Endocrinology. Philadelphia: Elsevier Science, 2002, pp 211–288. **This chapter reviews GH physiology and pathophysiology.**
4. Wilson TA, Rose SR, Cohen P, et al: Update of guidelines for the use of growth hormone in children: The Lawson Wilkins Pediatric Endocrinology Society Drug and Therapeutics Committee. J Pediatr 143:415–421, 2003. **This paper reviews guidelines and recommendations for treating patients with GH.**
5. Wit JM: Growth hormone therapy. Best Pract Res Clin Endocrinol Metab 16:483–503, 2002. **This chapter reviews treatment with GH: indications, side effects, and monitoring.**
6. Finkelstein BS, Imperiale TF, Speroff T, et al: Effect of growth hormone therapy on height in children with idiopathic short stature: a meta-analysis. Arch Pediatr Adolesc Med 156:230–240, 2002. **Meta-analysis of studies looking at the effect of growth hormone therapy in children with ISS.**

Thyroid Disorders

Thomas P. Foley, Jr.

KEY CONCEPTS

- Rarely, congenital hypothyroidism (CH) and acquired infantile primary hypothyroidism may be missed on routine newborn screening. Therefore, clinicians need to know the symptoms and signs, and, when these are present, order serum thyroid-stimulating hormone (TSH) and free thyroxine (FT_4) tests.
- Very few tests are needed during the initial evaluation of suspected thyroid disease in infants and children. These procedures include serum TSH, FT_4, thyroid antibodies, and thyroid imaging.
- In hyperthyroidism, TSH values should be undetectable or very low. If not, the clinician needs to determine if there is a laboratory error and/or hyperthyroidism, which is rarely caused by TSH-mediated diseases and requires additional tests or referral to a pediatric endocrinologist.
- In the evaluation of thyroid nodules on physical examination, thyroid imaging and fine-needle aspiration biopsy (FNAB) are necessary diagnostic tests to determine which patients require surgery.
- Solitary and multiple thyroid nodules are less common during the first 2 decades of life, but, when present, they are more likely to be caused by thyroid cancer than in adult patients.
- During infancy, full replacement doses of levothyroxine (L-thyroxine, T_4) are indicated whenever the FT_4 values are low. During childhood and adolescence in patients with moderate to severe hypothyroidism, T_4 therapy should be initiated at the lowest daily dose available (25 µg) and gradually increased over months to the full replacement dose to avoid undesirable symptoms and signs of thyrotoxicosis that develop even when biochemical hypothyroidism persists.

BOX 1 Classification of Thyroid Diseases

Abnormalities of Thyroid Function
- Hypothyroidism
  - Congenital hypothyroidism of fetal, neonatal, or infantile onset: Sporadic, genetic, or transient
  - Acquired hypothyroidism with onset during infancy, childhood, or adolescence: Autoimmune (Hashimoto disease; toxic thyroiditis); environmental, and iatrogenic diseases
- Hyperthyroidism
  - Congenital hyperthyroidism: Genetic, maternal transplacental mediated
  - Acquired hyperthyroidism with thyrotoxicosis (Graves disease)
  - Acquired hyperthyroidism without thyrotoxicosis (thyroid hormone resistance)
  - Acquired thyrotoxicosis without hyperthyroidism (factitious thyrotoxicosis)

Structural Changes in the Thyroid
- Diffuse thyromegaly (goiter)
  - Autoimmune (Hashimoto thyroiditis and/or Graves disease)
  - Familial thyroid dyshormonogenesis (hypothyroidism)
  - Exposure to goitrogens through medications or the environment
- Nodular thyroid disease: Solitary and multiple thyroid nodules
  - Thyroid neoplasia: Benign (thyroid adenoma, thyroid cysts), malignant (epithelial thyroid carcinoma: papillary and follicular, familial and sporadic medullary thyroid carcinoma, and MEN syndromes), and other malignancies (lymphoma, histiocytoma)
  - Embryonic remnants and thyroid cysts

MEN, multiple endocrine neoplasia.

BOX 2 Clinical Presentation of Acquired Thyroid Diseases during Infancy, Childhood, and Adolescence

- Abnormal thyroid gland on examination
  - Thyromegaly: Diffuse versus nodular, smooth versus granular, soft versus firm versus hard
  - Atrophic or fibrotic gland
- Growth retardation in chronic hypothyroidism
- Symptoms of thyrotoxicosis
- Abnormal thyroid function test on screening

Disorders of the thyroid gland are the most common of the endocrine and metabolic diseases when iodine-deficiency disorders are included. Among iodine-sufficient populations, thyroid disease is only second in frequency after diabetes mellitus. Additionally, 25% to 30% of children with type 1 diabetes mellitus develop autoimmune thyroid disease during childhood or adolescence. Certain thyroid diseases often pose a diagnostic and therapeutic challenge (e.g., Graves disease and thyrotoxicosis, and thyroid cancer). Furthermore, the onset of hypothyroidism is often subtle, with minimal and nonspecific symptoms and signs that often cause a delay in diagnosis. For these reasons, newborn screening programs are mandated in most populations to detect congenital hypothyroidism (CH) shortly after birth because detecting the disease in early infancy can help prevent permanent mental retardation and neurobehavorial disabilities that otherwise occur when the diagnosis is delayed beyond 3 to 6 months of age.

Two broad categories of thyroid disorders—secretory versus anatomic disease—are based on the clinical presentation and pathogenesis, and they may manifest anytime during fetal or postnatal life. Thyroid diseases are further classified as familial or sporadic, congenital or acquired, diffuse or nodular thyroid enlargement on examination, and by the state of thyroid secretion and metabolism as hypothyroidism, thyrotoxicosis with or without hyperthyroidism, and euthyroidism (Box 1).

Acquired thyroid diseases often manifest as a midline anterior cervical mass noticed by the patient, family members, or friends. They also may be found by accident during an evaluation for another medical problem or during a careful routine annual physical examination by a primary care physician (Box 2). The diffusely enlarged gland (Box 3) with granular and firm texture usually represents autoimmune thyroiditis,

---

BOX 3 Etiologies of Thyromegaly

Etiology of Diffuse Thyromegaly
- Autoimmune (Hashimoto) thyroiditis
  - Thyrotoxicosis
  - Graves disease
  - Toxic thyroiditis
  - TSH-secreting pituitary adenoma
  - Resistance to thyroid hormone
- Iodine deficiency
- Goitrogen ingestion: antithyroid drugs, chemicals, and foods
- Familial dyshormonogenesis (defective thyroxine synthesis)
- Acute and subacute thyroiditis (bacterial or viral)
- Idiopathic (simple goiter)

Etiology of Nodular Thyromegaly
- Thyroid neoplasia
- Thyroid cyst(s)
- Autoimmune (Hashimoto) thyroiditis

TSH, thyroid-stimulating hormone.

BOX 4 Thyroid Function in Thyroid Diseases

- Primary hypothyroidism
  - Elevated serum or filter paper TSH value
  - Low serum-free thyroxine
- Primary hypothyroidism, compensated
  - Elevated serum or filter paper TSH
  - Normal serum free thyroxine
- Non–TSH-mediated thyrotoxicosis
  - Undetectable serum TSH value
  - Elevated serum free thyroxine
  - Elevated serum total and free triiodothyronine
  - Measurable TSH receptor autoantibodies (TRAbs)
- TSH-mediated thyrotoxicosis
  - Normal or mildly elevated serum TSH
  - Elevated serum free thyroxine
  - Elevated serum total and free l-triiodothyronine
  - Elevated serum alpha subunit in pituitary adenomas

TSH, thyroid-stimulating hormone.

---

the most common cause of acquired thyroid diseases. The same disease with a different pathologic process causes a small atrophic, firm gland, and the patient usually has symptoms of hypothyroidism. A solitary smooth, hard nodule with a history of increasing size is thyroid malignancy until proven benign. A tender thyroid gland indicates an inflammatory process that usually is subacute (viral) thyroiditis. During the first 2 decades of life it is uncommon, but thereafter peaks in frequency during the third and fourth decades. Rarely, a perithyroidal bacterial infection causes a very tender gland with an acute septic presentation that requires urgent medical and surgical management. During childhood, a diffusely enlarged, smooth, soft thyroid gland is almost invariably present in children with Graves disease; in contrast to the presentation in adults, the absence of a diffusely enlarged thyroid gland rarely is associated with Graves disease.

Deceleration in linear growth often is the first clue of hypothyroidism and one of many reasons in support of annual accurate measurements of height and weigh plotted on growth charts. The onset of hyperthyroidism also may be subtle initially, but the symptoms in children become more pronounced and characteristic of the hypermetabolic state: hyperactivity, deteriorating school performance, onset of nocturia and enuresis, restless sleeping with fatigue by the afternoon, increasing appetite without weight gain and even weight loss. Symptoms more typical of adults with hyperthyroidism may also develop, including palpitations. Ophthalmic symptoms and signs usually are mild and not prominent early in the disease.

Congenital hypothyroidism nearly always is identified within the first 2 weeks of life through mandatory newborn screening. Most programs measure thyroid-stimulating hormone (TSH) alone, thyroxine (T_4) initially followed by TSH on the lower 10% to 20% of T_4 values, and TSH plus T_4 on every newborn. Abnormal screening tests must be confirmed by serum determinations of TSH and free thyroxine (FT_4). The total T_4 is not a useful test and may even cause misleading

information when performed in an infant. Patients with certain diseases associated with an increased risk for thyroid diseases are screened at defined intervals. Hypothyroidism or hyperthyroidism often are first detected by these programs. Patients with Down syndrome, type 1 diabetes mellitus, Addison disease and other autoimmune diseases, Turner syndrome, juvenile rheumatoid arthritis, and myasthenia gravis should be tested annually by measuring serum TSH to detect an elevation, suggestive of primary hypothyroidism and, less commonly, thyroid antibodies and FT_4.

Once a thyroid disease is suspected and a detailed history obtained, the initial laboratory evaluation is based on the clinical presentation:

- Thyroid function and antibody tests are obtained when there is evidence of a secretory abnormality of the thyroid gland: hypothyroidism versus hyperthyroidism.
- When a structural or anatomic abnormality is found, such as diffuse thyromegaly or goiter verus solitary or multiple thyroid nodules versus no palpable thyroid tissue, imaging tests of the thyroid (thyroid ultrasound, radionuclide scan) may be indicated in addition to serum tests for thyroid function (TSH, FT_4) and thyroid antibody titers.

The laboratory tests in children with suspected thyroid disease are limited to serum TSH, FT_4, and thyroid antibodies (thyroid peroxidase and thyroglobulin antibodies) (Box 4). Additional blood tests are not usually needed. Thyroid image tests are rarely required in the evaluation of children with a diffusely enlarged thyroid (Box 5), but those with one or more discrete nodules and no detectable thyroid antibodies should have further evaluation. Because a pure thyroid cyst is more common in children than adults, the initial image usually is a thyroid ultrasound. If the nodule is solid on ultrasound, many elect to obtain a radionuclide image with ^{123}I-iodine or ^{199m}Tc pertechnetate before proceeding with a fine-needle aspiration biopsy (FNAB) of the nodule. A definitive diagnosis of benign or malignant lesion is needed to determine the need for thyroidectomy (Box 6).

BOX 5 Treatment and Management of Diffuse Thyromegaly

- Graves disease with thyrotoxicosis
  - Antithyroid drug therapy: methimazole or propylthiouracil.
  - β-Adrenergic blockade: propranolol, atenolol, others.
  - Radioiodine ablation therapy when antithyroid therapy fails.
  - Subtotal thyroidectomy when other therapy fails.
  - Monitor serum TSH, free thyroxine, gland size, and TRAbs.
- Primary hypothyroidism
  - L-Thyroxine therapy: 1–3 µg/kg once daily.
  - Maintain serum TSH in the normal range.
  - Annual tests with no change in therapy or clinical disease.
  - Test 1–3 mo after changes in therapy or concerns about compliance.
  - Monitor linear growth and pubertal development.

TRAb, thyrotropin receptor autoantibody; TSH, thyroid-stimulating hormone.

BOX 6 Treatment and Management of Juvenile-Onset Thyroid Cancer

Papillary and Follicular Thyroid Carcinoma
Diagnosis by FNAB

- If malignant:
  - Total thyroidectomy
  - Lobectomy recommended by some for solitary papillary cancer: small, encapsulated, well-differentiated cancer, <20 mm; no evidence of contralateral lobe or isthmus; no evidence of metastatic disease
- Suspicious or inconclusive malignancy:
  - Lobectomy
  - Completion thyroidectomy if final pathology confirms malignancy

Therapy

- Radioiodine scan and remnant ablation therapy
- Therapy with L-thyroxine at doses to maintain serum TSH approximately 0.3–0.5 mU/L.

Management

- Monitoring serum thyroglobulin (valid only if thyroglobulin antibodies are negative)
- Repeat of radioiodine scan, 6 mo–1 yr: after cessation of thyroxine therapy until TSH > 25 mU/L, after treatment with recombinant TSH (Thyrolar), serum thyroglobulin, and TSH just prior to administration of isotope

Medullary Thyroid Carcinoma (MTC): Sporadic and Familial (MEN Syndromes)

- Positive family history
  - Genetic analysis of *RET* proto-oncogene very early in life.
  - If positive, total thyroidectomy and serial calcitonin monitoring.
  - Evaluate for other diseases in the MEN syndromes.
- Baseline calcitonin value during evaluation of solitary nodule.
  - Negative family history for MTC and MEN.
- FNAB; if malignant:
  - Total thyroidectomy and serial calcitonin monitoring.
  - Genetic analysis of *RET* proto-oncogene.
  - Evaluate for other diseases in the MEN syndromes.

FNAB, fine-needle aspiration biopsy; MEN, multiple endocrine neoplasia; TSH, thyroid-stimulating hormone.

Expert Opinion on Management Issues

CONGENITAL HYPOTHYROIDISM AND HYPERTHYROIDISM

Congenital Hypothyroidism

The management of the neonate with thyroid disease usually begins with reviewing the results of mandatory screening tests for hypothyroidism. These tests are collected before discharge of the neonate from the nursery or during the first week of life for small infants who remain in the nursery. Blood is collected by heel prick, placed on special filter paper specimens, and allowed to air dry at room temperature. Screening programs usually test only TSH, initially T_4 and subsequently TSH, on the lowest 3% to 20% of the T_4 values, or both TSH and T_4 simultaneously. An elevated TSH value with either a low or normal T_4 value requires serum confirmation tests of thyroid function that should be performed the next working day after the physician is notified. These tests should include serum TSH and FT_4. A history of maternal thyroid disease, familial thyroid disease, exposure to excess iodine, or iodine deficiency provide important information in determining transient versus permanent disease and familial versus sporadic disease.

Additional tests may be indicated to define the etiology and determine transient versus permanent disease. When the TSH is elevated on the newborn screen, a thyroid scan or ultrasound is useful to obtain at the same time that serum confirmation tests are drawn. Because an anatomic abnormality is the most common cause, a technetium scan is the most cost-effective method to promptly diagnose athyreosis, ectopic thyroid dysgenesis, or a eutopic gland that is small (hypoplastic), normal, or enlarged (goiter). A bone age radiograph may be useful to estimate the fetal age of onset of hypothyroidism for infants with severe hypothyroidism. If the skeletal maturation is comparable to a newborn infant, no fetal hypothyroidism of significant duration occurred, and the prognosis for normal intellectual, neurobehavioral, and physical development is excellent. Conversely, skeletal maturation of an infant less than 36 fetal weeks for a full-term infant indicates fetal hypothyroidism with an onset before 8 months of age gestation for an undermined duration. Fetal hypothyroidism of several weeks or months of duration has a guarded prognosis and an increased risk for abnormal intellectual and neurobehavioral development.

In newborn screening programs that test total T_4, other conditions may be identified, such as thyroxine-binding protein deficiencies, which do not require therapy, and hypothalamic or pituitary hypothyroidism that requires further investigation and therapy. The differential diagnosis depends on the FT_4 value; the most accurate and definitive FT_4 test is the direct dialysis method. A diagnosis in the neonate should not depend on indirect determinations of FT_4, unless those methods were validated against the direct dialysis FT_4

method in healthy and ill preterm and term infants. When the total T_4 is elevated, some screening programs evaluate infants for conditions, such as excessive T_4 binding proteins, not requiring therapy, and thyroid hormone resistance syndromes and hyperthyroidism that require further investigation.

Once the diagnosis of congenital primary hypothyroidism is suspected and specimens are collected for confirmation of the diagnosis, L-thyroxine (LT_4) therapy should be started promptly, even before the results of serum confirmation tests are obtained. Therapy is not harmful and can be stopped at any time should the confirmatory tests be normal.

The usual starting LT_4 dose is 10 to 15 µg/kg given once daily at least 30 minutes before food intake. Infants with athyreosis and very low or undetectable FT_4 and elevated TSH values should start with 13 to 15 µg/kg/day. In children with a TSH greater than 20 mU/L and normal T_4 values, a LT_4 dose of 37.5 µg/day for term infants of normal weight should be sufficient. Because the absorption of T_4 varies from patient to patient, the correct dose for each child should be determined by serial measurements of FT_4 and TSH. The TSH value should be suppressed below 10 mU/L by 2 weeks of therapy and kept above 0.1 mU/L to prevent excessive thyroid hormone effect. Blood specimens for TSH and FT_4 should be collected at weekly intervals for the first month, at monthly intervals until 6 months of age, and at 3-monthly intervals until 2 years of age. To monitor therapy in Switzerland, TSH and T_4 are measured in eluates from dried blood stain (DBS) filter paper specimens mailed to the screening laboratory, thus avoiding venipuncture and enabling the family to have their primary care physician collect the specimens at a convenient location.

LT_4 is available for infants in 25-, 50-, 75-, and higher µg tablets. During infancy, 25-µg tablets should be prescribed; $1\frac{1}{2}$ tablets provide a daily dose of 37.5 µg, and $2\frac{1}{2}$ tablets provide a daily dose of 62.5 µg. Adjustments in dosage can be achieved by an increase or decrease in the LT_4 dose by one tablet per week or by 12.5-µg increments daily. The addition of one 25-µg tablet per week provides approximately 3.5 µg daily, and one 50-µg tablet increase per week provides approximately 7 µg of LT_4 daily. Minor dose adjustments can be achieved by the addition or omission of one dose per week. Medication should be administered at least 30 minutes before feeding and never with substances that may interfere with its absorption, such as medications containing iron, possibly calcium, and some soy-containing formulas or fiber-containing foods.

Liquid preparations of LT_4 in the United States are not stable on storage. If the medication cannot be swallowed as a tablet, it should be crushed in a spoon with water or another liquid. LT_4 only needs to be administered once daily. If a dose is missed or thought to be missed, a double dose should be given the next day. Substances that affect T_4 metabolism or absorption need to be eliminated or higher doses prescribed (Box 7).

BOX 7 Medications, Foods, and Chemicals that Interfere with Thyroid Function Tests, Thyroid Hormone Metabolism, or Thyroid Hormone Absorption

Medications that Alter the Binding of T_4 and T_3 in Serum
- Decreased total T_4 and/or T_3
  - Androgens
  - Anabolic steroids
  - Glucocorticoids
  - Nicotinic acid
  - Salicylates
  - Furosemide
  - Phenytoin
- Increased total T_4 and T_3
  - Estrogens (oral, not transdermal)

Medications that Increase the Metabolism of T_4 and T_3
- Rifampin
- Phenobarbital
- Carbamazepine
- Phenytoin

Medications, Foods, and Chemicals that Decrease Absorption of Ingested Thyroid Hormones
- Iron salts
- High dietary fiber
- Soy-milk formulas
- Calcium salts
- Cholestyramine
- Activated charcoal
- Sucralfate
- Preparations containing aluminum hydroxide

T_3, triiodothyronine; T_4, thyroxine.

Acquired Hypothyroidism of Infancy

Infants with acquired hypothyroidism caused by autoimmune thyroiditis may present with symptoms and signs of congenital hypothyroidism that develop after 6 months of age. These infants are asymptomatic during the first 6 months of life, but at diagnosis they have symptoms and signs similar to infants with congenital hypothyroidism not detected by screening. These important clinical features as in untreated congenital hypothyroidism may be seen: dry skin and constipation, deceleration in linear growth beginning late in the first year or early in the second year of life, and a delay or arrest in developmental milestones. If hypothyroidism begins around 2 years of age, there may be some symptoms and signs characteristic of hypothyroidism in older children, such as muscular pseudohypertrophy. Delay in skeletal maturation or in eruption of primary teeth may not be evident when first seen because hypothyroidism often develops rapidly in these young infants. If the duration of hypothyroidism is not prolonged and LT_4 treatment is adequate, the delay in developmental milestones should not be permanent.

An occasional infant, often with Down syndrome, has mildly elevated TSH values (<20 mU/L), persistently normal FT_4 values, negative thyroid antibodies, and, if measured, normal FT_3 (free triiodothyronine) levels. During infancy and childhood the TSH values do not further increase, often decrease, and eventually normalize. There is no evidence that LT_4 therapy is beneficial as long as the free hormone values do not decrease. Treatment, however, certainly would not cause harm if thyroid function is carefully monitored to avoid iatrogenic thyrotoxicosis. The cause of the abnormality in TSH feedback control is unknown.

Congenital Hyperthyroidism

Neonatal thyrotoxicosis usually is caused by transplacental transfer of thyroid-stimulating immunoglobulins (TSIs) from the mother (see Box 5). The disease occurs in 1 neonate of approximately every 70 infants born to mothers known to have active Graves disease either before or during pregnancy, Graves disease previously treated with thyroidectomy or radioiodine ablation, or Hashimoto disease. However, mothers with detectable TSI usually give birth to normal infants, especially when maternal serum TSI activity is only mildly elevated.

Neonatal thyrotoxicosis may occur in infants without detectable TSI (see Box 5). In these infants, the disorder is caused either by the syndrome of generalized resistance to thyroid hormone with mild thyrotoxicosis (autosomal dominant inheritance) or germ-line mutations in the TSH receptor gene that cause constitutive activation of the TSH receptor. The mutations in the transmembrane domains of the receptor keep the receptor in the activated state so G protein and adenylate cyclase are constitutively activated, causing hyperthyroidism. In this situation, TSI does not play a role, serum FT_4 and FT_3 are elevated, and serum TSH is unmeasurable.

Infants, children, and adolescents with the clinical symptoms and signs of thyrotoxicosis and hyperthyroidism caused by Graves disease and confirmed by abnormal serum thyroid function tests (unmeasurable TSH, elevated FT_4 and FT_3) are treated with antithyroid drugs initially. If unsuccessful, radioiodine ablative therapy or subtotal thyroidectomy are selected. Those patients with a measurable serum TSH should have further diagnostic tests to establish the definitive diagnosis and treatment based on the diagnosis. Because of the complexity of these diseases, the patient should be referred to a pediatric endocrinologist with experience in the diagnosis and treatment of the causes of hyperthyroidism in infancy, childhood, and adolescence. Toxicity to the antithyroid medications rarely occurs in infancy but must be remembered when unexplained illnesses develop (Box 8).

ACQUIRED THYROID DISORDERS OF CHILDHOOD AND ADOLESCENCE

Autoimmune Thyroiditis without and with Primary Hypothyroidism

Primary hypothyroidism usually is caused by autoimmune thyroiditis: either thyroiditis with goiter or nongoitrous thyroiditis with the chronic fibrous variant of autoimmune thyroiditis. Iatrogenic causes of primary hypothyroidism include radiation-induced and postsurgical thyroidectomy. Globally, iodine deficiency is the most common cause. When the onset of hypothyroidism occurs after 3 years of age, treatment should be initiated slowly, beginning with a 25-µg daily dose for 2 to 4 weeks and increasing by a 12.5- to 25-µg daily dose every 2 to 4 weeks until thyroid function tests are normal. Patients corrected more rapidly experience very disturbing and uncomfortable symptoms of thyrotoxicosis that interfere with schoolwork, sleep, and daily activities. The reason is unknown, but the metabolic correction toward euthyroidism is recognized systemically as hyperthyroidism, presumably mediated in part through hypersensitive adrenergic receptors. Small doses of β-adrenergic blocking drugs, if not otherwise contraindicated, may provide some relief until readjustment occurs, usually within 6 to 12 months. LT_4 should be given at least 30 minutes before a meal to avoid impaired absorption of thyroxine by certain foods and infant formulas, and it should not be given at the same time of day as foods that contain fiber and medications containing iron, calcium, or resins. Serum TSH is the test of choice to monitor adequacy and compliance of therapy unless symptoms of hyperthyroidism develop; in this situation, FT_4 and FT_3 measurements are useful.

Acute Suppurative Thyroiditis

Acute suppurative thyroiditis, a rare disease, is easy to recognize but difficult to manage. The disease is a perithyroidal inflammation usually because of a persistent left-sided embryonic perilymphatic fistulous tract that becomes infected with oral pathogens. The thyroid is very tender, and the child appears toxic from the infection but is not thyrotoxic. Serial thyroid ultrasound examinations are very important to detect abscess formation early, so proper incision and drainage can be performed. Intravenous antibiotics and fluids are essential. No residual thyroid disease is expected. Once the infection has subsided, to prevent recurrence, imaging studies are needed to identify the fistula so it can be excised.

BOX 8   **Side Effects of Antithyroid Drugs**

- Granulocytopenia
- Hypoprothrombinemia
- Dermatitis, urticaria, edema
- Conjunctivitis
- Arthralgia, arthritis
- Hepatitis
- Sensorineural hearing loss
- Thrombocytopenia
- Peripheral neuritis
- Lupus-like syndrome
- Loss of taste sensation
- Lymphadenopathy
- Fever
- Disseminated intravascular coagulation
- Toxic psychosis

Subacute Thyroiditis

Subacute thyroiditis also is rarely diagnosed during childhood and adolescence, because either it rarely occurs or is so mild that an underlying upper respiratory infection could mask its clinical presentation. The disease presumably results from a viral infection of the thyroid gland, which typically is tender but not always. During the early phase of the disease, the child may have mild hyperthyroidism with elevated levels of total and FT_4 and FT_3, normal or undetectable levels of TSH, either negative or low titers of thyroid antibodies, and a low or absent uptake of radioactive iodine. The erythrocyte sedimentation rate usually is markedly elevated but may be normal to slightly elevated when the thyroid is not tender. Mild thyrotoxicosis is controlled with low-dose β-adrenergic blockade. The clinical course of subacute thyroiditis is variable but often progresses through three phases (mild hypothyroidism, euthyroid goiter, and mild hypothyroidism) before the patient finally recovers and has normal thyroid function. The transient phase of hypothyroidism during recovery varies in length and severity and may require a course of FT_4 therapy. Full recovery is expected, although late recurrences may occur but are rare.

MANAGEMENT OF JUVENILE THYROTOXICOSIS

Management of thyrotoxicosis during childhood is challenging and difficult. Factors such as age and severity of disease influence the mode and duration of therapy. For most children and adolescents, the antithyroid medication methimazole (MTZ), preferably, or propylthiouracil (PTU) is prescribed to bring the disease under control. β-Adrenergic blocking drugs, such as propranolol or atenolol, promptly exert effective control of clinical symptoms in moderately to severely affected patients, reduce the risk for the development of thyroid storm should another serious intervening illness develop, and provide symptomatic relief in days. For mildly affected children, β-adrenergic blockade is not needed unless school performance is affected or sleeping habits are disturbed; a single morning dose could improve an adjustment in school, or an evening dose could improve problems with restless sleeping. The major contraindication is asthma.

The antithyroid medications available in North America are MTZ and PTU. They are equally effective and probably have comparable frequency and severity of side effects. PTU is prescribed initially in divided doses three or four times daily for patients with moderate to severe thyrotoxicosis. MTZ may be given once daily. The PTU dose is 5 to 10 mg/kg/day, and MTZ is 0.5 to 1 mg/kg/day. A starting dose for children is usually 5 mg three times per day for MTZ or 50 mg three times per day for PTU; for older children and adolescents, the starting doses are 20 mg to 40 mg daily for MTZ and 100 to 150 mg for PTU—both drugs in three divided doses daily. Serious side effects from MTZ and PTU are uncommon (see Box 8). Approximately 5% of children experience mild and reversible side effects, such as rashes, arthralgia, and neutropenia, that disappear on discontinuation of therapy. If the side effect is not serious, the other available antithyroid medication can be tried; however, very close monitoring is most important because rarely the same problem may recur with the other drug.

When higher doses are used, hypothyroxinemia is induced in most patients within the first 4 to 12 weeks of therapy, depending on the severity and duration of the disease at diagnosis. Often the serum TSH remains undetectable even when FT_4 levels have decreased into the hypothyroid range. Serum T_3 should be monitored because some patients have normal or low FT_4 but persistently elevated serum T_3 levels. Once the serum TSH is measurable or elevated, either LT_4 therapy can be initiated or the dose of MTZ or PTU decreased. The definite advantage of MTZ therapy is that it can be changed to a once-daily regimen once euthyroidism is achieved. Activity of Graves disease can be judged by serum TSI activity and, more accurately, by reduction in size of the thyroid gland to normal, for a normal size thyroid gland is the most reliable indicator of remission. If the gland size is normal, the continual presence of TSI would indicate the high likelihood of relapse, and antithyroid drugs should be continued. A normal or small thyroid gland with persistently detectable thyrotropin receptor autoantibody (TRAb) by thyroid-binding inhibitory immunoglobulin (TBII) methods may indicate the presence of TSH receptor blocking antibodies (TRBAbs); in this situation, a trial off antithyroid drugs would be worthwhile. If the thyroid gland size remains normal and the TSI test is negative, a trial off medication is indicated, although a negative TSI titer has a relatively low predictive value for remission (50%). If relapse occurs in children after cessation of antithyroid therapy, it usually occurs within 6 to 9 months after therapy is discontinued.

If relapse occurs after cessation of therapy, the patient and family have two options: another course of MTZ or PTU or an alternate form of therapy such as radioiodine ablation or subtotal thyroidectomy. In prepubertal children, most endocrinologists prefer to continue MTZ or PTU therapy into the adolescent age unless a serious idiosyncratic reaction with the medication occurs or an enlarging thyroid nodule is present. The reason for the preference of antithyroid drugs in childhood is the limited experience with radioiodine therapy in young children and the concern about the potential carcinogenesis of ^{131}I-iodine therapy during the growth phase of the thyroid gland if nonablative doses are administered. However, it should be acknowledged that large studies in the United States and Europe have failed to document any increased risk for thyroid malignancy after radioiodine therapy in adults and some adolescents. Because there are risks for serious complications from thyroidectomy during childhood, especially when surgeons have limited experience with thyroid surgical in children, radioiodine ablation therapy is the second treatment of choice after failure of antithyroid drug therapy for older children and adolescents and for any child with an idiosyncratic reaction to medication. The morbidity, cost, and mortality of radioiodine therapy are lower than surgery. Within 6 to 12 months, permanent hypothyroidism usually develops, necessitating LT_4 replacement therapy.

For the rare patient with thyrotoxicosis caused by a hypersecreting thyroid adenoma, surgical excision of the tumor cures the disease. The surgery is not associated with the known risks of thyroidectomy because only resection of the tumor or a lobectomy usually is performed. The indications for surgery are clinical thyrotoxicosis associated with elevated levels of serum FT_4 and FT_3, undetectable levels of TSH, an enlarging mass, and lack of homogeneity on ultrasound or radionuclide imaging. Because this cause of thyrotoxicosis is rare, other forms of therapy (e.g., radioiodine, ethanol injections) are not advocated because of the lack of experience in their use in children.

MANAGEMENT OF NODULAR THYROMEGALY

Infants, children, and adolescents with thyroid nodules not caused by autoimmune thyroiditis are very uncommon. The diagnostic evaluation usually includes thyroid function tests, thyroid antibodies, thyroid ultrasound and/or radionuclide image, and FNAB. If the FNAB is inconclusive, follicular, suspicious, or indicative of thyroid cancer, total thyroidectomy is indicated, followed by other diagnostic and therapeutic procedures. Because of the complexity of these diseases, the patient should be referred to a pediatric endocrinologist with experience in the diagnosis and treatment of the neoplastic thyroid diseases that manifest during the first two decades of life.

The clinical presentation, diagnostic evaluation, and management of children and adolescents with medullary thyroid carcinoma (MTC) are the same as described for adults. Where there is a family history of familial MTC or multiple endocrine neoplasia (MEN) IIa or IIb syndromes, every member of the family is tested for the *RET* proto-oncogene mutations including infants. Depending on the mutation identified, infants should have a total thyroidectomy before 6 months of age in MEN IIb with *RET* codon mutations 883, 918, or 922 because MTC is very aggressive; with other *RET* codon mutations, total thyroidectomy is recommended by 2 years of age for certain *RET* codon mutations and by 5 years of age with other mutation because the specific mutations dictate the age of onset of MTC. The opportunity for a cure is best achieved by total thyroidectomy during the preclinical stage of the disease when C-cell hyperplasia without tumors is seen.

Common Pitfalls

The child with abnormalities in thyroid function who requires additional studies or dose alterations should be monitored with serum concentrations of TSH and FT_4 performed by methods validated for accuracy and reliability in infancy. Examples of occasionally encountered problems, summarized by the abnormality of thyroid function, are:

■ *Undetectable TSH concentrations with consistently normal FT_4 and T_3 values*: If the child has clinical thyrotoxicosis, the dose of LT_4 should be reduced until the TSH is measurable and the clinical symptoms subside. If the child is clinically euthyroid and the serum TSH value is unmeasurable, it is advisable to decrease the dose of LT_4 only slightly by half to one tablet per week to retain normal FT_4 and T_3 values with a normal, measurable TSH value.

■ *Persistently elevated serum TSH and normal serum FT_4 concentrations*: Usually a persistent elevation in serum TSH indicates the need for an increase in the LT_4 dose followed by repeat thyroid function tests in 4 to 6 weeks. Factors that influence the absorption or metabolism of LT_4 need to be excluded, or the dose increased as long as these factors persist (see Box 7). The expected upper normal values for serum TSH and FT_4 are highest during the first 9 months of age and gradually decline to adult TSH values later in childhood. The serum TSH usually is the best indicator of normal thyroid function at this age.

■ *Intermittent elevations of serum TSH on the same LT_4 dose*: Fluctuations in serum TSH while the child receives the same dose of LT_4 usually are caused by inconsistent compliance with medication, inconsistent absorption, or, least likely, variable potency of the medication. Parents who forget to give the medication or do not supervise their child while taking medication may decide to give their child excessive amounts of LT_4 just prior to blood testing. This causes the serum TSH to still be elevated, but the FT_4 will be normal or mildly elevated. At other times, when compliance is satisfactory, TSH and FT_4 values will be normal. When LT_4 is given with medications that interfere with absorption, such as iron, possibly calcium, or with foods that prevent complete absorption, such as fiber-containing foods, inconsistent thyroid function tests are observed. In these circumstances, when education fails, it may be necessary to increase the dose, realizing there may be episodes of better compliance and/or improved absorption associated with mild thyrotoxicosis.

■ *An increase in serum TSH, FT_4, and T_3*: Children with these results are rare and the most difficult to manage. Data in experimental animals indicate that intrauterine hypothyroidism may be associated with abnormal feedback control of pituitary TSH secretion. In the experimental animal or child, excessive amounts of thyroid hormone are necessary to normalize serum TSH values. Elevated FT_4 and T_3 are required to reduce serum TSH to normal, and the patient may have clinical signs and symptoms of thyrotoxicosis. Once this situation can be documented clinically, the dose of LT_4 should be reduced until the patient is clinically euthyroid and FT_4 and T_3 levels are normal, regardless of serum TSH levels. This abnormality in the feedback control of TSH usually subsides during childhood. Chronic thyrotoxicosis in the infant may cause deleterious effects on intellectual development and skeletal maturation.

In the clinically euthyroid child with normal linear growth and serum TSH and FT_4 values, no additional laboratory tests are needed. After 3 years of age in euthyroid children with normal growth and thyroid function tests, only an annual evaluation is needed, unless other clinical conditions develop that could interfere with the oral administration and absorption of clinically. After 3 years of age, if the diagnosis of hypothyroidism was not clearly established at initiation of LT_4 therapy, and serum TSH values remained normal or suppressed on the same dose of LT_4 since 3 months of age, LT_4 therapy should be discontinued or decreased and serum TSH and FT_4 measured to establish the diagnosis of permanent primary hypothyroidism and determine if lifelong LT_4 therapy is needed.

There are specific management issues for infants with familial inborn errors of thyroid hormone synthesis and metabolism, a group of disorders known collectively as familial thyroid dyshormonogenesis. These autosomal recessive conditions are usually detected on newborn screening with elevations in TSH, and they comprise approximately 10% to 15% of the newborn hypothyroid population, depending on the frequency of the mutation in the population. They are suspected in the newborn period by palpable or enlarged thyroid glands. Thyromegaly can be documented with thyroid ultrasound or scan. The parents should be advised about the possibility of a 25% chance of the disease in subsequent children that is easiest to document by measuring TSH in cord serum. In those with partially reduced enzymatic activities, the dose of LT_4 replacement therapy often is less than usually prescribed for infants with athyreosis.

Communication and Counseling

At diagnosis, parents of infants must be educated about the importance and proper techniques in the administration of levothyroxine. The tablet must be crushed, and not until immediately before dosing can it be suspended in a small amount of liquid. At no age should T_4 be given with food or with medications that contain iron, calcium, soy-containing food or beverage, or fiber; T_4 should be given orally at least 30 minutes and preferably 1 hour before food intake. Parents should be told never to miss a dose of T_4; if they forget, or are uncertain if the dose was given, the missed dose in its entirety should be given without delay.

The prognosis for intellectual and neurobehavorial development is very good for infants with CH who are diagnosed and treated when asymptomatic very soon after birth, and it is guarded when clinical symptoms and signs are evident during fetal life or at birth. If the diagnosis of symptomatic primary hypothyroidism is delayed longer than 1 to 3 years and little FT_4 is measured in serum, the child may not achieve an adult target height based on parental height. The common forms of thyroid cancer (papillary and follicular) have an excellent prognosis when diagnosis and treatment begins during the first two decades of life. Parents can be offered the following websites for additional information: http://www.thyroid.org; http://www.magicfoundation.org; http://www.thyroidmanage.org (thyroid textbook for sophisticated readers).

SUGGESTED READINGS

1. Dorman JS, Foley TP Jr: Epidemiology of chronic autoimmune thyroiditis type I diabetes. In Gill RG (ed): Immunologically Mediated Endocrine Diseases. New York: Lippincott Williams & Wilkins, 2001, Chapter 17, pp 351–368. **Autoimmune diseases are the most common etiology of thyroid diseases and type 1 diabetes mellitus and autoimmune thyroid diseases are the most common endocrine diseases during the first 2 decades of life. This review provides a detailed review of the etiology, pathogenesis, and epidemiology of these diseases.**
2. Fisher DA, Brown RS: Thyroid physiology in the perinatal period during childhood. In Braverman LE, Utiger RD (eds): Werner and Ingbar's The Thyroid, 8th ed. Philadelphia: Lippincott Williams & Wilkins, 2000, pp 959–972. **This chapter covers pediatric thyroid physiology.**
3. Foley TP Jr: Hypothyroidism in infants children. Congenital hypothyroidism. In Braverman LE, Utiger RD (eds): Werner and Ingbar's The Thyroid, 8th ed. Philadelphia: Lippincott Williams & Wilkins, 2000, pp 977–983. **This chapter reviews congenital hypothyroid disease in infants and children.**
4. Foley TP Jr: Hypothyroidism in infants children. Acquired hypothyroidism in infants, children and adolescents. In Braverman LE, Utiger RD (eds): Werner and Ingbar's The Thyroid, 8th ed. Philadelphia: Lippincott Williams & Wilkins, 2000, pp 983–988. **This chapter reviews acquired hypothyroid disease in infants and children.**
5. Foley TP Jr, Abbassi V, Copeland KC, Draznin MB: Acquired autoimmune mediated infantile hypothyroidism: A pathologic entity distinct from congenital hypothyroidism. N Engl J Med 330:466–468, 1994. **A clinical description of acquired hypothyroidism during infancy, a newly recognized variant of autoimmune thyroiditis with primary hypothyroidism that manifests with symptoms and signs similar to congenital hypothyroidism.**
6. Klein RZ, Mitchell ML: Hypothyroidism in infants children. Neonatal screening. In Braverman LE, Utiger RD (eds): Werner and Ingbar's The Thyroid, 8th ed. Philadelphia: Lippincott Williams & Wilkins, 2000, pp 973–977. **This chapter reviews neonatal screening for hypothyroidism.**
7. LaFranchi S, Hanna CE: Graves' disease in the neonatal period childhood. In Braverman LE, Utiger RD (eds): Werner and Ingbar's The Thyroid, 8th ed. Philadelphia: Lippincott Williams & Wilkins, 2000, pp 989–997. **This chapter provides a review of pediatric Graves disease.**
8. Newborn screening for congenital hypothyroidism: Recommended guidelines. AAP Section on Endocrinology; AAP Committee on Genetics; ATA Committee on Public Health. Pediatrics (in press). **The most recent update on congenital hypothyroidism—newborn screening, diagnosis, treatment, outcome—are provided as guidelines for clinicians.**
9. Refetoff S, Dumont JE, Vassart G: Thyroid disorders. In Scriver CR, Beaudet AL, Sly WS, Valle D (eds): The Metabolic Molecular Bases of Inherited Disease, Vol. 3, 8th ed. New York: McGraw-Hill, pp 4029–4075. **Provides the most comprehensive discussion and data on familial diseases of the thyroid that manifest during the first two decades of life.**
10. Rivkees SA, Sklar C, Freemark M: The management of Graves' disease in children, with special emphasis on radioiodine treatment. J Clin Endocrinol Metab 83:3767–3776, 1998. **Comprehensive review of the treatments for juvenile Graves disease and their expected outcomes and complications.**

11. Williams D: Science and society: Cancer after nuclear fallout: Lessons from the Chernobyl accident. Nat Rev Cancer 2:543–549, 2002. **The most authoritative clinical scientist in the field discusses what is known and what more needs to be learned about radiation-induced endocrine and nonendocrine diseases following radiation exposure from the Chernobyl accident.**

Disorders of the Parathyroids, Hypocalcemia, and Hypercalcemia

Harald W. Jüppner and Thomas O. Carpenter

KEY CONCEPTS

- The parathyroid hormone (PTH) is the major peptide hormone regulator of calcium/phosphate homeostasis.
- PTH-related peptide (PTHrP), which has limited structural homology with PTH, is the most frequent cause of the syndrome of humoral hypercalcemia of malignancy in adults.
- Treating hypocalcemia and hypercalcemia preemptively may prevent major morbidity.

Parathyroid Physiology and Its Relation to Clinical Disease

Through its actions on bone and kidney, parathyroid hormone (PTH) is the major regulator of calcium/phosphate homeostasis. PTH-related peptide (PTHrP), which has limited structural homology with PTH, is the most frequent cause of the syndrome of humoral hypercalcemia of malignancy in adults. Both peptides bind to and activate the PTH/PTHrP receptor, which is most abundantly expressed in kidney, bone, and growth plate chondrocytes. Unlike PTH, which is synthesized and secreted only by the parathyroid glands, PTHrP is expressed in a large variety of normal fetal and adult tissues. The homozygous ablation of the genes encoding PTHrP or the PTH/PTHrP receptor is perinatally lethal and leads to a dramatic acceleration of the endochondral bone formation process; other developmental defects include abnormal breast and nipple development.

Increased circulating concentrations of intact PTH, which is usually measured by two-site immunometric assays, may be associated with hypercalcemia (primary or tertiary hyperparathyroidism) or with frank or relative hypocalcemia (e.g., pseudohypoparathyroidism or uncompensated secondary hyperparathyroidism, caused by renal failure or vitamin D deficiency). Inappropriately elevated levels of PTH are also observed in familial benign hypocalciuric hypercalcemia, an inherited autosomal dominant disorder caused by inactivating mutations in the calcium-sensing receptor. Decreased PTH secretion, as in one of the different forms of hypoparathyroidism, is usually associated with hypocalcemia.

Expert Opinion on Management Issues

DISORDERS WITH HYPOCALCEMIA

In comparison to maternal blood calcium concentration, fetal calcium is considerably higher through an active fetus-directed calcium transport in the placenta that depends on the midregional portion of PTHrP. Because of this relative hypercalcemia and an increased set point of the parathyroid calcium sensor, PTH concentration is low in fetal blood. After delivery, the cessation of maternal calcium supplies results in a rapid decrease in neonatal blood calcium concentration. This leads to an increase in PTH secretion, which in turn mobilizes calcium from bone, enhances the reabsorption of calcium in the maturing kidney, and stimulates the renal 1α-hydroxylase to increase the synthesis of the biologically active 1,25-dihydroxyvitamin D_3 (1,25[OH]$_2D_3$).

Early Neonatal Hypocalcemia

Early neonatal hypocalcemia with total calcium concentrations below 7 mg/dL usually occurs during the first 3 days of life and is associated with increased concentrations of plasma PTH; the incidence is considerably higher in premature infants and in newborns of mothers with diabetes mellitus or hyperparathyroidism. Symptomatic hypocalcemia requires immediate treatment with intravenous calcium (Table 1), and prolonged intravenous or oral therapy may be necessary until the mechanisms for renal tubular calcium reabsorption and intestinal absorption are fully adapted.

Hypocalcemia Later in Infancy and Childhood

Hypocalcemia that develops after several weeks or months may be associated with a variety of causes, including phosphate loading, magnesium or vitamin D deficiency, parathyroid hypoplasia or aplasia with associated immunologic deficiencies (DiGeorge syndrome), polyglandular autoimmune disease, thyroid or parathyroid surgery, renal tubular disease (i.e., cystinosis), or renal failure. Splicing defects of the PTH pre-mRNA (messenger RNA) or mutations in the prepro sequence of PTH are described for familial forms of hypoparathyroidism. Hypocalcemia can also be caused by activating mutations in the calcium-sensing receptor. Despite hypocalcemia, patients affected by this autosomal dominant disorder show inappropriately increased urinary excretion of calcium and normal or suppressed PTH in the circulation. It is important to recognize this disorder because overly aggressive treatment of affected individuals with calcium salts and vitamin D analogues causes a further

TABLE 1 Hypocalcemia

Onset	Comments
Newborn Period	
"Early" neonatal hypocalcemia	Associated with perinatal asphyxia, preeclampsia, maternal diabetes, maternal hyperparathyroidism
"Late" neonatal hypocalcemia	Associated with parathyroid agenesis (as in DiGeorge syndrome, phosphate loading, maternal vitamin D deficiency)
Later Onset	
Abnormalities in Availability or Activity of PTH	
Hypoparathyroidism	Congenital, acquired (autoimmune or postsurgical), calcium-sensing receptor mutations resulting in increased affinity for calcium
Pseudohypoparathyroidism type I	Blunted renal cAMP and phosphate generation in response to PTH (see text)
Pseudohypoparathyroidism type II	Normal cAMP but blunted phosphate response to PTH
Abnormalities in Availability or Action of Vitamin D	
Vitamin D deficiency	Occurs in breast-fed infants in winter; more common in blacks
Defect in 1α-hydroxylation	Autosomal recessive defect in metabolism of vitamin D to active metabolite, 1,25(OH)$_2$D
Hereditary vitamin D resistance	Mutation in vitamin D receptor with resultant absence or low affinity of receptor for DNA or 1,25(OH)$_2$D
Hypomagnesemia	Impaired PTH secretion and action
Dietary calcium deficiency	Can be associated with diminished vitamin D stores
Selective Calcium Malabsorption	
Acute pancreatitis	
Blood transfusion	Low ionized calcium may occur with normal total calcium
Acute phosphate load	
Hungry bone syndrome	Seen in treatment phase of severe vitamin D deficiency or postoperatively in hyperparathyroidism
Acute illness	
Chronic renal failure	

cAMP, cyclic adenosine monophosphate; PTH, parathyroid hormone.

increase in urinary calcium excretion, often leading to renal stone formation and nephrolithiasis.

Hypocalcemia caused by pseudohypoparathyroidism (PHP) develops usually during childhood, but some patients may not become symptomatic until much later in life. PHP comprises several forms of only partially understood disorders, which are characterized by hypocalcemia and hyperphosphatemia despite elevated concentrations of circulating PTH. Because of renal resistance, exogenous biologically active PTH fails to increase the urinary excretion of cyclic adenosine monophosphate (cAMP) and phosphate (PHP-Ia and PHP-Ib); in a few cases, urinary excretion of phosphate seems to be affected alone (PHP-II). In addition to PTH-resistant hypocalcemia and hyperphosphatemia, patients affected by PHP-Ia often present with other endocrine deficiencies (e.g., hypothyroidism caused by thyroid-stimulating hormone [TSH] resistance and/or hypogonadism caused by luteinizing hormone/follicle-stimulating hormone [LH/FSH] resistance) and with characteristic clinical features, including short stature, round face, varying degrees of intellectual impairment, and multiple bone abnormalities (e.g., short metacarpals and metatarsals); these latter changes are collectively termed Albright hereditary osteodystrophy (AHO). Hormonal resistance occurs only if a mutation is inherited from a female. Thus inheritance of the genetic defect from a female carrier results in PHP-Ia, and inheritance from a male carrier results in pseudo-pseudohypoparathyroidism (pPHP), that is, AHO without hormonal resistance. Both disease forms, PHP-Ia and pPHP, are caused by heterozygous inactivating mutations in *GNAS*, a highly complex gene that gives rise to several different coding and noncoding mRNAs. One of these mRNAs encodes the stimulatory G protein (Gsα); additional alternatively spliced transcripts encode several other proteins, including XLαs and NESP55. Mutations in the Gsα-specific exons lead to an approximately 50% reduction in Gsα protein/activity.

Patients with PHP-Ib show renal PTH resistance leading to hypocalcemia and hyperphosphatemia, but they usually lack associated endocrine disorders and have a normal phenotypical appearance. Furthermore, individuals affected by PHP-Ib often show hyperparathyroid bone disease (a form of the disorder often referred to as pseudohypohyperparathyroidism), indicating that the actions of PTH on bone are not impaired. The genetic defect leading to PHP-Ib was mapped to a region on the telomeric end of chromosome 20q, which comprises *GNAS*, and several different microdeletions were identified that reside either upstream of or within *GNAS*. PTH resistance develops only if these microdeletions are inherited from a female (i.e., its mode of inheritance is identical to the hormonal resistance in kindreds with PHP-Ia/pPHP). Furthermore, there are methylation changes affecting one or several exons and their promoters, which affect Gsα expression in the renal proximal tubules. Duplication of paternal chromosome 20q with an associated loss of the maternal allele (i.e., paternal uniparental isodisomy) leads to a disorder similar to PHP-Ib.

DISORDERS WITH HYPERCALCEMIA

Synthesis and secretion of PTH by the parathyroid glands is tightly regulated by extracellular calcium. The calcium-dependent regulation of PTH production is mediated by a calcium-sensing receptor, a G protein–coupled receptor (its gene is located on chromosome 3q) that is most abundantly expressed in the parathyroid glands and in kidney. Other important regulators of PTH secretion include 1.25(OH)$_2$D$_3$, magnesium (Mg^{2+}), and phosphate. Primary hyperparathyroidism (HPT) as the cause for hypercalcemia is very rare in young children and adolescents, but it can be an acutely life-threatening disease, particularly in the neonate. Neonatal HPT is usually caused by homozygous inactivating mutations in the calcium-sensing receptor and requires immediate parathyroidectomy (possibly with reimplantation of small portions of parathyroid tissue into the forearm). Heterozygous mutations in this receptor are the cause of benign familial hypocalciuric hypercalcemia (FHH), a disorder that usually requires no surgical intervention. Two other less frequent forms of FHH are mapped to the long and the short arm of chromosome 19, respectively; the defective genes have not yet been identified.

Other causes of hypercalcemia include the treatment with or accidental ingestion of vitamin D preparations (the accidental fortification of milk with exceedingly high concentrations of vitamin D was reported), tumor-associated hypercalcemia secondary to humoral or osteolytic mechanisms, multiple endocrine neoplasia (MEN) I and II, McCune-Albright syndrome, hereditary hyperparathyroidism/jaw tumor syndrome, Williams-Beuren syndrome, Jansen metaphyseal chondrodysplasia, sarcoidosis, immobilization, subcutaneous fat necrosis, or autonomous hyperparathyroidism caused by prolonged renal failure.

TREATMENT OF HYPOCALCEMIA AND TETANY

Serum calcium is normally maintained within a very narrow range (8.5–10.5 mg/dL at our institution) by an exquisitely sensitive homeostatic system. The clinically relevant component of the total serum calcium is the ionized, or free, fraction, which comprises 45% to 50% of the total. Approximately 45% to 50% of the total calcium is protein bound (predominantly to albumin), and a small portion is complexed to anions such as phosphate, citrate, or bicarbonate. *True hypocalcemia* refers to a reduction in the concentration of ionized calcium. Low serum calcium may occur with normal ionized fractions in the special situations of hypoproteinemia or acidosis. Various formulas were devised to "correct" the serum calcium: a decrement in serum albumin of 1 g/dL below the lower limit of normal allows the total calcium concentration to be adjusted upward by 1 mg/dL; ionized calcium concentrations decrease by 0.2 mg/dL for an incremental rise in pH by 0.1 U. Such estimates are not precise and should be confirmed by measurement of ionized calcium levels when possible. Ionized calcium determinations, however, can be difficult to perform accurately, particularly in infants, because the use of a tourniquet and prolonged crying associated with restraint can influence the determination. Many methods require anaerobic collection into a 2 mL or greater tube and performance immediately following sample collection. Most normal ranges for ionized calcium run approximately 50% of the range for total calcium.

Tetany may be defined as the heightened degree of neuromuscular excitability that occurs during symptomatic hypocalcemia. The classic features of this phenomenon include perioral tingling and cyanosis, which may extend to the entire face or occur at the fingertips with progression upward in the arm. Tetany may manifest as a so-called writer's cramp, or rigid spasm of the muscles of the upper and lower extremities (carpopedal spasm). Fixation of the wrist in flexion with extension of the thumb is typical of carpal spasm. The generalized spastic phenomenon may progress to generalized tonic-clonic activity of the extremity or even generalized convulsions. In infants, signs are less specific, so only jitteriness and irritability are evident. A diagnosis of croup was entertained when laryngospasm was the presenting manifestation of hypocalcemia. Generalized seizures may also develop from hypocalcemia in this age group. *Latent tetany* is precipitated by maneuvers of pressure or ischemia. Percussion of the facial nerve, just anterior to the ear, with a finger or reflex hammer may result in twitching of the facial muscles around the eye and mouth. This response is referred to as the Chvostek sign, and it is generally interpreted to represent hypocalcemia, although some 20% of normocalcemic individuals may demonstrate this finding. Induction of ischemia for 2 to 3 minutes by inflation of a blood pressure cuff over the brachial artery at pressures just above systolic blood pressure readings can precipitate carpal spasm; this response is referred to as the Trousseau sign.

Although tetany is most often associated with hypocalcemic symptomatology, it may occur with hypomagnesemia or hyperkalemia. Signs of hypocalcemia may be accentuated when these other disturbances are also present. Unlike calcium, magnesium is predominantly an intracellular ion, and serum levels may not reflect intracellular magnesium status. If questions regarding symptomatic hypomagnesemia are present, documentation can be performed by a magnesium retention test, done as follows:

- Obtain initial spot urinary magnesium-to-creatinine ratio.
- Infuse 2.4 mg elemental magnesium in 50 mL in dextrose 5% in water (D5W) over 4 hours.
- Collect 24-hour urine, beginning with magnesium infusion, for determination of magnesium and creatinine (Cr).
- Calculate percentage retention as follows: % Mg retention = 1 − [24-hour urine Mg − (spot Mg/Cr × 24-hour urine Cr)/total elemental magnesium infused] × 100. Retention of greater than 25% is considered definite deficiency; retention greater than 50% is considered probable deficiency.

ACUTE MANAGEMENT OF HYPOCALCEMIA

Newborns

Early neonatal hypocalcemia should be treated in preterm infants when the total serum calcium is less than 5 to 6 mg/dL or if specific signs of hypocalcemia are present. Term infants are usually treated at slightly higher total serum calcium levels (less than 6 to 7 mg/dL). Treatment of acute symptomatic hypocalcemia consists of a slow intravenous infusion (less than 1 mL/min) of calcium gluconate in a 10% solution (calcium gluconate is 9% elemental calcium). Observation for extravascular infiltration should be performed and the infusion stopped if any infiltration is suspected, so to avoid toxicity to surrounding tissues. Likewise, calcium should never be administered intramuscularly.

Cardiac monitoring and careful observation during acute infusions should be performed. An infusion of 1 to 3 mL usually arrests convulsions; the maximum single dose is 2 mg of elemental calcium/kg body weight. This dose may be repeated up to four times in a 24-hour period; however, with persistent severe hypocalcemia it is more effective to infuse calcium gluconate until oral calcium can maintain adequate serum levels. We suggest infusion of 20 to 50 mg of elemental calcium/kg over 24 hours. A third of the total amount may be infused over 8 hours, and the necessity to continue therapy can be reevaluated at that time. If chronic infusions are necessary, assessment should be repeated when oral intake is implemented. Calcium chloride is less preferential for intravenous use because it is more irritating than calcium gluconate. Bicarbonate and phosphate should not be infused with calcium because calcium salts of these anions may precipitate in tubing or the patient's intravascular space.

Beyond the Newborn Period

Acute therapy consists of intravenous infusion of 10% calcium gluconate, at a dose of 1 mL/kg. This dose should be infused at a rate of 1 mL/min up to a maximum of 20 mL of calcium gluconate per bolus infusion. For a longer term infusion, 4 to 6 mL of 10% calcium gluconate per kilogram per 24 hours can be used, providing 36 to 54 mg of elemental calcium per kilogram. In the setting of acute exacerbations of calcium malabsorption, which occurs in patients with hypoparathyroidism and associated gastrointestinal disorders, nocturnal nasogastric supplementation of calcium carbonate or calcium gluconate is sometimes used, such that up to 20 mg of elemental calcium per kilogram of body weight per 8 hours is provided, until the acute exacerbation of intestinal malabsorption has resolved.

Magnesium

Correction of low serum calcium levels may be refractory to the therapeutic approaches just described in the setting of hypomagnesemia. Therefore magnesium therapy may be required to restore PTH secretion and peripheral activity. Before any administration of magnesium, renal function and urinary output should be assessed. Magnesium levels should be monitored to avoid toxicity. Examination of deep tendon reflexes can be performed acutely, and therapy can be halted if reflexes significantly decrease in briskness. Intravenous calcium gluconate is an antidote for magnesium intoxication and should be available at the bedside. As with calcium therapy, cardiac monitoring should be performed and therapy stopped if electrocardiographic changes become evident. In infancy, 5 to 10 mg of elemental magnesium per kg is given slowly intravenously or intramuscularly. Magnesium sulfate heptahydrate ($MgSO_4 \cdot 7H_2O$) is available as a 50% solution, containing 48 mg of elemental magnesium per milliliter. The dose may be repeated every 12 to 24 hours. In older individuals, up to 2.4 mg of elemental magnesium per kilogram body weight can be given over a 10-minute period (to a maximum of 180 mg). A continuous infusion of 576 mg of elemental magnesium over 24 hours may also be used. Reassessment of calcium and magnesium status should be performed at regular intervals to determine the necessity of continuing the dose. Duration of intravenous requirements varies, and transition to oral magnesium supplementation may be necessary.

GOALS OF CHRONIC THERAPY OF HYPOCALCEMIA: IMPLICATIONS OF DIAGNOSIS

Hypocalcemia may be a manifestation of numerous underlying disorders (see Table 1). Specific goals of chronic therapy depend on the specific clinical setting in which the disturbance occurs, and management decisions often require individual attention to the underlying physiology of each patient's underlying disorder.

The transition from acute management of hypocalcemia to chronic maintenance in the newborn period depends highly on the individual clinical situation. It is often possible to begin oral supplementation within a few days of intravenous therapy. As a general rule, we prefer to use calcium salts alone (usually calcium glubionate) and monitor the course of hypocalcemia. Addition of vitamin D compounds prior to the knowledge of the patient's vitamin D status may confuse the diagnosis and may be inappropriate for an unestablished underlying problem (e.g., $1,25[OH]_2D_3$ may act to suppress PTH synthesis in a parathyroid gland recovering from perinatal insults or maternal hyperparathyroidism). A specific cause of transient hypocalcemia is usually not identified, and the course of such cases results in gradual diminution of the calcium dose until no supplementation is required. However, it is also possible that partial hypoparathyroidism may still be present, particularly in the setting of DiGeorge-like features. Therefore, monitoring of serum calcium should be performed after cessation of calcium therapy, particularly if an intermittent gastrointestinal illness occurs. We have observed the capacity of several children with DiGeorge syndrome and partial hypoparathyroidism to maintain normal serum calcium when healthy, but their parathyroid reserve is sufficiently limited so that hypocalcemia ensues when held nothing by mouth (NPO) for greater than 12 hours or during an episode of gastroenteritis. Thus it is important to evaluate such individuals periodically and specifically to document appropriate maintenance of hypocalcemia and PTH reserve during conditions of limited calcium availability. It has been suggested that all patients with a documented abnormality of chromosome 22 undergo PTH provocative testing with citrate or ethylenediaminetetraacetic acid (EDTA) to identify latent hypoparathyroidism.

If the child is identified to have a specific cause of hypocalcemia, such as vitamin D deficiency or hypomagnesemia, these abnormalities should be appropriately treated, and if persistent, investigation of the etiology of the underlying disorder should be undertaken.

TABLE 2 Oral Calcium Preparations

Preparation	Calcium Content
Calcium glubionate	115 mg/5 mL
Calcium gluconate	
500-mg tablet	45 mg/tablet
Calcium carbonate	
500-mg tablet	200 mg/tablet
650-mg tablet	260 mg/tablet
Alka-Mints	340 mg/tablet
Calci-Chew	500 mg/tablet
Calci-Mix	500 mg/capsule
Caltrate	600 mg/tablet
Chooz	200 mg/tablet
Equilet	200 mg/tablet
Nephro-Calci	600 mg/tablet
Os-Cal 500, 1250 mg tablet	500 mg/tablet
Rolaids-Calcium Rich	220 mg/tablet
Titralac	168 mg/tablet
Tums	200 mg/tablet
Tums-EX	300 mg/tablet
Suspension	500 mg/5 mL
Calcium lactate	
325-mg tablet	42 mg/tablet
650-mg tablet	84 mg/tablet

TABLE 3 Vitamin D and Related Agents

Name	Formulation	Typical Dose*
Vitamin D (Calciferol)		
Drisdol	Solution: 8000 IU/mL	2000 IU/day
	Tablet: 25,000 IU	1 tablet/day
	50,000 IU	1 tablet/day
Dihydrotachysterol (DHT)		
	Solution: 0.2 mg/5 mL	0.5 mg/day
	Tablets: 0.125 mg	0.5 mg/day
	0.2 mg	0.5 mg/day
	0.4 mg	0.4 mg/day
1,25 Dihydroxyvitamin D (Calcitriol)[†]		
Rocaltrol	0.25-μg capsule	0.5 μg/day
	0.5-μg capsule	0.5 μg/day
	Solution: 1 μg/mL	0.5 μg/day

*1 μg vitamin D = 40 IU

[†]Calcijex solution: Ampules for IV use containing solutions with 1 or 2 μg/mL of drug.

Table 2 lists various oral calcium preparations and their costs. Table 3 outlines therapeutic preparations of vitamin D and its metabolites.

Hypoparathyroidism

Frequently, because of the absence of the calcium-retaining effect of PTH in hypoparathyroidism, there is a greater degree of calciuria at normal serum calcium values than that seen in normal individuals. Therefore, the goals of chronic therapy in this disorder are not necessarily to normalize serum calcium. We prefer to maintain fasting serum calcium in an asymptomatic range, which may vary with individuals, but is generally between 7.8 to 8.5 mg/dL. In addition, patients generally have elevated serum phosphate (P) levels, and a secondary goal of management is to maintain a serum phosphocalcic product (total serum Ca × serum P, both in mg/dL) less than 60 mg^{2}/dL^{2}. We are often forced to use two medications to achieve this balance: calcium and $1,25(OH)_2D_3$ (Rocaltrol). When confronted with the therapeutic decision to increase circulating calcium levels, when both compounds are already being administered, we find that an increment in the $1,25(OH)_2D_3$ dose may also increase the serum P. If a markedly elevated serum P is of concern, supplementation with calcium salts is preferred; if given close to meals, a phosphate-binding effect may also occur. Hypoparathyroidism may be caused by a mutation in the calcium-sensing receptor located on parathyroid cell membranes and in the renal tubule. Although clinical experience with such individuals is scarce, it is thought that these patients may be distinguished from patients with parathyroid agenesis by a more exaggerated degree of calciuria at low to normal serum calcium levels. It is important to identify such individuals and adjust therapy accordingly so as not to risk iatrogenic renal damage. Although vitamin D and dihydrotachysterol (DHT) are used to treat hypoparathyroidism, $1,25(OH)_2D_3$ is the preferred metabolite. It is more consistently effective at nontoxic doses, has a shorter half-life, and allows more rapid correction of hyper calcemic complications after withdrawal, should they develop. The active fragment of PTH is currently being studied as yet another form of treatment for this disorder.

Pseudohypoparathyroidism

As outlined earlier, there are two major forms of type I pseudohypoparathyroidism (PHP). In these forms of the disease, urinary cAMP and phosphate excretion after infusion of exogenous PTH is blunted; in type II, cAMP response is normal, but phosphate excretion remains abnormal. In general, the principles of therapy described earlier for hypoparathyroidism apply for pseudohypoparathyroidism. However, there is a lesser tendency to develop hypercalciuria in PHP; in fact, patients who may be relatively hypocalciuric because of elevated PTH levels appear to have normalized distal tubular calcium reabsorption. Because of the variable degree of PTH resistance at the skeleton, hyperparathyroid bone disease may be present in PHP. We approach management with a goal of achieving normocalcemia without causing hypercalciuria and effectively lowering circulating PTH levels. Because the renal production of $1,25(OH)_2D_3$ is usually impaired, this vitamin D metabolite is the drug of choice for treating PHP. Calcium carbonate should be added as well because it helps lower blood phosphate concentration in addition to supplying calcium. Vitamin D in high dosages (up to 100,000 U daily) is also used.

Vitamin D Deficiency

In most situations, modest doses (1000 to 2000 U daily) of vitamin D adequately treat vitamin D deficiency states. This form of therapy runs little risk of complications, and if there is any question about the diagnosis, the response to this therapy may help in re-establishing the correct one. Alternatively, in situations where follow-up is unlikely, large doses of vitamin D can be given (higher dose or so-called Stoss therapy). It is recommended that 600,000 units of vitamin D be given in two to three oral doses in 1 day or as an intramuscular injection. It is important to ensure that adequate calcium intake complements the vitamin D administration because rapid mineralization of the skeleton may follow initial treatment, potentially causing a precipitous drop in serum calcium (hungry bone syndrome). If dietary intake is less than 40 mg of elemental calcium per kilogram per day, calcium supplementation should be employed to achieve that minimum daily intake. We have observed that spontaneous tetany can occur following Stoss therapy and asymptomatic hypocalcemia following standard daily vitamin D treatment. We do not recommend $1,25(OH)_2D_3$ as a treatment of this condition.

1α-Hydroxylase Deficiency and Vitamin D Resistance

$1,25(OH)_2D_3$ in physiologic doses (0.25 to 1.0 μg/day) is the treatment of choice for 1α-hydroxylase deficiency, also referred to as vitamin D–dependent rickets, type I. Higher dosages (up to 3 μg/day) may be required initially. *Hereditary vitamin D resistance* may require very high dosages of $1,25(OH)_2D_3$. Variable degrees of resistance can exist, so patients may show variable responsiveness. In complete resistance, $1,25(OH)_2D_3$ is not effective, and long-term intravenous calcium infusions are indicated. Management of this rare disorder should be performed by specialists in pediatric bone disease.

Hypomagnesemia

Chronic magnesium supplementation may be required in individuals with ongoing renal or intestinal losses. Oral magnesium is available as salts of citrate, lactate, oxide, sulfate, chloride, hydroxide, and glycerophosphate. Provision of 3 to 6 mg of elemental magnesium per day divided into three or four daily dosages is recommended. No more than 500 mg should be administered routinely per 24-hour period. If the cathartic effects of magnesium are encountered, dosing can be more frequent, with less of the salt administered at each dose. If any decrement in glomerular filtration rate is present, half the calculated dose should be administered. Monitoring of serum magnesium is essential, especially in the setting of renal disease. Table 4 lists various magnesium salts for therapeutic use.

Calcium Malnutrition

Calcium deficiency caused by diet is rare in the United States but may occur as part of the avoidance learned in individuals with lactose intolerance. It is suggested that such individuals be supplemented with calcium so their total daily calcium intake is 30 to 50 mg/kg up to a maximum of 1500 mg/day. If calcium malabsorption is present, larger doses may be given. If maintenance of calcium via the oral route is not possible, other

TABLE 4 Oral Magnesium Salts

Preparation	Magnesium Content
Magnesium Chloride	
Slow-Mag 535 mg	64 mg
Magnesium Citrate	
Magnesium citrate solution	9.8 mg/mL
Magnesium Gluconate	
Magtrate 500 mg	29 mg
Generic magnesium gluconate (500 mg)	29 mg
Magnesium Oxide	
Uro-Mag 140 mg	84.5 mg
Mag-Ox 400 mg	240 mg
Generic magnesium oxide (500 mg)	300 mg
Other	
Magnesium sulfate solution (Unformulated)	6.25 mg/mL
	12.5 mg/mL
Chelated magnesium (500 mg) (Chelated to soy-derived amino acids)	100 mg

measures need to be entertained, depending on the clinical situation at hand. Use of overnight nasogastric infusions can be performed; home parenteral nutrition is used in certain settings. The experience with severe forms of hereditary vitamin D resistance indicates that the gastrointestinal tract can be entirely bypassed to deliver adequate calcium, although the measures required are intensive.

MANAGEMENT OF HYPERCALCEMIA

Hypercalcemia is defined as a persistent elevation in total serum calcium above 11 mg/dL, which can be associated with little or no symptomatology, or more severe symptoms (more than 13 mg/dL), generally accompanied by failure to thrive, abdominal pain (vomiting), somnolence, stupor, constipation, muscle weakness, polydipsia, and polyuria. The complications of long-standing hypercalcemia include nephrocalcinosis, renal stones, and renal failure.

Treatment of persistent mild hypercalcemia consists of dietary restriction of calcium (to less than 400 mg/day, which is less than half the recommended daily allowance), elimination of vitamin D supplementation, and avoidance of excessive exposure to sunlight. Special formula low in calcium and vitamin D is available. Corticosteroids (prednisone, 1 to 2 mg/kg/day) may be effective in the treatment of hypercalcemia resulting from increased intestinal calcium absorption, but long-term steroid treatment is not indicated because of possible adverse effects. In most situations, idiopathic hypercalcemia is a transient phenomenon; therefore, long-term therapy of any modality is generally not necessary, and attempts to discontinue therapy should be made regularly. Individuals with Williams syndrome, even those who are normocalcemic, should avoid markedly excessive calcium intake because hypercalcemia has recurred under such circumstances.

Extremely severe hypercalcemia (more than 15.0 mg/dL) should be treated with intravenous fluids and

14

BOX 1   Drug Therapy for Hypercalcemia

Acute Treatment of Life-Threatening Hypercalcemia

- Forced diuresis with normal saline and appropriately added potassium at 1.5 times maintenance; after achieving adequate hydration, furosemide may be given at 1 mg/kg BW IV q6h if necessary.
- Calcitonin, 2–8 U/kg BW IV, SC, or IM; repeat q6–12h.
- Bisphosphonates:
  - Pamidronate (APD, Aredia), 35–50 mg/m^2 or 0.5–2.0 mg/kg BW as a single dose (a single dose of 60–90 mg IV normalizes serum calcium levels in 80%–100% of adult patients).
  - Plicamycin (Mithracin), 15–25 µg/kg BW/day IV over 4–8 hours (beware of toxicity).
  - Etidronate (EHDP, Didronel), 5–10 mg/kg BW/day IV over 3 consecutive days.
- Peritoneal dialysis or hemodialysis with low-calcium dialysate.

Supportive Therapy

- Glucocorticoids to decrease intestinal calcium absorption (prednisone, 1–2 mg/kg BW/day).
- Cellulose sodium phosphate to reduce intestinal calcium absorption (Calcibind given PO in 3–4 doses).
- Reduction of dietary calcium and vitamin D$_3$.

BW, body weight; IM, intramuscular; IV, intravenous; PO, by mouth; q*x*h, every *x* hours; SC, subcutaneous.

---

furosemide (up to 1 mg/kg every 6 hours), as needed. Hypercalcemia secondary to excess bone resorption can be treated with calcitonin (salmon calcitonin, 4 IU/kg every 12 hours intramuscularly or subcutaneously) or with bisphosphonate preparations. There is increasing experience with intravenous pamidronate in children, and it is generally well tolerated. The authors have found this agent useful in the therapy of humoral hypercalcemia of malignancy, Williams syndrome, subcutaneous fat necrosis, and as a temporal measure in managing hyperparathyroidism, if surgery is not imminently available. In general, hypercalcemia related to abnormally increased bone resorption should respond well to this drug. Box 1 lists therapies for hypercalcemia.

Common Pitfalls

- Overtreatment of some hypocalcemic conditions with calcium and vitamin D analogues leading to nephrocalcinosis and nephrolithiasis
- Renal failure as a cause of hypocalcemia and hyperphosphatemia
- Too aggressive treatment with bisphosphonates for the treatment of hypercalcemic conditions resulting in significant hypocalcemia

Communication and Counseling

Numerous disorders affecting the regulation of mineral ion homeostasis are now being explored at the molecular level. Appropriate testing should therefore be considered to establish a diagnosis if possible.

SUGGESTED READINGS

1. Bastepe M, Jüppner H: The GNAS locus and pseudohypoparathyroidism. Horm Res 63:65–74, 2005. **Summary of the different forms of pseudohypoparathyroidism and their molecular causes.**
2. Brown EM: Physiology of calcium homeostasis. In Bilezikian JP, Levine MA, Marcus R (eds): The Parathyroids. Basic and Clinical Concepts. New York: Raven Press, 2001, pp 167–181. **Review of the regulation of calcium homeostasis with particular emphasis on the calcium-sensing receptor.**
3. Jüppner H, Gardella TJ, Brown EM, et al: Parathyroid hormone and parathyroid hormone–related peptide in the regulation of calcium homeostasis and bone development. In DeGroot LJ, Jameson JL (eds): Endocrinology, 5th ed. Philadelphia: Elsevier Inc, 2006, pp 1377–1417. **Review of the biology of PTH.**
4. Kovacs CS, Kronenberg HM: Maternal-fetal calcium and bone metabolism during pregnancy, puerperium, and lactation. Endocr Rev 18:832–872, 1997. **Review of the regulation of fetal and maternal calcium regulation.**
5. Marx SJ: 1,25-Dihydroxyvitamin D$_3$ receptors resistance: Implications in rickets, osteomalacia, and other conditions. In Glorieux FH (ed): Rickets. New York: Raven Press, 1991, pp 167–184. **Role of the vitamin D receptor in the development of certain forms of rickets.**
6. Philbrick WM: Parathyroid hormone-related protein: Gene structure, biosynthesis, metabolism, regulation. In Bilezikian JP, Levine MA, Marcus R (eds): The Parathyroids. Basic and Clinical Concepts. New York: Raven Press, 2001, pp 31–51. **Review of the biology of PTHrP.**
7. Rude RK: Magnesium homeostasis. In Bilezikian JP, Raisz LG, Rodan GA (eds): Principles of Bone Biology. New York: Academic Press, 1996, pp 277–293. **Review of the regulation of magnesium homeostasis and its biologic roles.**
8. Thakker RV, Jüppner H: Genetics disorders of calcium homeostasis caused by abnormal regulation of parathyroid hormone secretion or responsiveness. In DeGroot LJ, Jameson JL (eds): Endocrinology, 5th ed. Philadelphia: Elsevier Inc, 2006, pp 1511–1531. **Review of those disorders affecting calcium homeostasis that are defined at the molecular level.**

Disorders of the Adrenal Gland

Mary Min-Chin Lee and Lynne L. Levitsky

KEY CONCEPTS

- Adrenal disease can be caused by either inadequate or excess production of one or more types of the hormones produced by the adrenal gland.
- The symptoms of chronic adrenal insufficiency are nonspecific, but the accompanying electrolyte abnormalities of hyponatremia alone, or with hyperkalemia, point to adrenal dysfunction. The presence of hyperkalemia is suggestive of primary rather than secondary adrenal insufficiency.
- An acute adrenal crisis is a life-threatening condition that requires immediate resuscitation with dextrose-containing fluids and administration of stress doses of hydrocortisone.
- All patients on chronic steroids or within 6 to 12 months of discontinuation of daily steroids are at risk for adrenal suppression and acute adrenal insufficiency. Such families require education and counseling about when and how to administer stress steroids for acute illnesses and other physiologic stresses.

- The evaluation of Cushing disease in childhood is challenging because of the difficulty in diagnosis and the risks associated with its diagnostic evaluation and management. In children, 50% of adrenocorticotropic hormone (ACTH)-producing pituitary tumors are malignant; thus long-term follow-up is essential.

Adrenal disease is characterized by either insufficient or excess production of its biosynthetic end products and can be classified as primary disease of the adrenal cortex and/or medulla or a central process associated with hypothalamic or pituitary dysfunction. The adrenal cortex produces three classes of steroids: glucocorticoids (cortisol), mineralocorticoids (aldosterone), and sex steroids (testosterone and estradiol). Cortisol secretion is tightly regulated via negative feedback through hypothalamic corticotropin-releasing hormone (CRH) and pituitary adrenocorticotropic hormone (ACTH). Aldosterone production is modulated largely by the renin-angiotensin system and therefore responsive to vascular volume, renal blood flow, and serum sodium. The regulation of adrenal sex steroid production is not established. The adrenal medulla and its associated tissues produce catecholamines and are under neuroendocrine control.

In the neonate, the most frequent etiology of adrenocortical insufficiency is congenital adrenal hyperplasia (CAH) caused by inherited enzymatic defects in cortisol biosynthesis. Rarer causes during infancy include congenital adrenal hypoplasia (*DAX1* gene mutations), familial glucocorticoid deficiency (ACTH receptor defects), adrenoleukodystrophy (peroxisomal very-long-chain fatty acid disease), isolated ACTH or multiple pituitary hormone deficiencies, and traumatic or hemorrhagic injury to the adrenal glands. Iatrogenic adrenal insufficiency has become more common in premature infants who require prolonged glucocorticoid therapy for respiratory disease. Beyond infancy, autoimmune adrenalitis becomes the predominant cause of acquired adrenal insufficiency, although congenital, iatrogenic, and infectious or infiltrative causes of adrenal dysfunction must also be considered. Secondary or tertiary adrenal insufficiency can occur with any process that disrupts hypothalamic or pituitary function, including structural central nervous system (CNS) abnormalities (i.e., septo-optic dysplasia); craniopharyngiomas, gliomas, and other brain tumors; infiltrative disease (histiocytosis and sarcoidosis); infections; autoimmune hypophysitis; pituitary apoplexy; and CNS irradiation or trauma.

Congenital deficiency disorders of the adrenal medulla are not yet described. Adrenalectomized individuals do not seem to suffer unduly from loss of medullary function because of compensation from non-adrenal autonomic nervous system release of norepinephrine. Children with CAH, however, have dysplastic adrenal medullae with decreased secretion of catecholamines, suggesting a role of glucocorticoids in maintenance of the adrenal medulla.

Glucocorticoid excess leading to increased weight gain, growth attenuation, hypertension, myopathy, centripetal distribution of body fat, skin striae, and other components of the cushingoid habitus is most commonly attributable to exogenous glucocorticoid therapy. Hyperfunction of the adrenal gland caused by adrenal tumors, McCune-Albright syndrome, ACTH-secreting pituitary tumors (Cushing disease), and ectopic ACTH- or CRH-producing tumors is less common in children and adolescents. Isolated mineralocorticoid excess may result from an aldosterone-producing adrenal tumor, from dexamethasone-suppressible aldosterone secretion, or from the condition of apparent mineralocorticoid excess. Adrenal etiologies of excess sex steroid production causing virilization or, more rarely, feminization include ACTH-driven stimulation of adrenal activity because of cortisol deficiency in CAH and functioning adrenal tumors. The virilization or feminization caused by adrenal tumors typically occurs at a rapid pace, and the tumors are generally large enough to be palpable at the time of diagnosis; thus abdominal distention or an abdominal mass may be found on examination.

Overproduction of catecholamines by adrenal medullary tumors (pheochromocytomas, neuroblastomas) causes an array of symptoms, of which hypertension is usually the most significant. In children, pheochromocytomas are often associated with familial disorders, such as neurofibromatosis, von Hippel-Lindau syndrome, multiple endocrine neoplasia syndrome, or isolated familial pheochromocytoma. Approximately 35% of pheochromocytomas are extra-adrenal.

14

INADEQUATE HORMONE PRODUCTION

Adrenal Insufficiency

Expert Opinion on Management Issues

The symptoms of cortisol and aldosterone deficiency are initially subtle and nonspecific. Feeding intolerance with emesis, irritability, and poor weight gain are early features in newborns. In female infants with virilizing CAH, the diagnosis is usually recognized before signs of adrenal insufficiency are evident. The effects of CAH on genital development are discussed in the chapter "Gonadal Disorders." Older children with chronic glucocorticoid deficiency have generalized malaise, lethargy, easy fatigability, poor weight gain, and vague gastrointestinal complaints. Hyperpigmentation is present in primary adrenal insufficiency, whereas hypoglycemia is more often associated with a central defect. Isolated mineralocorticoid deficiency leads to decreased intravascular volume and dehydration that may initially manifest as postural hypotension.

If the deficiency is untreated, an acute adrenal crisis can develop with persistent vomiting, dehydration, hypotension, tachycardia, and cardiovascular shock. In patients on maintenance corticosteroid therapy, an intercurrent illness or other form of physiologic stress may precipitate an acute adrenal crisis. Laboratory testing may reveal azotemia, hyperchloremic acidosis, hyponatremia, hyperkalemia, hypoglycemia, and elevated plasma renin activity (PRA). If the child has secondary or tertiary adrenal insufficiency, hyperkalemia is unusual, but hyponatremia may still occur because of increased vasopressin secretion in response to intravascular volume contraction.

An acute adrenal crisis is a life-threatening emergency that requires immediate restoration of intravascular volume and correction of electrolyte abnormalities. Rapid volume expansion with 10 to 20 mL/kg of isotonic saline is essential and should be followed by rehydration with 5% to 10% dextrose and half-normal saline at 3000 mL/m^2/day (twice maintenance). Potassium is withheld until serum potassium normalizes and urine output is documented. In new patients without established adrenal disease, blood should be drawn for diagnostic studies before initiating glucocorticoid therapy, although therapy should not be delayed. A stress dose of hydrocortisone sodium succinate (Solu-Cortef) is given as an initial intravenous bolus and then provided as a continuous infusion for at least 24 hours or until the patient is stable (Table 1). The hyperkalemia may warrant cardiac monitoring but will correct with hydrocortisone, which at high doses has mineralocorticoid activity. If the patient is symptomatic, a slow intravenous infusion of 10% calcium gluconate (0.5 mL/kg over a 10-minute period) or sodium bicarbonate (3 mEq/kg) lowers the serum potassium concentration. Fludrocortisone acetate (Florinef) is added when stress doses of steroids are no longer required.

Physiologic replacement of glucocorticoids and mineralocorticoids is necessary as maintenance therapy in adrenal insufficiency. In children, hydrocortisone is used most often at a dose of 10 to 15 mg/m^2/day. Hydrocortisone has a short half-life, so it is typically given as a twice- or thrice-daily regimen, often with a larger dose in the morning to mimic the diurnal secretory pattern (Table 1). The aims of therapy are to prevent chronic symptoms of malaise and decreased energy, to downregulate ACTH sufficiently to minimize hyperpigmentation, and to permit good weight gain and normal growth. Infants requiring small doses may need to be treated with prednisone liquid (see Table 1) or have special preparations formulated by a compounding pharmacy. Mineralocorticoid deficiency is treated with fludrocortisone at doses of 0.05 to 0.2 mg/day, which are unrelated to weight or size. Fludrocortisone doses are adjusted by monitoring blood pressure, serum electrolytes, and PRA. NaCl (salt) supplementation is not usually needed, except in occasional infants, who may benefit from the addition of 500 mg of salt daily to compensate for their low salt intake. Free access to salt with food, particularly in hot weather, allows the child to self-regulate salt needs. In children with CAH, the adrenal gland is initially hyperplastic; thus higher doses are needed transiently to achieve adequate adrenal suppression. Children with CAH also typically require NaCl supplementation (5 mL 10% NaCl or $\frac{1}{4}$ to $\frac{1}{2}$ tsp of table salt [2.3 g NaCl/tsp]) twice a day, especially during infancy and in hot weather, even in the absence of clinical manifestations of salt loss. In these patients, subclinical mineralocorticoid deficiency can stimulate the secretion of ACTH and make it more difficult to achieve control with glucocorticoids.

Children with any form of adrenal insufficiency and those who receive chronic glucocorticoid therapy are unable to mount an adrenal response to stress. After discontinuation of steroids, it may take as long as 6 to 12 months to fully recover from chronic adrenal suppression and regain a normal hypothalamic-pituitary-adrenal (HPA) axis. Therefore, stress doses of glucocorticoids should be administered for any

TABLE 1 Medications for Adrenal Insufficiency

Drug	Dose	Formulation	Pharmacokinetics/Indications
Glucocorticoid Replacement			
Hydrocortisone (Cortisol)	10–15 mg/m^2/day for adrenal insufficiency. 10–20 mg/m^2/day for CAH. q8–12h. Usual dose may be doubled or tripled for stress of fever or for minor surgery.	5-, 10-, 20-mg tablets	Half-life is 80 min when levels are within the binding capacity of corticosteroid binding globulin.
Prednisone	Four times the potency of cortisol. Dose twice daily.	2.5-, 5-, 10-, 20-, and 50-mg tablets Liquid preparation of 1 mg/mL	Must be metabolized to prednisolone in the liver.
Hydrocortisone sodium succinate	1.5–2 mg/kg IV or IM; or, for ease of use, 25 mg for infants, 50 mg for young children, 100 mg in older children.	100-mg vial; 100-, 250-, 500-, 1000-mg vials with ready-to-mix diluent	Stress dose to be administered q6h or as continuous infusion. Replacement dose is $\frac{2}{3}$ of oral dose.
Mineralocorticoid Replacement:			
Fludrocortisone (Florinef)	0.05–0.2 mg/day daily or twice daily.	0.1-mg scored tablet	Effective daily. May be better as twice daily dose.

CAH, congenital adrenal hyperplasia; IM, intramuscularly; IV, intravenously; qxh, every x hours.

significant physiologic stress in such patients. Hydrocortisone can be given orally at 30 to 50 mg/m^2/day for minor events such as acute febrile illnesses or minor surgical procedures. For major surgery, trauma, or other catastrophic events, hydrocortisone, 50 to 100 mg/m^2/day, is administered parenterally divided every 6 hours or as a continuous infusion (see Table 1). The dose can be tapered quickly to physiologic replacement doses and discontinued as the acute stress resolves and the clinical condition stabilizes.

For diagnostic evaluation, a low early morning serum cortisol and elevated ACTH are consistent with primary adrenal insufficiency, whereas low levels of both cortisol and ACTH are suggestive of central disease or suppression by exogenous steroids. With the latter conditions, potassium abnormalities are rare because aldosterone secretion is intact. With acquired adrenal insufficiency, adrenal antibodies should be assayed but are often negative at the time of clinical evaluation, even with autoimmune disease. Assessment of antibodies to other endocrine organs may help establish the diagnosis of an autoimmune endocrinopathy. An ACTH stimulation test may be necessary to distinguish pituitary dysfunction from primary adrenal disease. Pituitary imaging is recommended in central adrenal insufficiency to exclude tumors, infiltrative disease, or structural abnormalities of the pituitary gland. In patients receiving high-dose corticosteroid therapy, assessment of adrenal function after tapering the steroids to an every-other-day regimen is a better predictor of HPA recovery. An early morning serum cortisol and ACTH obtained 24 to 48 hours after the last dose of steroids provides a measure of basal adrenal function; low-dose ACTH stimulation testing helps evaluate pituitary recovery. Additional testing with insulin-induced hypoglycemia or overnight metyrapone suppression may be indicated to diagnose central adrenal insufficiency of recent onset, such as after pituitary surgery.

Common Pitfalls

The onset of an adrenal crisis occurs rapidly; thus recognition of the acute illness and timely provision of stress glucocorticoid coverage is essential. Morbidity and mortality in adrenal insufficiency arises from delayed or inadequate treatment of acute adrenal insufficiency because of lack of recognition of an impending adrenal crisis. Long-term therapy for a child with 21-hydroxylase deficiency, the most common form of CAH, poses special challenges because of difficulty balancing suppression of the hyperplastic adrenal gland with the growth-inhibitory effects of glucocorticoids. For chronic management, the doses of hydrocortisone needed are often higher than those required for other causes of adrenal insufficiency, and a three-times-daily or every-8-hour rather than a twice-daily regimen may be necessary (see Table 1). If control is poor, administration of a larger fraction of the dose at bedtime or the use of a longer acting glucocorticoid, such as prednisone or dexamethasone, may help inhibit the

nocturnal rise in ACTH. The efficacy of treatment is monitored clinically and by measuring serum 17-hydroxyprogesterone, androstenedione, and testosterone levels and/or urinary concentrations of 17-ketosteroids. A number of investigative approaches are being used to optimize linear growth and improve final adult height in children with CAH. Pharmacologic interventions include the combined use of growth hormone, antiandrogens, and gonadotropin-releasing hormone analogue therapy. Alternatively, prophylactic adrenalectomies are performed for patients with poorly controlled CAH.

Patients with 11β-hydroxylase deficiency (P450c11) may have hypertension caused by excess production of deoxycorticosterone. When treated with glucocorticoids to suppress adrenal steroidogenesis, a salt-losing tendency may develop that requires supplementation with fludrocortisone. In contrast, in individuals with P450c17 gene (17-hydroxylase deficiency) defects, a rare cause of hypertension also associated with genital ambiguity in boys or delayed puberty in girls, only glucocorticoid therapy is needed. Children with 3β-hydroxysteroid dehydrogenase deficiency associated with undervirilized males and mildly virilized females manifest both glucocorticoid and mineralocorticoid deficiency and therefore require replacement with hydrocortisone and fludrocortisone.

Communication and Counseling

We advise families of patients receiving chronic glucocorticoid therapy to have the child wear a medical information bracelet. Parents and frequent caregivers are counseled about the subtle symptoms and risks of acute adrenal insufficiency and are taught to recognize situations in which stress coverage with steroids is needed. For minor viral infections associated with low-grade fevers, parents are instructed to double the oral dose of hydrocortisone. For febrile and more severe illnesses, parents are taught to triple the hydrocortisone dose and administer it thrice daily. Parents and caregivers are instructed to keep an updated vial of parenteral hydrocortisone (Solu-Cortef) for use in case of nausea and vomiting or impending cardiovascular collapse. Except in the most severe shock associated with adrenal insufficiency, subcutaneous administration with an insulin syringe is effective and obviates parental concern about giving an intramuscular injection.

Isolated Mineralocorticoid Deficiency

Expert Opinion on Management Issues

Isolated mineralocorticoid deficiency is an uncommon condition characterized by poor feeding, irritability, formula intolerance, vomiting, failure to thrive, and intermittent low-grade fevers. At diagnosis, affected infants are usually dehydrated and have hyponatremia, varying degrees of hyperkalemia, and hyperchloremic metabolic acidosis. PRA is elevated, and urinary excretion of salt is high. Measurement of serum aldosterone and aldosterone precursors serves to distinguish an enzymatic defect in aldosterone synthesis from mineralocorticoid resistance (pseudohypoaldosteronism). Despite high aldosterone concentrations suggestive of tissue resistance to mineralocorticoids, abnormalities in the mineralocorticoid receptor are identified in only a minority of patients with mineralocorticoid resistance (pseudohypoaldosteronism type 1a). A few patients are now found to have genetic defects in the epithelial sodium channel (ENaC) (pseudohypoaldosteronism type 1b).

Acute therapy consists of restoration of fluid volume and salt deficit with infusions of normal saline. Patients with a defect in aldosterone production require fludrocortisone (.05 to 0.1 mg/day) and salt supplementation during infancy and with acute diarrheal illnesses. Patients with mineralocorticoid resistance already have elevated serum concentrations of aldosterone; thus fludrocortisone therapy is superfluous, and treatment consists primarily of adequate fluid intake, salt replacement, and potassium restriction. Occasional children with mineralocorticoid resistance and acidosis also require chronic oral sodium bicarbonate supplementation (5 to 10 mEq/day). For most patients, the salt wasting abates during childhood, and therapy is not necessary beyond infancy except during acute gastrointestinal illnesses. The effectiveness of therapy is monitored by following growth and blood pressures and measuring serum electrolytes and PRA.

Common Pitfalls

The clinical features of isolated mineralocorticoid deficiency resemble that of adrenal insufficiency; thus care must be taken to differentiate this condition from CAH to avoid inappropriate therapeutic intervention. Both inadequate replacement and excess doses of salt and/or fludrocortisone can manifest as poor growth and irritability. Close attention to blood pressures, serum electrolytes, and PRA is essential to titrate the salt intake appropriately and adjust fludrocortisone dosing.

Communication and Counseling

Parents are counseled to be attentive to fluid and salt intake during infancy when infants are unable to self-regulate their intake. Throughout childhood, illnesses or strenuous activities that result in excess fluid or salt loss require extra supplementation.

Adrenal Medullary Deficiency

Functional deficiencies of catecholamine secretion are present in children with tightly controlled diabetes and recurrent hypoglycemia. Adrenal medullary catecholamine release gradually diminishes with loss of "hypoglycemia awareness," which is restored after avoidance

of hypoglycemia for only a few weeks. Primary deficiencies of catecholamine secretion are not described.

EXCESS HORMONE PRODUCTION

Glucocorticoid Excess (Cushing Syndrome)

Expert Opinion on Management Issues

Cushing disease is usually secondary to a small ACTH-producing pituitary adenoma of clonal cell origin and rarely caused by diffuse corticotroph hyperplasia. Treatment is generally directed toward removal or ablation of the hyperplastic cells. MRI to localize these small tumors, which are often less than 1 cm in diameter, is successful only 40% of the time. Inferior petrosal sinus sampling with CRH administration to ensure that the ACTH is of pituitary origin and to assist in localizing the tumor is generally recommended.

Transsphenoidal surgery to resect the tumor and reestablish normal neuroendocrine function is successful in more than 80% of cases in children and adolescents. In the hands of experienced surgeons, long-term cure rates are greater than 90% in adults and may be similar in children. A harbinger of excellent long-term outcome is adrenal insufficiency lasting for a year or more, as documented by suppressed levels of urinary free cortisol. If the initial surgery is not curative, alternative approaches can be considered. Bilateral adrenalectomy, now usually performed laparoscopically, carries relatively low risk, but the outcome is lifetime adrenal insufficiency. Adrenalectomy also increases the potential for the development of Nelson syndrome, an aggressive pituitary corticotroph tumor. Repeat transsphenoidal surgery increases the risk of anterior or posterior hypopituitarism (or both), but lifetime replacement of pituitary hormones must be weighed against the morbidity of Cushing disease or complete adrenalectomy. Conventional orthovoltage, proton beam, and gamma irradiation (gamma knife) are all used successfully to treat pituitary Cushing disease. The experience at Massachusetts General Hospital since 1990 is with the proton beam, which offers tightly targeted pituitary irradiation and typically leads to remission over a 3- to 6-month period. The development of anterior hypopituitarism over a span of several years is an anticipated common side effect. Irradiation by any method slowly induces remission of the hypercortisolism and often leads to gradual loss of other anterior pituitary function and a small increase in the risk of secondary CNS tumors. Our approach is to present the various therapeutic options and assist the patient and family to make an informed decision.

If the treatment plan selected does not lead to immediate resolution of symptoms, a number of drugs can reduce adrenal production of glucocorticoids and provide symptomatic relief. Ketoconazole, the initial treatment of choice, suppresses cortisol production by

TABLE 2 Treatment of Glucocorticoid Excess

Drug	Dose	Formulation	Pharmacokinetics/Indications
Ketoconazole	5–32 mg/kg/day q12h	200-mg scored tablets	Inhibits cholesterol side chain cleavage P450 and other P450 steroid synthetic enzymes
Metyrapone	15–30 mg/kg/day q8–12h	250-mg tablets	Inhibits 11β-hydroxylase enzyme so that levels of 11-desoxycortisol and desoxycorticosterone (DOC) increase
Aminoglutethimide	0.5–2 g/day q6h (adult dose = 2 g)	250-mg tablets	Inhibits adrenal steroid biosynthesis
o-p-DDD (mitotane)	0.5–1 g daily, higher as tolerated up to 20 g in adults	0.5-g tablets	Cytotoxic to adrenal; inhibits steroidogenesis

DDD, dichlorodiphenyldichloroethane; q*x*h, every *x* hours.

inhibiting P450scc ([cholesterol] side chain cleavage) and other P450 steroidogenic enzymes and also inhibits the ACTH response. Doses above 8 mg/kg/day are more likely to produce side effects such as nausea, pruritus, and gastrointestinal discomfort (Table 2). Liver and kidney function should be monitored to screen for hepatic and renal toxicity. Ketoconazole reduces protein binding of warfarin (Coumadin), so the dose of warfarin required for anticoagulation therapy may need to be decreased. Ketoconazole is marketed as an antifungal agent and not approved by the U.S. Food and Drug Administration (FDA) for use in hyperadrenalism. Metyrapone blocks cortisol synthesis by inhibiting 11β-hydroxylase, but excess 11-deoxycortisol and deoxycorticosterone are produced, which can cause hypertension, volume expansion, edema, and hypokalemia. Gastrointestinal distress is a common side effect and may be ameliorated by giving metyrapone with food. Metyrapone was withdrawn from the commercial market in the United States and is only available on request from the manufacturer. Aminoglutethimide inhibits adrenal steroid biosynthesis by binding to cytochrome P450 enzymes and can lead to mineralocorticoid and glucocorticoid deficiency. Side effects include rash, nausea, and dizziness. In the United States, o,p'-DDD (2,4'-dichlorodiphenyldichloroethane, or mitotane) is seldom used to ablate the adrenal glands in individuals with this condition. This drug is both cytotoxic to the adrenal gland and a steroidogenic inhibitor. Side effects include anorexia, nausea, vomiting, diarrhea, dizziness, other CNS problems, and transient rash.

More than 50% of adrenal tumors causing Cushing syndrome in childhood are malignant. The prognosis is directly related to the age of the patient, tumor size, and the presence of capsular and vascular invasion. Surgical removal is the most effective therapy. Perioperative supplementation with glucocorticoids is essential because the residual adrenal and the HPA axis are usually suppressed in children with cortisol-secreting adrenal tumors. Other adjuvant treatments are not particularly successful in enhancing longevity in children with malignant or metastatic disease. Mitotane is sometimes used for adjunctive chemotherapy, but examples of the curative use of this agent are few. Ketoconazole, metyrapone, and other agents can sometimes be helpful in ameliorating the hypercortisolism in children with incurable adrenal carcinoma and debilitating symptoms from hypercortisolism. Long-term management of children with adrenal tumors after surgery includes careful clinical and biochemical monitoring to detect recurrence and adjustment of the glucocorticoid dose on return of adrenal function.

Several rare causes of primary adrenal hyperfunction require adrenal ablation for the resolution of symptoms. In bilateral micronodular adrenal dysplasia (also known as adrenocortical nodular dysplasia), a rare cause of cortisol excess in children, both adrenals function autonomously or express anomalous receptors for gastrointestinal hormones. Adrenal hyperplasia associated with McCune-Albright syndrome is caused by an activating G protein mutation coupled to the ACTH receptor. The treatment of choice in both disorders is adrenalectomy plus lifelong supplementation with glucocorticoids and mineralocorticoids as described earlier.

Common Pitfalls

Determination of the cause of Cushing syndrome can be difficult in some instances. Localization to the pituitary using MRI or even transsphenoidal sampling is not always clear-cut because of the small size of the tumor or variable blood flow from the transsphenoidal sinuses. Ectopic ACTH or corticotropin-releasing hormone—secreting tumors can be extremely difficult to identify. Repetitive imaging and the use of octreotide scanning may increase the chances of identifying an ectopic source of ACTH or CRH. If the source cannot be readily identified, often the best choice is bilateral adrenalectomy with careful follow-up.

Successful transsphenoidal pituitary surgery in Cushing disease requires a very experienced neurosurgeon and an experienced support team. Referral to a specialty center may be indicated. In successfully treated children, adrenal replacement therapy may be required postoperatively for a year or more; thus patients are at long-term risk for acute adrenal insufficiency.

Cushingoid children are in a hypercoagulable state and more susceptible for venous thrombosis, which was observed in the course of investigation and therapy. Complaints that might be explained by deep vein thrombosis or pulmonary embolism should be investigated carefully.

Mood and learning disorders may be found in some children and adolescents with Cushing disease and may worsen after therapy, requiring specialized psychiatric and neurocognitive support. Children with this disorder should be followed carefully and for many years because of the risk of recurrence or potential loss of other endocrine function.

Children with short stature after many years of growth suppression may never attain their full height potential.

Exposure to excess endogenous glucocorticoid decreases bone mineral density. If bone density is abnormal, it should be followed at yearly or biennial intervals after treatment.

Communication and Counseling

We counsel parents about the risks of the various types of treatment, of adrenal insufficiency, and of the risk of recurrence. We discuss the possibility of mood and neurocognitive disorders that may take some years to remit. We discuss height potential in treated children, depending on the degree of stunting during the period of glucocorticoid excess. Until the children are fully recovered from adrenal insufficiency, they are counseled about stress supplementation like other children with adrenal insufficiency (see earlier). Bone mineral density may be diminished by hyperadrenocorticism, and we counsel careful follow-up of bone density.

Disorders of Androgen Or Estrogen Excess

Expert Opinion on Management Issues

The diagnosis of CAH relies on a characteristic profile of adrenal steroids and steroid precursors, and it may require ACTH stimulation testing for a definitive diagnosis. A nonspecific elevation in serum adrenal androgens and estrogens and urinary 17-ketosteroids is concerning and warrants abdominal imaging studies to exclude an adrenal tumor. Head imaging may also be necessary if a central process is suspected.

Management of CAH was discussed earlier. In late-onset CAH, as opposed to classic CAH, lower doses of glucocorticoid are often successful in controlling the excessive secretion of androgens.

Adrenal tumors are generally palpable at the time of diagnosis; thus abdominal distention or an abdominal mass may be found on examination. The finding of coexisting cushingoid or feminizing features is indicative of an adrenal tumor with mixed hormonal excess. Estrogen excess is manifested as accelerated growth in conjunction with early breast development or vaginal bleeding in girls (or both) and gynecomastia in boys. Feminizing adrenal or ovarian tumors are exceedingly rare in children. The primary therapy for adrenal tumors is surgical resection, usually unilateral adrenalectomy. Tumor size is the major consideration

in designating the tumor as benign or malignant. Other prognostic factors are local lymphatic and vascular invasion and distant metastases. Chemotherapy is still considered experimental, but o,p′-DDD (mitotane) is reported to control local tumor regrowth and distant metastases. Mitotane produces adrenocortical necrosis but is associated with considerable toxicity. Patients generally have adrenal insufficiency after tumor resection and require both glucocorticoid and mineralocorticoid replacement.

Common Pitfalls

Removal of an adrenal tumor often results in transient adrenal insufficiency; thus adequate postoperative and short-term glucocorticoid replacement may be necessary. If the tumor is secreting glucocorticoids, long-term hydrocortisone replacement is needed; otherwise, the corticosteroids should be tapered rapidly to avoid further iatrogenic suppression of adrenal function. Assessment of the HPA axis may be needed to assess the ability to respond to stress and determine the need for stress steroids.

Communication and Counseling

If HPA axis suppression is identified, parents should be counseled about recognition of situations in which stress steroids are needed and the appropriate doses (as discussed earlier in the section on adrenal insufficiency).

Mineralocorticoid Excess

Clues to the diagnosis of aldosteronoma and dexamethasone-suppressible aldosterone secretion include hypertension, which is associated in most instances with relative hypokalemia, hyporeninemia, and an elevated aldosterone level. In apparent mineralocorticoid excess, the hyporeninemia is associated with normal or suppressed levels of aldosterone. Imaging studies to localize an aldosteronoma are followed by curative surgical resection for these generally benign tumors. Dexamethasone-suppressible aldosteronism, also called glucocorticoid-responsive aldosteronism, is often treated with glucocorticoids because aldosterone synthesis is under ACTH regulation in this disorder. Some patients are treated with potassium-sparing diuretics and antihypertensives. However, not all individuals with the defect are symptomatic, and these individuals are not treated. The underlying genetic defect is a gene conversion with fusion of the 11β-hydroxylase promoter to the aldosterone synthase gene.

Apparent mineralocorticoid excess is caused in most cases by a mutation in the gene encoding 11β-hydroxysteroid dehydrogenase 2, the enzyme that converts cortisol to cortisone in the kidney. If cortisol is not converted to cortisone, it interacts with the mineralocorticoid receptor in the kidney and causes apparent mineralocorticoid excess.

Interval therapy (Table 3) for all these disorders can be undertaken with high doses of spironolactone.

TABLE 3 Treatment of Mineralocorticoid Excess

Drug	Dose	Formulation	Pharmacokinetics/Indications
Spironolactone	1.5–5 mg/kg/day q12h	25-, 50-, 100-mg tablets	Competitively inhibits aldosterone at the distal renal tubule, inhibits other steroids at the receptor as well. May cause gynecomastia, irregular menses, increased digoxin half-life, hyperkalemia. Half-life is 1.5 h, but metabolites with longer half-lives are also active.
Amiloride	0.625 mg/kg/day maximum in children, to 40 mg/kg/day in adults	5-mg tablets	Competitively inhibits mineralocorticoid at the distal renal tubule.

qxh, every x hours.

TABLE 4 Disorders of Catecholamine Excess

Drug	Dose	Formulation	Pharmacokinetics/Indications
α-Adrenergic Blocking Agents (Preparation for Surgery)			
Phenoxybenzamine HCl	Adult: Titrate from 10 mg q12h to 20–40 mg q8–12h. Children: 0.2 mg/kg daily, increase by 0.2 mg/kg/day every 4 days to maintenance of 0.4–1.2 mg/kg/day divided every 6–8 hours (max 10 mg/dose); doses up to 4 mg/kg/day have been used.	10-mg capsules	α-Adrenergic blocker Long half-life (20%–30% gut absorption)
Prazosin	Adult: 1 mg q8h up to 20 mg daily. Children: Initial 6 µg/kg/dose every 6h, increase to 25 µg/kg/dose q6h (max 15 mg/dose or 0.4 mg/kg/day).	1-, 2-, and 5-mg capsules	Selective α_1-antagonist has a short half-life.
β-Adrenergic Blocking Agent (Use only after patient's α-adrenergic system is fully blocked.)			
Propranolol	1 mg/kg/dose q8–12h.	10-, 20-, 40-, 60-, 80-mg tablets	Nonselective β-adrenergic blocker; biologic half life is 4 h. May induce asthma in reactive airway disease.
Combined α/β-Blocker (Preparation for Surgery)			
Labetalol HCl	Titrate from 1–3 mg/kg to 10–12 mg/kg q12h (max 1200 mg/day).	100-, 200-, and 300-mg capsules	α- and β-adrenergic blocker Long half-life (30%–40% gut absorption) May induce wheezing in reactive airway disease
Long-acting			
Propranolol	1 mg/kg daily.	60-, 80-, 120-mg capsules	
Atenolol	1–2 mg/kg daily.	25-, 50-, 100-mg tablets	Selective β_1-adrenergic blocker, only 50% absorbed orally. Peak levels at 2–4 h, half-life of 6–7 h; duration PO is 24 h.

PO, orally; qxh, every x hours.

Amiloride is also a useful adjunct to therapy, although side effects, including gastrointestinal distress, headache, and dizziness, may limit its usefulness.

Catecholamine Excess (Pheochromocytoma and Neuroblastoma)

Expert Opinion on Management Issues

Treatment of benign pheochromocytoma is almost always surgical. After localization of the tumor or tumors with CT or MRI or, at times, with more specific imaging with ^{131}I-MIBG (metaiodobenzylguanidine), patients are usually prepared for surgery with α-blockade or, in some centers, with the combined α/β-blocker labetalol (Table 4). The most commonly used agent for such blockade is phenoxybenzamine. The dose is titrated from 10 mg twice daily up to 40 mg three times daily over a period of 7 to 10 days until recumbent blood pressure normalizes and postural hypotension is achieved. This titration was traditionally done in the hospital but may be accomplished at home with supervision. Phenoxybenzamine has a long half-life (more than 25 hours when given intravenously), and approximately 20% to 30% is absorbed from the gut. Major adverse effects are those of α-adrenergic blockade and include orthostatic hypertension, tachycardia, vomiting, and lethargy. Epinephrine can induce hypotension in treated patients because it stimulates both α- and β-adrenergic receptors. Prazosin, a selective $α_1$-antagonist with a shorter half-life, can also be used and is administered as 1 mg every 8 hours up to 20 mg as necessary and titrated to achieve postural hypotension. Such dosing permits withdrawal of α-blockade after surgery when severe hypotension secondary to α-blockade can require fluid loading after removal of the pheochromocytoma. If tachycardia is significant after the patient is fully α-blocked, a β-blocker such as propranolol or atenolol can be added. Alternatively, labetalol may be used.

Neuroblastomas rarely secrete sufficient catecholamines to necessitate similar medical preparation for surgery. Hypertension and tachycardia occurring during removal of tumor may on occasion require perisurgical administration of rapidly acting α- or β-blocking agents by the anesthesiologist. In addition, some patients who are fully blocked by medication may require fluid resuscitation intraoperatively once the tumor has been removed because their blood pressure may drop precipitously.

Common Pitfalls

Pheochromocytomas may be multifocal and may recur. They may be only one manifestation of another disorder, such as neurofibromatosis, von Hippel-Lindau disease, or a multiple endocrine neoplasia syndrome. If it is necessary to remove both adrenal glands during surgery for this condition, lifelong replacement for adrenal insufficiency must begin at the time of surgery.

Communication and Counseling

Families must be aware of the risk of recurrence and of associated disorders. They must understand the need for long-term follow-up and for adrenal steroid supplementation if bilateral adrenalectomy is necessary for cure of the disorder.

Disorders of the adrenal gland are relatively rare and may involve hypofunction or hyperfunction of the adrenal cortex or medulla. With the widespread use of glucocorticoids for the management of many pediatric illnesses, the side effect of iatrogenic adrenal suppression with its associated complications is important to keep in mind. Understanding the etiology and physiology of adrenal disorders allows targeted diagnostic evaluation and appropriate decision making regarding medical, surgical, and adjunctive therapies.

SUGGESTED READINGS

1. Ghizzoni L, Mastorakos G, Vottero A: Adrenal hyperandrogenism in children. J Clin Endocrinol Metab 84:4431–4435, 1999. **Brief review of hyperandrogenism with a focus on benign premature adrenarche, adrenal tumors, and glucocorticoid resistance.**
2. Moshang T: Cushing's disease, 70 years later . . . and the beat goes on. J Clin Endocrinol Metab 88:31–33, 2003. **Editorial regarding the management controversies for children with Cushing disease (see reference 4).**
3. Speiser PW, White PC: Congenital adrenal hyperplasia. N Engl J Med 349:776–788, 2003. **A comprehensive up-to-date review of 21-hydroxylase CAH, including a discussion of clinical features, genetic diagnosis, prenatal diagnosis and treatment, and standard and novel therapies.**
4. Storr HL, Plowman PN, Savage MO: Clinical endocrine responses to pituitary radiotherapy in pediatric Cushing's disease: An effective second-line treatment. J Clin Endocrinol Metab 88:34–37, 2003. **The experience of the group from St. Bartholomew's Hospital with the treatment of pediatric Cushing disease from 1983 to 2000.**
5. Stowasser M, Gordon RD: Primary aldosteronism: Learning from the study of familial varieties. J Hypertens 18:1165–1176, 2000. **Review of the evaluation and features of primary aldosteronism with a more detailed discussion of familial forms.**
6. Teeger S, Papanicolaou N, Vaughan ED Jr: Current concepts in imaging of adrenal masses. World J Urol 17:3–8, 1999. **Review of the imaging features of adrenal masses on CT and MRI and the relative merits of each imaging modality.**
7. Ten S, New M, Maclaren N: Addison's disease 2001. J Clin Endocrinol Metab 86:2909–2922, 2001. **This review includes a description of adrenal gland development and a detailed discussion of different causes of adrenal insufficiency.**
8. Thaler LM, Blevins LS: The low dose (1 mcg) adrenocorticotropin stimulation test in the evaluation of patients with suspected central adrenal insufficiency. J Clin Endocrinol Metab 83:2726–2729, 1998. **Review of literature comparing the efficacy of low and standard dose testing to evaluate central adrenal insufficiency.**
9. Young WF Jr: Pheochromocytoma and primary aldosteronism: Diagnostic approaches. Endocrinol Metab Clin North Am 26:801–827, 1997. **This article reviews the clinical features and differential diagnosis of catecholamine-secreting tumors and primary aldosteronism. It also presents a logical approach with flow charts for the evaluation of these two conditions and includes useful tables and figures, such as a list of medications that may alter the levels of catecholamines.**

Gonadal Disorders

Elka Jacobson-Dickman and Madhusmita Misra

Gonadal disorders include primary hypogonadism (abnormalities in the gonads) or secondary hypogonadism (dysfunction in the hypothalamus or the pituitary gland). These disorders become apparent during infancy and adolescence, two periods of life when the gonadal axis is active. Sex determination depends on the sex chromosome complement of the embryo and is established by multiple molecular events that direct the development of germ cells, their migration to the urogenital ridge, and the formation of either testis, in the presence of the Y chromosome, or an ovary, in the absence of a Y chromosome. Sex determination sets the stage for sex differentiation, the sex-specific response of tissues to hormones produced by the gonads after they have differentiated in a female or male pattern. A functional testis is essential for both male differentiation in utero and secondary sexual maturation at puberty. In contrast, an intact ovary is not necessary for differentiation of female genitalia, but it is required for the development of later secondary sexual characteristics. Conversely, conditions that expose a female fetus to androgens in utero virilize the female genitalia, whereas in a male fetus, genital ambiguity is not observed.

Hypogonadism manifests as delayed puberty in adolescence and as infertility in adult men and women.

AMBIGUOUS GENITALIA (INTERSEX DISORDERS)

KEY CONCEPTS

- Any divergence from normal development of the external genitalia results in genital ambiguity.
- Intersex disorders can be categorized into disorders in the primary process of gonadal formation, virilization in a genetic female, and undervirilization in a genetic male.
- Disorders of gonadal morphogenesis include pure and partial gonadal dysgenesis, mixed gonadal dysgenesis, true hermaphroditism, and sex-reversal syndromes.
- Virilization in a genetic female is characterized by a 46,XX karyotype. The most common etiology is congenital adrenal hyperplasia (CAH).
- Undervirilization in a genetic male is characterized by a 46,XY karyotype and the presence of testes. Androgen resistance syndromes, both androgen insensitivity and 5α-reductase deficiency, are the most frequently diagnosed etiologies of undervirilized males.
- The practice of caring for patients with ambiguous genitalia has encountered much controversy and some degree of reform. Gender assignment and the timing of reconstruction surgery are major ethical dilemmas.

Table 1 describes the classification and features of various intersex disorders, and Table 2 lists syndromes associated with genital ambiguity.

Expert Opinion on Management Issues

In cases of sexual ambiguity, gender assignment or reassignment is a significant ethical dilemma. The principles and paradigms underlying gender assignment decisions have undergone major shifts over the last 5 to 10 years. Traditionally, gender assignment was based on the assumption of gender neutrality in infancy. Potential for future sexual and reproductive function, in addition to etiology and capabilities and limitations of reconstructive surgery, were initially taken into account in assigning gender. However, reports emphasizing the role of androgen imprinting on the fetal brain in gender-role and sexual identity introduced the necessity to include in utero androgen exposure as an important consideration in gender assignment. The necessity and timing of reconstructive surgery to allow appearance of external genitalia to match the assigned gender has also become controversial. Proponents of delayed surgery argue that genital surgery is a cosmetic procedure and may affect genital sensation and not be congruent with sexual identity, and therefore they urge that the decision be deferred until the patient can actively participate in the decision-making process. Box 1 and Figure 1 describe the evaluation of patients with ambiguous genitalia.

In conditions of gonadal morphogenesis, dysgenetic gonads are usually removed at a young age because of the increased risk of malignancy (5% to 20%). In adolescence, sex steroid replacement therapy is necessary to induce secondary sexual maturation. In girls, hormone replacement is provided for initiation and maintenance of feminization and to protect against osteoporosis (Box 2). We initiate low-dose estrogen therapy in girls at 10 to 12 years of age to initiate breast budding without advancing bone age unduly and inadvertently causing stunting of adult height potential. In complete androgen sensitivity, testosterone is aromatized to estrogen and allows for breast development and a female habitus; gonadectomy may be delayed until pubertal development is complete. In addition to individual counseling and general support groups for individuals with intersex disorders, etiology-specific support groups may be helpful.

If unrecognized at birth, the salt-losing form of congenital adrenal hyperplasia (CAH) manifests as vomiting, hyponatremic dehydration, hyperkalemia, and hypoglycemia in the second week of life and is more likely seen in male infants. These clinical scenarios are less frequent with the institution of newborn screening for CAH. Female infants with CAH (except for the milder forms) usually present with some degree of virilization at birth. Prenatal dexamethasone therapy shows efficacy in reducing virilization when compared to untreated affected siblings; however, it is associated with significant steroid effects in the mothers. Box 3 describes the management of neonatal CAH.

In addition to the conditions described in Table 1, defects in the gene for müllerian-inhibiting substance (MIS) or the MIS receptor may rarely occur, resulting in the persistent müllerian duct syndrome, in which müllerian derivatives persist and development of the wolffian structures is normal with varying degrees of hypospadias or normal genitalia. Testicular ectopia with torsion generally brings this condition to medical attention. In an undervirilized male, corrective surgery for hypospadias, chordee, or genital anomalies may be necessary after the initial trial of androgens. Such surgery is usually performed at 6 to 18 months of age. Cryptorchid testes are at increased risk for functional damage and malignancy, so orchiopexy is recommended during late infancy to optimize testicular function and facilitate long-term monitoring. At puberty, supplemental sex steroids are needed for secondary sexual maturation (see Box 2). Too rapid a growth rate or advancing bone age should prompt dose reduction to avoid early epiphyseal closure and ultimate stunting of adult height potential. Local side effects of testosterone administration include tenderness at the site of injection and allergy to the vehicle carrying the testosterone ester (sesame or cottonseed oil). Large testosterone doses can cause severe acne, prolonged and painful erections, gynecomastia, fluid retention, and behavioral aberrations. Development of these features should prompt a reduction in dose or in the frequency of administration.

Transdermal testosterone preparations are also available and have an attractive pharmacokinetic

TABLE 1 Classification and Features of Intersex Disorders

Disorder	Genotype	Gonads	Müllerian Structures	Gonado-tropins	MIS	Testoste-rone
Disorders of Gonadal Morphogenesis						
Complete gonadal dysgenesis	46,XY Female, no pubertal development	Streak Undescended	Rudimentary	↑↑	Absent	↓↓
Partial gonadal dysgenesis	46,XY Female/ ambiguous	Dysgenetic	Absent	↑	↓ for males or absent	↓
Mixed gonadal dysgenesis	45,X/46,XY Usually male; may be ambiguous or rarely female	Testis and streak or dysgenetic testis	Present on side of streak gonad	Normal or ↑	↓ for males or normal	↓ or normal
True hermaphroditism	46,XX, 46,XX/46,XY, 46,XY Ambiguous	Ovary/ovotestis B/L ovotestes Ovary/testis	Present on side of ovary	Normal	↓ for males or normal	↓ or normal
Virilization of a Genetic Female						
Congenital adrenal hyperplasia (CAH)	46,XX Ambiguous	Ovaries	Present	Normal	Female range	↑ for females
21-Hydroxylase	Defect in CYP21, ↑ 17-hydroxyprogesterone, most common CAH, ± salt wasting					
11β-Hydroxylase	Defect in CYP11B1,↑ deoxycorticosterone, second most common CAH, no salt wasting, hypertension					
3β-Hydroxysteroid dehydrogenase	Defect in HSD3B2, ↑ DHEA and 17-hydroxypregnenolone, rare, ± salt wasting, mild ambiguity					
In utero exposure to androgens and progestational agents; placental aromatase deficiency	46,XX Ambiguous	Ovaries	Present	Normal	Female range	Female range
Undervirilization of a Genetic Male						
Complete androgen insensitivity	46,XY Female; breast development at puberty, no menses	Testes Undescended or descended	Rudimentary in approximately one third	↑↑	Normal or ↑	↑ or normal
Partial androgen insensitivity	46,XY Varying degrees of ambiguity	Testes Undescended or descended	Absent	↑	Normal or ↑	↑ or normal
5α-Reductase deficiency	46,XY Varying degrees of ambiguity; ↑ virilization at puberty	Testes Descended or inguinal	Absent	↑	Normal	↓ DHT ↓ Ratio of DHT to T
Disorders of testosterone biosynthesis	46,XY Varying degrees of ambiguity	Testes Descended or undescended	Absent	↑/↑↑	Normal	↓
Steroidogenic acute regulatory protein	Defect in stAR; female genitalia or mild ambiguity; adrenal insufficiency and salt-losing state; ↓ in all precursors and products					
17-Hydroxylase	Defect in CYP17; varying degrees of ambiguity; not a salt losing state; hypertension; ↓ ratio of 17-hydroxyprogesterone to progesterone and 17-hydroxypregnenolone to pregnenolone					
3β-Hydroxysteroid dehydrogenase	Defect in HSD3B2; ↑ DHEA and 17-hydroxypregnenolone, rare; may be salt wasting					
17-Ketosteroid reductase	Defect in HSD17B3; ↑androstenedione and ↑ ratio of androstenedione to testosterone; ↑ virilization at puberty					
Inactivating mutations of the LH receptor	46,XY Varying degrees of ambiguity	Testes (small) Undescended or descended	Absent	↑/↑↑	Normal	↓

B/L, bilateral; DHEA, dehydroepiandrosterone; DHT, dihydrotestosterone; LH, luteinizing hormone; MIS, müllerian-inhibiting substance; stAR, steroid acute regulatory protein; T, testosterone.

TABLE 2 Syndromes Associated with Genital Ambiguity

Syndrome	Gene	Clinical Characteristics
Pure gonadal dysgenesis; Swyer syndrome	SRY	46,XY sex reversal, streak gonads.
Camptomelic dysplasia	SOX9	46,XY sex reversal, gonadal dysgenesis, severe skeletal malformation.
Sex reversal with adrenal insufficiency	SF-1	
Fraser syndrome	WT1	46,XY sex reversal, gonadal dysgenesis, nephrotic syndrome.
Denys-Drash syndrome	WT1	Gonads affected later in differentiation, MIS produced, testosterone synthesis impaired, undervirilized genitalia, varying degrees of hypospadias, undescended testes; high incidence of Wilms tumor.
Androgen insensitivity syndromes	AR	External genitalia fail to respond to testosterone and dihydrotestosterone, testes may be undescended, varying degrees of undervirilization.
Hand-foot-genital syndrome	HOXA13	Vaginal abnormalities, deformities of hands and feet, spinal abnormalities, and exstrophy of bladder and cloaca.

MIS, müllerian-inhibiting substance.

profile. These require daily replacement and provide a more consistent concentration of serum testosterone than do parenteral depot preparations. Scrotal testosterone patches generate supraphysiologic blood dihydrotestosterone levels, which is not the case with nonscrotal testosterone patches. Dosing is monitored by measuring serum testosterone concentrations 2 to 4 hours after applying the Testoderm patch or the morning after applying the Androderm patch. Transdermal testosterone gel causes less skin irritation than the patch and offers greater flexibility in dosage. Secondary to risks and benefits of various testosterone replacement options, the patient should be involved in the selection of type of testosterone preparation when possible.

Common Pitfalls

Gender assignment or reassignment represents an emotional and controversial ethical dilemma. The emergence of patient and parent support groups, the interchange of information via the Internet, and increased media attention all contribute to a climate in which past medical decisions and management of intersex conditions are now the subject of increasingly close and critical scrutiny. In past decades, standard pediatric practice was to recommend surgery for infants with ambiguous genitalia in early infancy. Many parents, with the advice of medical providers, raised children in a scenario of strict gender unambiguity with the help of corrective surgery, and in this vein, many patients were never candidly informed about their medical histories. Certain patient groups have expressed frank outrage at their prior surgical intervention and management. Limited data are available regarding long-term psychosexual outcomes of early versus late surgery. There is widespread recognition of the need for long-term functional and psychosexual outcome studies to formulate a more evidence-based approach.

Communication and Counseling

Management of a child with genital ambiguity involves a team of physicians, including the family's pediatrician, a geneticist, endocrinologist, urologist or pediatric surgeon, and a child psychiatrist or counselor. Parental involvement is essential, and it is important for parents to observe the genitalia of their infant. They need to be reassured that their child's genital ambiguity is a problem in embryonic development like other disorders in development. The emotional tone established by health care professionals in conveying this information can have a lasting influence on how parents conceptualize the abnormal genital development and how they initiate their relationship with their child. Ongoing emotional support is critical, and introduction to support groups and other families with similar problems may be helpful. In past decades, when intersex infants were raised as unambiguous boys or girls following corrective surgery, caregivers and parents often concealed aspects of surgical and medical history from the patient. This secrecy can be damaging to the patient, and parents should be counseled that at an appropriate developmental stage, the patient is entitled to full disclosure.

HYPOGONADISM

KEY CONCEPTS

- Hypogonadism can occur as a result of impaired secretion or action of gonadal steroids or from impaired gonadotropin secretion or action.
- Hypogonadotropic hypogonadism (secondary/tertiary hypogonadism) is caused by dysfunction at the level of the pituitary gland or hypothalamus, resulting in impaired gonadotropin secretion.
- Causes of hypogonadotropic hypogonadism include Kallmann syndrome (hypogonadotropic hypogonadism with anosmia), idiopathic hypogonadotropic hypogonadism, constitutional delay of growth and puberty, and structural lesions and other insults to the hypothalamus and pituitary gland.
- Primary gonadal failure, or hypergonadotropic hypogonadism, may be caused by congenital and genetic disorders that affect gonadal development and differentiation or be acquired in later life.
- The most common genetic cause of gonadal failure is Klinefelter syndrome in males and Turner syndrome in females.

14

KEY CONCEPTS—cont'd

- Autoimmune ovarian failure is the most common acquired cause of primary gonadal failure in girls. Acquired causes of primary gonadal failure include gonadal trauma, vascular damage from torsion, infection, and use of chemotherapeutic agents or irradiation.
- Sex steroid replacement at puberty is necessary to optimize development of secondary sexual characteristics and bone mass accrual.

Box 4 describes the causes of gonadal failure. Hypogonadism may manifest as undervirilization of the external genitalia in males or as absent secondary sexual maturation at puberty in both males and females. When the defect is severe or occurs early in gestation, ambiguous genitalia and microphallus result, with or without hypospadias. These conditions are often associated with midline defects. Milder defects, or those occurring in late gestation, cause isolated microphallus. Acquired hypogonadism may manifest as interrupted sexual development, secondary amenorrhea, or infertility.

Secondary hypogonadism is less common than primary hypogonadism and differs from the latter in males in two main characteristics. First, secondary hypogonadism is usually associated with an equivalent decrease in sperm and testosterone production. This occurs because the primary reduction in luteinizing hormone (LH) secretion results in a decrease in testicular testosterone production and therefore intratesticular testosterone, which is a principal hormone stimulus for sperm production. In contrast, there is a greater decrease in sperm production than testosterone secretion in primary hypogonadism because the seminiferous tubules are damaged to a greater extent than are Leydig cells. A second major difference is that secondary hypogonadism is less likely to be associated with gynecomastia, presumable because serum follicle-stimulating hormone (FSH) and LH concentrations are not high and therefore do not stimulate testicular aromatase to increase conversion of testosterone to estradiol.

Expert Opinion on Management Issues

HYPOGONADOTROPIC HYPOGONADISM (SECONDARY/TERTIARY GONADAL FAILURE)

Evaluation and management can be separated into management of issues in infancy and at puberty.

BOX 1 Evaluation of Ambiguous Genitalia

History

- Intrauterine exposure to androgens or progestational agents.
- Family history of ambiguous genitalia, unexplained neonatal deaths, primary amenorrhea, infertility, or inguinal hernias with prolapsed gonads.
- Parental consanguinity.

Physical Exam

- Genital examination for gonadal position,* size of phallus,[†] location of urethral opening, extent of chordee, and labiosacral fusion.
- Syndromic features.
- Per rectal palpation: Uterus appreciated as a firm, midline, pencil-width structure in neonates.

Laboratory Workup

- Karyotype and evaluation for Y chromosome material; mutations in specific genes.
- Evaluation for CAH and testosterone biosynthetic defects: Electrolytes, 17-hydroxyprogesterone, 17-hydroxypregnenolone, pregnenolone, deoxycortisol, DHEA, androstenedione, testosterone, and dihydrotestosterone (baseline values and following an ACTH stimulation test).

- Müllerian-inhibiting substance: Secreted by Sertoli cells and highly predictive for the presence of testicular tissue.
- Testosterone: Basal levels elevated at 4–12 weeks of age in the presence of functional testicular tissue.[‡]
- hCG stimulation test[§] (useful for identifying functional testicular tissue in postinfancy prepubertal years, for diagnosis of 5α-reductase deficiency and testosterone biosynthetic defects): 1500 U/m^2 administered on days 1 and 3, testosterone ± dihydrotestosterone ± steroid precursors measured at baseline, day 3, and day 6.
- Genital tissue biopsy for androgen receptor studies.
- Gonadal biopsy for suspected disorders of gonadal morphogenesis.

Imaging

- Sonogram or MRI to identify gonads and müllerian structures.

Testosterone Trial as a Measure of Androgen Responsiveness

- Short course of testosterone cypionate or enanthate in undervirilized genetic males to assess capacity for phallic growth.[¶]
  - 10–25 mg IM monthly for 3 months.
  - 50–100 mg IM monthly for another 3 to 4 months if necessary.

*Gonads located below the external inguinal ring invariably contain some testicular tissue. Asymmetrical positioning of gonads is suggestive of a disorder of gonadal morphogenesis.

[†]Third percentile for stretched phallic length in a full-term male infant is 2.8 cm. A small phallus with minimal corporeal tissue raises concerns of impaired phallic response to androgens, testosterone biosynthetic defects, inadequate conversion of testosterone to dihydrotestosterone, or deficient gonadotropin secretion.

[‡]After the initial neonatal period, testosterone levels are indistinguishable between prepubertal males and females.

[§]In hCG stimulation testing, testosterone is expected to double from baseline to day 3 and double again from days 3 to 6. A longer period of stimulation (i.e., every other day for 2 weeks) is sometimes necessary to elicit a response.

[¶]Testosterone response assessed by measuring the stretched phallic length. An increase of >0.5 cm/mo is considered a positive response. A negative response suggests androgen insensitivity or insufficient corporeal tissue, and it can be further evaluated with a trial of a higher dose of testosterone. A positive response suggests partial androgen insensitivity syndrome (PAIS), and absence of a response implies complete androgen insensitivity syndrome (CAIS).

ACTH, adrenocorticotropic hormone; CAH, congenital adrenal hyperplasia; DHEA, dehydroepiandrosterone; hCG, human chorionic gonadotropin; IM, intramuscular.

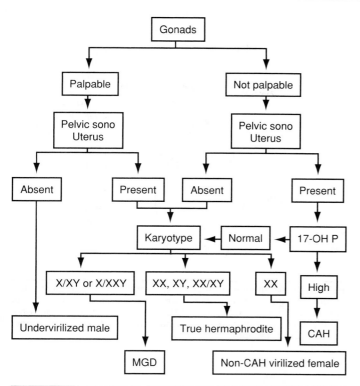

FIGURE 1. A systematic approach to the evaluation of ambiguous genitalia. CAH, congenital adrenal hyperplasia; MGD, mixed gonadal dysgenesis; 17-OH P, 17-hydroxyprogesterone. (From Grumbach MM, Hughes IA, Conte FA: Disorder of sex differentiation. In Williams RH, Larsen PR, Kronenberg HM, et al [eds]: Williams Textbook of Endocrinology, 10th ed. Philadelphia, WB Saunders, 2002, p 964.)

BOX 2 Steroid Replacement Doses for Hypogonadism

Males

- Infancy (to increase penile length)
  - Testosterone enanthate/cypionate: 10–25 mg/mo IM × 3
  - If no initial response, 50–100 mg/mo IM × 3 additional months
- Induction of puberty
  - Testosterone enanthate/cypionate: 50 mg/mo IM × 6–12 mo; increase by 25–50 mg/mo q6–12mo to reach a dose of 200 mg q2–3wk
  - Testosterone patches (adult dose): Androderm, 5 mg/day used nightly on nonscrotal skin; Testoderm, 4–6 mg/day used once a day (Testoderm TTS for nonscrotal skin, Testoderm for scrotal skin)

Females

- Induction of puberty
  - Conjugated estrogen (Premarin): 0.3 mg qod for 6–12 months; increase to 0.3 mg/day for another 6–12 mo; increase to 0.625 mg/day (days 1 to 26 of each month); or
  - Ethinyl estradiol: 50 ng/kg/day; increase by 50–100 ng/kg/day q6–12mo to a dose of 20–35 μg/day; or
  - Estrogen patches: 0.025 mg/day patch twice a week for 6–12 mo; increase to 0.0375 mg/day patch twice a week for 6–12 mo; increase to 0.05 mg/day patch twice a week for 6–23 mo and
  - Medroxyprogesterone acetate (Provera): 5–10 mg/day (days 15–26); added after full estrogen replacement when the uterus is present.

IM, intramuscular; qod, every other day.

14

BOX 3 Management of Congenital Adrenal Hyperplasia

Prenatal Therapy

- Maternal dexamethasone* therapy initiated before 5 to 6 weeks' gestation (before sexual differentiation occurs).
- Affected females identified by chorionic villous sampling or amniocentesis.

Therapy in the Neonate

- Initial vigorous volume expansion with isotonic saline.
- Intravenous hydrocortisone† begun in stress doses and rapidly tapered to physiologic replacement (10 to 15 mg/m²/day divided in two to three doses).
- Fludrocortisone begun at 0.05 to 0.2 mg/day.‡

*Dexamethasone is discontinued if the fetus is a male or an unaffected female; continued throughout pregnancy if the fetus is a female with CAH.
†Glucocorticoid replacement suppresses secretion of ACTH, thereby reducing androgen production and avoiding progressive virilization.
‡Even in children without overt salt wasting, some aldosterone deficiency is present and control of CAH and linear growth improves with addition of fludrocortisone.
ACTH, adrenocorticotropic hormone; CAH, congenital adrenal hyperplasia.

Congenital and genetic conditions that cause decreased gonadotropin secretion are rare but well recognized. Various known gene defects are associated with hypogonadal disorders (Fig. 2). Sexual differentiation in boys with these disorders is normal male because in the first trimester of pregnancy, when sexual differentiation occurs, testosterone secretion by fetal Leydig cells is stimulated by placental human chorionic gonadotropin (hCG). However, phallic development during the third trimester is suboptimal because testicular testosterone secretion at this stage depends on fetal LH secretion, which is subnormal, resulting in microphallus. Midline defects, such as midfacial hypoplasia and a cleft palate, may coexist. The association of microphallus with hypoglycemia and jaundice should prompt an immediate evaluation for panhypopituitarism. Microphallus resulting from hypogonadotropic hypogonadism shows excellent response to androgen therapy, and a short trial of testosterone after birth is warranted to assess response and to increase phallic size.

Kallmann syndrome is characterized by hypogonadotropic hypogonadism of varying severity and one or more nongonadal congenital anomalies, including anosmia, red-green color blindness, midline facial abnormalities, urogenital abnormalities, and neurosensory hearing loss. Most cases are sporadic, but X-linked autosomal dominant and autosomal recessive inheritance is also described. In X-linked Kallmann syndrome, deletions are observed in the *KAL-1* gene (Xp22.3), which encodes anosmin, a neural cell adhesion-like molecule, resulting in the inability of gonadotropin-releasing

---

BOX 4 Hypogonadism: Etiology and Associated Genes

Hypergonadotropic Hypogonadism (Primary)

- Gonadal dysmorphogenesis
  - Compete/partial gonadal dysgenesis (*SRY, SOX-9, SF-1, WT-1*)
  - Mixed gonadal dysgenesis
  - True hermaphroditism
- Undervirilized males
  - Complete and partial androgen insensitivity (*AR* gene)
  - 5α-Reductase deficiency
  - Defects in testosterone biosynthesis
  - Inactivating mutations of the LH receptor
  - Congenital anorchia/vanishing testes (bilateral in utero testicular torsion)
- Others
  - Turner syndrome (45,X or 45,X/46,XX or other mosaics)
  - Klinefelter syndrome (47,XXY)
  - Chemotherapy
  - Ovarian or testicular irradiation
  - Autoimmune ovarian or testicular failure
  - Viral oophoritis or orchitis

Hypogonadotropic Hypogonadism (Secondary or Tertiary)

- Idiopathic (often associated with gene defects)
  - Idiopathic hypogonadotropic hypogonadism
  - Kallmann syndrome (*KAL-1* gene)
  - Constitutional delay in puberty
  - Adrenal hypoplasia congenita (*DAX-1* gene)
- Structural
  - Congenital pituitary hypoplasia (*PIT-1, PROP-1, LHX-3* and *-4* genes), septo-optic dysplasia (*HESX-1*)
  - Hypothalamic-pituitary tumors, trauma, surgery
  - Infiltrative disorders
  - Radiation therapy
- Functional
  - Starvation, anorexia nervosa, depression, excessive exercise (particularly gymnasts and marathon runners)
- Miscellaneous
  - Autoimmune hypophysitis
  - Prader-Willi syndrome
  - Bardet-Biedl syndrome

LH, luteinizing hormone.

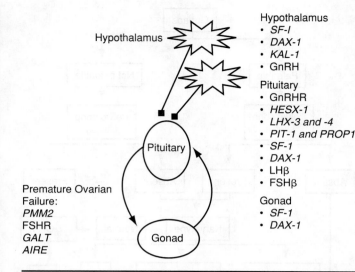

FIGURE 2. Mutations in several genes involved in the hypothalamic-pituitary gonadal axis cause impaired gonadotropin and sex steroid release or function. FSH, follicle-stimulating hormone, FSHR, FSH receptor; GnRH, gonadotropin-releasing hormone; GnRHR, GnRH receptor; LH, luteinizing hormone.

---

hormone (GnRH)-secreting neurons to migrate from the olfactory placode to the arcuate nucleus of the hypothalamus. Idiopathic hypogonadotropic hypogonadism is not associated with anosmia, but the two conditions may coexist within the same family.

Evaluation of hypogonadism is described in the chapter "Disorders of Puberty" and in Box 1. In addition, when hypogonadotropic hypogonadism is evident in infancy, evaluation should include a detailed family history, an examination for syndromic features, an evaluation of penile size with respect to future function, identification and location of the gonads (by palpation or by imaging studies), and assessment of the degree of hypospadias. The minipuberty of infancy allows useful information to be gleaned from levels of gonadotropins and gonadal steroids in boys with microphallus and/or hypospadias. In children of pubertal age, eunuchoid body proportions (arm span greater than height, lower segment longer than upper segment) and prepubertal-sized testes in boys or sexual infantilism in girls are characteristic.

In boys, the goal of management is induction of secondary sexual maturation, including adequate phallic growth and development of a male habitus. If normal function cannot be restored with treatment of the underlying functional abnormality, testosterone replacement is the mainstay of treatment (see Box 2). Therapy is started at 14 years of age or at the time of diagnosis, if later. As an alternative to testosterone, low-dose hCG is successful in boys with hypogonadotropic hypogonadism with intact and functional testes. A dose of 200 to 500 U of hCG is administered on alternate days. The therapy has the advantage of not only producing virilization by normalizing testosterone levels but also inducing an increase in testicular size. Excessive Leydig cell stimulation may cause excessive estrogen production and gynecomastia. This situation is avoided by using the lowest dose of hCG that maintains testosterone in the normal range for age. Girls with hypogonadotropic hypogonadism have primary amenorrhea and lack breast development. Estrogen therapy begins at 10 to 12 years of age as described in Box 2 to induce pubertal maturation and optimize bone mineralization.

When gonads are intact and the defect is at the hypothalamic-pituitary level, fertility may be induced when desired with the use of hCG or with human menopausal gonadotropin (hMG)/recombinant FSH and hCG in combination. Gonadotropins are preferred over pulsatile GnRH when the abnormality lies in the pituitary gland. Although both methods are generally effective in inducing spermatogenesis, women treated with pulsatile GnRH have higher conception rates and fewer multiple pregnancies than women treated with gonadotropins.

HYPERGONADOTROPIC HYPOGONADISM (PRIMARY GONADAL FAILURE)

Hypergonadotropic hypogonadism, or primary gonadal failure, is characterized by low levels of sex steroids and elevations in levels of FSH and LH. In males, Leydig cell function may be preserved longer than spermatogenesis, and consequently, such males have low to normal testosterone but elevated gonadotropins. General management principles involve initiation of sex steroid therapy in early adolescence, as for other forms of hypogonadism (see Box 2). If gonadal failure occurs at a more advanced stage of puberty, androgen therapy can be started at higher doses appropriate for the stage of sexual maturation.

Premature ovarian failure (POF) results from the depletion of functional ovarian follicle secondary to accelerated atresia or reduced number of oocytes at birth. A total depletion of ovarian follicles differentiates POF from the potentially treatable disorder termed *resistant ovary syndrome,* in which ovarian biopsy demonstrates primordial and immature follicles. Although Turner syndrome and autoimmune ovarian failure are the most common etiologies presenting at puberty, galactosemia and other forms of gonadal dysgenesis need to be excluded. Autoimmune ovarian failure can occur as an isolated disorder or as part of an autoimmune polyglandular syndrome. Laboratory evaluation should include FSH, LH (elevated to menopausal levels), estradiol, and a karyotype. Cytogenetic analysis should be considered for females presenting with unexplained POF, even when no other clinical features suggest chromosomal abnormality, particularly when onset is in adolescents and women younger than 30 years. Thyroid function tests, early-morning cortisol, measurements of antithyroid peroxidase, and antiadrenal antibodies are useful to determine whether associated endocrinopathies are present.

Treatment includes replacement of estrogen to induce breast development and, later, cyclical estrogen and progesterone to maintain secondary sexual characteristics without causing continuous endometrial stimulation (see Box 2). Before radiotherapy, transposition of the ovaries to a protected site reduces the radiation dose to the ovaries and helps preserve ovarian function. The use of GnRH analogues, antiestrogens, and birth control pills before chemotherapy may help maintain ovarian function. Immunosuppressive doses of steroids successfully restore fertility in the rare women with autoimmune ovarian failure. The only means of achieving pregnancy in patients with POF is fertilization of donor oocytes. Harvesting and cryopreservation of oocytes is successful in animals but awaits refinement before it can be applied to humans with early signs of POF.

TURNER SYNDROME

Turner syndrome is the most common sex chromosome anomaly and cause of primary hypogonadism in females. The incidence in live-born females is 1 in 2500 to 3000. Approximately half have X monosomy (45,X), 5% to 10% have duplication of the long arm of one X (46,X,i[Xq]), and mosaics make up the majority of the remainder. The Turner phenotype includes short stature, gonadal dysgenesis, a broad chest with hypoplastic nipples, congenital lymphedema of the hands and feet, a low posterior hairline with excess nuchal skin and webbing (pterygium coli), and cubitus valgus. Associated features include multiple pigmented nevi, bicuspid aortic valves, aortic coarctation, hypoplastic left heart, renal anomalies, idiopathic hypertension, recurrent otitis media, a high arched palate, short fourth metacarpals, Madelung deformity of the wrist, defective dentition, and scoliosis. Overall cognitive development is usually normal, although visuospatial and visuoperceptual organization may be affected; attention-deficit disorder is not uncommon. In addition to short stature and gonadal failure, endocrine manifestations include autoimmune thyroiditis, glucose intolerance, insulin resistance, and osteoporosis.

One fifth to one third of affected girls are diagnosed as newborns because of puffy hands and feet or redundant nuchal skin, the residual effect of cystic hygromas in utero. Approximately one third are diagnosed in mid-childhood in the course of investigation for short stature. The diagnosis should be excluded in any teenage girl with primary or secondary amenorrhea. Growth failure and short stature are almost uniformly present. Without growth hormone treatment, adult height is almost 20 cm less than that of population norms. Adult height correlates with mid-parental height. The growth velocity typically decelerates to levels below normal between 2 to 4 years of life, although growth failure may be evident even during infancy. Scoliosis occurs in approximately 10% of girls with Turner syndrome and may contribute to short stature. Turner growth charts are available to monitor growth in girls with this disorder. Growth hormone therapy is recommended to optimize stature, but it may be associated with disproportionate growth of the hands and feet, more frequent episodes of otitis media, and an increase in the size and number of pigmented nevi. Box 5 provides details regarding management of various clinical aspects of Turner syndrome.

KLINEFELTER SYNDROME

Klinefelter syndrome (47,XXY), the most common sex chromosome disorder in males, affects 1 in 500 men and is caused by nondisjunction of the maternal or paternal X chromosome. Mosaicism occurs in one in three individuals with this syndrome, and infrequent cases with three or more X chromosomes are reported with more severe pathology. The syndrome includes primary testicular failure with severely impaired spermatogenesis and varying degrees of hypogonadism. Although gonadal failure may be present at birth, more often

---

BOX 5 Management of Turner Syndrome

Prenatal Management

- Fetal echocardiography to identify cardiac structural abnormalities.
- Fetal ultrasonography to identify renal anomalies, cystic hygromas.
- Parental counseling regarding the wide variety of somatic features and high probability of short stature and ovarian failure.

Management in Infancy and Childhood

- Short stature and pubertal development:
  - Short stature is a consequence of haploinsufficiency of *SHOX*.
  - Provocative growth hormone testing not indicated.
  - Early initiation of rhGH therapy necessary to optimize height potential: 0.35 to 0.375 mg/kg/week SC.
  - Duration of rhGH treatment before initiation of estrogen replacement is a positive predictor of adult height.
  - Estrogen replacement delayed until at least 12 years of age to avoid early epiphyseal fusion and stunting of height potential.
  - Benefits of further delaying estrogen replacement must be weighed against the psychosocial stress of delayed puberty and the advantageous effects of estrogen on bone mineralization.
- Risk of gonadoblastoma:
  - Approximately 5% of girls with Turner syndrome have Y chromosome material (5%–20% risk for gonadoblastoma); possibility of Y mosaicism should be considered.
  - Prophylactic removal of gonads advised in the presence of Y chromosome material.
- Osteoporosis:
  - Long-term growth hormone treatment optimizes bone mineral density and may be beneficial for attainment of peak bone mass when estrogen is provided.
  - Long-term treatment with estrogen, adequate calcium intake (1.3 g/day), and weight-bearing activities all help to optimize bone density.

- Other endocrinopathies:
  - TSH (and possibly thyroid antibodies) should be monitored annually (10%–30% develop autoimmune thyroiditis).
  - Glucose intolerance and insulin resistance are common and worsened by growth hormone treatment; weight control is to be encouraged.
- Cardiac and renal anomalies:
  - Echocardiography or MRI at diagnosis to assess cardiac and aortic status (50% have bicuspid aortic valves, 20% have coarctation of the aorta).
  - Repeat echocardiography every 5 years to monitor the diameter of the aortic root because dilation of the aortic root can occur even without structural abnormalities.
  - Dental and surgical procedures in those with cardiac abnormalities require coverage with prophylactic antibiotics.
  - Renal ultrasound at diagnosis to identify abnormalities in the structure and position of the kidneys (e.g., horseshoe kidney), aberrant vasculature, and abnormalities of the collecting system.
- Ear, nose, and throat abnormalities:
  - Aggressive management of recurrent otitis media because of the association with conductive hearing loss.
  - Continued screening for auditory deficits; progressive sensorineural hearing loss in the 500–2000-Hz range may occur as the patient gets older.
- Reproductive potential:
  - Contraception and genetic counseling should be discussed and offered to girls who achieve spontaneous puberty (up to one third in mosaic karyotypes).
  - Amniocentesis should be offered to all pregnant women with Turner syndrome because of the high rate of congenital abnormalities. Of pregnancies surviving to term, 30% have major anomalies, including Down syndrome, spina bifida, and congenital heart disease; 35% of liveborn fetuses have Turner syndrome.
  - In vitro fertilization using donated oocytes has achieved as high as 50%–60% success rates.

rhGH, recombinant human growth hormone; SC, subcutaneous; TSH, thyroid-stimulating hormone.

---

testicular function is not impaired until puberty. If gonadal failure occurs prior to or in early puberty, the individual has pubertal delay or stalled pubertal development, and eunuchoid proportions develop. If testicular function is preserved during puberty, normal pubertal changes occur, and the diagnosis may be missed until the person seeks medical assistance for impotence or infertility. Findings include tall stature, gynecomastia, small testes, and a small phallus. Germ cells in the testes are reduced from infancy, but at puberty, hyalinization and fibrosis occur, and the testes become atrophic. The prevalence of breast cancer is 20 times higher in patients with Klinefelter syndrome than healthy men, especially when gynecomastia is present, and Klinefelter syndrome accounts for 4% of breast cancer cases in men. A higher incidence of extragonadal germ cell tumors, autoimmune connective tissue disorders, insulin resistance, and learning disabilities (particularly verbal cognitive deficits and poor impulse control) are reported. Osteoporosis may occur from testosterone deficiency.

Laboratory analysis shows low or low-normal testosterone and elevated gonadotropins (FSH greater than LH concentrations). Diagnosis is confirmed with a karyotype. Testosterone replacement helps improve libido, bone density, and quality of life. Gynecomastia is treated with cosmetic surgery after androgen replacement has begun. Recent advances in the treatment of male infertility, including intracytoplasmic injection of sperm aspirated from testes of men with Klinefelter syndrome, are reported. However, some Klinefelter syndrome patients do not have viable sperm, and analysis of their intratesticular germ cells shows spermatozoa with extra X chromosomes. For these reasons, artificial insemination with donor sperm or adoption are better options for fertility for most patients.

Common Pitfalls

The diagnosis of certain gonadal disorders may be difficult or delayed. For example, constitutional delay in puberty, the most common cause of pubertal delay and a form of hypogonadotropic hypogonadism, is a diagnosis of exclusion that is difficult to differentiate from other causes of hypogonadotropic hypogonadism. A diagnosis of true hypogonadotropic hypogonadism may thus be missed or delayed, particularly in the setting of a family history consistent with constitutional delay. In girls with Turner syndrome, the diagnosis may not be evident from the clinical phenotype. For this reason, we recommend a karyotype for every girl with short stature even in the absence of any features suggestive of Turner syndrome. In situations in which short stature is the only presenting sign, the diagnosis of Turner syndrome is often delayed, and the short time available before growth plate fusion occurs limits the efficacy of GH therapy in improving height potential.

Communication and Counseling

Many patients and parents feel a major sense of loss when informed about limits to their or their child's reproductive capabilities. Although it is important to acknowledge and legitimize these emotions, reproductive assistance options and future directions of reproductive medicine must be mentioned. Parents and children may benefit from counseling and from participating in support groups and meeting others who can personally relate to their situation. Many hypogonadal syndromes are associated with stigmata that may be of concern to parents regarding their child's potential for a normal life. It is, of course, advisable to be honest regarding associated physical and medical problems so the child receives required medical attention. However, also emphasizing the quality of life the child can achieve with proper attention to medical and psychological well-being is essential.

SUGGESTED READINGS

Ambiguous Genitalia (Intersex Disorders)

1. American Academy of Pediatrics Committee on Genetics, Section on Endocrinology, Section on Urology: Evaluation of the newborn with developmental anomalies of the external genitalia. Pediatrics 106:138–142, 2000. **Comprehensive review of diagnosis and management of the neonate with external genitalia abnormalities.**
2. Faisal AS, Hughes I: The genetics of male undermasculinization. Clin Endocrinol 56:1–18, 2002. **A review of the genetics of undermasculinization, the embryology of the genital system, and the investigation of disorders associated with male undermasculinization of prenatal onset.**
3. Gooren LJ, Bunck MC: Androgen replacement therapy: Present and future. Drugs 64:1861–1891, 2004. **Review of general considerations of androgen therapy, available preparations, biochemical and clinical endpoints, and potential negative side effects.**
4. Kipnis K, Diamond M: Pediatric ethics and the surgical assignment of sex. J Clin Ethics 9:398–409, 1998. **Reviews the ethics of surgery and gender assignment.**
5. Lee M, Misra M, Donahoe P, MacLaughlin DT: MIS/AMH in the assessment of cryptorchidism and intersex conditions. Mol Cell Endocrinol 21:91–98, 2003. **Discusses the role of MIS/antimüllerian hormone (AMH) in delineating gonadal pathology and facilitating the differential diagnosis and management of children with various gonadal disorders.**
6. Lerman SE, McAleer IM, Kaplan GW: Sex assignment in cases of ambiguous genitalia and its outcome. Urology 55:8–12, 2000. **A synthesis of available data to aid clinicians in counseling parents regarding decisions of sex of rearing and sex assignment procedures.**
7. MacLaughlin D, Donahoe P: Sex determination and differentiation. N Engl J Med 350:367–378, 2004. **Reviews the molecular**

basis of intersex disorders and the influence on diagnosis and management of these conditions.
8. Sybert VP, McCauley E: Turner's syndrome. N Engl J Med 351:1227–1238, 2004. **Review of the clinical features, diagnosis, management, and genetics of Turner syndrome.**
9. Thomas DFM: Gender assignment: Background and current controversies. BJU Int 93:47–50, 2004. **Discussion of the background of gender assignment and some important unresolved questions and issues.**

Hypogonadism

1. Achermannn J, Weiss J, Lee E, Jameson JL: Inherited disorders of the gonadotropin hormones. Mol Cell Endocrinol 179:89–96, 2001. **A characterization of the molecular basis of gonadotropin deficiency.**
2. Amory JK, Bradley A, Paulsen A, Bremner WJ: Klinefelter's syndrome. Lancet 356:333–335, 2000. **Case presentation and discussion of Klinefelter syndrome: clinical features, laboratory analysis, pathophysiology, and new developments.**
3. Laml T, Preyer O, Umek W, et al: Genetic disorders in premature ovarian failure. Hum Reprod Update 4:483–491, 2002. **Review of the relationship between genetic disorders and premature ovarian failure. Turner syndrome, carriers of fragile X permutation, and certain autosomal disorders are discussed.**
4. Pitteloud N, Hayes FJ, Boepple P, et al: The role of prior pubertal development, biochemical markers of testicular maturation, and genetics in elucidating the phenotypic heterogeneity of idiopathic hypogonadotropic hypogonadism. J Clin Endocrinol Metab 87:152–160, 2002. **Study examining historical, clinical, biochemical, histologic, and genetic features in 78 men with idiopathic hypogonadotropic hypogonadism.**
5. Schlessinger D, Herrer L, Crisponi L, et al: Genes and translocations involved in POF. Am J Med Genet 111:328–333, 2002. **Review of current studies and models demonstrating autosomal defects and X-chromosome changes resulting in POF.**

14

Diabetes Mellitus in Children and Adolescents

Britta M. Svoren and Lori M. B. Laffel

KEY CONCEPTS

- Diabetes mellitus is characterized by inappropriate hyperglycemia that is caused by either impaired insulin secretion or increased insulin resistance.
- Symptoms of marked hyperglycemia include polyuria, polydipsia, and weight loss.
- The diagnosis of diabetes rests on the measurement of plasma glucose levels.
- The tempo of presentation is highly variable for each patient.
- Clinicians should be alert to the possibility of diabetes to prevent progression to diabetic ketoacidosis.
- Since the mid 1980s, there has been an alarming increase in the prevalence of pediatric type 2 diabetes mellitus.

Diabetes mellitus (DM) is a group of metabolic disorders characterized by inappropriate hyperglycemia due to either an absolute deficiency of insulin secretion or a reduction in the biologic effectiveness of insulin (or both). Patients with diabetes frequently present with

BOX 1 Criteria for the Diagnosis of Diabetes Mellitus

- Symptoms of diabetes plus casual plasma glucose concentration ≥200 mg/dL (≥11.1 mmol/L). *Casual* is defined as any time of day without regard to time since last meal. The classic symptoms of diabetes include:
  - Polyuria
  - Polydipsia
  - Unexplained weight loss
  or
- FPG ≥126 mg/dL (≥7.0 mmol/L): Fasting is defined as no calorie intake for at least 8 h.*
  or
- Two-hour plasma glucose ≥200 mg/dL (≥11.1 mmol/L) during an oral glucose tolerance test. The test should be performed as described by the World Health Organization with a glucose load containing the equivalent of 75 g anhydrous glucose dissolved in water* or 1.75 g/kg up to the maximum dose of 75 g.

*Criteria 2 and 3 should be confirmed by repeating testing on separate day.
FPG, fasting plasma glucose.
From Diabetes Care 25:S5–S20, 2002. Copyright © 2002 American Diabetes Association. Reprinted with permission from the American Diabetes Association.

BOX 2 Classification of Diabetes Mellitus

- Type 1 diabetes
  - Immune-mediated
  - Idiopathic
- Type 2 diabetes
  - May range from predominantly insulin-resistant to predominantly insulin-deficient
- Gestational diabetes
- Other specific types
  - Genetic defects of beta-cell function
  - Genetic defects in insulin action
  - Diseases of exocrine pancreas
  - Endocrinopathies
  - Drug- or chemical-induced diabetes
  - Infections
  - Uncommon forms of immune-mediated diabetes
  - Other genetic syndromes sometimes associated with diabetes

From Diabetes Care 25:S5–S20, 2002. Copyright © 2002 American Diabetes Association. Reprinted with permission from the American Diabetes Association.

polyuria, polydipsia, fatigue, and weight loss. Because the timeline of progression from glucose intolerance to overt disease varies for each child, it is important for the clinician to maintain a high index of suspicion for diabetes, as early identification is important to prevent progression to ketoacidosis.

The diagnosis of diabetes rests on the measurement of plasma glucose levels. The diagnostic criteria for diabetes were changed in 1997. One of the most significant changes was that the level of fasting plasma glucose (FPG), recognized as diagnostic for diabetes, was decreased from 140 to 126 mg/dL. Box 1 shows the diagnostic criteria for diabetes.

Different types of diabetes may occur in children and adolescents. The new classification system of diabetes is based on etiology (Box 2). The terms *type 1 diabetes* (T1DM) and *type 2 diabetes* (T2DM) have now eliminated the terms *insulin-dependent* and *non–insulin-dependent* diabetes. T1DM is characterized by absolute insulin deficiency resulting from immune-mediated destruction of beta cells. By comparison, T2DM, often associated with obesity and a family history of the disease, manifests with varying degrees of insulin resistance and relative insulin secretory deficiency. Since the mid 1980s, there has been an alarming increase in the prevalence of pediatric T2DM. Other known causes of diabetes fall into a third category known as "other specific types," which includes the various forms of maturity-onset diabetes of the young (MODY).

Expert Opinion on Management Issues

DIABETIC KETOACIDOSIS

Diabetic ketoacidosis (DKA) constitutes a medical emergency. Severe insulin deficiency causes unrestrained lipolysis and ketoacid production that leads to an anion-gap acidosis characterized by nausea, vomiting, abdominal pain, and hyperpnea. If DKA occurs, the initial goals of therapy are to stabilize the metabolic state using insulin, fluid, and electrolyte replacement.

The initial clinical evaluation is meant to establish the diagnosis, determine the precipitating event (especially to seek evidence of infection), and assess the patient's hydration and baseline neurologic status. Blood samples for measurement of plasma glucose, electrolytes, total carbon dioxide, blood urea nitrogen, serum osmolality, venous pH, partial pressure of carbon dioxide (P_{CO_2}), complete blood count, calcium, magnesium, and phosphorus should be obtained. A urinalysis and appropriate specimens for culture (blood, urine, throat) should be obtained as dictated by the history and physical examination.

To initiate fluid and electrolyte treatment, 10 mL/kg of isotonic saline solution is administered as a bolus. In the severely dehydrated patient or the patient in shock, an additional 10mL/kg may be indicated. Once the circulation has been stabilized, the intravenous fluids are adjusted with the aim of achieving slow correction of the serum hyperosmolality and avoiding rapid fluid shifts. An intravenous infusion of regular insulin diluted in normal saline (50 units in 50 mL) is recommended. Intravenous insulin is given at a rate of 0.1 U/kg/hour, controlled by an infusion pump. With the administration of fluid and insulin, close attention must be paid to the serum potassium with the goal of maintaining it in the normal range. All patients with DKA are potassium depleted on presentation and are therefore predisposed to cardiac arrhythmias without adequate replacement. After urine output is established, potassium replacement should begin (Table 1). Once DKA treatment has been initiated, the patient's clinical and laboratory data (including an electrocardiogram (EKG) when potassium levels are abnormal), details of fluid and electrolyte therapy, administered

TABLE 1 Recommended Potassium Replacement during Treatment of Diabetic Ketoacidosis

Plasma Potassium (mEq/L) (normal 3.0–4.5)	Infusate Potassium Concentration (mEq/L)
<3.0	40–60
3.0–4.5	30–40
4.5–5.0	20
>5.0	0

insulin, and urine output should be meticulously recorded in a flowchart so that timely adjustments in the treatment regimen can be made when necessary.

When DKA has resolved (venous pH >7.32, total carbon dioxide >18 mEq/L), the change to subcutaneous insulin is planned. The first injection should be given 60 to 90 minutes before stopping the insulin infusion, to allow sufficient time for the injected insulin to be absorbed.

CEREBRAL EDEMA

Cerebral edema is an uncommon complication of DKA that can occur before or at any time during treatment. It typically manifests as headache, vomiting, gradual deterioration in level of consciousness, slowing of the heart rate, and an increase in blood pressure. When cerebral edema is suspected, the rate of fluid administration should be reduced, intravenous mannitol (0.25 to 1 g/kg) should be administered, and transfer to an intensive care setting should be arranged.

INSULIN THERAPY

Subcutaneous insulin is started in a child with newly diagnosed T1DM who is not significantly dehydrated, is not vomiting, and does not have ketoacidosis. Insulin therapy is also used for youth with T2DM presenting with metabolic instability. The aim of insulin replacement in the treatment of diabetes is to simulate the fluctuations in plasma insulin levels that are normally seen in nondiabetic individuals. A generally acceptable insulin regimen for children with newly diagnosed diabetes is two or three injections per day consisting of a mixture of human intermediate-acting Neutral Protamine Hagedorn (NPH) and regular or rapid-acting analogues such as lispro or aspart insulin. When a two-dose regimen is used, the total daily dose is typically divided so that approximately two thirds is given before breakfast and one third is given before supper. With a three-dose regimen, short- or rapid-acting insulin is administered before supper, and the second dose of intermediate-acting insulin is given at bedtime rather than before the evening meal. The initial ratio of short/rapid- to intermediate-acting insulin at both times is approximately 1:2. With the current understanding of the link between intensive insulin therapy and prevention of microvascular complications, many would advocate beginning a multiple (>2) daily injection program from the time of initial diagnosis.

Although insulin has been available for more than 80 years, major advances in its clinical use have been made over the past two decades. Much of the progress is a result of three factors:

1. The introduction of self-monitoring of blood glucose
2. A change in the philosophy of diabetes management, such that patient self-management and flexibility in lifestyle have come to drive treatment approaches
3. The development of insulin analogues that have time-action profiles aligned with physiologic insulin secretion.

Table 2 summarizes the action profiles of the various insulin preparations currently available for use in the United States.

More aggressive insulin treatment with a combination of long-acting (Ultralente or Lantus), intermediate-acting (NPH), and short/rapid-acting (regular, lispro, aspart) insulin; three to four injections per day; or continuous subcutaneous insulin infusion (CSII) with a portable pump can provide means to more closely simulate normal insulin profiles and avoid some of the problems with the standard two-shot schedule. However, intensified insulin therapy takes more effort and commitment on the part of patients and their parents, and much support is required from the treatment team. Nevertheless, the results from the Diabetes Control and Complications Trial (DCCT) indicate that such an effort is worth the investment in terms of reduced risk of microvascular complications.

ORAL HYPOGLYCEMIC THERAPY

For youth with T2DM, some clinicians initiate oral pharmacologic therapy upon diagnosis. Others prescribe insulin until stable metabolic control is achieved and then transition the patient to oral therapy. In the United States, the only oral agent currently approved for the treatment of T2DM in children and adolescents is metformin. Metformin is a biguanide that decreases hepatic glucose production and increases insulin-mediated glucose uptake in peripheral tissues. Metformin may aid weight loss because it has a mild anorectic effect in some patients and has the additional benefit of modestly lowering triglyceride and low-density lipoprotein (LDL) concentrations. Lactic acidosis is a rare, potentially fatal side effect of metformin. Provided that metformin is not administered to patients with renal insufficiency, poor tissue perfusion, or those undergoing procedures requiring contrast agents or anesthesia, the risk of lactic acidosis is not increased compared with that of other antihyperglycemic agents.

DIABETES CARE IN THE OUTPATIENT SETTING

One of the most important factors determining whether young patients with diabetes go on to develop late degenerative complications is the adequacy of diabetes care received during childhood. However, the rapid

14

TABLE 2 Time Course of Action of Human Insulin Preparations

Insulin Preparation	Onset of Action	Peak Action	Effective Duration of Insulin Preparation
Rapid-Acting Insulin Analogues			
Insulin lispro	5–15 min	30–90 min	3–5 h
Insulin aspart	5–15 min	30–90 min	3–5 h
Insulin glulisine*	5–15 min	30–90 min	3–5 h
Short-Acting Insulin			
Regular	30–60 min	2–3 h	5–8 h
Intermediate-Acting Insulins			
NPH[†]	2–4 h	4–10 h	10–16 h
Lente[‡]	3–4 h	4–12 h	12–18 h
Long-Acting Insulins			
Ultralente	6–10 h	10–16 h	18–24 h
Insulin glargine	2–4 h	Peakless	20–24 h
Insulin detemir*	2–4 h	6–14 h	16–20 h
Insulin Mixtures			
70/30 human mix (70% NPH, 30% regular)	30–60 min	Dual	10–16 h
75/25 lispro analogue mix (75% intermediate, 25% lispro)	5–15 min	Dual	10–16 h
70/30 aspart analogue mix (70% intermediate, 30% aspart)	5–15 min	Dual	10–16 h
50/50 human mix (50% NPH, 50% regular)	30–60 min	Dual	10–16 h

*FDA approval 2005 for use in adults.
[†]NPH, Neutral Protamine Hagedorn.
[‡]Lente insulin production terminated in 2005.

physiologic and psychosocial changes that occur during childhood and adolescence often make these patients among the most challenging to manage. Children with diabetes should, therefore, be managed by a multidisciplinary diabetes team consisting of a pediatric endocrinologist or pediatrician with training in diabetes, a pediatric diabetes nurse educator (DNE), a dietitian, and a mental health professional.

Education is necessary not only for new diabetes patients and their families but also for patients with diabetes of any duration. The importance of self-monitoring of blood glucose (SMBG) should be emphasized and instructions on recording of data should be provided. Patients and their families should be taught to adjust the timing and quantity of their insulin dose, food, and exercise in response to their recorded blood glucose values, so that optimal blood glucose control is achieved.

Diet and physical activity play critical roles in successful management for both T1DM and T2DM. Involvement of a registered dietitian who is knowledgeable about and comfortable working with children is strongly recommended. An individualized meal plan, using carbohydrate-counting and/or a system of exchanges, should be formulated for each child. Regular exercise and active participation in organized sports have positive implications concerning the psychosocial and physical well-being of young patients and should be encouraged. Patients must be educated that different types of exercise may have different effects on blood glucose levels.

Regular follow-up on a 3-month basis is recommended for each child. The main purpose of these visits is to ensure that the patient is achieving the primary treatment goals of normal growth and development in the absence of significant symptomatic complaints related to hyperglycemia or hypoglycemia. Additionally, 3-month intervals allow for the timely adjustment of insulin dosages.

GOALS OF THERAPY

The American Diabetes Association (ADA) has recommended treatment goals for adolescents 13 years of age or older and for adults with diabetes mellitus: glycosylated hemoglobin (HbA_{1c}) less than 7% (nondiabetic range 4% to 6%), preprandial plasma glucose 90 to 130 mg/dL, and peak postprandial plasma glucose less than 180 mg/dL. Because there are no clinical trial data available for children younger than 13 years of age, clinical judgment is required to determine appropriate goals for children of various ages. It is important to avoid recurrent, severe hypoglycemia in a child younger than 7 years of age whose central nervous system is still developing. Recent treatment recommendations have been published by the ADA.

HYPOGLYCEMIA

Occasional episodes of hypoglycemia are an unavoidable consequence of insulin therapy aimed at maintaining blood glucose levels as close to normal as possible. Patients and family members must be taught to recognize the early symptoms of hypoglycemia and to treat it promptly with a suitable form of concentrated carbohydrate. Most episodes of hypoglycemia are satisfactorily treated with 10 to 20 g of glucose. If the child is unconscious or unable to swallow or retain ingested carbohydrate, glucagon (0.02 to 0.03 mg/kg, maximal dose 1.0 mg) is injected intramuscularly or subcutaneously to raise blood glucose.

SCREENING FOR OTHER AUTOIMMUNE DISEASES AND LONG-TERM COMPLICATIONS

Children with T1DM are at increased risk for the development of autoimmune thyroid disorders and celiac disease. It is suggested that all asymptomatic individuals be screened annually with a thyroid-stimulating hormone (TSH) assay. It has also been suggested that children with T1DM should be screened annually for celiac disease with either antiendomysial or tissue transglutaminase antibodies. If the screening is not routine, the possibility of celiac disease should be considered in any child presenting with poor glycemic control, diarrhea, abdominal pain, or recurrent hypoglycemia. Celiac screening is sometimes complicated by concomitant immunoglobulin (Ig) A deficiency. Referral to a pediatric gastroenterologist may be warranted in the patient with IgA deficiency and any of these clinical concerns.

Diabetic complications develop insidiously. Retinopathy is rare before the onset of puberty or in patients who have had T1DM for less than 5 years. Therefore, annual dilated retinal examinations should begin 5 years after diagnosis or at puberty. Renal disease is first detected by persistent albuminuria. After 5 years of diabetes, an annual screening measurement of urine albumin and creatinine concentrations should be performed to detect microalbuminuria. To monitor for macrovascular disease, blood pressure should be checked at each office visit. A lipid panel should be checked shortly after diagnosis when metabolism has been restored toward normal and repeated as necessary.

Common Pitfalls

- Psychological and social factors influence a patient's or family's success in adhering to any prescribed diabetes regimen.
- Following the diagnosis of diabetes in a child or adolescent, parents grieve the loss of their healthy child. While grieving, they are expected to acquire an understanding of the disease and skills necessary to manage the illness at home.
- Occasional episodes of hypoglycemia are an unavoidable consequence of insulin therapy aimed at maintaining blood glucose levels near normal.
- Children or adolescents with long-standing diabetes or medical complications are subject to "burnout" and have a higher prevalence of depression, anxiety, and eating disorders.

Communication and Counseling

Diabetes is a chronic disease that requires lifelong therapy. However, the overall goals of treatment in children and adolescents have changed substantially over the years. The treatment regimen is adjusted to minimize symptoms of hypoglycemia and hyperglycemia while promoting normal growth and development. Increasing effort is being directed toward maintaining blood glucose profiles as close to normal as possible.

SUGGESTED READINGS

1. American Diabetes Association: Type 2 diabetes in children and adolescents (consensus statement). Diabetes Care 23:381–389, 2000. **Describes treatment goals for children and adolescents with T2DM.**
2. DCCT Research Group: The effect of intensive treatment of diabetes on the development and progression of long-term complications in insulin-dependent diabetes mellitus. N Engl J Med 329:977–986, 1993. **Demonstrates the importance of lowering HbA$_{1c}$ values to reduce the risk of development and progression of microvascular complications.**
3. DCCT Research Group: Effect of intensive diabetes treatment on the development of long-term complications in adolescents with insulin-dependent diabetes mellitus. J Pediatr 125:177–188, 1994. **Shows that adolescents benefit from intensive insulin therapy with a reduction in the occurrence and progression of microvascular complications.**
4. Diabetes Control and Complications Trial/Epidemiology of Diabetes Interventions and Complications Research Group: Effect of intensive therapy on the microvascular complications of type 1 diabetes mellitus. JAMA 287:2563–2569, 2002. **Shows that improved glycemic control is associated with a sustained decreased rate of development of diabetic complications.**
5. Diabetes Prevention Trial-Type 1 Diabetes Study Group: Effects of insulin in relatives of patients with type 1 diabetes mellitus. N Engl J Med 346:1685–1691, 2003. **Shows that insulin therapy does not delay or prevent diabetes in persons at high risk for diabetes.**
6. Fagot-Campagna A, Pettitt DJ, Engelgau MM, et al: Type 2 diabetes among North American children and adolescents: An epidemiologic review and a public health perspective. J Pediatr 136:664–672, 2000. **Describes the increase in the prevalence of pediatric T2DM in North America.**
7. Jones KL, Arslanian S, Peterokova VA, et al: Effect of metformin in pediatric patients with type 2 diabetes: A randomized controlled trial. Diabetes Care 25:89–94, 2002. **Shows that metformin is safe and effective for the treatment of T2DM in pediatric patients.**
8. Laffel LMB, Vangsness L, Connell A, et al: Impact of ambulatory, family-focused teamwork intervention on glycemic control in youth with type 1 diabetes. J Pediatr 142:409–416, 2003. **Shows that successful family involvement assists in the preservation of health and the prevention of long-term diabetes complications for youth with diabetes.**
9. Plotnick LP, Clark LM, Brancati FL, et al: Safety and effectiveness of insulin pump therapy in children and adolescents with type 1 diabetes. Diabetes Care 26:1142–1146, 2003. **Shows that pump therapy is safe and effective in selected children and adolescents with T1DM.**
10. Silverstein J, Slingensmith G, Copeland K, et al: Car of children and adolescents with type 1 diabetes: A statement of the American Diabetes Association. Diabetes Care 28:186–212, 2005. **Provides treatment recommendations including glycemic control guidelines for children and adolescents of all ages with T1DM.**
11. Weissberg-Benchell J, Antisdel-Lomaglio J, Seshadri R: Insulin pump therapy: A meta-analysis. Diabetes Care 26:1079–1087, 2003. **Describes how with appropriate education, training, and support, many children can manage the responsibility of using an insulin pump and benefit from its advantages.**

14

Hypoglycemia

William L. Clarke

KEY CONCEPTS

- The signs and symptoms of hypoglycemia may be confused with those of other disorders, such as epilepsy, tetany, sepsis, or intoxication.
- Hypoglycemia is always the result of an imbalance between glucose production and glucose use.
- Obtaining the critical samples of blood and urine during the hypoglycemic episode are essential to determining the specific cause and, therefore, the specific treatment needed.

Hypoglycemia, or low blood glucose (BG), is a medical emergency requiring immediate recognition and treatment. Unfortunately, the signs and symptoms of this metabolic imbalance can be relatively nonspecific and, therefore, delay its recognition, along with the performance of critical diagnostic tests on samples of blood and urine and immediate therapy. Pediatricians need to include hypoglycemia among the differential diagnoses of many acute problems seen in the emergency department. Prolonged hypoglycemia and/or recurrent asymptomatic hypoglycemic episodes are associated with substantial permanent cognitive and motor deficits.

Definition

A precise (mg/dL) definition of hypoglycemia remains somewhat elusive because various sources suggest different minimal BG levels for infants and children of different ages. Recommendations are often made on BG and symptom associations and/or whether the source of the measurement was plasma or whole blood. It seems reasonable here to assign the term *hypoglycemia* to any BG level 50 mg/dL (2.8 mmol/L) or less, with the understanding that some infants and children are not symptomatic at this level, whereas others may be symptomatic at even higher BG levels. Treatment should be designed to keep BG levels above 60 mg/dL (3.3 mmol/L).

Expert Opinion on Management Issues

The BG level in infants, children, and adults is always the result of the balance between glucose use and glucose production. Intermediary metabolism is carefully tuned to maintain this balance, and thus *any* hypoglycemia represents a pathologic state requiring an investigation of etiology. Hypoglycemia cannot just be treated acutely and dismissed as a variation of normal; whenever hypoglycemia is suspected or identified, it is crucial to obtain critical samples of blood and urine

---

BOX 1 The Critical Samples

When hypoglycemia occurs (either spontaneously or during a diagnostic fast):
- Obtain urine for ketones and reducing substances; store excess for organic acids.
- Obtain sufficient blood for determination of glucose, insulin, cortisol, growth hormone, lactate, and amino acids. Store excess for ketone bodies, free fatty acids, and carnitine.

(Box 1) prior to treatment to aid in the diagnostic evaluation.

GLUCOSE USE

In infants, more than 90% of glucose produced is consumed by the brain. This percentage drops to approximately 40% in adults. With the exception of the brain and red blood cells, all tissues require *insulin* to initiate glucose transport and metabolism. Thus the most common cause of excess glucose use is *hyperinsulinism*, either endogenous or exogenous (as occurs with excess administration of injected insulin; see chapter "Diabetes Mellitus in Children and Adolescents"). Although hyperinsulinism resulting from maternal hyperglycemia or dysregulation of endogenous insulin secretion occurs in the newborn period, occasionally congenital hyperinsulinism (persistent hyperinsulinemic hypoglycemia of infancy [PHHI]) is not identified until later in infancy or childhood. Four different gene defects on chromosome 11 are responsible for PHHI:

1. Sulfonyl urea receptor defects (*SUR1*)
2. Defects in the inward-rectifying potassium channel *Kir6.2* gene
3. Regulatory mutations in the glutamate dehydrogenase (*GDH*) gene
4. An activating glucokinase mutation.

Defects in the *GDH* gene are often associated with a hepatic enzyme disorder and manifest with an associated hyperammonemia. Islet cell adenomas or other islet cell secreting tumors (such as occur with the MEN-1 [multiple endocrine neoplasia] syndrome) are rare in childhood and not discussed here. Any measurable insulin level concurrent with hypoglycemia is evidence of hyperinsulinism and should be treated accordingly. Insulin secretion can also be increased in salicylate intoxication.

GLUCOSE PRODUCTION

Glucose production is the result of gluconeogenesis and/or glycogenolysis. In children, glycogen stores may provide glucose from 4 to 8 hours. After that time, stores are depleted, and glucose must be provided by gluconeogenesis. Gluconeogenesis requires precursors, primarily the amino acids alanine and glutamate; an intact gluconeogenic system; and intact hormonal modulation/direction. Alanine comes primarily from muscle stores, and some children may exhibit a reduced ability to generate this glucose precursor. These children typically present with fasting ketotic hypoglycemia around 2 years of age. Children with ketotic hypoglycemia may require frequent high-carbohydrate feedings, especially when ill, but typically they outgrow this disorder by 8 to 10 years of age. Hypoglycemia with substrate deficiency is also seen with prolonged starvation and severe diarrhea.

Four rate-limiting hepatic enzymes are necessary to convert alanine to glucose: glycogen-6-phosphatase, fructose-1,6-diphosphatase, pyruvate carboxylase, and phosphoenolpyruvate carboxy kinase. Absence or deficiency of any of these results in fasting hypoglycemia and lactic acidosis. Fructose-1-phosphate aldolase deficiency (hereditary fructose intolerance) also interferes with gluconeogenesis and leads to liver and kidney failure as well as hypoglycemia.

Gluconeogenic hormones—cortisol, growth hormone, epinephrine, and glucagon—modulate or direct the process. Deficiencies of cortisol and/or growth hormone are associated with fasting hypoglycemia. Deficiencies of epinephrine and/or glucagon are associated with defective counter-regulation to insulin-induced hypoglycemia in type 1 diabetes.

Gluconeogenesis can be impaired by the ingestion of ethanol. An estimated 5% of children with alcohol intoxication present with hypoglycemia.

Three glycogen storage diseases (GSDs) are associated with hypoglycemia: glucose-6-phosphatase deficiency (type I), amylo-1,6-glucosidase deficiency (debrancher deficiency, type III), and liver phosphorylase deficiency (types VI and IX). GSD type I is the most common. All can be associated with lactic acidosis during prolonged fasting. Glycogen synthetase deficiency, sometimes called GSD 0, an inability to synthesize glycogen, is a rare disorder, associated with ketosis and hypoglycemia during fasting but not lactic acidosis. Galactose-1-phosphate uridyltransferase deficiency (galactosemia) causes postprandial hypoglycemia following the ingestion of galactose, by inhibiting glycogenolysis.

ALTERNATIVE FUELS

During fasting or severe illness, free fatty acids (FFAs) can be mobilized from adipose tissue and used directly or oxidized by the liver to ketone bodies to be used for fuel by muscle. Defects in fatty acid oxidation, such as medium-chain acyl–coenzyme A dehydrogenase (MCAD) deficiency, result in severe hypoglycemia with absence of hyperketonemia/ketonuria. The diagnosis is often made by measurement of plasma acyl carnitine profiles and urinary organic acids and dicarboxylic aciduria. Valproic acid may interfere with FFA oxidation and be associated with hypoglycemia in infants.

INITIAL DIAGNOSTIC EVALUATION

When hypoglycemia is suspected, the initial evaluation may give important clues to its etiology and may make it unnecessary for the child to undergo a diagnostic fast. The history should identify whether or not the episode is related to eating specific substances, to prolonged fasting, or not related to eating. If the examination of the first voided urine reveals reducing substances, galactosemia or hereditary fructose intolerance may be present. Ketonuria with hepatomegaly points to a glycogen storage disease or a hepatic enzyme deficiency. Ketonuria without hepatomegaly suggests an endocrine or substrate deficiency (ketotic hypoglycemia). Absence of ketonuria suggests hyperinsulism or defects in fatty acid oxidation. The additional evidence acquired from the initial critical blood sample should confirm or deny immediate suspicions.

THE DIAGNOSTIC FAST

A diagnostic fast should be undertaken in children for whom the etiology of the hypoglycemic episode is not readily apparent from the history and physical exam and for whom the critical samples were not obtained when the child was hypoglycemic. The fast should occur under carefully monitored circumstances because there is a significant risk of provoking an episode of severe encephalopathy if a defect in fatty acid or carnitine metabolism is present. The fast should include baseline and hypoglycemic critical samples as listed in Box 1. During the fast, which should not exceed 24 to 30 hours, BG should be measured hourly, all urine should be sampled for ketones, and neurologic checks should be performed at least hourly. The fast should be terminated when the stabilized (laboratory) BG is less than 40 mg/dL (2.2 mmol/L) or the child exhibits symptoms of severe hypoglycemia (i.e., severe lethargy, extreme jitteriness, etc.). If feasible and safe, the fast should be terminated with an intravenous glucagon challenge. If glucagon (0.03 mg/kg) elicits a glycemic response (20 to 30 mg/dL rise in BG) within 10 to 20 minutes, hyperinsulinism is the likely cause of the hypoglycemia. A rise in lactate levels strongly suggests a defect in either the glycogenolytic or gluconeogenic pathways.

TREATMENT

The treatment of childhood hypoglycemia, which varies depending on the etiology of the process, is detailed in Box 2.

Common Pitfalls

- Failure to consider hypoglycemia in the differential diagnosis of the extremely ill or lethargic-appearing infant or child
- Failure to obtain an adequate history from caregivers relating to eating patterns and associated symptoms

---

BOX 2 Treatment of Hypoglycemia

Acute Therapy: To Restore Blood Glucose Level to 60 mg/dL or Higher

- Administer 0.2 g/kg bolus of $D_{10}W$, followed by continuous infusion of 0.5 mL/kg/h.
- Repeat bolus if BG level is not restored within 15 minutes.
- Adjust continuous IV glucose rate as needed.

Chronic Therapy: Based on Specific Etiology of Hypoglycemia

- Hyperinsulinism
  - Diazoxide: 5–15 mg/kg/day in 3 doses; start with maximum dose and reduce.
  - Octreotide: 2–5 µg/kg/day and increase to 20 µg/kg/day SC q6–8h as needed.
  - Cornstarch (uncooked): 1–2 g/kg/day q4–6h.
  - Partial pancreatectomy.
- Hormonal deficiencies
  - Cortisol: hydrocortisone, 6–10 mg/m²/day.
  - Growth hormone: 0.3 mg/kg/wk in 7 daily doses each week.
- Substrate deficiencies: Frequent feedings consisting of high-carbohydrate diet
- Glycogen storage diseases (particularly GSD I)
  - Cornstarch: 1–2 g/kg q4–6h.
  - Overnight nasogastric glucose (~8 mg/kg/min).
- MCAD deficiencies
  - Avoid prolonged fasting.
  - ±Oral carnitine. 100 mg/kg/day in 3–4 doses.
- Disorders of gluconeogenesis
  - Fructose-1-phosphate aldolase deficiency (hereditary fructose intolerance): Avoid all fructose-containing foods.
  - Fructose-1,6-diphosphatase deficiency: Avoid prolonged fasting; reduce fructose intake.
  - Other enzyme defects: Avoid prolonged fasting.

BG, blood glucose; $D_{10}W$, 10% aqueous dextrose solution; GSD, glycogen storage disease; IV, intravenous; MCAD, medium-chain acyl-coenzyme A dehydrogenase; qxh, every x hours; SC, subcutaneous.

- Failure to obtain critical urine and blood samples prior to the initiation of glucose-containing intravenous fluids

Communication and Counseling

Hypoglycemia is always a medical emergency requiring immediate treatment. Long-term management requires a treatment strategy based on identifying the underlying cause of the problem. Care should be taken to collect critical samples of blood and urine when the child is experiencing hypoglycemia. Should this not be possible, it is advisable to undertake a controlled, closely monitored diagnostic fast. Treatment of rare metabolic causes of hypoglycemia or persistent hyperinsulinism may require the consultation of experts in specialized centers.

SUGGESTED READINGS

1. Aynsley-Green A, Hussain K, Hall J, et al: Practical management of hyperinsulinism in infancy. Arch Dis Child Fetal Neonatal Ed 82:F98–F107, 2000. **Provides detailed information on the management of hyperinsulinism in infants.**
2. De Lonlay P, Fournet J, Touati G, et al: Heterogeneity of persistent hyperinsulinaemic hypoglycemia. A series of 175 cases. Eur J Pediatr 161:37–48, 2002. **Presents clinical experience in the classification and management of infants with hyperinsulinism.**
3. Finegold D, Stanley C, Baker L: Glycemic response to glucagon during fasting hypoglycemia: An aid in the diagnosis of hyperinsulinism. J Pediatr 96:257–259, 980. **Describes how and when to perform this diagnostic maneuver and how to interpret the results.**
4. Hale D, Bennett M: Fatty acid oxidation disorders: A new class of metabolic diseases. J Pediatr 121:1–9, 1992. **Describes the spectrum of fatty acid disorders and their clinical presentations.**
5. Haymond MW: Hypoglycemia in infants and children. Endocrinol Metab Clin North Am 18:211–252, 1989. **Excellent review of the pathophysiology of childhood hypoglycemia and strategies for identifying its causes.**
6. Stanley C: Advances in diagnosis and treatment of hyperinsulinism in infants and children. J Clin Endocrinol Metab 87:4857–4859, 2002. **Describes the recent progress in identifying and understanding this group of disorders.**
7. Touma E, Charpentier C: Medium chain acyl-CoA dehydrogenase deficiency. Arch Dis Child 67:142–145, 1992. **Discusses the natural history of children with this diagnosis.**
8. Wolfsdorf J, Holm I, Weinstein D: Glycogen storage diseases. Phenotypic, genetic, and biochemical characteristics, ADM therapy. Endocrinol Metab Clin North Am 28:801–823, 1999. **Good source for reviewing the pathophysiology and clinical characteristics of these disorders.**

Diabetes Insipidus, SIADH, and Cerebral Salt Wasting

Rebecca P. Green and Louis J. Muglia

KEY CONCEPTS

- Regulation of arginine vasopressin (AVP) secretion and thirst occur in concert, to maintain serum osmolality within a restricted range.
- Abnormalities in AVP secretion can result in significant and potentially life-threatening perturbations in serum osmolality.
- Diabetes insipidus (DI) is caused by deficient AVP production or action, producing polyuria and polydipsia if thirst is intact; DI can result in hypernatremia when access to water is restricted or thirst response is not normal.
- Excessive nonphysiologic AVP production (syndrome of inappropriate antidiuretic hormone [SIADH]) can result in hyponatremia because of inability to produce a dilute urine and therefore excrete free water adequately.
- If electrolyte imbalance is nonacute, both hyponatremia and hypernatremia should be corrected slowly to protect the brain.

Although water intake and excretion can vary widely in normal individuals, plasma osmolality is normally maintained within the restricted range of 275 to 295 mOsm/L. To limit excursions in osmolality, the thirst mechanism controls water intake and the action of the posterior pituitary hormone arginine vasopressin (AVP), also known as antidiuretic hormone, on the kidney controls urine concentration and, therefore, water excretion. Under normal physiologic conditions, the most important regulator of AVP secretion is plasma osmolality. In healthy persons, the normal set point for initiation of AVP secretion occurs at a plasma osmolality of approximately 280 mOsm/L, although this can vary somewhat. When serum osmolality falls below the osmotic threshold for AVP release, plasma AVP concentration falls, and this reduction in AVP action on the kidney serves to promote excretion of a maximally dilute urine. The resultant loss of free water serves to increase serum osmolality and limit further fluid accumulation. Once the serum osmolality exceeds the threshold for AVP release, increasing AVP release promotes renal water retention, thereby reducing urinary water excretion. Thirst, the conscious sensation of the need to drink, is the essential mechanism by which water losses are replaced. Thirst is regulated by many of the same physiologic factors that regulate AVP release, of which plasma osmolality is the most potent. These two systems typically work in concert to preserve fluid balance and maintain plasma osmolality within a narrow range. When the

regulation of AVP secretion and thirst are perturbed, significant abnormalities of plasma osmolality can occur, and the consequences can be life-threatening.

Expert Opinion on Management Issues

AVP DEFICIENCY: DIABETES INSIPIDUS

Deficiencies in AVP secretion or action, known as diabetes insipidus (DI), result in polyuria, characterized by excretion of abnormally large volumes of dilute urine (exceeding 2 L/m^2/day). In the presence of an intact thirst mechanism, modest increases in plasma osmolality produce an intense thirst response, and the resultant increased water intake (polydipsia) prevents significant increases in serum sodium or osmolality. However, when access to water is restricted or the thirst mechanism is impaired, DI can quickly result in hypernatremia.

The most common form of diabetes insipidus results from primary deficiency of AVP secretion. This is

TABLE 1 Management of Diabetes Insipidus

Generic Name (Trade Name)	Dosage/Route/ Regimen	Maximum Dose	Dosage Formulation	Common Adverse Reactions
Drugs				
Desmopressin (dDAVP)	0.1–2 µg/SC/qd or bid	4 µg/day.	4 µg/mL	Flushing, headache, rhinitis, abdominal pain, dizziness, cough
	2.5–20 µg/IN/qd or bid	40 µg/day.	10 µg/spray; 10 µg/0.1 mL solution	
	0.05–0.6 mg/PO/qd, bid, or tid	1.2 mg/day.	Tablets: 0.1, 0.2 mg	
Vasopressin (Pitressin)	0.5 mU/kg/h, double dose prn q30min to desired effect	10 mU/kg/hr.	20 U/mL	Cramps, nausea, sweating
Hydrochlorothiazide (HCTZ)	2–4 mg/kg/PO/div bid-tid	Age <2 yr: 37.5 mg; age 2–12 yr: 100 mg; age >12 yr: 200 mg.	Solution: 50 mg/5 mL Tablets: 12.5, 25, and 50 mg	Hyponatremia, hypokalemia, metabolic alkalosis, hyperuricemia
Amiloride	0.2–0.4 mg/kg/PO/div tid		Tablets: 5 mg; with HCTZ: 5 mg/50 mg	Headache, weakness, nausea, diarrhea, hyperkalemia
Fluids with dDAVP				
IV or PO fluids	≈1 L/m^2/day IV or PO	Determined by UOP; monitor Na to make adjustments.		Hyponatremia
Fluids Alone				
IVF: 0.225% saline and D5W	0.225% saline at 1 L/m^2/day *plus* D5W to replace urine volumes >40 mL/m^2/ hr	Initial limit of 4–5 L/m^2/ day total fluids, adjusted to maintain Na 145–155 mEq/L.		Hypernatremia; increasing urine volumes if excessive sodium
PO	Normal dietary fluids, added water; limit salt			

bid, twice daily; D5W, dextrose 5% in water (solution); div, divided; IN, intranasal; IV, intravenous; IVF, intravenous fluid; Na, sodium; PO, by mouth; prn, as needed; qd, every day; tid, three times per day; UOP, urinary output.

14

TABLE 2 Identification and Evaluation of Diabetes Insipidus

Important Clinical Information to Identify Diabetes Insipidus	Expected with Diabetes Insipidus
What is the child's intake (and output if this can be quantitated)?	> 2 L/m^2/day.
Is the need to drink and urinate interfering with other activities or waking the child at night?	Need to drink and urinate is unremitting, and may result in bedwetting.
What is the preferred fluid?	Cold water.
What is the appearance of the child's urine?	Light colored to clear.
Is there a psychological component to the need to drink?	Important to exclude psychogenic polydipsia.
Important Clinical Information to Determine Etiology	**What Information Suggests**
Family history of DI?	Familial central or nephrogenic DI.
History or physical exam suggesting deficit or excess of other pituitary hormones?	Central DI caused by structural, invasive, or destructive process.
Are there any signs or symptoms suggestive of CNS mass?	Central DI caused by CNS tumor/mass lesion.
Is there any bone pain or rash?	Langerhans cell histocytosis.
Any known kidney disease or risk factor for kidney dysfunction?	Nephrogenic DI.
Other ongoing medical problems?	CNS structural abnormalities, infection, hypoxic injury, head injury, autoimmune disease.
Evaluation of Possible DI	**Interpretation**
Random serum sodium and osmolality *plus* urinalysis and urine osmolality	Serum Na usually normal if unrestricted access to water and normal thirst. However, serum Na >145 and Osm >300 in presence of urine Osm <600 suggests DI.
First-morning urine specific gravity/osmolality	Greater than 600 mOsm/kg not consistent with DI.
BUN/creatinine	Evidence of an ongoing kidney disease that could produce nephrogenic DI.
Potassium, calcium, and glucose	Hypokalemia, hypercalcemia, and hyperglycemia associated with AVP-resistant polyuria and polydipsia.
Water deprivation test	Allows confirmation of suspected diagnosis and differentiation of central and nephrogenic DI.

AVP, arginine vasopressin; BUN, blood urea nitrogen; CNS, central nervous system; DI, diabetes insipidus; Na, sodium.

known as central diabetes insipidus (CDI). The degree of polyuria and polydipsia depend on the extent of the deficiency, level of renal function, dietary salt load, and function of other endocrine systems. CDI responds well to treatment with aqueous AVP (Pitressin) or the longer lived AVP analogue desmopressin acetate (dDAVP). dDAVP can be administered by subcutaneous injection, by nasal spray, or by mouth, and it is the preferred therapy for CDI in the outpatient setting (Table 1). In the context of dDAVP therapy, excessive fluid intake should be avoided, because hyponatremia may result. However, in some settings it may be more practical to manage CDI with fluids alone. This is true in the setting of acute CDI following central nervous system (CNS) surgery, a situation in which the DI may be transient or may be followed by a period in which ADH secretion is inappropriately high (syndrome of inappropriate antidiuretic hormone [SIADH]). Infants with CDI, who have large obligate fluid requirements for nutrition, may be at risk of fluid overload and hyponatremia if treated with dDAVP; thus managing them with fluids alone may be the best strategy. If AVP or dDAVP are not being used, any unnecessary salt intake should be avoided because it will result in increased urine volumes.

Nephrogenic diabetes insipidus is caused by renal resistance to the action of AVP, and it is characterized by impaired urinary concentrating ability, despite normal or elevated AVP levels. As expected in this setting, Pitressin and dDAVP do not prevent the associated polyuria, and providing adequate fluid intake is critical. Urine volumes can be reduced by minimizing dietary solute load and, if polyuria is severe, addition of thiazide diuretics with or without amiloride. These medications may also be useful in infants with CDI who are being managed without dDAVP.

Table 2 lists the pertinent clinical details to look for when considering a diagnosis of DI. Diagnosis often involves the use of a water deprivation test (Box 1). Once the diagnosis of central or nephrogenic DI is made, a critical component of the initial management is a careful search for the cause (Box 2). When hypernatremia has developed in the setting of DI, it is corrected by administering free water, as detailed in Box 3.

SYNDROME OF INAPPROPRIATE ANTIDIURETIC HORMONE

The body's primary defense against developing hyponatremia is the kidney's ability to generate dilute urine and excrete free water, a process inhibited by AVP. Figure 1 illustrates an approach to hyponatremia. When AVP secretion is increased, maximally dilute

---

BOX 1 Water Deprivation Testing for Suspected Diabetes Insipidus

Water Deprivation Phase

- Obtain initial weight, vital signs.
- Place IV line to assist with repeated blood drawing. Place Foley catheter in children too young to provide hourly voided urine specimens.
- Draw baseline serum sodium, vasopressin, and collect urine for osmolality and specific gravity.
- Begin water deprivation.
- Measure and record hourly on flow sheet:
  - Weight, HR, BP, urine output, and urine specific gravity.
  - Stat laboratory testing: serum sodium and urine osmolality.
- If Na <145 mEq/L, urine osmolality <600 mOsm/L, and there is no evidence of significant symptomatic hypovolemia, continue water deprivation.
- If urine osmolality is >1000 mOsm/L or >600 mOsm/L and stable over two measures, stop test. Patient does not have diabetes insipidus.
- If serum osmolality is >300 mOsm/L and urine osmolality is <600 mOsm/L, the patient has diabetes insipidus. Proceed to vasopressin response phase.

Vasopressin Response Phase

- Collect blood for vasopressin level.
- Administer Pitressin SC, 1 U/m^2.
- Allow the patient to eat and drink, limiting fluid intake to the volume of urine produced during the entire testing period.
- Measure vital signs, urine output, and urine specific gravity and send urine to laboratory for osmolality 30 and 60 min after Pitressin.
  - A twofold increase in urine osmolality indicates central diabetes insipidus.
  - An increase of less than twofold in urine osmolality is consistent with nephrogenic diabetes insipidus.

BP, blood pressure; HR, heart rate; IV, intravenous; Na, sodium; SC, subcutaneous.

BOX 2 Causes of Diabetes Insipidus

Central Diabetes Insipidus: Deficiency of AVP Secretion

Genetic Causes

- Mutations in AVP-neurophysin gene
  - Familial autosomal dominant
  - Familial autosomal recessive (rare)
- Wolfram syndrome
- Congenital absence of posterior pituitary

Acquired

- Tumors
  - Craniopharyngioma
  - Germinoma
  - Pinealoma
  - Leukemia/lymphoma
- Traumatic injury: may see "triple phase" (DI→SIADH→DI)
  - CNS surgery
  - Head trauma
  - Hypoxia
- CNS infection
  - Meningitis
  - Encephalitis
  - Congenital infection
- Inflammatory/infiltrative
  - Langerhans cell histiocytosis
  - Systemic lupus erythematosus
  - Neurosarcoidosis
  - Lymphocytic neurohypophysitis
- Idiopathic

Nephrogenic DI: Deficiency of AVP Action

Genetic Causes

- Mutations in AVP V2R: X-linked
- Mutations in aquaporin-2 water channel
  - Autosomal recessive
  - Autosomal dominant (rare)

Acquired

- Drug induced:
  - Lithium
  - Foscarnet
  - Many others (rarely)
- Metabolic causes
  - Hypokalemia
  - Hypercalcemia
  - Protein malnutrition
- Kidney injury/disease
  - Chronic renal failure
  - Ischemic injury
  - Medullary damage
  - Obstruction

AVP, arginine vasopressin; CNS, central nervous system; DI, diabetes insipidus; SIADH, syndrome of inappropriate antidiuretic hormone; V2R, vasopressin receptor.

---

urine cannot be produced. SIADH results from an abnormality in the regulation of AVP, resulting in excessive, nonphysiologic AVP secretion. If water intake is not reduced sufficiently to match the reduction in urine output, free water accumulates, resulting in the development of hypotonic hyponatremia. When the expansion of body water exceeds 5% to 6%, plasma renin activity and aldosterone are suppressed, atrial natriuretic peptide levels increase, and urine sodium excretion begins to increase. These compensatory mechanisms interrupt further increase in the extracellular volume expansion but aggravate the hyponatremia.

When hyponatremia is mild or develops slowly, it usually produces few or no symptoms and may go unrecognized for long periods of time. When symptoms occur, they can include anorexia, headache, nausea, emesis, muscle cramping, weakness, altered responsiveness, obtundation, and/or seizures. In its most severe form, hyponatremia may progress to frank cerebral edema and herniation. Children appear to be more susceptible to symptomatic hyponatremia after closure of the fontanelles, presumably because of a greater brain-to-skull size, which leaves less room for brain expansion.

SIADH is one of many causes of hyponatremia (Box 4). Determining the etiology of the hyponatremia is critical because management of the various etiologies of hyponatremia differ dramatically, and inappropriate management may worsen the hyponatremia. In addition, not only the etiology of the hyponatremia but also its duration, degree, and the presence or absence of symptoms are important considerations when deciding on the optimal management of hyponatremia.

BOX 3 Correction of Hypernatremia in Diabetes Insipidus

- The net increase in body water that must be achieved to correct the deficit can be estimated by this formula: $\Delta H_2O = [(P_{Na} - 140)/140] \times 0.6 \times BW$, where H_2O is the estimated water deficit in liters; P_{Na} is the plasma sodium concentration expressed in mEq/L; and BW is the body weight in kg.
- Nonacute hypernatremic dehydration (present for >12 h) or hypernatremic dehydration of uncertain duration should be corrected over a minimum of 24–48 h, avoiding changes greater than 0.5–1 mEq/h to prevent cerebral edema and the resultant herniation, which can be devastating.
- The fluid administration rate is determined by the free water deficit, divided by the desired time over which the deficit is to be replaced, added to fluid administration sufficient to replace estimated or measured renal and GI output and estimated insensible losses.
- The portion of the fluids used for correction of the free water deficit (and to replace urine output in nephrogenic DI or central DI not treated with dDAVP) should have minimal solute, ideally enteral water, if this route is available, or D5W, if it is not.
- During the correction of hypernatremia, fluid intake, output, and plasma sodium should be monitored frequently, and the treatment plan adjusted as necessary to achieve the desired rate of correction.

dDAVP, desmopressin acetate; D5W, dextrose 5% in water (solution); DI, diabetes insipidus; GI, gastrointestinal.

If SIADH is present, the underlying cause should be identified and treated when possible and the excess in body water should be corrected. If the primary abnormality in AVP secretion is caused by ectopic production by a tumor, excessive dDAVP, deficiency of glucocorticoid or thyroid hormone, or release from the posterior pituitary in response to drugs that can be discontinued, the AVP excess can be corrected. However, much of the time, the abnormal secretion of AVP must be allowed to run its course until spontaneous recovery occurs. Fortunately, SIADH is generally temporary, and therapy is only necessary until the SIADH remits.

When the sodium is above 120 mEq/L and significant symptoms are not present, fluid restriction is the optimal therapy by which the hyponatremia can be corrected and sodium stabilized. To promote an increase in serum sodium, fluid restriction to amounts less than obligate urine and insensible losses is required, generally 600 to 800 mL/m²/day. The goal is to promote a gradual increase in plasma sodium, followed by stabilization in the normal range. When hyponatremia is not acute, rapid correction can be associated with central pontine myelinolysis, a rare and sometimes fatal neurologic demyelinating disorder. Patients in whom hyponatremia has been present for more than 48 hours may have few symptoms but are more likely to have serious complications from rapid correction of their hyponatremia. The target is to increase the sodium at most to 0.5 mEq/hour or 12 mEq/day. Once the sodium rises into the desired range, maintenance of sodium in that range can generally be achieved with a fluid restriction of

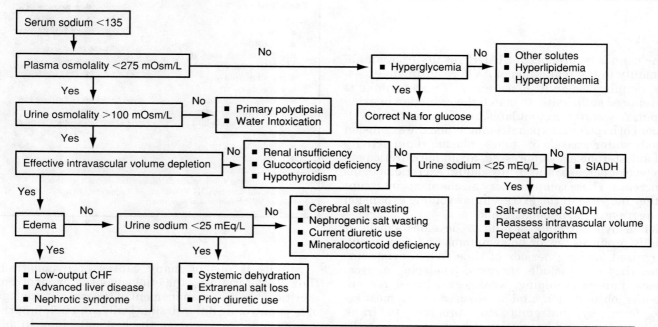

FIGURE 1. Diagnostic approach to hyponatremia. CHF, congestive heart failure; Na, sodium; SIADH, syndrome of inappropriate antidiuretic hormone.

BOX 4 Causes of Hyponatremia

Decreased AVP Secretion

- Water intoxication
  - Primary polydipsia
  - Infants fed dilute formula
- Renal failure

Increased AVP Secretion

Euvolemic State: SIADH

- Neoplasms (rare in children)
  - Bronchogenic carcinoma
  - Other lung tumors
  - Head and neck tumors
- Respiratory disease
- CNS disorders
  - Inflammatory processes: SLE, sarcoidosis, Guillain-Barré syndrome
  - Infection: Tuberculous meningitis, other meningitis or encephalitis, CNS abscess
  - Injury: may be part of triple phase (DI→SIADH→DI)
- Drugs/Medications
  - Carbamazepine
  - Chlorpropamide
  - Vinblastine
  - Vincristine
  - Tricyclic antidepressants
  - Ecstasy
- Postsurgical stress
- Glucocorticoid deficiency
- Severe hypothyroidism

Hypovolemic State

- Systemic dehydration
  - Gastroenteritis
  - NG suction
- Salt loss
  - Diuretic use
  - Renal disease
  - Diarrhea
  - Burns
  - Cystic fibrosis
  - Cerebral salt wasting

Hypervolemic State

- Nephrotic syndrome
- Congestive heart failure
- Cirrhosis with ascites

ADH, antidiuretic hormone; AVP, arginine vasopressin; CNS, central nervous system; DI, diabetes insipidus; NG, nasogastric; SIADH, syndrome of inappropriate antidiuretic hormone; V2R, vasopressin receptor.

---

the aim of raising serum sodium more quickly. Because of the risk of central pontine myelinolysis, hypertonic saline should be used only to the extent necessary to raise plasma sodium to levels above those that cause symptoms. Normal saline alone is not appropriate for the treatment of severe hyponatremia in SIADH because the sodium infused will be rapidly excreted while water is retained, potentially worsening the hyponatremia.

CEREBRAL SALT WASTING

Following CNS injury or surgery, a syndrome of polyuria associated with increased urine sodium, volume depletion, and hyponatremia is described and known as cerebral salt wasting (CSW). This form of hyponatremia is associated with primary renal salt losses in the absence of primary renal disease, and it is now postulated to be caused by excessive secretion of natriuretic peptide. It is critical to distinguish CSW from the other two major disturbances of water metabolism that can occur associated with CNS injury: CDI and SIADH. All of these syndromes share some clinical features (Table 3), yet the distinction between the disorders is of considerable clinical importance, given the divergent nature of the treatments.

Common Pitfalls

- Rapid correction of nonacute hypernatremia or hyponatremia can result in life-threatening complications.
- Excessive administration of sodium, such as sodium-containing intravenous fluids, can drive up urine output and worsen hypernatremia when managing CDI without dDAVP.
- When dDAVP is being used to manage CDI, excessive fluid administration or intake must be avoided to prevent hyponatremia.
- Adequate clinical assessment of the cause of hyponatremia is critical because SIADH requires a markedly different treatment approach than other causes of hyponatremia.
- Administration of isotonic saline can worsen hyponatremia in the setting of SIADH if provided at greater than the rate of insensible and urine volume loss.

Communication and Counseling

In the setting of DI or SIADH, the dissociation between urine output and hydration status is counterintuitive for both physician inexperienced with these diseases and for parents of affected children. Therefore, parents need to be carefully educated about the disease process, so they can play an active role in helping

---

0.8 to 1 $L/m^2/day$. Fluid restriction can be difficult in infants and young children because the water content of formula or infant food is relatively high, and fluid restriction may result in unintentional caloric restriction.

Symptomatic hyponatremia is a medical emergency requiring prompt treatment to prevent permanent brain damage or death. Therefore symptomatic or severe hyponatremia should be treated by administration of hypertonic saline in addition to fluid restriction, with

TABLE 3 Distinguishing Characteristics of Central Diabetes Insipidus, SIADH, and Cerebral Salt Wasting

Feature	CDI	SIADH	CSW
Plasma volume	Decreased	Increased	Decreased
Clinical signs of volume depletion	Present	None	Present
Serum sodium/osmolality	High	Low	Low
Urine sodium/osmolality	Low	High	High
Urine flow rate	Increased	Decreased	Increased
Plasma renin activity	High	Low	Low
Plasma aldosterone	High	Low or normal	Low
Plasma AVP	Low	High	Low or normal
BUN/creatinine	Low/high	Low/low	High/high
Hematocrit	Increased	Decreased	Increased
Albumin	Increased	Decreased	Increased
Serum uric acid	High	Low	Low or normal
Atrial or brain natriuretic peptide	High	High	High
Treatment	Salt-poor fluid replacement	Fluid restriction	Salt and fluid replacement

AVP, arginine vasopressin; BUN, blood urea nitrogen; CDI, central diabetes insipidus; CSW, cerebral salt wasting; SIADH, syndrome of inappropriate antidiuretic hormone.

to avoid fluid overload or severe dehydration in their children.

SUGGESTED READINGS

1. Baylis PH: The syndrome of inappropriate antidiuretic hormone secretion. Int J Biochem Cell Biol 35:1495–1499, 2003. **Review of SIADH, its etiologies and management.**
2. Betjes MG: Hyponatremia in acute brain disease: The cerebral salt wasting syndrome. Eur J Intern Med 13:9–14, 2002. **Review of CWS, suggesting it is relatively common.**
3. Cheetham T, Baylis PH: Diabetes insipidus in children: Pathology, diagnosis and management. Pediatr Drugs 4:785–796, 2002. **Current review of pathogenesis, evaluation, and therapy for diabetes insipidus.**
4. Decaux G, Soupart A: Treatment of symptomatic hyponatremia. Am J Med Sci 326:25–30, 2003. **Reviews brain adaption to hyponatremia and treatment of acute and chronic hyponatremia.**
5. Maghnie M, Cosi G, Genovese E, et al: Central diabetes insipidus in children and young adults. N Engl J Med 343:998–1007, 2000.

Review of 26 years of CDI characterizing common clinical presentations.
6. Morello JP, Bichet DG: Nephrogenic diabetes insipidus. Ann Rev Physiol 63:607–630, 2001. **Current review of biology of nephrogenic diabetes insipidus.**
7. Oh MS: Pathogenesis and diagnosis of hyponatremia. Nephron 92(Suppl 1):2–8, 2002. **Describes the classifications of hyponatremia and their distinctions.**
8. Pogacar PR, Mahnke S, Rivkees SA: Management of central diabetes insipidus in infancy with low renal solute load formula and chlorothiazide. Curr Opin Pediatr 12:405–411, 2000. **Description of use of salt restriction and thiazide diuretic to manage CDI in infancy.**
9. Singh SK, Unnikrishnan AG, Reddy VS, et al: Cerebral salt wasting syndrome in a patient with a pituitary adenoma. Neurol India 51:110–111, 2003. **Review of CSW, suggesting it is not common.**
10. Smith DM, McKenna K, Thompson CJ: Hyponatremia. Clin Endocrinol (Oxf) 52:667–678, 2000. **Reviews classifications of hyponatremia and management.**
11. Verbalis JG: Disorders of body water homeostasis. Best Pract Res Clin Endocrinol Metab 17:471–503, 2003. **Describes regulation of total body water balance and disorders that perturb it.**

15 Metabolic Disorders

An Approach to the Treatment of Metabolic Disease

Russell W. Chesney

KEY CONCEPTS

- Metabolic diseases represent inborn errors of metabolism and are usually recessive.
- Metabolic diseases often manifest with acidosis.
- Many metabolic diseases are evaluated by means of the neonatal genetic screenings.
- Tandem mass spectrometric methods currently may detect 40 disorders.
- Severe acute metabolic diseases of infancy often present in a fashion similar to neonatal sepsis or congenital heart disease.
- Neonates or infants with a metabolic disease may have a peculiar odor.
- Rapid diagnosis may be lifesaving.

If one suspects that a neonate or young child suffers from a metabolic disease, the imperative is to make a rapid diagnosis and initiate early therapy so as to forestall considerable morbidity and/or mortality. This chapter discusses the fundamental cause of these disorders and how to rapidly screen for disease.

Although the term *metabolic disease* may denote diabetes mellitus or chronic renal insufficiency, in this context it denotes an acute disorder, also termed an *inborn error of metabolism*. These metabolic diseases usually manifest acutely and are due to a monogenic mutation that affects the protein products synthesized by the particular mutated genes. Structural proteins, enzymes, receptors, transport systems, or intracellular structure can be affected, and the given mutation may result in attenuation of the quantity of protein synthesized or in the amino acid sequence of the primary protein. The fundamental consequences of these mutations are that they interrupt the process of intermediary metabolism, depriving the body of energy. These mutated proteins fail to function to remove excess metabolites, built up from prior steps, or fail to produce other metabolites at distal steps in metabolic pathways.

For this reason, disorders of virtually each step in metabolism may manifest in a stereotypic fashion. While most mutations are polymorphisms and do not confer appreciable clinical consequences, some mutations result in severe or potentially lethal disease. Most of these severe disorders have a neonatal or infantile presentation. Often evident is an abnormal urinary and/or plasma value of a specific metabolite (amino acid, organic acid, fatty acid, or ammonia). Less often these conditions manifest in childhood after the stress of a viral infection or sepsis.

Expert Opinion on Management Issues

The clinical features of metabolic disorders are broad and may resemble neonatal sepsis or congenital heart disease. Lethargy, coma, hypotonia, failure to thrive, metabolic acidosis with a high or normal anion gap, reduced serum glucose levels and, often, a strange odor are features. Other features are tachycardia, hyperpnea, rash, cardiomegaly, hepatomegaly, corneal opacity, cataract formation, retinitis, optic atrophy, deafness, and various dysmorphic features. Hepatic disease may progress to jaundice, cirrhosis, and hepatic failure.

When metabolic disease occurs in the neonatal period, it can be life-threatening. Hence, a high index of suspicion is necessary. Screening for symptoms of a metabolic disease can be performed prenatally (for those at risk based upon a family history), neonatally, and after death (metabolic autopsy). Although only a few disorders are detected with standard screening procedures, many states are converting to tandem mass spectrometry (Table 1). This methodology is so valuable that it will likely be used worldwide.

A simple starting point when confronted with an ill neonate is a family history along with a physical examination, and measurement of electrolytes, glucose, bicarbonate, ammonia and pH. If ammonia is elevated and the pH and bicarbonate are normal (or slightly alkalotic), a urea cycle defect should be suspected. If the pH is low, in the face of hyperammonemia, then an organic acidemia is more likely. With jaundice, galactosemia or fructosemia are possible. Likewise, the determination of urinary ketonuria is important, especially as a clue of organic or fatty acid acidosis. Other useful laboratory tests for initial evaluation are plasma

TABLE 1 Newborn Screening

Genetic Disorder	Estimated Incidence	Prevention of Morbidity by Early Diagnosis	Conventional Screening Program	Detectable By MS/MS Analysis
Classic phenylketonuria (PKU)	1:10,000	+++	Yes	Yes
Other hyperphenylalaninemias	1:20,000	+	Yes	Yes
Homocystinuria	1:150,000	+++	Yes	Yes
Maple syrup urine disease (MSUD)	1:180,000	+++	Yes	Yes
Biotinidase deficiency	1:100,000	+++	Yes	Yes
Hemoglobinopathies	1:2,000	+++	Yes	Yes
Congenital adrenal hyperplasia	1:12,000	+++	Yes	Possible
Congenital hypothyroidism	1:4,000	+++	Yes	No
Galactosemias	1:50,000	+++	Yes	No
Cystic fibrosis	1:2,000	+	Yes	No
MCAD deficiency	1:17,000	+++	No	No
Glutaric acidemia type I	1:30,000	+++	No	No
Tyrosinemias	1:100,000	+++	No	No
CPS deficiency	1:80,000	+	No	Possible
OTC deficiency	1:80,000	+	No	Possible
Citrullinemia	1:80,000	+	No	Yes
Argininosuccinic aciduria	1:80,000	+	No	Yes
Arginase deficiency	1:100,000	+	No	Possible
HHH syndrome	Unknown	+	No	Possible
Nonketotic hyperglycinemia	1:250,000	−	No	Yes
Propionic acidemias	1:50,000	+	No	Yes
Methylmalonic acidemias	1:50,000	+	No	Yes
Isovaleric acidemia	1:50,000	+	No	Yes
Methylcrotonyl-CoA carboxylase deficiency	Unknown	+	No	Yes
HMG-CoA lyase deficiency	Unknown	+	No	Yes
Glutaric acidemia type II, severe form	1:100,000	−	No	Yes
Glutaric acidemia type II, mild form	1:100,000	+	No	Yes
Carnitine uptake defect	Unknown	+++	No	Possible
Translocase deficiency	Unknown	+	No	Yes
CPT II deficiency	Unknown	+	No	Yes
VLCAD deficiency	1:50,000	+	No	Yes
TFP/LCHAD deficiency	1:40,000	+	No	Yes
SCAD deficiency	Unknown	+	No	Yes

CPS, carbamoylphosphate synthetase; CPT, carnitine palmitoyltransferase; HHH, hyperornithinemia-hyperammonemia-homocitrullinuria; HMG-CoA, 3-hydroxy-3-methylglutaryl-coenzyme A; LCHAD, long-chain 3-hydroxyacyl-CoA dehydrogenase; MCAD, medium-chain acyl-CoA dehydrogenase; OTC, ornithine transcarbamylase; SCAD, short-chain acyl-CoA dehydrogenase; TFP, trifunctional protein; VLCAD, very-long-chain acyl-CoA dehydrogenase; +, treatment is available but the prognosis is guarded in most patients; +++, effective treatment is available; −, disorders that will be detected by MS/MS but are currently considered untreatable.

From Rinaldo P, Matern D: Biochemical diagnosis of inborn errors of metabolism. In Rudolph CD, Rudolph AM, Hostetter MK, et al. (eds): Rudolph's Pediatrics, 21st ed. New York: McGraw-Hill, 2004.

pyruvate and lactate, which are elevated in several mitochondrial disorders.

Early and accurate diagnosis is imperative in the treatment of metabolic disorders so that appropriate treatment can be initiated. This therapy may include dietary protein restriction, specific nutritional supplements, amino acid–deficient formula, and supraphysiologic amounts of certain vitamins for cofactor-dependent metabolic disorders.

Drug therapy (and dietary intervention) depends on which metabolic pathway and which step is abnormal. Only then can an appropriate diet be chosen.

Common Pitfalls

Upon occasion a neonate or an infant with metabolic disease will become comatose with evidence of severe acidosis and hypoventilation. The following key sequence of therapies should be tried:

1. Stop all dietary sources of protein.
2. Begin D_{10} at 1.5 to 2 times maintenance dose to block catabolism, add Na^+, K^+, and Cl^- (sodium, potassium, and chloride) as needed.
3. Provide $NaHCO_3$ (sodium bicarbonate) replacement if blood pH is greater than 7.1. In the event of hyperammonemia, use sodium benzoate (5.5 g/m^2), sodium phenylacetate (5.5 g/m^2) and arginine HCl (hydrochloride; 10% solution) at 12 g/m^2. If the patient fails to respond, initiate hemodialysis.

The latter two steps should be performed only under the care of a pediatric biochemical geneticist and a nephrologist.

Communication and Counseling

If a diagnosis of an inborn error of metabolism is established, it is imperative to involve the patient's family. Several messages are crucial. First, these are lifelong disorders. Second, treatment should be lifelong. Third, a failure to treat may result in severe morbidity, illness, mental retardation, and death. Fourth, if a child develops an intercurrent infection, the underlying metabolic disease may worsen. Fifth, communication and contact is important, even lifesaving. Thus, all phone numbers, fax numbers, and e-mail addresses should be exchanged between parents and the staff in the genetic unit (or other caring unit). Sixth, dietary restrictions must be maintained on trips out of the home, at summer camp, or during sleepovers.

These patients require extensive genetic counseling because of recurrence risks (usually one in four births), and because of the need to rapidly evaluate a neonate should a sibling be found to have one of these metabolic disorders. Family members should also be alerted to the presence of one of these disorders in the family.

In these disorders, communication and counseling must be conveyed in a clear and logical fashion. Such sessions should not be rushed. The messages provided may need to be repeated often both within these sessions and at additional sessions.

SUGGESTED READINGS

1. American Academy of Pediatrics: A report from the newborn screening task force. Pediatrics 106:383–427, 2000. **This is an updated and comprehensive statement about this group of diseases from the American Academy of Pediatrics Council on Genetics.**
2. Gunn VL, Nechyba C (eds): Genetics Inborn Errors of Metabolism: Abnormalities of Biochemical Pathways in the Harriet Lane Handbook—The Johns Hopkins Hospital, 16th ed. Philadelphia: Mosby, 2002, pp 267–275. **A succinct and practical guide to many of these disorders with emphasis on screening and urine and plasma assays.**
3. Rezvani I: Metabolic diseases: An approach to inborn errors of metabolism. In Richard E, Behrman RM, Kliegman HB, et al (eds): Nelson Textbook of Pediatrics, 17th ed. Philadelphia: WB Saunders, 2004. **This overview of neonatal metabolic disorders emphasizes their clinical similarity.**
4. Rinaldo P, Matern D: Biochemical diagnosis of inborn errors of metabolism. In Colin D, Rudolph AM, Rudolph MK, et al (eds): Rudolph's Pediatrics, 21st ed. New York: McGraw-Hill, 2004. **This chapter defines the four basic forms of newborn screening and is very practical.**
5. Scriver CR, Beaudet AL, Sly WS, et al (eds) The Metabolic and Molecular Bases of Inherited Disease, 8th ed. New York: McGraw-Hill, 2001. **This three-volume set is the encyclopedia of metabolic disorders and is a text written by "experts."**

15

16 Musculoskeletal System and Connective Tissue

Pediatric Systemic Lupus Erythematosus

Polly J. Ferguson

KEY CONCEPTS

- Systemic lupus erythematosus (SLE) is a phenotypically heterogeneous disease, making diagnosis difficult.
- Autoantibody production to nuclear antigens is a unifying disease manifestation.
- Severity of disease varies widely from individual to individual.
- Pediatric SLE is often more severe than adult SLE.
- Prompt diagnosis and treatment is essential to optimize outcome.
- Treatment must be tailored to the individual.
- There continues to be significant disease- and treatment-associated morbidity and mortality.

Systemic lupus erythematosus (SLE) is an autoimmune disease characterized by antinuclear antibody (ANA) production with widespread immune dysregulation, often resulting in multiorgan system inflammation. Fifteen percent of all lupus cases have onset in childhood. The clinical features of the disease are extremely variable. Not only is there variability in presentation among individuals, but there can also be variability in disease manifestations over time in a single individual. This variability in phenotype has made uncovering the etiology of this multifaceted disease very difficult. Although the etiology of SLE is unknown, it is clear that genetic and environmental factors play an important role in the pathogenesis of the disease. Disease outcomes have improved over the past several decades, but many patients continue to have significant disease- and/or treatment-related morbidity and mortality. The heterogeneity in the phenotype and waxing and waning nature of the disease have made new drug development difficult. In fact, there has not been a new U.S. Food and Drug Administration (FDA)-approved drug for the treatment of lupus for more than 40 years.

Expert Opinion on Management Issues

The treatment of SLE in children must be tailored to maximize disease control, minimize treatment-related side effects, and maintain normal growth and development. Maintaining normal physical and psychological development can be very challenging in pediatric SLE because of the increased disease severity. Most children with SLE require treatment with glucocorticoids at some point in the disease course, which adversely affects linear growth. Additionally, the physical side effects of corticosteroids are poorly tolerated, particularly by adolescents, as the development of exogenous Cushing syndrome in these patients is often accompanied by problems with low self-esteem and other psychosocial issues. Therefore, glucocorticoids should be used in the lowest dose possible to achieve clinical improvement, and a steroid-sparing agent is usually added early in the treatment of pediatric SLE.

Disease manifestations and severity guide the choice of therapeutic agents used to treat lupus in childhood (Box 1). Constitutional symptoms including arthralgia, fatigue, malaise, and weight loss are treated with nonsteroidal anti-inflammatory drugs (NSAIDs) and hydroxychloroquine. When this approach is not efficacious, low-dose steroids may be added (≤ 5 mg prednisone or its equivalent), typically with good results. Cutaneous manifestations of the disease, when present in isolation, can be treated with hydroxychloroquine and topical medications. However, isolated cutaneous disease is infrequent in pediatric SLE. In general, the medications used to treat major organ involvement will control the cutaneous manifestations of the disease. Serositis is usually treated with a short course of low-dose steroids and a NSAID. If the serositis recurs when the steroids are discontinued, a steroid-sparing agent such as azathioprine or methotrexate is typically added to the treatment regimen. Hydroxychloroquine is beneficial in treating arthritis in SLE but may require several months before the maximal benefit is seen. Central nervous system (CNS) inflammation in childhood lupus requires aggressive therapy, often requiring high-dose steroids and cyclophosphamide. Cytopenia in SLE usually responds to low- to moderate-dose corticosteroids; however, occasionally a child

BOX 1 Management of Pediatric Systemic Lupus Erythematosus

General

- Use high-SPF sunscreen throughout the year.
- Encourage good sleep and nutritional patterns.
- Address psychological aspects of disease/treatment.
- Prescribe calcium and vitamin D supplements (especially if on corticosteroids).
- Immunize against pneumococcus.
- Treat with anticoagulant if evidence of antiphospholipid antibody is present (agent depends on if the child has had a clot or not).
- Perform annual ophthalmologic evaluations (especially if on hydroxychloroquine).
- Treat dyslipoproteinemia when present.
- Maintain good blood pressure control in those with hypertension.

Noncytotoxic

- Nonsteroidal anti-inflammatory medications:
  - Prescribe for constitutional symptoms (arthralgia, fatigue, malaise).
  - Avoid ibuprofen (associated with aseptic meningitis in SLE).
- Use hydroxychloroquine (<6.5 mg/kg/day, not to exceed 400 mg/day) for:
  - Arthritis.
  - Cutaneous disease.
- Low-dose methotrexate may be useful with mild disease and when arthritis is a prominent feature.

Glucocorticoids

- Use topical steroids for cutaneous disease.
- Use low-dose oral (< 0.5 mg/kg/day) for:
  - Arthritis.
  - Serositis.
  - Mild cytopenia.
- Use moderate-dose oral (0.5 to 1 mg/kg/day) for mild nephritis (mesangial, focal proliferative, membranous).
- Use high-dose oral (1 to 2 mg/kg/day) for:

- Diffuse proliferative lupus nephritis and membranous disease with nephrotic syndrome.
  - CNS disease.
  - Acute hemolytic anemia.
- Use pulse intravenous for:
  - Severe, life-threatening or organ-threatening disease.
  - Severe, hematologic abnormalities.
  - Catastrophic antiphospholipid syndrome.

Cytotoxic

- Azathioprine can be used as a steroid-sparing drug for:
  - Arthritis.
  - Serositis.
  - Following induction therapy with cyclophosphamide to maintain remission.
- Mycophenolate mofetil can be used as a steroid-sparing drug, especially if patient does not tolerate azathioprine, for:
  - Following induction therapy with cyclophosphamide to maintain remission.
  - Induction therapy in nephritis for patients who do not want the toxicity associated with cyclophosphamide.
- Cyclophosphamide is used for:
  - Major renal involvement, particularly diffuse proliferative glomerulonephritis.
  - CNS lupus.
  - Catastrophic antiphospholipid syndrome.

Other

- Use plasmapheresis for catastrophic antiphospholipid syndrome.
- Use IVIG for refractory thrombocytopenia.

Experimental Therapies*

- Anti-CD20 B-cell depletion therapy.
- Autologous stem cell transplantation.
- CTLA4Ig.

---

*Currently used only for severe disease unresponsive to standard therapies or in clinical trials.
CNS, central nervous system; CTLA4Ig, cytotoxic T lymphocyte–associated protein 4 immunoglobulin; IVIG, intravenous immunoglobulin; SLE, systemic lupus erythematosus; SPF, sun protection factor.

---

will present with acute hemolytic crisis that may require pulse intravenous (IV) corticosteroids to gain rapid control of the hemolytic process. The presence of antiphospholipid antibodies requires attention. The primary treatment in these patients is anticoagulation as antiphospholipid antibody levels are resistant to immunosuppressive or cytotoxic agents. Its treatment depends on whether or not there is a history of a clot. It is advisable to involve a pediatric hematologist in the care of these children.

The treatment of lupus nephritis varies depending on the renal lesion present. In mesangial disease, low-dose steroids are usually adequate. Treatment of focal proliferative glomerulonephritis often consists of moderate doses of corticosteroids plus a cytotoxic agent such as azathioprine. The treatment of diffuse proliferative glomerulonephritis is in transition. The current trend in treatment of this serious renal lesion is sequential therapy designed to induce and then maintain disease remission with the goal of improving the rate of remission although at the same time minimizing

the long-term toxicity of the treatment. The most common approach is to induce remission with monthly IV cyclophosphamide combined with high-dose corticosteroids (IV pulses followed by high-dose daily oral glucocorticoids) for 3 to 6 months, followed by a less-toxic treatment regimen to maintain remission. Maintenance therapy typically consists of either less-frequent (quarterly) IV cyclophosphamide or, more commonly, discontinuing cyclophosphamide and replacing it with either azathioprine or mycophenolate mofetil. Using this approach, renal outcomes have improved in diffuse proliferative glomerulonephritis (GN). Yet, despite the improvement in the treatment, many children with diffuse proliferative glomerulonephritis (DPGN) go on to end-stage renal disease (ESRD).

Membranous lupus nephritis continues to be difficult to treat. This type of lesion is less responsive to immunosuppressive therapy and a substantial proportion of individuals with membranous disease develop nephrotic syndrome and ESRD. Despite the poor response to treatment, those individuals with membranous disease who develop nephrotic syndrome are treated with IV pulse cyclophosphamide and glucocorticoids. This treatment can be debated, but until well-controlled trials are performed, the optimal therapy for membranous nephritis remains unknown.

Drug-induced lupus requires special mention as discontinuation of the offending drug is a critical step in management. Children with drug-induced lupus usually present with fever, serositis, and rash. CNS and renal disease are rare. Most will have a positive ANA with a homogeneous pattern with specificity toward histone antigens. Antibodies to double-stranded DNA are rarely present. Serum complement levels are typically normal. The list of drugs that have been implicated in drug-induced lupus is too long to review, but the drugs that are frequently implicated include multiple anticonvulsants, hydralazine, isoniazid, procainamide, minocycline, D-penicillamine, penicillin, and multiple sulfonamides. Treatment typically involves low-dose corticosteroids that are weaned over time. Cytotoxic drugs are rarely needed.

The medications used to treat pediatric SLE typically result in a relative immunodeficient state. Additionally, lupus patients may develop splenic dysfunction over time, which increases their risk of serious infection with encapsulated organisms, particularly pneumococcus. Together, this puts children with SLE at risk for significant infectious complications from a wide range of organisms. As survival has improved over the decades with more aggressive therapy, infections have emerged as an important cause of mortality in SLE. Given that a lupus flare and an infection in an immunosuppressed lupus patient can manifest with similar clinical presentations, caution must be exercised in therapeutic decision-making in this setting. Further immunosuppression, in the absence of treating a potential infection, can have life-threatening consequences. In short, it is essential to include infection in the differential diagnosis when caring for a seriously ill lupus patient. Preventive measures include the recommendation for routine pneumococcal vaccination.

The disease itself and its treatment often result in the development of significant atherosclerotic disease in children with lupus. Although it is rare to have a symptomatic cardiovascular disease during the pediatric years, significant complications of atherosclerotic disease do occur in young adulthood. Attention to dyslipoproteinemia is warranted but optimal treatment has not yet been established. Clinical trials are currently being conducted to assess the efficacy of statins in preventing atherosclerosis in this patient population.

The psychological impact of this disease cannot be underestimated. Chronic illness, treatment-related side effects (becoming cushingoid) and disease-related cosmetic issues (alopecia, facial rash) make this an especially difficult disease to have as a child and is even worse for an adolescent. Low self-esteem and depression frequently occur. Additionally, CNS disease can result in neurocognitive dysfunction that adversely affects school performance. Overt psychosis can occur as part of CNS lupus.

Common Pitfalls

- Failing to consider SLE as a diagnostic possibility in children and thus delaying diagnosis
- Not realizing that pediatric SLE is more severe than adult SLE and undertreating
- Misdiagnosing an infection as a disease flare
- Underestimating the psychological impact of the disease and its treatment for the child

Communication and Counseling

Lupus in childhood is a serious disease that remains difficult to treat. Although current treatment regimens have improved the disease outcome for patients with lupus, most children continue to develop significant treatment-associated side effects including, but not limited to, an increased susceptibility to infections, increased infertility (associated with cyclophosphamide treatment), and increased risk of malignancy. A shift in treatment strategy that is more in line with the strategy used by oncologists to treat cancer (i.e., induction followed by maintenance therapy) shows promise in improving renal outcomes while minimizing treatment-associated morbidity and mortality. In the future, this sequential strategy may be the way that we treat all aspects of the disease, not just nephritis. New treatments are on the horizon. Anti–B-cell therapies show promise but further study is needed to determine the efficacy and safety of this approach.

SUGGESTED READINGS

1. Cassidy JT, Petty RE: Systemic lupus erythematosus. In Cassidy JT, Petty RE (eds): Textbook of Pediatric Rheumatology, 3rd ed. Philadelphia: WB Saunders, 1995, pp 260–322. **Comprehensive review of pediatric SLE.**
2. Cassidy JT: Systemic lupus erythematosus. In Harris ED Jr, Budd RC, Genovese MC, et al (eds): Kelley's Textbook of Rheumatology, 7th ed. Philadelphia: WB Saunders, 2005, pp 1597–1600. **Concise summary of pediatric SLE.**
3. Hochberg MC: Updating the American College of Rheumatology revised criteria for the classification of systemic lupus erythematosus. Arthritis Rheum 40:1725, 1997. Available online at http://www.rheumatology.org/publications/classification/SLE/1982 SLEupdate.asp (accessed October 4, 2005). **Summary of updated criteria for the classification of SLE.**
4. Houssiau FA: Management of lupus nephritis: An update. J Amer Soc Neph 15(10):2694–2704, 2004. **This article reviews the treatment of proliferative and membranous lupus nephritis.**
5. Klein-Gitelman M, Reiff A, Silverman ED: Systemic lupus erythematosus in childhood. Rheum Dis Clin N Am 28:561–577, 2002. **Concise reference for clinical and laboratory features of pediatric lupus.**
6. Milojevic DS, Ilowite NT: Treatment of rheumatologic diseases in children: Special considerations. Rheum Dis Clin N Am 28:461–482, 2002. **Concise reference for the drugs used to treat rheumatologic diseases in children, including pediatric SLE, with special emphasis on specific pediatric issues such as growth and development, immunization, and toxicity.**
7. Schandberg LE, Sandborg C: Dyslipoproteinemia and premature atherosclerosis in pediatric systemic lupus erythematosus. Curr Rheum Reports 6(6):425–433, 2004. **Comprehensive review of atherosclerosis in pediatric SLE.**

8. Tan EM, Cohen AS, Fries JF, et al: The 1982 revised criteria for the classification of systemic lupus erythematosus. Arthritis Rheum 25:1271–1277, 1982. Available online at http:// www.rheumatology.org/publications/classification/SLE (accessed October 4, 2005). **Summary of the 1982 criteria.**

Disorders of the Spine and Shoulder Girdle

J. Scott Doyle

KEY CONCEPTS

- Scoliosis may be congenital or idiopathic.
- Patients with congenital scoliosis frequently have renal, cardiac, or spinal cord abnormalities.
- Renal ultrasounds and a good cardiac examination should be done on all patients with congenital scoliosis.
- Scoliosis greater than 20 degrees should be referred for treatment.
- Back pain is uncommon in younger children.
- Younger children are more likely to have demonstrable pathology than adolescents.

Expert Opinion on Management Issues

THE SPINE

Scoliosis

Scoliosis is defined as a lateral curvature of the spine exceeding 10 degrees. The major divisions of scoliosis are congenital scoliosis, idiopathic scoliosis, and scoliosis associated with neuromuscular or connective tissue diseases. The cause of the spinal deformity and the consequences to the patient are different for each etiologic category.

Congenital Scoliosis

Congenital scoliosis is a curvature that, by definition, is a consequence of abnormal formation or failure of proper separation of the bony elements of the spine. Depending on the magnitude of the curve, the clinical deformity may or may not be apparent in the first year of life. The vertebral anomalies are usually easily appreciated on plain radiographs. Periodic radiographic reevaluation is important once the diagnosis is made because the curve may be static or may be relentlessly progressive. Marked progression can produce a significantly disfigured trunk and, in extreme cases, compromised pulmonary function secondary to restrictive lung disease. During the first several years of life, radiographic monitoring and a clinical examination should be done every 6 months. Radiographic measurement of all curves is crucial because it is the most sensitive and accurate means of determining progression. When normal growth velocity slows, visits can be less frequent.

Congenital scoliosis is often accompanied by other abnormalities. Renal and cardiac anomalies are seen in approximately 15% to 20% of patients. Spinal cord abnormalities and other intraspinal lesions may be seen in up to 20% of patients. Other associated conditions may include VATER abnormalities (vertebral, anus, tracheoesophageal, radial, and renal), Klippel-Feil syndrome (congenital fusion of the cervical vertebrae), and Sprengel deformity. A child with congenital scoliosis should at the very least have a good clinical cardiac examination and a screening renal ultrasound to rule out anomalies. Most orthopaedic surgeons would also recommend an MRI of the spine when a good quality study can be safely undertaken.

Curves that are progressive usually require surgery. Bracing of the congenitally abnormal portion of the spine is an ineffective means of arresting progression. When worsening is documented, a fusion of the anomalous portion of the spine (even at a very young age) is indicated. To preserve stature and spinal motion, attempts are made to fuse as short a segment of the spine as is compatible with arresting the forces of progression. The purpose of the fusion is to eliminate the deforming growth of the anomalous portion of the spine. Bracing of compensatory curves in the more normally formed portions of the spine may be effective at preventing progressive curvature of these segments.

Idiopathic Scoliosis

Idiopathic scoliosis is a lateral curvature greater than 10 degrees in a spine with normally formed elements. Affected individuals are usually otherwise normal. Using this definition, the overall incidence is approximately 2% to 3%. For curves greater than 20 degrees, the incidence falls to approximately 0.3%. At present the root cause of idiopathic scoliosis remains a mystery. Genetics clearly plays a role. A family history is often positive, and the risk to an individual with an affected parent is significantly greater than the general population. Studies of monozygotic twins show a high correlation, but the lack of 100% concordance indicates that there are influences other than genetics.

Once scoliosis has developed, growth, gender, and curve magnitude are the most important determinants of risk for progression of the curve. Several natural history studies exist that allow rough calculations of the risk of progression based on the curve magnitude and growth remaining. In general, the risk of progression is greater with larger curve magnitude at presentation and the further the patient is from skeletal maturity. The proximity to maturity is best judged by menarchal history, Tanner staging, and radiographic assessment of the iliac apophysis growth center (Risser staging). Curves less than 20 degrees are at low risk for progression and are observed. Curves between 20 and 45 degrees are at high risk for progression during growth. Curves of this magnitude are generally braced. Once curve magnitude reaches 50 degrees, progression is probable even after maturity and is usually an indication for surgery. Female gender is another risk factor. The incidence of small curves is roughly equal between the sexes (1.4:1.0 female-to-male ratio). This ratio increases to 5:1 for curves greater than 20 degrees. For curves large enough to require surgery (>50 degrees), the ratio increases to approximately 8:1.

Since the 1990s, there has been a reassessment of the long-term consequences of untreated scoliosis. In the past, it was felt that thoracic deformity caused restrictive lung disease, cor pulmonale, and premature mortality. Studies looking specifically at adolescent idiopathic scoliosis (as opposed to scoliosis from other etiologies and early-onset disease) do not show significant increases in expected mortality. Adults with thoracic curves greater than 100 degrees demonstrate a restrictive pattern of pulmonary dysfunction, but premature mortality or cardiopulmonary symptoms are rare. When there is a severe deformity of the chest cage during the formative years of the bronchopulmonary system (before age 8 years), there can be significant cardiopulmonary consequences. Fortunately, this is rare and most curves that come to the attention of physicians are adolescent idiopathic curves.

Patients usually present with a painless truncal deformity. The Adams forward bend test detects rotational deformity from the curve. A scoliometer reading of 7 degrees is advocated as a threshold for referral to reduce the number of false positives and to reduce the radiographs for insignificant curves. A careful history and neurologic exam are important to rule out abnormalities in "idiopathic-like" curves. Intraspinal abnormalities may cause idiopathic-like curves and should be ruled out in cases of early onset, in left thoracic curves, and in patients with neurologic findings or symptoms.

Most curves are nonprogressive. For curves at risk for progression, bracing is the only nonoperative measure that alters the natural history of scoliosis. For curves large enough to require surgery, a posterior spinal fusion with instrumentation is the usual treatment. Techniques are evolving, and there is an increased use of anterior surgery and, in some instances, thoracoscopic surgery. The type of surgery is determined by curve pattern and surgeon preference.

A comment on infantile scoliosis is needed. An infant with scoliosis merits referral. It is important to rule out congenital scoliosis and to evaluate the patient for the likelihood of progression. If the scoliosis progresses rapidly, lung development may be impeded. Technologies such as an expandable artificial rib cage or rods that allow the spine to continue to grow can be employed in certain high-risk patients.

Other Scoliosis

Scoliosis is more common in connective tissue diseases and neuromuscular conditions. The muscular dystrophies, Frederich ataxia, and spinal muscular atrophy are the most common neuromuscular causes of scoliosis apart from cerebral palsy. Loss or imbalance of the muscular support to the bone column is probably a major factor in the development of curves in these patients. The incidence and severity of curves increase as the diseases progress. Surgery to improve sitting may make a significant difference in the quality of life of these patients, but clear-cut evidence that it improves life expectancy or pulmonary health is lacking.

Scheuermann Kyphosis

Kyphosis, a forward (sagittal plane) curvature of the spine, is a pathologic curvature that should be distinguished from postural roundback. The thoracic spine normally has between 20 and 45 degrees of kyphosis. This is considered physiologic and varies widely among individuals. Patients with *postural* kyphosis may have a rounded appearing back but are asymptomatic and can reverse their kyphosis with active extension.

Scheuermann kyphosis is a progressive, often painful condition seen in late childhood and adolescence. It typically involves the thoracic spine but may involve the lumbar spine with loss of the normal lumbar lordosis. Clinically, the patient may complain of mild to moderate back pain an increasing roundback deformity. The kyphosis is relatively rigid.

Scheuermann kyphosis may be recognized radiographically by anterior wedging of three adjacent vertebrae, end plate irregularities, and Schmorl nodes (intrusions of the disc into the vertebra). The pain and progression of this condition tend to arrest after maturity. Although there is an increase in the incidence and severity of back pain in adulthood, the natural history of this condition is relatively benign. Pulmonary compromise is not seen. Brace treatment is indicated for progressive deformity and symptoms. Surgery is occasionally indicated for bigger curves that are not amenable to brace treatment.

Spondylolysis/Spondylolisthesis

Spondylolysis is an acquired (not congenital) defect in the pars region of the posterior arch of a vertebra. It is most common in the low lumbar region and develops secondary to repetitive stress (especially with extension of the lumbar spine). The lesion rarely heals and usually progresses to a pseudarthrosis. Hyperextension of the spine increases the biomechanical stress on the pars region of the arch and in a susceptible individual can result in a chronic stress fracture. Gymnasts and other athletes who repeatedly hyperextend the spine have a higher incidence of spondylolysis than the general population. In adolescence and adulthood the incidence is approximately 5%. The spinal lesion is an acquired defect secondary to repetitive stress in a genetically susceptible individual. It may be a cause of back pain, but it is often asymptomatic. In the absence of symptoms, it requires no treatment or activity restriction. If a child has significant low back pain, activity modification or a brace is employed to try to ameliorate the symptoms. Surgical repair of the par interarticularis is rare and reserved for unremitting symptoms.

Spondylolisthesis is a forward slippage of one vertebra on the vertebra below. In children, spondylolisthesis is usually secondary to spondylolysis. The defect in the arch dissociates the vertebra from its inferior facet and posterior ligamentous restraints. This separation may allow for a slow forward slippage of the vertebra on the vertebra below. Progression occurs in approximately 5% to 7% of patients with spondylolisthesis. It is more likely in girls and in patients who have greater than 50% forward slippage at diagnosis. Progression and symptoms are most likely to occur during the adolescent growth spurt. Low back pain is the most common symptom. Some cases are diagnosed because the patient has an abnormal gait or postural deformity. Only 10% to 15% of patients develop symptoms. The pain is believed to result from motion and stress on the pseudarthrosis at the pars defect. Nociceptive receptors have been found in the tissue in the pars defect. Adjacent nerve root irritation may occur in more significant slippages. Radicular symptoms are not indicative of a neurologic deficit per se and usually resolve with treatment of the spondylolisthesis. Disc herniation in adolescents is rare.

Treatment typically is aimed at the alleviation of back pain. This usually may be accomplished with activity restrictions or a period of bracing. A posterior fusion of the involved vertebra to the sacrum is reserved for refractory symptoms that fail nonoperative management. Documented progression and slippages greater than 50% are the other principle indications for surgery. As this is a chronic condition, the spine is not acutely unstable and the risk to the neural elements is low. Patients without symptoms and with less than 50% slippage may continue in sports without restriction. Asymptomatic patients with greater than 50% slippage should be restricted from contact sports to decrease the risk of traction injury to the lumbosacral nerve roots.

Back Pain in Children

Although it has been traditionally taught that back pain was uncommon in children, recent studies show that more than half of adolescents report back pain but seldom seek medical attention. In younger children back pain is uncommon and deserves a higher index of suspicion.

Fortunately, most episodes of back pain are brief and nonspecific. The older the patient, the more likely it is that the pain is musculoskeletal. If the results of all examinations are normal, a course of nonsteroidal anti-inflammatory drugs and observation are appropriate. If symptoms persist or worsen, re-examination is prudent.

THE SHOULDER GIRDLE

Sprengel Deformity

Sprengel deformity is a congenital anomaly that results from a failure of scapular descent during the early fetal period. The scapula forms adjacent to the mid-cervical region and normally descends to its normal posterior thoracic position by week 10 of gestation. A failure of this descent results in an elevated scapula.

The abnormality of the scapula is not limited to its position at birth. Usually the scapula is hypoplastic and malrotated. Often a persistent band of tissue (termed an *omovertebral bone*) connects the scapula to cervical structures. The band is usually incomplete but restricts the motion of the scapula. The cause of the deformity is unknown. Its occurrence is sporadic and without risk of transmission. The deformity is usually unilateral and thought to worsen with growth, although there is no good documentation of this in the literature.

It is important to recognize other anomalies that can be associated with Sprengel deformity. Cervical spine anomalies, congenital scoliosis, renal, cardiac, and intraspinal anomalies are not infrequent. Patients with Sprengel deformity should have neck and back radiographs and a renal ultrasound.

The clinical presentation depends on severity. Some patients have little cosmetic deformity and no functional loss of motion of the shoulder. These patients are best left alone. Other patients have severe deformity and a loss of shoulder abduction. These patients may benefit from resection of the bony bar and a caudal transfer of the trapezial origin to lower the scapula.

Congenital Pseudarthrosis of the Clavicle

Congenital pseudarthrosis is usually obvious at birth as anterior prominence over the right clavicle. It represents a failure of the two ossification centers of the clavicle to unite. This failure to unite is believed to be caused by pulsation of the subclavian artery subjacent to the clavicle disrupting the normal ossification sequence. The subclavian artery is higher on the right, accounting for the consistent right sided presentation of congenital pseudarthrosis of the clavicle. Ten percent may be bilateral. The only cases of isolated left-sided presentation have been seen in association with dextrocardia.

The condition may be distinguished from a clavicle fracture by the absence of pain, swelling, or tenderness. A clavicle fracture at birth usually heals with abundant callous, whereas in this condition the ends of the bone have a wispy, atrophic appearance. In addition to the prominence, some painless mobility of the ends of the clavicle may be noted. The prominence may increase and the shoulder may look foreshortened. Surgical repair is done for symptoms but parents usually want the pseudarthrosis repaired (even in the absence of symptoms) for cosmetic reasons. Repair with bone grafting and internal fixation is usually successful.

SUGGESTED READINGS

1. Nachemson AL, Peterson LE: Effectiveness of treatment with a brace in girls who have adolescent scoliosis: A prospective controlled study based on data from the Scoliosis Research Society. J Bone Joint Surg Am 77:815–822, 1995. **Critically evaluates brace treatment and effect on natural history during growth.**
2. Payne WK, Olgivie JW, Resnick MD, et al: Does scoliosis have a psychological impact and does gender make a difference? Spine 22:1380–1384, 1997. **Discusses the psychosocial impact of spine deformity.**

3. Pehrsson K, Larsson S, Nachemson A, et al: A long-term follow-up of patients with untreated scoliosis: A study of mortality, causes of death, and symptoms. Spine 17:1091–1096, 1991. **Demonstrates a lower morbidity from late onset spinal deformity than early onset disease.**

4. Weinstein SL, Zavala DC, Ponsetti, IV: Idiopathic scoliosis: Long-term follow-up. J Bone Joint Surg Am 702–712, 1983. **Elucidates risks for progression in adulthood and the long-term clinical consequences of scoliosis.**

Rotational Orthopedic Problems of the Extremities

Jeffrey R. Sawyer and Amy L. Drendel

KEY CONCEPTS

■ Almost all children are born with some degree of internal rotation of the lower extremities that resolves over the first 8 to 10 years of life.

■ A thorough understanding of the normal development of the lower extremities is essential in identifying pathologic conditions from normal development.

■ Plain radiographic studies are rarely helpful in the diagnosis of rotational deformities.

■ Most cases of intoeing and out-toeing resolve spontaneously without intervention.

■ Surgical treatment is reserved for older patients with severe rotational abnormalities that significantly affect function.

Intoeing and other rotational malalignments are one of the most common sources of parental concern and physician visits regarding their children's extremities. There are a wide variety of conditions—most of which are self-limiting and part of normal growth and development—that can give the appearance that the child's leg is rotated. In 90% or more of children, the condition is a function of normal development and will resolve spontaneously without formal treatment. It is essential to have a thorough understanding of the normal developmental process of the lower extremities to determine which conditions are part of this normal development and which require further evaluation and possible treatment.

Rotational deformities in children 1 year of age or younger usually occur at the level of the foot. Metatarsus adductus is the most common congenital foot deformity, with an incidence of 1 in 1000 live births, although it is not usually detected until 2 to 3 months of age. Many investigators believe intrauterine positioning plays a role in this condition as it is seen more frequently in conditions of intrauterine "packing" such as twin pregnancies, oligohydramnios, uterine fibroids, and maternal diabetes. It has been associated with other packing disorders such as developmental dysplasia of the hip and torticollis. Any child with metatarsus adductus should be evaluated for these other conditions.

Internal tibial torsion is the most common cause of intoeing between the ages of 1 and 4 years. This is often associated with frequent falls, especially in the early ambulator. These children walk with the patella facing forward and the foot internally rotated (Fig. 1). This

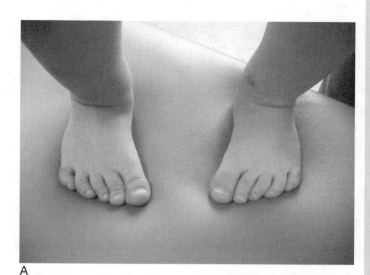

A

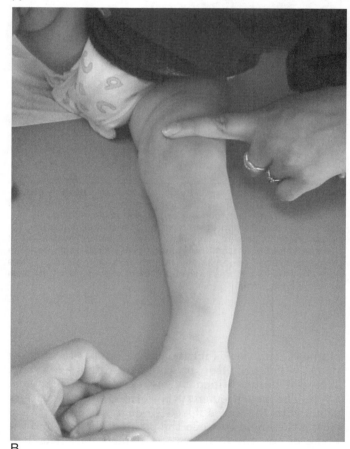

B

FIGURE 1. *A,* Metatarsus adductus in a 1-year-old. Note the internal rotation of the forefoot. *B,* Internal tibial torsion in a 2-year-old. Note the internal rotation of the tibia. The rotational alignment for both of these children is within the range of normal development.

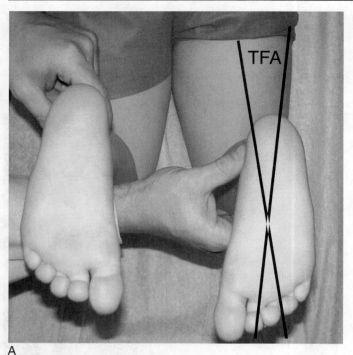

A

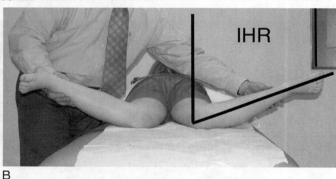

B

FIGURE 2. Rotational measurements commonly used in evaluation of rotational alignment. *A,* The thigh–foot angle (TFA) is the angular difference between the axis of the foot and thigh. In this case the TFA is 15 degrees internally rotated, indicating internal tibial torsion is present. This also allows excellent evaluation of the foot shape. *B,* Internal hip rotation (IHR) is the angle between the vertical and the maximally rotated axis of the tibia. In this case the IHR is 70 degrees, which indicates that increased femoral anteversion is present.

painless condition is felt not to be related to growing pains, which are also very common in this age group. This can be quantified by measuring the thigh–foot angle. The measurement is performed with the patient prone with the knees flexed 90 degrees (Fig. 2). Measuring the angle between the plane of the foot and the plane of the thigh allows the determination of how much rotation of the tibia is present. Plain radiographs are typically not helpful in evaluation of tibial torsion. Special CT scans can be used to quantify the rotation of the tibia, but this is usually reserved for preoperative planning and complex deformities.

TABLE 1 Common Rotational Problems

Condition	Peak Ages	Foot Direction	Patella Direction
Metatarsus adductus	0–1 yr	Adducted	Forward
Internal tibial torsion	1–4 yr	Straight	Forward
Femoral anteversion	4–8 yr	Straight	Internally rotated

Intoeing after 3 years of age is usually caused by increased femoral anteversion. This, like tibial torsion, is part of the normal limb development and rarely requires treatment. Femoral anteversion describes forward tilt of the femoral neck relative to the femoral shaft in the axial plane. Physical examination findings show increased internal and decreased external rotation of the hip measured with the child prone and knees flexed (see Fig. 2). This, like tibial torsion, usually occurs bilaterally. In contrast to patients with tibial torsion, patients with femoral anteversion ambulate with the patella and foot rotated inward (Table 1). These children commonly sit in the "W" position, which, although not the cause of this condition, should be discouraged. This condition, in most cases, will resolve over time with no treatment.

Unresolved intoeing in the child older than 10 years of age is rare and usually requires further examination and possible orthopaedic referral. At this age parents should be counseled that little if any spontaneous correction can be expected and surgical treatment may be necessary. Plain radiographs are typically not helpful in the evaluation of the older child with unresolved intoeing.

Out-toeing is much less common than intoeing and can be thought of in a similar age-related fashion. External rotation contracture of the hips or newborn contracture of the hips affects most children younger than 1 year of age and is felt to be related to having the hips held in external rotation in utero. This will gradually resolve by the time the child begins to stand, and occasionally physical therapy can be used should these contractures interfere with early gait development. External tibial torsion can also occur in the 1- to 4-year-old child although much less commonly than internal torsion. The evaluation and treatment are the same as for internal torsion and most cases gradually correct as well. Femoral retroversion, unlike femoral anteversion, is very uncommon and usually requires orthopedic evaluation. The most common cause of femoral retroversion in the older child is slipped capital femoral epiphysis.

Expert Opinion on Management Issues

In general, these conditions are very common in the pediatric population and gradually correct with age. Spontaneous correction occurs with the vast majority of patients. Plain radiographic studies are rarely needed to diagnose rotational deformities; history and physical examination are sufficient. Treatment consists of observation, parental teaching, reassurance, and encouraging activity for the child. Even when deformities persist, they rarely lead to functional disabilities and commonly are cosmetic concerns. Surgical treatment, which consists of rotational osteotomies, in which the bone is cut and rotated into the corrected position, is reserved for older patients with severe rotational abnormalities that do not correct with growth and significantly affect function.

Treatment for metatarsus adductus depends on the flexibility of the foot. Careful observation is advocated in mild cases. Some authors recommend treatment as soon as possible regardless of severity, but 85% to 95% of these cases resolve without treatment by 1 year of age and only 4% of cases persist at 16 years of age without intervention. Simple home stretching programs may be used if the deformity is mild and fully correctable. Parents hold the hindfoot in one hand and stretch the midfoot, opening the C-shaped curve and overcorrecting the deformity. This can be done in conjunction with a physical therapist if necessary. Custom molded, reverse-lace shoes and wearing shoes on the opposite foot have been used extensively in the past but have not been shown to be of any benefit. Children who have severe metatarsus adductus that does not resolve spontaneously or who have rigid deformity may benefit from a short course of serial casting or use of an ankle–foot orthosis, a removable plastic version of the stretch cast. There is some controversy regarding the effectiveness of casts or braces, the best timetable for treatment approaches, and the utility of stretching exercises with no reliable evidence-based comparisons. For older children with fixed deformities, operative treatment may be necessary to restore normal foot alignment and allow for comfortable shoe wear.

Tibial torsion resolves spontaneously in 90% of cases by the time the child is 8 years old, most within the first full year of ambulation. Bracing, night splints, shoe wedges, and orthotics have been tried in the past for this condition; however, long-term studies have failed to show any beneficial effect. Newer studies suggest there may be a negative psychological effect with bracing and for these reasons it should be avoided. Eliminating prone sleeping and the child sitting on their feet enhances resolution. Surgical treatment with osteotomy can be associated with compartment syndrome and peroneal nerve injury and is reserved for children older than 8 years of age with severe functional deformity and significant thigh–foot angles.

As with internal tibial torsion, femoral anteversion spontaneously resolves in more than 80% of cases by age 10 years. Some experimental models show that increased load of the hip (like that which occurs when sitting in the "W" position) can increase femoral version and should be discouraged. Hip range of motion can be followed every 6 to 12 months to document resolution. Surgery should be considered only in older patients with severe deformity and cosmetic or functional disability. Long-term studies have shown no

beneficial effect of bracing on the natural history of this condition.

Femoral retroversion causing out-toeing should resolve by 10 to 12 years of age. An orthopedic evaluation is recommended for persistent physical findings at this age because of an increased incidence of osteoarthritis, stress fractures, and slipped capital femoral epiphysis later in life. External tibial torsion requires surgical evaluation if symptoms persist at 10 years of age with thigh–foot angles greater than 40 degrees. These patients have an increased likelihood of patellofemoral instability and pain.

Common Pitfalls

Toddlers may have intoeing that is unilateral or bilateral, but femoral anteversion is nearly always bilateral and symmetric. Asymmetry in an older child is unusual and should be investigated. These deformities are typically structural and recognized when the patient is at rest. Gait dysfunction, especially falls, in patients with rotational deformities do tend to worsen with fatigue; this historical point is reassuring to parents. They commonly demonstrate a familial tendency that can be elicited in the history. Rotational deformities are rarely painful.

Because lower extremity alignment changes with age, it is important to be able to separate pathologic conditions from normal developmental patterns. Normal assessment of height and weight makes skeletal dysplasia and metabolic bone disease less likely. Questions about perinatal events and motor development can identify risk factors for the diagnosis of cerebral palsy. A careful spine and neurologic examination reduces the possibility of a neuromuscular disorder and spinal dysraphisms.

Metatarsus adductus must be differentiated from clubfoot or congenital talipes equinovarus, which is a foot disorder characterized by ankle plantar flexion, hindfoot varus, and forefoot adduction. In patients with metatarsus adductus the forefoot is abnormal whereas in clubfoot the forefoot, hind foot, and ankle are all abnormal. The treatment and prognosis for clubfoot is very different from metatarsus adductus. In late childhood and early adolescence, rotational deformities can lead to abnormalities about the knee, including knee pain and patellar instability, so vigilance in the preteen years for these deformities is important.

Communication and Counseling

In general, these conditions are part of normal lower extremity development and are, therefore, very common in the pediatric population. Spontaneous correction occurs in the vast majority of patients. Treatment consists of careful observation and parental reassurance. Having the parents photograph or videotape their children at time intervals for comparison is helpful as well. Surgical treatment is reserved for a few older patients with severe rotational abnormalities that significantly affect function. Interestingly, intoeing may be beneficial for sports that require quick direction shifts like tennis, soccer, and baseball.

SUGGESTED READINGS

1. Dietz FR: Intoeing: Fact, fiction and opinion. Am Fam Physician 50(6):1249–1258, 1994. **Review of examination findings.**
2. Sass P, Hassan G: Lower Extremity Abnormalities in Children. Am Fam Physician 68(3):461–468, 2003. **Review with tables including ranges for measured angles.**
3. Staheli LT, Corbett M, King H: Lower extremity rotational problems in children. Normal values to guide management. J Bone Joint Surg Am 67:39–47, 1985. **Angle measurement values.**
4. Staheli LT: Torsion: Treatment indications. Clin Orthop 247:61–66, 1989. **Discussion of surgical options.**

The Hip

Suken A. Shah and Lawrence M. Stankovits

KEY CONCEPTS

- Septic arthritis
  - Septic arthritis of the hip is a surgical emergency. Suspicion of a septic hip should trigger immediate laboratory and radiologic investigation and orthopedic consultation.
  - Frequently, diagnosis is narrowed down to septic arthritis versus transient synovitis. Four independent multivariate clinical predictors can be used to predict the probability of septic arthritis versus transient synovitis of the hip.
  - Diagnosis is confirmed by image-guided hip aspiration.
  - Treatment for septic arthritis consists of hip arthrotomy and age-directed empirical antibiotic therapy. Cultures guide organism-specific therapy.
  - Hip pain in a child is a problem that commonly faces the clinician, and the differential diagnosis can be extensive. In this chapter, we attempt to shed some light on the more common conditions and their treatment.
- Developmental dysplasia of the hip
  - Screening for developmental dysplasia of the hip begins in the nursery and continues at each well visit during the first year of life. A complete understanding of the physical tests and signs is necessary to prevent both undertreatment and overtreatment.
  - Most of the bony elements of the hip are not calcified at birth. Ultrasound is the best diagnostic tool available for evaluating the newborn hip until the ossific nucleus of the femoral head appears (4 to 6 months).
  - Hip "clicks" are usually caused by synovial folds or by snapping tendons. These are of no consequence and do not indicate hip instability. A hip click that does not resolve by 3 weeks of age should be evaluated with a dynamic ultrasound of both hips.
  - The goal of treatment for developmental dysplasia is a reduced hip and a normally formed acetabulum. This can be achieved in most cases with early brace treatment, avoiding the need for surgery.
  - In late presenting cases or failed brace treatment, surgery is usually necessary.

- Legg-Calvé-Perthes disease
  - The Legg-Calvé-Perthes disease process can take 18 to 24 months. Among factors determining the prognosis are the child's age at presentation and how much of the femoral head is involved. If the femoral head is abnormally shaped after the healing process, limitation of motion and premature degenerative joint disease are the usual sequelae. Children presenting at older than age 8 years have a guarded prognosis.
  - Age and physical examination findings are keys to recognizing Legg-Calvé-Perthes disease.
  - Legg-Calvé-Perthes disease is a self-limited disease in which the epiphysis undergoes necrosis, revascularization, removal of necrotic bone, and reossification. The primary goal of treatment is to maintain range of motion. Containment of the epiphysis in the acetabulum enhances the ability of the femoral head to regain its spherical shape.
  - Treatment is generally nonsurgical. However, these children require close observation by an orthopedic surgeon experienced in treating Legg-Calvé-Perthes disease.
- Slipped capital femoral epiphysis
  - The age at presentation of a slipped capital femoral epiphysis in boys is most often between 10 and 16 years (average 13.5 years), and in girls it is between 9 and 15 years (average 12.1 years).
  - If a patient with slipped capital femoral epiphysis presents outside these ranges, one should exclude an underlying endocrine or systemic disease, such as hypothyroidism, panhypopituitarism, and renal osteodystrophy.
  - Bilateral symptomatic involvement is found in approximately 50% of cases, with half of those presenting with bilateral involvement and the other half showing sequential onset. However, recent evidence shows that bilateral sequential involvement may often be asymptomatic prior to the end of growth.
  - The etiology of slipped capital femoral epiphysis remains unknown.

Transient Synovitis

Transient synovitis of the hip (TSH), or toxic synovitis, is a self-limited, postinfectious inflammatory arthritis. The peak incidence is in boys (70%) between 3 and 10 years of age. Its etiology is unknown, but it is frequently preceded by a nonspecific upper respiratory tract infection, and trauma may be a predisposing factor.

Of concern to the clinician is the problem that TSH may mimic early septic arthritis. The differential diagnosis also includes trauma, juvenile idiopathic arthritis, acute rheumatic fever, Lyme disease, malignancy, and other inflammatory arthritides. Guidelines for differentiating TSH from septic arthritis are given in the following section. The child with TSH presents with the gradual onset of pain that is focused to the hip, thigh, or knee (referred) and typically lasts up to 6 days, as well as a limp or an inability to walk. The hip is usually held in flexion, abduction, and external rotation. A low-grade fever may be present, and the erythrocyte sedimentation rate (ESR), C-reactive protein (CRP), and serum white blood cell (WBC) count are normal to mildly elevated. Plain radiographs are usually normal, and ultrasound is useful to evaluate the presence of an effusion, which is small and not loculated, if present at all. A small number of cases (4%) are bilateral.

Most cases resolve completely with rest and non-steroidal anti-inflammatory drugs (NSAIDs) within 2 weeks. Children's ibuprofen (40 to 50 mg/kg/day, divided into three or four daily doses, with maximum of 2400 mg/day) is effective and generally well tolerated. These patients can be treated as outpatients with very close follow-up to determine the resolution of symptoms. TSH is usually a single event, but up to 17% of children have a recurrence within 6 months of the initial event. The prognosis is generally excellent.

SEPTIC ARTHRITIS

Septic arthritis of the hip can be the result of hematogenous spread of bacteria to the joint or spread of osteomyelitis from the metaphyseal bone of the proximal femur. In neonates, blood vessels cross the physis (growth plate) of the proximal femur and allow spread of bacteria from an osteomyelitic focus in the metaphyseal bone into the hip joint. Degradative enzymes are released from leukocytes, synovial cells, and cartilage, and proteolytic enzymes are liberated from certain organisms, both of which damage the matrix and collagen of articular cartilage very quickly (as early as 8 hours in experimental models). Clinical predictors are listed in Box 1.

The most common presenting sign is pain, or in the younger, nonverbal child, refusal to bear weight. Symptoms begin shortly after the inflammatory reaction in the joint (12 to 24 hours), but may be blunted in children who have already received antibiotics. The child with septic arthritis will hold the hip in flexion, abduction. and slight external rotation, and resist passive motion of the limb because it is painful.

Expert Opinion on Management Issues

The suspicion of septic arthritis should prompt one to obtain an emergency consultation with an orthopedic surgeon to evaluate the child, examine the laboratory data, and direct further treatment, The orthopedist's goal is to differentiate septic arthritis from transient synovitis. When hip aspiration is performed, the fluid is sent for cell count, fluid analysis, Gram stain, and culture. In cases of septic arthritis, the fluid will reveal a high leukocyte count (>80,000 cells/mL), elevated protein, and decreased glucose, and the Gram stain will demonstrate the microorganisms.

If the fluid aspiration reveals pus, an immediate surgical arthrotomy should be performed to drain the joint of remaining fluid and decompress the hip capsule. The joint is then irrigated to remove the necrotic debris, inflammatory mediators, leukocytes, and bacteria, which can damage the cartilage cells, matrix, or ossific nucleus, leading to degenerative joint disease and permanent disability. Antibiotics should be started intravenously as soon as the diagnosis is made and cultures are obtained. Empirical therapy (Table 1), based on the child's age and the most likely causative organisms, can be modified when culture and sensitivity results are obtained. Duration depends on the response to treatment; in the typical case of a quick response to treatment, 5 days of intravenous antibiotics can be followed by 3 to 6 weeks of oral therapy.

Common Pitfalls

Delay in diagnosis can lead to rapid, permanent destruction of both the femoral head and acetabular cartilage. Outcome is optimized when treatment is initiated within 8 hours of symptoms. Therefore, septic hip arthritis should be the leading diagnosis in the child who presents with a painful hip or refusal to bear weight.

Although the clinical predictors are helpful to differentiate septic hip arthritis from transient synovitis, other causes of lower extremity pain should be ruled

---

BOX 1 Clinical Predictors of Septic Arthritis Versus Transient Synovitis

- Fever
- Refusal to bear weight
- Sedimentation rate >40 mm/h
- White blood cell count >12,000 cells/mm^3

TABLE 1 Empiric Antibiotic Therapy in Septic Arthritis in Children

Age	Common Organisms	Antibiotic
Premature neonates	Staphylococcus aureus, group B streptococcus, gram-negative bacilli	Oxacillin plus gentamicin or cefotaxime, or vancomycin (MRSA)
Term neonates	Group A, B streptococcus, Streptococcus pneumoniae, Escherichia coli, S. aureus	Cefotaxime, ceftriaxone, methicillin
6 mo–4 yr	S. aureus, Haemophilus influenzae	Ceftriaxone, cefuroxime
4 yr–12 yr	S. aureus	Cefazolin, cefuroxime, oxacillin
12 yr–18 yr	S. aureus, Neisseria gonorrhoeae	Cefazolin, cefuroxime, oxacillin

MRSA, methicillin-resistant *Staphylococcus aureus*.

out. Anteroposterior (AP) pelvis and, if tolerated, frog-leg lateral radiographs should be obtained.

Identification of the causative organism is critical. Intravenous antibiotics should be started only after hip aspiration has been performed to improve the yield.

Communication and Counseling

Children may recover from septic hip arthritis with minimal long-term effects. Full activities may be resumed after antibiotic treatment has ended and symptoms allow. It must be made clear to parents that despite appropriate treatment, devastating loss of function is possible. Long-term effects include postinfectious arthritis, hip subluxation or dislocation, physeal disturbances, and limb-length discrepancy, so these children need long-term follow-up care.

DEVELOPMENTAL DYSPLASIA OF THE HIP

Developmental dysplasia of the hip (DDH), previously known as congenital dislocation of the hip, affects as many as 10 in 1000 children in the U.S. DDH represents a spectrum of conditions, from hip instability or subluxation (loss of the tight fit between the femoral head and acetabulum, and made to slide in and out of the acetabulum) to dislocation (no contact between the femoral head and acetabulum). The condition is not always present at birth, and dysplasia (a shallow, more vertical acetabular socket) may be diagnosed many years after birth. Risk factors for DDH are listed in Box 2.

In the newborn, maternal hormones induce ligamentous laxity, and when combined with neonatal positioning of hip flexion and adduction and knee extension (such as in the breech position), they seem to contribute to formation of a hypertrophied ridge of acetabular cartilage, called the neolimbus. The left hip is more commonly involved because it is this hip that is most usually forced into adduction against the mother's sacrum in the common fetal positions. In rare cases, DDH may be irreducible at birth, also called a teratologic dislocation, and in these cases the clinician should suspect a neuromuscular condition such as myelomeningocele or arthrogryposis.

BOX 2 Risk Factors for Developmental Dysplasia of the Hip

- Breech position
- Female gender
- Family history or ethnic background (Native American or Laplander)
- Lower limb deformity (e.g., clubfoot, dislocated knee)
- Torticollis
- Metatarsus adductus
- Oligohydramnios

Expert Opinion on Management Issues

Ultrasound can evaluate the morphology and dynamic characteristics of the newborn hip, but is operator dependent. Ultrasound screening of all newborns is controversial; it is probably not cost-effective and leads to overtreatment. However, ultrasonography of the hips in children with certain risk factors (see Table 1), an abnormal examination, or a persistent click beyond 3 weeks of age is reasonable.

Radiographs of the pelvis are effective after development of the femoral ossific nucleus (age 4 to 6 months), and can be used to aid in diagnosis or to evaluate the outcome of treatment. In DDH, an AP view of the pelvis may indicate a more oblique acetabular slope, a smaller ossific nucleus than the contralateral normal side, or a femoral metaphysis displaced laterally and superiorly (Fig. 1).

A prompt diagnosis and referral to an orthopedic surgeon is essential for successful treatment. The Pavlik harness is a lightweight brace that has been used with over a 95% success rate in the management of DDH in newborns. It is a safe, inexpensive, and comfortable treatment that acts by keeping the hip gently abducted and flexed, guiding the femoral head into the acetabulum, and promoting concentric development of the hip joint. It allows the baby to move the legs, but only within a zone of safety. The earlier treatment is initiated, the more likely the outcome will be successful. The harness is generally worn full-time for a period of months and then weaned to be worn less time during the waking hours until it is discontinued.

If the child is older than 6 months or fails the Pavlik harness, a reduction of the hip is performed under general anesthesia (closed reduction), usually with a lengthening of the adductor longus tendon, and then prolonged immobilization in a cast. Older children, those who fail closed reductions, or those with teratologic

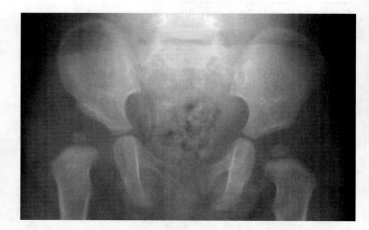

FIGURE 1. Developmental dysplasia of the right hip in a 16-month-old. This child has been treated with a Pavlik harness, closed reduction, and open reduction, but has persistent acetabular dysplasia. Note the smaller ossific nucleus that has migrated superiorly and laterally. The acetabulum is more shallow than the normal left side.

dislocations (usually because of a syndrome) require open reductions in which the hip capsule is opened, any impediments removed, the femoral head reduced in the acetabulum, the capsule tightened, and casting to immobilize the hip in the reduced position. Sometimes this procedure is accompanied by various bony procedures of the femur or pelvic osteotomies. The complications of avascular necrosis and degenerative joint disease are increased in older children and those requiring more involved surgery.

Common Pitfalls

The Barlow and Ortolani tests should be performed gently in a relaxed child. Forceful manipulation may overstretch an already lax hip capsule. A child who is not relaxed may mask subtle instability.

An infant treated in a Pavlik harness is likely to present for well-child visits during the bracing period. Excessive hip flexion (beyond 100 degrees) or abduction (beyond 60 degrees) can be harmful and should prompt the clinician to immediately consult with the treating orthopedist.

Recognize the entity of acetabular dysplasia with located hips. These older infants may present with limited abduction.

Communication and Counseling

The goals of treatment of DDH are a painless hip with full range of motion, a well-located femoral head, and a well-formed acetabulum. Recurrence and late acetabular dysplasia are not uncommon; the clinician and parents must understand that a child with DDH should be followed until the cessation of growth. DDH is the most common cause of early degenerative arthritis of the hip. Residual subluxation or acetabular dysplasia may cause accelerated destruction of the hip joint as early as the third decade of life.

LEGG-CALVÉ-PERTHES DISEASE

Legg-Calvé-Perthes disease (LCPD) is an idiopathic avascular necrosis of the femoral head. It occurs most commonly in the age range of 4 to 8 years and is up to 5 times more common in boys than girls. The incidence of bilaterality is 10% and occurs asynchronously in each

hip; synchronous involvement suggests the possibility of other causes (skeletal dysplasia).

Epidemiologically, genetic factors are lacking, but children with LCPD have shown various associations with delayed bone age, anthropometric abnormalities, urban environments, and deficiencies in somatomedin C (insulin-like growth factor-1 [IGF1]). The current theories about etiology of LCPD center around interruption of the blood supply to the femoral head by some transient mechanism; the roles of hypercoagulability, thrombophilia, and a disorganization of the physeal plate are controversial. Prognostic factors are listed in Box 3.

Diagnosis is confirmed by radiographs in the anteroposterior and frog-lateral position. Very early in the disease, the x-rays may be normal. Thereafter, there are four radiographic stages (Fig. 2).

Expert Opinion on Management Issues

Controversy exists regarding whether the outcome of LCPD can be altered by treatment because of the lack of long-term natural history data and the variability of treatment given by various authors in retrospective studies. Restriction of weight-bearing, bedrest, or immobilization seem to have no beneficial effect on the outcome. Patients with known poor prognostic signs should be treated. The current treatment protocols center around preservation of motion and containment of the femoral head within the acetabulum.

Restoration and preservation of abduction can be performed with bedrest, traction, and progressive abduction to relieve muscle spasms through physiotherapy. Occasionally, surgical lengthening of the contracted adductors is necessary. Good results were obtained in long-leg abduction plaster casts in earlier series, but currently, abduction braces such as the Atlanta Scottish Rite orthosis are widely used. This brace

---

BOX 3	Prognostic Factors in Legg-Calvé-Perthes Disease

- Deformity of the femoral head
- Hip joint incongruity
- Age at disease onset older than 8 years
- Extent of epiphyseal involvement
- Premature physeal closure
- Stage at treatment initiation
- Protracted disease course

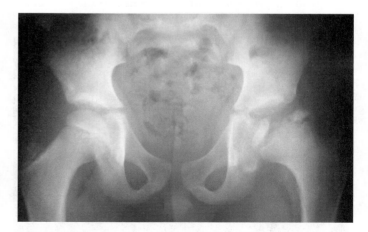

FIGURE 2. Left hip Legg Calvé Perthes disease (LCPD), reossification phase. This 9-year-old had been treated with range of motion and bracing. The lateral femoral epiphysis has lost significant height. During abduction, the epiphysis impinges on the acetabulum.

obtains containment, allows weight bearing, preserves hip motion, and permits ambulation because the knee and ankle are free. The brace should be worn full time for 6 to 18 months, until the reossification stage, and hence requires considerable compliance by the family. Other experts use traction, nighttime abduction bracing, or stretching exercises in lieu of full-time bracing.

Surgical methods of providing containment are advocated by many centers and offer the advantages of earlier mobilization and the avoidance of prolonged cast immobilization or brace treatment. The most common procedures are a varus femoral osteotomy (to redirect the avascular femoral head into the acetabulum), a pelvic osteotomy (to redirect the acetabulum), both procedures simultaneously, or a shelf acetabuloplasty (to extend the lateral edge of the acetabulum and contain the enlarged femoral head).

Common Pitfalls

The pain of LCPD is usually localized to the hip, but it may be referred to the medial thigh or knee. The diagnosis may be delayed with failure of the clinician to recognize that thigh or knee pain may indicate hip pathology.

Certain conditions, such as multiple epiphysial dysplasia, can mimic LCPD on radiographs. Full-length radiographs of the lower extremities are necessary to rule out such conditions.

SLIPPED CAPITAL FEMORAL EPIPHYSIS

Slipped capital femoral epiphysis (SCFE), the most common hip disorder in adolescents, is characterized by displacement of the femoral neck from the capital epiphysis through the physeal plate. The femoral neck moves anteriorly and proximally, and the epiphysis displaces posteriorly and medially (Fig. 3). It is generally a gradual process of slippage from chronic abnormal

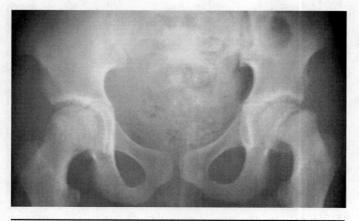

FIGURE 3. Left slipped capital femoral epiphysis (SCFE). This 13-year-old presented with an acutely painful left hip following a minor fall. Note the widening of the physis and displacement of the femoral neck.

shear forces on the physis before it closes during late puberty.

Expert Opinion on Management Issues

Once the diagnosis is made, the patient should be kept non–weight-bearing and hospitalized immediately. The goals of treatment include prevention of further slippage by surgically stabilizing the diseased physis, thereby reducing the onset of osteoarthrosis and avoiding iatrogenically induced avascular necrosis and chondrolysis. This is usually done with fixation in situ with a single threaded screw across the physis into the center of the femoral epiphysis. Attempts at reducing the deformity prior to fixation should be avoided to decrease the risk of avascular necrosis. Redirectional osteotomy of the proximal femur is only rarely necessary subsequently to treat persistent deformity after physeal closure or avascular necrosis of the femoral head.

Common Pitfalls

Knee or medial thigh pain is commonly the only presenting complaint, which may mislead many clinicians into delaying the treatment of SCFE. The anatomic basis for this pattern of referred pain is the course of the anterior branch of the obturator nerve.

In patients who present with synchronous, bilateral slips or fall outside of the common age range (male 10 to 16 years, female 9 to 15 years), and endocrine workup should be initiated. Children who have received total body radiation or steroid therapy may be at increased risk for SCFE.

Accommodations for immediate non–weight-bearing should be made at the time of diagnosis and immediate referral for surgical stabilization should be initiated. A stable slip that becomes unstable carries a much worse prognosis.

Communication and Counseling

Following in situ pinning of an SCFE, many patients are anxious to return to previous levels of activity, including contact sports. Most patients are eventually able to return to full activities, although an extended period of restriction may be necessary. In more severe slips, degenerative changes in the hip may occur in early adulthood secondary to impingement. In situ pinning closes the proximal femoral physis, which grows at a rate of approximately 4 mm per year. Children who present early may develop a significant limb-length discrepancy.

SUGGESTED READINGS

1. Kocher MS, Zarakowski D, Kasser JR: Differentiating between septic arthritis and transient synovitis of the hip in children: An evidence-based clinical prediction algorithm. J Bone Joint Surg

[Am] 81:1662, 1999. **An algorithm for the clinician to differentiate septic arthritis from toxic synovitis based on evidence-based probabilities.**

2. Morrissy RT, Weinstein SL (eds): Pediatric Orthopaedics, 5th ed. Philadelphia: Lippincott, Williams & Wilkins, 2001. **Comprehensive textbook on pediatric orthopedic conditions and treatment.**

3. Wenger DR, Ward WT, Herring JA: Current concepts review: Legg-Calvé-Perthes disease. J Bone Joint Surg [Am] 73:778, 1991. **A thorough review of Perthes disease and its treatment alternatives.**

Torticollis

Benjamin D. Roye and David P. Roye

KEY CONCEPTS

- Torticollis is a symptom with a large number of underlying etiologies that often require a multidisciplinary approach to properly diagnose and treat.
- Congenital muscular torticollis is the most common form of torticollis and responds favorably to therapy when diagnosed in a timely fashion.
- As many as 20% of children with congenital muscular torticollis have hip dysplasia.
- Delay in diagnosis and treatment of any cause of torticollis can result in fixed deformities and unsightly molding abnormalities of the face and skull.
- Torticollis outside of infancy requires an aggressive approach to rule out dangerous neurologic causes and to prevent fixed deformities.

Torticollis (twisted neck or wry neck) is a deformity characterized by a combined head tilt and rotation of the neck (Fig. 1). When examining a child with torticollis, it is important to think of torticollis as a symptom and not a diagnosis in and of itself. The diagnoses associated with torticollis range from the benign positional torticollis of infancy to posterior fossa brain tumors (Table 1). Therefore, the history and physical are critical first steps to determine how to carry out the workup. A referral to one or more specialists is often required, including orthopedists, ophthalmologists, neurologists, neurosurgens, and otolaryngologists.

Expert Opinion on Management Issues

NONOSSEOUS TORTICOLLIS

Congenital muscular torticollis (CMT) accounts for approximately 80% of torticollis in children. The etiology of CMT remains unknown and is likely multifactorial; suspected causes include compartment syndrome secondary to venous obstruction, hemorrhage, abnormal intrauterine positioning, and difficult deliveries. Pathologically there is shortening and fibrosis of the sternocleidomastoid muscle.

On examination, the short sternocleidomastoid muscle causes the head to tilt toward the involved side and the chin to rotate toward the uninvolved side. When attempting to rotate the head opposite the direction of the deformity, motion will be limited by the involved muscle, which can be palpated as a tight band in the neck. Additionally, a palpable mass often develops within the substance of the sternocleidomastoid muscle during the perinatal period; this mass usually resolves after the first year of life even if the torticollis persists. Finally, look for flattening and asymmetry of the skull and face (plagiocephaly), which can develop if the torticollis is not effectively treated. In addition to the neck examination, a careful hip examination including an ultrasound is mandatory because approximately 20% of children with CMT have developmental hip dysplasia. Radiographs of the cervical spine may also be required to rule out bony abnormalities, especially in atypical cases.

If detected in the first 6 months of life, up to 95% of cases of CMT can be managed with a stretching

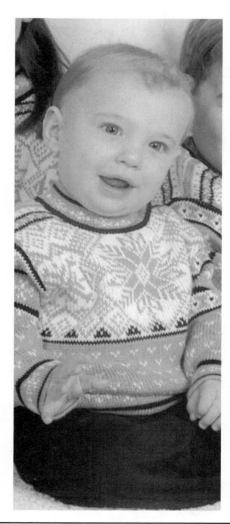

FIGURE 1. Typical appearance of torticollis in a 10-month-old baby.

16

TABLE 1 Common Causes of Torticollis

Diagnosis	CMT	Paroxysmal/ Positional Torticollis	Ocular Dysfunction	Sandifer Syndrome	Neurogenic	Atlantoaxial Rotatory Displacement
History	Present at birth. Head tilt always present and always to the same side.	Manifests early in life. Comes and goes. Deformity to different sides at different times.	Can manifest in infancy or childhood. Head tilt always to same side.	Manifests in infancy. Head tilt episodic and can be to either side. Head tilt seen with arching of back and extension of arms.	Can manifest at any time in life, but always suspect this cause in older child. Rapid and progressive onset of symptoms. Pain and irritability.	Manifests in childhood. Head tilt always to same side. Ask for history of upper respiratory tract infection or head/neck surgery (Grisel syndrome).
Physical examination	Limited rotation and lateral tilt of neck to one side. Tight mass in SCM.	Full passive ROM of neck. SCM not tight. Can see abnormal eye movements and lateral trunk shift.	Full active and passive ROM of neck. May see occulomotor deficits. Tilt may disappear when child supine.	Full passive ROM of neck. SCM not tight.	Rigid or flexible head tilt. Abnormalities in gait and/or balance.	Painful, limited neck motion.
Studies	Ultrasound of hips.	None required.	X-rays and possibly head CT if manifests outside of infancy.	None typically required unless in evaluation of reflux.	X-ray of neck. Head CT and MRI.	X-rays of neck including open-mouth views. Dynamic CT of neck.
Referrals	Orthopedics.	Orthopedics if confirmation of diagnosis required.	Ophthalmology. Possibly neurology.	Gastroenterology.	Neurology, neurosurgery.	Orthopedics. Otolaryngology for Grisel syndrome.
Treatment	Stretching exercises. Bracing or molding helmets in advanced cases.	Observation.	Typically surgical.	Treatment for gastroesophageal reflux.	Typically surgical. Traction if symptoms of more than 1 week duration.	Bracing and muscle relaxants. Surgery for failed conservative treatment.
Complications	Plagiocephaly.	None.	Plagiocephaly. Vision problems.	Related to reflux, not torticollis.	Depends on pathology. Can develop permanent neurologic deficit.	Plagiocephaly. Permanent, locked torticollis.

CMT, congenital muscular torticollis; ROM, range of motion; SCM, sternocleidomastoid (muscle).

program performed by parents with oversight by a physical therapist. The results are even more favorable for positional torticollis (0% failure rate), which is not associated with any tightness of the sternocleidomastoid muscle. However, children with a palpable mass are slightly more likely to fail nonoperative treatment (7.5% failure rate). Older babies with significant molding problems (plagiocephaly) may benefit from molding helmets to reshape the head. Surgical release of the contracted sternocleidomastoid muscle is indicated for children who fail physical therapy or present after 1 year of age. Surgery is followed by physical therapy and bracing.

Sandifer syndrome involves abnormal posturing of the back, arms, and neck associated with gastroesophageal reflux. The torticollis is probably a response to the pain of the esophagitis and is not associated with sternocleidomastoid tightness. Treatment of the reflux is usually curative for the torticollis and other postural abnormalities.

Ocular dysfunction can also cause torticollis. Weakness of the fourth cranial nerve can cause eye deviation to which the child responds by tilting the head (without rotation) to maintain visual acuity and binocularity. An ophthalmologist should evaluate torticollis not associated with sternocleidomastoid tightness. Treatment usually requires surgery to restore muscle balance around the eye.

Neurogenic causes must be considered in the diagnosis of any torticollis, especially one that is unusual or recalcitrant to therapy. These include central nervous system tumors (of the posterior fossa or spinal cord), syringomyelia, and Arnold-Chiari malformations. In these children the initial diagnosis may be CMT; however, on closer evaluation they are often found to have pain, spinal rigidity, irritability, and rapid progression of their spinal deformity. There can be other neurologic abnormalities as well, such as disturbances in gait or balance. Children with a suspected neurogenic cause need to be evaluated radiographically with plain films, CT scan, and MRI in addition to being assessed by a neurologist and neurosurgeon familiar with these problems. Treatment usually requires neurosurgical correction of the underlying pathology.

Paroxysmal torticollis of infancy is a rare, episodic form of torticollis that is usually self-limiting. It is characterized by periods of torticollis, usually in the morning, that last from minutes to a few days and have a frequency of one to four episodes per month. It is often associated with abnormal eye movements, lateral trunk shifts, and alternating sides of torticollis. No specific treatment is necessary as paroxysmal torticollis is usually a self-limiting disease.

Inflammatory conditions affecting the neck and cervical spine can also manifest as torticollis. Local irritation of any of the soft tissues of the neck can lead to torticollis, including viral myositis, cervical adenitis, retropharyngeal abscess, pharyngitis, cellulitis, sinusitis, or minor soft tissue trauma. Treatment of the underlying focus of inflammation is usually curative. Depending on the etiology, treatment may require use of nonsteroidal anti-inflammatory drugs (NSAIDs),

antibiotics, or surgery. A pediatric otolaryngologist can be helpful in many of these cases.

Spontaneous disc calcification, phenomenon of unknown etiology, is most frequently seen in the cervical spine. Clinical symptoms include pain, muscle spasm, low-grade fever, and occasionally torticollis. Laboratory studies are typically normal. Symptoms are acute in onset and may be related to trauma or an upper respiratory tract infection. The calcification typically disappears in 2 to 3 months. A cervical collar and mild analgesics are usually adequate therapy.

OSSEOUS TORTICOLLIS

Atlantoaxial rotatory displacement (subluxation) is one of the most common causes of torticollis outside of infancy. Increased ligamentous and capsular laxity from inflammation or trauma have been implicated as etiologic factors. Although often occurring after minor trauma, when atlantoaxial rotatory displacement occurs with an upper respiratory tract infection or after head and neck surgery, it is termed *Grisel syndrome*.

Prompt diagnosis is critical to avoid a locked dislocation that requires surgical reduction. Children usually present with painful torticollis and severely limited motion and are often not able to rotate their head past midline. Because of the position of the neck, plain radiographs are difficult to interpret. Dynamic CT scanning is currently the best imaging study to confirm the diagnosis.

Management depends on the duration of symptoms. Symptoms of less than 1 week's duration can be managed with a soft cervical collar, anti-inflammatory medication, and rest. If this fails, or if the child presents after 1 week of symptoms, the child should be hospitalized for halter or halo traction and muscle relaxants (e.g., diazepam). Fixed deformities may require open reduction and fusion of the upper cervical spine.

Approximately 25% of children with juvenile rheumatoid arthritis develop involvement of their cervical joints and can present with a torticollis. This entity can manifest similarly to atlantoaxial rotatory displacement and needs to be differentiated from other causes listed above. Symptoms usually respond to nonoperative measures—anti-inflammatory medications, heat, and a soft collar. The underlying systemic disease should also be addressed medically.

A variety of congenital vertebral anomalies can cause torticollis. The most common of these include occipitocervical synostosis, basilar impression, and odontoid anomalies, with an incidence of 1.4 to 2.5 per 100 children. Basilar impression may also be secondary to softening of the osseous structures at the base of the skull from metabolic bone disease, chronic inflammatory conditions, or a bone dysplasia. In addition to torticollis, these children may have low hairlines, restricted neck motion, neck webbing, and a high scapula. They need to be closely monitored clinically and radiographically by an orthopedist for signs of cervical instability and neurologic changes. Treatment varies widely depending on the severity of the deformity and the degree of instability, but may include surgical correction and stabilization.

Osteoid osteoma is the most common neoplasm in childhood causing torticollis. These children present with a painful torticollis and decreased neck motion. The pain classically is worst at night and responds dramatically to NSAIDs. Osteoid osteomas are often not readily visible on plain x-rays and frequently require a radionuclide bone scan to identify the pathology. A CT scan is then used to precisely confirm and localize the lesion. Although these lesions may spontaneously regress over years, the vast majority of orthopedists recommend surgical resection to prevent pain, complications associated with chronic NSAID use, and the development of a fixed deformity.

Common Pitfalls

The treating physician must be cognizant of the many diagnoses that share the common endpoint of torticollis to avoid the most common pitfall: failure to promptly diagnose and institute treatment. With congenital muscular torticollis, a delay in diagnosis can lead to unsightly flattening of the face and skull (plagiocephaly). In children with atlantoaxial rotatory displacement, delays in treatment can result in a rigid deformity requiring surgical correction. Although rare, neurologic causes for torticollis do exist, and failure to suspect and diagnose them in a timely manner can result in severe, permanent disability.

Another potential pitfall is failure to adequately examine the hips of a child with congenital muscular torticollis, as nearly 20% have hip dysplasia, half of which require treatment.

Communication and Counseling

Although most children with torticollis are successfully treated by nonoperative means, the treating physician must be aware of the different causes of torticollis because the proper treatment cannot be initiated unless the proper diagnosis is made. Most treatment regimens require cooperation from the family to assist in home therapy, monitor braces, or administer medications. Family members providing care must be instructed on the importance of their role in securing a successful outcome and avoiding potential complications.

SUGGESTED READINGS

1. Cheng JC, Tang SP: Outcome of surgical treatment of congenital muscular torticollis. Clin Orthop 362:190–200, 1999. **A retrospective review of surgically treated congenital muscular torticollis documenting excellent results, even for older children.**
2. Hensinger RN: Congenital anomalies of the cervical spine. Clin Orthop 264:16, 1991. **Reviews the findings and natural history of congenital cervical spine anomalies and associated comorbidities.**
3. Phillips WA, Hensinger RN: The management of rotatory atlantoaxial subluxation in children. J Bone Joint Surg Am 71(5):664–668, 1989. **This retrospective review of rotatory atlantoaxial subluxation found nonoperative therapy initiated before 1 month of symptoms eliminated the need for surgery.**
4. Tien YC, Su JY, Lin GT, et al: Ultrasonographic study of the coexistence of muscular torticollis and dysplasia of the hip. J Pediatr Orthop 21(3):343–347, 2001.

Muscular Dystrophies

Estanislao Bachrach, Antonio Luis Perez, and Louis M. Kunkel

KEY CONCEPTS

- Skeletal muscle is a normally regenerative tissue.
- Mature muscle cells of mammalian skeletal muscle, known as myofibers, are multinucleated syncytia formed by the fusion of mononucleated precursors, named myoblasts.
- The muscular dystrophies are a heterogeneous group of inherited disorders characterized by progressive muscle wasting and weakness caused by loss of the linkage between the extracellular matrix and the actin cytoskeleton.
- Successive rounds of degeneration and regeneration of muscle fibers eventually result in necrosis and replacement of muscle with fatty and fibrous tissue.
- The most common and severe form of muscular dystrophy is Duchenne muscular dystrophy, which affects 1 in 3500 live male births.

The muscular dystrophies are a heterogeneous group of genetic disorders characterized by progressive muscle weakness and wasting because of degeneration of muscle fibers and infiltration of connective and adipose tissue. Dystrophic muscle shows variation in muscle fiber size and centrally located nuclei. To date, mutations in more than 25 genes have been identified in human muscular dystrophies, the majority of which have been identified in recent years. These genes encode structural proteins at the muscle fiber membrane and the contractile apparatus, and potential signaling and enzymatic molecules. Muscular dystrophy includes a spectrum of disorders caused by loss of the linkage between the extracellular matrix and the actin cytoskeleton. These distinct disorders vary in degree of severity, the muscle groups affected, the mode of inheritance, and the age of onset (Table 1).

Muscle is known to be a regenerative tissue; this regeneration is accomplished via a heterogeneous population of muscle-resident cells, which include putative stem cells called satellite cells and myoblasts. On damage to muscle, these cells divide, fuse to one another and with existing myofibers, and create new muscle fibers, replacing the necrotic ones. In patients with muscular dystrophies the regeneration-degeneration cycle of muscle fibers is much more frequent than in normal individuals. This process causes muscle tissue to remain inflamed and become rich in cytokines and cell-signaling molecules. These signals are hypothesized to

TABLE 1 List of Muscular Dystrophies

Disease	Disease Subtype	Inheritance Pattern	Gene Product
DMD/BMD		XR	Dystrophin
EDMD		XR	Emerin
		AD/AR	Lamin-A/C
LGMD	1A	AD	Myotilin
	1B	AD	Lamin-A/C
	1C	AD	Caveolin-3
	1D	AD	Unknown
	1E	AD	Unknown
	2A	AR	Calpain-3
	2B	AR	Dysferlin
	2C	AR	γ-sarcoglycan
	2D	AR	α-sarcoglycan
	2E	AR	β-sarcoglycan
	2F	AR	δ-sarcoglycan
	2G	AR	Telethonin
	2H	AR	TRIM32
	2I	AR	Fukutin-related protein
	2J	AR	Titin
CMD	1A	AR	Lamini α2 chain
	1B	AR	Unknown
	1C	AR	Fukutin-related protein
	Fukuyama	AR	Fukutin
	Integrin α7	AR	Integrin α7
	MEB deficiency	AR	O-mannose β–1,2-*N*-acetylglucosaminyl transferase
Distal	Miyoshi myopathy	AR	Dysferlin
	Tibial MD	AD	Titin

AD, autosomal dominant; AR, autosomal recessive; BMD, Becker muscular dystrophy; CMD, congenital muscular dystrophy; DMD, Duchenne muscular dystrophy; EDMD, Emery-Dreifuss muscular dystrophy; XR, X chromosome recessive.

BOX 1 Duchenne Muscular Dystrophy Mutations

- 70% Duchenne muscular dystrophy (DMD) cases with affected relatives
- 30% DMD de novo mutations
- 60% large deletions
- 5% duplications
- 35% point mutation/small deletion/insertions

---

be able to recruit progenitor cells into the damaged tissue for repair processes.

The most common and severe form of muscular dystrophy is Duchenne muscular dystrophy (DMD). DMD is an X-linked recessive disease characterized by a mutation in the gene encoding dystrophin, a muscle myofiber-stabilizing protein (Box 1). Cloning of this gene and subsequent protein studies have enabled significant diagnostic and therapeutic advances for muscular dystrophies. Dystrophin forms a complex with other several sarcolemmal and subsarcolemmal proteins known as the dystrophin-associated protein complex (DAPC) (Fig. 1). The DAPC is constituted by the sarcoglycan-sarcospan complex and three groups of proteins: dystroglycan, dystrobrevin, and syntrophin.

Approximately 1 out of 3500 live male births is affected by DMD. These children suffer bilateral weakness in the proximal muscles of the hip girdle and legs in early childhood, progressing by age 11 to widespread weakening of the musculature and loss of ambulation. DMD patient life expectancy is in the third decade, with death resulting most frequently from cardiac complications or respiratory failure (Table 2). Dystrophin is also compromised in another less frequent and milder disease, Becker muscular dystrophy (BMD), which affects only 1 out of 30,000 males. These patients present a much broader variation of symptoms, rate of progression and life expectancy. There is another diverse group of muscle-wasting disorders, less frequent than DMD and BMD, which characteristically affect the large muscles of the pelvic and shoulder girdles, known as the limb-girdle muscular dystrophies (LGMD). Onset of LGMD often occurs in the second or third decade and has a mild progression relative to the DMD. Mutations affecting LGMD are found in many different genes whose products are components of the myofiber, such as the contractile apparatus, the nuclear lamina, the sarcolemma, and the cytoplasm.

Expert Opinion on Management Issues

Curative therapies do not yet exist for muscular dystrophies. Thus, current treatments are intended to maintain muscle flexibility and strength and to provide mechanical and respiratory support. Muscular dystrophy patients annually undergo electrocardiography, pulmonary function studies, and chest radiographs,

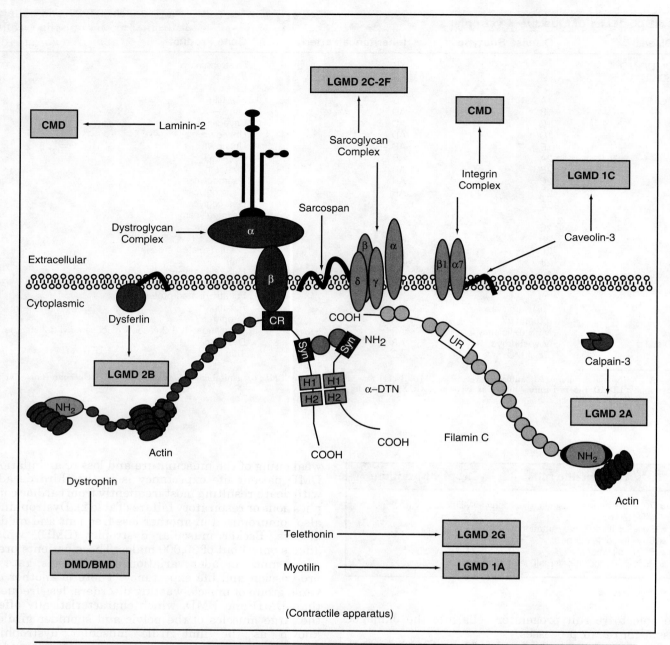

FIGURE 1. Dystrophin-associated protein complex (DAPC) and associated subtypes of muscular dystrophies. αDTN, dystrobrevin; BMD, Becker muscular dystrophy; CMD, congenital muscular dystrophy; DMD, Duchenne muscular dystrophy; LGMD, limb-girdle muscular dystrophies.

along with tests to monitor the swallowing function. Physical therapy is used to prevent contractures, a condition in which shortened muscles around joints cause abnormal and sometimes painful positioning of the joints and orthoses. In some cases corrective orthopedic surgery may be needed to improve the quality of life. These palliative treatments help to slow functional impairment but cannot prevent disability, which usually begins by the end of the first decade in DMD patients, or death, which on average occurs in the third decade. Today, several treatment approaches—including pharmacologic, gene therapy, cell-based therapy, RNA, and

down- or upregulation of gene therapies—are being explored. Additionally, several nutritional supplements (e.g., creatine, glutamine, and coenzyme Q) have been studied in a series of clinical trials, some showing mild increases in arm-muscle strength and time until fatigue (Box 2).

The pharmacologic therapies involve the use of steroids, antibiotics, and anabolic agents, which may slow the progression of the disease. So far, clinical trials using such agents have shown poor or negative results. Although the benefits of glucocorticoid steroid use in DMD are well documented, there is only emerging

TABLE 2 Duchenne Muscular Dystrophy Clinical Symptoms and Diagnosis

Age	Most Common Symptoms	Diagnosis
1–5 yr	Motor delays Tripping or falling Toe walking	Patient's family history Pattern of muscle involvement Age of onset Gower sign Muscle pseudohypertrophy
6–10 yr	Worsening of tripping and falling	Increased serum levels of muscle enzymes (CK, aldolase, ALT, AST, LDH) DNA examination (multiple PCR testing [hot spots]) Protein examination (immunohistochemistry/ Western blot)
11–15 yr	Loss of ambulation Scoliosis Lung atelectasis Possible cardiomyopathy	Histologic examination (muscle fiber size, necrosis, phagocytosis, regenerating fibers, connective and adipose tissue infiltration)
20–25 yr	Decreased lung capacity Difficulty clearing respiratory secretions Increase risk of pneumonia and respiratory failure Worsening cardiomyopathy	

ALT, alanine transaminase; AST, aspartate transaminase; CK, creatine kinase; LDH, lactate dehydrogenase; PCR, polymerase chain reaction.

BOX 2 Current Treatments and Research

- Physical therapy—prevents contractures
- Corrective orthopedic surgery—slows functional impairment
- Nutritional supplements—creatine, glutamine, and coenzyme Q
- Pharmacologic—steroids, antibiotics, and anabolic agents
- Gene therapy—lentiviral and adeno-associated vectors (AAV) coding muscle-specific promoters
- Cell-based therapy—myoblasts, myogenic progenitor cells, and pluripotent stem cells
- RNA therapy—exon-skipping to correct the transcript reading frame, down- or upregulation of genes myostatin, utrophin

---

consensus on the best dose, dosage regimen, and age at which treatment should be initiated. Prednisone and its derivatives are the most widely used in the United States. Steroids have been reported to improve muscular dystrophy symptoms potentially through anti-inflammatory effect, stabilization of the sarcolemma, protection from Ca^{2+} influx, and immunosuppression. However, side effects include stunting of growth, loss of bone density, behavioral changes, weight gain, and cataracts. Recently, aminoglycoside antibiotics, such as gentamicin, have been shown to partially restore expression of genes with a premature stop codon allowing translational read-through in mammalian cells. Those drugs have already been approved for use in humans and clinical trials are now under way in DMD patients.

Gene therapy, which involves the introduction of functional copies of genes into mutated cells, is an attractive approach given that most of the muscular dystrophies are caused by single-gene defects. For example, the restoration of normal dystrophin expression in murine models for DMD has been shown to reverse the mutant phenotype. Because of the large size of some of the genes involved in muscular dystrophies and the size-limited capacity of transportation of viral vectors used in studies of gene therapy, mini and micro genes are being designed with already some promising results. Current generations of lentiviral and adeno-associated vectors (AAV) coding muscle specific promoters have demonstrated highly efficient gene transduction into skeletal muscle. Expression cassettes must not only include the gene to be delivered but also the DNA elements that control the activity of the gene.

Introduction of cells bearing a functional gene is an attractive method for treating the muscular dystrophies. Any effective cell therapy must target delivery of functional donor cells to all areas of muscle regeneration. For muscle diseases, the donor cells currently under investigation as candidates for clinical trials include myoblasts, myogenic progenitor cells, and pluripotent stem cells isolated from different tissues, mostly skeletal muscle and the hematopoietic compartment. Three routes for delivery of these donor cells to damaged muscles are being studied. These methods allow the evaluation of the ability of donor cells to fuse with existing myofibers and to produce absent gene products. Intramuscular transplantation allows for the direct delivery of cells to sites of interest in damaged tissue. It was shown in animal models for muscular dystrophies that donor cells introduced into the venous system can be delivered to damaged muscle. Degree of tissue injury appears to correlate with cellular uptake and engraftment into muscle. Finally, transplantation into arteries that feed myogenic tissue allows injected cells to be delivered directly to the muscle, bypassing circulation through lungs and heart. This recent approach has yielded promising early results with much higher efficiency of engraftment in mouse models than both intramuscular and intravenous delivery. Importantly, both intravenous and intra-arterial injections are safe, common clinical procedures.

Recently, the use of RNA to induce exon-skipping to correct the transcript reading frame has shown some success. Similar techniques use antisense oligoribonucleotides directed against the splice site of the affected intron or chimeric DNA or RNA oligomers, which induce base pair changes in the genome using a cellular mismatch repair mechanisms. Although still inefficient, these emerging treatment methods have potential. The efficiency of these procedures will depend on precise knowledge of the gene mutation in each patient.

Finally, studies including down- or upregulation of different muscle genes or their protein products are being investigated. Myostatin, a transforming growth factor-β (TGF-β) family member, acts as a negative regulator of muscle growth, suggesting that inhibition of this protein, for example with antibodies, may benefit patients at all stages of the disease. Utrophin, a sarcolemmal protein, is upregulated in DMD patients. It may provide a similar link between the cytoskeleton and extracellular matrix. Different agents, such as ADAM12 (a *d*istintegrin *a*nd *m*etallo) or calcineurin, are being used to upregulate endogenous utrophin.

Common Pitfalls

- Curative therapies do not yet exist for muscular dystrophies.
- Prednisone, the most used drug in the United States to alleviate muscular dystrophy symptoms, has side effects including stunting of growth, loss of bone density, behavioral changes, weight gain, and cataracts.
- Because the rate of spontaneous mutations is high, some muscular dystrophies, such as DMD and BMD, are difficult to prevent.

Communication and Counseling

Muscular dystrophies can affect people of all ages. Although some forms first become apparent in infancy or childhood, others may not appear until middle age or later.

Since the discovery of the dystrophin gene in the late 1980s, important progress has been made in understanding the genetics and pathogenesis of DMD. This has led to the identification of a number of genetic defects, which give rise to other muscular dystrophies. Unfortunately, there is still no curative treatment for any muscular dystrophy; however, advances in ventilation, surgical, and pharmacologic methods that can alleviate disease symptoms have greatly increased patient lifespan over the last decade. The use of a variety of animal models and transgenic technology are important tools for the development of novel therapies. In combination, these advances may have the potential to move research closer to the ultimate objective of finding curative treatments. Advances in diagnostic methods have already provided significant benefits to the management of these diseases by physicians, patients, and their families.

SUGGESTED READINGS

1. Dubowitz V: Therapeutic efforts in Duchenne muscular dystrophy; the need for a common language between basic scientists and clinicians. Neuromuscul Disord 14(8–9):451–455, 2004. **Detailed differences between animal models and human patients.**
2. Lapidos KA, Kakkar R, McNally EM: The dystrophin glycoprotein complex: Signaling strength and integrity for the sarcolemma. Circ Res 94(8):1023–1031, 2004. **Describes the dystrophin glycoprotein complex.**
3. Manzur AY, Kuntzer T, Pike M, Swan A: Glucocorticoid corticosteroids for Duchenne muscular dystrophy. Cochrane Database Syst Rev (2):CD003725, 2004. **Assesses glucocorticoid corticosteroids treatments.**
4. Mukherjee M, Mittal B: Muscular dystrophies. Indian J Pediatr 71(2):161–168, 2004. **Reviews all muscular dystrophies.**
5. Laval SH, Bushby KM: Limb-girdle muscular dystrophies—from genetics to molecular pathology. Neuropathol Appl Neurobiol 30(2):91–105, 2004. **Gives detailed review of limb-girdle muscular dystrophy.**
6. Mathews KD: Muscular dystrophy overview: Genetics and diagnosis. Neurol Clin 21(4):795–816, 2003. **Indicates importance of genetics and diagnosis in muscular dystrophies.**
7. Riggs JE, Bodensteiner JB, Schochet SS Jr: Congenital myopathies/dystrophies. Neurol Clin 21(4):779–794; v–vi, 2003. **Reviews congenital dystrophies.**
8. Sohn RL, Gussoni E: Stem cell therapy for muscular dystrophy. Expert Opin Biol Ther 4(1):1–9, 2004. **Indicates importance of stem cells in future treatments.**
9. Bogdanovich S, Perkins KJ, Krag TO, Khurana TS: Therapeutics for Duchenne muscular dystrophy: Current approaches and future directions. J Mol Med 82(2):102–115, 2004. **Reviews therapeutic approaches for DMD.**
10. Collins CA, Morgan JE: Duchenne's muscular dystrophy: Animal models used to investigate pathogenesis and develop therapeutic strategies. Int J Exp Pathol 84(4):165–172, 2003. **Indicates importance of animal models studies.**
11. Hoffman EP, Brown KJ, Eccleston E: New molecular research technologies in the study of muscle disease. Curr Opin Rheumatol 15(6):698–707, 2003. **Describes new technologies for diagnosis.**

Myasthenia Gravis

Peter B. Kang and Richard S. Finkel

KEY CONCEPTS

- There are three basic forms of myasthenia gravis in children: neonatal, congenital, and juvenile.
- The neonatal and juvenile forms are autoimmune, the congenital is genetic in origin.
- With supportive therapy, the neonatal form resolves spontaneously. Congenital myasthenia syndrome may be difficult to treat, as immune-modulating therapies are ineffective
- The therapeutic approach to juvenile myasthenia gravis is similar to that in adult autoimmune myasthenia gravis.
- Drug therapy should be tailored to the subtype and may sometimes worsen symptoms.

Myasthenia gravis (MG) in its various forms, although best known as an adult illness, can affect children of all ages. Weakness is caused by ineffective acetylcholine transmission at the neuromuscular junction (NMJ). MG should be considered whenever ptosis; ophthalmoparesis; or weakness of bulbar, respiratory, or limb muscles is present. Current classification is based on distribution (ocular, bulbar, generalized), age at onset (neonatal, congenital, juvenile), and mechanism (autoimmune, genetic). These distinctions have important implications for therapy. In MG, weakness tends to fluctuate, with worsening of symptoms as the day advances, and painless fatigue occurs during acute exercise with improvement after rest. Autoimmune MG is typically idiopathic; rare iatrogenic cases in children are seen following bone marrow transplant or from D-penicillamine or interferon use. Associated autoimmune disorders may also be seen: hyperthyroidism and collagen vascular disorders. By comparison, fixed weakness suggests a myopathy or neuropathy, although poor endurance is often also seen.

The prognosis in children varies with the type of MG, the age at onset, human leukocyte antibody (HLA) status, ethnicity, and gender. Treatment modalities include symptomatic management with acetylcholinesterase (AChE) inhibitors, immune-modulating medications and thymectomy, acute medical management of myasthenic and cholinergic crises, genetic counseling, and ongoing psychological support. Although death from MG is now rare, chronic physical and psychological disabilities remain challenges.

Expert Opinion on Management Issues

The goals of treatment are to provide symptomatic relief, prevent generalization of ocular MG, anticipate and prevent exacerbations, stabilize and reverse acute deterioration, restore function, and avoid chronic impairment from the disease or its treatment. Certain medications are useful in childhood MG (Table 1). Acute worsening of symptoms may be triggered by such events as intercurrent illnesses and cessation of medications.

SYMPTOMATIC TREATMENT

Cholinesterase inhibitors such as pyridostigmine bromide (Mestinon) and neostigmine prolong the effect of acetylcholine at the NMJ and lessen symptoms in MG, especially in the neonatal and juvenile forms. The short half-life of edrophonium (Tensilon) makes it useful only for diagnostic purposes. Pyridostigmine bromide is typically the first medication tried in both ocular and generalized disease. The extended-release preparation is used infrequently in children, apart from an adolescent with bulbar symptoms who may benefit from a dose before bedtime. Oral neostigmine is rarely used because of greater muscarinic side effects. *Intravenous or intramuscular doses are one thirtieth of the usual oral dose.* On occasion, an oral antimuscarinic agent (e.g., glycopyrrolate) is used adjunctively to reduce hypersalivation. During labor, a woman with MG should receive a parenteral dose of pyridostigmine bromide, which improves the strength of uterine contractions and may also benefit the infant at delivery. The patient and parent must understand that cholinesterase inhibitor medications improve, but rarely fully resolve, myasthenic symptoms and that the dosage should not be increased without direction from a physician. Prepubertal children may have a spontaneous remission of MG.

IMMUNE-MODULATING THERAPY

If the maximum tolerated dose of a cholinesterase inhibitor does not adequately control acute or chronic symptoms, immunosuppressive medications may result in further improvement and help modulate the course of disease.

For those with bulbar symptoms, respiratory distress, severe limb weakness, and residual ophthalmoparesis (but usually not in those with purely ocular manifestations), immunosuppressive therapy should be considered. Oral prednisone is traditionally the first medication added to a cholinesterase inhibitor in adults, although chronic side effects may limit its use, especially in growing children. During the first few weeks of steroid therapy, symptoms may worsen, sometimes to the point of myasthenic crisis. Once control is established, the patient should be switched to an alternate-day schedule and the dosage slowly tapered over a period of several months while watching closely for a flare in disease activity and monitoring for infection and chronic steroid side effects. On occasion, pulse intravenous methylprednisolone is used to treat acute decompensation in a patient already receiving steroids, is used in a monthly chronic treatment regimen in a steroid-dependent patient who cannot tolerate prednisone, or is used in conjunction with monthly intravenous immune globulin (IVIG) infusions. In childhood ocular myasthenia, the ptosis is more responsive than oculomotor palsies to drug therapy.

Cytotoxic agents are added if steroids are not adequately effective, if the dosage cannot be tapered to a low alternate-day schedule, or if side effects are excessive. In some cases, steroids may be bypassed entirely in favor of a cytotoxic agent. Azathioprine is the mildest agent and is often used first, but it may take several months to take effect. Cyclosporine acts more quickly but has a higher toxicity profile. Cyclophosphamide is not commonly used in children with juvenile MG (JMG) and may cause hemorrhagic cystitis. Chronic immunosuppressive medications increase the risk of hematopoietic, renal, hepatic, and reproductive (sterility and teratogenicity) toxic effects, and infections and late malignancies. Newer agents that have had anecdotal success include rituximab and mycophenolate mofetil (CellCept).

IVIG and plasmapheresis can be important emergency treatments during acute deterioration. On a chronic basis, IVIG is given every 4 to 8 weeks (as often as every 2 weeks during exacerbations) when the other medications mentioned previously do not control the symptoms or while waiting for them to take effect. Side effects include transient leukopenia, aseptic meningitis, and renal failure. Plasmapheresis and IVIG are used before or after thymectomy (or both) to minimize postoperative complications. The effect of plasmapheresis usually lasts 6 to 8 weeks; complications include hypotension, hypoalbuminemia, coagulopathies, and hypocalcemia.

TABLE 1 Medications Useful in Childhood Myasthenia Gravis*

Generic Name (Trade Name) OTC/Rx	Dosage/Route/Regimen	Maximum Dose	Dosage Formulations	Common Adverse Reactions	Therapeutic Concentrations	Comments
Cholinesterase inhibitors: Inhibit metabolism of acetylcholine at neuromuscular junction						
Edrophonium chloride (Tensilon) Rx; used only for diagnostic purposes	Neonates and infants IV: 0.01 mg/kg test dose × 1 0.1 mg/kg; may repeat every min to maximum of 0.5 mg.	0.5 mg	10 mg/mL (15 mL) injectable, dilute 1:10 in normal saline	Arrhythmias, increased secretions, dizziness, headache, gastrointestinal distress	N/A	Patient must be on cardiac monitor during test; have atropine ready in case of overdose. Most sensitive in NMG and JMG, but also positive in some cases of CMS.
	Children > 1 year and < 34 kg: 1 mg IV; may repeat every min to maximum of 5 mg.	5 mg				
	Children > 1 yr and > 34 kg: 2 mg IV; may give additional 1 mg every min to maximum of 10 mg.	10 mg				
Pyridostigmine bromide (Mestinon) Rx	0.5–1.0 mg/kg/dose PO q4–6h; IV dose is 1/30th of PO dose.	7 mg/kg/day (pediatric) or 300 mg/day (adult)	12 mg/mL syrup; 60 mg tablet; 180 mg LA tablet; 5 mg/mL (2 mL) injectable			Most effective in NMG and JMG, variable in CMS (may not be effective at all).
Neostigmine methylsulfate Rx	0.03 mg/kg/dose IM or SC q3–6h.	0.03 mg/kg/ dose	1 mg/mL (2 mL) injectable			Oral formulation not recommended. Renal adjustment required.
Immunosuppressants: Reduce autoimmune activity at the neuromuscular junction						
Prednisone (Deltasone) Rx	0.5–2.0 mg/kg/day PO, initially given bid, then qd, then qod.	2 mg/kg/day (pediatric), 100 mg/day (adult)	1, 5, 10, 20, 50 mg tablets	Weight gain, hypertension, hyperglycemia, immunosuppression, behavioral changes, insomnia, growth retardation, cataracts, gastritis, osteopenia	N/A	80% response in JMG in 2–8 weeks.
Prednisolone (Prelone) Rx			15 mg/5 mL (240 mL), 5 mg/5 mL (120 mL)			
Methylprednisolone (Solu-Medrol) Rx	10–30 mg/kg/day divided q6h for 3 days, or given as a single pulse.	1 g/day	Various injectable formulations		N/A	

IVIG (Gamunex, Sandoglobulin) Rx	2 g/kg total divided over 2–5 days; 5 days recommended for initial course. Infusion rate must be increased slowly according to hospital protocol.	150 g	10% = 100 mg/mL injectable (10, 50, 100, 200 mL)	Aseptic meningitis, renal failure, hypertension, transient leukopenia, contraindicated in IgA deficiency (can cause anaphylaxis), stroke (rare in children).	N/A	73% of JMG patients improve within 5 days; can be used q 4–8 wk chronically and q 2–3 wk during exacerbations.
Plasmapheresis Rx	250 mL/kg total divided into 4 or 5 sessions over 7–14 days.	250 mL/kg	N/A	Hypotension, coagulopathies, hypoalbuminemia, hypocalcemia.	N/A	Especially useful before thymectomy or during acute crisis.
Azathioprine[†] (Imuran) Rx	1 mg/kg/dose qd; increase by 0.5 mg/kg/dose q4–8 weeks.	3 mg/kg/dose qd	50 mg tablet, 50 mg/mL liquid 100 mg/20 mL injection	Bone marrow suppression, rash, hepatotoxicity, alopecia, serum sickness, gastrointestinal distress	N/A	Very slow onset of action (months); liquid prepared in pharmacy.
Cyclosporine (Neoral, Sandimmune) Rx	3–5 mg/kg/day divided q12h; IV dose is 1/3 PO dose.	10 mg/kg/day	25, 100 mg caps, 100 mg/mL liquid, 50 mg/mL injectable (5 mL)	Renal insufficiency, hypertension, headache, hirsutism, gastrointestinal distress	Serum level therapeutic at 150–250 ng/mL; lower levels may suffice.	More rapid onset than azathioprine, but more side effects; Neoral and Sandimmune are not bioequivalent.
Cyclophosphamide[†] (Cytoxan) Rx	2 mg/kg PO daily; 50 mg/kg IV daily × 4 days, repeat as needed (typically once a month); PO regimen usually more effective than IV.	4 mg/kg PO daily	25 mg tablet, 20 mg/mL injectable	Hemorrhagic cystitis, alopecia, sterility, gastrointestinal distress, leukopenia, late malignancy including bladder carcinoma and lymphoma.	N/A	Hemorrhagic cystitis is potentially a fatal reaction and can be avoided with adequate hydration; most aggressive therapy, not first-line.

*Therapeutic concentrations not routinely used with these medications.
[†]Azathioprine and cyclophosphamide formulations are mixed in individual pharmacies.
bid, two times daily; CMS, congenital myasthenic syndrome; IM, intramuscularly; IV, intravenously; JMG, juvenile myasthenia gravis; LA, long acting; NMG, neonatal myasthenia gravis; qd, every day; qod, every other day; qph, every x hours; PO, orally; Rx, prescription; SC, subcutaneously.
From Andrews PI: Autoimmune myasthenia gravis in childhood. Semin Neurol 24:101–110, 2004.

In neonatal MG, exchange transfusion is used instead of plasmapheresis.

The thymus is a significant source of the antibodies that cause JMG, possibly via removal of thymic CD4+ helper T cells that modulate B-cell antibody production. Thymomas are rare in children, but even the suspicion of a tumor on chest CT is an absolute indication for thymectomy. Otherwise, the decision about surgery rests on the probability of achieving remission, which is more likely if thymectomy is performed early, within two years of diagnosis. It is not usually performed for pure ocular JMG. Approximately 50% of the patients with JMG who undergo thymectomy improve significantly, with reduction or elimination of the need for medications. The entire thymus should be removed whenever possible, because even a small amount of thymus tissue can produce large quantities of antibodies. The standard approach is trans-sternal, but some centers have reported equally favorable results in children with a video-assisted thoracoscopic approach. Often, corticosteroids are given preoperatively to reduce the size of the gland, followed by a slow taper. The response to thymectomy may take over a year. Because thymectomy can trigger a myasthenic crisis, postoperative patients need to be monitored carefully.

CRITICAL CARE MANAGEMENT

MG can deteriorate quickly into a medical emergency characterized by respiratory failure and dysphagia. When caused by accentuation of underlying disease, it is termed *myasthenic crisis* and must be distinguished from a cholinergic crisis resulting from excessive cholinesterase inhibitor medication. Common triggers include infection, initiation of steroid therapy, abrupt cessation of medication, and thymectomy. Respiratory failure can be caused by airway obstruction, diaphragmatic weakness, or both. Airway obstruction, often heralded by increased bulbar symptoms (dysphagia and dysarthria) or aspiration, is caused by weakness of the pharyngeal muscles. Objective respiratory measurements include forced vital capacity (normal, >15 mL/kg; hard to measure in young children, especially if lip weakness creates a poor seal), negative inspiratory force (normal, below −20 cm H_2O), and arterial blood gas testing for CO_2 retention. Clinical assessments include counting during one exhalation (older children should be able to count past 30 on one breath), peak cough flow, watching the child swallow water, and testing of neck flexion and extension strength. Complications during acute exacerbations include sleep apnea, aspiration, and weight loss.

A potentially unstable patient should be placed in a critical care unit with frequent forced vital capacity and negative inspiratory force measurements and cardiac monitoring. In this closely monitored setting, a test dose of edrophonium (0.015 mg/kg) is given 1 hour after the usual dose of oral cholinesterase inhibitor medication and may be repeated once if tolerated and no improvement is seen. Improvement in respiratory status indicates an exacerbation of MG, whereas worsening suggests a cholinergic crisis. When the latter is present, all cholinesterase inhibitor therapy should be discontinued until the patient is stabilized. A myasthenic or cholinergic crisis may require intubation, mechanical ventilation, and enteral tube feedings if gastrointestinal motility remains intact. In crises triggered by infection, medical therapy should be restricted to cholinesterase inhibitors whenever possible and the acute use of corticosteroids or aminoglycoside antibiotics should be avoided. Oral feedings are best

---

BOX 1 Medications Contraindicated in Myasthenia Gravis*

Absolute Contraindication: These drugs should never be administered

- D-penicillamine
- Interferon

Relative Contraindication: These drugs should be avoided whenever possible

- Aminoglycoside antibiotics
  - Amikacin
  - Gentamicin
  - Neomycin
  - Streptomycin
  - Tobramycin
- Anesthetic agents, including ethanol
- Antiarrhythmics
  - Procainamide
  - Quinidine
  - Quinine
  - Lidocaine
  - Procaine
- Antibiotic agents, other (check individual antibiotic before prescribing)
- Anticonvulsants
  - Gabapentin
  - Phenytoin
- β-blockers
  - Propranolol
  - Timolol maleate eyedrops
- Calcium-channel blockers
  - Verapamil
- Fluoroquinolone antibiotics
  - Norfloxacin
  - Ofloxacin
  - Pefloxacin
- Iodinated contrast agents
- Magnesium compounds
  - Certain antacids
  - Epsom salts
  - Milk of magnesium
- Neuromuscular blocking agents
  - Botulinum toxin
  - D-tubocurarine
  - Succinylcholine
  - Vecuronium
- Thyroid preparations

---

*This list is not exhaustive. Any new medication should be checked against an up-to-date drug database. A number of medications not listed here have been reported to cause worsening of myasthenia gravis (MG) in rare cases. As with other cases in which relative contraindications exist, clinical judgment should be exercised; if alternative medications are not available and the clinical situation is serious enough, some of these may need to be administered under close supervision. Corticosteroids initially worsen symptoms, so should be used with caution for indications other than MG in affected patients.

From Andrews PI: Autoimmune myasthenia gravis in childhood. Semin Neurol 24:101–110, 2004.

deferred until swallowing and gastrointestinal motility are evaluated.

Common Pitfalls

- The intravenous or intramuscular dose of the acetylcholinesterase inhibitors (physostigmine and neostigmine) is one-thirtieth the oral dose.
- Certain medications are contraindicated in MG (Box 1) (check all drugs against a medication database).
- Undertreatment and overtreatment with acetylcholinesterase inhibitors may both manifest with increased weakness and may be difficult to distinguish.
- Symptoms may worsen for the first week after initiating steroid therapy; chronic therapy may cause significant side effects. Alternate-day regimens may reduce side effects.

Communication and Counseling

Close follow-up by an ophthalmologist is necessary to minimize the risk of amblyopia. Sometimes, lid surgery or lid crutches for the ptosis are helpful. Physical therapy can help maintain activity levels. Children with MG, much like adults, are often fragile psychologically and benefit from ongoing counseling. Micromanagement of medication by patients or parents can present a challenge to treating physicians. The role of the primary care physician is critical in maintaining the well-being of a child with MG. Coordinated specialty care is available in the United States at a Muscular Dystrophy Association-sponsored neuromuscular clinic. The Muscular Dystrophy Association (http://www.mdausa. org), the Myasthenia Gravis Foundation of America (800–541–5454, http://www.myasthenia.org), and the Myasthenia Gravis Association of Canada (416–444–8357) provide excellent resources.

ACKNOWLEDGMENT

The authors thank Kwang S. Kang, R.Ph., for assistance with medication information.

SUGGESTED READINGS

1. Andrews PI: Autoimmune myasthenia gravis in childhood. Semin Neurol 24:101–110, 2004. **Recent review of pediatric MG.**
2. Harper CM: Congenital myasthenic syndromes. Semin Neurol 24:111–123, 2004. **Recent review of congenital myasthenic syndrome.**
3. Kim JH, Hwang JM, Hwang YS, et al: Childhood ocular myasthenia gravis. Ophthalmology 110:1458–1462, 2003. **Series of 24 children with ocular MG.**
4. Kolski HK, Kim PC, Vajsar J: Video-assisted thoracoscopic thymectomy in juvenile myasthenia. J Child Neurol 16:569–573, 2001. **Series of patients with JMG treated with minimally invasive thymectomy.**
5. McConville J, Farrugia ME, Beeson D, et al: Detection and characterization of MuSK antibodies in seronegative myasthenia gravis. Ann Neurol 55:580–584, 2004. **Describes presence and pathophysiology of MuSK antibodies in pediatric and adult MG patients.**
6. Meriggioli MN, Ciafaloni E, Al-Hayk KA, et al: Mycophenolate mofetil for myasthenia gravis: An analysis of efficacy, safety, and tolerability. Neurology 61:1438–1440, 2003. **Retrospective analysis of an alternative immunosuppressive agent in children and adults.**
7. Midelfart J, Daltveit AK, Gilhus NE: Myasthenia gravis: Consequences for pregnancy, delivery, and the newborn. Neurology 61:1362–1366, 2003. **Investigates complications of maternal MG for the child, including neonatal MG.**
8. Palace J, Vincent A, Beeson D: Myasthenia gravis: Diagnostic and management dilemmas. Curr Opin Neurol 14:583–589, 2001. **Discusses diagnostic and therapeutic problems.**
9. Wylam ME, Anderson PM, Kuntz NL, et al: Successful treatment of refractory myasthenia gravis using rituximab: A pediatric case report. J Pediatr 143:674–677, 2003. **Report of antibody therapy for MG.**

16

17

K. Robin Carder

Skin Diseases of the Neonate, Including Diaper Dermatitis

KEY CONCEPTS

- Familiarity with and recognition of newborn dermatoses is important for avoiding extensive laboratory workups and unnecessary parental anguish. These conditions can be benign and transient, but they can also be fatal, so an accurate and prompt diagnosis is crucial.
- Infants presenting with cutaneous blisters or pustules should be closely evaluated for signs of underlying illness. In addition to herpes and varicella infections, blisters or pustules can be seen in the setting of other potentially serious infections, such as cytomegalovirus, staphylococcal scalded skin syndrome or bullous impetigo, *Listeria monocytogenes, Pseudomonas, Aspergillus*, syphilis, or systemic candidiasis.
- In the evaluation of a newborn with blisters or pustules, bedside laboratory tests including cultures of lesional fluid and skin scrapings for Wright, potassium hydroxide (KOH), and/or Gram stains are essential and valuable tools. These simple tests can provide immediate confirmation of the diagnosis.
- Herpes or varicella infection in the newborn should be considered a medical emergency.
- A variety of skin conditions may manifest in the diaper area, including fungal or yeast infections, bacterial infections, chronic dermatoses, and systemic diseases. Close clinical evaluation, an accurate history, and knowledge of the differential diagnoses are essential for proper diagnosis and therapy.
- Mid- to high-potency topical steroids should be avoided in the diaper area as the risk of skin atrophy and systemic absorption are enhanced by diaper occlusion.

Neonatal Skin Diseases

Skin diseases of newborns vary from benign, transient conditions requiring no therapy to life-threatening diseases, which can be fatal if unrecognized and untreated. The majority of fatal diseases involve infection, most notably with herpes simplex virus (HSV), and for this reason, blistering eruptions in the newborn should be considered a medical emergency. Fear of missing a more serious condition may prompt a prolonged and costly evaluation and result in unnecessary worry for the family. An efficient, accurate, and cost-effective approach to the diagnosis of neonatal dermatoses, including diaper dermatitis, is therefore essential.

The most common benign transient dermatosis of the newborn is *erythema toxicum neonatorum*. Typically, term infants are affected. Lesions appear at 24 to 48 hours of life and last from 1 to a few days. Onset at birth or as late as 10 to 14 days of life has been reported. Lesions consist of blotchy erythema, often with a central vesicle or pustule, giving a "flea-bitten" appearance. The face, buttocks, trunk, and proximal extremities are most commonly affected; palms and soles are spared. Diagnosis can often be made clinically, but a Wright-stained skin scraping (Tzanck preparation) revealing a predominance of eosinophils provides rapid confirmation.

Transient neonatal pustular melanosis is the second most common benign newborn skin disease affecting term infants, but it differs from erythema toxicum in that skin lesions are usually present at birth. Lesions begin as small pustules (Fig. 1), which rupture, leaving peripheral scale or crusts, followed by small hyperpigmented macules (see Fig. 1). The pustules may rupture in utero, so only hyperpigmented macules, or a combination of pustules and macules, may be noted at birth. Lesions may appear on any body site, including the genitalia, palms, and soles. Pustules resolve in a few days, but the hyperpigmentation fades slowly over weeks to months. Like erythema toxicum, the diagnosis is usually clinical, but it can be confirmed with a Wright stain showing a predominance of neutrophils. The differential diagnosis includes other conditions causing pustules on the palms and soles, such as neonatal candidiasis and acropustulosis of infancy.

Congenital candidiasis in full-term infants is usually a benign condition with spontaneous resolution. The eruption is characterized by diffuse erythema and fine white scaling, commonly with scattered red papules or pustules. Pustules may be multiple and commonly involve the palms and soles. Nail discoloration or thickening and oral thrush may also be noted. Diagnosis is made by potassium hydroxide (KOH) preparation from a skin smear of a pustule or area of scale.

Infantile acropustulosis (Fig. 2) is an uncommon newborn eruption. Pustules appear on the palms and

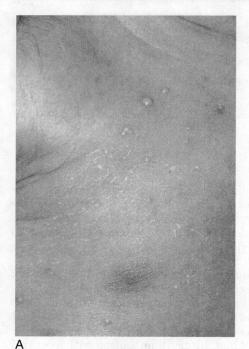

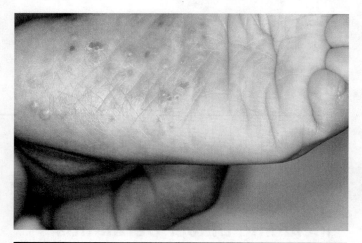

FIGURE 2. Crops of pruritic pustules on the soles are characteristic features of acropustulosis of infancy, but they must be distinguished from scabies, which can have an identical appearance. See color insert.

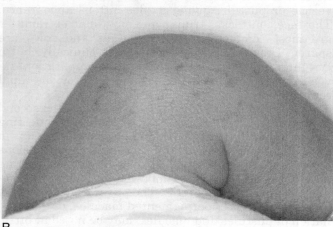

FIGURE 1. Transient neonatal pustular melanosis may present with either *A*, small flaccid pustules or *B*, residual 2- to 4-mm hyperpigmented macules, or a combination of both lesions. See color insert.

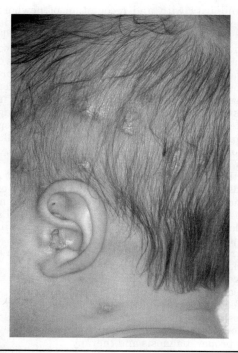

FIGURE 3. Pustules and crusted papules on the face and scalp of an infant with eosinophilic pustular folliculitis. See color insert.

soles, with occasional extension onto the proximal extremities, at a few weeks to a few months of life. The lesions are extremely pruritic and closely resemble the pustules seen with scabies infestation. A distinguishing feature is that the lesions of acropustulosis come and go, appearing in crops every few weeks, whereas scabies lesions persist and continue to progress without therapy. A skin scraping is essential to rule out scabies. Neutrophils and eosinophils are expected, but no mites should be present in acropustulosis. Spontaneous resolution within 1 to 2 years is typical.

Another uncommon pustular eruption affecting newborns is *eosinophilic pustular folliculitis* (Fig. 3). Although the condition is benign and noninfectious, the appearance of multiple crusted, pruritic pustules on the scalp and face often causes concern for possible bacterial infection. Onset is from birth to the first year of life. Like acropustulosis, the lesions may wax and wane over months to several years before resolving spontaneously. A negative Gram stain and a Wright stain showing multiple eosinophils aid diagnosis.

Miliaria ("prickly heat") occurs fairly commonly in neonates and manifests as either small pustules with peripheral erythema (miliaria rubra) or as fragile, flaccid, clear blisters (miliaria crystallina) (Fig. 4). The lesions are caused by blockage of the sweat ducts

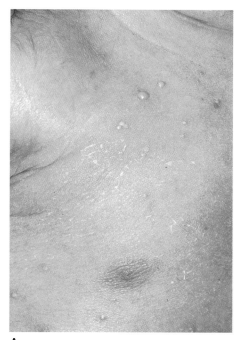

A

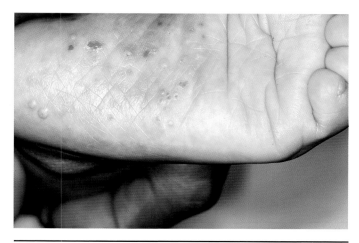

FIGURE 2. Crops of pruritic pustules on the soles are characteristic features of acropustulosis of infancy, but they must be distinguished from scabies, which can have an identical appearance.

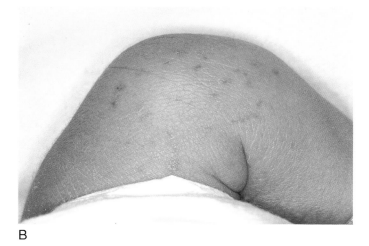

B

FIGURE 1. Transient neonatal pustular melanosis may present with either *A*, small flaccid pustules or *B*, residual 2- to 4-mm hyperpigmented macules, or a combination of both lesions.

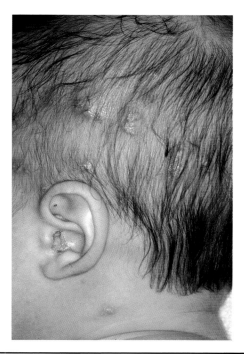

FIGURE 3. Pustules and crusted papules on the face and scalp of an infant with eosinophilic pustular folliculitis.

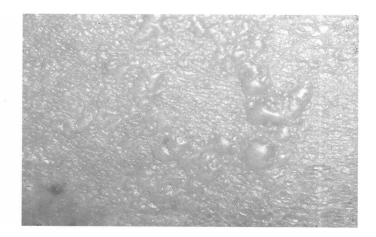

FIGURE 4. Case of congenital miliaria crystallina with typical flaccid, "dewdrop" vesicles.

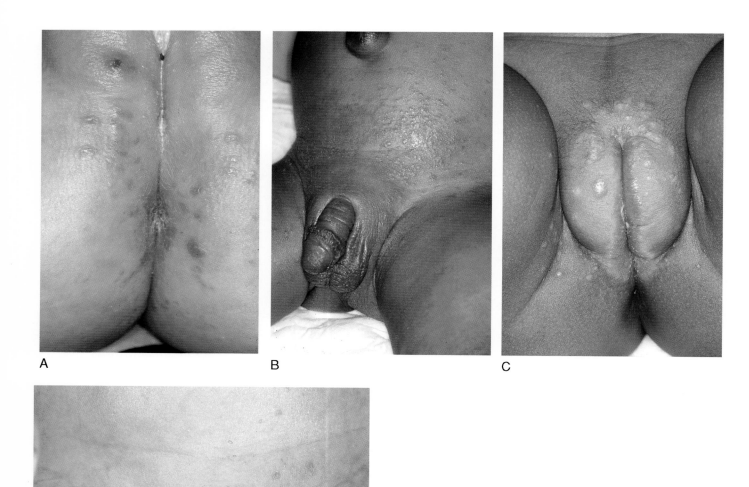

A

B

C

D

FIGURE 5. Forms of diaper dermatitis: *A*, Jacquet erosive diaper dermatitis, *B*, seborrheic dermatitis, *C*, psoriasis, *D*, bullous impetigo (note that erosions may predominate because the blisters are flaccid and rupture easily).

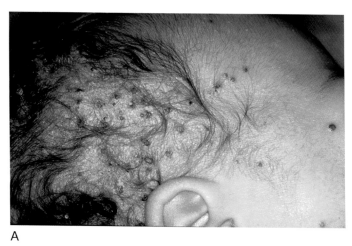

A

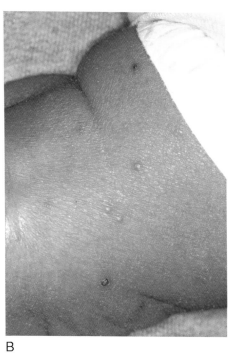

B

FIGURE 6. Neonatal varicella with lesions at varying stages: *A*, crusted papules on the scalp and *B*, intact vesicles on the extremities.

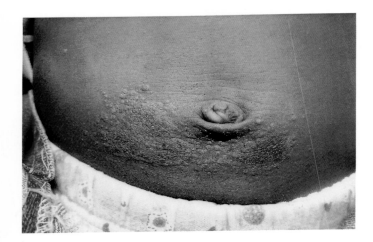

FIGURE 1. Allergic contact dermatitis from nickel-containing metal snaps.

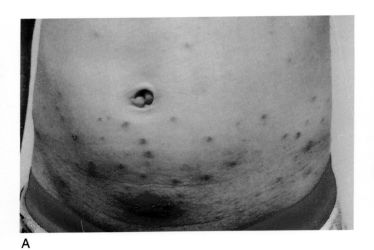

A

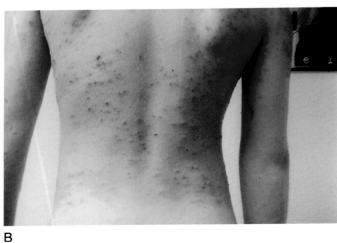

B

FIGURE 2. In this case of nickel dermatitis, there is an intense id reaction located near the primary site *(A)* and on a distant site on the patient's back *(B)*.

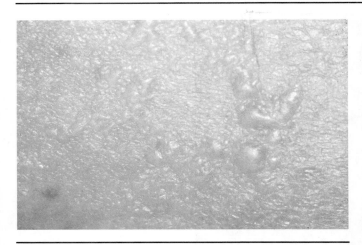

FIGURE 4. Case of congenital miliaria crystallina with typical flaccid, "dewdrop" vesicles. See color insert.

following exposure to warm environments, occlusive dressings, fever, or excess bundling. Miliaria is most common after the first week of life. Congenital cases of miliaria crystallina have been reported and are often associated with maternal fever preceding delivery. The diagnosis can usually be made by history and clinical examination, but a biopsy may occasionally be needed for confirmation.

A final benign cause of pustules in the newborn period is *neonatal acne.* Red papules and pustules appear at a few weeks of age and are most common on the cheeks and forehead but may also involve the upper trunk. It often appears concurrently with the greasy yellow scale and erythema of seborrheic dermatitis ("cradle cap"), and both conditions are thought to be associated with sebaceous gland responses to the presence of maternal androgens. Some believe that both conditions may also be partly caused by *Malassezia furfur.* The timing, distribution, and clinical appearance of the lesions are usually sufficient to make the diagnosis of neonatal acne. Spontaneous resolution at 2 to 3 months of life is the usual course.

Diaper Dermatitis

A discussion of newborn skin disease must also include a discussion of diaper dermatitis. Because of the advent of superabsorbent disposable diapers, the frequency and severity of *irritant diaper dermatitis*, the most common type of diaper rash, have greatly decreased. Irritant diaper dermatitis is the result of skin irritation from moisture, friction, and fecal enzymes. Onset is between a few weeks of age to 1 to 2 years, but the most severe cases occur after 6 months of age when infants are sleeping through the night and diaper changes are performed less frequently. Classic findings include redness and scaling or maceration of the groin with sparing of the skin creases. Severe cases may follow diarrhea illnesses. When diaper dermatitis is severe, a noduloulcerative form of diaper dermatitis, called *Jacquet erosive diaper dermatitis* (Fig. 5), with

nodules, erosions or ulcerations on the labia, penis, or buttocks, may occur.

Candida diaper dermatitis is the second most common cause of diaper dermatitis in neonates and may be accompanied by oral thrush. *Candida* thrives in the warm, moist environment of the diaper area, especially if oral antibiotics are used. Unlike irritant diaper dermatitis, *Candida* involves the skin creases. Diffuse redness and scaling with peripheral (satellite) red papules or pustules is the classic presentation.

Another form of diaper dermatitis is *seborrheic dermatitis* (see Fig. 5). This condition usually begins during the first 4 to 6 weeks of life and resolves by 6 months of age. Lesions consist of confluent erythema with greasy, white-yellow scale, most notably on the scalp (cradle cap) but often on the eyebrows and creases of the ears, nose, neck, axillae, and groin as well. The intertriginous areas are often moist or macerated. Less commonly, generalized involvement of the scalp, face, trunk, and groin may be seen. Diagnosis can usually be made clinically by the appearance and distribution of the lesions. Differential diagnosis includes atopic dermatitis, which differs in that it spares the diaper area, and psoriasis.

Psoriasis is an uncommon cause of diaper dermatitis in neonates. The lesions of psoriasis differ from seborrheic dermatitis in that they are deep pink or red with very well-defined borders (see Fig. 5). The thicker silver-white scale typical of plaque-type psoriasis may or may not be present in the diaper area. The presence of nail pitting or a positive family history of psoriasis can be helpful diagnostic clues.

A final cause of diaper dermatitis is *bullous impetigo*, which, although uncommon in the newborn period, has a predilection for the diaper area (groin and lower abdomen) in this age group. Onset is typically in the first 2 weeks of life, and the affected infant often appears well. The cause is coagulase positive *Staphylococcus aureus*, phage group 2, which produces epidermolytic (exfoliative) toxins causing blister formation. Lesions of bullous impetigo may appear pustular, similar to *Candida*, but more typically consist of clear blisters. These blisters are superficial and flaccid and rupture easily; therefore, it is not uncommon for only shallow erythematous erosions to be present with no intact blisters (see Fig. 5).

Expert Opinion on Management Issues

The most important aspect of management is to obtain a correct diagnosis as efficiently as possible. The most valuable diagnostic tools for diagnosing neonatal dermatoses are a good history and physical examination, with close attention to time of onset, clinical appearance of the lesions, assessment of whether the infant is well or ill, and a skin scraping, if indicated.

Tzanck smear or Wright stain of blisters and pustules in the newborn is very useful to confirm a diagnosis. This is easily performed by scraping an intact blister or pustule with a No. 15 scalpel blade, after

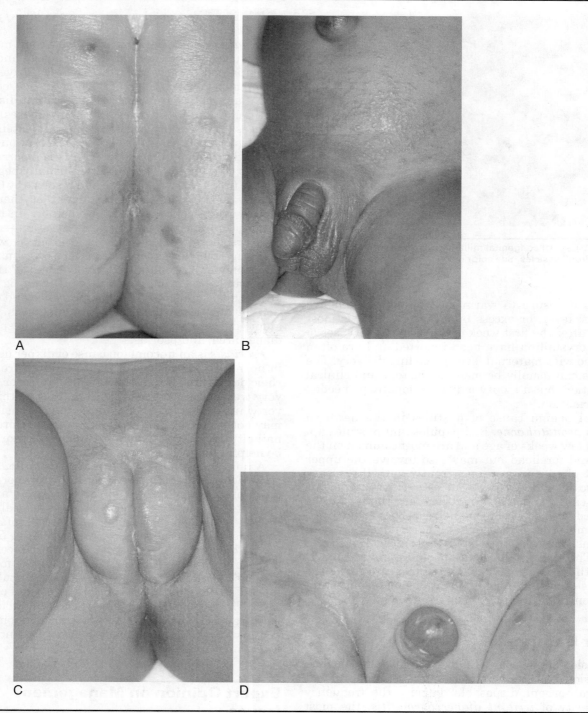

FIGURE 5. Forms of diaper dermatitis: *A*, Jacquet erosive diaper dermatitis, *B*, seborrheic dermatitis, *C*, psoriasis, *D*, bullous impetigo (note that erosions may predominate because the blisters are flaccid and rupture easily). See color insert.

cleansing the site with alcohol. Gentle force should be used, as it is crucial to scrape the moist blister base (some discomfort and slight bleeding are to be expected). The material on the blade is smeared in a thin layer on a clean glass slide and allowed to air dry. If the slide must be transported to the lab and cannot be immediately stained, the slide should be fixed with 95% ethanol, 100% methanol, or Pap smear fixative spray

prior to transport. After mineral oil and a cover slip are placed on the slide, it can be examined under the microscope for multinucleated giant cells (indicating HSV or varicella virus infection), and also for the presence of neutrophils and eosinophils.

A predominance of neutrophils suggests transient neonatal pustular melanosis, infantile acropustulosis, or bullous impetigo. Further confirmation of impetigo

TABLE 1 Medications for Neonatal Skin Diseases

Generic (Trade) OTC/Rx	Dosage/Route/Regimen	Max. Dose	Formulations	Common Adverse Reactions	Concentrations
Neonatal Acne Medication*					
Benzoyl peroxide (Benzac, Desquam-E, Brevoxyl, PanOxyl, Oxy, Triaz, Fostex BPO, others) OTC, Rx	Topical qd-bid	None	Cream, gel, lotion, wash, soap	Contact dermatitis, stinging, dryness, erythema	2.5%, 5%, 10%
Candidiasis and Neonatal Acne (*Malassezia furfur*) Antifungal Medication†					
Clotrimazole (Lotrimin, Mycelex, Cruex) OTC	Apply topically twice daily	None	Cream, troche, Solution, Vaginal tablet	Erythema, pruritus, urticaria, irritation, stinging/burning	Cream/solution 1%, Vaginal cream 2%, Troche 10 mg, Vaginal tablet 10 mg
Irritant Diaper Dermatitis Medication					
Nystatin† (Mycostatin, Nystop, Pedi-Dri) Rx	Apply topical bid, Oral susp 50,000 units to each side of mouth qid	None	Capsule, cream, lozenge, tablet, ointment, powder, suspension	Contact dermatitis, Stevens-Johnson syndrome, irritation, nausea, vomiting, diarrhea	100,000 units/mL, 100,000 units/g, 200,000 units, 500,000 units
Zinc oxide§ (Balmex, Desitin, others) OTC	Topical	None	Paste, ointment	None	10%, 11.3%, 16%20%, 40%
Seborrheic Dermatitis, Psoriasis, Severe Irritant Diaper Dermatitis Topical Corticosteroid Medication					
Hydrocortisone acetate or as base (Cortaid, Cortizone, Hytone, Caldecort, many others) OTC, Rx	Topical bid	None	Cream, ointment, lotion, gel, suppository, solution	Atrophy, hypertension, acne, dermatitis, striae, Cushing syndrome, HPA suppression, cataracts	0.5%, 1%, 2.5%
Bullous Impetigo Medications					
Cephalexin‖ (Keflex, Biocef, Keftab)	PO, qid 25–100 mg/kg/day (child) 250–500 mg/dose qid (adult)	4 g/day	Capsule, Suspension, Tablet	Dizziness, headache, fever, rash, nausea, pseudomembranous colitis, vomiting, diarrhea	125 mg/5 mL, 250 mg/5 mL, 250 mg, 500 mg
Dicloxacillin¶ (Dycill, Pathocil)	PO, qid 25–50 mg/kg/day (child) 125–500 mg/dose qid PO (adult)	2 g/day	Capsule	Rash, fever, nausea, vomiting, diarrhea, elevated liver enzymes, leukopenia, thrombocytopenia, neutropenia, serum sickness-like reaction	62.5 mg/5mL, 250 mg, 500 mg

*Antiacne medication releases free-radical oxygen, oxidizes bacterial proteins; keratinolytic, comedolytic.
†Antifungal (azole) blocks ergosterol synthesis.
‡Medication class is antifungal (polyene); binds cell membrane sterols causing cell leakage.
§Medication class is barrier cream.
‖Medication class is cephalosporin (β-lactamase resistant); inhibits enzymes involved in cell wall synthesis.
¶Medication class is antibiotic (β-lactamase–resistant penicillin); inhibits bacterial cell wall synthesis.
bid, two times a day; HPA, hypothalamic-pituitary axis; OTC, over the counter; PO, orally; qd, daily; qid, four times a day; Rx, prescription.

can be obtained with a Gram stain from a culturette swab of the lesion. A predominance of eosinophils suggests erythema toxicum, eosinophilic pustular folliculitis, or an uncommon syndrome called incontinentia pigmenti. No significant infiltrate will be seen with miliaria. *Candida* can be confirmed with a KOH preparation of a scraping from a pustule or scaling area of skin. Lastly, mineral oil preparation of a skin scraping (preferably of a burrow or crusted papule) can diagnose scabies. Fungal, bacterial, or viral culture, or a viral direct fluorescent antibody (DFA) test, should also be performed if infection is suspected. In most cases a skin biopsy is not necessary for diagnosis.

Most newborn skin eruptions are benign and require no therapy. Spontaneous resolution is expected for erythema toxicum, transient neonatal pustular melanosis, and miliaria. The skin and nail findings of most cases of congenital candidiasis and most cases of neonatal acne also do not routinely require therapy. For persistent or severe cases of neonatal acne, benzoyl peroxide cream one to two times daily can be helpful (Table 1).

Although eosinophilic pustular folliculitis and infantile acropustulosis also resolve spontaneously, pruritus can be severe. Pruritus can usually be alleviated with a combination of oral antihistamines and high-potency topical steroids.

For persistent cutaneous or diaper candidiasis, nystatin cream or other topical antifungal with anti-*Candida* activity is usually sufficient (see Table 1) Preterm infants weighing less than 1000 g or infants with a burn-like dermatitis, respiratory distress immediately after birth with laboratory evidence of sepsis, or positive blood, urine, or cerebrospinal fluid (CSF) cultures should be treated parenterally.

Treatment of irritant or Jacquet erosive diaper dermatitis consists of eliminating occlusion, friction, and prolonged exposure to moisture, urine, and fecal material. This is most easily achieved with frequent diaper changes and liberal application of a zinc oxide–based barrier cream with every diaper change. Avoidance of wipes containing alcohol or fragrance is also helpful as they are irritating to the skin. Use of a moist damp cloth for cleansing is preferred. Changing to cloth diapers does not seem to be helpful, as the incidence of diaper dermatitis is greatly decreased with use of the newer superabsorbent disposable diapers. If the dermatitis is not improving, a topical antifungal, such as clotrimazole or nystatin (see Table 1) for possible secondary *Candida* infection, or brief use of a mild topical steroid, such as 1% hydrocortisone (see Table 1), can be useful. In most cases, a topical steroid is not necessary, but if one is used, the medication should be discontinued immediately once the eruption begins to improve. Use of potent topical steroids or topical steroid/antifungal combination medications is contraindicated on the diaper area.

Psoriasis and persistent cases of seborrheic dermatitis involving the diaper area usually respond to emollients and mild topical steroids such as 1% or 2.5% hydrocortisone ointment (see Table 1). Mid- or high-potency topical steroids (including combination antifungal/steroid preparations) are not recommended for use in the diaper area as the delicate skin in this area combined with occlusion from the diaper increases the risk of systemic absorption and atrophy or striae. Topical immunomodulators have been used, but at this time they are not yet approved by the U.S. Food and Drug Administration (FDA) for use in infants. There have also been no studies to date evaluating the safety of these medications when applied to intertriginous areas or under occlusion in infants.

Bullous impetigo requires therapy with β-lactamase–resistant antibiotics (see Table 1). Infants with no fever or clinical evidence of sepsis or soft tissue infection may be treated with oral antibiotics, such as cephalexin or dicloxacillin. Because of the increased

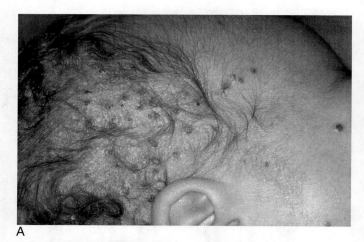

A

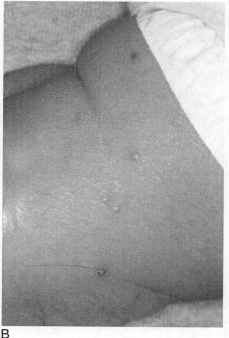

B

FIGURE 6. Neonatal varicella with lesions at varying stages: *A*, crusted papules on the scalp and *B*, intact vesicles on the extremities. See color insert.

risk of sepsis, cellulitis, or omphalitis in neonates, many physicians advocate initial parenteral antibiotic therapy. A blister should be cultured for antibiotic susceptibility and for the possibility of methicillin-resistant *S. aureus* (MRSA). The recommended duration of antibiotic therapy is 10 days.

Common Pitfalls

■ Failure to recognize neonatal herpes simplex or varicella virus infection is the most feared pitfall. Tzanck smear or direct fluorescent antibody testing and/or viral culture should be considered for any blister in the newborn, particularly grouped blisters or crusts on an erythematous base (Fig. 6).
■ Persistent or recalcitrant diaper dermatitis in the setting of chronic diarrhea and failure to thrive may be a sign of an underlying immune, metabolic, or nutritional disorder; these infants should be closely evaluated.
■ Petechiae in the diaper area may be the first sign of histiocytosis and should not be overlooked.

Communication and Counseling

Many neonatal skin eruptions are benign and transient and, therefore, require no therapy. Nevertheless, careful clinical evaluation is essential to exclude a potentially life-threatening infection or underlying systemic disease. If detected early and treated promptly and aggressively, neonatal infections often resolve with little to no adverse effects to the infant, but lack of recognition and therapy can be devastating. Parents should be advised to have their infant evaluated immediately if blisters or pustules are noted. Physicians should consider blisters in the newborn a medical emergency, until the possibility of a serious infection can be ruled out. Also, children with persistent diaper dermatitis not improving with standard therapy, particularly in the presence of petechiae or failure to thrive, merit a thorough clinical evaluation for an underlying systemic disease, such as histiocytosis, or for nutritional deficiency.

SUGGESTED READINGS

1. Buckley DA, Munn SE, Higgins EM: Neonatal eosinophilic pustular folliculitis. Clin Exp Dermtol 26:251–255, 2002. **Review of the clinical and histologic features and differential diagnoses of eosinophilic pustular folliculitis.**
2. Darmstadt GL, Dinulos JG, Miller Z: Congenital cutaneous candidiasis: Clinical presentation, pathogenesis, and management guidelines. Pediatrics 105:438–444, 2000. **Reviews the clinical presentations of congenital cutaneous candidiasis including risk factors for systemic involvement.**
3. Frieden IJ, Howard R: Vesicles, pustules, bullae, erosions, and ulcerations. In Eichenfield LF, Frieden IJ, Esterly NB (eds): Textbook of Neonatal Dermatology, 1st ed. Philadelphia: WB Saunders, 2001. **Detailed differential diagnosis of vesiculopustular dermatoses of the newborn.**
4. Krafchik BR: Eczematous disorders. In Eichenfield LF, Frieden IJ, Esterly NB (eds): Textbook of Neonatal Dermatology, 1st ed. Philadelphia: WB Saunders, 2001. **Clear discussion of diaper dermatitis in the newborn period with excellent clinical photographs.**

Allergic Contact Dermatitis
Fred E. Ghali

KEY CONCEPTS

■ Allergic contact dermatitis manifests only after sensitization to an allergen has occurred.
■ A key clinical feature to diagnosing allergic contact dermatitis is the well–defined margins corresponding to areas of contact.
■ Allergic contact dermatitis may manifest as an acute eruption (with blistering and weeping) or as a chronic eruption (with lichenification and dyspigmentation).
■ Of the potential allergens causing an acute allergic contact dermatitis, poison ivy is the most common.
■ Nickel dermatitis, a very common form of chronic allergic contact dermatitis, may occur in several affected sites that the clinician should recognize.
■ An idiosyncratic reaction appears distant from the primary site of exposure and is the result of chronic antigen exposure.

Contact dermatitis can be either irritant or allergic in nature; this chapter focuses on the latter. Allergic contact dermatitis (ACD) is a type IV delayed hypersensitivity response that is elicited when the skin comes in contact with an allergen to which an individual has previously been sensitized.

To properly diagnose and treat ACD, the physician needs to maintain an appropriate level of suspicion and be familiar with its varying clinical presentations. The diagnosis of ACD is often suggested by the linear or well–demarcated distribution of the eruption, which corresponds to the area of contact. Acute ACD is characterized by erythema, edema, blisters, and crusting; chronic ACD is characterized by lichenification, scaling, excoriations, and dyspigmentation.

The most common cause of acute ACD is poison ivy. Dermatitis occurs after exposure to the urushiol contained in the plants either by direct or indirect (e.g., exposure to burning plant material) contact. Despite common belief, the fluid content of the lesions is not contagious. Sequential outbreak of the skin occurs as a result of differential exposure on various parts of the body or failure to completely remove the allergen from contaminated sources (e.g. clothing, animal hair, toys, sports equipment).

Other common childhood contact allergens are nickel, neomycin, chromates, thimerosal, formaldehyde and related preservatives, and lanolin. Of these, nickel is the most commonly encountered allergen and the clinician should be aware of the common sites of nickel dermatitis as follows:

1. Bellybutton region—from metal snaps, zippers, belt buckles (Fig. 1)
2. Neck—from necklaces
3. Wrist—from watches or bracelets
4. Earlobes—from earrings
5. Thighs (bilateral, flexural)—from metal screws in wooden–type classroom seats

17

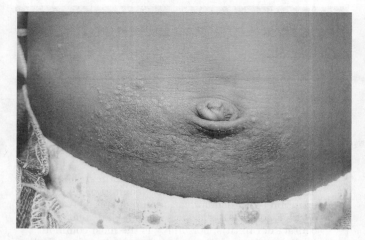

FIGURE 1. Allergic contact dermatitis from nickel-containing metal snaps. See color insert.

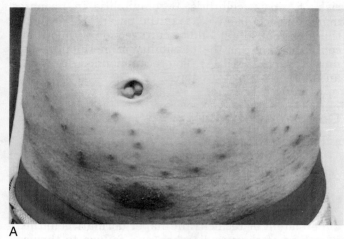

A

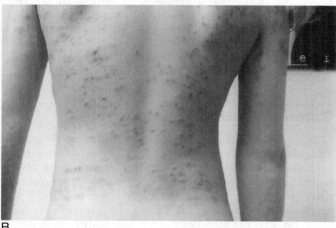

B

FIGURE 2. In this case of nickel dermatitis, there is an intense id reaction located near the primary site *(A)* and on a distant site on the patient's back *(B)*. See color insert.

Some patients have an associated generalized dermatitis, termed an *id* (idiosyncratic) reaction, auto-eczematization, "sympathy" rash, or "secondary" rash. The eruption typically consists of pruritic, monomorphic papules distributed symmetrically on the arms and legs, or less commonly on the trunk (Fig. 2). The id reaction appears distant from the primary site of exposure and is the result of chronic antigen exposure. The clinician needs to understand the direct correlation between the primary contact dermatitis and the secondary id reaction.

Expert Opinion on Management Issues

Treatment of allergic contact dermatitis primarily focuses on the identification and avoidance of the causative allergen(s). Sometimes the source is easily identified based on history or distribution of the dermatitis; however, some cases require more investigation. Patch testing, which involves applying allergen-impregnated patches to nonaffected skin, may be used to objectively screen for potential allergens. Once the allergen is known, patients should be educated on avoidance.

In addition to prompt removal of the suspected allergen, treatment of allergic contact dermatitis usually involves various interventions (Box 1). Cool compresses with tap water, saline (1 teaspoon/pint), aluminum acetate (1:40 dilution), or lukewarm oatmeal baths help dry lesions and decrease symptoms. Antipruritic lotions (e.g., calamine lotion, Eucerin cream combined with 0.25% menthol) and sedating systemic antihistamines (e.g., diphenhydramine, hydroxyzine) can be helpful for diminishing pruritus. Topical or systemic antibiotics may be needed if secondary infection is present.

Corticosteroids are the mainstay of treatment. The choice of corticosteroid should be based on the severity and extent of the eruption. For mild to moderate

---

BOX 1 Management of Allergic Contact Dermatitis

Identification and avoidance of allergen(s)
Symptomatic treatment

- Tap water, saline (1 tsp salt/pint water), or aluminum acetate (Burow solution; 1:40 dilution) compresses for acute dermatitis
- Oatmeal baths
- Topical antipruritic lotions (calamine lotion, Eucerin with 0.25% menthol)
- Sedating antihistamines (diphenhydramine, hydroxyzine)
  - Topical or systemic antibiotics for secondary infection
  - Corticosteroids
- Acute allergic contact dermatitis (ACD)
  - Localized: Medium-to-high potency topical corticosteroids applied bid until resolution
  - Generalized: Prednisone 1 to 2 mg/kg/day for 7 days followed by a taper over 7 to 10 days
- Chronic ACD
  - Medium potency topical corticosteroid applied bid until resolution

---

bid, two times a day.

cases that are relatively localized or chronic ACD, a medium- to high-potency topical corticosteroid can be applied twice daily until the condition improves. For more widespread or severe cases of acute ACD, short-term systemic corticosteroids are indicated. Prednisone at a dose of 1 to 2 mg/kg/day given once in the morning for 7 to 10 days is advisable, with gradual tapering of the dose over the next 7 to 10 days. Steroid courses shorter than 14 days may result in rebound dermatitis.

Physicians should always look for a possible secondary id reaction, and therapy should be aimed at both the primary dermatitis and the secondary id reaction. Generally, if both optimal avoidance of the responsible allergen is combined with adequate therapy of the primary contact rash, the secondary id reaction should improve. In the majority of cases, topical corticosteroids are most effective in treating both the primary rash and the id reaction. For patients who present with an intense id reaction, a short tapering course of oral corticosteroids can be effective.

Common Pitfalls

- A high probability of recurrence of the dermatitis occurs in those cases in which no etiologic source can be identified.
- Even in cases in which the etiology is known, recurrence and presumed treatment failure may occur unless the patient strictly adheres to avoidance of the source on a continual basis.
- For severe cases of acute allergic contact dermatitis requiring oral steroids, rapid rebound may occur if the oral steroids are tapered too quickly.
- Failure to recognize a superimposed id reaction (autosensitization) on the background of a preexisting allergic contact dermatitis can create a pitfall in both diagnosis and treatment.

Communication and Counseling

The physician needs to possess an appropriate level of suspicion to properly diagnose a case of an allergic contact dermatitis. Next, it is important for the clinician to provide patients with education on this condition. An emphasis is made on identification and avoidance of the allergen(s). When patients adhere to the recommended avoidance measures and are compliant with their appropriate topical and/or systemic therapy, allergic contact dermatitis is manageable.

SUGGESTED READINGS

1. Hurwitz S: Eczematous eruptions. In Hurwitz S (ed): Childhood. Philadelphia: WB Saunders, 1993. **Provides an authoritative discussion of contact dermatitis, including clinical features and management in children.**
2. Shah M, Lewis FM, Gawkrodger DJ: Patch testing in children and adolescents: Five years' experience and follow-up. J Am Acad Dermatol 37:964–968, 1997. **Provides benefits of performing patch testing in pediatric population.**
3. White IR: Allergic contact dermatitis. In Harper J, Prose N (eds): Pediatric Dermatology, vol 1. Malden, Mass: Blackwell Science, 2000. **Detailed chapter review of allergic contact dermatitis focusing on allergens of particular importance in children.**

Atopic Dermatitis

Ivan Cardona, Mark Boguniewicz, and Donald Y. M. Leung

KEY CONCEPTS

- Atopic dermatitis is the most common chronic skin disease of young children, and nearly 80% will develop asthma or allergic rhinitis, suggesting that atopic dermatitis is often the first step in the "atopic march."
- In up to 40% of children with moderate to severe atopic dermatitis, a food allergen may contribute to their skin disease.
- The skin of atopic dermatitis patients is more susceptible to bacterial, viral, and fungal infections.
- Frequent skin hydration followed immediately by application of moisturizers to unaffected skin ("soak and seal" method) or topical anti-inflammatory agents to affected skin is fundamental to effective maintenance care of atopic dermatitis.
- Systemic glucocorticoids, although often providing rapid clinical improvement, should be avoided, except in rare instances, because of the associated rebound flaring of atopic dermatitis when coming off the steroid and potential for adverse events.
- Patient education and an individualized step-wise approach to acute and maintenance care should be provided to all patients and caregivers.

Atopic dermatitis (AD) is a chronic, relapsing, highly pruritic inflammatory skin disease, affecting 10% to 20% of children worldwide. Epidemiologic studies demonstrate that the prevalence of this disease, particularly in industrialized countries, has increased twofold to threefold during the past 3 decades. Although AD can occur at any age, it is one of the most common skin disorders of childhood, with 60% of affected individuals presenting by the first year of life, and up to 85% of affected individuals presenting by 5 years of age.

AD is characterized by pruritic eczematous skin lesions, which significantly affect the quality of life of the child, the parent, and other caretakers. Of note, AD is a leading cause of school absenteeism and loss of work time for caregivers. It is a genetically determined skin disease that is strongly associated with risk for developing asthma and allergic rhinitis (first step in the atopic march). Although AD is a common skin disorder, it is important to consider other diseases in the differential diagnosis of AD (Box 1). Pruritus, the cardinal feature of this disorder, along with the age-specific distribution and morphology of the lesions, constitute the essential features needed for

---

BOX 1 Differential Diagnosis of Atopic Dermatitis

Immunodeficiencies
- Wiskott-Aldrich syndrome
- Severe combined immunodeficiency
- Hyper-IgE syndrome

Chronic Dermatoses
- Seborrheic dermatitis
- Contact dermatitis (allergic or irritant)
- Psoriasis
- Nummular eczema
- Ichthyosis

Autoimmune Disorders
- Graft-versus-host disease
- Pemphigus foliaceus
- Dermatitis herpetiformis
- Dermatomyositis

Malignant Diseases
- Letterer-Siwi disease
- Cutaneous T-cell lymphoma (mycosis fungoides/Sézary syndrome)

Congenital Disorders
- Netherton syndrome
- Familial keratosis pilaris

Infections and Infestations
- Scabies
- Dermatophytosis
- HIV-associated dermatitis

Metabolic Disorders
- Zinc deficiency
- Phenylketonuria
- Pyridoxine (vitamin B_6) and niacin deficiency
- Multiple carboxylase deficiency

HIV, human immunodeficiency virus.

BOX 2 Clinical Criteria of Atopic Dermatitis*

Essential Features
- Pruritus (cardinal feature)
- Typical morphology (chronic or relapsing dermatitis)
- Acute
- Poorly defined erythematous patches, papules, and plaques (with or without scale)
- Excoriations (as a result of scratching)
- Chronic
- Lichenification (thickening of skin with accentuation of skin markings)
- Fissures
- Alopecia (as a result of scratching)
- Typical distribution and age-specific pattern
- Infants and children: facial, neck, and extensor surfaces
- Older children, adolescents, and adults: flexural surfaces
- Sparing of the groin

Frequently Associated Features
- Atopy (personal or family history)
- Xerosis
- Early age of onset
- Raised serum IgE concentrations
- Peripheral blood eosinophilia
- Positive immediate-type allergy skin tests
- Cutaneous infections
- Nonspecific dermatitis of the hands or feet

Other Features
- Facial erythema or pallor
- Perifollicular accentuation
- Dennie-Morgan infraorbital folds, periorbital darkening
- White dermatographism and delayed blanch response
- Nipple eczema
- Pityriasis alba
- Ichthyosis, Palmer hyperlinearity, keratosis pilaris
- Anterior subcapsular cataracts, keratoconus

---
*Other skin conditions that mimic atopic dermatitis should be excluded (see Box 1).
IgE, immunoglobulin E.

---

the diagnosis. Box 2 presents clinical criteria used in the diagnosis of AD.

Expert Opinion on Management Issues

Management of AD requires a comprehensive approach to skin care that includes hydration and moisturizers, identification and elimination of irritants and specific triggers, treatment with anti-inflammatory medications with selective use of antimicrobial therapy, and patient education with a personalized action plan for maintenance care and flares (Box 3).

Skin barrier function is defective in AD. Atopic skin is more susceptible to evaporative water loss and this leads to dry skin (xerosis), which promotes cracks and microfissures. Moreover, this skin barrier defect creates a portal of entry for irritants, allergens, and microbial pathogens. Hydration and the use of moisturizers help to maintain normal barrier function and are fundamental components of AD therapy.

Soaking in a warm bath for 15 to 20 minutes, then lightly patting dry and immediately applying an occlusive or moisturizer, serves to soak and seal and prevents evaporation that leads to skin damage. While the patient is in the tub, hydration of the face can be achieved by applying a wet washcloth with holes cut out for the eyes and mouth. Showering may be sufficient for mild disease; however, moderate to severe AD requires soaking baths to maintain skin hydration. The frequency of soaking baths can vary from one to three baths a day, depending on the severity of the AD flare. It is important that an occlusive, moisturizer, or topical medication be applied immediately after bathing.

Moisturizers come in lotions, oils, creams, and ointments. Ointments usually have the fewest additives and are the most occlusive, although in hot climates they may trap perspiration and increase pruritus. In these situations, less occlusive creams or, rarely, lotions may be preferred, keeping in mind that they may be irritating because of added preservatives and fragrances. Crisco shortening is an inexpensive

BOX 3 Management of Atopic Dermatitis*

Conventional Management

- Hydration and moisturizer ("soak and seal")
- Topical corticosteroids
- Topical calcineurin inhibitors
- Antipruritics, sedatives, antiallergic oral medications
- Antimicrobial therapy
- Irritant elimination
- Food and inhalant allergen elimination when proven by challenge or convincing history
- Stress reduction
- Education with action plan

Recalcitrant Disease Management

- Wet dressing
- Phototherapy
- UVA (broad-band and UVA–1)
- UVB (broad-band and narrow-band)
- PUVA
- Systemic immunomodulatory agents
- Cyclosporin A
- Recombinant human IFN-γ
- Tacrolimus
- IVIG
- Mycophenolate mofetil
- Methotrexate
- Azathioprine
- Hospitalization

*Consultation with an allergy and immunology or dermatology specialist is recommended if patient fails to respond to basic treatment measures or for question of allergic triggers.

IFN, interferon; IVIG, intravenous immunoglobulin, PUVA, psoralen plus ultraviolet light of A wavelength; UV, ultraviolet light.

17

and effective moisturizer. Petroleum jelly is not a moisturizer but can be used as an occlusive agent after hydrating baths. Topical medications should not be mixed with moisturizing or occlusive agents or applied in layers, because this can decrease the efficacy of the treatment.

AD skin is more susceptible to irritants than the skin of normal individuals. Detergents, chemicals, soaps, alcohol, and astringents in skin care products are potential irritants and should be avoided. Sensitive-skin cleansers are usually tolerated and may be helpful in removing irritants such as chlorine after swimming (moisturizers should then be applied). Temperate, moderately humid weather, loose-fitting cotton (or cotton-blend) clothing, and air-conditioned environments help minimize perspiration, which can act as an irritant. Hypoallergenic or facial sunscreen products are often best tolerated, and they should be applied when patients are outside for extended periods of time.

Food and aeroallergens have been shown to trigger AD in a subset of patients. Up to 40% of children with moderate to severe AD may have food allergies that trigger their disease. Therefore, a food allergy workup consisting of skin prick testing, ImmunoCAP assay, and selective food challenges can help to identify clinically relevant allergens that can be eliminated. Furthermore, environmental controls, such as reducing

house dust exposure with allergen-proof covers and possibly eliminating animal allergens can help minimize allergen exposure and subsequent flares in patients who are sensitized.

The skin of AD patients is also more susceptible to bacterial (e.g., *Staphylococcus aureus*), viral (e.g., herpes simplex, molluscum), and fungal (e.g., *Malassezia furfur, Pityrosporum ovale*) infections than the skin of normal individuals. More than 90% of patients with chronic AD skin lesions are colonized with *S. aureus*. Hydration, cleansers, and topical anti-inflammatory therapies, by healing the skin barrier, are enough to reduce *S. aureus* colonization and improve clinical status. AD exacerbations that are slow to respond to these therapies or show signs of overt bacterial superinfection should prompt further evaluation for the presence of an infectious agent. Based on the results of skin lesion cultures including antibiotic sensitivities, appropriate antibiotic, antiviral, or antifungal therapy should be started.

Pruritus is the cardinal feature of AD. It is critical to eliminate triggers to maintain normal sleep patterns and avoid scratch-induced skin damage. Measures that heal the skin barrier all lead to reduced pruritus. Additionally, oral sedating or antiallergy medications may be useful adjuvants. Keeping nails cut short and using cotton gloves or socks over the hands at night can help reduce scratch-induced skin damage, which often occurs unbeknownst to the restless sleeping AD patient.

Topical corticosteroids have long been the mainstay of therapy for AD. They are available in potencies ranging from extremely high (class I) to low (class VII). Be aware that the vehicle of the preparation can alter potency such that ointments are most occlusive, have better delivery, have the fewest additives, and decrease evaporative losses. The choice of topical corticosteroid preparations depends on the severity and distribution of the flare. Fortunately most AD flares can be controlled with a low- to mid-potency topical corticosteroid in conjunction with the soak and seal method described. Although side effects, such as the development of striae or thinning of the skin, are infrequent with low- to mid-potency topical corticosteroids when used once daily, they can occur when the frequency of application or potency of steroid is increased. Ultimately, the least potent corticosteroid that is effective should be used.

The development of the topical calcineurin inhibitors, tacrolimus, and pimecrolimus has provided more treatment options. Randomized, double-blind, placebo-controlled studies of these nonsteroidal topical immunosuppressants have demonstrated their efficacy, long-term safety profile, and tolerability in children 2 years of age or older. The calcineurin inhibitors can be a safe steroid-sparing agent especially useful for the treatment of the thinner skin of the face, neck, groin, and axillae. Moreover, because even normal-appearing skin in AD is immunologically abnormal, these agents are an appealing choice for first-line therapy, with topical steroids used for short courses as rescue therapy. A minority of patients complain of stinging and local irritation in the first few days of use. Usually this passes and this class of medications is well tolerated.

Recently the FDA issued a Public Health Advisory for this class of medications, stating that they should be used only as labeled (i.e., in children ≥2 years of age) and for patients who have failed treatment with other therapies. This stemmed from increasing off-label use and animal data suggesting a potential risk for lymphoma and skin cancer. At the same time, it is important to note that the rate of lymphoma formation reported to date for topical calcineurin inhibitors is lower than that predicted in the general population. In addition, the animal data were based on 26 to 47 times the maximum recommended human dose. On the basis of these data, the Task Force Committee assembled by the American Academy of Allergy, Asthma and Immunology and the American College of Allergy, Asthma and Immunology have concluded that the risk-to-benefit ratio of these medications is similar to that of conventional therapies for the treatment of AD.

When all of the aforementioned therapies are insufficient in controlling AD, the use of wet dressings can augment the soak-and-seal process, improving penetration of the topical steroid and improve sleep disturbance, by serving as a protective barrier from scratch-induced skin trauma. Cultures (with antibiotic sensitivities) of the skin to evaluate for infection should be performed. Those who are erythrodermic or appear toxic may require hospitalization and intravenous antibiotics. Consultation by a specialist such as a dermatologist or allergist should be considered because they may advocate the use of other therapies such as phototherapy or systemic immunomodulators for control of severe AD.

As in asthma, the management of AD requires patient education including a personalized (preferably written) action plan, which provides instructions for maintenance care and flares. A step-wise approach to therapy based on mild, moderate, or severe exacerbations should be outlined. Additionally, action plans should spell out potential and known allergic triggers.

Common Pitfalls

Reliance on oral steroids is a significant pitfall. Although oral steroid therapy can be highly effective, it should be used only in the rare patient as rebound flaring of AD can occur even when medication is tapered carefully, thus resulting in a vicious cycle leading to oral steroid dependence.

Historically the *dry method* approach, in which patients avoid bathing and hydration, has been widely advocated. Supporters of this method have argued that frequent bathing promotes skin moisture loss, as water evaporates off the skin. Although this is true to an extent, the water loss that occurs can be prevented if an occlusive or moisturizer is applied within a few minutes after bathing. In the authors' experience, the *wet method* approach is preferred because hydration of the stratum corneum is maintained.

Despite its role in allergic rhinitis and atopic asthma, immunotherapy is not proven to be efficacious in the treatment of AD. Well-controlled studies are still needed to determine the role of immunotherapy in this disease.

Lack of proper patient education can lead to confusion and nonadherence. For example, explaining the differences in topical steroid potencies is important, as patients often confuse the percentage on the label with the potency of the topical steroid compound; fluticasone propionate 0.005% ointment, for example, is actually more potent than hydrocortisone 2.5% ointment. Additionally, topical antihistamines and anesthetics can induce cutaneous sensitization. And finally, applying a topical medication on top of moisturizer, or vice versa, decreases the effectiveness of the medicine and is unnecessary for maintaining hydration. Topical medications should be reserved for use in affected areas and moisturizer for use in unaffected areas.

Communication and Counseling

With identification of triggers, proper skin care, appropriate topical anti-inflammatory use, and patient understanding and adherence, most forms of AD can be controlled. The disease often becomes less prominent as the child becomes older; however, the prognosis is poorer in children with severe disease and an atopic family history. Parents need to be reassured that often a multitude of foods are falsely associated as being allergenic, especially when the disease is not well controlled. This leads to detrimental and unnecessary restriction diets. Finally, given the significant impact of AD on the quality of life of patients and families, psychosocial issues should not be ignored because stress can serve as an added trigger, leading to habitual scratching.

ACKNOWLEDGMENTS

We would like to thank Maureen Sandoval for assistance with the manuscript.

SUGGESTED READINGS

1. Boguniewicz M, Eichenfield L, Hultsch T: Current management of atopic dermatitis and interruption of the atopic march. J Allergy Clin Immunol 112:S140–S150, 2003. **A recent and comprehensive review of conventional therapy principles, including the newer topical calcineurin inhibitors, and systemic therapies.**
2. Boguniewicz M, Nicol N: Conventional therapy for atopic dermatitis. Immunol Allergy Clin North Am 22(1):107–124, 2002. **A practical review of atopic dermatitis (AD) management including detailed descriptions and pictures of patients with wet dressings.**
3. Eichenfield LF, Lucky AW, Boguniewicz M, et al: Safety and efficacy of pimecrolimus (ASM 981) cream 1% in the treatment of mild and moderate atopic dermatitis in children and adolescents. J Am Acad Dermatol 46:495–504, 2002. **Study showing the safety and efficacy of pimecrolimus 1% in children and adolescents.**

4. Fonacier L, Spergel J, Charlesworth EN, et al: Report of the Topical Calcineurin Inhibitor Task Force of the American College of Allergy, Asthma and Immunology and American Academy of Allergy, Asthma and Immunology. J Allergy Clin Immunol 115 (6):1249–1253, 2005. **A critical review of the available data on the risk-to-benefit ratio of using topical calcineurin inhibitors.**

5. Friedlander SF, Hebert AA, Allen DB: Safety of fluticasone propionate cream 0.05% for the treatment of severe and extensive atopic dermatitis in children as young as 3 months. J Am Acad Dermatol 46:387–393, 2002. **Study showing the safety and efficacy of a class V potency topical steroid in young infants.**

6. Paller AS, Eichenfield LF, Leung DY, et al: A 12-week study of tacrolimus ointment for the treatment of atopic dermatitis in pediatric patients. J Am Acad Dermatol 44:S47–S57, 2001. **Study showing the safety and efficacy of tacrolimus 0.03% and 0.1% in young infants and children.**

Urticaria and Angioedema

Ilan Dalal

KEY CONCEPTS

- Urticaria is classified as acute or chronic according to its duration (less or more than 6 weeks, respectively) because the causes and mechanisms of urticaria formation are different, as are the therapeutic approaches.
- Approximately 50% of patients with urticaria also have angioedema, and these patients tend to have more severe disease.
- Recurrent episodes of angioedema without urticaria should be evaluated with specific complement studies to exclude hereditary or acquired C1 esterase inhibitor deficiency.
- Acute urticaria and angioedema is more common in children and most often is caused by immunoglobulin (Ig) E–mediated reaction to allergens such as drugs, foods, and insect stings. In contrast, chronic urticaria is rare in the pediatric population.
- A special form of acute urticaria in children is papular urticaria, which represents an ectoparasite hypersensitivity reaction, usually to dog or cat fleas or mites.
- Despite the high perception in the population, particular ingestants (foods, food additives and coloring agents, herbs, supplements) or contactants (soaps, lotions, detergents, cosmetics, toiletries, hair or nail products, and latex) are rare causes of chronic urticaria.
- Because histamine is the most important mast cell mediator in the pathogenesis of hives, antihistamines are the cornerstone in treatment of these conditions.
- Acute urticaria is a self-limited illness requiring only a short course of antihistamines in most cases. In partial response, a substitution to another class or a combination of first- and second-generation antihistamines can be of benefit.
- The second-generation antihistamines are often used in children because of negligible sedative and anticholinergic effects as compared to first-generation antihistamines. However, first-generation drugs are still widely used because of lower cost and large

availability (many of theses drugs are available over the counter).
- Intramuscular or subcutaneous epinephrine should be used in cases of severe facial angioedema associated with airway obstruction.

Urticaria and angioedema (hives) is a common disorder affecting at least 20% of the population at some point during their lives. Urticaria occurs as raised intensely pruritic papules that are usually pale wheals surrounded by an erythematous flare. The lesions are roughly circular and discrete but can be of varying sizes and irregular in shape when lesions coalesce. Urticaria is caused by vasodilation and increased vascular permeability of blood vessels in the superficial dermis. Angioedema is caused by a similar process in blood vessels but involves the deeper dermis and subcutaneous tissues. The lesions are characterized by asymmetric, localized, nondependent, and transient edema and are usually less pruritic than urticarial lesions. Approximately 50% of patients with urticaria also have angioedema, and these patients tend to have more severe and prolonged disease. Angioedema may involve the upper airway and can cause life-threatening obstruction. A patient presenting with recurrent episodes of acute angioedema of the face, tongue, or lips, associated with bouts of severe abdominal pain, without urticaria, should be evaluated with specific complement studies to exclude hereditary or acquired C1 esterase inhibitor deficiency. Acquired C1 esterase inhibitor deficiency can be associated with malignancies, autoimmune disorders, or drugs, especially angiotensin-converting enzyme (ACE) inhibitors or nonsteroidal anti-inflammatory drugs (NSAIDs).

Urticaria is usually classified as acute or chronic according to its duration (less or more than 6 weeks, respectively) because the causes and mechanisms of urticaria formation are different, as are the therapeutic approaches. Acute urticaria and angioedema is more common in children and is often caused by an immunoglobulin (Ig) E–mediated reaction to allergens such as foods, drugs (particularly antibiotics) and stinging insect venoms. Acute urticaria can also result from direct non–IgE-mediated stimulation of mast cells by certain agents, including radiocontrast media, viruses, opiates, vancomycin, and NSAIDs. However, a specific cause may not be identified in up to 50% of cases of acute urticaria. A special form of acute urticaria in children is papular urticaria (lesions are typically on the extremities on exposed skin), which represents an ectoparasite hypersensitivity reaction usually to dog or cat fleas, mosquitoes, or lice.

If symptoms have persisted for more than 6 weeks the patient is considered to have chronic urticaria. The two largest groups of chronic urticaria (which is rare in childhood) are the physical urticaria and autoimmune urticaria. Physical urticarias share the common property of being induced by environmental factors. It is common for patients to present with several physical urticarias. This includes cold, cholinergic, dermographism, pressure, vibration, solar, and aquagenic urticaria. The autoimmune urticaria is caused by functional autoantibodies to the high affinity receptor for IgE (FcεRI) or in few cases to IgE.

Expert Opinion on Management Issues

ACCEPTED INTERVENTIONS

A careful history is of most importance in uncovering the possible cause of a patient's hives. Identification of the etiologic factor(s) and removal of factors that may augment or induce hives such as NSAIDs, aspirin-containing medications, or alcohol ingestion may result in significant improvement.

Because histamine is the most important mast cell mediator in the pathogenesis of hives, antihistamines are the cornerstone in treatment of these conditions. Histamine exerts its effect through binding with one of its three receptors: H_1 through H_3. The H_1 receptor is the most relevant in the allergic inflammation. The H_1 antihistamines prevent the effect of histamine through a reversible, competitive inhibition of histamine by binding to the receptor. As a result these drugs work best when taken prophylactically rather than reversing the actions of histamine after it has been released. These drugs are traditionally divided into six classes based on differences in their chemical structures. They are further divided into first-generation antihistamines, which cross the blood–brain barrier (BBB) because of their lipophilicity and cause sedation, which may interfere with cognitive, motor, and intellectual performance. Young children may occasionally suffer from paradoxical agitation. In contrast, the second-generation drugs do not cross the BBB owing to their size, charge, and lipophilicity. As a result of their selective engineering, the second-generation antihistamines do not bind muscarinic receptors and therefore do not have anticholinergic side effects. The anticholinergic adverse effects include dry mouth and eyes, urinary retention, constipation, excitation, nervousness, palpitations, and tachycardia. Prolongation of the QT interval and ventricular tachycardia (torsades de pointes) was reported in association with the use of two second-generation antihistamines that have since been removed from the market (terfenadine and astemizole). The drugs currently in use are safe and such a phenomenon has not been reported.

Antihistamines are well absorbed, reaching peak serum concentrations within 2 hours. Most drugs are metabolized by the hepatic cytochrome P450 enzyme system. As a result, elimination may be reduced in patients with hepatic impairment or by simultaneous ingestion of other inhibitors of this pathway, such as erythromycin, macrolides, ciprofloxacin, ketoconazole, and some antidepressants (nefazodone, fluvoxamine).

The second-generation antihistamines are often used in children because of negligible sedative and anticholinergic effects as compared to first-generation antihistamines. Additionally, most of these drugs can be prescribed as once-a-day dosing, which is a well-known factor in increasing the compliance. However, first-generation drugs are still widely used because of lower cost and large availability (many of theses drugs are available over the counter). In more severe cases, a reasonable approach is to prescribe a low-sedation second-generation antihistamine in the morning and first-generation such as hydroxyzine at night. If optimal doses of H_1 antihistamines do not provide adequate control, an H_2 antagonist may be added, although the benefit of this regime in children is unclear. Ranitidine (Zantac) may have an advantage over cimetidine (Tagamet) because of higher potency and a lack of interference with hepatic microsomal enzymes and androgen receptors. Doxepin is a tricyclic antidepressant, which has potent H_1- and H_2-antihistamine activity (H_1-receptor affinity nearly 800 times that of diphenhydramine). This drug may be used in much smaller doses than those typically needed for antidepressant effects. Despite dosing at night, using doxepin is limited substantially by significant side effects of sedation, increased appetite, and weight gain (Table 1).

URGENT INTERVENTIONS

β-Agonists should be used only for patients presenting with episodes of severe facial angioedema associated with airway obstruction. Rapid therapy with subcutaneous epinephrine or (the preferred option) intramuscular injection of epinephrine (1:1000, 0.01 mL/kg, maximum of 0.3 mL) every 15 to 20 minutes is critical for immediate relief. Patients with recurrent episodes of life-threatening urticaria/angioedema should carry an emergency epinephrine kit (EpiPen Jr., 0.15 mg, or adult, 0.3 mg). In cases of severe airway obstructions emergent tracheotomy is required.

CONTROVERSIAL INTERVENTIONS

The use of systemic glucocorticoids in the treatment of acute urticaria is rarely necessary. However, systemic glucocorticoids are useful in the management of patients with pressure urticaria, vasculitic urticaria (especially with eosinophil prominence), idiopathic angioedema with or without urticaria, or chronic urticaria that responds poorly to conventional treatment. If glucocorticoids are administered, only short tapering courses should be employed. Topical antihistamines or glucocorticoids are of no value in the management of urticaria and/or angioedema. A number of other drugs may be useful in selected nonresponsive or steroid-dependent cases of chronic urticaria. Ketotifen, zileuton, and montelukast—drugs that alter the leukotriene pathway either by inhibiting production or blocking receptor binding—have been shown to be effective in some patients with urticaria, particularly in aspirin-induced urticaria/angioedema. Thyroxine has been used in patients with chronic urticaria and associated autoimmune thyroiditis. Severe nonresponsive cases have been treated with plasmapheresis,

TABLE 1 Antihistamine Receptor Antagonists

Generic Name (Trade Name) OTC/Rx	Dosage/Route/ Regimen	Maximum Dose	Dosage Formulations	Common Adverse Reactions	Comments
Diphenhydramine (Benadryl)	PO, IV, IM: 5 mg/kg/day q4–6h	50 mg/dose 300 mg/day	Tablet: 12.5, 25, 50 mg Capsule: 25, 50 mg Syrup: 2.5 mg/mL Injection: 50 mg/1 mL	Sedation, dizziness, dry mouth, nose and throat, dyskinesias, thickening of bronchial secretions	Marked sedation. Anti–motion sickness activity.
Chlorpheniramine (Chlor-Trimeton)	PO: 2 mg q4–6h IM, SC: 87.5 µg/kg q6h	12 mg/day	Tablet: 4, 12 mg Syrup: 2 mg/5 mL Injection: 10, 100 mg/1 mL	Drowsiness, sedation, dry mouth, nose and throat, GI symptoms	Slight sedation. Common component of OTC "cold" medication.
Hydroxyzine (Atarax, Vistaril IM)	PO: 2–5 mg/kg/day q6–8h IM: 1.1 mg/kg/dose	400 mg/day	Tablet: 10, 25, 50, 100 mg Syrup: 2 mg/mL Injection: 25, 50 mg/mL	Sedation, dizziness, dry mouth, nose and throat, dyskinesias	Marked sedation. IM solution must NOT be given IV or SC.
Promethazine (Phenergan)	PO: 2 mg/kg/day q6–8h IV, IM: 0.5–1 mg/kg/dose		Tablet: 12.5, 25, 50 mg Syrup: 6.25 mg/5 mL Injection: 25, 50 mg/1 mL Suppl: 12.5, 25, 50 mg	CNS depression, drowsiness, extra-pyramidal symptoms, dermatitis, dry mouth, nasal stuffiness	Not recommended in children <2 yr. Antiemetic.
Cyproheptadine (Periactin)	PO: 2–4 mg q8–12h	12–16 mg/day	Tablet: 4 mg Syrup: 2 mg/5 mL	CNS depression, drowsiness, dry mouth, weight gain, GI symptoms	Moderate sedation. In pediatric population used also as appetite stimulation.
Loratadine (Claritin)	PO: 5 mg/day (2–5 yr), 10 mg/day for >6 yr	10 mg/day	Tablet: 10 mg Syrup: 1 mg/1 mL	Dry mouth, fatigue, headache, somnolence	Not recommended in children <2 yr. Approved for OTC use. Metabolized by the cytochrome P450 system.
Cetirizine (Zyrtec)	PO: 2.5–10 mg/day q12–24 h	10 mg/day	Tablet: 5, 10 mg Syrup: 1 mg/1 mL	Dry mouth, fatigue, headache, somnolence	Not recommended in <6 months. The active metabolite of hydroxyzine. Not metabolized by the liver.
Fexofenadine (Allegra)	PO: 60 mg/day (6–11 yr), 120–180 mg/day 12 yr and more	180 mg/day	Capsule: 30, 60, 180 mg	Dry mouth, fatigue, headache, somnolence, dysmenorrhea, dyspepsia, flu-like symptoms	The active metabolite of terfenadine. not metabolized by the liver
Desloratadine (Clarinex)	PO: 5 mg/day	5 mg/day	Tablet: 5 mg	Dry mouth, fatigue, headache, somnolence, flu-like symptoms	The primary active metabolite of Loratadine
Doxepin (Sinequan, Zonalon, Adapin)	PO: 10–30 mg/day at bedtime	30 mg/day	Capsule: 10, 25, 50, 75, 100, 150 mg; Cream: 50 mg/g Solution: 10 mg/mL	Severe CNS depression, blurred vision, dry mouth, constipation, urinary retention, cytopenia	Not recommended in children <12 yr. Used in higher doses (up to 150–300 mg/day) in psychiatric disorder such as depression and anxiety.
Ranitidine (Zantac)	PO: 2–4 mg/kg/day q12h IV: 2–4 mg/kg/day q6–8h	300 mg/day	Tablet: 150, 300 mg Syrup: 15 mg/1 mL Injection 25 mg/1 mL	GI symptoms, bradycardia, hypotension, fatigue, somnolence, agitation	In severe chronic urticaria in combination with H$_1$ antagonists.

CNS, central nervous system; GI, gastrointestinal; IM, intramuscularly; IV, intravenously; qxh, every x hours; PO, orally.

17

intravenous immunoglobulin, and low-dose cyclosporine. These agents should be restricted only to centers familiar with these modalities.

Common Pitfalls

- Failure to identify the etiology or to remove factors that may augment or induce hives such as NSAIDs, aspirin-containing medications, or alcohol ingestion is a pitfall.
- Patients should be aware that the main goal of antihistamine administration is to relieve the intense pruritus and not to cause the lesions to fade out.
- Some cases respond to systemic steroids, but the potentially serious side effects, especially in the pediatric population, preclude their safe chronic use.
- Intercurrent viral infections may cause flare-ups of chronic urticaria and parents should be warned about this.
- Restriction diets are of little value if a suspected food has not been identified.
- Any atypical aspects of urticarial lesions (lesions that last for more than 24 to 36 hours, painful more then pruritic, do not blanch, leave permanent pigmentation, or are associated with purpura) suggest urticarial vasculitis, and a skin biopsy should be performed.

Communication and Counseling

Most cases of acute urticaria/angioedema recover spontaneously or with a short course of antihistamines. The prognosis of chronic urticaria is relatively good, but 10% to 20% of patients have symptoms lasting 20 years. Because the current treatment for this condition is not satisfactory, either because of limited efficacy (antihistamines) or significant side effects (steroids), there is a pressing need to search for better options. Better knowledge of mast cell biology and other mediators involved in this disease might yield insights into new modalities of treatment.

Evaluation, diagnosis, and management of acute and especially chronic urticaria may be challenging, and therefore cases for which the inciting triggers are not clear and easily avoided or for which initial therapy is not optimally effective might be considered for referral to an allergy/immunology specialist.

SUGGESTED READINGS

1. Dibbern DA Jr, Dreskin SC: Urticaria and angioedema: an overview. Immunol Allergy Clin N Am 24:141–162, 2004. **An extremely detailed review of the issue, focusing on chronic urticaria as an autoimmune disorder.**
2. Ehlers I, Niggemann B, Binder C, et al: Role of nonallergic hypersensitivity reactions in children with chronic urticaria. Allergy 53:1074–1077, 1998. **This study (in contrast to many other articles) shows that food additives such as coloring agents and preservatives might play a role in chronic urticaria in children.**
3. Greaves MW: Chronic urticaria in childhood. Allergy 55:309–320, 2000. **A detailed description of the different types of chronic urticaria and other similar lesions.**
4. Horowitz R, Reynolds S: New oral antihistamines in pediatrics. Pediatr Emerg Care 20:143–146, 2004. **A detailed review on antihistamines with focusing on second-generation drugs.**
5. Joint Task Force on Practice Parameters: The diagnosis and management of urticaria: A practice parameter; Part I: Acute urticaria/angioedema; Part II: Chronic urticaria/angioedema. Ann Allergy Asthma Immunol 85:521–544, 2000. **A comprehensive review of the issue, focusing on practical approach and management, including many common questions raised by patients and physicians.**
6. Leung DYM: Urticaria and angioedema (hives). In Behrman RE, Kliegman RM, Jenson HB (eds): Nelson Textbook of Pediatrics. Philadelphia: WB Saunders, 2004. **A detailed summary of the issue in the pediatric population, including a therapeutic approach and description of diagnostic testing for the different types of urticaria.**
7. Leznoff A, Sussman GL: Syndrome of idiopathic chronic urticaria and angioedema with thyroid autoimmunity: A study of 90 patients. J Allergy Clin Immunol 84:66–71, 1989. **This is the first study that showed the association between chronic urticaria and autoimmunity, particularly thyroid disorders.**

Drug Reactions and the Skin
Michael J. Rieder

KEY CONCEPTS

- The skin is commonly involved in adverse drug reactions. These often produce major morbidity and can be associated with a significant risk for mortality.
- Management is dependent on accurate diagnosis. Discontinuing the offending drug and symptomatic management is often the only treatment required.
- For very serious adverse drug reactions involving the skin, there are a limited number of therapeutic options, including the use of corticosteroids and intravenous immunoglobulin. Little data support this, and consultation with an expert in the management of adverse drug reactions is advised in this case.

Drug therapy has provided some of the significant advances in the medical care of children. However, the ready availability of effective specific therapy has come at a price. This price includes the economic cost—in many regions, drugs cost more than physician services. Another major price is the risk of adverse drug reactions (ADRs). ADRs complicate the course of approximately 5% of the course of therapy for most drugs, with the risk being higher in certain populations and some disease states. Known risk factors for ADRs germane to children include developmental immaturity or disease of the liver or kidney (organs of drug elimination), multidrug therapy, prematurity and female gender.

ADRs can be predictable or unpredictable (Box 1, Box 2). Many predictable ADRs such as side effects can be treated, with the reasonable expectation that the symptoms of the adverse event will decline and disappear over time. However, many unpredictable ADRs—such as drug allergy and drug hypersensitivity—require both discontinuation of the offending drug and therapy for symptomatic relief. Although ADRs can involve many different systems, many of the most severe and worrisome ADRs involve the skin. Skin involvement is one of the commonest manifestations of ADRs in children, a problem compounded by the frequent involvement of the skin in infections and the subsequent difficulty in diagnosis.

Expert Opinion on Management Issues

The first step in managing cutaneous ADRs is an accurate diagnosis. As noted previously, the differential diagnosis of cutaneous signs in the presence of drug therapy includes infectious rashes. Thus, an accurate diagnosis is essential, notably in determining if the cutaneous manifestations troubling the patient are etiologically related to drug therapy or if an alternate explanation is likely. The diagnosis of a cutaneous ADR is almost entirely clinical.

There are a limited number of clinical manifestations of cutaneous ADRs. The management is largely predicated on the clinical presentation of the ADR. As a general principle, the offending drug should be discontinued; in the case in which the therapeutic goal for which the drug was prescribed has not been achieved, the consideration needs to be made regarding what would constitute reasonable alternative therapy. This is frequently overlooked in the management of ADRs, and the primary diagnosis for which therapy was

prescribed must always be considered when planning the evaluation and therapy of the adverse event.

CONTACT DERMATITIS

Contact dermatitis is a delayed-type hypersensitivity reaction that is characterized by the development of plaques, which may be bullous, erythematous, papular, or urticarial, on the skin where the drug of interest has been applied. Onset occurs within 24 hours of exposure, typically following a sensitizing exposure, which usually must be at least 5 days. Accompanying pruritus is common. Agents that commonly induce contact dermatitis include benzocaine, paraben, neomycin, and some topical antihistamines. Therapy includes the use of topical corticosteroids and an oral antihistamine such as diphenhydramine 1 mg/kg/dose three or four times a day if pruritus is a problem. Although rare, contact dermatitis has been described in association with prolonged use of topical corticosteroids, and this should be suspected if symptoms worsen after therapy with topical corticosteroids.

FIXED DRUG ERUPTIONS

Fixed drug eruptions are an uncommon cutaneous ADR in children. A fixed drug eruption is characterized by the development of a single or several plaques, which may be erythematous, bullous or eczematous, at the same location after systemic exposure to a drug. The indicated management is discontinuation of the offending agent; rarely, local pruritus may be sufficiently troubling to require brief therapy with an oral antihistamine such as diphenhydramine 1 mg/kg/dose three or four times a day. Following resolution of the rash, postinflammatory hyperpigmentation is common.

EXANTHEMS

Exanthems associated with therapy include maculopapular rashes, erythematous exanthems, and morbilliform rashes. Nonspecific maculopapular rashes are commonly associated with therapy and represent a diagnostic problem, in that the issue most commonly raised is whether the rash is because of an infectious cause or to the suspect drug. In the case in which the etiology is unclear the usual management is to discontinue the offending agent; symptomatic therapy is rarely required.

URTICARIA

Urticaria is a common cutaneous ADR, notably in the context of drug allergy. Therapy for urticaria relies on the use of systemic antihistamines, typically administered orally. The newer selective antihistamines appear to be less effective for this indication than the older, nonselective agents. The usual first-line agent is diphenhydramine, typically given in a 1 mg/kg dose four times a day as needed. In the event that adequate symptomatic relief is not obtained, a brief course of hydroxyzine should be considered, in a dose of 10 mg three or four times a day for children under 6 years old and 10 to 20 mg three to four times a day for older children.

ANAPHYLAXIS

The therapy of anaphylaxis is covered elsewhere, and anaphylaxis constitutes a true pediatric emergency, with urgent attention to airway, breathing, and circulation being critical in ensuring the best outcome for the patient. The principle cutaneous manifestation of anaphylaxis is urticaria, which may be accompanied by significant pruritus. As in the case of isolated urticaria, diphenhydramine, typically given in a 1 mg/kg dose four times a day as needed, is the first-line therapy.

ERYTHEMA MULTIFORME MINOR

Erythema multiforme minor can be an isolated cutaneous ADR or can be a cutaneous manifestation of multisystemic ADRs, such as sulfonamide-induced hepatitis or aromatic anticonvulsant hypersensitivity. Supportive and symptomatic therapies are the mainstays of management, and the intensity and nature of symptomatic therapy depend on the associated symptoms; for example, ibuprofen therapy for small joint arthritis associated with cefaclor associated serum sickness-like reactions. Therapy for the cutaneous manifestations of these events is rarely needed, but vigilance is required, as progression of the cutaneous involvement may include evolution to Stevens-Johnson syndrome or toxic epidermal necrolysis. When symptoms include pruritus, diphenhydramine may be a useful agent for symptomatic relief.

STEVENS-JOHNSON SYNDROME/TOXIC EPIDERMAL NECROLYSIS

The most severe cutaneous ADRs are Stevens-Johnson syndrome and toxic epidermal necrolysis (SJS-TEN). SJS-TEN are serious cutaneous ADRs characterized by the development of a central macular exanthema associated with mucous membrane involvement. These conditions are the most severe cutaneous ADRs and are associated with a great deal of morbidity and a significant risk for mortality. Historically, the mortality from SJS-TEN has been in the range of 15% for SJS and 30% for TEN, although a recent retrospective experience of the analysis of a large tertiary care center has demonstrated only a 2% mortality rate, presumably on the basis of improved supportive care. Drug-induced SJS-TEN is most commonly seen in association with therapy with antimicrobials or anticonvulsants.

The natural history of these disorders is progression, and the clinician caring for children with drug-induced SJS-TEN should anticipate that progression of the lesions despite discontinuing the offending drug.

The development of a serious cutaneous ADR is likely to be uncommon in the context of the individual practitioner and consultation with an expert in the area is highly recommended. There are three key elements in the care of patients with drug-induced SJS-TEN following discontinuation of the offending drug.

The first element is symptomatic care. These reactions are often accompanied by severe pain, and the physician should not hesitate to use morphine, in the form of a bolus, intravenous drip, or patient-controlled analgesia, for pain relief. Fentanyl or other opiates can also be used if these agents are more commonly used at the treating institution. Patients may also have complaints of pruritus, and diphenhydramine in a dose of 1 mg/kg/dose three or four times a day may be helpful.

The second element of care is supportive, the importance of which cannot be overstated. Key issues for supportive care include skin care, fluid and electrolyte balance, and nutrition. The major improvement in mortality associated with SJS-TEN, although difficult to define in detail, is probably largely due to better skin care and decreased rates of opportunistic infections, notably sepsis. Patients with SJS, and especially patients with TEN, should be cared for by nursing staff expert in skin care, ideally staff with considerable experience with burns. Skin care with burn care regimens is associated with a reduced risk of serious infection. Good mouth care is also important when there are oral lesions. In the care of ophthalmic involvement, the patient should be evaluated by an ophthalmologist; treatment with topical agents is usually necessary in these cases. Fluid and electrolyte status must be carefully monitored, notably if there is extensive skin loss. In addition to expert skin care, attention should be given to nutrition. Mucous membrane involvement may be severe and is usually fairly painful, and consideration should be given to early use of total parental nutrition in addition to use of liquid nutrition such as PediaSure.

The final element of care is definitive care. The pathogenesis of drug-induced SJS-TEN appears to involve altered immunity, with recent work focusing on the role of reactive drug intermediates in the initial pathogenesis of the events and alterations in immune response being key in the clinical manifestations of the reaction. Recent work has pointed to a key role for activation of death receptors via activation of the CD95 receptor by the association of soluble Fas ligand and the Fas receptor, leading to apoptosis of epithelial cells.

A number of interventions aimed at altering the immune response have been described in case reports and short series. These have included thalidomide, plasmapheresis, and cyclophosphamide. Issues with respect to availability, toxicity, and potential adverse events are major concerns with these therapies, notably in the absence of controlled trials demonstrating efficacy. Definitive therapy for SJS-TEN over the past two decades has primarily been by the use of pulse corticosteroid therapy, with intravenous immunoglobulin (IVIG) being a more recent therapy. The major controversy with respect to the management of drug-induced

SJS-TEN relates to whether to treat patients with pulse corticosteroid therapy IVIG.

Several studies, including small comparative studies, have examined the use of pulse corticosteroid therapy for SJS-TEN. The usual dose is 1 to 2 mg/kg/day of prednisone or prednisolone for 5 days. There is some evidence of efficacy in reducing the severity of symptoms if given early in the evolution of symptoms. However, there is also some evidence that the risk of infection increases when corticosteroids are given later in the course of infection. One of the principle causes of mortality in drug-induced SJS-TEN is infection, and this suggests that corticosteroids should be used with caution, if at all, in well-established cases of SJS-TEN and that corticosteroids should be reserved for early cases of drug-induced SJS-TEN.

The potential role of soluble FAS ligand in the pathogenesis of drug-induced SJS-TEN had been the stimulus for the use of IVIG to arrest disease progression. Although there are only a small number of cases in the comparative studies of IVIG, there are a number of small series that suggest that IVIG is effective in reducing the severity and duration of SJS-TEN. Not all the experience is positive; one European study did not demonstrate benefit, although the majority of studies to date have suggested benefit. The experience with IVIG has not suggested that there are few adverse effects associated with therapy. There have been no dose-finding studies, but the dose of IVIG used has been in the range of 1 to 2 g/kg given in a single dose or daily spread out for as many as 4 days. I use 2 to 3 g/kg of IVIG in divided doses given daily over 3 days.

Common Pitfalls

A major pitfall in the management of cutaneous ADRs is an incorrect diagnosis. If a cutaneous ADR is diagnosed as something else, notably when therapy is continued and when the ADR is severe such as SJS-TEN, there is the potential for a more severe ADR with a more prolonged duration of illness.

Another major pitfall is underestimating the severity of the ADR, especially for drug-induced SJS-TEN. Given the current thoughts with respect to the pathogenesis of these reactions, notably the concept that immunity is a key element, this helps to understand why symptoms continue to develop and evolve after the offending drug is discontinued.

Prevention

Severe cutaneous ADRs are typically defined as unpredictable ADRs, and thus prevention would seem problematic. However, in the case of severe cutaneous ADRs such as drug-induced SJS-TEN there is good evidence that there may be cross-class sensitivity, that is, children who react to one sulfonamide are highly likely to react to other sulfonamides. As well, it appears that some children who react to one of the aromatic anticonvulsants, such as carbamazepine, are likely to have reactions to other aromatic anticonvulsants such as phenytoin.

Communication and Counseling

When adverse events occur in the context of therapy there are two distinctly different views commonly taken: Physicians commonly look to the disease being treated, and patients commonly look to the drug being taken. This cultural difference needs to be remembered when a cutaneous ADR has occurred, and the child health care practitioner needs to clearly communicate to patient and family what has occurred, what the plan for managing this will be, and counseling on how this will affect future care. It is probable that having a child sustain a serious ADR will affect the extent to which families will comply with future therapy, and thus dealing with the ADR as a separate clinical problem and having a clear dialogue about causes and future care is important in fostering the ongoing relationship between the patient and family and the health care team. In addition to communicating with the family, it is important that the adverse event and the responsible drug be communicated to other health care practitioners involved in the patient's care, notably when children have chronic or complex illness and may be seen by multiple caregivers. Clear and comprehensive communication is important in the common goal of providing children with optimal care.

Counseling should focus on the drug(s) responsible for the patient's adverse event and the drugs that the patient should avoid. In the context of children who require chronic or ongoing therapy, counseling should also address the issue of what drugs are likely to be tolerated without adverse events.

SUGGESTED READINGS

1. Abe R, Shimizu T, Shibaki A, Nakamura H: Toxic epidermal necrolysis and Stevens-Johnson syndrome are induced by soluble Fas ligand. Am J Patho 162:1515–1520, 2003. **An elegant study using material from controls and patients with SJS-TEN supporting the role of interactions between Fas and soluble Fas ligand as key elements in the pathogenesis of the syndrome.**
2. Forman R, Koren G, Shear NH: Erythema multiforme, Stevens-Johnson syndrome and toxic epidermal necrolysis in children: A review of 10 years' experience. Drug Safety 25:965–972, 2002. **A good review of the clinical presentation and complications of these serious cutaneous ADRs based on the experience of a large tertiary care hospital.**
3. Fritsch PO, Sidoroff A: Drug-induced Stevens-Johnson syndrome/toxic epidermal necrolysis. Am J Clin Dermatol 1:349–360, 2000. **A well-written review of the clinical presentation and therapeutic controversies in the treatment of these serious cutaneous ADRs.**
4. Kakourou T, Klontza D, Soteropoulou F, Kattamis C: Corticosteroid treatment of erythema multiforme major (Stevens-Johnson syndrome) in children. Eur J Pediatr 156:90–93, 1997. **A comparative study of corticosteroids versus supportive therapy demonstrating reduced duration of fever and rash in children treated with corticosteroids.**
5. Metry DW, Jung P, Levy ML: Use of intravenous immunoglobulin in children with Stevens-Johnson syndrome and toxic epidermal necrolysis: Seven cases and review of the literature. Pediatrics

112:1430–1436, 2003. **A small case series and thoughtful review of the literature on the use of IVIG in SJS-TEN.**

6. Patterson R, DeSwarte RD, Greenberger PA, et al: Drug allergy and protocols for management of drug allergies. Allergy Proceedings 15:239–264, 1994. **A clinically relevant system for classifying and approaching adverse drug reactions.**

7. Roujeau JC: Treatment of severe drug eruptions. J Dermatol 26:718–722, 1999. **A thoughtful review of the controversy with respect to use of corticosteroids for cutaneous ADRs by one of the international experts in the field.**

Erythema Nodosum

Samuel Chachkin, Judy W. Cheng, and Albert C. Yan

KEY CONCEPTS

- Erythema nodosum is a self-limited inflammatory skin disorder of the subcutaneous fat.
- The most common identifiable cause in children is infection with β-hemolytic streptococci, although erythema nodosum has been associated with a number of other infections, medications, and inflammatory disorders.
- Classic findings are painful, erythematous, and bilateral nodules and plaques on the extensor surfaces of the lower extremities.
- Lesions typically resolve in less than 2 weeks in children but can last as long as 3 to 6 weeks.
- Therapy is focused on symptomatic relief, parental reassurance, and focused treatment of any underlying disorder associated with erythema nodosum.

Erythema nodosum (EN) is an inflammatory skin disorder of the subcutaneous fat (panniculitis). Affected patients typically present with painful, tender, erythematous, subcutaneous nodules on the extensor surfaces of the lower extremities.

Essentially a reactive phenomenon, EN may represent a hypersensitivity reaction to one of a number of possible offending stimuli: infectious agents (such as mycobacteria and β-hemolytic streptococci), autoimmune disorders (such as sarcoidosis, inflammatory bowel disease, and Behçet disease), malignancies (such as lymphoma), pregnancy, and medications (such as oral contraceptives and sulfonamides). EN has historically been associated with tuberculosis, although currently most childhood cases of EN with an identifiable etiology appear to be caused by infection with β-hemolytic streptococci. Other infectious causes of EN vary in incidence by region and include fungal infections, yersiniosis, hepatitis B, mycoplasma, and the zoonotic diseases. Given the female preponderance of EN among adolescents and adults, estrogen has been postulated to play a role in the pathogenesis of EN. In children, however, the disease is distributed equally among both sexes.

EN generally manifests with the acute onset of painful and tender, red, bilateral lower extremity plaques and nodules located on the extensor surfaces. Some patients experience prodromal symptoms that may include fever, arthralgias, arthritis, and fatigue up to 8 weeks before eruption of skin lesions. Nodular lesions may occur on the upper extremities or face, a feature more commonly observed in children. The nodules gradually flatten and affected areas may develop post-inflammatory hyperpigmentation. The lesions neither ulcerate nor scar, and lesions that do so should raise the suspicion of alternative diagnoses, such as nodular vasculitis (erythema induratum) or Sweet syndrome (acute febrile neutrophilic dermatosis). Cutaneous findings of EN may persist for 2 weeks in younger children, although in older patients, lesions last an average of 3 to 6 weeks and may be influenced by the duration of the underlying disease process associated with EN.

Expert Opinion on Management Issues

This inflammatory skin condition is usually a self-limited, nonscarring disease without long-term dermatologic sequelae. Appropriate screening for underlying disorders based on careful history-taking and physical examination, symptomatic management, and patient and parental reassurance are recommended.

Chronic and recurrent cases of EN should prompt a thorough re-evaluation to investigate underlying causes, including a detailed history and review of systems, a review of administered medications, and complete physical examination. Special attention to symptoms or signs of infection, such as diarrhea, pharyngitis, respiratory symptoms, and changes in weight or growth patterns, may indicate a potential cause.

Laboratory evaluations where appropriate may include:

- Rapid strep testing or bacterial culture (throat or perianal)
- Antistreptolysin antibody
- Erythrocyte sedimentation rate
- Chest radiography
- Partial purified derivative (PPD)
- If diarrhea is present, stool culture for agents such as yersinia, *Campylobacter*, and salmonella.

Erythema nodosum may resolve more promptly if its associated underlying cause is treated appropriately.

To reduce associated pain and edema, bed rest, compression stockings, and elevation of the affected extremity may be helpful. Additionally, several medications have traditionally been used to treat the condition:

- *Nonsteroidal anti-inflammatory drugs (NSAIDs)*: Can be effective for pain management in many patients but do not appear to significantly alter the course of the underlying disease. In children, ibuprofen, naproxen, and indomethacin have been used safely for various indications including erythema nodosum, although aspirin has been sometimes favored in adults for EN. These can be used as long as symptoms persist.

■ *Supersaturated potassium iodide (SSKI)*: Included here mostly for historical reasons, this drug is rarely used in pediatric EN. Although effective for EN, use of SSKI is limited by its adverse effects, particularly gastrointestinal effects of diarrhea, abdominal pain, and vomiting. Additionally, long-term use of SSKI can lead to alterations in thyroid hormone activity, producing either hypothyroid or hyperthyroid states.

■ *Corticosteroids*: Although effective by systemic or intralesional administration, these agents are rarely needed for this self-limited disease. Corticosteroid use appears to be suppressive, and lesions may recur after cessation of therapy. These medications may also be contraindicated in the context of an underlying infection, particularly tuberculosis or a fungal infection.

■ *Other therapies*: Mycophenolate mofetil, dapsone, colchicine, and hydroxychloroquine have been reported as possible treatments for severe or recurrent EN, but they have limited use in children. Additionally, some therapies used for the management of underlying etiologies, such as infliximab in Crohn disease, may affect the course of erythema nodosum.

Common Pitfalls

■ Chronic or recurrent cases of EN should always prompt a thorough re-evaluation for an underlying disorder.
■ Scarring or ulcerating lesions should raise suspicion for alternative diagnoses.
■ The lesions of EN are more likely to present in atypical locations (e.g., upper extremities, face) in pediatric patients than in adults.
■ If an underlying cause is unclear after evaluation (as described earlier), or if there is uncertainty about the diagnosis of EN, patients should be referred to a dermatologist for further evaluation.

Communications and Counseling

Patients and families should be reassured that EN is a self-limited disorder that usually resolves in less than 2 to 4 weeks without scarring or recurrence. Although there are many possible associated disorders, the most common association in children is infection with β-hemolytic streptococci.

SUGGESTED READINGS

1. Cribier B, Caille A, Heid E, Grosshans E: Erythema nodosum and associated diseases. A study of 129 cases. Int J Dermatol 37:667–672, 1998. **This retrospective study examines the underlying diseases associated with EN.**
2. Kakourou T, Drosatou P, Psychou F, et al: Erythema nodosum in children: A prospective study. J Am Acad Dermatol 44:17–21, 2001. **This prospective study follows the course of 35 children with EN.**
3. Psychos DN, Voulgari PV, Skopouli FN, et al: Erythema nodosum: The underlying conditions. Clin Rheumatol 19(3):212–216, 2000. **This prospective study of 153 adult patients examines the identifiable underlying causes of EN.**

Erythema Multiforme

Sarah L. Stein

KEY CONCEPTS

■ Erythema multiforme (EM) is a distinct disorder differentiated from Stevens-Johnson syndrome (SJS) and toxic epidermal necrolysis (TEN) by the clinical presentation of target lesions, minor mucosal involvement, and a benign course. EM does not progress to SJS or TEN.
■ EM has a strong association with infectious precipitants, particularly herpes simplex virus. Frequent recurrences of EM may be controlled with use of prophylactic antiviral therapy. Antiviral therapy during an acute episode of EM is not likely to shorten the course.
■ SJS is most commonly a reaction to drugs and less commonly a reaction to an infectious agent. The clinical presentation is of severe mucosal involvement and variably extensive atypical targetoid lesions with epidermal necrosis. Significant morbidity and mortality are associated.
■ TEN is a severe drug reaction that presents with extensive rapidly progressive epidermal necrosis, with or without significant mucosal involvement. There is a high mortality rate associated with this syndrome.
■ Supportive care is indicated for all of these acute bullous disorders. The use of systemic corticosteroids is highly controversial. Encouraging retrospective reports of a benefit of intravenous immunoglobulin in cases of SJS and TEN suggest that this therapy may be valuable to interrupt the progression and facilitate healing.

17

Erythema multiforme (EM) is an acute self-limiting eruption of targetoid papules and variably developing bullae that commonly involves the face, extensor surfaces of the extremities, and palms and soles. Mucous membranes may be involved with erythema and erosions, although this tends to be of lesser extent than in Stevens-Johnson syndrome (SJS). Controversy has existed over the association of EM with the conditions of SJS and toxic epidermal necrolysis (TEN). Some authors have proposed that all three of these conditions exist within a spectrum, although most would now agree that EM is a distinct entity, whereas SJS and TEN may be considered on a continuum. EM is generally thought to be a reaction pattern that develops in some individuals in relation to certain infections, most commonly herpes simplex virus infections. More rarely, some drugs have been reported to precipitate EM. SJS and TEN, however, are mainly, perhaps exclusively, caused by drugs (Box 1) and result in significantly

---

BOX 1 Medications Frequently Associated with SJS and TEN

- Aminopenicillins
- Aromatic anticonvulsants (e.g., carbamazepine, phenobarbital, phenytoin)
- Lamotrigine
- Sulfasalazine
- Trimethoprim-sulfamethoxazole

SJS, Stevens-Johnson syndrome; TEN, toxic epidermal necrolysis.

BOX 2 Treatment of Erythema Multiforme

Symptomatic Care

- Systemic antihistamines
- Systemic analgesics
- Wound care
- Systemic antimicrobials as indicated

Prevention of Herpes Simplex

- Avoiding midday sun exposure
- Wearing sun-protective clothing
- Applying sunscreens (SPF 15 or higher)

For Frequently Recurring EM

- Prophylactic acyclovir:
  - <40 kg: 20mg/kg/day in 2 divided doses
  - >40 kg: 400 mg bid
- 6- to 12-month trial, stopping periodically to reassess
- Acyclovir during an acute episode of EM will not alter the episode.

bid, twice daily; EM, erythema multiforme; SPF, sun protection factor.

BOX 3 Treatment of Stevens-Johnson Syndrome and Toxic Epidermal Necrolysis

- Admit to pediatric ICU or burn unit.
- Discontinue potential inciting drugs.
- Manage fluids and electrolytes.
- Provide nutritional support.
- Control pain.
- Perform ophthalmologic evaluation.
- Perform surveillance cultures with antimicrobial therapy if indicated.
- Care for wounds with nonadherent dressings.
- Use antacids and antimicrobial washes for mouth care if needed.
- Provide physical therapy.
- Consider use of IVIG, 0.5–1g/kg/day × 3 days.

ICU, intensive care unit; IVIG, intravenous immunoglobulin.

---

more epidermal detachment and subsequent morbidity and mortality. Cases of typical EM do not progress to SJS.

Classic EM has been attributed to herpes simplex virus in 80% of childhood cases. A clinically recognizable lesion of herpes labialis or progenitalis may or may not be present at the time of EM onset. Often the preceding herpetic lesion will have already healed, or may even have been subclinical. EM tends to be recurrent, as herpes lesions tend to be recurrent. The skin lesions of EM are believed to be the result of the host immune response to the herpes simplex virus, genetic particles, and proteins that have been found in and on lesional keratinocytes by molecular techniques.

Expert Opinion on Management Issues

Management of EM is predominantly supportive as most episodes are self-limited. Symptomatic treatment may include systemic antihistamines for itching or burning sensation, topical antibacterials for open erosions to prevent secondary bacterial infection, acetaminophen for pain relief, and bland emollients. There is no evidence that oral or topical corticosteroids are efficacious. There is no evidence that oral or topical acyclovir is efficacious, because viral replication has likely already ceased with the onset of EM. Frequently recurrent EM can be treated with oral acyclovir at suppressive doses (Box 2).

Morbidity and mortality from SJS and TEN are much greater and therapy that might interrupt the progression of these conditions is being actively sought. Supportive care is critical and involves close monitoring of fluid and electrolyte status, nutritional support, wound care, pain control, pulmonary toilet, and antimicrobial therapy when indicated. Surveillance bacterial cultures of skin, eyes, and mucosal sites should be performed regularly. Antacids and mouth rinses are helpful with extensive oral involvement. Potential offending drugs should be discontinued. Ophthalmologic evaluation is indicated when there is ocular involvement. Physical therapy to prevent contractures may be necessary. Care may be best achieved in an intensive care unit or burn unit when epidermal necrosis is extensive (Box 3).

The use of systemic corticosteroids in SJS and TEN is controversial. Some authors suggest that early use in drug-induced cases is beneficial, but other retrospective studies do not demonstrate an improvement in outcome. Complications such as sepsis and gastrointestinal tract hemorrhage are attributed in some cases to use of systemic corticosteroids in this setting. Unfortunately there have not been controlled prospective clinic trials investigating the use of systemic corticosteroids in these diseases.

Intravenous immunoglobulin (IVIG) interrupts the progression of these severe blistering reactions in children, with subsequent rapid recovery. Published reports are retrospective, and controlled prospective clinical trials have not been done. In vitro experiments show the capacity of IVIG to block binding of the apoptotic ligand to the keratinocyte cell surface and prevent the programmed cell death that is observed in TEN. Retrospective data have demonstrated the use of IVIG in adult and pediatric SJS and TEN patients to be safe, well tolerated, and likely effective in improving outcome. Most authors recommend doses of 0.5 to

1.0 g/kg/day for 3 days. Concomitant use of corticosteroids may lead to longer time to response as observed in some of the retrospective reports.

Common Pitfalls

- Failure to discontinue an offending drug may prolong the course of SJS and TEN.
- A child maintained on chronic systemic corticosteroids may develop recurrent, overlapping, or apparent continuous episodes of EM.
- Confusion has arisen regarding the appropriate classification of these acute bullous disorders, leading to misdiagnoses such as EM in the setting of urticaria and SJS in the setting of EM. Patients may become mislabeled allergic to certain medications if EM is misdiagnosed as SJS. Overly aggressive treatment of EM may even occur out of the mistaken concern that EM can progress to SJS.
- The controversy in the literature regarding the benefits of systemic corticosteroids and IVIG in these acute bullous disorders may lead to confusion over the optimal management course. Vigilant supportive care of all affected systems remains the fundamental basis of therapy.

Communication and Counseling

If a drug was likely involved as a precipitant of SJS or TEN, families need to be clearly informed so this and related drugs are avoided in the future.

Pigmentary changes are very common sequelae to EM and SJS/TEN and can last for months following the acute episode. Patients and their families should be counseled to expect these changes and advised to follow strict sun-protection guidelines to facilitate resolution of these changes.

SUGGESTED READINGS

1. Assier H, Bastuji-Garin S, Revuz J, et al: Erythema multiforme with mucous membrane involvement and Stevens-Johnson syndrome are clinically different disorders with distinct causes. Arch Dermatol 131:539–543, 1995. **Study demonstrating distinct clinical patterns of EM and SJS and associating the syndromes with specific causes.**
2. Bastuji-Garin S, Rzany B, Stern RS, et al: Clinical classification of cases of toxic epidermal necrolysis, Stevens-Johnson syndrome, and erythema multiforme. Arch Dermatol 129:92–96, 1993. **Study defining five clinical classes in which to categorize acute severe bullous disorders.**
3. Metry DW, Jung P, Levy ML: Use of intravenous immunoglobulin in children with Stevens-Johnson syndrome and toxic epidermal necrolysis: Seven cases and review of the literature. Pediatrics 112:1430–1436, 2003. **A comprehensive review of the use of IVIG for SJS and TEN in children.**
4. Weston WL, Morelli JG: Herpes simplex virus-associated erythema multiforme in prepubertal children. Arch Pediatr Adolesc Med 151:1014–1016, 1997. **Study of the role of herpes simplex virus in pediatric EM and the effect of acyclovir therapy on the course of EM in children**
5. Weston WL: What is erythema multiforme? Pediatr Ann 25:106–109, 1996. **A detailed description of the entity of EM and differentiation of EM from commonly misdiagnosed conditions.**

Psoriasis and Other Papulosquamous Disorders

David A. Dasher and Dean S. Morrell

KEY CONCEPTS

- Psoriasis occurs in all ages, including infancy. Children make up one third of cases.
- The disorder typically has a chronic and relapsing course, with frequent remissions and exacerbations.
- Common causes of exacerbation include infection, stress, trauma, and certain medications.
- Topical treatment options include corticosteroids, keratolytics, and nonsteroidal immunomodulators.
- The overall goal in topical treatment is to use the least potent corticosteroid possible, especially in intertriginous (axillary, inframammary, and inguinal) and facial skin sites.
- As understanding of the pathophysiology of psoriasis becomes clearer, treatments will likely continue to become more narrowly targeted.

The papulosquamous disorders have diverse causes, typical ages of onset, and associated clinical features; their shared feature is the presence of raised scaling lesions. The elevation of the lesions is caused by thickening of the epidermis or underlying dermal inflammation. Scale represents thickened stratum corneum. Despite the diverse causes, topical steroids, with potency dictated by location on the body, are used in the treatment of many of these disorders. This section will be devoted primarily to the management of psoriasis, followed by discussion of seborrheic dermatitis, lichen planus, and pityriasis rosea.

Psoriasis

Psoriasis is a common papulosquamous condition notable for well-demarcated, erythematous, scaling papules and plaques. The exact pathophysiology of the disease is not completely understood. However, evidence suggests that psoriasis is an immunologically mediated disease, with a dysfunctional response by T-lymphocytes in the skin to internal or external stimuli leading to many of its clinical features. Psoriasis occurs at all ages including infancy; one third of cases have an onset during childhood. The disease is characterized by a chronic and relapsing course, although spontaneous remissions can occur. Bacterial or viral infection, psychological stress, injury, and certain medications are known to cause disease exacerbations. It also tends to worsen during the fall and winter, probably secondary to decreased humidity within the environment and to decreased ultraviolet light (UVL) exposure.

Various forms of psoriasis exist. The most common variety is psoriasis vulgaris, which can be localized or generalized in its distribution. Symmetrically distributed, round, well-demarcated, erythematous, scaling plaques, most often located on the elbows, knees, and scalp characterize psoriasis vulgaris. Umbilical and lumbosacral regions, and the intergluteal cleft, are also commonly involved, and can be clues to the underlying diagnosis of psoriasis. The so-called micaceous scale is distinctive in its silvery appearance, with pinpoint bleeding points (Auspitz sign) revealed on their removal. Nail plate involvement is common and includes pitting, onycholysis, subungual hyperkeratosis, and oil staining (yellowish-brown subungual macular discoloration).

In comparison to other forms of psoriasis, guttate psoriasis is most commonly seen in children. Numerous drop-like, scaling, erythematous papules and small plaques in a generalized distribution typify this type of psoriasis. Many reports attribute the onset of guttate psoriasis to prior streptococcal infections.

Inverse psoriasis describes the presence of marginated, bright red, scaling patches and plaques in the axillary and inguinal regions. Scale may be less apparent because of the moisture in intertriginous areas. Distinction from seborrheic dermatitis, candidiasis, and noninfectious intertrigo can be difficult to an inexperienced observer.

Erythrodermic and pustular forms of psoriasis are severe and potentially fatal generalized forms of psoriasis that are less common in the pediatric populations. Acute onset of generalized erythema with subsequent exfoliative scaling typifies erythrodermic psoriasis, although spreading erythematous patches with a sudden onset of fine, 2- to 3-mm sterile pustules at the periphery of the lesions characterize pustular psoriasis. Patients can have fever, leukocytosis, and toxicity. High output cardiac failure may also rarely occur. Progression to widespread "lakes of pus" on erythematous backgrounds can occur.

Expert Opinion on Management Issues

Multiple treatment options for psoriasis are available. These can be broadly divided into topical therapy, phototherapy, and systemic therapy (Table 1).

TOPICAL THERAPY

The cornerstone of topical therapy is corticosteroids. Because of the risk of atrophy, striae, and telangiectasias, especially when potent fluorinated corticosteroid preparations are chronically employed, the overall goal is to use the least potent corticosteroid possible, especially in intertriginous and facial skin sites. Nonfluorinated corticosteroids (e.g., 1% or 2% hydrocortisone) are preferred for use in these particularly sensitive areas. Short duration (twice daily, 1 to 2 months) of medium-potency (e.g., triamcinolone) to high-potency (e.g., fluocinonide, clobetasol) corticosteroids are frequently necessary for thick, inflammatory plaques of the torso and extremities. Generalized psoriasis vulgaris, pustular psoriasis, and erythrodermic psoriasis can usually be effectively treated with inpatient intensive application of topical steroids, followed by application of tap water compresses, for 1 to 2 hours, 3 to 4 times per day. Tap water compresses should be used with caution in infants and small children because of the risk of inducing hypothermia if too much surface area is treated simultaneously. Instead, it is usually most prudent to treat only limited areas (the arms, for example, or the trunk) at any one time, and to cover the wet wraps with sufficient blankets to reduce chilling as much as possible. Systemic retinoids are also often employed in the treatment of severe erythrodermic and pustular psoriasis. Isolated, recalcitrant plaques are amenable to intralesional steroids (triamcinolone

TABLE 1 Topical Agents Used in the Treatment of Psoriasis

Treatment	Advantages	Disadvantages
Topical corticosteroids	Mainstay of treatment related to immunosuppressive and antiproliferative effects.	Atrophy, striae, telangiectases. Risk of growth retardation. Possible effect on pituitary-adrenal axis. Tachyphylaxis may occur with repeated use of superpotent agents.
Intralesional steroids	Effective for isolated recalcitrant plaques.	Painful. Poorly tolerated by children. Possibility of systemic toxicity.
Keratolytics (salicylic acid)	Decreases scale. Optimizes topical steroid treatment.	
Calcipotriene	No risk of atrophy when used alone. May combine with topical steroids for an effect greater than either used alone.	Cost. Irritation. Limited data on use in children.
Tacrolimus	Effective in facial and intertriginous areas where steroids should be avoided. No risk of atrophy.	Not effective in other areas. Cost.
Tazarotene	No risk of atrophy.	Irritation. Limited data on use in children. Potential teratogen.

2 to 5 mg/mL) via multiple injections every 6 weeks, although this is usually poorly tolerated by children, even if the skin is preanesthetized with a topical anesthetic. Considering the many potential side effects of intralesional corticosteroids, these should be administered only by a dermatologist who is experienced with their use.

Keratolytics can be effective in decreasing scale. This is not only cosmetically desirable, especially when the scalp is involved, but it will also optimize topical corticosteroid delivery into otherwise recalcitrant psoriatic plaques. Salicylic acid (2% to 5%) can be compounded into petrolatum and applied nightly. Widespread application of salicylic acid should be avoided, however, especially in infants and small children, because systemic toxicity is possible. Topical solutions (e.g., P & S liquid; Derma-Smoothe FS) are useful overnight preparations for the scalp, particularly if excessive scale is present.

Although irritating to some patients, calcipotriene (vitamin-D derivative) and tazarotene (topical retinoid) are topical agents that may spare psoriatic skin from chronic exposure to corticosteroids. Although probably safely used in children, there are limited published data available on the safety of their long-term use in this particular patient population. Additionally, the topical nonsteroidal immunomodulator tacrolimus is another agent with no risk of atrophy that has been shown to be effective on facial and intertriginous areas, in which more potent topical steroids should be avoided. Unfortunately, its effectiveness is limited elsewhere on the body.

PHOTOTHERAPY

Many psoriatic patients will relate a history of improvement during the summer months. UVL has an immunomodulatory effect on the inflammatory cells in psoriatic plaques. Although it is well known that chronic ultraviolet exposure causes photoaging and increases the risk of skin cancer, exposure to natural sunlight 15 to 30 minutes per day can be therapeutic for a patient with generalized psoriasis vulgaris or guttate psoriasis. Inconvenience, difficulty in keeping a child standing motionless in a phototherapy unit, and the risk of skin cancer make phototherapy difficult to use in children. Narrowband ultraviolet B (UVB) offers promising results but still carries the risk of chronic ultraviolet exposure.

SYSTEMIC THERAPY

Systemic therapies in children should be reserved for only severe and recalcitrant cases. Agents such as methotrexate, acitretin, and cyclosporine can dramatically improve psoriasis, but they need frequent medical and hematologic monitoring for potentially serious side effects. Additionally, there are multiple systemic immunomodulatory agents that are approved by the U.S. Food and Drug Administration (FDA) or are being investigated for the treatment of moderate to severe plaque psoriasis. These biologic agents act either by depleting T cells (alefacept), inhibiting T-cell trafficking from the circulation into dermal and epidermal tissues (efalizumab), or by inhibiting tumor necrosis factor (adalimumab, infliximab, etanercept). Ideally, all systemic therapies used for psoriasis should be administered under the strict supervision of a dermatologist who has extensive experience with their use and monitored for potential side effects.

Common Pitfalls

- Periods of remissions and exacerbations can occur independently of ongoing treatment. Therefore one should be cautious in attributing clinical improvement to therapy.
- Excessive use of topical corticosteroids may result in the development of atrophy, striae, and telangiectasias.
- Long-term use of topical corticosteroids can lead to tachyphylaxis.
- Systemic corticosteroids, oral or intramuscular, have no role in the treatment of psoriasis, as their use can induce a severe pustular eruption.
- Pustular psoriasis may also rarely occur as a patient is being weaned from potent topical corticosteroids.
- Great care must be given to the topical use of corticosteroids in children, especially if widespread areas are to be treated for prolonged periods of time, because significant systemic side effects (which include growth retardation and alterations in the pituitary-adrenal axis) may occur.

Communication and Counseling

Initially, a thorough investigation into the patient's medications should be performed to uncover any potentially exacerbating drugs (Box 1). In cases of new onset and flares of guttate psoriasis, the possibility of concurrent streptococcal infection (including perianal streptococcal cellulitis) should be investigated. Parents and patients should be counseled about the typical course of the disorder, which involves the possibility

---

BOX 1 Drugs that May Unmask or Exacerbate Psoriasis

- Nonsteroidal anti-inflammatory agents
- Systemic corticosteroids
- β-blockers
- Antimalarials
- Lithium
- Tetracyclines

of relapses. Patients who do not respond adequately to topical agents should be referred to a dermatologist.

The concept of total care is especially important when treating childhood psoriasis because it can have a significant negative impact on the child's quality of life. Total care includes developing a close physician–child/parent relationship, education regarding the chronicity of this disease and the treatment options that are available, controlling stress and providing psychological support if necessary, and maintaining good skin care and overall physical wellness. The National Psoriasis Foundation (1–800–723–9166 or http://www.psoriasis.org) has some very good educational materials for children.

OTHER PAPULOSQUAMOUS DISORDERS

Seborrheic Dermatitis

Seborrheic dermatitis is an inflammatory disease that is common in all age groups. In infancy, cradle cap is the most common presentation. Extension to forehead and postauricular areas is often seen. Diaper and intertriginous areas can have sharply demarcated erythematous patches with yellowish, "greasy" or waxy-appearing scale. The eruption lacks pruritus, satellite pustules, and purpura to differentiate it from atopic dermatitis, *Candida* infection, and Langerhans cell histiocytosis, respectively. In adolescence, involvement of the eyebrows, nasal bridge, and nasolabial folds is more typical. Waxy scale on an erythematous patch predominates in seborrheic dermatitis after childhood; however, intertriginous involvement still occurs in some. Rarely, progression to generalized erythematous exfoliation is seen. Although the exact pathogenesis of the disorder is not completely understood, evidence suggests a causal role for *Malassezia furfur* (formerly *Pityrosporum ovale*), a skin saprophyte, which has been shown to colonize the skin of patients. Treatment is directed at decreasing the yeast, the inflammation it causes, or both.

Other than cradle cap, seborrheic dermatitis is a chronic dermatosis with exacerbations and remissions. Cradle cap is self-limited and resolves during the first year of life. Treatment for 3 to 5 days is usually adequate to clear flares. In all ages, shampooing with zinc pyrithione (Head and Shoulders, SHS Zinc), selenium sulfide 1% to 2.5%, salicylic acid (TSal), or ketoconazole (Nizoral) can treat scalp scale. Cases with copious scale can be treated prior to shampooing with a 10-minute application of mineral oil or P & S liquid in infants. After childhood, overnight application of P & S liquid or Derma-Smoothe FS can assist in decreasing scale. Facial and intertriginous areas typically respond to periodic application of hydrocortisone 1% to 2.5%, ketoconazole 2% cream, or sulfur-based products (Klaron, Sulfacet-R). Resistant cases may need brief application (twice daily, 5 to 7 days) of medium potency corticosteroids and should be evaluated for possible secondary bacterial or fungal infections.

Lichen Planus

Lichen planus is an uncommon dermatosis in childhood, with children accounting for less than 5% of cases. The primary lesion is a pruritic, flat-topped, polygonal, violaceous papule that most often arises on the flexor wrists, lower extremities, and genitalia. Close inspection of the surface of the papule reveals a fine whitish reticulation or streaking called Wickham striae. Mucous membranes are involved in 50% of the cases, with Wickham striae seen on the buccal mucosa and infrequently on the palate, lips, and tongue. At times, painful erosive oral lesions can occur. Nail involvement may occur; characteristic findings include nail plate ridging, dystrophy, subungual hyperkeratosis, or pterygia.

Lichen planus is a chronic disorder, lasting, on average, approximately 12 to 15 months. More chronic cases can persist for years, with episodes of remissions and exacerbations. Postinflammatory hyperpigmentation can persist for months to years after resolution of papules and plaques.

The underlying etiology of lichen planus is unknown, although numerous systemic medications have been associated with lichen planus-like rashes. A review of the patient's medications is an important part in the patient's evaluation prior to treatment initiation. Similarly, diabetes mellitus and hepatitis C may be associated with generalized lichen planus and, therefore, should be excluded as a possible cause.

Treatment approach includes the use of systemic antihistamines (hydroxyzine, diphenhydramine) for pruritus and corticosteroids (topical, intralesional, and systemic). Medium-potency (e.g., triamcinolone, fluocinonide) and higher-potency(e.g., clobetasol) corticosteroids are indicated for oral (triamcinolone in Orabase) and cutaneous lesions. Intralesional injections (triamcinolone 3 to 5 mg/mL) can be effective for symptomatic intraoral and isolated hypertrophic cutaneous lesions, particularly those that do not respond to conventional topical corticosteroid therapy. There is growing evidence that topical tacrolimus ointment can be quite effective in the treatment of oral lichen planus. In cases of generalized and recalcitrant eruptions with incessant pruritus, tapering (4 to 8 weeks) doses of systemic prednisone (starting at 1 mg/kg/day) may be necessary. Painful oral lesions usually can be treated symptomatically with the frequent (4 to 6 times daily) use of compounded oral rinses that contain diphenhydramine and viscous lidocaine with or without additional hydrocortisone.

Regular monitoring of oral lesions is indicated, especially those that become chronic, as reports suggest oral lichen planus to be a possible precursor for intraoral squamous cell carcinoma.

Pityriasis Rosea

Pityriasis rosea is a benign, self-limited eruption occurring at all ages, with peak incidence during adolescence. There is a probable viral etiology considering the seasonal clustering of cases, rare involvement of multiple family members, reports of prodrome, and the tendency for lifelong immunity (although rare reports of recurrent episodes exist).

There may be mild constitutional symptoms followed by a solitary 2- to 5-cm scaling plaque with an active border on the torso or proximal extremity. This "herald patch" is often misdiagnosed as fungal or eczematous in origin. One to 2 weeks later, multiple oval-to-oblong, erythematous or fawn-colored macules with fine, bran-like scale erupt on the torso and proximal extremities in a characteristic arrangement parallel to skin tension lines (Christmas tree pattern). Papular and papulovesicular variants are more commonly seen in infants, young children, pregnant women, and more highly pigmented races. Usually the condition is asymptomatic, but pruritus can be present in approximately 25% of cases. The eruption lasts 4 to 14 weeks, with gradual resolution and occasional residual hyperpigmentation or hypopigmentation that can take additional months to clear. The differential diagnosis includes secondary syphilis, drug eruption, and viral exanthem.

Usually treatment is unnecessary. However, pruritus can be managed with oral antihistamines (hydroxyzine or diphenhydramine), phototherapy (UVB or natural sunlight), and low-strength (hydrocortisone 2.5%) to medium-strength (triamcinolone 0.1% mixed 1:1 with Eucerin) topical corticosteroids.

SUGGESTED READINGS

1. Farber EM: Total care of psoriasis. Cutis 66:318, 2000. **Outlines the concept of "total care" for the pediatric patient with psoriasis.**
2. Gupta AK, Madzia SE, Batra R: Etiology and management of seborrheic dermatitis. Dermatology 208:89–93, 2004. **A discussion of etiology and treatment strategies in seborrheic dermatitis.**
3. Morris A, Rogers M, Fischer G, et al: Childhood psoriasis: A clinical review of 1262 cases. Pediatric Dermatol 18:188–198, 2001. **A clinical review of a large number of pediatric patients with psoriasis referred to a tertiary care center.**
4. Sharma R, Maheshwari V: Childhood lichen planus: A report of fifty cases. Pediatric Dermatol 16:345–348, 1999. **A clinical review of a large number of pediatric patients with lichen planus.**

Chronic, Nonhereditary Bullous Diseases of Childhood

Denise W. Metry and Reena Moza Vaid

KEY CONCEPTS

- The chronic, nonhereditary bullous diseases of childhood are a rare group of disorders, of which dermatitis herpetiformis, linear immunoglobulin A bullous dermatosis of childhood, pemphigus vulgaris, pemphigus foliaceus, and bullous pemphigoid are among the best known.

- The management approach to the pediatric bullous diseases, as with any chronic disorder, must be individualized, with risks and benefits of potential therapies carefully weighed.
- With the exception of dermatitis herpetiformis, systemic corticosteroids are often necessary to achieve rapid control of the bullous diseases. However, the ultimate goal of therapy should be to reduce cumulative steroid exposure with the use of steroid-sparing agents when medically indicated.

Expert Opinion on Management Issues

DERMATITIS HERPETIFORMIS

Dermatitis herpetiformis (DH) is an autoimmune bullous disease that can occur at any age during childhood. Because of the intense pruritus associated with DH, primary lesions are rarely found intact, with excoriated lesions most commonly seen (Table 1). Eighty-five percent to 95% of children with DH have an associated gluten-sensitive enteropathy, in which a varying degree of villous atrophy of the small intestine can be demonstrated. The recognition of the association of DH with gluten-sensitive enteropathy is essential in order that a gluten-free diet be initiated. This reverses the intestinal abnormalities in all patients and prevents potential growth retardation because of chronic malabsorption.

A gluten-free diet also effectively controls skin lesions in the majority of children. (Management approaches are listed in Box 1.) Potent topical corticosteroids are useful adjunctive therapy until dietary control is achieved, and in refractory patients with limited cutaneous disease or contraindications to systemic therapy. In severe cases, dapsone may be used for cutaneous involvement, but provides no benefit for the enteropathy. Dapsone is generally initiated at doses of 0.5 to 2.0 mg/kg/day until disease control is attained, then gradually tapered either by reducing the daily dose, or increasing the time interval between doses. Adequate control may be possible with doses as low as 0.125 mg/kg/day, or with single weekly dosing.

The most common side effects (Table 2) of dapsone therapy are hemolysis and methemoglobinemia. The majority of patients treated with dapsone will develop some degree of hemolysis, but patients with hereditary glucose-6-phosphate dehydrogenase (G6PD) deficiency are at particular risk for clinically significant hemolytic anemia. For this reason, baseline G6PD screening is essential prior to dapsone initiation. Patients treated with dapsone also commonly develop some increase in methemoglobin levels, although clinically significant methemoglobinemia, characterized by the development of bluish discoloration of the lips and tongue, is rare. The "sulfone syndrome," a rare, idiosyncratic mononucleosis-like hypersensitivity reaction to dapsone, occurs in less than 1% of patients, generally 4 or more weeks into therapy. In dapsone hypersensitivity,

17

TABLE 1 Disease Features of the Chronic, Nonhereditary Bullous Diseases of Childhood

Clinical Presentation	Associations	Histology	Immunopathology	Differential Diagnosis
Dermatitis herpetiformis				
Intensely pruritic, papulovesicles or urticarial plaques. Symmetrically distributed: Extensor knees and elbows Sacrum, and buttocks Posterior neck and scalp Scarring unusual. No mucous membrane involvement.	Gluten-sensitive enteropathy. Most children asymptomatic at time of presentation, though some will have history of chronic or relapsing diarrhea.	Subepidermal blister with neutrophilic microabscesses within dermal papillae.	Granular deposition of IgA within dermal papillae.	Scabies Atopic dermatitis
Linear IgA bullous dermatosis of childhood				
Most common among children < age 5. New bullae classically arise at the margins of older ones, producing rosette patterns described as "cluster of jewels" or "string of pearls." Perioral, genital, chest involvement most common. May be mildly pruritic. Mucous membrane involvement may lead to scarring.	Preceding: Prodromal illness. Antibiotic or NSAID use. Vaccination.	Subepidermal bullae with dermal papillary edema. Dermal infiltrate with neutrophils and eosinophils.	Linear IgA deposit at dermal-epidermal junction.	Herpes simplex virus Bullous impetigo
Pemphigus vulgaris				
Painful oral erosions precede cutaneous vesiculobullous eruption by several weeks to months. Blisters flaccid, fluid filled; rupture quickly with positive Nikolsky sign (application of pressure to blister edge results in peripheral extension). Severe pain with pruritus. Scarring unusual.	Genetic susceptibility. Environmental triggers: Drugs (penicillamine, captopril, enalapril, rifampicin). Certain plant foodstuffs.	Acantholysis, individual keratinocytes floating in suprabasal plane, with basal keratinocytes remaining attached.	IgG deposition around keratinocytes, "chicken wire" appearance. Autoantibody to desmoglein 1 and 3.	Stevens-Johnson syndrome Drug eruption
Pemphigus foliaceus				
Superficial, crusted erosions and polycyclic lesions most common to sun-exposed areas of head and neck. No scarring Oral involvement uncommon.	Environmental triggers: Drugs. Infections. Sun exposure. Blackfly insect, a disease vector in certain endemic regions of Brazil.	Subtle acantholysis. Cleavage plane at stratum granulosum.	IgG around keratinocytes. Autoantibody to desmoglein 1.	Seborrheic dermatitis Psoriasis Impetigo Staphylococcal scalded skin syndrome
Bullous pemphigoid				
Large tense bullae with oral lesions. Urticarial in annular or polycyclic pattern. Predilection for flexural and plantar/palmar areas, face.	Possible triggers: vaccines, second organ transplantation, chronic renal allograft rejection	Subepidermal blister with intact epidermis. Eosinophils, with some neutrophils and lymphocytes.	Linear deposition of IgG and C3. Autoantibody to hemidesmosome proteins.	Systemic lupus erythematosus CBDC Epidermolysis bullosa acquisita

CBDC, chronic bullous dermatosis of childhood; IgA, immunoglobulin A; IgG, immunoglobulin G; NSAID, nonsteroidal anti-inflammatory drug.

multiorgan involvement can occur, with a higher risk of liver complications than with other drug hypersensitivity syndromes. Agranulocytosis, another rare, idiosyncratic side effect of dapsone, occurs in 0.01% to 0.10% of patients and, although usually reversible, it can also be fatal. Other rare potential side effects of dapsone include hepatotoxicity and distal motor neuropathy, mostly of the hands. Such reversible side effects can occur months to years after therapy initiation.

Dapsone tolerance may be improved by the simultaneous administration of cimetidine, which reportedly decreases headache, lethargy, and methemoglobin production. Dapsone should be used with extreme caution in patients with known sulfa allergy, those with signs of megaloblastic anemia, and those already on other potentially hemolytic drugs, especially in patients with G6PD deficiency. Dapsone prescribers should also be aware of potential drug interactions, including antacids that decrease dapsone absorption, other medications with potential bone marrow toxicity, sulfa drugs that increase the risk of hemolysis and methemoglobinemia, and any drug metabolized by the cytochrome P450 system which may influence the metabolism of dapsone.

DH has a variable prognosis. Although short- and long-term remissions are common, so are recurrences late in adolescence or early adulthood, especially without adequate dietary control.

LINEAR IMMUNOGLOBULIN A BULLOUS DERMATOSIS OF CHILDHOOD

Linear IgA bullous dermatosis (LABD) of childhood, also known as chronic bullous dermatosis of childhood (CBDC), has a generally good prognosis, with natural remission occurring in the majority of patients within 5 years of disease onset. Disease features are listed in Table 1. In LABD, systemic corticosteroids are often necessary to achieve acute disease control, with dapsone the steroid-sparing agent of choice. In many cases, systemic corticosteroids and dapsone are started concomitantly; as soon as control of blistering is achieved, the corticosteroid is gradually tapered, followed by a gradual reduction in dapsone to the lowest possible dose necessary to adequately control the disease (see section on dermatitis herpetiformis). Ophthalmologic monitoring throughout childhood is also advisable given that conjunctival scarring in LABD can lead to entropion and corneal damage. Management approaches are listed in Box 1.

Systemic corticosteroids are best administered in a once-daily dose in the early morning (between 6 and 8 AM), which correlates with the normal daily physiologic surge of cortisol and thus minimizes suppression of the hypothalamic-pituitary axis (HPA). Although the average corticosteroid dose varies from 0.5 to 2 mg/kg/day for most conditions, it is best to begin with a dose high enough to control the disease, with gradual tapering once the condition improves. Ideally, corticosteroid tapering should include the goal of achieving alternate-day dosing, which has the least amount of HPA axis suppression and minimizes other adverse effects, such as weight gain and growth retardation. It is our practice to gradually decrease (by a small increment weekly) the dose taken every other day until the medication is only given every 48 hours. For example, with a 40-mg daily regimen, one could begin tapering by administering 40 mg on day 1 and 35 mg on day 2 for the first week, 40 mg on day 1 and 30 mg on day 2 the second week, and so forth.

Systemic corticosteroid therapy longer than 1 month will result in HPA suppression for up to 6 to 12 months (see Table 2). Slow tapering in patients on prolonged therapy is thus essential to avoid steroid withdrawal, as is stress dose replacement therapy for major surgeries, trauma, or illness. The low-dose adrenocorticotropic hormone (ACTH) stimulation test is the standard criterion in the assessment of HPA suppression and the need for stress doses of steroids.

Numerous other side effects are associated with prolonged systemic corticosteroid therapy. Children are particularly more susceptible than adults to growth suppression and posterior subcapsular cataracts. It may be necessary to treat certain adverse sequelae, such as diabetes or high blood pressure, concomitantly. Children on long-term therapy who are exposed to varicella should receive prophylactic therapy with varicella zoster immunoglobulin (VZIG) and treated with acyclovir if cutaneous manifestations develop. Additionally, children on prolonged corticosteroids should not receive live vaccines,

TABLE 2   Most Commonly Used Medications for the Pediatric Bullous Diseases: Potential Side Effects and Monitoring Recommendations

Therapy	Mechanism of Action	Formulation	Potential Side Effects	Monitoring Recommendations

Systemic corticosteroids	Immunosuppressive, anti-inflammatory, vasoconstrictive	1-, 5-, 10-, and 20-mg tablets; 5 mg/5 mL and 15 mg/5 mL suspension; intramuscular; intravenous	HPA suppression
			Cutaneous effects
			  Acne
			  Striae
			  Hirsutism
			  Easy bruisability
			Altered body habitus
			  Truncal obesity
			  Moon face
			  Buffalo hump
			Hypertension
			Hyperglycemia
			Growth suppression
			Osteoporosis
			Aseptic necrosis of bone
			Ocular effects
			  Posterior subcapsular cataracts
			  Glaucoma
			Decreased cell-mediated immunity/increased risk of infections
			Hematologic abnormalities
			  Neutrophilia
			  Lymphocytopenia
			  Monocytopenia
			Delayed wound healing
			Behavioral and personality changes
			  Increased appetite
			  Insomnia
			  Nervousness
			  Euphoria
			  Hyperkinesis
			Myopathy
			Pseudotumor cerebri
				Baseline:
				  Blood pressure
				  Height/weight plotted on growth curve
				  PPD (purified protein derivative of tuberculin) skin testing for tuberculosis
				  Electrolytes
				  Urine and blood sugars
				  Fasting triglycerides
				  Ophthalmologic examination
				Every 3 mo:
				  Blood pressure
				  Height/weight plotted on growth curve
				  Electrolytes
				  Urine and blood sugars
				  Fasting triglycerides
				  Ophthalmologic examination

Azathioprine	Immunomodulatory		Hematologic
			  Pancytopenia
			  Leukopenia
			  Anemia
			  Coagulopathy
			Gastrointestinal
			  Nausea
			  Vomiting
			  Elevation in liver enzymes
			Dermatologic
			  Rash
			  Increased risk for squamous cell carcinoma
			Idiosyncratic
			  Azathioprine hypersensitivity syndrome
			Renal insufficiency
			Opportunistic infections
			Birth defects
				Baseline:
				  CBC with differential
				  Liver function studies
				  Urinalysis
				  Pregnancy test in females of childbearing age
				During therapy:
				  CBC with differential and liver function studies monthly for 3 mo; if stable, then every 2 mo
				  Pregnancy test monthly in females of childbearing age

TABLE 2—cont'd

Therapy	Mechanism of Action	Formulation	Potential Side Effects	Monitoring Recommendations

Dapsone	Antimicrobial and anti-inflammatory	25- and 100-mg tablets	Hemolytic anemia
			Methemoglobinemia
			Neuropathy (rare)
			Agranulocytosis
			Hepatitis
				Baseline:
				  G6PD level
				  CBC with differential
				  Liver function tests
				  Blood urea nitrogen
				  Creatinine
				  Urinalysis
				During therapy:
				  CBC with differential every wk for 4 wk; if stable, then q 2 wk for 8 wk; if stable then q 3 mo
				  Liver function tests, blood urea nitrogen, creatinine, urinalysis every mo for 3 mo; if stable, then every 3 mo
				  Reticulocyte count and methemoglobin levels as clinically indicated

Intravenous immunoglobulin (IVIG)	Immune replacement, immunomodulatory, anti-inflammatory		Contraindicated in those with known IgA deficiency
			Flu-like and gastrointestinal symptoms may occur during or persist after infusion
			May be improved or prevented by slowing the rate of infusion, premedication with acetaminophen, diphenhydramine, and/or intravenous hydrocortisone.
				Baseline:
				  Liver and renal function tests
				  CBC with platelets
				  Immunoglobulin levels to exclude IgA deficiency
				  Screen for hepatitis A, B, C and HIV antibodies
				Follow-up:
				  Liver and renal function tests
				  CBC with platelets
				  HIV and hepatitis screening annually for those with known risk factors.

Mycophenolate mofetil			Nausea
			Diarrhea
			Anorexia
			Abdominal cramps
			Vomiting
			Leukopenia
			Elevations in liver transaminases
				Baseline:
				  CBC with platelets and differential
				  Electrolytes
				  Glucose
				  Liver function tests
				During therapy:
				  CBC with platelets and differential once per wk for 1 mo; if stable then every 2 wk for 2 mo; if stable then once monthly.
				  Liver function tests monthly.

CBC, complete blood count; G6PD, glucose-6-phosphate dehydrogenase; HIV, human immunodeficiency virus; HPA, hypothalamic-pituitary axis; IgA, immunoglobulin A; PPD, purified protein derivative; q, every.

which include varicella-zoster, measles, mumps, and rubella.

PEMPHIGUS VULGARIS

Pemphigus vulgaris (PV) is the most potentially serious of the bullous diseases, although the prognosis in children tends to be better than in adults, and fatalities are rare. Characteristics of PV are listed in Table 1. First-line therapy for PV in children is concomitant systemic corticosteroid therapy and mycophenolate mofetil (MMF), with gradual tapering of the corticosteroid once disease control is achieved (see section on linear IgA bullous dermatosis of childhood). Management approaches are given in Box 1.

There are a growing number of reports suggesting that MMF is effective therapy for a number of autoimmune blistering disorders, including PV, pemphigus foliaceus, and bullous pemphigoid. The typical dose is approximately 1 to 2 g/day, although there may be a need for higher doses in more severe cases of PV. Overall, MMF is well-tolerated with a low incidence of adverse effects. Gastrointestinal symptoms are most common, although infrequent complications include urinary frequency or urgency, dysuria, sterile pyuria, and hematologic abnormalities, most commonly lymphopenia. MMF should be decreased or discontinued if the leukocyte count falls below 4000 cells/mm^3. Occasional elevations in liver transaminases may also be observed, but MMF does not appear to cause significant renal or hepatic toxicity.

Intravenous immunoglobulin (IVIG) is another potential adjunctive therapy that may be useful in helping to achieve acute disease control in more severe autoimmune bullous cases. Although relatively safe, IVIG is very expensive to manufacture and administer, and it is not always readily available.

Alternative steroid-sparing agents to MMF in PV include azathioprine and cyclophosphamide. Azathioprine is an effective therapy for the immunobullous disorders, but is considered second-line therapy in children because of potential adverse effects involving multiple organ systems. Although gastrointestinal side effects are most common, the most serious potential complication of azathioprine is myelosuppression, which can occur even years after therapy is initiated (see Table 2). Azathioprine is also associated with an increased risk of opportunistic infections and the development of certain malignancies. Cyclophosphamide has a side effect profile similar to azathioprine's, with the addition of potential hemorrhagic cystitis and male/female infertility, which are both dose- and duration-dependent. Transitional cell carcinoma of the bladder is another potential side effect, generally seen only with high doses and prolonged use. For these reasons, cyclophosphamide is also considered a second-line steroid-sparing agent to MMF in the pediatric bullous diseases.

PEMPHIGUS FOLIACEUS

Pemphigus foliaceus (PF) is considered by many to be a "benign" form of pemphigus vulgaris, with a typically more limited course. Characteristics of PF are listed in Table 1. Because patients lack intact blisters and can present with findings that mimic several other common disorders, the diagnosis requires a high index of suspicion.

Mid- to high-potency topical corticosteroids may be sufficient to control mild cases of PF with limited areas of cutaneous involvement. Antihistamines are often needed to control symptoms of pruritus, and adamant photoprotection is also essential in photodistributed cases. For more severe/extensive cases of PF, the management approach is similar to that outlined for PV (see Box 1).

BULLOUS PEMPHIGOID

Bullous pemphigoid (BP) is uncommon in children and generally has a better prognosis than in adults, with the majority of cases lasting 1 year or less. Similar to PF, limited cases can be managed with topical corticosteroids alone, although more severe cases may be managed similar to PV.

Common Pitfalls

- Risks of medication side effects, especially those of chronic systemic corticosteroids, which may result in greater morbidity/mortality than the disease itself
- Failure to appropriately monitor patients for medication side effects, especially potential long-term complications

The rapid effectiveness of systemic corticosteroid therapy is often necessary to achieve acute disease control in more extensive bullous disease cases. However, alternative immunosuppressive agents should be considered as early as possible in the course of therapy in order to avoid long-term corticosteroid side effects. Serious complications may arise from any long-term immunosuppressive therapy, and thus frequent monitoring is necessary. Regardless of which cytotoxic agent is used, it is generally recommended that monitoring be continued for at least 3 to 6 months after the discontinuation of therapy, and then as clinically indicated, as some side effects may manifest even months after medication discontinuation. Furthermore, because susceptibility to infection is a major cause of morbidity and mortality among immunosuppressed patients, timely treatment of suspected infection is essential.

Communication and Counseling

The management of the pediatric bullous diseases generally requires a cooperative, multidisciplinary approach, of which psychosocial support is often an important aspect. Support groups such as the Pemphigus Foundation (http://www.pemphigus.org) and the Dermatitis Herpetiformis online community (http://www.dermatitisherpetiformis.org.uk) are important sources of education and networking for affected patients and their families.

SUGGESTED READINGS

1. Anhalt GJ: Pediatric Bullous Diseases. Presented at the Society for Pediatric Dermatology meeting in Santa Fe, New Mexico; July 13–17, 2002. **An in-depth discussion of the management of the childhood bullous diseases.**
2. Fry L: Dermatitis herpetiformis: Problems, progress and prospects. Eur J Dermatol 12:523–531, 2002. **Detailed description of the history, clinical manifestations, and treatment of dermatitis herpetiformis.**
3. Swords S, Lauer SJ, Nopper AJ: Systemic treatment. In Schachner LA, Hansen RC (eds): Pediatric Dermatology, 3rd ed. Philadelphia: Elsevier, 2003. **Extensive information on the systemic medications most commonly used for the pediatric bullous diseases.**

4. Wolverton S: Comprehensive Dermatologic Drug Therapy. Philadelphia: WB Saunders, 2001. **Detailed description of the medications used for the childhood bullous diseases, including medication side effects and monitoring guidelines.**

Fungal Infections of the Skin, Hair, and Nails

Elizabeth Alvarez Connelly and
Sheila Fallon Friedlander

KEY CONCEPTS

- Tinea capitis is the most common fungal infection of preschool age children in the United States.
- Many children present with alopecia, scale, and head/neck lymphadenopathy, but some patients will not exhibit appreciable hair loss.
- Fungal cultures should be obtained, to confirm a diagnosis of tinea capitis, prior to committing the child to long-term oral antifungal treatments.
- Treatment of tinea capitis with griseofulvin 20 to 25mg/kg/day microsize remains the standard of care in the United States; however, newer antifungal agents have been shown to be safe and effective and may offer an alternative to current therapy.
- Tinea corporis is common in children.
- *Trichophyton rubrum, T. tonsurans,* and *M. canis* are the most common pathogens causing tinea corporis.
- A simple potassium hydroxide (KOH) stain examination may be performed to confirm the diagnosis of tinea corporis, or a culture may be obtained if the diagnosis is in question.
- Tinea pedis can occur in children. History often reveals that other family members are affected with the same condition.
- Prophylactic use of medicated talcs or creams on a daily basis may prevent reinfection. Ensuring that feet are completely dry is essential and should be part of daily foot care.
- Candidiasis is common in infancy and most commonly occurs in the diaper or intertriginous areas of the body.
- Keeping these areas dry and protected with barrier creams, such as zinc oxide, will protect against recurrent infections.
- A second form of candidiasis in children and adolescents is perlèche or angular stomatitis. A less common form of cutaneous candidal infection (chronic mucocutaneous candidiasis) can involve the nails and mucous membranes and may be associated with underlying endocrinologic abnormalities.

Fungal infections are common in infancy and childhood. The usual offending organisms are yeasts (e.g., diaper dermatitis) and dermatophytes (e.g., tinea capitis). Dermatophytes may infect the hair shaft of the scalp (tinea capitis), the skin (tinea corporis, pedis, and cruris), or the nails (onychomycosis). Candidiasis and pityriasis (tinea) versicolor both result from invasion of the skin by yeasts.

Expert Opinion on Management Issues

TINEA CAPITIS

Accepted Interventions

Table 1 shows treatment options for patients with tinea capitis. Recent advancements in the treatment of tinea capitis show that newer antifungal agents such as oral terbinafine, itraconazole, and fluconazole are effective and safe. Additionally, these agents have the advantage of shorter treatment durations and increased patient compliance; however they are not yet approved by the U.S. Food and Drug Administration (FDA) for this indication. Oral griseofulvin, therefore, remains the standard of care for tinea capitis in the United States at the present time.

Griseofulvin is poorly absorbed after oral ingestion. Absorption is improved by micronization of the medication. As a result, two forms of the medication exist, micronized and ultramicronized. Dosing varies depending on the form of the medication used (see Table 1). In a small study performed by Sharpe and Smith, a clear relationship between dose and recurrence rate was shown. Patients who received 15 mg/kg/day of griseofulvin were more likely to relapse; however, no recurrences were noted in children treated with 25 mg/kg/day. Regardless of the form of griseofulvin used, giving the medication with fatty foods, which improve the uptake of the drug, may optimize absorption. Toxicities are generally minimal, and include gastrointestinal disturbance, photosensitivity eruptions, and headache. If duration of therapy exceeds 8 weeks, laboratory monitoring is recommended.

The duration of therapy ranges between 6 to 8 weeks. Treatment must be continued until there is clinical and mycological cure. Zoophilic fungi infections, such as those caused by *Microsporum canis*, may require longer durations of therapy compared with *Trichophyton tonsurans*.

Terbinafine is a tertiary allylamine with a high bioavailability. It is lipophilic and fungicidal via inhibition of the production of ergosterol, an essential constituent of the fungal cell membrane. Comparative studies between terbinafine and griseofulvin have shown that treatment with terbinafine for 4 weeks is as effective as griseofulvin for 8 weeks. Like griseofulvin, cure rates with terbinafine appear to be dose-dependent. Studies of patients infected with both *Trichophyton* and *Microsporum* species, have shown that patients treated with more than 4.5 mg/kg/day of terbinafine had a higher clinical and mycological cure rate compared with patients who were treated with less than 4.5 mg/kg/day of terbinafine. Additionally, terbinafine may be more efficacious against tinea capitis caused by *T. tonsurans* than by *M. Canis*. Conversely, there appears to be a better response to griseofulvin than to terbinafine in patients with *Microsporum* infections. Therefore, higher doses of terbinafine and/or longer duration of treatment may be required for *M. Canis* infections.

TABLE 1 Treatment of Tinea Capitis

Drug	Formulation	Daily Dose	Scheduled Dosing	Duration of Therapy
Griseofulvin microsize (Grifulvin V)	Tablet: 250 or 500 mg Suspension: 125 mg/5 mL	20–25 mg/kg/day		6–8 wk
Griseofulvin ultramicrosize (Fulvicin P/G, Gris-PEG)	Tablet: 125, 165, 250, 330 mg No oral suspension	10–15 mg/kg/day		6–8 wk
Terbinafine	Tablet: 250 mg No oral suspension	4–6 mg/kg/day*	Classic dosing regimen: <20 kg: 62.5 mg/day 20–40 kg: 125 mg/day >40 kg: 250 mg/day or 5 mg/kg/day, max 250 mg/day	4 wk
Itraconazole	Tablet: 100 mg Oral solution: 10 mg/mL†	5 mg/kg/day 3 mg/kg/day	Pulsed dosing: 5 mg/kg/day for 1 wk, each pulse separated by 2–3 wk, for a total of 2–4 pulses	4 wk
Fluconazole	Tablet: 50, 100, 150, 200 mg Oral suspension: 10 mg/mL, 40 mg/mL	6 mg/kg/day		3 wk

*Higher dosing (>4.5 mg/kg/day) has been associated with higher cure rates

†Contains cyclodextrin, which has been shown to cause pancreatic adenocarcinomas in rats, at human exposure doses, and may also induce gastrointestinal symptoms including diarrhea; lower dosing used for liquid formulation.

Note: Only griseofulvin is FDA approved for this indication in children; fluconazole, itraconazole, and terbinafine are not.

BOX 1 Drugs that Increase the Metabolism of Itraconazole and May Lead to Treatment Failures

- Rifampin
- Isoniazid
- Phenobarbital
- Carbamazepine
- Phenytoin

BOX 2 Drugs whose Levels Increase When Taken Concomitantly with Itraconazole

- Terfenadine
- Astemizole
- Midazolam
- Triazolam
- Simvastatin
- Lovastatin
- Cyclosporine
- Oral hypoglycemic agents
- Warfarin
- Phenytoin
- Cisapride

Optimal dosing for terbinafine is still under investigation as pharmacokinetic studies are currently under way. Until clear guidelines are set, the practitioner may use the standard dosing regimen listed in Table 1, with the caveat that such dosing regimens are not FDA-approved. Lastly, terbinafine is only available as a tablet, which may be crushed and sprinkled over food if necessary.

Terbinafine has some significant drug interactions but no significant contraindications. Plasma levels of terbinafine are increased by cimetidine and reduced by rifampin. The most common side effects are headache, gastrointestinal symptoms, and rash. Although clinically significant hepatobiliary dysfunction is rare, transient elevated serum transaminases have been reported in 3% to 7% of patients.

Itraconazole is a triazole antifungal agent with fungistatic activity. It has broad in vitro spectrum activity against dermatophytes, *Candida*, and some molds. Capsules should be taken with food, but not with antacids, H₂ antihistamines or proton pump inhibitors, for optimal absorption. A liquid formulation is available; however, it contains cyclodextrin that has been shown to cause pancreatic adenocarcinomas in rats at human exposure doses. Gastrointestinal disturbances, such as diarrhea, have also been associated with its use. When prescribed, the liquid formulation should be taken while fasting and at lower doses because of greater bioavailability. Itraconazole is metabolized by the liver and significant drug interactions exist (Boxes 1 and 2).

Fluconazole is a hydrophilic azole and as such more than 90% absorbed. Because of this high bioavailability, fluconazole does not need to be taken with food, nor does gastric acidity play a role in its absorption. Fluconazole is excreted primarily by the kidneys and dose adjustments may be required for patients with renal impairment.

Table 1 lists dosing recommendations for fluconazole for the treatment of tinea capitis. Fluconazole is available in both tablet and liquid form, an advantage over terbinafine. Like itraconazole, fluconazole is

BOX 3 Drugs Contraindicated with the Use of Fluconazole

- Terfenadine
- Astemizole
- Midazolam
- Triazolam
- Cisapride

metabolized by the liver and certain drug interactions exist. Refer to Box 3 for a list of contraindicated medications.

Urgent Interventions

A kerion is an inflammatory form of tinea capitis. Plaques and nodules may be oozing and boggy and may demonstrate severe tenderness on palpation. Usually hair loss has occurred within the lesion and pustules may be present at follicular orifices. A scarring alopecia may result after healing and thus hair loss may be permanent. The use of oral steroids in the treatment of kerions is controversial because studies have failed to show an improvement in cure rates or improvement of the scarring alopecia. However, steroids may be considered if the patient is bothered by the itch, pain, and scaling or if significant inflammation persists beyond 2 weeks of antifungal therapy. Surgical drainage and excision of kerions should be avoided. Lastly, systemic antibiotics may be considered if an overlying, secondary bacterial infection is suspected.

Adjunctive Therapy

Added measures to decrease the fungal load, decrease the spread of the infection, and lead to a more rapid cure, include the use of multiple treatment modalities. Use of 2% ketoconazole or 1% selenium sulfide shampoo reduces the surface colony counts of dermatophytes. The use of an oral antifungal agent plus a medicated shampoo presumably decreases the risk of infection to another individual and allows the patient to return to work or school once on the appropriate regimen. These medicated shampoos should be applied to the scalp and left in place for at least 5 minutes prior to rinsing. The regimen should be repeated two to three times per week until mycological cure is achieved. Lastly, patients should not share items such as combs or caps with others because fomites may play a role in the spread of the infection.

Asymptomatic carriers may play a role in the spread of the disease, especially in families in which children are cycling through repeated infections. In these cases it is important to culture all suspected family members and treat accordingly. One study showed that adult female caregivers can be infected, and may well serve to transmit or perpetuate infection in a household.

In cases in which *M. canis* is the infectious agent, then the family pet (cat or dog) is likely the carrier. Families should be made aware of this and have their pet seen by a veterinarian for examination and treatment if deemed necessary.

TINEA CORPORIS/PEDIS/CRURIS AND ONYCHOMYCOSIS

Standard therapy of tinea corporis, tinea pedis, and tinea cruris is with topical antifungals (Table 2). Topical agents are often ineffective for the treatment of onychomycosis and long-term use of oral antifungals is indicated (Table 3). Newer antifungal agents such as terbinafine, itraconazole, and fluconazole have replaced griseofulvin in the treatment of onychomycosis, but are not yet approved in children for this purpose. Daily prophylactic use of medicated creams or talc is recommended to prevent re-infection of tinea pedis and onychomycosis.

Ciclopirox (Penlac nail lacquer) is sometimes effective in adults with onychomycosis, with cure rates of approximately 30%. Studies on children are currently under way and, pending results, ciclopirox may offer an alternative for children with less extensive involvement.

CANDIDIASIS

Accepted Interventions

Topical treatment is usually sufficient for the treatment of candidiasis (see Table 2). In addition to the medications included in Table 2, nystatin cream, applied twice daily to affected areas, is effective for the treatment of candidiasis.

Adjunctive Therapy

Topical medications combining both antifungal agents and topical steroids should be used with caution because such medications contain potent topical steroids with significant side effects, especially when applied to thin, intertriginous skin. When the use of a topical steroid is necessary, in combination with a topical antifungal agent, it is recommended that a low-potency topical steroid be used, such as 1% or 2.5% hydrocortisone cream, and that it be used for a short period of time (2 to 3 days).

PERLÈCHE

Perlèche or angular stomatitis is common in children and in adolescents undergoing isotretinoin therapy. Retainers and orthodontia also may exacerbate the condition. Patients usually present with fissures, erosions, and crusting at the corners of the mouth.

Treatment with a topical antifungal agent with antiyeast and antibacterial properties such as clotrimazole and econazole creams is recommended.

PITYRIASIS VERSICOLOR

Pityriasis versicolor is caused by the yeast *Malassezia furfur*. Older textbooks often inappropriately use the term "tinea" for this disorder. Discrete and confluent pink, brown, or hypopigmented macules or patches develop, which scale on scratching. They most commonly involve the upper back, chest, and arms in adolescents but are frequently noted on the forehead and temple areas in younger children.

TABLE 2 Topical Treatment Recommendations for Tinea Corporis/Pedis/Cruris

Drug	Dosing Frequency	Duration of Therapy
Over the counter		
Azoles (Clotrimazole, miconazole)	twice daily	2 wk
Terbinafine (Lamisil)*	twice daily	1 wk
Prescription		
Azoles (econazole, oxiconazole, ketoconazole 2%), naftifine, butenafine	daily	2 wk

*Terbinafine is not effective against yeast infections.

TABLE 3 Treatment Recommendations for Onychomycosis

Drug	Dose	Duration of Therapy	Site of Infection
Terbinafine*	4–6 mg/kg/day	6 wk	Fingernails
	4–6 mg/kg/day	12 wk	Toenails
Itraconazole			
Daily dosing	5 mg/kg/day	6 wk	Fingernails
	5 mg/kg/day	12 wk	Toenails
Pulse dosing	5 mg/kg/day	1 wk/mo × 2 mo	Fingernails
	5 mg/kg/day	1 wk/mo × 3 mo	Toenails
Fluconazole	6 mg/kg/wk	4 mo	Fingernails
	6 mg/kg/wk	8 mo	Toenails
Griseofulvin†	15–20 mg/kg/day	4–9 mo	Fingernails
	15–20 mg/kg/day	6–18 mo	Toenails
Ciclopirox (Penlac nail lacquer)	Daily application to affected nail		Fingernails, toenails

*Refer to Table 1 for classic dosing guide for terbinafine.
†Refer to Table 1 for different formulations of griseofulvin; decrease dose for ultramicronized form.
Note: These drugs are not yet FDA approved for this indication in children.

Topical treatment usually suffices; however, recurrence is common, especially during the summer. Topical antifungal agents with antiyeast activity are effective (see Table 2). Ketoconazole 2% shampoo may also be effective in treating this condition. It can be applied to wet skin for 5 to 15 minutes daily for 3 days, and then washed off in the shower. Selenium sulfide lotions and shampoos are also used for this purpose; a number of therapeutic regimens have been developed, including leaving the medication on overnight for several days, but drying and irritation may develop. A number of therapeutic regimens have been developed with various antifungal agents, but recurrence is common regardless of which agent is used. Prophylaxis with 2.5% selenium sulfide shampoo or ketoconazole shampoo may be effective at preventing recurrences. It should be applied to the skin for 10 to 15 minutes once a week or once a month as needed to prevent recurrences. For extensive disease, oral ketoconazole may be used. The dose is two 200-mg tablets orally once, followed by exercise to induce sweating. Because ketoconazole is excreted in the sweat, the patient should avoid showering after exercising to allow the medication to reach the skin. Treatment can be repeated in one week.

Common Pitfalls

- Currently griseofulvin is considered the drug of choice for tinea capitis in the United States. It has a long safety record, but its prolonged duration of therapy and strict food requirements for administration may result in poor patient compliance.
- If patients fail treatment or develop adverse reactions to griseofulvin, then terbinafine, itraconazole, and fluconazole appear to be safe alternatives for the treatment of tinea capitis.
- Concurrent topical therapy most likely decreases spore shedding and eradicates spores, which might otherwise lead to reinfection. Although documentation of its efficacy is lacking, most experts recommend adjuvant topical therapy 2 to 3 times a week in addition to oral therapy. Hair care practices may decrease compliance with topical therapy.
- When treating fungal infections in the pediatric population it is prudent to question families regarding other symptomatic individuals or pets. Evaluation of such individuals may help to prevent re-infection and cycling of the disease from one family member to another. Some experts

recommend treating asymptomatic carriers with medicated shampoos.

■ Empirical treatment of tinea capitis, without a confirmed diagnosis is expensive and commits the patient to several weeks of therapy with the potential for side effects.

■ Following a course of oral antifungal for the treatment of onychomycosis, the patient should continue with a medicated topical regimen to prevent re-infection.

Communication and Counseling

The patient should be told the response rate to treatment may be slow, and the medication should be continued until the infecting organism is eradicated. It is important to counsel the patient and family on the possibility of reinfection with these organisms after successful treatment. Children should avoid sharing combs, headgear, pillows, towels, razors, and so on. Patients with tinea pedis and/or onychomycosis should be instructed to discard old worn shoes and to avoid walking barefoot over surfaces that may be infected with fungus. All household contacts with similar signs and symptoms should be evaluated and treated accordingly.

SUGGESTED READINGS

1. Allen HB, Honig PJ, Leyden JJ, McGinley KJ: Selenium sulfide: Adjunctive therapy for tinea capitis. Pediatrics 69:81–83, 1982. **Data showing that the use of therapy led to decreased spore shedding time.**
2. Chan YC, Friedlander SF: New treatments for tinea capitis. Curr Opin Infect Dis 17(2):97–103, 2004. **A comprehensive review of therapeutic options for tinea capitis.**
3. Friedlander SF, Aly R, Krafchik B, et al: Terbinafine in the treatment of *Trichophyton* tinea capitis: A randomized, double blind, parallel group, duration-finding study. Pediatrics 109:602–607, 2002. **This study shows that the duration of terbinafine treatment (1, 2, or 4 weeks) does not statistically change response to therapy; further evaluation of this data show that it was dose rather than duration that affected cure rate.**
4. Friedlander SF, Pickering B, Cunningham BB, et al: Use of the cotton swab method in diagnosing Tinea capitis. Pediatrics 104:276–279, 1999. **Study evaluating this simple method of obtaining cultures.**
5. Gupta AK, Adam P, Dlova N, et al: Therapeutic options for the treatment of tinea capitis caused by *Trichophyton* species: Griseofulvin versus the new oral antifungal agents, terbinafine, itaconazole, and fluconazole. Pediatr Dermatol 18:433–438, 2001. **Excellent results with the newer fungal agents are noted; however, such high cure rates have not been replicated in large multicenter studies.**
6. Gupta AK, Cooper EA, Ryder JE, et al: Optimal management of fungal infections of the skin, hair, and nails. Am J Clin Dermatol 5(4):225–237, 2004. **Excellent results with the newer fungal agents are noted; however, such high cure rates have not been replicated in large multicenter studies.**
7. Gupta AK, Solomon RS, Adam P: Itraconazole oral solution for the treatment of tinea capitis. Br J Dermatol 139:104–106, 1998. **Itraconazole is also efficacious for scalp tinea.**
8. Higgins EM, Fuller LC, Smith CH: Guidelines for the management of tinea capitis. British Association of Dermatologists. Br J Dermatol 143:53–58, 2000. **The British approach to this infectious disease.**
9. Hussain I, Muzaffar F, Rashid T, et al: A randomized, comparative trial of treatment of kerion lesions with griseofulvin plus oral prednisolone vs. griseofulvin alone. Med Mycol 37:97–99, 1999. **Systemic prednisone therapy did not significantly improve outcome for kerion therapy.**
10. Lipozencic J, Skerlev M, Orofino-Costa R, et al: A randomized, double blind, parallel group, duration-finding study of oral terbinafine and open-label, high-dose griseofulvin in children with tinea capitis due to *Microsporum* species. Br J Dermatol 146:816–823, 2002. **A trial showing that 12 weeks of high-dose griseofulvin was superior to 6 to 12 weeks of terbinafine therapy in the treatment of patients with *Microsporum* tinea capitis.**
11. Sharpe BA, Smith M: Investigation into the efficacy of conventional dose griseofulvin for treatment of tinea capitis. Poster presentation no. 3, Society for Pediatric Dermatology Annual Meeting. Santa Fe, New Mexico, July 12–15, 2000. **Study showing that high-dose griseofulvin was not associated with recurrences.**
12. Solomon BA, Collins R, Sharma R, et al: Fluconazole for the treatment of tinea capitis in children. J Am Acad Dermatol 37:274–275, 1997. **Initial findings regarding efficacy of fluconazole therapy at 6 mg/kg/day.**

Warts and Molluscum in Children

Nanette B. Silverberg

17

KEY CONCEPTS

■ Warts and molluscum are common mucocutaneous viral infections of childhood.

■ Warts are caused by the human papillomavirus (HPV), of which there are more than 100 subtypes; only approximately 20 are of clinical significance in childhood.

■ Molluscum contagiosum is caused by the molluscum contagiosum virus (MCV), a poxvirus infection limited to the skin and skin appendages.

■ Immune clearance of warts and molluscum generally occurs within 2 years by spontaneous immune-induced regression.

■ Clearance of warts and molluscum can be induced through destructive, immunologic, sclerosant, psychological, antiviral, and antimitotic therapies.

■ Increases in the incidence of cutaneous viral infections have been observed in children worldwide.

Warts are benign epithelial tumors of the skin and mucous membranes caused by infection with the human papillomavirus (HPV), of which there are more than 100 subtypes. Only approximately 20 subtypes, however, are of clinical significance in childhood. The location most commonly affected by HPV is the extremities (including the palms and soles); acral warts are primarily caused by HPV subtypes 1 and 2. Acquisition of disease occurs through contact of abraded skin with infected surfaces. At least 10% of children will be infected with HPV, with 4.5% of children

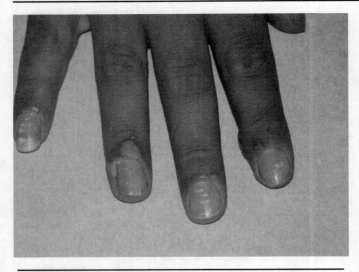

FIGURE 1. Common warts.

experiencing plantar warts. The peak age of infection is usually the preteen or teenage years. Clinically, warts appear as verrucous flesh-colored papules and plaques (Fig. 1). On average, two thirds of warts will be spontaneously cleared by the immune system in 2 years. A variety of immunologic mechanisms including cell-mediated immunity, anti-HPV immunoglobulin production, and antibody mediated cellular immunity contribute to wart clearance. On the mucosa, warts are termed condyloma acuminatum and appear as smooth flesh-colored to tan-brown plaques. Condyloma caused by certain HPV subtypes (HPV 16, 18, 31, and 33) may be associated with malignant conversion, but is rare in childhood, except for late adolescence. Warts may be more widespread and difficult to eradicate in immunosuppressed patients.

Molluscum contagiosum is a viral infection of the skin caused by the molluscum contagiosum virus (MCV) a poxvirus infecting only the skin and mucous membranes. MCV1 is the serotype causing childhood infection. Acquisition occurs via contact with infected skin or fomites. The incidence of MCV infection is rising in the general population. Children 2 to 11 years of age are most likely to be infected. Clinically, disease appears as pearly papules, 3- to 10-mm in size, with a central dell. Lesions usually appear on the chest wall, axillae, inner arms, chest and back, but can occur virtually anywhere, even on the mucous membranes. Typically children have between 11 and 20 lesions on the skin. Approximately one third of children experience atopic dermatitis-like symptoms with their MCV infection, including pruritus and erythema. Excoriation of lesions may cause extension of disease via mechanical spread of viral particles. Each individual lesion may only last up to 6 months; however, infection can take anywhere from 6 months to 5 years to clear completely. Immune clearance of MCV is similar in mechanism to that of HPV clearance, but may be prevented by a variety of factors produced by MCV that prevent immune induction. These molecules include MC54L, MC148, MC013L, and MC159.

Expert Opinion on Management Issues

DRUG THERAPY

Warts

A variety of drug options exist for HPV infections in childhood. Choice of treatment depends on the age of the patient, the location of the warts, the number of warts, duration of infection, underlying illnesses, and patient preference.

For warts, there are six types of treatments that can be used: destructive, immunologic, psychological, sclerosant, antiviral, and antimitotic. Often the clinician will choose moderately effective methods of therapy that have few side effects or no pain over a very effective but painful regimen of therapy.

Among destructive methods, salicylic acid has the best clinical trial data supporting its use, with a number of placebo-controlled trials documenting a 50% to 75% rate of cure with 6 weeks' use. Cantharidin has been described as a fairly effective therapy for warts. Donut warts around the original lesion tend to be very common when this drug is used. Cantharidin is almost as effective as liquid nitrogen and is best in young children as a therapy because its use is rarely associated with pain. Use of cantharidin mixed with other agents such as podophyllin is inadvisable in pediatric practice. Topical garlic has been used on a nightly basis as a homeopathic method of wart therapy and works over a 6-week time period. It is well-tolerated and very cheap.

Occlusional wart therapy is a standard mechanism of enhancing drug efficacy. Recently a small study documented the efficacy of weekly reapplied duct tape alone as a therapy for nonacral warts. The success rate was 85% in 6 weeks with limited side effects.

Immunotherapies hasten immune recognition of HPV by the body. Imiquimod 5% cream is an immune response modifier approved in the United States for the treatment of genital warts. When applied to the skin, imiquimod induces production of interferon-α, tumor necrosis factor-α (TNF-α), interleukin (IL)-1, IL-6, and IL-8. Many small case series or single case reports have anecdotally reported a variety of successful regimens of imiquimod application for common warts in children. The most effective regimen reported has been a twice-daily application. Use under a diaper is inadvisable, as severe ulceration may result. Other topical immunotherapies used in children include diphencyclopropenone (DCP) and squaric acid dibutylester (SADBE). SADBE has been described for office or home use, whereas DCP is generally used in the office. Clearance rates in published studies have varied from 58% to 90% with eczematous side effects being common and rarely urticaria. Oral cimetidine (30–40 mg/kg/day in two or three divided doses) can enhance wart clearance, but works in only about half of patients treated. Intralesional injections of mumps and Candida antigen are painful and cause flu-like side effects but may induce more than 60% wart clearance. Interferon injections can also be used as immunotherapy for warts and condyloma.

Vaccination against HPV is now coming into clinical trial. The target group for vaccination is young women who may acquire oncogenic strains of HPV through sexual intercourse. The candidate genes of promise from HPV have been the virus-like particles (VLPs), which induce a high titer of virion neutralizing antibodies and require little adjuvant. A large-scale phase III trial has recently been published, which demonstrated great efficacy of a VLP vaccine derived from HPV 16. In the college-age girls who received the vaccine over placebo, no cases of HPV 16 infection were noted in 17.4 months of follow-up, as opposed to placebo-receiving patients. This remarkable success holds tremendous promise for the future of cervical cancer prevention.

Pulsed dye laser destroys the extensive vascular supply required to maintain rapid cellular proliferation in warts. Pulsed dye laser can be effective for common and anogenital warts in children, but is painful and multiple treatment sessions are often necessary.

There are no anti-HPV medications, but patients with concurrent HIV will have less HPV-related morbidity when treated with antiretrovirals. Two antimitotic chemotherapeutic agents have been described as being helpful in wart therapy. Podophyllin can be used in office or at home as the extracted podophyllotoxin. 5-Fluorouracil in cream base can be used for common and genital wart therapy. This pyrimidine metabolite interferes with DNA and RNA synthesis. The medication is used locally on a daily basis. Data from a recent review of placebo-controlled clinical trials suggest comparable efficacy to agents such as salicylic acid.

Molluscum

Molluscum therapy begins with treatment of secondary pruritus and xerosis. Treatment is similar to that of atopic dermatitis. Topical corticosteroids are better for short-term management of symptoms.

Therapies for molluscum contagiosum may be destructive, immune-enhancing, or antiviral in nature. Appropriateness of the agent use in children is measured by the efficacy of the therapy and its side effect profile. Natural healing is associated with a 7% rate of scarring. Gentle local destruction is the typical approach to treating molluscum contagiosum. Cantharidin is a vesicant that when skillfully applied clears most molluscum. Although painless going on, the side effects a few hours later of blistering and pain may be disturbing, especially if this medication is injudiciously applied or left on too long. Tylenol may be used adjunctively at home to reduce any pain associated with vesiculation. Other topical therapies include topical retinoids, alpha hydroxy (lactic) and beta hydroxy (salicylic) acids. Tretinoin 0.025% gel may be used beginning every other day and advancing to twice a day as tolerated for 4 to 6 weeks. Silver nitrate, phenol, and trichloroacetic acid can help but may cause scarring even in the hands of the most experienced of practitioners.

Immune-enhancing agents speed up the immune clearance of MCV infection, whether through induction of antiviral cytokines or via influx of white blood cells (WBCs) capable of viral clearance. The data on the efficacy of imiquimod are limited; however, some studies have shown the drug to be beneficial against MCV virus. Furthermore, an analogue of imiquimod was effective in clearing MCV in a single investigation. A recently published double-blind, placebo-controlled trial showed superior efficacy with daily imiquimod over vehicle placebo. Oral cimetidine has been demonstrated to be effective in atopic dermatitis patients with MCV infection. Antiretrovirals can enhance T-cell activity and promote clearance of MCV in human immunodeficiency virus (HIV)-infected children.

Antiviral therapies are limited in number, as little pharmaceutical research with respect to MCV has been done in the past. Recently, acidified nitrite cream has been proposed as an effective therapy. The drug has direct antiviral effects as a nitric oxide donor. Topical cidofovir, an antiviral in the nucleoside analogue family, is a particularly useful alternative for patients whose lesions are recalcitrant to the conventional treatments, as in HIV and acquired immune deficiency syndrome (AIDS). Within the HIV and AIDS population, treatment with highly active antiretroviral therapy (HAART) has been shown to cause the resolution of molluscum contagiosum infections, even those resistant to standard treatment.

PSYCHOLOGICAL AND SURGICAL THERAPY

Immune response to warts can be controlled through the patient's psyche. There are multiple techniques to help harness the psyche as an effective wart-killing tool. A variety of suggestive techniques can be used; these include "purchasing" of warts and hypnosis. A recently published study shows that patients who receive placebo radiograph therapy have good wart clearance because of the power of suggestion.

Among the destructive therapies for warts and molluscum are surgical techniques including cryosurgery, curettage, and laser. Curettage and laser are very effective for molluscum but less so for warts, with a high recurrence and scar rate for the latter. Liquid nitrogen is a commonly used dermatologic office-based therapy for warts, with a 60% to 76% clearance rate with two to three sessions spaced 2 to 3 weeks apart. Side effects of therapy include pain, blisters, dyspigmentation and rarely, scars or nerve or vascular damage (when performed over the digital nervous and vascular bundle). Use of topical lidocaine tape may slightly reduce the pain of cryotherapy. Carbon dioxide laser has been a useful therapy in adult patients with recalcitrant warts. Use in children has been limited essentially by the issue of pain and scarring.

Light cryosurgery and curettage can be performed after application of topical anesthetics such as EMLA (*eu*tectic *m*ixture of *l*ocal *a*nesthetics—lidocaine and prilocaine) or LMX$_4$ (lidocaine 4% cream). Use of these substances should be limited based on the size and body surface area (BSA) of the patient. Methemoglobinemia and central nervous system toxicity can be observed with the use of prilocaine over a BSA in excess of the maximum area recommended.

PREVENTIVE MEASURES

Prevention is difficult with warts and molluscum, as they are caused by ubiquitous viruses. However, a number of public health efforts can reduce transmission of warts and molluscum. First, when using a public pool or health club, swim shoes should be worn for swimming, and public showering in bare feet should be avoided. Swim shoes have been successful in preventing acquisition of plantar warts in published studies. However, gym users who use public showers are 27 times more likely than those who don't to acquire plantar warts. HPV-infected patients should not share towels with family members. With regard to molluscum contagiosum, approximately 40% of patients acquire them from friends or family. Acquisition has been linked to crowded living conditions or to common bath or pool use. Thus MCV patients are advised to bathe separately, although this may not prevent sibling transmission. As fomites persist on surfaces, separate towels for drying infected skin are advisable. Additionally, because atopic dermatitis patients are more susceptible to MCV and wart infections, use of emollients and gentle skin care that would enhance the overall integrity of the skin barrier may reduce autoinfection and disease acquisition by atopics, although the latter is controversial. It is essentially unproven regarding whether atopics acquire HPV and MCV because of active atopic disease or underlying immunological abnormality. For HPV, sexual abstinence and condom use will reduce infection of the genitalia. As sexually transmitted MCV is often not covered by a condom, abstinence is the safest way to prevent acquisition.

Common Pitfalls

■ No therapy for warts or molluscum is completely effective and without side effects.

■ Treatments reported in the literature have rarely been investigated through double-blind, placebo-controlled trials.

■ Rare reports of genital warts in children younger than age 3 years transmitted by caretakers with HPV-infected hands, an infected maternal genital tract, or shared towels have been reported. Despite this, aggressive review of a child's life to rule out sexual abuse should be conducted in all childhood condyloma acuminata.

Communication and Counseling

Parents of children with warts and molluscum should be advised that therapy can be prolonged and that no therapy works in 100% of cases. In HPV infection, parents and children should be offered the options and allowed to choose the therapeutic modality right for them. In MCV infection, parents should be guided toward a painless method of therapy, whether it is active nonintervention, topical anesthetic and curettage, or application of cantharidin. No matter what therapy is chosen, parents should expect that new lesions of MCV may arise for a few months afterwards, and that a second session of treatment may be necessary. Use of pool shoes in HPV of the sole and separate bathing for MCV-infected children are advisable interventions.

SELECTED READINGS

Warts

1. Ciconte A, Campbell J, Tabrizi S, et al: Warts are not merely blemishes on the skin: A study on the morbidity associated with having viral cutaneous warts. Australasian J Dermatol 44:169–173, 2003. **A survey of the psychological morbidity of warts.**
2. Cobb MW: Human papillomavirus infection. J Am Acad Dermatol 22:547–566, 1990. **A good review of warts from a clinical perspective.**
3. Koutsky LA, Ault KA, Wheeler CM, et al: A controlled trial of a human papillomavirus type 16 vaccine. N Engl J Med 347:1645–1651, 2002. **The first clinical trial data on human papillomavirus (HPV) vaccination and HPV 16 prevention.**
4. Micali G, Dall'Oglio F, Nasca MR: An open label evaluation of the efficacy of imiquimod 5% cream in the treatment of recalcitrant subungual and periungual cutaneous warts. J Dermatol Treatment 14:233–236, 2003. **The clinical trial of imiquimod with the best results in common wart therapy.**
5. Silverberg NB, Lim JK, Paller AS, et al: Squaric acid immunotherapy for warts in children. J Am Acad Dermatol 42:803–808, 2000. **Study of immunotherapy for warts.**
6. Torrelo A: What's new in the treatment of viral warts in children? Pediatr Dermatol 19:191–199, 2002. **A pediatric dermatology perspective on wart therapy.**

Molluscum

1. Diven DG: An overview of poxviruses. J Am Acad Dermatol 44:1–16, 2001. **A broad overview of molluscum is included in this article.**
2. Silverberg NB, Sidbury R, Mancini AJ: Childhood molluscum contagiosum: Experience with cantharidin therapy in 300 patients. J Am Acad Dermatol 43:503–507, 2000. **In addition to data on the efficacy and tolerability of cantharidin, this article highlights some epidemiologic points about molluscum.**
3. Silverberg N: Pediatric molluscum contagiosum: Optimal treatment strategies. Paediatr Drugs 5:505–512, 2003. **A practical therapeutic strategy for treating molluscum.**
4. Theos AU, Cummins R, Silverberg NB, et al: Effectiveness of imiquimod cream 5% for treating molluscum contagiosum in a double-blind randomized pilot trial. Cutis 74:134–138, 141–142, 2004. **The first randomized, placebo-controlled trial of imiquimod for molluscum.**

Scabies and Pediculosis

Amy J. Theos

KEY CONCEPTS

■ Permethrin 5% cream is the treatment of choice for scabies, especially in infants and young children.

■ Lindane 1% lotion, especially if misused, may cause significant neurotoxicity.

■ In children younger than 2 years with scabies, the medication needs to also be applied to the scalp and face.

- Family members and close contacts of patients with scabies need to be treated, even if they are asymptomatic.
- Transmission of scabies or pediculosis from fomites is possible and needs to be addressed as part of the management plan.
- Nits in the eyelashes are usually from pubic lice and may be a sign of sexual abuse in children.
- Improper use of the prescribed medication, re-infestation, or resistance of the mite or louse to the prescribed chemical agent may cause treatment failures.

Scabies and pediculosis are common ectoparasitic infestations that occur worldwide and affect millions, especially children. They are obligate human parasites that can only survive a few days away from the human host. Both are acquired through direct contact with an infested individual, with transmission from fomites less common.

The mite *Sarcoptes scabiei hominis* causes scabies. The adult female mite burrows into the stratum corneum, in which she completes her life cycle. The incubation period between initial infestation in a naïve host and the onset of symptoms is 4 to 6 weeks; for reinfestation it can be as short as 48 hours. Patients with scabies usually complain of severe pruritus, especially at night, and a rash. The pathognomonic lesion of scabies is the burrow, a thin wavy line with a black dot (the mite) at one end. Other skin manifestations include papules, pustules, nodules, excoriations, and eczematous lesions. Lesions are usually concentrated in the axillae, periumbilical region, groin, and web spaces of the fingers. In infants and young children, involvement of the scalp, face, palms, and soles is common. Definitive diagnosis is made by identification of the mite, eggs, or feces on skin scraping. Crusted, or Norwegian, scabies manifests as crusted plaques in an immunocompromised or institutionalized individual. This type of scabies is highly contagious because of the large number of mites present.

Three species of lice can infest humans: *Pediculosis humanus capitis* (head louse), *Pediculosis humanus corporis* (body louse), and *Phthirus pubis* (pubic louse). Head lice generally affect children, primarily girls age 3 to 12 years, and are rare in African Americans. Patients with head lice may be asymptomatic, but scalp pruritus is the common chief complaint. Excoriations, cervical lymphadenopathy, conjunctivitis, secondary bacterial infection, and a generalized hypersensitivity rash (pediculi) may be seen. The diagnosis of active infestation is confirmed by identifying live lice on the scalp. Nits, the flask-shaped egg cases found close to the scalp, are also indicative of active infestation but alone are not diagnostic. Body lice primarily affect the homeless and cause bite reactions and pruritus. They are also important vectors of disease, such as trench fever and typhus. The diagnosis is confirmed by identifying the lice and nits in the seams of the patient's clothing. Pubic lice are usually spread as a sexually transmitted disease and are often associated with other sexually transmitted diseases. Nits may attach to the eyelashes. Pubic lice in children, especially in the eyelashes, should always raise the question of sexual abuse.

Several treatments are currently available for treating scabies and pediculosis, and in most cases, are effective. However, resistance to these chemical agents is a growing problem. The management of patients with infestation refractory to treatment can be challenging.

SCABIES

Expert Opinion on Management Issues

ACCEPTED INTERVENTIONS

Table 1 presents regimens for the treatment of scabies. Permethrin 5% cream is considered the treatment of choice, especially in infants and young children. Because the small amount of permethrin absorbed is metabolized by skin esterases into inactive forms, the potential for systemic toxicity is very low. The cure rate is 90% to 97% after a single application. See Box 1 for detailed instructions on use. Permethrin is approved by the U.S. Food and Drug Administration (FDA) for use in patients as young as 2 months of age. The safe use of permethrin in the treatment of a 23-day-old infant has been reported. Safety for pregnant women has not yet been evaluated. Infants younger than 2 months of age and pregnant or lactating women should only be treated if the benefit exceeds the risk and the diagnosis is confirmed by skin scraping.

Lindane 1% lotion was the standard treatment prior to permethrin but is now a second-line therapy because of a higher potential for neurotoxicity. Reported central nervous system (CNS) effects of lindane include headache, dizziness, irritability, paresthesias, seizures, and death. Most serious adverse events reported have been because of misuse, but there are case reports of serious reactions with apparently normal use. Populations at an increased risk for toxicity are neonates, children weighing less than 50 kg, or patients with a defective skin barrier, seizure disorder, or human immunodeficiency virus (HIV)/acquired immune deficiency syndrome (AIDS). Bathing prior to application may increase the absorption of lindane. The cure rate is 96% after two applications, but lindane-resistant scabies has been reported.

Other topical treatment for scabies includes precipitated sulfur 5% to 10% in petrolatum and crotamiton cream or lotion. Precipitated sulfur is reported to be safe in neonates and pregnant women but well-designed safety and efficacy studies are lacking. Crotamiton has proved much less reliable than permethrin, and five daily applications, instead of two, are recommended.

Recently, oral ivermectin has been used as a treatment for scabies, especially for outbreaks in institutional

TABLE 1   Treatment of Scabies*

Generic Name (Trade Name)	Route of Administration	Instructions	Formulation	Side Effects	Strength	Comments
Permethrin (Elimite, Acticin) Rx	Topical	Apply to whole body from neck down[†]; wash off in 8–14 h; optional reapplication in 1 wk.	Cream	Irritant or allergic contact dermatitis; may temporarily worsen erythema or itching.	5%	First-line treatment; FDA approved down to 2 mo of age; 96% cure rate after single application.
Lindane (Kwell) Rx	Topical	Apply to whole body from neck down[†]; wash off in 8–12 h; repeat in 1 wk.	Lotion	Irritant or allergic contact dermatitis; risk of neurotoxicity/ seizures.	1%	Do not use in children <2 years; caution in patients with extensive dermatitis, seizure disorders, or HIV/AIDS.
Crotamiton (Eurax) Rx	Topical	Apply to whole body from neck down for 2–5 days; bathe every 24 h.	Lotion or cream	Irritant dermatitis or allergic contact dermatitis	10%	High failure rate.
Precipitated sulfur in petrolatum compounded Rx	Topical	Apply nightly for 3 nights; wash off 24 h after each application.	Ointment	Allergic reaction, skin irritation.	6%–10%	Some authors claim treatment of choice in pregnant women and neonates; foul odor; messy; stains fabric.
Ivermectin (Stromectol) Rx	PO: 200 µg/kg; 2 doses spaced 2 wk apart		Tablet: 3 mg, 6 mg	Nausea, vomiting, abdominal pain, drowsiness.		Not an FDA-approved indication; not approved for children <5 years or <15 kg.

*All scabicide compounds listed are toxic to the *Sarcoptes scabiei* mite.
[†]In children ≤2 years old, also apply to scalp and face, avoiding the eyes, nose, and mouth.
AIDS, acquired immunodeficiency syndrome; FDA, Food and Drug Administration; HIV, human immunodeficiency virus; PO, orally; Rx, prescription.

BOX 1   Patient Instructions for Scabicidal Therapy

1. Bathe with warm water and dry thoroughly before applying medication. Trim and clean nails.
2. Remove all rings, watches, and bracelets.
3. Apply a thin layer of cream/lotion behind the ears and to the entire body surface from the chin down, including the nail edges, web spaces between the fingers and toes, groin, axillae, umbilicus, and buttock crease. Include the scalp, face, palms, and soles in children younger than 2 yr. Avoid the eye and mouth areas.
4. Do not wash hands after application.
5. Thoroughly remove medication after 8–14 hr (permethrin), 8–12 hr (lindane), or 24 hr (crotamiton or precipitated sulfur)
6. After bathing, wash and dry all bed linens, clothing worn during the treatment, and towels. For articles that cannot be washed, store in plastic trash bags for 7 days.
7. Treat all household members simultaneously.
8. Your doctor may have you repeat the above treatment in 1 wk.

Adapted from Hoke A, Maibach H: Scabies management: A current perspective. Cutis 64(suppl. 4): 2–14, 1999.

settings, in tropical countries in which scabies is endemic, and for crusted scabies in immunocompromised individuals. Two randomized controlled trials show a cure rate of 96% when two doses, spaced 2 weeks apart,

were given. Ivermectin is currently not FDA-approved for the treatment of scabies and is not approved for use in children younger than 5 years of age or weighing less than 15 kg.

GENERAL MEASURES

Although carefully controlled trials are lacking, most experts recommend that all household members and close contacts be treated simultaneously, even if asymptomatic. After completion of a treatment course, bedding, clothing, and towels should be washed in hot water. Items that cannot be washed immediately, such as comforters or stuffed animals, can be stored in plastic garbage bags for 1 week.

SYMPTOMATIC CARE

It is important to counsel patients that the pruritus may persist for up to 3 months after successful treatment. Mild to intermediate strength topical corticosteroids and oral sedating antihistamines may be of help in decreasing the pruritus. Secondary infections are usually caused by *Streptococcus pyogenes* or *Staphylococcus aureus* and should be treated with appropriate antibiotics.

TABLE 2 Treatment of Head Lice*

Generic Name (Trade Name)	Route of Administration	Instructions	Formulation	Side Effects	Strength	Comments
Permethrin (Nix) OTC	Topical	Apply to dry scalp for 5–10 min, rinse; repeat in 1 wk.	Creme rinse	Irritant or allergic contact dermatitis	1%	Favorable safety profile; evidence of increasing resistance.
Pyrethrins and piperidyl butoxide (RID, A-200, R and C, Pronto, Clear Lice) OTC	Topical	Apply to dry scalp for 5–10 min, rinse; repeat in 1 wk.	Shampoo, mousse, gel	Irritant or allergic contact dermatitis		
Lindane (Kwell) Rx	Topical	Apply to dry scalp for 5–10 min, rinse, repeat in 1 wk.	Shampoo	Irritant or allergic contact dermatitis; risk of neurotoxicity and seizures	1%	Less ovicidal than permethrin; do not use in children <2 yr; use with caution in patients with extensive dermatitis, seizure disorders, or HIV/AIDS.
Malathion (Ovide) Rx	Topical	Apply to dry scalp for 8–12 h, rinse, repeat in 1 wk.	Lotion	Irritant or allergic contact dermatitis	0.5%	Highly ovicidal; flammable—avoid open flames or electric heat sources; odor.

*All pediculicidal agents cause death of the head louse. AIDS, acquired immune deficiency syndrome; HIV, human immunodeficiency virus; OTC, over the counter; Rx, prescription.

17

Common Pitfalls

- Treatment failure is usually because of improper application of the medication or failure to treat all family members and close contacts simultaneously, and not drug resistance.
- Misuse of medications, especially lindane, can result in systemic toxicity.

Communication and Counseling

Clear written instructions for scabicidal therapy should be given to the patient. It is important to counsel the patient that the pruritus may persist for several weeks after successful treatment, but no new lesions should appear. It is important to counsel patients not to over bathe, as xerosis will lead to persistent pruritus and perceived continued infestation. Educate patients on the dangers of overusing the prescribed medication, especially lindane.

PEDICULOSIS

Expert Opinion on Management Issues

ACCEPTED INTERVENTIONS

Table 2 gives agents currently available for the treatment of head lice. All agents should be applied to a dry scalp to avoid dilution of the product, and repeated in 1 week to kill newly hatched nymphs. Permethrin, pyrethrin, and malathion are equally efficacious. Pubic lice are also usually sensitive to these agents. Infestation of eyelashes with pubic lice can be treated with petroleum jelly applied two times a day for 10 days. Body lice are eradicated by proper laundering of the infested clothing.

ALTERNATIVE AND UNCONVENTIONAL TREATMENTS

Occlusive agents such as petroleum jelly, mayonnaise, and hair gels "suffocate" the lice and may be of some benefit when added as an adjunctive measure. Permethrin 5% cream has been used in an effort to overcome relative resistance to the 1% cream. In several small studies, trimethoprim-sulfamethoxazole (TMP-SMX) was effective in eradicating head lice. It is thought to work by eradicating the gut flora of the lice, with death ensuing from a deficiency of B vitamins. The potential adverse reactions must be weighed carefully before a clinician considers such off-label use. Ivermectin, as described for the treatment of scabies, has also been reported.

NIT REMOVAL

Mechanical removal of all nits is an important adjunct to chemical treatment. This is accomplished with a plastic or metal nit comb. Wetting the hair and applying a conditioner, distilled vinegar, or a commercial nit remover can aid in removal.

GENERAL MEASURES

Avoidance of repeated infestation is critical to successful treatment. All family members and close contacts (e.g., classmates) need to be examined, and those with evidence of active infestation need to be treated. Hats, scarves, brushes, combs, headgear, linens, and stuffed animals need to be appropriately cleaned; washing in hot water, dry cleaning, vacuuming, or isolating in sealed bags for 2 weeks are all effective.

Common Pitfalls

Treatment failures are common and may result from improper use of the medication, failure to treat contacts and fomites, or resistance to the used chemical agent. See Box 2 for advice on managing refractory head lice.

Communication and Counseling

It is helpful to provide written instruction for the patient on the proper use of the selected medication. The patient needs to be counseled to repeat the treatment in 1 week. The importance of identifying and treating infested close contacts and fomites needs to be stressed.

SUGGESTED READINGS

1. Chouela EN, Abeldano AM, Pellerano G, et al: Equivalent therapeutic efficacy and safety of ivermectin and lindane in the treatment of human scabies. Arch Dermatol 135:651–655, 1999. **A randomized controlled trial (RCT) comparing the efficacy of ivermectin with lindane for the treatment of scabies.**
2. Hipolito RB, Mallorca FG, Zuniga-Macaraig ZO, et al: Head lice infestation: Single drug versus combination therapy with one percent permethrin and trimethoprim/sulfamethoxazole. Pediatrics 107:E30, 2001. **A randomized study that shows the combination of TMP-SMX and permethrin was more effective in eradicating head lice than either agent alone.**
3. Ko CJ, Elston DM: Pediculosis. J Am Acad Dermatol 50:1–12, 2004. **An updated review on the taxonomy, epidemiology, and treatment of the three major types of lice that infest humans.**
4. Usha V, Gopalakrishnan Nair TV: A comparative study of oral ivermectin and topical permethrin cream in the treatment of scabies. J Am Acad Dermatol 42:236–240, 2000. **A randomized controlled trial that addressed the relative efficacy of permethrin and ivermectin for the treatment of scabies.**
5. Wendel K, Rompalo A: Scabies and pediculosis pubis: An update of treatment regimens and general review. Clin Infect Dis 35:s146–s151, 2002. **An evidence-based review, updating the current treatments for scabies.**

Disorders of Pigmentation

Kord Honda and Robert Sidbury

KEY CONCEPTS

- Disorders of pigmentation can be divided into disorders of hyperpigmentation, hypopigmentation, and depigmentation. The nature of the pigment and its location are important in diagnosis and treatment.
- Familiarity with the use of the Wood lamp is helpful in examining and evaluating these patients.
- Genetic etiologies should be considered in neonates with pigmentary anomalies.
- Appropriate sun care with protective clothing and broad spectrum sunscreen is a critical component in the treatment of the disorders of pigmentation regardless of their etiology.
- When relevant, offending medications and exposures should be stopped as the first step.

Disorders of pigmentation encompass a wide range of pathologic mechanisms. The pigmentary anomaly may be an isolated finding or it may reflect an underlying syndrome. Dyspigmentation can present in a random pattern or conform to lines of melanocyte migration from the neural crest called lines of Blaschko. Melanocytes also migrate to the eye, brain, and inner ear, which accounts for some of the associated symptoms and signs of syndromic dyschromia. Many of these disorders lack effective therapies and can have significant psychological and cultural effects on patients and their families.

This group of acquired and congenital conditions can be divided into disorders of hyperpigmentation, hypopigmentation, or depigmentation. Hyperpigmentation may result from increased melanocytes, increased melanin production, or deposition of pigment within dermal macrophages. Disorders of hyperpigmentation may also be classified according to the location of excess pigment (dermal versus epidermal) and this can have a significant impact on therapy. Disorders of hypopigmentation and depigmentation reflect decreased or absent melanocytes or melanin production. When pigmentary loss or gain is subtle a Wood lamp examination may accentuate areas of abnormality. The Wood lamp is especially useful in distinguishing hypopigmentation from depigmentation and epidermal from dermal hyperpigmentation.

Expert Opinion on Management Issues

HYPERPIGMENTATION

Ephelides and Lentigines

Ephelides are commonly known as *freckles*. These hyperpigmented macules are more common in fair-skinned individuals. Ephelides darken with sun exposure and fade with sun avoidance, whereas lentigines are unaffected by sun exposure. Multiple lentigines may be isolated or may be associated with various syndromes such as:

- Xeroderma pigmentosum
- Nevi, atrial myxomas, myxomas, ephelides (NAME) syndrome; lentigines, atrial myxomas, myxomas, and blue nevi (LAMB) syndrome
- Lentigines, EKG changes, ocular hypertelorism, pulmonary stenosis, abnormal genitalia, growth retardation, and deafness (LEOPARD) syndrome

Oral and acral lentigines may be found in Peutz-Jeghers syndrome and Laugier-Hunziker syndrome. No treatment is required for lentigines, but successful treatment with lasers has been reported.

Melasma

Melasma, commonly called the mask of pregnancy, usually does not occur until after puberty. Adolescent girls taking oral contraceptive medication may develop the characteristic irregular, circumscribed hyperpigmented patches over the malar face. Individuals with darker skin type are more commonly affected. Gradual improvement is typically seen with discontinuation of hormonal medications and strict sun avoidance, but some degree of hyperpigmentation may persist indefinitely. Melasma that does not resolve may be treated with topical hydroquinone, topical retinoic acids, topical corticosteroids, and azelaic acid. Hydroquinone bleaches melanin and is available over-the-counter (OTC) as a 2% formulation. A 4% preparation is available by prescription and is approved by the U.S. Food and Drug Administration (FDA) for patients older than 12 years. A combination prescription cream containing tretinoin 0.05%, fluocinolone acetonide 0.01%, and hydroquinone 4% may improve the hyperpigmentation associated with melasma. Caution should be observed with long-term use of hydroquinone as it may cause exogenous ochronosis, a distinctive blue-gray pigment deposition in the treated areas. Azelaic acid is an acne medication that can cause iatrogenic pigment diminution through tyrosinase inhibition, resulting in decreased melanin formation.

Medication-Induced Hyperpigmentation

Various medications and toxins may cause hyperpigmentation. In most instances, the dyspigmentation will fade over months following discontinuation of the offending medication. Minocycline and the antimalarials hydroxychloroquine and chloroquine are the most likely agents to cause hyperpigmentation in children. Prolonged use of minocycline may cause a blue-gray pigment deposition in prior acne scars, mucosal surfaces, and the anterior tibia. Bleomycin may cause bizarre linear hyperpigmentation over the trunk. Lead exposure may induce gingival hyperpigmentation and can be a useful marker of suspected lead toxicity.

Erythema Dyschromicum Perstans

Ashy dermatosis (erythema dyschromicum perstans) is an idiopathic disorder characterized by ashy gray macules and patches (0.5 to 2.0 cm in diameter) that most commonly affect the trunk of Hispanic patients. Although in adults this disorder may persist, in children it often fades over 2 to 5 years. There have been reports of successful treatment with dapsone and clofazimine in adults. However, because the disease may spontaneously remit in children, watchful waiting is recommended.

Postinflammatory Hyperpigmentation

Postinflammatory hyperpigmentation (PIH) is more common in darkly pigmented individuals and may occur after trauma or any inflammatory dermatosis. PIH is not easily treated but will usually fade over months to years. A variety of topical treatments, including hydroquinone, retinoic acid, corticosteroids, and azelaic acid, have been used with varying degrees of success. Lesions of PIH will darken with sun exposure; therefore, the daily use of a broad spectrum sunscreen is mandatory. Treatment should also be aimed at controlling the underlying skin disease to prevent further PIH.

Acanthosis Nigricans

Acanthosis nigricans occurs on the sides of the neck, axillae, groin, and hands as velvety hyperpigmented plaques. In children, the most common association is obesity, which may be associated with insulin resistance. Weight reduction and correction of the hyperinsulinemic state can result in resolution of the lesions. Topical keratolytics (e.g., urea, salicylic acid) and topical retinoids have been reported to improve the appearance of the lesions.

Confluent and Reticulated Papillomatosis of Gougerot and Carteaud

Confluent and reticulated papillomatosis (CARP) of Gougerot and Carteaud is a dermatosis of unknown cause that presents with oval plaques composed of small scaly hyperpigmented papules usually over the neck, chest, and back. It is often confused for tinea versicolor or acanthosis nigricans, but unlike these other diseases it responds well to minocycline therapy.

HYPOPIGMENTATION

Nevus Depigmentosus

Nevus depigmentosus (ND) is an isolated hypopigmented patch that occurs in otherwise healthy children at birth or in early childhood. More extensive linear or swirled mosaic hypopigmentation, also called hypomelanosis of Ito, may be associated with central nervous system (CNS) and musculoskeletal abnormalities. Affected children should receive appropriate referrals to neurology and genetics. There are no effective therapies for these congenital disorders of pigment diminution. Sun protection is recommended and benign persistence is expected, although frequently some improvement in appearance is seen in later years. Nevus anemicus, caused by abnormal vascular tone, may be mistaken for a pigment disorder. No treatment is required

Pityriasis Alba

Pityriasis alba presents as oval poorly demarcated hypopigmented patches on the cheeks or arms, often in patients with atopic dermatitis. Treatment consists of the liberal use of emollients and sun protection. A mild topical corticosteroid can be used if erythema is present.

DEPIGMENTATION

Vitiligo

Vitiligo is an inflammatory condition of unknown cause that appears most commonly in the periocular and perioral areas, dorsal knuckles, elbows, and knees. Symmetrical pigment loss is the rule, but localized and segmental variants are also well described. A careful history and physical examination should screen for other autoimmune diseases such as diabetes and autoimmune thyroiditis, and laboratory assessment should be performed when appropriate. Circumferential depigmentation around a pigmented nevus is called a halo nevus and may be seen in vitiligo or as an isolated finding. Vitiligo may spontaneously repigment, starting with perifollicular hyperpigmented macules, although segmental vitiligo has a poorer prognosis for repigmentation.

Treatment is not required for vitiligo, but the variable pigmentation can be extremely distressing to patients and parents. First-line therapy is a medium- to high-potency topical corticosteroid twice daily for a 2- to 4-week trial. If a response is noted, continued safe use of topical corticosteroids will require close follow-up and treatment breaks to prevent cutaneous atrophy. The topical calcineurin inhibitors pimecrolimus and tacrolimus have shown promise and may be used in areas with thinner skin and around the eyes. Phototherapy is commonly used in adults

with vitiligo and can include ultraviolet B, ultraviolet A (UVA) with or without psoralen (PUVA), and newer modalities such as the 308-nm excimer laser. Phototherapy is not frequently employed to treat childhood vitiligo because of inconvenience related to the necessity for multiple treatment sessions and concerns for photocarcinogenicity. If large areas are involved without evidence of repigmentation on appropriate therapy, extensive discussion, education, and counseling should precede consideration of permanent total body depigmentation with topical 20% monobenzyl ether of hydroquinone.

Albinism

Oculocutaneous albinism is a heterogeneous group of disorders resulting from enzyme defects affecting melanin production. These patients have very light skin and hair and photophobia. Depending on the enzyme defect, the children may develop some degree of pigmentation with age. In Hermansky-Pudlak syndrome, patients have partial albinism with bleeding abnormalities. Treatment should be directed toward strict photoprotection and ophthalmologic follow-up.

Piebaldism

Piebaldism appears at birth with depigmented patches on the lower extremities, anterior chest, and the superior forehead with an associated white forelock. Characteristic hyperpigmented patches may be found within the depigmented patches. The back is commonly spared and these children are otherwise healthy. The depigmented areas are relatively static after birth. Infants should be screened for hearing loss to distinguish piebaldism from Waardenburg syndrome.

Waardenburg Syndrome

Waardenburg syndrome (WS) appears at birth with depigmented patches and a white forelock as in piebaldism. Associated anomalies may include hearing loss, heterochromic irides, synophrys, broadened nasal root, and dystopia canthorum (lateral displacement of the medial canthus). Melanocyte transfer has been reported to be successful, but this therapy is not widely available and in general treatment of skin in these disorders caused by abnormal melanin production or melanocyte migration is unsatisfactory.

Common Pitfalls

- Prolonged use of hydroquinone may cause an irreversible pigment deposition (exogenous ochronosis).
- Patients with vitiligo should be screened for autoimmune diseases during the history and physical examination.
- Syndromes such as neurofibromatosis and tuberous sclerosis should be considered in children with

multiple hyperpigmented or hypopigmented macules or patches, respectively.

- The psychosocial impact of these disorders can be marked and may be disproportionate to clinician perception of severity. Cultural context should be considered as pigmentary anomalies may cause variable degrees of social stigmatization.

Communication and Counseling

It is important to emphasize the chronic nature of the disorders of pigmentation while also acknowledging the impact of the disease. Cover-ups may be recommended to decrease unwanted attention. The importance of sun protection in reducing photodamage and accentuation of the pigmentary anomalies should be emphasized. The basics of sun avoidance during peak hours, protective clothing, and the judicious use of sunscreens should be reinforced. Appropriate genetic counseling is important if a syndrome is diagnosed or suspected.

SUGGESTED READINGS

1. Dimson O, Drolet BA, Esterly NB: Hermansky-Pudlak Syndrome. Pediatr Dermatol 16:475–477, 1999. **Review of the Hermansky-Pudlak syndrome.**
2. Dohil MA, Baugh WP, Eichenfield LF: Vascular and pigmented birthmarks. Pediatr Clin North Am 47:783–812, 2000. **Reviews café-au-lait macules and the multiple lentigines syndromes and many disorders of pigmentation.**
3. Kovacs SO: Vitiligo. J Am Acad Dermatol 38:647–668, 1998. **Great review of the epidemiology, etiology, clinical presentation, and treatment of vitiligo.**
4. Lee HS, Chun YS, Hann SK: Nevus depigmentosus: Clinical features and histopathologic characteristics in 67 patients. J Am Acad Dermatol 40:21–26, 1999. **Details the features of nevus depigmentosus.**
5. Njoo MD, Nieuweboer-Krobotova L, Westerhof W: Repigmentation of leukodermic defects in piebaldism by dermabrasion and thin split-thickness skin grafting in combination with minigrafting. Br J Dermatol 139:829–833, 1998. **Trial of grafting for one of the disorders of depigmentation.**
6. Schwartz RA: Acanthosis nigricans. J Am Acad Dermatol 31:1–19, 1994. **Review of acanthosis nigricans.**

Nevi and Nevoid Tumors

Robert L. Buka

KEY CONCEPTS

- Nevi are classified by cell type and location within the skin.
- A lesion's morphologic features may aid the clinician in discerning an early malignant process.
- A multitude of therapeutic options exist for the management of nevi and nevoid lesions; however, an astute clinical diagnosis is the first step toward any lesion's appropriate management.

A nevus is a proliferation of any dermal or epidermal cell type. The term has historically been reserved for lesions of a melanocytic origin that may vary widely in neoplastic behavior. Nevi differ from hamartomas insofar as the latter are strictly benign proliferations. Both nevi and hamartomas may result in compressive sequelae secondary to local growth; however, only nevi may undergo malignant transformation. Nevi are usually benign in children but may cause significant cosmetic deformity if large, hair-bearing, or present on the face. A clinician's primary responsibility rests with clinically discerning a nevus's malignant potential.

Expert Opinion on Management Issues

CONGENITAL MELANOCYTIC NEVI

Congenital melanocytic nevi (CMN) are present at birth in 1.6% of all infants. These lesions typically present as homogeneous, brown, ovoid lesions with sharply demarcated borders (Fig. 1). CMNs that are less than 1.5 cm in greatest diameter are classified as small; CMNs greater than 1.5 cm but less than 19.9 cm are designated as medium, and those that are 20 cm or greater are considered large.

The risk of developing melanoma in a CMN correlates roughly with the size of the nevus, with large congenital nevi carrying a lifetime risk between 4.5% and 10%. Early treatment of large CMNs is imperative because 70% exhibit malignant degeneration before the age of 10 years. Clinical evaluation is further complicated because two thirds of these CMN-derived melanomas arise in nonepidermal sites such as the central nervous system (CNS) and subcutis. Even a benign proliferation of nevomelanocytes in the leptomeninges

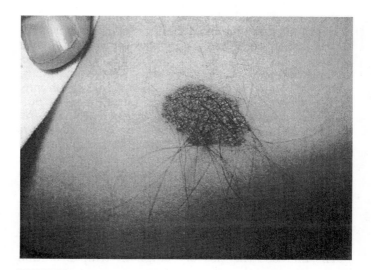

FIGURE 1. Note the homogenous brown color and regular borders of this small congenital melanocytic nevus, which measured 1.3 × 0.9 cm. Coarse terminal hairs are a common component of these nevi and may be cosmetically disfiguring.

TABLE 1 Guidelines for Management of Congenital Melanocytic Nevi

	Small and Medium CMNs	Large CMNs
Management standards	Expectant management Excision if rapid change	Prophylactic excision in infancy with expanders and grafts as necessary
Diagnostic aids	Baseline photography	Baseline photography MRI of CNS
Complications	Psychosocial/cosmetic Low risk of melanoma	High risk of melanoma Other malignancy (e.g., rhabdomyosarcoma)
Referrals	Dermatology Psychology prn	Dermatology Plastic surgery Pediatric neurology Psychology prn

CMN, congenital melanocytic nevi; CNS, central nervous system; prn, as needed.

BOX 1 Risk Factors for Dysplastic Nevi

<10 × Relative Risk
- Single first-degree relative with melanoma
- Excessive sun exposure
- Immunosuppression
- Lighter skin type (Fitzpatrick I/II)

>10 × Relative Risk
- Numerous (>30 by age 16) nevi
- Previous melanoma

>100 × Relative Risk
- Photosensitive genodermatoses
  - Xeroderma pigmentosa
  - BK mole syndrome

(leptomeningeal melanocytosis) can result in obstructive hydrocephalus and death. Lethargy, bulging fontanelles, and vomiting may be early indicia of leptomeningeal melanocytosis (LM), an especially common complication among midline, large CMNs. Patients with large posterior axial CMN, more than 3 medium-size CMN, and/or more than 20 satellite nevi are at an increased risk for LM—a screening MRI should be considered within the first 6 months of life. Although some experts encourage laser therapy, dermabrasion, and curettage for large CMNs, these modalities are fraught with high recurrence rates and are not currently standard of care. If excision of a large CMN is not possible or declined, baseline photography and biannual follow-up are essential.

The management of small and medium CMNs is far more controversial. The risk of melanoma in these patients may only be marginally higher than in unaffected individuals; however, indications for removal include disfiguring appearance and the anxiety associated with the continued potential for malignancy. The decision to excise these lesions hinges on any family history of melanoma, anticipated cosmetic outcome, or an appreciable change in the CMN. Careful measurement or in-office photography of CMNs is recommended because even subtle change may portend malignancy. Should a small or medium CMN change in color, size, or border or become symptomatic, excision with pathologic tissue examination is warranted. If a small or medium CMN remains unchanged over several years, annual examination (active nonintervention) is certainly reasonable. Clinicians must also stress the importance of sun protection techniques, because sunburns increase the risk of malignant transformation within congenital nevi.

In summary, treatment options range from clinical follow-up and monthly self skin examination for small and medium sized CMNs to staged excision with tissue expansion and skin grafts for large CMNs. Table 1 details general guidelines for CMN management.

ACQUIRED/DYSPLASTIC NEVI

Acquired nevi are extremely common proliferations of melanocytic cells that are not present at birth. These lesions develop in over 90% of white patients, typically in sun-exposed areas. Indications for removal range from poor cosmesis to frictional irritation to suspicion of malignant potential. Excision of these lesions may be performed with a shave biopsy or a full-thickness excision. Shave biopsies, although less invasive, carry a recurrence risk of roughly 20%. Evidence for malignant transformation in acquired nevi is similar to that observed in CMNs. Asymmetric *a*ppearance, irregular *b*orders, stark change in *c*olor or *d*iameter (>6 mm) over time, and *s*ymptomatic change have been affectionately termed the "ABCDs" of melanoma recognition. A family history of melanoma should lower the clinician's threshold for removal of an acquired, atypical-looking nevus. Lesions that may be difficult to effectively monitor, such as nevi on the scalp or back, may also be removed prophylactically.

Box 1 details the relative risk factors for melanoma arising from dysplastic nevi.

SPITZ NEVI

Spitz nevi typically appear as solitary, reddish, smooth papules on the head and neck; they are clearly differentiable from pigmented lesions but may be confused with mastocytomas, amelanotic melanoma, pyogenic granulomas, and even verrucae. These nevi share many features with melanoma, and the two are often difficult to differentiate histologically. Both entities consist of enlarged epithelioid melanocytes that extend ominously downward from the dermoepidermal junction. The majority of clinicians recommend complete excision with at least a 2-mm margin, because of their occasional erratic and aggressive behavior. A dermatopathologist is best equipped to comment on the potential for malignancy based on the lesion's histologic appearance.

TABLE 2 Dermal Melanocytoses

	Mongolian Spot	Nevus of Ota/Ito	Blue Nevus
Location	Lumbosacral	Face/shoulder.	Buttock or acral
Age	Congenital	Congenital.	Childhood
Associations	Hurler disease if multiple	Sensorineural deafness	Rarely, malignant degeneration
		Glaucoma	
		Rarely, malignant degeneration	
Natural course	Usually resolves spontaneously	Static	Static
Ethnic predilection	Black, Latino, Asian	Asian (Japanese)	None

DERMAL MELANOCYTOSIS

Dermal melanocytosis refers to lesions in which melanocytes are found within the reticular dermis. Melanin pigment within the dermis results in a bluish coloration observed clinically (the Tindel effect). Three common presentations of dermal melanocytosis include Mongolian spots, nevi of Ota/Ito, and blue nevi. Table 2 details their respective features. No treatment is medically necessary for any of these lesions; however, improved cosmesis may result from cosmetic camouflage (e.g., Dermablend), laser therapy, or excision. Pigmented lasers that penetrate deeply into the dermis are preferred. The Q-switched ruby (694 nm) and Q-switched Nd:YAG (1064 nm) lasers are the most commonly used for ameliorating the blue color of dermal melanocytosis.

EPIDERMAL NEVI

Epidermal nevi (EN) are the result of a hyper-proliferative epidermis that may occur at birth or during early childhood. They may be slightly hyperpigmented, owing to an increase in the amount of melanin pigment deposited at the dermoepidermal junction. An EN may be present anywhere on the body surface and commonly appears as a solitary, linear verrucous plaque with variable erythema. When multiple epidermal nevi are observed on the same patient, epidermal nevus syndrome should be considered with its attendant underlying musculoskeletal, CNS, and ocular defects. Treatment for EN is not medically necessary, because these lesions carry an infinitesimal risk of malignant transformation into squamous cell cancer. Should an EN become cosmetically deforming, clinicians may try topical keratolytics such as tretinoin preparations and the salicylates. More aggressive modalities such as cryotherapy, CO_2 laser ablation, and excision are usually more effective but carry additional risks of scarification. In lesions with significant erythema and inflammation, patients may complain of an itching or burning sensation. Mid-potency topical corticosteroids can be applied in this setting twice a day for a few weeks with good symptomatic relief.

NEVUS SEBACEOUS

Nevus sebaceous (NS) is a well-differentiated nevoid proliferation of normal sebaceous, eccrine, and apocrine structures beneath a hyperplastic epidermis. The lesion typically presents at birth or early infancy as a hairless, yellow-orange plaque on the scalp with a papillomatous appearance. NS follows a quiescent course until adolescence when an increase in circulating hormone levels causes this lesion to proliferate in a vertical fashion. In less than 10% of cases, NS eventuates into a second benign tumor, most commonly trichoblastoma or syringocystadenoma papilliferum. In exceedingly rare instances, NS has been reported to deteriorate into a malignant basal cell carcinoma. Because of its vertical growth phase, typical location on the scalp, and small risk of malignant transformation, this author routinely recommends full excision of NS (with 2-mm margins) sometime between late childhood and early adolescence.

BECKER NEVUS

Becker nevus (BN) is a relatively common nevoid proliferation of smooth muscle cells with overlying hypertrichosis and melanin deposition at the dermoepidermal junction. Like NS, BN is also hormonally responsive and typically appears during late childhood as a patch of hyperpigmented skin with overlying hypertrichosis on the chest or back. These lesions carry no risk of malignant potential, so indications for treatment are wholly cosmetic. The brown color of BN may be lightened with a pigmented laser such as the Q-switched ruby and Nd:YAG detailed above. Terminal hair growth can be retarded with a hair laser such as the long-pulsed alexandrite (755 nm). Excision is rarely an option as BN typically exceed 5 to 10 centimeters in diameter; however, a subcision (partial surgical removal) may achieve the desired "debulking" effect.

Common Pitfalls

- Failure to document an atypical lesion with either size parameters or in-office photography.
- Failure to sample (or refer) a lesion that fulfills one of the ABCD criteria for atypical behavior.
- Failure to review with both parent and child the importance of at-home monitoring and sunscreen practice.

Communication and Counseling

The overwhelming majority of pigmented lesions are benign. Do not alarm parents, but rather stress the importance of in-home monitoring of pigmented lesions with the ABCD guidelines. Yearly total body exams by a dermatologist are recommended, especially in families with a first-degree history of melanoma. Clinicians must stress the importance of sun protection and avoidance.

ACKNOWLEDGMENT

The author wishes to thank Dr. Bari Cunningham for her exceptional guidance throughout the preparation of this chapter.

SUGGESTED READINGS

1. Barnhill RL: Malignant melanoma, dysplastic melanocytic nevi, and Spitz tumors. Clin Plast Surg 27(3):331–360, 2000. **Discusses classification and histologic features of melanoma, dysplastic nevi, and Spitz tumors.**
2. Bittencourt FV, Marghoob AA, Kopf AW, et al: Large congenital melanocytic nevi and the risk for development of malignant melanoma and neurocutaneous melanocytosis. Pediatrics 106 (4):736–741, 2000. **Presents the cumulative 5-year risks for developing melanoma and CMN from the New York registry data.**
3. Buka RL: Sunscreens and insect repellents. Curr Opin Pediatr 16(4):378–384, 2004. **Reviews the use of sunscreens in children.**
4. Ceballos PI, Ruiz-Maldonado R, Mihm MC Jr: Melanoma in children. N Engl J Med 9; 332(10):656–662, 1995. **Discusses the clinical characteristics and predisposing factors of melanoma in children.**
5. Chamlin SL, Williams ML: Pigmented lesions in adolescents. Adolesc Med 12(2):195–212, 2001. **Reviews congenital and acquired pigmented lesions in children.**
6. Kinsler VA, Aylett SE, Coley SC, et al: Central nervous system imaging and congenital melanocytic naevi. Arch Dis Child 84 (2):152–155, 2001. **MRI findings in children with medium and large congenital nevi.**
7. Sahin S, Levin L, Kopf AW, et al: Risk of melanoma in medium-sized congenital melanocytic nevi: A follow-up study. J Am Acad Dermatol 39(3):428–433, 1998. **Short-term follow-up study that examines the risk of melanoma arising in medium-size CMN.**

Management of Genetic Skin Disorders

Mary Beth Dinulos and James G. H. Dinulos

KEY CONCEPTS

- Genetic skin disorders are often characterized by identifiable patterns of inheritance and malformations.
- For many of the genodermatoses, the skin findings are unique and often are the first presenting sign of the disorder.
- One of the most common cutaneous findings in inherited skin disease is alterations in pigmentation (hyperpigmentation and hypopigmentation).

- For the majority of genetic skin disorders, diagnosis is based on the clinical findings and genetic testing may be helpful in certain situations.
- Management of the vast majority of these conditions requires a multidisciplinary approach, depending on the nature of the condition.

Genetic skin disorders were once thought to be rare and infrequently encountered in general practice. To date, there are more than 300 cutaneous disorders with an identifiable genetic cause. The vast majority of the genodermatoses are multisystem disorders. Thus, a multidisciplinary approach to these patients is recommended. For this reason, it is important for all practitioners of medicine to understand core genetic concepts and the basic principles of managing families with inherited skin conditions. Management guidelines using an organ-based approach are available for many of the genodermatoses. In this chapter, we present the basic principles of management for selected common cutaneous disorders.

Expert Opinion on Management Issues

NEUROFIBROMATOSIS TYPE 1

Neurofibromatosis type 1 (NF1) is one of the most common neurocutaneous disorders, affecting 1 in 3500 live births. NF1 is an autosomal dominant disorder caused by mutations in the *NF1* gene. Typically, diagnosis is established by clinical diagnostic criteria. A child with multiple café au lait macules should be followed for suspected NF1, as other features may not be appear until later in life. Management of NF1 is preventative in nature and organ system-based (Table 1).

TUBEROUS SCLEROSIS COMPLEX

Tuberous sclerosis complex (TSC) is an autosomal dominant neurocutaneous disorder with an incidence of 1 in 10,000 live births worldwide. Mutations in both *TSC1* (hamartin) and *TSC2* (tuberin) genes cause the characteristic phenotype of TSC. Similar to NF1, clinical diagnostic criteria have been established. Multiple organ systems are involved, requiring a multidisciplinary approach to management. The following is a brief description of organ-based management of TSC.

- Cardiac system: Cardiac rhabdomyomas can be seen in utero or early in infancy. Affected patients can develop arrhythmias and congestive heart failure, requiring medical management. Fortunately, cardiac rhabdomyomas spontaneously remit.
- Nervous system: Infants can develop seizures such as infantile spasms or generalized seizures. Seizures in TSC can be difficult to control and often require multiple medications. Brain lesions include cortical tubers, subependymal nodules, and subependymal giant cell astrocytomas. These lesions may require surgical excision.

TABLE 1 Management of Neurofibromatosis Type 1

Feature	Management
Skin tumors	Dermal or plexiform neurofibromas that are painful or rapidly increasing in size should be evaluated for potential malignant transformation.
Optic pathway tumors	Annual ophthalmologic evaluation recommended in childhood.
Hypertension	Blood pressure monitoring with each visit, at least annually.
	Hypertension workup includes abdominal MRI/renal angiography, 24-h urine for catecholamines, HVA, VMA, creatinine.
Skeletal problems	Plot growth on NF1 growth grids for proper evaluation of short stature.
	Annual scoliosis screening.
	Early recognition of tibial bowing is important. Orthopedic referral as needed.
CNS abnormalities	Document head circumference at each visit.
	Developmental and behavioral assessments as needed.
	Special education if warranted.
	Evaluation for ADHD as needed.

ADHD, attention deficit hyperactivity disorder; CNS, central nervous system; HVA, homovanillic acid; NF1, neurofibromatosis type 1; VMA, vanillylmandelic acid.

From Dinulos MB: Chromosomal and single gene disorders. In Osborn LM, DeWitt TG, First LR, et al. (eds): Pediatrics. Philadelphia: Mosby, 2005, p 1059.

- Eye: Retinal hamartomas are helpful in diagnosis, but they don't place vision in jeopardy.
- Kidney: Multicystic kidneys and renal angiomyolipomas can cause hypertension, requiring medical management.

EPIDERMOLYSIS BULLOSA

Epidermolysis bullosa (EB) represents a broad spectrum of genetic skin disorders characterized by skin fragility and blistering. These "mechanobullous" disorders are produced by mutations in genes that produce proteins critical to the structural integrity of the skin. The hallmark of EB is friction-induced blistering. In general, blisters should be lanced and drained to avoid spreading of the blister. The roof of the blister should be left intact and the skin should be allowed to re-epithelialize under the blister roof. For skin that is eroded and open, a topical antibiotic such as bacitracin may be applied to the skin to avoid infection. Liberal application of petrolatum to blistering areas, covered by a nonadherent dressing and elastic netting, is helpful. Dressings should be changed only once per day. More frequent dressing changes may induce new blisters. Dressing changes are painful, and adequate oral pain medications should be administered. Extracutaneous complications of EB may include anemia, squamous cell carcinoma at sites of chronic ulceration, esophageal and urethral strictures, and joint contractures.

ICHTHYOSIS

Ichthyoses are a group of disorders characterized by thick, dry, and scaly skin. The majority of the ichthyoses are caused by alterations in genes responsible for the formation of the outermost layer of the skin, the stratum corneum. Most forms of ichthyosis can be managed with emollients that assist in the exfoliation of the stratum corneum. These "keratolytics" such as lactic acid, urea, and salicylic acid are useful to remove excess, thickened skin. These agents can sting when applied to cracked and fissured skin and they should be used with caution in young children. Newborns with ichthyosis can be encased in a thin layer of skin referred to as a collodion membrane. The vast majority of these infants have lamellar ichthyosis. These infants should be placed in a warm, humidified incubator. The skin is gently cleansed with a mild soap followed by thin application of a bland emollient, such as petrolatum. Cracks and fissures can predispose to sepsis and should be treated with a topical antibiotic. In the early newborn period, infants should be monitored closely for respiratory insufficiency because the collodion membrane can restrict respiratory movements.

Common Pitfalls

- Patients with genetic skin disorders can have involvement of multiple organ systems. Accurate diagnosis and attention to potential extracutaneous complications are essential in the management of these patients. Failure to look beyond the skin is a common pitfall, especially in high-volume clinical settings.
- Often many subspecialists are involved in the care of children with genetic skin disorders. Primary care providers are essential in the implementation of management protocols. Many centers have multidisciplinary clinics to assist in communication between subspecialists, primary care providers, and families.
- It is important to remember that the diagnosis and management of genetic skin disorders is a "family affair." In inherited conditions, one should look for subtle manifestations of the disorders in at-risk family members so that appropriate recurrence risk counseling and/or genetic testing can be offered to all family members at risk.

Communication and Counseling

Open and relaxed communication is essential in the management of families with inherited skin disorders. In many instances, the visits are emotionally charged and patients and parents may express guilt, denial, and anger when an inherited skin disorder is first diagnosed. Thus, enough time must be given to empathetically address all questions and concerns. Providers must be prepared to offer counseling regarding prognosis. Genetic counselors can be exceedingly helpful in the counseling of these families and providing support group information. Finally, it is paramount to outline a detailed management plan for these patients and their families.

17

SUGGESTED READINGS

1. Cassidy SB, Allanson JE (eds): Management of Genetic Syndromes, 2nd ed. New York: Wiley-Liss, 2005. **This is a standard textbook of the management of genetic syndromes and includes some of the more common genodermatoses.**
2. University of Washington: GeneTests. Available at http://www.genetests.org. **This National Institutes of Health–funded website, sponsored by the University of Washington, has up-to-date reviews of genetic syndromes and a list of laboratories that offer genetic testing.**
3. Sybert VP: Genetic Skin Disorders. New York: Oxford University Press, 1997. **This textbook is an excellent resource to assist in the diagnosis and management of genetic skin disease. It is written in a clear and concise manner.**

Disorders of the Hair and Scalp

Richard J. Antaya

KEY CONCEPTS

- Alopecia should be classified into two categories, congenital or acquired and localized or diffuse.
- The most common types of alopecia in childhood are the localized and acquired types: tinea capitis, alopecia areata, and traumatic alopecia.
- Alopecia is an emotionally distressing condition for children and parents that requires both medical and emotional support by the treating physician.
- Telogen effluvium presents with diffusely decreased hair density, and the chief complaint is increased hair falling out. A search for a preceding stressful event will aid in achieving the diagnosis.
- A large scalp scar or bullous-like lesion associated with a hair collar of hypertrichosis may suggest an intracranial connection and appropriate imaging and surgery may be needed.
- Midline scalp lesions, especially when associated with other skin abnormalities, should be promptly imaged for intracranial connections and if present surgically corrected.

Alopecia (hair loss) in children can be classified into disorders that are congenital or acquired and into diseases that are localized or diffuse. Most alopecia in children is acquired and localized and includes alopecia areata, tinea capitis, and traumatic alopecia. Acquired diffuse alopecia is most commonly caused by telogen effluvium.

Expert Opinion on Management Issues

LOCALIZED AND ACQUIRED ALOPECIA

Alopecia Areata

Alopecia areata (AA) is an inflammatory disorder involving the hair bulb with subsequent arrested hair growth. The etiology is unknown but infrequently can be associated with other autoimmune diseases such as thyroiditis, atopic dermatitis, and vitiligo. Children with trisomy 21 have an increased incidence of AA. Greater than 90% of cases remain localized, with complete resolution in less than 2 years, but a minority may have a prolonged severe course.

AA manifests with asymptomatic, acutely occurring, solitary or multiple, round to oval, smooth, noninflammatory, patches of complete or near complete hair loss. Close inspection may reveal hairs measuring only a few millimeters in length, which are tapered proximally (aptly termed exclamation point hairs) and usually indicate recent, active hair loss. Ten percent to 50% demonstrate tiny pits in the nail plates. On regrowth the hair is initially hypopigmented and has a smaller caliber. Other variants conferring a worse prognosis include alopecia totalis (entire scalp, eyebrows, and lashes) or universalis (entire body).

No single therapy is consistently effective, and nonintervention is rational for small patches. The most common treatments include topical, intralesional, or monthly pulsed oral glucocorticosteroids; topical short contact anthralin; topical immunotherapy (e.g., squaric acid dibutyl ester); and psoralen with ultraviolet A phototherapy (PUVA) (Table 1). Some of these may act by targeting infiltrative lymphocytes and altering the expression of key inflammatory cytokines (e.g., tumor necrosis factor). Minoxidil 5% solution twice daily appears to assist the newly growing hairs to mature faster but does not alter the course as monotherapy. Physicians should acknowledge and offer support for the consequent emotional suffering this disorder elicits. Referral to the National Alopecia Areata Foundation (www.naaf.org), for hair prosthesis, or to a dermatologist is recommended for children with more severe disease.

Tinea Capitis

Tinea capitis is covered in the chapter entitled, "Fungal Infections of the Skin, Hair, and Nails."

Traumatic Alopecia

Traumatic alopecia includes hair pulling, trichotillomania, and traction alopecia. Hair pulling is a self-limited habit tic response to a stressful life event.

Trichotillomania, alone or in association with other psychopathology such as depression or obsessive-compulsive disorder, may occur later in childhood and persist into adulthood. The presentation is similar in all hair pulling conditions with circumscribed, incomplete, and irregularly shaped alopecia, typically involving the frontal or parietal scalp. Eyelashes and eyebrows may also be affected less frequently. Close inspection may reveal twisted or broken tips and irregular short stubble. A skin biopsy is seldom necessary; however, it can be diagnostic in difficult cases. Parents and most children typically deny that the child is hair pulling because it is often done unwittingly in private. Individuals with trichotillomania have an irresistible urge to pull out their hair and derive pleasure and relief when pulling out their hair. Trichophagia (eating of one's pulled hair) can result in a trichobezoar

TABLE 1 Treatment for Alopecia Areata

Treatment	Medication (concentration, route)	Frequency/ Duration	Common Adverse Reactions	Clinical Trial Response Rates (%)	Clinical Trial Reference
Intralesional corticosteroids	Triamcinolone acetonide 5–10 mg/mL (total max 2 mL) inject 0.1 mL every 1 cm^2	4–6 wk; variable × several mo	Skin atrophy	64–86	Br J Dermatol 1971; 85:272–273 Br J Dermatol. 1973; 88:55–59
Topical corticosteroids	Fluocinolone cream 0.2%	qd-bid, occlusion hs × several mo	Skin atrophy, skin irritation	61	Dermatologica 1970; 141:193–202
Pulsed oral corticosteroids	Prednisolone PO 5 mg/kg/day (or 300 mg for 12–18 yr olds)	Single dose per mo × 3–8 mo	GI upset, headache, giddiness	60 in widespread AA/AT	Pediatr Dermatol 1998; 15:313–317
Short contact topical anthralin	Anthralin cream 0.5%–1.0%	10–60 min qd before shampoo out × several mo	Irritation, stains skin and bath fixtures	AA 29–75 AT: 20–25	Arch Dermatol 1987; 123:1491–1493 Arch Dermatol 1979; 115:1254–1255

AA, alopecia areata; AT, alopecia totalis; bid, twice daily; GI, gastrointestinal; hs, at bedtime; qd, daily.

(hairball) with symptoms ranging from weight loss and anorexia to intestinal obstruction.

Traction alopecia is characterized by thinning of the scalp hair in specific areas as a result of prolonged traction or friction. A history of prolonged wearing of a tight hairstyle (e.g., cornrows or ponytails, or using curlers) is necessary to confirm the diagnosis. This is characterized by hair thinning usually at marginal sites, a decrease in the caliber of the remaining hair, and the absence of broken hairs or inflammation. The presence of follicular papules can aid in the diagnosis.

Treatment for stress-related hair pulling is to determine the stressor and seek remediation of it. Frequently the stressor (a new family member, school, or home) is self-limited and requires no intervention; however, other more worrisome etiologies should be considered such as bullying at school and child abuse. Treatments proven effective for trichotillomania are behavioral therapy (including habit substitution such as pulling weeds instead), group and individual psychotherapy, and pharmacotherapy. The most effective approach may combine behavioral techniques and medication. Medications include the selective serotonin reuptake inhibitors, lithium, tricyclic antidepressants, pimozide, haloperidol, and monoamine oxidase inhibitors. Often symptoms return after withdrawal of medication, unless behavioral techniques are used. Psychiatry or psychology consultation should be sought if psychoactive drugs or psychotherapy is warranted.

DIFFUSE ACQUIRED ALOPECIA

Telogen Effluvium

Telogen effluvium (TF), literally "flowing out of telogen hair," is a form of incomplete alopecia, or, more aptly, hair thinning. TF results from the conversion of some of the growing anagen hairs into the resting telogen hairs following acutely stressful events, such as high fever, systemic illness, surgery, acute psychiatric disease,

nutritional or iron deficiencies, or hormonal alteration (changes in oral contraceptive medications, thyroid disease, or birth). Increased hair shedding, often first associated with grooming, is noticed approximately 2 to 4 months following the acute event. The hair density decreases but never proceeds to bald patches. The diagnosis is confirmed with the appropriate history; negative laboratory evaluation for endocrinopathy, nutritional or iron deficiency; lack of other scalp or hair shaft abnormality; and a forcible hair pluck of approximately 25 hairs revealing more than 20% white club-like telogen hairs. Treatment is directed at the underlying etiology if one is identified. Reassure the patient and family that hair density will improve over the subsequent months in the vast majority of patients. Topical minoxidil solution 2% or 5% twice daily may hasten regrowth of anagen hairs.

Loose Anagen Syndrome

Loose anagen syndrome (LAS) is a sporadic or less commonly autosomal dominant disorder of unknown etiology that is diagnosed primarily in children. The classic patient with LAS is a girl age 2 to 5 years with blonde hair; however, cases of LAS in boys, in individuals with dark hair, and in adults have been reported. LAS is characterized by slow-growing hair that seldom requires cutting. On examination, there is diffuse or patchy alopecia without inflammation or scarring; the hair is often dull, matted, or unruly in appearance. With gentle hair pull, numerous hairs can be easily and painlessly extracted from the scalp. These hairs (termed *loose anagen hairs* ([LAH]), when viewed under light microscopy, have an absent outer root sheath, a misshapen bulb, and a ruffled hair cuticle. The presence of LAH is not diagnostic for LAS, as one or two LAH can be a normal finding in children; children with LAS will usually have at least ten LAH on the pull test. Although there is no treatment for this disorder, it is reassuring to parents that it is most often seen in otherwise healthy children and often improves spontaneously with time.

Diffuse and Localized Congenital Alopecia

Congenital or infantile alopecia can be caused by many rare syndromes, ranging from hair shaft abnormalities to ectodermal dysplasias. Many are associated with genetic diseases with no specific treatment. The scope of this text precludes further discussion.

LOCALIZED CONGENITAL ALOPECIA: APLASIA CUTIS CONGENITA

Aplasia cutis congenita (ACC) is a developmental skin defect, either because of failure of the skin to form in utero or secondary to intrauterine injury. Regardless of the etiology, the result is a focal defect and subsequent scarring alopecia. There are several associated syndromes; however, the vast majority of ACC are isolated. Most are located on the paramedian vertex scalp although they can occur anywhere on the body, and are usually sharply demarcated, round to oval, 1- to 2-cm erosions, ulcers, or scars. Some have a thin translucent membrane over the defect (membranous ACC). The lesions that manifest with open wounds or membranes will heal spontaneously over the first several weeks to months to a hairless scar. A thorough history and physical examination to rule out any associated conditions is recommended. Radiological imaging to rule out an underlying skull or brain defect is rational for large, deep lesions. Treatment, if desired, is surgical excision with primary closure for small lesions. For large defects, hair transplantation has been successful. If the lesion is not adequately covered by hair, the patient should be counseled about sun protection to reduce the risk of skin cancer.

Common Pitfalls

- Failure to acknowledge the emotional impact alopecia has on the family
- Failure to differentiate alopecia areata from tinea capitis, which leads to inappropriate treatment with oral antifungals
- Failure to screen for endocrine disorders, especially thyroid disease, in children with alopecia areata and telogen effluvium

Communication and Counseling

Alopecia of any origin can be distressing for both children and parents, and physician reassurance regarding the benign and self-limited nature of many of these conditions is important. Parents of children who are likely to have more long-term hair loss or have suffered a loss of self-esteem should consider prosthetic hair pieces. There are two nonprofit organizations that provide real hair prosthetics for children (Locks of Love, www.locksoflove.org and Wigs for Kids, www.wigsforkids.org). For children with AA, the National Alopecia Areata Foundation (www.naaf.org) is a valuable resource.

SUGGESTED READINGS

1. Porter D, Burton JL: A comparison of intralesional triamcinolone hexacetonide and triamcinolone acetonide in alopecia areata. Br J Dermatol 85:272–273, 1971. **After injection of 34 sites with the listed glucocorticosteroids, hair growth occurred at the sites in 97% and 64%, respectively, for 18 months after injection.**
2. Schmoeckel C, Weissmann I, Plewig G, et al: Treatment of alopecia areata by anthralin-induced dermatitis. Arch Dermatol 115:1254–1255, 1979. **Application of 0.2% to 0.8% anthralin cream produced cosmetically acceptable hair growth in 18 of 24 cases of alopecia areata and 2 of 8 cases of alopecia totalis.**
3. Sharma VK, Muralidhar S: Treatment of widespread alopecia areata in young patients with monthly oral corticosteroid pulse. Pediatr Dermatol 15(4):313–317, 1998. **Sixteen children with widespread alopecia areata received pulsed monthly oral corticosteroids with excellent regrowth in 60% at 6 months without significant adverse events.**

Acne Vulgaris

Robert Sidbury

KEY CONCEPTS

- Acne therapy should be matched to acne phenotype.
- Education is as important as pharmacologic therapy. Essential points that patients must grasp are:
  - Acne response to medication can be slow and any new therapy must not be abandoned prior to 4 to 6 weeks of treatment absent adverse effects.
  - Acne may transiently worsen after starting a new therapy.
  - Avoid greasy cosmetics or hair care products that can exacerbate acne.
  - Patient compliance can be variable particularly in adolescents and an honest self-appraisal regarding likelihood of taking an oral or topical medication may prevent frustration and allow optimal therapy earlier in the course.
  - "Perfect skin" is an unrealistic expectation.
  - Isotretinoin is the most effective medication for nodulocystic scarring acne. Careful patient selection, education, and follow-up are essential for safe use of this medication.

Acne vulgaris is a multifactorial skin condition affecting up to 50 million individuals in the United States including 85% of those between the ages of 12 and 25 years. The cause of acne is not known but contributing factors include abnormal cornification of follicular epithelium, *Propionibacterium acnes* resident in the hair follicle, androgen-dependent sebum overproduction, and individual host response.

TABLE 1 Treatment of Acne Based on Phenotype

Acne Phenotype	Treatment Options
Noninflammatory: open and closed comedones	Topical retinoids Adapalene Salicylic acid Benzoyl peroxide
Inflammatory: papules/pustules	Topical antibiotics Oral antibiotics Benzoyl peroxide Hormonal therapy
Nodulocystic	Isotretinoin Hormonal therapy Oral antibiotics

The initial pathologic event is abnormal shedding of follicular epithelial cells, leading to obstruction of sebaceous outflow. These earliest noninflammatory stages progress from simple obstruction (microcomedones) to varying degrees of ostial dilatation (closed and open comedones).

Inflammatory stages of acne occur as androgen dependent sebum continues to be produced and metabolized behind a follicular plug leading to the production of chemotactic and pro-inflammatory metabolites including free fatty acids. The expanding sebaceous hair follicle may ultimately rupture extending the inflammatory process into the surrounding dermis. This clinical spectrum of inflammatory acne ranges from red papules and pustules to deep cysts and nodules with scarring potential. Acne therapy should be primarily predicated on acne phenotype (Table 1).

Expert Opinion on Management Issues

NONINFLAMMATORY ACNE

Topical retinoids are the most appropriate initial therapy for comedonal acne. Retinoids are derivatives of vitamin A that prevent follicular plugging by normalizing desquamation of follicular epithelium. There are three commonly prescribed topical retinoids: tretinoin (Retin A, Avita), adapalene (Differin), and tazarotene (Tazorac).

Tretinoin (all-*trans*-retinoic acid) is available in a variety of formulations including the most commonly prescribed creams (0.025%, 0.05%, and 0.1%), gels (0.01%, 0.025%), solution (0.05%), and a microemulsion form (0.04%, 0.1%) designed to decrease side effects. The most common adverse effect caused by all topical retinoids is dryness, which is dose-related, and is more apt to occur with gels and liquids. Photosensitization may also occur particularly in the initial weeks of therapy, and photoprotection with noncomedogenic sunscreens is indicated. The choice of retinoid depends on the patient's skin type, specifically the degree of oiliness and the tendency toward irritation. Sparing application to affected areas is indicated once daily at bedtime after washing and thorough drying of skin.

Adapalene is a derivative of naphthoic acid that has retinoid activity and is available as a 0.1% cream, gel, or solution all with similar efficacy.

Tazarotene is indicated for psoriasis but can be quite efficacious for comedonal acne. Tazarotene is available as a 0.05% and 0.1% cream or gel.

Randomized, controlled trials demonstrate reduction of comedones and inflammatory lesions in the range of 40% to 70% for all topical retinoids, with adapalene the least likely to cause irritation and tazarotene appearing to be the most efficacious.

Salicylic acid is also a useful comedolytic and is available in preparations ranging from 0.5% to 5.0%. Sulfur products and benzoyl peroxide–based products also have mild comedolytic activity and could serve as an alternative for patients intolerant of topical retinoids.

INFLAMMATORY ACNE

Topical Antimicrobial Agents

Mild inflammatory acne composed of papules and occasional pustules may respond to topical therapy. Currently available topical antimicrobial agents include benzoyl peroxide, clindamycin, erythromycin, tetracycline, and azelaic acid. Benzoyl peroxide confers some advantage over other agents because it can reduce *P. acnes* organisms by as much as 95% without the development of bacterial resistance. It is available in a variety of formulations including washes, soaps, lotions, gels, and solutions, in concentrations from 2.5% to 10%. Local irritation, redness, and scaling can occur with benzoyl peroxide use, as well as bleaching of clothing and hair. Benzoyl peroxide can be used as monotherapy but is often used in concert with a topical retinoid to improve comedolytic and antibacterial effects, and as a combination product with a topical antibiotic (clindamycin; BenzaClin) (erythromycin; Benzamycin). Topical clindamycin or erythromycin alone can be effective but increasing resistance of *P. acnes* is now being seen. Two randomized, controlled trials demonstrate that after 11 weeks a greater percentage of patients using a combination clindamycin–benzoyl peroxide gel had a good or excellent response (66%) compared with patients using benzoyl peroxide alone (41%), clindamycin alone (36%), or vehicle (10%).

Oral Antibiotics

Oral antibiotics are the most commonly prescribed systemic medications for moderate to severe acne. Oral antibiotics have both antibacterial and anti-inflammatory properties that function to lower lesion counts, improve appearance, and reduce scarring potential. Tetracycline, doxycycline, minocycline, and erythromycin are prescribed most frequently, although amoxicillin, azithromycin, and trimethoprim-sulfamethoxazole may also benefit acne.

Tetracycline doses range from 250 to 500 mg twice daily, whereas doxycycline and minocycline generally range from 50 to 100 mg twice daily. A recent randomized, controlled trial has shown that doxycycline may be efficacious at submicrobicidal doses (20 mg twice daily) versus placebo (52% vs. 18%). Lower doses could limit potential adverse effects.

Adverse effects experienced with all members of this antibiotic class may include gastrointestinal upset, yeast infections in female patients, and photosensitivity. Minocycline has structural characteristics that may cause more significant side effects including vestibular effects such as vertigo, bluish pigment staining of teeth, nails, and scars, a lupus-like reaction, hepatitis, and hypersensitivity syndrome. Children younger than 8 years of age should not take tetracycline class antibiotics because of risks of dental staining and decreased bone growth. Erythromycin can safely be used in this population when systemic therapy is indicated.

Hormonal Therapy

Female patients with evidence of acne flaring in association with menstrual cycles or with androgen excess may be candidates for hormonal therapy. Anti-androgenic medications such as oral contraceptives, spironolactone, flutamide, and cyproterone acetate can effectively reduce androgen-dependent sebum overproduction and resulting inflammatory acne. Randomized, controlled trials involving women with moderate acne show that triphasic norgestimate and ethinyl estradiol (Ortho TriCyclen) significantly decreased inflammatory acne lesions versus placebo (50% vs. 30%). Additional trials demonstrate the efficacy of other oral contraceptive formulations (20 μg ethinyl estradiol plus 100 μg levonorgestrel; Alesse) (30 μg ethinyl estradiol plus 3 mg drospirenone; Yasmin). All of the oral contraceptives used for acne have 35 μg or less of ethinyl estradiol although counseling regarding possible cardiovascular and breast cancer risks is essential.

Spironolactone is an androgen receptor blocker at doses of 50 to 200 mg/day, and studies have demonstrated 50% to 70% improvement when used alone or adjunctively.

Isotretinoin

Isotretinoin is indicated for severe nodulocystic acne unresponsive to conventional therapy. Isotretinoin functions primarily by decreasing sebum production and has a response rate approaching 87%. Standard dosing is 1 mg/kg/day for 4 to 6 months and some evidence suggests improved long-term remission rates if a cumulative dose of 120 to 150 mg/kg is achieved. Some prescribers start patients at a lower dose such as 0.5 mg/kg/day to minimize side effects which do tend to lessen over time.

Isotretinoin is teratogenic and it is essential that patients do not become pregnant during or for 1 month following treatment. Provider registration is now required to prescribe isotretinoin, primarily to prevent pregnancies in female patients taking isotretinoin. Isotretinoin has been linked with mood disturbance, violent behavior, depression, and suicide, but as yet this association is unproven despite extensive study. Common side effects include xerosis of skin and mucous membranes, hypertriglyceridemia, mild elevation of liver function tests, headache and musculoskeletal pain. To lessen the risk of pseudotumor cerebri, isotretinoin should not be used in conjunction with tetracycline or its derivatives. It is important that the patient avoid concomitant use of vitamin A.

Baseline and monthly laboratory monitoring including pregnancy tests in female patients and a complete blood count, liver function tests, and fasting triglyceride levels should be obtained. Careful patient education, selection, and follow-up are necessary for use of this uniquely effective acne medication.

ACNE VARIANTS

Distinctive subpopulations exist and may require adjustment of the therapeutic paradigm. Neonatal acne occurs primarily on the face in the first months of life in response to maternal androgens. Neonatal acne resolves spontaneously as these androgens naturally wane generally in 2 to 3 months. Infantile acne occurs beyond this initial window and may persist for several years. It is more common in males and can range in severity from mild comedones to scarring cysts. Treatment should be appropriate for the type of lesion, starting with topical antibacterial agents such as benzoyl peroxide and progressing to systemic agents such as erythromycin as indicated. Rarely intralesional Kenalog and/or isotretinoin may be required to prevent permanent scarring. Most infants have normal hormone levels and no signs of precocious puberty, but ruling out an underlying endocrinologic disorder may be warranted.

Pomade acne manifests with closed comedones along the forehead and hairline resulting from oily skin and the use of occlusive hair care products. Education regarding the role of those products is generally sufficient.

Acne excoriée occurs most commonly in adolescent girls and presents as angulated excoriated acne lesions that may cause scarring because of manipulation. This may represent a habitual behavior. Insight and potential intervention are as important as pharmacologic acne therapy.

Drug-induced acne presents as monomorphous crops of pustules most commonly on the trunk, and has been linked to systemic or potent topical corticosteroids, anabolic steroids, methotrexate, and anticonvulsants. Cessation of the offending medication and topical therapy are generally sufficient.

Common Pitfalls

- Failure to recognize the potential psychosocial impact of acne
- Delay in appropriate treatment of nodulocystic acne until after scarring has occurred
- Failure to match acne therapy to acne phenotype
- Inadequate counsel of the patient
- Failure to consider hormonal triggers (monthly flares with menses) in female patients

Communication and Counseling

Acne affects most teenagers and it can generally be treated successfully. Providers must realize that even mild acne can have a huge impact on a child's self-image, and early intervention can make a big difference. Discussion about patient compliance and willingness to use a certain treatment regimen, counseling patience regarding effect, and vigilance regarding side effects, can lessen frustration with therapy. Isotretinoin is reserved for the most severe or refractory patients and its safe use depends on ongoing counsel, communication, and follow-up.

SUGGESTED READINGS

1. Elkayam O, Yaron M, Capsi D: Minocycline induced autoimmune syndromes: An overview. Semin Arthritis Rheum 28:392–397, 1999. **Thorough review of potential side effects of this commonly prescribed acne antibiotic.**
2. Haider A, Shaw JC: Treatment of acne vulgaris. JAMA 292:726–735, 2004. **Recent evidence-based review of available acne therapies.**
3. Leyden JJ: Therapy for acne vulgaris. N Engl J Med 336:1156–1162, 1997. **Excellent review of acne pathogenesis and good correlation with therapeutic choices.**
4. Lucky AW, Henderson TA, Olson WH, et al: Effectiveness of norgestimate and ethinyl estradiol in treating moderate acne vulgaris. J Am Acad Dermatol 37:746–754, 1997. **Study of hormonal therapy in female acne patients.**
5. Sidbury R, Paller AS: The diagnosis and management of acne vulgaris. Ped Annals 29:17–24, 2000. **Thorough discussion of different acne subtypes.**
6. Sidbury R: Drug watch. Isotretinoin. Journal Watch: Pediatrics and Adolescent Medicine 3(10):77, 2004. **Recent review of isotretinoin indications, clinical trials, and adverse effects.**

Sun Protection in the Pediatric Patient

Latanya T. Benjamin, Elizabeth Alvarez Connelly, Leslie Baumann, and Lawrence A. Schachner

KEY CONCEPTS

- Sunlight is composed of both visible light and invisible light. It is the invisible rays that are harmful. An individual does not have to be burned to be harmed by the sun's rays.
- Acute and chronic sun exposure can result in erythema, sunburns, tanning, wrinkles and other signs of skin aging, cataracts, melanoma and nonmelanoma skin cancers, and photosensitivity to certain chemicals or medications.
- A history of severe childhood sunburns is a risk factor for malignant melanoma.
- Sun protection factor (SPF) measures the ultraviolet radiation protection afforded in sunscreens. This factor is a ratio of the dose of ultraviolet required, with and without sunscreen, to produce skin redness.
- Ultraviolet protection factor ratings describe the capability of a fabric to prevent ultraviolet radiation from reaching the skin. This rating is regarded as equivalent to sun protection factor in describing the level of sun protection offered.

It is estimated that nearly two thirds of an individual's lifetime ultraviolet radiation dose is received by 18 years of age. Recent statistical analysis reveals that a child born in the 1930s had a 1 in 1500 lifetime risk for melanoma, as opposed to those born in 1990, whose risk is more on the order of 1 in 100, or a child born today, whose risk is now estimated as 1 in 71. Indeed, melanoma is the most rapidly increasing cancer in incidence over the past 2 decades. More than one fourth of melanomas develop in patients younger than 40 years of age, and melanoma is the most frequent cancer of women ages 25 to 29 years and the second most frequent in women ages 30 to 35 years. On average, young people are receiving more ambient ultraviolet (UV) radiation, resulting in an increase in melanoma and nonmelanoma skin cancer.

Children are particularly susceptible to ultraviolet radiation. For the average child, evidence suggests that there are age-related structural and immunologic differences that make sunburns and other acute and chronic sun exposures more dangerous to humans in the first 2 decades of life. Myriad intrinsic factors and inherited and acquired disorders can heighten susceptibility. These factors include skin that easily burns and does not tan, light eyes and hair color, the presence of multiple nevi, and a tendency toward freckling.

Throughout the years, increased knowledge and heightened awareness resulted in universal precaution against UV exposure in children. In 1989, the National Institutes of Health convened a consensus development conference on sunlight, ultraviolet radiation, and the skin. Key issues relevant to pediatric health care providers were reviewed, including (1) whether there are specific factors that influence children's susceptibility to solar UV radiation that make them particularly vulnerable to its adverse effects and (2) whether adverse UV induced changes can be prevented. In 1995, the American Academy of Dermatology and the Centers for Disease Control and Prevention co-hosted a national multidisciplinary consensus meeting to develop a skin cancer prevention and early detection agenda. Several points were stressed, including the need for physicians to integrate sun protection counseling into well-child visits to begin skin cancer prevention at an early age. In 1999, a publication by the American Academy of Pediatrics addressed safety concerns regarding the use of sunscreens in infants younger than 6 months of age. The committee concluded that sunscreens were safe to use in this age group.

Expert Opinion on Management Issues

Acute signs of sunburn usually appear 6 to 12 hours after exposure. Sunburns can range from temporary mild discomfort to life-threatening complications. If a child displays minimal signs such as redness, warmth, and mild pain, this type of burn may be treated in the home with cool compresses, a bath in cool water, and/or acetaminophen to relieve pain. However, treatment by a health professional should be sought if the child experiences blisters or a general feeling of illness such as fever, chills, or headaches. Young babies are at further risk for dehydration and heatstroke because they are not fully mobile and have impaired functional sweating. If the burn is severe, hospitalization may be required. The burn may be treated like other burns, and antibiotics may be warranted for infected blisters.

Prevention geared toward children, by modification of extrinsic factors, can allow for greater protection against the sun's harmful rays. If one can establish appropriate guidelines for clothing and sunscreens and modify time of sun exposure, the current mortality rate of one American dying each hour from skin cancer can be dramatically decreased.

SUNSCREENS

Sunscreens should be used during appropriate times of the year on a daily basis. Choose a sunscreen that offers both UVB/UVA protection with a sun protection factor (SPF) of at least 15 that is both sweatproof and waterproof. It should be applied 30 minutes before exposure and reapplied every 3 to 4 hours depending on the amount of perspiration, water activity, and prolonged exposure during the course of the day.

For children who have sensitive skin, such as those with atopic dermatitis, sunscreens that contain physical blockers rather than chemical blockers (such as "contains only titanium dioxide and zinc oxide [COTZ]") are recommended.

CLOTHING

The tighter weave of cotton clothing (as compared to that made from synthetic fibers) offers increased protection by permitting less UV radiation to pass through. Additionally, its light weight will be better tolerated both in long-sleeved shirts and long pants. The use of high socks is also suggested. All families may benefit from laundry treatments that help block additional sun rays. For example, a typical white cotton T-shirt rated UPF 5 can be increased to a UPF rating of 30 with a single treatment of Rit Sunguard. Families at particular risk for skin cancer may benefit from sun-protective clothing such as Solumbra.

Caps and hats with visors protect more than 70% of the face and offer photoprotection of the skin and eyes alike. Wide-brimmed hats provide additional protection to the ears from cancer. The use of well-fitted UV protective sunglasses is also encouraged in children.

POLICIES OF SUN EXPOSURE

The regional policies that reduce or stop the forced sun exposure of children during the peak sun hours in day care centers, schools, camps, and so on, should be encouraged. On a sunny May or June day, more than 60% of solar UVB radiation reaches the surface of the Earth between 10:00 AM and 3:00 PM. *Scheduling physical education classes, marching bands, and other outdoor activities before 10:00 AM and after 3:00 PM can greatly diminish a child's daily UV radiation dose.* A more practical approach is to allow the use of wide-brimmed hats while engaging in physical activity while outdoors at school. Older children can also be encouraged to apply sunscreen while outdoors at school.

AVOIDANCE OF ARTIFICIAL TANNING DEVICES

There are no safe, healthy tans and no safe, healthy tanning devices. Physicians should address these myths, especially with their female adolescent patients. In a survey of 1013 tanning parlor customers, the majority were found to be young women between the ages of 16 and 30 years. A study from Sweden looked at 400 patients with melanoma and found tanning bed use to be a significant risk factor in melanoma patients younger than 30 years of age. Despite the known risks of indoor tanning, more than 1 million Americans visit tanning salons on a given day. The pediatrician should lead the campaign to educate the public that artificial tanning devices are a hazard to young people's health.

Common Pitfalls

- Dark-skinned individuals are not immune to the sun's burning rays; educate all children about sun protection, regardless of complexion.
- The Skin Cancer Foundation recommends practicing sun protection year-round, not just during the summer months.

Communication and Counseling

Remind all patients and families:

- The sun can also be dangerous even when it is not shining brightly. Staying out longer on foggy or hazy days may expose the child to more UV rays, despite the fact that clouds scatter 20% of UV light.
- Seek shade under beach umbrellas, trees, and so on during peak sun hours.
- Be aware of reflective surfaces (water, sand, snow, cement). These surfaces can reflect up to 85% of sunlight.
- Never seek a tan, either naturally or at an artificial tanning salon.
- Teach the child sun safety, including self-examinations, and caregivers should model the behaviors themselves.
- If anything looks suspicious, see a dermatologist immediately.

The pediatric age seems to be a very important time in the evolution of skin cancer from sun exposure. It is believed that 75% of all skin cancers can be prevented by the use of appropriate sunscreen, clothing, and behavior that avoids peak sun exposure.

SUGGESTED READINGS

1. American Academy of Pediatrics: Committee on Environmental Health: Ultraviolet light: A hazard to children. Pediatrics 104:328–333, 1999. **A review of the effects of ultraviolet light on the skin and the recommended preventative measures for children.**

2. Rigel D: The incidence of malignant melanoma in the United States: Issues as we approach the 21st century. J Am Acad Dermatol 34:839–847, 1996. **Examines the rising incidence of malignant melanoma in the United States.**

3. Schachner LA, Hansen RC: Pediatric Dermatology, 3rd ed. Philadelphia: Elsevier, 2003, pp 96–97 and 1229–1230. **Provides details regarding photoprotection and strategies to minimize sun exposure in children.**

4. Schachner LA: Current issues in photosusceptibility and protection. Pediatr Derm 9:351–352, 1992. **A review of childhood factors affecting photosusceptibility.**

5. Spencer J: Indoor tanning: Risks, benefits, and future trends. J Am Acad Dermatol 33:288–298, 1995. **Provides a comprehensive review of the operation and effects of indoor tanning.**

Amblyopia

Monte D. Mills and Leila M. Khazaeni

KEY CONCEPTS

- Amblyopia results from abnormal or asymmetric visual input during visual development.
- Causes of abnormal or asymmetric input include:
  - Optical blur from uncorrected refractive error
  - Strabismus
  - Anatomic defects in the optics of the eye including cataract, corneal opacity, vitreous hemorrhage
  - Ptosis, especially if asymmetric
  - Iatrogenic, from therapeutic or perioperative patching or medications that affect focus
- The sensitive period for development of amblyopia, and for treatment of amblyopia, is birth until 8 to 10 years of age.
- The earlier the abnormal input, the greater the likelihood and severity of amblyopia.
- Asymmetrical input between the two eyes (unilateral cataract, unequal refraction) is much more likely to cause amblyopia than symmetrically poor images.
- Bilateral amblyopia may result from severe, symmetrical bilateral image degradation such as bilateral cataract, bilateral high ametropia (high refractive error), and bilateral ptosis.
- Visual acuity in amblyopic eyes varies from minimal impairment (20/25) to legal blindness (<20/200). Other significant impairments in amblyopic eyes include reduced contrast sensitivity, reduced or absent binocularity and depth perception, and impaired or distorted spatial perception. Peripheral visual fields are preserved, and vision is never completely lost (no light perception) from amblyopia alone.
- Treatment of amblyopia involves reversing the asymmetry by eliminating optical or refractive blur and penalizing the better-seeing eye.
- Treatment may involve occlusion (patching), medication (atropine), optics (glasses), or a combination.

Amblyopia is poor vision, usually just in one eye, resulting from poor visual input during early childhood (the critical period for visual development). Although the cause of amblyopia (refractive blur, strabismus, cataract) may be correctable, vision is not restored immediately because of poor development of the central visual pathways and connections. The earlier the abnormality

in visual input occurs, the greater the potential for amblyopia.

Equal, focused visual input from each eye is necessary for the visual system to develop normally. Anything that interferes with a clear image that can be fused (integrated in the brain) during the first 8 to 10 years of life may cause amblyopia. Amblyopia is almost always a unilateral problem, but in some children with abnormalities in both eyes, bilateral amblyopia can develop.

Expert Opinion on Management Issues

The most important factor in visual outcome in amblyopia is the age at detection. The younger the patient is at the time amblyopia is detected, the more likely treatment will improve vision. After approximately 8 to 10 years of age, amblyopia treatment is usually not successful.

Children with amblyopia are usually asymptomatic. Unless there is an associated ocular or visual abnormality (strabismus, cataract, ptosis), amblyopia may only be detected through routine vision screening. Visual fixation, alignment, and ocular screening (up to age 3 years) and recognition vision testing (usually possible at age 3 years and older) are critical to detect amblyopia in young children and should be done universally for well-child examinations in early childhood.

Reversal of the causative factors may include prescribing glasses, correcting cataract or ptosis with surgery, or other ophthalmic interventions. After the underlying cause is addressed, amblyopia therapy involves reversing the asymmetric input by "penalizing" the previously better-seeing eye (Box 1). This can be accomplished by occlusion with a patch, intentional blurring with glasses, or blurring with

---

BOX 1 Amblyopia Therapies

- Occlusion—adhesive patches or overspectacle occlusion
- Optical—spectacles that over- or undercorrect the penalized eye, or optical films over a lens that cause blurring; rarely, opaque or overcorrective contact lenses
- Pharmacologic penalization—atropine or other topical cycloplegic agent, given to the penalized eye to prevent accommodative focusing and cause blurring

cycloplegic eye drops such as atropine. Recent studies suggest that patching and atropine penalization have similar results, and selection of the therapy should be guided by factors including patient and parental acceptance and compliance.

The length of time and amount of penalization necessary to restore or optimize vision in an amblyopic eye depend on many factors including the age of the patient, degree of amblyopia, and intensity of treatment. In general, amblyopia therapy should continue until vision in the two eyes is equal or until vision in the amblyopic eye has been maximally improved and shows no further improvement with persistent treatment.

Recurrence of amblyopia after stopping active treatment is common, especially in young patients. Close monitoring, and in some cases low-grade maintenance treatment, is necessary to maintain long-term results. In general, after 8 to 10 years of age, the maturity of the visual system will no longer allow recurrence and treatment and monitoring can safely be discontinued.

In unusual cases with bilateral amblyopia, treatment consists of optimizing the optical and refractive components in both eyes, without penalization of either eye. Depending on the cause, depth of bilateral amblyopia, and age of the patient, gradual bilateral improvement of vision is seen.

Common Pitfalls

The most important consideration in management of amblyopia is early detection and treatment. Amblyopia can only be treated during early childhood, and delay or failure to detect amblyopia may result in permanent, irreversible vision loss.

Reversal of the underlying cause of amblyopia may involve compliance with glasses, surgical treatment, or other management issues before amblyopia treatment can begin.

Compliance with treatment, whether glasses, patching, medications, or other treatments, may be difficult. Patching and atropine penalization have similar effectiveness in patients with mild or moderate amblyopia, and compliance should be a major consideration in planning treatment.

Treatment must be monitored closely. It is possible to reverse amblyopia by overtreating with patches, atropine, or other amblyopia therapies. Vision should be measured frequently during and after treatment, to avoid overtreatment and detect recurrence early.

Communication and Counseling

Early detection and referral are critical for successful management of amblyopia, which can only be treated during early childhood. Primary care providers who are involved in health maintenance and screening examinations during early childhood must screen vision, and promptly refer patients suspected of amblyopia. Parents must understand that the success of treatment depends on the age, and delays in treatment may

limit the potential benefit in this treatable cause of vision loss.

Compliance with amblyopia therapy may be difficult. The choice of treatments should be individualized to optimize compliance and parental acceptance of the treatment, and allow the best outcomes. When therapy is not effective, reevaluation and consideration of alternative treatments is important. Treatment of amblyopia is most successful when parents and the treating provider have a shared understanding of the treatment options and expected outcomes, and jointly agree on the best treatment strategy.

SUGGESTED READINGS

1. American Academy of Ophthalmology: Preferred Practice Pattern: Amblyopia. San Francisco: American Academy of Ophthalmology, 2002. **Clinical summary of best practice in amblyopia treatment for eye care professionals, including screening recommendations and treatment guidelines**
2. Pediatric Eye Disease Investigators Group: A comparison of atropine and patching treatments for moderate amblyopia by patient age, cause of amblyopia, depth of amblyopia, and other factors. Ophthalmology 110(8):1632–1637, 2003. **A large, multicenter, randomized trial of therapy for moderate amblyopia, reporting outcomes of patching and atropine penalization in various clinical subcategories**
3. Pediatric Eye Disease Investigator Group: A randomized trial of atropine vs. patching for treatment of moderate amblyopia in children. Arch Ophthalmol 120(3):268–278, 2002. **A large, multicenter, randomized trial of therapy for moderate amblyopia, which demonstrates the clinical equivalence of patching and atropine penalization.**
4. Repka MX, Beck RW, Holmes JM, et al., and the Pediatric Eye Disease Investigator Group: A randomized trial of patching regimens for treatment of moderate amblyopia in children. Arch Ophthalmol 121(5):603–611, 2003. **A large, multicenter, randomized trial of therapy for moderate amblyopia, demonstrating equivalent effectiveness of atropine penalization and patching.**

Strabismus

Monte D. Mills and Leila M. Khazaeni

KEY CONCEPTS

- Any misalignment of the eyes, even if only intermittent, may be a sign of significant strabismus in childhood.
- Eye alignment should be straight by 8 weeks of age in normal term infants. Misalignment after 8 weeks of age is always abnormal.
- Early detection and prompt treatment of strabismus will minimize the effects on the developing visual system, including amblyopia.
- Strabismus is detected by close examination of the eyes during fixation with Hirschberg testing (examination of the corneal light reflex as children watch a light), alternate cover testing, and the Bruchner test (simultaneous bilateral red reflex test). Of these tests, alternate cover, corneal light reflex, and Bruchner tests are the most reliable.
- Strabismus is frequently associated with other visual developmental problems including amblyopia, lack of binocularity, refractive errors, nystagmus, and reduced vision.

- Treatment for strabismus must be individualized, and may involve prescribing glasses, amblyopia therapy (patching, pharmacologic penalization), and surgery, depending on the situation.
- Wide epicanthal folds and eyelid shape may give infants the appearance of strabismus even when the eyes are straight. This is known as "pseudostrabismus" or "pseudoesotropia."

> ### BOX 1 Treatment for Strabismus
>
> - Amblyopia treatment—patching, optical, pharmacologic penalization
> - Orthoptic eye exercises—to develop convergence (effective only in certain situations)
> - Optical treatment—glasses with optical correction or prisms to optically improve eye alignment
> - Surgery—anatomic adjustment of the extraocular muscles to realign eyes

Strabismus is misalignment of the eyes. The misalignment may be constant or intermittent, and it may occur in any direction.

In children, the most common types of strabismus are esotropia (eyes crossing inward) and exotropia (eyes drifting outward). Strabismus in childhood is frequently associated with developmental visual abnormalities including amblyopia and lack of binocularity. Detection and treatment of strabismus, and related problems including amblyopia, are primary goals of early childhood vision screening and should be considered in all early childhood well-child evaluations.

The pathophysiology of the most common forms of childhood strabismus is poorly understood. Infants with strabismus demonstrate subtle abnormalities in both motor function and binocular sensory function, even after successful strabismus treatment. Neuroanatomic abnormalities have not been consistently demonstrated in infants with idiopathic strabismus, although strabismus is frequently seen in children with neurologic abnormalities, including cerebral palsy and nonspecific developmental delay.

Accommodative esotropia, a common strabismus syndrome, is caused by abnormalities in the reflexive convergence that is necessary for looking at near objects. Focusing causes an abnormal amount of convergence and esotropia. In many patients, accommodative esotropia can be treated successfully with glasses alone.

Less often, strabismus syndromes are caused by anatomic restriction to extraocular rotation (Graves disease, Brown syndrome), congenital or acquired paresis or palsy of extraocular muscles (III, IV, or VI palsy, Duane syndrome, Möbius syndrome), or abnormalities of vision (sensory strabismus).

Expert Opinion on Management Issues

Strabismus management must be individualized to the particular patient and situation. Treatment options are listed in Box 1. Nonsurgical treatments that may be useful in certain cases include optical correction (glasses or contact lenses), orthoptic exercises, and amblyopia therapy with patching, pharmacologic penalization, or optical penalization. In general, any measure that will improve the vision in either or both eyes, including refractive correction and amblyopia therapy, will improve the potential for normal eye alignment. In many cases, it is only after other measures are completed that a final decision about potential surgical therapy can be made.

Surgery for strabismus involves adjusting the relative strength of antagonistic extraocular muscle pairs to realign the eyes. Using empirical guidelines, muscles can be "weakened" (recessed) or "tightened" (resected) surgically by shifting the position of the extraocular muscle on the sclera, accessible immediately beneath the conjunctiva on the surface of the eye. Extraocular muscle surgery is generally done in an ambulatory surgical setting, usually under general anesthesia in children. Specifics of the individual patient, associated abnormalities including amblyopia and refractive error, and surgeon preference may determine which of several potential approaches may be best for a particular patient, including whether to operate on muscles of one or both eyes.

In addition to nonsurgical ophthalmic treatments, which may include glasses, patching, and exercises, perioperative management of strabismus patients is similar to management for other elective pediatric procedures. Postoperatively, children are generally expected to have mild discomfort and conjunctival redness, and to be able to return to normal activities within 48 to 72 hours. Topical antibiotics are usually prescribed for 7 to 10 days postoperatively, with resolution of redness and stabilization of eye alignment within 7 to 14 days.

The most significant surgical risk is residual or recurrent misalignment, which may occur in 5% to 20% of children treated surgically, and may require reoperation. Children with strabismus also frequently need additional refractive or amblyopia treatment, even after successful surgery for strabismus.

Common Pitfalls

Early detection and treatment of strabismus are essential to minimize the impairment and optimize visual function. Eye alignment should be a part of every well-child evaluation. Alternate cover, corneal light reflex, and simultaneous bilateral red reflex tests are the best way to evaluate eye alignment in infants and young children.

Pseudostrabismus is the appearance of misalignment, usually esotropia, because of epicanthal skin folds and eyelid shape and position. Patients with pseudostrabismus have normal corneal light reflex, bilateral red reflex, and alternate cover tests. Patients with intermittent strabismus may also appear normal on routine testing, and they may require full eye examinations to detect the full extent of strabismus.

Strabismus is frequently associated with other eye and vision problems. Correction of the eye alignment does not always correct all the treatable associated problems. Children may still need glasses, patching, or exercises even after successful strabismus surgery.

Patients with strabismus are frequently unstable after treatment, and recurrence after nonsurgical and surgical treatments requires vigilance and regular reexamination.

Communication and Counseling

The significance of early treatment to long-term vision and visual function must be explained to parents when discussing strabismus. Even though most parents are bothered most by the appearance of the misalignment, normal visual development with binocularity are the most important long-term goals, and will require long-term monitoring during childhood. Successful nonsurgical treatment including wearing glasses and patching may help avoid the need for surgery, and may also improve surgical outcome. Surgery is generally not an alternative to patching or glasses, but is complimentary.

SUGGESTED READINGS

1. Elston J: Concomitant strabismus. In Taylor D (ed): Paediatric Ophthalmology, 2nd ed. Oxford, England: Blackwell Science, 1997, pp 925–936. **A concise chapter reviewing the common forms of concomitant childhood strabismus, including an overview of nonsurgical and surgical therapy.**
2. Robb RM: Strabismus in childhood. In Albert DM, Jakobiec FA (eds): Principles and Practice of Ophthalmology, 2nd ed. Philadelphia: WB Saunders, 2000, pp 4358–4378. **A well-written chapter discussing pediatric strabismus detection, evaluation, and treatment.**
3. Von Noorden GK, Campos EC: Binocular Vision and Ocular Motility, 6th ed. St Louis: Mosby, 2002. **A dense basic and clinical text on normal and abnormal eye movements.**

Nasolacrimal Duct Obstruction

Monte D. Mills and Leila M. Khazaeni

KEY CONCEPTS

- Nasolacrimal duct obstruction may manifest as a chronically sticky eye.
- It should be differentiated from congenital glaucoma on the basis of history and symptoms.
- Most congenital dacryostenosis is caused by an imperforate valve of Hasner.
- Most cases of nasolacrimal duct obstruction spontaneously resolve by 1 year of age.
- Lacrimal sac massage is often the only intervention required.

- If necessary, probing and irrigation may be performed at 1 year of age.
- The presence of a dacryocele may require early probing and irrigation.
- In cases of nasolacrimal duct obstruction acquired as a result of trauma, probing and irrigation with silastic intubation are often required.

Nasolacrimal duct obstruction, or dacryostenosis, refers to partial or complete obstruction of the nasolacrimal duct that drains tears from the eyes to an opening in the nasal mucosa. It can be a congenital condition, or can be acquired through trauma. The nasolacrimal drainage system begins with puncta located medially in the upper and lower eyelids. These puncta deliver tears to the canalicular system, leading to the lacrimal sac, which is then drained by the nasolacrimal duct through an anastomosis with the nasal mucosa of the inferior nasal meatus. In most cases of congenital dacryostenosis, a membrane covers this opening, creating the obstruction and resulting clinically in epiphora, or tearing. Infants generally begin tear production after the first few weeks of life. Patency of the nasolacrimal duct is often only 50% at birth; however, in most infants the persistent membranous obstruction of the nasal end breaks down quickly. One study of 181 full-term infants reported a symptomatic nonpatency rate of 15%. Thus despite the frequency of a nonpatent nasolacrimal duct at birth, relatively few infants develop symptoms.

The infant with a congenital nasolacrimal duct obstruction characteristically develops epiphora, or tearing, at 2 to 6 weeks, as well as recurrent conjunctivitis, discharge, and occasionally dacryocystitis. The condition is bilateral in approximately one third of infants. A thorough history should be obtained and the specific symptoms of the "sticky eye" should be elicited, such as crusting, mucous discharge, and redness of the eye and the eyelids in addition to tearing. Furthermore, the chronicity of the symptoms should be probed. Other symptoms, such as photophobia and blepharospasm, should be investigated. These three symptoms (tearing, photophobia, and blepharospasm) are typical for congenital glaucoma and may be confused with nasolacrimal obstruction. The medial canthal area should be examined for the presence of a blue mass, which may indicate the presence of a dacryocele (a dilated lacrimal sac containing a sterile accumulation of mucus or even amniotic fluid). Dacryoceles require immediate probing and irrigation to prevent secondary infections.

Expert Opinion on Management Issues

The most useful physical examination maneuver is palpation of the lacrimal sac with the forefinger. Firm pressure should be applied over the area of the medial canthus to express discharge through the puncta.

Reflux of material from the puncta demonstrates the upper lacrimal drainage system to be patent and indicates an obstruction distal to the lacrimal sac. Although this test is specific, it is not very sensitive, and the absence of reflux from the puncta does not rule out an abnormality of the lower system. Diagnosis can also be supported by the fluorescein dye disappearance test. Fluorescein dye is instilled in the inferior conjunctival sac of each eye. The patient is then checked after 2 minutes and again after 5 minutes post instillation using a cobalt blue light from a distance of a few feet. The amount of fluorescein left in the conjunctival sac is graded at each of these intervals on a scale of 0 to 3. A negative dye disappearance test is a good indicator of a patent nasolacrimal duct. A positive test indicates poor outflow but does not further localize the problem.

Dacryostenosis should be managed conservatively whenever possible. The initial treatment strategy of choice is a combination of antibiotic drops and lacrimal sac massage. Antibiotic drops are preferred to ointments because they are believed to penetrate more quickly. Erythromycin or a polymyxin B–gramicidin combination are the agents of choice as they are well tolerated and complications have not been observed with long-term use (6 to 9 months). There is, however, a role for antibiotic ointment in performing the Crigler method of lacrimal sac massage. Parents should be instructed in the office to apply the antibiotic ointment to the pad of one forefinger, and this finger should then be placed over the medial canthal area on the inferior lacrimal crest. The finger should be moved in a sliding motion inferiorly with moderate pressure over the sac and duct.

Further diagnostic testing consists of probing of the nasolacrimal duct in the operating room and possibly irrigating the duct to ensure patency. The timing of initial probing is a controversial subject. Delaying surgical probing until after 12 months of age allows a period of time for spontaneous resolution to occur, because 90% of congenital obstructions resolve by 1 year of age. Furthermore, waiting beyond 1 year of age may be associated with an increased number of subsequent procedures and more complex procedures. Nasolacrimal probing is often both diagnostic and therapeutic. Patency can usually be judged within days of the procedure.

If medical management followed by diagnostic probing and irrigation have failed to establish a patent nasolacrimal duct, the next step becomes intubation of the nasolacrimal duct with tube stents. This is a surgical procedure whereby a silicone tube attached to a metal probe at each end is maneuvered into the nasolacrimal duct and secured. The tube is left in place for 3 to 6 months so that patency can be established. In rare instances, a dacryocystorhinostomy (DCR) must be performed. This is a surgical procedure in which a fistula is created between the lacrimal sac and the nasal mucosa. It is indicated in cases in which epiphora persists despite prior silicone intubation and there is an inability to establish patency with probing and intubation and acquired dacryostenosis because of trauma.

As previously mentioned, most congenital nasolacrimal duct obstruction cases resolve by 1 year of age. Patients who continue to be symptomatic at 1 year of age and undergo a therapeutic probing and irrigation generally do well and do not require further intervention. In most cases, initial probing and irrigation are successful and children do not suffer sequelae. It is only in the rare and traumatic cases that repeat procedures and surgical intervention become necessary.

WHEN DO YOU NEED A REFERRAL?

Tearing that persists up to 1 year of age despite lacrimal sac massage necessitates referral to a pediatric ophthalmologist for further management, including probing and irrigation. Tearing in an infant who presents with a dacryocele (a bluish mass in the medial canthal area) requires referral for possible early probing. Also, tearing accompanied by conjunctival injection, photophobia, blepharospasm, or is associated with a history of trauma should prompt urgent referral for ophthalmologic evaluation.

SUGGESTED READINGS

1. Katowitz JA, Welsh MG: Timing of initial probing and irrigation in congenital nasolacrimal duct obstruction. Ophthalmology 95:698, 1987. **A report of the effect of age on success of initial probing.**
2. Katowitz JA, Low JE, Covici SJ, Goldstein JB: Management of pediatric lower system problems: Probing silastic intubation. In Katowitz JA (ed): Principles of Pediatric Oculoplastic Surgery. New York: Springer, 2002, pp 309. **A chapter-length review of the management of nasolacrimal duct obstruction.**
3. Kushner B: Congenital nasolacrimal system obstruction. Arch Ophthalmol 100:597, 1982. **A report of surgical management of nasolacrimal obstruction.**
4. MacEwen CJ: The fluorescein disappearance test (FDT): An evaluation of its use in infants. J Pediatr Ophthalmol Strabismus 28:302, 1991. **A description of the fluorescein dye disappearance test for nasolacrimal patency.**
5. Nelson LB, Calhoun JH, Menduke H: Medical management of congenital nasolacrimal duct obstruction. Ophthalmology 92:1187, 1985. **A report of nonsurgical management including nasolacrimal duct massage.**

18

Red Eye

Monte D. Mills and Leila M. Khazaeni

KEY CONCEPTS

- Conjunctivitis must be differentiated from other causes of a pediatric red eye including trauma and foreign bodies.
- In all cases of neonatal conjunctivitis, conjunctival swabs and scrapings must be performed. Treatment is

Conjunctivitis is the most common cause for a red eye in infancy and childhood. The conjunctiva may become inflamed as a result of viral or bacterial infections, exposure to allergens, autoimmune processes, or toxicity to medications. Furthermore, the conjunctiva may be secondarily hyperemic as a result of inflammation of other ocular structures such as the cornea, the episclera, the sclera, and the anterior chamber of the eye. Historical clues such as the age of the patient, nature of the discharge, onset and laterality of symptoms, and contact with infected individuals are very important in making the diagnosis.

Conjunctivitis during the newborn period, referred to as ophthalmia neonatorum, is categorized as a distinct pathologic entity. The etiologic agents include chemical irritants (silver nitrate), *Neisseria gonorrhoeae*, *Chlamydia trachomatis*, herpes simplex virus (HSV), and other bacteria. Classically, the various etiologic agents of neonatal conjunctivitis have been differentiated on the basis of age of onset and quality of discharge or presenting symptoms (Table 1). These

TABLE 1 Etiologic Agents in Neonatal Conjunctivitis

Etiologic Agent	Age of Onset	Characteristics
Silver nitrate	1 day	Conjunctival erythema, mild serous discharge
Neisseria gonorrhoeae	3–5 days	Conjunctival erythema, chemosis, lid edema may be present. Hyperacute, copious purulent discharge
Chlamydia trachomatis	5–14 days	Conjunctival erythema: palpebral > bulbar involvement. Moderate thick, purulent discharge
Herpes simplex virus	5–30 days	Mild conjunctival erythema, serosanguineous discharge. Vesicular rash may be present on eyelids.
Bacteria*	5–14 days	Conjunctival erythema. Purulent discharge; specific characteristics vary by organism.

*Most frequently isolated organisms are *Staphylococcus aureus*, *Staphylococcus epidermidis*, *Streptococcus pneumoniae*, *Streptococcus viridans*, *Haemophilus influenzae*, *Escherichia coli*, and *Pseudomonas aeruginosa*.

features may overlap, however, and so diagnosis and treatment must be guided by cultures and laboratory testing. Chemical conjunctivitis resulting from exposure to silver nitrate historically occurs in the first 1 to 2 days of life. It does not require topical or systemic treatment and is self-limited. *N. gonorrhoeae* conjunctivitis classically manifests during the first week of life with a purulent discharge. The danger of *N. gonorrhoeae* infection lies in the organism's ability to rapidly penetrate intact epithelial cells, leading to corneal infection with possible scarring and even perforation, thus making gonococcal conjunctivitis a true ocular emergency. Conjunctivitis caused by *C. trachomatis* can occur during the first 3 weeks of life and is often bilateral. Systemic chlamydial infection can occur in conjunction with the conjunctival infection; therefore, infants should be assessed for pharyngitis, otitis media, and pneumonia. Chlamydial conjunctivitis requires both topical and systemic treatment. HSV conjunctivitis is usually acquired at the time of delivery from the maternal cervix; however, symptomatic disease in the neonate can occur at any time during the first month of life. Neonatal infection may be disseminated in two thirds of cases, and confined to the central nervous system (CNS), mouth, eyes, or skin in one third of cases.

Most cases of conjunctivitis in school-age children are caused by viruses or bacteria. Adenovirus infections of the conjunctiva are acute and self-limited although highly contagious. Children present with acute onset of watery discharge, photophobia, and foreign body sensation. Symptoms of an upper respiratory tract infection are often present as is a palpable preauricular or submandibular lymph node. Bacterial conjunctivitis in children is a result of either direct contact with an infected individual's eye discharge or from the spread of infection from the organisms colonizing the patient's own nasal mucosa and sinuses. The incidence is higher in winter months, and the most common pathogens include *Haemophilus influenzae*, *Streptococcus pneumoniae*, and *Moraxella* species. *Staphylococcus aureus* is less common except after surgical or accidental eye trauma. Children present with burning, stinging, foreign body sensation, and a mild to moderate mucoid or purulent discharge. They often complain of morning crusting and difficulty opening the eyelids; however, unlike viral conjunctivitis, there is typically no lymphadenopathy. Suspected bacterial conjunctivitis should be cultured and treated empirically with broad-spectrum antibiotic drops such as trimethoprim/polymyxin B until culture results are available to tailor therapy.

Allergic conjunctivitis is associated with mucus discharge, lid edema, conjunctival chemosis, and hyperemia. Patients usually have intense pruritus. Treatment with topical mast cell stabilizers and topical antihistamines (e.g., olopatadine) may relieve symptoms. HSV can cause a blepharoconjunctivitis associated with a periorbital vesicular dermatitis. Keratitis (with dendritic corneal lesions) and iritis (causing photophobia) may develop and these patients should be promptly referred to an ophthalmologist.

Juvenile rheumatoid arthritis (JRA) may also cause an iritis, which presents with a red eye and photophobia. Patients with a history of JRA who present with a red eye should be referred to an ophthalmologist promptly.

Expert Opinion on Management Issues

Any case of conjunctivitis during the neonatal period should be cultured to tailor antibiotic therapy. Treatment of nondisseminated gonococcal conjunctivitis consists of hospitalization and administration of ceftriaxone, one intravenous (IV) or intramuscular (IM) dose of 25 to 50 mg/kg, not to exceed 125 mg. Disseminated infections should be treated with 10 to 14 days of parenteral antibiotics. Because of the risk of corneal perforation, the eyes should be irrigated with saline frequently until the discharge is eliminated. The newborn, the mother, and her sexual partner are treated for *Chlamydia* as well, because of the high incidence of concomitant *Chlamydia* infection in women who contract gonococcus. Infants with chlamydial conjunctivitis should be treated systemically with oral erythromycin (50 mg/kg/day in four divided doses) for 14 days. Topical treatment is not necessary in infants. The parents of the child should also be treated. Disseminated HSV infection should be treated with acyclovir or vidarabine. Eye involvement including conjunctivitis and epithelial keratitis can be treated with topical antiviral agents such as vidarabine, trifluridine, and idoxuridine, or debridement.

Adenovirus conjunctivitis is a self-limited infection, and treatment is supportive only. Cold compresses and topical vasoconstrictors may provide symptom relief. Little clinical evidence supports the use of topical antibacterial drops. The peak intensity of the conjunctivitis occurs 5 to 7 days after onset and the fellow eye becomes involved in at least 50% of cases.

WHEN DO YOU NEED A REFERRAL?

Any patient with neonatal conjunctivitis should be evaluated by an ophthalmologist. Conjunctivitis in an older child that persists beyond 2 weeks' duration or is associated with severe pain, decrease in vision, or a history of trauma necessitates immediate evaluation by an ophthalmologist. Cases of suspected herpes simplex or herpes zoster conjunctivitis or keratitis should be referred to an ophthalmologist promptly. Suspicion of uveitis in a patient with a history of JRA or other inflammatory diseases should also prompt urgent referral.

SUGGESTED READINGS

1. Jackson WB: Differentiating conjunctivitis of diverse origins. Surv Ophthalmol 38:91–104, 1993. **Review of clinical characteristics of conjunctivitis in children and adults.**

2. O'Hara MA: Ophthalmia neonatorum. Pediatr Clin North Am 40:715–725, 1993. **Review of the diagnosis and treatment of neonatal conjunctivitis.**

Intraocular and Extraocular Retinoblastoma

Eric F. Grabowski

KEY CONCEPTS

- Treatment for intraocular tumor is directed toward saving useful vision, not life, and risks of fever and neutropenia and other chemotherapy side effects should be minimized.
- On the other hand, systemic chemotherapy has a special role in potentially allowing for the avoidance of radiation therapy altogether in children harboring the germinal mutation. Such children are at high risk of second, nonocular tumors, a risk that is made especially high in children who receive radiation therapy, which generally includes the orbital bones in the radiation field.
- Children with tumor invading the optic nerve but not the surgical margin (when an eye is enucleated and globe and optic nerve pathology is available) are at low to moderate risk (10% to 15%) of developing extraocular tumor weeks to months later. These children require systemic chemotherapy but not radiation.
- Children with tumor extending to or beyond the surgical margin require radiation in addition to systemic chemotherapy.
- Children with tumor extending regionally (into the orbit or preauricular lymph nodes) also require radiation in addition to systemic chemotherapy.
- Children with tumor extending to the central nervous system (CNS) and/or bone and bone marrow should undergo remission induction with systemic chemotherapy followed by myeloablative chemotherapy and autologous stem cell transplantation. Long-term survival is limited (<30% at most centers) in the absence of such an aggressive approach.

The management of retinoblastoma has seen striking advances in the past decade. These include the now widespread use of chemotherapy, with or without conventional radiation therapy, for intraocular tumors; the identification of children who, based on globe and optic nerve pathology, may be at high risk for micrometastases; the successful use of chemotherapy for localized bulky tumor (orbital recurrence, optic nerve tumor at the margin of surgical section) or cerebrospinal fluid (CSF) tumor only; and the successful application of combination chemotherapy followed by autologous stem cell rescue for bone and bone marrow disease. For intraocular tumor, a new staging system is gaining widespread acceptance and has been adopted internationally and by the Children's Oncology Group (COG).

Expert Opinion on Management Issues

BILATERAL OR UNILATERAL INTRAOCULAR TUMOR, GROUP A

Children with group A tumor(s) (Box 1) can generally be managed by local measures carried out by an ophthalmologist and do not need chemotherapy. These measures include photocoagulation, cryotherapy, and diathermy.

BILATERAL INTRAOCULAR TUMOR, WITH AT LEAST ONE GROUP B EYE

For bilateral intraocular tumor, with at least one group B eye, our group in Boston believes that a combination of upfront systemic chemotherapy and proton beam radiation, each of lower intensity than if offered alone, can afford improved eye salvage with useful vision together with fewer and/or less severe side effects from *both* chemotherapy and radiation therapy. Accordingly, our carboplatin-vincristine–based protocol does not employ etoposide, a measure that may reduce the risk of hospitalizations for fever and neutropenia and eliminate a small risk of myelodysplasia, a potentially fatal condition. The elimination of etoposide is unlikely to lead to undertreatment of intraocular tumors for several reasons. First, such tumors do respond to carboplatin alone. Second, local treatment modalities remain in place to enhance the durability of responses to carboplatin and vincristine. Third, should these responses be considered insufficient (see next paragraph), provision for proton beam radiation is in place. Fourth, the importance of etoposide to chemotherapy responses in retinoblastoma has not been established.

For tumors that are equivalent to 3 mm or for any smaller tumors if the macula is involved or the tumors are peripapillary, we recommend a two-agent regimen: carboplatin and vincristine (Table 1 provides dosing information), given at 3-week intervals for a total of six courses, with consolidation with proton beam radiation for tumors that do not fully respond (see below). Twenty-four hours after completion of a course of chemotherapy, granulocyte colony-stimulating factor (G-CSF) is started at 5 μg/kg subcutaneously (SC) daily until the absolute neutrophil count (ANC) is greater than 1000/μL. The reason for including in this approach tumors that involve the macula or are peripapillary is that such tumors lack pigment, rendering them relatively poorly responsive to photocoagulation. All smaller tumors 3 mm or more away from the macula are treated by local measures, as for group A eyes. If any tumors fail to fully respond—defined as a reduction in size to less than 3 mm before the completion of chemotherapy at week 18, or failure of any tumors to continue to respond at or after week 6—the child should go on to have involved field proton beam radiation therapy (40 cGy), which largely spares the orbital bones and minimizes the risks of radiation-induced bone tumors (Wong et al., 1997) and radiation-associated

impairment of orbital bone growth (Imhof et al., 1996; Kaste et al., 1997).

Three-agent regimens, which include the above agents plus etoposide, have as a major aim the

---

BOX 1 International Classification System for Intraocular Retinoblastoma

Group A

Small intraretinal tumors away from foveola and disc:
- All tumors are 3 mm or smaller in greatest dimension, confined to the retina.
- All tumors are located further than 3 mm from the foveola and 1.5 mm from the optic disc.

Group B

All remaining discrete tumors confined to the retina:
- All other tumors confined to the retina not in group A.
- Tumor-associated subretinal fluid less than 3 mm from the tumor with no subretinal seeding.

Group C

Discrete local disease with minimal subretinal or vitreous seeding:
- Tumor(s) are discrete.
- Subretinal fluid, present or past, without seeding involving up to one fourth of the retina.
- Local fine vitreous seeding may be present close to discrete tumor.
- Local subretinal seeding less than 3 mm (2 disk diameters) from the tumor.

Group D

Diffuse disease with significant vitreous or subretinal seeding:
- Tumor(s) may be massive or diffuse.
- Subretinal fluid present or past without seeding, involving up to total retinal detachment.
- Diffuse or massive vitreous disease may include "greasy" seeds or avascular tumor masses.
- Diffuse subretinal seeding may include subretinal plaques or tumor nodules.

Group E

Presence of any one or more of these poor prognosis features:
- Tumor touching the lens.
- Tumor anterior to anterior vitreous space involving ciliary body or anterior segment.
- Diffuse infiltrating retinoblastoma.
- Neovascular glaucoma.
- Opaque media from hemorrhage.
- Tumor necrosis with aseptic orbital cellulitis.
- Phthisis bulbi.

TABLE 1 Doses of Chemotherapy Used in Retinoblastoma

Drug	Route	Dose	Days (of course)
Vincristine	IV push	0.05 mg/kg	1
Carboplatin	IV over 6 h	8.35 mg/kg	1, 2
Etoposide	IV over 1 h	3.3 mg/kg	1, 2, 3

Criteria for starting carboplatin cycle: ANC > 1000 μL; platelet count >100,000 μL; ALT less than 10 times the upper limits of normal; normal GFR.

ALT, alanine transaminase; ANC, absolute neutrophil count; GFR, glomerular filtration rate; IV, intravenously.

elimination, where possible, of radiation therapy altogether. Nonproton beam radiation therapy has a recognized contribution to secondary nonocular malignancies in children with germline RB1 mutations. Additionally, radiation therapy causes and/or contributes to transient retinopathy (incidence of 15% to 25%), vitreous hemorrhage (10% to 20%), neovascular glaucoma (0% to 5%), lacrimal gland/duct injury (diminished tear production with dry and sometimes photophobic eyes [2% to 50%]), cataracts (10% to 25%), and impaired orbital bone growth (up to 100%). Toward this end, Friedman and associates (2000) used six cycles of vincristine, carboplatin, and etoposide to treat 39 eyes that were chiefly group B eyes, and avoided enucleation or external beam radiation in all. G-CSF was used as previously discussed. Jubran and associates (2001) treated 11 eyes in this fashion, and avoided enucleation and external beam radiation in 9. Nonetheless, the COG is now studying a two-agent (vincristine-carboplatin) regimen for group B eyes with the same aim of avoiding radiation.

BILATERAL INTRAOCULAR TUMOR, WITH AT LEAST ONE GROUP C OR D EYE

Where proton beam radiation is available, our group believes that the protocol described for group B eyes is also to be recommended for groups C and D eyes, given that proton radiation therapy is an integral part of the treatment plan. Three out of three group C and D eyes have no active tumor after 18 or more months of follow-up (and have not required enucleation).

COG has piloted a protocol that uses courses of vincristine, carboplatin, and etoposide given every 28 days for a total of six courses for group C eyes, and for eight courses (with a dose escalation) for group D eyes. For each group C or D eye and for courses 2 through 4, subtenon carboplatin is also given, at a dose of 1 mL of 10 mg/mL at each of two sites in two quadrants of each group C or D eye. G-CSF is used as previously described. Children with eyes that fail to respond to this chemotherapy are considered "off study," and go on to either enucleation of a failed eye or radiation therapy to that eye. Twelve of 22 eyes after 24 months or more of follow-up have not required enucleation and/or external beam radiation.

UNILATERAL TUMOR WITH HIGH-RISK FEATURES ON HISTOPATHOLOGIC EXAMINATION

Children with unilateral tumor may have high-risk features on histopathologic examination that place them at risk for developing CNS and/or bone and bone marrow disease at a later time. These children have one or more of the following:

- One or both eyes enucleated and tumor involvement of the optic nerve beyond the lamina cribrosa, but not to the line of surgical section
- Massive choroidal tumor defined as posterior uveal invasion

- Any posterior uveal involvement with any optic nerve disease (optic nerve head, prelamina and postlamina cribrosa)

Excluded from this category are those with extraocular tumor, including disease at the surgical margin, and those with tumor in an emissary vein and/or on the episcleral surface. The former children have an estimated 10% to 15% mortality from recurrent tumor and, therefore, should receive chemotherapy, which includes vincristine, carboplatin, and etoposide given every 28 days for six courses (see Table 1 for dosing).

In view of our experience in having seen four cases of tumor involving the CSF only (each case had a repeat positive CSF cytology), we recommend a diagnostic lumbar puncture in cases of retinoblastoma involving or obscuring the optic nerve. If the CSF cytology is positive (preferably confirmed by means of a repeat lumbar puncture for CSF cytology), we recommend including intrathecal chemotherapy with methotrexate and cytosine arabinoside at weeks 0, 1, 2, and 3 with age-related (and therefore, CSF volume-related) dosing. Doses for methotrexate are 6 mg for ages 4 to 11 months, 8 mg for ages 12 to 23 months, 10 mg for ages 24 to 36 months, and 12 mg for children older than 37 months. Corresponding doses for cytosine arabinoside are 20, 30, 50, and 70 mg. For ages 0 to 3 months, we recommend half-doses of methotrexate and cytosine arabinoside of 3 and 10 mg, respectively. (In this situation, the extraocular tumor is technically no longer regional.)

We consider radiation therapy to be unnecessary for high-risk features. Of 12 children we have treated in this manner, none developed extraocular tumor after 48 months or more of follow-up.

REGIONAL EXTRAOCULAR TUMOR

Children with regional extraocular tumor, for whom mortality is in the range of 20%, are those with measurable or microscopic extraocular tumor, which may include:

- Orbital recurrence (orbital mass)
- Presence of episcleral tumor following enucleation
- Positive preauricular lymph nodes

Excluded are children with central nervous system (CNS), and/or bone and bone marrow disease.

All patients should receive an induction, according to a new COG protocol for extraocular tumor, with four courses of vincristine, cisplatin, cyclophosphamide with mesna, and etoposide. G-CSF is given as previously described. Orbital radiation therapy (RT) (stereotactic or proton beam) should begin at week 6 for orbital recurrence.

A good outcome in 5 of 6 patients following orbital recurrence was reported by Goble and associates (1990), who used vincristine-carboplatin-etoposide alternating with vincristine-doxorubicin-ifosfamide for a total of three courses of each, with orbital radiation and with or without intrathecal chemotherapy. GCSF was used as described previously. Our group has had a similarly good outcome in two out of two patients with orbital recurrence using the same chemotherapy combined with proton beam radiation.

EXTRAOCULAR TUMOR WITH CNS AND/OR BONE AND BONE MARROW INVOLVEMENT

Children with extraocular tumor with CNS and/or bone and bone marrow involvement, for whom mortality in the absence of aggressive treatment approaches 100%, are those with measurable extraocular tumors, which may include:

- Isolated meningeal disease, with absence of disseminated meningeal tumor (two or more foci)
- Ectopic intracranial retinoblastoma,
- Bone and/or bone marrow tumor (bilateral bone marrow aspirates and biopsies)

An exception appears to be the rare case of a child with an isolated CSF tumor. Such cases have been treated effectively by us as described previously for tumors with high-risk features.

Although extraocular retinoblastoma is usually very chemosensitive and a number of long-term survivors exist (Grabowski & Abramson, 1987), durable remission rates (at 3 to 5 years) with bone and bone marrow disease at most centers are only 20% to 30%, indicating the need to offer myeloablative chemotherapy followed by stem cell rescue (Dunkel, et al., 2000) to this subgroup.

All patients should receive the same induction with four courses of vincristine, cisplatin, cyclophosphamide with mesna, and etoposide as is done for regional extraocular tumors. In addition and according to the same COG extraocular tumor protocol described previously, patients in this category should go on to consolidation with myeloablative chemotherapy with carboplatin, thiotepa, and etoposide, followed by autologous stem cell rescue. G-CSF is used as previously described. This approach can be taken provided a child has adequate stem cell yield on collection of stem cells following induction chemotherapy, and adequate remission status. Children with regional extraocular tumors should *not* receive consolidation because they have a good prognosis with induction chemotherapy alone.

External beam radiation therapy should be administered to sites that initially harbored bulky disease on or about day +42 after stem cell rescue.

All patients should be followed with audiograms or brain stem auditory evoked responses (BAERs), and echocardiograms.

Common Pitfalls

- Failure to provide a comprehensive care team. The treatment of any child with non–group A retinoblastoma should be undertaken only by a comprehensive health care team, which includes a pediatric hematologist/oncologist, an ophthalmologist who is a retinal specialist, a radiation oncologist, a neuroradiologist, a pediatric surgeon for insertion of central venous access devices, a genetics counselor, and a social worker for the child and family, and an outstanding nursing staff.
- Failure to follow a carefully considered treatment plan. The recommendations provided here are guidelines only. A specific and complete treatment protocol should be followed in any particular instance, such as one from COG or, for proton beam therapy with or without systemic chemotherapy, that of our group in Boston.

Communication and Counseling

Retinoblastoma, the most common primary ocular malignancy of childhood, is a condition for which the pediatrician and pediatric hematologist/oncologist can now play a much more significant role in therapy. Developments in molecular biology have now made carrier testing and prenatal diagnosis feasible. These developments augment the pediatrician's and pediatric hematologist/oncologist's ability to offer accurate and appropriate genetic counseling for affected families.

Chemotherapy and radiation therapy options now exist that make possible preservation of many more eyes for useful vision, and long-term survival for the overwhelming majority of children with retinoblastoma, even those with high-risk features for micrometastases and those with regional extraocular tumor. Those who develop CNS and/or bone and bone marrow tumor, however, require intensive chemotherapy followed by autologous stem cell rescue to have reasonable hope of long-term survival. Finally, 40% of all children with retinoblastoma (those with the germinal mutation) are at lifelong risk for second, nonocular malignancies. The recognition that one third to half of these children will actually develop second tumors by the fourth decade of life makes vigilant follow-up care for these patients a necessity.

SUGGESTED READINGS

1. Chantada G, Fandino A, Casak S, et al: Treatment of overt extraocular retinoblastoma. Med Pediatr Oncol 40:158–161, 2003. **This article points out a poor outcome with CNS tumor and bone and bone marrow tumor when treated with conventional combination chemotherapy.**
2. Dunkel IJ, Aledo A, Kernan NA, et al: Successful treatment of metastatic retinoblastoma. Cancer 89:2117–2121, 2000. **This paper describes a series of patients with bone and bone marrow tumor who did well with intensive chemotherapy combined with autologous stem cell rescue.**
3. Friedman DL, Himelstein B, Shields CL, et al: Chemoreduction and local ophthalmic therapy for intraocular retinoblastoma. J Clin Oncol 18:12–17, 2000. **This paper summarizes success in using chemotherapy to avoid external beam radiation in principally stage B intraocular tumors.**
4. Goble RR, McKenzie J, Kingston JE, et al: Orbital recurrence of retinoblastoma successfully treated by combined therapy. Brit J Ophthalmol 74:97–98, 1990. **This paper describes early success in managing orbital recurrence of tumor.**
5. Grabowski EF, Abramson DH: Intraocular and extraocular retinoblastoma. Hematol Oncol Clin North Am 1(4):721–735, 1987. **This work outlines a clinical and histopathologic staging system for extraocular tumor, reports successful treatment of tumor extending into the optic nerve, and also reports a**

group of long-term survivors with bone and bone marrow tumor treated with combination chemotherapy.

6. Imhof SM, Mouritis MP, Hofman P, et al: Quantification of orbital and mid-facial growth retardation after megavoltage external beam irradiation in children with retinoblastoma. Ophthalmology 103:263–268, 1996. **This paper describes impairment of orbital bone growth associated with external beam radiation.**

7. Jubran RF, Murphree AL, Villablanca JG: Low dose carboplatin/etoposide/vincristine and local therapy for intraocular retinoblastoma group II-IV eyes. Proceedings of the 10th International Symposium on Retinoblastoma, May 4, 2001. **This report supports the preceding reference.**

8. Kaste SC, Chen G, Fontanese J, et al: Orbital-development in long-term survivors of retinoblastoma. J Clin Oncol 15:1183–1189, 1997. **This article ia a good companion to the proceeding.**

9. Wong FL, Boice JD, Abramson DH, et al: Cancer incidence after retinoblastoma. JAMA 278:1262–1267, 1997. **This is a good review of second, non-ocular tumors seen with germinal retinoblastoma.**

19 Ear, Nose, and Throat

Choanal Atresia

Joseph Haddad, Jr. and Erich N. Mussak

KEY CONCEPTS

- Bilateral choanal atresia is more common than unilateral and manifests as acute respiratory distress at birth.
- In bilateral cases, the airway is secured by intubation or oral airway and a CT scan is performed to plan surgical repair.
- Endoscopes and endoscopic instruments, along with the development of small drills, have improved the ease and success of transnasal repairs.
- The transpalatal repair remains an excellent option for difficult cases and transnasal surgical failures.
- The application of mitomycin C has become a useful adjunctive therapy in preventing restenosis of the choana.
- Most surgeons favor the use of postoperative stenting of the choana for 4 to 6 weeks, to maintain patency and help prevent restenosis.

Choanal atresia is a congenital malformation of the nasal airway in which no communication exists between the nasal cavity and the nasopharynx. This anomaly occurs in 1 in 5000 to 8000 live births (female-to-male ratio of 2:1); atresia may be bilateral (67%) or unilateral (33%), complete or incomplete, completely bony (30%) or a combination of bone and membrane (70%). Most cases of choanal atresia are isolated malformations, but association with other deformities can occur in the CHARGE syndrome (a congenital syndrome that includes *colo*boma, *h*eart disease, *a*tresia of choana, *r*etarded development, *g*enital hypoplasia, and *e*ar anomalies). In addition, syndromes with midface hypoplasia and nasal stenosis may manifest in a similar fashion.

Neonates are obligate nasal breathers, and bilateral choanal atresia constitutes a medical emergency. Acute respiratory distress is present with a characteristic pattern of normal breathing and skin color while crying, and cyanosis and apnea when quiet. These infants require upper airway management with intubation, a McGovern nipple, or an oral airway. A feeding tube often is necessary until the problem is corrected. Diagnosis is suggested when a catheter cannot be passed from the nose to the pharynx; flexible fiberoptic scoping may confirm a lack of choana patency. High-resolution CT gives a definitive diagnosis and allows for preoperative planning because it defines the overall anatomy of the nose and nasopharynx and demonstrates the thickness, composition, and location of the atresia plate.

Unilateral choanal atresia is not associated with respiratory compromise and usually manifests during childhood in association with unilateral mucoid rhinorrhea and nasal congestion. Differential diagnosis includes foreign body or nasal mass (Table 1).

Expert Opinion on Management Issues

Choanal atresia may be associated with life-threatening conditions such as congenital heart disease; these defects need to be ruled out or addressed before surgical repair is performed. Ranges of surgical procedures to repair choanal atresia have been described in the literature. The most common approaches are transnasal and transpalatal, with transnasal being the most common initial approach in uncomplicated cases. The transnasal technique has improved in the past decade with development of pediatric endoscopes, as well as microsurgical and powered instruments, which allow better visualization of the infant nose and removal of bone and soft tissue. The transpalatal route is generally favored for complete bony atresia, association with other abnormalities such as bony septal deviation, or when the transnasal approach has failed. Advantages of this approach include excellent visualization and exposure of the atresia plate and ample room through the mouth to drill away the bone of the plate and bony nasal septum. Disadvantages to the transpalatal approach include increased operative time, greater pain, difficulties with feeding, possible increased blood loss, and potential for palate fistula (Table 2).

Other advances include the topical application of mitomycin C, an antibiotic and fibroblast inhibitor that may help to minimize scarring and improve healing time. Some practitioners have reported success with the use of a KTP (potassium titanyl-phosphate) laser, and CT-assisted choanal atresia repair. The individual surgeon bases decisions for repair on the type of atresia and which instruments are available and most suitable for each patient.

TABLE 1 Diagnosis of Choanal Atresia

Feature	Unilateral Choanal Atresia	Bilateral Choanal Atresia
Key initial observations	Mucoid rhinorrhea Unilateral congestion	Acute respiratory distress
Typical age of diagnosis	Early childhood	Immediately after birth
% of total choanal atresias	≈33%	≈67%
Final diagnostic criteria	CT showing bony and soft tissue blockage of one choana	CT showing bony and soft tissue blockage of both choana

TABLE 2 Transnasal and Transpalatal Approaches to Choanal Atresia Repair

Transnasal	Transpalatal
Advantages	
No incision necessary to achieve repair.	Better visualization of and access to the choanal region and posterior septum.
May have less associated morbidity, e.g., pain, bleeding.	Easier to drill and remove bone of the atresia plate and septum.
Disadvantages	
Repair is done blindly, or by visualizing through an endoscope in a small nasal airway, which may limit the surgeon.	Incision of the palate required. Potential for increased bleeding and higher morbidity (pain, feeding difficulties).
Higher risk for stenosis if access or visualization is limited.	Palate fistulas may occur.

Stents are placed at the time of surgery to maintain the nasal airway and to prevent stenosis. Pediatric endotracheal tubes or red rubber catheters are commonly used for stenting and are often left in place for 3 to 6 weeks. Frequent suctioning, application of saline to the nose, and oral antibiotics can help maintain stent patency and improve nasal hygiene with lower chance for infection. Antireflux therapy can help to prevent gastroesophageal reflux, which can contribute to the development of granulation tissue and stenosis of the choana.

Common Pitfalls

- Stenosis of the choana has been reported in as many as one third of cases, associated with nasal obstruction and congestion. Leaving stents in place for 4 to 6 weeks may prevent stenosis.
- Poor nasal hygiene may develop after stent placement unless appropriate measures are taken. Antibiotics, saline, and frequent suctioning are recommended.
- If a transnasal surgical approach fails, the transpalatal approach may allow better access to the area of atresia and lead to improved success.

Communication and Counseling

When the diagnosis of choanal atresia is made in a newborn, the parent needs to understand that further testing needs to be performed to rule out associated abnormalities or underlying conditions. Once the child is cleared for surgery, the parent should understand options for surgery and the need for supportive care postoperatively. Before the infant is discharged, appropriate equipment and medications must be ordered for the home, including a portable suction machine. The parent is instructed in the instillation of nasal saline and the use of the suction to maintain stent patency and to keep the nose clean. Discharge should not take place until the parent is comfortable with the infant's care; a visiting nurse at home may help in supportive care. Instruction is given for follow-up and when to call for emergencies. The parent should understand that there is a significant risk of stenosis after the initial surgery, and that further surgeries may be necessary to achieve patency of the choana.

SUGGESTED READINGS

1. Gujrathi CS, Daniel SJ, James AL, Forte V: Management of bilateral choanal atresia in the neonate: An institutional review. Int J Ped Otorhinolaryngol 68:399–407, 2004. **A 10-year, 54-patient retrospective review that concludes that the puncture, dilation, and stenting technique is preferred despite advances in endoscopic technology.**
2. Josephson GD, Vickery CL, Giles WC, et al: Transnasal endoscopic repair of congenital choanal atresia: Long-term results. Arch Otolaryngol Head Neck Surg 124:537–540, 1998. **Supports the endoscopic transnasal route and suggests that the use of newer powered instrumentation further improves efficacy.**
3. Khafagy YW: Endoscopic repair of bilateral congenital choanal atresia. Laryngoscope 112:316–319, 2002. **Transnasal endoscopic treatment is safe and effective treatment for bilateral choanal atresia.**
4. Prasad M, Ward RF, April MM, et al: Topical mitomycin as an adjunct to choanal atresia repair. Arch Otolaryngol Head Neck Surg 128:398–400, 2002. **Study showing that mitomycin used as an adjunct can improve patency and decrease the need for stenting and revision surgery.**
5. Rahbar R, Jones DT, Nuss RC, et al: The role of mitomycin in the prevention and treatment of scar formation in the pediatric aerodigestive tract: Friend or foe? Arch Otolaryngol Head Neck Surg 128:401–406, 2002. **Concludes that topical mitomycin is effective in the prevention of scar formation in the aerodigestive tract.**
6. Samadi DS, Shah UK, Handler SD, et al: Choanal atresia: A twenty-year review of medical comorbidities and surgical outcomes. Laryngoscope 113:254–258, 2003. **A review of 78 patients to assess outcomes and morbidities in choanal atresia. This report has the largest series of patients with choanal atresia studied to date.**

7. Van Den Abbeele T, Francois M, Narcy P: Transnasal endoscopic treatment of choanal atresia without prolonged stenting. Arch Otolaryngol Head Neck Surg 128:936–940, 2002. **A report that asserts transnasal endoscopic repair with some postoperative revision can avoid prolonged stenting and is a safe and successful technique.**

Tumors and Polyps of the Nose

Udayan K. Shah and Lawrence W.C. Tom

KEY CONCEPTS

- Management of nasal polyposis requires medical therapy in addition to endoscopic surgery.
- Radiologic image guidance for surgical excision of nasal tumors may allow for more complete excision and less morbid surgery.
- The techniques of skull base and craniofacial surgery permit less morbid surgical management of extensive lesions of the paranasal sinuses and nasopharynx.
- Postoperative surveillance for recurrence may require imaging or examination under anesthesia.

Most tumors and polyps of the nose and nasopharynx in children are benign and limited, and surgical management is both straightforward and curative. Rarely, malignant and/or extensive lesions require therapy and are accompanied by a guarded long-term prognosis.

History, Examination, and Radiologic Examination

HISTORY

Gradual nasal airway obstruction accompanied by loss of smell and taste are common complaints. Rhinitis and sinusitis may be seen. Cheek pressure, tearing, or blurry vision may be reported by patients with extensive lesions. Epistaxis is seen with vascular lesions.

EXAMINATION

Physical examination by anterior rhinoscopy may be performed with a nasal speculum or an otoscope. Optimal examination requires a flexible or rigid endoscope. Palpation may differentiate a cystic from a solid lesion. Office biopsy is not recommended. Large ethmoid or congenital midline nasal lesions may cause widening of the nasal dorsum. Large maxillary or lateral nasal wall lesions may cause bulging of the anterior wall of the maxillary sinus (identified by cheek fullness or by obliteration of the sulcus between the upper lip and gum), hypesthesia of the cheek, and/or epiphora. Lesions extending into the nasopharynx may displace the soft palate or may be visible behind the uvula.

RADIOLOGIC EXAMINATION

Diagnostic imaging demonstrates the extent of a lesion and permits tissue characterization. CT without intravenous contrast is the current standard for imaging most lesions of the paranasal sinuses. CT scanning may be performed in anticipation of upcoming surgery, using specific protocols designated for image-guided surgery. MRI is less useful unless there is a concern for intracranial or ophthalmic complications. MRI with contrast enhancement using gadolinium is indicated for such complicated lesions.

Postoperative radiologic imaging for surveillance of recurrence may be required because of the aggressiveness of some lesions, or because of the difficulty and limited visibility of the office examination.

Benign Tumors/Nasal Polyps

The most common nasal tumor in children is a nasal polyp (NP) consisting of a sac of respiratory epithelium encasing a viscous fibromucoid stroma. Nasal airway obstruction and loss of smell and taste are common complaints. Symptoms of environmental allergies should be sought. A history of aspirin sensitivity, along with asthma and nasal polyps, indicates Samter triad, a more aggressive form of nasal polyposis.

Physical examination shows a pale, grape-like translucent rounded mass in the nose. Although a single NP may occur, more commonly NPs are multiple and bilateral. An NP may also be extensive, in the form of an antrochoanal polyp, which originates from the medial wall of the maxillary sinus and extends into the nose and then the nasopharynx. A large antrochoanal polyp may be seen behind the soft palate by oral examination.

Because up to two thirds of children with cystic fibrosis have NP, a test for cystic fibrosis should be performed for children with NP, by genetic testing or a sweat chloride test. Radiologic imaging shows medial bowing of the maxillary sinus walls. Poor pneumatization of the maxillary and ethmoid sinuses is seen because of chronic inflammation. Nasal obstruction, mouth breathing, snoring, chronic cough, and worsening pulmonary function despite maximal medical therapy are indications for endoscopic sinus surgery (ESS). Pulmonary function improves following ESS for NP in children with cystic fibrosis.

Expert Opinion on Management Issues

Medical management of NP is rarely curative but may alleviate symptoms of facial pain or pressure, headache, nasal obstruction, and loss of smell; it also may reduce the frequency and severity of acute sinusitis related to NP. Nasal and oral steroids, immunotherapy (shots), and antihistaminic or antileukotriene medications may be useful prior to considering surgery.

Medical management reduces surgical morbidity by reducing the amount of bleeding during surgical dissection and by reducing postoperative scarring.

19

SURGICAL MANAGEMENT

Removal of NP is accomplished by ESS. Removed tissue should be sent for histopathologic evaluation. Antrochoanal polyps require surgical removal of the origin of the polyp from the maxillary sinus. Extensive polyposis may require an open surgical approach.

After surgery, nasal saline and topical nasal steroids are used to reduce scarring and recurrence of polyps. An overall recurrence rate for NP of approximately 20% indicates the need for careful office evaluation after surgery.

CONGENITAL NASAL TUMORS

Encephaloceles, gliomas, and nasal dermoids are embryonic remnants that usually manifest in the nasal midline. Encephaloceles manifest as cystic masses that may enlarge with crying or straining and that contain cerebrospinal fluid. Gliomas represent persistent neural crest tissue that failed to resorb into the cranial vault. Dermoids usually present as a hair-bearing midline nasal pit. Both gliomas and dermoids have up to a 25% incidence of intracranial extension. Radiologic imaging determines the extent of intracranial involvement. The treatment is surgical.

FIBRO-OSSEOUS TUMORS

Fibromas, osteomas, giant cell granulomas, fibrous dysplasia, and the brown tumor of hyperparathyroidism are benign lesions that may occur in the nose and cause nasal obstruction, and facial or nasal deformity. Endocrinologic evaluation is required in cases of hyperparathyroidism and for the McCune-Albright syndrome (polyostotic fibrous dysplasia, precocious puberty, and cutaneous hyperpigmentation). Surgical resection may be curative; debulking of the tumor may allow for symptomatic palliation.

VASCULAR TUMORS

Benign vascular neoplasms such as hemangiomas are common on the skin of the nasal dorsum. Management is usually expectant, as their natural history is involution by 6 years of age. Immediate treatment is required for hemangiomas that cause visual impairment, airway obstruction, platelet-trapping coagulopathy (Kasabach-Merritt syndrome), or high-output cardiac failure. These lesions usually respond to high-dose corticosteroid treatment. Hemangiomas, which are refractory to systemic corticosteroids, may be treated with intralesional corticosteroid injections, interferon, laser therapy, or surgery.

Lymphangiomas also occur in the nasal region and do not involute. Lymphangiomas usually require surgical excision to maintain the airway and reduce cosmetic deformity.

ANGIOFIBROMA

Juvenile nasal angiofibroma (JNA) is a tumor that usually manifests with unilateral nasal obstruction and epistaxis in a teenage boy. Physical examination reveals a lobulated, red-pink mass. A contrast-enhanced CT scan shows the bony limits of the tumor, and MRI with gadolinium allows better prediction of CNS or orbital invasion. The vascularity of this lesion precludes safe biopsy before surgical resection. Surgical resection is required for cure. Angiographic embolization is usually performed before surgery to reduce intraoperative bleeding. Estrogen treatment may reduce the vascular component but is not curative.

MALIGNANT TUMORS

A unilateral nasal mass that is irregular and friable is suggestive of malignancy. The patient may experience severe facial pain, cranial neuropathy, or overlying bone or skin changes. A less common presentation of nasal malignancy is persistent opacification of a single paranasal sinus on CT or MRI. Constitutional symptoms of lethargy, malaise, weight loss, night sweats, and low-grade fevers may also be present. Unilateral serous otitis media may be seen because of eustachian tube obstruction. Radiographic characterization and tissue biopsy are required before definitive therapy. A wide range of tumors may occur in the nasal region. In addition to the lesions detailed below, children may require treatment for fibrosarcoma, leiomyosarcoma, chondrosarcoma, and adenocarcinoma. Metastatic spread to the nasal vault from other tumors may also occur. Appropriate therapy requires consideration of histopathologic and anatomic stage and grade, comorbid conditions, and the effects of therapies on adjacent organs (CNS and the eyes). The goal of treatment is to optimize long-term survival while maintaining the quality of life and to permit normal growth and function of craniofacial structures.

Nasopharyngeal Carcinoma

Nasopharyngeal carcinoma (NPCa) is an Epstein-Barr virus (EBV)-related malignancy that accounts for one third of pediatric nasopharyngeal neoplasms. Tumors manifest with nasal obstruction, epistaxis, rhinorrhea, otalgia and hearing loss from eustachian tube obstruction, and, because of advanced stages at presentation, often with a neck mass. Cranial neuropathies are common.

Physical examination may show only mucosal bulging, although extensive lesions are lobulated and may be friable. CT and MRI provide complementary information on the extent of disease, and tissue biopsy allows histopathologic classification of the neoplasm into the World Health Organization's staging system for NPCa that is predictive of survival. EBV markers of a specific tumor also may guide therapy. Following tissue diagnosis, chest, abdomen, and bone scanning allow for an assessment of metastasis. CNS involvement may require an examination of the cerebrospinal fluid.

Radiotherapy of the primary site and nodal pathways is the primary mode of therapy. Chemotherapy is used for systemic disease. Surgery is reserved for residual or recurrent disease and may have a greater role in the future, as skull-base surgical techniques are refined.

Rhabdomyosarcoma

Most pediatric rhabdomyosarcoma (RMS) manifests in the head and neck, particularly in the parameningeal sites, such as the paranasal sinuses. Accurate histopathologic evaluation requires assessment of tumor markers. Combined chemotherapy and radiotherapy with the selective use of surgery for excision or debulking has resulted in improved survival rates, with more than a 70% survival rate for the most common types of pediatric head and neck RMS. Although all children require some combination of chemotherapy and radiotherapy, surgical excision is most often advocated for small tumors, cancers that are responding poorly to chemotherapy and radiotherapy, and residual or recurrent disease. There is no routine role for surgical removal of lymph nodes in the neck. Improved supportive care, with parenteral nutrition and better antibacterial and antifungal medications, in addition to advanced surgical techniques for excision and reconstruction are credited with the reduced morbidity of treatment. Careful surveillance post-treatment is essential because of the risk of recurrence.

Esthesioneuroblastoma

Endoscopic and intracranial techniques are used to surgically resect this tumor at the superior aspect of the nasal vault, at the junction between the sinonasal cavity and the brain. Radiotherapy is required postoperatively.

Common Pitfalls

The correct histopathologic diagnosis is critical to the management of tumors of the nasal region. In some cases, repeat biopsy and consultative review of histopathologic specimens by pathologists experienced in otolaryngic pathology may be warranted.

Physical examination of subtle lesions may be difficult. Repeated examinations, under anesthesia if necessary, and tissue biopsy of selected nasopharyngeal sites may be warranted when there is a high index of suspicion of neoplasia.

Communication and Counseling

Medical management must be stressed for most lesions of the nose. Inappropriate use of adrenergic agents such as oxymetazoline or phenylephrine nasal sprays, in an attempt to treat nasal obstruction, may instead worsen nasal congestion. Inadequate use of nasal saline may allow allergens and secretions to block the nasal airway and limit the transmucosal delivery of other nasal sprays.

Families' concerns over the likelihood of malignancy must be realistically addressed from the outset. This requires an understanding by the provider of the variable clinical presentations of the wide variety of possible nasal lesions. Similarly, families benefit from understanding early on in the management of nasal lesions that surgical biopsy and therapy are likely, that surgery often can be accomplished today by endoscopic rather than by open techniques (limiting morbidity and allowing for a faster return to activities), and that recurrence of benign lesions such as NP may be seen.

SELECTED READINGS

1. Constantinidis J, Steinhart H, Koch M, et al: Olfactory neuroblastoma: The University of Erlangen-Nuremberg experience 1975–2000. Otolaryngol Head Neck Surg 130:567–574, 2004. **This series spans a long time frame, during which advanced surgical techniques and chemotherapeutic regimens have changed.**
2. Daya H, Chan HSL, Sirkin W, Forte V: Pediatric rhabdomyosarcoma of the head and neck. Arch Otolaryngol Head Neck Surg 126:468–472, 2000. **Recent update on management and morbidities.**
3. Halvorson DJ: Cystic fibrosis: An update for the otolaryngologist. Otolaryngol Head Neck Surg 120:502–506, 1999. **This review article summarizes cystic fibrosis as it pertains to the otolaryngologic role, particularly with respect to sinus surgery.**
4. Rahbar R, Resto VA, Robson CD, et al: Nasal glioma and encephalocele: Diagnosis and management. Laryngoscope 113:2069–2077, 2003. **This review article presents a well-written discussion of the pathophysiology and clinical presentation of nasal gliomas and encephalocele. Endoscopic views of these lesions are complemented by histopathologic and radiographic images.**

19

Foreign Bodies in the Ears, Nose, and Pharynx

Lawrence W. C. Tom and Udayan K. Shah

KEY CONCEPTS

- The first attempt at removal is the one most likely to be successful. If the foreign body cannot be removed easily, referral is recommended.
- A superior light source is necessary. A hand-held light or otoscope may be used for diagnosis, but a fiberoptic head light or operating microscope is preferred for the removal because it provides superior illumination and frees both hands.
- Children must be adequately immobilized. This may be accomplished with parental or nursing help, a papoose board, sedation, and/or general anesthesia.
- The proper instruments for removal must be readily available before attempting removal.
- To ensure optimal visualization, the orifice should be cleaned thoroughly before beginning the removal.
- With a suspected pharyngeal foreign body, the physician must first assess the adequacy of the airway.

Children are naturally inquisitive, and this curiosity often leads to the insertion of foreign bodies into the ears, nose, and mouth. Although most of these objects do not pose serious problems, some require immediate removal and others can be life-threatening. Regardless of the object or anatomic site, following basic principles increases the chances of safe, successful removal. Box 1 lists the clinical presentation of foreign bodies.

The first attempt at removal is the most likely to be successful. Initially, children tend to be more cooperative, but once they have experienced discomfort, they become apprehensive and less cooperative. The site may become traumatized, causing bleeding and edema. This may reduce visualization and increase the risk of complications. Once the diagnosis of a foreign body has been made, the physician must decide whether it can be easily and safely removed. If it cannot, referral to an emergency department or otolaryngologist is recommended.

Proper planning and preparation are essential for safe removal, and the key elements are illumination, immobilization, visualization, and instrumentation. Before beginning the removal, all of these conditions should be met.

Expert Opinion on Management Issues

EAR FOREIGN BODIES

Ear foreign bodies are common in children. Most are asymptomatic and are usually discovered during an otoscopic examination. They include beads, earrings, small toys, paper, cotton, pieces of earplugs, beans, insects, and disc batteries.

Because most ear foreign bodies are not emergencies, the physician should optimize the conditions to facilitate removal. An otoscopic examination establishes the shape and location of the object. With a superior light source and the child immobilized, the physician can assess the ease of and the best method for removal. Objects lateral to the isthmus of the ear canal are easier to remove. Objects medial to the isthmus are more difficult to remove, and there is a greater risk for injury to the ear canal, tympanic membrane, and middle-ear structures. Foreign bodies with a leading edge may be grasped with an alligator or Hartman forceps. Round objects are difficult to grasp. A curette or hook can be advanced beyond the object that is rolled out with the instrument. Suctioning and irrigation are other techniques. If attempted removal is likely to be difficult, to cause injury, or to require special instruments such as a microscope, the child should be referred to an otolaryngologist.

Disc and button batteries must be removed emergently. The electrical current and alkaline leakage from the battery causes liquefaction necrosis and damage to the surrounding tissue. Irrigation is contraindicated because it will accelerate the leakage of alkaline solution. Live insects may enter the ear canal causing irritation and pain. If an insect is forcibly removed,

body parts may become embedded within the canal skin. Prior to removal, the insect is killed by instilling mineral oil, alcohol, or lidocaine into the canal.

A child with an ear foreign body who complains of vertigo or demonstrates nystagmus should be immediately referred to an otolaryngologist. There is a good possibility that the cochlea or vestibular apparatus has been injured. In addition to removing the object, the middle ear may have to be explored for a fistula.

After the foreign body is removed, the entire ear is carefully examined. Small abrasions and lacerations usually heal spontaneously, whereas infections should be treated with antibiotic otic drops. Children with tympanic membrane perforations, infections, and significant soft tissue injury must be re-examined. If a perforation persists or there is a suspicion of hearing loss, an audiologic evaluation is performed.

NASAL FOREIGN BODIES

Nasal foreign bodies in children are common. The insertion may be witnessed, but often it is suspected only after the development of the classic symptoms of unilateral obstruction and foul-smelling, purulent rhinorrhea. Any child with these symptoms (unilateral or bilateral) must be assumed to have a nasal foreign body.

The patient is first immobilized, usually with a papoose board. The child's head is elevated to decrease the chances of aspiration of the foreign body, blood, and secretions. Using a headlight, the nasal cavities are examined. Blood and secretions must be suctioned. Topical decongestants may help reduce mucosal swelling and improve visualization. Nasal foreign bodies should be removed either by grasping with a forceps or pulling the object, or by rolling it out of the nasal cavity with a hook or curette. If no object is identified, a flexible fiberoptic scope is introduced into the nasal cavities and advanced to the foreign body or until the

---

BOX 1 Clinical Presentation of Foreign Bodies

Ear
- Asymptomatic (most common)
- Aural fullness
- Pain
- Discomfort
- Hearing loss
- Vertigo
- Nystagmus

Nose
- Unilateral obstruction
- Unilateral, foul smelling, purulent rhinorrhea

Pharynx
- Choking
- Drooling
- Dysphagia
- Odynophagia
- Refusal to eat
- Hoarseness
- Aphonia
- Respiratory distress

nasopharynx is visualized. No attempt is made to remove a posterior nasal foreign body in the office or emergency department.

After the foreign body is removed, the other nostril is examined. Any epistaxis is controlled. Infection or secondary inflammation should resolve after the object is removed. If there has been significant trauma or infection, antibiotics are administered.

PHARYNGEAL FOREIGN BODIES

Foreign bodies of the pharynx are uncommon. The tongue and gag reflex expel many of them, and others pass into the esophagus or tracheobronchial tree. Children younger than 6 years of age are at greater risk because they lack molars for chewing. When pharyngeal foreign bodies occur, there is the potential for fatal consequences from airway obstruction. Conforming objects such as latex balloons and spherical objects such as pieces of hot dog, grapes, popcorn, and small balls are the most dangerous. These objects remain a leading cause of accidental deaths in children under 6 years.

The clinical presentation of a pharyngeal foreign body includes choking, stridor, respiratory distress, hoarseness, aphonia, drooling, odynophagia, dysphagia, and refusal to eat. The initial step in the evaluation of a child with a pharyngeal foreign body is an assessment of the airway. Respiratory distress and difficulty with phonation are signs of airway compromise, and attempts must be made to dislodge the object immediately. If the child is able to stand, a subdiaphragmatic thrust (Heimlich maneuver) should be tried. In young children, blows to the back followed by blows to the chest may expel the object.

If the airway is adequate, the child should be positioned and secured properly, and with adequate illumination, the oral cavity and pharynx should be examined. A flexible fiberoptic scope aids in examination of the distal pharynx and helps to establish the relationship between the object and the laryngeal inlet. If the object is accessible and will not compromise the airway, it may be removed with the proper instruments. This often applies to fish bones that lodge in the tongue or tonsils and can be removed with forceps. Care must be taken to avoid pushing the foreign body farther into the airway and causing obstruction. If the object may potentially obstruct the airway or cannot be visualized, the patient should be referred to an otolaryngologist.

Common Pitfalls

Although irrigation can be used to remove foreign bodies of the ear, it is contraindicated in children with perforated eardrums and ventilating tubes; for hydrophilic, organic objects such as dried beans and peas, which swell with moisture; and for batteries, for which moisture enhances the leakage of the alkaline solution, increasing tissue injury. If the stream of water is directed at the eardrum, a perforation may occur.

Nasal foreign bodies should never be pushed or irrigated. The object may be dislodged posteriorly and aspirated into the larynx or tracheobronchial tree, converting a nonemergent condition into an airway emergency. Irrigation causes hydroscopic objects to swell, and with batteries increases the leakage of alkaline solution and the likelihood of soft tissue and cartilage injury. As in the ear, batteries in the nasal cavity are removed immediately.

Although conscious sedation has been used to facilitate the removal of nasal foreign bodies, sedation decreases the laryngeal reflexes, increasing the risk of aspiration. If the foreign body is difficult to remove, has associated granulation tissue, or is suspected but not visualized, it is safer to remove the object under general anesthesia.

With pharyngeal foreign bodies, the greatest risk is life-threatening airway obstruction. No attempt should be made to remove objects that may potentially obstruct the airway in patients without airway compromise.

Communication and Counseling

Although insertion of foreign bodies into the ears and nose may be unavoidable, pharyngeal foreign bodies may be prevented. Education and counseling may increase parental awareness of the dangers of certain foods and toys such as hot dogs, popcorn, grapes, and balloons.

Once a foreign body is diagnosed, the physician must have the appropriate instruments and control of the patient necessary for removal. If not, attempted removal is unlikely to succeed. At best, this will result in patient apprehension making future attempts more difficult; at worst, it will lead to serious or even life-threatening complications.

SUGGESTED READINGS

1. Bressler K, Shelton C: Ear foreign-body removal: A review of 98 consecutive cases. Laryngoscope 103:367–370, 1983. **Reviewing 98 consecutive cases of ear foreign bodies managed in a tertiary care emergency room by otolaryngologists, the authors found that 61% of patients with previous attempt at removal suffered ear canal trauma. They recommend referral to an otolaryngologist when the object is not easily removed.**
2. Jones NS, Lanigan FJ, Salama NY: Foreign bodies in the throat: A prospective study of 388 cases. J Laryngol Otolaryngol 105:104–108, 1991. **A prospective study of 388 cases indicates that careful examination of the oral cavity and oropharynx and laryngoscopy are the best means for evaluation of a pharyngeal foreign body. Radiography is rarely helpful.**
3. Lin VYW, Daniel SJ, Papsin BC: Button batteries in the ear, nose and upper aerodigestive tract. Int J Pediatr Otolaryngol 68:473–479, 2004. **This review of button batteries in the ear, nose, and throat emphasizes the need for rapid diagnosis and treatment for prevention of serious complications.**
4. Rimell FL, Thome A Jr, Stool S, et al: Characteristics of objects that cause choking in children. JAMA 274:1763–1766, 1995. **This study analyzes two distinct groups of children. In the group 165 children who underwent endoscopy for foreign body aspiration or ingestion, food, or coins were most common. In the group of 449 children who died from asphyxiation of foreign bodies, conforming objects, particularly balloons, were responsible for the majority of deaths.**

5. Tong MC, Van Hasselt CA, Woo JK: The hazards of button batteries in the nose. J Otolaryngol 21:458–460, 1992. **This is an analysis of the complications occurring in 7 children who had button battery impaction in the nose.**
6. Tong MC, Ying SY, Van Hasselt CA: Nasal foreign bodies in children. Int J Pediatr Otolaryngol 35:207–211, 1996. **This study investigated 147 children with nasal foreign bodies. Most children had successful, uneventful removal. Most complications were related to attempts at removal. Ten percent of the objects were button batteries.**

Pediatric Rhinitis and Acute and Chronic Sinusitis

Mark G. Shrime and Jeffrey L. Keller

KEY CONCEPTS

- Allergic rhinitis is a clinical diagnosis based on symptoms of rhinorrhea, nasal pruritus, nasal congestion, and sneezing. Treatment includes allergen avoidance, antihistamines, topical steroids, and possible immunotherapy.
- Acute bacterial sinusitis is diagnosed based on the presence of major and minor criteria and the duration of symptoms. Its treatment includes antibiotics and decongestants. Adjuvant therapy is controversial, although potentially helpful.
- Imaging is of limited use in the pediatric patient with rhinitis or sinusitis.
- Surgery is reserved for patients with complications of sinusitis or those for whom medical therapy has failed.
- Parents should be counseled regarding the natural course of upper respiratory illnesses, the directed use of antibiotics, and the problem of increasing resistance.

Upper respiratory tract symptoms are the most common reason for visits to the pediatrician's office, with acute sinusitis now the fifth most common diagnosis leading to the prescription of antibiotics in children. In addition, the prevalence of atopy and its related respiratory diseases (asthma, allergic rhinitis) has increased in the last few decades.

Rhinitis manifests with a range of symptoms in children: cough, sneezing, rhinorrhea, nasal congestion, nasal pruritus, halitosis, and hyponasality. Its pathophysiology can be divided into conditions of allergic origin and those without (e.g., vasomotor rhinitis, ciliary dysmotility); the latter are beyond the scope of this chapter. Allergic rhinitis, in addition to affecting quality of life, has been postulated to be a distinct manifestation of the same inflammatory process that causes asthma. In population studies, allergic rhinitis often precedes asthma, and effective treatment of allergic rhinitis correlates with a decrease in the use of health care resources (including visits to the emergency department) for asthma.

Of the four paranasal sinuses, only the maxillary and anterior ethmoid sinuses are present at birth; they are, unsurprisingly, the most common site of sinus-related pathophysiology in children. The sphenoid sinus begins its development at the second or third year of life and the frontal sinus by the age of eight. Both are not completely pneumatized until late adolescence. The functions of the paranasal sinuses are disputed. Possibilities include air exchange, shock absorption, olfaction, humidification of inspired air, a lessening of the weight of the skull, and vocal resonance.

Normal function of the paranasal sinuses requires three elements: patent ostia, functioning cilia, and normal quantity and quality of mucoid secretions. Impairment in any of the three can lead to sinusitis. Reviews of sinus computed tomography (CT) scans in children with and without sinusitis have demonstrated no consistent difference in the bony anatomy of the affected patients—the pathophysiology of sinusitis, therefore, has more to do with functional obstruction of the ostia and deficits in mucociliary clearance than it does with anatomic anomalies.

The clinical diagnosis of acute sinusitis is often complicated by the increased incidence of acute upper respiratory tract infections in children and the prevalence of asymptomatic *Streptococcus pneumoniae* carriage (in up to 8.5% of healthy children). Children have between 6 and 10 episodes of viral rhinosinusitis a year, with any of several symptoms, including nasal congestion, sneezing, rhinorrhea, hyposmia/anosmia, facial pressure, postnasal drip, sore throat, cough, otalgia/aural fullness, fever and myalgia; many of these symptoms are classically associated with the diagnosis of sinusitis. Bacterial superinfection may occur at any point in the course of a viral rhinosinusitis—a change in the color of the mucus does not correlate with a sensitive predictor of superinfection, but it is most likely if the symptoms have persisted for more than 10 days. As a result, most authors favor this cutoff for the definition of acute sinusitis.

Formal diagnosis of acute sinusitis requires the presence of two major criteria or one major criterion and two minor criteria (Box 1). Note that facial pain/pressure alone does not constitute a good history of sinusitis in the absence of other criteria. There are five manifestations of sinusitis, divided by time course (Box 2). The proposed five-axis system for the classification of sinusitis is:

1. Clinical presentation (acute, subacute, and chronic)
2. Location (ethmoid, frontal, sphenoid, and maxillary)
3. Organism (bacterial, viral, and fungal)
4. Complications by extra-sinus involvement
5. Aggravating factors

A patient could have a diagnosis of acute bacterial ethmoid sinusitis complicated by periorbital extension, aggravated by immunosuppression. It is important to note that rhinitis and sinusitis often exist together.

<table>
<tr><td>

BOX 1 Major and Minor Criteria in the Diagnosis of Sinusitis

Major Criteria
- Facial pain/pressure
- Facial congestion/fullness
- Nasal obstruction
- Discolored nasal discharge/postnasal drip
- Hyposmia/anosmia
- Purulence on nasal examination
- Fever (acute sinusitis only)

Minor Criteria
- Headache
- Fever (all nonacute sinusitis)
- Halitosis
- Fatigue
- Dental pain
- Cough
- Otalgia/aural fullness

</td></tr>
</table>

BOX 2 Definitions of Sinusitis

Acute sinusitis: Symptoms present between 10 days and 4 weeks.
Subacute sinusitis: Symptoms present between 4 and 12 weeks.
Recurrent acute sinusitis: Episodes of acute sinusitis (each episode lasting <4 weeks) separated by symptom-free intervals of at least 10 days.
Chronic sinusitis: Symptoms persistent >12 weeks.
Acute-on-chronic sinusitis: The development of new symptoms of sinusitis in patients with the diagnosis of chronic sinusitis.

Expert Opinion on Management Issues

ALLERGIC RHINITIS

Because of the possible risks that steroids pose, a treatment stratagem that minimizes their use as much as possible is preferred. First-line therapy for any allergic disease is avoidance of the allergen. Because dust mites and pet dander are the most common culprits, the corpus of the literature has been focused on them. Unfortunately, the avoidance of pets is often unacceptable, and the various conservative measures for avoidance of dust (e.g., pillow and mattress covers) have not had significant clinical utility. Regardless, the avoidance of cockroach antigens (through frequent house cleaning), animal dander, cigarette smoke, fresh paint, perfumes, fog, smog, and pollen can halt the development of allergic rhinitis symptoms. It is interesting to note, however, that exposure during early childhood to a large family, pets, and farm animals protects against the development of allergic rhinitis.

In the absence of avoidance, appeal is then made to pharmacotherapy. The classic pharmacologic trinity includes antihistamines, decongestants, and corticosteroids, and, although some patients benefit from single-modality therapy, the majority require a combination approach. Decongestants are of limited long-term use secondary to tachyphylaxis and are fraught with complications including tachycardia, rebound nasal congestion, and rhinitis medicamentosa.

Antihistamines are generally effective for the symptoms of itching, rhinorrhea, and sneezing. However, the first-generation antihistamines are notoriously sedating and correlate with a decrease in the low quality of life in patients with rhinosinusitis. Second-generation antihistamines are largely, though not reliably, nonsedating. Desloratadine and cetirizine have been approved for use in children as young as 6 months of age, and fexofenadine and loratadine are approved for children older than the ages of 6 and 2, respectively. Nasal antihistamines are of theoretical benefit as well, but their clinical utility has not been assessed.

Systemic corticosteroids have multiple potentially serious side effects, including avascular femoral necrosis, glaucoma and cataracts, immunosuppression, suppression of the hypothalamic-pituitary-adrenal axis, and, most worrisome in children, growth retardation. In short-, intermediate-, and long-term studies, however, intranasal and inhaled corticosteroids have had no significant effect on lower-leg growth in children. There is a concern, however, in children with atopy who are also taking inhaled and transdermal corticosteroids. In a prospective cohort study of children with asthma treated with inhaled budesonide, approximately 30% also used intranasal budesonide for rhinitis. There was no significant change in the adult height in patients who used budesonide versus those who had never used it, nor was there a difference between predicted target and actual adult heights in the budesonide users. Because of the possibility (and occasional case report) of adverse side effects, however, the lowest possible dose of steroids should be used.

The cromones (sodium cromoglycate is the intranasal version) are less effective in the treatment of symptoms than intranasal corticosteroids, but may be beneficial in patients in whom the possible dysphonia that can result from intranasal and inhaled corticosteroids is unacceptable.

SINUSITIS

CT has become the accepted imaging modality in the diagnosis of acute or chronic sinusitis. CT scanning has approximately a 90% negative predictive value, but a positive predictive value of only 40% to 85% in children with clinical sinusitis. Moreover, the correlation between CT findings of sinusitis (mucosal thickening, hyperostosis, air-fluid levels) and the presence of symptoms has been difficult to establish. Therefore, most authors and the American Academy of Pediatrics (AAP) favor limiting the use of adjunct imaging studies to children older than the age of 6 years or those for whom operative intervention is planned.

Treatment for sinusitis encompasses surgical and nonsurgical modalities. The microbiology of acute, subacute, and chronic sinusitis, however, has been well described. In children with acute sinusitis, *S. pneumoniae* is recovered in 35% to 42% of aspirates, nontypeable *Haemophilus influenzae* in 21% to 28%, *Moraxella catarrhalis* in 21% to 28%, *Streptococcus pyogenes* in 3% to 7%, and anaerobes in 3% to 7%. The microbiology changes in favor of the anaerobes with increased chronicity of disease. In a study of aspirates of acutely and chronically infected sphenoid sinuses, 43% of aspirates contained anaerobes alone, 14% contained aerobic and facultative organisms alone, and 43% contained mixed aerobic and anaerobic isolates. Predominant aerobes included *Klebsiella pneumoniae*, *Escherichia coli*, and *Pseudomonas aeruginosa*; whereas *Peptostreptococcus* species, *Prevotella* species, and *Fusobacterium* species were the most common anaerobes. The aerobic bacteria implicated in acute sinusitis, as well as *Staphylococcus aureus*, coagulase-negative *Staphylococcus*, and *Neisseria* have been isolated from aspirates of maxillary sinuses in children with chronic sinusitis.

In the choice of an antimicrobial agent, it is important to remember that the majority of isolates of *S. pneumoniae* (45%–55%), *H. influenzae* (50%), and *M. catarrhalis* (100%) are resistant to penicillin. Although 60% to 80% of acute sinusitis episodes resolve within 4 weeks without antibiotics, there is strong consensus in the literature that acute rhinosinusitis should be treated with an antibacterial to increase the speed of resolution and decrease the amount of mucosal damage sustained. The Sinus and Allergy Health Partnership and the AAP both recommend amoxicillin/clavulanate, high-dose amoxicillin (80–90 mg/kg/d), cefpodoxime proxetil, or cefuroxime axetil as initial therapy for children with acute sinusitis who have not received antibiotics in the previous 4 to 6 weeks (the AAP recommendations also include amoxicillin at 40–45 mg/kg/day, although in the presence of documented high rates of resistance this treatment should probably be avoided). In the presence of type I hypersensitivity to penicillin derivatives, the recommendations include azithromycin, clarithromycin, erythromycin, or sulfamethoxazole/trimethoprim. Failure rates with these modalities run from 20% to 38%.

In children with prior antibiotic use, clindamycin should be added. Children with moderate disease should receive coverage for gram-positive organisms in the form of high-dose amoxicillin/clavulanate plus gram-negative coverage in the form of cefpodoxime proxetil or cefixime. The duration of any therapy should extend at least 10 to 14 days, although some published recommendations extend therapy as long as 6 weeks.

The pathophysiology of chronic sinusitis is more complicated, with bacteriology playing only a contributory role. As a result, treatment with antimicrobials is more controversial. Two placebo-controlled trials have addressed this issue in children (one unfortunately assessing low-dose amoxicillin and the other cefaclor). In neither study was there significant difference in improvement with antibiotics versus placebo. Because of the chronic inflammatory nature of this disease process, intranasal corticosteroids could be of potential benefit, although there is no placebo-controlled randomized clinical trial evaluating their effectiveness. Referral to an otolaryngologist should be considered.

The use of adjuvant therapy (nasal saline irrigations, decongestants, intranasal steroids) in either acute or chronic sinusitis is controversial. One prospective study evaluating fluticasone propionate (two puffs of 50 μg/100 mL in each nostril once daily), 0.05% oxymetazoline (one puff in each nostril three times a day), 3% sodium chloride, and 0.9% sodium chloride nasal irrigations against placebo on mucociliary clearance in adults with acute sinusitis did demonstrate an increase in mucociliary clearance in the 3% saline and oxymetazoline groups, but no correlation was made to clinical improvement. Other studies have suggested a benefit in acute bacterial sinusitis from the adjunct use of intranasal steroids, but the benefit is moderate at best.

SURGERY

A consensus statement on pediatric sinus surgery, published in 1996, delineates extranasal complications of sinusitis (see later), sinonasal malformations, and the need for access to the skull base as absolute indications for sinus surgery; a diagnosis of chronic sinusitis is listed as only a possible indication. Sinus surgery should be reserved for patients who have demonstrably failed maximal medical therapy. Many authors also recommend adenoidectomy prior to formal endoscopic sinus surgery.

COMPLICATIONS

Acute sinusitis can be complicated by extension intracranially and intraocularly. Intracranial complications are rare but can include subdural/epidural abscesses, meningitis, and intraparenchymal abscesses. Ocular complications have been classified by Chandler (Box 3). These manifest with gradually worsening eyelid edema and erythema, cheilosis, limitation of extraocular mobility, proptosis, decreasing vision, and pupillary defects, secondary to both direct extension and hematogenous spread through valveless veins in the face. Both intracranial and ocular complications are indications for aggressive treatment, including surgical drainage.

Other, less emergent complications of sinusitis include oroantral fistulae and dental sequelae.

BOX 3 Ocular Complications of Acute Sinusitis

Stage I: Preseptal cellulitis
Stage II: Orbital cellulitis
Stage III: Subperiosteal abscess
Stage IV: Orbital abscess
Stage V: Cavernous sinus thrombosis

Common Pitfalls

- The overuse of antibiotics, especially in patients without actual sinusitis, and inappropriate choices of antimicrobials promote the selection of resistant organisms.
- Undertreatment prior to referral for surgery places patients at undue risk for a potentially medically treatable condition.
- Overuse of local decongestants leads to rhinitis medicamentosa and rebound nasal congestion.
- Delay in the recognition of extranasal complications of sinusitis is potentially fatal.

Because of the difficulty in diagnosis surrounding pediatric rhinosinusitis, the clinician is faced with two potential pitfalls, both surrounding the use of antibiotics. There is the temptation among many primary care physicians to prescribe antibiotics for any child presenting with "purulent" (usually defined by color) rhinorrhea. This practice leads to increased resistance. On the other hand, referring a patient to surgery who has yet to receive maximal medical therapy subjects the patient to undue risk. Failure to recognize and aggressively treat intracranial or ocular complications also puts patients at undue risk. The progression from preseptal cellulitis to cavernous sinus thrombosis, which has a significant mortality rate, can be rapid.

Communication and Counseling

Most children with acute viral upper respiratory infections resolve without any intervention. Those who continue to be symptomatic after 10 days or whose symptoms worsen after approximately 5 to 7 days are candidates for antibiotic therapy. Parents need to be educated about the increasing problem of antimicrobial resistance and the natural course of viral respiratory illnesses. In addition, clinicians should familiarize themselves with over-the-counter options (oxymetazoline, cromolyn, saline, zinc) and advise parents regarding their proper use.

SUGGESTED READINGS

1. American Academy of Pediatrics: Clinical practice guideline: Management of sinusitis. Pediatrics 108:798–808, 2001. **Recommendations for sinusitis treatment in children, with a focus on acute sinusitis.**
2. Chandler JR, Langenbrunner DJ, Stevens ER: The pathogenesis of orbital complications in acute sinusitis. Laryngoscope 80:1414–1428, 1970. **The initial classification of orbital complications of acute sinusitis.**
3. Conrad DA, Jenson HB: Management of acute bacterial rhinosinusitis. Curr Op Pediatr 14:86–90, 2002. **A review of the data available on microbiology, diagnosis, and treatment of acute sinusitis in children.**
4. Fuhlbrigge AL, Adams RJ: The effect of treatment of allergic rhinitis on asthma morbidity, including emergency department visits. Curr Op Allergy Clin Immunol 3:29–32, 2003. **Reviews the clinical evidence for the putative correlation between atopic rhinitis and asthma.**
5. Lack G: Pediatric allergic rhinitis and comorbid disorders. J Allergy Clin Immunol 108:S9–S15, 2001. **An overview of allergic rhinitis in children and the diseases with which it clusters.**
6. Morris P, Leach A: Antibiotics for persistent nasal discharge (rhinosinusitis) in children (Cochrane Review). Cochrane Database Syst Rev 4:CD001094 2002. **A meta-analysis examining the strength of evidence available for recommendations on treatment of sinusitis in children.**
7. Poole MD, Jacobs MR, Anon JB, et al: Antimicrobial guidelines for the treatment of acute bacterial rhinosinusitis in immunocompetent children. Int J Pediatr Otorhinolaryngol 63:1–13, 2002. **Discusses anatomy, development, and physiology in addition to treatment.**
8. Scadding GK: Corticosteroids in the treatment of pediatric allergic rhinitis. J Allergy Clin Immunol 108:S59–S64, 2001. **Reviews the multiple treatment modalities (not limited to corticosteroids) employed in allergic rhinitis.**
9. Sinus and Allergy Health Partnership: Antimicrobial treatment guidelines for acute bacterial sinusitis. Otolaryngol Head Neck Surg 123:S1–S32, 2000. **A thorough discussion of the pathophysiology, microbiology, and treatment algorithms for acute sinusitis in adults and children.**
10. Skoner D: Update of growth effects of inhaled and intranasal corticosteroids. Curr Op Allergy Clin Immunol 2:7–10, 2002. **Summarizes data available on the long- and short-term effects on growth of topical airway steroids.**
11. Terreehorst I, Hak E, Oosting AJ, et al: Evaluation of impermeable covers for bedding in patients with allergic rhinitis. N Engl J Med 349:237–246, 2003. **Impermeable mattress covers were shown to reduce the levels of exposure to dust mite allergen but effected no clinical improvement of allergic rhinitis symptoms. A companion article in the same issue confirms this finding in patients with asthma.**

19

Bacterial Infections of the Neck
Eric D. Baum and Lisa M. Elden

KEY CONCEPTS

- Any neck swelling or mass can compromise the airway.
- When radiologic studies are needed, contrast-enhanced neck CT is preferred.
- Empiric therapy with ampicillin/sulbactam is usually begun.
- Surgical drainage may be required.

Bacterial infections of the neck in children generally occur in lymphoid tissue following a viral upper respiratory illness. Usually, pediatric upper respiratory infections are self-limited viral infections, but these entities occasionally lead to bacterial superinfection in their respective draining nodal basins. Less common causes include dental infection (spontaneously or after dental work); pharyngeal trauma; and spread of an infectious source from the face, mediastinum, or blood stream.

Although much has been written about the detailed anatomy of the numerous fascial planes and spaces in the neck, suppurative bacterial infections in this area can be broadly thought of as external (cervical adenitis), deep (retropharyngeal and parapharyngeal), and peritonsillar (in the soft palate, lateral and superior to the tonsil). The signs and symptoms and the actual pathologic processes can overlap.

Presentation

Age ranges vary widely, but retropharyngeal infections typically occur in a younger group (2–5 years) because lymph nodes in the posterior pharyngeal wall tend to involute as children grow. Conversely, peritonsillar abscess is more common in young teenagers and is not usually associated with deep space lymph nodes. Many authors have noted a general increase in the incidence of bacterial neck infections over the last few years, and for unclear reasons these infections are more common in boys than in girls.

The most common presenting symptoms are neck pain, fever, anorexia, and sore throat. Some patients develop symptoms rapidly (within 48 hours), but most present with a history of an upper respiratory tract infection that progresses despite a trial of observation or a course of antibiotics. To identify possible causes, the initial history should include questions regarding recent dental work, animal exposure (especially cats), recent travel, and exposure to persons with tuberculosis. In addition, it is important to determine if breathing has worsened with the onset of illness, and specific questions should be asked about snoring and sleep apnea.

All patients require a complete physical examination, with particular attention to the head and neck. As always, general appearance, body position, and vital signs serve as important clues to the patient's overall level of illness and remind the clinician that urgent action (in the form of hemodynamic support or respiratory intervention) may be required even before a firm diagnosis is made.

Children with retropharyngeal infections usually present with nasal congestion, drooling, and dysphagia. Those with a parapharyngeal or peritonsillar infection frequently have trismus, muffled speech, and an altered voice and complain of odynophagia and dysphagia. Patients with larger or more lateral neck infections (cervical adenitis) often display an obvious asymmetry and tender swelling of the neck, sometimes with overlying skin erythema and edema. Peritonsillar abscesses in particular are often seen in the setting of an exudative pharyngitis, and asymmetric swelling of the soft palate just superior and lateral to the tonsil is obvious. In these cases, the uvula and soft palate may be deviated toward the uninfected side (Fig. 1).

Expert Opinion on Management Issues

DIAGNOSTIC STUDIES

Laboratory studies should be ordered judiciously. Although they may be helpful as a gauge of the patient's general level of illness, they do not routinely aid in the management of these specific conditions. Thus, a complete blood count and serum electrolytes may be useful

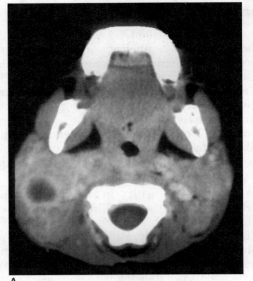

A

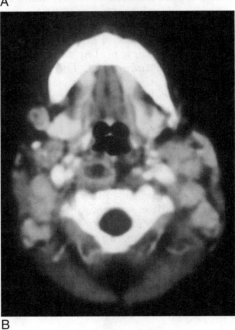

B

FIGURE 1. Contrast-enhanced axial computed-tomography (CT) scans of lateral neck *(A)* and retropharyngeal *(B)* abscesses.

initially, but further tests should be performed based on clinical findings and the importance of ruling in or out likely diagnoses (Table 1).

Plain films of the neck rarely add information beyond the initial examination, but they can be very helpful in ruling out infection in the difficult-to-examine retropharyngeal space. Lateral soft tissue neck films have excellent sensitivity, but their specificity suffers because even slightly improper patient positioning can result in a falsely thickened retropharyngeal shadow. Thus, a negative radiograph in a patient exhibiting "mixed signals" is very valuable. Occasionally, plain films also help to identify other entities in

TABLE 1 Differential Diagnosis: Selected Etiologies of Pediatric Neck Masses

Pediatric Neck Mass	Some Features Suggesting the Diagnosis
Viral cervical adenitis	Multiple bilateral, similar-sized nodes; no skin change or fluctuance
Non-TB mycobacteria tuberculosis	Painless lump, overlying blue skin discoloration, no fever Exposure history, overlying erythema, other TB symptoms
Cat-scratch disease	Exposure history, inoculation site papule, positive serology
Kawasaki disease	Conjunctivitis, strawberry tongue, desquamation
Parasitic infection	Recent immigration from tropics
Sarcoidosis	Hilar lymphadenopathy, black female
Malignancy	Firmness, rapid enlargement
Fungal infection	Immunocompromise
Drug reaction	Phenytoin, isoniazid, pyrimethamine, allopurinol, phenylbutazone

TB, tuberculosis.

the differential diagnosis (epiglottitis, foreign body), and they can give an estimate of the patency of the airway.

Contrast-enhanced CT of the neck is the most valuable radiologic tool to diagnose, assess, and even follow the progression of deep neck infections. Although studies vary in their results, the sensitivity and specificity of contrast CT in the detection of a purulent collection in the neck have been reported to be above 80%. CT is also useful for operative planning, differential diagnosis, and assessment of potential complications independent of its accuracy in confirming the presence of a collection.

The role of ultrasound has not been as thoroughly studied in these conditions, but it is more useful (and more tolerated by young patients) in superficial lateral neck infections. Ultrasound can reliably differentiate an inflamed node from a fluid-filled collection, thus sparing the patient risks of ionizing radiation, intravenous contrast, and exacerbation of respiratory symptoms from sedation.

TREATMENT

All patients should be started on antibiotics that provide broad coverage for gram-positive organisms, specifically group A streptococci and *Staphylococcus aureus*. Patients who have not improved in 48 hours or who present severely ill should also be treated with antibiotics active against anaerobes. Ampicillin/sulbactam is a popular first-line therapy because it is well tolerated, is effective, and has a good oral equivalent (amoxicillin/clavulanate). Clindamycin is a useful alternative, especially in penicillin-sensitive patients

and in areas with a high prevalence of methicillin-resistant *S. aureus*. A second-generation cephalosporin requires the addition of metronidazole for anaerobic coverage, but the combination would be acceptable and is often less expensive.

Because the patient with a peritonsillar abscess is usually a bit older and has a more physically accessible infection, transoral drainage is often possible. Even when such abscesses are partially or completely drained, trismus and odynophagia may preclude immediate hospital discharge, and full-course antibiotic therapy is still recommended. Very superficial external neck infections (deep to the skin but superficial to the sternocleidomastoid muscle) may also be aspirated in cooperative patients if marked fluctuance is noted.

Many authors recommend aerobic and anaerobic culture of all aspirated purulent material, noting that cultures are often positive despite prior antibiotic therapy. Although such test results may be helpful, these infections are frequently polymicrobial, and not all microbes are consistently cultured. For this reason, aggressive narrowing of antibiotic coverage based on laboratory findings is discouraged.

The most common organisms found in bacterial neck infections include *S. aureus* and β-hemolytic streptococci. Anaerobic organisms are less common; when present, species include *Bacteroides, Prevotella,* and *Peptostreptococcus.*

Patients with cellulitis or small or early CT-confirmed abscesses usually improve on medical therapy alone, most often within 48 hours of antibiotic treatment. Patients who present with impending airway compromise, enlarging masses, significant comorbidities, or spontaneously draining areas should be treated operatively without a 48-hour medical trial.

The optimal duration of antibiotic therapy is not known in bacterial neck infections, but many physicians recommend a 10- to 14-day course of antibiotics. Patients who remain afebrile for 24 hours, continue to improve, and tolerate an oral diet can be safely switched to an oral agent and discharged from the hospital.

Tonsillectomy is rarely indicated in the patient with peritonsillar abscess. When such children also have a history of recurrent strep throat, obstructive sleep apnea, or, rarely, recurrent peritonsillar abscesses, tonsillectomy may be appropriate. If surgical extirpation is to be performed, it is generally better to treat the infection and delay the tonsillectomy at least a few weeks. Although studies have confirmed the safety of performing the procedure in the setting of active infection (the quinsy tonsillectomy), the operation is generally easier and quicker and involves less bleeding in patients without an active infection.

When symptoms do not resolve, or recur despite antibiotic or surgical therapy, unusual diagnoses should be considered (see Table 1). Treatment failures occur more commonly in patients with an infected congenital cyst or tract, an unusual organism (e.g., atypical mycobacteria, cat-scratch disease), or even a rare noninfectious cause (e.g., retained foreign body).

19

Common Pitfalls

- Airway safety is paramount. Patients with neck infections may present with noisy breathing or frank respiratory distress requiring urgent intervention. Mild airway distress may be exacerbated by the sedation and positioning required for CT scan. Careful monitoring is imperative.
- Cellulitis and early abscesses generally respond to antibiotic coverage of *Staphylococcus* and *Streptococcus*. Additional coverage of anaerobic organisms may be required in polymicrobial infections.
- Progressive abscesses and lack of improvement in 48 hours indicates the need for surgical drainage.

Communication and Counseling

Most patients with bacterial infections of the neck have excellent outcomes with appropriate treatment, but clinicians in a modern era of powerful antibiotics and sophisticated imaging tools should not be complacent. These infections can spread to the skull base and chest and even to other distant locations, they can cause sepsis and septic thrombophlebitis, and of course they always have the potential to lead to life-threatening airway compromise. Medically complicated patients and those who do not improve quickly require thorough reevaluation; they may require repeat imaging, altered antimicrobial coverage, or more urgent surgical intervention.

Parents should be reminded that dyspnea, worsening pain, enlarging mass, high fever, and anorexia require prompt reevaluation, but that residual palpable lymphadenopathy after fully treated infections may last for many weeks. Furthermore, overlying skin changes generally resolve without further intervention. The importance of completing the full course of antimicrobial therapy should be emphasized.

SUGGESTED READINGS

1. Craig FW, Schunk JE: Retropharyngeal abscess in children: Clinical presentation, utility of imaging, and current management. Pediatrics 111:1394–1398, 2003. **Details presenting signs and symptoms and examines the relationship between CT findings and surgical versus medical intervention.**
2. Kirse DJ, Roberson DW: Surgical management of retropharyngeal space infections in children. Laryngoscope 111:1413–1422, 2001. **Despite the title, this article includes both retro- and parapharyngeal space infections. Correlates CT and intraoperative findings and provides valuable information on microbiology, medical treatment, and epidemiology.**
3. Rosenfeld RM: Cervical adenopathy. In Bluestone CD, Stool SE (eds): Pediatric Otolaryngology, 4th ed. Philadelphia: WB Saunders, 2004, pp 1665–1680. **Comprehensive overview of pediatric cervical lymphadenopathy.**
4. Vural C, Gungor A, Comerci S: Accuracy of computerized tomography in deep neck infections in the pediatric population. Am J Otolaryngol 24:143–148, 2003. **One of many studies in the literature investigating the accuracy of CT in distinguishing abscess versus cellulitis in deep neck infections.**
5. Yellon RF: Head neck space infections. In Bluestone CD, Stool SE (eds): Pediatric Otolaryngology, 4th ed. Philadelphia: WB Saunders, 2004, pp 1681–1701. **Anatomist's classic perspective on the various deep neck spaces.**

Tonsillectomy and Adenoidectomy

David Henry Hiltzik and Lianne M. de Serres

KEY CONCEPTS

- Clinical evaluation and decision making for tonsillectomy and adenoidectomy relies heavily on a thorough history of infections of both the ears and the throat as well as careful questioning about breathing, sleeping, and behavioral patterns. Polysomnography is useful but not necessary.
- There are absolute and relative indications for tonsillectomy, adenoidectomy, and adenotonsillectomy. Adenotonsillectomy is absolutely indicated when hypertrophy causes dysphagia, extreme breathing difficulties, and significant obstructive sleep apnea.
- Tonsillectomy alone is absolutely indicated with the appropriate number of documented tonsillar infections, considerable obstructive symptoms, and recurrent peritonsillar abscesses. Most indications for adenoidectomy are relative.
- There are few contraindications to adenotonsillectomy, tonsillectomy, and adenoidectomy. Appropriate preoperative evaluation is necessary, with attention to medical and surgical history.
- Adenoidectomy and/or tonsillectomy should be considered in the treatment of decreased olfaction, dental-facial abnormalities, and attention deficit hyperactivity disorder.
- Clear communication and understanding between the otolaryngologist and parents regarding possible complications and postoperative care is paramount.

Diseases relating to the tonsils and adenoids are among those most commonly faced by the pediatrician. Although they are often grouped together, the tonsils and adenoids are distinct entities responsible for different diseases, most often related to general categories of infection and obstruction. These lymphoid masses occupy the lateral walls of the oropharynx and the midline nasopharynx; they contribute to the pathology and the pathophysiology of pharyngotonsillitis, sleep-related breathing disorders, recurrent acute and chronic otitis media, nasal congestion and sinusitis; and now they are linked to behavioral disturbances. Although they function as a part of the immune system by providing a large surface area for antigen presentation at the entrance of the aerodigestive tract, no specific adverse effects are documented after their removal. Regardless, the tonsils and adenoids must be removed only for clearly defined clinical disease.

The clinical evaluation for potential tonsillectomy and/or adenoidectomy relies heavily on a thorough history that focuses on documenting the frequency and severity of the episodes of infections of both the ear and the throat and the history of peritonsillar abscess; and symptoms such as rhinorrhea, cough, postnasal drip, mouth breathing, and snoring; in addition to irregular sleeping and breathing patterns, nocturnal coughing and choking, daytime somnolence, and inattentiveness. Although direct examination of the adenoids is best performed by fiberoptic nasopharyngoscopy, adenoid hypertrophy can be inferred by the presence of open mouth breathing, copious nasal discharge, and hyponasal speech resonance. A lateral soft-tissue film of the neck can easily be obtained for confirmation. Examination of the tonsils includes the measurement of the tonsil size and degree of obstruction based on a scale of 1+ to 4+, as well as the presence of erythema, exudates, debris, and halitosis, along with tender palpable lymph nodes. Polysomnography can be used to document obstructive sleep apnea but is not warranted if clinical evaluation is supportive. Alternatively, obtaining a tape or video recording of the child sleeping can demonstrate obstructive sleep symptoms such as loud snoring, gasping or struggling for air, or overt apneas.

Expert Opinion on Management Issues

INDICATIONS

Table 1 presents the general indications for tonsillectomy and/or adenoidectomy. However, it is crucial to stratify these indications into the categories of *absolute* *relative*. Adenotonsillectomy is absolutely necessary when massive adenotonsillar hypertrophy causes dysphagia, extreme breathing difficulties, and clinically significant obstructive sleep apnea. In the cases of apparent obstruction as determined by the history and physical, a course of antibiotics may first be administered to lessen possible edema secondary to subacute infection before the decision for surgery is made. Antibiotics may actually reduce the size of tonsils and adenoids by 15% to 20%. Similarly, in the cases of nasal obstruction, at least a month's trial of nasal steroids should be given as a medical therapy directed at alleviating symptoms.

Physician-documented recurrent pharyngotonsillitis of more than seven infections per year for 2 years, five infections per year for 2 years, or three infections per year for 3 years (preferably with confirmation of streptococcus) and obstructive symptoms such as nighttime awakening, "hot potato" voice, and recurrent peritonsillar abscess are considered absolute indications for tonsillectomy. Chronic tonsillitis unresponsive to medical management, tonsillolithiasis, halitosis, and acute peritonsillar abscess are relative indications for surgery. Adenoidectomy is recommended in the context of obstructive adenoidal hypertrophy that persists after medical treatment, recurrent or chronic otitis media that failed to respond to tympanostomy tube placement (adenoidectomy is not effective as a first-line surgical treatment in otitis media), and chronic sinusitis that was treated maximally with nasal steroids, antibiotics, and possibly cromolyn and antihistamines. Other underlying causes, such as ciliary dysmotility syndromes and immunodeficiencies, should be ruled out. Importantly, adenoidectomy as an isolated procedure may help avoid more invasive sinus surgery.

CONTRAINDICATIONS

Absolute contraindications to adenotonsillectomy are rare. Medically necessary adenotonsillectomy can be performed in the face of additional medical conditions, as long as appropriate precautions are taken. These conditions relate to velopharyngeal, hematologic, immunologic, and infectious causes. In patients with a history of cleft palate, neurologic disease, and/or neuromuscular disease, postoperative velopharyngeal insufficiency may lead to hypernasal speech resonance. The surgeon needs to be aware of the anatomic issues, and a partial adenoidectomy should be performed. This technique preserves the lower portion of the adenoid bed, which is important in speech production and can prevent postoperative sequelae. Patients with a family history of blood disorders, anemia (hemoglobin less than 10 g/dL and/or a hematocrit less than 30%), and coagulopathies should have a hematology consultation. Patients with acute streptococcal infections should be treated with a minimum of 72 hours of antibiotics before undergoing anesthesia. Children with acute upper respiratory infections should have their surgery postponed by 2 to 3 weeks to lessen the chance of perioperative bronchospasm. Otherwise healthy patients do not require routine preoperative blood testing. In the case of patients with a history of congenital heart disease, a preoperative cardiology evaluation should be obtained. In children with trisomy 21, care is taken not to hyperextend the neck during

19

TABLE 1 Indications for Tonsillectomy and/or Adenoidectomy

Indication	Tonsillectomy	Adenoidectomy
Recurrent tonsillitis	√	
Chronic tonsillitis	√	
Recurrent otitis media with prior tube placement and antibiotics		√
Chronic/recurrent sinusitis		√
Obstruction unresponsive to medical therapy ± apnea, dysphagia, failure to thrive		
With adenoid hypertrophy		√
With tonsillar hypertrophy	√	
With adenotonsillar hypertrophy	√	√
Recurrent peritonsillar abscess	√	
Chronic tonsillolithiasis	√	

surgery because of the possibility of atlantoaxial instability.

POSTOPERATIVE CARE

Postoperatively, children undergoing adenotonsillectomy for moderate to severe obstructive sleep apnea documented by sleep study should be observed overnight in a monitored setting. Postoperative edema, residual anesthetic agents, decreased respiratory drive, and postobstructive pulmonary edema may cause respiratory distress on the first night. Additionally, children younger than 3 years, those with craniofacial syndrome (including trisomy 21), and/or those with significant medical problems (neuromuscular, respiratory, and hematologic disorders) should be admitted for overnight observation.

Common Pitfalls

Adenoidectomy and/or tonsillectomy may be overlooked as an additional treatment modality for other conditions such as decreased olfaction and dental-facial abnormalities. Children evaluated for attention deficit hyperactivity disorder (ADHD) should have a careful examination, and children with open-mouth breathing or tonsillar hypertrophy should be considered for polysomnography as part of the evaluation. Ten percent of these patients have obstructive sleep apnea as the etiology of their ADHD. In addition, tonsillectomy can be effective in treating pediatric autoimmune neuropsychiatric disorders associated with streptococcal infections (PANDAS). Adenoidectomy may play a role in the pathophysiology of chronic otitis media with effusion. Every patient with nasal congestion should also have a complete allergy workup before surgery is considered. All the preceding scenarios warrant a thorough exam for adenoid and tonsillar hypertrophy and possible tonsillectomy and/or adenoidectomy.

Communication and Counseling

Parents must be fully informed about the most common risks of adenotonsillectomy, including severe postoperative pain, the potential for bleeding, dehydration, fever, and temporary voice changes. Much rarer complications include nasopharyngeal stenosis, velopharyngeal insufficiency, symptomatic adenoid regrowth, and a 1 in 15,000 chance of death. Parents must maximize pain management and monitor their child's fluid intake and urine output in the first postoperative week. Significant bleeding occurs 1% of the time in the first 24 hours and 3% of the time between days 5 and 10 after surgery in normal children.

In general, the physician should communicate to the parent the need for initial medical treatment of adenotonsillar disorders, even in instances when parents are strong proponents of surgery. Adenotonsillectomy performed for appropriate indications is very successful in general, but it does carry some small risks that must be weighed in the decision-making process.

SUGGESTED READINGS

1. Bluestone CD: Controversies in tonsillectomy, adenoidectomy, and tympanostomy tubes. In Bailey B (ed): Head and Neck Surgery-Otolaryngology, 3rd ed. Philadelphia: Lippincott, Williams, and Wilkins, 2001. **Overview of early landmark articles defining the parameters for tonsillectomy and adenoidectomy by a leader in pediatric otolaryngology.**
2. Brodsky L: Adenotonsillar disease in children. In Cotton R, Myer C (eds): Practical Pediatric Otolaryngology. Philadelphia: Lippincott-Raven, 1999. **Textbook overview of indications, complications, and outcomes of adenotonsillectomy.**
3. Darrow DH, Siemens C: Indications for tonsillectomy and adenoidectomy. Laryngoscope 112(8 Pt 2 Suppl 100):6–10, 2002. **Evidence-based approach reviews clinical trials addressing indications for adenotonsillectomy, tonsillectomy, and adenoidectomy. This article provides a foundation on which clinicians can base decisions regarding adenotonsillar surgery for their patients.**
4. Goldstein NA, Pugazhendhi V, Rao SM, et al: Clinical assessment of pediatric obstructive sleep apnea. Pediatrics 114(1):33–43, 2004. **Clinical study examining whether children with a clinical assessment suggestive of obstructive sleep apnea but with negative polysomnography have improvement in their clinical assessment score after tonsillectomy and adenoidectomy as compared with similar children who do not undergo surgery.**
5. Paradise JL: Pittsburgh tonsillectomy and adenoidectomy study: Differences from earlier studies and problems of execution. Ann Otol Rhinol Laryngol (2 Pt 2 Suppl. 19):15–19, 1975. **Review and critique of previous large prospective studies regarding tonsillectomy and adenoidectomy.**
6. Paradise JL, Bluestone CD, Rogers KD, et al: Efficacy of adenoidectomy for recurrent otitis media in children previously treated with tympanostomy-tube placement. Results of parallel randomized and nonrandomized trials. JAMA 263(15):2066–2073, 1990. **Landmark study describing clinical relationship of adenoidectomy to otitis media and tympanostomy tube placement with regard to pathophysiology and treatment.**
7. Paradise JL, Bluestone CD, Bachman RZ, et al: Efficacy of tonsillectomy for recurrent throat infection in severely affected children. Results of parallel randomized and nonrandomized clinical trials. N Engl J Med 310(11):674–683, 1984. **Landmark, randomized, controlled study investigating the indications for tonsillectomy as a treatment for recurrent tonsillitis.**
8. Richards W, Ferdman RM: Prolonged morbidity due to delays in the diagnosis and treatment of obstructive sleep apnea in children. Clin Pediatr (Phila) 39(2):103–108, 2000. **Query of patients undergoing tonsillectomy and adenoidectomy demonstrating that patients with underdiagnosed obstructive sleep apnea experienced severe and discomforting symptoms with all describing severe or moderate snoring. The symptoms included chronic mouth breathing, frequent otitis media, sinusitis, sore throat, choking, and daytime drowsiness in addition to poor school performance, enuresis, poor appetite and/or weight gain, dysphagia, and vomiting.**

Otitis Media

Richard M. Rosenfeld

KEY CONCEPTS

- Acute otitis media (AOM) is the presence of middle-ear effusion (MEE) with the rapid, usually abrupt, onset of one or more signs or symptoms of inflammation of the middle ear.
- Otitis media with effusion (OME) is MEE without signs or symptoms of acute ear infection.

- Children in the United States have 5 million AOM episodes and 2 million OME episodes annually.
- Appropriate oral antibiotic use is essential to limit bacterial resistance because 50% of all oral antibiotics in preschoolers are prescribed for otitis media.
- Strategies for appropriate antibiotic use include watchful waiting for OME, the observation option for AOM, surgical prevention, and antibiotic eardrops for AOM with tympanostomy tubes.
- Children with OME, who are at risk for delays in speech, language, learning, or development, should have prompt evaluation of hearing and the need for intervention.

An evidence-based approach to managing otitis media is optimally based on current best research evidence blended with provider experience and patient preference. This chapter summarizes best evidence using meta-analysis, when available, or individual randomized, controlled trials. Clinical practice guidelines from national organizations are also discussed. Research evidence, however, rarely applies to individual patients with any degree of certainty, so that clinician experience and judgment are essential aspects of any management plan. There is also ample room to incorporate patient preference, particularly when using the observation option for AOM or when contemplating typanostomy tube insertion.

Expert Opinion on Management Issues

WATCHFUL WAITING

The favorable natural history of acute otitis media (AOM) (Table 1) suggests that most children improve (eventually) regardless of management. Rather than endorse nihilism, these data suggest a careful need to balance nature's accomplishments against potential therapeutic benefits. For example, although antimicrobials have proven efficacy for AOM, initial observation of selected children can also achieve excellent outcomes (as described later). Similarly, delaying interventions for recurrent AOM by 6 months often provides relief. Otitis media with effusion (OME) is initially managed with watchful waiting for 3 months, but extending this to 6 months increases resolution by 30% to 50%.

The *observation option* for AOM allows selected children to fight the infection on their own for 48 to 72 hours before starting antibiotics. The paradigm initially proposed in New York in 2002 (Table 2), later adopted by the American Academy of Pediatrics (AAP) and American Academy of Family Physicians (AAFP) in 2004, allows clinicians to use the observation option based on current best evidence. Children are best suited for observation if they are 2 years of age or older with nonsevere AOM or an uncertain diagnosis. In contrast, observation is not advised for children younger than 6 months, those who had AOM treatment failures or AOM relapses (within 30 days), or in patients with immune deficiency, craniofacial anomalies, or coexisting streptococcal pharyngitis or bacterial sinusitis.

Observing AOM differs from not treating it. All children should receive adequate analgesics (acetaminophen or ibuprofen), especially for the first 24 hours after diagnosis. Analgesics, not antibiotics, are the cornerstone of initial pain relief because the incremental benefit of antibiotics over placebo or natural history is not apparent until day 2 or later (Table 3). Children

19

TABLE 1 Natural History of Otitis Media

Clinical Situation	Time Point	N*	Rate†	(95% CI)
Symptomatic relief of pain and fever caused by AOM in children randomized to placebo	24 h	3	.61‡	(.50, .72)
	2–3 d	5	.80	(.69, .90)
	4–7 d	8	.74	(.64, .85)
Resolution of OME persisting after AOM in children randomized to placebo or no drug	4 wk	4	.59	(.50, .68)
	12 wk	2	.74	(.68, .80)
Resolution of newly diagnosed OME of unknown duration by ear	1 mo	2	.22	(.16, .29)
	3 mo	4	.28	(.14, .41)
	6 mo	4	.42	(.35, .49)
		3		
Clinical resolution of documented OME lasting ≥3 mo by ear	6 mo	4	.25	(.17, .34)
	12 mo	4	.31	(.19, .43)
Future incidence of AOM episodes/mo for children with a history of recurrent AOM	up to 2 yr	14	.23	(.18, .28)
Future chance of having no AOM episodes for children with recurrent AOM	6 mo median	13	.41	(.32, .51)
Future chance of having ≤2 AOM episodes for children with recurrent AOM	6 mo median	8	.83	(.74, .91)

*Number of studies from which data were combined to derive the overall resolution rate.
†Estimate based on random effects meta-analysis.
‡Based on children 2 years or older; resolution may be poorer for younger children.
AOM, acute otitis media; CI, confidence interval; OME, otitis media with effusion.
Data from Rosenfeld RM, Kay DJ: Natural history of untreated otitis media. Laryngoscope 113:1645–1657, 2003.

TABLE 2 Criteria for Initial Antibiotics vs. Observation with Acute Otitis Media

Child Age	Certain Diagnosis or Definite Acute Otitis Media*	Uncertain Diagnosis or Suspected Acute Otitis Media[†]
<6 mo	Antibiotics	Antibiotics
6 mo–2 yr	Antibiotics	Antibiotics if severe[†] illness Observe[‡] if nonsevere[†] illness
≥2 yr	Antibiotics if severe[†] illness Observe[‡] if nonsevere[†] illness	Observe[‡]

*Certain diagnosis implies definitive middle-ear effusion plus recent onset of signs and symptoms of middle-ear inflammation; uncertain diagnosis implies nondefinitive effusion or signs and symptoms.

[†]Nonsevere illness is mild otalgia and fever <102°F (39°C) orally or <103.1°F (39.5°C) rectally in the past 24 hours; severe illness is higher fever, moderate to severe otalgia, or both.

[‡]Observation option is appropriate *only* when follow-up can be assured (by telephone or office visit) and antibiotics started if symptoms worsen or persist by 48–72 hours.

Adapted from the American Academy of Pediatrics/American Academy of Family Physicians Clinical Practice Guideline: Lieberthal AS, Ganiats TG, Cox EO, et al: Clinical practice guideline: Diagnosis and management of acute otitis media. Pediatrics 113:1451–1465, 2004.

TABLE 3 What to Expect from Antibiotic Therapy for Otitis Media

Clinical Situation and Outcome	Time Point	N*	RD[†]	(95% CI)	NNT[‡]	(95% CI)
Symptomatic relief AOM in RCTs of antibiotic vs. placebo or no drug	24 h	3	0	(−.07, .08)	—	
	2–3 days	5	.04	(.02, .07)[¶]	25	(14, 50)
	4–7 days	6	.09	(.01, .18)[¶]	11	(6, 333)
Incidence of suppurative complications of AOM in RCTs of antibiotic vs. placebo or no drug	7–14 days	9	.001	(−.007, .008)	—	
Resolution of persistent OME after treatment of AOM in RCTs of antibiotic vs. placebo	4–6 wk	6	.03	(−.02, .08)	—	
	3 mo	2	.05	(−.08, .17)	—	
Complete resolution of OME in blinded RCTs of antibiotic therapy vs. placebo	4 wk median	9	.15	(.06, .24)[¶]	7	(4, 17)
Complete resolution of OME in RCTs of steroid and antibiotic vs. placebo and antibiotic	Up to 2 mo	5	.25	(.02, .47)[¶]	4	(2, 43)
Incidence of AOM episodes/patient-month in RCTs of antibiotic prophylaxis vs. placebo	Up to 2 yr	10	−.09	(−.12, −.05) NT only for statistically significant outcomes.[¶]	11	(8, 19)
Having no further AOM episodes in RCTs of antibiotic prophylaxis vs. placebo	6 mo median	10	.21	(.13, .30)[¶]	5	(3, 8)
Having ≤2 AOM episodes in RCTs of antibiotic prophylaxis vs. placebo	6 mo median	5	.08	(.04, .12)[¶]	13	(8, 24)

*Number of studies from which data were combined to derive the overall treatment effect.
[†]RD is the absolute change in outcome for treatment vs. control groups.
[‡]NNT is the number of children who must be treated for one additional successful outcome and is relevant only for statistically significant outcomes.
[¶]$P < .05$ when the 95% CI does not contain zero.
AOM, acute otitis media; CI, confidence interval; OME, otitis media with effusion; RCT, randomized controlled trial; RD, absolute rate difference; NNT, number needed to treat; NT, no test.
From Rosenfeld RM, Bluestone CD (eds): Evidence-Based Otitis Media, 2nd ed. Hamilton, Ontario, Canada: BC Decker, 2003.

who are initially observed should receive antibiotics if symptoms worsen or fail to improve at 48 to 72 hours, which occurs in approximately 25% to 35% of cases. A convenient way to implement the observation option is with a safety net antibiotic prescription, given to the family at the initial encounter with instructions to wait 48 to 72 hours before obtaining medication and to call the physician's office if the prescription is filled.

ORAL ANTIBIOTICS

The primary role of oral antibiotic therapy for AOM is to reduce the risk of suppurative complications in at-risk children. Suppurative complications have an incidence of approximately 1:600 and include mastoiditis, meningitis, facial paralysis, and brain abscess. The guidelines for antibiotic therapy in Table 2 are intended to ensure that children at greatest risk for suppurative complications from AOM receive initial antibiotic therapy.

Antibiotics are *not* pain relievers or antipyretics, and the majority of symptomatic relief for AOM (especially during the first 24 hours) results from analgesics and spontaneous resolution. By 4 to 7 days (see Table 3), the impact of antibiotics is significant but modest: Approximately 11 children need treatment (number needed to

TABLE 4 Recommended Antibiotics for Children with Acute Otitis Media

Clinical Situation	Nonsevere Illness*	Severe Illness*
Initial antibiotic therapy of AOM or clinical failure of observation option at 48–72 h	Amoxicillin, 80–90 mg/kg/day PCN allergy non–type I: cefdinir, cefuroxime, cefpodoxime[†] PCN allergy type I: azithromycin, clarithromycin[†]	Amoxicillin-clavulanate, 90 mg/kg/day of amoxicillin with 6.4 mg/kg/day of clavulanate PCN allergy non–type I: ceftriaxone 1 or 3 days[†]
Clinical failure of antibiotic therapy at 48–72 h	Amoxicillin-clavulanate, 90 mg/kg/day of amoxicillin with 6.4 mg/kg/day of clavulanate PCN allergy non–type I: ceftriaxone 3 days[†] PCN allergy type I: clindamycin[†]	Ceftriaxone 3 days PCN allergy type I: tympanocentesis, clindamycin[†]

*Nonsevere illness is mild otalgia and fever <102°F (39°C) orally or <103.1°F (39.5°C) rectally in the past 24 hours; severe illness is higher fever, severe otalgia, or both.
[†]Type I PCN allergy, or hypersensitivity, is urticaria or anaphylaxis.
AOM, acute otitis media; PCN, penicillin.
Adapted from the American Academy of Pediatrics/American Academy of Family Physicians Clinical Practice Guideline: Lieberthal AS, Ganiats TG, Cox EO, et al: Clinical practice guideline: Diagnosis and management of acute otitis media. Pediatrics 113:1451–1465, 2004.

treat [NNT] = 11) to increase by 1 child the number with symptomatic relief beyond spontaneous resolution. The impact of initial antibiotics on school or work absence is also modest, ranging from no impact in some studies to between 0.5 and 1.5 days in others.

When a decision is reached to treat AOM with antibiotics, a drug should be used that is most likely to eradicate common pathogens (Table 4). Approximately 25% to 50% of AOM is caused by *Streptococcus pneumoniae*, 15% to 30% by nontypeable *Haemophilus influenzae*, and 3% to 20% by *Moraxella catarrhalis*, of which an estimated 0%, 50%, and 100%, respectively, produce β-lactamase. The prevalence of pneumococcal resistance to penicillin is approximately 30% (range 15% to 50%), of which 50% are highly resistant strains. Risk factors for resistant pneumococcus are antibiotic use, young age, daycare attendance, and prior hospitalization.

The optimum duration of AOM therapy is controversial. Short-course therapy (3 days of azithromycin, 5 days of other antibiotics) is an option for children 2 years or older, and full-course treatment (5 days of azithromycin, 7 to 10 days of other antibiotics) is better for younger children (especially when attending group child care). Better outcomes with full-course therapy are also demonstrated for children with AOM in the preceding month.

Oral antibiotics increase absolute resolution rates of OME by 15% over placebo (see Table 3), but the benefits are short term. Consequently, antibiotic therapy for OME is not recommended, unless there are significant associated symptoms or surgery is imminent. Adding an oral steroid to antibiotic therapy for OME increases short-term resolution to 25% (see Table 3), but the unfavorable harm-to-benefit ratio argues against routine therapy. Similarly, antibiotic prophylaxis should rarely be used to prevent recurrent AOM because the risk of accelerated bacterial resistance far exceeds the small benefits (see Table 3) of daily low-dose antibiotics beyond the already favorable natural history (see Table 1).

INTRAMUSCULAR ANTIBIOTICS

A single intramuscular dose of ceftriaxone has comparable efficacy to a 7- to 10-day course of oral antibiotics for AOM, but use of ceftriaxone as *initial* therapy should be discouraged. Liberal use of this drug may accelerate bacterial resistance and compromise efficacy as a backup for suppurative complications (for which oral alternatives do not exist). Ceftriaxone is appropriate for severe AOM associated with penicillin allergy or clinical failure of oral antibiotics (see Table 4).

SURGERY

Children with recurrent AOM who receive tympanostomy tubes have 67% less AOM than controls, and they can generally be managed with antibiotic eardrops. Children with chronic OME who receive tympanostomy tubes have 161 fewer days with effusion during the first year of intubation, a relative decrease of 72% versus no surgery or myringotomy alone. Tubes also improve hearing. Studies on the effects of ventilation tubes on language developmental outcomes show no or only marginal beneficial effects.

Surgical candidacy for otitis media (Table 5) depends largely on associated symptoms (e.g., otalgia, hearing loss); frequency and severity of AOM; the child's risk of developmental delays; and the chance of timely spontaneous resolution of OME. Duration of OME *should not* be the sole operative criterion. A healthy child with chronic bilateral OME but normal development could be safely observed for months (or even years) until spontaneous resolution occurs, but a child with developmental delays could be a surgical candidate after weeks or months depending on individual circumstances.

When a decision is made to proceed with surgery for otitis media, *initial surgery* consists of myringotomy and tympanostomy tube placement; adenoidectomy is withheld unless nasal obstruction is present. *Repeat surgery* consists of adenoidectomy and myringotomy, with or without tube placement. Adenoidectomy reduces

TABLE 5 Factors Influencing the Threshold for Surgical Intervention in Children with Otitis Media

Prognostic Factor	Lowers Surgical Threshold	Raises Surgical Threshold
Developmentally at-risk child*	Yes (major factor)	No
Hearing and auditory function	Abnormal	Normal
Language/academic achievement	Abnormal or delayed	Normal
Tympanic membrane structure	Abnormal[†]	Normal
Recurrent acute otitis media	Present	Absent
Imbalance, clumsiness, vertigo	Present	Absent
Environment	Unfavorable[‡]	Favorable
Quality of life[¶]	Poor	Good

*Cleft palate, Down syndrome, autism-spectrum disorder, or other pervasive developmental disorder, attention deficit or hyperactive disorder, speech or language delays, syndrome or craniofacial disorder, sensorineural hearing loss, psychomotor retardation or sensory defects, intellectual impairment, cognitive deficits, school problems.
[†]Atelectasis, retraction pocket, or thickened and hypervascular tympanic membrane.
[‡]Environmental tobacco smoke; group daycare (4–6 children or more); less responsive home or child-care environment.
[¶]Physical symptoms, sleep disturbance, emotional distress, activity limitations, etc.

the need for future surgery by approximately 50%. Tonsillectomy alone (without adenoidectomy) and myringotomy alone (without tube insertion) are ineffective.

ANTIBIOTIC EARDROPS

Acute tympanostomy tube otorrhea (TTO) in children 2 years or younger is usually caused by typical AOM pathogens. Conversely, *Pseudomonas aeruginosa* and *Staphylococcus aureus* are more prevalent in older children, when TTO is related to water exposure or when ear odor is present. Because most acute TTO is painless, initial management should consist of daily cleaning of the ear canal by the parents with a cotton wick or a nasal aspirator to remove secretions.

Topical antibiotic eardrops are the treatment of choice for persistent or symptomatic TTO, unless another bacterial infection warrants oral antibiotics (streptococcal pharyngitis, bacterial rhinosinusitis). Antibiotic drops have comparable clinical efficacy to oral antibiotics, yet they offer higher pathogen eradication and fewer adverse effects. Moreover, topical antibiotics achieve middle-ear drug levels that are 1000 times higher than those attainable orally, which maximizes efficacy and minimizes selective pressure for bacterial resistance.

Quinolone eardrops containing ofloxacin or ciprofloxacin are the only products approved by the U.S. Food and Drug Administration (FDA) for topical therapy of TTO. Eardrops containing neomycin and polymyxin are not recommended because they are ototoxic and have limited efficacy against common pathogens. Eardrops with a steroid (ciprofloxacin plus dexamethasone) are preferred for TTO with significant otalgia, severe inflammation, or granulation tissue. Overuse of antibiotic eardrops can result in fungal overgrowth in the ear canal.

Common Pitfalls

- Antihistamine or decongestant preparations are ineffective for AOM or OME and should not be used as primary therapeutic agents.

- The observation option for AOM should not be used unless provisions are made to start an antibiotic if the child worsens or fails to improve at 48 to 72 hours.
- Antibiotic therapy is not recommended for routine management of OME.
- Oral antibiotics should not be used for routine therapy of TTO because antibiotic eardrops are more effective and have fewer side effects.
- Eardrops with ototoxic antibiotics (e.g., neomycin, tobramycin) should not be used to treat AOM with a tympanostomy tube or perforated tympanic membrane.

Communication and Counseling

Parents should understand that otitis media is an occupational hazard of early childhood, one that disappears gradually between 3 and 8 years of age. Most management of otitis media can be summed up in the words of Voltaire as "amusing the patient while nature cures disease." Judicious use of antibiotics and surgery improves quality of life for children with frequent or persistent illness. Educational materials for parents include excellent brochures from the AAP, Centers for Disease Control and Prevention, and the New York State Department of Health. Complementary and alternative medicine cannot be recommended for treating otitis media until well-designed studies show benefits beyond the already favorable natural history.

SUGGESTED READINGS

1. Goldblatt EL, Dohar J, Nozza RJ, et al: Topical ofloxacin versus systemic amoxicillin/clavulanate in purulent otorrhea in children with tympanostomy tubes. Int J Pediatr Otorhinolaryngol 46:91–101, 1998. **Study showing comparable clinical efficacy, but better bacteriologic efficacy, for eardrops.**
2. Lieberthal AS, Ganiats TG, Cox EO, et al: Clinical practice guideline: Diagnosis and management of acute otitis media. Pediatrics 113:1451–1465, 2004. **Official AAP/AAFP guideline.**
3. New York Regional Otitis Project: Observation Option Toolkit for Acute Otitis Media. State of New York, Department of Health. Publication 4894, March 2002. **Contains a laminated decision chart and parent education materials.**

4. Roberts JE, Rosenfeld RM, Ziesel SA: Otitis media and speech and language: A meta-analysis of prospective studies. Pediatrics 113: e238–e248, 2004. **Meta-analysis of prospective studies and randomized trials.**

5. Roland PS, Kreisler LS, Reese B, et al: Topical ciprofloxacin/dexamethasone otic suspension is superior to ofloxacin otic solution in the treatment of children with acute otitis media with otorrhea through tympanostomy tubes. Pediatrics 113:e40–e46, 2004. **Comparative efficacy study of two FDA-approved eardrops for treating TTO.**

6. Rosenfeld RM: A Parent's Guide to Ear Tubes. Hamilton, Ontario, Canada: BC Decker, 2005. **Educational guide for parents that emphasizes shared decision making and appropriate antibiotic use.**

7. Rosenfeld RM, Bluestone CD (eds): Evidence-Based Otitis Media, 2nd ed. Hamilton, Ontario, Canada: BC Decker, 2003. **Comprehensive overview including extensive evidence tables.**

8. Rosenfeld RM, Culpepper L, Doyle KJ, et al: Clinical practice guideline: Otitis media with effusion. Otolaryngol Head Neck Surg 130:S95–S118, 2004. **Official AAP/AAFP/AO-HNS (American Academy of Otolaryngology-Head and Neck Surgery) guideline.**

9. Rosenfeld RM, Kay DJ: Natural history of untreated otitis media. Laryngoscope 113:1645–1657, 2003. **Meta-analysis of cohort studies and placebo groups from randomized trials.**

Labyrinthitis

John A. Germiller and Ken Kazahaya

19

KEY CONCEPTS

- Labyrinthitis is almost always secondary to a primary infectious or inflammatory disorder.
- The most serious long-term complication is permanent sensorineural hearing loss.
- Labyrinthitis can be classified as:
  - Tympanogenic: Serous or suppurative, usually unilateral, and associated with otitis media.
  - Meningitic: Secondary to bacterial meningitis, commonly bilateral, with high incidence of severe hearing loss and cochlear ossification.
  - Hematogenic: Secondary to a systemic viral or inflammatory condition.
- Treatment is mainly directed at the primary disorder:
  - Tympanogenic: Systemic antibiotics combined with myringotomy and tube; mastoidectomy is reserved for recalcitrant infection and labyrinthectomy for severe, life-threatening infection with intracranial extension.
  - Meningitic: Systemic antimicrobials combined with early dexamethasone provides best preservation of hearing.
  - Hematogenic: Viral and autoimmune labyrinthitis respond to symptomatic care for vertigo, and oral corticosteroids may help preserve hearing.
- Early otolaryngology and audiology consultation and follow-up are critical.

Labyrinthitis is an infectious or other inflammatory process occurring within the labyrinth, the fluid-filled chambers of the inner ear. It is manifest by sensorineural hearing loss (SNHL) and vertigo, which result from injury to the sensory neuroepithelial elements of the inner ear. Labyrinthitis is nearly always a secondary event, and treatment approaches are strongly influenced by the primary infectious or inflammatory process. Therefore, it is helpful to classify labyrinthitis according to source.

Tympanogenic labyrinthitis results from middle-ear disease and thus is most commonly unilateral. It results from acute otitis media (most common) or chronic otitis media, with inflammation entering the middle ear via the oval or round windows or through a defect or fistula. The latter can occur secondary to trauma (e.g., temporal bone fracture), surgery, or from the bony erosion caused by cholesteatoma. Tympanogenic labyrinthitis can be serous or suppurative. Serous labyrinthitis is more common and is a sterile inflammation of the labyrinth resulting from accumulation of bacterial toxins or inflammatory mediators in the inner ear. Dysequilibrium and vertigo in a child with otitis media is a typical presentation. Suppurative labyrinthitis is a more acute and destructive form of tympanogenic labyrinthitis and results from direct bacterial invasion of the inner ear. It is characterized by severe, rapidly progressive SNHL and vertigo. Complete deafness and loss of vestibular function in the affected ear are not uncommon. Aggressive treatment is needed because infection can spread intracranially.

Meningitic labyrinthitis is usually a complication of bacterial meningitis resulting from spread of infection in the reverse direction, from the meninges or cerebrospinal fluid (CSF) directly into the inner ear. A suppurative and most commonly bilateral labyrinthitis, it is the most frequent cause of acquired SNHL in childhood. Permanent hearing loss occurs in 5% to 35% and is often profound. The most common pathogens are *Haemophilus influenza* and *Streptococcus pneumoniae*.

Hematogenic labyrinthitis is a heterogeneous group of conditions in which labyrinthitis is secondary to a systemic infectious or inflammatory disorder.

Viral labyrinthitis can result from systemic mumps, measles, cytomegalovirus (CMV), influenza, parainfluenza, or herpes simplex infections. A typical presentation is the onset of hearing loss and vertigo in the setting of an otherwise unremarkable viral infection. Mumps is the most common cause of acquired viral hearing loss and is most often unilateral. Fortunately, viral labyrinthitis is quite rare in children. It is often confused with vestibular neuronitis (also rare in children), which is an idiopathic but likely viral inflammation of the vestibular nerve that causes vertigo but no hearing loss. Prenatal or perinatal infections with CMV, rubella, or toxoplasmosis are important causes of congenital hearing loss. CMV is particularly devastating; the incidence of hearing loss is high—up to 30% to 60% in cytomegalic inclusion disease—and can progress throughout childhood.

Syphilitic labyrinthitis results most commonly from congenital infection, but can also result from acquired systemic disease in later childhood. The presentation and course of hearing loss and vestibular symptoms can vary from sudden to fluctuating to progressive.

Autoimmune labyrinthitis is rare in children. It is associated with systemic disease, including Wegener granulomatosis, vasculitides, rheumatoid arthritis, and Cogan syndrome. Importantly, hearing loss may be the first manifestation of one of these systemic autoimmune disorders.

Diagnosis

Because labyrinthitis is a secondary condition, the first element of diagnosis is recognition of the primary disorder (e.g., acute otitis media, cholesteatoma, meningitis, viral illness). The diagnosis of labyrinthitis can then be made if there is evidence for SNHL, vestibular dysfunction, or both. Vestibular dysfunction is often not recognized in children, especially the very young, however, because the symptoms are difficult to verbalize and the only signs may be subtle dysequilibrium or clumsiness. Spontaneous nystagmus is a hallmark of the acute vestibular inflammation or destruction of labyrinthitis and is also readily observable on physical examination. Hearing loss should be confirmed via audiometry with both air and bone conduction testing. Although labyrinthitis can be diagnosed by gadolinium uptake on MRI, it is seldom necessary.

Expert Opinion on Management Issues

MEDICAL AND SURGICAL THERAPY

Treatment approaches for labyrinthitis are dictated by the primary source of infection or inflammation. Early otolaryngology and audiology consultations are essential.

Tympanogenic Labyrinthitis

The presence of active otitis media should first be determined. In the setting of acute otitis media, treatment starts with aggressive systemic antimicrobials directed empirically at common acute otitis media pathogens, especially *S. pneumoniae*, *H. influenzae*, and *Moraxella catarrhalis*. A wide-field myringotomy, or standard myringotomy with tube, is essential to provide drainage, ventilate the middle-ear space, and obtain material for culture. Systemic antibiotics should be tailored accordingly. In severe forms of suppurative labyrinthitis, the patient should be admitted for intravenous antibiotics and close observation for further sequelae, such as an ascending infection (e.g., meningitis or intracranial abscess). In all forms of tympanogenic labyrinthitis, lack of response to treatment or signs of further complications, such as meningeal signs, mental status changes, facial nerve involvement, or postauricular fluctuance, may require urgent mastoidectomy. CT imaging should be performed preoperatively. In severe cases of suppurative labyrinthitis with documented or impending intracranial involvement, a labyrinthectomy with cochleostomy should be considered at the time of mastoidectomy as a lifesaving measure. Although this procedure sacrifices all hearing and vestibular function in the affected ear, the suppurative labyrinthitis will likely have already destroyed it.

In the setting of chronic otitis media or trauma, early imaging with high-resolution temporal bone CT is essential to determine the presence of cholesteatoma and bony erosion or defects that may have provided entry of organisms into the inner ear. Systemic antimicrobials are essential. If chronic otitis media exists, broadening the antibiotic coverage to include *Pseudomonas aeruginosa* and other gram-negative organisms should be considered. Mastoidectomy should be performed to remove cholesteatoma if present, and cultures should be obtained. If erosion of the bony otic capsule is found, it is commonly through the lateral semicircular canal and may cause a perilymph fistula. A fistula secondary to trauma (most commonly a temporal bone fracture), with progressive symptoms, should prompt middle-ear exploration and fistula repair.

Meningitic Labyrinthitis

Systemic antibiotic treatment should be directed at the primary bacterial meningitis, which is discussed in the chapter "Bacterial Meningitis and Septicemia." Systemic corticosteroids not only reduce mortality and neurologic sequelae but also dramatically reduce the risk of severe postmeningitic hearing loss. In one large review, dexamethasone reduced the risk of severe hearing loss by 58%. Dexamethasone should be given at 0.4 to 0.6 mg/kg/day divided every 6 hours for 4 days and started as soon as possible. If possible, for maximal effectiveness, steroid should be started prior to starting antibiotics.

After recovery, an important sequela of meningitic labyrinthitis is labyrinthitis ossificans, ossification of the inner ear. This is a frequent complication, especially when profound hearing loss has occurred (up to 80%), and progresses over several months. This is significant because many of these patients become candidates for cochlear implantation, and implant insertion becomes progressively more difficult with continued ossification. Urgent cochlear implantation is indicated in some cases, and thus prompt referral of patients with severe hearing losses is essential. Corticosteroids, now becoming part of primary therapy for meningitis (dexamethasone, 0.5 to 0.6 mg/kg/day for 4 days) also reduce labyrinthine ossification after recovery.

Hematogenic Labyrinthitis

Labyrinthitis secondary to viral illness or suspected autoimmune conditions requires prompt otolaryngology and audiologic evaluation because early treatment may preserve hearing. These conditions may not be distinguishable clinically, but initial management is similar and primarily involves corticosteroids. Most data come from adults. If the patient presents within 14 days of onset of deafness or if hearing loss is still progressing, oral prednisone is generally started at 1 mg/kg/day and then tapered. There is no agreement in the literature on duration of therapy. Courses range from 10 days to 3 months. Audiograms are used to monitor progress. Cyclophosphamide is beneficial in adult patients with autoimmune labyrinthitis who respond poorly to steroids; however, it has not been studied in children. Treatment for CMV labyrinthitis remains problematic, with ganciclovir showing some benefit. Syphilitic labyrinthitis requires penicillin in high doses to obtain inner ear penetration and should be combined with high-dose systemic steroids for 4 weeks to maximize chances of hearing preservation.

MANAGEMENT OF DIZZINESS

Vertigo and dysequilibrium are common to all types of labyrinthitis. Vertigo results from an imbalance in the signals coming from the vestibular apparatuses on each side. With an acute presentation, the brain does not have time to compensate for the disparity. This can occur when there is acute inflammation of one inner ear, asymmetrical involvement of both ears, or sudden complete loss of function on one side. Importantly, vertigo ultimately resolves in most patients as central compensation occurs over several weeks, although the time course is highly variable. Thus management of dizziness is twofold: supportive management for acute vertigo and long-term therapy to optimize central compensation. The former should include bed rest and fluids; vestibular suppressants, such as diazepam and meclizine, should be used only as needed. Importantly, both bed rest and medications should be discontinued as soon as possible because they interfere with the ongoing process of central compensation. Compensation can be enhanced by vestibular rehabilitation therapy, a specialized form of physical therapy. In the rare event that incapacitating vertigo persists long term (e.g., after 6 months), ablative neurotologic procedures are available, which include labyrinthectomy, aminoglycoside ablation, and vestibular nerve section. Fortunately, these procedures are rarely necessary in children. Unremitting vertigo should also prompt consideration for further workup, particularly high-resolution gadolinium-enhanced MRI of the temporal bones and brainstem, to detect underlying neoplasms or other unusual lesions.

PREVENTIVE MEASURES

In labyrinthitis, the only preventive measure of importance is prompt recognition of the primary infection or inflammatory process before it can spread into the chambers of the inner ear. Prompt diagnosis and management of acute otitis media is an obvious example. Patients with chronic otitis media are at risk for cholesteatoma and its complications, including labyrinthitis, and so they need close monitoring by an otolaryngologist for development of cholesteatoma and symptoms such as episodic vertigo or fluctuating hearing loss and tinnitus. Prevention measures for meningitic labyrinthitis naturally include immunization for pathogens such as *H. influenzae*. Immunizations against mumps, measles, and rubella may reduce the incidence of viral labyrinthitis.

Common Pitfalls

The most significant complication surrounding labyrinthitis is permanent deafness, which is particularly common after suppurative labyrinthitis. The degree of loss is frequently severe at presentation; and although hearing may improve somewhat after treatment, it rarely returns to normal. Serous labyrinthitis can result in permanent SNHL, but total deafness in the involved ear is uncommon.

Meningitic labyrinthitis deserves special mention because hearing losses are often very severe and bilateral. Hearing can continue to worsen progressively, even after resolution of the infection, and thus these patients need audiometric evaluation as soon as their disease is stabilized and require subsequent follow-up for several years. If bilateral involvement progresses to severe or profound hearing loss, the patient may become a candidate for cochlear implantation. This procedure currently is performed routinely as early as 12 months of age, but postmeningitic deafness often dictates urgent implantation of even younger infants because of the progressive nature of labyrinthitis ossificans, as described earlier.

Communication and Counseling

If hearing loss is identified, immediate audiologic referral is essential to begin hearing rehabilitation. The audiologist evaluates for amplification (e.g., hearing aids) and helps recommend special educational interventions, such as teacher/room-amplification systems and preferential seating in the classroom. Special educational services should be coordinated with the schools as soon as possible. The importance of early amplification should be emphasized to all caregivers and educators because evidence clearly indicates that it benefits speech acquisition. This is true even for unilateral deafness because bilateral input is important for hearing in a noisy environment. Finally, parents should be reminded that hearing losses can progress, and therefore they have to take their child for regular audiometric follow-up. In patients with hearing loss, speech and language pathology evaluations should be considered at intervals to ensure proper development of speech and timely initiation of therapy if necessary.

SUGGESTED READINGS

1. Chan YM, Adams DA, Kerr AG: Syphilitic labyrinthitis—an update. J Laryngol Otol 109(8):719–725, 1995. **Long-term study of treatments for syphilitic labyrinthitis.**
2. Goldstein NA, Casselbrant ML, Bluestone CD, et al: Intratemporal complications of acute otitis media in infants and children. Otolaryngol Head Neck Surg 119(5):444–454, 1998. **Retrospective study of otitis media complications and treatment, including five children with labyrinthitis.**
3. Hartnick CJ, Kim HY, Chute PM, et al: Preventing labyrinthitis ossificans; the role of steroids. Arch Otolaryngol Head Neck Surg 127:180–183, 2001. **Retrospective study suggesting steroids may prevent labyrinthitis ossificans in patients with meningitis.**

4. Irving RM, Ruben RJ: The acquired hearing losses of childhood. In Lalwani AK, Grundfast KM (eds): Pediatric Otology Neurotology. Philadelphia: Lippincott-Raven, 1998, pp 375–385. **Review of acquired hearing loss including meningitic and viral etiologies.**

5. Jacobs IN, Todd NW: Regional intracranial complications of otitis media. In Wetmore RF, Muntz HR, McGill TJ (eds): Pediatric Otolaryngology: Principles and Practice Pathways. New York: Thieme, 2000, pp 305–326. **Practical overview of otitis media complications including labyrinthitis.**

6. Stone JH, Francis HW: Immune-mediated inner ear disease. Curr Opin Rheumatol 12(1):32–40, 2000. **Comprehensive review of autoimmune labyrinthitis and its treatment.**

7. Strauss M: Human cytomegalovirus labyrinthitis. Am J Otolaryngol 11(5):292–298, 1999. **Review of clinical and pathologic findings in CMV labyrinthitis.**

8. van de Beek D, de Gans J, McIntyre P, et al: Corticosteroids in acute bacterial meningitis. Corticosteroids in acute bacterial meningitis. Cochrane Database Syst Rev 3:CD004305 2003. **Systematic review of steroids for meningitis, showing clear benefit in preserving hearing.**

Disorders of the Neck and Parotid

Sezelle Gereau and Eli Grunstein

KEY CONCEPTS

- Neck masses in children are common.
- The differential diagnosis of a pediatric neck mass usually falls under the categories of congenital masses, inflammatory processes, both benign and malignant neoplastic masses, and other noncategorized masses.
- Less than one third of pediatric neck masses are found to be malignant neoplasms.
- Important elements of the history include age of onset, change in size, pain, history of malignancy, and associated symptoms and diseases.
- A systematic and thorough head and neck exam, including examination of all mucosal surfaces of the upper aerodigestive tract, is essential. This may necessitate referral to an otolaryngologist.
- Most pediatric neck masses occur in the anterior triangle and have a lower incidence of malignancy compared with masses in the posterior triangle.
- Diagnostic testing may include complete blood count, thyroid-function tests, liver-function tests, purified protein derivative, and serology.
- Plain films, chest x-ray, ultrasound, magnetic resonance imaging, magnetic resonance angiography, and positron-emission tomography scanning may be necessary for further evaluation of the mass.
- Fine-needle aspiration biopsy (FNAB) can be helpful in differentiating benign from malignant disease, directing antibiotic therapy for infectious masses, and may be therapeutic for abscesses.
- Open biopsy is the gold standard technique for the diagnosis of a neck mass. It should be employed if the diagnosis is unclear after a noninvasive workup or if response to treatment is inadequate.

Expert Opinion on Management Issues

The most common neck mass in the pediatric patient is inflammatory cervical lymphadenopathy, usually secondary to a viral or bacterial upper respiratory tract infection (URTI). Patients generally present with history of a recent URTI, systemic symptomatology associated with infection (e.g., fever, malaise), and tender adenopathy on exam. A trial of observation or oral antibiotics for 10 to 14 days may be appropriate for a recent onset of symptomatology and mild or moderate exam findings. More extensive adenopathy on exam warrants intravenous antibiotic therapy. Fluctuation on examination is highly suspicious for an abscess and should be confirmed with a CT scan. Incision and drainage should be considered for inflammatory processes that do not improve after 48 hours of intravenous antibiotics and for abscesses.

Inflammatory adenopathy may also be secondary to both tuberculous (TB) and nontuberculous (NTM) mycobacterial disease. A purified protein derivative (PPD) test may be helpful, but the diagnosis usually requires aspiration and positive cultures. NTM should be treated with excision, whereas TB can be treated with antituberculous chemotherapy. Epstein-Barr virus (EBV) adenopathy should be confirmed with heterophile antibodies and serology. Conservative therapy is the standard of care for EBV adenopathy. *Bartonella*, cytomegalovirus (CMV), human immunodeficiency virus (HIV), toxoplasmosis, brucellosis, and tularemia are all in the differential of inflammatory adenopathy; diagnosis can be made with serology and treated with appropriate medical therapy. Referral to an otolaryngologist should be considered for masses that do not respond to conservative therapy, particularly for those larger than 2 cm.

Congenital lesions are the most commonly excised pediatric neck mass. Branchial anomalies may manifest as a fistula (an epidermal-lined tract from the pharynx to the skin), a sinus tract (a tract that communicates externally or internally, but not both), or a cyst (an epidermal-lined mass without a communication between the skin or pharynx). First branchial anomalies usually appear in the preauricular region, with a variable relationship to the facial nerve. These can also manifest with otorrhea or submandibular drainage in the setting of a URTI. Second branchial anomalies are most common, accounting for greater than 90% of all branchial anomalies. These usually occur at the anterior border of the sternocleidomastoid muscle (SCM), at or below the level of the hyoid bone. Second branchial fistulas or external sinus tracts may manifest with external drainage in the setting of a URTI, whereas infected cysts can manifest with dysphagia, dyspnea, stridor, neck pain, and neck fullness. The internal communication of second branchial fistulas or sinus tracts is usually in the region of the tonsillar fossa. Third and fourth branchial anomalies are rare; they drain internally in the region of the pyriform sinus and externally at the anterior border of the SCM. These can manifest

TABLE 1 Congenital Masses

Mass	Diagnosis	Treatment
Thyroglossal duct cyst	Midline neck mass, moves with swallowing, must document thyroid in normal location	Excision (Sistrunk), antibiotics if infected, avoid I & D
Dermoid	Midline neck mass, usually submental, no movement with swallowing, moves with skin	Surgical excision
Branchial anomalies: fistula, cyst, sinus	Mass or sinus at anterior border of SCM, may have associated syndrome, CT: cyst, course of fistula/sinus tract	Surgical excision, antibiotics if infected, avoid I & D
Thymus abnormalities	Cystic mass or ectopic rest anywhere along the embryologic path of the thymus, CT or MRI diagnostic, 50% extend into the mediastinum	Observation, surgical excision
Teratoma	Cystic mass in anterior or posterior triangle of neck, CT/MRI diagnostic	Surgical excision
Fibromatosis coli (SCM tumor of infancy)	Lateral neck mass in first 10 days of life, torticollis	Massage, stretching exercises, excision if not improved after 1 yr
Hemangioma	Present in first year of life, can occur in any region in the head and neck, rapid growth then involution, MRI diagnostic	Conservative management unless complicated, systemic/intralesional steroids, interferon, excision ± embolization
Lymphatic malformation	First 2 years of life, slow growing, fluctuant, painless, can occur in any region in the head and neck, rapid enlargement with URTI, evaluation with CT/MRI	Excision, sclerotherapy
Vascular malformation	Present at birth, can occur in any region in the head and neck, steady growth, rapid enlargement with infection/trauma, pulsatile neck mass, MRA diagnostic	Excision ± preoperative embolization
Jugular vein phlebectasia	Cystic swelling anterior to SCM, muscle enlarges with crying/Valsalva, MRI, CT with contrast, or angiography diagnostic	Observation once diagnosis confirmed
Carotid aneurysm	Pulsatile lateral neck mass, usually after trauma or surgery, unilateral headache, cranial neuropathy, MRA or angiography diagnostic	Anticoagulation, then definitive surgical repair

I & D, incision and drainage; MRA, magnetic resonance angiography; SCM, sternocleidomastoid muscle; URTI, upper respiratory tract infection.

19

with suppurative thyroiditis, dysphagia, dyspnea, stridor, neck pain, and neck fullness. The diagnosis of a branchial anomaly can be made with CT scan, and the treatment of choice is surgical excision because of the risk of infection and malignant degeneration. Acutely infected lesions should be treated with a course of antibiotics before excision, and incision and drainage should be strenuously avoided. Aspiration of an infected cyst may be helpful by decompressing the lesion, as well as identifying the causative organisms.

Thyroglossal duct cysts (TGDCs) and dermoid cysts are the most common midline neck masses. A TGDC usually manifests as a firm midline mass, thought to form from a remnant of embryonic thyroid tissue. It moves with swallowing and can become secondarily infected. An ultrasound or radionuclide scan should be done to confirm the presence of thyroid tissue in the normal location before excision so as not to remove the patient's only functioning thyroid tissue. The standard of care is to excise the central portion of the hyoid bone and a core of the base of the tongue (Sistrunk procedure) in an effort to minimize recurrence. As with branchial anomalies, infected lesions should be treated with antibiotics prior to excision, with an effort

to avoid incision and drainage. Dermoids usually attach to and move with the skin, but they do not move with swallowing. Excision is the treatment of choice for dermoids as well.

Hemangiomas are the most common congenital vascular masses in the pediatric population. They typically appear during the first year of life with rapid growth during the proliferative phase. MRI is diagnostic. With time, they undergo involution, and they completely resolve in 50% of patients by 5 years of age and in 70% by 7 years of age. A conservative approach is therefore warranted unless the lesion causes functional impairment, compromises vital structures (e.g., airway obstruction), bleeds, or causes consumptive coagulopathy (Kasabach-Merritt syndrome). Treatment options include systemic steroids, intralesional steroids, systemic interferon-alfa, and excision with or without preoperative embolization.

Vascular malformations are present at birth, enlarge steadily as the body grows, do not regress, and may rapidly enlarge after infection, trauma, or hormonal surges. The diagnosis can be made with magnetic resonance angiography (MRA). Treatment involves early resection with consideration for preoperative embolization.

TABLE 2 Inflammatory Masses

Mass	Diagnosis	Treatment
Infectious cervical lymphadenitis	Palpable cervical adenopathy, tender, systemic symptoms and signs of infection, elevated WBC count Lyme disease: tick bite, serology, tularemia: milk exposure, serology. *Bartonella*: cat bite/scratch	Viral: observation Bacterial: β-lactamase stable antibiotics Tuberculous: TB medications Nontuberculous: excision *Bartonella*: azithromycin Fungal: antifungal medications
Abscess	Fluctuant lateral neck mass, systemic signs and symptoms of infection, CT (ring-enhancing hypodense lesion), elevated WBC count	Incision and drainage
Kawasaki disease	<5 yr, fever, nonexudative conjunctivitis, strawberry tongue, fissured lips, rash, erythema of palms/soles, periungual desquamation, cervical adenopathy, coronary artery aneurysms	IV γ-globulin, aspirin, possibly steroids
Kikuchi-Fujimoto disease	Usually young Asian female, unilateral or bilateral lymphadenopathy not responsive to antibiotics, biopsy diagnostic	Spontaneous regression
Kimura disease	Young Asian male, lymphadenopathy and tender subcutaneous swelling, elevated IgE and eosinophils, biopsy diagnostic	Complete excision, irradiation for older patients
Sarcoidosis	Children rarely affected, adenopathy or parotid enlargement, CXR with bilateral hilar lymphadenopathy, elevated ACE level, biopsy diagnostic	Steroids, low-dose methotrexate
Rosai-Dorfman disease	Massive nontender adenopathy, children <10 yr may have extranodal disease (sinonasal region common), biopsy diagnostic	Observation; surgery, radiation, or chemotherapy for disseminated disease
Castleman disease	Chronic asymptomatic enlarging lateral neck mass, biopsy diagnostic	Complete excision
Autoimmune disease	Cervical adenopathy in association with autoimmune disorder (e.g., rheumatoid arthritis, lupus, etc.)	Treatment of primary disease
Sialoadenitis: viral, bacterial, granulomatous	Swollen and tender salivary gland, fever, purulent discharge from parotid or submandibular duct, elevated WBC count, needle biopsy for suspicion of granulomatous lesion, PPD	Viral: conservative management Bacterial: hydration, broad-spectrum antibiotics, sialogogues, warm compresses Granulomatous: chemotherapy vs. surgical excision
Thyroiditis (infectious)	Fever, neck pain, tender midline neck mass, hyper, hypo, or euthyroid, elevated WBC count	Hydration, observation if suspect viral, antibiotics if bacterial, incision and drainage for abscess

ACE, angiotensin-converting enzyme; CXR, chest radiograph; Ig, immunoglobulin; IV, intravenous; PPD, purified protein derivative; TB, tuberculosis; WBC, white blood cell.

Lymphatic malformations are slow growing, fluctuant, and painless lesions that can cause significant cosmetic and functional deformities, including airway obstruction. They usually appear before 2 years of age and can become acutely enlarged during a URTI. As part of the diagnostic evaluation, CT or MRI is essential in noting the characteristics of the lesion, as well as its relationship to the adjacent anatomy. Surgical excision is the traditional method of treatment, with careful attention to sparing critical adjacent structures. Sclerotherapy using OK432 may have shown promise in macrocystic (cystic hygroma) lesions.

Fibromatosis coli usually manifests in the first 10 days of life as torticollis and a lateral neck mass within the sternocleidomastoid muscle. The etiology is not completely understood but is thought to be secondary to intrauterine positioning or birth trauma. Diagnosis is made by history but may require CT or biopsy. The initial treatment should be conservative, including massage and stretching exercises. If improvement is not noted after 1 year, surgical excision may be appropriate.

Malignant lesions usually manifest as asymptomatic neck masses. Solid masses increase in size within weeks to months, and associated systemic symptoms, such as fever, night sweats, and fatigue, should raise the suspicion of malignancy. Lymphomas are the most common pediatric head and neck malignancy. Although non-Hodgkin lymphoma is more common, Hodgkin disease more often occurs in the neck. Associated symptoms may include fever, weight loss, and night sweats. The diagnosis should be confirmed with a tissue biopsy and treated with a combination of radiation and chemotherapy, depending on the disease stage.

Rhabdomyosarcoma is the second most common head and neck malignancy and can occur in the orbit, sinonasal region, nasopharynx, temporal bone, parotid,

TABLE 3 Neoplastic Masses

Mass	Diagnosis	Treatment
Benign		
Pilomatrixoma	Solitary, firm, nontender dermal or subcutaneous nodule	Surgical excision
Benign salivary gland tumor	Enlargement of respective gland, FNA often helpful, CT/MRI to define anatomy	Excision of respective gland, observation for hemangioma
Benign thyroid disease	Central neck mass, hyper, hypo, or euthyroid	Observation or excision
Paraganglioma: jugular, carotid, vagal	Solitary tumor in lateral neck, carotid most common, cranial neuropathy, CT/MRI to define anatomy, angiography for both diagnosis and preoperative embolization	Observation for tiny asymptomatic lesions; otherwise resection with preoperative embolization
Schwannoma	Solitary tumor in lateral neck, vagus and sympathetic nerves most common, cranial neuropathy, CT/MRI diagnostic and to define anatomy	Surgical excision
Neurofibroma	Sporadic or, as part of NF1 or NF2, can involve any nerve, subcutaneous nodules (NF 1/2), CT/MRI helpful to define anatomy	Surgical excision
Malignant		
Hodgkin and non-Hodgkin lymphoma	Neck mass, fever, weight loss, night sweats, need pathologic specimen for diagnosis	Radiation ± chemotherapy
Post-transplantation lymphoproliferative disease	Immunosuppressed transplant recipients, solid tumor or diffuse lymphoid enlargement, airway obstruction if massive hypertrophy of Waldeyer ring, biopsy diagnostic	Reduction in immunosuppression
Rhabdomyosarcoma	Head or neck mass, weight loss, fever, cranial neuropathy, need pathological specimen for diagnosis	Chemotherapy + radiation, surgery for very limited disease or salvage
Other sarcomas	Neck mass, cranial neuropathy, need pathological specimen for diagnosis	Wide local excision, possible radiation/chemotherapy
Salivary gland malignancies	Mass in respective gland, neck mass, facial nerve paralysis, FNA helpful, CT/MRI define anatomy	Excision of respective gland, neck dissection and radiation for high-grade lesions
Neuroblastoma	<10 yr of age, firm mass in lateral neck, cranial neuropathy, compression of upper aerodigestive tract, possible distant metastasis, CT/MRI to define anatomy, FNA helpful	Surgical excision for localized disease, chemotherapy for incomplete resection or distant metastasis
Nasopharyngeal cancer	Adolescents, metastatic lateral neck mass, unilateral otitis media, rhinorrhea, nasal obstruction, cranial neuropathy, CT/MRI to define anatomy, biopsy for diagnosis at primary site, FNA helpful for metastatic neck disease	Radiation and chemotherapy, ± surgery for neck disease
Malignant thyroid disease	Central or lateral neck mass, history of radiation exposure, family history of medullary carcinoma or MEN, FNA helpful	Surgery ± radioactive iodine
Malignant cervical adenopathy	Nontender, hard lateral neck mass, head and neck primary vs. distant metastasis: lung, esophageal, renal, testicular, FNA helpful CT/MRI to document anatomy	Treatment of the primary malignancy; treatment of the neck may involve surgery, radiation, chemotherapy, or any combination

FNA, fine-needle aspiration; MEN, multiple endocrine neoplasia; NF, nasopharyngeal fibroma.

and neck. Diagnosis must be confirmed with tissue biopsy. Depending on the extent of the disease, therapeutic options include surgical resection or a combination of radiation and chemotherapy.

Thyroid cancer manifests as a palpable anterior or lateral neck mass in adolescence, and it is more common in females than males. Up to 55% of palpable nodules in the pediatric population harbor malignancy, most commonly papillary carcinoma. A history of radiation exposure is a critical risk factor for the development of a thyroid malignancy. Although children with well-differentiated thyroid cancer tend to present with more advanced locoregional disease than adults, their prognosis is still excellent. Fine-needle aspiration (FNA) can be helpful in making the diagnosis, and the treatment of choice is thyroidectomy, often with postoperative radioactive iodine. Patients with multiple endocrine neoplasias IIa and IIb are at considerable risk for developing medullary carcinoma of the thyroid and should undergo prophylactic thyroidectomy.

TABLE 4 Other Masses

Mass	Diagnosis	Treatment
Plunging ranula	Cystic midline neck mass, associated compressible floor of mouth mass, CT/MRI notes penetration of mylohyoid muscle	Surgical excision with removal of sublingual gland
Lipoma	Slowly enlarging, painless, subcutaneous mass, deeper lesions may compress upper aerodigestive tract	Surgical excision
Laryngocele	Air filled lateral neck mass, CT: air filled mass originating in larynx	Observation, laryngoscopic or open excision

Acute sialoadenitis usually manifests with swelling, pain, and tenderness in either the preauricular (parotid gland) or submandibular (submandibular gland) regions, usually in association with a concurrent illness or dehydration. A purulent discharge can often be expressed from the papilla of the parotid (Stensen) duct opposite the second upper molar or the submandibular (Warthin) duct opposite the frenulum of the tongue. The treatment of choice is intravenous antibiotics with coverage for staphylococcus, warm compresses, hydration, and sialogogues, such as lemon drops. Any signs of cellulitis or deep neck infection are indications for intravenous antibiotics. Incision and drainage are warranted if an abscess develops. Chronic and recurrent parotitis usually manifest similarly to acute parotitis but with a less fulminant course. The treatment is supportive, with warm compresses, hydration, massage, antibiotics, and analgesia. Parotidectomy is reserved for patients with symptoms refractory to conservative management.

Ten percent of children with human immunodeficiency virus (HIV) present with lymphoepithelial changes of the parotid gland. Treatment is supportive. Antibiotics may be required for infections. Repeat aspiration with or without low-dose radiation may provide relief. The incidence of parotid lymphoma is increased in these patients and should be suspected for any sudden increase in gland size.

Salivary gland neoplasms in the pediatric population are not common. The parotid gland is the most frequent location, with hemangioma accounting for approximately 40% of the cases. Lymphomas and pleomorphic adenomas are the next most common neoplasms. Mucoepidermoid carcinoma is the most common malignant salivary epithelial lesion in children, usually of the low-grade histologic type. Treatment of salivary gland neoplasms often involves surgery. Radiation and chemotherapy are reserved for lymphomas and high-grade malignancies.

Tables 1 through 4 summarize the diagnosis and management of the various pediatric neck masses.

Common Pitfalls

- Consider a congenital cystic mass if a deep neck infection recurs.
- Confirm thyroid tissue in usual location before thyroglossal duct cyst excision.
- Simple excision of a thyroglossal duct cyst is associated with a high rate of recurrence; perform the Sistrunk procedure instead.
- Follow and excise entire tract for branchial abnormality to minimize recurrence.
- Ensure that initial surgery for lymphoma and rhabdomyosarcoma involves biopsy and not heroic attempts at complete resection because these disease processes are initially treated with radiation with or without chemotherapy.
- Do not resect uncomplicated hemangiomas because of the high likelihood of spontaneous resolution.
- Avoid incision and drainage of a potential mycobacterial collection because of the increased incidence of chronic fistula formation in these cases.
- Be aware that preoperative embolization for vascular tumors may reduce intraoperative bleeding.
- Lymphatic malformations, although benign, can cause upper aerodigestive tract compression; consider surgical excision in these cases.
- The facial nerve is at risk for injury during incision and drainage of a parotid abscess; make the incision parallel to the expected course of the nerve branch to minimize the risk of nerve transection.
- Avoid open biopsy of metastatic malignant cervical adenopathy at all costs. FNA may be helpful in making the diagnosis in these cases.

Communication and Counseling

Most pediatric neck masses are benign. Malignant neck masses are usually associated with a good prognosis. Parents need to be educated about the signs and symptoms of aerodigestive tract compromise, which may be the result of a progressing inflammatory neck process or an enlarging neck mass. A multidisciplinary approach to patients with these masses yields the best outcomes. Thus treatment involves the surgeon and pediatrician and occasionally the oncologist, radiation oncologist, rheumatologist, and infectious disease specialist.

SUGGESTED READINGS

1. Bauer PW, Lusk RP: Neck masses. In Bluestone CD, Stool SE, Casselbrant ML, et al (eds): Pediatric Otolaryngology, 4th ed. Philadelphia: WB Saunders, 2001. **Overview of the diagnosis and management of pediatric neck masses.**

2. Cunningham MJ: Congenital malformations of the head and neck. In Cotton RT, Myer CM (eds): Practical Pediatric Otolaryngology. Philadelphia: Lippincott-Raven, 2003. **Detailed description of the diagnosis and management of congenital neck masses.**

3. Cunningham MJ: Neoplastic disorders: Benign and malignant. In Cotton RT, Myer CM (eds): Practical Pediatric Otolaryngology. Philadelphia: Lippincott-Raven, 2003. **Detailed description of the diagnosis and management of neoplastic pediatric neck masses.**

4. Karmody CS: Developmental anomalies of the neck. In Bluestone CD, Stool SE, Casselbrant ML, et al (eds): Pediatric Otolaryngology, 4th ed. Philadelphia: WB Saunders, 2001. **Detailed description of the diagnosis and management of pediatric developmental anomalies.**

5. Rosenfeld RM: Cervical adenopathy. In Bluestone CD, Stool SE, Casselbrant ML, et al (eds): Pediatric Otolaryngology, 4th ed. Philadelphia: WB Saunders, 2001. **Detailed description of the diagnosis and management of cervical adenopathy, with particular emphasis on inflammatory neck disease.**

6. Shott SR: Salivary disease in children. In Cotton RT, Myer CM (eds): Practical Pediatric Otolaryngology. Philadelphia: Lippincott-Raven, 2003. **Detailed description of the diagnosis and management of pediatric salivary gland diseases and masses.**

Serum Sickness

Seema S. Aceves

KEY CONCEPTS

- Serum sickness represents an immune complex–mediated process.
- Symptoms consist of fevers, rash (usually urticarial), lymphadenopathy, arthralgias, and edema.
- Serum sickness usually begins 1 to 2 weeks following initiation of the inciting agent; it can begin earlier and with increased severity if the reaction is a secondary immune response.
- Symptom resolution occurs 1 week to 1 month following removal of the offending antigen.
- Common inciting antigens are protein antigens from another species (e.g., horse, rabbit, and humanized mouse antitoxins), antivenoms, and monoclonal antibodies. Molecules that act as haptens, such as antibiotics, are also common causes of serum sickness.
- The most important therapeutic intervention is removal and future avoidance of the offending antigen.

Von Pirquet and Schick first described serum sickness in 1905 as an illness that developed 8 to 12 days following the injection of horse diphtheria antitoxin in children. The illness consisted of a clinical constellation of fever, urticaria, lymphadenopathy, arthralgias, and peripheral edema, and it is now known to result from the formation and deposition of immune complexes, which cause a type III hypersensitivity reaction.

Clinical features of serum sickness include fevers, malaise, headaches, myalgias, arthralgias, and gastrointestinal upset, starting 1 to 2 weeks after initiation of the offending agent. The rash associated with serum sickness can sometimes precede fever, and it is usually urticarial and/or morbilliform, with biopsy findings of a leukocytoclastic vasculitis with neutrophils and immune complex deposition on immunofluorescence. In patients treated with antithymocyte globulin, the finding of a serpiginous linear erythema at the dorsolateral surface of the palmar or plantar skin is often the initial rash. Arthritis (occurring in 10% to 50% of patients) is usually symmetrical and involves the

metacarpophalangeal joints and knees. Lymphadenopathy can be regional or diffuse and can be associated with splenomegaly. Serious complications include acute renal failure and peripheral neuropathies, including peripheral neuritis and Guillain-Barré syndrome, as well as central processes including myelitis, cranial nerve palsies, and encephalitis. Subsequent antigenic exposures result in a secondary antibody response, which elicits a more rapid and clinically severe course. Symptoms usually remit 1 week to 1 month following removal of the inciting agent, reflecting the removal of immune complexes by the reticuloendothelial system. Complete clinical recovery is the norm.

The key feature in the history is identification of the offending agent, which allows its subsequent removal and avoidance. Common inciting antigens are proteins from other species and small molecules that function as haptens, such as antibiotics. Classically, antitoxins and antivenoms are common causes of serum sickness. Patients are more likely to suffer from serum sickness if they are given higher doses of antivenom or antitoxoid. Newer humanized monoclonal antibodies, such as anti–tumor necrosis factor (TNF)-α, are also reported to cause immune complex–mediated disease in humans. In addition, proteins from other species that are therapeutic agents (e.g., streptokinase and hormones) can cause serum sickness, as can envenomation by toxins from hymenoptera and ticks. Antibiotics can act as haptens to induce serum sickness, with cefaclor the most commonly cited offending agent in children (Box 1).

Children with serum sickness caused by cefaclor tend to be younger and have a history of exposure to multiple antibiotics. Many cases of cefaclor-induced serum sickness are not associated with hypocomplementemia and thus are labeled serum sickness–like reaction (SSLR). SSLR is a clinical syndrome that does not present with the full clinical picture of serum sickness or lacks the laboratory findings of proteinuria and circulating immune complexes. However, distinguishing between serum sickness and SSLR can be difficult because often laboratory studies for circulating immune complexes are not drawn, and even true serum sickness can present without the full clinical syndrome. The same treatment guidelines apply to both serum sickness and SSLR.

BOX 1 Proteins and Medications that Cause Serum Sickness*

Proteins from Other Species
- Antithymocyte globulin
- Antitetanus toxoid
- Antivenin (Crotalidae) polyvalent (horse serum based)
- Crotalidae polyvalent immune Fab (ovine serum based)
- Antirabies globulin
- Infliximab
- Rituximab
- Etanercept
- Anti-HIV antibodies ([PE]HRG214)
- Hymenoptera stings
- Streptokinase

Drugs

Antibiotics
- Cefaclor

Penicillins
- Trimethoprim-Sulfa
- Minocycline
- Meropenem

Neurologic
- Bupropion
- Carbamazepine
- Phenytoin
- Sulfonamides
- Barbiturates

*Based on review of most current literature. Other medications that are not listed are also cited to cause serum sickness.
HIV, human immunodeficiency virus.

TABLE 1 Medications Used to Treat Serum Sickness or SSLR

Medication	Dose
Prednisone	1–2 mg/kg/day, max 60 mg qd
Cetirizine (sedating in a subset of patients)	6–23 mo: 2.5 mg qd 2–5 yr: 2.5–5 mg qd ≥6 yr: 5–10 mg qd
Fexofenadine	6–12 yr: 30 mg bid ≥12 yr: 180 mg qd
Loratadine	2–5 yr: 5 mg qd ≥6 yr: 10 mg qd
Hydroxyzine (sedating)	2 mg/kg/day div q6–8h
Diphenhydramine (sedating)	5 mg/kg/day div q6h

bid, twice daily; div, divided; qd, every day; qxh, every x hours; SSLR, serum sickness–like reaction.

Expert Opinion on Management Issues

LABORATORY STUDIES

Although studies such as cryoglobulins and Raji cell assays can detect the presence of circulating immune complexes, the diagnosis of serum sickness is made clinically. During the peak of symptoms, patients have decreased C_3, C_4, and CH_{50} (complement levels), which reflects the consumptive nature of the process. In addition, inflammatory markers are elevated, such as the erythrocyte sedimentation rate and C-reactive protein. Transient elevations in liver function tests can also occur, but the importance in checking liver function tests is more relevant if hepatitis is a clinical concern. An analysis of renal function to assess for evidence of renal failure and urinalysis for proteinuria is also warranted, especially if peripheral edema is present.

MEDICAL MANAGEMENT

There are no clinical trials evaluating the effectiveness of medication use in the type III immune response characterized by serum sickness. Existing clinical trials evaluating the prevention of complications following snake antivenoms focus on the role of adrenaline and antihistamines in preventing the immediate hypersensitivity response of anaphylaxis to animal sera.

The most important first step is to remove the offending antigen. Once this is done, serum sickness follows a typical clinical course of resolution within 7 to 28 days. Mild to moderately symptomatic patients with fevers and musculoskeletal complaints benefit from nonsteroidal anti-inflammatory medications. Antihistamines are used to alleviate the pruritus associated with urticaria. If the urticarial rash has a large vasculitic component, corticosteroids may be needed for therapy. Patients who are significantly debilitated by symptoms of serum sickness should be treated with prednisone. In addition, patients with evidence of renal impairment should be treated with oral corticosteroids. A reasonable dose of prednisone is 1 to 2 mg/kg/day as a single dose with a maximum dose of 60 mg daily (Table 1). Given the natural history of spontaneous resolution, a prednisone course of 5 to 14 days is usually sufficient.

Common Pitfalls

Potential pitfalls in the treatment of serum sickness include not eliminating the offending antigen and not coming to the correct diagnostic conclusion. Failure to eliminate the inciting agent results in continued symptoms. The differential diagnoses for serum sickness should include infections such as hepatitis, endocarditis, and rheumatic fever as well as rheumatologic and autoimmune illnesses such as juvenile rheumatoid arthritis, mixed connective tissue diseases, and Kawasaki disease. Case reports document that the treatment of presumed serum sickness with prednisone delays the diagnosis of hepatitis. If risk factors, symptoms, and signs of hepatitis are present, appropriate laboratory evaluation should be performed. In addition, patient follow-up to document resolution of symptoms and laboratory abnormalities is important. If symptoms do not resolve in 1 week to 1 month following removal of the presumed inciting agent or if prolonged steroid courses are required, other rheumatologic or infectious diagnoses must be considered (Box 2).

BOX 2   Differential Diagnoses for Serum Sickness

Infections
- Hepatitis
- Endocarditis
- Rheumatic fever
- Lyme disease

Other Drug-Induced Reactions
- Drug hypersensitivities syndrome (refers to a specific severe idiosyncratic reaction of rash, fever, hepatitis, arthralgias, lymphadenopathy, and hematologic abnormalities most commonly seen with anticonvulsant medications)
- Drug-induced vasculitis

Rheumatologic/Autoimmune Diseases
- Kawasaki disease
- Systemic-onset juvenile rheumatoid arthritis (Still disease)
- Mixed connective tissue disease

Communication and Counseling

The most important issue in counseling patients with a diagnosis of serum sickness is to educate the patient to avoid the inciting antigen in the future. Reintroduction of the same medication or animal serum results in quicker onset and exaggerated symptoms during a secondary immune response. Patients should also be informed that serum sickness is a self-limited process and will resolve within the month and that continued symptomatology beyond this time frame warrants evaluation for other etiologies. Lastly, if symptoms progress or involve neurologic manifestations, such as weakness or mental status changes, immediate medical attention should be solicited.

SUGGESTED READINGS

1. King B, Geelhoed G: Adverse skin and joint reactions associated with oral antibiotics in children: The role of cefaclor in serum sickness–like reactions. J Pediatr Child Health 39:677–681, 2003. **Large retrospective study of children with serum sickness–like reactions to antibiotics in Australia that demonstrates common inciting agents.**
2. Roujeau JC, Stern RS: Severe adverse cutaneous reactions to drugs. N Engl J Med 331:1272–1285, 1994. **Review of drug-induced hypersensitivities (includes photographs).**

Allergic Gastrointestinal Disorders

Anthony M. Loizides and Barry K. Wershil

KEY CONCEPTS

- True gastrointestinal allergies must be properly diagnosed before treatment is instituted to avoid malnutrition, vitamin deficiencies, and the undue monetary as well as emotional expense of therapy.
- Immunoglobulin (Ig) E-based tests are appropriate for IgE-mediated disorders such as immediate hypersensi-

tivity or the oral allergy syndrome. Evidence-based levels of IgE radioallergosorbent test (RAST) results can predict the presence of a food allergy with a high probability.
- An oral food challenge, ideally a double-blind placebo-controlled food challenge, is the gold standard in the diagnosis of non–IgE–mediated food allergy and should be used to document problematic foods, particularly when multiple foods allergies are thought to be present.
- The hallmark of eosinophilic disorders of the gastrointestinal tract is an increase in the number of tissue eosinophils, even though absolute criteria are not yet established. Biopsies are therefore necessary for diagnosis, and often serial biopsies are performed for management.
- Education of patients and parents regarding testing, diagnosis, and therapy is crucial for compliance and successful treatment.

An authentic hypersensitivity reaction to food typically involves the gastrointestinal tract but can also have extraintestinal manifestations, most commonly in the skin and the lungs. A wide variety of symptoms are attributed to food allergies, sometimes without even a rudimentary investigation. However, true food allergic reactions can be serious and even life-threatening.

Food allergy is defined as an immunologic response to ingested food antigens, and it must be differentiated from *food intolerance*, which is characterized by symptoms or signs resulting from a nonimmunologically based reaction to a food or food component (e.g., lactose intolerance). This distinction leads to some confusion when examining the prevalence of the problem. In infants younger than 2 years, the incidence of food allergy is reported to be between 6% and 8%, mostly based on clinical response to formula changes. In some series, as many as 20% of adults report having food allergies, but when tested by a double-blind food challenge, the real incidence in this population was only 1.4%.

Hypersensitivity reactions to food are typically categorized on the basis of the immunologic response involved, either immunoglobulin (Ig) E mediated or non–IgE mediated. Immediate-type hypersensitivity reactions (occurring seconds to minutes after ingestion) and the oral allergy syndrome are primarily IgE based. Eosinophilic esophagitis, gastritis, and gastroenterocolitis may involve a combination of IgE- and non–IgE-mediated mechanisms and dietary protein–induced enterocolitis, proctitis, and enteropathy, which are primarily non–IgE mediated (Box 1). Celiac disease is also a food allergy but not discussed in this chapter.

The diagnosis of food allergy is often suggested by a clinical reaction associated with a particular food. In some food-allergic individuals, however, there may not be a clear temporal relationship between the ingestion of the offending agent and symptoms. Often the diagnosis is made by some type of food challenge and/or histologic findings on biopsy of the gastrointestinal tract (usually eosinophilia). The gold standard remains the double-blind, placebo-controlled foods challenge. A more practical diagnostic test is the single-blind food challenge, which permits objective reporting of symptomatology. This approach is also helpful when several foods are considered, and it can be used in individuals who have already eliminated foods from their diet, not only to verify the allergy but also to expand the diet when there are multiple allergies. A much less stringent procedure is an open-label food challenge, which can be useful particularly in infants or to screen for reactions that can then be tested by blinded challenges.

A variety of in vitro and in vivo tests are available, but they tend to be useful for only a limited number of foods where reliable criteria are established (Table 1). Skin prick tests are slightly more sensitive than IgE radioallergosorbent test (RAST) testing. Atopy patch testing may be useful in the future to detect food allergy, but standards currently do not exist.

Expert Opinion on Management Issues

Therapy is tailored to the specific entity encountered. Dietary protein–induced proctitis/proctocolitis usually occurs in infants, who may present with bloody stools, diarrhea, and abdominal pain. It is treated by the elimination of cow's milk protein in the diet (including the maternal diet if breast-feeding). Approximately 30% of patients are also allergic to soy protein, so the preferred approach is to begin a so-called hypoallergenic formula, which typically has either hydrolyzed protein or protein in the form of elemental amino acids. This strategy usually leads to the resolution of gross bleeding within 3 to 5 days and of microscopic bleeding within 2 to 3 weeks. The entity itself typically resolves by 1 to 2 years of age.

Dietary protein enteropathy or a more severe presentation, dietary protein enterocolitis, may manifest with vomiting, diarrhea with or without blood, or even shocklike with acidosis. It is essential to rule out other causes of diarrhea and vomiting. The diagnosis often requires endoscopy and biopsies to confirm villus injury, most commonly atrophy. IgE-based tests are typically negative. A history of eczema, seasonal allergies, or asthma in the patient and a family history of atopy and food allergies help support the diagnosis but are not necessarily seen in every case. Ultimately, avoidance of the most common offenders, cow's milk and soy proteins, is necessary. In young infants, this is accomplished by initiating a hypoallergenic formula. The introduction of solids should also be delayed until 6 months of age and then each food introduced with a lag period to observe for symptoms. Most children outgrow this condition by 2 years of age, but caution needs to be used in reintroducing offending foods, particularly if the child initially presented with shock or anaphylactic-like symptoms.

IgE-mediated disorders, such as immediate-type gastrointestinal hypersensitivity and oral allergy syndrome, are usually diagnosed by history and physical exam, and they are confirmed by specific IgE testing; either in vitro RASTs or in vivo skin prick testing (see Table 1). If there is still uncertainty, blinded food challenges are helpful. Immediate-type gastrointestinal hypersensitivity is usually associated with the onset of nausea, vomiting, and abdominal pain within minutes to 1 to 2 hours after ingestion of the offending agent, and diarrhea within 2 to 6 hours. The most common foods causing this condition are usually milk, egg, peanuts, wheat, and seafood.

Oral allergy syndrome produces symptoms confined to the oral cavity (pruritus, burning, erythema, and angioedema) and is usually triggered by fresh fruits—apples, peaches, and cherries—and vegetables. There is usually a concomitant history of seasonal allergic rhinitis and positive skin tests to certain pollens. Skin

---

BOX 1 Categorization of Food Allergies and Typical Ages of Presentation

IgE
- Immediate hypersensitivity (infancy, childhood)
- Oral allergy syndrome (beyond infancy)

Combination of IgE/non–IgE
- Allergic eosinophilic esophagitis (infant to adolescent)
- Allergic eosinophilic gastritis (infant to adolescent)
- Allergic eosinophilic gastroenterocolitis (infant to adolescent)

Non–IgE
- Dietary protein enterocolitis (younger than 1 year)
- Dietary protein proctitis (younger than 1 year)
- Dietary protein enteropathy (younger than 1 year)

Ig, immunoglobulin.
From Sampson HA, Anderson JA: Summary and recommendations: Classification of gastrointestinal manifestations due to immunologic reactions to foods in infants and young children. J Pediatr Gastroenterol Nutr 30:S88, 2000.

TABLE 1 In Vitro IgE Values Used to Determine Need for Food Challenges*

	Egg	Milk	Peanut	Fish	Soy	Wheat
Reaction highly probable (no challenge needed)	>7	>15	>14	>20	>60	>80
Young children (reaction highly probable)	>2 (<2 yr)	>5 (<1 yr)				
Reaction unlikely (home or physician challenge)	<0.35	<0.35	<0.35	<0.35	<0.35	<0.35

*Values are expressed in kilo units of antibody/liter (kUA/L). Values above the cutoff levels indicate a >95% probability that food challenges will be positive and therefore need not be performed. If the measurement is in between these levels, the challenge should be performed under physician supervision. Even if no antibody is detectable, the history may dictate the need for physician-supervised challenge.
Ig, immunoglobulin.
From Bock SA: Diagnostic evaluation. Pediatrics 111(6):1641, 2003. Used with permission of the American Academy of Pediatrics.

prick tests for fresh fruits or vegetable extracts are usually positive. In both of these IgE-mediated conditions, avoidance of the offending food antigen is key, but injectable epinephrine should be carried at all times in case of accidental exposure.

The pathogenesis of eosinophilic enteropathies (eosinophilic esophagitis, gastritis, and gastroenterocolitis) is not well understood and may not necessarily be the result of food hypersensitivity. Symptoms and signs of eosinophilic gastrointestinal disorders include failure to thrive, abdominal pain, irritability, vomiting, diarrhea, dysphagia, microcytic anemia, and hypoproteinemia. The presence of peripheral eosinophilia is variable, so the hallmark of these diseases is an "abnormal" number of tissue eosinophils. Other causes of hypereosinophilia such as drug hypersensitivity, collagen-vascular disease, malignancy, or parasitic infection should be ruled out. Once the diagnosis is made, treatment with corticosteroids can improve symptoms, but symptoms frequently recur when the medication is stopped. Depending on the form of the disease, an attempt should be made at dietary therapy, usually by initiating an elimination diet. Dietary elimination can be of all but a defined group of so-called oligoantigenic foods, such as meats, vegetables, fruits, water (possibly also enriched rice milk), salt, sugar, olive oil, and a grain like corn or rice. More commonly, an elemental diet of an amino acid–based formula is started and the symptoms and histologic findings monitored. Thereafter, foods may then be added back one at a time to identify problematic as well as acceptable foods. Other forms of immunosuppressive therapy (e.g., 6-mercaptopurine therapy) have not been extensively studied. Cromolyn and leukotriene antagonists appear to have a limited role in the treatment of eosinophil-associated disease. Finally, patients with refractive disease may benefit from total parenteral nutrition.

Some promising therapies on the horizon include biologic agents such as anti–interleukin-5, adhesion molecule antagonists (to prevent eosinophils from tracking into target organs) and anti-IgE antibodies when IgE-mediated reactions are involved. Chemokine and chemokine receptor antagonist-based therapies directed at eosinophil-specific targets such as eotaxin are also being developed.

Common Pitfalls

There are many myths about food allergy. It is important to appreciate the difference between allergy and intolerance. A wide variety of complaints are attributed to food allergies, including chronic rhinitis and sinusitis, recurrent/chronic otitis media, chronic fatigue syndrome, migraine headaches, and various behavioral disorders. The role of food allergy in these conditions is controversial, and labeling a patient "food allergic" without proper testing should be avoided. Although food hypersensitivity may be involved in any particular individual with these complaints, no convincing evidence shows that it plays a dominant etiologic role in any of these conditions.

An unsubstantiated diagnosis of food allergy in children may lead to malnutrition, failure to thrive, and vitamin deficiencies when a restrictive diet is initiated. If an offending food is not identified by history, some type of food challenge, ideally a double-blind, placebo-controlled study, is necessary to diagnose true food hypersensitivity as well as to identify the offending food(s). Thereafter, an appropriate elimination diet can be selected. When testing is done in suspected cases of oral allergy syndrome, fruit and vegetable antigens must be freshly extracted because these proteins are extremely labile, and challenge with processed antigens may cause a false-negative test.

Some non–IgE-mediated processes, such as food protein–induced enterocolitis, can have an anaphylactic or shocklike presentation. In such cases, the diagnosis may not be considered or missed if only IgE-based testing is performed.

Eosinophilic diseases of the gastrointestinal tract remain difficult conditions to diagnose and treat. A complaint of dysphagia or food impaction should alert the physician to the possibility of eosinophilic esophagitis. There are no good standards for how many eosinophils need to be present in tissues to make this diagnosis. A high index of suspicion must be maintained and appropriate biopsies performed in patients with what otherwise might seem to be functional complaints.

Communication and Counseling

Educating the patient/parents is a key component of the therapy for these disorders. If an elimination diet is prescribed, avoidance of manufacturing cross contamination must be explained. Also, instruction on selecting appropriate food substitutes and nutritional follow-up to avoid undernutrition is important. Grandparents, babysitters, and family friends must be taught about food allergen avoidance, and schools and daycare sites must be notified to assist with food allergy management. The rationale and side effects of any medications prescribed should be explained, and when an epinephrine pen is indicated, the patient must be instructed in its use and the need to carry it at all times.

The participation of a trained dietician can be invaluable in assessing and maintaining nutritional status, teaching patients/parents what to look for on food labels, and providing sound food substitution.

Finally, discussions concerning preventive measures may be indicated. For high-risk infants (strong family history or an affected sibling), it is recommended to avoid the introduction of milk and/or soy before 1 year of age; eggs before 2 years of age; and peanuts, tree nuts, and shellfish before 3 years of age.

SUGGESTED READINGS

1. Bock SA: Diagnostic evaluation. Pediatrics 111(6):1638–1644, 2003. **Discussion of the diagnosis of adverse food reactions.**

2. De Boisseau D, Waguet JC, Dupont C: The atopy patch test for detection of cow's milk allergy with digestive symptoms. J Pediatr 142:203–205, 2003. **Atopy patch testing to enhance yield of cow's milk allergy detection in children.**

3. Eigenmann PA: Future therapeutic options in food allergy. Allergy 58:1217–1223, 2003. **Comprehensive discussion of ongoing trials and possible therapies.**

4. Eigenmann PA: Do we have suitable in-vitro diagnostic tests for the treatment of food allergy? Curr Opin Allergy Clin Immunol 4:211–213, 2004. **Up-to-date assessment of available in vitro testing for food allergy.**

5. Heine RG: Pathophysiology, diagnosis, and treatment of food protein–induced gastrointestinal diseases. Curr Opin Allergy Clin Immunol 4:221–229, 2004. **Insight into the pathophysiology of food protein–induced disease.**

6. Molfidi S: Nutritional management of pediatric food hypersensitivity. Pediatrics 111(6):1645–1653, 2003. **Management of food allergy using dietary manipulation.**

7. Rothenberg M: Eosinophilic gastrointestinal disorders. J Allergy Clin Immunol 113:11–28, 2004. **Excellent review of the mechanism, diagnosis, and treatment of eosinophilic disorders.**

8. Sampson HA, Anderson JA: Summary and recommendations: Classification of gastrointestinal manifestations due to immunologic reactions to foods in infants and young children. J Pediatr Gastroenterol Nutr 30:S84–S94, 2000. **Excellent review that breaks down entities by mediators of disease and comments on diagnosis as well as treatment.**

9. Sampson HA, Sicherer SH, Birnbaum AH: AGA technical review on the evaluation of food allergy in gastrointestinal disorders. Gastroenterology 120:1026–1040, 2001. **Consensus statement from American Gastroenterological Association (AGA) Clinical Practice and Practice Economics Committee.**

10. Zeiger RS: Food allergen avoidance in the prevention of food allergy in infants and children. Pediatrics 111(6):1662–1671, 2003. **Thoughtful comparison of preventive recommendations of several international nutrition committees.**

Adverse Drug Reactions

Christine J. Kubin and Lauren M. Robitaille

KEY CONCEPTS

- An adverse drug reaction (ADR) is any noxious, unintended, and undesired effect of a drug that occurs at doses used for prevention, diagnosis, or treatment.
- ADRs are a significant public health problem.
- ADRs are under-reported. Providers should maintain a high index of suspicion and report all suspected and confirmed ADRs.
- Type A reactions relate to the pharmacologic action of the drug. They are considered dose related and predictable.
- Type B reactions are unpredictable and unpreventable, including drug intolerance, idiosyncratic reactions, and hypersensitivity reactions.
- Factors contributing to the likelihood of an ADR are dose, route of administration, polypharmacy, patient's age, disease state, organ function, gender, and genetics.
- Management of ADRs relies on a high index of suspicion. A thorough history, clinical evaluation, and laboratory workup are essential to identifying the suspect drug, classifying the adverse reaction, and minimizing patient harm.

A number of established definitions are used to describe an adverse drug reaction, but most simply stated, an adverse drug reaction (ADR) is any unexpected, unpredictable, and undesired reaction that occurs from the normal use of a medication (i.e., within accepted doses and indications). Conversely, a side effect is a reaction that is known and expected, which may or may not require modification to the patient's regimen.

Adverse drug reactions are classified into type A and type B reactions. Type A reactions are the more common of the two (80%) and are often dose-dependent reactions that arise because of an extension of the medication's pharmacologic properties. Alternatively, type B reactions are uncommon and unexpected and include intolerance, idiosyncratic, allergic, and pseudoallergic reactions. Allergic reactions require previous drug exposure and develop rapidly upon reexposure. Allergic reactions manifest as clinical syndromes related to the immunologic mechanism that is activated (Table 1). Clinicians must attempt to make the distinction among the various types of reactions to better direct their management.

Because ADRs are a significant part of our health care system, organizations such as the Joint Commission on the Accreditation of Healthcare Organizations (JCAHO) and the U.S. Food and Drug Administration (FDA) have put systems into place to encourage reporting. The JCAHO requires hospitals to have a definition for an adverse drug reaction and requires that all ADRs be reported and tracked. The FDA has set up the MedWatch program and the Vaccine Adverse Event Reporting System (VAERS) for use by health care professionals, manufacturers, and consumers. Both the MedWatch and VAERS programs can be easily accessed via the Internet.

ADRs are regarded as an important public health problem. Despite attempts to increase reporting, ADRs are still under-reported. Recognizing the effect of ADRs on our health care system and appreciating the importance of accurate and thorough reporting of such reactions are the first steps in gaining further insight into their true incidence and impact. The overall incidence of ADRs in the general population is an estimated 15%, and roughly one tenth of these are classified as allergic reactions. In the United States, ADRs are cited as the fourth to sixth leading cause of death, accounting for approximately 106,000 deaths each year, and they are responsible for an estimated 5.1% and 2.1% of all hospital admissions among the general and pediatric populations, respectively.

In children, the reported overall incidence of ADRs averages approximately 10%. Pediatric patients are particularly vulnerable to severe reactions because of differences in physiologic maturity, differences in disease patterns, and their smaller size. Additionally, approximately one third of the medications used in children are prescribed in a way that differs from their approved indication and/or dosing "off label," and nearly 75% of ADRs classified as severe result from the use of a medication in an off-label manner.

TABLE 1 Gell and Coombs Classification of Hypersensitivity

Class	Mechanism	Common Manifestations	Usual Timing
Type I (anaphylaxis)	IgE mediated	Anaphylaxis, urticaria, angioedema	Within minutes to hours after exposure (provided initial antigen exposure and sensitization have occurred)
Type II (cytotoxic)	IgG or IgM mediated	Hemolytic anemia, thrombocytopenia, granulocytopenia	Variable, typically at least 7 days after exposure
Type III (immune complex)	IgG or IgM mediated	Serum sickness	7–21 days after exposure
Type IV (cell mediated)	Drug-specific T lymphocytes	Contact dermatitis	2–7 days after exposure

Ig, immunoglobulin.

Expert Opinion on Management Issues

ADRs tend to occur more frequently in seriously ill patients who require multiple drug therapies, but they can occur in any patient receiving prescription, over-the-counter, and herbal products. Providers must recognize the broad array of possible reactions and understand the distinction among the types of ADRs.

RISK FACTORS

Predisposing factors for ADRs are either patient or drug related. The most reliable risk factor for developing an allergic reaction is a previous history of hypersensitivity to a drug or one that is chemically similar. Such is the case in patients with a reported penicillin allergy, where administration of other β-lactam antibiotics increases the possibility of a reaction. A family history of a drug allergy is also a risk factor for developing an allergic drug reaction. Adverse drug reactions occur more commonly in females. Children tend to experience fewer reactions, presumably because of less cumulative drug exposure. Viral infections may be a risk factor for the development of an ADR. Patients infected with human immunodeficiency virus (HIV) experience ADRs more frequently than HIV-negative patients. In addition, the incidence of rash in children and young adults following the administration of amoxicillin or ampicillin in patients with infectious mononucleosis (Epstein-Barr virus) is increased. Certain comorbid conditions, such as renal insufficiency, liver disease, systemic lupus erythematosus, and asthma, are also risk factors. Finally, specific genetic polymorphisms that affect the metabolism of drugs may affect the incidence of ADRs.

Drug-related risk factors include the dose, duration of therapy, frequency of exposure, route of administration, concomitant drug therapy, and factors related to the chemical nature of the drug itself. Higher doses and prolonged therapy are more often associated with cytopenias, interstitial nephritis, and serum sickness reactions. Anecdotal reports also indicate that patients may tolerate a drug at a certain dose but then experience an acute immunoglobulin (Ig) E-mediated allergic reaction at higher dosages. Frequent, repetitive courses of therapy are also associated with more allergic reactions. The route of administration affects the likelihood of sensitization and the subsequent development of a reaction in a previously sensitized patient. Topical administration of drugs appears to be the most sensitizing; the oral route is the least. The risk of developing an allergic reaction in a previously sensitized patient is greatest when a drug is administered intravenously and least when administered orally. Polypharmacy is a risk factor among all age groups. In the hospitalized pediatric population, for each additional drug prescribed, the likelihood of an ADR increases approximately 1.7-fold. Finally, large molecular weight drugs are more likely to be immunogenic. Smaller molecular weight drugs may also become immunogenic by binding well to large molecular weight carriers, usually proteins, resulting in drug-carrier complexes called haptens.

CLINICAL MANIFESTATIONS

The clinical manifestations of ADRs vary depending on the immune mechanism and the organ involved (Table 2). Similarly, the time to onset varies according to the immune mechanism involved.

EVALUATION

The patient experiencing an adverse reaction must be carefully evaluated. The initial evaluation should include a medical history and careful physical examination. To determine whether a reaction is potentially drug related, a detailed drug history should be obtained. This history should include previous and current drug usage, drug dosages, temporal relationship between initiation of therapy and onset of symptoms, and symptoms experienced. This information is reviewed in the context of previous reports in the medical literature of similar reactions with the same or similar drugs. The physical examination may provide important information, especially if the patient is still experiencing the drug reaction. An evaluation of all organ systems is essential to

TABLE 2 Common Clinical Manifestations

Type of Reaction	Examples
Generalized, systemic reactions	Anaphylaxis, serum sickness, drug fever, autoimmune reactions, vasculitis
Organ-specific reactions	Cutaneous: urticaria and angioedema, maculopapular rashes, fixed eruptions, toxic epidermal necrolysis, Stevens-Johnson syndrome, erythema multiforme, vasculitis, exfoliative dermatitis, erythroderma, contact dermatitis, photodermatitis
	Hematologic: eosinophilia, anemia, granulocytopenia, thrombocytopenia
	Pulmonary: airway obstruction, interstitial/alveolar pneumonitis, edema, fibrosis
	Hepatic: cholestasis, hepatocellular damage
	Renal: interstitial nephritis, glomerular nephritis, nephrotic syndrome

---

BOX 1 Management of the Drug-Allergic Patient

- Select alternative, non–cross-reacting drugs.
- Consider premedication with antihistamines and corticosteroids if premedications are effective in preventing reactions.
- Consider graded drug rechallenge for reactions that are not IgE mediated.
- Consider drug desensitization for IgE-mediated reactions where no alternative drug therapy exists (*potentially dangerous and should be done with close observation by an allergist experienced with desensitization*).

Ig, immunoglobulin.

---

determine those involved. The clinician must initially rule out the presence of an immediate, life-threatening, generalized reaction. Urticaria, laryngeal or upper airway edema, wheezing, tachycardia, and hypotension may signal the potential for cardiovascular collapse. More serious reactions may include fever, mucous membrane lesions, lymphadenopathy, hepatosplenomegaly, joint tenderness or swelling, or an abnormal pulmonary examination. Because the skin is the organ most frequently affected, cutaneous lesions should be described according to gross appearance and distribution.

Laboratory evaluation depends on the immune mechanism of the ADR and the organs involved. Some drug reactions may be accompanied by eosinophilia, proteinuria, liver enzyme abnormalities, or the presence of antinuclear antibodies. Consideration should be given to obtaining a complete blood count with differential, liver enzymes, renal function tests, urinalysis, and urine eosinophil count. Other laboratory tests specific to organs affected may also be useful. Occasionally, biopsies of the liver, kidney, or skin may assist in the histopathologic diagnosis, but they are not able to implicate a specific drug.

CLINICAL MANAGEMENT OF ACUTE REACTIONS

The management of an ADR begins with a high index of suspicion that a clinical manifestation may be a component of a hypersensitivity reaction. A drug–disease connection must be established. Treatment of an allergic reaction should include discontinuation of the suspected drug and implementation of usual therapy to treat the clinical manifestations. Acute anaphylaxis requires the early and appropriate use of epinephrine and subsequent treatment to maintain an effective airway and circulatory system. For type A reactions, dosage modification prior to readministration rather than discontinuation of therapy may be adequate to alleviate symptoms. For type B drug intolerance reactions, the suspect drug may be readministered if the adverse reaction was mild. This may not be possible in idiosyncratic reactions, and the suspect drug should not be readministered following severe or life-threatening reactions. For type B immunologically mediated reactions, management depends on the mechanism. Skin testing may be helpful to determine the allergic status of the patient. If an alternative agent is available, readministration of the suspect drug may not be necessary. If an alternative agent is not available, a graded challenge with the suspect drug by an experienced allergist may be attempted, provided the reaction was not IgE mediated and not life-threatening. In other cases, desensitization may be necessary (Box 1).

PREVENTION

To prevent future adverse events, ADRs should be well documented in the patient's medical chart and pharmacy records. In addition, reactions should be well described to distinguish drug intolerance from true allergic reactions.

Common Pitfalls

Adverse drug reactions are widely under-reported in the literature. This is problematic, considering the medical literature serves as a warning system for clinicians about adverse reactions, both common and rare, and helps identify patients at higher risk of experiencing such reactions.

In many instances, it is difficult to determine causality and the pharmacologic relationship of drug to clinical syndrome. Limited reliable laboratory tests are available to confirm a drug allergy, making the diagnosis dependent on clinical evaluation. In addition, ADRs are often difficult to classify. Taken together, these aspects make optimal management strategies less clear.

Adverse drug reactions occurring in patients receiving multiple medications are difficult to evaluate. A systematic approach to better define the suspect drug while avoiding additional patient harm is necessary.

Communication and Counseling

It may be warranted to educate parents about common presenting clinical manifestations of drug hypersensitivity because many children may be treated at home or in other out-of-hospital settings. As health care professionals it is imperative to report ADRs through a medical institution's reporting system, through the FDA's MedWatch program, or via publication in the medical literature.

SUGGESTED READINGS

1. Demoly P, Bousquet J: Epidemiology of drug allergy. Curr Opin Allergy Clin Immunol 1(4):305–310, 2001. **Describes potential problems with the epidemiologic data associated with the incidence, mortality, and socioeconomic impact of drug allergies.**
2. deShazo RD, Kemp SF: Allergic reactions to drugs and biologic agents. JAMA 278(22):1895–1906, 1997. **Review of the clinical manifestations of allergic reactions; includes a detailed table of presentations associated with various drugs.**
3. Gruchalla RS: Drug allergy. J Allergy Clin Immunol 111:S458–S459, 2003. **Describes the reactions and immune mechanisms associated with classes of drugs more commonly linked to adverse reactions.**
4. Impicciatore P, Choonara I, Clarkson A, et al: Incidence of adverse drug reactions in paediatric in/out-patients: A systematic review and meta-analysis of prospective studies. Br J Clin Pharmacol 52(1):77–83, 2001. **Meta-analysis of prospective studies on ADRs in children.**
5. Joint Task Force on Practice Parameters, the American Academy of Allergy, Asthma and Immunology, the American Academy of Allergy, Asthma and Immunology, and the Joint Council of Allergy, Asthma and Immunology: Executive summary of disease management of drug hypersensitivity: A practice parameter. Ann Allergy Asthma Immunol 83(6 Pt 3):665–700, 1999. **Comprehensive discussion of the immunology, risk factors, clinical evaluation, and management of drug hypersensitivity.**
6. Nagao-Dias AT, Barros-Nunes P, Coelho HL, et al: Allergic drug reactions. J Pediatr (Rio J) 80(4):259–266, 2004. **Review of drug allergies and the need for aggressive management, highlighting the importance to the health-care system.**

Treatment of Juvenile Dermatomyositis

Ilona S. Szer

KEY CONCEPTS

- Early recognition of juvenile dermatomyositis (JDM) is based on classic rash and documentation of weakness using manual muscle testing and all muscle enzymes, including aspartate transaminase (AST), alanine transaminase (ALT), lactate dehydrogenase (LDH), creatine phosphokinase (CPK), and aldolase.

- Aggressive early management of weakness is advocated with intravenous administration of corticosteroids, subcutaneous injections of methotrexate, with or without intravenous immunoglobulin (IVIG). Cyclosporine A (CSA) is used, even though it is an oral medication, as plasma levels are available. Focus is on rapid normalization of all muscle enzymes and subsequently of strength and function.
- Muscle strength and enzymes should be monitored monthly and no changes made unless all are normal.
- Patience is key; it takes a while to address the problems associated with JDM.
- Passive range of motion exercises are recommended during the initial inflammatory phase.
- Active strengthening as soon as possible and return to normal function is recommended.
- Calcinosis heralds ongoing muscle disease and should be treated as such.

Juvenile dermatomyositis (JDM) is a rare autoimmune pediatric illness manifested by a classical rash and progressive muscle weakness. In the untreated child, the muscle weakness may progress over time to inability to clear secretions and the risk of death from profound weakness. Before the steroid era, a third of children with JDM died, another third recovered almost completely, and the rest recovered but were disabled to a certain extent. The early recognition and aggressive treatment by a team expert in the management of chronic childhood rheumatic diseases and led by the pediatric rheumatologist are imperative and have changed the outcome of this disease. Multiple studies document excellent prognosis for children treated early and aggressively, underscoring the fact that any delay in treatment leads to unnecessary complications and increased morbidity and mortality. Diagnosis of dermatomyositis is based on demonstration of classic rash (Gottron papules, cuticle hyperemia, and dry, scaly erythema over extensor surfaces of elbows and knees) as well as demonstration of weakness (by manual muscle testing and muscle enzyme levels, including aspartate transaminase [AST], alanine transaminase [ALT], lactate dehydrogenase [LDH], creatine phosphokinase [CPK], and aldolase, or in the absence of supportive physical findings or muscle enzyme elevation by electromyelogram [EMG], MRI, or muscle biopsy). It is important to remember that 10% of children who are weak have normal muscle enzymes.

Expert Opinion on Management Issues

DRUG THERAPY

Corticosteroids

The corticosteroids are the mainstay of JDM treatment, and experts concur that all children with JDM should be so treated. However, both the dose and mode of administration are controversial, with most in agreement that high-dose intravenous (IV) administration is preferable (Box 1). Evidence suggests that children

BOX 1 Medications Used to Treat Dermatomyositis

- Corticosteroids
  - Initial: IV methylprednisolone 30 mg/kg/dose for 3 consecutive days, then weekly for several weeks until muscle enzymes are almost normal, in addition to oral prednisone 1–2 mg/kg/day divided qid or tid.
  - During the course: gradual reduction in oral prednisone by approximately 10% per month, usually maintained for at least 2 years and always managed using muscle enzymes that must be as normal as possible.
- Methotrexate, used SC, IM, or IV only, 0.5–1 mg/kg/week with monthly liver function monitoring.
- Hydroxychloroquine, used mostly for rash, 6 mg/kg/day with annual monitoring of color vision.
- Cyclosporine A, 3.5 mg/kg/day or dose that achieves a trough level of 100–140.
- IVIG, 1–2 g/kg/dose, given monthly.
- Azathioprine, 2 mg/kg/day.
- MMF, 20–30 mg/kg/day in two divided doses.
- Cyclophosphamide, 0.5–1 mg/m^2/dose, given as monthly pulses with bladder protection.
- Calcium and vitamin D supplementation as recommended for age.

IM, intramuscular; IV, intravenous; IVIG, intravenous immunoglobulin; MMF, mycophenolate mofetil; qid, four times per day; SC, subcutaneous; tid, three times per day.

with JDM, particularly those who have cutaneous vasculitis, experience decreased gastrointestinal (GI) absorption of oral medications and thus may respond poorly to oral corticosteroids.

Children who are strong enough to remain outside the hospital should be seen frequently and evaluated with both manual muscle exams and laboratory studies. Monitoring of several muscle enzymes (CPK, aldolase, AST, ALT, and LDH) aids in the decision-making process, although the use of methotrexate with its potential for liver toxicity presents a challenge because the same enzymes become elevated, suggesting both liver and muscle involvement. Inclusion of more specific liver enzymes, such as γ-glutamyltransferase (GGT), is helpful.

Treatment of severe JDM early in the disease course with both methylprednisolone and methotrexate appears to be more useful than when either agent is used alone. Most pediatric rheumatologists administer IV pulses of methylprednisolone at 30 mg/kg/dose per day for 3 consecutive days while starting methotrexate at approximately 0.5 to 1 mg/kg/dose per week and continuing weekly pulses of corticosteroids for many weeks depending on the child's response. Daily oral steroid, 1 to 2 mg/kg/day, initially divided into several daily doses, is also administered early in the course, but it is preferable to administer intermittent IV steroid pulses in addition to oral medications. Children who are unable to clear secretions and/or who require ventilatory support or are at risk for repeated trauma from falling should be admitted to the hospital and receive IV medications until they are safe. A dynamic swallow study is useful in recognizing children at risk for aspiration. Although respiratory problems are reported in a third of children, intubation is rarely needed, whereas nasogastric feeding is a frequent occurrence in hospitalized children with JDM.

Children with severe cutaneous manifestations may benefit from the addition of hydroxychloroquine (6 mg/kg/day). All patients must avoid ultraviolet (UV) light with hats and sunblock lotions. Topical corticosteroids are not particularly useful in this illness; the response is variable and frequent administration may cause skin atrophy. Skin care is particularly important in children who may develop fissures and breakdown when immunosuppression is particularly aggressive and predisposes the patient to infection.

Prolonged use of corticosteroids leads to accumulation of side effects. Virtually all children develop the Cushing stigmata and obesity; with exercise and attention to a healthy low fat/salt/carbohydrate diet, these side effects can be minimized and do eventually go away. More difficult complications include osteoporosis, which may lead to vertebral compression fractures (worsened by inactivity from weakness); cataract formation; avascular necrosis; and opportunistic infections. Some children develop diabetes, gastric irritation, tremulousness, mood swings, and poor sleep. At times it may seem the treatment is worse than the underlying disease. To lessen these side effects, the use of steroid-sparing immunosuppressive therapies is common. The most commonly recommended is methotrexate, followed by cyclosporine A, mycophenolate mofetil (MMF) or azathioprine, and, lastly, cyclophosphamide.

Methotrexate

Weekly subcutaneous administration of methotrexate is the first choice of steroid-sparing treatment, although no controlled studies have ever been done to prove its efficacy over other immunosuppressive drugs. Most pediatric rheumatologists agree that methotrexate should be started at the same time as IV corticosteroids and maintained for several years. Monthly monitoring of liver function tests and urinalysis as well as blood counts is imperative. Most children tolerate a dose of 0.5 to 1 mg/kg/week, but many require folic or folinic acid supplementation, and some children may have to split the dose to avoid nausea, mouth sores, or abdominal pain.

Cyclosporine A

Several studies suggest the efficacy of cyclosporine A (CSA) in controlling JDM. Some studies suggest CSA should be used as first-line therapy, before methotrexate; however, renal side effects often preclude chronic administration of CSA, and attention to blood pressure and renal function are of paramount importance. Hirsutism and gingival hyperplasia may lead to noncompliance, especially in girls concerned about their appearance. Hackman reported a study of 14 children with JDM who failed to respond to steroids and were given CSA. Most had a good response to a dose of 2.5 to 7.5 mg/kg and were able to discontinue steroids.

Intravenous Immunoglobulin

Intravenous immunoglobulin (IVIG), used in adults with severe skin disease and only moderate muscle involvement, is associated with improvement. In children, however, the results of treatment seem to be temporary and require repeated infusions for maintenance of control. No studies are available to inform the decision of when and how to use IVIG and/or when to stop. Retrospective observations suggest improvement when IVIG is given in monthly intervals of 1 g/kg. From those studies it is not clear when and how to begin eliminating the treatments. Whereas some physicians admit patients for overnight infusions, others work with outpatient infusion centers. In some centers, children are admitted overnight; in others, the infusions are given in outpatient areas. These infusions take many hours to administer and are at times associated with a syndrome of headache, emesis, and fever.

Cyclophosphamide, Azathioprine, and Mycophenolate Mofetil

There are no studies evaluating the efficacy of the cytotoxic drugs cyclophosphamide, azathioprine, and MMF in children with JDM; however, many pediatric rheumatologists are increasingly using either azathioprine or MMF in individual patients as steroid-sparing agents with good anecdotal success. IV cyclophosphamide is reserved for the most profoundly ill children—those with gastrointestinal ulcerations and respirator dependence or lack of improvement despite the standard measures just described.

PHYSICAL AND OCCUPATIONAL THERAPY

Most children with JDM should participate in an exercise program from the earliest sign of illness, but in practice the referral to physical therapy (PT) and occupational therapy (OT) services is inadvertently delayed. Initially, patients need to perform passive range of motion exercises to remain flexible. Over time, as they move through the healing phase of illness, they are able to participate in muscle strengthening (resistive exercise program). It is not recommended to start strengthening during the inflammatory phase, particularly if there is profound weakness. However, once the child has been treated, participating in therapy is both rewarding and successful. Premature referral to the physical therapist may lead to frustration, in addition to contributing to pain, disability, and fragmentation of care. The overall goal of PT and OT is to normalize function and return the child to regular school and community life.

CALCINOSIS

Approximately a third of children with JDM develop calcinosis during the course of the illness. There is no treatment for this complication, and although the literature is replete with unsuccessful trials of various regimens, none offer benefit. Ample evidence now indicates that calcinosis occurs in the context of smoldering, uncontrolled muscle disease and may be prevented by aggressive early treatment and by normalization of muscle enzymes initially in the illness. Once calcinosis is first recognized, treatment of underlying JDM not only continues but may need to be stepped up, on the premise that calcinosis is a sign of active muscle inflammation.

Common Pitfalls

- Mistaking eczema for Gottron papules and the dry scaly erythema of JDM seen over extensor surfaces of elbows and knees. Although eczema is a common skin condition of young children, it is found on opposite parts of the body, namely, on the flexor surfaces of joints and not on the extensor surfaces where it classically affects the child with JDM.
- Mistaking swollen eyelids (heliotrope) seen in JDM for the nephrotic syndrome affecting similarly aged children. Children with fluid overload (nephrotic syndrome) wake up with swollen eyelids but do not have the classic violaceous erythema in addition to swelling, which together is the cutaneous manifestation of JDM.
- Confusing the malar rash of JDM with that of systemic lupus erythematosus (SLE). Malar rash seen in JDM classically travels down the nasolabial folds, whereas the malar rash of SLE, by definition, spares the nasolabial folds. In addition, JDM tends to be an illness of young children and boys as equally as girls, whereas SLE affects primarily teenagers, with girls outnumbering boys 8:1.
- Mistaking weakness for fatigue. Unless the manual muscle exam is done, the physician is unable to diagnose weakness. In addition, the patients may not be able to describe their difficulties in terms that use weakness as an explanation for the inability to function normally. A simple maneuver of observing every patient complete an unassisted sit-up when going from supine to sitting position will reveal weakness in affected children.
- Mistaking weakness for laziness. Parents, unaware of the process of inflammation and resultant muscle injury, may describe their children as not wanting to do their chores or being obstinate when told to help carry groceries. Some youngsters may refuse to sit on the floor and earn the reputation of acting out in class. Yet others are accused of not wanting to run during physical education. As they lose their balance and fall, other children may call them names. The physician must perform a minimal manual muscle exam on every child who has stopped doing some regular activities no matter how convincing the interpretation of the observers may be.
- Diagnosing mononucleosis based on history of fatigue and available laboratory data. The routine

metabolic panel includes the AST and ALT but not CPK and aldolase. This leads the physician on a path to hepatitis and related infectious disorders without the consideration of muscle breakdown as the source of elevated transaminases. This assumption is common and based on the fact that most of the time the source of elevated AST and ALT is indeed the liver. Not so in children with JDM, who routinely have elevated AST and ALT levels in addition to high CPK, LDH, and aldolase.

■ Frequent falling and a changed gait in young children with JDM is too often assumed to be of neurologic origin, and the workup is then aimed inappropriately at ruling out central nervous system (CNS) and spinal pathology. Focusing on strength, even in the youngest children, improves outcome and avoids this inappropriate use of precious resources.

Communication and Counseling

Children with JDM generally do not improve quickly and almost always become cushingoid, overweight, and frustrated with the seeming lack of progress. Frequent visits to the pediatric rheumatologist, counseling, and the use of the entire interdisciplinary team with each visit are very helpful. Community programs, such as summer camps for children with rheumatic diseases, offer the child with JDM an opportunity to meet other like-affected children, thus lessening the burden of living with a rare and chronic illness. It may take weeks to gain control of elevated muscle enzymes and months or even years to return to regular function and endurance. In addition, systemic complications, such as GI bleeding, may be life-threatening, especially early in the course of the disease, and for some children, the initial hospitalization may last for weeks. Emotional support is always needed when the children flare after complete remission. Flares are predictably unpredictable, and their impact on the family as a unit is indescribable.

SUGGESTED READINGS

1. Al-Mayouf S, Al-Mazyed A, Bahabri S: Efficacy of early treatment of severe juvenile dermatomyositis with IV methylprednisolone and methotrexate. Clin Rheum 19:138–141, 2000. **Original study of treatment of JDM using IV modalities, underscoring the appropriateness of early and aggressive interventions. Our current practice of using IV treatments is substantiated.**
2. Goldsmith A, Feldman B, Singh G, et al: Aseptic meningitis following IVIG in children. Arthritis Rheum 34:S121, 1991. **Retrospective review of reactions to IVIG over a number of years.**
3. Grau JM, Herrero C, Casademont J, et al: CSA as first choice therapy for DMS. J Rheumatol 21:381–382, 1994. **Original study of the superiority of CSA in the treatment of JDM. A previous study published in *Lancet* reported the same findings and made the same recommendations.**
4. Malleson P: Controversies in JDM. J Rheumatol Suppl 23:1–2, 1990. **Thoughtful discussion of available treatment modalities in JDM with a focus on evidence-based recommendations for management. Well written and important.**
5. Pachman LM, Hayford JR, Chung A, et al: Juvenile dermatomyositis at diagnosis: Clinical characteristics in 79 children. J Rheumatol 25:1198–1204, 1998. **Large cohort prospective study of children with JDM registered in a national database. Descriptive and excellent.**
6. Reiff A, Rawlings D, Shaham B, et al: Preliminary evidence of cyclosporine A as an alternative in the treatment of recalcitrant JRA and JDM. J Rheumatol 24:2436–2443, 1997. **Further support for the use of CSA, this one in a retrospective review of patients treated at one large institution.**
7. Ryder L: Calcinosis as harbinger of active dermatomyositis. J Rheumatol (in press). **Original study examining pathologic specimens obtained from the muscle of children with calcinosis, who are thought to be in remission from JDM, documenting acute and chronic inflammation in the affected muscles. These data have changed previous practice, and currently children with calcinosis are assumed to have ongoing muscle inflammation. An important paper.**
8. Rider L, Miller FW: Classification and treatment of the juvenile idiopathic inflammatory myopathies. Rheum Dis Clin North Am 23:619–655, 1997. **Important review by experts in pediatric inflammatory muscle disorders. It is a must read.**
9. Tsai MJ, Lai CC, Lin SC, et al: IVIG therapy in juvenile dermatomyositis. Chung Hua Min Kuo Hsiao Erh Ko I Hsueh Hui Tsa Chih 38:111–115, 1997. **Review of a cohort of children with severe JDM recalcitrant to methotrexate, treated successfully with IVIG.**

Juvenile Rheumatoid Arthritis and Spondyloarthropathy Syndromes

Philip J. Kahn and Lisa Imundo

KEY CONCEPTS

■ Despite improved therapeutics and increased awareness, arthritis is still an important cause of disability in children.

■ Early referral to a pediatric rheumatologist for JRA is recommended to prevent disability.

■ The goal of therapy is to alleviate symptoms and prevent joint destruction and disability.

■ A diagnosis of JRA requires that all known causes of arthritis be ruled out, including infectious, malignant, and traumatic etiologies.

■ Characteristics not typically associated with the arthritis of JRA include severe pain, inability to bear weight, nocturnal wakening, and hot, erythematous joints.

■ Systemic JRA should always be included in the differential for fever of unknown origin, after ruling out infection and malignancy.

■ The characteristic features of juvenile-onset spondyloarthritis are:
  ■ High frequency of HLA-B27 antigen.
  ■ Seronegativity (no antinuclear antibodies [ANA], and rheumatoid factor [RF]).
  ■ Frequent enthesitis.
  ■ More axial disease than JRA.
  ■ Asymmetrical peripheral arthritis with propensity for lower extremities.

Chronic childhood arthritis is defined by the onset of arthritis at or prior to 16 years of age that persists for at least 6 weeks in at least one joint. Arthritis is defined as fluid within a joint on palpation or pain with limitation of motion.

Juvenile rheumatoid arthritis (JRA) affects approximately 80,000 children in the United States. At the time of this writing there is an international discussion to reclassify this syndrome as juvenile idiopathic arthritis, although the reclassification has not gained wide acceptance as of yet in the United States. We chose to continue using the more familiar JRA classification. Children with JRA may be classified as oligoarticular (four or fewer joints); polyarticular (five or more joints); or systemic onset, characterized by fever, serositis, and a characteristic rash (Table 1).

Growth and development must be carefully monitored during treatment. Arthritis may cause local growth disturbances, such as a shorter leg in a child with arthritis of the knee. Systemic JRA often results in short stature, the etiology of which is multifactorial, including poor caloric intake, the catabolic state of chronic inflammation, and use of medications (e.g., corticosteroids).

In addition to the pharmacotherapeutic treatment of JRA, the clinician must also address the psychosocial, financial, educational, and growth factors that affect a child with a chronic illness. Therefore, a multidisciplinary approach is recommended with a team including physical therapy, social work, psychology, orthopedics, and ophthalmology, with the aim of returning the patient to normal independent functioning.

Juvenile-onset spondyloarthritis (Jo-SpA) consists of a group of disorders that includes arthritis, enthesitis, HLA-B27 association, and a variety of extra-articular features. Jo-SpA is often associated with a prior infection, and there is a suggested role for ineffective clearance of infectious arthrogenic pathogens in the pathogenesis. Frequently there is a family history of SpA in a first- or second-degree relative and a slight male predominance. The spondyloarthritides include differentiated and undifferentiated forms (Table 2). Enthesitis is inflammation of tendons, ligaments, joint capsule, or fascial insertions into bone. Although adult SpA is an aggressive disease, the majority of Jo-SpA cases consist of mild enthesitis, and at least 50% of children achieve remission. Jo-SpA may be the most common form of childhood arthritis. In contrast to JRA, the arthritis of Jo-SpA is typically asymmetrical, commonly affecting the lower extremities, as well as the spinal column and sacroiliac joints. Jo-SpA is also known as the seronegative spondyloarthritis because ANA and RF factor are not present. Extra-articular features that may be seen in Jo-SpA include systemic features, such as fever, anemia, leukocytosis, lymphadenopathy, serositis, and weakness, as well as mucocutaneous lesions, uveitis, arrhythmias, nonspecific inflammatory bowel disease, and aortic regurgitation.

TABLE 1 Clinical Features of Juvenile Rheumatoid Arthritis Onset Subtypes

Onset Type (%)	Clinical Features	Subtypes	Associated Features
Oligoarticular (60%)	Four or fewer joints	Early childhood onset	Usually females, large joints, high incidence of uveitis (20%–30%), ANA + (up to 60%)
Polyarticular (30%)	Five or more joints	Late childhood onset RF negative RF positive	Usually boys, RF/ANA⁻, higher incidence of sacroiliitis Early or late childhood onset; rheumatoid nodules Later childhood onset (>8 yr); similar to adult rheumatoid arthritis (symmetrical, erosive arthritis); rheumatoid nodules
Systemic (10%)	Quotidian fever, salmon-colored evanescent rash, poly/pauciarticular arthritis	Any age	Anemia, serositis, lymphadenopathy, hepatosplenomegaly, MAS; typically negative ANA/RF

ANA, antinuclear antibody; MAS, macrophage activation syndrome; RF, rheumatoid factor.

TABLE 2 The Spondyloarthropathies

Differentiated Forms	Clinical Features
Juvenile ankylosing spondylitis	Characterized by persistent axial involvement (sacroiliitis, spondylosis), and enthesitis.
Juvenile-onset psoriatic arthritis (Jo-PsA)	Presence of psoriasis and arthritis in children younger than 16 years. Although there is a weaker HLA antigen association, there is usually a strong family history of psoriasis. Most psoriatic lesions are mild and found in characteristic locations, such as the scalp, umbilicus, and extensor surfaces. Dactylitis is common, as is nail psoriasis manifesting as pitting, striae, thickening, or oncolysis.
Reactive arthritis (Reiter syndrome)	Reactive arthritis (ReA) is a sterile arthritis that is preceded by a gastrointestinal or genitourinary infection with arthrogenic organisms. Reiter syndrome is a form of reactive arthritis, complicated by uveitis, conjunctivitis, and urethritis or cervicitis. Children often have only one or two manifestations.
Arthritis of inflammatory bowel disease (IBD)	Classically pauciarticular arthritis of the lower extremities, often preceding the gastrointestinal manifestations. The gastrointestinal manifestations often do not parallel the arthritis.

Expert Opinion on Management Issues

JUVENILE RHEUMATOID ARTHRITIS

There is no universal approach to treatment of JRA. Treatment components include controlling symptoms, suppressing inflammation, and preventing progression of disease. In addition to older medications such as methotrexate that have been used in the past, newer agents are now used. There have been many recent advances in pharmacotherapy including new biologic agents such as etanercept, which specifically targets tumor necrosis factor-α (TNF-α), a pathogenic cytokine in JRA.

Pharmacotherapy

Nonsteroidal Anti-Inflammatory Drugs

Initial therapy in the majority of patients with JRA is nonsteroidal anti-inflammatory drugs (NSAIDs), which are conventional prostaglandin inhibitors that block cyclooxygenase-1 (COX-1) and COX-2. In general, NSAIDs have similar efficacy and toxicity. Choice of NSAID may be based on dosing schedule and the availability of liquid preparations. Only three NSAIDs are approved by the U.S. Food and Drug Administration (FDA) in children: ibuprofen, naproxen, and tolmetin (Table 3). Most children tolerate NSAID therapy well, with few associated gastric ulcers. COX-2 inhibitors, such as celecoxib, selectively inhibit COX-2, allowing the continued production of COX-1, which is involved in the cytoprotective regulatory functions of the gastrointestinal mucosa, platelets, and red blood cells. At present there are some issues with NSAIDs and COX-2 inhibitors regarding the possible increased risk of stroke and heart attacks in adult patients. A COX-2 inhibitor may be considered for patients who do not tolerate nonselective NSAIDs.

Corticosteroids

Intra-articular steroids can be a first-line therapeutic option in JRA, because they are a safe, effective, inexpensive, well-tolerated medication, providing immediate and sustained anti-inflammatory effects on the synovium for 6 months to 1 year. With intra-articular injections one may avoid the need for daily oral medication. This is ideal in the young oligoarticular JRA patient with one swollen knee, although sedation is required for children younger than 8 years. Systemic corticosteroids are necessary for the majority of patients with systemic JRA to control the characteristic fever, anemia, and fatigue. Corticosteroids are powerful, fast-acting, anti-inflammatory medications that block the synthesis of prostaglandin via the COX pathway as well as inhibit the nuclear factor κB (NF-κB) signaling pathway. High-dose intravenous pulse corticosteroids (methylprednisolone 30 mg/kg/day for 3 days) are used for life-threatening complications, such as macrophage activation syndrome (MAS) (see later). Corticosteroids may also be used sparingly for severe polyarticular JRA until the therapeutic effects of other medications are achieved, which can take 4 to 6 weeks. Corticosteroids have many side effects, including increased risk of infection, avascular necrosis, osteoporosis, and growth suppression, among others (see Table 3).

Disease-Modifying Antirheumatic Drugs

Early joint damage in patients with RF-positive polyarticular JRA supports the use of early, intensive disease-modifying antirheumatic drugs (DMARDs). Only three DMARDs have demonstrated efficacy in JRA in double-blind, placebo-controlled trials: methotrexate (MTX), sulfasalazine (SSZ), and etanercept (ETA).

For more than 10 years, low-dose MTX, a folic acid analogue, has been considered the gold standard DMARD in JRA. An estimated 72% of patients experience at least 30% clinical improvement, with less arthritis and improved function. MTX takes 4 to 6 weeks to reach full therapeutic effect. Although side effects include marrow suppression, teratogenicity, and gastrointestinal intolerance, MTX is generally well tolerated, especially with the addition of folic acid. The more serious side effects of liver or lung fibrosis have not been described in children. As with all patients on immunosuppressive therapy, live-virus vaccines should be avoided. Furthermore, patients with fever should always be evaluated for infection. MTX is often discontinued after a period of "sustained" remission, although a significant number of patients flare upon withdrawal.

Biologic Therapy

The therapeutic armamentarium of chronic arthritis was expanded by the introduction of biologics that target cytokines involved in the pathogenesis of arthritis. TNF-α is elevated in the synovium of patients with active JRA and is believed to initiate the pathogenic inflammatory cascade. Available TNF-α inhibitors are etanercept, infliximab, and adalimumab. These biologics are generally well tolerated and demonstrate efficacy in the treatment of JRA; 74% of patients have at least a 30% improvement, often with a rapid response within two weeks, which is sustained. Currently very little long-term data are available regarding toxicity, and there is a clear association with anti-TNF therapy and the reactivation of tuberculosis. It is therefore recommended to place a purified protein derivative (PPD) and update vaccinations before initiating anti-TNF therapy. The addition of anti-TNF therapy to MTX appears to have a synergistic benefit in adults, although the data in children are not available. Additional biologic therapies are in development and being tested in JRA. Some are listed in Table 3.

Although there is no widely established approach to therapy in a child with chronic arthritis, we have included the algorithms used at our center that outline our early and intensive treatment of arthritis, with the goal of a rapid return to normal function and suppression of all inflammation (Figs. 1–3). Medications used in the past, including gold, penicillamine, and hydroxychloroquine, are not efficacious in JRA.

TABLE 3 Pharmacotherapy for Chronic Childhood Arthritis

Medication	Dose (max/day)	Side Effects
NSAIDs		
Ibuprofen (Motrin, Advil)	10 mg/kg qid (max 2400 mg/day)	GI intolerance, platelet dysfunction, renal insufficiency, anemia, rash, rare: pseudoporphyria
Naproxen (Naprosyn)	10 mg/kg bid (max 1000 mg/day)	Same as for ibuprofen
Indomethacin (Indocin)*	1–3 mg/kg div bid/tid (max 200 mg/day)	Same as for ibuprofen
Diclofenac (Voltaren)*	2–3 mg/kg div bid (max 200 mg/day)	Same as for ibuprofen
Tolmentin (Tolectin)	15–30 mg/kg div tid/qid (max 2000mg/day)	Same as for ibuprofen
COX-2 Inhibitor		
Celecoxib (Celebrex)*	(>17 yr) 100–200 mg qd-bid (max 400 mg/day)	Sulfa allergy, GI intolerance, headache, weight gain, rash
Corticosteroids		
Intra-articular-triamcinolone hexacetonide (Aristospan)	Large joint: 1 mg/kg (max 40 mg); small joint: 0.5 mg/kg	Skin atrophy at injection site, some systemic absorption
Systemic	Oral vs. intermittent intravenous bolus	Weight gain, osteoporosis, growth retardation, striae, mood/personality changes/psychosis, avascular necrosis, infection risk, hypertension, gastritis, pancreatitis, diabetes, cataracts, glaucoma
Topical eye drops	qd to q1h for uveitis	Cataracts, glaucoma
Traditional DMARDs		
Methotrexate (Trexall)*	30 mg/m² or 1 mg/kg once per wk SC/PO (up to 50 mg)	GI intolerance, stomatitis, myelosuppression, fatigue, increased risk of infection, teratogenic, headache, rare: B cell lymphoma; pneumonitis and liver toxicity not described in children
Sulfasalazine (Azulfidine)*	40 mg/kg div bid (max 3 g/day, as tolerated)	GI intolerance, rash, rare: agranulocytosis
Cyclosporine A (Neoral)*	2–5 mg/kg/d (max 200 mg/day). *Follow trough levels*	Nephrotoxic (elevated creatinine, hypertension), GI intolerance, tremors, hypertrichosis, paresthesias, gum hyperplasia, increased risk of infection, possible increased risk of cancer
Leflunomide (Arava)*	Loading dose: 100 mg/day × 3 days; maintenance: 10–20 mg/day	Diarrhea, nausea, hepatotoxicity, myelosuppression, reversible alopecia, and rash
Other possible DMARDs: Azathioprine, Thalidomide, Cyclophosphamide		
Biologic DMARDs		
Etanercept (Enbrel)	(>2 yr) 0.4 mg/kg SC every wk (up to 25 mg/dose) or one weekly dose up to 50 mg/dose	Injection site reaction, headaches, rash, GI intolerance, increased risk of infection, tuberculosis reactivation, hypersensitivity reaction, rare: reversible lupus-like illness, autoantibody production, possible increased risk of lymphoma. Relative contraindication: CHF and demyelinating disorder
Infliximab (Remicade)*	3–10 mg/kg/dose IV q2–8wk	Same as for etanercept
Adalimumab (Humira)*	40 mg SC every other wk	Same as for etanercept
Other biologic DMARDs undergoing clinical trials in JIA: Anakinra (Kineret) (anti-IL1 antagonist) MRA (Atlizumab) (anti-IL6-receptor antagonist) Rituximab (anti-CD-20) Anti-CTLA-4 Ig (Abatacept)		

*Not currently approved by the U.S. Food and Drug Administration for treating JRA.

bid, twice daily; CHF, congestive heart failure; COX, cyclooxygenase; div, divided; DMARD, disease-modifying antirheumatic drug; GI, gastrointestinal; max, maximum; Ig, immunoglobulin; IL, interleukin; JRA, juvenile rheumatoid arthritis; NSAID, nonsteroidal anti-inflammatory drug; PO, by mouth; qd, daily; qid, four times per day; qxh, every x hours; SC, subcutaneous; tid, three times per day.

Physical and Occupational Therapy

Physical and occupational therapy should be incorporated into the therapeutic regimen for JRA at diagnosis. The goal of physical therapy is to reduce pain, increase function, and prevent disability, such as contractures or muscle atrophy. Therapeutic interventions involving muscle strengthening, flexibility, and aerobic conditioning may be supplemented by the

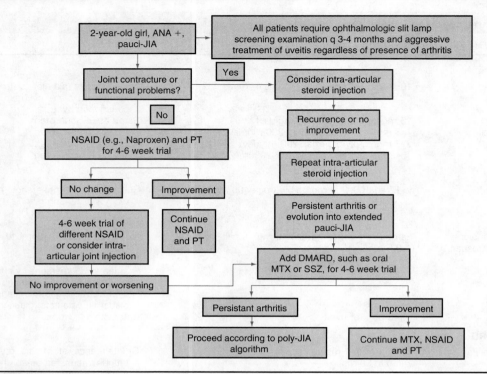

FIGURE 1. Treatment algorithm for oligoarticular juvenile rheumatoid arthritis. ANA, antinuclear antibody; DMARD, disease-modifying antirheumatic drug; JRA, juvenile rheumatoid arthritis; MTX, methotrexate; NSAID, nonsteroidal anti-inflammatory drug; q, every; PT, physical therapy; SSZ, sulfasalazine.

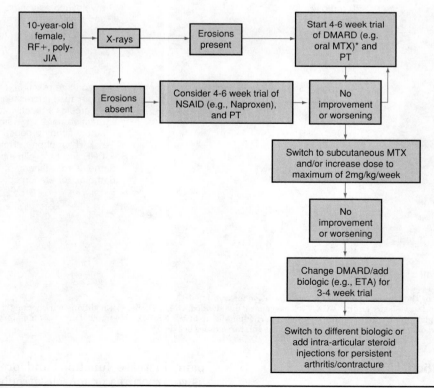

FIGURE 2. Treatment algorithm for polyarticular juvenile rheumatoid arthritis. DMARD, disease-modifying antirheumatic drug; ETA, etanercept; JRA, juvenile rheumatoid arthritis; MTX, methotrexate; NSAID, nonsteroidal anti-inflammatory drug; PT, physical therapy; RF, rheumatoid factor.
*Some clinicians now advocate using TNF inhibitors as a first line DMARD in children.

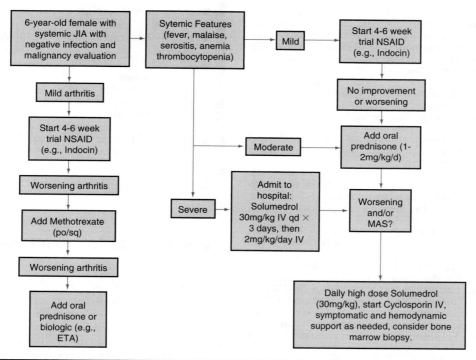

FIGURE 3. Treatment algorithm for systemic juvenile rheumatoid arthritis. ETA, etanercept; IV, intravenously; MAS, macrophage activation syndrome; NSAID, nonsteroidal anti-inflammatory drug; qd, daily; sc,subcutaneous.

use of splints or orthotics at a center with experience with children.

Special Treatment Considerations

Features unique to childhood arthritis include the increased risk of uveitis and MAS. Uveitis is the often asymptomatic inflammation of the uveal tract, most commonly seen in 20% to 30% of girls with ANA-positive oligoarticular JRA. Such high-risk patients require screening slit-lamp examinations every 3 to 4 months, with aggressive treatment of any intraocular inflammation to prevent possible blindness. Often the uveitis does not parallel the arthritis course, which reveals the importance of regular ophthalmologic exams despite quiescent arthritis. A potentially life-threatening complication of systemic JRA is MAS, an idiopathic condition of overwhelming cytokine activation resulting in possible coagulopathy, encephalopathy, respiratory distress syndrome, renal failure, and worsening serositis. Although there are no clear diagnostic criteria, bone marrow biopsy may reveal the presence of histiocytes actively phagocytizing red cells and platelets. The presence of MAS necessitates aggressive treatment with high-dose prednisone and cyclosporine.

SPONDYLOARTHROPATHY SYNDROMES

The medications used in Jo-SpA are similar to those cited in the algorithms for JRA. In contrast to adults, most children have mild disease and improve with NSAIDs and physical therapy. These mild syndromes are termed *spondyloarthropathy*. For children with persistent disease, DMARD therapy is initiated. Research suggests that anti-TNF therapy may be more effective than standard DMARDs, such as MTX, in retarding the radiographic progression of axial disease in adults with ankylosing spondylitis. Many therefore may consider anti-TNF therapy earlier in the treatment of severe Jo-SpA.

Communication and Counseling

Patients with JRA and Jo-SpA currently have a relatively good prognosis because of increased awareness and detection of childhood arthritis among pediatricians, active screening and treatment of uveitis, and intensive early pharmacotherapy. Unfortunately, a small fraction of children with severe arthritis still progress to permanent articular damage. Joint replacements are currently limited to hips and knees. Other surgical procedures have limited success in JRA. Although there is no cure for childhood arthritis, pediatric rheumatologists now have better tools to treat arthritis more effectively. By using a team approach to therapy and close monitoring, the clinician is able to minimize or prevent disability and provide the patient a return to full normal functioning.

SUGGESTED READINGS

1. Burgos-Vargas R: The juvenile onset spondyloarthritis. Rheum Dis Clin North Am 28(3):531–560, 2002. **A thorough review of JoSpA, including in-depth clinical manifestations, presumed pathogenesis, and approach to therapy.**

2. Emery H: Pediatric rheumatology: What does the future hold? Arch Phys Med Rehabil 85(8):1382–1384, 2004. **A thoughtful manuscript that emphasizes the importance of early and intensive rehabilitation in pediatric rheumatology, focusing on the prevention deformity and disability in JRA patients, and a brief discussion regarding pharmacotherapy.**

3. Fleischmann R, Iqbal I, Nandeshwar P, Quiceno A: Safety and efficacy of disease modifying anti-rheumatic drugs: Focus on the benefits and risks of etanercept. Drug Safety 25(3):173–197, 2002. **This paper discusses the risks and benefits of NSAIDs, DMARDs, and new biologic therapy in the treatment of rheumatoid arthritis, with an emphasis on safety issues of etanercept in several studies.**

4. Haskes PJ, Laxer RM: Medical treatment of juvenile idiopathic arthritis. JAMA 294(13):1671–1684, October 2005. **A thorough review of the prior studies of juvenile idiopathic arthritis (JIA) with the intent to provide an evidence-based approach to the treatment of JIA.**

5. Ilowite N: Current treatment of juvenile rheumatoid arthritis. Pediatrics 109(1):109–115, 2002. **JRA prognostic features and pharmacotherapy are the focus of this paper, including recent trials involving anti-TNF therapy in JRA.**

6. Munro JE, Murray KJ: Advances in paediatric rheumatology beyond NSAIDs and joint replacement. J Paediatric Child Health 40(4):161–169, 2004. **The use of new therapeutics available to clinicians is detailed in this paper, which also stresses the need to continue to investigate pathogenic factors and prognostic factors in children with rheumatologic diseases such as JRA.**

7. Schanberg LE, Anthony KK, Gil KM, Maurin EC: Daily pain and symptoms in children with polyarticular arthritis. Arthritis Rheum 48(5):1390–1397, 2003. **This paper investigates the biopsychosocial aspects of chronic pain in children with JRA and suggests more intensive treatment, including pharmacologic and psychosocial therapy, in order to preserve function by preventing deformity and disability.**

8. Schneider R, Passo M: Juvenile rheumatoid arthritis. Rheum Dis Clin North Am 28(3):503–530, 2002. **In addition to reviewing past classifications of JRA and features unique to childhood arthritis, this paper stresses the importance of reaching an international consensus regarding the possible classification as juvenile idiopathic arthritis, through which we may be able to gain a better understanding of childhood arthritis.**

9. Wilkinson N, Jackson G, Gardner-Medwin J: Biologic therapies for juvenile arthritis. Arch Dis Child 88(3):186–191, 2003. **This paper reviews autoimmune pathways that become aberrant in JRA and therefore can be specifically targeted with new biologic therapy, emphasizing the anti-TNF therapeutics.**

Primary Immunodeficiency Syndromes

Sophie Hambleton and Andrew R. Gennery

KEY CONCEPTS

- Primary immunodeficiencies are a heterogeneous group of genetically determined, life-limiting disorders in which susceptibility to infection is a major feature.
- Early diagnosis is critical to successful therapy.
- Optimal therapy includes immune replacement where available.

- Potentially harmful infectious exposures should be avoided.
- Prophylaxis has an important place in selected circumstances.
- Patients and caregivers should be alert to early signs of infection; these should be investigated and treated promptly and vigorously.
- Clinicians should be alert to noninfectious complications, particularly malignancy and autoimmune phenomena.
- Therapy is often demanding for patient and family. Education and support are important for successful outcome.

Defects of Cellular and Humoral Immunity

Primary immunodeficiency (PID) was classified by the World Health Organization (WHO) Working Party on Immunodeficiency and can be divided into four main categories: combined T- and B-lymphocyte disorders, B-lymphocyte and antibody disorders, phagocyte disorders, and disorders of the complement system. The overall incidence of any significant immunodeficiency disorder (excluding selective immunoglobulin [Ig] A deficiency) is estimated at 1 in 10,000 births. Most of the PIDs are genetically determined, and the molecular basis of many is defined (Table 1). Although many of the interventions described in this chapter are supportive and apply to the broad range of disorders, identification and clarification of the precise genetic defect enables more focused and specific treatment for the patient, as well as facilitating genetic counseling, antenatal diagnosis, and screening of other potentially affected but asymptomatic family members.

In the past, PIDs were often undiagnosed, and affected children died young from multiple and persistent infections with progressive end-organ damage. Modern diagnostic techniques, in conjunction with new, more efficacious antibacterial, antiviral, and antifungal agents and improved intensive care, now allow us to rescue many such children from what were previously fatal infections. Prophylactic therapy can both improve quality of life and prevent infection-related end-organ damage and death. Permanent cure of many severe PIDs is possible through hematopoietic stem cell transplantation (HSCT), considered separately in the chapter entitled, "Blood and Marrow Transplantation." Gene therapy remains at a research stage at present but appears promising as a possible curative therapy for certain disorders in the future. To benefit from these advances, children with immunodeficiency must be recognized, worked up, and treated appropriately pending definitive therapy. Box 1 briefly summarizes indicators of the diagnosis of PID, and Table 1 groups some of the major disorders by pattern of presentation and outlines their main features and therapy. Complement disorders are discussed in a separate chapter.

TABLE 1 Presentation and Therapy of Selected Primary Immunodeficiencies

Presentation	Disease Type	Examples				Treatment						
		Disorder	Inheritance	Genetic Defect	Additional Features	PCP Prophylaxis	Antifungal Prophylaxis	Antibacterial Prophylaxis	Immunoglobulin Replacement	HSCT	Gene Therapy†	Other
Failure to thrive, diarrhea, severe opportunistic infections in infancy	SCID	TB and SCID	XL	IL2RG	T lymphopenia, normal or increased B cells (but hypogammaglobulinemia)	•					•	Antiviral agents as suppressive/preemptive therapy
			AR	Jak3, IL7RA, CD45, CD3D			•		•	•	±	
		TB without SCID	AR	RAG1, RAG2, Artemis + unknown	T lymphopenia, decreased B-cell numbers	•	•		•			
			AR	ADA	Progressive decline in all lymphocyte subsets	•	•		•	•	•	PEG-ADA
		Defective MHC class II expression	AR	MHC2TA, RFXANK, RFX5, RFXAP	Selective loss of CD4+ T cells, severely immunodeficient phenotype	•	•		•	•	±	
Recurrent/refractory bacterial infections (often sinopulmonary)	Antibody deficiency	Agammaglobulinemia	XL / AR	Btk; μ, Igα, λ5, BLNK, LRRC8	Early onset (6–18 mo); B cells ~ absent; susceptibility to enteroviral meningitis and Giardia lamblia as well as bacterial infections			±	•	±	±	
		Hyper IgM syndrome	XL / AR	CD40L, CD40	A combined immunodeficiency: risk of PCP, GI infections, especially Cryptosporidium parvum (with cholangitis and liver involvement); also autoimmune phenomena, including neutropenia, thrombocytopenia	•		•	•	±		G-CSF for neutropenia, boiled water to reduce risk of C. parvum
		Common variable immunodeficiency	AR*	Most unknown	Onset beyond infancy; associated with T-cell hyporesponsiveness in many patients; autoimmune phenomena including neutropenia			±	•			
		Other antibody deficiencies	AR*	UNG, AID*	Various phenotypes			±	•			

TABLE 1—cont'd

Presentation	Disease Type	Disorder	Inheritance	Genetic Defect	Additional Features	Treatment						
						PCP Prophylaxis	Antifungal Prophylaxis	Antibacterial Prophylaxis	Immunoglobulin Replacement	HSCT	Gene Therapy[†]	Other
Recurrent skin infections/ulcers, abscesses, periodontitis, unusual wound healing	Hyper-IgE syndrome		Sp AD	Unknown	Coarsening facies; dermatitis; bacterial infections, particularly *Staphylococcus*, affecting skin and lungs (with abscess formation, pneumatoceles); fungal infections			●	●			IFN-γ may be helpful; surgery often necessary for pulmonary complications; HSCT not curative
	Phagocyte disorder	Chronic granulomatous disease	XL AR	*CYBA* *CYBB* *NCF1* *NCF2*	Deep-seated fungal infections, especially *Aspergillus*; *Staphylococcus aureus*, *Burkholderia* septicemia and pneumonia, colitis		●	●		●	±	Surgery often necessary for deep abscesses (e.g., liver).
		Leukocyte adhesion deficiency	AR	*INTG2* Others	Delayed cord separation; leukocytosis; necrotizing infections without pus			±		●		
	Neutropenia	Severe congenital neutropenias	AD XL	*ELA2* *WASP*	Associated gingivitis, other cytopenias; late progression to myelodysplasia/AML		●	●		±		G-CSF helpful; full vaccination important, especially conjugate vaccines.
Recurrent, severe bacterial infections	Hyposplenia	Familial, syndromic, and sporadic forms			May occur in association with cardiac defect; NB: splenectomy sometimes required in other PIDs (e.g., WAS)			●				Pneumococcal sepsis a particular risk.
	Complement deficiency		AR	Defects of individual complement components	Neisserial infection; SLE association			±				Risk of late autoimmune disease.
Disseminated/ refractory NTM or *Salmonella* infection	Defects of T-cell monocyte interaction (IFN-α: IL-12 pathway)		AR AR AD	*IL12p40* *IL12Rβ1* *IFN-γ R1* *IFN-γ R2* *STAT1*				●		±		IFN-γ, antimycobacterial therapy.

Category	Disease	Inheritance	Gene defect	Clinical/associated features	Treatment
Overwhelming viral infection, lymphoproliferative disease and/or hemophagocytosis	X-linked lymphoproliferative disease	XL	*SAP/SH2D1A*	Symptoms provoked by EBV; lymphoma follows	Antiviral and cytotoxic therapy; Rituximab for LPD.
	Familial hemophagocytic lymphohistiocytosis	AR	*PRF1* *MUNC13-4**	Cytotoxic functions of NK and T cells impaired; often presents with fever, lymphadenopathy, hepatosplenomegaly, and cytopenias	
Associated features predominant in initial presentation	Monogenic disorders: WAS	XL	*WASP*	Thrombocytopenia, small platelets; eczema; hypogammaglobulinemia; recurrent sinopulmonary infections; risk of lymphoma	Splenectomy for intractable symptomatic thrombocytopenia.
	Anhydrotic ectodermal dysplasia with immunodeficiency	XL AD	*NEMO* *IKBA*	Recurrent severe bacterial infections from infancy; specific antibody deficiency; marked T-cell defect in AD form	
	DNA repair disorders	AR	*ATM* + others	Variable immune defect; susceptibility to lymphoreticular malignancies	
Chromosomal disorders	DGS	Sp AD	22q11-ter deletion	Cardiac defects, hypocalcemia, abnormal facies; thymic aplasia with variable T-cell deficiency (ranges from SCID to no immune phenotype)	Thymic transplantation in complete DGS (not widely available).
Chronic superficial fungal infection	Chronic mucocutaneous candidiasis	AR*	*AIRE**	Some forms associated with autoimmune polyendocrinopathy, ± ectodermal dysplasia	Endocrine replacement therapy.

*Others unknown.

†Gene therapy is not routinely available. In this column, bullets indicate previous trials in therapy (some have been performed in animal models). In this column, bullets indicate previous trials in therapy (●, previous trials in humans; ±, possible candidate for gene therapy (some have been applied in animal models)).

AD, autosomal dominant; AML, acute myeloid leukemia; AR, autosomal recessive; bullet (●), previous trials in humans; DGS, DiGeorge syndrome; EBV, Epstein-Barr virus; G-CSF, granulocyte colony-stimulating factor; GI, gastrointestinal; HSCT, hematopoietic stem cell transplantation; Ig, immunoglobulin; LPD, lymphoproliferative disease; MHC, major histocompatibility complex; NTM, nontuberculous mycobacteria; PCP, *Pneumocystis jiroveci* (formerly *carinii*) pneumonia; PEG-ADA, polyethylene glycol-adenosine deaminase; SCID, severe combined immune deficiency; SLE, systemic lupus erythematosus; Sp, sporadic; TB, tuberculosis; WAS, Wiskott-Aldrich syndrome; XL, X-linked.

Expert Opinion on Management Issues

GENERAL AND PREVENTIVE MEASURES

The aims of therapy are to improve quality of life, lengthen survival, prevent end-organ damage, and optimize the chances of successful cure. Education and support of the patient and family are critical to this process. The management of acute infection is considered separately in the chapter "The Immunocompromised Host."

AVOIDANCE OF EXPOSURE TO INFECTION

Sensible measures to avoid exposure to infectious agents should be adopted, in proportion to the nature and severity of the immunodeficiency; these must be balanced against the social and developmental needs of the child. Many milder immunodeficiencies require no special precautions, whereas others call for rather specific measures (e.g., drinking water should be boiled for individuals at risk for *Cryptosporidium* infection because of deficiency of CD40L or CD40). In the case of severe combined immune deficiency (SCID), however, the risks posed by ubiquitous pathogens such as respiratory viruses are often considered sufficient to warrant admission to a laminar flow cubicle in the hospital. Strict attention to infection-control measures is essential for these patients, including hand washing and provision of clean food, clean water, and clean air. Exposure to potentially infectious persons should

be strenuously avoided. Despite these measures, the accumulation of opportunistic and other infections is inevitable over time, hence the importance of early stem cell transplantation where possible.

IMMUNIZATIONS INCLUDING POSTEXPOSURE PROPHYLAXIS

Immunodeficient children who are able to respond to active vaccination potentially have more to gain than their immunocompetent peers because it may circumvent their immune defect. For example, asplenic children should be vaccinated against *Streptococcus pneumoniae* because they are particularly vulnerable to this organism. Conversely, live vaccines (Bacille Calmette-Guérin [BCG], measles, varicella zoster virus [VZV], live polio) represent a significant risk to many immunodeficient children because of their susceptibility to infection with low-virulence organisms. This risk is greatest in, but not confined to, those with T-cell defects; therefore general advice is to avoid live vaccines in children with immunodeficiency. (There are certain exceptions to this rule: For example, live vaccines are probably safe in partial DiGeorge syndrome; expert advice should always be sought, however.) Nonlive vaccines may safely be given, depending on the likelihood of any protective response; indeed, measurement of the resulting antibody titers may assist in diagnostic evaluation. However, vaccination should not be undertaken if the child's disease or therapy precludes development of adaptive immunity, and it is not usually considered necessary for those receiving Ig replacement.

Passive immunization may be appropriate as postexposure prophylaxis against infection with some pathogens, notably VZV, but also measles and cytomegalovirus (CMV). Once established, these viruses are life-threatening and difficult to treat in children with T-cell defects. As an adjunct, preemptive antiviral therapy may also be considered where the risk of infection is high.

CONTINUOUS ANTIMICROBIAL THERAPY

Although antimicrobial prophylaxis is not a panacea, in selected conditions it can be highly effective in reducing the burden of infections. In broad terms, three sets of circumstances may call for continuous antimicrobial therapy:

1. Specific susceptibility to overwhelming infection with a restricted set of pathogens (e.g., pneumococcal sepsis in asplenia, *Pneumocystis jiroveci* pneumonia in T-cell defects).
2. Vulnerability to recurrent, end-organ–damaging infection (e.g., chronic lung disease of hypogammaglobulinemic states, chronic granulomatous disease [CGD]).
3. Requirement for ongoing suppressive therapy when eradication of low-virulence organisms cannot be achieved (e.g., superficial fungal infection in chronic mucocutaneous candidiasis, staphylococci in hyper IgE syndrome,

mycobacteria in interleukin (IL)–12 and interferon (IFN)-γ defects, zoster in cellular immunodeficiency).

Prophylactic therapy must be tailored to the individual and vigilance maintained with respect to adverse effects and emerging microbial resistance. Table 2 offers information on commonly used agents and their indications; as with many aspects of these rare conditions, the evidence base for these therapies is small.

CHEST PHYSIOTHERAPY

Children with defects of humoral immunity are at risk of developing chronic lung disease including bronchiectasis. Once established, this requires the same therapy as bronchiectasis of any other cause: regular physiotherapy and postural drainage, monitoring of respiratory flora, treatment of infective respiratory exacerbations, and close monitoring of respiratory function, together with appropriate radiologic imaging. An expert in pediatric pulmonology should oversee these aspects of care.

NUTRITIONAL SUPPORT

Children with primary immunodeficiencies are at risk of suboptimal nutrition because of a number of factors, including poor appetite and catabolism during infection, special diets, hospitalization, and malabsorption because of infective or autoimmune gut inflammation. Malnutrition may compound existing immunocompromise and increase morbidity related to HSCT. Strategies to optimize nutrition should be tailored to the child but may include dietary supplements, nasogastric feeding, or total parenteral nutrition according to the circumstances.

CORRECTIVE THERAPY

Immunoglobulin Replacement

The availability of immunoglobulin replacement therapy has transformed the prospects for children with Ig deficiency, even in its most severe form (X-linked agammaglobulinemia [XLA]). Ig is also useful in the therapy of combined immunodeficiencies and an ever-growing number of other disorders. Clearly, patient selection is important to avoid wasting time and resources, as well as preventing unnecessary exposure to a human blood product (albeit one subject to stringent safety standards).

The primary aim of Ig replacement in PID is to reduce the incidence and severity of infections, which delays respiratory disease and prolongs life. Intravenous immunoglobulin (IVIG) is most commonly used, but preparations suitable for subcutaneous infusion are also available in Europe. The latter route has several advantages over IVIG, notably increased patient autonomy, ease of administration in patients with poor venous access, and more consistent Ig levels, but it requires more frequent administration.

Although the life-enhancing effect of Ig replacement therapy is not in doubt, few data inform the issues of dose and schedule. This is important because individuals with XLA in whom Ig therapy is begun prior to the establishment of bronchiectasis nonetheless succumb to chronic lung disease over time. Small trials suggest that standard doses, which elevate plasma IgG to 500 mg/dL or above, may be suboptimal; however, consensus is as yet lacking on whether to titrate dose to some predetermined higher trough level (e.g., 800 to 1000 mg/dL) or to clinical effect.

Hematopoietic Stem Cell Transplantation

HSCT, which offers the possibility of cure of many primary immunodeficiencies, is considered in a separate chapter. Table 1 indicates the role of HSCT in the treatment of a number of PIDs.

Polyethylene Glycol–Conjugated Adenosine Deaminase

Adenosine deaminase (ADA) deficiency, a disorder of purine metabolism leading to the toxic destruction of lymphocytes, is unusual in that the faulty enzyme can be replaced by injection of its pegylated form. Although inconvenient and expensive, this therapy is remarkably effective and represents the treatment of choice in those children for whom a suitable marrow donor cannot be found.

Colony-Stimulating Factors and Cytokines

The immune system represents a complex and dispersed network within which intercellular communication is mediated through both cell contact and soluble mediators. Some of the latter molecules—cytokines, chemokines, and colony-stimulating factors (CSFs)—can be of clinical use in specific immunodeficiencies when administered by injection. In some cases, therapy can be easily understood as a means of correcting abnormally low levels of cytokine activity; one such example would be IFN-γ therapy of IL-12R deficiency (in which T cells fail to respond to an important stimulator of IFN-γ production). The mechanism of action is not always so clear, however, as in the case of IFN-γ therapy of CGD (not in routine use in Europe). Because these agents are costly to produce and difficult to administer, therapy should not be undertaken lightly.

Therapeutic Monoclonal Antibodies

A related immunomodulatory therapy exists in the form of rituximab, a monoclonal antibody against B cells. This can be useful in circumstances of uncontrolled Epstein-Barr virus (EBV) infection leading to lymphoproliferative disease (LPD) (e.g., X-linked LPD [XLP] disease, post-transplant B-cell LPD [BLPD]). Another useful agent in highly immunocompromised patients is the humanized monoclonal antibody preparation palivizumab, which offers protection against respiratory syncytial virus (RSV) infection.

TABLE 2 Selected Agents Useful In the Long-Term Therapy of Primary Immunodeficiency

Generic Name	Dosage/Route/Regimen	Maximum Dose	Common or Severe Adverse Reactions	Indications
PCP Prophylaxis				
Trimethoprim-sulfamethoxazole (TMP-SMX)	150/750 mg/kg/day PO, preferably in 2 div doses, at least × 3/wk	320 mg trimethoprim	Erythema multiforme, Stevens-Johnson syndrome, neutropenia	Significant T-cell defect
Dapsone	2 mg/kg PO qd or 4 mg/kg PO weekly	100 mg/daily dose 200 mg/weekly dose	Hemolysis, methemoglobinemia, neuropathy, allergic dermatitis, GI intolerance, hepatitis, and numerous others	Criteria for first-degree PCP prophylaxis in HIV infection (on basis of T-cell numbers/%) of unclear usefulness in PIDs
Pentamidine	300 mg inhalation (nebulizer) monthly 4 mg/kg IV q2–4wk		Risk of severe reaction (hypotension, hypoglycemia, pancreatitis, and arrhythmias); numerous other toxicities*	
Atovaquone	45 mg/kg PO qd (4–24 mo of age) 30 mg/kg PO qd (1–3 mo of age or >24 mo of age)		Rash, nausea, diarrhea, vomiting, headache, insomnia, fever, anemia, hyponatremia, neutropenia	
Antifungal Prophylaxis				
Fluconazole	3–6 mg/kg PO qd	12 mg/kg	GI intolerance, rash, Stevens-Johnson syndrome, hepatotoxicity	SCID, CMC
Itraconazole	<13 yr of age, <50 kg: 100 mg qd >13 yr of age, >50 kg: 200 mg qd		As above plus edema, headache, hypokalemia, blood dyscrasias	CGD; measure serum levels
Voriconazole	Loading dose: 6 mg/kg bid × 2, then: 4 mg/kg bid IV/PO		Nausea, vomiting, transient visual disturbance, rash, deranged LFTs, cheilitis	Maintenance therapy following invasive fungal infection (e.g., aspergillosis) (also effective as first-line therapy)
Liposomal amphotericin	1 mg/kg qd IV (prophylaxis) 3–10 mg/kg qd IV (treatment)	10 mg/kg	Fever, rigors, nausea, vomiting, renal and liver toxicity	High-risk patients unable to tolerate oral therapy
Antibacterial Agents				
TMP-SMX	5 mg/kg/day PO in 1 or 2 div doses	320 mg TMP	Erythema multiforme, Stevens-Johnson syndrome, neutropenia	CGD; Wiskott-Aldrich syndrome
Phenoxymethyl-penicillin (Penicillin V)	<6 yr: 125 mg PO bid 6–12 yr: 250 mg PO bid >12 yr: 500 mg PO bid			Hyposplenism (including postsplenectomy)
Azithromycin	10 mg/kg qd (on days 1–3 of a 10-day cycle) or 20 mg/kg once weekly or 5 mg/kg qd	20 mg/kg 1200 mg 250 mg	GI upset, hepatotoxicity	Antibody deficiency with breakthrough infection despite adequate Ig replacement therapy
Flucloxacillin or Dicloxacillin	25–50 mg/kg/day PO in 2–4 div doses		Cholestasis (rarely)	Recurrent/refractory staphylococcal infection, especially Hyper IgE syndrome (TMP-SMX provides anti-*Staphylococcus* cover in CGD)
Antiprotozoal Agents				
Nitazoxanide	100 mg PO bid × 3/7 (1–3 yr of age) 200 mg PO bid × 3/7 (4–11 yr of age)	500 mg	Abdominal pain, nausea, vomiting, headache	Use in immunocompromised patients not evidence based
Paromomycin	25–35 mg/kg/day PO in 3 div doses		GI upset, hearing problems	
Azithromycin	10 mg/kg PO qd	20 mg/kg	Nausea, abdominal pain, vomiting, diarrhea	

Antiviral Agents

Agent	Dose	Toxicity/Side Effects	Indication/Comments
Acyclovir	5–15 mg/kg IV tid (420–1350 mg/m²/day) or <2 yr, 100–200 mg PO q6h; >2yr, 200–400 mg PO q6h	GI disturbance, headache, fatigue, rash, pruritus, photosensitivity, nephrotoxicity; IV: fever, severe local inflammation	Severe T-cell defects; active against α-herpesviruses and, to a lesser extent, CMV
Ganciclovir	5 mg/kg (150 mg/m²) IV qd, given × 5–7 wk (suppressive dose) 90–120 mg/kg IV qd	Neutropenia: major side effect, but many toxicities*	Suppressive therapy for CMV in severe T-cell defect
Foscarnet	80 mg/kg/day	GI disturbance, neurologic problems, nephrotoxicity*	CMV suppression (not first-line therapy because highly toxic); possible role in adenovirus therapy in SCID
Cidofovir	3 mg/kg/wk IV with hydration/probenecid	Nephrotoxicity, neutropenia, fever, weakness, alopecia, nausea, vomiting, hypotony*	Case reports of successful IV therapy of adenoviral infection in children with profound immunocompromise
Ribavirin	IV: Loading: 33 mg/kg then 16 mg/kg IV q6h or: Aerosolized: 2 g in 33 mL water over 2 hr, tid; or 6g/300 mL over 18h qd	Hemolysis, myelosuppression; inhaled therapy difficult and isolating to administer	also has activity against RSV; preemptive aerosolized therapy may have a role
Oseltamivir	<15 kg: 30 mg PO bid; 15–23 kg: 45 mg PO bid; 23–40 kg: 60 mg PO bid; >40 kg: 75 mg/kg PO bid	GI disturbance; headache, fatigue, insomnia, dizziness; conjunctivitis, rash, epistaxis	Postexposure prophylaxis of influenza in SCID (treatment doses are quoted)

Immunomodulators

Agent	Dose	Toxicity/Side Effects	Indication/Comments
Immunoglobulin	300–800 mg/kg monthly as single dose (IV) or div doses (IV/SC/IM); 1 g/kg	Headache, malaise, fever, rigors, anaphylaxis	Combined immunodeficiencies; primary antibody deficiencies; various secondary immune deficiencies
γ-Interferon	50 µg/kg/m²SC ×3/wk (1.5 µg/kg if <0.5m²)	Fever, headache, chills, myalgia, fatigue; nausea, vomiting, arthralgia, rashes, and injection-site reactions	CGD (standard therapy in United States); Defects of IL12, IFN-γ pathway
G-CSF	5 µg/kg SC qd (but titrated to response); 120 µg/kg	Risk of late evolution to AML in congenital neutropenia (link to G-CSF therapy unclear)	Severe chronic neutropenias; Neutropenia complicating X-linked hyper IgM syndrome
PEG-ADA	Initially 30 U/kg IM twice weekly; maintenance: 15–30 U/kg IM weekly	Transient platelet abnormalities; antibodies to PEG-ADA commonly develop (leading to increased enzyme clearance in 10%)	ADA deficiency (pending HSCT)

*Significant toxicity substantially limits use of asterisked agents.

ADA, adenosine deaminase; AML, acute myeloid leukemia; bid, twice daily; CGD, chronic granulomatous disease; CMC, chronic mucocutaneous candidiasis; CMV, cytomegalovirus; div, divided; G-CSF, granulocyte colony-stimulating factor; GI, gastrointestinal; HIV, human immunodeficiency virus; HSCT, hematopoietic stem cell transplantation; Ig, immunoglobulin; IM, intramuscular; IV, intravenous; LFT, liver function test; PCP, *Pneumocystis jiroveci* (formerly *carinii*) pneumonia; PEG-ADA, polyethylene glycol-adenosine deaminase; PID, primary immunodeficiency; PO, by mouth; q, every; qd, every day; qxh, every x hours; RSV, respiratory syncytial virus; SC, subcutaneous; SCID, severe combined immune deficiency.

Note: Drug doses and regimens are based on published evidence but rarely have these been subjected to controlled trials.

Gene Therapy

An enormous effort has been put into the development of gene therapy for primary immunodeficiencies, culminating in the successful correction of common γ-chain deficiency by this means in 10 human subjects. The principle of this therapy is to purify hematopoietic stem cells from the immunodeficient patient, introduce into them a wild-type copy of the affected gene, and return the transduced cells to the host. A number of practical requirements currently limit the applicability of this approach: The affected gene must be known, retrovirally driven expression must correct the gene defect, and constitutive expression must be tolerated within the hematopoietic compartment. In addition, the gene-corrected cells are more likely to persist if their phenotype confers a survival advantage over uncorrected cells. This is the case in many forms of SCID and in XLA, but it is not so in many other significant immunodeficiencies. A further major hurdle in the development of gene therapy is the recognition of two cases of lymphoid malignancy that were directly attributable to retroviral insertional mutagenesis. It is as yet unclear to what extent modified gene delivery technologies may circumvent this complication.

Thymus Transplantation

Complete DiGeorge syndrome (DGS) is characterized by a profound deficiency of T cells owing to thymic aplasia. This defect cannot be corrected by stem cell transplantation; patients lack not T-cell precursors but only the appropriate microenvironment for them to mature. Surprisingly, engraftment of minimally manipulated thymic tissue (from infants undergoing cardiac surgery) restores T lymphopoiesis in such children. In the future, this may become standard therapy for complete DGS.

MANAGEMENT OF ACUTE INFECTIONS

The large topic of acute infections is discussed in the chapter "The Immunocompromised Host." Key features of successful management include:

- Early recognition (education of patient and/or caregivers, screening measures in some circumstances).
- Aggressive pursuit of microbiologic diagnosis in close liaison with clinical laboratory colleagues, bearing in mind the possibility of mixed infection (serologic tests are often unhelpful, increasing reliance on direct antigen detection, e.g., polymerase chain reaction [PCR] and tissue diagnosis).
- Prompt and vigorous therapy; optimization of drug levels, use of multiple agents, and prolonged courses where appropriate.

Common Pitfalls

Failure to consider the diagnosis of primary immunodeficiency early connotes a missed opportunity to institute therapy. The results of such delay may range from preventable significant infections through irreversible lung disease to death (particularly in late-diagnosed SCID). Simple investigations (e.g., complete blood count with low lymphocyte count, interpreted in relation to age-appropriate normal values) often give valuable clues to PID and should not be overlooked. Where suspicions of PID are aroused, early discussion with an expert is advised.

Many PIDs carry with them a greatly increased risk of hematologic malignancy, and some are associated with autoimmune phenomena. In addition, the immunologic phenotype may itself evolve over time, as occurs classically in common variable immune deficiency but also in other disorders (hypogammaglobulinemia, Wiskott-Aldrich syndrome). These possibilities need to be borne in mind when evaluating new symptoms.

Communication and Counseling

The diagnosis of PID has tremendous implications for the affected children and for their parents and siblings. The psychological and emotional work required of these families should not be underestimated. First, they are confronted with a diagnosis that frequently implies life-limiting illness, the possibility of chronic ill health, frequent or prolonged hospitalization (possibly far from home), and long-term therapy. Second, this information may be imparted at a time when the child is already severely ill, following a period of diagnostic uncertainty. Third, the genetic dimension of many of these conditions introduces added complexity to the emotional responses of both parents and siblings, who may feel very guilty. Beyond the analysis of parental carrier status, there may be issues of carrier detection for female relatives (sisters, aunts) of boys with X-linked PIDs; genetic counseling may therefore be needed for the wider family. Finally, the possibility of curative HSCT, although offering hope in desperate circumstances, is itself a risky and highly stressful undertaking (for the patient, parents, and siblings, especially the donor).

In recognition of these factors, it is clearly important to establish a trusting, open, and sustained relationship between family and caregiving team. Families have different needs in terms of information, practical help (including money), and social support; some of these, particularly long-term social support, may be addressed by voluntary groups such as the Immune Deficiency Foundation (http://www.primaryimmune.org), the Primary Immunodeficiency Association (http://www.pia.org.uk), and similar organizations (useful links through http://www.ipopi.org).

SUGGESTED READINGS

1. Antoine C, Muller S, Cant A, et al: Long-term survival transplantation of haemopoietic stem cells for immunodeficiencies: Report of the European experience 1968–99. Lancet 361(9357):553–560, 2003. **Documents the improved outcome in SCID and other PIDs following early HSCT (and trimethoprim-sulfamethoxazole prophylaxis).**

2. Berger M: Subcutaneous immunoglobulin replacement in primary immunodeficiencies. Clin Immunol 112(1):1–7, 2004. **Compares IVIG with SCIG from a U.S. perspective.**

3. Bonilla FA, Geha RS: Primary immunodeficiency diseases. J Allergy Clin Immunol 111(2 Suppl):S571–S581, 2003. **Succinct up-to-date introduction to PIDs with background on their molecular genetics.**

4. Chinen J, Puck JM: Successes and risks of gene therapy in primary immunodeficiencies. J Allergy Clin Immunol 113(4):595–603, 2004. **Excellent and detailed review of the current status of gene therapy.**

5. Gallin JI, Alling DW, Malech HL, et al: Itraconazole to prevent fungal infections in chronic granulomatous disease. N Engl J Med 348(24):2416–2422, 2003. **One of the few double-blind, randomized, controlled trials in the field, which established the important place of itraconazole prophylaxis in CGD.**

6. Gennery AR, Cant AJ: The immunocompromised host: The patient with recurrent infection. Adv Exp Med Biol 549:109–117, 2004. **How to recognize the child with immunodeficiency.**

7. Kaplan JE, Masur H, Holmes KK: Guidelines for preventing opportunistic infections among HIV-infected persons—2002. Recommendations of the U.S. Public Health Service the Infectious Diseases Society of America. MMWR Recomm Rep 51(RR-8):1–52, 2002. **Many of the sensible recommendations here apply equally to individuals with combined PIDs.**

8. Plebani A, Soresina A, Rondelli R, et al: Clinical, immunological, and molecular analysis in a large cohort of patients with X-linked agammaglobulinemia: An Italian multicenter study. Clin Immunol 104(3):221–230, 2002. **Important study documenting the natural history of treated XLA; the earlier therapy is begun, the later bronchiectasis develops.**

9. Stiehm ER: Human intravenous immunoglobulin in primary and secondary antibody deficiencies. Pediatr Infect Dis J 16(7):696–707, 1997. **Thorough review of the development and use of IVIG, with suggested guidelines for patient selection.**

10. Stiehm ER, Ochs HD, Winkelstein JA (eds): Immunologic Disorders in Infants and Children, 5th ed. Philadelphia: Elsevier Saunders, 2004. **The definitive text, with excellent review chapters on general and specific features of the immunodeficiencies by experts in the field.**

■ Complement-targeted therapy (soluble complement receptor 1 [CR1] and antibodies against C5 or C5a receptor [C5aR] antagonists) will become important tools in the near future for adjuvant treatment in ischemia-reperfusion injury, transplantation medicine, and inflammatory disease.

The complement system consists of more than 35 soluble and plasma membrane proteins that interact to recognize, opsonize, and clear or kill invading microorganisms or altered host cells (e.g., apoptotic or necrotic cells). Soluble complement system proteins make up approximately 5% of the total protein content of human blood plasma. They are also present at lower concentrations in other body fluids. Complement is a major part of the innate immune system.

The three different routes of complement activation (classical, alternative, and lectin pathway) involve several proteins (Fig. 1), most of which are produced in the liver by hepatocytes and secreted in plasma constitutively or induced by inflammatory cytokines during the acute phase response (APR). Some proteins, such as C1q, C7, and factor D, are mainly produced extrahepatically—C1q is mainly synthesized by cells of the monocyte-macrophage lineage and factor D by adipose and renal tubular cells. Local synthesis of complement proteins by resident or infiltrating cells is pivotal for driving inflammatory processes, such as for the kidney.

The first and main physiologic activity of the complement system is the host defense against infections. As part of innate immunity, complement is able to immediately respond to invading pathogens and thus prevent microorganisms from damaging the host. Complement activation has to take place to exert protection

Complement Disorders and Lectin Pathway

Taco W. Kuijpers

KEY CONCEPTS

■ The complement system plays a role in the recognition, opsonization, and killing or clearance of invading microorganisms, immune complexes, and altered host cells.

■ There are three main pathways of complement activation: the classical pathway (C1-dependent), lectin route (mannose-binding lectin [MBL]/ficolin and MBL-associated serine proteases [MASP]-dependent) in which both C4 and C2 play a role, and the alternative pathway (factors B and D and properdin).

■ MBL deficiency is frequent (25%) and acts as a disease-modifying factor. All other complement deficiencies are infrequent and result in pyogenic infections or autoimmune disease reminiscent of systemic lupus erythematosus.

■ C1-INH replacement therapy is available for hereditary (or acquired) angioedema (HAE). Regarding all other soluble complement components, replacement therapy is available only for MBL.

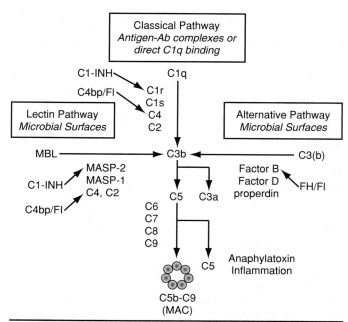

FIGURE 1. The three routes of complement activation (classical, alternative, and lectin).

through complement-mediated opsonization (C3 deposition) for recognition and uptake by phagocytes, or by direct killing (via the membrane attack complex [MAC], C5b-C9). During complement activation, anaphylatoxins such as C3a and C5a are released to attract and stimulate cells of the immune system such as granulocytes, neutrophils, and monocytes. The final formation of the terminal complement complex C5b-C9 leads to the lysis of invading pathogens. Moreover, sublytic C5b-C9 is also known as a proinflammatory mediator.

Recognition proteins such as C1q and lectins (e.g., mannose-binding lectin (MBL) and ficolins) bind to targets via charge or sugar arrays. In the circulation, C1q is associated with the serine proteases C1r and C1s, whereas MBL associates with the MBL-associated serine proteases (MASP) 2 and 1 (–3). Recognition by the classical and lectin pathways leads to conformational changes in these associated serine proteases that cleave complement components C4 and C2, itself a serine protease, leading to the formation of the protease complex C4b2a. Activity of $C1r_2s_2$ and MASPs can be inhibited by C1-inhibitor (C1-INH), a plasma protein of the serine protease inhibitor (SERPIN) family; whereas C4-binding protein (C4bp) acts as a cofactor to the serine protease factor I, in the proteolytic inactivation of C4b, which prevents the formation of the classical C3-convertase (C4b2a).

Any active C3-convertase complex cleaves C3 into C3a and C3b. C3b is a central component of the complement system because of its many effector functions.

The alternative pathway route recognizes targets bearing surface clusters of both charged and neutral sugar. There is continuous spontaneous activation: C3 undergoes hydrolysis of its internal thiolester at a low rate to form C3i (or C3[H_2O]). When in complex with the serine protease factor B, factor B is cleaved by the serine protease factor D to form C3bBb, stabilized by properdin, thus causing C3b to fix in clusters to the target surface. This complex produces strong opsonization and functioning as C5-convertase, cleaving C5 and initiating the assembly of the MAC. At this level of C3b, plasma factor H accelerates decay of the alternative pathway C3 convertase and acts as cofactor for the plasma factor I–mediated proteolytic inactivation of C3b into iC3b and further into C3d(g). The inactivated iC3b remains covalently bound to the surface and still is opsonically active.

A second important function of the complement deals with the capacity of complement to bridge innate and adaptive immunity. This has great impact on our strategies to protect patients with known complement deficiencies from further recurrent attacks of bacterial infections. Depletion of C3 in an animal model resulted in an impaired humoral response to T-dependent and T-independent antigens. Extensive studies demonstrate the important role of C3 fragments in modulating the response of B cells and follicular dendritic cells (FDCs) in the spleen and lymph nodes via the specific complement receptors CD21 for C3dg and CD35 for C3b and C4b. First, by FDC-mediated trapping of antigen (CD35), the B cells may generate a high-avidity antibody response (CD35). Second, by lowering the threshold for B-cell activation via combined specific antigen recognition (BcR) and C3dg binding (CD21), such a response is allowed by low antigen concentrations.

The third major role for complement is demonstrated in the disposal of immune complexes and apoptotic cells. This function is pivotal because the persistence and precipitation of immune complexes associated with an altered clearance of wasted self material is one of the major hypotheses for the pathogenesis of systemic lupus erythematosus (SLE), the prototype autoimmune disease.

Thus, humans deficient for complement proteins such as C3, MBL, factor B, C4, or C1q are more susceptible to bacterial infections and autoimmunity.

Blood levels of MBL are affected by structural mutations in exon 1 and promoter polymorphisms in the *MBL2* gene. MBL deficiency is present in approximately 25% of the general population. Although sometimes more prevalent in certain racial or ethnic groups, in general the remainder of complement defects are rare. Some of the complement deficiencies are secondary to other mechanisms. For instance, congenital deficiency of factor H or I results in unrestrained complement activation followed by depletion of C3. Acquired C3 deficiency may be the consequence of nephritic factors, autoantibodies responsible for the stabilization of the C3-convertase activity of the alternative pathway (C3bBb), and unrestricted complement consumption.

Tissue cells of the host are protected from exaggerated complement activation by several soluble or cell-associated regulatory proteins like factor H, factor I, complement receptor–1 (CR1) (CD35), membrane cofactor protein (MCP) (CD46), decay-accelerating factor (DAF) (CD55), and homologous restriction factor (HRF) (CD59), which are usually not found on microorganisms.

Paroxysmal nocturnal hemoglobinuria (PNH) is an acquired clonal stem cell disorder characterized by intravascular hemolysis, cytopenias, frequent infections, and high incidence of severe venous thrombosis. The somatic mutation of the *PIG-A* gene disturbs lipid anchorage of several surface membrane proteins to hematopoietic cells. In the case of the red cell, the absence of CD55 and CD59 may lead to hemolytic attacks, hemoglobinuria, and the need for regular transfusions.

Uncontrolled complement activation caused by C3-nephritic factor or factor H deficiency, for example, results in membranoproliferative glomerulonephritis (MPGN) type II. However, the heterozygous factor H mutations associated with atypical familial hemolytic uremic syndrome (aHUS) rarely results in hypocomplementemia or decreased factor H plasma levels. Most of these missense mutations cluster within the tail of the protein (domains SCR19 and SCR20), a region that is critical to control activation complement on cell surfaces but not required to regulate complement activation in plasma. Apart from heterozygous factor H mutations, both hetero- and homozygous MCP46-deficiencies have been defined as other causes of aHUS, each accounting for approximately 20% of aHUS cases.

Expert Opinion on Management Issues

The infectious organisms predominating in the clinical spectrum include mostly encapsulated bacterial pathogens. An MBL phase II study in children by Kuipers and colleagues is ongoing (results are as yet unpublished); it will allow future treatment as adjuvant therapy in selected disease conditions. Substitution of any other single component is not yet feasible to date, apart from C1-INH. Curing a congenital complement deficiency is only possible with liver transplantation. In the case of CD46 deficiency, renal transplantation does not end in relapse of HUS, in contrast to the situation with factor H mutations. A realistic option in recurrent HUS caused by factor H deficiency may consist of a combined liver/kidney transplant.

ACCEPTED INTERVENTIONS

Patients with the rare complement deficiencies suffer from meningococcal disease with a relative risk of 5000 compared to persons without a complement deficiency. Factors B and D and properdin deficiency results in early and often severe disease, while the late complement components of the terminal pathway give rise to a relatively mild yet recurrent presentation of meningococcal (or gonococcal) disease starting late during childhood and adolescence.

Preventive measures consist of vaccination against the most common encapsulated pathogens. Vaccination against the common meningococcal strains and pneumococci is possible in children older than 2 years of age. For patients younger than 2 years, the antibody responses cannot be relied on for protection. In these children, prophylactic antibiotics (oral penicillin or cotrimoxazole) are effective. The meningococcal (Men) C and pneumococcal conjugate vaccines can be used from the age of 2 months onward but have major drawbacks, including incomplete coverage (MenA, MenW135, MenY, and many pneumococcal strains) as well as the incomplete humoral response inherent to the complement defect per se. Antibody responses should be tested. Immunization ought to be repeated every 2 to 5 years depending on the potential risk of exposure. The alternative option of antibiotic prophylaxis should be considered.

In HAE, three sites can be affected: skin, the gastrointestinal mucosa, and the upper airways. Larynx edema makes the disease life-threatening when it goes unrecognized. The main cause of HAE is the increased vascular permeability caused by bradykinin, similar to rare side effects with angiotensin-converting enzyme (ACE) inhibitors. These are strictly prohibited in HAE. Long-term prophylaxis should be reserved for the ones with frequent (more than 1 or 2) attacks per month. Prophylaxis consists of antifibrinolytic drugs (tranexamic acid 50–100 mg/kg in three doses) or, in young adulthood, attenuated androgens such as stanozolol or danazol. The induction of benign or malignant liver neoplasia is extremely rare; the most common complaints include weight gain, minimal signs of virilization, and menstrual irregularities.

CONTROVERSIAL INTERVENTIONS

One report indicates that during acute infection, fresh-frozen plasma accelerates the inflammatory response in a complement-deficient patient, presumably by

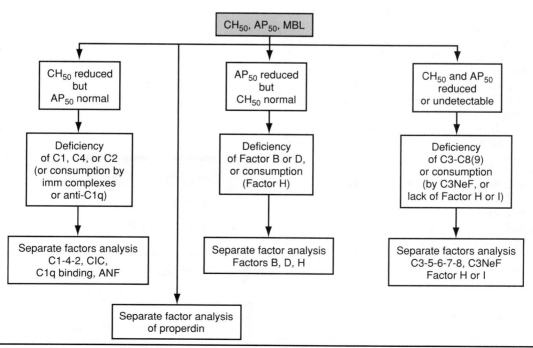

FIGURE 2. Algorithm for testing complement components.

complement activation subsequent to substitution. The danger of supplementation of a missing complement factor remains an unsettled issue. In fact, the diagnosis of a rare inherited complement defect cannot be made at clinical presentation because of the consumption of components during complement activation. The low incidence of these inherited defects does not allow for further clinical consideration and, in practice, plasma will be administered in case of meningococcemia with concomitantly disseminated intravascular coagulation.

FUTURE INTERVENTIONS

Administration of humanized anti-C5 svFc (pexelizumab) decreases overall patient morbidity and mortality in patients undergoing coronary bypass grafting. Soluble CR1 (TP10) binds and displaces C4b and C3b from the C3/C5 convertase complexes and assists in factor I–mediated cleavage of both factors. The inhibitor TP10 has been beneficial in cardiopulmonary bypass patients as well. These studies (phases II and III) also offer potential use of these drugs under conditions of concomitant ischemia-reperfusion injury (cardiogenic or hypovolumic shock, sepsis, multitrauma, head injury). Moreover, anti-C5 (eculizumab) is highly effective in reducing hemolysis, hemoglobinuria, and the need for transfusions in PNH, and it is potentially relevant for the treatment of fulminant transfusion reactions as well.

Common Pitfalls

Complement components should be tested in a logical manner (Fig. 2). Suspicion should rise when less virulent strains are being cultured from cerebrospinal fluid or blood, such as the W135 or Y-serogroups. The standard screening consists of the CH_{50} and AP_{50} hemolysis assays, which are not very sensitive. When screening tests are abnormal or of serious clinical doubt, separate analysis of the various complement factors should be performed. If there are factor H or I deficiencies or C3 nephritic factors, the individuals show very low levels of C3 and factor B. With primary C3 deficiency, factor B is normal (as well as factors H and I). C1-INH deficiency results in low C4 and C2 (with normal C1q in HAE and low C1q in the acquired forms in elderly persons because of lymphoproliferative disease).

Symptoms in HAE are unpredictable in frequency and severity, and some individuals have HAE without a single attack. C1-INH plasma levels are largely below the 50% of normal that one would not expect in a heterozygous defect (HAE type I). An explanation is still lacking. In 15% of persons with HAE, levels are normal (type II) and C1-INH is dysfunctional, which can be missed when only antigen levels are tested.

Communication and Counseling

Parents and family members should be informed about the increased risk of infections. Early start of empirical treatment with small-spectrum antibiotics in case of febrile illness is advised when a rare complement defect is diagnosed. Genetic counseling, carrier detection, and prenatal diagnosis are possible when the defect is elucidated at the level of DNA.

SUGGESTED READINGS

1. Barrington R, Zhang M, Fischer M, Carroll MC: The role of complement in inflammation and adaptive immunity. Immunol Rev 180:5–15, 2001. **Looks at host protection, inflammation, and regulation of B lymphocytes.**
2. Frank MM: Complement deficiencies. Pediatr Clin North Am 47:1339–1354, 2000. **The role of complement proteins in immunity.**
3. Granger CB, Mahaffey KW, Weaver WD, et al: Pexelizumab, an anti-C5 complement antibody, as adjunctive therapy to primary percutaneous coronary interventions in acute myocardial infarction. Circulation 108:1184–1190, 2003. **The mortality rate of patients with myocardial infarction was significantly lower in patients treated with pexelizumab.**
4. Hillmen P, Hall C, Marsh JCW, et al: Effect of eculizumab on hemolysis and transfusion requirements in patients with paroxysmal nocturnal hemoglobinuria. New Engl J Med 350:552–559, 2004. **Eculizumab reduces intravascular hemolysis, hemoglobinuria, and transfusion requirements.**
5. Lehner PJ, Davies KA, Walport MJ: Meningococcal septicaemia in a C6-deficient patient and the effects of plasma transfusion on lipopolysaccharide release. Lancet 340:1379–1381, 1992. **C6-deficient patients have reduced mortality from meningococcal infection, possibly because their serum cannot cause the pathogen to release endotoxin.**
6. Manderson AP, Botto M, Walport MJ: The role of complement in the development of systemic lupus erythematosus. Annu Rev Immunol 22:431–456, 2004. **Complement may have a role in the physiological waste-disposal mechanisms of dying cells and immune complexes. Complement deficiency could also cause incomplete maintenance of peripheral tolerance.**
7. Turner MW: The role of mannose-binding lectin in health and disease. Mol Immunol 40:423–429, 2003. **MBL deficiency increases a person's overall susceptibility to infection. However, MBL deficiency may protect against some intracellular parasites.**
8. Walport MJ: Complement. First of two parts. N Engl J Med 344:1058–1066, 2001.
9. Walport MJ: Complement. Second of two parts. N Engl J Med 344:1140–1144, 2001. **Comprehensive discussion of complement and the immune system.**

Blood and Marrow Transplantation

Gustavo Del Toro, Erin Morris, and Mitchell S. Cairo

KEY CONCEPTS

- Blood and/or marrow transplantation (BMT) is curative in a number of pediatric malignant and nonmalignant diseases.
- Donor sources for BMT include autologous (self) and allogeneic (another human) and may consist of bone marrow, peripheral blood, or cord blood.

- Limitations to BMT include inadequate donor source, human leukocyte antigen (HLA) incompatibility, failure to engraft, graft-versus-host disease (GVHD), infectious morbidity, and late effects.
- BMT is successful through a variety of mechanisms, including myeloablation, immune suppression, gene replacement, graft-versus-tumor effect, and graft-versus-autoimmune effect.
- Children and families undergoing BMT require multidisciplinary psychosocial consulting and support prior to, during, and after BMT.

A number of malignant and nonmalignant conditions are successfully treated with either autologous or allogeneic blood and/or marrow transplantation (BMT) (Tables 1 and 2). Cure rates vary from 10% to 80%, depending on the condition of the patient, type of hematopoietic stem/immune cells used, disease status, and specific preparative regimen used. Among the childhood malignant conditions, the most common diseases treated with BMT include acute lymphoblastic leukemia, acute nonlymphoblastic leukemia, chronic myelogenous leukemia, juvenile chronic myelogenous leukemia, non-Hodgkin lymphoma, Hodgkin disease, neuroblastoma, Wilms tumor, high-risk sarcomas, high-risk brain tumors, and a variety of other less-common tumors.

Nonmalignant conditions that require BMT early in the disease course include conditions such as severe combined immune deficiency, Wiskott-Aldrich syndrome, and lethal inborn errors of metabolism such as adrenoleukodystrophy, Hurler syndrome, and Marateaux-Lamy syndrome. Diseases that fail standard medical management may, alternatively, be cured with BMT; these include chronic granulomatous disease, Kostmann syndrome (congenital neutropenia), sickle cell disease, thalassemia, Diamond-Blackfan syndrome, and others.

Patient Eligibility

The traditional myeloablative (marrow ablative) transplant has a high risk of post-transplant complications. Thus the potential recipient of myeloablative therapy must be able to tolerate the intense doses of chemotherapy and/or radiation. Pretransplant evaluation routinely includes determining the Lansky/Karnofsky score and obtaining echocardiogram, pulmonary function testing, renal function evaluation, and liver function evaluation. Although the actual test results that make a patient eligible vary with treatment plan and/or transplant center, organ function must be high enough to allow the patient to tolerate the conditioning regimen and post-transplant complications without excessive morbidity and/or mortality.

The patient's psychosocial situation should be considered as part of the eligibility criteria:

- Financial cost to the parents: One parent may drop out of the workforce to take care of the patient during the intense post-transplant months; many items may not be covered by the family's medical insurance carrier. Sometimes even the transplant itself is not covered.
- Separation of patient and parent(s) from home for prolonged periods of time. Home may be very far from the transplant center; siblings may be left at home without the same attention paid to the

TABLE 1 Malignant Diseases Successfully Treated with BMT

Disease	Autologous or Allogeneic BMT
Acute lymphoblastic leukemia	Autologous/allogeneic
Acute myeloid leukemia	Autologous/allogeneic
Myelodysplastic syndrome	Autologous/allogeneic
Chronic myelogenous leukemia	Allogeneic
Juvenile myelomonocytic leukemia	Allogeneic
Hodgkin lymphoma	Autologous
Non-Hodgkin lymphoma	Autologous/allogeneic
Central nervous system tumors	Autologous
Neuroblastoma	Autologous
Wilms tumor	Autologous
Germ cell tumor	Autologous
Ewing sarcoma	Autologous
Rhabdomyosarcoma	Autologous
Retinoblastoma	Autologous
Hemophagocytic lymphohistiocytosis	Allogeneic

BMT, blood and/or marrow transplantation.

TABLE 2 Nonmalignant Diseases Successfully Treated with BMT

Disease	Autologous or Allogeneic BMT
Aplastic anemia	Allogeneic
Thalassemia	Allogeneic
Sickle cell disease	Allogeneic
Fanconi anemia	Allogeneic
Severe combined immunodeficiency syndrome	Allogeneic
Combined immunodeficiency syndrome	Allogeneic
Wiskott-Aldrich syndrome	Allogeneic
Osteopetrosis	Allogeneic
Hurler syndrome	Allogeneic
Maroteaux-Lamy syndrome	Allogeneic
Sly syndrome	Allogeneic
Cerebral X-adrenoleukodystrophy	Allogeneic
Globoid-cell leukodystrophy	Allogeneic
Metachromatic leukodystrophy	Allogeneic
α-Mannosidosis	Allogeneic
Aspartylglycosaminuria	Allogeneic
Kostmann syndrome	Allogeneic
Reticular dysgenesis	Allogeneic
Chédiak-Higashi syndrome	Allogeneic
Chronic granulomatous disease	Allogeneic
Griscelli syndrome	Allogeneic
Multiple sclerosis	Autologous
Juvenile idiopathic arthritis	Autologous
Systemic lupus erythematosus	Autologous
Immune thrombocytopenic purpura	Autologous
Systemic sclerosis	Autologous

BMT, blood and/or marrow transplantation.

transplant recipient; separation may exacerbate marital stress for the parents.

■ The feasibility of home care must be assessed early on, including the safety of the home, likelihood of adherence to medical therapy, and availability of support necessary to carry out complex home care in the months after transplantation.

Within the past year or more, several transplant centers began to perform allogeneic reduced-intensity transplantation in children. This new type of transplant uses reduced doses of conditioning chemotherapy/radiation and compensates by using higher doses of immunosuppression to ensure engraftment. Reduced-intensity allogeneic transplantation in adult patients has led to a significant reduction in acute toxicity. Thus it is being offered to patients whose overall condition may not otherwise have allowed them to become eligible for a conventional myeloablative transplant.

Donor Sources for Blood and Marrow Transplantation

ALLOGENEIC BMT

Matched Family Donors

In the beginning, siblings identical for the human leukocyte antigen (HLA) type were the only source of normal hematopoietic progenitor cells for allogeneic BMT. Allogeneic BMT (from another individual) is the only effective source of hematopoietic progenitor cells for patients with inherited diseases or marrow failure. For patients with malignancies, the use of allogeneic hematopoietic progenitors ensures lack of contamination by tumor cells. For patients with leukemia or lymphoma, the use of allogeneic progenitor cells has the additional benefit of providing antileukemic activity, termed *graft-versus-leukemia* (GVL). Hematopoietic progenitor cells from HLA-identical siblings lack malignant cells and, additionally, they are closely matched with the recipient's cells. This results in a low rate of severe acute graft-versus-host disease (GVHD) as compared to family donors who are less well matched. Unfortunately, only 25% of potential recipients have an HLA-identical sibling donor. Therefore, efforts are being made to develop alternative sources of hematopoietic progenitor cells for transplantation.

Mismatched Family Donors

For patients who lack an HLA-identical sibling, a number of alternative sources exist for allogeneic progenitor cells. Partially matched family members (disparate for no more than one HLA antigen) can be used. Using marrow from family member donors who are disparate for two or more HLA antigens results in a higher incidence of severe GVHD or graft failure. The use of these mismatched family donors usually requires some form of immune cell depletion from the donor hematopoietic progenitor cells to prevent severe acute GVHD in the recipient. T cell depletion may result in a lower incidence of severe GVHD but a higher incidence of graft

failure, malignancy recurrence, and/or delayed immune reconstitution.

Unrelated Adult Donors

With computerized registries of potential volunteer adult donors, such as the National Marrow Donor Program, more than 6 million potential adult donors are currently available. Unrelated-donor transplantation is associated with a higher incidence of severe GVHD, even if donor and recipient are HLA identical. Identifying, screening, and consenting an unrelated adult donor require a minimum of 2 to 3 months. After identifying a donor using a computer search, the donor's HLA type must be confirmed by additional testing. Once the donor is confirmed as a suitable match, the volunteer donor must undergo a thorough medical evaluation. During the time required to identify unrelated donors, patients are at risk for developing complications such as infection or malignancy relapse that are relative contraindications to proceeding with BMT. Another limitation of the adult unrelated donor registries is that ethnic minorities are underrepresented.

Unrelated Umbilical Cord Blood

Placental umbilical cord blood is enriched with early hematopoietic progenitor cells, and, additionally, cell-mediated immunity is immature when compared with adult peripheral blood or bone marrow. Over the past 12 years, a number of cord blood banks were established worldwide and cryopreserved more than 110,000 U of umbilical cord blood. More than 2000 unrelated and related cord blood transplants have been performed as an alternative to allogeneic BMT in recipients who lack an HLA-matched family donor or who cannot wait a minimum of 2 to 3 months for an unrelated matched-adult donor to be found and evaluated. Results suggest that cell dose and HLA disparity are important predictors of rapidity of allogeneic engraftment, severity of GVHD, morbidity, and mortality. Unrelated cord blood transplantation is associated with decreased severity of both acute and chronic GVHD, but it is also associated with delayed hematopoietic engraftment. In addition, the cell dose of a particular donor unit may prove inadequate to a large recipient because the cell dose is based on recipient size. Finally, it is not possible to reacquire cord blood from the donor when there is graft failure or relapse.

AUTOLOGOUS BMT

Bone Marrow Hematopoietic Progenitor Cells

Autologous BMT (autologous means "from the self") is used in the treatment of malignancies and autoimmune diseases. It is far more established in those malignancies that do not arise from the bone marrow. Bone marrow is commonly harvested (collected) from the posterior iliac crests during anesthesia and subsequently cryopreserved in dimethylsulfoxide (DMSO) while the patient is in remission. At a later time, the patient receives myeloablative therapy and is infused with his or her bone marrow precursor cells. The main advantage of autologous BMT is that GVHD rarely occurs. The major disadvantage of autologous BMT, however, is the potential for contamination of the marrow by the original disease, and in the case of malignancies, the lack of a graft-versus-malignancy effect.

Peripheral Blood Hematopoietic Progenitor Cells

Autologous peripheral hematopoietic progenitor cell transplantation (HPCT) has essentially replaced autologous bone marrow transplantation. After high-dose chemotherapy, small numbers of hematopoietic progenitors can be detected circulating in the peripheral blood, especially in patients who receive hematopoietic growth factors such as granulocyte colony-stimulating factor (filgrastim) or granulocyte-macrophage colony-stimulating factor (sargramostim). As the hematopoietic progenitor cells circulate in the peripheral blood, peripheral blood hematopoietic progenitor cells are collected by apheresis over a 1- to 2-day period. In older patients, the progenitor cells can often be collected using peripheral venous access. Those without suitable venous access or younger patients may require the temporary placement of a dialysis catheter to perform the apheresis. After collection, the cells are cryopreserved in DMSO until the day of transplant. The numbers of early hematopoietic progenitor cells collected from the peripheral blood often exceed those that could be obtained from harvesting bone marrow. Peripheral blood HPCT results in more rapid restoration of neutrophil and platelet numbers, thus reducing the likelihood of bleeding or developing infectious complications. Peripheral blood hematopoietic progenitor cell collection is subject to the same concerns about contamination with tumor cells as autologous bone marrow transplantation. Tables 3 and 4 summarize the commonly used sources of hematopoietic progenitor cells and their advantages and disadvantages.

Procedure

Patients undergoing HPCT and myeloablative therapy are usually isolated in rooms in which the air is filtered to remove potentially dangerous infectious particles. Patients receive chemotherapy with or without radiation therapy before receiving hematopoietic progenitor cells (conditioning regimen). This therapy serves two purposes. For patients undergoing allogeneic HPCT for treatment of cancer, the high-dose chemotherapy kills residual malignant cells and must be sufficiently immunosuppressive to allow allogeneic engraftment. The conditioning regimen for autologous HPCT only needs to provide antimalignancy effects because rejection is quite unlikely. For patients undergoing allogeneic HPCT for nonmalignant diseases, the therapy only needs to be sufficiently immunosuppressive to allow engraftment of allogeneic donor hematopoietic progenitor cells. In patients undergoing autologous HPCT for nonmalignant diseases (autoimmune diseases), the

TABLE 3 Allogeneic Sources of Hematopoietic Progenitor Cells

Source/ Donor	Advantages	Disadvantages
HLA-identical relative	Low risk of GVHD. High rates of engraftment.	Available in <30% of recipients
HLA-mismatched relative	Many recipients have a readily available donor.	High risk of GVHD High risk of graft failure
Unrelated adult donor	Rapid engraftment. Relatively easier to find donor for whites.	High risk of GVHD 2–3 mo lag time
Unrelated cord blood donor	Readily available. Low risk of GVHD. More choices for minorities.	Delayed engraftment Cell dose a limiting factor

GVHD, graft-versus-host disease; HLA, human leukocyte antigen.

TABLE 4 Autologous Sources of Hematopoietic Progenitor Cells

Source/ Donor	Advantages	Disadvantages
Bone marrow	No GVHD	Potential tumor/disease contamination No graft vs. malignancy
Peripheral blood	Readily available Faster engraftment than bone marrow	Potential tumor/disease contamination No graft vs. malignancy

GVHD, graft-versus-host disease.

20

conditioning regimen only needs to provide the ability to adjust the imbalance of an autoaggressive immune system. Preparative therapies vary greatly among institutions and according to protocols (Tables 5 and 6). Many preparative therapies used for autologous HPCT consist of chemotherapy only. Total body irradiation (TBI) is commonly used in preparative therapies for leukemias and in recipients of T-cell–depleted hematopoietic progenitor cell transplants. Total lymphoid irradiation and thoracoabdominal irradiation are highly immunosuppressive and can used in combination with cyclophosphamide in allogeneic HCPT for patients with severe aplastic anemia or Fanconi anemia. The use of reduced intensity conditioning for allogeneic transplants, in which myeloablation is limited but compensated for by increased immunosuppression, is commonly used in adults now and reported as a viable option in pediatrics.

Infusion of hematopoietic progenitor cells is usually carried out at the bedside. Freshly obtained or thawed hematopoietic progenitors are infused intravenously in a central venous catheter. For thawed progenitor cell infusions, nausea and vomiting secondary to the cryopreservative agent DMSO are common side effects. Less common side effects include hypotension or

TABLE 5 Common Conditioning Regimens for Hematopoietic Progenitor Cell Transplantation

Type of Transplant	Regimen
Myeloablative, allogeneic	Total body irradiation/cyclophosphamide
Myeloablative, allogeneic	Busulfan/cyclophosphamide
Autologous	Thiotepa/etoposide ± carboplatin
Autologous	Melphalan ± total body irradiation
Autologous	Cyclophosphamide/carmustine/etoposide
Autologous	Carmustine/etoposide/cytarabine/melphalan
Autologous	Carmustine/cytarabine/cyclophosphamide
Reduced intensity, allogeneic	Fludarabine/busulfan
Reduced intensity, allogeneic	Fludarabine/total body irradiation

TABLE 6 Common Doses Used in Pretransplant Conditioning Regimens

Treatment	Dose
Total body irradiation	Myeloablative: 10–16 Gy
Total body irradiation	Reduced intensity: 2 Gy
Cyclophosphamide	120–200 mg/kg
Busulfan	Myeloablative: 10 to 16 mg/kg
Busulfan	Reduced intensity: 8 mg/kg
Thiotepa	500 mg/m^2
Etoposide	60 mg/kg
Carboplatin	1400 mg/m^2
Melphalan	110–140 mg/m^2
Carmustine	300–600 mg/m^2
Cytarabine	800–1600 mg/m^2
Fludarabine	180 mg/m^2

hypertension, allergic reactions, and hematuria. After the infusion of the hematopoietic progenitors, patients may receive additional anti-infection prophylaxis, blood product support, hematopoietic growth factors, and narcotics for painful mucositis. Patients who receive allogeneic progenitor cells receive GVHD prophylaxis.

Complications

The major complications of HPCT are those caused by the toxicities of the preparative therapy and, in the case of allogeneic transplants, those because of GVHD.

Pancytopenia

Pancytopenia is expectable and routine after a myeloablative conditioning regimen during the first few weeks after transplantation until marrow function is reconstituted. During this time patients are dependent on erythrocyte and platelet transfusions and at risk for developing life-threatening infections. Prophylactic

platelet transfusions are given to prevent severe bleeding. Blood products contain viable donor lymphocytes, and therefore they must be irradiated to prevent transfusion-associated GVHD. The duration of pancytopenia may be reduced in patients who receive higher hematopoietic progenitor cell doses (e.g., recipients of peripheral blood hematopoietic progenitor cells). The use of cytokines such as filgrastim or sargramostim during the early post-transplant period is effective in reducing the duration of neutropenia after transplantation.

Gastrointestinal Toxicity

Nausea and vomiting are common, especially while receiving chemotherapy and/or radiation. Chemotherapy-induced enteritis may last several weeks after transplantation. Common symptoms include abdominal pain, diarrhea, nausea, vomiting, and anorexia. Most patients require parenteral nutrition during this period and may continue to receive parenteral nutrition at home. Chemotherapy-induced mucositis commonly manifests as oral ulcerations and/or gingivitis. Patients often require narcotic therapy as treatment for pain from mucositis.

Infectious Complications

Neutropenia, together with the disruption of mucosal barriers, the presence of indwelling central venous catheters, and prolonged immunosuppression, predisposes the transplant recipient to infection, usually by endogenous flora. Bacterial infections are common during the period of neutropenia. Invasive fungal infections, usually *Candida* or *Aspergillus* species, are common after prolonged pancytopenia, immunosuppression, and use of antibiotics. Viral infections can occur throughout the course of transplantation. Reactivation of latent herpes simplex virus commonly presents as severe mucositis and can be prevented by treatment with acyclovir. Reactivation of cytomegalovirus (CMV) can produce disease of variable severity, ranging from mild, self-limited manifestations to potentially fatal ones like interstitial pneumonia. CMV can be acquired from leukocytes contaminating blood products. This can be prevented by using blood from CMV seronegative donors or by using filtration to remove leukocytes before infusion. The use of ganciclovir and/or foscarnet is effective for prophylaxis and treatment of CMV disease after HPCT. The incidence of *Pneumocystis carinii* pneumonia is reduced through the use of cotrimoxazole prophylaxis. Pentamidine is also effective for patients who cannot tolerate cotrimoxazole (Table 7).

Sinusoidal Obstruction Syndrome

Sinusoidal obstruction syndrome (SOS) is caused by obliterative fibrosis within the hepatic sinusoid that results in hepatomegaly, fluid retention, weight gain, and hyperbilirubinemia. SOS is believed to be a toxic reaction to the chemoradiotherapy used in pretransplant conditioning regimens. Patients who receive

TABLE 7 Infectious Prophylaxis in Hematopoietic Progenitor Cell Transplantation

Organism	Agent
Herpes simplex	Acyclovir
Fungal infection	Fluconazole, amphotericin B, or derivatives
CMV	Ganciclovir, foscarnet
PCP	Cotrimoxazole, pentamidine

CMV, cytomegalovirus; PCP, *Pneumocystis carinii* pneumonia.

myeloablative doses of cyclophosphamide or busulfan are at particularly high risk of developing SOS. Gemtuzumab, an antibody to CD33, is another drug with a high risk for SOS. SOS can vary from a mild self-limited disease to a severe disease in which reversal of portal blood flow can be seen using ultrasonography. The diagnosis of SOS is often based on clinical parameters, including hyperbilirubinemia, painful hepatomegaly, and fluid retention. Treatment consists of salt and fluid restriction with aggressive use of diuretics and repeated paracenteses for ascites that is associated with discomfort or pulmonary compromise. Infusions of thrombolytic agents such as alteplase or heparin reverse severe cases of SOS in a small proportion of cases. In uncontrolled trials, defibrotide, a drug with thrombolytic, antithrombotic, and anti-ischemic properties, reversed SOS in up to 60% of moderate to severe cases.

Hemorrhagic Cystitis

Hemorrhagic cystitis is a common complication of high-dose cyclophosphamide-containing regimens. Acrolein, a metabolite of cyclophosphamide, irritates the bladder mucosa, causing hemorrhagic cystitis. Prevention of cyclophosphamide-induced hemorrhagic cystitis is accomplished through aggressive hydration while receiving chemotherapy together with the use of 2-mercaptoethane sulfonate (Mesna). Hemorrhagic cystitis can also be caused by adenovirus, CMV, BK virus, or other polyoma viruses.

Graft-versus-Host Disease

GVHD is caused by T lymphocytes from the donor that recognizes the recipient tissue as foreign. Although GVHD is most commonly seen after allogeneic HPCT, GVHD can also occur after autologous HPCT or after infusion of unirradiated blood products into susceptible hosts such as patients with severe T cell immunodeficiencies and recipients of intensive chemotherapy. GVHD occurs in approximately 50% of recipients of hematopoietic progenitor cells from HLA-identical siblings. The incidence of severity of GVHD is significantly higher after partially matched related donor or unrelated donor transplants.

There are two forms of GVHD: acute and chronic. Acute GVHD starts about the time of engraftment or around 2 weeks after transplantation. Patients commonly present with a skin rash, but diarrhea and/or hyperbilirubinemia are common manifestations. The diagnosis of acute GVHD is made using clinical criteria: the extent of skin disease, volume of diarrhea, and degree of hyperbilirubinemia. Biopsies of the skin, rectum, and liver can sometimes be helpful in confirming the diagnosis of acute GVHD and distinguishing GVHD from viral infections or drug reactions. Prednisone is the preferred treatment for severe acute GVHD. Survival after mild to moderate GVHD is excellent. Patients with severe GVHD often do not respond to prednisone therapy and require additional immunosuppression. Death from progressive organ dysfunction or opportunistic infection is more common in patients with severe GVHD.

Chronic GVHD is classified as either limited or extensive and usually begins approximately 100 days after the transplant. Chronic GVHD usually occurs in patients who had acute GVHD, but it can develop de novo. Limited chronic GVHD is defined as a rash together with elevation of hepatic transaminase levels. Extensive chronic GVHD is more common. Cutaneous manifestations are seen in at least 80% of patients. Cholestasis and oral manifestations (dryness) are seen in approximately 80% of patients.

Less common manifestations of chronic GVHD include sicca syndrome, infection, weight loss, joint contractures, obstructive lung disease, polyserositis, and myositis. Autoimmune thrombocytopenia is common. Prednisone and cyclosporine A is the preferred therapeutic combination for extensive chronic GVHD. Patients with chronic GVHD have a higher incidence of pneumococcal sepsis and require penicillin prophylaxis as well as *P. carinii* prophylaxis.

Because GVHD is associated with significant morbidity and mortality, efforts focus on its prevention (Box 1). Immunosuppressive therapy with drugs such as methotrexate and cyclosporine A (or both), immediately after hematopoietic progenitor cell transplantation, is the most common method used to prevent GVHD. Combinations using newer agents, such as tacrolimus and mycophenolate mofetil, are effective in GVHD prophylaxis. Another approach to GVHD prophylaxis is removal of T lymphocytes from the donor marrow immediately before infusion. T-cell depletion is usually performed when a high incidence of severe GVHD is likely, such as in partially matched donors. For patients undergoing unrelated donor HPCT, the use of T-cell depletion is being studied in a prospective randomized trial to determine its usefulness. The majority of recipients of progenitor cells from HLA-identical siblings do not require T-cell depletion because the incidence of severe GVHD is low compared to other donor sources, and there are concerns about increasing the likelihood of graft rejection and leukemic relapse.

Long-Term Complications

Long-term complications of HPCT include decreased linear growth and chronic sinusitis (often secondary to radiation therapy). Cataracts and hypothyroidism

BOX 1 Common Graft-versus-Host Disease Prophylactic Agents and Combination Regimens

Individual Agents with Proven Efficacy

- Methotrexate
- Cyclosporine
- Tacrolimus
- Prednisone
- Mycophenolate mofetil
- Ursodeoxycholic acid
- Sirolimus
- Fludarabine
- Trimetrexate
- Antithymocyte globulin during pretransplant conditioning
- Alemtuzumab during pretransplant conditioning
- Intravenous immunoglobulin

Effective Combinations

- Methotrexate + cyclosporine
- Methotrexate + tacrolimus
- Tacrolimus + mycophenolate mofetil
- Cyclosporine + prednisone
- Methotrexate + cyclosporine + prednisone
- Methotrexate + antithymocyte globulin (pretransplant) + prednisone

Procedures

- T-cell depletion of donor progenitor cells
- Ultraviolet irradiation

are common in patients who receive total body irradiation. Patients who have undergone hematopoietic progenitor cell transplants are more likely to develop secondary malignancies. The secondary malignancies can be solid tumors in previous areas of radiation therapy, hematologic malignancies, or skin cancer. Infertility and gonadal failure requiring hormone replacement therapy are also common long-term complications.

Common Pitfalls

- Inadequate hematopoietic progenitor cell dose following progenitor cell harvesting, resulting in nonengraftment
- Low number of viable progenitors upon thawing of umbilical cord blood unit, resulting in nonengraftment
- Inability to find an adequately matched donor, delaying or preventing transplantation
- Failure to recognize donor/recipient ABO incompatibility prior to transplantation, resulting in severe hemolytic anemia
- Inadequate donor screening for infectious and/or genetic diseases, leading to disease transmission to the host
- Inadequate progenitor cell selection/purging during autologous harvesting, leading to tumor contamination of the autologous graft
- Failure to maintain adequate levels of post-transplant immunosuppression, leading to severe GVHD
- Failure to maintain adequate post-transplant infectious disease prophylaxis, leading to opportunistic infections

Communication and Counseling

Successful hematopoietic progenitor cell transplantation requires a cooperative and educated family/caregiver and/or patient. The transplantation process is long and does not end upon the patient's discharge after transplantation. The patient/family must have a solid understanding of the process prior to starting. Immune system deficiencies persist for prolonged periods after transplantation, way beyond the return of a white blood cell count to the normal range. The risk of late infectious complications may persist even beyond the return of normal immune function on in vitro testing. Even harmless-appearing symptoms must be discussed with members of the transplant service in a timely fashion.

HPCT is a highly challenging experience for the patient and/or family/caregiver. The members of the transplant service must be aware of the patient's emotional needs and quality of life. A multidisciplinary team, consisting of social workers, psychologists, psychiatrists, transplant nurse educators, nurses, nurse practitioners, and transplant physicians, must be accessible to all patients.

SUGGESTED READINGS

1. Atkinson K: Reconstruction of the hemopoietic and immune systems after marrow transplantation. Bone Marrow Transplant 5:209–226, 1990. **Excellent discussion of immune reconstitution after transplantation.**
2. Baker KS, Gordon BG, Gross TG, et al: Autologous hematopoietic stem-cell transplantation for relapsed or refractory Hodgkin's disease in children and adolescents. J Clin Oncol 17:825–831, 1999. **This study shows the benefits of autologous HPCT in pediatric Hodgkin disease.**
3. Blanche SM, Caniglia M, Girault D, et al: Treatment of hemophagocytic lymphohistiocytosis with chemotherapy and bone marrow transplantation: A single-center study of 22 cases. Blood 78:51–54, 1991. **This report shows benefits for allogeneic HPCT in hemophagocytic lymphohistiocytosis.**
4. Boulad F, Steinhertz P, Reyes B, et al: Allogeneic bone marrow transplantation versus chemotherapy for the treatment of childhood acute lymphoblastic leukemia [ALL] in second remission: A single-institution study. J Clin Oncol 17:197–207, 1999. **This retrospective single-institution study favors the use of allogeneic HPCT for ALL.**
5. Buckley RH, Schiff SE, Schiff RI, et al: Hematopoietic stem-cell transplantation for the treatment of severe combined immunodeficiency [SCID]. N Engl J Med 340:508–517, 1999. **This prospective single-institution study confirms the long-term efficacy of HPCT in SCID.**
6. Cairo MS, Wagner J: Placental and/or umbilical cord blood: An alternative source of hematopoietic stem cells for transplantation. Blood 90:4665–4678, 1997. **One of the first reports of the effective use of umbilical cord blood as a source for HPCT.**
7. Del Toro G, Satwani P, Harrison L, et al: A pilot study of reduced intensity conditioning and allogeneic stem cell transplantation from unrelated cord blood and matched family donors in children and adolescent recipients. Bone Marrow Transplant 33:613–622, 2004. **One of the first reports of reduced-intensity allogeneic HPCT in pediatrics.**

8. Driessen GJ, Gerritsen EJ, Fischer A, et al: Long-term outcome of hematopoietic stem cell transplantation in autosomal recessive osteopetrosis: An EBMT report. Bone Marrow Transplant 32:657–663, 2003. **Large retrospective analysis of the HPCT experience for osteopetrosis.**

9. Dunkel IJ, Finlay JL: High-dose chemotherapy with autologous stem cell rescue for brain tumors. Crit Rev Oncol Hematol 41:197–204, 2002. **Comprehensive review of the use of autologous HPCT for pediatric brain tumors.**

10. Gluckman E, Auerbach AD, Horowitz MM, et al: Bone marrow transplantation for Fanconi anemia. Blood 86:2856–2862, 1995. **Large retrospective study of HPCT in patients with Fanconi anemia.**

11. Ho VT, Soiffer RJ: The history and future of T-cell depletion as graft-versus-host disease prophylaxis for allogeneic hematopoietic stem cell transplantation. Blood 98:3192–3204, 2001. **Provides a comprehensive review of the use of T cell depletion for GVHD prophylaxis.**

12. Kernan NA, Bartsch G, Ash RC, et al: Analysis of 462 transplantations from unrelated donors facilitated by the National Marrow Donor Program. N Engl J Med 328:593–602, 1993. **Landmark article that emphasizes the benefits of matched-unrelated adult-donor HPCT.**

13. Lucarelli G, Galimberti M, Polchi P, et al: Bone marrow transplantation in patients with thalassemia. N Engl J Med 322:417–421, 1990. **Landmark article that presents the use of allogeneic HPCT for thalassemia.**

14. Matthay KK, Villablanca JG, Seeger RC, et al: Treatment of high-risk neuroblastoma with intensive chemotherapy, radiotherapy, autologous bone marrow transplantation, and 13-cis-retinoic acid. Children's Cancer Group. N Engl J Med 341:1165–1173, 1999. **Landmark article that presents the benefits of autologous HPCT in neuroblastoma.**

15. Osunkwo I, Bessmertny O, Harrison L, et al: A pilot study of tacrolimus and mycophenolate mofetil graft-versus-host disease prophylaxis in childhood and adolescent allogeneic stem cell transplant recipients. Biol Blood Marrow Transplant 10:246–258, 2004. **Describes a single center's experience with the combination of tacrolimus and mycophenolate mofetil for GVHD prophylaxis.**

16. Peters C, Steward C: National Marrow Donor Program; International Bone Marrow Transplant Registry; Working Party on Inborn Errors, European Bone Marrow Transplant Group: Hematopoietic cell transplantation for inherited metabolic diseases: An overview of outcomes and practice guidelines. Bone Marrow Transplant 31:229–239, 2003. **Excellent review and update on the use of allogeneic HPCT for various inborn errors of metabolism.**

17. Petersdorf EW, Hansen JA, Martin PJ, et al: Major-histocompatibility-complex class I alleles and antigens in hematopoietic-cell transplantation. N Engl J Med 345:1794–1800, 2001. **Discusses important issues in class I HLA matching for transplantation.**

18. Philip T, Guglielmi C, Hagenbeek A, et al: Autologous bone marrow transplantation as compared with salvage chemotherapy in relapses of chemotherapy-sensitive non-Hodgkin's lymphoma. N Engl J Med 333:1540–1545, 1995. **Prospective randomized study showing benefits for autologous HPCT for non-Hodgkin lymphoma.**

19. Socie G, Stone JV, Wingard JR, et al: Long-term survival and late deaths after allogeneic bone marrow transplantation. Late effects working committee of the International Bone Marrow Transplant Registry. N Engl J Med 341:14–21, 1999. **Excellent report on the long-term survival rates after myeloablative allogeneic HPCT.**

20. Stucki A, Leisenring W, Sandmaier BM, et al: Decreased rejection and improved survival of first and second marrow transplants for severe aplastic anemia (a 26-year retrospective analysis). Blood 92:2742–2749, 1998. **Large single-institution study that provides information on some of the common complications of transplantation for aplastic anemia.**

21. Truitt RL, Johnson BD: Principles of graft-vs.-leukemia reactivity. Biol Blood Marrow Transplant 1:61–68, 1995. **Explains the concept of graft-versus-malignancy in allogeneic HPCT.**

22. Tyndall A, Koike T: High-dose immunoablative therapy with hematopoietic stem cell support in the treatment of severe autoimmune disease: Current status and future direction. Intern Med 41:608–612, 2002. **Comprehensive review of the use of autologous HPCT for refractory autoimmune diseases.**

23. Vogelsang GB, Lee L, Bensen-Kennedy DM: Pathogenesis and treatment of graft-versus-host disease after bone marrow transplant. Ann Rev Med 54:29–52, 2003. **Comprehensive review of GVHD.**

24. Walters MC, Patience M, Leisenring W, et al: Bone marrow transplantation for sickle cell disease. N Engl J Med 335:369–376, 1996. **Landmark article describing the American experience with allogeneic HPCT in sickle cell disease.**

25. Woods WG, Neudorf S, Gold S, et al: A comparison of allogeneic bone marrow transplantation, autologous bone marrow transplantation, and aggressive chemotherapy in children with acute myeloid leukemia [AML] in remission. Blood 97:56–62, 2001. **Landmark article that shows the benefit of allogeneic HPCT in pediatric AML.**

Solid Organ Transplantation*

Julie R. Ingelfinger

KEY CONCEPTS

- Transplantation of solid organs is no longer rare, and children with end-stage disease are routinely considered candidates.
- Data indicate that children, particularly young children, have excellent renal and hepatic allograft survival and are essentially restored to normal life. Data are improving for other solid organ transplants.
- Pretransplant preparation optimally should involve coordination between the primary care physician (PCP) and the specialty team. The PCP can be a major support to the child and family undergoing transplantation.
- Children receiving a solid organ transplant need full medical assessment. They should be caught up on immunizations pretransplant and preimmunosuppression whenever possible. Other health issues should be identified and a pretransplant plan made to deal with these.
- Children with transplants need preemptive and rapid care if they get ill, and PCPs should be aware of particular needs.

Children are now routinely recipients of solid organ transplants. Kidney transplantation in children began in the late 1950s, and pediatric liver transplantation was first performed in 1967. Many renal and liver transplant recipients have now reached adult life and have children of their own. Children currently also receive heart, lung, heart-lung, kidney-pancreas, and intestinal transplants. Virtually all young recipients are managed by a multidisciplinary transplant team

---

*Sections of this chapter were adapted from chapters in the last edition of this book: "Heart Transplantation" by Linda Addonizio and F. Jay Fricker; "Liver Transplantation" by Ajoke Sobanjo, Debora Kogan-Liberman, and Margaret Burroughs; and "Renal Transplantation" by Demetrius Ellis.

both initially and for follow-up care. However, the primary care physician (PCP) needs to know some common elements about transplantation. This chapter provides a brief overview with suggested resources for further reading.

Expert Opinion on Management Issues

PRETRANSPLANT EVALUATION OF THE CHILD WITH ENDSTAGE ORGAN DISEASE

The child receiving a solid organ transplant should undergo a major review of health issues that goes far beyond the failing organ. Other conditions should be carefully sought and worked up. Whether the child is fully immunized must be considered early enough to complete necessary immunizations before the child is immunosuppressed. Further, some assessment of growth and development and secondary metabolic effects caused by the failure of a major organ system should take place. The pediatric transplant candidate needs to undergo an assessment of previous viral infections as well as current susceptibilities because the results will inform therapy.

Planning for the transplant should include whether it is possible to schedule the transplant in a semielective fashion, as with preemptive transplant for a child with failing kidneys for whom the likely timing for dialysis is possible to calculate. Sometimes, however, solid organ transplantation must be performed on an urgent basis (e.g., with fulminant hepatic failure).

DECISION ABOUT DONOR TYPE

Certain transplants, such as heart transplants, can only occur with deceased donor organs. Transplants of other organs may come from either deceased donors or living donors. Today the living donor no longer needs to be a relative because immunosuppressive therapy has made it possible to transplant organs successfully from living unrelated donors. Thus family, extended family, friends, or anonymous living donors are possible.

TRANSPLANTATION OF SPECIFIC ORGANS

Kidney Transplantation

See the chapter "Managing End-Stage Renal Disease," which discusses renal transplantation in some detail. Much information and the latest report (2005) from the North American Pediatric Renal Transplant Cooperative Study (NAPRTCS) may be found at the NAPRTCS website (http://spitfire.emmes.com/study/ped/announce.htm). Another useful website for kidney and other organs is the United Network for Organ Sharing (UNOS) site (http://www.unos.org/).

Liver Transplantation

Various diseases necessitate liver transplantation in a child, but the decision to transplant generally arises from one of four indications:

1. Progressive primary liver disease leading to end-stage liver failure
2. Stable liver disease that is, nonetheless, associated with significant morbidity or mortality
3. Metabolic defects that affect the liver and would be improved or reversed by transplantation
4. Fulminant hepatic failure

Urgent liver transplantation may be needed for children with end-stage liver disease accompanied by hepatorenal or hepatopulmonary syndrome, encephalopathy, recurrent infection, variceal hemorrhage, or intractable ascites. The diseases that lead to transplantation can be classified as metabolic diseases, acute and chronic hepatitis, intrahepatic cholestasis, obstructive biliary diseases, and miscellaneous illnesses such as congenital hepatic fibrosis and cystic fibrosis. Extrahepatic biliary atresia accounts for approximately 50% of children needing a liver transplant. More information can be found at the website of the Liver Foundation (http://www.liverfoundation.org).

Heart Transplantation

More than 2600 children received heart transplants in the past decade, and the 10-year survival rate of 65% is improving. A heart transplant is indicated in children with advanced (end-stage) heart disease unresponsive to maximal medical therapy and with no surgical procedure that could restore them to a productive, active life. Cardiomyopathy and complex congenital heart disease (CHD) are the two most common reasons for heart transplantation. Infants have received heart transplants successfully, with congenital heart disease the most common indication. This diagnosis drops to 40% among those between 1 to 10 years of age, a group in which 50% have myopathies as the diagnosis. In adolescence, cardiomyopathy is the indication for transplantation in 65%. The International Society for Heart and Lung Transplantation (ISHLT) (http://www.ishlt.org) publishes much information about heart and lung transplantation.

Other possible treatment options should be weighed in children referred for heart transplantation. If none are possible, the optimal timing and management of the child awaiting transplantation should be the focus.

Lung Transplantation

Lung transplantation in children has been a reality since the early 1990s. The indications for lung transplant in a child are similar to those in adults. The most common cause leading to lung transplant in older children and adolescents is end-stage lung disease caused by cystic fibrosis (CF). Developmental abnormalities and certain congenital heart diseases are rather commonly associated with severe pulmonary vascular, rather than idiopathic pulmonary, hypertension. Thus isolated lung transplant in such children is rare. Combined heart-lung transplantation is now also performed.

Intestine Transplantation

It is more difficult to transplant the intestine compared to other solid organs. In a report from 61 programs using data on 989 grafts in 923 patients, 61% of the recipients were 18 years of age or younger. Relatively more combined intestinal and liver transplants were carried out in this group. More than 80% of reported survivors were able to stop parenteral nutrition and resume normal daily activities. One-year graft survival rates of 81% were achieved in patients who were induced with antithymocyte globulin and maintained on tacrolimus. Thus intestinal transplantation appears to be an effective therapy for the treatment of patients with end-stage intestine failure who cannot tolerate or are not doing well on parenteral nutrition. This type of transplant is clearly in its early days, and a great deal remains to be learned. The Intestinal Transplant Registry can be accessed online at http://www.intestinal-transplant.org.

Pancreas Transplant and Kidney-Pancreas Transplant

Both pancreas transplants and kidney in combination with pancreas transplants are performed, as well as islet cell transplants. Few children are recipients, although some adolescents with long-standing diabetes have received transplants. More information may be found at the International Pancreas Transplant Registry: http://www.med.umn.edu/IPTR/home.html.

TRANSPLANTS AND REJECTION

The signs and symptoms of rejection vary somewhat, depending on the organ, but there are some similarities. Rejection episodes are common. Hyperacute rejection fortunately now occurs very rarely because multiple tests are done prior to transplantation to minimize the occurrence of this serious complication, which usually leads to allograft loss. Episodes of acute rejection are usually reversible, and the protocol depends to some extent on the organ. Chronic rejection is more insidious but too often progressive.

The mechanisms of rejection remain incompletely elucidated. As these mechanisms are better understood, highly specific immunosuppressive drugs ideally will be developed to allow for tolerance of the transplanted organ while decreasing the risk of infections, other drug side effects, and post-transplant lymphoproliferative disorder (PTLD).

Present immunosuppressive regimens are intended to lower antigen-induced CD4+ T-cell and cytokine production and to diminish allo-major histocompatibility complex recognition.

Immunosuppression

Except for the case in identical twins or tolerance protocols, which currently are all experimental, children and adolescents with transplants require immunosuppressive medication. The agents used vary somewhat depending on the organ, the center doing the transplant, and the specific needs of the child. Generally, there are several phases. First is an induction phase, often using high-dose steroids and either a monoclonal antibody or antilymphocyte globulin plus immunosuppressive medications. Then there is an early post-transplant phase, followed by a maintenance phase. Table 1 lists current immunosuppressive agents, but the immunosuppressive regimen is generally determined and adjusted by the transplant group involved with the patient. There are some center-to-center variations.

Post-transplant Concerns

In addition to rejection and preventing it, a variety of issues affect organ transplant recipients. These include adverse effects from the necessary immunosuppressive agents, recurrence of original diseases in certain cases, infections, hypertension, hyperlipidemia, and other metabolic problems. Some of these issues are discussed here.

Drug Side Effects

Most long-term difficulties following transplantation involve immunosuppressive medications or problems related to them. Allograft loss may occur because of too little immunosuppression, but there is a high incidence of post-transplant malignancy, hypertension, renal failure, or diabetes related to immunosuppression. Age-related differences affect both biologic and psychological aspects of post-transplant function. These may be anticipated and should feature importantly in optimizing post-transplant treatment.

The handling of medications varies with age, and substantial age-related differences are evident in pharmacokinetics of the drugs used—in absorption, distribution, metabolism, and elimination. Despite this, there is not a great deal of evidence on this point for many immunosuppressive medications. The various immunosuppressive agents used carry with them a number of side effects, some of which are listed in Table 1. Generally, the transplant team goes over these side effects and adverse effects at length, but the list of the most common problems is provided as a reference.

Infections

Because of the post-transplant immunosuppressed state, recipients are susceptible to certain infections. Many centers now place children on prophylactic Bactrim for a period of time (typically 6 months) post-transplant to avoid *Pneumocystis carinii,* and the frequency of that infection is, accordingly, less common than in prior eras. Many programs use antiviral therapy in an effort to prevent primary or secondary recrudescence of cytomegalovirus. Other viral complications include herpes simplex virus syndromes, adenovirus hepatitis, varicella, and enterovirus-induced gastroenteritis.

TABLE 1 Immunosuppressive Agents Commonly Used in Pediatric Renal Transplantation

Agent*	Action	Side Effects	Comments
Glucocorticoids	Inhibit T- and B-cell lymphocyte growth and differentiation. Nonspecific anti-inflammatory action. Inhibit monocyte migration into sites of inflammation. Inhibit cytotoxic cells. Inhibit IL-1 and IL-6 transcription in macrophages and mononuclear cells. Block IL-1-dependent release of IL-2.	Hypertension, glucose intolerance. Lymphopenia and increased risk of infection. Impair linear growth. May cause cataracts, osteopenia, osteonecrosis of the femoral head, poor wound healing, hypertrichosis, peptic ulcers, psychosis, acne, cushingoid appearance.	Withdrawal or alternate-day use of cyclosporine-based or other regimens allows for better linear growth, less hypertension, and fewer other side effects. Whether this leads to more acute rejection is being studied.
Azathioprine	Inhibits proliferation of actively replicating cells in nonspecific fashion. Purine analogue that impairs DNA and RNA synthesis in actively dividing cells. Competitively inhibits conversion of inosinic acid to adenylic and guanylic acids.	Generalized myelosuppression, liver dysfunction, pancreatitis, nausea, vomiting, alopecia.	Of questionable value in increasing graft tolerance when combined with tacrolimus. Dosage should be adjusted if leukopenia or thrombocytopenia occurs.
Mycophenolate mofetil (CellCept)	Antimetabolite inhibits purine/DNA synthesis.	Bone marrow suppression, GI intolerance.	
Cyclosporine (Neoral)	Calcineurin inhibitor. Prevents helper T-cell activation in response to antigen-presenting cells. Prevents T-cell proliferation. Binds to specific cytoplasmic cyclophilin, which then binds and neutralizes the action of the calcium-calmodulin-calcineurin complex and prevents signal transduction events leading to transcription of IL-2 in T cells.	Nephrotoxicity (reversible and irreversible forms). Neurotoxicity including insomnia, headache, tremors, dysesthesias. Hypertension in as many as 80% of patients. Hepatotoxicity, cholelithiasis. Susceptibility to viral, bacterial, protozoan, and fungal infections. Increased risk of EBV-related lymphoma and other malignancies. Gingival hyperplasia and hirsutism are common.	Wide intrapatient and interpatient variability in absorption and bioavailability mandates close whole blood level monitoring. This may improve with use of a microemulsion preparation (Neoral). Low therapeutic index. Bile acids are needed for absorption. Faster elimination in children than in adults. Possible multiple drug interactions.
Tacrolimus (FK506) (Prograf)	Calcineurin inhibitor. Similar to cyclosporine. Mechanism of action similar to cyclosporine's but binds to a specific cytoplasmic binding protein (FKBP–12) and is approximately 100 times more potent than cyclosporine.	Bile acids and diarrhea have little effect on absorption. Better bioavailability than cyclosporine but large intrapatient variability in dosing. Important drug interactions similar to cyclosporine.	More steroid sparing than cyclosporine, which allows withdrawal of steroids and optimized growth. Reverses many steroid- and OKT3-resistant rejections in cyclosporine recipients. Similarly nephrotoxic and neurotoxic but less hypertension and no gingival hyperplasia or hirsutism when compared with cyclosporine. EBV-related disorders and reversible insulin-dependent diabetes mellitus may be seen more frequently with tacrolimus use.
Thymoglobulin and antilymphocyte globulin (ATG, ALG)	Depletes T cells.	Allergic reactions, serum sickness, leukopenia, thrombocytopenia. Increases rate of CMV and EBV infections.	Polyclonal antibody against multiple antigens on lymphocyte surface. Similar to OKT3 (see later) except for absence of systemic "cytokine release syndrome."
Anti-CD25 antibodies (daclizumab, basiliximab)	Blocks T cell proliferation induced by IL–2.		Monoclonal antibodies specific against α-chain of IL–2R expressed only on activated T cells. Used for induction to protect against CsA or tacrolimus nephrotoxicity while reducing the incidence of acute rejection. No cytokine release syndrome and little neutralizing antibody response.

TABLE 1—cont'd

Agent*	Action	Side Effects	Comments
OKT3 (monoclonal antibody)	Binds to CD3 receptor and inactivates T-cell function by shedding or internalizing CD3 T-cell receptor.	Anaphylaxis, pulmonary capillary leak, meningoencephalitis, PTLD.	
Sirolimus (rapamycin)	Target of rapamycin inhibitor. Inhibition of T-cell activation and proliferation by preventing translation of mRNA.	Nephrotoxicity, hyperlipidemia, thrombocytopenia, leukopenia, GI intolerance.	

*Other agents and protocols are under development. These include everolimus, which is a derivative of sirolimus; FK 778 and malonitrile (derivative of tacrolimus); molecules to inhibit cytokine signaling, such as CP-690, 550 and tyrphostin AG 490, and steroid-withdrawal protocols.
CMV, cytomegalovirus; CsA, cyclosporine A; EBV, Epstein-Barr virus; GI, gastrointestinal; IL, interleukin; mRNA, messenger RNA; PTLD, post-transplant lymphoproliferative disease.

Post-transplant Lymphoproliferative Disease

PTLD may first manifest with benign complaints such as upper respiratory tract infection symptoms, sinusitis, or gastrointestinal symptoms such as diarrhea. Thus in the child with a transplant who has lymphadenopathy, unexplained fever, graft dysfunction, or a mass lesion, PTLD should be suspected and an evaluation should be done promptly. PTLD in children is related to the Epstein-Barr virus (EBV). Most children who receive transplants are EBV seronegative, but most adults, who are the donors, are EBV seropositive. Thus pediatric recipients should be monitored for potential change in their EBV status. EBV titers should be followed. It may be helpful to carry out serial monitoring of EBV DNA using polymerase chain reaction (PCR); a value exceeding 200 EBV genomes per 105 peripheral blood lymphocytes is considered positive for the presence of EBV. Biopsy confirmation of changes in lymph nodes, abnormal lesions found on endoscopy, or tumors noted on computed tomography suggest PTLD. EBV-related PTLD is often managed by decreasing or stopping immunosuppression and administering IgG, ganciclovir intravenously, followed by oral ganciclovir for 2 months so the EBV levels as measured by PCR decrease to below those associated with PTLD. Immunosuppression is then reintroduced, with the dosage kept considerably lower than that before EBV infection. This sort of strategy is associated with resolution of the lymphoma and maintenance of the graft. However, recipients who fail to respond to decreased immunosuppression may respond to chemotherapy, surgical resection, or monoclonal antibody treatment directed against CD20 receptors present on EBV-transformed lymphocytes.

THE FUTURE

The ideal outcome for solid transplantation is tolerance, so recipients would not require immunosuppressive agents, with their side effects and attendant allograft damage.

Common Pitfalls

- Not communicating that transplantation is now widely available and generally highly successful.

Patients and families needing such care should be referred to appropriate teams that can consider together with the family, the patient, and the PCP what the options are in a given situation.
- Failing to assess the post-transplant patient who is on immunosuppressive medications and feeling ill more quickly than a child who has not had a transplant.
- Failing to consider drug-drug interactions in a child receiving immunosuppressive medications, the levels of which may be altered by other medications.

Communication and Counseling

More than most situations in pediatrics, the amount of time and effort needed for the coordination, education, and evaluation of the child needing a solid organ transplant or being followed after such a procedure is huge. The PCP and staff can be enormously important in ensuring follow-through and restoration of health.

SELECTED REFERENCES

1. Alonso EM: Long-term renal function in pediatric liver and heart recipients. Pediatr Transplant 8(4):381–385, 2004. **Looking at renal function in nonrenal transplant patients.**
2. Fine RN, Alonso EM, Fischel JE, et al: Pediatric transplantation of the kidney, liver and heart: Summary report. Pediatr Transplant 8(1):75–86, 2004. **Review of pediatric transplantation.**
3. Fouquet V, Alves A, Branchereau S, et al: Long-term outcome of pediatric liver transplantation for biliary atresia: A 10-year follow-up in a single center. Liver Transplant 11(2):152–160, 2005. **Data on pediatric liver transplantation for biliary atresia.**
4. Grant D, Abu-Elmagd K, Reyes J, et al: on behalf of the Intestine Transplant Registry: 2003 report of the intestine transplant registry: A new era has dawned. Ann Surg 241(4):607–613, 2005. **Report from the Intestine Transplant Registry with recent data.**
5. Halloran PF: Immunosuppressive drugs for kidney transplantation. N Engl J Med 351:2715–2729, 2004. **Review of immunosuppressive medications with helpful diagrams. Applicable to other organs as well.**
6. Herrington CS, Tsirka AE: Pediatric cardiac transplantation. Semin Thorac Cardiovasc Surg 16(4):404–409, 2004. **Review of pediatric heart transplantation.**

7. Hsu DT: Biological and psychological differences in the child and adolescent transplant recipient. Pediatr Transplant 9(3):416–421, 2005. **Psychological issues in children with transplants.**

8. Magee JC, Bucuvalas JC, Farmer DG, Harmon WE, et al: Pediatric transplantation. Am J Transplant, 4(Suppl)9:54–71, 2004. **Review of pediatric transplantation.**

9. Mallory GB, Spray TL: Paediatric lung transplantation. Eur Respir J 24(5):839–845, 2004. **Recent data on lung transplantation in children.**

10. McDiarmid SV, Anand R, SPLIT Research Group: Studies of Pediatric Liver Transplantation (SPLIT): A summary of the 2003 Annual Report. Clin Transplant 119–130, 2003. **Useful information on pediatric liver transplantation.**

11. Mintzer LL, Stuber ML, Seacord D, et al: Traumatic stress symptoms in adolescent organ transplant recipients. Pediatrics 115(6):1640–1644, 2005. **Psychological issues in children with transplants.**

12. Uejima T: Anesthetic management of the pediatric patient undergoing solid organ transplantation. Anesthesiol Clin North Am 22(4):809–826, 2004. **Good summary of issues about anesthesia in the child receiving a solid organ transplant.**

The Immunocompromised Host

Karoll J. Cortez and Thomas J. Walsh

KEY CONCEPTS

- Immunocompromised pediatric patients present with specific infections related to underlying immune deficits.
- The underlying immune deficits define the risk for specific infections, allowing for early therapeutic intervention pending results of diagnostic evaluation.
- Quantitative and qualitative defects in neutrophils result in increased risk for aerobic gram-negative and gram-positive bacteria, as well as opportunistic fungi, such as *Candida* species and *Aspergillus* species.
- Deficits in cellular immunity lead to increased risk of infection caused by organisms such as *Pneumocystis jiroveci*, atypical mycobacteria, *Cytomegalovirus*, *Toxoplasma gondii*, *Cryptococcus neoformans*, and *Histoplasma capsulatum*.
- Quantitative and qualitative defects in immunoglobulins or B cells result in increased risk of infections with encapsulated bacteria, such as *Streptococcus pneumoniae*. Functional or anatomic splenectomy also may result in increased susceptibility to infection caused by encapsulated bacteria.

Infectious diseases are major causes of morbidity and mortality in immunocompromised pediatric patients. Advances in supportive care of infectious diseases have contributed substantially to the improved survival, outcome, and reduction of suffering and pain due to infectious complications.

Host defenses against bacterial, fungal, viral, and parasitic pathogens can be considered innate or adaptive. Innate host defenses include mucocutaneous barriers, phagocytic cells, cytokine regulatory networks, the toll-like receptor system, natural killer cells, and nonclonal T and B cells. Adaptive immunity encompasses the production of pathogen-specific antibodies and T-lymphocyte cell-mediated immunity.

Expert Opinion on Management Issues

IMMUNOCOMPROMISED HOST

The risk of development of infection and strategies for management of infections in immunocompromised children can be understood through a practical classification of the types of immune impairment and associated pathogens.

Normal host response depends on the coordinated activity of several arms of innate and adaptive host response; an intact phagocytic system consisting of polymorphonuclear leukocytes, monocytes, macrophages, and dendritic cells; T lymphocytes, B lymphocytes, and NK cells; intact mucocutaneous barriers; and intact peritoneal hollow viscera as well as intact circulating and innate mucosal immune defense molecules. Quantitative and qualitative deficits in any of these components of the immune system may lead to an increased risk of infection. Table 1 lists these deficits and associated immunodeficiencies.

Among the common conditions associated with immunocompromised pediatric patients are those with a quantitative defect associated with cancer chemotherapy (neutropenia); inherited immunodeficiencies (e.g., chronic granulomatous disease); hypogammaglobulinemia (e.g., Bruton agammaglobulinemia, X-linked agammaglobulinemia); and T-lymphocyte depletion (e.g., human immunodeficiency virus [HIV] infection). Cystic fibrosis is associated with obstruction of the tracheobronchial tree leading to recurrent pneumonias; solid tumors in pediatric oncology patients may obstruct the gastrointestinal and urinary tract, creating the conditions for severe infections; deficits in complement may result in increased infections caused by encapsulated bacteria; splenectomy resulting in loss of opsonization and tissue macrophages also may result in increased susceptibility to potential fatal infections caused by encapsulated bacteria.

Although a detailed discussion of the management of infections of the multiple types of immunocompromised hosts is beyond the scope of this chapter, this standardized approach to management of infections in neutropenic patients, hematopoietic stem cell transplant recipients, and HIV-infected patients serves as a useful model. The basic algorithms for management of neutropenic patients are well established and predicated on the known risk factors and associated organisms for the development of life-threatening infections during the course of neutropenia (Table 2 and Box 1).

Neutropenic patients are at risk for infections caused by aerobic enteric gram-negative bacilli, *Pseudomonas aeruginosa*, and opportunistic fungi (e.g., *Candida* species and *Aspergillus* species). Thus the new onset of fever in the setting of neutropenia warrants the empirical administration of antibacterial therapy directed at the most lethal pathogens. Monotherapy or combination therapy with selected agents may be used in the initial treatment of empirical antibacterial therapy of febrile neutropenic children. Monotherapy with ceftazidime or cefepime is effective in settings where the frequency of gram-negative bacilli expressing extended-spectrum β-lactamases (ESBLs) or stably derepressed (type 1 or Amp C) β-lactamases is uncommon. Meropenem or imipenem may be used for treatment of these β-lactamase producers as well as for mixed aerobic-anaerobic infections. The combination of an acyl-ureidopenicillin plus aminoglycoside also is used for empirical antibacterial therapy, particularly in settings in which infections caused by gram-negative bacilli expressing ESBLs are common. The increasing frequency of gram-positive infections resistant to standard initial antibacterial therapy may warrant the use of vancomycin. However, the use of vancomycin must be tempered with the potential for selection of resistant organisms (vancomycin-resistant *Enterococcus species*) and for infusion-related toxicity.

Risks for invasive fungal infections as such increase in relationship to the duration of neutropenia and mucosal disruption. Prophylactic and empirical strategies have evolved for the development of infections caused by *Candida* species, *Aspergillus* species, and other life-threatening pathogens because the establishment of invasive fungal infections during the period of neutropenia carries considerable morbidity and mortality. However, despite these early interventions to preempt development of overwhelming infections during profound neutropenia, the initial evaluation of neutropenic patients requires a careful history, meticulous physical examination, and a comprehensive laboratory assessment, including diagnostic imaging and blood cultures.

In a profoundly neutropenic patient, the presence of pulmonary infiltrates that do not resolve or respond to initial antibacterial therapy warrants further assessment with bronchoalveolar lavage (BAL). Patients undergoing hematopoietic stem cell transplantation (HSCT) have a similar risk during the neutropenic phase of transplantation. However, there is increased immunosuppression in the postengraftment period. This is associated with severe impairment of T-cell function in order to prevent graft-versus-host disease (GVHD). The use of corticosteroids further adds to the immune suppression at multiple levels of host response, including phagocytic function, T-cell function, and B-cell function. Hence patients in the postengraftment period of HSCT are at increased risk for invasive fungal infections, DNA viruses/herpesvirus infections (e.g., varicella-zoster virus [VZV], cytomegalovirus [CMV]). Thus prophylactic acyclovir is administered as prophylaxis for VZV antibody–positive patients who may be at risk for reactivation. Preemptive therapy with ganciclovir or foscarnet is used to prevent development of disease because of the CMV. Preemptive therapy is guided under these circumstances by the detection of the PP65 antigen in peripheral neutrophils and/or a positive polymerase chain reaction (PCR) at a certain threshold of DNA copies (genome copies per

mL). HSCT recipients are also at high risk for invasive fungal infections, often caused by uncommon but emerging pathogens including *Aspergillus* species and Zygomycetes. Antifungal therapy directed at specific pathogens is particularly important.

HIV infection may cause profound depletion of CD4+ cells and severe impairment of cellular immune response. This quantitative and qualitative impairment of T-cell–mediated immunity puts these patients at high risk for the development of infections caused by *Pneumocystis jiroveci* (*P. carinii*), atypical mycobacteria (especially *Mycobacterium avium* complex), *Cryptococcus neoformans*, cytomegalovirus, and *Toxoplasma gondii*. Well-defined strategies for the prevention and treatment of these infections are defined in a series of guidelines. The intervention of prophylaxis, such as that for *P. jiroveci,* or for early detection and appropriate therapeutic intervention, such as for *Cryptococcus neoformans*, may significantly reduce the morbidity and mortality associated with these infections that typify profound impairment of cell-mediated immunity.

Inherited defects of the phagocytic system classically exemplified by chronic granulomatous disease (CGD) are characterized by recurrent infections caused by *Staphylococcus aureus, Nocardia* species, and filamentous fungi, particularly *Aspergillus* species. These infections may present as severe and extensive in a patient with no prior history of immunosuppression. Such patients should be carefully evaluated for the possibility of CGD or a similar defect in neutrophil function. Intervention with appropriate antistaphylococcal therapy (oxacillin, trimethoprim-sulfamethoxazole) and for *Aspergillus* species (e.g., voriconazole).

Common Pitfalls

- Failure to recognize that emerging conditions, such as fever complicating neutropenia, represent a life-threatening process that may result in refractory infection if not managed urgently.
- Management of febrile neutropenic patients requires a careful assessment for antimicrobial therapy directed at specific clinical manifestations. One antibiotic alone may not be sufficient for management of concomitant infections or complicated conditions.
- Recognition of other ensuing complications in neutropenic, HSCT, and other severely immune-impaired patients may result in misdiagnosis and progressive infection.
- Neutropenic patients with abdominal symptoms and no fever are at high risk for septic complications. Neutropenic patients with a clinical documented infection but no fever should be treated as if they are febrile and managed as appropriate with antimicrobial therapy. Fever may be delayed at onset or nonexistent until septic complications ensue.
- During the course of antimicrobial therapy in neutropenic patients, resistant bacterial and

TABLE 1 Concepts of Immune Impairment: Cellular Targets, Mechanisms, Associated Pathogens, and Therapeutic Interventions

Cellular Target of Immune Impairment	Mechanism or Etiology of Immune Impairment	Diagnosis (Disease or Syndrome)	Typical Associated Pathogens	Representative Therapeutic Intervention
Phagocytic cells Neutrophils ↓Quantity	Cytotoxic chemotherapy Aplastic anemia Bone marrow failure Defective adhesion	Neutropenia Myelodysplasia Leukocyte adhesion deficiencies	Staphylococcus aureus Escherichia coli Pseudomonas aeruginosa Streptococcus aureus, Aspergillus species Nocardia asteroides	Ceftazidime Meropenem Imipenem ± Vancomycin
↓Quality	Impaired oxidative metabolism	CGD		
Monocytes	Corticosteroids	Cushing syndrome/disease		
Macrophages	Corticosteroids Corticosteroids	Infants of very low birth weight	Intracellular pathogens (Listeria monocytogenes)	For Listeria: Ampicillin Trimethoprim-sulfamethoxazole Penicillin
Splenectomy	Functional/anatomic splenectomy	Sickle cell disease	Encapsulated bacteria: Streptococcus pneumoniae, Haemophilus influenzae	Ampicillin/clavulanate Ceftriaxone Levofloxacin Vancomycin
Macrophages B lymphocytes	Impaired antibody production	MDS Lymphoid malignancies		Penicillin
B lymphocytes	Hypogammaglobulinemia Dysgammaglobulinemia	Lymphoid malignancies Multiple myeloma X-linked agammaglobulinemia SCID Common variable hypogammaglobulinemia	Encapsulated bacteria: S. pneumoniae H. influenzae Neisseria meningitidis	Ampicillin/clavulanate Ceftriaxone Levofloxacin Vancomycin

T lymphocytes CD4+ NK cells	TH1/TH2 dysregulation Corticosteroids	HIV GVHD SOT Corticosteroids SCID DiGeorge syndrome	Herpesviruses: HSV-1, -2, VZV, HHV-6, CMV; *Pneumocystis jiroveci (carinii)* *Mycobacteria* species *Cryptococcus* species *Toxoplasma gondii*	Acyclovir, foscarnet specific IVIG, HAART (HIV specific) Anti-tuberculous antimicrobials Trimethoprim-sulfamethoxazole
Mucocutaneous integrity	Cytotoxic chemotherapy Radiation	Mucositis	Gram-positive cocci: *Streptococcus mitis* group Enterobacteriaceae (GNRs and anaerobic bacteria) *P. aeruginosa*	Vancomycin Ceftazidime Ceftriaxone Fluoroquinolone Fluoroquinolone
Obstruction of hollow viscera (e.g., caused by tumor, metastatic disease, calculus formation, extrinsic obstruction)	CFTR: bronchial and pancreatic obstruction Urinary tract Infection (stone) Small/large bowel obstruction: Peritonitis Postobstructive pneumonia	Cystic fibrosis Solid tumors (primary or metastatic) Metabolic abnormalities (e.g., hypercalcuria, hyperoxalemia)	Enterobacteriaceae: *Klebsiella* species, *E. coli*, etc. Respiratory pathogens, anaerobic mouth or enteric flora, enteric aerobes: GNR	Third-generation cephalosporin
Innate immune defense molecules	Complement Lectins Ficolins Surfactants Toll-like receptors	Sepsis	*Neisseria* species CMV *Candida* species *Aspergillus* species	Penicillin Third-generation cephalosporin Amphotericin B (deoxycholate, lipid formulations) Azoles: fluconazole, voriconazole Echinocandins: caspofungin

CFTR, cystic fibrosis transmembrane conductance regulator; CGD, chronic granulomatous disease; CMV, cytomegalovirus; GNR, gram-negative rod; GVHD, graft-versus-host disease; HAART, highly active antiretroviral therapy; HHV, human herpesvirus; HIV, human immunodeficiency virus; HSV, herpes simplex virus; IVIG, intravenous immunoglobulin; MDS, myelodysplastic syndrome; SCID, severe combined immune deficiency; SOT, solid organ transplant; VZV, varicella-zoster virus.

TABLE 2 Diagnostic Approach in Suspected Immunocompromised Children

History of Current Illness	Duration/Progression of Symptoms
Timing of developmental milestones	Infancy: Umbilical cord separation Dentition
Environmental exposures	Recent travel Insect bites Indoor and outdoor activities
History of previous infections	Bacterial Fungal Viral Recurrent infections Hospitalizations
Surgical history	Implants Prosthesis Catheters
Current medication list	Dose Length of therapy Last dose
Complete physical exam	Facial features Organomegaly
Laboratory studies	**Host evaluation:** CBC/differential Urinalysis C3, C4, CH$_{50}$ Quantitative immunoglobulins and subtypes CD4+ (if lymphopenia) HIV–1 and –2 ELISA NBT (or FACS for oxidative metabolism) **Other investigations:** Electrolytes BUN/creatinine Liver function tests CRP, ESR LDH **Microbiological evaluation:** Blood Cx Urine Cx Sputum: Gram stain and Cx
Radiologic imaging	Chest radiograph, CT scan of head, chest, abdomen, pelvis (as indicated) MRI as indicated

BUN, blood urea nitrogen; CBC, complete blood count; CH$_{50}$, (total serum) hemolytic complement; CRP, C-reactive protein; Cx, culture; ELISA, enzyme-linked immunoabsorbent assay; ESR, erythrocyte sedimentation rate; FACS, fluorescence-activated cell sorter; HIV, human immunodeficiency virus; NBT, nitroblue tetrazolium.

BOX 1 Diagnostic Approach to the Immunocompromised Host

- History of current illness
  - Onset of symptoms
  - Recent antibiotic, antifungal, antiviral therapy (prophylaxis, preemptive, ongoing)
  - End of last chemotherapy cycle
  - Type of antineoplastic drug use, dose, reactions
  - Amount of radiation therapy, dose, body site
  - Recent treatment with IVIG (if applicable)
- Environmental exposures
  - Recent travel, insect bites, indoor and outdoor activities
- History of previous infections
  - Bacterial, fungal, or viral
- Surgical history
  - Implants, prosthesis
- Complete physical exam
- Laboratory studies
  - Complete WBC/differential
  - Urine analysis
  - Stool for WBC and O+P
  - Electrolytes, BUN, creatinine
  - Liver function test
  - CRP, LDH
  - NPW for respiratory virus culture
  - Swabs of suspicious drainages for gram stain and culture
  - If cough/pulmonary infiltrates in CXR or CT scans: Sputum for gram stain and routine bacterial Cx, DFA for *Pneumocystis*, PCR *for Chlamydia, Legionella, Mycoplasma*
  - If negative initial evaluation: prompt bronchoalveolar lavage for Gram stain, wet mount; EIA for RSV, influenza virus; routine cultures; DFA and PCR for *Pneumocystis*; PCR for *Legionella, Mycoplasma*; fungal cultures; viral cultures (respiratory, HSV, CMV)
  - As indicated: lumbar puncture for CSF examination and cultures
- Radiologic imaging
  - Chest radiograph
  - CT scan of head, chest, abdomen, pelvis (as indicated)
  - MRI as indicated

BUN, blood urea nitrogen; CMV, cytomegalovirus; CRP, C-reactive protein; CSF, cerebrospinal fluid; Cx, culture; CXR, chest radiograph; DFA, direct fluorescence antibody; EIA, enzyme immunoassay; HSV, herpes simplex virus; IVIG, intravenous immunoglobulin; LDH, lactate dehydrogenase; NPW, nasopharyngeal wash; O+P, ova and parasites; PCR, polymerase chain reaction; RSV, respiratory syncytial virus; WBC, white blood cells.

fungal infections may develop. Early recognition and modification of existing antimicrobial therapy may be lifesaving pending results of cultures and other diagnostic studies.

- Pulmonary infiltrates refractory to conventional antibacterial therapy require evaluation with invasive procedures such as BAL or percutaneous fine-needle aspiration (FNA) to establish a definitive diagnosis.
- Evaluation of all patients for vaccination is an important component of overall management of immunocompromised children.

Communication and Counseling

The successful long-term management of immunocompromised children requires close cooperation, communication, and counseling with family members, caretakers, and the total health care team. To the greatest extent possible, the child should be engaged in these discussions so all members recognize the importance of the manifestations of infections and the need for close monitoring and reporting of any new developments suspicious of an ensuing infection. Recognition of the need for evaluation by qualified medical staff is imperative for making early interventions possible. Good practices of personal hygiene and environmental precautions to reduce acquisition of pathogens are also important in the general management of immunocompromised children.

SUGGESTED READINGS

1. Buckley RH: Pulmonary complications of primary immunodeficiencies. Paediatr Respir Rev 5:S225–S233, 2004. **Comprehensive review of more than 100 additional immunodeficiency syndromes described since Ogden Bruton discovered agammaglobulinemia 50 years ago.**
2. Burchett SK, Pizzo PA: HIV infection in infants, children, and adolescents. Pediatr Rev 24:186–194, 2003. **Detailed review of infections in HIV-positive children.**
3. Clark R, Powers R, White R, et al: Prevention and treatment of nosocomial sepsis in the NICU. J Perinatol 24:446–453. 2004. **Describes how implementing simple changes can reduce nosocomial infection rates in neonates and improve outcomes.**
4. Groll AH, Walsh TJ: Fungal infections in pediatric patients. In McGinnis M, Pfaller M, Anaissie E (eds): Clinical Mycology. Philadelphia: Churchill Livingstone, 2003, pp 417–442. **General review of risk factors, host defenses, and management of invasive mycoses.**
5. Keough WL, Michaels MG: Infectious complications in pediatric solid organ transplantation. Pediatr Clin North Am 50: 1451–1469, 2003. **Complete issue dedicated to infectious complications in pediatric immunosuppressed patients.**
6. Paller AS: Genetic immunodeficiency disorders. Clin Dermatol 23:68–77, 2005. **Immunodeficiency should be considered in children with a history of infections that are recurrent, respond poorly to antibiotics, are of increased duration and severity, and/or result from unusual organisms.**
7. Panitch HB: Evaluation of recurrent pneumonia. Pediatr Infect Dis J 24:265–266, 2005. **Children with recurrent pneumonia have an identifiable underlying cause.**
8. Prober CG: Pediatric infectious diseases. Pediatr Clin North Am 52:699–948, 2005. **Comprehensive issue dedicated to pediatric infectious diseases.**
9. Rosenzweig SD, Holland SM: Phagocyte immunodeficiencies and their infections. J Allergy Clin Immunol 113:620–626, 2004. **Detailed review of infections in phagocytic deficiencies.**
10. Walsh TJ, Roilides E, Groll A, et al: Infectious complications in pediatric cancer patients. In Pizzo PA, Poplack DG (eds): Principles and Practice of Pediatric Oncology, 5th ed. Philadelphia: Lippincott Williams & Wilkins (in press). **General review of risk factors, host defenses, and management of immunocompromised pediatric oncology patients.**

21

Neuroblastoma

Carola A. S. Arndt

KEY CONCEPTS

- Neuroblastoma is the most common extracranial solid tumor in children.
- Presenting signs and symptoms depend on the location of the primary tumor.
- Opsoclonus myoclonus syndrome is often missed as a presenting paraneoplastic syndrome of neuroblastoma.
- Therapy depends on appropriate risk group assignment, depending on clinical factors such as age and stage of tumor and biological prognostic factors such as DNA ploidy of the tumor, histologic classification, and amplification of the N-*myc* gene.
- Most patients with low- and intermediate-risk neuroblastoma can be cured, whereas more than half of patients with high-risk disease will not survive their disease despite very aggressive treatment.
- New approaches including stem cell transplant and use of biologic agents are being evaluated for patients with high-risk disease.

Neuroblastoma, ganglioneuroblastoma, and ganglioneuroma are derived from primordial neural crest cells. Neuroblastoma arises from postganglionic sympathetic neuroblasts. It is the most common extracranial solid tumor in children, accounting for 8% to 10% of all childhood cancers. There are approximately 550 new cases of neuroblastoma annually in the United States. Approximately one third of patients are younger than 1 year of age at diagnosis and 97% of cases are diagnosed by 10 years of age.

Signs and Symptoms

Signs and symptoms at diagnosis are variable and depend on the location of the primary tumor. Most primary tumors occur within the abdomen and may manifest with abdominal pain or fullness. Primary thoracic tumors are often discovered incidentally when a chest radiograph is performed for other reasons. Neuroblastoma located in the high cervical or thoracic region

may cause Horner syndrome. Paraspinal lesions may extend into neural foramina and cause symptoms of spinal cord compression. Widespread metastatic disease may cause fever, bone pain, irritability, limping, anemia, and the classic "raccoon eyes" secondary to periorbital ecchymoses resulting from retrobulbar infiltration. A unique paraneoplastic syndrome of opsoclonus-myoclonus can be seen and is sometimes mistaken for benign cerebellar ataxia or middle ear dysfunction. Bluish skin nodules are seen exclusively in infants with stage 4S tumors.

The most commonly used staging system is the International Neuroblastoma Staging System (INSS) (Table 1). To evaluate a patient appropriately, the extent of primary disease and the presence of metastatic disease should be determined. Appropriate evaluation involves performing CT or MRI scanning of the primary site, a chest CT scan, bone marrow aspirates and biopsies from at least two sites, a bone scan, and additional radionuclide imaging with metaiodobenzylguanidine (MIBG). Because most neuroblastomas secrete high levels of catecholamines, urinary levels of homovanillic acid and vanillylmandelic acid should be obtained and should aid in both establishing the diagnosis and monitoring the response to treatment. Tumor tissue must be obtained for pathologic confirmation, and for determination of histologic subtype (Shimada classification), N-*myc* studies, and DNA ploidy, as these factors are prognostic and help classify patients into risk groups for appropriate therapy.

Expert Opinion on Management Issues

Treatment of neuroblastoma depends on assigning risk group according to a number of well-defined biologic characteristics of the tumor and the age of the patient at time of diagnosis. Table 2 shows the categories of current risk group assignment, which determines therapy. Patients with clinically and biologically defined low-risk disease generally undergo only resection of tumor, followed by observation alone if more than 50% of the tumor has been resected. In the majority of such patients, a residual tumor will regress spontaneously, but close observation is mandatory to monitor regression. In case of tumor regrowth or progression,

TABLE 1 International Neuroblastoma Staging System (INSS)

Stage	Features
1	Localized tumor with complete gross excision, with or without microscopic residual disease; representative ipsilateral lymph nodes are negative for tumor microscopically (nodes attached to and removed with the primary tumor may be positive).
2A	Localized tumor with incomplete gross resection; representative ipsilateral nonadherent lymph nodes are negative for tumor microscopically.
2B	Localized tumor with or without complete gross excision, with ipsilateral nonadherent lymph nodes positive for tumor; enlarged contralateral lymph nodes must be negative microscopically.
3	Unresectable unilateral tumor infiltrating across the midline, with or without regional lymph node involvement, or localized unilateral tumor with contralateral regional lymph node involvement, or midline tumor with bilateral extension by infiltration (unresectable) or by lymph node involvement.
4	Any primary tumor with dissemination to distant lymph nodes, bone, bone marrow, liver, skin, and/or other organs (except as defined for stage 4S).
4S	Localized primary tumor (as defined for stage 1, 2A, or 2B) with dissemination limited to skin, liver, and/or bone marrow (limited to infants <1 yr of age). *Marrow involvement in stage 4S* should be minimal (less than 10% of total nucleated cells identified as malignant on bone marrow biopsy or marrow aspirate). More extensive marrow involvement would be considered to be stage 4. The MIBG scan (if performed) should be negative in the marrow.

MBIG, metaiodobenzylguanidine.

reoperation and/or chemotherapy in selected cases are recommended. Low-risk patients for whom chemotherapy is recommended immediately include patients in whom less than 50% of the tumor can be initially resected, patients whose tumors are not resectable and threaten life or function owing to spinal cord compression, or respiratory compromise because of huge intra-abdominal or hepatic masses. For low-risk patients requiring chemotherapy, multiagent chemotherapy with carboplatin, cyclophosphamide etoposide, and doxorubicin is administered. Patients with low-risk disease have a greater than 90% chance of survival 3 years after diagnosis.

Intermediate-risk patients, as defined by the criteria in Table 2, have overall survival rates of more than 90% but require surgery and multiagent chemotherapy to achieve cure. Four to eight cycles of chemotherapy with the agents discussed previously are given. The number of cycles administered depends on the biological characterization of the tumor (favorable or unfavorable). Patients in this risk group have an overall survival of approximately 70% at 3 years from diagnosis.

Patients with high-risk disease remain a challenge. The survival rate for patients with the highest risk is only approximately 35% at 3 years from diagnosis. Very aggressive multiagent chemotherapy followed by autologous stem cell transplant and treatment with the differentiating agent *cis*-retinoic acid is promising in improving the outcome of this group of patients. Current studies are exploring the value of purging the stem cell product to eliminate contaminating tumor cells. Other clinical studies for high-risk neuroblastoma include evaluation of a fusion protein, which consists of a humanized monoclonal antibody recognizing the GD2 disialoganglioside on neuroblastoma linked

TABLE 2 Risk Group and Protocol Assignment Schema*

INSS stage	Age	N-myc Status	Shimada Histology	DNA Ploidy	Risk Group/Study
1	0–21 yr	Any	Any	Any	Low
2A/2B	<365 days	Any	Any	Any	Low
	≥365 days–21 yr	Non-amp	Any	—	Low
	≥365 days–21 yr	Amp	Favorable	—	Low
	≥365 days–21 yr	Amp	Unfavorable	—	High
3	<365 days	Non-amp	Any	Any	Intermediate
	<365 days	Amp	Any	Any	High
	≥365 days–21 yr	Non-amp	Favorable	—	Intermediate
	≥365 days–21 yr	Non-amp	Unfavorable	—	High
	≥365 days–21 yr	Amp	Any	—	High
4	<365 days	Non-amp	Any	Any	Intermediate
	<365 days	Amp	Any	Any	High
	≥365 days–21 yr	Any	Any	—	High
4S	<365 days	Non-amp	Favorable	>1	Low
	<365 days	Non-amp	Any	=1	Intermediate
	<365 days	Non-amp	Unfavorable	Any	Intermediate
	<365 days	Amp	Any	Any	High

*Biology is defined by: N-*myc* status: Amplified (amp) vs. non-amplified (non-amp). Shimada histopathology: Favorable vs. unfavorable. DNA ploidy: DNA index (DI) > 1 or = 1; hypodiploid tumors (with DI < 1) is treated as a tumor with a DI > 1. (DNA index < 1 [hypodiploid] to be considered favorable ploidy.) INSS, International Neuroblastoma Staging System.

genetically to the human recombinant interleukin (IL)-2 lymphokine, and evaluation of the use of radioactive ^{131}I-MIBG.

Common Pitfalls

The importance of obtaining adequate tissue at diagnosis from the primary tumor to be able to stratify patients into risk groups for therapy cannot be overemphasized. This strategy allows low-risk patients to avoid excessive or unnecessary therapy, and high-risk patients to receive appropriately aggressive therapy. Referral to centers with a multidisciplinary pediatric oncology team is required for optimal therapy of this and other childhood cancers. Careful follow-up of all patients is required to monitor for recurrence and for late effects of therapy.

Communication and Counseling

The diagnosis of cancer in a child is always devastating for families. Emotional support for families and patients from appropriately trained professionals is critical. The health care providers need to make available to the family educational materials about the disease, information about the importance and role of clinical trials, and information on informed consent. Counseling about side effects of treatment and importance of adequate long-term follow-up should be provided.

SUGGESTED READINGS

1. Matthay KK, Villablanca JG, Seeger RC, et al: Treatment of high-risk neuroblastoma with intensive chemotherapy, radiotherapy, autologous bone marrow transplantation, and 13-*cis*-retinoic acid. Children's Cancer Group. N Engl J Med 341 (16):1165–1173, 1999. **Results of clinical trial for high-risk neuroblastoma showing importance of myeloablative chemotherapy and differentiating therapy with cis-retinoic acid.**
2. Nickerson HJ, Matthay KK, Seeger RC, et al: Favorable biology and outcome of stage IV-S neuroblastoma with supportive care or minimal therapy: A Children's Cancer Group study. J Clin Oncol 18(3):477–486, 2000. **Supports minimal therapy for selected infants with stage 4S disease.**
3. Perez CA, Matthay KK, Atkinson JB, et al: Biologic variables in the outcome of stages I and II neuroblastoma treated with surgery as primary therapy: A Children's Cancer Group study. J Clin Oncol 18(1):18–26, 2000. **Describes good outcome with surgery alone for patients with stage 1 or 2 neuroblastoma and the need for additional therapy in certain stage 2 patients with unfavorable biologic characteristics.**
4. Schmidt ML, Lukens JN, Seeger RC, et al: Biologic factors determine prognosis in infants with stage IV neuroblastoma: A prospective Children's Cancer Group study. J Clin Oncol 18(6):1260–1268, 2000. **This study shows the importance of N-myc amplification as a prognostic factor for infants with stage 4 neuroblastoma.**
5. Shimada H, Ambros IM, Dehner LP, et al: The International Neuroblastoma Pathology Classification (the Shimada system). Cancer 86(2):364–372, 1999. **Describes the prognostic significance of morphology in conjunction with age.**

Pediatric Brain Tumors

Torunn I. Yock and Nancy J. Tarbell

KEY CONCEPTS
- Low-grade gliomas and medulloblastomas are the most common brain tumors of childhood.
- Tissue diagnosis is usually necessary to guide treatment decisions.
- All brain lesions require MRI with gadolinium enhancement for full delineation of the tumor, and some require spinal imaging if the tumor has the potential to seed the cranial-spinal axis.
- Neurologic findings on physical examination should prompt an MRI for workup.
- Many childhood brain tumors are curable but require a multidisciplinary team to manage the disease and the side effects of treatment.

Brain tumors are the most common solid tumor of childhood. In 2004, more than 2000 pediatric patients in the United States were diagnosed with brain tumors. Approximately 60% can be cured through a variety of treatment approaches including radiation, surgery, and chemotherapy. Surgery plays an important role in the management of children with brain tumors, either for definitive diagnosis and/or for resection. Patients with aggressive tumors or incompletely resected tumors may require definitive radiotherapy with or without chemotherapy. The optimal management of a child with a brain tumor involves a multidisciplinary team that includes a pediatric oncologist, a pediatric neurosurgeon, and pediatric radiation oncologist. A brain tumor and its treatment can affect cognition, behavior, hormonal function, and vision. Therefore, important health care providers may also include rehabilitation specialists, pediatric neurologists, social work specialists, neuroendocrinologists, and neuroophthalmologists, and child psychiatrists or psychologists.

The symptoms associated with a brain tumor depend largely on its location and the age of the child. The most common symptoms associated with a posterior fossa tumor include headache, morning nausea and vomiting, ataxia, and diplopia. Most of these symptoms are related to a relative obstruction of the flow of cerebrospinal fluid (CSF), causing hydrocephalus. Nystagmus and papilledema are two important signs to look for when a brain tumor is suspected. In an infant the symptoms might be a bulging fontanel and increasing head size and varying degrees of failure to thrive. Because of open cranial sutures, papilledema may be absent in infants. Supratentorial tumors are more likely to manifest with focal abnormalities such as long track signs and seizures. However, alterations in behavior or personality are often the first symptoms of any brain tumor. Lethargy, irritability, hyperactivity, and poor ability to concentrate can all be manifestations of a brain tumor. Usually such behavioral changes are reversible once the tumor is adequately treated.

In children between the ages of 2 and 12 years, two thirds of the brain tumors occur in the posterior fossa. The most common tumors in the posterior fossa include astrocytomas and medulloblastomas. In teenagers and infants younger than 2, 50% of tumors occur in the posterior fossa and 50% occur supratentorially. The most common tumor of the supratentorial region is an astrocytoma. Astrocytomas in children are more likely to be low-grade, whereas in adults, high-grade lesions are more common. A gadolinium-enhanced MRI of the brain is essential to delineate the tumor margins and differential diagnosis. Once a lesion is identified, the subsequent workup depends on the characteristics of the lesion found. A neurosurgeon should always be consulted to discuss obtaining tissue for definitive diagnosis and, if possible, surgical removal of the lesion. Children with medulloblastomas, ependymomas, primitive neuroectodermal tumors (PNETs), or germ cell tumors will also need gadolinium-enhanced MRI imaging of the spine to rule out CSF spread of disease. Additionally, patients with suspected germ cell tumors in the pineal or suprasellar regions should have serum and CSF levels of alpha-fetoprotein (AFP) and β-human chorionic gonadotropin (β-HCG) performed.

Expert Opinion on Management Issues

MEDULLOBLASTOMA AND PRIMITIVE NEUROECTODERMAL TUMORS

Medulloblastomas are undifferentiated tumors that belong to the class of embryonal tumors. Medulloblastomas arise from primitive neuroectodermal tissue located in the external granular layer of the cerebellum. Tumors that arise from the same tissue in the cerebrum or spinal cord are related and require similar aggressive treatment. Pineoblastomas and ependymoblastomas are also embryonal tumors that behave aggressively. These similar tumor types all require a multimodality approach consisting of surgery, radiation, and chemotherapy, but the medulloblastomas fare somewhat better than the other types. Pathologically, these tumors typically consist of immature small round blue cells that share a tendency toward subarachnoid dissemination. The most common of this group of tumors is the medulloblastoma arising in the posterior fossa. There are in excess of 400 cases per year in the United States, and this class of tumor accounts for 20% of all pediatric brain tumors. The four most common presenting symptoms include vomiting, headache, ataxia, and nausea. A gadolinium-enhanced brain and spine MRI are required to evaluate the entire central nervous system (CNS) for disease. Cytology in CSF obtained from a lumbar puncture is also required to rule out micrometastases in the CSF after any herniation risk has been mitigated with resection, ventricular-peritoneal (VP) shunting, or external ventricular drain. Between 10% and 30% of patients have subarachnoid metastases at presentation.

Surgery, radiation, and chemotherapy provide the backbone of treatment. A total resection of the grossly visible posterior fossa tumor is possible in more than 70% of cases. Cranial-spinal axis radiation is required postoperatively even in the setting of negative CSF cytology and spinal MRIs because of the high propensity of these tumors to recur without irradiation. Standard-risk patients are defined as those patients with less than 1.5 cm^2 of tumor after resection and no evidence of CNS metastasis. The higher-risk patients are defined as those with spinal or cerebral metastases or incomplete resection (greater than 1.5 cm^2) residual. Risk stratification is prognostic and determines the intensity of treatment. Standard-risk patients older than 3 years of age receive 23.4 Gy of cranial-spinal irradiation, whereas the high-risk children generally receive 36 Gy. In both cases the posterior fossa is boosted to 54 to 55.8 Gy. The active chemotherapeutic agents include platinum-based chemotherapies, lomustine [CCNU], etoposide, cyclophosphamide, and vincristine.

LOW-GRADE GLIOMAS

Almost 40% of pediatric brain tumors are low-grade astrocytomas. In children the most common histology is juvenile pilocytic astrocytoma (grade I/IV). Fibrillary or gemistocytic or protoplasmic (grade II/IV) astrocytomas and oligodendrogliomas (grade II to III/IV) occur with much less frequency. The juvenile pilocytic astrocytomas (JPA) have the most favorable prognosis. Multiple grading systems are used, but the World Health Organization (WHO) system of grading glial tumors is widely accepted. Grading is based on anaplasia, nuclear atypia, mitotic activity, presence of necrosis, and vascular proliferation. Grades I and II are classified as low-grade tumors; grades III and IV tumors are classified as high-grade.

When low-grade astrocytomas occur in the posterior fossa, they usually can be fully resected and no radiation or chemotherapy is needed. Where possible, gross total resection is the treatment of choice. Patients with pilocytic astrocytomas that have undergone a gross total resection can enjoy 10-year progression-free survival rates of up to 100%. When these tumors occur in the supratentorium, they tend to arise in the diencephalon and involve the hypothalamus, the optic chiasm, or the thalamus, which renders them generally unresectable or only partially resectable. Low-grade astrocytomas generally require treatment only when they cause symptoms. It is standard practice to follow a patient with regular MRI scans after an incomplete resection or if the tumor is found incidentally on imaging, especially if the patient is very young or asymptomatic. However, potential risks of expectant management include the possibility of irreversible neurologic impairment because of tumor growth or malignant degeneration. If a patient is very young, generally younger than 7 years of age and symptomatic, then chemotherapy using carboplatin and vincristine is typically administered with a high rate of response or stabilization of the tumor. Second-line chemotherapy includes newer drugs such as temozolomide. Delaying radiation allows time for more development and diminishes negative effects on cognition from the radiation. In some cases chemotherapy can delay radiation for many years.

Low-grade astrocytomas lend themselves well to highly conformal radiation techniques such as stereotactic radiotherapy, intensity-modulated radiotherapy, or proton radiotherapy, all of which minimize the dose to the normal brain. (Please refer to "Current and Future Developments in Radiotherapy" later in this chapter for more details on the types of conformal radiation.)

The disease-free survival for patients with pilocytic astrocytomas treated with radiation therapy is between 60% and 100% at 10 years depending on the series reported and the location of the tumor. The outcome for other histologies is not quite as favorable. After definitive radiation therapy these patients are followed with MRI. Within months to 2 years after treatment up to 40% of the MRIs done in routine follow up demonstrate increase in tumor size, increased signal intensity, and increased enhancement characteristics or cavitations, but these findings are not usually associated with symptoms and generally resolve with time. However, these radiation changes can mimic tumor progression. Furthermore, these tumors are typically very slow to respond to radiation change. The median time to a 50% partial radiographic response in one series was 62 months.

Patients with neurofibromatosis type 1 (NF1) commonly (11% to 19%) develop low-grade tumors of the optic tract, which may remain quiescent without therapy for many years. These lesions are so typical that most do not require a biopsy for confirmation. However, these children must be followed carefully with MRI scans and regular ophthalmologic examinations. Treatment must commence as soon as there is a clinical change.

HIGH-GRADE GLIOMAS

High-grade gliomas (also called malignant gliomas) in children consist mostly of high-grade astrocytomas and represent approximately 10% of all pediatric brain tumors. Children tend to do somewhat better than their adult counterparts but the prognosis is considerably worse when compared with the low-grade astrocytomas. Although very few low-grade astrocytomas disseminate through the CSF, 15% to 30% of high-grade gliomas will over the course of the disease. The WHO classifies grade III tumors as anaplastic astrocytomas and grade IV tumors as glioblastoma multiforme. On MRI these lesions appear poorly marginated, with significant edema. These lesions infiltrate surrounding brain tissue much more than the lower grade astrocytomas. Usually because of disease extent and location, gross total resection is possible in only 25% of patients. A gross total resection is associated with longer disease-free survival of approximately 60% at 3 to 5 years. Postoperative radiation is administered after resection but can generally be delayed with chemotherapy in children younger than 3 years. Patients with

anaplastic astrocytomas may survive 2 to 5 or more years. Patients with glioblastoma multiforme fare worse with a median survival of less than a year. Chemotherapy improves survival in patients with high-grade glial tumors. Agents with activity include lomustine, carmustine [BCNU], vincristine, VP-16, thiotepa, and temozolomide.

BRAIN STEM GLIOMAS

Brain stem gliomas constitute approximately 10% of intracranial tumors in children. The peak age incidence is between the ages of 6 and 10 years, and males are more commonly affected than females. The most common and devastating brain stem glioma is the diffusely infiltrating pontine glioma, accounting for approximately 70% of these brain stem tumors. Biopsy of diffuse pontine lesions is generally unnecessary. Studies have shown that approximately 50% are low grade and 50% are high grade, but the histology and grade do not correlate with survival. Median survival is approximately 1 year. Radiation therapy is the mainstay of treatment and improves symptoms and prolongs life. Concurrent chemotherapy with temozolomide and radiation to 54 Gy is currently standard treatment. However, because of the dismal prognosis, multiple phase I studies are under way in this population. Surgery essentially plays no role for the diffuse brain stem gliomas except for placement of a VP shunt if obstructive hydrocephalus becomes a problem.

Lesions arising in the medulla and midbrain have a more favorable prognosis. They are also more commonly focal instead of diffuse and often exophytic instead of intrinsic to the brain stem. Management of these more favorable tumors mirrors that of low-grade gliomas occurring in the posterior fossa or supratentorially.

CRANIOPHARYNGIOMAS

Craniopharyngiomas are benign tumors of epithelial origin arising from the remnants of the Rathke pouch in the suprasellar region. They usually present by causing visual field deficits and symptoms of raised intracranial pressure, and hormonal deficits. Surgical resection was the mainstay of treatment for many years. Craniopharyngiomas have clearly defined margins, and a total resection is potentially curative treatment but possible in only 50% to 80% of patients. Even in patients with a gross total resection, a significant proportion will recur. Additionally, approximately 10% of patients suffer a significant visual or neurological deficit after radical surgery. The tumor is often adherent to the optic nerves or chiasm or the major vessels around the circle of Willis.

Diabetes insipidus occurs in 80% to 90% of patients postoperatively and morbid hypothalamic obesity develops in 50% of patients. In contrast, limited surgery, consisting of debulking and immediate postoperative radiation, has excellent disease control (between 83% and 96% at 10 years) and may be somewhat less morbid. Additionally, diabetes insipidus is rarely caused by radiotherapy for these tumors. However, there are late neuroendocrinologic effects from radiation that commonly manifest with time. In the pediatric population, growth hormone secretion is often diminished over time and thyroid hormone production is the second most likely to be affected. However, sexual development and glucocorticoid production can also be affected and may require replacement as well. Hypothalamic obesity may also be induced by tumors in this region, requiring surgery or radiation, and can be a very troublesome side effect of treatment. Additionally, late vascular events are much more rare, but they have been reported as a complication of radiotherapy. There is a trade-off between the immediate side effects of surgery and the delayed side effects from radiation. However, a neuroendocrinologist can adequately correct most of the hormonal aberrations that may arise from the surgery or radiation therapy.

INTRACRANIAL GERM CELL TUMORS

Intracranial germ cell tumors occur within the diencephalic structures, almost exclusively as midline third ventricular lesions. Fifty percent to 60% of germ cell tumors are located in the pineal region, whereas 30% to 35% are located in the suprasellar region. Occasionally they arise in the basal ganglia or thalamic nuclei. Germ cell tumors represent only 1% to 3% of pediatric CNS neoplasms. Most germ cell tumors are germinomas (60% to 70%), but there are other more malignant germ cell types such as embryonal carcinomas, endodermal sinus tumors, or choriocarcinomas accounting for 15% to 20%. The remaining 15% to 20% are teratomas, which can be benign or malignant. The necessity of pathologic diagnosis is debated when tumor markers do not definitively establish the diagnosis but is generally indicated to better tailor the treatment.

Radiation therapy is the standard treatment for germinomas and plays a significant role in malignant germ cell tumors. Germinomas can be treated with radiation alone or with a combination of chemotherapy and radiation therapy. Surgery is generally reserved for biopsy diagnosis. Germinomas are very sensitive to chemotherapy and radiation therapy and the 5-year disease control rates are more than 90%. Chemotherapy alone is not recommended because it has resulted in high rates of failure.

Surgery plays a more important role in establishing a firm diagnosis and in resection of nongerminoma histologies, such as teratomas, that do not respond well to radiation alone or to combined modality therapy. However, surgery in the pineal region is especially challenging because of the vascular plexus surrounding it and should only be performed by a neurosurgeon who has a good experience with lesions in this region. The chemotherapeutic agents that are active in germ cell tumors include platinum-based chemotherapy, VP-16, cyclophosphamide, ifosfamide, and bleomycin.

EPENDYMOMAS

Ependymomas are tumors that arise from the ependymal cells lining the ventricles and the central canal of the spinal cord. Intracranial ependymomas represent up to 10% of brain tumors in children; two thirds occur in the posterior fossa. They can also occur supratentorially or within the spinal cord. Ependymomas typically occur in young children, 50% of whom are younger than 5 years old. The WHO recognizes two grades of ependymoma, anaplastic ependymomas (WHO grade III, deemed malignant), which fare worse than the classic ependymoma (WHO grade II, deemed benign) and have an even greater propensity to disseminate via the CSF. CSF cytology and full-spine MRI should be obtained to rule out dissemination at presentation.

Surgery is an important component of treatment, with the goal of a gross total resection whenever feasible. Disease control is markedly improved with fractionated postoperative radiation therapy. Durable disease control is achieved in 60% to 80% of patients treated with radiotherapy after a gross total resection of a classic ependymoma and drops to approximately 30% to 50% in patients with gross residual disease or anaplastic histology.

In very young patients chemotherapy has been used in the postoperative setting to delay radiation therapy with limited success. However, the delay does result in a compromise in disease control. Currently, conformal radiation therapy is given to patients even as young as 1 year old. Merchant and associates reported excellent neurocognitive outcome at 2 years in patients treated with highly conformal photon radiation therapy. Craniospinal irradiation should be reserved for patients who present with disseminated disease. In patients with supratentorial ependymomas, there is controversy about the need for postoperative radiotherapy, as tumors in these areas tend to do better than those in the posterior fossa.

Current and Future Developments in Radiotherapy

The 1990s witnessed a new era of MRI- and CT-based radiation treatment planning that better targeted the tumor and more effectively spared normal brain and nerves. The goal of treatment has become twofold—first, to control the primary tumor, and second, to decrease the complications of treatment. The latest versions of highly conformal treatment that are now being used have taken the form of stereotactic radiosurgery (γ-knife or linear accelerator [LINAC]-based), stereotactic radiotherapy, intensity-modulated radiotherapy (IMRT), or proton radiotherapy.

Stereotactic radiosurgery (SRS) is the process by which a single large dose (usually >10 Gy) is delivered to the tumor with a γ-knife, with a linear accelerator, or by proton beam. This approach is very effective but has some technical limitations. The target must be relatively small, with very little normal tissue included in the high-dose field. Therefore, tumor involvement with critical structures, such as optic nerves, the speech center, or the brain stem, generally precludes this technique from being used. Metastatic tumors to the brain are ideally suited for this kind of treatment but rarely occur in children. There are very few indications for radiosurgery in the child who has not already been treated by fractionated radiation therapy and has a form of recurrent tumor. A patient's head must be precisely immobilized with an invasive frame anchored onto the skull and a CT obtained with the frame in place for planning. High doses to the tumor are achieved by using many different fields or arcs of irradiation. The dose to the normal brain is usually clinically inconsequential. Although this approach is rarely used in children, it led to the genesis of stereotactic radiotherapy (SRT). SRT can only be delivered by a LINAC-based system (not γ-knife) and has resulted in our ability to more safely and precisely treat children with selected types of brain tumors with conventionally fractionated radiotherapy, which is better tolerated by normal brain tissue. SRT allows a much smaller volume of tissue to be treated when compared with conventional CT-based 3D conformal approaches that ultimately decrease the incidence and severity of the acute and late side effects from treatment.

Another innovative method of delivering conformal radiotherapy is IMRT. IMRT uses dynamic leaves that move across a field and modulate the dose within a given field. This treatment technique is especially useful for irregularly shaped tumors that are intimately involved with nearby critical structures such as the brain stem, and gives comparable dose distributions to stereotactic radiotherapy but can be used in even more clinical situations.

Proton radiation techniques constitute another therapeutic development that will have a tremendous impact on children. Proton radiation has the physical property of entering tissue at relatively low levels of energy and depositing all of its energy in a burst—known as the Bragg peak. In contrast, standard photon-based radiotherapy involves the beam entering the body, treating normal tissue as it traverses to the tumor (entrance dose) and then subsequently dosing normal tissue as it exits the body (exit dose) after treating the tumor. Proton radiation is especially attractive because there is no exit dose, which spares normal tissue better than any form of photon (x-ray) radiation by approximately 50%. Currently the availability of protons is limited to three institutions in the United States located in Boston, Massachusetts; Loma Linda, California; and Bloomington, Indiana. However, more proton centers are planned in the United States and throughout the world.

Common Pitfalls

The majority of children with brain tumors can be treated with durable disease control, but some require a combined approach of radiation, surgery, and chemotherapy (Table 1). These three modalities can have lasting side effects. The outcome for these children is getting better as new surgical and radiation techniques are developed and more effective chemotherapeutic regimens are developed. Better surgical techniques and approaches have improved the rates of total

TABLE 1 Summary of Treatment Modalities Used for Treatment of Selected Primary Brain Tumors

Tumor	Surgery	Radiation	Chemotherapy
Medulloblastoma/ PNET	+	+	+
Craniopharyngioma	+/−	+/−	
Ependymoma	+	+	(On protocol only)
Low-grade astrocytoma	+	+/−*	+/−†
High-grade astrocytoma	+	+	+

*If patients have a subtotal resection and have persistent/progressive clinical symptoms.
†Often used in neurofibromatosis patients and young children to delay the use of radiation for further neural development.
PNET, primitive neuroectodermal tumor.

resection, with a decrease in the risk of devastating neurocognitive or functional effects. Pediatric brain tumors are sufficiently rare and should be handled in centers of excellence that see adequate numbers of patients so that they can manage the nuances of the often complicated therapy.

Radiation therapy is a potent and necessary tool but also comes with a price in neurocognitive functioning that is more profound with younger age of treatment. Historically, radiation therapy for brain tumors during childhood has impaired intellectual development, impeded growth, and interfered with normal hormone functioning. Additionally, radiation-induced second malignancies seen in some patients decades after treatment are a concern. Such treatment complications have resulted from previously unavoidable treatment to normal tissues to adequately treat the tumor. However, the costly side effects of brain tumor treatment in children are changing dramatically in the face of new radiation and surgical technologies that better target tumor and spare normal brain. Better surgical techniques are leaving children more intact prior to starting radiation or chemotherapy. Chemotherapy effectively puts off radiation therapy in very young children with selected tumor types to allow the brain to develop more fully with good success.

Communication and Counseling

The effective treatment of pediatric brain tumors continues to improve as a result of advances in the fields of neurosurgery, chemotherapeutic agents, and radiation therapy. The cure rates continue to climb and the incidence and severity of treatment sequelae continue to diminish. However, prognosis depends heavily on the tumor type. Typically, imaging studies never fully normalize after treatment of a brain tumor, but stable imaging indicates tumor control. Additionally, advances in related medical fields such as rehabilitation medicine and endocrinology have also improved the outcome and quality of life in children with brain tumors.

SUGGESTED READINGS

1. Jemal A, Tiwari RC, Murray T, et al: Cancer statistics, 2004. CA Cancer J Clin 54:8–29, 2004. **A good cancer statistic reference.**
2. Halperin EC, Constine LS, Tarbell NJ, Kun LE (eds): Pediatric Radiation Oncology, 4th ed. New York: Raven Press. **An excellent resource for more in-depth discussion of pediatric brain tumors.**
3. Keating RF, Goodrich JT, Parker RJ (eds): Tumors of the Pediatric Central Nervous System. New York: Thieme, 2001. **An excellent resource for more in-depth discussion of pediatric brain tumors.**
4. McLean TW: Medulloblastomas and central nervous system primitive neuroectodermal tumors. Curr Treat Options Oncol 4:499–508, 2003. **A good review article on medulloblastoma.**
5. Packer RJ, Ater J, Allen J, et al: Carboplatin and vincristine chemotherapy for children with newly diagnosed progressive low-grade gliomas. J Neurosurg 86:747–754, 1997. **A landmark article on the use of chemotherapy for low-grade gliomas.**
6. Bakardjiev AI, Barnes PD, Goumnerova LC, et al: Magnetic resonance imaging changes after stereotactic radiation therapy for childhood low grade astrocytoma. Cancer 78:864–873, 1996. **Describes response and imaging changes after treatment.**
7. Tao ML, Barnes PD, Billett AL, et al: Childhood optic chiasm gliomas: Radiographic response following radiotherapy and long-term clinical outcome. Int J Radiat Oncol Biol Phys 39:579–587, 1997. **Describes response and imaging changes after treatment.**
8. Duffner PK, Horowitz ME, Krischer JP, et al: Postoperative chemotherapy and delayed radiation in children less than three years of age with malignant brain tumors. N Engl J Med 328:1725–1731, 1993. **Landmark article describing the use of chemotherapy to delay radiation therapy in pediatric brain tumor patients.**
9. Fischer EG, Welch K, Shillito J Jr, et al: Craniopharyngiomas in children. Long-term effects of conservative surgical procedures combined with radiation therapy. J Neurosurg 73:534–540, 1990. **Describes the outcome of treatment for craniopharyngiomas.**
10. Merchant TE, Kiehna EN, Sanford RA, et al: Craniopharyngioma: The St. Jude Children's Research Hospital experience, 1984–2001. Int J Radiat Oncol Biol Phys 53:533–542, 2002. **Describes the outcome of treatment for craniopharyngiomas.**
11. Lustig RH, Post SR, Srivannaboon K, et al: Risk factors for the development of obesity in children surviving brain tumors. J Clin Endocrinol Metab 88:611–616, 2003. **Describes the endocrine side effects of treatment for brain tumors.**
12. Merchant TE, Mulhern RK, Krasin MJ, et al: Preliminary results from a phase II trial of conformal radiation therapy evaluation of radiation-related CNS effects for pediatric patients with localized ependymoma. J Clin Oncol 22:3156–3162, 2004. **Describes treatment sequelae and outcome in a large modern series.**
13. Yock TI, Tarbell N: Technology Insight: proton beam radiotherapy for treatment in pediatric brain tumors. Nature Clin Pract Oncol 1:97–103, 2004. **A review of innovative radiotherapy treatments for pediatric brain tumor patients.**

Histiocytosis

Robert J. Arceci

KEY CONCEPTS

- Langerhans cell histiocytosis
  - Langerhans cell histiocytosis (LCH) is a clonal, myeloproliferative disorder of immature Langerhans cells with variable clinical behavior.
  - Diagnosis is made by biopsy of involved site.
  - Although some forms of LCH may be limited and self-resolving, others may be progressive and fatal.
  - Systemic chemotherapy significantly improves the outcome for patients with multisystem LCH.
  - Recurrent disease is common in patients with multisystem disease.
  - A poor response to the initial 6 to 12 weeks of treatment portends a very poor prognosis.
  - Adverse long-term sequelae are common and may include endocrinologic, skeletal, dental, liver, lung, neurocognitive, and neurodegenerative problems.
- Hemophagocytic lymphohistiocytosis
  - Hemophagocytic lymphohistiocytosis (HLH) is caused by an immune deficiency of cytolytic T-lymphocyte or natural killer cell functions that regulate macrophage responses.
  - HLH may be primary (inherited) or secondary (usually associated with infections or malignancy).
  - The diagnosis of HLH is based on clinical, laboratory, and genetic criteria.
  - Some patients present with initial central nervous system signs and symptoms.
  - Prompt treatment with immunochemotherapeutic approaches is critical.
  - The only known curative treatment for primary HLH is allogeneic bone marrow transplantation.
  - Genetic counseling is critical for families with primary HLH.
  - Long-term follow-up is required for patients with HLH.

Cell types and origins lead to biologically based classification of the histiocytoses. The histiocytoses are a diverse group of heterogeneous disorders that primarily involve cells of the mononuclear phagocytic system. The generic and historic term *histiocyte* derives from the Latin *histion* meaning "little web" and *kytos* meaning "cell." The histiocyte is thus a resident tissue (meaning "web") mononuclear phagocyte.

Although the two main types of histiocytes, namely dendritic cells and macrophages, are derived from a common hematopoietic progenitor cell, they can be distinguished by differences in their morphology, lineage, distinctive markers. and function. Dendritic (from the Greek *dendros,* referring to the cell's arborization) cells, and particularly Langerhans cells, are the principal antigen-presenting cells responsible for stimulating primary T-lymphocyte responses and are especially important in host immunity to virus as well as tumor or self antigens. When activated by antigen, they migrate from their primary location along lymphatic channels to parafollicular regions of lymph nodes, where they interact and stimulate antigen-specific T lymphocytes. In addition to activating T lymphocytes, Langerhans cells are capable of secreting a variety of important inflammatory cytokines, which in turn contribute to mounting immune responses.

In contrast, macrophages (from the Greek referring to "large eaters") play important roles in innate immunity through the phagocytosis of large particulate antigens, including bacteria. Following ingestion of these antigens, macrophages process and then display antigen fragments on their cell surface in order to stimulate T-lymphocyte responses. Similar to Langerhans cells, macrophages are also potent producers of immune and inflammatory cytokine-soluble mediators that act to attract lymphocytes, eosinophils, neutrophils, and other mononuclear phagocytes. In such an "inflammatory" microenvironment, macrophages can often be found to become multinucleated giant cells as well as to nonspecifically ingest red cells (erythrophagocytosis) or other hematopoietically cellular elements (hemophagocytosis). Of note, although Langerhans cells and macrophages are potent stimulators of lymphocytes, there are specific subsets of T lymphocytes that in turn suppress macrophage activation and proliferation to contain and eventually turn off immune responses.

The histiocytoses were separated in 1985 into three major classes (Box 1). These included the Langerhans cell histiocytoses (LCHs), which included the historic eponyms of eosinophilic granuloma, Hand-Schüller-Christian disease, and Abt-Letterer-Siwe disease; the non-LCHs, which included primary and secondary hemophagocytic lymphohistiocytoses (HLHs) as well as macrophage activation syndromes; and malignant histiocytoses, including disorders such as monocytic leukemia and rare malignant tumors of the mononuclear phagocytic system.

The accurate diagnosis and classification of the histiocytic disorders is of critical importance in terms of performing the proper staging workup, selecting appropriate treatment, and evaluating responses and follow-up, as well as patient and family counseling.

BOX 1 Classification of Histiocytic Disorders

I.   Histologically nonmalignant, dendritic cell proliferative disorders
   A. Langerhans cell histiocytosis
   B. Juvenile xanthogranulomatous disease
II. T-lymphocyte/macrophage activation disorders (immune reactive disorders)
   A. Hemophagocytic syndromes associated with immune deficiency
     ■ Primary or familial hemophagocytic lymphohistiocytosis
     ■ Chediak-Higashi syndrome
     ■ Griscelli disease
     ■ X-linked lymphoproliferative disease (XLP)
   B. Hemophagocytic syndromes associated with infection
     ■ Secondary or nonfamilial hemophagocytic lymphohistiocytosis
     ■ Infection-associated hemophagocytic syndrome (IAHS)
   C. Hemophagocytic syndromes associated with malignancy
     ■ Malignancy-associated hemophagocytic syndrome (MAHS)
   D. Sinus histiocytosis with massive lymphadenopathy (Rosai-Dorfman disease)
   E. Solitary histiocytoma (macrophage phenotype)
   F. Multicentric reticulohistiocytosis (frequently associated with arthritis)
   G. Generalized eruptive histiocytoma
III. Malignant disorders
   A. Monocytic leukemia (FAB classification M5)
   B. Malignant monocytic cell neoplasm
   C. Malignant dendritic cell neoplasm
   D. Malignant macrophage cell neoplasm

This chapter focuses on the most frequently encountered disorders, namely LCH and HLH.

LANGERHANS CELL HISTIOCYTOSIS

Biology, Pathophysiology, and Epidemiology

Although the cause of LCH remains unknown, the disease is demonstrated to be a clonal proliferation of immature and abnormal Langerhans cells, which further display DNA microsatellite instability and characteristic regions of chromosome loss and gain. The cytokine environment, which contributes to the local and systemic pathophysiology of LCH, is a result of the activity of the Langerhans cells, lymphocytes, and macrophages. No consistent immunologic abnormalities are identified in patients with LCH, suggesting, along with the preceding information, that the Langerhans cell is the primary cell responsible for LCH.

The estimated incidence of LCH is between 4 and 8 patients per million children. There may be as many cases in adults as well. Rare instances of familial cases are reported, particularly in identical twins but also in fraternal twins and parent/child combinations.

Diagnosis

The diagnosis of LCH should always be based on a biopsy of involved tissue, which shows characteristic Langerhans cells that are typically rounded with pale cytoplasm and folded nuclei. These cells should stain positive for expression of the surface antigen CD1a and the cytoplasmic marker S100. There is also a mixed cellular infiltrate composed of lymphocytes, eosinophils, neutrophils, macrophages, and sometimes multinucleated giant cells. The most easily accessible site should be used for biopsy. This usually means the skin or gums, but sometimes lymph nodes and bone lesions need to be biopsied to make the diagnosis.

Expert Opinion on Management Issues

CLINICAL PRESENTING FEATURES

The clinical presentation of LCH can occur at any age and be quite variable, with nearly every organ being at some risk of involvement. In addition, in some patients, the disease may be self-limited and resolve spontaneously; in others, LCH can be relentlessly progressive and fatal.

The historic eponyms of eosinophilic granuloma (usually unifocal LCH), Hand-Schüller-Christian disease (skull lesions, exophthalmos, and diabetes insipidus or, more typically, multifocal involvement) and Abt-Letterer-Siwe disease (systemic LCH) all describe various presentations of a disease that is pathologically similar. Eosinophilic granuloma usually occurs as a solitary lesion of bone associated with pain and swelling. Although the calvaria is most commonly affected, other sites include the mandible, long bones, ribs, scapulae, and vertebrae. The small bones of the hands and feet are usually spared. Lesions appear as punched-out holes and sometimes have sclerotic edges as observed by plain radiograph. Vertebra plana often manifests with back pain, and radiograph examination shows a collapsed vertebral body. MRI may also show a soft tissue component that can rarely lead to spinal cord compression. Multifocal bone involvement and eczematoid skin rash, usually involving the scalp, axillae, and groin, are characteristic of LCH in the young child, but they also can appear in adults of any age. The oral cavity is commonly involved as well as lymph nodes. Lung, liver, and brain involvement can also occur and should be carefully considered in the workup. The acute changes observed in the lung include the development of micronodular infiltrative disease, cyst formation, and pneumothoraces. Acute liver involvement includes elevated transaminases and increased bilirubin that can proceed to sclerosing cholangitis.

The most common type of brain involvement is diabetes insipidus, which may occur at any time before or during the course of the disease. LCH can also manifest with extensive systemic involvement characterized by rash, gum disease, hepatosplenomegaly, bone lesions, gastrointestinal involvement, and pancytopenia caused by splenic sequestration as well as bone marrow replacement by histiocytes. This most severe presentation of LCH most commonly occurs in infants, who may present with failure to thrive. Progression from disease that has limited involvement to severe, systemic disease is rare.

DIAGNOSTIC WORKUP AND STAGING

Once a diagnosis is made by biopsy of an involved site, the extent of disease should be determined to decide on the type of treatment that will be most useful and the likely outcome. There is no consensus for a standard workup for patients with LCH, in part because of the variable clinical presentation and course that different patients may follow.

A complete blood count and differential and liver and kidney function tests should be done in all patients to assess systemic involvement of these organs. Although the estimated sedimentation rate often correlates with the extent and activity of disease, it is nonspecific and fluctuates similar to that of other acute-phase reactants, such as fibrinogen and C-reactive protein. A urinalysis with specific gravity should be done to establish that the patient does not have diabetes insipidus. However, if there is any question of diabetes insipidus, a proper water deprivation test to document serum and urine osmolality as well as antidiuretic hormone levels is needed.

A chest radiograph should be obtained as baseline as a means of detecting clinically silent disease such as bullous cysts. An MRI with gadolinium contrast of the brain is being more frequently recommended at the time of diagnosis in order to establish baseline findings, especially in terms of the hypothalamus and pituitary region but also other areas of central nervous system (CNS) involvement, especially in patients with lesions of the skull, which may be associated with an increased incidence of subsequent adverse brain sequelae. Most patients should have a skeletal survey and a technetium bone scan because these two studies are complementary: The former study detects primarily active and older healed lesions and the latter study is better at detecting very early lesions. These studies may also be useful in following the response of patients to therapy, but both plain radiograph and bone scan may remain abnormal for months after initial presentation.

Additional diagnostic tests, such as bronchoscopy or chest CT, lumbar puncture, endocrinologic workup, bone marrow aspirate and biopsy, or gastrointestinal biopsy should be done only when there is clinical evidence for organ involvement or dysfunction.

TREATMENT AND PROGNOSIS

Patients with limited involvement of LCH usually have an excellent prognosis and may not require systemic therapy, whereas patients with multifocal skeletal lesions, refractory skin disease, or other organ involvement usually benefit substantially from systemic treatment. Although this latter group of patients has an excellent overall survival, disease recurrence is common, along with adverse long-term sequelae. The prognosis for patients with systemic disease and organ dysfunction who do not show a good response to the first 6 to 12 weeks of treatment is poor, with survival of approximately 20%.

MANAGEMENT OF PATIENTS WITH LIMITED DISEASE

Limited disease localized to the skin can be observed for regression. Nonregressing skin lesions can usually be effectively treated with topical steroids or, in more refractory cases, with the use of topical tacrolimus, nitrogen mustard, or psoralen ultraviolet-A (PUVA) phototherapy. Patients with isolated bone lesions (eosinophilic granuloma) often only require curettage of the lesion. Extensive surgery should not be done to accomplish a complete resection if that will involve potential adverse long-term outcomes. Curettage is usually sufficient to eradicate the disease, although recurrence at the same site can occur. The subsequent development of other skeletal lesions should not require more surgery or biopsy. If such a lesion is relatively asymptomatic, it may regress without treatment over a period of weeks to months. Lesions that cause significant pain but do not threaten vital structures and are not in risk sites as noted earlier can be effectively treated with local injection of corticosteroids or with oral nonsteroidal anti-inflammatory drugs such as indomethacin or ibuprofen over several weeks. When isolated lesions threaten organ function or cosmetic appearance, they may require immediate intervention with relatively low-dose radiation (usually between 400 and 1200 cGy).

MANAGEMENT OF PATIENTS WITH MULTISYSTEM DISEASE

The Italian cooperative AIEOP-CNR-HX 83 and the Austrian/German DAL-HX 83/90 trials, using such agents as vinblastine and etoposide in conjunction with prednisone, achieved 60% to 90% complete response rates, depending on the extent of involvement that patients presented. The rate of complete response was greater in patients with multifocal bone disease as compared to patients with extensive organ involvement and/or dysfunction. Overall survival was greater than 90% for patients without organ dysfunction and approximately 45% to 65% for patients with extensive disease involvement and organ dysfunction. The recurrence rate was also highest in patients with more extensive disease involvement. The first international cooperative group study, LCH-I, was a prospective, randomized trial that compared the response and outcome for patients treated with prednisone plus either vinblastine or etoposide (VP-16). This study showed no difference in response rate or outcome for patients randomized to receive vinblastine compared to those who received etoposide during the first 6 weeks of therapy. Secondly, the response of patients after 6 to 12 weeks of therapy was predictive of overall survival. Third, patients who were 2 years of age or older and who did not have pulmonary, hepatosplenic, or hematopoietic involvement had a response rate of approximately 90% and an overall survival of 100%.

A comparison of the results from the DAL-HX 83/90 study to the LCH-I study suggested that the more aggressive therapeutic approach of DAL-HX 83/90 resulted in a lower recurrence rate as well as a lower rate of diabetes insipidus. The LCH-II study was thus designed to test in a randomized fashion whether high-risk patients with multisystem LCH benefit from more aggressive treatment with VP-16, vinblastine, and corticosteroid compared to only vinblastine plus corticosteroid. The outcome results of this trial are not yet officially reported. The current LCH-III study is examining whether the addition of intermediate-dose methotrexate to prednisone and vinblastine during initial therapy and low-dose methotrexate during continuation therapy improves outcome for multisystem risk patients (Box 2).

These studies show that a subset of patients requires very minimal therapeutic interventions, whereas other patients clearly benefit from systemic treatment. Whether more aggressive multiagent therapy is the optimal approach or whether maintenance therapy significantly reduces the risk of significant recurrent disease requires further study. More effective chemotherapeutic therapies have decreased the role of radiation therapy, which now should only be used in patients with lesions that could cause acute organ damage and dysfunction, as well as cosmetic disfigurement.

ADVERSE LONG-TERM SEQUELAE AND FOLLOW-UP

Over half the patients with multisystem and/or relapsing disease have significant late effects, commonly

---

BOX 2 Stratification of Patients with Langerhans Cell Histiocytosis

Group I: Multisystem "risk" patients (eligible for randomizations)
- Multisystem patients with involvement of one or more risk organs (hematopoietic system, liver, lungs, or spleen)

Group II: Multisystem "low-risk" patients (not eligible for randomization)
- Multisystem patients with multiple organs involved but without involvement of "risk" organs

Group III: Single system "multifocal bone disease" and localized "special site" involvement
- Patients with multifocal bone disease (i.e., lesions in two or more different bones)
- Patients with localized special site involvement (e.g., "CNS-RISK" lesions with intracranial soft tissue extension or vertebral lesions with intraspinal soft tissue extension)

CNS, central nervous system.
Adapted from Histiocyte Society LCH-III Study. Description available at http://histio.org/society/protocols/trials-protocols.html (accessed November 5, 2005).

---

orthopedic problems, including arthritis; hearing loss; and dental abnormalities. CNS problems include diabetes insipidus, and approximately half of these patients develop panhypopituitarism. As patients are followed for longer periods of time, an increasing number are developing neurocognitive deficits and psychological problems as well as neurologic complications characterized by a distinctive neurodegenerative pattern of CNS involvement. Pulmonary or hepatic fibrosis may progress in some patients to such an extent that solid organ transplantation becomes necessary. Patients with LCH appear to have a lifelong susceptibility of increased risk of pulmonary disease associated with cigarette smoking. The development of secondary malignancies is also reported in patients with LCH. Similar to survivors of childhood cancer, patients with LCH require long-term follow-up by a multidisciplinary team of caretakers with knowledge of LCH.

TREATMENT OF RECURRENT LCH

Patients with recurrent disease often respond to the same drugs with which they initially were treated and showed response. However, for patients with progressive disease while on therapy, alternative approaches such as immunomodulatory therapies as well as alternative cytolytic agents are necessary. Reported responses (anecdotal) to immunosuppressive agents, such as cyclosporin A or antithymocyte immunoglobulin, appear to be transient at best. Several studies using 2-chlorodeoxyadenosine (2-CdA; Cladribine), including an international phase II trial, showed remissions in over a third of patients. Some patients with refractory disease responded to the synergistic combination of 2-CdA plus cytosine arabinoside, a regimen with proven benefit in patients with relapsed acute myelogenous leukemia. Hematopoietic stem cell transplantation is also used successfully in patients with refractory disease with variable results and significant treatment-related toxicity. Nonmyeloablative bone marrow transplantation is now being tested to try to reduce treatment-related morbidity and mortality. Targeted immunotherapy, for example with anti-CD52 antibodies (Campath) and anti-CD1a antibodies, is an interesting approach but not yet fully tested in clinical trials.

Common Pitfalls

The diagnosis and treatment of patients with LCH is exceedingly challenging. The first pitfall to avoid is not making the correct diagnosis because LCH is not included as part of the differential diagnosis of more common disorders such as malignancies, immune deficiencies, and different forms of cancer. Biopsy is required for diagnosis, but the anatomic site that is biopsied should always be the one associated with the least morbidity. For instance, it makes little sense to biopsy a skull lesion when a skin or oral lesion can be more easily biopsied.

Once a diagnosis is made, the proper approach to treatment needs to be initiated. For some patients, their disease may be self-resolving and thus not require therapeutic intervention. Unfortunately, there is no definitive test to predict which patients will have disease that self-resolves or progresses. Close follow-up is therefore required to assure that treatment can be initiated as soon as it becomes clear that the disease is not self-resolving or progressive. The use of radiation therapy should not be considered unless a vital organ is being threatened because of the increased risk of secondary malignancies. Doing surgery on a recurrent lesion when less invasive therapeutic approaches would be helpful should be avoided.

The lack of recognition of pulmonary fibrosis, sclerosing cholangitis, and neurodegenerative disease as part of the spectrum of clinical manifestations of LCH is a significant pitfall and has resulted in delays in diagnosis and therapy, even if that therapy is only supportive care.

Communication and Counseling

Patients and parents need to be made aware of the potential short- and long-term complications of having multisystem LCH. For patients with lack of response following 6 to 12 weeks of initial therapy, the prognosis is quite poor. Patients should be told that recurrent disease may be a lifelong issue in some cases, but these recurrences are usually not life-threatening. Exceptions to this include the development of significant liver and/or pulmonary disease associated with fibrosis and organ failure. To this end, hepatic toxins should be avoided, and patients should be counseled strongly never to smoke. Finally, patients need to be followed closely for long-term endocrinologic, neurocognitive, psychological, and neurodegenerative signs and symptoms.

HEMOPHAGOCYTIC LYMPHOHISTIOCYTOSIS

Biology, Pathophysiology, and Epidemiology

Although the HLH syndromes usually are the result of an immune deficit and/or dysregulatory defect, the common final pathway is the proliferation of lymphocytes and, particularly, hemophagocytic macrophages. HLH may be inherited (primary) or acquired (secondary). Several genetic causes are described that give rise to inherited syndromes that result in HLH (Table 1). A wide variety of associated etiologies are reported to be in part responsible for secondary HLH, which historically was referred to as infection-associated hemophagocytic syndrome (IAHS), viral-associated hemophagocytic syndrome (VAHS), or malignancy-associated hemophagocytic syndrome (MAHS).

Decreased numbers or defective natural killer (NK) cells or cytolytic T lymphocytes (CTLs) are fundamental to the initiation and pathophysiology of the HLH disorders. This deficiency or lack of cytolytic regulation of macrophage activity is believed to lead to extensive macrophage activation, proliferation, and hemophagocytosis along with systemic hypercytokinemia. The increased cytokine production involves excess production of a variety of inflammatory cytokines, including interleukin (IL)-2, IL-6, IL-10, IL-12, tumor necrosis factor-α (TNF-α), and interferon-γ (IFN-γ). The infiltrative lesions of such syndromes are characterized by the presence of nonclonal accumulations of activated macrophages and lymphocytes along with hemophagocytosis. The function of most organs, but particularly the liver, spleen, lymph nodes, bone marrow, and CNS, can be adversely affected as a result of such lymphohistiocytic infiltrates and the hypercytokinemia. Whether caused by an inherited or acquired immune deficiency, a variety of infectious agents, notably viruses such as Epstein-Barr virus or cytomegalic virus, can trigger or exacerbate these disorders.

Diagnosis

The diagnosis of HLH is based on clinical, laboratory, and pathologic criteria and, more recently, the

TABLE 1 T-Cell/Macrophage Activation Syndromes

Disorder	Inheritance	Gene Defect
Chediak-Higashi syndrome	AR	LYST
Griscelli syndrome	AR	Myonin Va
XLP	X	SAP
HLH	AR	Perforin, MUNC13–4

AR, autosomal recessive; HLH, hemophagocytic lymphohistiocytosis, X-linked; XLP, X-linked lymphoproliferative disease.

Adapted from Arceci RJ: The histiocytoses: The fall of the Tower of Babel. Eur J Cancer 35(5):747–767; discussion 767–769, 1999.

identification of mutations in specific genes (Box 3). In 1991, the Histiocyte Society published consensus criteria to guide in the diagnosis of HLH. Five criteria were required, including fever; hepatosplenomegaly; at least two cytopenias, hypertriglyceridemia and/or hypofibrinogenemia; and hemophagocytosis. Subsequently, additional criteria were added: hyperferritinemia, low or absent NK cell activity, and elevated CD25 levels. Thus current diagnostic criteria require five out of the eight criteria or the identification of specific gene mutations or the presence of familial disease.

Expert Opinion on Management Issues

CLINICAL PRESENTING FEATURES

Patients with primary HLH commonly present at younger than 1 year; patients with secondary HLH usually present at older ages. Patients most commonly present with fever, hepatosplenomegaly and sometimes lymphadenopathy, and skin rash characterized as eczematoid on the scalp or maculopapular on the torso. Pulmonary involvement caused by lung lymphohistiocytic infiltrates as well as the effects of hypercytokinemia leading to capillary leak can present with tachypnea and poor oxygenation. Pancytopenia secondary to hepatosplenomegaly and/or bone marrow infiltration with hemophagocytic macrophages may lead to pallor, increased bruising, and increased susceptibility to infection. In infants, failure to thrive is a common finding. Some infants present with CNS involvement, most often seizures and/or hydrocephalus.

A complete blood count and differential diagnosis demonstrate cytopenias and often pancytopenia. The

---

BOX 3 Diagnostic Criteria for Hemophagocytic Lymphohistiocytosis*

Clinical
- Fever
- Hepatosplenomegaly

Hematologic
- Cytopenias (≥2 of 3 lineages in peripheral blood)
- Hemophagocytosis

Laboratory
- Hypertriglyceridemia (fasting triglycerides ≥2 mmol/L or ≥3 standard deviations [SD] above normal)
- Hypofibrinogenemia (≤1.5 g/L or ≤3 SD below normal)
- Hyperferritinemia

Immunologic
- Low or absent natural killer (NK) function
- Elevated soluble CD25 serum levels

Additional
- Molecular demonstration of known gene mutation
- Presence of familial disease

*Diagnosis requires five out of the eight clinical and laboratory criteria or the identification of specific gene mutations or presence of familial disease.

---

hyperferritinemia and increased serum CD25 (IL-2 receptor) serum levels are surrogate markers of the inflammatory response, and the hypertriglyceridemia is believed to be secondary to cytokine down-regulation of lipoprotein lipase activity. The hypofibrinogenemia may be secondary to macrophage activity as well as a consumptive coagulopathy that is observed in these patients. Elevated liver transaminases and increased serum bilirubin is caused by hepatic dysfunction secondary to hypercytokinemia as well as lymphohistiocytic infiltration. Hemophagocytosis can be observed in any organ, but characteristically it is found in the bone marrow, liver, and spleen. Several bone marrow samples may need to be obtained before hemophagocytosis is detected. When there is CNS involvement, the cerebrospinal fluid shows a mononuclear pleocytosis. Immunologic studies show decreased or absent NK cell activity, although NK cell numbers may not be decreased. Brain MRI may show infiltrative disease as well as involvement of the leptomeninges and hydrocephalus. The identification of specific infections or concomitant cancer, especially lymphoid malignancies and particularly cutaneous T-cell lymphoma or γ/δ T-cell lymphomas, should be pursued.

TREATMENT AND PROGNOSIS

HLH is usually rapidly fatal without prompt initiation of effective treatment. Optimal initial therapy should include a combination of cytotoxic and immunosuppressive agents to obtain a complete remission. The Histiocyte Society HLH-94 and HLH-2004 international trials combined the use of VP–16, high-dose steroids, and cyclosporin A. When patients have CNS involvement, intrathecal methotrexate is recommended. Although this type of combination therapy is quite effective at achieving disease remission, the only truly curative treatment for primary HLH is allogeneic bone marrow transplantation, giving a 3-year overall survival of approximately 50% when combined with initial chemo-immunosuppressive treatment; for patients who get through bone marrow transplantation, the 3-year probability of survival is approximately 60%. The prognosis is worse for patients who go to transplant with evidence of active disease, but this is not a contraindication to going to transplant.

Patients with severe and/or persistent secondary HLH should be treated with the initial therapy as recommended by the HLH–94/HLH–2004 clinical trials, including VP–16, high-dose steroids, and cyclosporin A. If viral- or malignancy-associated etiologies are identified, specific therapies should be initiated to test for them. Patients who achieve a complete remission of their disease after the initial 8 weeks of treatment can be observed off therapy and may not require prolonged continuation therapy. However, when patients with secondary HLH show recurrence and/or progression, they may also require allogeneic bone marrow transplantation. In cases of mild, secondary HLH, less intensive therapy can be tried, such as a course of corticosteroids or intravenous gammaglobulin.

ADVERSE LONG-TERM SEQUELAE AND FOLLOW-UP

Long-term adverse sequelae may include a variety of bone marrow transplantation–associated problems, such as growth abnormalities, sexual maturation, and fertility issues, as well as secondary malignancies and the consequences of graft-versus-host disease. Neurocognitive, psychological neurologic problems (e.g., seizures) may develop as a result of HLH involvement as well as bone marrow transplantation. In addition, secondary leukemias may result from VP-16 exposure. Long-term follow-up is critical for these patients.

Common Pitfalls

The prompt and accurate diagnosis of HLH is extremely important along with the rapid initiation of appropriate treatment. In many cases, the diagnosis and treatment of these patients should be considered a medical emergency. Failure to pursue a complete diagnostic workup promptly may lead to a delay in therapy and poor outcome. It is also critical to always take a good family history to determine if consanguinity or other individuals in the family have had similar disorders, even those family members who might have died from unknown causes during infancy.

Communication and Counseling

Patients and families must be informed of the gravity of the diagnosis of HLH and an overview of the treatment, including the possible need for bone marrow transplantation and long-term adverse sequelae. In addition, it is critical to provide genetic counseling for cases of primary HLH. At the current time, no approved prenatal diagnostic test is available.

Current Controversies and Future Directions

- Determining the etiology of LCH: Neoplasia? Immune dysregulation? Something in between?
- Improving therapy and outcome for patients with refractory and/or progressive LCH.
- Reducing the frequency of disease recurrence and late complications of LCH, including lung, liver, and CNS involvement.
- Defining additional genetic causes for HLH and how they can be used for early diagnosis and genetic counseling as well as possible future therapies.
- Development of new treatment approaches to improve the approximately 50% survival plateau currently achieved.

SUGGESTED READINGS

1. Arceci RJ: The histiocytoses: The fall of the Tower of Babel. Eur J Cancer 35(5):747–767; discussion 767–769, 1999. **Detailed review of the history, biology, clinical features, and treatment of the histiocytoses.**
2. Arceci RJ, Longley BJ, Emanuel PD: Atypical cellular disorders. Hematology (Am Soc Hematol Educ Program): 297–314, 2002. **Describes the clinical features and treatment of LCH in children and adults.**
3. Arico M, Nichols K, Whitlock JA, et al: Familial clustering of Langerhans cell histiocytosis. Br J Haematol 107(4):883–888, 1999. **Characteristics of familial cases of LCH are described.**
4. Egeler RM, Neglia JP, Arico M, et al: Acute leukemia in association with Langerhans cell histiocytosis. Med Pediatr Oncol 23 (2):81–85, 1994. **Describes the types and timing of leukemias associated with LCH.**
5. Egeler RM, Neglia JP, Puccetti DM, et al: Association of Langerhans cell histiocytosis with malignant neoplasms. Cancer 71 (3):865–873, 1993. **Detailed description of the cancers associated with LCH.**
6. Feldmann J, Callebaut I, Raposo G: Munc13–4 is essential for cytolytic granules fusion and is mutated in a form of familial hemophagocytic lymphohistiocytosis (FHL3). Cell 115(4):461–473, 2003. **First description of the alternative gene mutation and pathway as a cause of primary HLH.**
7. Henter JI: Biology and treatment of familial hemophagocytic lymphohistiocytosis: Importance of perforin in lymphocyte-mediated cytotoxicity and triggering of apoptosis. Med Pediatr Oncol 38(5):305–309, 2002. **Describes the link between perforin defects and the pathophysiology of HLH.**
8. Henter JI, Arico M, Elinder G: Familial hemophagocytic lymphohistiocytosis. Primary hemophagocytic lymphohistiocytosis. Hematol Oncol Clin North Am 12(2):417–433, 1998. **Detailed description of the clinical characteristics and treatment of patients with HLH.**
9. Henter JI, Samuelsson-Horne A, Arico M: Treatment of hemophagocytic lymphohistiocytosis with HLH-94 immunochemotherapy and bone marrow transplantation. Blood 100(7):2367–2373, 2002. **Report of the outcomes of the HLH-94 clinical trial.**
10. Histiocyte Society: LCH-III Study. http://histio.org/society/protocols/trials-protocols.html (accessed November 5, 2005). **Description of an international multicenter, prospective clinical study.**
11. Laman JD, Leenen PJ, Annels NE: Langerhans-cell histiocytosis "insight into DC biology." Trends Immunol 24(4):190–196, 2003. **Detailed update on dendritic cell biology and cytokines as the information relates to the pathophysiology of LCH.**
12. Nanduri VR, Bareille P, Pritchard J, Stanhope R: Growth and endocrine disorders in multisystem Langerhans' cell histiocytosis. Clin Endocrinol (Oxf) 53(4):509–515, 2000. **Description of the long-term endocrinologic problems that patients with LCH experience.**
13. Nanduri VR, Lillywhite L, Chapman C: Cognitive outcome of long-term survivors of multisystem Langerhans cell histiocytosis: A single-institution, cross-sectional study. J Clin Oncol 21 (15):2961–2967, 2003. **Describes the long-term neurocognitive and neurologic problems encountered by patients with LCH.**
14. Stepp SE, Dufourcq-Lagelouse R, Le Deist F: Perforin gene defects in familial hemophagocytic lymphohistiocytosis. Science 286(5446):1957–1959, 1999. **First description of perforin mutations in primary HLH.**

Burkitt Lymphoma

Leslie E. Lehmann

KEY CONCEPTS

- Burkitt lymphoma (BL) is a rapidly growing tumor. The interval between the first appearance of signs or symptoms and presentation to medical attention is usually short and expeditious workup is essential.

- BL can manifest with rapidly enlarging, painless lymphadenopathy, usually involving the cervical region or Waldeyer ring. Abdominal pain (often because of ileocecal intussusception) and/or swelling or neurologic symptoms such as weakness, paresthesias, or paraplegia because of spinal cord compression from an epidural mass are other common manifestations of BL.
- Patients with abnormal immune function are known to be at an increased risk for the development of lymphoma. Thus, BL may be the first manifestation of a congenital or acquired immunodeficiency syndrome or may occur in the context of the prolonged immunosuppressive therapy required after solid organ or marrow transplantation.
- Correct diagnosis is the cornerstone of management. Diagnosis requires a tissue sample of adequate size and subsequent evaluation of morphology, flow cytometry, and both cytogenetic and fluorescent in situ hybridization evaluation looking for characteristic chromosomal abnormalities.
- The stage of disease determines therapy, and a thorough staging evaluation includes CT scans of neck/chest/abdomen/pelvis, bone marrow aspirate, lumbar puncture, and functional imaging with gallium and/or positron emission tomography scan.
- Therapy is of relatively short duration and consists of cycles of multiagent chemotherapy. Radiation is not a routine aspect of therapy for BL.
- Overall survival is good, and more than 90% of limited stage and 75% to 80% of advanced stage patients are cured. Central nervous system involvement at diagnosis is an adverse prognostic factor and only approximately 60% of those patients will be cured. Most relapses occur within months of completing therapy and patients are closely monitored during this time. There are few long-term sequelae of therapy.

Burkitt lymphoma (BL) or small noncleaved cell lymphoma (SNCCL) is an aggressive, rapidly growing neoplasm that accounts for more than one third of cases of pediatric non-Hodgkin lymphoma (NHL). BL was first described by Dennis Burkitt in 1958 when he noted an endemic tumor of the jaw among children of equatorial Africa. It was soon recognized that a pathologically identical but epidemiologically distinct tumor occurred sporadically in other parts of the world. In Africa, the tumor almost universally contains evidence of Epstein-Barr virus (EBV) DNA, and EBV infection is thus believed to be at least a contributory factor in development of malignancy. Evidence of EBV is found in less than 20% of sporadic cases of BL, however, suggesting that other factors are involved in nonendemic areas.

Histologically, BL is composed of intermediate-size lymphocytes with a very homogeneous appearance. BL has the most rapid doubling time of any neoplasm and cells undergoing mitosis are plentiful. Lighter colored macrophages are scattered among the blue lymphoma cells, resulting in the "starry sky" appearance characteristic of all rapidly dividing tumors. The lymphocytes are always of B lineage and derive from germinal center cells. Clonal immunoglobulin (Ig), usually IgM, is expressed on the cell surface. Analysis by flow cytometry reveals other B-lymphocyte specific surface markers such as CD 10, 20, and 22. Almost all cases demonstrate a chromosomal translocation between the C-*myc* oncogene on chromosome 8 and one of the Ig loci on chromosome 14 (heavy chain locus), 22 (λ light chain locus), or 2 (κ light chain locus). These translocations, by placing an oncogene adjacent to a constitutively expressed Ig constant region, presumably allow uncontrolled cellular proliferation to occur.

Expert Opinion on Management Issues

BL, perhaps because of its rapid rate of growth, is very responsive to chemotherapy. The duration and intensity of therapy depends on the stage of the disease at presentation (Box 1). Patients with limited stage disease (Murphy stage I or II), including those presenting with intussusception and undergoing complete surgical resection, are treated with three courses of moderate intensity chemotherapy, including alkylating agents such as cyclophosphamide. There is a greater than 90% chance of cure, and patients generally have minimal if any long-term complications from therapy. Patients with advanced stage disease (Murphy stage III or IV) are treated with very intensive multiagent chemotherapy including high doses of cyclophosphamide and methotrexate and administration of intrathecal chemotherapy. The duration of treatment is still

---

BOX 1 Staging System for Pediatric Non-Hodgkin Lymphoma

Stage I
- A single tumor (extranodal) or involvement of a single anatomic area (nodal), with exclusion of the mediastinum and abdomen

Stage II
- A single tumor (extranodal) with regional node involvement
- Two or more nodal areas on the same side of the diaphragm
- Two single (extranodal) tumors, with or without regional node involvement on the same side of the diaphragm
- A primary gastrointestinal tract tumor (usually in the ileocecal area) that is completely resectable, with or without involvement of associated mesenteric nodes

Stage III
- Two single tumors (extranodal) on opposite sides of the diaphragm
- Two or more nodal areas above and below the diaphragm
- Any primary intrathoracic tumor (mediastinal, pleural, or thymic)
- Extensive primary intra-abdominal disease
- Any paraspinal or epidural tumor, regardless of whether other sites are involved

Stage IV
- Any of the findings defined in stages I, II, and III with initial involvement of the central nervous system, bone marrow, or both

Based on the classification proposed in Murphy SB: Classification, staging and end results of treatment of childhood non-Hodgkin's lymphomas: Dissimilarities from lymphomas in adults. Semin Oncol 7:332–339, 1980.

quite short, however, lasting approximately 3 to 4 months. Patients can experience significant infections during this time but, as with limited stage disease, there are generally few long-term sequelae. With such therapy approximately 80% of patients are cured, including those with Burkitt or L3 leukemia (i.e., more than 25% involvement with BL cells in the bone marrow).

Patients with central nervous system (CNS) involvement at diagnosis have historically been very refractory to therapy with survival of less than 10%. The role of cranial irradiation has been examined but has not been shown to improve outcome and is not a component of current protocols. More recently, these patients have received additional therapy with drugs such as etoposide and ifosfamide and preliminary data indicate that, although survival has improved, CNS involvement remains an adverse prognostic factor.

Rituximab, a monoclonal antibody directed against CD20, has been shown in multiple studies to be active against follicular and large cell lymphomas of B cell origin. BL cells always express CD20 and current multi-institutional trials are investigating the role of rituximab in the treatment of BL (Box 2).

PREVENTION OF TUMOR LYSIS SYNDROME

A variety of methods are used to treat tumor lysis syndrome (TLS), and anticipatory care is among the most important. The patient's pretherapy tumor burden, electrolytes, renal function, and uric acid levels must be assessed. The typical findings in TLS include hyperuricemia, hyperkalemia, and hyperphosphatemia with secondary hypocalcemia. In some cases, preemptively adding allopurinol or rasburicase plus brisk intravenous hydration and urinary alkalinization may prevent the full-blown syndrome. It may be necessary to employ dialysis to treat established TLS.

Common Pitfalls

- Given the rapid proliferation characteristic of BL and the large tumor burden in those with advanced stage disease, many patients are seriously ill at presentation. Despite improvements in supportive care, fatal complications are still reported in up to 10% of patients during induction; thus, meticulous management during this time can significantly affect overall survival.
- Common problems include involvement of the gastrointestinal tract or genitourinary tract, causing symptoms of bowel obstruction or renal dysfunction. When chemotherapy is initiated, there is rapid lysis of tumor cells and patients require very close monitoring during this time.
- Complications include hyperkalemia, hyperuricemia, hyperphosphatemia with associated hypocalcemia, and even renal failure necessitating dialysis.
- Given the intensity of the therapy for advanced stage patients, infection is another serious complication and should be aggressively treated with intravenous antibiotics. Prophylaxis against Pneumocystis pneumonia is routine for this group of patients.
- If relapse occurs, cure is much more difficult to achieve. If a second remission can be attained with salvage chemotherapy and the bone marrow is uninvolved with lymphoma, high-dose chemotherapy with autologous stem cell support is the standard approach. Long-term survival has been reported in up to 50% of patients in remission at the time of transplant. In cases in which the lymphoma develops in the setting of an underlying immunodeficiency or when the bone marrow is persistently involved with lymphoma allogeneic transplant may be considered.

BOX 2 Evaluation of Patients with Small Noncleaved Cell Lymphoma

- History and physical examination including evaluation for immunodeficiency
- Complete blood count
- Serum chemistry panel: BUN, Cr, electrolytes, uric acid, calcium (Ca^{++}), PO$_4$, LDH, ALT, AST, bilirubin
- HIV testing
- Urinalysis
- Bone marrow examination (aspiration and biopsy) sent for histology/flow cytometry/cytogenetics/FISH
- CSF examination (including cell count and cytocentrifuge examination)
- Imaging studies
  - Chest radiograph
  - CT scans: chest and abdomen/pelvis, head and neck (if indicated by symptoms and physical findings)
  - Abdominal ultrasound (may be useful in initial rapid evaluation)
  - Gallium scan and/or PET scan

ALT, alanine transaminase; AST, aspartate transaminase; BUN, blood urea nitrogen; CR, creatinine; CSF, cerebrospinal fluid; HIV, human immunodeficiency virus; LDH, lactate dehydrogenase; PET, positron emission tomography; FISH, fluorescent in-situ hybridization.

Communication and Counseling

Parents are understandably devastated when a malignancy such as BL is diagnosed in their child. It is important to review with the family, ideally on multiple occasions, that the cause of BL is not known and thus there are no preventive measures that could have been taken. Additionally, there does not appear to be a genetic predisposition, so other family members are not at increased risk for developing lymphoma. The association of BL with EBV is intriguing but there is not a simple causal relationship, especially in the sporadic cases. Some, but not all, studies have suggested that exposure to pesticides is associated with the development of pediatric non-Hodgkin lymphomas, including BL, but again the relationship is not straightforward.

Therapy for BL is of short duration. For patients with limited disease, therapy can usually occur in the outpatient setting. Therapy for advanced disease is very intensive and may involve prolonged periods of hospitalization. In both situations, cure is likely and the long-term side effects associated with current regimens are minimal. If relapse occurs it is usually within the first year after therapy is finished. During that period children are seen for monthly physical examinations and screening laboratory tests such as blood counts and lactate dehydrogenase (LDH).

SUGGESTED READINGS

1. Atra A, Imeson J, Hobson R, et al: Improved outcome in children with advanced stage B-cell NHL: Results of the United Kingdom Children Cancer Study Group 9002 protocol. Br J Cancer 82:1396–1402, 2000. **More recent results of treatment of advanced stage patients excluding those with central nervous system involvement. The authors report an 87% disease-free survival and only 2.7% toxic death rate.**

2. Bowman W, Shuster J, Cook B, et al: Improved survival for children with B-cell acute lymphoblastic leukemia stage IV small noncleaved-cell lymphoma: A pediatric oncology group study. J Clin Oncol 14:1252–1261, 1996. **Results and toxicities associated with short-term intensive chemotherapy in children with advanced stage Burkitt lymphoma (BL).**

3. Buckley J, Meadows A, Kadin M, et al: Pesticide exposures in children with non-Hodgkin's lymphoma. Cancer 89:2315–2321, 2000. **The authors found a statistically significant association between risk of non-Hodgkin lymphoma and reported pesticide use in the home. No specific agents were implicated.**

4. Link M, Shuster J, Donaldson S, et al: Treatment of children and young adults with early stage non-Hodgkin's lymphoma. N Engl J Med 337:1259–1266, 1997. **This report reviews the data supporting a 9-week-only chemotherapy regimen without irradiation for children and young adults with early-stage non-Hodgkin lymphoma.**

5. Sandlund J, Downing J, Crist W: Non-Hodgkin's lymphoma in childhood. N Engl J Med 334:1238–1248, 1996. **A comprehensive review of the epidemiology, clinical features, and therapy of the most common types of childhood non-Hodgkin lymphomas.**

Visceral Tumors

William S. Ferguson

KEY CONCEPTS

- Malignant tumors of the abdominal viscera are uncommon, but often grow rapidly with only nonspecific symptoms (if any) other than a mass.
- Palpation of a mass, or unexplained abdominal or systemic symptoms, should lead to appropriate radiographic imaging; if the result is positive, a tissue diagnosis is mandatory.
- Surveillance screening is appropriate for children with certain inherited syndromes.
- With proper treatment, cure rates are generally excellent. However, because current multimodal treatments are complex and have many associated toxicities,

optimal care should be delivered by an experienced multidisciplinary team.
- Late effects of treatment remain a significant problem and require specific long-term surveillance strategies.

Malignant tumors arising primarily within the abdominal viscera are uncommon, accounting for approximately 15% of all childhood malignancies, an annual incidence of approximately 1 out of 50,000 children in the United States. These tumors often grow rapidly and frequently cause few local or systemic symptoms until they have disseminated. Thus, palpation of a large mass—either by a parent or during a routine physical examination—is often the first clue that a tumor is present. The detection of an abdominal mass obviously warrants further evaluation; however, the possibility of an occult intra-abdominal mass should also be considered in children with unexplained abdominal or systemic symptoms.

Abdominal ultrasound is probably the best initial imaging study, insofar as it provides good data about the organ from which a mass arises and whether it is solid or cystic, and also some data regarding local extension. A computed tomography (CT) scan is often superior to ultrasound in determining the exact extent of tumor and whether regional nodes are involved, which can be especially important in planning subsequent surgery. An MRI is best reserved for cases in which CT does not adequately distinguish infiltrating neoplasm from normal tissue, such as some soft tissue sarcomas. Additional imaging studies—most commonly CT of the chest and bone scan—are usually required to determine whether there is metastatic disease.

In some instances measuring serum or urine tumor markers can be diagnostically valuable. β-Human chorionic gonadotropin (β-hCG) and/or α-fetoprotein (AFP) can be elevated in some germ cell tumors, and AFP is also elevated in many liver tumors. Urinary catecholamines are elevated in many cases of neuroblastoma. It is reasonable to test for these markers even before biopsy if the appropriate tumor is suspected, because they may provide both an early clue to the correct diagnosis—thus facilitating the timely initiation of treatment—and serve as a baseline for measuring the tumor's response to therapy.

Neuroblastoma and Wilms tumor represent the most common malignant abdominal tumors, with liver tumors, germ cell tumors and retroperitoneal soft tissue sarcomas being considerably less common. Lymphomas (particularly Burkitt lymphoma), can also manifest with primary abdominal masses. Table 1 outlines the more common tumors and their associated markers and predisposing risk factors.

Expert Opinion on Management Issues

Although imaging studies may provide a clue regarding the nature of a mass, precise diagnosis requires histologic examination. In addition to obtaining sufficient

TABLE 1 Risk Factors and Tumor Markers Associated with Intra-abdominal Tumors

Tumor	Location	Markers	Risk Factors
Neuroblastoma Ganglioneuroblastoma Ganglioglioma	Adrenal/sympathetic chain	Urinary catecholamines (VMA, HVA)	Family history of neuroblastoma
Wilms tumor	Kidney		WAGR syndrome Aniridia Hemihypertrophy Neurofibromatosis type 1 Beckwith-Wiedemann syndrome Denys-Drash syndrome Perlman familial nephroblastomatosis Genital abnormalities (especially males)
Clear cell sarcoma	Kidney		
Rhabdoid tumor	Kidney		
Renal cell carcinoma	Kidney		Tuberous sclerosis Von Hippel–Landau syndrome
Hepatoblastoma	Liver	AFP	Familial adenomatous polyposis Beckwith-Wiedemann syndrome Infants of very low birth weight
Hepatocellular carcinoma	Liver	AFP	Hepatitis Viral Chemical (e.g., anabolic steroids) Metabolic (α-1-antitrypsin deficiency, tyrosinemia)
Germ cell tumors	Gonadal or extragonadal	AFP β-hCG	Familial testicular carcinoma Undescended testis
Rhabdomyosarcoma	Retroperitoneal soft tissue		Li-Fraumeni syndrome
Soft-tissue sarcomas	Liver, gallbladder Abdominal wall Intestine (rare)		Neurofibromatosis type 1 Retinoblastoma gene mutation Werner syndrome
Lymphomas	Lymph nodes Peyer patches	LDH (nonspecific)	

AFP, α-fetoprotein; β-hCG, β subunit of human chorionic gonadotropin; HVA, homovanillic acid; LDH, lactate dehydrogenase; VMA, vanillylmandelic acid; WAGR, *W*ilms tumor, *a*niridia, *g*enitourinary abnormalities or *g*onadoblastoma, mental *r*etardation.

material for conventional microscopy, immunohistochemical, biochemical, and cytogenetic characteristics are increasingly important in establishing both a precise diagnosis and in assigning a prognostic and therapeutic risk category. Although sufficient diagnostic material can sometimes be obtained by needle biopsy, either open or laparoscopic biopsy or total excision of the mass is often preferable.

With the exception of lymphomas, surgical resection remains vitally important in the successful treatment of these tumors and in some cases is curative. Complete removal with negative margins is the ideal goal, and if technically feasible it is usually performed either as the initial surgical procedure or soon after diagnostic biopsy. However, in situations in which initial resection would run the risk of unacceptable morbidity, neoadjuvant chemotherapy and/or radiation therapy can often shrink primary tumors enough to facilitate secondary resection. Thus, proper surgical management requires not only experience with pediatric tumor surgery but also careful coordination with pediatric oncology and radiation therapy, and so should be performed by pediatric surgeons as part of a multidisciplinary oncology team.

The presence of measurable metastatic disease is often of prognostic significance and usually mandates more intensive therapy. Thus, careful screening for distant spread is required once a diagnosis of malignancy is established. However, because a majority of patients have at least microscopic dissemination of their tumor at the time of diagnosis, additional adjuvant therapy is typically required even if careful staging shows no evidence for overt metastatic disease. Common metastatic sites include the liver and lungs, which are best imaged by CT. Other metastatic sites can include cortical bone (for which ^{99m}Tc bone scan is the usual screening test), bone marrow (evaluated by bone marrow aspiration and biopsy), and brain (imaged by CT or, preferably, MRI). Radioactive iodine-131-meta-iodobenzylguanidine (^{131}I-MIBG) is used for imaging neuroblastomas. Innovative imaging techniques such as rapid whole-body MRI and positron emission tomography (PET) scanning are currently being evaluated and in the future may become the modalities of choice for determining the precise extent of disease.

NEUROBLASTOMA

Neuroblastomas exhibit a tremendous variation in natural behavior and response to treatment, ranging from indolent localized tumors to aggressive disseminated disease. In addition to histologic grade, the most important prognostic features currently used to guide therapy include stage of tumor, age at diagnosis, amplification of the N-*myc* oncogene, and (among infants but not older children) DNA index. Analysis of survival data over the last 20 years suggests that neuroblastomas fall into three relatively distinct groups:

1. *Low-risk* patients are typically infants (<18 months old) with localized, hyperdiploid, N-*myc* unamplified tumors; they have a very high survival and usually require only surgical excision of the primary tumor.

2. *Intermediate-risk* patients tend to be older and have locally invasive tumors, but still without N-*myc* amplification. With moderately aggressive multiagent chemotherapy—usually including cyclophosphamide, vincristine, doxorubicin, etoposide, cisplatin and carboplatin—they will have a long-term survival rate of 80% to 90%.

3. *High-risk* patients have either distant metastases or locally invasive tumors with adverse biologic features (in particular, amplification of the N-*myc* oncogene). Traditionally this group of patients has had a dismal prognosis, with fewer than 10% being long-term survivors. More recently, the combination of very intensive chemotherapy regimens (requiring autologous stem cell support), sequential surgery, and radiation followed by maintenance therapy with *cis*-retinoic acid (which induces differentiation and apoptosis of malignant neuroblasts) has markedly improved survival, although the long-term outcome of these patients is still uncertain. The use of monoclonal antibody therapy directed against the GD2 molecule present on the surface of neural cells is also being actively investigated.

WILMS TUMOR

Surgery remains the cornerstone of the management of Wilms tumor. In the United States, complete excision of the involved kidney at the time of diagnosis is the usual practice, with four exceptions: the presence of bilateral disease, extensive tumor thrombus in the inferior vena cava (IVC), patients with a single kidney, and those with such extensive local invasion that resection would be difficult or impossible. For these patients, there is a clear-cut benefit to reducing the tumor size with chemotherapy prior to attempting surgical resection.

Postresection chemotherapy and radiation therapy are based on both the extent of tumor and the histologic appearance of the tumor. The most commonly used drugs include vincristine, actinomycin-D, and doxorubicin; cyclophosphamide and etoposide are added for the approximately 5% of children with anaplastic tumors. The prognosis for patients with either favorable histology or focal anaplasia is excellent, with 4-year survivals of approximately 95% for stage I, 90% for stages II and III, and 80% for stage IV tumors. The outcome for patients with diffuse anaplasia is poorer, with an overall survival of approximately 50% despite more intensive therapy. For patients who relapse,

intensive chemotherapy (including high-dose regimens followed by autologous bone marrow support) can be curative in some instances.

CLEAR CELL SARCOMA OF THE KIDNEY

Originally described as a variant of Wilms tumor, clear cell sarcoma of the kidney (CCSK) is now considered a completely separate entity. It is an uncommon diagnosis, comprising slightly less than 5% of patients entered on the National Wilms Tumor Study. In addition to pulmonary and hepatic metastases, this tumor has a propensity to spread to bone, brain, and soft tissue. Postsurgical treatment with vincristine, actinomycin-D, and doxorubicin plus irradiation of all tumor sites results in a 6-year survival of approximately 60%.

RHABDOID TUMOR OF THE KIDNEY

This is a rare but highly aggressive tumor of younger children (median age at diagnosis is 13 months). It can metastasize to the brain, and there is also a relatively high risk of developing second primary tumors of the CNS (usually some variety of primitive neuroectodermal tumors). This tumor usually responds poorly to chemotherapy although there have been some long-term survivors.

RENAL CELL CARCINOMA

Less than 5% of all malignant kidney tumors in children are renal cell carcinomas, although with a median age at diagnosis of 11 years they are about as common as Wilms tumor during the second decade of life. Pain and hematuria are common presenting symptoms; often the tumor cannot be palpated. Nonspecific symptoms such as malaise, fever, and nausea may be present.

The overall long-term survival of children with renal cell carcinoma is approximately 50% to 60%, but the probability of survival is strongly related to tumor stage and the ability to achieve complete surgical excision. Traditional chemotherapy has little beneficial effect. Immunotherapy with interleukin-2 and/or interferon-α appears to benefit a minority of patients.

LIVER TUMORS

Hepatoblastomas commonly arise in early childhood (median age of diagnosis is 1 year), whereas hepatocellular carcinoma tends to affect older children and often arises in the context of chronic liver disease. For both tumors, complete surgical resection is essential for cure, but can be accomplished initially for only approximately half of children with hepatoblastoma and approximately one third of those with hepatocellular carcinoma. Even with complete removal, liver tumors have a substantial risk of local or distant relapse; thus, adjuvant chemotherapy is commonly used to prevent recurrence after surgery. The most commonly used drugs are cisplatin, vincristine, and fluorouracil, although carboplatin and doxorubicin also show activity against these tumors. Chemotherapy can sometimes convert an unresectable lesion into one amenable to surgical removal.

Patients with metastatic liver tumors clearly have a worse prognosis than those with localized resectable disease, but aggressive use of surgery, chemotherapy, and radiation can lead to long-term survival in some patients. In general, hepatocellular carcinomas are more likely to manifest with local or distant invasion and are much less sensitive to chemotherapy, and so have a much poorer prognosis than hepatoblastomas. Liver transplantation is also an alternative for patients with persistent (and unresectable) disease confined to the liver, with a reported survival in small series of 20% to 40%.

GERM CELL TUMORS

Germ cell tumors (GCTs) include a wide range of tumors, ranging from benign teratomas to the very aggressive malignant germ cell tumors. GCTs are somewhat more common in girls than boys. Girls generally present during adolescence, whereas a substantial proportion of boys present during early childhood. Approximately half of childhood GCTs arise in nongonadal sites (most commonly sacrococcygeal). Serum markers can be useful in predicting the presence of malignant elements and in subsequently following response to therapy, with AFP being elevated in yolk sac/endodermal sinus tumors and in some embryonal carcinomas, and β-hCG in choriocarcinoma, some embryonal carcinomas, and some germinomas.

Overall, teratomas compose the largest group of germ cell tumors; surgery alone is usually curative for benign teratomas and probably of the majority of immature teratomas, even when small foci of malignant elements are present (with the possible exception of testicular teratomas in postpubertal males, which appear to be potentially malignant lesions regardless of stage and histologic appearance). In contrast, most patients with malignant germ cell tumors require adjuvant chemotherapy, and platinum-based therapy (most frequently a combination of cisplatin, etoposide, and bleomycin) results in 3-year event free survival over 90% for gonadal tumors and 80% for extragonadal tumors; this is superior to the results obtained in adult studies. Additional chemotherapy (including high-dose chemotherapy with autologous stem cell support) will salvage some of the small number of patients who relapse after combined surgery and chemotherapy.

RHABDOMYOSARCOMA AND OTHER SOFT-TISSUE SARCOMAS

Rhabdomyosarcoma can arise from the retroperitoneum and elsewhere in the abdomen and pelvis, including liver, uterus, bladder, and abdominal wall. Many other soft-tissue sarcomas can also arise in this part of the body and be radiographically indistinguishable from rhabdomyosarcoma. Surgery is the mainstay of treatment for these tumors, regardless of histologic type. The most important determinants of survival include degree of resection and presence or absence of metastatic disease; for rhabdomyosarcoma, patients with alveolar histology have a poorer prognosis than those with embryonal histology.

Rhabdomyosarcoma has a high propensity for metastatic spread and so invariably requires adjuvant therapy. The standard criterion is combination therapy with vincristine, actinomycin-D, and cyclophosphamide, along with radiation to any sites of gross or microscopic residual disease following initial surgery. Although children with rhabdomyosarcomas of the trunk or retroperitoneum were identified as a poor-prognosis group in the first Intergroup Rhabdomyosarcoma Study, the survival of patients with nonmetastatic tumors increased to approximately 65% in subsequent studies, presumably a result of more intensive chemotherapy.

Adjuvant therapy for nonrhabdomyosarcoma soft tissue sarcomas is less well defined. Patients with a complete gross resection, particularly with low-grade tumors, have an excellent outcome with either no additional therapy, or local radiation if there are positive surgical margins. Patients with unresectable primaries or distant metastases generally have a poor prognosis. Although doxorubicin-based chemotherapy is commonly used for these patients, its efficacy in providing long-term tumor control is unclear.

Common Pitfalls

- Although the overall incidence of malignant solid tumors in children is very low, there are clearly populations at significantly increased risk (see Table 1). These children may benefit from regular radiographic surveillance in an effort to detect malignancies at an earlier (and more easily managed) stage in their growth.
- Despite its rarity, the possibility of intra-abdominal malignancy should be kept in mind for patients with unexplained local or systemic symptoms to avoid a delay in diagnosis that may have medical or legal ramifications.
- With appropriate management, overall the cure rate for these tumors is excellent. Because treatment plans are complex and associated with many potentially serious toxicities, early referral to a center with multidisciplinary experience is essential.
- Current treatments also can cause many serious long-term effects. Patients who cannot receive long-term follow-up in an oncology center should have an individualized surveillance schedule to detect and treat these potential problems.

Communication and Counseling

Although the diagnosis of cancer is very frightening for patients and families, they should be reassured that the majority of children can be treated and cured—although the necessary treatment is often very intensive and prolonged, and the potential for long-term adverse effects cannot be ignored. Psychosocial and emotional support for these patients and families is often as valuable as the direct medical care.

Families also need education and support in terms of potential participation in clinical trials. The markedly improved outcome for children with cancer has been the direct result of carefully planned multi-institutional trials, and multiple studies have consistently shown a superior outcome for children enrolled in cooperative group treatment protocols.

SUGGESTED READINGS

1. Green DM, D'Angio GJ, Beckwith JB, et al: Wilms' Tumor. Ca Cancer J Clin 46:46–63, 1996. **A good overview of the diagnosis, staging, and treatment of Wilms tumor in children. Although several years old, the treatment guidelines are still fairly current.**
2. Kushner BH, Cheung N-KV, LaQuaglia MP, et al: Survival from locally invasive or widespread neuroblastoma without cytotoxic therapy. J Clin Oncol 14:373–381, 1996. **A series from Memorial–Sloan Kettering Cancer Institute describing the institution's successful use of surgery alone in the treatment of some intermediate-stage neuroblastomas.**
3. Lindor NM, Greene MH, and the Mayo Familial Cancer Program: The concise handbook of family cancer syndromes. J Natl Cancer Inst 90:1039–1071, 1998. **A detailed description of inherited syndromes predisposing to cancer, along with some screening recommendations.**
4. Matthay KK, Villablanca JG, Seeger RC, et al: Treatment of high-risk neuroblastoma with intensive chemotherapy, radiotherapy, autologous bone marrow transplantation, and 13-*cis*-retinoic acid. N Engl J Med 341:1165–1173, 1999. **A report from the Children's Cancer Group demonstrating improved outcome with intensive therapy augmented with retinoic acid.**
5. Pappo AS, Shapiro DN, Crist WM: Rhabdomyosarcoma: Biology and treatment. Pediatr Clin North Am 44:953–972, 1997. **An overview of rhabdomyosarcoma.**
6. Raney B: Hepatoblastoma in children: A review. J Pediatr Hematol/Oncol 339:605–615, 1998. **A concise review of hepatoblastoma, including treatment outcomes.**

Acute leukemia is the most common form of childhood cancer. There are approximately 3500 new cases every year in the United States. Acute lymphoblastic leukemia (ALL) accounts for 75% of the cases with acute myeloid leukemia (AML) making up the remainder. Acute leukemia was once an incurable disease. However, because of major advances in chemotherapy and supportive care, up to 80% of children with ALL and up to 50% of those with AML can now be cured.

Expert Opinion on Management Issues

ACUTE LYMPHOBLASTIC LEUKEMIA

The treatment of ALL consists of three phases: induction, consolidation. and maintenance. Therapy directed at the central nervous system (CNS) is a part of each phase. The intensity of therapy is determined by considering prognostic factors that help predict which patients are at high risk for relapse (Table 1).

The goal of induction chemotherapy is to induce a complete remission and restore normal hematopoiesis. This phase usually lasts 28 days. The mainstays of induction chemotherapy are glucocorticoids (prednisone or dexamethasone), vincristine and L-asparaginase. An anthracycline, such as daunorubicin, may be added for high-risk patients. A bone marrow aspirate is performed on day 7 or day 14 to determine early response. Complete remission is achieved by more than 95% of patients by the end of the induction phase.

Consolidation (also called intensification) is a period of intensified therapy immediately after the induction of remission. The drugs used in this phase vary widely by protocol. Drugs with little cross-resistance to those drugs used during induction are often used. Intermediate- or high-dose methotrexate is frequently employed

21

Acute Leukemia

Anna Keating Franklin and Peter G. Steinherz

KEY CONCEPTS

- Children with acute leukemia should be referred to a tertiary care center and treated under the supervision of a pediatric oncologist. Ideally, treatment should be administered according to a clinical research protocol.
- Up to 85% of children with acute lymphoblastic leukemia (ALL) survive more than 5 years after the diagnosis.
- Relapsed or refractory acute myeloid leukemia (AML) carries a poor prognosis.
- Allogeneic bone marrow transplantation is considered during a second complete remission in ALL and in the first complete remission in AML.
- Survivors of childhood leukemia should be followed closely because treatment-related side effects can occur months to years after treatment.

TABLE 1 Characterization of Risk Factors for Treatment Failure in ALL

Characteristic	High Risk	Low Risk
WBC at diagnosis	$\geq 50,000/mm^3$	$<50,000/mm^3$
Age	<1 year or $\geq$10 years	1 to 9 years
Cytogenetics	t(9;22) BCR-ABL t(4;11), MLL hypodiploidy (<45 chromosomes)	trisomy 4, trisomy 10 t(12;21) TEL-AML1 Hyperdiploidy (>50 chromosomes)
Response to therapy	Late responder (not in complete remission at end of induction)	Rapid early responder (<5% blasts by day 7)
Immunophenotype	T cell, mature B cell	Precursor B cell
CNS status	Positive	Negative
Ethnic background	African American, Hispanic	White, Asian
Gender	Male	Female

ALL, acute lymphoblastic leukemia; CNS, central nervous system; MLL, mixed lineage leukemia; WBC, white blood cell.

during this phase. Use of L-asparaginase is usually continued into the consolidation phase.

The maintenance phase consists of less intensive chemotherapy to minimize the risk of a late relapse. The two mainstays of this phase are oral methotrexate and 6-mercaptopurine (6-MP). Methotrexate is ideally administered intermittently and is typically given once weekly, whereas 6-MP is most effective when administered continuously, so it is dosed daily. The doses of these drugs are adjusted to maintain an absolute neutrophil count of between 1000 and 2000/μL. "Pulses" of vincristine and prednisone are often added as well. The total duration of therapy for ALL is 2.5 to 3 years. Boys are treated longer than girls because boys have a higher rate of late relapse, even when testicular relapse is excluded.

CNS therapy may consist of cranial irradiation or the intrathecal administration of chemotherapy. Cranial irradiation is reserved for the highest-risk patients (those with hyperleukocytosis or T-cell ALL) because of its severe long-term side effects. Intrathecal methotrexate is the mainstay of CNS prophylaxis and therapy. Intrathecal cytarabine and hydrocortisone may be added for certain patients. The chemotherapy is dosed according to age, which correlates with cerebrospinal fluid (CSF) volume. Systemic administration of dexamethasone is thought to have better CNS penetration than prednisone, but this benefit must be balanced with the adverse effects of dexamethasone.

Seventy-five percent of children with ALL will survive at least 5 years from diagnosis with chemotherapy alone. Because of this, allogeneic stem cell transplantation is not recommended for patients in a first remission. The exceptions are patients with the Philadelphia chromosome or those who fail to achieve remission at the end of the induction phase, both of which confer a very high risk of relapse. Children with ALL who relapse should be referred for allogenic stem cell transplantation once they achieve a second complete remission. However, HLA typing of the patient and siblings should begin as soon as a relapse is diagnosed. This allows adequate time for an unrelated donor search, if necessary.

Mature B-cell ALL is a rare form of ALL. The blasts in this type of ALL are identical to those in Burkitt lymphoma. Because of the rapid doubling time of these blast cells, patients may have an extensive disease burden at the time of diagnosis and are at high risk of developing tumor lysis syndrome (see section "Supportive Care"). These patients do very well with abbreviated intensive chemotherapy, as opposed to the prolonged therapy of other forms of ALL.

ACUTE MYELOID LEUKEMIA

Treatment of AML is divided into two stages: induction and consolidation. CNS prophylaxis is also a part of therapy for AML. However, maintenance therapy is not a part of most pediatric AML protocols because it has not been shown to reduce the risk of relapse or prolong survival. Therapy for AML is much more intensive than therapy for ALL. Five percent to 10% of

children with AML die of complications, such as hemorrhage or infection, so they require intense supportive care.

The two most effective drugs in AML are cytarabine and anthracyclines. The most commonly used anthracycline in children with AML is daunorubicin. Induction chemotherapy consists of cytarabine and daunorubicin in combination with other drugs, such as etoposide and/or thioguanine. The intensity of induction chemotherapy is very important in the overall outcome of children with AML. Increasing the intensity of therapy can be achieved by decreasing the interval between courses of chemotherapy, prolonging the duration of therapy or by using high-dose cytarabine. Consolidation therapy may include intensive chemotherapy. However, patients with a human leukocyte antigen (HLA)-matched related donor should be referred for allogeneic stem cell transplantation after remission has been achieved.

Unfortunately, up to half of children with AML relapse. The length of the first remission is an important prognostic factor. Patients with a first remission of less than 1 year have a lower rate of achieving a second remission and a lower overall survival. Treatment of relapsed AML consists of high-dose cytarabine in combination with other agents, which may include mitoxantrone, fludarabine, and idarubicin, or L-asparaginase. Consolidation therapy after a second remission is attained may include allogeneic stem cell transplantation or additional intensive chemotherapy.

Acute promyelocytic leukemia (APL) is a distinct subtype of AML. It has a characteristic chromosomal abnormality, a translocation between chromosomes 15 and 17, which produces PML-RARa fusion protein. This fusion protein makes APL very sensitive to differentiating agents, such as all-*trans*-retinoic acid (ATRA) and arsenic trioxide. Treatment of APL consists of ATRA alone or in combination with chemotherapy for remission induction. Patients with APL have a very high risk of severe hemorrhagic complications with induction therapy. Maintenance therapy with retinoic

TABLE 2 Late Complications of Treatment for Childhood Leukemia

Complication	Associated Treatment
Brain tumor	Cranial irradiation
Acute myeloid leukemia	Epipodophyllotoxins, alkylating agents, anthracyclines
Cardiomyopathy	Anthracyclines
Encephalopathy	Cranial irradiation, methotrexate, glucocorticoids
Avascular necrosis of bone	Glucocorticoids, local irradiation
Osteoporosis	Cranial irradiation, glucocorticoids, antimetabolites
Short stature	Cranial irradiation, intensive chemotherapy
Obesity	Cranial irradiation, glucocorticoids
Thyroid dysfunction	Cranial and neck irradiation, intensive chemotherapy
Ovarian or testicular failure	Intensive chemotherapy

TABLE 3 Medication Tables

Generic Name (Trade Name) OTC/Rx	Dosage/Route/ Regimen	Maximum Dose	Dosage Formulations	Common Adverse Reactions	Comments
Acute Lymphoblastic Leukemia Chemotherapy					
Vincristine (Oncovin) Rx	1.5 mg/m^2 IV	2 mg		Peripheral neuropathy	Induction, consolidation, maintenance
Prednisone (multiple) Rx	40–180 mg/m^2 PO tid	None	Tablets: 1, 2.5, 5, 10, 20, 25, 50 mg Liquid: 5 mg/5 mL, 5 mg/mL	Immunosuppression, hypertension, hyperglycemia, obesity, mood changes, cataracts, osteoporosis	Induction, consolidation, maintenance
Dexamethasone (Decadron) Rx	6–10 mg/m^2 PO qd	None	Tablets: 0.25, 0.5, 0.75, 1, 4, 6 mg Elixir: 0.5 mg/ 0.5 mL Solution: 4, 10, 20 mg/mL	Immunosuppression, hypertension, hyperglycemia, obesity, mood changes, cataracts, osteoporosis, avascular necrosis	Induction, consolidation, maintenance
L-Asparaginase (Elspar) Rx	6000 U/m^2 IM q MWF	None	10,000 units powder for injection	Hypersensitivity, pancreatitis, hemorrhage, thrombosis, hyperglycemia	Induction, consolidation
PEG-Asparaginase (Oncaspar) Rx	2500 IU/m^2 IM q 14 days	3750 units		Hypersensitivity, pancreatitis, hemorrhage, thrombosis, hyperglycemia	Induction, consolidation
Daunorubicin Rx	20 to 60 mg/m^2 IV	Cumulative 350 mg/m^2 Hemorrhagic cystitis, hair loss, myelo-suppression		Vesicant, cardiomyopathy, arrhythmias	Induction for high risk patients
Cyclophosphamide (Cytoxan) Rx	1000 mg/m^2 IV	None			Consolidation
Mercaptopurine	75 mg/m^2 PO qd				Maintenance
Methotrexate Rx	20 mg/m^2 PO q wk			Nausea/vomiting, stomatitis, myelosuppression	Maintenance
Acute Myeloid Leukemia Chemotherapy					
Daunorubicin Rx	20 to 45 mg/m^2 IV	Cumulative 350 mg/m^2		Vesicant, cardiomyopathy, arrhythmias	Induction
Cytarabine (Cytosar) Rx	100–200 mg/m^2 or 1–3 g/m^2 IV	None		Nausea/vomiting, stomatitis, myelosuppression, alopecia	Induction, consolidation
Thioguanine Rx	50 to 100 mg/m^2 PO bid	None		Myelosuppression	Induction, consolidation
Etoposide Rx	100 mg/m^2 IV	None		Nausea/Vomiting, myelosuppression, hypotension during infusion	Induction
Dexamethasone (Decadron) Rx	2 mg/m^2 PO/IV tid	None		Immunosuppression, hypertension, hyperglycemia, obesity, mood changes, cataracts, osteoporosis, avascular necrosis	Induction
Central Nervous System Leukemia Intrathecal Chemotherapy					
Methotrexate	<1 yr: 6 mg; 1–2 yr: 8 mg; 2–3 yr: 10 mg; >3 yr: 12 mg	12 mg		Nausea/vomiting, headache	
Cytarabine (Cytosar) Rx	<1 yr: 20 mg; 1–2 yr: 30 mg; 2–3 yr: 50 mg; >3 yr: 70 mg	70 mg		Fever, nausea/vomiting, headache	

bid, twice daily; IM, intramuscularly; IV, intravenously; PO, orally; q, every; qd, each day; Rx, prescription; tid, three times daily.

acid has been shown to reduce the risk of relapse and improve overall survival, unlike other forms of AML.

SUPPORTIVE CARE

Children with leukemia require intensive supportive care at diagnosis and during treatment. Tumor lysis syndrome is an emergency and may be present at diagnosis. It is a constellation of metabolic abnormalities that occur when leukemia cells die and release their intracellular contents into the circulation. It can result in hyperkalemia, hyperuricemia, hyperphosphatemia, and hypocalcemia. Renal failure and cardiac arrest may occur as a result. Tumor lysis syndrome can be prevented with aggressive intravenous hydration, urinary alkalinization with sodium bicarbonate, allopurinol, or urate oxidase (Elitek [rasburicase]) to lower serum uric acid levels and phosphate binders to lower serum phosphorus levels.

Chemotherapy-induced neutropenia places a child with leukemia at very high risk for infection. When patients are neutropenic and have a fever, intravenous broad-spectrum antibiotics should be started promptly because of the risk of overwhelming sepsis. During this time, granulocyte-colony stimulating factor (G-CSF) can be administered to decrease the duration of the neutropenia. Anemia and thrombocytopenia caused by chemotherapy may require transfusion support. All blood products should be irradiated and leukocyte-depleted. Patients who do not have positive cytomegalovirus (CMV) immunoglobulin (Ig) G levels at diagnosis should receive CMV-negative blood products.

Prophylaxis against *Pneumocystis carinii* pneumonia should be administered to all patients undergoing treatment for leukemia. Trimethoprim-sulfamethoxazole can be given 3 days per week. Alternatives include dapsone, atovaquone, or inhaled pentamidine.

Patients should have varicella zoster titers drawn at the time of diagnosis. Nonimmune patients with significant exposure to varicella or zoster should receive varicella-zoster immune globulin as soon as possible. Patients who develop primary varicella or zoster while they are receiving therapy for leukemia require therapy with acyclovir or other antiviral to prevent disseminated infection.

Common Pitfalls

Although chemotherapy and radiation therapy can cure children of the life-threatening disease of acute leukemia, these treatments also affect normal tissues. One of the primary reasons leukemia patients undergo risk stratification is to balance efficacy and toxicity of therapy (Table 2). Glucocorticoids have many adverse effects. Acutely, they can cause gastrointestinal distress, hypertension, hyperglycemia, and increased susceptibility to infection. Long-term effects of glucocorticoids can include avascular necrosis of bone, osteoporosis, short stature, and obesity. Anthracyclines can cause congestive heart failure, which may occur years after the end of treatment. This can be minimized by

not exceeding a cumulative dose of 350 mg/m^2. Dexrazoxane is a free-radical scavenger that is currently being studied as a cardioprotectant to be administered immediately prior to the anthracycline (Table 3).

The most serious late effects are secondary malignancies. Epipodophyllotoxins (such as etoposide), anthracyclines, and alkylating agents can all cause secondary AML. Remission is more difficult to achieve and maintain in these patients compared to those with de novo AML. Cranial irradiation at doses up to 2400 cGy used in previous eras increases the risk of brain tumors. Lower doses of 1200 to 1800 cGy are currently being used in hopes of decreasing the risk of brain tumors.

Communication and Counseling

A diagnosis of leukemia can be very frightening to the patient and the family. Although intensive therapy will be required, a multidisciplinary team of pediatric oncologists, nurse practitioners, a psychologist or psychiatrist, pharmacists, and social workers can help the family through this time. It is important to assure the family that it was not anything they did to cause the leukemia and there was nothing that could have been done to prevent the leukemia. The leukemia is usually not familial or inherited.

SUGGESTED READINGS

1. Ebb DH, Weinstein HJ: Diagnosis and treatment of childhood acute myelogenous leukemia. Pediatr Clin North Am 4:847–862, 1997. **A comprehensive review of the diagnosis and management of AML for primary care physicians.**
2. National Cancer Institute online: Childhood acute lymphoblastic leukemia (PDQ): Treatment. Available at http://www.cancer.gov/cancerinfo/pdq/treatment/childALL/healthprofessional (accessed November 3, 2005). **An evidence-based summary of ALL that is updated regularly by pediatric oncology specialists.**
3. National Cancer Institute online: Childhood acute myeloid leukemia/other myeloid malignancies (PDQ): Treatment. Available at http://www.cancer.gov/cancerinfo/pdq/treatment/childAML/healthprofessional (accessed November 3, 2005). **An evidence-based summary of AML that is updated regularly by pediatric oncology specialists.**
4. Pui CH, Evans WE: Acute lymphoblastic leukemia. New Engl J Med 339:605–615, 1998. **A review of the biology and therapy of ALL.**

Malignant Tumors of Bone and Limb Salvage

Brian E. Brigman and Mark C. Gebhardt

KEY CONCEPTS

- Malignant bone tumors are the third most common childhood malignancy behind leukemias and lymphomas. Most patients with a malignant bone tumor present with pain or a mass.

- The workup of a suspected malignant bone tumor should include plain radiographs of the bone in question, an MRI of the entire bone in question, a CT scan of the chest, and a whole body bone scan. A biopsy is necessary for diagnosis but should be deferred until the rest of the workup is complete.
- The biopsy of suspected malignant bone tumors should be performed by an experienced musculoskeletal surgical oncologist, as an incorrectly performed biopsy may limit limb salvage options.
- Treatment of osteosarcoma and Ewing sarcoma should include systemic chemotherapy and local control (surgery for osteosarcoma, surgery or radiation for Ewing sarcoma). Approximately 90% of limbs with malignant bone tumors can be salvaged.

Malignant bone tumors are rare, but they represent the third largest group of malignancies in childhood, following behind lymphomas and leukemias. Osteosarcoma and Ewing sarcoma make up approximately 90% of the cases of malignant bone tumors in children and adolescent patients. Changes in treatment over the last 30 years have resulted in significant increases in both life expectancy and function in patients with malignant tumors of bone. Prior to the institution of chemotherapy in the treatment of these tumors, the treatment was a radical amputation or disarticulation above a tumor. This resulted in 5-year survival in approximately 20% of osteosarcoma patients and 10% of Ewing sarcoma patients. The use of chemotherapy, starting in the 1970s, increased survival to 60% to 70%. At the same time, advancing imaging modalities have permitted improved staging, and improvements in surgical techniques have allowed for wide resection of malignant tumors with salvage of the limb without an increase in local recurrence of tumor or a decrease in patient survival.

Expert Opinion on Management Issues

SIGNS AND SYMPTOMS

Patients with malignant bone tumors typically present with pain or with pain and a mass. In general, they do not appear to be ill. A deep ache, frequently worse at night, is often described. Tumors in the lower extremity often cause a limp and, in the spine or pelvis, may mimic a disc herniation. The duration of symptoms prior to diagnosis averages approximately 3 months. Rarely, a pathologic fracture may be the initial presentation.

EVALUATION

After a history and physical examination, the initial step in the evaluation is orthogonal plain radiographs of the entire bone in question. Nearly all malignant bone tumors can be recognized on radiograph. A permeative osseous lesion with both radiodense and radiolucent areas and cortical destruction is typical of osteosarcoma. A Codman triangle (elevation of the periosteum at the upper or lower edge of the tumor) is often present but is not pathognomonic of a malignant bone tumor. Cortical soft-tissue extension may produce radiating spicules of bone resulting in the characteristic "sun-ray" appearance.

Ewing sarcomas typically manifest as permeative lesions with cortical destruction and a predominantly radiolucent component. Layers of periosteal reactive bone, a so-called onion skin appearance, may be present.

STAGING

Staging evaluates both local and distant extent of disease. Evaluation of the local extent of tumor is best seen by MRI. The relation of the soft-tissue extent of the tumor to the surrounding neurovascular structures is best seen on the axial images and aids in the planning of local control. The entire affected bone should be imaged to evaluate the intraosseous extent of tumor, and skip lesions (metastatic foci within the bone containing the primary tumor). The MRI should be obtained prior to biopsy of a lesion, as the edema from a biopsy may alter the ability to interpret the staging studies.

When sarcomas metastasize, they typically do so via the hematogenous route. The lungs, therefore, are the most common site of metastatic disease. A CT of the chest is used to evaluate the patient for pulmonary metastatic disease. A ^{99m}Tc bone scintigraphy (bone scan) is used to evaluate for the less common metastatic disease to bone.

More than 75% of patients with osteosarcoma present with local soft-tissue extension of the tumor outside the bone. Approximately 10% to 20% have detectable metastatic disease at presentation. The figures for Ewing sarcoma are similar: There is almost uniformly a soft-tissue mass. Roughly 25% of patients have metastatic disease at presentation.

BIOPSY

Following appropriate staging studies, the lesion must be biopsied for a tissue diagnosis. Because an improperly placed biopsy incision may compromise the subsequent local treatment, biopsy of musculoskeletal tumors should generally be done by the surgeon who will be responsible for the final management of the tumor. The biopsy should be planned with the definitive surgical procedure in mind, because the biopsy tract will be considered contaminated and will necessarily be removed en bloc with the tumor at the time of tumor resection.

Core needle biopsy has the advantages of less morbidity and lower cost compared to open biopsy, but it may not provide sufficient tissue for special studies such as molecular diagnostic studies and is subject to sampling error. Core needle biopsy may be done under CT or fluoroscopic guidance for lesions that are difficult to reach.

If an open biopsy is undertaken, transverse incisions should be avoided in the extremity and the biopsy should traverse the minimum number of anatomic compartments. Neurovascular structures should be avoided. The biopsy specimen should be taken from the periphery of the soft-tissue mass. If there is no soft-tissue extension, a small round or oval window in the cortex should be fashioned to decrease the risk of pathologic fracture. Meticulous hemostasis must be obtained to avoid a hematoma or ecchymosis that may spread tumor cells through previously uninvolved planes.

OSTEOSARCOMA

Osteosarcoma, a sarcoma in which malignant cells produce osteoid, or immature bone, is the most common malignant tumor of bone in childhood. Osteosarcomas are a heterogeneous group of tumors, and may be divided into subgroups based on location in the bone, intramedullary versus surface (parosteal and periosteal) or histologic subtype. The most common osteosarcoma is the high-grade intramedullary osteosarcoma.

The peak incidence of osteosarcoma is in the second decade of life (approximately 0.7 cases per 100,000 persons). Osteosarcoma occurs across all racial lines and affects males and females in a ratio of 1.5:1.

Osteosarcomas occur most commonly in the metaphyseal segment adjacent to rapidly growing physes. The most common locations are therefore the distal femur (35%), proximal tibia (20%), and proximal humerus (10%).

The etiology of osteosarcoma is unknown, but several risk factors are now delineated. Osteosarcoma is the most common secondary malignancy in children with retinoblastoma and patients with osteosarcoma often show loss of heterozygosity in the Rb locus on chromosome 13. Alterations in the p53 locus, such as occurs in the Li-Fraumeni syndrome, are also common in osteosarcoma patients. Ionizing radiation and alkylating chemotherapeutic agents each increase the risk of developing osteosarcoma.

Therapy

Treatment of high-grade osteosarcoma includes systemic therapy for control of presumed micrometastatic or measurable metastatic disease, coupled with local control of the tumor by amputation or limb salvage surgery. Low-grade osteosarcomas such as parosteal osteosarcoma are usually treated with surgery alone. Radiation therapy is seldom used for local control of an osteosarcoma.

The use of adjuvant chemotherapy in the treatment of patients with osteosarcoma has increased survival from approximately 10% to 20% to approximately 60% to 70% at 5 years. Current protocols involve multiagent chemotherapy including doxorubicin, cisplatin, and high-dose methotrexate with leucovorin rescue. This is typically given in a neoadjuvant (preoperative) fashion over the course of 8 to 12 weeks, at which time local control is achieved after staging studies are repeated. Following surgery, tumor response (necrosis) to the preoperative chemotherapy can be assessed histologically; the chemotherapy regimen may be altered if response is poor. Tumor response to chemotherapy, as measured at the time of resection, is the most important predictor of survival in osteosarcoma patients. To date, however, changing chemotherapy in patients who have not had good histologic necrosis has not led to improved survival.

Patients with metastatic disease at presentation are also treated with chemotherapy and resection of pulmonary metastases and the primary tumor if possible. Those that can be rendered surgically disease-free have an approximately 30% to 40% chance of long-term survival.

EWING SARCOMA

Ewing sarcoma is a high-grade small round blue cell tumor of uncertain histogenesis that arises in bone or soft tissue. Ewing sarcoma is the second most common malignant tumor of bone in the pediatric age group. The peak incidence of 0.5 cases per 100,000 patients occurs in the second decade of life. There is a 1.5:1 male to female ratio. Ewing sarcoma almost never occurs in patients of African descent and is rare in patients of Asian descent.

The most common location for Ewing sarcoma is the metaphyseal or metadiaphyseal region of long bones, but it can occur in the diaphyses. The femur is the most common site (25%), followed by the pelvis (20%), tibia (15%), and shoulder (10%).

A consistent reciprocal chromosomal translocation, t(11;22)(q24;q12), is seen in 90% of Ewing sarcoma cases. This translocation is also seen in peripheral neuroectodermal tumors (PNET), which have a similar histologic appearance and clinical behavior. This similarity has led most investigators to conclude that Ewing sarcoma is of neuroectodermal origin, and currently these tumors are treated with identical protocols.

Therapy

As with other high-grade sarcomas, therapy is a combination of systemic and local control. In the absence of chemotherapy for systemic control, survival at 5 years following local control of the tumor is approximately 10%. Chemotherapeutic protocols for Ewing sarcoma typically include vincristine, dactinomycin, cyclophosphamide, and doxorubicin. Therapy is delivered both pre- and postoperatively, and changes in therapy are dictated by tumor response to chemotherapy as measured histologically at the time of tumor resection.

Local control of Ewing sarcomas can be achieved with either surgery, radiation therapy, or, in certain circumstances, both. Some studies have shown that the recurrence rate in patients treated with radiation is higher than in those treated with surgery for extremity lesions. This, coupled with the late effects of radiation, including limb-length discrepancy, joint fibrosis, and risks of radiation-induced secondary malignancy, has made surgery a more attractive option for accessible lesions. No differences in recurrence rates or survival have been demonstrated for pelvic lesions between surgical and radiation therapies. Doses of 50 to 65 Gy are used for treatment.

LIMB-SALVAGE SURGERY

Surgery for malignant bone tumors involves resection of the tumor with a margin of normal tissue surrounding the tumor—a wide margin. If this can be done sparing the neurovascular bundle of the extremity, thereby leaving a functional limb following reconstruction, then limb salvage can be attempted. If a wide margin cannot be obtained, an amputation should be considered. As mentioned, limb salvage is possible in approximately 90% of pediatric malignant bone tumors. The goal of limb salvage is to give the patient a *functional* extremity. Patients must be helped to understand that their limb will not be *normal*, that they will be subject to limitations of activity and that complications of limb-salvage surgery, including infection, fractures, and revision of prostheses, are common.

Reconstruction options following tumor resection depend on the bone involved, the location of the tumor within the bone, the extent of bony and soft-tissue resection, the age of the patient and the expertise of the surgeon. Lesions in *expendable* bones such as the fibula, ilium, ribs, metacarpals and metatarsals, clavicle, and scapular body can be resected without a bony reconstruction. Diaphyseal lesions in which the articular surfaces can be preserved can be reconstructed with fresh-frozen allograft or autograft bone. Allografts are procured sterilely from donors who are screened for transmissible diseases such as human immunodeficiency virus (HIV), hepatitis, and bacteria and kept frozen in bone banks until needed. Autograft bone (the patient's own bone) is in more limited supply and generally is harvested from the iliac crest or fibula with or without a vascular pedicle.

Because of their common metaphyseal location, most malignant bone tumors require resection of an articular surface for an adequate margin. Reconstruction options include creating a mobile joint or performing an arthrodesis. Reconstruction of a mobile joint requires the use of a metal prosthesis, an osteoarticular allograft or a combination of allograft and prosthesis to replace resected bone and joint.

In the pediatric patient, limb length discrepancy following reconstruction should be considered. This is particularly an issue in patients less than 10 years of age with tumors in the distal femur, the most active physis in the body. Expandable metallic prostheses, which require interval surgical procedures for lengthening, are being developed, but few long-term outcome studies are available. More recently a temporary prosthesis that can be expanded without surgical intervention has become available; however, no long-term studies on this prosthesis are available. Another option in this patient group is the Van Nes rotationplasty. A rotationplasty fuses the tibia to the remaining proximal femur after rotation of the tibia 180 degrees to allow the ankle joint to function as a knee joint in a prosthesis. In patients with a rotationplasty, the reconstructed leg functions like a below-the-knee amputation; thus, an external prosthesis is required.

The results of these reconstruction options vary with the age of the patient, the type of reconstruction, the location of the tumor, and the amount of tissue resected. In general, both allografts and metallic prostheses provide functional outcomes in approximately 70% of children with osteosarcoma and Ewing sarcoma. The parents and child must weigh the treatment options and must be helped to appreciate that amputation and rotationplasty are less complicated procedures with fewer potential complications. For very athletic and very young children, amputation may be preferable. With modern prostheses in the lower extremity, patients can have good function without the risk of injury to the reconstruction.

Common Pitfalls

- Failure to recognize a patient with a malignant bone tumor is a serious and avoidable pitfall. Patients with a mass or continued complaints of pain deserve radiographic evaluation. Patients with spine or pelvic tumors may have atypical pain patterns.
- An improperly done biopsy may not only provide insufficient tissue for diagnosis, but may compromise the ability to perform limb-salvage surgery safely, necessitating an amputation.
- Patients should understand that a salvaged limb will not be a normal limb. If the patient is not willing to accept limitations of activities, then he or she should consider an amputation or rotationplasty, or be prepared for earlier failure or revision of the salvaged limb.

Communication and Counseling

Counseling patients and families of patients with malignant bone tumors is sobering. It is important to help both child and family understand that although in the past a diagnosis of a malignant bone tumor meant an amputation followed by an 80% chance of succumbing to their disease, these figures are now nearly reversed; currently 60% to 70% of patients who present with sarcoma and osteosarcoma without metastases can expect long-term survival with a functional extremity. Both the patient and family should be counseled, however, that the results of limb-salvage surgery are not perfect and that salvaged limbs are not normal limbs. There will be limitation of activity, and probably additional surgery will be required for patients electing limb salvage options. There is still much to be learned and achieved to decrease tumor drug resistance and to develop chemotherapeutic agents and better reconstruction methods.

SUGGESTED READINGS

1. Brigman BE, Hornicek FJ, Gebhardt MC, Mankin HJ: Allografts about the knee in young patients with high-grade sarcoma. Clin Orthop Rel Res 421:232–239, 2004. **Results of allograft reconstructions after resections of osteosarcoma and Ewing sarcoma in patients 18 years old or younger.**

2. Doubousset J, Missenard G, Kalifa C: Management of osteogenic sarcoma in children and adolescents. Clin Orthop Rel Res 270:52–59, 1991. **Review of one institution's results with various reconstruction methods after sarcoma resection in young patients.**

3. Eckardt JJ, Kabo JM, Kelley CM, et al: Expandible endoprosthesis reconstruction in skeletally immature patients with tumors. Clin Orthop Rel Res 373:51–61, 2000. **One institution's experience with expandable prosthetic reconstructions in the skeletally immature.**

4. Enneking WF, Spanier SS, Goodman MA: Current concepts review: The surgical staging of musculoskeletal sarcoma. J Bone Joint Surg 62A:1030–1980, 1980. **Description of the staging system used for bone sarcomas.**

5. Mankin HJ, Mankin CJ, Simon MA: The hazards of the biopsy, revisited: Members of the Musculoskeletal Tumor Society.

J Bone Joint Surg 78A:656–663, 1996. **Description of problems associated with improper biopsy of musculoskeletal tumors.**

6. Rougraff BT, Simon MA, Kneisl JS, et al: Limb salvage compared with amputation for osteosarcoma of the distal end of the femur: A long-term oncological, functional and quality-of-life study. J Bone Joint Surg 76A:649–656, 1994. **Article indicates there is no significant difference in outcomes seen between amputees and limb-salvage patients.**

7. Widhe B, Widhe T: Initial symptoms and clinical features in osteosarcoma and Ewing sarcoma. J Bone Joint Surg 82A:667–674, 2000. **A mass and pain are the most common presenting symptoms of Ewing sarcoma.**

8. Winkelmann WW: Rotationplasty. Orthop Clin N Am 27:503–523, 1996. **Overview of rotationplasty as a reconstruction option.**

22 Mental Development and Behavioral Disorders

Psychiatric Disorders and Mental Health Disorders

Lee I. Ascherman, James T. Cullinan, Dominic J. Maxwell, Laura Montgomery-Barefield, and Francisca Okolo MgBodile

KEY CONCEPTS

- Psychotic disorders
  - Accurate diagnosis of psychotic disorders involves a careful history and knowledge of the required symptoms.
  - Treatment of psychotic illnesses involves a multimodal approach and careful monitoring.
  - Referral to a mental health professional is appropriate for assistance in diagnosis and treatment of these complex disorders.
  - Schizophrenia is rare in young children and may manifest with a more gradual onset and with developmental disruptions.
  - Adolescents with schizophrenia have a presentation similar to that of adults with the disorder.
  - Hallucinations and delusional symptoms can be a feature of other psychiatric conditions such as mood disorders, as well as those caused by medical conditions and substance use.
- Elimination disorders
  - Elimination disorders include enuresis and encopresis.
  - Parent guidance is an essential component of treatment of both to interrupt dysfunctional struggles, to help protect the child's esteem, and to provide education regarding the symptoms and treatment.
  - Invasive studies may exacerbate symptoms and should be avoided unless clearly indicated.
  - Pharmacologic intervention should be deferred to initial behavioral interventions and parent education.
- Depressive disorders
  - Forty percent to 90% of adolescents with depression have other comorbid psychiatric disorders.
  - Twenty percent to 40% of adolescents with depression develop bipolar disorder within 5 years of the onset of depression.
  - Ongoing assessment of suicide risk is a critical component of care for adolescents with a diagnosis of depression.
  - Suicide is the third leading cause of death in adolescents and young adults between 15 and 24 years of age.

- Treatment of depression in children and adolescents with selective serotonin reuptake inhibitors (SSRIs) remains clinically appropriate as long as monitoring for increased suicidal ideation is adequate.
  - Medication and psychotherapy are more effective in treating adolescent depression than medication alone.
- Anxiety disorders
  - Anxiety disorders in children and adolescents are distinguished from more common experiences of anxiety in childhood by severity, duration, and the degree of disability imposed by the illness.
  - Separation anxiety disorder is the only anxiety disorder specific to childhood.
  - Behavioral therapies, including exposure and desensitization, are effective in the treatment of specific phobias, social phobia, and obsessive-compulsive symptoms.
  - SSRIs typically constitute the first line of medication treatment.
  - Limiting treatment to pharmacologic intervention often proves inadequate. Attention to environmental factors and family dynamics is often key.
  - Parent guidance and individual psychotherapy for the child often maximize and sustain benefit from medication.

Psychiatric disorders in children and adolescents encompass a broad spectrum of disturbances in development and mental functioning. A potentially perplexing array of clinical manifestations is often first reported in the pediatrician's office. Categorization as exemplified in the *Diagnostic and Statistical Manual of Mental Disorders, Fourth Edition (DSM-IV)* attempts to provide a diagnostic coherence useful for clinical, training, and research purposes.

Psychiatrists for children and adolescents organize disturbances in their patient population by criteria outlined in the *DSM-IV*. These criteria are largely descriptive and therefore carry inherent limitations. As noted in the *DSM-IV*,

Although this manual provides a classification of mental disorders, it must be admitted that no definition adequately specifies precise boundaries for the concept of "mental disorder." The concept of mental disorder, like many other concepts in medicine and science, lacks a consistent operational definition that covers all situations . . . . Mental disorders have also been defined by a variety of concepts (e.g., distress, dyscontrol, disadvantage, disability, inflexibility, irrationality, syndromal pattern, etiology, and statistical deviation). Each is a useful indicator for a mental disorder, but none is equivalent to the concept, and different situations call for different definitions.

The *DSM-IV* further notes,

Despite these caveats, the definition of mental disorder ... is presented here because it is as useful as any other available definition and has helped to guide decisions regarding which conditions on the boundary between normality and pathology should be included in *DSM-IV*. In *DSM-IV*, each of the mental disorders is conceptualized as a clinically significant behavioral or psychological syndrome or pattern that occurs in an individual and that is associated with present distress (e.g., a painful symptom) or disability (i.e., impairment in one or more important areas of functioning) or with a significantly increased risk of suffering death, pain, disability, or an important loss of freedom.

It is important to communicate that, as noted in *DSM-IV*, "the provision of a separate section for disorders that are usually first diagnosed in infancy, childhood, or adolescence is for convenience only and is not meant to suggest that there is any clear distinction between childhood and adult disorders. Although most individuals with these disorders first come to clinical attention during childhood or adolescence, the disorders sometimes are not diagnosed until adulthood." The *DSM-IV* distinguishes these disorders as "disorders usually first diagnosed in infancy, childhood or adolescence."

This chapter discusses four major categories of psychiatric disorders of childhood and adolescence: depressive disorders, anxiety disorders, psychotic disorders, and elimination disorders. Other areas of child and adolescent psychiatry, such as mental retardation and specific developmental disorders (including learning disabilities), are reviewed elsewhere.

Treatment Recommendations

Because psychiatric disorders in children and adolescents are often the product of multiple forces and comorbidity is not unusual, the treatment plan is rarely one dimensional. Treatment often includes multiple modalities of intervention in an effort to address biologic issues; psychological issues; and social, family, and educational/vocational concerns. Clinicians are often challenged to formulate treatment recommendations that address the multiplicity of factors influencing the course while remaining attentive to what may be realistic within the resources of the family and community. Recommendations may include a trial of medication and one or more types of psychotherapy (individual, family, group, cognitive-behavioral). The thoughtful clinician also addresses broader issues relevant to a child's course, including the degree of structure needed for the child to function optimally (outpatient, day treatment, inpatient), school placement issues, and other interventions that can influence the course, such as vocational guidance.

When to Refer

The potential variety of psychiatric presentations in the pediatrician's office is enormous. Psychiatric emergencies such as suicidal ideation or a suicide attempt clearly warrant immediate psychiatric evaluation and close supervision of the child until that evaluation can be accessed. Less urgent disturbances may be marked by subjective distress (anxiety or depression); disruptive behaviors at home, at school, or in the community; substance abuse; academic difficulties; parent-child discord; disturbance in thought processes; elimination problems (enuresis, encopresis); or developmental problems.

Most presentations warrant a thorough, comprehensive psychiatric evaluation. On occasion, the pediatrician may be comfortable treating a focused target symptom with medication, such as the use of a psychostimulant for symptoms of attention deficit hyperactivity disorder. When such interventions fail to yield the desired results, it is reasonable to suspect that other variables are at play, and referral to a child and adolescent psychiatrist is appropriate.

Pediatricians should not feel obligated to treat psychiatric disorders or target psychiatric symptoms beyond their level of comfort. Neither do they need to be an authority on psychiatric disorders of children and adolescents to know when a child is in distress. In addition to the child's subjective report of well-being, children are expected to function reasonably at home, at school, in the community, and with peers. When significant disturbances in any of these areas occur, it is reasonable to pursue a more thorough diagnostic psychiatric evaluation.

Pediatricians may be reluctant to suggest a psychiatric evaluation out of concern that parents may be offended, perhaps hearing the recommendation as a criticism of them or their child. When the pediatrician can reframe the referral away from the language of psychopathology to a concern about a difficulty in functioning or well-being, the referral can be accepted more easily. The psychiatric evaluation can be presented as an effort to try to understand what forces may be preventing the child from functioning at his or her potential. The stigma of mental illness and parents' fears they are responsible for their child's difficulties, through either biologic inheritance or their failure as parents, are nonetheless barriers to accepting a referral for psychiatric evaluation. Pediatricians can do a great deal to allay these anxieties by presenting the recommendation in a calm and gentle fashion, highlighting the complexity of forces that affect development while emphasizing the importance of understanding factors that may interfere with the child's potential.

DEPRESSIVE DISORDERS

Depression as a symptom can be seen in a diverse array of psychiatric disorders, ranging from adjustment disorder with depressed mood to severe depression with psychotic features. Depression is common among youth, with a prevalence of 2% in children and 4% to 8% in adolescents. To complicate the picture further, 40% to 90% have other comorbid psychiatric illnesses, such as conduct disorder and anxiety disorder. Children with chronic medical illness are particularly prone to depressive episodes. Factors such as environment, genetics, and gender also play a role in the expression of depressive symptoms. After puberty there is an increased incidence of depression, particularly in females. The median duration of depression is 7 to 9 months for clinically referred youths. Forty percent to 60% of youths with depression have a relapse after successful treatment. Further, 20% to 40% develop bipolar disorder within 5 years of the onset of depression.

Expert Opinion on Management Issues

The first step toward the accurate treatment of depression is a thorough psychiatric assessment. Collateral information should be obtained from parents, caregivers, and often teachers. Assessment of the patient's safety is the paramount priority. If the patient describes imminent suicide, an inpatient evaluation for stabilization and assessment is indicated.

Historically, tricyclic antidepressants such as imipramine were the standard pharmacologic intervention for the treatment of depression in children and adolescents. Today, selective serotonin reuptake inhibitors (SSRIs) are the first line of pharmacologic treatment. Studies show that an antidepressant in conjunction with individual therapy is superior to either alone. A landmark study, the Treatment for Adolescents with Depression Study (TADS), confirmed that cognitive-behavioral therapy (CBT), a type of psychotherapy that focuses on managing negative emotions and thoughts, and fluoxetine (Prozac) can result in the successful treatment of moderate to severe adolescent depression. Seventy-one percent of the patients responded positively to the combination treatment of fluoxetine and therapy, a rate double the 35% response rate for patients on placebo. More than 60% of those assigned to fluoxetine alone responded by the end of the 12-week trial.

Controversy has emerged over the safety of the use of SSRIs with children and adolescents, however. The U.S. Food and Drug Administration (FDA) required the pharmaceutical industry to place a black box warning on all SSRIs to alert prescribers to increased suicidal thinking and behavior that can occur in children and adolescents during the early phase of treatment. It is believed this may be caused by the activating effect of the SSRIs on these patients. The American Academy of Child and Adolescent Psychiatry recommends the continued use of SSRIs when clinically appropriate as long as adequate monitoring can occur. The FDA outlines recommendations for monitoring when SSRIs are initiated. Observation for clinical worsening, suicidal tendencies, or unusual changes in behavior during the initial few months of antidepressant drug therapy is advised. The FDA specifies that this monitoring "ideally would include at least weekly face-to-face contact with patients or their family members or caregivers during the first four weeks of treatment, then biweekly visits for the next eight weeks, then as clinically indicated beyond 12 weeks."

Common Pitfalls

The treatment of depression is an ongoing process that requires a therapeutic relationship with the patient and family and ongoing reassessment of symptoms. Untreated, depression can progress to suicidal ideation and completed suicide. Currently, suicide is the third leading cause of death in adolescents and young adults between 15 and 24 years of age. In addition to the risk of suicide, depression carries significant morbidity related to an overall deterioration in functioning and notable suffering.

Treatment-resistant depression should prompt reassessment of the accuracy of the diagnosis. Augmentation with other antidepressants and mood stabilizers such as lithium carbonate and valproic acid (Depakote) is often useful. Medical problems that can mimic depression such as hypothyroidism must also be explored. Depression with psychotic features requires concurrent treatment with antipsychotics.

Communication and Counseling

The successful treatment of depression requires education and support for the patient and the family. Parents are often ambivalent about using medication or accepting psychotherapy. Spending time to educate the parent and child and to discuss their concerns is a solid investment in compliance. Informed consent that includes review of the risks and benefits of recommended treatment and alternatives should be obtained and documented.

ANXIETY DISORDERS

Anxiety disorders in children and adolescents are distinguished from more common experiences of anxiety in childhood by the severity of symptoms, duration of symptoms, and degree of disability imposed by the illness. By definition, symptoms must result in a significant impairment in social, family, or occupational (school) functioning. The *DSM-IV* lists several distinct anxiety disorders: panic disorder (with or without agoraphobia), specific phobia, social phobia, obsessive-compulsive disorder, post-traumatic stress disorder, generalized anxiety disorder, and separation anxiety disorder. Of these, only separation anxiety disorder is specific to childhood.

Panic disorder is heralded by discrete episodes (panic attacks) of acute anxiety. By definition, these occur without provocation or stimulus ("out of the blue") and are short lived, usually lasting less than 5 minutes. The distinction between panic attacks and panic disorder is made on whether or not the patient engages in behavior with the intent of preventing future attacks or if there is prominent anxiety about a future attack. As in adults, panic disorder may be associated with or without agoraphobia, a fear of being in places from which escape may be difficult. When severe, it may lead to an inability to leave the house altogether.

Specific phobia is a marked and persistent fear of specific objects or situations. By definition, the fear is excessive and unreasonable, and it may be cued by exposure or mere anticipation. Unlike adults with this disorder, children may not have the insight to realize their degree of fear is unreasonable. Some common examples of specific phobia in children include fear of certain animals (snakes, spiders) as well as exposure to storms, water, and blood. Exposure to the offending object or situation is avoided at all costs. If exposure is threatened, it results in severe distress, often manifesting in crying, panic attacks, and tantrums.

Social phobia (social anxiety disorder), a marked and persistent fear of social or performance situations, is distinguished from normal shyness by its degree and the associated level of disability. The stimulus involves exposure to unfamiliar people and/or potential scrutiny by others. Insight that the degree of fear is excessive or unreasonable may not be present in younger children. The anxiety is present in situations with peers and not limited to interactions with adults.

Obsessive-compulsive disorder is more common in males than females in childhood. The illness consists of either persistent and disruptive obsessions (intrusive thoughts and ideas) or compulsions (repetitive actions designed to alleviate or reduce anxiety) or both. The disorder is distinguished from the ritualistic games and obsessional habits common in some children by their degree, time consumption (at least 1 hour per day), and associated level of disability. In children, symptoms may not cause discomfort and may at times be revealed only with careful questioning of both the child and caregivers.

Post-traumatic stress disorder (PTSD) may manifest with a wide range of symptoms and signs, especially in younger children. The diagnosis requires exposure to a traumatic event that threatens the physical integrity of the individual or others and a duration of symptoms of at least 1 month (if symptoms are short lived, acute stress disorder is diagnosed). Whereas adolescents may present with the classic symptoms of flashbacks and dissociation commonly seen in adults with PTSD, younger children may not. Common symptoms in prepubertal children include disturbed sleep, irritability of mood, aggression, and nightmares.

Generalized anxiety disorder is associated with nonspecific, free-floating anxiety without any apparent cause. These children tend to be overly conforming and perfectionistic. Examples may include fear of a catastrophic event or natural disaster befalling themselves or loved ones or excessive and undue concern about school performance.

Separation anxiety disorder is generally seen in prepubertal children in whom anticipation of or separation from the primary caregivers generates excessive and undue fear. Anxiety about separation is frequently present in the caregivers themselves. The anxiety may manifest as somatic symptoms, such as stomachaches, nausea, or headaches. It may culminate in school refusal, an inability to sleep away from home, or the persistent fear that an untoward event will lead to separation from a primary caregiver. Separation anxiety may emerge as part of a regression associated with a significant life stressor (death in family, divorce, relocation) in a child who previously functioned well.

Expert Opinion on Management Issues

Successful treatment of anxiety disorders may consist of psychotherapy, pharmacologic interventions, or both. The goals of treatment are to educate the family and child about the nature of the disorder, to identify and reduce potentially provocative stimuli, to reduce the severity and duration of symptoms, and to restore premorbid functioning.

Behavioral therapies, including exposure and desensitization, are very effective in the treatment of specific phobias, social phobia, and obsessive-compulsive symptoms. More traditional forms of psychotherapy may offer substantial benefit to individuals with panic disorder, post-traumatic stress disorder, generalized anxiety disorder, and separation anxiety disorder. The successful treatment of more severe separation anxiety disorder may require concurrent treatment of the caregiver.

Severe forms of anxiety, regardless of type, frequently benefit from judicious and thoughtful psychopharmacologic interventions. SSRIs typically constitute the first line of medication treatment. The first FDA indication for the use of these medications in children was for obsessive-compulsive disorder. Tricyclic antidepressants, especially clomipramine (Anafranil), may be effective in the treatment of more refractory cases of obsessive-compulsive disorder. Clonidine (Catapres) and guanfacine (Tenex), both α_2-adrenergic agonists, can be very effective in reducing adrenergic tone in children with anxiety from a wide range of causes. In addition, the newer atypical antipsychotics, although not specifically FDA approved for such use in children, may offer considerable benefit in the treatment of the most severe and treatment-resistant anxiety disorders. Despite their relatively frequent use in the adult population, benzodiazepines should generally be avoided as long-term agents in children and adolescents. The careful and time-limited use of these agents in the treatment of acute anxiety may be justified.

Common Pitfalls

Limiting treatment to pharmacologic intervention often proves inadequate. Careful attention to environmental factors and family dynamics is often key to more comprehensive and effective intervention. Caretakers often need significant support of their efforts to help the child contain and master anxiety effectively.

Parent guidance and individual psychotherapy for the child often maximize and sustain any benefit from medication.

Communication and Counseling

Adequate attention to the education and support of patients and caretakers is key, both in enhancing compliance with treatment recommendations and ultimately in addressing sources of anxiety adequately. The management of anxiety is often a long-term prospect with likely episodes of symptom exacerbation warranting more intensive phases of treatment.

PSYCHOTIC DISORDERS

Psychotic symptoms occurring during childhood and adolescence can vary from the very subtle to the dramatic. They can manifest as a main symptom of a psychotic disorder, such as in schizophrenia, or they can be an associated feature of other disorders, such as depression or bipolar disorder. Psychosis can also be induced by substance intoxication or withdrawal or by medical disorders. Screening for psychotic symptoms is essential when assessing any youth with psychiatric complaints. When psychotic symptoms are identified, a determination of their source is critical because diagnosis, treatment, and prognosis are all based on it.

The psychotic disorders listed in the *DSM-IV-TR* (Text Revision of the *DSM-IV*) are schizophrenia, schizophreniform disorder, schizoaffective disorder, delusional disorder, brief psychotic disorder, shared psychotic disorder, psychotic disorder caused by a general medical disorder, substance-induced psychotic disorder, and psychotic disorder not otherwise specified. Schizophrenia, the prototypical psychotic disorder, can manifest during early childhood, although this is rare. More commonly its symptoms are first seen during late adolescence and young adulthood.

The symptoms of schizophrenia can vary based on whether the individual is in a prodromal phase or active phase of the illness. Characteristic active-phase symptoms required for a diagnosis of schizophrenia include delusions, hallucinations, disorganized speech, grossly disorganized or catatonic behavior, and the presence of negative symptoms such as a flat affect or impoverishment of speech. To diagnose schizophrenia, two or more of these characteristic symptoms must be present over at least a 1-month period. However, only one of these symptoms is required for the diagnosis if the delusions are bizarre, the hallucinations are of a voice keeping a running commentary of the individual's thoughts or behaviors, or multiple voices are talking with each other. There must also be at least 6 continuous months of disturbance, which may include milder prodromal or residual symptoms in addition to at least 1 month of active symptoms. The symptoms of schizophrenia must also lead to impairments in functioning in one or more major areas such as school or interpersonal relations. This may manifest as the child or adolescent not achieving age-appropriate developmental levels. Mood disorders with psychotic features and schizoaffective disorder need to be ruled out to give a diagnosis of schizophrenia.

A diagnosis of schizophreniform disorder is given when the criteria for schizophrenia are met, *except* the total duration is at least 1 month but less than 6 months. Schizoaffective disorder is diagnosed when the main criteria for schizophrenia are present along with mood symptoms of either a major depressive, manic, or mixed episode, if during that same period there are at least 2 weeks of delusions or hallucinations without mood symptoms and the mood symptoms are present for a significant portion of the total active and residual phases of the illness.

Psychotic symptoms that occur as part of a mood disorder can sometimes be difficult to distinguish from the active-phase symptoms of schizophrenia. However, in contrast to schizophrenia, psychotic symptoms that are a feature of a mood disorder are only present during active episodes of the mood disturbance. For example, youths with major depressive disorder may report hearing voices calling their name or may believe their peers are making fun of them, but these symptoms are present only during active depressive episodes and not during periods of normal mood. Similarly, during a manic episode, an individual may have grandiose delusions and disorganized, agitated behavior that may appear to be like those observed in schizophrenia. However, these symptoms are not present when the manic episode resolves. A careful history will clarify that the psychotic symptoms were not present prior to the onset of mania.

Expert Opinion on Management Issues

Proper management of psychotic disorders in children and adolescents begins with an accurate diagnosis based on a careful history. The treatment of psychotic disorders in youth involves a multimodal approach, which should include psychological, social, educational, and family interventions. Referral to or consultation with a child and adolescent psychiatrist is generally indicated. Medication treatment of psychotic symptoms varies depending on whether the psychotic symptoms are associated features of a mood disorder or part of a primary psychotic illness. Primary psychotic illnesses such as schizophrenia and schizophreniform disorder may require ongoing antipsychotic medication. Major depression with psychotic features generally requires treatment with an antidepressant and the temporary use of antipsychotic medication. Failure to recognize and treat psychotic features in depressive illness may result in a less than optimal recovery. In bipolar disorder, the mainstay of pharmacologic treatment is mood-stabilizing agents, although antipsychotic medications may be used to treat acute mania, even in the absence of psychotic features. Mania with psychotic features may require both a mood stabilizer and an antipsychotic medication.

Most of the atypical or next-generation antipsychotic medications currently used as first-line treatment for adult schizophrenia do not have formal FDA approval for the treatment of psychosis in the pediatric age group. Nonetheless, the use of these newer antipsychotic medications in young people may be preferred over the older "typical" antipsychotics because of a lower potential for extrapyramidal (dystonia, akathisias, Parkinson-like features) and other undesirable side effects. Further research is needed to help clarify the safety and efficacy of these medications.

Common Pitfalls

Schizophrenia and other psychotic disorders are complex and serious disorders interfering with the development and functioning of young people in many areas. Behavioral symptoms, for example, can lead to misdiagnosis and inappropriate consequences, such as legal system involvement. Symptoms often interfere with academic and social functioning. Unless school officials have some knowledge of the illness and treatment plan, the student may be viewed as simply unmotivated or disruptive. Substance abuse is a common comorbid condition in psychotic illness that can interfere with treatment and expected improvements unless it is recognized and addressed. Failure to identify the presence of a primary mood disorder such as depression or mania can result in a misdiagnosis of schizophrenia and inaccurate treatment. Underinvolvement of the patient's family in the treatment of the illness or the family's misunderstanding of the nature or severity of the symptoms can result in poor compliance, monitoring, and outcome.

Communication and Counseling

Adequate communication and education of the child or adolescent, the family, and school officials is essential for the optimal treatment of psychotic disorders. Psychotic illness in young people is extremely taxing for both that individual and the family. Referral of the patient and family for counseling, psychoeducation, and therapy is indicated. Support groups, such as the National Alliance for the Mentally Ill (NAMI), can help families cope with the challenges inherent to having a child with a psychotic illness.

ELIMINATION DISORDERS

Child psychiatrists, family practitioners, and pediatricians are often faced with significant challenges when evaluating and treating children with elimination disorders encopresis and enuresis. Although it is important to consider organic etiologies for either enuresis or encopresis, invasive studies should generally be avoided unless unequivocal indications are present. Enuresis is defined as the repeated voiding of urine into the bed or clothes at least twice a week for at least 3 consecutive months in a child who is a least 5 years of age. Encopresis is the repeated passage of feces into inappropriate places occurring at least once a week for 3 months in a child who is at least 4 years of age.

Encopresis is also more common in boys and may be manifested as constipation and overflow incontinence. Patients often respond to behavioral interventions that avoid struggle and provide structure and positive reinforcement for the regular use of the toilet. Sometimes patients can benefit from a toileting schedule. On occasion, a child may benefit from the judicious use of oral laxatives, stool softeners, or both. Rectal stimulation should be avoided when it is clear that organic factors are not primary. Encopresis may relate to family disturbances, underlying psychiatric difficulties in the child, or both. Depression, anxiety disorders, difficulties with anger, and disruptive behavior disorders may coexist. Parent guidance is often an essential component of treatment, supporting the parent's efforts to avoid more entrenched struggles that exacerbate symptoms. Younger children with encopresis may benefit from some education about how their body functions.

Enuresis is more common in males than females. A family history of primary relatives with enuresis is common. Most children with enuresis struggle with wetting restricted to when they are asleep (nocturnal enuresis), although some have diurnal enuresis. Children with attention deficit hyperactivity disorder have comorbid nocturnal enuresis more than the general population. Difficulty with enuresis generally improves with age. Enuresis is not predictive of any long-term psychiatric disorder.

When a child has an acute onset of enuresis or encopresis without previous difficulties, underlying stressors such as a recent change in environment, family system, or trauma should be considered. Enuresis or

TABLE 1 Expert Opinion on Management of Elimination Issues

Strategy	Enuresis	Encopresis
Organic cause	Rule out.	Rule out.
Behavior intervention	Provide structure.	Educate both parent and child about bowel function and toileting approaches.
	Give positive reinforcement.	Diffuse psychological tension that may have developed around bowel control.
	Try moisture-sensitive pads.	
	Avoid beverages close to bedtime.	
	Void before going to bed.	Encourage bowel training.
Medication	Use desmopressin (DDAVP).	Use oral laxatives judiciously.
	Use low-dose tricyclic antidepressants (TCAs).	Use cathartics (rare) occasionally.

encopresis may be a manifestation of anxiety or depression. Whenever possible it is best to attempt behavioral interventions first. Pharmacologic interventions may be used when behavioral interventions fail or to augment behavioral interventions if they are partially successful (Table 1).

Common Pitfalls

Invasive studies that are performed prematurely and without clear indications can worsen symptoms and add to their entrenchment. Pharmacologic interactions without attention to dynamics between the child and caretakers are often ineffective and can lead to an intensification of symptoms. Behavioral interventions should be attempted along with parent/caretaker guidance before pharmacologic interventions are tried. Enuresis is not predictive of longer term psychopathology. Encopresis usually suggests significant a comorbid psychiatric disturbance that should be assessed and treated.

Communication and Counseling

Elimination disorders almost always require significant education for the child and parent/caretaker. Parent guidance should focus on how to best support the child's efforts to achieve bladder or bowel control and how to avoid approaches that can worsen symptoms. More intensive family treatment can be indicated in cases reflecting more seriously disturbed family relationships. An encouraging, patient approach is often extremely helpful, modeling a constructive approach to the elimination disorder for both caretaker and child.

SUGGESTED READINGS

1. American Academy of Child and Adolescent Psychiatry: Message to AACAP members by President Richard Sarles, October 2004. **AACAP workgroup letter to its members supporting use of SSRIs.**
2. American Academy of Child and Adolescent Psychiatry: Practice parameter for the assessment and treatment of children and adolescents with schizophrenia. J Am Acad Child Adolesc Psychiatry 40(7), (Suppl) 4S–23S, 2001. **Reviews the current information available regarding the diagnosis and treatment of schizophrenia in children and adolescents.**
3. American Academy of Child and Adolescent Psychiatry: Practice parameters for the assessment and treatment of children and adolescents with depressive disorders. J Am Acad Child Adolesc Psychiatry 37:1–45, 1998. **Discussion of the epidemiology and guidelines for evaluation of depressed children and adolescents.**
4. American Academy of Child and Adolescent Psychiatry: Practice parameter for the assessment and treatment of children and adolescents with bipolar disorder. J Am Acad Child Adolesc Psychiatry 36:1–38, 1997. **Criteria for diagnosis.**
5. American Academy of Child and Adolescent Psychiatry: Practice parameters for the psychiatric assessment of children and adolescents. J Am Acad Child Adolesc Psychiatry 36:10 (Suppl):4S–20S, 1997. **Describes evaluation standards for child and adolescent psychiatrists.**
6. American Academy of Child and Adolescent Psychiatry: Practice parameters for the psychiatric assessment of infants and toddlers (0–36 months). J Am Acad Child Adolesc Psychiatry 36:10 (Suppl), 1997. **Describes evaluation standards for child and adolescent psychiatrists.**
7. American Psychiatric Association: Diagnostic and Statistical Manual of Mental Disorders, Fourth Edition, Text Revision. Washington, DC: American Psychiatric Association, 2000. **Explains the diagnostic criteria for the psychotic disorders and other psychiatric illnesses with psychotic features.**
8. Engel G: The clinical application of the biopsychosocial model. Am J Psychiatry 137:535–544, 1980. **Introduces and explains the biopsychosocial model.**
9. FDA News Public Health Advisory: FDA launches a multipronged strategy to strengthen safeguards for children treated with antidepressant medications. October 15, 2004. Available at http://www.fda.gov/bbs/topics/news/2004/NEW01124.html (accessed November 25, 2005). **FDA directive that all SSRI medication labeling be revised to include black box warning.**
10. Lewis M: Enuresis encopresis. In Child and Adolescent Psychiatry Comprehensive Textbook, 3rd ed. Philadelphia: Lippincott Williams & Wilkins, 2002, pp 700–711. **Clinical diagnosis of elimination treatment and progress.**
11. Rimm DC, Masters JC: Behavior Therapy Techniques and Empirical Findings. Orlando, Fla: Academic Press, 1979. **Comparison of drug techniques in treatment of elimination disorders.**
12. Twardosz S, Nordquest VM: Parent training. In Herson M, Van Hasselt VB (eds): Behavior Therapy with Children Adolescents: A Clinical Approach. New York: John Wiley, 1987, pp 75–105. **History and encouragement of appropriate behavior is the key to management of elimination disorders.**
13. Wright L, Walker CE: Behavioral treatment of encopresis. J Pediatr Psychol 4:35–37, 1976. **Behavior interventions in management of encopresis.**

22

Autism

Ditza A. Zachor

KEY CONCEPTS

- Autism spectrum disorder (ASD) spans a broad continuum of deficits in social interaction; communication; and restricted, repetitive, and stereotyped behaviors ranging in degree of severity, developmental level, and language skills.
- Early diagnosis and early intervention for children with ASD improves the long-term outcome. Implementation of early, consistent, and appropriate intervention at home or in center-based programs should include behavioral and educational (communication, occupational, social skills) interventions tailored to the needs of the children and their parents.
- Behavior management reduces problem behaviors and improves adaptation.
- Medication trials should be considered when the problem is not responsive to nonpharmacologic intervention, behavioral causation or environmental problems are excluded, the behavior has a negative impact on function and learning, benefits outweigh risks and side effects, and the problem responds to medical intervention. Newer and safer medicines are now available and can improve behaviors such as aggression, self-injurious behavior, anxiety, obsessive-compulsive disorder (OCD), and sleep difficulties.

Autism is a neurodevelopmental disability characterized by severe and persistent deficits in three functional areas: social reciprocity and social interaction, language and communication, the presence of circumscribed interests, and repetitive and stereotyped behaviors. Autism is now viewed as a spectrum of conditions—termed *autism spectrum disorder* (ASD)—that range in severity of symptoms and functioning. Under the definition of pervasive developmental disorder (PDD), according to the *Diagnostic and Statistical Manual of Mental Disorders, Fourth Edition (DSM-IV)*, criteria are classic autism, Asperger syndrome, Rett syndrome, childhood disintegrative disorder, and PDD not otherwise specified (PDD-NOS).

Autism was once thought to be a rare condition, but now ASD is considered one of the most common developmental disorders. Prevalence rates for ASD are estimated around 2 to 4 per 1000 in the United States when all the disorders on the spectrum are included. Part of the apparent increase in the number of individuals diagnosed with ASD may relate to changed criteria, improved diagnostic tools, and better detection of milder forms. Autism is four times more prevalent in males than females, and the prevalence is even higher at the milder end of the spectrum (Asperger syndrome). Diagnosis of autism requires a thorough caregiver interview and an interactive assessment of the child. Two gold standard instruments based on *DSM-IV* criteria for autism are currently widely used to obtain reliable and valid diagnosis of autism: the Autism Diagnostic Interview—Revised (ADI-R) and the Autism Diagnostic Observation Schedule (ADOS). There is clear evidence that autism is a disorder with a significant genetic component (recurrence rates of approximately 6% to 8%). Probably several susceptible genes interact with each other to cause the autism phenotype.

Symptoms

SOCIAL INTERACTION AND RECIPROCITY

Individuals with autism exhibit impairments in initiating social interactions and in interpersonal relatedness (coordinating affective perspectives with others). They also show deficits in using gaze and facial expression to communicate and in joint attention (drawing another person's attention to a distant object). The degree and type of the social deficits vary among individuals, and they are affected by developmental level and change over time. Some patients are aloof and withdrawn; some show a desire to engage socially but have difficulties grasping social codes.

LANGUAGE AND COMMUNICATION

Most children with ASD have delays in reaching speech milestones, which is the main reason for their referral for an evaluation. The nature of the language deficit in autism is semantic-pragmatic, meaning the use of language for communication purposes is particularly impaired. Immediate echolalia (repeating what have been just heard) and delayed echolalia (verbalizing fragments of language or citation heard in the past) are quite common. Individuals with Asperger syndrome have higher IQs and mild or no early speech delay. Their language can become functional and even sophisticated (using "big words"). Delay or absence of imitation, imaginative, and pretend play are common.

RESTRICTED, REPETITIVE, AND STEREOTYPIC BEHAVIOR AND INTERESTS

Behavior tends to be perseverative and repetitious and tends to reflect the desire for sameness and rigid routines. It includes stereotypic motor and verbal behavior (flapping hands, finger mannerisms) or a tendency to be preoccupied with limited objects, activities, or circumscribed interests (traffic lights, flushing toilets). Interest in parts of objects and stereotypic behavior (turning wheels, doll's eyes, lining up objects in identical patterns), adherence to routines, compulsions, and rituals are commonly described.

Expert Opinion on Management Issues

Management of autism requires a multimodal approach that typically involves special education, behavioral interventions, and pharmacologic treatment of problematic behaviors and comorbidities. Intervention focuses on improving social and language skills and reduction of maladaptive behaviors. The goals are to improve the child's overall functional and adaptive status and provide support for the family.

The treatment of choice for the core symptoms of autism tend to be educational and behavioral. At present no treatment guidelines are available for ASD because few empirical studies are focused on treatment effectiveness. However, it is now accepted that any child with ASD should be enrolled in an intensive early intervention program that promotes development of communication, social, adaptive, behavioral, and academic skills and decreases maladaptive and repetitive behaviors. Early diagnosis resulting in early appropriate and intensive intervention improves the long-term outcome of ASD.

BEHAVIORAL TEACHING APPROACHES

Applied behavior analysis (ABA) employs methods based on scientific principles of behavior aimed at building socially useful repertoires and reducing behavior problems. ABA focuses on teaching small measurable units of behavior using discrete trial treatment

(DTT) in mass trials for 30 to 40 hours a week for at least 2 years in home-based or center-based programs. Simple responses are then built systematically into complex age-appropriate skills with emphasis on teaching how to learn from the normal environment. For more advanced children, ABA is implemented in relatively unstructured situations to enhance generalization, increase motivation, and develop social skills. Common behavioral instructional strategies include incidental teaching (child-initiated natural interactions), pivotal responses training (certain behaviors are seen as central for development), and peer-mediated teaching (children with autism are instructed by their peers). Follow-up studies showed that approximately half of the children receiving behavioral treatment made substantial gains in the targeted areas and on standardized tests. They were indistinguishable from typically developing children at the same ages, were included in regular educational settings, and maintained this level of functioning into adolescence. However, the rest of the children made only mild to moderate progress. In the case of maladaptive behaviors, functional behavioral analysis should be used.

TREATMENT AND EDUCATION OF AUTISTIC AND RELATED COMMUNICATION-HANDICAPPED CHILDREN

One of the best-known approaches is the treatment and education of autistic and related communications handicapped children (TEACCH) program, originally a statewide project in North Carolina. This approach focuses on the use of visual cues, schedules, and work stations to teach individuals with ASD. The program emphasizes improving communication skills. The structure of the environment is important in TEACCH because it may increase the likelihood that individuals with autism will be able to understand and predict their surroundings and the expectations for their behavior. A few controlled studies show gains with the use of these methods over control groups.

DEVELOPMENTAL, INDIVIDUAL DIFFERENCE, RELATIONSHIP MODEL

The developmental, individual difference, relationship (DIR) model, developed by Greenspan, is used as the basis for a comprehensive intervention approach emphasizing the child's affect and relationships, developmental level, and individual differences (in motor, sensory, affective, cognitive, and language functioning). Intervention approaches using the DIR model are based on the theory that symptoms of a child with autism may be related to underlying biologically based processing difficulties that cause the child to have problems with relationships and affective interactions. The intervention strategy is informally referred to as "floor time" because the approach may include a component that encourages the therapist and parent to spend a great deal of time on the floor interacting with the child. At home, parents are asked to spend from 6 to 10 daily sessions lasting 20 to 30 minutes each, working on the child's ability for affective-based interactions, using the child's individual differences and developmental level as a starting point. Parents receive training and feedback on working with their child. There is currently no empirical support for the effectiveness of this approach.

DEVELOPMENTAL APPROACHES

Additional approaches include the Denver model, which involves approximately 20 hours per week of center-based developmental intervention and emphasizes play, language, cognition, and social relationships. This approach results in gains in cognition and language.

COMMUNICATION

Speech and language intervention is important and should be provided by personnel with experience in autism. The work of Koegel and colleagues shows that incorporating the child's choice and interest in the selection of language intervention results in greater language learning (the naturalistic approach) than in traditional approaches. The picture exchange communication system (PECS) is widely used in nonverbal children. The system consists of numerous picture symbols printed on small cards that the child can give to someone to communicate. The exchange portion of the program teaches the children that giving someone something (pictures and, later, words) results in receiving something back (the item they want).

SENSORY INTEGRATION

Sensory integration (SI) therapy conducted by occupational therapists is often recommended for children with autism but has limited empirical support. Therapy focuses on combining tactile, vestibular, and proprioceptive input to increase attention and arousal. It is based on the theory that disturbances in sensory modulation are the primary problem in autism and therefore may result in improved communication and social relation. Based on clinician reports, it may be useful to incorporate SI therapy for children who display sensory defensiveness or appear to seek unusual, excessive, or harmful sensory input. SI may include a "sensory diet" designed to provide the children with a range of materials addressing their sensory needs.

MEDICAL MANAGEMENT

The role of medication in autism is quite limited. However, pharmacotherapy can improve certain behavioral problems and comorbidities. Interestingly, the behaviors and symptoms that are most effectively addressed with medication are typically not the core features of autism (communication and social deficits) but rather include overactivity, inattention, aggression, tantrums, self-injurious behavior, anxiety, depression, obsessive-compulsive traits, sleep disturbances, and seizures (Table 1).

TABLE 1 Common Comorbid Disorders in Autism

Behavior	Manifestation	Group of Drugs	Examples
ADHD: hyperactivity: inattention	High activity level, restlessness, on the go, impulsivity; difficulties with attention and listening, joint attention deficits, overfocusing, disorganization	Stimulant medications Atypical neuroleptics Neuroleptics α-Adrenergic agonists	Methylphenidate, amphetamines Risperidone Haloperidol Guanfacine
Disruptive behavior: self-injury, aggression, tantrums	Head banging, pinching, poking, and biting of self; biting and hitting others; episodic physical and verbal outbursts that disrupt function	Atypical neuroleptics SSRIs α-Adrenergic agonists β-Blockers Mood stabilizers	Risperidone, olanzapine, ziprasidone Fluoxetine, fluvoxamine Guanfacine Propranolol Carbamazepine
Obsessive-compulsive traits	Resistance to change in routine, recurrent and persistent obsessive tendencies (stuck on a thought or an activity), rituals, repetitive behaviors with rules that cause distress	SSRIs Atypical neuroleptics α-Adrenergic agonists	Fluoxetine, fluvoxamine Risperidone, olanzapine, ziprasidone Guanfacine
Mood problems	Depression; mood swings (bipolar tendencies)	SSRIs Tricyclic antidepressants Anticonvulsants	Fluoxetine, sertraline, paroxetine Imipramine Carbamazepine, valproic acid
Anxiety	Unrealistic apprehension, fear or terror, inability to relax	SSRIs Anxiolytics	Sertraline, paroxetine Lorazepam, buspirone
Sleep problems	Impaired initiation/induction of sleep; impaired maintenance and early arousal	Melatonin Benzodiazepines Antihistamines Antidepressant α-Adrenergic agonists	 Lorazepam, diazepam, clonazepam Diphenhydramine Trazodone Clonidine, guanfacine
Seizures	Generalized, partial, infantile spasm, epileptic aphasia	Anticonvulsants Ketogenic diet	

ADHD, attention deficit hyperactivity disorder; SSRI, selective serotonin reuptake inhibitor.

TABLE 2 Medications for ADHD Symptoms in Autism: Hyperactivity, Inattention

Drug	Dose	Max Dose	Formulation	Side Effects	Comments
Selected Stimulants* (Increases dopamine or norepinephrine availability in neuronal synapses by inhibition of dopamine or norepinephrine reuptake)					
Methylphenidate (Ritalin, Concerta)	PO: 0.3–0.6 mg/kg		Tablet:	Poor appetite, insomnia, headache, tics, emotional instability	See chapter on ADHD where medications are listed in more detail.
Ritalin	IR tid	60 mg/day	5, 10, 20 mg		
Concerta	ER qd at AM	54 mg/day	18, 36, 54 mg; do not crush		
Amphetamine mixture (Adderall)	PO: 0.15 mg/kg	30 mg/day	Tablets IR: 5, 7.5, 10, 12.5, 15, 20, 30 mg	Poor appetite, insomnia, headache, tics, emotional instability	
Adderall	bid				
Adderall XR	qd		ER: 5, 10, 15, 20, 25, 30 mg		
Selected α-Adrenergic Agonists (Central α-2A receptor agonist in postsynaptic frontal cortex)					
Guanfacine (Tenex)	PO: 1–3.5 mg/day	Max: 4 mg/day	Tablet: 1, 2 mg	Lethargy, headache, stomachache, decreased appetite, xerostomia	

*May benefit attention and hyperactivity but may worsen symptoms; may cause irritability and increase stereotypic behavior.

ADHD, attention deficit hyperactivity disorder; bid, twice daily; ER, extended release; IR, immediate release; max, maximum; PO, by mouth; qd, every day; tid, three times per day.

When attention deficit hyperactivity disorder (ADHD) is suspected, the first step is to exclude other etiologies (such as affective problems, social withdrawal, lack of interest or understanding). The use of medications that stimulate dopamine activity for ADHD symptoms in autism is controversial. Some children become more agitated and engage in more stereotyped behaviors. However, some children with ASD, especially those with Asperger syndrome and PDD-NOS, may respond well by exhibiting reduced distractibility and inattention. Therefore, a short trial with stimulants (short or long acting) that have relatively minimal

TABLE 3 Medications for Disruptive Behavior in Autism: Self-injury, Aggression, Tantrums

Drug	Dose	Max Dose	Formulation	Side Effects	Comments
Selected Atypical Neuroleptics (Dopamine and serotonin antagonists)					
Risperidone (Risperdal)	PO: 0.25–5 mg/day	8 mg/day	Tablet: 0.25, 0.5, 1, 2, 3, 4 mg Oral suspension: 1 mg/mL	Weight gain, sedation, drowsiness movement problem, drooling, tardive dyskinesia, hyperprolactinemia	The most studied neuroleptic drug in autism.
Olanzapine (Zyprexa)	PO: 8–20 mg/day	20 mg/day	Tablet: 2.5, 5, 7.5, 10, 15, 20 mg	Weight gain, ECG changes, drowsiness, headache, insomnia, tardive dyskinesia, hyperprolactinemia	Follow with ECG.
Ziprasidone (Geodon)	PO: 10–100 mg/day	100 mg/day	Capsule: 20, 40, 60, 80 mg	QTc prolongation (rare), drowsiness, extrapyramidal syndrome	Take with food. Follow with ECG.

ECG, electrocardiogram; max, maximum; PO, by mouth.

TABLE 4 Medications for Mood Problems in Autism: Anxiety, Depression, OCD Symptoms

Drug	Dose	Max Dose	Formulation	Side Effects	Comments
Selected SSRIs (Specific serotonin reuptake inhibitors)					
Fluoxetine (Prozac)	PO: 5–40 mg/day	40 mg/day	Caps: 10, 20, 40 mg Oral suspension: 20 mg/ 5 mL (mint flavor) Tablet: 10 mg	GI disturbances, fatigue, weakness, insomnia, headache, nervousness, hypomania	The most studied SSRI in autism.
Fluvoxamine (Luvox)	PO: 12.5–200 mg/day	200 mg/day	Tablet: 25, 50, 100 mg	Somnolence, insomnia, headache, nervousness, tremor, GI upset, agitation, weight loss, dry mouth	Divide total daily dose >50 mg into two. Give larger portion at bedtime; should not be given with astemizole or cisapride for risk of increased QT interval.

GI, gastrointestinal; max, maximum; PO, by mouth; OCD, obsessive-compulsive disorder; SSRI, selective serotonin reuptake inhibitor.

side effects and are cleared out rapidly is recommended (Table 2). When disruptive behavior (aggression, tantrums, self-injurious behavior) is the predominant target, atypical (second-generation) neuroleptics (Table 3) are the drugs of choice, but SSRIs (selective serotonin reuptake inhibitors), α-adrenergic agonists, and β-blockers are good alternatives. These drugs can be used in combination, thereby allowing for the use of lower doses of each. The atypical neuroleptics block dopamine and serotonin receptors and have a reduced risk of tardive dyskinesia (a common side effect of first-generation neuroleptics such as haloperidol). These medicines also seem to help with agitation and high activity levels and improve social withdrawal, lack of motivation, and language.

Risperidone was extensively studied in autism in large double-blind studies (Research Units on Pediatric Psychopharmacology Autism Network) and found to be very effective in improving significant behavior problems (see Table 3). The α-adrenergic agonists (guanfacine, clonidine), once used to lower blood pressure, can improve aggressive outbursts, hyperactivity, and agitation. However, tolerance is reported, and data on their effect and use in ASD are quite limited (see Table 2).

The SSRIs, which stimulate serotonin, a neurotransmitter under research in autism, have attracted interest for treating ASD because they seem to affect the prominent behavioral rigidity, ritualistic behaviors, and rituals as well as depression, lack of motivation or interest, and anxiety symptoms. Studies on the effects of SSRIs (mostly using fluoxetine) show that individuals with ASD have variable responses to these medicines, but those who respond show marked improvement (Table 4).

Children with ASD may show anxiety symptoms, especially when they encounter new situations. There is no research on the effect of anxiolytic drugs in autism, but SSRIs, minor tranquilizers (lorazepam, buspirone), and β-blockers can be used to reduce anxiety (Table 5).

The occurrence of mood disorders in ASD is controversial. Children with cyclic patterns of mood problems, irritability associated with insomnia, overactivity, and family history of bipolar disorder may respond well to mood stabilizers (see Table 1), mainly to anticonvulsants (valproic acid, carbamazepine).

Sleep problems are frequent in ASD (40% to 70%). Treatment consists of using a regular routine approach

TABLE 5 Medications for Anxiety Symptoms in Autism

Drug	Dose	Max Dose	Formulation	Side Effects
Selected Anxiolytics				
Lorazepam (Ativan)*	PO: 0.5–2 mg /day bid or tid	2 mg/day	Oral solution: 2 mg/mL Tablet: 0.5, 1, 2 mg	Dizziness, sedation, weakness, unsteadiness
Buspirone (BuSpar)†	PO: 2.5–20 mg/day	20 mg/day	Tablet: 5, 7.5, 10,15, 30 mg	Dizziness, GI upset, headache, drowsiness (more common with 20 mg/day)

*Benzodiazepine that enhances the inhibitory action of GABA in the CNS.
†Azaperone that causes downregulation of the 5-HT_2 receptors.
bid, twice daily; CNS, central nervous system; 5-HT_2, 5-hydroxytryptamine (serotonin); GABA, γ-aminobutyric acid; GI, gastrointestinal; max, maximum; PO, by mouth; tid, three times per day.

to sleep disorders, analysis of triggers, and medication only as the last resort. Commonly used nonprescription medicines are diphenhydramine (an antihistamine) and melatonin (which controls and resets the sleep cycles). Medications such as benzodiazepines, clonidine, and trazodone can alleviate the symptoms temporarily, but no long-term studies are available that prove their effectiveness (see Table 1).

Naltrexone, a potent opioid antagonist, is shown only in case reports but not in well-controlled double-blind studies to improve self-injurious behavior and rituals (the theory suggests self-injurious behavior induces opiate-like compounds in the brain). It may worsen the outcome in Rett syndrome and in rare cases cause hepatotoxicity.

Seizures occur in 20% to 30% of the children with ASD. Common seizure types are generalized (tonic-clonic, absence, myoclonic, atonic), complex partial, infantile spasm, and Landau-Kleffner syndrome (epileptic aphasia with language regression). Anticonvulsant medications are the preferred treatment and adjusted according to the seizure type. If seizures are intractable to multiple medicines, a ketogenic diet can be used (see Table 1).

ALTERNATIVE THERAPIES

Dietary Interventions

At present no scientific data support special diets such as gluten-free, casein-free, antiyeast, or Feingold diets. Several anecdotal reports found an association between gluten and casein sensitivities and autism. Although nonspecific gastrointestinal (GI) abnormalities were described in autism, studies found no increase in specific antibody titers to gluten or casein.

Vitamins, Minerals, and Supplements

Treatment with pyridoxine, magnesium megavitamins, and mineral supplements was reported to improve sleep, tantrums, aggression, and socialization and to decrease stereotypies in early reports, but lack of efficacy is revealed in more recent double-blind studies. Dimethylglycine treatment is based on its immune system enhancement effects. Again, data are lacking, although anecdotal reports described better eye contact, improved communication, and decreased tantrums in family-oriented literature such as *The Autism Review International* (San Francisco, Calif.).

Drug Treatment

Antiyeast therapy was based on the theory that intestinal *Candida* or bacterial overgrowth produces central nervous system toxins. It was claimed that abnormal metabolic products can be detected by urine organic acid analysis. No peer review studies exist to support the relationship between the biochemical findings and the immune theory. Secretin is a hormone in the gut that causes the pancreas to secrete bicarbonate and bile. Secretin receptors are also present in the hippocampus. The media and a relatively obscure journal reported a "dramatic cure" of three patients with autism and GI problems after injection of secretin during GI endoscopy procedure. More careful scientific studies including both single and multiple doses of secretin on several hundred children have all so far failed to show significant improvement. Immune system deficits are described in autism (altered interferon, interleukin, and transfer factor actions). The use of intravenous immunoglobulin therapy was suggested, but no good scientific data to support it are available.

Other Treatments

Facilitated communication claimed that providing physical support by a trained facilitator under the arm of a child with ASD to allow the child to type messages on a keyboard improves communication. Research provided no validation and showed the facilitator was the source of the messages. Auditory integration training was based on the unproven theory that autism is caused by disturbances in the auditory system. Treatment includes sessions of listening to music when some frequencies of sounds are filtered. Although no scientific support exists, it can alleviate the unpleasant sensation that originates from some sounds in children with autism. The Option Institute method grew out of the experience of two parents who treated their autistic child. The philosophy of this approach is controversial because it is assumed part of the cause of autism is psychological. No solid scientific evidence supports this expensive and time-consuming method.

Common Pitfalls

- Educational programs vary in their philosophy, curricula, and implementation. Pediatricians and parents should be aware of the differences and long-term outcome studies and should make sure the program provides the child with structure, facilitates functional communication and social skills, addresses behavior concerns, and provides parents' training.
- In general, polypharmacy is not recommended. It is difficult to assess which medicine works, there is more potential for side effects and drug interactions, and some combinations simply do not work and might be risky together.
- It is important to be familiar with the category of complementary and alternative treatments for ASD. Because autism has no known cure and is a heterogeneous disorder with diverse outcomes, families and professionals are inclined to try alternative approaches. One must be careful to not accept therapy based solely on semiscientific interpretation of the condition and relying mostly on case reports without well-controlled studies to support it.
- Parents should be cautioned about the possibility of misinformation, especially from the Internet, regarding etiology (e.g., the alleged association with measles, mumps, rubella [MMR] vaccines) and miracle cures (secretin, vitamins, diets, etc.).

Communication and Counseling

The family is a critical component in the success of early intervention for a child with ASD. Parents should be actively involved in the treatment planning and treatment implementation. By including parents in the interventions with children, greater maintenance and generalization of skills can be achieved. It can increase parents' feeling of relatedness with their child and improve their sense of competence as parents, thereby decreasing emotional stress. Some intervention programs require significant time commitments from parents and endorse their use of specific behavior strategies to increase the children's skills and to solve behavioral problems in the home setting. The care of a child with autism can sometimes be confusing for parents because it requires the involvement of multiple disciplines, from educators and developmental therapists (speech, motor, behavior) to developmental and behavioral pediatricians, child psychiatrists, and child neurologists. A regional center for diagnosis and treatment of autism can greatly assist parents in navigating all these resources. It is important to be involved in local support groups and advocacy organizations such as the American Autism Society (1-800-3-AUTISM or http://www.autism-society.org).

SUGGESTED READINGS

1. American Academy of Pediatrics—Committee on Children with Disabilities: The pediatrician's role in the diagnosis and management of autistic spectrum disorder in children. Pediatrics 107:1221–1225, 2001. **AAP recommendations for diagnostic approach and treatment plan of ASD for pediatricians in clinical practices.**
2. American Psychiatric Association: Diagnostic and Statistical Manual of Mental Disorders, Fourth Edition. (DSM-IV). Washington, DC: American Psychiatric Association, 1994. **Manual used for diagnosis of all pervasive developmental disorders, including autism, by providing strict criteria in the three impairment areas (social, communication, and restricted behavior).**
3. DeLong GR, Ritch CR, Burch S: Fluoxetine response in children with autistic spectrum disorders: Correlation with familial major affective disorder and intellectual achievement. Dev Med Child Neurol 44:652–659, 2002. **Describes response of a large group of children with ASD to fluoxetine treatment and analyzes variables affecting this response.**
4. Hansen RL, Ozonoff S: Alternative theories: Assessment and therapy options. In Ozonoff S, Rogers SJ, Hendren RL (eds): Autism Spectrum Disorders: A Research Review for Practitioners. Washington, DC: American Psychiatry Association Press, 2003. **Excellent review of variety of alternative treatments in ASD, the rationale behind their use, and evidence-based data regarding their effectiveness.**
5. Koegel LK: Interventions to facilitate communication in autism. J Autism Dev Disord 30:383–391, 2000. **This article discusses several areas of intervention that may improve assessment and intervention practices and produce greater long-term communicative outcomes for individuals with autism.**
6. McCracken JT, McGough J, Shah B, et al: Risperidone in children with autism and serious behavioral problems. N Engl J Med 347:314–321, 2002. **Comprehensive study that describes the effects and side effects of risperidone in children with autism.**
7. McEachin JJ, Smith T, Lovaas OI: Long-term outcome for children with autism who received early intensive behavioral treatment. Am J Ment Retard 97:359–372, 1993. **This follow-up study supports the effectiveness and long-lasting effects of early intensive intervention based on behavioral concepts.**
8. Volkmar FR: Pharmacological interventions in autism: Theoretical and practical issues. J Clin Child Psychol 30:80–87, 2001. **Comprehensive review of the rationale for medication use in autism and the mechanism of action of selected drugs. The review describes brain areas and neurotransmitters related to autism symptoms and comorbidities.**
9. Volkmar FR, Weisner LA: Common challenging behaviors. In Harris LS (ed): Healthcare for Children on the Autism Spectrum. Bethesda, Md: Woodbine House, 2004, pp 201–218. **Describes in detail the common behavior problems and comorbidities in autism and approaches for diagnosis and treatment.**
10. Weiss MJ, Harris SL: Teaching social skills to people with autism. Behav Modif 25:785–802, 2001. **Provides detailed description of various strategies to teach social competence.**
11. Wieder S, Greenspan SI: Climbing the symbolic ladder in the DIR model through floor time/interactive play. Autism 7:425–435, 2003. **This case report presents the principles of the developmental, individual-difference, relationship-based model (DIR), a comprehensive intervention model for children with autism. The report examines the functional developmental capacities of children in the context of their unique biologically based processing profile and their family relationships and interactive patterns.**
12. Wolery M, Garfinkle AN: Measures in intervention research with young children who have autism. J Autism Dev Disord 32:463–4781, 2002. **A comprehensive review of the different intervention approaches commonly used to treat autism that provides analysis of the outcome measures used in each reviewed study.**

13. Yeargin-Allsopp M, rice C, Karapurkar T, et al: Prevalence of autism in a US metropolitan area. JAMA 289:49–55, 2003. **This study examines the prevalence of autism among children aged 3 to 10 years in Atlanta, confirming the rise in rates of autism documented since the early 1990s around the world.**

Tourette Syndrome

Lawrence W. Brown

KEY CONCEPTS

- Tourette syndrome is characterized by the presence of waxing and waning motor tics plus at least one verbal tic over a period of more than a year.
- The first approach in treating Tourette syndrome should include multimodal support with family education, behavioral counseling, and school intervention.
- Many children require no medication; pharmacotherapy is reserved for functionally disabling symptoms.
- No broad-spectrum drug is available, and combination therapy is sometimes required.
- Adverse reactions should not discourage other drug trials.
- Periodic evaluation is required to determine if treatment is still appropriate.

Tourette syndrome is a neuropsychiatric disorder beginning in childhood characterized by chronic motor and phonic mannerisms with or without other features that commonly include attention deficit hyperactivity disorder (ADHD), obsessive-compulsive disorder (OCD), anxiety disorders, and other behavioral problems. It is not a functional disorder, although tics are often exacerbated by stress, disappear (for the most part) in sleep, and are usually suppressible for brief periods of time. A wide spectrum of tics and behavioral symptoms typically vary over time in a waxing and waning fashion. Although infection can precipitate or exacerbate tics, it is an unproven theory that Tourette syndrome is caused by a reaction to streptococcal infection or other autoimmune disorder.

It is now accepted that Tourette syndrome is a relatively common, biologically determined disorder with a very strong genetic predisposition in most cases. A fundamental understanding of the pathophysiology of Tourette syndrome has been as elusive as the search for the underlying gene or genes. However, clinical advances now provide new directions in understanding basic mechanisms as well as therapeutic implications. Treatment is available for most affected individuals, although side effects often limit otherwise effective intervention. Pharmacologic treatment should be limited to symptoms with significant impact on daily functioning. Medication is only indicated when the tics cause pain, interfere with ability to concentrate, disrupt others, or are socially disabling. It is often more important to first address coexisting neuropsychiatric

problems such as ADHD, although the possibility must be taken into account that treatment could further exacerbate the tic disorder.

Expert Opinion on Management Issues

ACCEPTED INTERVENTIONS

Overwhelming evidence indicates that the spectrum of tic disorders including Tourette syndrome have a neurobiologic basis rather than a purely psychological origin. This statement might lead to the erroneous conclusion that pharmacologic treatment is indicated for most affected children. Although medications are appropriate for many affected individuals, the majority do not require drug treatment if tics do not interfere with the child's ability to function at home or in school. However, all individuals with tic disorder should be offered guidance to understand the basis of their condition and its potential impact on daily life. The child, his or her family, and others in the environment need to understand which symptoms can be considered involuntary and which are within voluntary control. It can be very difficult to separate compulsive mannerisms from impulsive behaviors from tics. For example, a child may impulsively make inappropriate comments but insist, "I had to do it." It is important to educate the teacher and provide instruction to the entire class if a child's tics are severe enough to be noticed in school; this will lead to a greater understanding about Tourette syndrome and ideally more acceptance of differences and less ridicule from peers. School issues in children with Tourette syndrome are often much more difficult when compounded by ADHD, learning disabilities, OCD, or behavioral disorders. Some affected children benefit from special education to treat associated psychological or educational problems. Many also require formal counseling or family therapy.

As stated earlier, the decision to treat with medication must be guided by clear indications that the symptoms are interfering with daily life, which may include adverse impact on academic performance, peer relationships, socialization, or activities of daily living. The choice of drug should be based on the target symptom that is the source of the most significant impairment. This varies from child to child: usually one of the triad of tics, obsessive-compulsive mannerisms, or ADHD. The complex patient with more than one disabling symptom may eventually require more than one approach, but treatment should still begin by addressing the most severe problem. Because the natural history of the disease includes wide variability over time (waxing and waning of symptoms), an adequate trial should be given for each dosage of every medication.

The goal of treating tics should be better tic control as well as reduction of discomfort or social embarrassment sufficient to allow normal functioning, and not the complete elimination of all symptoms. The most effective agents to reduce tics include the typical and atypical neuroleptics. Haloperidol and pimozide are the only neuroleptic drugs approved by the U.S. Food and Drug Administration (FDA) for the treatment of Tourette syndrome. Comparative studies are few, but one randomized, double-blind controlled study found pimozide to be superior to haloperidol in terms of efficacy and tolerability. However, warnings were later raised about the safety of pimozide in terms of prolongation of the QT interval. Many clinicians prefer risperidone or one of the other newer atypical neuroleptics, such as quetiapine, olanzapine, ziprasidone, or aripiprazole. All of these typical and atypical neuroleptic drugs are potent dopamine blockers, and they all help in approximately 75% of cases. Undesirable side effects may include cognitive blunting, restlessness, weight gain, psychomotor retardation, and depressed mood. There is also the long-term risk of tardive dyskinesia with these drugs, although typical neuroleptics that specifically target dopamine (e.g., haloperidol and pimozide) are more likely to produce this adverse outcome. The atypical neuroleptics like risperidone are theoretically safer, but the clinical experience in children is very limited, particularly over long periods of exposure. Many clinicians obtain an electrocardiogram (ECG) with all of these drugs, but it is specifically recommended that ECG be performed prior to treatment with pimozide, 3 months after initiating the drug, and then yearly.

Although many clinicians have switched from haloperidol or pimozide to risperidone as the first-line agent for severe tics, the scientific basis remains limited. The first placebo-controlled trial of risperidone was not published until 2003, and this well-designed study suffers from small numbers and a short period of observation over only 8 weeks. Risperidone was clearly effective without any extrapyramidal side effects or cardiac abnormalities. However, the mean weight increase was 2.8 kg (compared to no change on placebo) even during that brief trial, and acute social phobia was induced in one subject. Clearly, more data over more extended periods of observation are needed.

Clonidine, originally developed as an antihypertensive agent, has proved to be somewhat less effective in controlling tics (50% to 60%). Many clinicians find it useful, however, because it can address other common coexisting issues, such as sleep resistance, anxiety disorders, and ADHD. Side effects typically include sedation and irritability, with rare reports of orthostatic hypotension. Clonidine is most effective when administered at least three times per day unless provided as the patch preparation, which only needs to be changed every 5 to 7 days. Typical doses range from 0.1 to 0.6 mg daily. Guanfacine is a similar α_1-adrenergic antagonist, but it has a longer half-life and a lower incidence of sedating side effects. Doses are approximately 10 times higher, usually 1 to 4 mg daily provided twice daily; a long-acting preparation is under development but not yet approved.

Other drugs reported to be useful in controlling tics include clonazepam, the nicotine patch, the nicotine receptor antagonist mecamylamine, and dopamine agonists including pergolide. However, none of these drugs has been adequately studied with well-designed trials. Attention has been directed at initial positive reports with antiepileptic drugs including topiramate and levetiracetam, but double-blind placebo-controlled trials are not yet completed.

There is recent successful experience with controlling intractable focal motor and vocal tics with local injection of botulinum toxin into the affected muscles. This toxic denervation can ameliorate involuntary tics for months, and evidence indicates it can also eliminate the premonitory sensation that may be an integral part of the tic pathology. Enormous interest was generated about the possibility of surgical treatment, but it is far too preliminary to consider in the pediatric population. There was a single-case report of successful treatment of a patient 42 years of age whose severe motor and phonic tics were controlled by deep brain stimulation of the thalamus.

TREATMENT OF NEUROBEHAVIORAL COMORBIDITY

It is impossible to discuss treatment of Tourette syndrome without directly incorporating approaches to other integral coexisting behavioral symptoms. As mentioned earlier, behavioral modification strategies and academic or behavioral supports in the classroom should be the first steps in controlling the psychological effects or associated behavioral problems with Tourette syndrome. It is often critically important to raise the child's self-esteem and improve motivation in addition to direct treatment of tics. However, a comprehensive discussion of the nonpharmacologic and drug management of behavioral problems is beyond the scope of this chapter.

Stimulants, including the various immediate- and extended-release preparations of methylphenidate and amphetamines, are the standard first-line treatment for ADHD, and they often improve other associated symptoms, from academic productivity to impulsive aggression, noncompliance, and poor socialization. The problem is that ADHD and Tourette syndrome commonly coexist with a prevalence rate of approximately 60%. ADHD almost always precedes the appearance of tics with a mean age of presentation before 5 years of age, whereas tics typically present several years later. This leads to a dilemma in the determination of the role of stimulants in inducing tics. Because stimulants are the first-line agents for the treatment of ADHD, many children destined to develop tics at a later age are first treated with methylphenidate or amphetamines. Certainly, conventional wisdom (and the *Physician's Desk Reference*) states that stimulants are potentially unsafe in children with a personal history of tics or a family history of Tourette syndrome. Most experts continue to recommend stimulants as a first-line treatment when all is taken into account, as long as families provide informed consent. They need to be aware of the possibility that medication can transiently induce or worsen tics, and sometimes the tics may be severe and chronic; it is necessary to emphasize the issue of relative risk and consider the safety and efficacy of alternative drug strategies as well as the risk of not treating.

Atomoxetine was released in early 2003 as a non-stimulant alternative for the treatment of ADHD in children and adults. A single randomized, placebo-controlled study was published in children with comorbid tic disorder and ADHD. The primary efficacy end point was improvement in the core symptoms of ADHD. In recognition of the waxing and waning nature of tics, the goal of the study was to demonstrate that the drug was no worse than placebo in worsening of tics. The study succeeded in both goals, with a marked improvement in ADHD symptoms and no worsening in tics. Indeed, a large minority had statistically improved tic rating scales over the course of the study.

Clonidine, although less effective than stimulants in controlling the core symptoms of ADHD (60% vs. 80%), may also directly treat tics. A randomized controlled trial not only addressed the role of clonidine in children with Tourette syndrome and ADHD but compared it to methylphenidate alone or in combination. Both clonidine and methylphenidate were individually effective in improving the primary outcome ADHD measure, and the combination produced the most robust effect. Interestingly, tic severity lessened in all active treatment groups, with the combination of clonidine and methylphenidate also being the most effective. However, side effects were common with clonidine administration. Guanfacine, another presynaptic α_2-agonist, has a longer half-life, weaker effects on blood pressure, and appears to have a lower incidence of sedative side effects. Both drugs are associated anecdotally with tic exacerbation, either with introduction of the medication or during drug withdrawal.

Tricyclic antidepressants can be used to treat ADHD, and they were once the drugs of second choice after stimulants. Little evidence indicates they are helpful in controlling tics, and there are even reports of tic exacerbation as well as the induction of other drug-induced movement disorders (dyskinesias). Safety concerns limit their use except under special circumstances; all have potential cardiac toxicity (QT prolongation), and sudden death was reported from desipramine. Sedation, weight gain, and anticholinergic side effects are also common side effects.

Selective serotonin reuptake inhibitors (SSRIs) are the most effective drugs to treat obsessive-compulsive disorder in children and adults. The greatest pediatric experience is with fluoxetine, but similar benefits (and side effects) are seen with other drugs in the class, including fluvoxamine, sertraline, paroxetine, citalopram, and escitalopram. Not only can these drugs treat OCD, but they are also effective in controlling associated anxiety symptoms and social phobias. Clomipramine was the first agent shown to be effective in childhood OCD, and it may actually have the most effectiveness. However, it also has all of the potential side effects of tricyclics, including sedation, weight gain, tachycardia, dry mouth, and other anticholinergic toxicity. Venlafaxine, with combined serotonin and noradrenergic reuptake inhibition properties, is also effective in treating OCD symptoms. There are no long-term comparison trials of any of these drugs in children with comorbid OCD and Tourette syndrome, and clinicians must rely on experience with other populations. Although there was much public discussion of the increased risks when SSRIs are prescribed for children and adolescents with depression, little was written about the risk of suicidal ideation in those with OCD. It is clear these drugs can produce overactivation, irritability, agitation, and even hypomania if introduced too quickly or administered at high doses; prudence would suggest careful risk-benefit analysis and a slow titration schedule.

Common Pitfalls

There is little information to guide clinical practice on the combination of drugs in children with Tourette syndrome, whether for intractable psychiatric symptoms or more complex patients with multiple disabling problems. Certainly, the one study in children with Tourette syndrome and ADHD that compared methylphenidate, clonidine, and dual therapy to placebo showed both safety and efficacy and even favored the combination treatment. Although there was much public concern several years ago about the safety of combining methylphenidate with tricyclic antidepressants, careful analysis demonstrated no cumulative toxicity. Combining SSRIs with other drugs, however, may require more caution. Atypical neuroleptics, for example, have serotonin-reuptake inhibiting properties as well. This can lead to the so-called serotonin syndrome, with excessive sweating, tremor, myoclonus, diarrhea, and fever, in addition to agitation, confusion, and hypomania.

It is important to maintain a clear vision of risk and benefit even when there is a prevailing public outcry against the dangers of treatment. Tourette syndrome is a model disorder of the interaction of developmental, genetic, neurobiologic, and behavioral influences. No entirely safe psychopharmacologic agent exists, but the risks of not treating must also be considered. Children with severe Tourette syndrome have difficulty learning because of the adverse impact of constant tics as well as other coexisting conditions, and they are often socially ostracized. Tic reduction and efforts to address serious comorbid conditions can dramatically improve quality of life. Adverse drug reactions should not discourage the clinician from consideration of other medication trials.

Communication and Counseling

The natural history of Tourette syndrome in most cases includes stabilization or spontaneous remission during adolescence or young adulthood. Many patients are able to stop medication by this time. Although tics may improve with maturity, other symptoms associated with the disorder may continue and even become more problematic. It is not uncommon for depression, mood swings, and rage attacks to worsen during adolescence. Symptoms of OCD, ADHD, and learning disabilities do not typically improve even when tics go into remission. Older, long-term outcome studies are not encouraging; in one review of more than 400 adult patients, only 36% had full-time employment and 34% were totally unemployed. There is much optimism in the field that these negative findings will be overturned by the combination of research advances in the underlying pathophysiology, effective treatment, and genetic basis of Tourette syndrome coupled with the demystification and growing recognition of the disorder as a medical condition.

SUGGESTED READINGS

1. Jancovic J: Medical progress: Tourette's syndrome. N Engl J Med 345:1184–1192, 2001. **Excellent, succinct review of the recent advances in diagnosis, pathogenesis, and treatment of the disorder.**
2. Kurlan R, Kaplan EL: The pediatric autoimmune neuropsychiatric disorders associated with streptococcal infections (PANDAS) etiology for tics and obsessive-compulsive symptoms: Hypothesis or entity? Practical considerations for the clinician. Pediatrics 113:883–886, 2004. **The most recent summary of the conflicting data on this intriguing hypothesis, which concludes there is insufficient evidence to support routine laboratory testing or treatment with antibiotics or immunomodulatory agents.**
3. Leckman JF, Zhang H, Vitale A, et al: Course of tic severity in Tourette syndrome: The first two decades. Pediatrics 102:14–19, 1998. **Results from this cohort study can be used by clinicians to reassure families that tic severity generally peaks at 10 years of age and then improves steadily so that half are virtually tic free by late adolescence.**
4. Robertson MM, Stern JS: Gilles de la Tourette syndrome: Symptomatic treatment based on evidence. Eur Child Adolesc Psychiatry 9(Suppl 1):160–175, 2000. **Concise compendium of the scientific basis for treating the various symptoms of Tourette syndrome.**
5. Scahill L, Leckman JF, Schultz RT, et al: A placebo-controlled trial of risperidone in Tourette syndrome. Neurology 60:1130–1135, 2003. **First controlled study of the drug that has become the current standard treatment for Tourette syndrome.**
6. Tourette's Syndrome Study Group: Treatment of ADHD in children with tics: A randomized controlled trial. Neurology 58:527–536, 2002. **Results of a large multicenter trial sponsored by the Tourette Syndrome Association and National Institutes of Health that demonstrated the safety and efficacy of stimulants and clonidine.**

Psychosomatic Illness

Melvin D. Oatis, Eraka Bath, and Harold S. Koplewicz

KEY CONCEPTS

- Psychosomatic illness is characterized by a pattern of recurring, multiple, and clinically significant complaints.
- The most common symptoms reported are headache, abdominal pain, back pain, and fatigue.
- The presence of a psychosomatic illness often indicates underlying psychosocial stressors such as family discord and academic and social difficulties.

- Genetic factors contribute to risk of illness.
- Multiple hypotheses regarding etiology suggest biopsychosocial underpinnings.
- Psychosomatic illness includes medical illness with psychological manifestations as well as physical symptoms that occur in the absence of medical illness.
- Laboratory testing is often nonspecific.
- Collaboration between primary care providers and mental health professionals is the key to management.

The notion of psychosomatic illness stems from an emerging realization in the medical community regarding the interplay between the biology and psychology of illness. Many medical illnesses have biologic and psychological underpinnings, and increasingly the exploration of these facets leads to the development of effective treatment interventions and improved clinical outcomes. Psychosomatic illness can represent medical disorders that have psychological manifestations as well as physical symptoms in the absence of medical illness. This definition for somatization is particularly useful: "the tendency to experience and communicate somatic distress and symptoms accounted for by pathologic findings, to attribute them to physical illness and to seek medical help for them."

Under the rubric of psychosomatic illness is the cluster of disorders known as the somatoform disorders. Somatoform disorders are characterized by a pattern of recurring, multiple, and clinically significant complaints. These symptoms are not produced voluntarily, and the pain and discomfort is very real to the child. When physical complaints have no apparent medical basis, they may be a reflection of stress, such as nervousness in social situations or in the context of family discord or academic difficulties.

History

Patients who have physical symptoms without apparent physical cause are not new to medicine. The Greeks first used the term *hysteria* to describe such persons. The term *Briquet syndrome* emerged in the 19th century when Paul Briquet studied patients with multiple unexplained physical symptoms. Charcot, Bernheim, Janet, and Freud studied what they called "hysterical" symptoms using hypnosis, and their work resulted in the development of the concept of dissociation. As the *Diagnostic and Statistical Manual of Mental Disorders (DSM)* has evolved, so too has the terminology and the classification of these disorders.

Incidence

In a general population study, recurrent distressing somatic symptoms were found to be present in as many as 11% of girls and 4% of boys from 12 to 16 years of age. The gender differences are striking when comparing postpubertal girls to boys, typically a 5:1 ratio. This difference is not found in most studies of prepubertal children, where a 1:1 ratio between the sexes seems to be most common. Additionally, it is

BOX 1 Factors in Somatization

Risk Factors

- Low socioeconomic status
- Low educational attainment
- Chaotic household with high levels of family distress
- History of sexual or physical abuse
- Presence of chronic medical illness in child or family member
- Parental reaction and perception of illness

Demographic Factors

- An estimated 25% of all children and adolescents suffer from chronic and recurrent pain.
- 10% to 30% of school-age children report weekly psychosomatic symptoms.
- Prepubertal children usually report one symptom.
- Postpubertal girls report somatic symptoms five times more often than boys.

important to recognize the influence of development when examining the expression of pain symptoms because certain somatic perceptions are clustered by age group. In prepubertal children, complaints are more likely to be monosymptomatic, with recurrent abdominal pain and headaches registering as the most common complaints (see later). An astonishing 10% to 30% of school-age children report psychosomatic symptoms as often as weekly. Neuromuscular symptoms and fatigue seem to increase with age (Box 1).

Genetic data suggest somatoform disorders tend to run in families, with an occurrence of 10% to 20% in first-degree female relatives of patients with somatization disorder. A higher frequency of anxiety and depressive disorders is present in the families of somatizing children. One study involving family members of subjects with somatization disorder demonstrated a higher incidence of physical illness in those family members as well as higher levels of psychosocial dysfunction and substance abuse. These family members also exhibited an increased likelihood to use illness for stress reduction as compared with controls.

In addition to the genetic contributions toward psychosomatic illness, possible psychosocial and environmental potentiators must also be considered. Psychosomatic illness is thought to occur more often in less-sophisticated or less-educated populations and in lower socioeconomic groups. Although the studies highlighting the relationships between childhood somatization disorder and the demographic variables of race, ethnicity, and class are limited, there are reported associations with histories of nonintact families, marital discord, and family conflict. Children living in homes with high levels of chaos and familial distress are more likely to use somatic complaints as a coping mechanism. Adolescents with histories of physical and sexual victimization score higher in measures of somatic symptoms than their counterparts without abuse histories.

Etiology

Hypotheses for the genesis of somatoform disorders abound, but the exact cause remains unknown.

Psychosocial theories view somatic symptoms as a form of social communication to express emotions or to symbolize feelings. Psychoanalytic interpretations view symptoms as representations of instinctual impulses, whereas biologic studies suggest that these patients may have faulty perceptions of and abilities to screen somatosensory inputs. The learning theory suggests that children who learn the benefits of the sick role may be hesitant to recover because the subsequent rewards (e.g., increased parental attention and absolution from responsibilities such as attending school) are potent reinforcers of sick-role behavior. Similarly, children who observe an ill sibling receiving extra parental attention may mimic the sibling's symptoms in an attempt to recoup that attention for themselves.

Symptoms

The most common reported symptoms in somatizing children are headaches, abdominal distress, back pain, fatigue, and sore muscles. Many of these children are subjected to myriad laboratory tests and evaluations that can sometimes be counterproductive by inadvertently rewarding the sick role. Therefore, the extensive investigative process poses a challenge because ruling out a psychosomatic illness requires that underlying medical causes also must be effectively ruled out. Conversely, when searching for a medical explanation of recurrent abdominal pain or headache in children, physicians often uncover associated anxiety and depressive symptoms. Not surprisingly, school-age children with anxiety symptoms have a higher incidence of unexplained chest pain than children with benign heart murmurs.

HEADACHE

Pediatric headache is a frequently occurring pain syndrome in approximately 2.5% of the child and adolescent population; an estimated 1 million children suffer from migraines. Pediatric results in several hundred thousand days of school absences per month, according to Holden and colleagues. Recurrent pediatric headache is rarely linked to underlying medical conditions that result in significant physical impairment, so the need for psychological approaches in their management is essential. Headaches that only occur on weekdays are often a symptom of separation anxiety disorder and social phobia in the school-age population.

Diagnostic challenges abound with respect to clarifying circumscribed symptomatology. An evolving discourse in the literature debates how to classify headaches in general but primarily as they relate to adults. Different models are proposed, and the notion of "chronic daily headaches" is used because its central feature is the characterization of daily headache that varies in duration and intensity of accompanying symptoms. Etiology remains undetermined, but genetic factors appear to play a role for tension and migraine headaches as well as for those with significant autonomic nervous system involvement.

Most headaches involve activation of the central and peripheral nervous system. Biologic treatment primarily focuses on unstable serotonergic pathways. The principal psychological interventions include relaxation therapies and biofeedback. Relaxation techniques typically focus on a form of progressive or imagery-guided relaxation appropriate to age level and practiced daily. Two types of biofeedback are helpful in managing pediatric headache: electromyographic (EMG) or thermal biofeedback. EMG consists of monitoring auditory and visual (A/V) signals from electrical impulses generated from the frontalis region of the head. Thermal biofeedback involves monitoring A/V signals that resonate from a thermistor placed on the fingers. It is thought to be useful in the treatment of migraine headache because of the strong vascular components involved and the well-documented impact of voluntary control of body temperature on vasoconstriction and vasodilation.

RECURRENT ABDOMINAL PAIN

Recurrent abdominal pain (RAP) is a common pediatric problem noted to occur in 10% to 30% of children and adolescents. It is currently defined as three or more episodes of abdominal pain over a period of at least 3 months that are severe enough to affect a child's social functioning by imposing limitations on activities. RAP may represent the paradigm of psychosomatic illness because it occurs commonly without a clear-cut etiology, yet numerous developmental pathways are associated with its onset, and a number of psychological and environmental factors are important in developing and sustaining the symptoms. Studies indicate that girls with RAP may be predisposed to having the same symptoms in adulthood or be at risk for developing irritable bowel syndrome.

Psychological and environmental factors associated with recurrent abdominal pain are not always consistent; however, personality traits of perfectionistic tendencies, shyness, and anxiety, along with negative life events and stress, are observed in these patients. Higher levels of anxiety and depressive symptoms are noted in children with RAP and their mothers compared with healthy controls. Parents of children with RAP report increased somatization and pain syndromes.

Maintenance of the sick role with reinforcements of staying home from school or escaping chores can perpetuate symptoms. Effective treatments include operant rewarding of nonpain behaviors, increased fiber in patients with constipation and abdominal pain, and cognitive-behavioral therapy using relaxation and imagery after obtaining a thorough history of the symptoms.

Diagnosis

The term *somatoform disorders* is used in the to describe a group of illnesses characterized by physical symptoms that cannot be fully explained by a neurologic or general medical condition. The diagnostic criteria defined by the fourth edition of the *Diagnostic and Statistical Manual of Mental Disorders (DSM-IV)* were established for adults and do not necessarily cover the psychosomatic illnesses encountered in children. Nevertheless, recurring complaints of somatic symptoms are commonplace in the pediatric population, and some studies estimate that 1.3% to 5% of children in outpatient clinics report somatic complaints. Although many children report recurrent physical symptoms with no physical cause, the actual diagnosis of a somatoform disorder in children continues to be rare, probably because the current diagnostic criteria outlined by the *DSM-IV* are extensive and require 13 physical symptoms from a list of 35, 8 of which are appropriate for postpubertal patients. This suggests that the development of more age-appropriate diagnostic criteria that take developmental considerations into account would yield higher prevalence rates in the pediatric population given the frequency with which young children report somatic complaints.

Assessment Instruments

A useful assessment tool for evaluating children who raise the suspicion of psychosomatic illness is the Children's Somatization Inventory (CSI), which assesses the occurrence of somatization symptoms in children and adolescents. Given the limited utility of the *DSM-IV* in effective screening for somatization disorder in pediatric patients, the CSI can be an important adjunct in screening and risk assessment.

The Living with a Chronic Illness Scale (LCI) was devised to measure impairments in social functioning in children and adolescents who experience a chronic illness. The LCI scale gathers information from both parents and children to ascertain a more comprehensive understanding of social functioning, with the hope that a multiple informant strategy can increase early detection of at-risk youth who may need psychological treatment.

Understanding the components of chronic recurrent pediatric pain has important implications in developing a model to assess and treat the psychosocial issues and dynamics of these children, who have social and academic dysfunction, higher emotional distress, and increased health care use. The numbers of children suffering from chronic and recurrent pain are staggering, estimated at 25% of all children and adolescents.

Interaction of Biologic and Psychosocial Factors

Viewing psychosomatic illness as it is defined along the two dimensions of an interplay between mind and body helps in understanding the medical illnesses, which have psychiatric sequelae that may or may not manifest with somatizing symptoms. Studies find that children with chronic medical conditions—in particular, asthma, diabetes, seizures, and hematologic disorders—have fairly well documented psychiatric manifestations of their illnesses. The etiology of comorbid psychiatric illness occurring with medical illness is multifactorial yet heavily depends on the interplay between biologic and psychosocial factors.

ASTHMA

The perception that children with asthma may have a higher incidence of depression and anxiety is hotly debated. One biologic theory suggests that co-occurrence of these physical and emotional symptoms may emerge as a consequence of dysregulated biochemical pathways, and the control of the processes of inflammation, bronchoconstriction, and mood regulation may share a common locus. In addition, children with asthma can experience anxiety related to anticipatory fear of having another asthma attack, particularly when exposed to environmental triggers known to precipitate asthmatic episodes. Being excluded from activities that require aerobic capacities beyond their abilities, not getting chosen by peers to play because of the perception of inferior physical abilities, or being restricted from the play by parents who fear their child's participation in sports maybe deleterious to their health are the psychosocial factors that may contribute to the development of this comorbidity. The parent's and child's knowledge about asthma and their perception of the severity of the illness play an important role in the potential development of psychiatric sequelae.

EPILEPSY

Emerging studies of epilepsy show it to be a disorder that overlaps with psychiatric conditions. School-age children with epilepsy have higher rates of learning, attention, and behavior problems that can affect their psychological development and self-esteem. In families with epileptic children, parents seem to have increased rates of marital discord and psychiatric difficulties.

Pseudoseizures, also known as psychogenic seizures, are a type of conversion disorder that can develop in an attempt to assume the sick role and achieve the secondary gain associated with it. Pseudoseizures can occur in children with or without epilepsy and are the most commonly reported conversion symptom in the child and adolescent psychiatry literature. Approximately 25% to 40% of patients with pseudoseizures also have epileptic seizures. Pseudoseizure resembles a convulsion but lacks the characteristic electroencephalogram (EEG) findings typical of a known seizure disorder.

DIABETES MELLITUS

The psychological ramifications of diabetes mellitus (DM) are numerous. Children and adolescents with diabetes often grapple with anxiety, depression, and eating disorders. The comorbidity of psychiatric illness with a diagnosis of diabetes can significantly increase the problems of managing diet and stabilizing glucose. Prevalence rates of depression in children and adolescents with type 1 DM are two to three times higher than those rates in adolescents without diabetes, according to population-based studies. There appears

to be a direct correlation between the development of depressive symptoms and the emergence of diabetic complications. Depression can often result in decreased personal and social functioning and can compromise a youth's ability to adhere to the diet, which is necessary for achieving psychological and physiologic well-being. Some studies indicate that depressed children with type 1 DM have poorer metabolic control, decreased quality of life, and impaired self-esteem.

TRANSPLANT RECIPIENTS

Although limited studies are available on children who are transplant recipients and suffer from oncologic disorders, evidence suggests these children also are at higher risk for developing psychological difficulties. Pediatric heart transplant recipients have greater academic difficulties compared to healthy controls. In a study of a limited sample of pediatric heart transplant patients, the majority of patients experienced adjustment difficulties after the transplant, manifested by anxiety and depression symptoms as well as behavior problems. A larger study conducted by Uzark, which gathered data using the Childhood Behavior Checklist, showed that pediatric heart transplant patients had more behavior problems and less social competence than healthy controls. Furthermore, the degree of their behavior problems correlated with greater degrees of family stress. Demaso's study revealed that 35% of cardiac transplant patients in the pretransplant phase met criteria for having psychological symptoms affecting their medical condition. This study also noted that 13% of this same cohort met criteria for mood disorder secondary to a general medical condition. These results resonate with other studies examining pediatric patients with cancer and with hematologic disorders.

A number of indications for clinical practice and management for the primary care physician and medical specialist can be inferred from these data. First, a pretransplant assessment of children covering the domains of psychological, cognitive, emotional, and behavioral functioning should be completed. This screening measure allows for early detection of possible underlying vulnerabilities so mental health practitioners can be brought on board prior to significant psychosocial decline as a preventive strategy. Additionally, these assessments should be coupled with family-based interventions that focus on disease psychoeducation.

Family Response

Parents' response to pain typically falls into two categories, the minimizing type or the reinforcing/encouraging type. Preponderance of either style of response can be problematic for certain youth depending on the biologic and environmental vulnerabilities. Increased sick-role behavior is associated with children whose parents are more solicitous in encouraging responses to pain. Additionally, psychological distress is linked to children with recurrent pain as a predictor of functional disability, and several studies have found elevated rates of depression and anxiety. In essence, in children suffering from recurrent pain syndromes who demonstrate greater psychological distress, parents' solicitous behavior was associated with greater childhood functional disability.

Parents of children with chronic health problems are at risk for emotional disturbances and impaired adjustment to the demands of caring for children with special needs, particularly if they are from lower socioeconomic strata. The family's ability to promote their child's health and wellness decreases as the psychological burden of caring for special needs children increases. Because pediatricians are often the first line of contact for these families, they are in an ideal position to provide the necessary psychosocial interventions, education, and support that can empower families to navigate the vagaries and complexities of the health care system. Pediatricians are in a unique position to coordinate the health care services for these children and their families.

There is a high prevalence of unmet needs among families of children with chronic health conditions identified in the primary care setting, particularly in the domains of effective care coordination and mental health services. These factors highlight the need for primary care physicians and pediatricians to collaborate frequently with mental health and other community professionals to provide additional support and resources. Appraisal of family burden should become a routine process of assessment and can be an effective screening method to ascertain which families are at high risk. Pediatric and psychiatric research has shown that a partnership among pediatricians, primary care physicians, and child mental health professionals can significantly enhance the levels of social support experienced by these families while fostering a more positive appraisal of the impact of the child's illness.

Expert Opinion on Management Issues

Collaboration between medical and mental health disciplines is essential. Referrals should be made early when medical workup is noncontributory and symptoms persist. Primary care providers should routinely triage families for distress because stressful home or school environments often precipitate psychosomatic illnesses. This evaluation should include assessing the presence of mental disorders or medical conditions in the family. In addition, the job of the primary care physician may include the management of parental stress and anxiety with psychoeducation and reassurance or referral for the parent if need be. As the gatekeeper of medical care, the primary care physician can also serve as the team leader by coordinating the different disciplines that may be involved in the care of the child. In addition to mental health providers, the team may include specialists in social service agencies, such as case workers or case managers, who may function as additional supports regarding the treatment

plan. It is critical that the collaboration among disciplines be consistent and synchronous when formulating the objectives for the treatment plan because it is extremely detrimental when families receive contrasting messages from different providers. The psychological aspects of managing psychosomatic illnesses require that all involved caregivers and supports try to be on the same page. Maintaining a daily routine by establishing consistent limits and boundaries is among the most beneficial of interventions (e.g., returning to school, continuing chores, and doing homework).

Providing a comprehensive treatment plan for children with chronic disease state is a surmountable challenge if the health provider is willing to use a multidimensional format (i.e., biopsychosocial), which undoubtedly requires the collaboration of different disciplines. In managing children with chronic pain, innovative psychosocial programs should be instituted in primary care settings to decrease indiscriminate and overuse of medical services and to promote child health and well-being.

Common Pitfalls

- Extensive and exhaustive medical workup yielding little information and exacerbating the sick role
- Neglecting to contact mental health professionals to reinforce treatment plan or directives to the family
- Failure to obtain adequate social and family history to understand the dynamic factors that may contribute to ongoing symptomatology
- Rewarding sick-role behavior by allowing the child to avoid routine activities (e.g., school attendance, homework, chores)
- Underdiagnosing depressive and anxiety symptoms that can contribute to the development and potentiation of psychosomatic illness

SUGGESTED READINGS

1. Adams CD, Streisand RM, Zawacki T, Joseph KE: Living with a chronic illness: A measure of social functioning for children and adolescents. J Pediatr Psychol 27:593–605, 2002. **Examines the ways children with chronic illness may have diminished functioning in social, academic, and interpersonal contexts.**
2. Campo J, Jansen-McWilliams L, Comer D, Kelleher K: Somatization in pediatric primary care: Association with psychopathology, functional impairment, and use of services. J Am Acad Child Adolesc Psychiatry 38:1093–1099, 1999. **Focuses on the role of the pediatrician in understanding that general and recurrent physical complaints may be associated with a psychosomatic illness in children.**
3. Drotar D: Psychological Interventions for Children with Chronic Physical Illness Their Families: Toward Integration of Research and Practice. Handbook of Psychotherapies with Children and Families. New York: Kluwer Academic/Plenum, 1999, pp 447–459. **Handbook written for health-care providers to quickly access useful interventions in children with chronic physical ailments.**
4. Franks R: Psychiatric issues of childhood seizure disorders. Child Adolesc Psychiatric Clin North Am 12:551–565, 2003.

Comprehensive review on the psychological and social sequelae of childhood seizure disorders.

5. Fritz G, Fritsch S, Hagino O: Somatoform disorders in children and adolescents: A review of the past 10 years. J Am Acad Child Adolesc Psychiatry 36:1329–1337, 1997. **This comprehensive peer-reviewed article discusses the need for better criteria in recognizing somatic symptoms in children and adolescents and also features epidemiologic and statistical data.**

6. Gallagher R, Koplewicz H: Treatment of adolescent precursors of adult anxiety disorders. Presented at the annual meeting of the American Association of Anxiety Disorders, Chicago, April 1991, 1991. **Highlights the significant need for early detection and treatment of anxiety disorders during adolescence to prevent later onset psychiatric morbidity.**

7. Holden EW, Deichamnn M, Levy J: Empirically supported treatments in pediatric psychology: Recurrent pediatric headache. J Pediatr Psychol 24:91–109, 1999. **Reviews the relative efficacy of different therapeutic modalities in managing recurrent pediatric headache.**

8. Lipsitz JD, Masia-Warner C, Apfel H, et al: Anxiety and depressive symptoms and anxiety sensitivity in youngsters with noncardiac chest pain and benign murmurs. J Pediatr Psychol 29:607–612, 2004. **Underscores the importance of screening for anxiety and mood disorders in children who present with somatic complaints of chest pain.**

9. Meesters C, Muris P, Ghys A, et al: The Children's Somatization Inventory: Further evidence for its reliability and validity in a pediatric and a community sample of Dutch children and adolescents. J Pediatr Psychol 28:413–422, 2003. **Examines the usefulness of using a rating scale to measure the presence of somatic symptoms in children.**

10. Mrazek D: Psychiatric symptoms in patients with asthma: Causality, comorbidity, or shared genetic etiology. Child Adolesc Psychiatric Clin North Am 12:459–471, 2003. **Comprehensive review of studies exploring the overlap between medical and psychiatric symptoms that may help clinicians deliver better care to their patients.**

11. Peterson CC, Palermo TM: Parental reinforcement of recurrent pain: The moderating impact of child depression and anxiety on functional disability. J Pediatr Psychol 29:331–341, 2004. **Helps clinicians appreciate how different parenting styles may potentiate psychiatric symptoms and somatic complaints in children.**

12. Szydlo D, Joost van Wattum P, Woolston J: Psychological aspects of diabetes mellitus. Child Adolesc Psychiatric Clin North Am 12:439–458, 2003. **Comprehensive review on the psychological and social sequelae in children and adolescents with diabetes mellitus.**

Common Sleep Disorders

Christopher M. Makris

KEY CONCEPTS

- Obstructive sleep apnea syndrome
  - Peak age for the development of obstructive sleep apnea syndrome (OSAS) is 2 to 7 years of age.
  - Hypertrophy of adenotonsillar tissue is the primary factor leading to OSAS in children.
  - A second peak occurs during adolescence and is frequently associated with obesity.
  - OSAS is more common in children with craniofacial anomalies, skeletal dysplasia, Down syndrome, neuromuscular disorders, and cerebral palsy.
  - OSAS often results in alterations in daytime function; children with OSAS may have decreased academic performance, hyperactivity, behavioral difficulties, excessive daytime sleepiness, irritability, or depression.
  - Most often a sleep study is required to make the diagnosis of OSAS in children; history alone is inadequate to base a recommendation for surgical intervention.
  - The majority of children with OSAS respond to surgical removal of the tonsils and adenoids.
  - For obese children with OSAS, weight loss should be a priority.
  - Children not "cured" with an adenotonsillectomy can be successfully treated with positive airway pressure therapy (continuous positive airway pressure [CPAP] or bilevel positive airway pressure [BiPAP]).
  - With the aid of a trained pediatric psychologist, almost all children can be successfully treated with positive airway pressure treatment.
- Sleep-onset association disorder and limit-setting disorder
  - Good sleep hygiene habits should be emphasized.
  - The environment at sleep onset should not require the presence of the caregiver to recreate. Rocking, holding, and other activities that depend on a parent's presence should be avoided.
  - Consistency in the sleep environment and the parental response to arousals is paramount.
- Narcolepsy
  - Prior to making a diagnosis of narcolepsy, other causes of daytime sleepiness must be ruled out.
  - A structured sleep/wake cycle and good sleep hygiene practices should be stressed.
  - Thirty-minute scheduled naps are often restorative.
  - Daytime sleepiness can be treated with an awake-promoting agent and/or stimulants.
  - The ancillary symptoms of narcolepsy (cataplexy, sleep paralysis, and hypnagogic hallucinations) may respond to selective serotonin reuptake inhibitors (SSRIs) or tricyclic antidepressants.
- Delayed sleep phase
  - The morning rise time should be set.
  - Napping must be avoided.
  - Early morning exposure to sunlight or a light box (2500 to 10,000 lux) for 30 minutes may reset the internal circadian clock.
  - Melatonin, 3 to 6 g, 1 hour prior to bedtime for 4 to 6 weeks, may be tried.
  - Substance abuse and depression must be ruled out.
  - The child *must* be committed to changing the sleep/wake schedule for interventions to be effective.
- Disorders of arousal
  - Parents should be educated regarding the benign nature and natural history of this disorder.
  - A structured sleep/wake cycle and appropriate sleep hygiene are paramount.
  - Sleep deprivation should be avoided.
  - During episodes, the child should not be awakened but gently guided back to his or her room and not overstimulated.
  - If events are severe, if the child may harm self or others, or if the events occur several times per night, a trial of clonazepam should be considered.

In general, children have few problems with sleep and are recognized as the gold standard for sleep quality. When tired, a child is able to fall asleep without difficulty, sleeps soundly despite outside stimuli, and awakens refreshed and ready to face the day. Unfortunately, not all children live up to this standard. An estimated one fourth of all children have sufficient difficulties with sleep to interfere with the quality of life of the child, the parent, or both. Sleep disorders such as narcolepsy, circadian rhythm disturbances, and obstructive sleep apnea, frequently thought of as adult sleep disorders, often originate in childhood. Sleep-onset association disorder and limit-setting disorder are sleep disorders unique to children. All too often, children's sleep difficulties are overlooked or not addressed adequately during encounters with health professionals.

Obstructive sleep apnea syndrome (OSAS) occurs when there is either partial or complete obstruction of the airway during sleep, resulting in increased resistance to airflow and nonrestorative sleep. The primary factor leading to OSAS in children is hypertrophy of adenotonsillar tissue, which is most prominent in children 3 to 7 years of age. A number of medical syndromes and conditions are associated with a functional narrowing of the upper airway. These include neuromuscular disorders, Down syndrome, Pierre Robin sequence, Treacher Collins syndrome, sickle cell anemia, Prader-Willi syndrome, and skeletal dysplasias.

In the infant or toddler, the most common etiology of sleeplessness is sleep-onset association disorder. The infant or toddler with sleep-onset association disorder typically falls asleep being rocked, held, or taking a bottle without difficulty. Nocturnal arousals, however, are often prolonged, occur every 2 to 3 hours, and require the parent to recreate the bedtime environment. Limit-setting disorder is characterized by bedtime struggles between the parent and child regarding bedtime routines and sleep onset. The child is unable or unwilling to go to sleep at the set bedtime. Battles between the child and parent become a nightly occurrence, with the child leaving the bedroom with complaints of hunger, thirst, headache, and so on, in efforts to avoid going to sleep. Inability of the parent to set limits and enforce appropriate bedtime routines and a defiant child are the primary factors leading to this disorder.

Disorders of arousal include confusional arousals, night terrors, and sleepwalking. Each of these disorders occurs as a partial arousal out of slow-wave sleep, typically in the first third of the night. During events the child appears confused or disoriented, has minimal response to outside stimulation, and often exhibits automatic behavior. The events are relatively brief, generally lasting less than 10 minutes, and they are not recalled by the child the following morning.

Disturbance in the timing of an individual's sleep patterns occurs in circadian rhythm disorders, the most common of which is delayed sleep phase syndrome. This syndrome can occur in children of all ages; however, it is seen most frequently in adolescence. Delayed sleep phase syndrome is characterized by a shift of the sleep/wake cycle to a much later hour. These individuals have difficulty falling asleep at bedtime, often staying awake until well after midnight, and then they have difficulty arising in the morning. When allowed to sleep on their own schedule, other than being delayed, sleep is unremarkable. This schedule, however, makes it very difficult for the child who is attending school, and referral to a sleep specialist often occurs after the child develops academic failure.

Excessive daytime sleepiness (EDS) in children is often overlooked by parents, teachers, and health care workers. Children with EDS are often labeled as lazy or as having a behavioral or attention disorder. Identifying EDS in children can be difficult because children may not appear somnolent but instead are inattentive, impulsive, and/or hyperactive. Too often children are referred only when their daytime sleepiness is profound and they are experiencing academic failure. The etiology of daytime sleepiness frequently is the result of poor-quality sleep, insufficient sleep, or delayed sleep phase. Narcolepsy is a relatively rare (incidence of 0.05%), lifelong, and often debilitating disorder characterized by excessive daytime sleepiness, cataplexy (brief loss of muscle tone, partial or complete, following emotional stimuli such as laughter or anger), sleep paralysis (loss of muscle tone at sleep onset or when awakening usually associated with a feeling of difficulty breathing), and/or hypnagogic hallucinations (vivid visual or tactile hallucinations occurring at sleep onset or offset).

Expert Opinion on Management Issues

The majority of children with OSAS respond to surgical intervention, with the procedure of choice being removal of the tonsils and adenoids. In a small percentage of patients, adenotonsillectomy does not result in a satisfactory "cure." For these children, continuous positive airway pressure (CPAP) or bilevel positive airway pressure (BiPAP) may be required. The use of a nasal positive pressure device in a child can be quite challenging, but with a high level of commitment by family and staff, successful therapy is possible in most children. Titration of CPAP or BiPAP should be carried out in the sleep laboratory every 6 to 12 months because changes in airway size and shape may occur abruptly in the growing child. Obstructive sleep apnea is a familial disorder, and children who were once declared cured by adenotonsillectomy may develop OSAS later in adolescence or adulthood and should therefore receive appropriate follow-up. Occasionally a child is unable to tolerate positive airway pressure, and other surgical procedures, including maxillary and/or mandibular distraction or placement of a tracheotomy, may be required. Fortunately, placement of a tracheotomy tube is now a rare event.

Treatment for sleep-onset association disorder involves behavioral techniques that teach children to initiate sleep on their own without the presence of a caretaker. Good sleep hygiene practices should be

---

BOX 1 Tips for Good Sleep Hygiene

- Maintain a structured sleep/wake cycle with fixed bedtime and rise times; these should not vary by more than 1 hour from day to day.
- Maintain an appropriate bedtime routine, a set of calming rituals repeated nightly.
- Provide adequate time for sleep; insufficient sleep time is a major problem for school-age children.
- Make sure the sleep environment is conducive to sleep. The room should be a comfortable temperature, free from excessive stimulation, and *quiet*.
- Advise that televisions, phones, and computers *not* be in the bedroom.
- Limit daily caffeine intake.
- Explain that naps should be age appropriate; younger children should take regularly scheduled naps; children older than 6 years should avoid napping altogether.
- Establish a daily exercise routine.

---

reinforced (Box 1). This includes a structured sleep/wake cycle, elimination of caffeine from the diet, and a consistent bedtime routine. At bedtime children should be comforted by the parent until sleepy. Once the child appears sleepy, they should be placed in their own bed and allowed to fall asleep on their own without the caregiver present. If the child cries, the parent may return to the room after 1 to 2 minutes and comfort them verbally but should avoid picking them up. After 1 to 2 minutes of soothing, the parent once again leaves the room, returning after 3 to 4 minutes if crying continues. The process should be continued with the time the parent spends outside of the room gradually lengthening. Once the child learns to make the transition from wakefulness to sleep on their own, problems with nocturnal awakenings resolve.

The diagnosis of limit-setting disorder is relatively easy; however, management is often more difficult and may require the assistance of a behavioral psychologist. In this disorder, bedtime is often a battle that provokes anxiety in both the child and the parent. A set of well-defined bedtime rules should be developed and written down. The rules should include appropriate nighttime routines with time limits, an appropriate bedtime, and developmentally appropriate responses to the child's opposition to the rules. The child should be aware of the bedtime rules, and positive reinforcement, using a reward system, should be used to help reinforce appropriate behaviors. Through positive feedback, bedtime should become a more enjoyable experience for both the child and the parent. If bedtime rules are adhered to consistently, without discussion or bartering, bedtime conflicts generally resolve without difficulty. The key to the successful treatment of this disorder is consistency because even minor deviations result in significant setbacks. Limit-setting disorder may be associated with deeper family conflicts or poor parenting skills, and evaluation and treatment by a trained psychologist or psychiatrist may be warranted.

Treatment of narcolepsy in children is similar to that in adults. The first step is to educate the child, family, and school about narcolepsy and its clinical manifestations and treatment. Everyone involved must understand that narcolepsy is a medical disorder and should be treated as such. Too often children with narcolepsy are labeled as lazy or as having behavioral problems. Good sleep hygiene practices with structured bedtime and rise times should become routine. Scheduling naps at school can be helpful, but it often requires the insistence of the family or physician to arrange.

Most children with narcolepsy require pharmacologic intervention to maintain wakefulness and to control the ancillary symptoms of the disorder (Table 1). Modafinil (Provigil), an agent approved by the U.S. Food and Drug Administration (FDA) for the treatment of narcolepsy, promotes wakefulness in adults and is used successfully in children with narcolepsy. Modafinil is associated with fewer side effects and has less potential for abuse than conventional stimulants, and it is now the drug of choice for this disorder. The starting dose of modafinil is 100 to 200 mg/day, with the dose titrated up to 400 mg/day as needed. Once-daily dosing is generally sufficient; however, some children benefit from a morning and noon dosing schedule. Methylphenidate or dextroamphetamine may be added if daytime sleepiness is not adequately controlled with modafinil alone. Doses start at 5 to 10 mg/day and are titrated upward as needed to control daytime sleepiness. Stimulants may be given two to three times per day, depending on the child, schedule, and the time of day he or she is most sleepy.

Ancillary symptoms of narcolepsy, including cataplexy, hypnagogic hallucinations, and sleep paralysis, are treated with nonsedating tricyclic antidepressants or selective serotonin reuptake inhibitors (SSRIs). Sodium oxybate (Xyrem) is now approved by the FDA for the treatment of cataplexy. This agent is associated with serious side effects and has significant potential for abuse, and it should only be prescribed by a sleep disorder specialist. Narcolepsy is often associated with depression, poor school performance, and altered social interactions; therefore counseling for the child and the family is a very important aspect of the treatment of this disorder.

Disorders of arousal are generally benign and self-limited and rarely require pharmacologic intervention. The family should receive appropriate education regarding the natural history of the disorder and strategies for decreasing the frequency and severity of the episodes. The nocturnal arousals in this disorder typically diminish in frequency and intensity as the child grows older. Sleep deprivation or an irregular sleep/wake cycle can exacerbate partial arousals. During the episodes the child should be gently directed back to the bedroom. Efforts to arouse the child should be avoided because they may exacerbate or prolong the episodes. For the child who experiences sleepwalking, safety measures must be addressed. Windows should be covered with heavy drapes and locked. Outside doors should be locked and, if need be, fitted with alarms to alert the family the child is attempting to leave the home. In severe cases when the child is in danger of self-injury or when episodes recur several times per night, drug therapy may be warranted. A benzodiazepine such as clonazepam is usually effective.

TABLE 1 Medication for Sleep Disorders

Generic Name (Trade Name) OTC/Rx	Dosage/Route/ Regimen	Maximum Dose	Dosage Formulations	Common Adverse Reactions	Comments
Narcolepsy Awake-Promoting Agents/Stimulants					
Modafinil (Provigil) Rx	PO: 100–400 mg/day May give single morning dose or divide into morning and noon dose	400 mg	Tablet: 100, 200 mg	Not a controlled substance. Fewer side effects than conventional stimulants. May write for refills. Less potential for abuse.	
Amphetamine/ dextroamphetamine (Adderall) Rx	PO: 10–80 mg/day May give single morning dose, bid or tid	80 mg	Tablet: 5, 7.5,10, 12.5, 15, 20, 30 mg Long-acting ER tablet: 5, 10, 15, 20, 25, 30 SR	Controlled substance; risk for abuse.	
Methylphenidate (Ritalin) Rx	PO: 10–80 mg/day May give single morning dose, bid or tid	80 mg	Tablet: 5, 10, 20 mg Long-acting capsule: 20, 20 SR, 30, 40 SR	Controlled substance; risk for abuse.	
Medications for Ancillary Symptoms of Narcolepsy: Cataplexy, Hypnagogic Hallucinations, Sleep Paralysis					
Venlafaxine (Effexor) Rx	PO: 37.5–150 mg/day	150 mg	Tablet: 25, 37.5, 50, 75, 100 mg Capsule, long acting: 37.5, 75, 150 mg	Nausea, headache, dry mouth, somnolence	
Fluoxetine (Prozac) Rx	PO: 10–20 mg/day	60 mg	Tablet: 10, 20, 40 mg	Nausea, headache, insomnia	
Sodium oxybate (Xyrem) Rx	PO: 6–9 g/day div in two equal doses	9 g	Solution: 0.5 g/mL	Nausea, headache, dizziness, somnolence	Only agent approved for treatment of cataplexy. Restricted access.
Other Sleep Medications					
Clonazepam (Klonopin) Rx	PO: 0.25–2 mg qhs	2 mg	Tablet: 0.5, 1.0, 2.0 mg	Drowsiness, ataxia, confusion	Used for disorders of arousals. May have rebound effect when discontinued.
Melatonin OTC	PO: 1–6 mg qhs	6 mg	Tablet: 1, 3, 5 mg	May reduce seizure threshold	Used to reset circadian clock; purity may be inconsistent.

bid, twice daily; div, divided; ER, extended release; OTC, over the counter; PO, by mouth; qhs, at bedtime; Rx, prescription; SR, slow release; tid, three times per day.

The family should be cautioned about the possibility of a rebound effect, with more severe events occurring upon discontinuation of the medication.

Treatment for delayed sleep phase syndrome is best carried out by maintaining a strict sleep/wake cycle, eliminating caffeine from the diet, and practicing good sleep hygiene. Bedtime and rise time on weekends and vacations should be within 1 hour of school day bedtime and rise time. Late night reading, talking on the phone, watching television, listening to music, and using the computer should be eliminated. Early morning light therapy, either with natural sunlight or a light box (2500 to 3000 lux for 30 minutes), can be quite helpful in advancing the sleep phase back to a more desired time. Successful treatment for delayed sleep phase syndrome requires a strong commitment by the adolescent and the family and will not be successful until the child is an active participant in the treatment process.

Common Pitfalls

Prevention is the single most important aspect in the treatment of behavioral pediatric sleep disorders. Parental education regarding the importance of a structured sleep/wake cycle, appropriate sleep hygiene, and appropriate responses to nocturnal arousals prevents the development of most behavioral sleep problems. Once sleep problems are identified, the primary care provider can usually manage most of the behavioral sleep disorders. In severe cases, referral to a sleep psychologist may be warranted. Physicians should have access to a sleep disorder center that has experience performing and interpreting pediatric sleep studies and multiple sleep latency tests (MSLTs). Children undergoing surgery for OSAS should be appropriately monitored postoperatively because they are at much higher risk for postoperative complications. Children with narcolepsy and OSAS who remain symptomatic following surgery should be referred to a sleep specialist for further evaluation and treatment.

Communication and Counseling

Sleep is a dynamic, vital process that can have a significant impact on the mental and physical health of children. Sleep disorders occur in approximately 25% of children and often go unrecognized by parents, teachers, and health care providers. Many sleep problems can be prevented by appropriate counseling regarding age-appropriate sleep requirements and sleep hygiene. Pediatricians should therefore use each encounter to address sleep concerns and provide appropriate counseling.

SUGGESTED READINGS

1. Clinical practice guidelines: Diagnosis and management of childhood obstructive sleep apnea syndrome. Pediatrics 109:704–712, 2000. **Consensus guidelines from the American Academy of Pediatrics regarding OSAS in children.**
2. Littner M, Johnson SF, McCall WV, et al: Practice parameters for the treatment of narcolepsy: An update for 2000. Sleep 23:451–466, 2001. **Very good review of the current treatment recommendations for excessive daytime sleepiness and ancillary symptoms associated with narcolepsy.**
3. Meltzer LJ, Mindell JA: Nonpharmacologic treatments for pediatric sleeplessness. Pediatr Clin North Am 51:135–151, 2004. **Excellent review of behavioral treatments for children experiencing difficulty sleeping through the night.**
4. Mindell JA, Owens JA: A Clinical Guide to Pediatric Sleep; Diagnosis and Management of Sleep Problems. Philadelphia: Lippincott Williams & Wilkins, 2003. **Excellent reference source with a CD containing disease-specific handouts.**

Breath-Holding Spells

Nathan J. Blum

KEY CONCEPTS

- Breath-holding spells have their onset before 30 months of age and their peak frequency between 13 and 24 months of age.
- Breath-holding spells are associated with a clear provoking event.
- The child should be evaluated for iron deficiency and anemia.
- An electrocardiogram (ECG) should be checked for prolonged QT syndrome in children with severe pallid breath-holding spells.

Breath-holding spells are involuntary (reflexive) events in which a child becomes apneic in response to a provoking event that causes anger, frustration, fear, or minor injury. The provoking event typically leads to crying that may be brief or prolonged. The crying ends at end expiration when the child becomes apneic and cyanotic or pale. If the event continues, the child loses consciousness and falls to the ground. On occasion a brief convulsion occurs. Often the child seems drowsy after the event.

Breath-holding spells usually begin between 3 and 18 months of age, although 5% to 10% of cases may begin before 3 months, and a slightly greater percentage of children do not have their first episode until after 18 months. It is unusual for breath-holding spells to begin after 30 months of age. At their peak frequency, which is most commonly between 13 and 24 months of age, the spells may occur more than once a day. It is very rare for breath-holding spells to continue past 7 years of age.

Breath-holding spells are classified depending on whether the child loses consciousness during the spell and whether the child is cyanotic or pallid during the spell. Simple breath-holding spells occur when the spell resolves before the child loses consciousness, whereas severe breath-holding spells are associated with loss of consciousness and sometimes a convulsion. Severe breath-holding spells occur in less than 5% of children, but simple spells are reported to occur in up to 27% of children. Cyanotic spells are more common than pallid spells, and some children have both types.

Pallid spells are thought to result from an overactive vagal response leading to bradycardia or brief asystole. Children with pallid spells appear to be at increased risk for having syncopal episodes as adolescents or adults. The etiology of cyanotic spells is less well understood, but it appears that a combination of autonomic dysregulation and pulmonary reflexes leads to expiratory apnea and intrapulmonary right to left shunting of blood or ventilation perfusion mismatches leading to cyanosis. Family genetic studies found that both types of breath-holding spells can occur in one family, suggesting the underlying pathophysiology of pallid and cyanotic spells may be related.

Making the diagnosis requires differentiating breath-holding spells from seizures and other causes of loss of consciousness. Usually the history of a provoking event and the presence of crying and color change before the loss of consciousness allow one to distinguish breath-holding spells from seizures without further medical evaluation. When the history is not clear, an electroencephalogram (EEG) may be helpful in distinguishing breath-holding spells from seizures. Children with breath-holding spells should have hemoglobin and iron studies because the spells are associated with iron deficiency and anemia. If a child has pallid spells or particularly severe spells, an electrocardiogram (ECG) should be obtained to distinguish the spells from conditions associated with cardiac arrhythmias, such as long QT syndrome. In infants, one should consider the possibility of gastroesophageal reflux resulting in apnea. In very rare cases, breath-holding

TABLE 1 Medication Used to Treat Breath-Holding Spells

Generic Name	Dosage/Route/ Regimen	Maximum Dose	Dosage Formulations	Common Adverse Reactions	Comments
Ferrous sulfate	5–6 mg iron/kg/day PO	60 mg	Drops: 15 mg of iron/0.6 mL Elixir: 44 mg of iron/5 mL Tablet: 60 mg	Nausea, vomiting, diarrhea, black stools	Discuss risk of overdose.

PO, by mouth.

spells are associated with brain stem dysfunction caused by tumors or Arnold-Chiari malformation. Investigation of these possibilities is indicated when breath-holding spells are progressive, occur outside of the usual age ranges for these spells, or other signs of brain stem dysfunction are apparent. Breath-holding spells are reported to occur with increased frequency in some more generalized disorders, such as Rett syndrome and familial dysautonomia, but they are not the sole manifestation of these disorders. Finally, the possibility of Munchausen syndrome by proxy as a form of child abuse should be considered.

Expert Opinion on Management Issues

In most cases, treatment primarily involves demystification and reassurance. The clinician should explain the sequence of events leading to the color changes and, if applicable, the loss of consciousness. When the child loses consciousness, parents should allow the child to remain in a horizontal position and resist the tendency to hold the child upright against their chest because this position may decrease cerebral perfusion. Parents should be encouraged to maintain appropriate expectations and limits for the child and can be reassured that breath-holding spells are not a sign of a severe behavior disorder or the result of inappropriate parenting practices.

The anemic child should be treated with iron, which decreases the frequency of breath-holding spells in many children. Although much less well investigated, treatment with iron (Table 1) is also reported to decrease the frequency of breath-holding spells in children who are not anemic. Thus it could be considered in these children if the breath-holding spells are severe.

CONTROVERSIAL INTERVENTIONS

On rare occasions, children with frequent severe breath-holding spells are found to have periods of bradycardia or brief asystole associated with the event. Anticholinergic medications may decrease the frequency of seizures in these children. A small series of children unresponsive to medications were treated with pacemaker implantation with improvement in symptoms. Although individual children may benefit from

these interventions, the vast majority can be managed without them.

Common Pitfalls

- Severe breath-holding spells with an unusual age of onset or natural history should prompt further evaluation.
- Attempts to perform cardiopulmonary resuscitation in children with breath-holding spells can cause aspiration.
- Holding the child upright decreases blood flow to the brain and prolongs the period of unconsciousness.

Communication and Counseling

Clinicians should inquire about the parents' response to the breath-holding spells. Although parents may be able to avoid some provoking events, it is not possible for them to prevent all episodes of fear or minor injury or desirable to try to prevent all experiences of anger or frustration. These are normal experiences for young children as they begin to express their autonomy. If children learn that emotional outbursts prevent parents from setting firm limits or cause parents to provide increased attention, the frequency of the outbursts and thus the breath-holding spells are likely to increase. If, after attempts at education and reassurance, parents are unable to set firm limits because they fear breath-holding spells or are unable to remain calm during the spells, referral to a mental health professional should be pursued.

SUGGESTED READINGS

1. Daoud AS, Batieha A, Al-Sheyyab M, et al: Effectiveness of iron therapy on breath-holding spells. J Pediatr 130:547–550, 1997. **Placebo-controlled study evaluating the efficacy of ferrous sulfate in the treatment of breath-holding spells.**
2. DiMario FJ: Prospective study of children with cyanotic and pallid breath-holding spells. Pediatrics 107:265–269, 2001. **Prospective study of the natural history of breath-holding spells.**
3. DiMario FJ: Breath-holding spells in childhood. Curr Probl Pediatr 29:281–299, 1999. **In-depth review of the natural history, pathophysiology, and treatment of breath-holding spells.**
4. McWilliam RC, Stephenson JDP: Atropine treatment of reflex anoxic seizures. Arch Dis Child 59:473–485, 1984. **Describes the use of an anticholinergic medication in the treatment of seven children.**

Attention Deficit Hyperactivity Disorder

Heidi M. Feldman and Irene M. Loe

KEY CONCEPTS

- Diagnosis of attention deficit hyperactivity disorder (ADHD) requires explicit descriptive information from one or both parents and also from one other informant, usually a teacher.
- Diagnostic evaluation should include review of core symptoms of ADHD and symptoms of commonly associated conditions, including anxiety, depression, oppositional defiant disorder, conduct disorder, learning disorders, and tic disorders.
- The diagnosis of ADHD requires functional impairments in multiple settings, usually at home and at school.
- Stimulant medications are the mainstay of psychopharmacologic treatment and are highly effective in reducing core behavioral symptoms.
- Behavior therapy is extremely helpful for reducing associated problems, such as family discord, academic failure, poor peer relationships, and low self-esteem.
- ADHD is a chronic condition and therefore requires long-term management in a medical home (a comprehensive, coordinated plan of care provided by a continuity provider).
- Adolescents and adults with persistent ADHD symptoms can have continued educational difficulties, as well as problems in the areas of employment, driving, and personal relationships.
- As adults, many individuals with ADHD can achieve at levels comparable to those of their siblings. Many individuals turn their rapid shifts of attention and high-energy level into assets in higher education and work settings.
- The ultimate goal of treatment is to facilitate positive adjustment to the individual's traits while minimizing adverse educational, occupational, social, or emotional consequences.

Attention deficit hyperactivity disorder (ADHD) is the most common neurobehavioral disorder in childhood. It is characterized by inability to sustain concentration and may be accompanied by hyperactivity and impulsivity. Attention deficits can be conceptualized as a spectrum, ranging from mild variations of normal to severe, chronic conditions. Studies suggest that approximately 4% to 12% of school-age children meet diagnostic criteria for the clinical disorder ADHD. This chapter provides practice guidelines for evaluating ADHD, choosing treatment interventions, and prescribing medications for ADHD, based primarily on the guidelines recommended by the American Academy of Pediatrics.

Management of ADHD is predicated on accurate diagnosis. Diagnosis requires that the child meet criteria from the *Diagnostic and Statistical Manual of Mental Disorders*, 4th edition *(DSM-IV)* in terms of

---

BOX 1　Common Coexisting Conditions

Learning Disorders
- Mild mental retardation
- Learning disabilities
- Poor academic performance
- Communication disorders

Neurobehavioral Conditions
- Oppositional defiant disorder
- Conduct disorder
- Anxiety
- Depression or dysthymia
- Tic disorders (e.g., Tourette syndrome)
- Substance use

---

core symptoms, onset, duration, and functional impairment in more than one setting. ADHD is often accompanied by other neurobehavioral disorders (Box 1).

Expert Opinion on Management Issues

Treatment options fall into two general categories, medication and behavior management. Studies show consistently that stimulant medications improve the core symptoms of ADHD. The dose and schedule of medication (Table 1) should be individualized based on target outcomes, and there are few contraindications. Tics and seizures are not absolute contraindications to the use of stimulant medications. However, children should be monitored closely for exacerbations of tics and seizures while on medication. Short-term side effects of stimulant medications include appetite suppression, sleep disturbance, headache, or stomachache. Irritability and emotionality are common when medication is wearing off in the late afternoon and can be managed with minor adjustments of the dosing schedule, planned after-school activities, or a small afternoon dose. Somatic complaints, prevalent in the first days of use, typically resolve within 1 to 2 weeks. Rarely, children become extremely unresponsive, socially withdrawn, or extremely focused on nonessential information. The side effects are more common in young children and those with mental retardation than in older children of normal intelligence. Reductions in the dose of stimulant medication often preserve benefits and eliminate side effects.

The optimal dose of a stimulant is the dose that provides maximal benefit with minimal side effects. The treating clinician should test several doses of medication to determine the optimal dose. The degree of improvement can be evaluated by repeating the baseline assessment after initiation of treatment. Many clinicians arrange for this reassessment within a month of initiating treatment. In a multisite randomized clinical trial, most of the children with ADHD showed reduction of rating scale scores to the normal range with the optimal medication dose. For children who do not benefit from first-line stimulant medication or who have significant side effects, the treating clinician should try another stimulant medication. The majority of children properly diagnosed with ADHD who fail to respond to one stimulant benefit from a different medication in this same category. Children can typically be maintained on the same dose for months to years.

Other medications may be considered in children who fail multiple types and formulations of stimulant medications. Two tricyclic antidepressants (TCAs), imipramine and desipramine, are effective for ADHD, but their use in children has declined because of the low margin of safety, possible cardiac side effects, and the requirements for careful monitoring of levels and adverse effects. Atomoxetine, a selective norepinephrine reuptake inhibitor, is another nonstimulant treatment option for ADHD approved for treatment of the condition in children by the U.S. Food and Drug Administration (FDA). Advantages of atomoxetine include long duration of action, little or no abuse potential, and good tolerability. Atomoxetine may be useful in children with tics. Atomoxetine carries a warning of increased risk of suicidal thinking in children and adolescents being treated with this medication. Although the half-life of atomoxetine is approximately 5 hours, clinical effects appear long lasting. Consequently, 2 to 4 weeks of therapy may be required before maximal response is achieved, and a taper is necessary when discontinuing the medication. Other antidepressants and α-adrenergic agents are not well studied in the treatment of ADHD and are not considered first-line therapies.

Behavior management therapy is not as effective as stimulant medications in reducing the core symptoms of hyperactivity, impulsivity, and inattention. Behavior management therapy is extremely useful for addressing associated symptoms of ADHD, including academic difficulty, poor peer or family relationships, and low self-esteem. Behavior management involves providing rewards and consequences for desired or undesired behavior, respectively. A behavior-management plan that coordinates the home and school interventions is ideal. Some children with ADHD are eligible for special education services, including academic support and behavior management. For children who do not meet eligibility criteria for special education, federal legislation through the Rehabilitation Act Section 504 provides a mechanism for implementing specialized plans at school, including behavior management.

Common Pitfalls

- Inaccurate diagnosis, including failure to obtain direct information from the school or to use the *DSM-IV* criteria
- Failure to diagnose coexisting conditions (see Box 1)

- Failure to assess baseline sleep disturbance, appetite, and irritability prior to initiating stimulant mediations, and failure to monitor these side effects after prescribing medication
- Failure to perform an adequate medication trial
- Shifting to second-line medications before trying multiple stimulant medications
- Failure to investigate reasons for poor effectiveness of medication or deterioration, including poor adherence, reduced use of behavior management, or presence of psychosocial stress
- Medication use without adequate psychosocial and educational interventions
- Use of ineffective psychosocial counseling techniques, such as psychodynamic or cognitive-behavioral therapies, for school-age children with ADHD, rather than evidence-based behavior management techniques
- Inadequate monitoring over time, especially after developmental, educational, or major environmental changes

Communication and Counseling

ADHD is a chronic condition. Management strategies should include all of the components of care that are required as part of the medical home. Parents and children need ready access to a clinician who monitors the condition over time. This clinician can provide current and unbiased information about the condition, its natural history, and its impact on child and family life. Parents may benefit from referral to parent support networks or national organizations to remain current about the condition and to learn strategies for care of their child. Coordination of educational, social, and medical services is likely to improve outcomes and simplify the burden on families. Regular monitoring is important because the condition and its manifestations may change with changes in the environment and with developmental progress of the child.

Appropriate family counseling includes education and support of families; recommendations to increase the structure of home life, such as initiating regular mealtimes and bedtimes; and rewards and consequences for behavior or compliance. Parents and teachers should use developmentally appropriate techniques, such as giving clear instructions, establishing age-appropriate rules, and using positive attention and praise in the home and classroom. Time-out and loss of privileges are appropriate consequences for noncompliance.

Additional classroom interventions include modifications of the school environment to reduce distractions. It may be necessary to make changes in the curriculum or testing procedures at school, such as testing children in quiet places with minimal distractions and eliminating time constraints. A strategy for coordinating home and school behavior management is the "Daily Report Card." The teacher sends home each day a report on the child's success or failure on specific

TABLE 1 Stimulant Medication Management Information

Active Ingredient	Drug Name	Dosing	Duration of Behavioral Effects*	Contraindications
Immediate Release				
Mixed salts of amphetamine (dextroamphetamine/ levoamphetamine)	Adderall Tablet (scored): 5 mg (blue), 7.5 mg (blue), 10 mg (blue), 12.5 mg (orange), 15 mg (orange), 20 mg (orange), 30 mg (orange)	Start with 5 mg 1–2 times per day and increase by 5 mg each week until good control achieved. Max dose: 40 mg.	4–6 h depending on dose	MAO inhibitors within 14 days. Glaucoma. Symptomatic cardiovascular disease. Hyperthyroidism. Moderate to severe hypertension.
Dextroamphetamine	Dexedrine Tablet: 5 mg (orange) Dextrostat Tablet (scored): 5 mg (yellow), 10 mg (yellow)	Tablet: Start with 5 mg 1–2 times per day and increase by 5 mg each week until good control achieved. Max dose: 40 mg.	Tablet: 4–5 h	MAO inhibitors within 14 days. Glaucoma.
Methylphenidate	Ritalin Tablet (scored): 5 mg (yellow), 10 mg (green), 20 mg (yellow) Methylin Tablet (scored): 5, 10, 20 mg Chewable tablets: 2.5, 5, 10 mg Oral solution: 5 mg/5 mL, 10 mg/5 mL Focalin (dexmethylphenidate) Tablet: 2.5 mg (blue), 5 mg (yellow), 10 mg (white)	Start with 5 mg (2.5 mg for Focalin) 1–2 times per day and increase by 5 mg each week until good control is achieved. May need third reduced dose in the afternoon. Max dose: 60 mg.	3–4 h	MAO inhibitors within 14 days. Glaucoma. Preexisting severe gastrointestinal narrowing. Use caution when prescribing concomitantly with anticoagulants, anticonvulsants, phenylbutazone, and tricyclic antidepressants.
Sustained Release				
Mixed salts of amphetamine (dextroamphetamine/ levoamphetamine)	Adderall XR Capsule (can be sprinkled): 5 mg (clear/blue), 10 mg (blue/blue), 15 mg (blue/white), 20 mg (orange/orange), 25 mg (orange/white), 30 mg (natural/orange)	Start at 10 mg in the morning and increase by 10 mg each week until good control is achieved. Max dose: 40 mg.	8–12 h	MAO inhibitors within 14 days. Glaucoma. Symptomatic cardiovascular disease. Hyperthyroidism. Moderate to severe hypertension.

Drug	Forms	Duration	Dosing	Contraindications
Dextroamphetamine	Dexedrine spansule (can be sprinkled): 5, 10, 15 mg (orange/black)	8–10 h	Start at 5 mg in the morning and increase by 5 mg each week until good control is achieved. Max dose: 45 mg.	MAO inhibitors within 14 days. Glaucoma.
Methylphenidate	Concerta Capsule (noncrushable): 18 mg (yellow), 27 mg (gray), 36 mg (white), 54 mg (reddish brown)	8–12 h	Start at 18 mg each morning and increase by 18 mg each week until good control is achieved. Max dose: 72 mg.	MAO inhibitors within 14 days. Glaucoma. Preexisting severe gastrointestinal narrowing. Use caution when prescribing concomitantly with anticoagulants, anticonvulsants, phenylbutazone, and tricyclic antidepressants.
	Ritalin SR Tablet: 20 mg SR (white) Ritalin LA Capsule (can be sprinkled): 10 mg (white/brown), 20 mg (white), 30 mg (yellow), 40 mg (light brown)	4–8 h	Start at 20 mg in the morning and increase by 10 mg each week until good control is achieved. May need second dose or regular methylphenidate dose in the afternoon. Max dose: 60 mg.	
	Metadate ER Tablet: 10, 20 mg ER Methylin ER Tablet: 10, 20 mg ER	4–8 h	Start at 10 mg each morning and increase by 10 mg each week until good control is achieved. May need second dose or regular methylphenidate dose in the afternoon. Max dose: 60 mg.	
	Metadate CD Capsule: 10 mg (green/white), 20 mg (blue/white), 30 mg (reddish brown/white) ER Focalin XR Capsule (can be sprinkled): 5 mg (blue), 10 mg (caramel), 20 mg (white)	4–8 h	Start at 10 or 20 mg each morning and increase by 10 or 20 mg each week until good control is achieved. Max dose: 60 mg. Start at 5 mg each morning and increase by 5 mg each week until good control is achieved. Max dose: 20 mg	

*These are estimates because duration may vary with the individual child.
ER, extended release; LA, long acting; MAO, monoamine oxidase; SR, sustained release; XR, extended release. Adapted from American Academy of Pediatrics, National Initiative for Children's Healthcare Quality. Caring for Children with ADHD: A Resource Toolkit for Clinicians. Elk Grove Village, Ill: American Academy of Pediatrics, 2002.

target goals. The parents provide appropriate rewards or consequences. Additional specific child interventions include focused work on problem-solving skills and social skills training.

SUGGESTED READINGS

1. American Academy of Pediatrics: The Classification of Child and Adolescent Mental Conditions in Primary Care: Diagnostic and Statistical Manual for Primary Care (DSM-PC), Child and Adolescent Version. Elk Grove Village, Ill: American Academy of Pediatrics, 1996. **Manual for primary care providers classifying neurobehavioral symptoms on a spectrum ranging from variants of normal, including symptoms subclinical for diagnosis, to full criteria for diagnostic disorder.**
2. American Academy of Pediatrics: The medical home. Pediatrics 110(1):184–186, 2002. **Policy statement issued by the American Academy of Pediatrics (AAP) advocating the use of a "medical home," a comprehensive, coordinated plan of care provided by a continuity provider to optimize the care of children with chronic conditions.**
3. American Academy of Pediatrics, National Initiative for Children's Healthcare Quality: Caring for Children with ADHD: A Resource Toolkit for Clinicians. Elk Grove Village, Ill: American Academy of Pediatrics, 2002. **Toolkit designed for primary care providers in accordance with the practice guidelines promulgated by the AAP. Clinical sheets, reminders, and handouts aid in efficient and effective diagnosis and management of children with ADHD.**
4. American Academy of Pediatrics, Committee on Quality Improvement, Subcommittee on Attention-Deficit/Hyperactivity Disorder: Clinical practice guideline: Diagnosis and evaluation of the child with attention-deficit/hyperactivity disorder. Pediatrics 105(5):1158–1170, 2000. **Evidence-based practice guideline issued by the AAP to aid the primary care provider in diagnosis and evaluation of children with ADHD.**
5. American Academy of Pediatrics, Committee on Quality Improvement, Subcommittee on Attention-Deficit/Hyperactivity Disorder: Clinical practice guideline: Treatment of the school-aged child with attention-deficit/hyperactivity disorder. Pediatrics 108(4):1033–1044, 2001. **Evidence-based practice guideline on treatment of ADHD that complements the guidelines on diagnosis and evaluation.**
6. American Psychiatric Association: Diagnostic and Statistical Manual of Mental Disorders, Fourth Edition. Text Revision. Washington, DC: American Psychiatric Association, 2000. **Manual from the American Psychiatric Association outlining diagnostic criteria for psychiatric disorders in infancy and childhood.**
7. Biederman J, Spencer T, Wilens T: Evidence-based pharmacotherapy for attention-deficit hyperactivity disorder. Int J Neuropsychopharmacol 7(1):77–97, 2004. **Comprehensive review of the evidence-based pharmacologic treatments for ADHD.**
8. MTA Cooperative Group: A 14-month randomized clinical trial of treatment strategies for attention-deficit/hyperactivity disorder. Arch Gen Psychiatry 56(12):1073–1086, 1999. **The Collaborative Multimodal Treatment Study of Children with ADHD is the largest randomized clinical trial of treatment options for ADHD, including medication, behavior management, and combined approaches.**
9. Wells KC, Pelham WE, Kotkin RA, et al: Psychosocial treatment strategies in the MTA study: Rationale, methods, and critical issues in design and implementation. J Abnormal Child Psychol 28(6):483–505, 2000. **Reviews the evidence basis for the design of the behavioral treatment strategies used in the Multimodal Treatment Study of Children with ADHD.**
10. World Health Organization: International Classification of Functioning [ICF], Disability, and Health. Geneva: World Health Organization, 2001. ICF framework also available online at http://www3.who.int/icf/icftemplate. Accessed November 26, 2005. **Textbook and website outline the dynamic framework proposed by the World Health Organization in classifying function, disability, and health.**

Dyslexia (Specific Reading Disability)

Sally E. Shaywitz, G. Reid Lyon, and Bennett A. Shaywitz

KEY CONCEPTS

- Dyslexia causes an unexpected difficulty with reading for children and adults who otherwise possess the intelligence, motivation, and reading instruction considered necessary for accurate and fluent reading.
- It is the most common and most carefully studied of the learning disabilities and affects 80% of all individuals identified as learning disabled.
- It is persistent and chronic and does not disappear over time.
- Diagnosis is established by unexpected difficulties in reading and associated linguistic problems at the level of phonologic processing.
- Treatment is based on evidence-based methods and reflects a life-span approach: remediation of the reading problem in early childhood and provision of accommodations in adolescents, young adults, and adults.

Developmental dyslexia is characterized by an unexpected difficulty in reading in children and adults who otherwise possess the intelligence and motivation considered necessary for accurate and fluent reading. The definition also assumes the individual has had the benefit of reasonably effective reading instruction. Dyslexia (or specific reading disability) is the most common and most carefully studied of the learning disabilities, affecting 80% of all individuals identified as learning disabled. Longitudinal studies indicate that dyslexia is a persistent, chronic condition; it does not represent a transient developmental lag. Among investigators in the field, a strong consensus now supports the phonologic theory. This theory recognizes that speech is natural and inherent, whereas reading is acquired and must be taught. To read, the beginning reader must recognize that the letters and letter strings (the orthography) represent the sounds of spoken language. To read, a child has to develop the insight that spoken words can be pulled apart into the elemental particles of speech (phonemes) and that the letters in a written word represent these sounds. Such awareness is largely missing in dyslexic children and adults.

At all ages, dyslexia is a clinical diagnosis. The clinician seeks to determine through history, observation, and psychometric assessment if there are unexpected difficulties in reading (i.e., unexpected for the person's age, intelligence, or level of education or professional status) and associated linguistic problems at the level of phonologic processing. No one single test score is pathognomonic of dyslexia. As with any other medical diagnosis, the diagnosis of dyslexia should reflect a thoughtful synthesis of all the clinical data available. In the preschool child, a history of language delay or of

---

BOX 1 Clues to Dyslexia from Second Grade On

Problems in Speaking

- Mispronunciation of long or complicated words
- Speech that is not fluent: pausing or hesitating often
- Use of imprecise language

Problems in Reading

- Very slow progress in acquiring reading skills
- Lack of a strategy to read new words
- Trouble reading *unknown* (new, unfamiliar) words sounded out
- The inability to read small function words such as *that, an, in*
- Oral reading that is choppy and labored
- Disproportionately poor performance on multiple-choice tests
- The inability to finish tests on time
- Disastrous spelling
- Reading that is very slow and tiring
- Messy handwriting
- Extreme difficulty learning a foreign language
- History of reading, spelling, and foreign language problems in family members

From Shaywitz S: Overcoming Dyslexia: A New Complete Science-Based Program for Reading Problems at Any Level. New York: Knopf, 2003, p 223 (with permission).

BOX 2 Critical Elements in an Effective Reading Program

- Phonemic awareness: the ability to focus on and manipulate phonemes (speech sounds) in spoken syllables and words
- Phonics: understanding how letters are linked to sounds to form letter-sound correspondences and spelling patterns
- Fluency
- Vocabulary
- Comprehension strategies

Note: These elements must be provided in a systematic, explicit, comprehensive manner.

---

not attending to the sounds of words (trouble learning nursery rhymes or playing rhyming games with words, confusing words that sound alike, mispronouncing words) and trouble learning to recognize the letters of the alphabet, along with a positive family history, represent important risk factors for dyslexia.

In the school-age child, presenting complaints most commonly center about school performance ("She's not doing well in school"), and often parents (and teachers) do not appreciate that the reason is a reading difficulty. A typical picture is that of a child who may have had a delay in speaking, does not learn letters by kindergarten, has not begun to learn to read by first grade, and has difficulty sounding out words consistently. The child progressively falls behind, with teachers and parents puzzled why such an intelligent child may have difficulty learning to read. The reading difficulty is unexpected with respect to the child's ability, age, or grade. Even after acquiring decoding skills, the child generally remains a slow reader. Thus bright dyslexic children may laboriously learn how to read words accurately, but they do not become fluent readers; that is, they do not recognize words rapidly and automatically. Dysgraphia and spelling difficulties are often present and accompanied by laborious note taking. Self-esteem is frequently affected, particularly if the disorder has gone undetected for a long period of time (Box 1).

In an accomplished adolescent or young adult, dyslexia is often reflected by slowness in reading or choppy reading aloud that is unexpected in relation to the person's level of education or professional status (e.g., graduation from a competitive college or completion of medical school and a residency). Thus, in bright adolescents and young adults, a history of phonologically based reading difficulties, requirements for extra time

on tests, and current slow and effortful reading (all signs of a lack of automaticity in reading) are the sine qua non of a diagnosis of dyslexia. In summary, at all ages, a history of difficulties getting to the basic sounds of spoken language, of laborious and slow reading and writing, of poor spelling, and of requiring additional time in reading and in taking tests provide indisputable evidence of a deficiency in phonologic processing, which, in turn, serves as the basis for, and the signature of, a reading disability.

Expert Opinion on Management Issues

The management of dyslexia demands a life-span perspective; early on, the focus is on remediation of the reading problem. As a child matures and enters the more time-demanding setting of secondary school, the emphasis shifts to also incorporate the important role of providing accommodations. Effective intervention programs provide children with systematic instruction in each of the critical components of reading (Box 2) and the practice aligned with that instruction. The goal is for children to develop the skills that will allow them to read and understand the meaning of both familiar and unfamiliar words they may encounter.

Just as in other areas of medicine, for the first time, a knowledge base is now developing to inform the practice of evidence-based education. In 1998, the U.S. Congress, concerned with what appeared to be an epidemic of poor reading nationally, mandated that a National Reading Panel (NRP) be formed. A major goal was to review the extant literature on teaching reading and to identify which specific methods and approaches are most effective. Based on an earlier consensus report from the National Research Council and on the results of its own analysis, the NRP reported five critical elements that are necessary to teach reading effectively:

1. Phonemic awareness (the ability to focus on and manipulate phonemes, elemental speech sounds, in spoken syllables and words)
2. Phonics (understanding how letters are linked to sounds to form letter-sound correspondences and spelling patterns)
3. Fluency

4. Vocabulary
5. Comprehension strategies

The NRP emphasized that these elements must be taught systematically and explicitly, rather than in a casual, fragmented, or implicit manner. Such systematic phonics instruction is more effective than whole-word instruction that teaches little or no phonics or teaches phonics haphazardly.

Fluency is of critical importance because it allows for the automatic, attention-free recognition of words, thus permitting these attentional resources to be directed to comprehension. Although fluency is generally recognized as an important component of skilled reading, it is often neglected in the classroom. The most effective method to build reading fluency is a procedure referred to as repeated oral reading with feedback and guidance; that is, the teacher models reading a passage aloud, the student rereads the passage repeatedly to the teacher, another adult, or a peer, receiving feedback until he or she is able to read the passage correctly. The evidence indicates that this process of repeated oral reading with feedback has a clear and positive impact on word recognition, fluency, and comprehension at a variety of grade levels and applies to all students—for good readers as well as those experiencing reading difficulties.

Where the evidence is less secure is for programs for struggling readers that encourage large amounts of independent reading, that is, silent reading without any feedback to the student. Thus, even though independent silent reading is intuitively appealing, at this time the evidence is insufficient to support the notion that in struggling readers, reading fluency improves. No doubt a correlation exists between being a good reader and reading large amounts; however, there is a paucity of evidence indicating a *causal relationship* (i.e., if poor readers read more they will become more fluent). In contrast to teaching phonemic awareness, phonics, and fluency, interventions for reading comprehension are not as well established. In large measure, this reflects the nature of the very complex processes influencing reading comprehension. The limited evidence indicates that the most effective methods for teaching reading comprehension involve teaching vocabulary and strategies that encourage an active interaction between reader and text.

Large-scale studies to date have focused on younger children; as yet, few data are available on the effect of these training programs on older children. The data on younger children are extremely encouraging, indicating that using evidence-based methods can remediate and may even prevent reading difficulties in children in primary school.

An essential component of the management of dyslexia in students in secondary school, and especially in college and graduate school, incorporates the provision of accommodations. High school and college students with a history of childhood dyslexia often present a paradoxical picture; they may be similar to their unimpaired peers on measures of word recognition and comprehension, yet they continue to suffer from the

---

BOX 3　Accommodations for People with Dyslexia

Providing extra time for reading is by far the most common accommodation for people with dyslexia. Other helpful aids include:

- Laptop computers with spelling checkers
- Tape recorders in the classroom
- Recorded books (materials are available from Recording for the Blind and Dyslexic, 800-221-4792; http://www.rfbd.org/)
- Access to syllabi and lecture notes
- Tutors to "talk through" and review the content of reading material
- Alternatives to multiple-choice tests (e.g., reports or orally administered tests)
- A separate, quiet room for taking tests

---

phonologic deficit that makes reading less automatic, more effortful, and slow.* Consequently, for these readers with dyslexia, providing extra time is an essential accommodation; it allows them the time to decode each word and to apply their unimpaired higher-order cognitive and linguistic skills to the surrounding context to get at the meaning of words they cannot entirely or rapidly decode. Other accommodations are listed in Box 3. With such accommodations, many students with dyslexia are now successfully completing studies in a range of disciplines, including medicine.

People with dyslexia and their families frequently consult their physicians about unconventional approaches to the remediation of reading difficulties; in general, very few credible data support the claims made for these treatments (e.g., optometric training, medication for vestibular dysfunction, chiropractic manipulation, and dietary supplementation). Pediatricians should be aware that no one magical program can remediate reading difficulties; a number of programs following the guidelines provided earlier are highly effective in teaching struggling children to read, provided they are implemented by knowledgeable teachers.

Common Pitfalls

- "Don't worry, she'll outgrow the reading problem." Dyslexia is a persistent problem and *not* a developmental lag. Reading problems in the early school years (grades 1 through 3) will *not* disappear over time.
- "He doesn't have a reading problem, he's just a slow reader." Problems in reading fluency may represent the most common problems in reading in later school years, and in adolescents and young adults, it may be the hallmark of dyslexia.
- "He should take his SATs [Scholastic Aptitude Tests] without accommodations—you don't want

---

*Neurobiologic data now provide strong evidence for the necessity of extra time for readers with dyslexia. Functional MRI data demonstrate a disruption in the left occipitotemporal word-form area, the region supporting rapid reading. At the same time, readers compensate by developing anterior systems bilaterally and the right homologue of the left word-form area. Such compensation allows for accurate reading but does not support fluent or rapid reading.

him labeled, do you?" In adolescents and young adults, accommodations in the form of extra time on standardized tests are as critical to the student with dyslexia as insulin is to a student with diabetes. Furthermore, flagging of scores (using a marker to denote the test was taken under special circumstances) is no longer used by the Educational Testing Service (ETS) for most standardized tests, including SAT.

SUGGESTED READINGS

1. Foorman BR, Brier JI, Fletcher JM: Interventions aimed at improving reading success: An evidence-based approach. Dev Neuropsychol 24:613, 2003. **More information about effective reading programs.**
2. Report of the National Reading Panel: Teaching Children to Read: An Evidence-Based Assessment of the Scientific Research Literature on Reading and its Implications for Reading Instruction. NIH Publication 00–4754. U.S. Department of Health and Human Services, Public Health Service, National Institutes of Health, National Institute of Child Health and Human Development, 2000. **Reviews the methodology for determining the most effective reading interventions for struggling readers.**
3. Shaywitz S: Overcoming Dyslexia: A New and Complete Science-Based Program for Reading Problems at Any Level. New York: Knopf, 2003. **Review the current scientific understanding of reading and dyslexia and its translation into approaches to diagnosis and evidence-based effective reading programs and accommodations.**

Child Maltreatment

John Stirling

KEY CONCEPTS

- Abuse should always be considered in the differential diagnosis of injury.
- Diagnosis requires a thorough medical evaluation.
- Most abuse reports are for neglect.
- Management of child abuse requires a multidisciplinary team effort.

Few other conditions carry so bleak a prognosis as untreated childhood abuse, and few are harder for the physician to diagnose with confidence. Certainly, few require such a comprehensive, multidisciplinary approach to treatment or so regularly threaten providers with the prospect of involvement with the legal system. Thus management of a maltreated child presents special challenges in recognition, diagnosis, and treatment.

In a volume on the therapy of pediatric illness, it is beyond the scope of this short chapter to fully explore all aspects of child maltreatment. The goal, instead, is to remind the practitioner of the requirements of successful intervention:

- Considering maltreatment as part of the differential diagnosis of injury
- Anticipating challenges to accurate diagnosis

- Recognizing acute and chronic sequelae of maltreatment
- Working effectively as a member of a multidisciplinary team

Expert Opinion on Management Issues

CONSIDERING THE DIAGNOSIS

To a large extent, the practical management of injuries caused by maltreatment of children is covered elsewhere in this volume. After all, bruises, broken bones, and other somatic injuries heal in much the same fashion whether the injuries happened accidentally or at the hand of another. Management of inflicted injuries, however, extends beyond merely approximating the wound edges or immobilizing a limb. To facilitate healing and to protect against future harm, the physician must accurately diagnose the nonaccidental nature of the injury and take steps to ensure that further abuse will not occur. To simply treat the injuries without taking steps to identify and eliminate their cause leaves the child, and perhaps others, open to future harm. Failure to make a timely diagnosis and to properly treat can have lifelong, or fatal, consequences. This consideration is equally important when the allegations involve neglect, as when a patient is receiving inadequate nutrition or not receiving needed health care. The majority of reports received by child protective services involve neglect, and the consequences can be just as serious as those of other types of abusive injury.

Given these considerations, it is surprising how little formal training in recognizing and treating child abuse is provided most practitioners. Medical schools and residency programs vary widely in their coverage of these issues, and there are as yet few fellowship programs, although the number continues to grow. Although child abuse was recognized by the ancients, modern medicine only began to take a scientific interest during the latter half of the 20th century. The pioneering work of C. Henry Kempe in 1962 describing the battered child syndrome led to the recognition that child abuse is in fact a widespread phenomenon in modern society. Subsequent literature built on this realization, and recent decades saw a virtual explosion of research-based literature, often published in the several journals devoted to the topic of child maltreatment. A well-established body of literature now describes the nature and appearance of child maltreatment, its causes and sequelae, and its horrible cost to society.

It can be hard to believe that a caregiver can so violate the bond of trust with a dependent child, but ample evidence indicates that many do. There can be no doubt of the serious consequences or of our responsibility to act on the child's behalf. The practitioner must work to overcome the natural reluctance to consider abuse when examining an injury or will lose a valuable opportunity to intervene on the child's behalf.

CHALLENGES TO DIAGNOSIS

Proper treatment of child abuse depends on proper diagnosis, but once abuse is considered among the possible etiologies for the injury in question, diagnosis becomes more difficult. Physicians are trained to rely on the history in making a diagnosis, but when the injury is caused by abuse, the history may be either absent (as when the nonoffending caretaker accompanies the child) or deliberately misleading (when given by the abuser or a compliant spouse). Examiners must persistently question unwitnessed injuries and be skeptical when the history fails to account for the extent of the damage. When the abuser is hiding the truth, the explanation for the injury may change over time. The practitioner should take pains to accurately document the history given because it may be compared to later versions.

As important as is consideration of abuse in the diagnosis, the physician in the office or hospital rarely has the resources to diagnose child abuse with complete certainty. Although the physical examination, imaging, and laboratory studies provide much information, much is still missing. The site of the injury must sometimes be visited (e.g., to measure the height of the stove or the temperature of the tap water in a scalding). Caregivers must be interviewed, but so must potential witnesses, who may not be present when the child presents to the doctor. Past medical records, often from other institutions, may be important, as may records of previous involvement with protective services or law enforcement.

REPORTING

When child abuse is considered as a diagnosis, the physician must act as a part of a multidisciplinary team to gather information and protect the child from further harm. Such a team is activated when the doctor reports the abuse to law enforcement or to child protective services. Reporting is best considered as a step in information gathering. Once the doctor raises the concern of abuse, the other team members can set about gathering the necessary social and environmental information to ensure more certain diagnosis. Law enforcement and protective services personnel can also help ensure that the victim does not suffer further harm during the investigation. A formal risk assessment after social investigation can help guarantee that the probable perpetrator is restrained or incarcerated or that the child is placed in foster care until safe. Although such actions are of paramount importance in the management of the abused patient, they cannot be achieved by the doctor alone.

Reporting suspected abuse can be difficult for the physician. Many feel it premature to report unless sure of abuse, although such assuredness is seldom, if ever, possible at the bedside. This fear is compounded by a concern that they may be open to reprisal if their fears prove unfounded. In fact, however, all states have long since passed laws indemnifying medical personnel (and most others who care for children) against such attacks, as long as the reports are made in good faith.

Other physicians fear loss of control, lacking confidence in others they may not know well or with whom they rarely communicate. Some worry that their relationship with the caregivers will suffer if an investigation commences. In both cases, the physician can act to minimize these concerns. A sensitive explanation of the reasons for reporting and of the mandated reporting statutes can serve to maintain relations with the caregivers. Efforts to get to know the caseworkers and investigators can be valuable and will help the physician continue to manage the patient as the case evolves.

THE PHYSICIAN'S ROLE

The composition of the investigatory team may vary from case to case. Law enforcement, for example, may be unable or unwilling to participate substantially in misdemeanors or cases where criminal charges cannot be brought, whereas child protective services workers are usually limited by statute to intrafamilial cases. As an individual whose global concern for the child's welfare is not circumscribed by jurisdictional considerations, the health care professional can play a key role in coordinating the team's initial plan of action.

Once a long-term safety plan is in place, the practitioner can continue to provide information about the plan's success and monitor the patient for sequelae. Children should be followed regularly, with careful attention to behavioral and developmental progress. Follow-up care of abused children, beyond ensuring that injuries heal properly, may involve referral to mental health professionals. Reactivation of the multidisciplinary team may be necessary when repeated abuse is suspected or a caregiver does not comply with the safety plan.

As the medical study of child maltreatment enters the 21st century, it has achieved the status of a true subspecialty, with ample literature, a research base, and fellowship training. When consultation is desired, it is usually possible to discuss the case with a pediatrician specially trained in child abuse evaluation or to refer for a second opinion. In remote communities, exchange of information via secure Internet channels may make it unnecessary for the family to travel long distances. The physician may also play a key role in the prevention of child maltreatment (discussed later).

COURT

The child's long-term safety may sometimes depend on the physician's testimony in court. Both civil proceedings, in which custody is determined, and criminal proceedings can derive from a report of abuse. Either may require the health care provider to supply the court with the information relevant to the decision to report and with other observations of the child's health. In court, advocacy for the child is best left to the attorneys involved in the case. The medical professional must remember that his or her role in court is to provide information objectively to the judge or jury and to help them understand the medical concerns relevant to the child's welfare.

A clinician may be asked to testify about a child's diagnosis and treatment months or years after the initial presentation and often must rely almost exclusively on medical records. That such records must be comprehensive, legible, and retrievable is common sense. As mentioned earlier, significant negatives must be recorded as well as positives, and comments on the child's development, speech, vocabulary, and demeanor may prove valuable as aids to recollection. Where possible, the caregiver's history—and certainly the child's—should be recorded as near verbatim as possible. Experienced physicians know that comprehensive and legible records may reduce the chances that a case will ever go to trial.

Common Pitfalls

- Failure to consider abuse in the differential diagnosis
- Missing significant injury by failing to do a complete evaluation
- Not asking for consultation when diagnosis is in question
- Failure to recognize abuse or neglect as the source of problem behavior
- Attempting to manage abusive injury in the medical setting alone
- Keeping inadequate records of the evaluation

Communication and Counseling

WHEN ABUSE HAS OCCURRED

Beyond communicating with other professionals, effective management of abuse demands sensitivity to the needs of child and to the nonoffending family members who will continue to act as caretakers. Whether acute or chronic, intra- or extrafamilial, the abuse or neglect of a child is a crisis that affects every member of the family. The alert practitioner anticipates the caregiver's feelings of guilt, anger, and bewilderment when faced with discovery of abuse. By acknowledging these emotions, and reassuring parents they are neither unique nor alone, the doctor can begin the healing process. Child victims may feel fear or guilt, and they may need reassurance they will recover. All family members may benefit from referral to an experienced counselor during these stressful times, and children suffering from chronic sequelae, such as post-traumatic stress disorder (PTSD) or attachment disorders, may require extensive therapy to minimize morbidity. The medical practitioner can help guide families through this unfamiliar territory by acting as a trustworthy resource and advocate.

PREVENTION

When a condition is as damaging and as difficult to treat as the abuse of a child, medical science always turns to the task of prevention. Immunization and programs to prevent accidental injury are effective in the fight to defend children against serious harm, and recent years have seen a swell of interest in prevention efforts directed against child maltreatment.

Successful prevention efforts recognize that child abuse, whether physical, sexual, or neglectful, is best considered a symptom rather than a disease, and they seek to address the underlying condition that impairs the bond between infant and parent. Prevention researchers agree with public health experts that the greatest risks for abuse occur in the presence of the three Ds: maternal depression, drug abuse, and domestic violence. When these conditions are recognized and addressed early in the dyad's career, both parent and child can build a healthier relationship, and abuse of all types decreases. Programs employing nurses as home visitors show the best results, especially when the visits begin during the pregnancy. Although physicians in practice have a unique opportunity to recognize these red flag conditions and to counsel and refer for appropriate treatment, their response is often inadequate or absent altogether. The large medical associations have all developed policies on these conditions, at least as separate issues, and it is hoped further progress will be seen.

A fourth D, lack of developmental awareness, can also correlate with maltreatment. When parents' expectations for the child's behavior exceed the child's abilities, they can become angry, resorting to harsher and harsher punishments. This pattern is most often seen in the context of toilet training and when parents are dealing with oppositional defiant behavior. Pediatricians and other physicians caring for families receive training in child development, and they have ample opportunity to help caregivers hold appropriate developmental expectations, but time constraints and other priorities often leave these opportunities unrealized. At the time of this writing, several efforts are under way to help address this failure. Some attempt to provide improved developmental training for practicing physicians and improving anticipatory guidance; others study the value of adding a developmental specialist to the pediatric office staff. All recognize the value of communicating accurate developmental expectations to the parent and the patient.

Our society is beginning to recognize the enormous penalty we pay when we fail to protect our children. From the level of the primary practitioner to that of the federal government, more attention than ever before is being paid to the prevention of child abuse. As the knowledge base grows with increased collaboration, it is to be hoped that prevention remains a priority.

SUGGESTED READINGS

1. Felitti VJ, Anda RF, Nordenberg D, et al: Relationship of childhood abuse and household dysfunction to many of the leading causes of death in adults: The adverse childhood experiences (ACE) study. Am J Prev Med 14:245–258, 1998. **Groundbreaking research into the consequences of abuse.**
2. Helfer MA, Kempe RS, Krugman RD (eds): The Battered Child. Chicago: University of Chicago Press, 1997. **Excellent**

reference text covering issues of physical sexual abuse and neglect.

3. Reece RM (ed): Treatment of Child Abuse. Baltimore: Johns Hopkins University Press, 2000. **Excellent reference text covering issues of physical sexual abuse and neglect.**

4. Reece RM, Ludwig S (eds): Child Abuse: Medical Diagnosis and Management. Baltimore: Johns Hopkins University Press, 2001. **Discusses proven interventions for abused children.**

Mental Retardation

Bruce K. Shapiro and Mark L. Batshaw

KEY CONCEPTS

- Mental retardation is a functional diagnosis that may result from many different etiologies.
- All children with mental retardation require standard well-child care; some have syndrome-specific health requirements.
- Mental retardation is associated with many different comorbidities.
- Successful management depends on a full delineation of the child's strengths and challenges.
- Environmental adjustments may be more effective than pharmacotherapy for behavioral dysfunction.

The diagnosis of mental retardation requires that three criteria be met:

1. Significantly subaverage intellectual functioning (an IQ standard score of 70 to 75 or below)
2. Concurrent deficits or impairments in adaptive functioning in at least two of the following areas: communication, self-care, home living, social and interpersonal skills, use of community resources, self-direction, health and safety, functional academic skills, leisure, and work
3. Onset before 18 years of age

The degrees of mental retardation include mild, moderate, severe, and profound, with each level representing an additional standard deviation (approximately 15 points) below the mean.

The identification of a child with intellectual deficits is a responsibility of the pediatrician. Most children do not come to the pediatrician's attention because of failed screening tests but rather as a result of dysmorphisms, the identification of a condition associated with developmental disabilities (e.g., Down syndrome), or failure to achieve early language and motor milestones. Mental retardation has no specific physical characteristics; most children with mental retardation have normal physical features and physical examination.

Mental retardation is not always a lifelong disorder. Children who meet the criteria for mental retardation at an early age may later evolve into a specific developmental disorder (e.g., communication disorder, autism, cerebral palsy). Others who have mild mental retardation during their school years may develop sufficient adaptive behavior skills so they no longer meet the criteria for the diagnosis of mental retardation as adolescents. Maturational effects may result in children moving from one diagnostic category to another (e.g., from moderate to mild mental retardation). Alternatively, some children with a specific learning disability or communication disorder may not maintain their rate of cognitive growth and may fall into the range of mental retardation over time. By adolescence, however, the IQ and the diagnosis generally are stable.

The long-term outcome of individuals with mental retardation depends on the underlying etiology, the degree of cognitive and adaptive deficits, the presence of associated medical and developmental impairments, the capabilities of the families, and the school/community supports, services, and training provided to the child and family. Life span is normal in all but the most severely affected individuals or in those with syndromes that have specific medical risks.

Expert Opinion on Management

Each child with mental retardation should have a medical home with a pediatrician who is readily accessible to the family to answer questions, help coordinate care, and discuss concerns. The role of the pediatrician includes involvement in prevention efforts, early diagnosis, identification of associated impairments, interdisciplinary management, provision of primary care, and advocacy for the child and family.

Although there are general principles of treatment, the management of each child with mental retardation requires a unique plan. A comprehensive plan of management should be designed to achieve goals in the areas of health care, social inclusion, behavioral independence, education, and productivity. Effective management requires the primary care provider to marshal resources that extend beyond the traditional medical role and interface with education and social services. A management plan should address the relevant specialized medical consultations, family support services (including counseling, financial planning, sibling support, and respite care), education and supplemental therapies (occupational therapy, physical therapy, speech and language therapy), assistive technology (e.g., computers, orthoses, augmentative communication devices), and other supports needed to achieve community inclusion. Successful management depends on a full delineation of the child's strengths and challenges, the setting of realistic long-term goals based on developmental levels rather than chronologic age, and the periodic readjustment of the program based on experience.

Management is a dynamic process. The objectives shift as the child advances in age. Initially, the focus is on diagnosis, etiology, and parental response to the diagnosis. Later, the focus shifts to academic achievement, socialization, and recreation/play. The academic focus continues through middle school but is supplemented by training directed toward increased community independence and prevocational skills. High school should focus on the transitions to work, the adult health care system, and long-term living accommodations.

GENERAL PEDIATRIC CARE

Most children with mental retardation do not have medical needs that extend beyond those of typically developing children. However, as a group, children with mental retardation are at greater risk for medical complications and use more medical services. In addition to ensuring that the care of children with mental retardation is in compliance with the American Academy of Pediatrics (AAP) Recommendations for Preventive Health Care, primary care providers should pay particular attention to oral health, growth (height, weight, and head circumference); vision (especially refractive errors and strabismus), and hearing. Mental retardation is not a contraindication to immunization or other established preventative measures.

Some children with genetic syndromes (e.g., fragile X and Down syndrome) have medical needs related to their underlying syndromes and not to their mental retardation. The AAP has developed policy statements about the care of children with a number of the more common causes of mental retardation (available online at http://aappolicy.aappublications.org/policy_statement/index.dtl).

ASSOCIATED IMPAIRMENTS

Although mental retardation is not treatable, many associated impairments are amenable to intervention and therefore should be identified early. Mental retardation is often associated with other deficits that may prove more limiting than the cognitive impairment itself. These include cerebral palsy, seizures, sensory impairments, autistic spectrum disorders, speech and flanguage disorders, attention deficit hyperactivity disorder (ADHD), and disorders of behavior and emotion. Formes frustes of these disorders include clumsiness, attentional peculiarities, articulation disorders, stubbornness, and tactile defensiveness that, if not addressed, can also lead to failed management programs.

EDUCATION

Education is the single most important discipline involved in the treatment of children with mental retardation. The educational program must focus on the child's needs and address the child's individual strengths and challenges. These management plans are called by different names: individualized family service plans (IFSPs) for infants and toddlers in early intervention programs, individualized education plans (IEPs) for children 3 to 21 years of age who receive special education, and individualized transition plans (ITPs) for adolescents receiving vocational rehabilitation services. The plans establish eligibility for services, delineate current and needed skills, identify supports that correspond to needs, and evaluate the success of the intervention.

BEHAVIOR/MENTAL HEALTH DISORDERS

Disorders of behavior and mental health in individuals with mental retardation are the primary causes for out-of-home placements, failure in community placements, reduced employment prospects, and reduced opportunity for social integration and leisure activities in community settings. Children with mental retardation experience the full spectrum of mental health disorders. Behavior disorders may result from organic problems, family difficulties, and/or a mismatch between the child's abilities and the demands of the situation.

Some behavior and emotional disorders are difficult to diagnose in children with more severe mental retardation because of their limited abilities to understand, communicate, interpret, or generalize what they are experiencing. Disordered behavior may represent attempts by the child to communicate, gain attention, or avoid frustration. It may also be an expression of a medical condition (e.g., ear infection, urinary tract infection, constipation). In assessing the challenging behavior, one must consider whether it is inappropriate for the child's mental age, rather than for his or her chronologic age. Other disorders may be masked by the mental retardation (e.g., anxiety disorder, depression, or ADHD). Finally, some behavioral conditions are unique to mental retardation (e.g., self-stimulatory, self-injurious, and stereotypic behaviors). Four major modalities are used to treat these disorders: educational-ecologic, behavior therapy, pharmacotherapy, and psychotherapy.

Common Pitfalls

- Before making the diagnosis of mental retardation, other disorders that affect cognitive abilities and adaptive behavior must be considered. Sensory deficits (severe hearing and vision loss), communication disorders, autistic spectrum disorders, specific learning disabilities, and poorly controlled seizure disorders may mimic mental retardation. Certain progressive neurologic disorders may manifest as mental retardation before regression is recognized.
- Often, pharmacologic treatment is tried, when adjusting the child's environment is what is really needed. Educational misplacement frequently is associated with onset of behavior disturbances. The new development of a behavior problem merits careful review of the educational program. Modification of the program may significantly improve both behavior and academic function.

Communication and Counseling

The pediatrician is responsible for consulting with other disciplines to make the diagnosis of mental retardation and to coordinate subsequent treatment services. Consultant services may include psychology, speech and language pathology, physical therapy, occupational therapy, audiology, nutrition, nursing, and social work, as well as medical specialties such as neurology, genetics, psychiatry, or surgical specialties. Contact with early intervention/school personnel is also important.

The family should be an integral part of the planning and direction of the process. Older children should participate in planning and decision making to whatever extent is possible. Care should incorporate sensitivity to cultural differences.

Although mental retardation is considered a static encephalopathy, periodic review is needed. Monitoring is the only way to ensure the management program is effective. As the child grows, new information must be imparted, goals revised, and programs adjusted. A periodic review requires information about health status, the child's functioning in the community, home, and school, and family function. Inquiry should be made about the use of respite care services. Other information, such as formal psychological or educational testing, may be needed. Reevaluation should be undertaken at routine intervals (6 to 12 months during early childhood and 1 to 2 years in older children), at any time the child is not meeting expectations, or when he or she is moving from one service delivery system to another. This is especially true during the transition to adulthood, beginning at 14 years of age. The pediatrician can play a number of advocacy roles.

SUGGESTED READINGS

1. Shapiro BK, Batshaw ML: Mental retardation. In Batshaw ML (ed): Children with Disabilities, 5th ed. Baltimore: Brookes, 2002, pp 287–305. **Overview to mental retardation diagnosis and management.**
2. Shapiro BK, Batshaw ML: Mental retardation. In Berman RE, Kliegman RM, Jenson HB (eds): Nelson Textbook of Pediatrics, 17th ed. Philadelphia: WB Saunders, 2004, pp 138–143. **Expanded discussion of pediatric aspects of mental retardation.**
3. Shevell M, Ashwal S, Donley D, et al: Practice parameter: Evaluation of the child with global developmental delay. Neurology 60:367–380, 2003. **Approach to etiologic evaluation as recommended by the American Academy of Neurology and the Child Neurology Society.**

Evidence-Based Practice in Communication Disorders: Language, Speech, and Voice Disorders

Richard G. Schwartz, Peggy F. Jacobson, and Frances L. V. Scheffler

KEY CONCEPTS

- Early communication disorders do not resolve themselves without intervention in the vast majority of cases.
- Even in cases in which early communication disorders may resolve without intervention, negative social and cognitive impact may be avoided.
- Early identification and intervention of communication disorders leads to improved outcomes.
- Successful intervention for communication disorders (language, phonology, voice, and fluency) consists of direct intervention focusing on speech or language.

Communication disorders affect approximately 12% to 15% of all children. Epidemiology studies have been conducted in the United States and Great Britain. We assume the prevalence to be similar internationally, with some variance due to environment, availability of early intervention, and other influences. The World Health Organization takes a broader approach to concerns about cognitive and social development.

A communication disorder occurs when speech, voice, or language deviates from the norm sufficiently to impair communication. These disorders include fluency disorders, phonologic (also called articulation or speech sound) disorders, language disorders, and voice disorders. Some are associated with more general developmental disabilities such as autism or developmental delay, syndromes such as Williams or fragile X, permanent or transitory hearing impairments, physical disabilities such as cleft palate, neuromotor disabilities such as cerebral palsy, or physical conditions such as vocal nodules. Even disorders that do not have obvious causes have identifiable neurobiologic bases and genetic origins. Regardless of their origins, these disorders can be described in terms of the affected aspect of speech, voice, or language.

One of the most important principles in treating communication disorders or related disabilities is early identification and early intervention. Early intervention improves the likelihood of a successful outcome. Hearing impairments can now be identified at birth. Language and speech impairments can be identified by 2 years of age, and fluency disorders may appear as early as 2 years of age. Voice disorders may emerge at any age. Individuals at risk may be identified by family history. Although some early deficits may resolve themselves without intervention, the vast majority do not. Furthermore, a period of communicative impairment may have long-lasting effects on cognitive and social development. Intervention can minimize negative outcomes and maximize the potential for learning.

A *language disorder* is a significant deficit in the production or understanding of one or more components of language. The components affected may include sentence length and structure (syntax); vocabulary development (lexicon, semantics); speech sound production (consonants, vowels, intonation) and the underlying system (phonology); word endings (e.g., morphology); conversation (discourse, pragmatics); or social interaction involving language (pragmatics). Standardized tests can reveal a child's language abilities.

A language disorder should not be described in terms of the number of months or years a child is behind his or her peers because a 6-month delay at 2 years of age is far more significant than a 6-month delay at 8 years of age. Instead, standard scores are preferred.

Language disorders vary in the pattern of deficits, depending on whether they occur independently of other developmental deficits or syndromes. One notable type of language impairment in children is specific language impairment (SLI). These children have significant deficits in one or more areas of language comprehension or production in the absence of autism, hearing impairment, or general developmental delay. This disorder may manifest itself differently at various points in development. For example, children with SLI exhibit late emergence of first words, slow vocabulary development during the period of the first 50 words (extending beyond 18 months of age), and late emergence of syntax (onset of two-word utterances after 24 months of age). Poor language comprehension, along with slow growth of vocabulary and limited sentence complexity, are continuing signs of SLI. A hallmark of SLI is the omission of verb endings such as third-person singular (e.g., "the girl walks") and past tense (e.g., "the girl walked"), symptomatic of more extensive grammatical deficits. Other populations may exhibit poor conversational skills, inappropriate repetition, and poor topic maintenance.

Phonologic disorders may occur in conjunction with or independently of language disorders. They involve errors in the production of consonants, vowel, syllables, or prosody (syllable stress and rhythm). The errors may involve omissions (e.g., absence of consonants at the ends of words, substitution of one sound for another, or distortion of correct sounds). Phonologic disorders range in severity from a few sounds in error that have a negligible effect on speech intelligibility to widespread errors resulting in speech that is difficult to understand, severely impairing communication. By 2 years of age, although a number of errors may remain, approximately half of what the child says can be understood by a person unfamiliar to the child. By 3 years of age, children should produce most sounds correctly, so approximately 75% can be understood.

A small subgroup of children may have developmental verbal apraxia (DVA), which is thought to be a motor-based rather than a cognitive-linguistic disorder. DVA is a controversial diagnosis that is often overapplied. Newer evidence suggests that the only feature differentiating DVA from other phonologic disorders is errors in syllable stress and speech rhythm in addition to more common speech errors.

Voice disorders involve congenital or acquired abnormalities in resonance, voice quality, pitch, or loudness that result from abnormalities of the vocal tract. Hoarseness, harshness, breathiness, and weakness are typical of voice quality disorders. Among the many causes are vocal fold hyperfunction, abuse, or paralysis; laryngeal stenosis; webbing; nodules; or contact ulcers. Hyper- and hyponasality are resonance disorders. Hypernasality may be caused by cleft palate or by an inadequate velopharyngeal mechanism due to physical or functional limitations. Hyponasality may be caused by an obstructed nasal pathway (e.g., nasal polyps, rhinitis).

Fluency disorders are disruptions in the fluent production of speech that involve whole-word or part-word distortions that may be repetitions, prolongations, and silent blocks. In some cases, the dysfluencies are accompanied by secondary behaviors, such as muscular tension, facial grimaces, extraneous movements of the extremities, and respiratory abnormalities. Many young children experience nonfluent episodes during early language acquisition. Normal nonfluency (e.g., whole-word repetitions) can be distinguished from stuttering (e.g., initial consonant repetitions, silent blocks). Normal nonfluency resolves as language skills mature. Stuttering persists. The onset of stuttering occurs by 3 years of age for 68% of all stutterers and by 4 years of age for 95% of all stutterers. The prevalence of stuttering is 2.5% among preschoolers; the prevalence is 1% across all ages. Furthermore, evidence indicates that although the onset of stuttering may be gradual for some children, nearly 40% of children who stutter have a sudden onset. The causes of stuttering appear to be genetic and underlying deficits in the cognitive-linguistic processes of language production (e.g., formulation, word and sentence frame access, and planning for speech) in addition to the neuromuscular control of speech.

Expert Opinion on Management Issues

STANDARD INTERVENTION APPROACHES

Two general principles are key in the treatment of communication disorders in children. First, early identification and intervention yield better outcomes and can prevent the negative social and cognitive impact of a prolonged delay in communication abilities. Second, treatment must focus on the aspect of communication (language, speech, voice, fluency) that is impaired to achieve improvements in those areas.

Treatment of language disorders involves a mixture of methods, including direct elicitation and training of target sentence structures, words, verb and noun endings, and language use. Procedures that use somewhat more indirect methods, such as systematically recasting the child's simple utterances into more complex utterances or providing focused stimulation of certain deficient aspects of language, are also effective methods. Often a combination of these approaches is the most effective. In addition, intervention may be delivered individually, in small or large groups, or in some combination of delivery methods. Also, intervention may be delivered by parents or by a speech-language pathologist. It appears to be most effective when the primary intervention is delivered by a speech-language pathologist with strong involvement of parents. Because of differences in symptoms and learning styles, individualized treatment plans are most successful.

Despite limited treatment evidence for children with autism, there is some consensus that strictly behavioral approaches (i.e., a highly structured environment with the use of reinforcers) combined with language intervention are most effective.

For phonologic disorders and developmental verbal apraxia, procedures that directly modify speech sound production through modeling, intensive stimulation, and directed production in communicative contexts are very effective approaches to intervention for speech disorders. This therapy may occur in individual sessions, group sessions, or a combination. Parents may also play a role in providing auditory input to facilitate correct production. A combination of these methods is the most effective. In contrast to long-standing practices, providing training on sounds that pose the greatest difficulty for the child promotes the greatest treatment results.

For voice disorders, there is general agreement that prevention (primary or secondary to vocal abuse) programs are time and cost effective. Voice disorders that cannot be fully treated with drug, surgical, or prosthetic therapies can be treated with direct voice therapy to modify vocal behavior. Similar to other communication disorders, a combination of behavioral techniques and modeling the desired behavior are the most effective treatments. Teaching vocal hygiene, providing biofeedback (e.g., visual displays of actual and desired pitch), and behavioral intervention combined with surgical treatment are also beneficial. The treatment of stuttering historically focused on modifications of the child's environment (indirect intervention) by either not calling attention to the child's normal dysfluencies or by controlling communicative situations. Newer research suggests that direct intervention to modify speech by reducing rate and prolonging productions is the most effective approach.

CONTROVERSIAL INTERVENTION APPROACHES

A number of intervention approaches are frequently employed for which there is no evidence or only questionable evidence of effectiveness. For language disorders, there are sensorimotor (sensory integration) approaches that involve gross motor movement and other sensory stimulation as a means of changing language. No evidence indicates that such approaches, independent of direct language intervention, have any effect on language. Computer-based approaches to language disorder treatment, such as those that use acoustically modified speech in computer-based tasks, are promising. However, they do not have any demonstrated impact on children's language beyond standardized tests that resemble the computer tasks. For DVA and phonologic disorders, oral motor approaches focusing on nonspeech oral motor abilities using whistles or other devices are also popular, but they are not supported by any evidence. Although nonspeech oral motor movements rely on the same physical mechanism, speech and nonspeech motor movements are controlled by separate and independent neuromotor systems. For

children with autism, controversial and non–evidence-based approaches include auditory integration therapy, music therapy, touch therapy, medication therapies, and dietary therapies. Although medication and dietary therapies may have some potential in the future, side effects and efficacy should be considered before any such therapies are used. Facilitated communication is discredited as a treatment for autism.

Communication and Counseling

Parents have an important role to play in the identification and treatment of children's communication disorders. They are often the first ones to observe unusual behavioral patterns or the absence of an expected skill. Thus parents must be aware of developmental milestones. They should understand the importance of early intervention and its positive effect on outcomes. Through increased awareness, parents can help prevent associated cognitive and social problems that arise when communication disorders go untreated. They can also play a role as providers of intervention in conjunction with direct intervention by a speech-language pathologist.

SUGGESTED READINGS

1. Gierut JA: Complexity in phonological treatment: Clinical factors. Lang Speech Hear Serv Sch 32:229–241, 2001. **Addresses the finding that working on more difficult aspects of phonology first yields greater gains than beginning treatment with "easier" goals. This principle is likely to be true for other components of language.**
2. Gierut J, Morrisette ML, Hughes MT: Phonological treatment efficacy and developmental norms. Lang Speech Hear Serv Sch 27: 215–230, 1996. **Reviews evidence concerning the relative efficacy of various approaches to the treatment of phonologic disorders.**
3. Hooper C: Treatment of voice disorders in children. Lang Speech Hear Serv Sch 35:320–326, 2004. **Reviews evidence-based current best practice for treatment of voice disorders in children. This is one article in an entire issue devoted to voice disorders in children.**
4. New York State Department of Health Early Intervention Program: Clinical Practice Guidelines: Report of the Recommendations. Autism/Pervasive Developmental Disorders: Assessment and Intervention for Young Children (Age 0–3 Years). Albany: New York State Department of Health, 1999. **Report from a panel of experts on evidence-based clinical practice for young children with autism and pervasive developmental disorders.**
5. New York State Department of Health Early Intervention Program: Clinical Practice Guidelines: Report of the Recommendations. Communication Disorders: Assessment and Intervention for Young Children (Age 0–3 Years). Albany: New York State Department of Health, 1999. **Report from a panel of experts on evidence-based practice and recommendations of best clinical practice for young children with communicative disorders.**
6. Yairi E, Ambrose N: Stuttering: Recent developments and future directions. ASHA Leader 9:4–5;14–15, 2004. **State-of-the-art review of stuttering research and clinical practice with additional resources.**

23 Dental Problems

Oral Health

Mark L. Helpin and Joel Howard Berg

KEY CONCEPTS

- Oral health is a vital component of good overall health.
- Dentistry strongly endorses for all children, healthy and medically compromised alike, the philosophy that primary prevention and treatment of the disease process, not its effects, are the best ways to address oral diseases.
- Establishment of a dental home by 12 months of age will do much to help ensure good oral health.
- A dentist with experience in treating special-needs children is best qualified to provide their care.

Oral health is an integral component of a child's overall health. A physician's knowledge of basic concepts of oral health can help in providing the highest level of comprehensive care for children. Medical providers should work in concert with dental colleagues to establish a partnership for care. This chapter attempts to familiarize physicians and other health care personnel with basic concepts on oral health, conditions, and techniques.

Expert Opinion on Management Issues

- The first visit to a dentist, based on risk assessment, is recommended for 12 months of age or within 6 months of the first tooth emerging into the mouth. Establishment of a dental home, primary prevention, and anticipatory guidance gives a child the best chance for remaining free of oral disease.
- Prevention of dental caries is aimed along multiple avenues including oral hygiene, diet, fluoride, sealant application, and attention to the mother's and/or primary caregiver's state of oral health.
- Periodontal disease is a continuum of a chronic disease process whose most severe presentation includes loss of bone and loss of teeth.
- Many pediatric dentistry emergencies can be initially managed by a physician or other health care

provider. Referral to a dentist is often helpful for diagnosis and treatment.
- Primary teeth that are avulsed should not be replanted.
- Permanent teeth that are avulsed should be replanted. The prognosis for an avulsed permanent tooth is directly related to the extraoral time. Replantation within 15 minutes offers the best prognosis of retention for an extended period of time.
- Special patients often require judicious timing of treatment. They may also require prophylactic antibiotic coverage to ensure that the dental care does not negatively affect their condition or general health status. Consultation with the dentist is often wise.

PREVENTION IN DENTISTRY

The Dental Home

The two major oral diseases, dental caries and periodontal disease, are both recognized as infectious diseases. In light of this, great emphasis is now placed on primary prevention. Principles of primary prevention in dentistry emulate the model already established in medicine, where major attention is placed on the disease process itself and not simply the effects of that disease.

Primary prevention is embodied in two concepts: the dental home and anticipatory guidance. Establishment of a "dental home" mirrors the recommendation by the American Academy of Pediatrics (AAP) for the "medical home." The goals of such homes include high-quality comprehensive care, continuous access to treatment, and cost-effective care. The benefits of educating families regarding oral health and principles of prevention, including oral hygiene, diet and dental caries, and the benefits of fluoride, can have significantly positive effects on the health of children.

Anticipatory guidance helps families understand dental and oral development, oral diseases and conditions, risk assessment, oral hygiene instruction, the use of fluorides, diet and its effect on teeth, nonnutritive sucking, injury prevention, and schedule of periodicity. It offers the framework for a plan of complete oral health care that maximizes the chances for a child to be free of oral disease.

The First Dental Visit

The AAP recommends establishment of a dental home by 1 year of age for children deemed at risk. Research has demonstrated that a first visit at the age of 3 years is too late for many children to avoid significant disease. In fact, the American Academy of Pediatric Dentistry (AAPD) recommends for all children that the first dental visit be scheduled by 12 months of age or within 6 months of the first tooth emerging into the mouth.

Diet and Dental Health

Diet is a major factor in the etiology of dental caries (tooth decay). An exposure to a carbohydrate source causes a decrease in oral pH from the normal 7.4 to below 5.5, the level where tooth demineralization (the initiation of dental decay) begins. It is organic acid, the bacterial metabolic process end-product, that causes this drop in pH and subsequent tooth demineralization. This low-pH condition can remain in the oral cavity for 30 to 60 minutes after eating. The appearance of caries (a cavity) in a tooth is based on a change in the balance between the processes of demineralization and remineralization. Prolonged and repeated exposure to an acid environment can cause the balance to shift toward demineralization, and as a result tooth integrity is compromised and ultimately frank cavitation (a hole) appears. Although parents may suggest that caries incidence in children is hereditary, most researchers agree that genetic influence is minor in relation to other etiologic factors, except in cases of heritable conditions that can cause gross malformation of teeth (for example, amelogenesis and dentinogenesis imperfecta).

Physicians should be aware that carbohydrate sources include not only the commonly recognized candy, cookies, and sweets, but also carbohydrates such as potato chips and pretzels. Physicians should also be aware that many medications they prescribe for children are sweetened with sugars.

Frequency of carbohydrate exposure and consistency of the carbohydrate are important factors in their cariogenicity. The higher the number of exposures, the longer a low pH can exist in the mouth. Frequency of exposure is, in fact, more important than the amount of carbohydrate ingested. Regarding food consistency, the stickier the carbohydrate, the more cariogenic it is, because it remains on the teeth and continues to be a substrate for bacteria to metabolize. Good nutritional counseling should stress healthy snacks such as fresh (not dried) fruits, vegetables, and cheese.

Physicians and families should be aware that an increasing number of schools are placing beverage and snack vending machines in their buildings. The AAPD views this with great concern and encourages medical and dental organizations, school officials, parent groups, and others to consider the importance of maintaining healthy choices in vending machines in schools. The Academy encourages promotion of beverages of high nutritional value, discourages use of bottles instead of cans (because bottles are convenient for consumption throughout the day), and recommends that bottled water always be available at the same place soft drinks are offered. Physicians should take an active role in educating and informing families and the public about the importance of nutritional habits as they relate to soft drinks.

Oral Hygiene

The goal of oral hygiene is to remove plaque (the organized bacterial ecosystem that leads to caries) and food debris from all surfaces of the teeth. This can be accomplished using a toothbrush for all exposed tooth surfaces and dental floss for between the teeth, where a brush cannot clean. Thorough cleaning minimizes risk of caries and also allows the gingiva (gums) to maintain a state of health and prevent the initiation of periodontal disease. Ideally, such cleaning occurs after each food exposure; however, it is not realistic to expect this to occur. During the day, when brushing is not possible, rinsing with water can help increase the speed with which oral pH returns to its normal level. Parents should select a brush that has soft nylon (not medium or firm) bristles with polished, rounded ends. If the family can afford an electric toothbrush, this may be recommended. Studies have shown electric toothbrushes to be extremely efficient and effective in removing plaque. Brushing should be augmented with flossing at least once a day where teeth are in contact and a brush cannot remove plaque. Because children generally do not have the manual dexterity to use a toothbrush effectively until 6 to 8 years of age, parents should be encouraged to assist their children with brushing. Flossing should be done for the child until he/she demonstrates they can do this themselves without injuring their gingiva. Caregivers should institute mouth cleaning during infancy, even before the first tooth is present. This helps the child become accustomed to this kind of activity in the mouth. During a bath, a damp facecloth can be rubbed on the gums.

Toothpaste should be used with great care. Until 2 to 3 years of age, parents should clean their child's teeth with only water or a fluoride-free toothpaste, unless otherwise specified by the dentist. Parents should be instructed that when they do begin to use toothpaste, they should place only a small, pea-sized amount across (not along) the brush. Because children tend to swallow toothpaste until 6 to 8 years of age, this will minimize the amount of fluoride that might be ingested from toothpaste; this, in turn, will minimize the risk of developing fluorosis (tooth malformation caused by the ingestion of too much fluoride). Caregivers should also be made aware that good positioning of a child for brushing and flossing can provide the best vision and head control.

Fluoride

Fluoride in drinking water has contributed significantly to the large reduction of dental caries in the U.S. population of school-age children. Numerous studies have shown that when fluoride is added to community water supplies to a level of 0.7 to 1.0 ppm, incidence of

TABLE 1 Intervention: Fluoride Supplementation*

Age	Fluoride Ion Level in Drinking Water		
	<0.3 ppm[†]	0.3–0.6 ppm	>0.6 ppm
Birth–6 mo	None	None	None
6 mo–3 yr	0.25 mg/day[‡]	None	None
3–6 yr	0.50 mg/day	0.25 mg/day	None
6–16 yr	1.0 mg/day	0.50 mg/day	None

*Indications: Children 6 months to 16 years of age living in areas with less than optimally fluoridated water; for example, the home or "primary" water supply is fluoride deficient. ADA Council on Scientific Affairs Recommendations, new dosage schedule approved April 1994.
[†]1.0 ppm = 1 mg/L.
[‡]2.2 mg sodium fluoride contains 1 mg fluoride ion.
From American Dental Association: Caries diagnosis and risk assessment: A review of prevention strategies and management. J Am Dent Assoc 126(Suppl):1S–24S, 1995. Copyright © 1997 American Dental Association. All rights reserved. Reproduced by permission.

dental caries is reduced by at least 40%. Systemic fluoride is provided either through community water fluoridation or daily prescription supplements in liquid or tablet form. Supplemental systemic fluoride should be recommended only when the fluoride content of the child's drinking water is known to be less than optimal. If the fluoride level in home water is not known (for example, water from a well), it should be analyzed before prescribing any fluoride or fluoride-containing vitamins. Each state board of health should be able to direct the physician or family to a state or private laboratory in which water analysis is performed.

Before prescribing supplemental fluoride, the physician should also take great care to inquire about alternative water sources and alternative sources of fluoride if the child spends time outside the home. Although a child may reside in a fluoride-deficient area, the child's daycare center or relatives may be located in a community with an optimally fluoridated water supply. In such cases, children may actually be receiving the optimal dose of fluoride, even though they reside in a nonfluoridated community. Physicians should be aware that some foods and beverages are processed with fluoridated water, and some children may be exposed to fluoride this way. In circumstances such as these, supplementation for a child may not be necessary or modification of the dosage schedule may be indicated.

After water analysis is complete, the physician should refer to Table 1 to determine the proper dosage of fluoride supplementation. Dental fluorosis, as discussed previously, is a discoloration and/or malformation of teeth that can occur if care is not taken in prescribing appropriate fluoride supplementation. Consideration of topical fluoride gel or fluoride gel rinse use is probably best done after consultation with a dentist. Topical application performed in a dental office should pose no increased risk for fluorosis.

Dental Sealants

Dental sealants are highly effective in preventing tooth decay. A dental sealant is a plastic resin coating placed on the biting surfaces of the posterior teeth. Its purpose is to prevent the initiation of dental caries in those areas that are most susceptible to decay—the pits and fissures, the rough areas on the occlusal surfaces of the teeth—in which plaque and food can easily become trapped and that are not easily cleaned, even with dental instruments. Sealants provide a physical barrier to the entry of food and plaque into the pits and fissures. Placement of a sealant uses the bonding technique and is completely noninvasive. Injection of local anesthesia is not required.

It is unfortunate that sealants are grossly underused, and parents should be encouraged to request their application by the dentist. Research has shown a large reduction in the prevalence of caries in teeth that have been sealed. The need for invasive restorative treatment, such as fillings or crowns, is then greatly reduced. One study has shown that 15 years after placement of sealant, 83% of unsealed first permanent molars had become decayed, whereas only 31% of sealed first permanent molars had experienced caries. It is important to note not only the remarkable benefit of sealant here, but also that in this study the sealants were applied only one time. It is reasonable to expect an even higher caries-preventive benefit when sealants are monitored and maintained because their rate of retention increases with periodic evaluation and maintenance.

Mouth Guards

The American Dental Association (ADA) and the AAPD strongly endorse the use of protective mouth guards for children who participate in active sports. Three types of mouth guards are available: stock, mouth-formed, and custom-made guards. Custom-made guards, similar to those worn by professional athletes, usually allow the wearer to speak most easily while the guard is in place. A dentist can fabricate custom mouth guards after taking an impression and making a model of the teeth. Stock and mouth-formed mouth guards are available in sporting goods stores. To prevent traumatic injury to the teeth, physicians are encouraged to discuss with parents and patients the wisdom and benefits of wearing protective mouth guards during all active sport activities, not just those where it is required. All health care providers should be advocates of requiring mouth protection in organized sports or in situations that pose a risk of facial injury.

ORAL CARE FOR INFANTS

The Centers for Disease Control and Prevention (CDC) has reported that the most prevalent infectious disease in America's children is dental caries, with caries found in more than 40% of children by the time they reach kindergarten. These findings have prompted a reassessment and new recommendations on timing of when the initial dental visit should be scheduled. The AAPD recommends the initial dental visit be scheduled as early as 6 months of age, 6 months after the first tooth emerges, and no later than 12 months of age.

Because physicians and other medical health care providers see infants regularly from birth, they are in an excellent position to share oral health information with families and to make the appropriate referrals for these initial dental visits, especially for children at high risk. All health care personnel should be very aware that their dental colleagues are trying to emulate their lead and follow medical models for disease prevention and care of children. The initial visit allows a family to establish a dental home and to be counseled regarding the principles of anticipatory guidance and primary prevention.

Early Childhood Caries (Baby Bottle Tooth Decay, Nursing Caries)

Dental caries (decay) is an infectious and transmissible disease. Although there are many bacteria in the oral cavity, specific bacteria involved with caries are *Streptococcus mutans*, *Streptococcus sobrinus*, and *Lactobacillus*. These bacteria are acquired by the infant through vertical transmission from their primary caregiver, usually the mother, from birth through 4 years of age.

Early childhood caries is a pattern of decay that is observed in very young children. It involves the smooth surfaces of teeth and/or many teeth in the mouth of a child who is younger than 6 years old. Early childhood caries affects 5% of children in Western countries, but it can affect up to 65% of children in socioeconomically disadvantaged or Native American populations. Caries itself is a multifactorial process that involves an imbalance in a tooth between demineralization and remineralization. When demineralization overwhelms remineralization, a carious lesion is formed. As the tooth becomes demineralized, its structural integrity is compromised, and ultimately its hard tissue breaks down and leaves a hole, what is commonly called a "cavity."

There are several avenues that can be used in preventing this disease. The teeth can be made more resistant to caries attack, the number of cariogenic bacteria can be reduced, diet can be modified, and the quality/quantity of saliva may be improved (if there is a saliva problem). Health care providers should be aware that emphasizing good prenatal and perinatal nutrition helps allow enamel to develop normally, free from defects that would be more susceptible to future caries attack. Additionally, exposure to optimal levels of systemic fluoride also makes the teeth more resistant to the initiation of caries. Lowering the mother's own bacterial load may assist in minimizing transmission of cariogenic bacteria to the infant. If the mother-to-be has a poor dentition, she should be referred to a dentist for consultation and formulation of a plan for her own oral health. It has been reported that children of mothers with a high caries rate are at greater risk of decay.

Caregivers should be advised not to put babies to sleep with a bottle or using a pacifier that has been dipped in a sweet substance (like honey) or to allow the child to carry a bottle or a sippy cup for prolonged periods during the day. Families should also be counseled that after feeding, it is helpful to clean the infant's mouth, even if this is done only with a damp facecloth. In the past, the role of breast milk in early childhood caries has been controversial. The AAPD now states that frequent bottle feeding at night, on-demand breast-feeding, and extended and repetitive use of a nonspilling training cup (sippy cup) are associated with, but not consistently implicated in, early childhood caries. When a caregiver assesses a child or family at high risk for caries, they should consider, within the realm of good clinical judgment, making the following recommendations:

- Avoid placing the child to sleep with a bottle.
- Water (water alone) may be placed in a bottle if child must sleep with a bottle.
- If the child is breast-fed, the mother should try to wipe the mouth out after each feeding to remove residual breast milk from the oral cavity.
- Use of a cup should begin at approximately 1 year of age.
- Juices and soft drinks should not be frequently placed in a bottle.
- Snacks should be healthy and noncariogenic (fresh fruits, vegetables, and cheese).
- Oral hygiene should begin before the first tooth emerges into the mouth.
- A dental home should be established by 12 months of age or within 6 months of the first tooth emerging into the mouth.

Oral Hygiene for Infants and Young Children

Oral hygiene measures should begin before the first tooth erupts into the mouth. This helps the child become accustomed to oral manipulations associated with cleaning. A damp facecloth or gauze pad can be used to rub the gingiva. When the incisors emerge into the mouth, parents can continue use of the previously mentioned methods or change to a small toothbrush. Use of water alone on the toothbrush is acceptable. Proper child positioning helps ensure effective mouth cleaning (see Early Childhood Caries section).

DENTAL CARIES

Dental caries (tooth decay) is the most common chronic infectious disease of childhood. The etiology of this disease and principles of primary prevention were discussed in the two previous sections of this chapter. According to the Surgeon General's Report on Oral Health in 2000, caries and dental-related illnesses were responsible for children missing 51,000,000 school hours each year. Although the focus of our attention has, to this point, been on etiology and primary prevention of caries and oral disease, it is helpful for physicians and other health care providers to be familiar with some basic concepts and techniques used to restore and repair carious teeth. In children, the most commonly used restorative materials are:

- Amalgam (silver fillings)
- Resin-based composites (tooth-colored plastics)
- Resin-modified glass ionomer (a tooth-colored combination of resin-based composite and glass ionomer, a material that has anticariogenic properties)
- Stainless steel crowns and esthetic variations of stainless steel crowns

Gold, other alloys, porcelain, and other types of ceramic restorations are generally not used for children. Selection of a material is based on several factors, including esthetics, size, and location of the carious lesion, and the material properties needed to ensure a long-lasting restorative result. Amalgam has been used for more than 150 years and has a long record of success. Resin-based composites, with their improved physical properties, are now being used a great deal and continue to increase in use because of the public's increased desire for esthetic restorations that offer good length of service. Resin-based composites must be bonded to teeth; therefore, meticulous technique is especially important. Resin-modified glass ionomers are extremely popular and often are the material of choice for filling-type restorations in children. This material releases fluoride over time and, therefore, combats the recurrence of decay in a tooth. Stainless steel crowns are the restoration of choice in children when a large portion of tooth structure has been lost to decay and when a filling will not predictably last for the life of a primary tooth. Stainless steel crowns have excellent retention and generally outlast other types of restorations.

Although minor, noncavitated areas of demineralization (the beginning of decay) can be remineralized and ultimately require no filling at all, health care providers should know that once frank cavitation (a hole) has appeared in a tooth, it cannot repair itself. Health care providers should also be aware that if caries is left untreated, it may progress to a point where the pulp tissue (dental nerve) becomes infected, not simply inflamed. If such infection occurs, pulp therapy (root canal treatment) or extraction is indicated. The type of pulp therapy needed depends on the extent of the infection. A pulpotomy procedure removes only the infected portion of the pulp tissue, whereas a pulpectomy removes all the pulp tissue in a tooth. In these circumstances, after the involved pulp tissue is removed, a root canal filling material is placed inside the tooth and tooth restoration is then completed. Postoperative discomfort and difficulty following root canal treatment, although often reported by adults, rarely occurs in children who have received pulp therapy.

Although dentists have many restorative techniques available, the trend in dentistry should continue to be on emphasizing principles of primary prevention, diagnosis, and treatment of the etiology of the caries disease process rather than its effects.

PERIODONTAL DISEASE IN CHILDREN

Periodontal disease is another major oral disease seen in children, and it, too, is an infectious process. Pathologic bacteria that cause periodontal disease are located in plaque, the complex, organized layer that adheres to teeth. (Plaque that becomes calcified and becomes firmly attached to teeth is called *calculus* or *tartar*.)

It is important to be aware that periodontal disease is a long-term, chronic process that begins as simple inflammation of the gingiva. If left untreated, it will progress to bone loss, which can ultimately lead to the loss of teeth. Studies indicate that gingivitis is nearly universal in children, and bone loss has now been reported in adolescents 12 to 17 years of age. Bone loss is occasionally observed in younger children; however, this is rarely the classic periodontal disease referred to here.

There are several types of gingivitis with which physicians and other health care providers should be familiar. Simple gingivitis is the type commonly encountered in children. This consists of only soft tissue inflammation with no bone involvement or bone loss. This condition is reversible with good oral hygiene techniques. Proper toothbrushing and flossing removes the plaque that is the irritant causing the inflammation. Increased observation of the oral soft tissues during routine medical examination might help with early diagnosis of this insidious disease. If the gingiva appears puffy or erythematous, or if a good deal of plaque is noted, a dental referral should be considered.

There are several distinct periodontal conditions that physicians or other health care providers may observe in children. Eruption gingivitis is an inflammatory condition that can occur as an anterior or posterior tooth emerges into the mouth. If a tooth is not fully erupted, a portion of gingiva often remains over a portion of that tooth. This situation can lead to irritation and/or food impaction and subsequent inflammation. This condition is generally self-limited and rarely requires intervention. As the tooth continues to emerge into the mouth, the tissue recedes into normal gingival architecture. It is rare that removal of tissue is necessary. Rinsing with dilute saline or 0.12% chlorhexidine gluconate (Peridex or PerioGard) might assist in combating the local inflammation.

Another common periodontal condition, usually noted in older children and generally associated with permanent teeth, is called pericoronitis. Here, a distal flap of tissue (the operculum) remains over a portion of the erupting tooth. If plaque, food, or other foreign body becomes lodged under the operculum, the removal of the food impaction or foreign body may be all that is needed. If there is no foreign body at all, the situation may resolve spontaneously, as seen in eruption gingivitis. If lymphadenopathy or suppuration is noted around the operculum, 0.12% chlorhexidine gluconate can be prescribed or a systemic antibiotic like penicillin or amoxicillin should be considered, with clindamycin the drug of choice for penicillin-allergic children. If the condition persists, surgical removal of the operculum might be indicated or, in the case of wisdom teeth, dental extraction might be indicated.

Recurrent aphthous ulcers (RAU), or canker sores, or recurrent aphthous stomatitis manifest with either local or generalized inflammation of the unattached mucous membranes. These ulcers are most frequently seen in children 10 to 19 years of age. The etiology of aphthous ulcers is unknown; however, physicians should be aware that such ulcers have been noted in patients with inflammatory bowel disease, neutropenia, immunodeficiency syndromes, Reiter syndrome, and systemic lupus erythematous (SLE). Treatment is usually palliative and focused on allowing the patient to continue adequate hydration and nutritional intake. Application of topical gels, creams, or ointments containing 0.5% fluocinonide or 0.25% triamcinolone along with additional placement of an oral bandage (Orabase) or a prepared combination of medication and bandage (Kenalog and Orabase) may have a salutary effect, especially when used before mealtimes and at bedtime.

Children present with several other common conditions associated with gingival inflammation. Acute primary herpetic gingivostomatitis and herpangina and other coxsackie-related viruses all can cause severe gingival inflammation with significant discomfort. Gingival inflammation associated with these infections will resolve as the primary disease runs its 10- to 14-day course. The important principles of care with these conditions are to keep the patient hydrated and to use analgesics as needed. Popsicles, ice chips, and cool foods, like milkshakes, help the mouth feel better and assist with hydration. Acetaminophen is usually an adequate analgesic, although ibuprofen might sometimes be indicated. Antibiotics are not routinely required in these situations; however, topical or systemic antiviral medications may be prescribed in severe cases. Having the child rinse with cool water or a prescription-formulated mouthwash ("magic mouthwash") might also be helpful in comforting what can be a very sore mouth. One such formulation is composed of one part diphenhydramine, two parts Kaopectate, and three parts water. Use of viscous lidocaine for oral rinsing, especially in young children, should be avoided because its systemic uptake places a child at risk for overdose.

Gingival Inflammation and Systemic Disease

Generalized gingival inflammation (also called stomatitis) may be seen with a number of systemic conditions. These include inflammatory bowel disease, neutropenia, immunodeficiency syndromes, Reiter syndrome, and SLE. The physician should focus on treatment of the primary disease and then turn the attention to specific oral involvement. Oral care may consist of a systemic antiviral, antimicrobial, or antifungal agent, depending on etiology. Additional local oral relief may be achieved by prescribing chlorhexidine gluconate rinse or topical application, a benzocaine topical anesthetic (not viscous lidocaine), magic mouthwash, or a formulation compounded by a local hospital or pharmacy. The physician may want to consider referral to a dentist for confirmation of diagnosis.

Physicians and other health care providers should be aware that gingival hyperplasia (mild, moderate, or severe) can be idiopathic or associated with several

therapeutic agents: cyclosporine, phenytoin, calcium channel blockers, and on rare occasions phenobarbital. Such tissues may not appear erythematous or otherwise inflamed. They may instead have a raised, pebbly, or berry-like appearance. Surgical removal of these tissues may be considered if the patient experiences difficulty with mastication and nutrition or proper mouth closure (occlusion) or if there are concerns with esthetics. Children with this gingival condition should be referred to a dentist who has had experience in dealing with medically compromised special-needs children. Medical prognosis, the child's general medical status, and the severity of the tissue overgrowth should all be factored into the decision regarding the need and/or timing of surgical removal of tissue. Observation of hyperplastic tissues is often a wise initial course to follow.

Periodontitis

Periodontitis is the late phase of the periodontal disease continuum. At this stage, there is loss of alveolar bone and tooth support structures. Although periodontal disease is most common in adults, it is encountered in 1% to 9% of 5- to 11-year-old children and can be seen in 1% to 46% of children 12 to 15 years of age. Periodontitis may be classified as chronic or aggressive, or it may be a manifestation of systemic disease. Chronic periodontitis is a type of bone loss commonly seen in the adult population. Aggressive periodontitis, localized or generalized, manifests with a history of rapid loss of bone and tooth attachment. This localized form is associated with virulent strains of *actinobacillus actinomycetemcomitans* and *bacteroides* species. The generalized form is associated with nonmotile, facultative, anaerobic, gram-negative rods like *Porphyromonas gingivalis*. Some systemic diseases associated with periodontal disease include Langerhans cell histiocytosis, hypophosphatasia, Papillon-Lefèvre syndrome, type 1 diabetes mellitus, cyclic neutropenia, acrodynia, Down syndrome, leukemias, and immunoglobulin deficiencies. These conditions may also cause premature loss of both primary and permanent teeth.

Oral Frenula

There are two types of oral frenula seen in children, the maxillary frenulum and the lingual frenulum. A frenulum itself consists of mucous membrane tissue with epithelial and connective tissue and muscle fibers. The maxillary frenulum runs from the inner aspect of the upper lip to the labial gingiva. Some of these frenula go between the maxillary central incisors and attach to the incisive papilla on the palate. It is rare that intervention needs to be recommended for this condition. However, if the frenulum interferes with good oral hygiene, prevents spontaneous closure of the midline diastema, or pulls the gingiva away from its attachment to the teeth, referral to a dentist should be considered. When revision is being considered for the maxillary frenulum, the physician should be advised that the surgical procedure is most often recommended for a time after the permanent canine teeth erupt and often after orthodontic therapy has been completed.

A lingual frenulum joins the ventral surface of the tongue or the tongue tip to the gingiva on the lingual surface of the mandibular incisors. Very few of these frenula require intervention. If this frenulum causes severe limitation of tongue movement, speech pathology, pulling away of the lingual gingiva from the incisors, or difficulty with oral hygiene, surgical revision should be considered. The final decision regarding surgery can be made in consultation with a dentist and a speech therapist. Even if surgery is indicated, the procedure itself may be postponed, depending on the severity of the problem and the patient's age. It might be prudent to wait until the child is older so treatment could be performed in an ambulatory setting and not in the operating room. Those surgeons with experience in revising frenula include ear, nose, and throat and plastic surgery specialists and periodontists and oral and maxillofacial surgeons.

DENTAL EMERGENCIES IN CHILDREN

A physician is often the first person to whom a family turns in case of a dental emergency. These acute situations most often involve pain, infection, or trauma. It should be helpful to the physician to have some familiarity with common dental emergencies.

Toothache

Dental decay (caries) initiates inflammation in the dental pulp, the neurovascular and connective tissue located inside the hard structure of a tooth. Mild-to-moderate pulpal inflammation may cause a complaint of pain when cold foods or sweets are eaten. Such pain is localized and disappears immediately or shortly after the stimulus is removed. Dental referral should be made in these circumstances. The objective of care should be not only relief of pain but also prevention of caries progression and risk of further infection. Occasionally analgesics such as acetaminophen or ibuprofen are needed to comfort the child with toothache. Often, however, these are not necessary.

If caries remains untreated, it will progress deeper into the tooth, create increased pulpal inflammation, and ultimately invade the pulp tissue itself. Although some children who present with obvious severe dental decay have no complaint of pain, many children experience spontaneous and/or severe discomfort during the day or at night. Those with pain generally find relief if given analgesics, as discussed previously. Referral to a dentist is an important component of treatment. Great care should also be taken to observe for local abscess or facial cellulitis in these children. Those who fall into this category may require systemic antibiotics.

Local Abscess

As mentioned previously, caries that are left untreated can cause frank bacterial invasion into the pulp tissue and that infection may lead to local dental abscess formation. If the degree of infection is not overwhelming and tracks a path of drainage superior to a muscle attachment, the patient presents with fistula and an intraoral abscess. (If drainage tracks inferior to the muscle attachment, it may manifest as a cellulitis.) This abscess may appear like a small pimple or "gum boil" on the gingiva, or it may occur as a more diffuse redness and swelling of an area of gingiva. Most often these two manifestations are seen on the buccal gingiva; however, they can occasionally be found on the lingual or palatal surfaces of the teeth. Suppuration may be seen when pressure is applied to the involved area.

When a local abscess and drainage occur, a patient may experience no pain at all or there may only be pain on mastication. Such teeth may, however, be mobile and sensitive to percussion. If drainage does not occur, the patient may experience severe spontaneous or stimulated pain. Patients with a local abscess should be referred for dental consultation within 1 week. Analgesics should be recommended as needed, although narcotics are rarely required for children with this condition. Antibiotics are not generally indicated for local, discrete, nondiffuse dental abscess. If infection is more diffuse, prescription of antibiotics should be considered. Amoxicillin, penicillin, or clindamycin for penicillin-allergic patients are the drugs of choice.

Occasionally a patient presents with a local infection that has been caused by periodontal infection. Although the picture may be identical to a slight to moderate dental infection, its etiology is most often a foreign body (often a popcorn hull) that is impacted into the gingival sulcus. In most cases, removal of the foreign body relieves the problem. Analgesics may be needed, but the need for antibiotics should be based on the degree of infection. Rinsing with chlorhexidine gluconate may assist in resolving this infection.

Cellulitis

Cellulitis secondary to dental infection may manifest as swelling of the cheek or lips or of the submandibular, infraorbital, or periorbital regions or as Ludwig angina. It may carry a risk of cavernous sinus thrombosis. Children with such a cellulitis can be lethargic and not feel well generally. They may be febrile. Antibiotics are indicated for these patients. The major questions that arise address how antibiotics should be delivered (by mouth, intramuscularly, or intravenously [IV]) and if admission to the hospital is necessary. Children with airway impingement or infraorbital or periorbital involvement should be strongly considered for admission and IV antibiotics. Referral for dental consult, either as an outpatient or inpatient, should be made. As the cellulitis resolves, definitive treatment of the involved tooth or teeth is needed. Treatment options include endodontic therapy (root canal treatment) or dental extraction.

Physicians or health care providers who see children with dental infection are urged to examine the mouth and try to assess the patient's risk for caries and future acute dental episodes. Referral for comprehensive dental evaluation and establishment of a dental home should also be encouraged.

Acute Primary Herpetic Gingivostomatitis

Acute primary herpetic gingivostomatitis (APHG) is a condition that is caused by the herpes simplex virus 1 (HSV-1). Initial exposure to HSV-1 usually occurs before 5 years of age and has an asymptomatic presentation. However, if full-blown APHG does occur, a child can become systemically ill, demonstrating lethargy, fever, and great discomfort. The oral involvement in these children consists of severe stomatitis with vesicles that can occur on the vermillion border of the lips, buccal mucosa, tongue, hard palate, soft palate, and gingiva. Vesicles tend to rupture quickly and may not be observed intact. Remnants of a vesicle may look very much like an aphthous ulcer (red, 2 to 3 mm in diameter). Larger lesions may be noted if several vesicles collapse. The gingiva, especially the interdental papillae, may be fiery red and bleed easily when touched.

Similar to other viral illnesses of childhood, APHG is self-limited and generally runs a 10- to 14-day course. Treatment may consist of systemic or topical antiviral agents such as acyclovir or penciclovir. Analgesics/antipyretics and local palliative and topical therapies can be helpful in making the child comfortable. Popsicles, ice chips, and milkshakes help the mouth feel better, as may sucking on a facecloth that was moistened and placed in the freezer or a frozen teething ring. These also help the child remain hydrated. A mouth rinse with both coating and analgesic characteristics, such as the previously described magic mouthwash, may also assist in obtunding the oral discomfort. Parents should be advised that APHG is contagious and other small children are at risk for infection if they are exposed to the patient and the patient's dinnerware or eating utensils. Parents should be warned to try to keep the child from placing his or her hands from mouth to eyes. Additionally, finger sucking during APHG can lead to a painful condition called herpetic whitlow, in which HSV–1 infection occurs in the nail bed.

Acute Necrotizing Ulcerative Gingivitis

Acute necrotizing ulcerative gingivitis (ANUG) is a fusospirochetal infection that usually affects children older than 12 years of age, although some patients 6 to 12 years of age may experience this disease. Stress is often a contributory factor. It is rare to see ANUG in a child younger than 5 years of age, and this helps in differentiating ANUG from APHG. Affected children generally have diminished resistance and malnutrition and are under psychological stress. Cardinal oral signs of ANUG are:

- Gingival tissues that are extremely tender and bleed easily
- Punched out interdental papillae
- A gray pseudomembrane on the gingiva
- Fetor oris (foul-smelling breath)

Systemically the child shows general malaise and fever. These children can feel very sick and have a very sore mouth. Treatment for these children should be both systemic and local. Penicillin or amoxicillin is the antibiotic of choice, with clindamycin recommended for penicillin-allergic patients; analgesics should be recommended. Local therapy may include rinses with dilute saline or chlorhexidine gluconate; short-term rinsing or topical application of 3% hydrogen peroxide may also help. Debridement of oral tissues and a thorough dental cleaning are indicated following the acute phase and when oral treatment can be tolerated. The primary factors of diminished resistance and psychological stress should be sought out and addressed by the physician.

Other Oral Infections

The varicella-zoster virus and coxsackie A viruses also may cause vesicle formation in the mouth and great discomfort for a child. These conditions should be treated in a manner similar to that for APHG, not ANUG.

Oral Bleeding

Oral bleeding following dental extraction is not an unusual occurrence. In most cases, hemorrhage is minimal; however, a small amount of blood in a volume of saliva can look like a lot of bleeding and can frighten a parent. Application of pressure usually controls the oozing. This can be achieved by having the patient bite on a 2- by 2-inch gauze pad or a facecloth or by having the parent apply pressure to the site. If these simple measures do not create hemostasis, a tea bag (with its tannic acid) can be used to apply pressure to the site. Parents should be advised not to let the child rinse the mouth vigorously and not to allow any use of mouthwash. They should also discourage the child from drinking through a straw. These measures help maintain the integrity of the clot in the extraction site. If bleeding is not controlled by local measures, the dentist who performed the extraction should be called or another dentist contacted, or the patient should be referred to an emergency department that has a dentist on call.

Complications Following Dental Local Anesthesia

Following administration of a dental local anesthetic, a child experiences the feeling that the lip, tongue, or cheek is big or tingling. Occasionally these children, especially the very young, chew or suck on the anesthetized oral mucosa. This can cause that area to swell and appear white or yellow and sloughing. These tissues are rarely infected, and physicians should be on the alert not to overdiagnose cellulitis secondary to dental treatment. This kind of postdental local anesthesia trauma is easily recognized by a dentist, and if there is some difficulty in diagnosis, the physician is encouraged to seek assistance. Once the etiology of the condition is recognized, treatment is relatively simple. The tissues can be cleaned with cool tap water or swabbed with dilute hydrogen peroxide; they heal uneventfully. The swelling resolves relatively quickly. Parents should be instructed to be vigilant in keeping the child from continuing to bite or suck on the anesthetized area.

DENTAL TRAUMA

General Medical Considerations

The physician is often the first health care provider to see a child who has sustained dental trauma. Traumatic injuries occur to primary teeth in 33% of children by the age of 5 years and to permanent teeth in 20% to 30% of children who have reached 12 years of age. In the primary dentition, the peak incidence is 2 to 3 years of age, as children begin to walk. In the permanent dentition, the peak incidence occurs around 9 to 10 years of age, with most of these injuries associated with athletic activities. Physicians should also be aware that more than 50% of abused children show signs of oral trauma.

When injury occurs, assessment of the child's general medical status and determination of the immunization status are primary concerns. Physical evaluation and identification of special medical considerations may influence dental treatment. (For example, many children with congenital heart disease or immunosuppressed children require antibiotic prophylaxis when dental treatment is performed.) Medical injuries generally take precedence over simple dental injuries; however, once the patient is stable, attention may then be turned to the mouth. If any teeth or pieces of teeth are missing, a concerted effort should be made to determine where they are located. In most instances, they are lost outside the mouth; at times, however, they may be lodged in soft tissue of the lip or may have been aspirated. When the location of missing teeth or pieces of teeth cannot be determined, a chest radiograph should be strongly considered to rule out possible aspiration. Evaluation for fracture of facial bones should also be performed, and examination for lacerations of intraoral and extraoral tissues should be completed.

Tooth Loosening (Subluxation)

In children younger than 5 years, loosening (subluxation) of a primary tooth following dental trauma is a common injury. The physician may or may not find bleeding in the gingival sulcus around the involved tooth. Unless these teeth are extremely mobile, treatment consists only of observation. Mobility usually resolves within 2 weeks and soft tissues usually heal uneventfully within this same period. If the injury has caused teeth to be extremely mobile or tissues have been lacerated, referral to a dentist is advisable. This tooth may need splinting or removal, and suturing may be necessary. If injury causes slight loosening in a permanent tooth, this, too, may resolve itself over a short period of time. If its mobility is moderate or severe, a splint may be indicated for 7 to 14 days. Patients with teeth loosened following traumatic injury, splinted or unsplinted, should maintain a soft diet for 14 days. Antibiotic coverage for these injuries is not routinely required. These injuries rarely cause acute pathology. Referral to a dentist for evaluation and follow-up is suggested because long-term injury can sometimes be associated with this type of injury.

Tooth Displacement (Lateral Luxation)

Tooth displacement in a lateral direction (lateral luxation) occurs commonly in children. Although many of these injuries are minor, some are more severe. The most critical of these injuries are those that interfere with normal occlusion (biting and closing). The dentist may be able to perform repositioning, splinting for stabilization, or both. Although heroic measures may be taken to save severely displaced permanent teeth, primary teeth with severe lateral luxation are often extracted. Extraction minimizes the risk of damage to the associated permanent tooth. For primary or permanent teeth that have only slight-to-moderate displacement, reposition the tooth with firm finger pressure. A follow-up visit should be made to a dentist to determine the need for splinting.

Tooth Displacement (Intrusion and Extrusion)

Primary teeth that are intruded may often be observed for spontaneous re-eruption. These teeth usually re-erupt fully within 6 months. If, however, the primary tooth is intruded to a position where it contacts or displaces its associated developing permanent tooth bud, that primary tooth should be extracted to maximize the healthy development of the permanent tooth. To perform the necessary full diagnosis, referral to a dentist for appropriate radiographs is necessary. Treatment of primary teeth that are extruded is based on the degree of displacement, interference with occlusion, and mobility. If extrusion is minor, there are no occlusal difficulties, and there is minimal mobility, the tooth may simply be observed. If displacement is moderate, repositioning with or without splinting may be considered. If there is severe displacement that cannot be corrected, occlusal interference, and/or severe mobility, extraction of the primary tooth should be strongly considered. Again, referral to a dentist is recommended. Treatment of permanent teeth that sustain intrusion or extrusion injuries is more complex than treatment for primary teeth; therefore, referral to a dentist is strongly advised.

Tooth Fractures

Tooth fractures are classified according to the degree of involvement of tooth structure and pulp tissue. A class I fracture involves only enamel and is a minimal emergency. The dentist might need only to smooth a sharp tooth edge for the child. A class II fracture involves enamel and dentin, the latter substance being located under the enamel and adjacent to and communicating with the pulp. To protect the pulp, maintain its integrity and health, and keep it from becoming infected, the dentist should place a protective cover on the dentin. If the tooth is sensitive to air, warm, moist gauze may be placed over it while the patient waits for dental treatment.

Classes III and IV both involve the pulp tissue directly, as well as tooth fracture and loss. A class III fracture involves a small area of pulp tissue, less than 3 mm. A class IV fracture involves a larger area of fractured tooth and pulp exposure. Injuries involving the pulp require immediate attention by a dentist to minimize contamination of the pulp. Again, warm, moist gauze may help keep patients comfortable until they are seen by a dentist. Successful treatment of classes III and IV fractures is possible and best performed as quickly as possible; however, permanent teeth with a class III or IV fracture have been successfully treated as many as 90 days after injury.

Tooth Avulsion

Treatment of avulsed primary and permanent teeth is very different. Avulsed primary teeth are not replanted in order to minimize risk to the normal development of the associated permanent tooth. Attempts to replant permanent teeth should almost always be made. The prognosis after avulsion of a permanent tooth is largely determined by the time it is out of the mouth. Teeth with an immature apex (root end) have a chance to revascularize if they are replaced within 60 minutes, with the best prognosis if they are replaced within 5 to 15 minutes extraoral time. A tooth with a mature apex is less likely to revascularize; however, the prognosis for long-term retention of this tooth following endodontic therapy is improved if it, too, is replanted within 5 to 15 minutes. Teeth with open or closed root ends that have been out of the mouth for longer than 60 minutes have a poor prognosis. This is especially true for the immature tooth, the tooth with an open apex.

In light of the importance of the extraoral time factor, replantation in a physician's office should proceed as quickly as possible. Before replacement, the tooth should be rinsed gently and cleansed to remove gross debris. It should be held by the crown and not along the root surface; it should not be scrubbed vigorously or placed in disinfectant because these actions kill cells that are along the root and that are vital to tooth reattachment. Before replanting the tooth, any clots within the avulsion site should be gently aspirated from the socket. Curettage or scraping of the socket is contraindicated to avoid damaging the viable cells that remain there. The tooth should be replanted with firm finger pressure. After the tooth is positioned, the alveolar bone should be gently compressed by applying finger pressure to the buccal and lingual alveolar plates around the tooth to place the bone into its proper position. The patient should be referred to a dentist for placement of a stabilizing splint.

Antibiotics should be prescribed for patients in whom a permanent tooth has been avulsed and replanted. Doxycycline is now the antibiotic of choice for those who are old enough to receive it without risk of tooth discoloration (usually after the age of 7 to 8 years of age). This antibiotic can be prescribed at a dose appropriate for weight, body surface area, or age. It should be given twice a day for 7 days. For patients who are too young to receive a tetracycline, penicillin should be appropriately dosed and administered, again for 7 days. Patients should also be instructed to rinse with chlorhexidine gluconate for 7 to 10 days. The aim of the antibacterial agents is to minimize bacterial invasion through the gingival sulcus (gum around the tooth) into the pulp of the injured tooth. Analgesics like acetaminophen may also be recommended. Lastly, the patient should be cautioned to eat a soft diet for 7 to 14 days. All patients who have experienced an avulsion should be seen by a dentist as quickly as possible. The physician should be aware that definitive endodontic therapy, when indicated, should begin within 7 to 10 days of the accident.

If the patient first contacts the physician by telephone, the parent or adult should be advised to try to replant the tooth immediately. If they are unable to do this, the tooth should be transported ideally in a Save-A-Tooth kit (if available) or in cold milk. Saliva or saline also may be used. Although saline is not an ideal transport medium, it is better than allowing the tooth to become dry. Plain tap water keeps the tooth moist, but is not as good as the other media. Regardless of the stage of development and the treatment provided, the long-term prognosis for all avulsed teeth is poor, with virtually all eventually being lost (although the tooth may remain in the mouth and benefit the patient for 10 to 20 years).

Physicians should be aware that when treatment decisions are made regarding primary teeth, the dentist considers very strongly the effect the injury may have on the healthy development of the permanent tooth under that primary tooth. If there is concern that the sequelae to the trauma of that primary tooth will harm the permanent tooth, the primary tooth will most often be extracted. Focusing only on the status of the primary tooth is not wise in developing a plan for treatment.

Alveolar Fractures

Fracture of the alveolar bone, the bone surrounding and supporting the teeth, can be of three types: simple, segmental, and comminuted. A simple fracture involves the buccal and/or lingual plate of alveolar bone. This may often be associated with moderate to severe tooth displacement. Diagnosis is made on visual inspection of the injured area.

A segmental type of fracture is diagnosed when there is involvement of a segment (block section) of alveolus. In these cases, an entire portion of the alveolus containing one or several teeth has a through and through buccal-lingual fracture and a segment of the bony arch can be moved or manipulated as a separate unit. Segmental fractures are often present not only with mobility but also with displacement. If this type of fracture is diagnosed, the physician or health care provider should try to reposition the entire segment as closely as possible to its anatomical position. The patient should then be referred to a dentist for immediate treatment. As mentioned previously, medical injuries take precedence; however, repositioning a displaced alveolus should rarely create undue delay in medical evaluation and care.

A comminuted fracture is the third type of alveolar fracture. This is more difficult to diagnosis than a simple or segmental fracture. This injury could be described as fracture of the alveolar bone that would look similar to the shell of a hard boiled egg after the egg was tapped on a countertop. The pieces of the alveolar bone all approximate each other and the overall form of that bone is undisturbed; however, the structural integrity is compromised by one or more fracture lines. This diagnosis is made by applying finger pressure on the buccal and lingual sides of the alveolus (not touching teeth) and observing for movement of the teeth within that bony segment. If teeth move when no direct force is applied directly to them and there is no frank segmental fracture, the diagnosis of a comminuted fracture can be made. Although this type of fracture is not as serious as a segmental type of injury, this patient should also be quickly referred to a dentist.

CHILDREN WITH SPECIAL MEDICAL NEEDS

Physicians and health care providers should be aware that treatment for special-needs children should be focused on the same principles of care as are embraced for healthy children: primary prevention and anticipatory guidance. The fact that modifications might be needed in some medical conditions should not overshadow these important cornerstones of care. Several specific medical conditions are discussed below.

Cardiac Anomalies

Many cardiac patients with cardiac anomalies are at risk for infective endocarditis (IE), with *S. viridans* the most commonly involved oral organism. Proper antibiotic prophylaxis minimizes, although it does not eliminate, the risk of its occurrence secondary to dental treatment. Amoxicillin, rather than penicillin, is now the antibiotic of choice because of its better absorption, higher blood level, and sustained serum levels. Physicians should also be aware that when antibiotic prophylaxis is required, the dentist should also have the patient rinse with chlorhexidine gluconate 0.12% (Peridex or PerioGard) immediately prior to the procedure. Indications, medication schedules, and dosages of antibiotics are recommended by the American Heart Association (AHA) and the American Dental Association (ADA) and should be closely followed (Box 1 and Table 2). Prophylaxis should be given for dental procedures known to cause gingival or mucosal bleeding, including even routine cleaning. Prophylaxis is not required for procedures that are not likely to induce gingival bleeding, such as pit and fissure sealants or adjustment of orthodontic appliances (although orthodontic appointments for tooth separation and placement of orthodontic bands should be covered). Exfoliation of primary teeth also does not require

---

BOX 1 Dental Procedures and Endocarditis Prophylaxis

Endocarditis Prophylaxis Recommended*

- Dental extractions
- Periodontal procedures, including surgery, scaling and root planing, probing, and recall maintenance
- Dental implant placement and reimplantation of avulsed teeth
- Endodontic (root canal) instrumentation or surgery only beyond the apex
- Subgingival placement of antibiotic fibers or strips
- Initial placement of orthodontic bands but not brackets
- Intraligamentary local anesthetic injections
- Prophylactic cleaning of teeth or implants when bleeding is anticipated

Endocarditis Prophylaxis Not Recommended

- Restorative dentistry[†] (operative and prosthodontic) with or without retraction cord[‡]
- Local anesthetic injections (nonintraligamentary)
- Intracanal endodontic treatment; postplacement and build-up
- Placement of rubber dams
- Postoperative suture removal
- Placement of removable prosthodontic or orthodontic appliances
- Taking of oral impressions
- Fluoride treatments
- Taking of oral radiographs
- Orthodontic appliance adjustment
- Shedding of primary teeth

*Prophylaxis is recommended for patients with high- and moderate-risk cardiac conditions.
†Includes restoration of decayed teeth (filling cavities) and replacement of missing teeth.
‡Clinical judgment may indicate antibiotic use in selected circumstances that may create significant bleeding.

Adapted from Dajani AS, Taubert KA, Wilson W, et al: Prevention of bacterial endocarditis: Recommendations by the American Heart Association. JAMA 277:1794–1801, 1997.

23

---

administration of antibiotics. Physicians should also be aware that if unanticipated bleeding occurs in a patient at risk, the AHA and ADA state that administering proper antibiotic prophylaxis within 2 hours will provide effective coverage.

The AHA and ADA emphasize that their recommendations are guidelines, not a standard of care; therefore, if questions arise regarding an individual patient, the physician should consult with the patient's cardiologist, dentist, or both. The physician should also be aware that poor oral hygiene and dental infection might produce bacteremia, with the magnitude of that seeding directly proportional to the degree of inflammation and infection. Most cases of bacterial endocarditis are not attributable to invasive procedures; however, if a procedure were suspected of being related to this illness, it would have had to occur within 2 weeks of onset of the disease.

It is important for the physician to note that if the patient is already taking penicillin or amoxicillin, a different antibiotic should be used for prophylaxis. Simply increasing the dose of current medication is not sufficient. If the dentist indicates that multiple visits will be necessary to complete all treatment in order to reduce the risk of emergence of resistant

TABLE 2 Prophylactic Regimens for Dental, Oral, Respiratory Tract, or Esophageal Procedures in Cardiac Patients

Situation	Agent*	Regimen*
Standard general prophylaxis	Amoxicillin	Adults: 2.0 g; children: 50 mg/kg PO 1 h before procedure
Unable to take oral medications	Ampicillin	Adults: 2.0 g IM or IV; children: 50 mg/kg IM or IV within 30 min before procedure
Allergic to penicillin	Clindamycin or	Adults: 600 mg; children: 20 mg/kg PO 1 h before procedure
	Cephalexin† or cefadroxil†or	Adults: 2.0 g; children: 50 mg/kg PO 1 h before procedure
	Azithromycin or clarithromycin	Adults: 500 mg; children: 15 mg/kg PO 1 h before procedure
Allergic to penicillin and unable to take oral medications	Clindamycin or	Adults: 600 mg; children: 20 mg/kg IV within 30 min before procedure
	Cefazolin†	Adults: 1.0 g; children: 25 mg/kg IM or IV within 30 min before procedure

*Children's dose should not exceed adult dose.
†Cephalosporins should not be used in individuals with immediate-type hypersensitivity reaction (urticaria, angioedema, or anaphylaxis) to penicillins.
IM, intramuscularly; IV, intravenously; PO, orally.
Adapted from Dajani AS, Taubert KA, Wilson W, et al: Prevention of bacterial endocarditis: Recommendations by the American Heart Association. JAMA 277:1794–1801, 1997.

organisms, there should be a 9- to 14-day interval between appointments.

Patients with Intravascular Catheters

Patients with vascular shunts and indwelling vascular catheters should receive antibiotic prophylaxis. Schedules and dosages are the same as for patients who have a cardiac anomaly. This group includes those with ventriculoatrial shunts, renal dialysis shunts, arteriovenous shunts, and IV access devices (e.g., Broviac and Hickman catheters, infusion ports, and peripherally inserted central catheter lines). Antibiotic prophylaxis is not generally recommended for patients with ventriculoperitoneal or ventriculopleural shunts. As with cardiac patients, the dentist should have the patient rinse the oral cavity with chlorhexidine gluconate prior to beginning a procedure.

Transplant Patients

Children who are candidates for transplantation (e.g., heart, liver, kidney, bone marrow) should receive a thorough oral examination before receiving a transplant. The evaluation should determine current and possible future sources of infection and should be performed by a dentist. Whenever possible, patients should receive any necessary dental treatment before the transplant procedure. Modification of dental care at that time may be required because of the individual's medical condition. For example, children with congenital heart disease are at risk for infective endocarditis; children with kidney disease may have a shunt.

The immune competence of the child is also an important consideration when determining the need for antibiotic prophylaxis. After transplantation, children are immunosuppressed, and the physician should be aware that the immunosuppressant agent, cyclosporin, can cause overgrowth of gingival tissue; if such overgrowth occurs, the child should be monitored by a dentist. Children who have received heart, lung, liver, or kidney transplants should plan to have antibiotic

prophylaxis administered for life. Children who have undergone successful bone marrow transplants may not require antibiotic coverage if their white blood cell (WBC) count and absolute neutrophil count (ANC) are within normal limits. If, however, the WBC count is less than 3500/mm^3 or the ANC is less than 1000/mm^3, patients may be at risk for orally induced bacteremia and should receive prophylaxis. When antibiotic coverage is prescribed, it should consist of the standard first dose according to the AHA recommendations. When the ANC is less than 500/mm^3, dental treatment should usually be postponed. Consultation with the child's hematologist, oncologist, dentist, or any combination of these specialists is strongly encouraged to determine whether long-term coverage might be necessary. Consultation with a patient's transplant team is also strongly urged.

Immunocompromised/Immunosuppressed Patients

Children who have compromised immunity because of a primary disease process or secondary to medications (steroids, chemotherapeutic agents, or transplant medications) are predisposed to infection. Because oral infection is a frequent cause of sepsis in immunocompromised children, physicians should emphasize the importance of primary prevention. They should strongly encourage their families to seek an early dental home, become involved with anticipatory guidance, be diligent in their dental visits, and be vigilant in performing routine oral hygiene measures at home. During acute medical episodes, oral hygiene routines may need to be modified. Consultation with a specialist or dentist can be valuable in helping guide care for these patients. Antibiotics are recommended for these children because it is not possible to predict when they might develop an infection following a bacteremia-producing procedure. As in cardiac patients, administration of appropriate antibiotic prophylaxis does not guarantee protection from infection; therefore, the patient should be observed and monitored during the post-treatment period. If infection does occur, medical treatment should begin, as indicated for each individual patient. Physicians should also consider extending the period of antibiotic coverage from the single dose to several days in this special population. Practitioners may consider giving antibiotics for a longer than usual period of time when faced with infection or a patient who has shown a high susceptibility to infection.

In general, these children should be covered as outlined by the AHA guidelines to prevent bacterial endocarditis. When ordering antibiotic prophylaxis for these children, the physician should follow coverage recommendations listed in the Cardiac Anomalies section. The physician is also encouraged to discuss specific care of these patients with both the dentist who can review the specifics of dental diagnosis and treatment plan and the specialist who is following the child.

Human Immunodeficiency Virus

Children with human immunodeficiency virus (HIV) may have oral manifestations and should be monitored jointly by the physician and dentist. In fact, oral lesions can be indicators of immune status and disease progress. Lesions commonly associated with pediatric HIV include oropharyngeal candidiasis (the most common oral manifestation), herpes simplex infection, linear gingival erythema (gingivitis), parotid enlargement (usually bilateral and symmetrical), recurrent aphthous stomatitis, and cervical lymphadenopathy. Lesions less commonly found in the pediatric population include bacterial infections (sinusitis, otitis media), severe periodontal disease, and viral infections. Oral conditions should be treated systemically and/or topically, depending on the specific situation. Palliative and supportive treatment is also appropriate. Physicians should be aware that some anti-HIV medications (zidovudine, interferon, ganciclovir, zalcitabine, and foscarnet) have been associated with development of oral ulcerations. In general, principles of oral health and primary prevention are the same in HIV-infected children as they are for well children. HIV-positive children do not require routine antibiotics prior to dental treatment. Factors that must be considered are ANC, immunoglobulin levels, CD4+ (cell count less than 200 may indicate neutropenia), and general health status. Consultation with the specialist monitoring the child's status is encouraged.

Sickle Cell Disease

In children with sickle cell disease, antibiotic coverage is not needed for routine dental procedures such as cleaning and restorative treatment. If extraction or pulp therapy is to be performed, standard AHA antibiotic prophylaxis should be administered. Because most children with sickle cell disease receive penicillin prophylaxis to prevent pneumococcal infection, prophylaxis for dental treatment should be provided with clindamycin, as recommended by AHA guidelines. This change in antibiotics takes into consideration the possible emergence of penicillin-resistant organisms. If the patient has a history of frequent infections, the need for increased antibiotic coverage, even for routine procedures, should be discussed with the hematologist. Whenever a patient with sickle cell disease is to receive dental treatment under general anesthesia, consultation with the child's hematologist and anesthesiologist should be done. These children generally require transfusion prior to the anesthesia, to increase their hemoglobin level to greater than 10 g/dL.

Orthopedic Hardware

The American Academy of Orthopaedic Surgeons and the ADA have formulated guidelines for patients who have received orthopedic devices. Antibiotic coverage is not indicated for most dental patients who have pins, plates, or screws. Antibiotics (Box 2) are recommended for patients who have an increased risk of infection (Box 3) and who have undergone total joint replacement, especially within the first 2 years following surgery. Because there remains some controversy surrounding these recommendations for dental treatment, consultation with the patient's orthopedist is strongly encouraged. The source of this controversy rests in the findings that two thirds of prosthetic joint infections have been found to be associated with *Staphylococcus*, whereas slightly less than 5% were associated with *S. viridans* and approximately 2% with *Peptostreptococcus* (another oral organism). This suggests that wound contamination or skin infection, not the oral cavity, is the source for the majority of joint infections in this patient population.

Neural Tube Defects/Latex Allergy

Children with neural tube defects, including myelomeningocele, may also have associated hydrocephalus and a ventricular shunt; therefore, consideration should be

---

BOX 2 Suggested Antibiotic Prophylaxis Regimens for Patients with Orthopedic Hardware*

- Patients not allergic to penicillin: cephalexin, cephradine, or amoxicillin
  - 2 g PO 1 h before dental procedure
- Patients not allergic to penicillin and unable to take oral medications: cefazolin or ampicillin
  - Cefazolin 1 g IV or ampicillin, 2 g IM or IV 1 h before the procedure
- Patients allergic to penicillin: clindamycin
  - 600 mg PO 1 h before the dental procedure
- Patients allergic to penicillin and unable to take oral medications: clindamycin
  - 600 mg IV 1 h before the procedure
  - Use children's doses per AHA/SBE guidelines in Table 2.

*No second doses are recommended for any of these dosing regimens.

Adapted from American Dental Association, American Academy of Orthopaedic Surgeons: Antibiotic prophylaxis for dental patients with total joint replacements. J Am Dent Assoc 128:1004–1007, 1997. Copyright © 1997 American Dental Association. All rights reserved. Adapted 2006 with permission.

IM, intramuscularly; IV, intravenously; PO; orally.

BOX 3 Patients at Potential Increased Risk of Hematogenous Total Joint Infection

Immunocompromised/Immunosuppressed Patients
- Inflammatory arthropathies, rheumatoid arthritis, systemic lupus erythematosus
- Disease-, drug-, or radiation-induced immunosuppression

Other Patients
- Insulin-dependent (type 1) diabetes
- First 2 years following joint placement
- Previous prosthetic joint infections
- Malnourishment
- Hemophilia

---

given to the need for antibiotic prophylaxis. Patients with ventriculoatrial or ventriculovenous shunts do require antibiotic prophylaxis according to AHA guidelines. The need for antibiotic coverage for patients with ventriculoperitoneal and ventriculopleural shunts is somewhat controversial, but antibiotic prophylaxis is not generally considered necessary. It would be best to consult with the patient's neurosurgeon for recommendations in this area. Additionally, physicians should recall that patients with myelomeningocele are considered to be at high risk for latex allergy, so appropriate precautions must be taken. The dentist must take precautions to avoid typical latex exposure that would occur in a dental office (latex gloves, prophylaxis rubber cups, rubber dam, and materials that are packaged with medicine droppers that may have a latex bulb included). Cross-sensitization and latex allergy in patients who have a known allergy to bananas, kiwis, avocados, and chestnuts must also be recognized.

Glucose-6 Phosphate Dehydrogenase Deficiency

Children with glucose-6 phosphate dehydrogenase deficiency do not require antibiotic prophylaxis before treatment. The dentist should be reminded that analgesics such as aspirin might trigger hemolysis in these children.

Common Pitfalls

- Postponing the initial dental visit and establishment of a dental home can place a child at risk for dental disease that is, in large part, preventable.
- Failure to provide appropriate antibiotic coverage for dental treatment can have enormously negative systemic effects in some children.
- Lack of adequate communication between the physician and dentist can place a child at risk for adverse dental and/or medical outcomes.

Communication and Counseling

Physicians should advocate for increased access to care and help foster a partnership of care with dental colleagues, family, and patients to minimize the onset and/or progression of pathologies associated with oral diseases. Familiarity with the nature of the two major oral diseases, dental caries and periodontal disease, will help physicians offer their patients the most comprehensive care possible.

SUGGESTED READINGS

Prevention in Dentistry

1. American Academy of Pediatric Dentistry: Reference Manual 25:11–12, 2003. **Policy statements regarding principles of prevention of dental disease.**
2. American Academy of Pediatrics: Section on Pediatric Dentistry Oral Health Risk Assessment, Timing and Establishment of the Dental Home 111:113–116, 2003. **Policy statement regarding establishment of a dental home and the timing of the initial dental visit.**
3. Simonsen RJ: Retention and effectiveness of dental sealant after 15 years. JADA 122:34–42, 1991. **Longest study on the retention and effectiveness of dental sealants.**
4. U.S. Department of Health and Human Services: Oral health in America: A report of the Surgeon General. Rockville, MD, 2000. U.S. Department of Health and Human Services, National Institute of Dental and Craniofacial Research, National Institutes of Health. **Status of oral health in U.S. children, the relationship between oral health and general health and well being, how oral health is promoted and maintained, and the needs and opportunities to enhance oral health.**

Oral Care for Infants

1. American Academy of Pediatric Dentistry Reference Manual: Reference Manual 25:11–12, 2003. **Policy statements regarding principles of care for infants and children.**
2. Pinkham JR: Pediatric Dentistry: Infancy through Adolescents. Philadelphia: WB Saunders, 1999, p 190. **Information on care of infants, with special emphasis on principles on anticipatory guidance.**

Dental Caries

1. American Academy of Pediatric Dentistry: Restorative Dentistry Consensus Conference. J Ped Dent, 24(5), 2002. **Historical perspective and specific recommendation on different treatment modalities.**
2. McDonald RE, Avery DR, Dean JA: Dentistry for the Child and Adolescent, 8th ed. Philadelphia: Mosby, 2004. **Information on epidemiology and treatment of dental caries in children.**
3. NIH Consensus Development Conference on Diagnosis and Management of Dental Caries throughout life. March 26–28, 2001. J Dent Educ 65:935–1179, 2001. **Recommendations for the treatment of dental caries.**
4. U.S. Department of Health and Human Services: Oral Health in America: A report of the Surgeon General, Rockville, MD, 2000. U.S. Department of Health and Human Services, National Institute of Dental and Craniofacial Research, National Institutes of Health. **Status of oral health in U.S. children, the relationship between oral health and general health and well-being, how oral health is promoted and maintained, and the opportunities to enhance oral health.**

Periodontal Disease in Children

1. American Academy of Pediatric Dentistry: Periodontal diseases of children and adolescents. Ped Dent Ref Man 25(7):117–127, 2004. **Information on the epidemiology, etiology, and the treatment of periodontal diseases in children.**
2. American Academy of Periodontics: Periodontal diseases of children and adolescents. J Perio 74:213–221, 2003. **Information on the epidemiology, etiology, and the treatment of periodontal diseases in children.**
3. McDonald RE, Avery DR, Dean JA: Dentistry for the Child and Adolescent, 8th ed. Philadelphia: Mosby, 2004. **Extensive and detailed information on the full range of gingival and periodontal diseases in children.**

Dental Emergencies in Children

1. Malamed SF: Handbook of Local Anesthesia, 5th ed. Philadelphia: Mosby, 2004. **Information on dosages of local anesthetics and management of local anesthesia overdose.**
2. McDonald RE, Avery DR, Dean JA: Dentistry for the Child and Adolescent, 8th ed. Philadelphia: Mosby, 2004. **Information on the management of dental emergencies in children.**

Dental Trauma

1. Andreasen JO, Andreasen FM: Traumatic Injuries: A Manual. Copenhagen: Muskgaard, 1999. **Summaries on the full range of traumatic dental injuries and their treatment.**
2. Barrett EJ, Kenny DJ: Recent developments in dental traumatology. Ped Dent 23(6):464–468, 2001. **Recent developments in the management of dental trauma.**
3. Florese MT, Andreasen JO, Bakland LK: Guidelines for the evaluation and management of traumatic dental injuries. Dent Traumatology 17:193–196, 2001. **Complete, comprehensive information on the full range of traumatic dental injuries, including pathophysiology and histology of each type of injury.**
4. Ram D, Cohenca N: Therapeutic protocols for avulsed permanent teeth: Review and clinical update. Ped Dent 26(3):251–255, 2004. **Recent developments in the management of dental trauma.**

Children with Special Medical Needs

1. American Academy of Pediatric Dentistry Reference Manual. Reference Manual 25:11–12, 2003. **Guidelines and recommendation for children with specific medical conditions, including patients with cardiac disease, those receiving chemotherapy, hematopoietic cell transplantation, and/or radiation therapy, and those with cleft palate and other craniofacial anomalies.**
2. Little JW, Fallace DA, Miller CS, Rhodus NL: Dental Management of the Medically Compromised Patient, 6th ed. St.Louis: Mosby, 2002. **Recommendations for medical and dental management of patients with medical disabilities.**

General

1. American Academy of Pediatric Dentistry: Periodontal diseases of children and adolescents. Ped Dent Ref Man 25(7):117–127, 2004. **Information on the epidemiology, etiology, and the treatment of periodontal diseases in children.**
2. American Academy of Pediatrics: Section on pediatric dentistry oral health risk assessment, timing and establishment of the dental home. 111:113–116, 2003. **Policy statement regarding establishment of a dental home and the timing of the initial dental visit.**
3. Andreasen JO, Andreasen FM: Traumatic Injuries: A Manual. Copenhagen: Muskgaard, 1999. **Summaries on the full range of traumatic dental injuries and their treatment.**
4. Florese MT, Andreasen JO, Bakland LK: Guidelines for the evaluation and management of traumatic dental injuries. Dent Traumatology 17:193–196, 2001. **Complete, comprehensive information on the full range of traumatic dental injuries, including pathophysiology and histology of each type of injury.**
5. McDonald RE, Avery DR, Dean JA: Dentistry for the Child and Adolescent, 8th ed. Philadelphia: Mosby, 2004. **General reference textbook on all aspects of pediatric dentistry.**
6. NIH Consensus Development Conference on Diagnosis and Management of Dental Caries throughout life, March 26–28, 2001. J Dent Educ 65:935–1179, 2001. **Thorough scientific examination of diagnosis and management of dental caries.**
7. Pinkham JR: Pediatric Dentistry: Infancy through Adolescence. Philadelphia: WB Saunders, 1999, p190. **General reference textbook on all aspects of pediatric dentistry.**
8. U.S. Department of Health and Human Services: Oral Health in America: A report of the Surgeon General, Rockville, MD, 2000. U.S. Department of Health and Human Services, National Institute of Dental and Craniofacial Research, National Institutes of Health. **Status of oral health in U.S. children, the relationship between oral health and general health and well being, how oral health is promoted and maintained, and the needs and opportunities to enhance oral health.**

Index

Note: Page numbers followed by the letter b refer to boxes, those followed by f refer to figures, and those followed by t refer to tables.

perléche, 1069
permethrin (Permanone)
    for babesiosis prevention, 859–860
    for lice and scabies, 906
    for pediculosis, 1077, 1077t
    for scabies, 1075, 1076t
permissive hypercapnia, for acute
    respiratory distress syndrome, 248, 467
peroxisomal disorders, 391
    genetics of, 389t
persistent pulmonary hypertension of the
    newborn (PPHN), 249–252
    common pitfalls with, 251
    communication for, 251
    congenital diaphragmatic hernia
        associated with, 251
    counseling on, 251
    diagnosis of, 250
    in infants of diabetic mothers, 266
    incidence of, 249
    key concepts of, 249
    management of, 250–251
    pathogenesis of, 249–250
    pulmonary vascular resistance regulation
        mechanisms in, 250
    septic shock and, 161, 161f
personal protective equipment (PPE),
    for health care-associated infections,
    694, 694t
personality disorders, suicide risk related
    to, 353
person-to-person transmission, of daycare
    environment infections, 904t
pertussis. See Bordetella pertussis;
    whooping cough
pertussis vaccines, 726, 726t
    acellular, 115
        new, 113
        schedule for, 109, 110f–111f
pervasive developmental disorder (PDD),
    1220, 1222
PET (positron emission tomography), for
    infantile spasms, 405, 406
petechiae, in diaper area, 1041
petroleum jelly
    atopic dermatitis and, 1045
    for epistaxis, 195
petroleum-based ointments, for
    transcutaneous evaporation
    prevention, 85
pets
    bites from (See mammalian bites)
    cat-scratch disease from, 701
    tinea capitis from, 1069
pexelizumab, for complement
    disorders, 1166
PF. See pemphigus foliaceus (PF)
PFGE (pulsed-field gel electrophoresis), for
    outbreak investigations, 694
PFLAG (Parents and Friends of Lesbians
    and Gays), 333
PFO (patent foramen ovale), 250
PGE₁ (prostaglandin E₁), for patent ductus
    arteriosus maintenance, with
    congenital heart disease, 256–257
PH. See primary hyperoxaluria (PH)
pH
    esophageal monitoring of, for
        gastroesophageal reflux, 533, 534
    in acid-base disorders, 78, 79t
        metabolic acidosis, 78, 80
        metabolic alkalosis, 82, 83, 84
    in metabolic disorder screening, 1003
    in pleural effusion classification,
        453, 453t

pH (Continued)
    oral, dental health and, 1256
PHA. See pseudohypoaldosteronism (PHA)
phagocytes
    in immunocompromised host, 1178, 1179,
        1180t
    primary disorder of, 1154, 1156t
phagocytic system, mononuclear, malignant
    tumors of, 1193
pharmacologic agents. See also specific
        classification or agent
    adverse drug reaction risk related to,
        1050, 1143. See also adverse drug
        reaction (ADR)
    anaphylaxis risks and, 140, 1052
    breastfeeding and, 77
    erythema multiforme associated with,
        1055, 1056b
    gynecomastia caused by, 339t, 340
    hematuria associated with, 609
    hyperpigmentation induced by, 1079
    iron absorption affected by, 911
    metabolism of, indomethacin impact
        on, 309–310
    review of
        for constipation evaluation, 52
        in abdominal pain differentiation, 40
    serum sickness related to,
        1137, 1138b
    systemic lupus erythematosus caused
        by, 1009
    therapeutic indications for (See also
        specific pathology)
pharyngitis
    group A streptococcal
        acute rheumatic fever and, 495
            treatment of, 495–496, 495t
                adherence importance, 496–497
        in daycare environments, 906
    infectious mononucleosis associated with,
        768, 769
pharyngotonsillitis, recurrent, 1121
pharynx
    carcinoma of, 1110–1111
    foreign bodies in
        clinical presentations of, 1112b
        communication/counseling for, 1113
        key concepts of, 1111–1112
        management of, 1113
phase-contrast microscopy, for hematuria
    evaluation, 608–609
PHD (paroxysmal hypnogenic
    dyskinesia), 387
phenazopyridine (Pyridium), for
    postoperative spasms, 20
phenobarbital
    for cholestasis, 562
    for infantile spasms, 405
    for intraventricular hemorrhage
        prevention, 275
    for neonatal seizures, 126–127, 126t
    for status epilepticus
        convulsive, 130, 130t
            refractory, 130t, 131
        nonconvulsive, 131
phenoxybenzamine, for
    pheochromocytomas, 979
phenoxymethyl penicillin, for anaerobic
    infections, 691t
phenytoin. See also fosphenytoin
    for neonatal seizures, 126–127, 126t
    for status epilepticus
        convulsive, 130, 130t
        nonconvulsive, 131
    in injury stabilization, 157

pheochromocytoma, excess catecholamine
    production with, 979–980, 979t
PHEX gene, 627
PHH. See posthemorrhagic hydrocephalus
    (PHH)
phimosis, circumcision and, 314
phlebectasia, of jugular vein, 1131t
phobia
    social, 1216
    specific, 1216
phonologic processing
    disorders of, 1252, 1253
        management of, 1253–1254
    dyslexia and, 1244–1245
phosphate
    decreased serum (See hypophosphatemia)
    for proximal renal tubular acidosis,
        625, 626t
phosphodiesterase inhibitors
    cGMP-specific, for pulmonary
        hypertension, 505t, 508–509
    for congenital heart disease, 257
    for persistent pulmonary hypertension of
        the newborn, 251
    for septic shock, 161f–162f, 162
phosphorus
    metabolic acidosis impact on, 79–80, 79t
    metabolism of
        in acute renal failure, 636, 636b
        in chronic dialysis, 649
        in chronic kidney disease, 641
photocoagulation
    for intraocular retinoblastoma, 1102
    laser, for retinopathy of prematurity,
        312, 313
phototherapy
    for neonatal hyperbilirubinemia, 120–122,
        121f, 270–271
        hemolytic disease-related, 285–286,
            286f
    for psoriasis, 1059
    for vitiligo, 1080
    ultraviolet-A
        for alopecia, 1086
        psoralen with, for Langerhans cell
            histiocytoses, 1194
PHP. See pseudohypoparathyroidism (PHP)
phylloquinone, 102
physeal fractures, tibial, distal, 179, 179t
    isolated, 181
physical activity(ies)
    emphysema cautions for, 450
    foot rotations and, 1015–1016
    for cerebral palsy, 382
    for weight loss, with obesity, 336–338
    limitations of, for cardiac
        arrhythmias, 520
    Marfan syndrome and, 477
    physical examination for, 346–349 (See
        also sports physical)
    pulmonary hypertension and, 507
    resting energy expenditure application
        to, 95, 95t
    systemic hypertension and, 512, 512f
physical countermaneuvers, for syncope,
    38, 38t
physical examination
    for abdominal pain, 41–42
    for acute renal failure, 634
    for adverse drug reaction evaluation,
        1143–1144
    for ambiguous genitalia, 984b, 985f
    for amenorrhea, 319, 321b
    for child maltreatment, 1248
    for cough, 1